D1608266

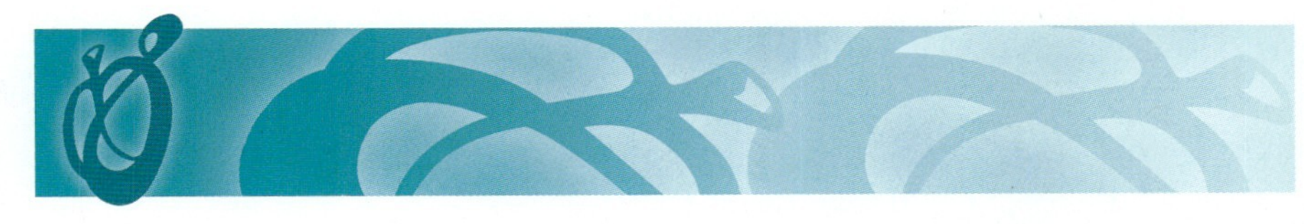

Clinical Arrhythmology and Electrophysiology

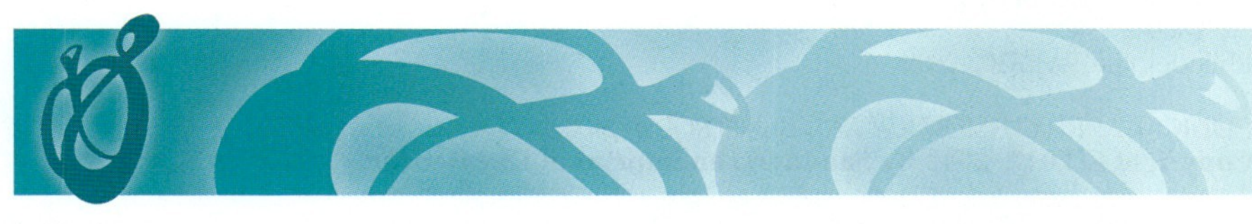

Clinical Arrhythmology and Electrophysiology

A Companion to Braunwald's Heart Disease

SECOND EDITION

Ziad F. Issa, MD
Clinical Assistant Professor
Internal Medicine
Southern Illinois University School of Medicine
Cardiac Electrophysiology
Prairie Cardiovascular Consultants
Prairie Heart Institute
St. John's Hospital
Springfield, Illinois

John M. Miller, MD
Professor of Medicine
Krannert Institute of Cardiology
Indiana University School of Medicine
Director
Clinical Cardiac Electrophysiology
Indiana University Health
Indianapolis, Indiana

Douglas P. Zipes, MD
Distinguished Professor
Professor Emeritus of Medicine, Pharmacology, and Toxicology
Director Emeritus
Division of Cardiology and the Krannert Institute of Cardiology
Indiana University School of Medicine
Indianapolis, Indiana

ELSEVIER
SAUNDERS

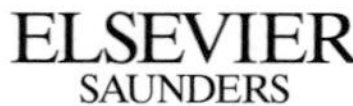

1600 John F. Kennedy Blvd.
Ste 1800
Philadelphia, PA 19103-2899

CLINICAL ARRHYTHMOLOGY AND ELECTROPHYSIOLOGY ISBN: 978-1-4557-1274-8

Notices

Knowledge and best practice in this field are constantly changing. As new research and experience broaden our understanding, changes in research methods, professional practices, or medical treatment may become necessary.

Practitioners and researchers must always rely on their own experience and knowledge in evaluating and using any information, methods, compounds, or experiments described herein. In using such information or methods they should be mindful of their own safety and the safety of others, including parties for whom they have a professional responsibility.

With respect to any drug or pharmaceutical products identified, readers are advised to check the most current information provided (i) on procedures featured or (ii) by the manufacturer of each product to be administered, to verify the recommended dose or formula, the method and duration of administration, and contraindications. It is the responsibility of practitioners, relying on their own experience and knowledge of their patients, to make diagnoses, to determine dosages and the best treatment for each individual patient, and to take all appropriate safety precautions.

To the fullest extent of the law, neither the Publisher nor the authors, contributors, or editors assume any liability for any injury and/or damage to persons or property as a matter of products liability, negligence or otherwise, or from any use or operation of any methods, products, instructions, or ideas contained in the material herein.

Library of Congress Cataloging-in-Publication Data
Issa, Ziad F.
Clinical arrhythmology and electrophysiology: a companion to Braunwald's heart disease / Ziad F. Issa, John M. Miller, Douglas P. Zipes.— 2nd ed.
p. ; cm.
Includes bibliographical references and index.
ISBN 978-1-4557-1274-8 (hardcover : alk. paper)
I. Miller, John M. (John Michael), 1954- II. Zipes, Douglas P. III. Braunwald's heart disease. IV. Title.
[DNLM: 1. Arrhythmias, Cardiac—diagnosis. 2. Arrhythmias, Cardiac—physiopathology.
3. Electrophysiologic Techniques, Cardiac. WG 330]
616.1′28—dc23 2012012441

Content Strategist: Dolores Meloni
Content Developmental Specialist: Andrea Vosburgh
Publishing Services Manager: Patricia Tannian
Project Manager: Linda Van Pelt
Design Direction: Steve Stave

Printed in China

Last digit is the print number: 9 8 7 6 5 4 3

We would like to thank our families for their support during the writing of this book, since it meant time away from them.

My wife Dana and my sons Tariq and Amr

Ziad F. Issa

My wife Jeanne and my children Rebekah, Jordan, and Jacob

John M. Miller

My wife Joan and my children Debbie, Jeff, and David

Douglas P. Zipes

We would also like to thank Julie Shelby, Leslie Ardebili, and Ralph Chambers for their help in preparing this manuscript.

FOREWORD

Disturbances in cardiac rhythm occur in a large proportion of the population. Arrhythmias can have sequelae that range from inconsequential to life-shortening. Sudden cardiac deaths and chronic disability are among the most frequent serious complications resulting from arrhythmias.

Braunwald's Heart Disease: A Textbook of Cardiovascular Medicine includes an excellent section on rhythm disturbances edited and largely written by Douglas Zipes, the most accomplished and respected investigator and clinician in this field. However, there are many subjects that simply cannot be discussed in sufficient detail, even in a 2000-page, densely packed book. For this reason, the current editors and I decided to commission a series of companions to the parent title. We were extremely fortunate to enlist Dr. Zipes' help in editing and writing *Clinical Arrhythmology and Electrophysiology*. Dr. Zipes, in turn, enlisted two talented collaborators, Drs. Ziad F. Issa and John M. Miller, to work with him to produce this excellent volume.

This second edition is superbly illustrated, with the number of figures and tables increasing by almost half from its predecessor. What has not changed, however, is the very high quality of the content, which is accurate, authoritative, and clear; second, it is as up-to-date as last month's journals; and third, the writing style and illustrations are consistent throughout with little, if any, duplication. As this important branch of cardiology has grown, so has this book.

The first seven chapters, on Molecular Mechanisms of Cardiac Electrical Activity, Cardiac Ion Channels, Electrophysiological Mechanisms of Cardiac Arrhythmias, Electrophysiological Testing, Conventional Intracardiac Mapping Techniques, Advanced Mapping and Navigation Modalities, and Ablation Energy Sources, provide a superb introduction to the field. This is followed by 24 chapters on individual arrhythmias, each following a similar outline. Here, the authors lead us from a basic understanding of the arrhythmia to its clinical recognition, natural history, and management. The latter is moving rapidly from being largely drug-based to device-based, although many patients receive combination device-drug therapy. These options, as well as ablation therapy, are clearly spelled out as they apply to each arrhythmia. The final chapter discusses the complications of catheter ablation of cardiac arrhythmias.

We are proud to include *Clinical Arrhythmology and Electrophysiology* as a Companion to *Braunwald's Heart Disease,* and we are fully confident that it will prove to be valuable to cardiologists, internists, investigators, and trainees.

Eugene Braunwald, MD
Peter Libby, MD
Robert Bonow, MD
Douglas Mann, MD

PREFACE

Readers' responses to the first edition of this textbook have been extremely gratifying, so much so that we were encouraged to update and revise the text relatively early after its initial publication in 2009. As all who work in this field know, however, the knowledge base is changing very rapidly at virtually all levels, from basic understanding of mechanisms to new ablation techniques, mapping, imaging advances, and development of new ablation energy sources. In addition, we are learning about new clinical states that have been "right under our noses" for a long time, such as the short QT and J wave syndromes. We have therefore added new chapters on those topics as well as on molecular mechanisms and ion channels, advanced mapping and navigation, and arrhythmias in congenital heart disease. For clarity, we have divided the idiopathic ventricular tachycardias (VTs) into adenosine- and verapamil-sensitive types and have written new chapters on both epicardial VTs and VTs in the different cardiomyopathies. The "old" chapters are no longer old; all have been totally revised and expanded with updated information. Additionally, we have included 27 new videos that vividly exemplify a variety of techniques and mapping observations.

As with the first edition, this book has been written by just the three of us, so that once again we can "explain, integrate, coordinate and educate in a comprehensive, cohesive fashion while avoiding redundancies and contradictions." Having lived through the changes of the past several years, we have been able to extract and write about those advances that we think are important and useful to the readers. This is similar to a travel guidebook written by someone who has actually stayed in that unique hotel or eaten in that special restaurant. We have experienced the progress firsthand and are able to pass on our experiences to you. In addition, as before—but expanded even further—readers have the option to delve deeper into basic mechanisms or invasive procedures... or not, depending on the level of interest. We have tried to keep the appeal for all levels of learners, from the beginner to the experienced electrophysiologist, so that you can stop reading with the fascinating array of ECGs or dig deeper into the mechanism of calcium handling—your call. We hope you enjoy learning from this second edition.

Ziad F. Issa
John M. Miller
Douglas P. Zipes

CONTENTS

VIDEO CONTENTS

Look for These Other Titles in the Braunwald's Heart Disease Family

Braunwald's Heart Disease Companions

PIERRE THÉROUX
Acute Coronary Syndromes

ELLIOTT M. ANTMAN & MARC S. SABATINE
Cardiovascular Therapeutics

CHRISTIE M. BALLANTYNE
Clinical Lipidology

DOUGLAS L. MANN
Heart Failure

HENRY R. BLACK & WILLIAM J. ELLIOTT
Hypertension

ROBERT L. KORMOS & LESLIE W. MILLER
Mechanical Circulatory Support

ROGER BLUMENTHAL, JOANNE FOODY, & NATHAN WONG
Preventive Cardiology

CATHERINE M. OTTO & ROBERT O. BONOW
Valvular Heart Disease

MARC A. CREAGER, JOSHUA A. BECKMAN, & JOSEPH LOSCALZO
Vascular Disease

Braunwald's Heart Disease Imaging Companions

ALLEN J. TAYLOR
Atlas of Cardiac Computed Tomography

CHRISTOPHER M. KRAMER & W. GREGORY HUNDLEY
Atlas of Cardiovascular Magnetic Resonance Imaging

AMI E. ISKANDRIAN & ERNEST V. GARCIA
Atlas of Nuclear Imaging

JAMES D. THOMAS
Atlas of Echocardiography

CHAPTER 1 Molecular Mechanisms of Cardiac Electrical Activity

Ionic Equilibrium

The lipid bilayer of the cell membrane is hydrophobic and impermeable to water-soluble substances such as ions. Hence, for the hydrophilic ions to be able to cross the membrane, they need hydrophilic paths that span the membrane (i.e., pores), which are provided by transmembrane proteins called ion channels. Once a hydrophilic pore is available, ions move passively across the membrane driven by two forces: the electrical gradient (voltage difference) and the chemical gradient (concentration difference). The chemical gradient forces the ions to move from a compartment of a higher concentration to one of lower concentration. The electrical gradient forces ions to move in the direction of their inverse sign (i.e., cations [positively charged ions] move toward a negatively charged compartment, whereas anions [negatively charged ions] move toward a positively charged compartment). Because the chemical and electrical gradients can oppose each other, the direction of net ion movement will depend on the relative contributions of chemical gradient and electrical potential (i.e., the net electrochemical gradient), so that ions tend to move spontaneously from a higher to a lower electrochemical potential.[1-3]

The movement of an ion down its chemical gradient in one direction across the cell membrane results in build-up of excess charge carried by the ion on one side of the membrane, which generates an electrical gradient that impedes continuing ionic movement in the same direction. When the driving force of the electrical gradient across the membrane becomes equal and opposite to the force generated by the chemical gradient, the ion is said to be in electrochemical equilibrium, and the net transmembrane flux (or current) of that particular ion is zero. In this setting, the electrical potential is called the equilibrium potential (E_{ion}) (reversal potential or Nernst potential) of that individual ion. The E_{ion} for a given ion depends on its concentration on either side of the membrane and the temperature, and it measures the voltage that the ion concentration gradient generates when it acts as a battery. At membrane voltages more positive to the reversal potential of the ion, passive ion movement is outward, whereas it is inward at a membrane potential (also known as transmembrane potential; E_m) more negative to the Nernst potential of that channel.[1,3]

When multiple ions across a membrane are removed from their electrochemical equilibrium, each ion will tend to force the E_m toward its own E_{ion}. The contribution of each ion type to the overall E_m at any given moment is determined by the instantaneous permeability of the plasma membrane to that ion. The larger the membrane conductance to a particular ion, the greater is the ability of that ion to bring the E_m toward its own E_{ion}. Hence, the E_m is the average of the E_{ion} of all the ions to which the membrane is permeable, weighed according to the membrane conductance of each individual ion relative to the total ionic conductance of the membrane.[1,2]

Transmembrane Potentials

All living cells, including cardiomyocytes, maintain a difference in the concentration of ions across their membranes. There is a slight excess of positive ions on the outside of the membrane and a slight excess of negative ions on the inside of the membrane, resulting in a difference in the electrical charge (i.e., voltage difference) across the cell membrane, called the membrane potential (E_m). A membrane that exhibits an E_m is said to be polarized.[2]

In nonexcitable cells, and in excitable cells in their baseline states (i.e., not conducting electrical signals), the E_m is held at a relatively stable value, called the resting potential. All cells have a negative resting E_m (i.e., the cytoplasm is electrically negative relative to the extracellular fluid), which arises from the interaction of ion channels and ion pumps embedded in the membrane that maintain different ion concentrations on the intracellular and extracellular sides of the membrane.[2]

When an ion channel opens, it allows ion flux across the membrane that generates an electrical current (I). This current affects the E_m, depending on the membrane resistance (R), which refers to the ratio between the E_m and electrical current, as shown in Ohm's law: $E = I \times R$ or $R = E/I$. Resistance arises from the fact that the membrane impedes the movement of charges across it; hence, the cell membrane functions as a *resistor*. Conductance describes the ability of a membrane to allow the flux of charged ions in one direction across the membrane. The more permeable the membrane is to a particular ion, the greater is the conductance of the membrane to that ion. Membrane conductance (g) is the reciprocal of R: $g = 1/R$.[1]

Because the lipid bilayer of the cell membrane is very thin, accumulation of charged ions on one side gives rise to an electrical force (potential) that pulls oppositely charged particles toward the other side. Hence, the cell membrane functions as a *capacitor*. Although the absolute potential differences across the cell membrane are small, they give rise to enormous electrical potential gradients because they occur across a very thin surface. As a consequence, apparently small changes in E_m can produce large changes in potential gradient and powerful forces that are able to induce molecular rearrangement in membrane proteins, such as those required for opening and closing ion channels embedded in the cell membrane. The capacitance of the membrane is generally fixed and unaffected by the molecules that are embedded in it. In contrast, membrane resistance is highly variable and depends on the conductance of ion channels embedded in the membrane.[2,3]

The sodium (Na^+), potassium (K^+), calcium (Ca^{2+}), and chloride (Cl^-) ions are the major charge carriers, and their movement across the cell membrane creates a flow of current that generates excitation and signals in cardiac myocytes. The electrical current generated by the flux of an ion across the membrane is determined by the membrane conductance to that ion (g_{ion}) and the potential (voltage) difference across the membrane. The potential difference represents the potential at which there is no net ion flux (i.e., the E_{ion}) and the actual E_m: current = $g_{ion} \times (E_m - E_{ion})$.[1,4]

By convention, an inward current increases the electropositivity within the cell (i.e., causes depolarization of the E_m [to be less negative]) and can result from either the movement of positively charged ions (most commonly Na^+ or Ca^{2+}) into the cell or the efflux of negatively charged ions (e.g., Cl^-) out of the cell. An outward current increases the electronegativity within the cell (i.e., causes hyperpolarization of the E_m [to become more negative]) and can result from either the movement of anions into the cell or the efflux of cations (most commonly K^+) out of the cell.[3]

Opening and closing of ion channels can induce a departure from the relatively static resting E_m, called a depolarization if the interior voltage rises (becomes less negative) or a hyperpolarization if the interior voltage becomes more negative. The most important ion fluxes that depolarize or repolarize the membrane are passive (i.e., the ions move down their electrochemical gradient without requiring the expenditure of energy), occurring through transmembrane ion channels. In excitable cells, a sufficiently large depolarization can evoke a short-lasting all-or-none event called an action potential, in which the E_m very rapidly undergoes specific and large dynamic voltage changes.[1]

Both resting E_m and dynamic voltage changes such as the action potential are caused by specific changes in membrane permeabilities for Na^+, K^+, Ca^{2+}, and Cl^-, which, in turn, result from concerted changes in functional activity of various ion channels, ion transporters, and exchangers.[3]

The Cardiac Action Potential

During physiological electrical activity, the E_m is a continuous function of time. The current flowing through the cell membrane is, at each instant, provided by multiple channels and transporters carrying charge in opposite directions because of their different ion selectivity. The algebraic summation of these contributions is referred to as net transmembrane current.[1]

The cardiac action potential reflects a balance between inward and outward currents. When a depolarizing stimulus (typically from an electric current from an adjacent cell) abruptly changes the E_m of a resting cardiomyocyte to a critical value (the threshold level), the properties of the cell membrane and ion conductances change dramatically, precipitating a sequence of events involving the influx and efflux of multiple ions that together produce the action potential of the cell. In this fashion, an electrical stimulus is conducted from one cell to all the cells that are adjacent to it.[2]

Unlike skeletal muscle, cardiac muscle is electrically coupled so that the wave of depolarization propagates from one cell to the next, independent of neuronal input. The heart is activated by capacitive currents generated when a wave of depolarization approaches a region of the heart that is at its resting potential. Unlike ionic currents, which are generated by the flux of charged ions across the cell membrane, capacitive currents are generated by the movement of electrons toward and away from the surfaces of the membrane.[2,3] The resulting decrease in positive charge at the outer side of the cell membrane reduces the negative charge on the intracellular surface of the membrane. These charge movements, which are carried by electrons, generate a capacitive current. When an excitatory stimulus causes the E_m to become less negative and beyond a threshold level (approximately −65 mV for working atrial and ventricular cardiomyocytes), Na^+ channels activate (open) and permit an inward Na^+ current (I_{Na}), resulting in a rapid shift of the E_m to a positive voltage range. This event triggers a series of successive opening and closure of selectively permeable ion channels. The direction and magnitude of passive ion movement (and the resulting current) at any given transmembrane voltage are determined by the ratio of the intracellular and extracellular concentrations and the reversal potential of that ion, with the net flux being larger when ions move from the more concentrated side.[3]

The threshold is the lowest E_m at which opening of enough Na^+ channels (or Ca^{2+} channels in the setting of nodal cells) is able to initiate the sequence of channel openings needed to generate a propagated action potential. Small (subthreshold) depolarizing stimuli depolarize the membrane in proportion to the strength of the stimulus and cause only local responses because they do not open enough Na^+ channels to generate depolarizing currents large enough to activate nearby resting cells (i.e., insufficient to initiate a regenerative action potential). On the other hand, when the stimulus is sufficiently intense to reduce the E_m to a threshold value, regenerative action potential results, whereby intracellular movement of Na^+ depolarizes the membrane more, a process that increases conductance to Na^+ more, which allows more Na^+ to enter, and so on. In this fashion, the extent of subsequent depolarization becomes independent of the initial depolarizing stimulus, and more intense stimuli do not produce larger action potential responses; rather, an all-or-none response results.[2]

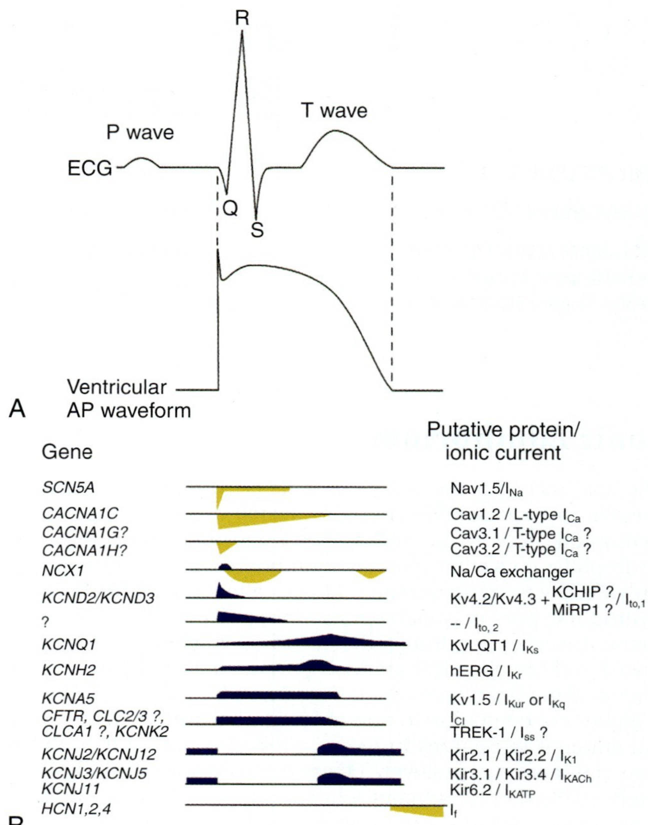

FIGURE 1-1 A, Depiction of a standard ECG tracing with respect to its underlying ventricular action potential (AP). B, The different ionic currents (see text) that contribute to action potential generation and the putative encoding genes are shown. Depolarizing currents are shown in yellow, repolarizing currents in blue. *(Modified with permission from Saenena JB, Vrints CJ: Molecular aspects of the congenital and acquired long QT syndrome: clinical implications. J Mol Cell Cardiol 44:633-646, 2007.)*

Electrical changes in the action potential follow a relatively fixed time and voltage relationship that differs according to specific cell types. Whereas the entire action potential takes several milliseconds in nerve cells, the cardiac action potential lasts several hundred milliseconds. The course of the action potential can be divided into five phases (numbered 0 to 4). Phase 4 is the resting E_m, and it describes the E_m when the cell is not being stimulated.

During the action potential, membrane voltages fluctuate in the range of −94 to +30 mV (Fig. 1-1). With physiological external K^+, the reversal potential of K^+ (E_K) is approximately −94 mV, and passive K^+ movement during an action potential is out of the cell. On the other hand, because the calculated reversal potential of a cardiac Ca^{2+} channel (E_{Ca}) is +64 mV, passive Ca^{2+} flux is into the cell.[5]

In normal atrial and ventricular myocytes and in His-Purkinje fibers, action potentials have very rapid upstrokes, mediated by the fast inward I_{Na}. These potentials are called fast response potentials. In contrast, action potentials in the normal sinus and atrioventricular (AV) nodal cells and many types of diseased tissues have very slow upstrokes, mediated by a slow inward, predominantly L-type voltage-gated Ca^{2+} current (I_{CaL}), rather than by the fast inward I_{Na} (Fig. 1-2). These potentials have been termed slow response potentials.[2,5]

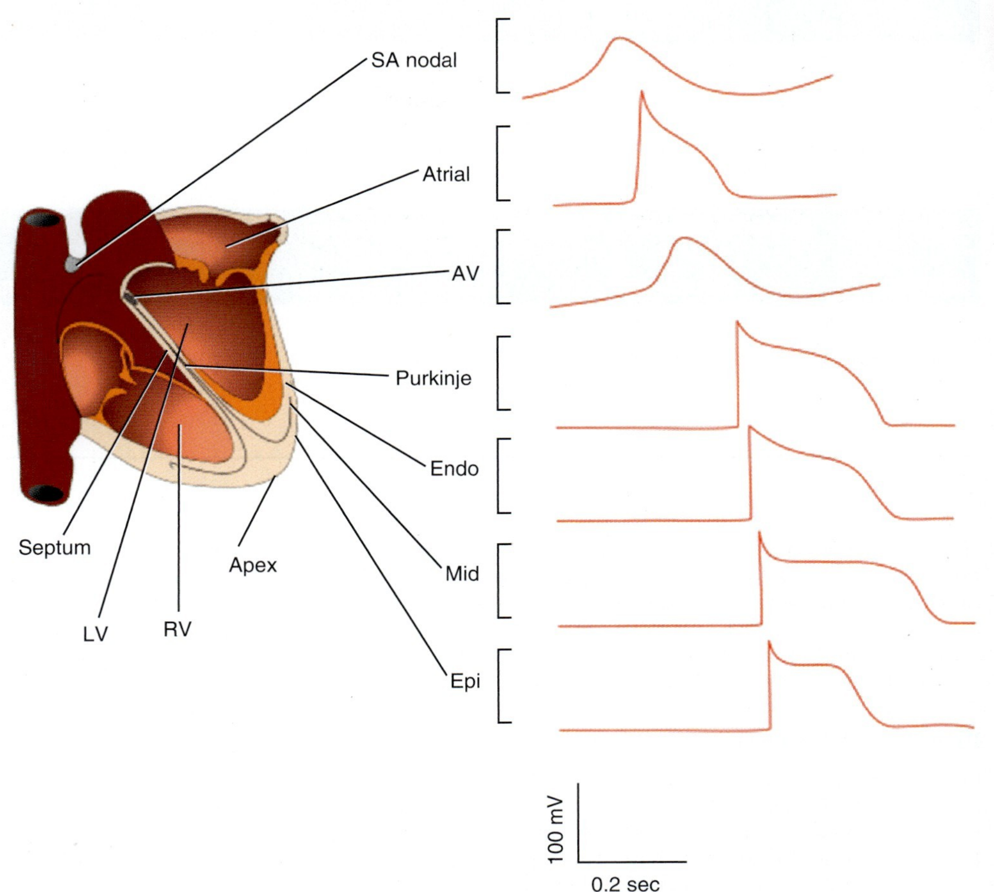

FIGURE 1-2 Action potential waveforms, displaced in time to reflect the temporal sequence of propagation, vary in different regions of the heart. AV = atrioventricular (node); endo = endocardial; epi = epicardial; mid = midmyocardial; LV = left ventricle; RV = right ventricle; SA = sinoatrial. *(Modified with permission from Nerbonne JM: Heterogeneous expression of repolarizing potassium currents in the mammalian myocardium. In Zipes DP, Jalife J, editors: Cardiac electrophysiology: from cell to bedside, ed 5, Philadelphia, 2009, Saunders, pp 293-305.)*

The Fast Response Action Potential

PHASE 4: THE RESTING MEMBRANE POTENTIAL

The E_m of resting atrial and ventricular cardiomyocytes remains steady throughout diastole. The resting E_m is caused by the differences in ionic concentrations across the membrane and the selective membrane permeability (conductance) to various ions. Large concentration gradients of Na^+, K^+, Ca^{2+}, and Cl^- across the cell membrane are maintained by the ion pumps and exchangers (Table 1-1).

Under normal conditions, the resting membrane is most permeable to K^+ and relatively impermeable to other ions. K^+ has the largest resting membrane conductance (g_K is 100 times greater than g_{Na}) because of the abundance of open K^+ channels at rest, whereas Na^+ and Ca^{2+} channels are generally closed. Thus, K^+ exerts the largest influence on the resting E_m. As a consequence, the resulting E_m is almost always close to the K^+ reversal potential (E_m approximates E_K). The actual resting E_m is slightly less negative than E_K because the cell membrane is slightly permeable to other ions.[2]

The inwardly rectifying K^+ (Kir) channels underlie an outward K^+ current (I_{K1}) responsible for maintaining the resting potential near the E_K in atrial, His-Purkinje, and ventricular cells, under normal conditions.[6,7] Kir channels preferentially allow currents of K^+ ions to flow into the cell with a strongly voltage-dependent decline of K^+ efflux (i.e., reduction of outward current) on membrane depolarization. As such, I_{K1} is a strong rectifier that passes K^+ currents over a limited range of E_m (see Chap. 2 for detailed discussion on the concept of rectification); at a negative E_m, I_{K1} conductance is much larger than that of any other current, thus, it clamps the resting E_m close to the reversal potential for K^+ (E_K). I_{K1} density is much higher in ventricular than in atrial myocytes, a feature that protects the ventricular cell from pacemaker activity. By contrast, I_{K1} is almost absent in sinus and AV nodal cells, thus allowing for relatively more depolarized resting diastolic potentials compared with atrial and ventricular myocytes (Table 1-2).[2]

A unique property of Kir currents is the unusual dependence of rectification on extracellular K^+ concentration. Specifically, on increase in extracellular K^+, the I_{K1} current-voltage relationship shifts nearly in parallel with the E_K and leads to a crossover phenomenon. One important consequence of such behavior is that at potentials positive to the crossover, K^+ conductance increases rather than decreases, against an expectation based on a reduced driving force for K^+ ions as a result of elevated extracellular K^+ concentration.[6-8]

The resting E_m also is powered by the Na^+-K^+ adenosine triphosphatase (ATPase) (the Na^+-K^+ pump), which helps establish concentration gradients of Na^+ and K^+ across the cell membrane. Under physiological conditions, the Na^+-K^+ pump transports two K^+ ions into the cell against its chemical gradient and three Na^+ ions outside against its electrochemical gradient at the cost of one adenosine triphosphate (ATP) molecule. Because the stoichiometry of ion movement is not 1:1, the Na^+-K^+ pump is electrogenic and generates a net outward movement of positive charges (i.e., an outward current). At faster heart rates, the rate of Na^+-K^+ pumping increases to maintain the same ionic gradients, thus counteracting the intracellular gain of Na^+ and loss of K^+ with each depolarization.

Although Ca^{2+} does not contribute directly to the resting E_m (since the voltage-activated Ca^{2+} channels are closed at the hyperpolarized resting E_m), changes in intracellular free Ca^{2+} concentration can affect other membrane conductance values. Increases in intracellular Ca^{2+} levels can stimulate the Na^+-Ca^{2+} exchanger

TABLE 1-1 Intracellular and Extracellular Ion Concentrations and Equilibrium Potentials in Cardiomyocytes

ION	EXTRACELLULAR CONCENTRATION (mM)	INTRACELLULAR CONCENTRATION (mM)	EQUILIBRIUM POTENTIAL (mV)
Na^+	135–145	10	+70
K^+	3.5–5.0	155	−94
Ca^{2+}	2	0.0001	+132

TABLE 1-2 Regional Differences in Cardiac Action Potential

PROPERTY	SINUS NODAL CELL	ATRIAL MUSCLE CELL	AV NODAL CELL	PURKINJE FIBER	VENTRICULAR MUSCLE CELL
Resting potential (mV)	−50 – −60	−80 – −90	−60 – −70	−90 – −95	−80 – −90
Action potential amplitude (mV)	60–70	110–120	70–80	120	110–120
Action potential duration (msec)	100–300	100–300	100–300	300–500	200–300

AV = atrioventricular.

(I_{Na-Ca}), which exchanges three Na^+ ions for one Ca^{2+} ion; the direction depends on the Na^+ and Ca^{2+} concentrations on the two sides of the membrane and the E_m difference. At resting E_m and during a spontaneous sarcoplasmic reticulum Ca^{2+} release event, this exchanger would generate a net Na^+ influx, possibly causing transient membrane depolarizations.[3]

PHASE 0: THE UPSTROKE—RAPID DEPOLARIZATION

On excitation of the cardiomyocyte by electrical stimuli from adjacent cells, its resting E_m (approximately −85 mV) depolarizes, leading to opening (activation) of Na^+ channels from its resting (closed) state and enabling a large and rapid influx of Na^+ ions (inward I_{Na}) into the cell down their electrochemical gradient. As a consequence of increased Na^+ conductance, the excited membrane no longer behaves like a K^+ electrode (i.e., exclusively permeable to K^+), but more closely approximates an Na^+ electrode, and the membrane potential moves toward the Na^+ E_{ion} (E_{Na}; see Table 1-1). Once an excitatory stimulus depolarizes the E_m beyond the threshold for activation of Na^+ channels (approximately −65 mV), the activated I_{Na} is regenerative and no longer depends on the initial depolarizing stimulus; the influx of Na^+ ions further depolarizes the membrane and thereby increases conductance to Na^+ more, which allows more Na^+ to enter.[2,9]

Normally, activation of Na^+ channels is transient; fast inactivation (closing of the pore) starts simultaneously with activation, but because inactivation is slightly delayed relative to activation, the channels remain transiently (less than 1 millisecond) open to conduct I_{Na} during phase 0 of the action potential before it closes. Additionally, the influx of Na^+ into the cell increases the positive intracellular charges and reduces the driving force for Na^+. When the E_{Na} is reached, no further Na^+ ions enter the cell.[9]

The rate at which depolarization occurs during phase 0, that is, the maximum rate of change of voltage over time, is indicated by the expression dV/dt_{max}, which is a reasonable approximation of the rate and magnitude of Na^+ entry into the cell and a determinant of conduction velocity for the propagated action potential.[2]

The threshold for activation of I_{CaL} is approximately −30 to −40 mV. Although I_{CaL} is normally activated during phase 0 by the regenerative depolarization caused by the fast I_{Na}, I_{CaL} is much smaller than the peak I_{Na}. The amplitude of I_{CaL} is not maximal near the action potential peak because of the time-dependent nature of I_{CaL} activation, as well as the low driving force ($E_m - E_{Ca}$) for I_{CaL}. Therefore, I_{CaL} contributes little to the action potential until the fast I_{Na} is inactivated, after completion of phase 0. As a result, I_{CaL} affects mainly the plateau of action potentials recorded in atrial and ventricular muscle and His-Purkinje fibers. On the other hand, I_{CaL} can play a prominent role in the upstroke of slow response action potentials in partially depolarized cells in which the fast Na^+ channels have been inactivated.[2]

PHASE 1: EARLY REPOLARIZATION

Phase 0 is followed by phase 1 (early repolarization) during which the membrane repolarizes rapidly and transiently to almost 0 mV (early notch), partly because of the inactivation of I_{Na} and concomitant activation of several outward currents. The transient outward K^+ current (I_{to}) is mainly responsible for phase 1 of the action potential. I_{to} rapidly activates (with time constants less than 10 milliseconds) by depolarization and then rapidly inactivates (25 to 80 milliseconds for the fast component of I_{to} [$I_{to,f}$], and 80 to 200 milliseconds for the slow component of I_{to} [$I_{to,s}$]). The influx of K^+ ions via I_{to} channels partially repolarizes the membrane, thus shaping the rapid (phase 1) repolarization of the action potential and setting the height of the initial plateau (phase 2; see Fig. 1-1). Additionally, an Na^+ outward current through the Na^+-Ca^{2+} exchanger operating in reverse mode likely contributes to early repolarization.[3,6,10]

PHASE 2: THE PLATEAU

Phase 2 (plateau) represents a delicate balance between the depolarizing inward currents (I_{CaL} and a small residual component of inward I_{NaL}) and the repolarizing outward currents (ultrarapidly [I_{Kur}], rapidly [I_{Kr}], and slowly [I_{Ks}] activating delayed outward rectifying currents; see Fig. 1-1). Phase 2 is the longest phase of the action potential, lasting tens (atrium) to hundreds of milliseconds (His-Purkinje system and ventricle). The plateau phase is unique among excitable cells and marks the phase of Ca^{2+} entry into the cell. It is the phase that most clearly distinguishes the cardiac action potential from the brief action potentials of skeletal muscle and nerve.[2]

I_{CaL} is activated by membrane depolarization, is largely responsible for the action potential plateau, and is a major determinant of the duration of the plateau phase. I_{CaL} also links membrane depolarization to myocardial contraction. L-type Ca^{2+} channels activate on membrane depolarization to potentials positive to −40 mV. I_{CaL} peaks at an E_m of 0 to +10 mV and tends to reverse at +60 to +70 mV, following a bell-shaped current-voltage relationship.[3]

Na^+ channels also make a contribution, although minor, to the plateau phase. After phase 0 of the action potential, some Na^+ channels occasionally fail to inactivate or exhibit prolonged opening or reopening repetitively for hundreds of milliseconds after variable and prolonged latencies, resulting in a small inward I_{Na} (less than

1% of the peak I_{Na}). This persistent or "late" I_{Na} (I_{NaL}), along with I_{CaL}, helps maintain the action potential plateau.[3,11,12]

I_{Kr} and I_{Ks} are activated at depolarized potentials. I_{Kr} activates relatively fast (in the order of tens of milliseconds) on membrane depolarization, thus allowing outward diffusion of K^+ ions in accordance with its electrochemical gradient, but voltage-dependent inactivation thereafter is very fast. Hence, only limited numbers of channels remain in the open state, whereas a considerable fraction resides in the nonconducting inactivated state. The fast voltage-dependent inactivation limits outward current through the channel at positive voltages and thus helps maintain the action potential plateau phase that controls contraction and prevents premature excitation. However, as the voltage becomes less positive at the end of the plateau phase of repolarization, the channels recover rapidly from inactivation; this process leads to a progressive increase in I_{Kr} amplitudes during action potential phases 2 and 3, with maximal outward current occurring before the final rapid declining phase of the action potential.[6,12,13]

I_{Ks}, which is approximately 10 times larger than I_{Kr}, also contributes to the plateau phase. I_{Ks} activates in response to membrane depolarization to potentials greater than −30 mV and gradually increases during the plateau phase because its time course of activation is extremely slow, slower than any other known K^+ current, and steady-state amplitude is achieved only with extremely long membrane depolarization. Hence, the contribution of I_{Ks} to the net repolarizing current is greatest late in the plateau phase, particularly during action potentials of long duration. Importantly, although I_{Ks} activates slowly compared with action potential duration, it is also slowly inactivated. As heart rate increases, I_{Ks} increases because channel deactivation is slow and incomplete during the shortened diastole. This allows I_{Ks} channels to accumulate in the open state during rapid successive depolarizations and mediate the faster rate of repolarization. Hence, I_{Ks} plays an important role in determining the rate-dependent shortening of the cardiac action potential.[6,12-14]

I_{Kur} is detected only in human atria but not in the ventricles, so that it is the predominant delayed rectifier current responsible for human atrial repolarization.[3,12] The Na^+-Ca^{2+} exchanger operating in forward mode and the Na^+-K^+ pump provide minor current components during phase 2.

Importantly, during the plateau phase, membrane conductance to all ions falls to rather low values. Thus, less change in current is required near plateau levels than near resting potential levels to produce the same changes in E_m. In particular, K^+ conductance falls during the plateau phase as a result of inward rectification of I_{Kr} and I_{K1} (that is, voltage-dependent decline of K^+ efflux and hence reduction of outward current) on membrane depolarization, in spite of the large electrochemical driving force on K^+ ions during the positive phase of the action potential (phases 0, 1, and 2). This property allows membrane depolarization following Na^+ channel activation, slows membrane repolarization, and helps maintain a more prolonged cardiac action potential. This also confers energetic efficiency in the generation of the action potential.[6,7,14]

PHASE 3: FINAL RAPID REPOLARIZATION

Phase 3 is the phase of rapid repolarization that restores the E_m to its resting value. Phase 3 is mediated by the increasing conductance of the delayed outward rectifying currents (I_{Kr} and I_{Ks}), the inwardly rectifying K^+ currents (I_{K1} and acetylcholine-activated K^+ current [I_{KACh}]), and time-dependent inactivation of I_{CaL} (see Fig. 1-1). Final repolarization during phase 3 results from K^+ efflux through the I_{K1} channels, which open at potentials negative to −20 mV.[6,12-14]

PHASE 4: RESTORATION OF RESTING MEMBRANE POTENTIAL

During the action potential, Na^+ and Ca^{2+} ions enter the cell and depolarize the E_m. Although the E_m is quickly repolarized by the efflux of K^+ ions, restoration of transmembrane ionic concentration gradients to the baseline resting state is necessary. This is achieved by the Na^+-K^+ ATPase (Na^+-K^+ pump, which exchanges two K^+ ions inside and three Na^+ ions outside) and by the Na^+-Ca^{2+} exchanger ($I_{Na\text{-}Ca}$, which exchanges three Na^+ ions for one Ca^{2+} ion).

Reduction of cytosolic Ca^{2+} concentration during diastole is achieved by the reuptake Ca^{2+} by the sarcoplasmic reticulum via activation of the sarco/endoplasmic reticulum Ca^{2+}-ATPase Ca^{2+} pump (SERCA), in addition to extrusion across the sarcolemma via the Na^+-Ca^{2+} exchanger. In the human heart under resting conditions, the time required for cardiac myocyte depolarization, contraction, relaxation, and recovery is approximately 600 milliseconds.[5,15,16]

REGIONAL HETEROGENEITY OF THE ACTION POTENTIAL

Substantial differences in the expression levels of ion channels underlie the substantial heterogeneity in action potential duration and configuration between cardiomyocytes located in different cardiac regions. The characteristics of the action potential differ in atrial versus ventricular myocardium, as well as across the ventricular myocardial wall from endocardium, midmyocardium (putative M cells), to epicardium (see Fig. 1-2).[3,12]

The density of I_{to} varies across the myocardial wall and in different regions of the heart. The markedly higher densities of I_{to}, together with the expression of I_{Kur}, accelerate the early phase of repolarization and lead to lower plateau potentials and shorter action potentials in atrial cells. In human ventricles, I_{to} densities are much higher in the epicardium and midmyocardium than in the endocardium. These regional differences are responsible for the shorter duration and the prominent phase 1 notch and the spike and dome morphology of epicardial and midmyocardial action potentials compared with endocardium. A prominent I_{to}-mediated action potential notch in ventricular epicardium but not endocardium produces a transmural voltage gradient during early ventricular repolarization that registers as a J wave or J point elevation on the ECG.[17] I_{to} densities are also reportedly higher in right than in left (midmyocardial and epicardial) ventricular myocytes, consistent with the more pronounced spike and dome morphology of right, compared with left, ventricular action potentials.[3,8,10,12]

Experimental studies in wedge preparations strongly suggest the presence of a subpopulation of cells in the midmyocardium (referred to as the M cells) that exhibits distinct electrophysiological (EP) properties, although the presence of M cells has not been consistently confirmed by intact heart experiments.[18-21] The putative midmyocardial cells appear to have the longest action potential duration across the myocardial wall, largely attributed to their weaker I_{Ks} current but stronger late I_{Na} and Na^+-Ca^{2+} exchanger currents. Hence, the M cells have been proposed to underlie the EP basis for transmural ventricular dispersion of repolarization and the T wave on the surface ECG, with the peak of the T wave (in wedge preparations) coinciding with the end of epicardial repolarization and the end of the T wave coinciding with the end of repolarization of the M cells. Although the role of M cells under physiological conditions remains controversial, these cells appear to have a significant role in arrhythmogenesis under a variety of pathological conditions, such as the long QT and Brugada syndromes, secondary to exaggeration of transmural repolarization gradients.[18,19]

As noted, I_{Kur} is detected only in human atria and not in the ventricles, so that it is the predominant delayed rectifier current responsible for human atrial repolarization and is a basis for the much shorter duration of the action potential in the atrium (see Table 1-2).[3,12]

I_{K1} density is much higher in ventricular than in atrial myocytes, and this explains the steep repolarization phase in the ventricles (where the more abundant I_{K1} plays a larger role in accelerating the terminal portion of repolarization) and the more shallow phase in the atria. The higher I_{K1} channel expression in the ventricle protects the ventricular cell from pacemaker activity.[6,7]

Changes in expression levels or gating properties of ion channels in pathological conditions can aggravate the regional heterogeneities in action potential duration and configuration that can be arrhythmogenic.[3,12]

The Slow Response Action Potential

In normal atrial and ventricular myocytes and in the His-Purkinje fibers, action potentials have very rapid upstrokes mediated by the fast inward I_{Na}. These potentials are called fast response potentials. In contrast, action potentials in the normal sinus and AV nodal cells and many types of diseased tissue have very slow upstrokes, mediated predominantly by the slow inward I_{CaL}, rather than by the fast inward I_{Na} (see Fig. 1-2). These potentials have been termed slow response potentials.[5]

As noted, the action potentials of pacemaker cells in the sinus and AV nodes are significantly different from those in working atrial and ventricular myocardium. The slow response action potentials are characterized by a more depolarized E_m at the onset of phase 4 (–50 to –65 mV), slow diastolic depolarization during phase 4, reduced action potential amplitude, and a much slower rate of depolarization in phase 0 than that in the working myocardial cells, thus resulting in slow conduction velocity of the cardiac impulse in the nodal regions (see Table 1-2). Cells in the His-Purkinje system can also exhibit phase 4 depolarization under special circumstances.[6,7]

PHASE 4: DIASTOLIC DEPOLARIZATION

In contrast to working atrial and ventricular myocytes and fibers in the His-Purkinje system, which maintain a steady diastolic E_m level of approximately –85 mV, sinus and AV nodal excitable cells exhibit a spontaneous, slow, progressive decline in the E_m during diastole (spontaneous diastolic depolarization or phase 4 depolarization) that underlies normal automaticity and pacemaking function. Once this spontaneous depolarization reaches threshold (approximately –40 mV), a new action potential is generated.[2,22,23]

The ionic mechanisms responsible for diastolic depolarization and normal pacemaker activity in the sinus node are still controversial. Originally, a major role was attributed to the decay of the delayed K^+ conductance (an outward current) activated during the preceding action potential (the I_K-decay theory). This model of pacemaker depolarization lost favor on the discovery of the "funny" current (I_f), sometimes referred to as the pacemaker current. Other ionic currents gated by membrane depolarization (i.e., I_{CaL} and T-type Ca^{2+} currents), nongated and nonspecific background leak currents, and a current generated by the Na^+-Ca^{2+} exchanger were also proposed to be involved in pacemaking.

Ic is a hyperpolarization-activated inward current (often referred to as the funny current because, unlike the majority of voltage-sensitive currents, it is activated by hyperpolarization rather than depolarization) that is carried largely by Na^+ and, to a lesser extent, K^+ ions. The I_f channels are deactivated during the action potential upstroke and the initial plateau phase of repolarization. However, they begin to activate at the end of the action potential as repolarization brings the E_m to levels more negative than approximately –40 to –50 mV, and they are fully activated at approximately –100 mV. Once activated, I_f depolarizes the membrane to a level where the Ca^{2+} current activates to initiate an action potential.[3] At the end of the repolarization phase of the action potential, because I_f activation occurs in the background of a decaying outward time-dependent K^+ current, the current flow quickly shifts from outward to inward, thus giving rise to a sudden reversal of voltage change (from repolarizing to depolarizing) at the maximum diastolic potential.[22-26]

On the other hand, several studies have shown that I_f is not the only current that can initiate the diastolic depolarization process in the sinus node. In addition to voltage and time, the electrogenic and regulatory molecules on the surface membrane of sinus node cells are strongly modulated by Ca^{2+} and phosphorylation, a finding suggesting that intracellular Ca^{2+} is an important player in controlling pacemaker cell automaticity. Newer evidence suggests that the sarcoplasmic reticulum, a major Ca^{2+} store in sinus node cells, can function as a physiological clock within the cardiac pacemaker cells and have a substantial impact on late diastolic depolarization.

The sarcoplasmic reticulum generates spontaneous, rhythmic, local Ca^{2+} releases (via ryanodine receptors, RyR2) beneath the surface of the membrane, in the absence of Ca^{2+} overload. Activation of the local oscillatory Ca^{2+} releases is independent of membrane depolarization and is driven by a high level of basal state phosphorylation of Ca^{2+} cycling proteins. Critically timed Ca^{2+} releases occur during the later phase of diastolic depolarization in the form of multiple locally propagating wavelets beneath the cell membrane, and they activate the forward mode of the Na^+-Ca^{2+} exchanger, thus resulting in an inward membrane current (I_{Na-Ca}). The I_{Na-Ca} causes the late diastolic depolarization to increase exponentially, driving the E_m to the threshold to activate a sufficient number of L-type Ca^{2+} channels and leading to generation of the upstroke of the next action potential. Although regulated by the E_m and submembrane Ca^{2+}, the Na^+-Ca^{2+} exchanger does not have time-dependent gating, as do ion channels, but generates an inward current almost instantaneously when submembrane Ca^{2+} concentration increases.[24,25,27,28]

Ca^{2+} influx via I_{CaL} during the action potential triggers Ca^{2+}-induced Ca^{2+} release from the sarcoplasmic reticulum. The resulting global sarcoplasmic reticular Ca^{2+} depletion synchronizes the sarcoplasmic reticulum throughout the cell in a Ca^{2+}-depleted state. Refilling of the sarcoplasmic reticulum ensures that the threshold of Ca^{2+} load required for spontaneous release is achieved at about the time when RyR2 inactivation is removed following prior activation; then the spontaneous local Ca^{2+} releases occur, thus activating I_{Na-Ca} to ignite the next action potential.[5,24,28]

Such rhythmic, spontaneous intracellular Ca^{2+} cycling has been referred to as the intracellular Ca^{2+} clock. Phosphorylation-dependent gradation of speed at which Ca^{2+} clock cycles is the essential regulatory mechanism of normal pacemaker rate and rhythm. The robust regulation of pacemaker function is ensured by tight integration of the Ca^{2+} clock and the classic sarcolemmal ion channel clock (formed by voltage-dependent membrane ion channels) to form the overall pacemaker clock. The action potential shape and ion fluxes are tuned by membrane clocks to sustain operation of the Ca^{2+} clock, which produces timely and powerful ignition of the membrane clocks to effect action potentials.[24,25,28]

There is some degree of uncertainty about the relative role of I_f versus that of intracellular Ca^{2+} cycling in controlling the normal pacemaker cell automaticity. Furthermore, the interactions between the membrane ion channel clock and the intracellular Ca^{2+} clock and cellular mechanisms underlying this internal Ca^{2+} clock are not completely elucidated. A further debate has arisen around their individual (or mutual) relevance in mediating the positive and negative chronotropic effects of neurotransmitters. Nevertheless, these interactions are of fundamental importance for understanding the integration of pacemaker mechanisms at the cellular level.[24,25,27]

PHASE 0: THE UPSTROKE—SLOW DEPOLARIZATION

I_{K1} is almost absent in sinus and AV nodal cells, thus allowing for relatively more depolarized resting diastolic potentials (–50 to –65 mV) compared with atrial and ventricular myocytes and facilitating diastolic depolarization mediated by the inward currents (e.g., I_f). At the depolarized level of the maximum diastolic potential of pacemaker cells, most Na^+ channels are inactivated and unavailable for phase 0 depolarization. Consequently, action potential upstroke is mainly achieved by I_{CaL}.[6,7]

L-type Ca^{2+} channels activate on depolarization to potentials positive to –40 mV, and I_{CaL} peaks at 0 to +10 mV. The peak amplitude I_{CaL} is less than 10% that of I_{Na}, and the time required for activation and inactivation of I_{CaL} is approximately an order of magnitude slower than that for I_{Na}. As a consequence, the rate of depolarization in phase 0 (dV/dt) is much slower and the peak amplitude of the action potential is less than that in the working myocardial cells.[5,15,29]

Excitability

Excitability of a cardiac cell describes the ease with which the cell responds to a stimulus with a regenerative action potential. A certain minimum charge has to be applied to the cell membrane to elicit a regenerative action potential (i.e., the stimulus should be sufficiently intense to reduce the E_m to the threshold value); excitability is inversely related to the charge required for excitation.[3]

Excitability of a cardiac cell depends on the passive and active properties of the cell membrane. The passive properties include the membrane resistance and capacitance and the intercellular resistance. The more negative the E_m, the more Na^+ channels are available for activation, the greater the influx of Na^+ into the cell during phase 0, and the greater the conduction velocity. In contrast, membrane depolarization to approximately −60 to −70 mV can inactivate half the Na^+ channels, and depolarization to −50 mV or less can inactivate all the Na^+ channels, thereby rendering Na^+ channels unavailable for mediating an action potential upstroke and reducing tissue excitability.[5]

On the other hand, supernormal excitability can be observed during a brief period at the end of phase 3 of the action potential. During the supernormal period, excitation is possible in response to an otherwise subthreshold stimulus; that same stimulus fails to elicit a response earlier or later than the supernormal period. Two factors are responsible for supernormality: the availability of fast Na^+ channels and the proximity of the E_m to threshold potential. During the supernormal phase of excitability, the cell has recovered enough to respond to a stimulus (i.e., an adequate number of Na^+ channels is available for activation). At the same time, because the E_m is still reduced, it requires only a little additional depolarization to bring the fiber to threshold; thus, a smaller stimulus than is normally required elicits an action potential.[30,31]

Reduced membrane excitability occurs in certain physiological and pathophysiological conditions. Genetic mutations that result in loss of Na^+ channel function, Na^+ channel blockade with class I antiarrhythmic drugs, and acute myocardial ischemia can cause reduced membrane excitability.[32]

Refractoriness

During a cardiac cycle, once an action potential is initiated, the cardiomyocyte becomes unexcitable to stimulation (i.e., unable to initiate another action potential in response to a stimulus of threshold intensity) for some duration of time (which is slightly shorter than the "true" action potential duration) until its membrane has repolarized to a certain level. This period of refractoriness to stimulation is physiologically necessary for the mechanical function of the heart; it allows only gradual recovery of excitability, thus permitting relaxation of cardiac muscle before subsequent activation. Additionally, the refractory period acts as a protective mechanism by preventing multiple, compounded action potentials from occurring (i.e., it limits the frequency of depolarization and heart rate). Therefore, this property is a determinant of susceptibility to arrhythmias.[33]

There are different levels of refractoriness during the action potential. During the *absolute refractory period* (which extends over phases 0, 1, 2, and part of phase 3 of the action potential), no stimulus, regardless of its strength, can reexcite the cell. After the absolute refractory period, a stimulus may cause some cellular depolarization, but it does not lead to a propagated action potential. The sum of this period (which includes a short interval of phase 3 of the action potential) and the absolute refractory period is termed the *effective refractory period* (ERP). The ERP is followed by the *relative refractory period*, which extends over the middle and late parts of phase 3. During the relative refractory period, initiation of a second action potential is *inhibited* but not impossible; a larger-than-normal stimulus can result in activation of the cell and lead to a propagating action potential. However, the upstroke of the new action potential is less steep and of lower amplitude, and its conduction velocity is slower than normal. As noted, there is a brief period in phase 3, the supernormal period, during which excitation is possible in response to an otherwise subthreshold stimulus (supernormal excitability).

The refractory period is determined, in part, by the action potential duration and the E_m, and the degree of refractoriness primarily reflects the number of Na^+ channels that have recovered from their inactive state. With repolarization, the Na^+ channel normally recovers rapidly from inactivation (within 10 milliseconds) and is ready to open again. The ERP extends from phase 0 to approximately −60 mV during phase 3 of the action potential, a time during which it is impossible for the myocardium to respond with a propagated action potential, or even to a strong stimulus. The relative refractory period extends from approximately −60 mV during phase 3 to the end of phase 3 of the action potential. During this period, a depressed response is possible to a strong stimulus. Therefore, when premature stimulation occurs during the relative refractory period (i.e., before full recovery and at less negative potentials of the cell membrane), a portion of Na^+ channels will still be refractory and unavailable for activation. Consequently, the I_{Na} and phase 0 of the next action potential will be reduced, and conduction of the premature stimulus will be slowed.[3,32]

In pacemaking tissues, I_{Na} is predominantly absent, and excitability is mediated by the activation of I_{CaL}. After inactivation, the transition of Ca^{2+} channels from the inactivated to the closed resting state (i.e., recovery from inactivation) is relatively slow. The time constant for recovery from inactivation depends on both the E_m and the intracellular Ca^{2+} concentration (typically 100 to 200 milliseconds at −80 mV and low intracellular Ca^{2+} concentration). This means that I_{CaL} must recover from inactivation between action potentials. As a result, excitability in pacemaking cells may not be recovered by the end of phase 3 of the action potential and full restoration of maximum diastolic potential, because L-type Ca^{2+} channels require longer time to recovery from inactivation to be able to mediate the upstroke of a new action potential. In other words, sinus and AV nodal cells remain refractory for a time interval that is longer than the time it takes for full voltage repolarization to occur, a phenomenon termed postrepolarization refractoriness.[5,29] This can also occur during some disease states such as myocardial infarction.

Conduction

Cardiac excitation involves generation of the action potential by individual cells, followed by propagation of the electrical impulse along each cardiac cell and rapidly from cell to cell throughout the cardiac tissue. The propagating electrical wavefront interacts with structural boundaries that exist at the cellular level (cell membranes, intercellular gap junctions), as well as at the more macroscopic level (microvasculature, connective tissue barriers, trabeculation).

Conduction velocity refers to the speed of propagation of the action potential through cardiac tissue and is determined by source-sink relationships, which reflect the interplay between the active membrane properties of cardiac cells (i.e., electrical excitability or refractoriness of the source generating the action potential, or both) and the passive properties determined by cell-to-cell coupling and tissue geometry (sink).[3,34]

During action potential propagation, an excited cell serves as a source of electrical charge for depolarizing neighboring unexcited cells. The requirements of adjacent resting cells to reach the threshold E_m constitute an electrical sink (load) for the excited cell. For propagation to succeed, the excited cell must provide sufficient charge to bring the E_m at a site in the sink from its diastolic value to the threshold. Once threshold is reached and action potential is generated, the load on the excited cell is removed, and the newly excited cell switches from being a sink to being a source for the downstream tissue, thus perpetuating the process of action potential propagation. Action potentials are "regenerative" because they can be conducted over large distances without attenuation.

The current provided by the source must reach the sink. The pathway between the source and the sink includes intracellular resistance (provided by the cytoplasm) and intercellular resistance (provided by the gap junctions). Extracellular resistance plays a role, but it can often be neglected. The coupling resistance is mainly determined by resistance of the gap junctions. Therefore, the number and distribution of gap junctions, as well as the conductance of the gap junction proteins (connexins) and the geometry of the source-sink relationship, are important factors for conduction of the action potential.

The safety factor for conduction predicts the success of action potential propagation and is based on the source-sink relationship. The *safety factor* is defined as the ratio of the current generated by the depolarizing ion channels of a cell (source) to the current consumed during the excitation cycle of a single cell in the tissue (sink). Thus, the safety factor for propagation is proportional to the excess of source current over the sink needs. By this definition, conduction fails when the safety factor drops to less than 1 and becomes increasingly stable as it rises to more than 1. This concept of propagation safety provides information about the dependence of propagation velocity on the state of the ion channels, cell-to-cell coupling, and tissue geometry.

An action potential traveling down a cardiac muscle fiber is propagated by local circuit currents, much as it does in nerve and skeletal muscle. Conduction velocity along the cardiac fiber is directly related to the action potential amplitude (i.e., the voltage difference between the fully depolarized and the fully polarized regions) and the rate of change of potential (i.e., the rate of rise of phase 0 of the action potential [dV/dt]). These factors depend on the amplitude of I_{Na}, which, in turn, is directly related to the E_m at the time of stimulation, the availability of Na^+ channels for stimulation, and the size of the Na^+ electrochemical potential gradient across the cell membrane. A reduction in I_{Na}, leading to a reduction in the rate or amplitude of depolarization during phase 0 of the action potential, can decrease axial current flow (and therefore capacitive current) and slow conduction or produce conduction block. Tissues with high concentration of Na^+ channels, such as Purkinje fibers, which contain up to 1 million Na^+ channels per cell, have a large, fast inward current. The large I_{Na} spreads quickly within and between cells to support rapid conduction (approximately 4 m/sec). In contrast, at a less negative resting E_m, Na^+ channel availability is limited because of the inactivation of a portion of the channels; hence, I_{Na} amplitude is attenuated, and the upstroke velocity is slowed. With progressive reduction of excitability, less Na^+ source current is generated, and conduction velocity and the safety factor decrease monotonically. When the safety factor falls to less than 1, conduction can no longer be sustained, and failure (conduction block) occurs. Action potentials with reduced upstroke velocity resulting from partial inactivation of Na^+ channels are called depressed fast responses.[35]

In tissues with slow response action potentials (sinus and AV nodes), the upstroke of the action potential is formed by I_{CaL} rather than I_{Na}. Because I_{CaL} has lower amplitude and slower activation kinetics than I_{Na}, slow response action potentials exhibit lower amplitudes and upstroke velocities. Hence, slow conduction (approximately 0.1 to 0.2 m/sec) and prolonged refractoriness are characteristic features of nodal regions. These cells also have a reduced safety factor for conduction, which means that the stimulating efficacy of the propagating impulse is low, and conduction block occurs easily.

Excitation-Contraction Coupling

Excitation-contraction coupling describes the physiological process by which electrical stimulation of the cardiomyocytes (the action potential) results in a mechanical response (muscle contraction). The contraction of a cardiac myocyte is governed primarily by intracellular Ca^{2+} concentration (Fig. 1-3). Ca^{2+} enters the cell during the plateau phase of the action potential through the L-type Ca^{2+} channels that line areas of specialized invaginations known as transverse (T) tubules. Although the rise in intracellular Ca^{2+} is small and not sufficient to induce contraction, the small amount of Ca^{2+} entering the cell via I_{CaL} triggers a massive release of Ca^{2+} from the sarcoplasmic reticulum (the major store for Ca^{2+}) into the cytosol by opening the RyR2 channels (present in the membrane of the sarcoplasmic reticulum) in a process known as Ca^{2+}-induced Ca^{2+} release (CICR). Approximately 75% of Ca^{2+} present in the cytoplasm during contraction is released from the sarcoplasmic reticulum.

Each junction between the sarcolemma (T tubule) and sarcoplasmic reticulum, where 10 to 25 L-type Ca^{2+} channels and 100 to 200 RyRs are clustered, constitutes a local Ca^{2+} signaling complex,

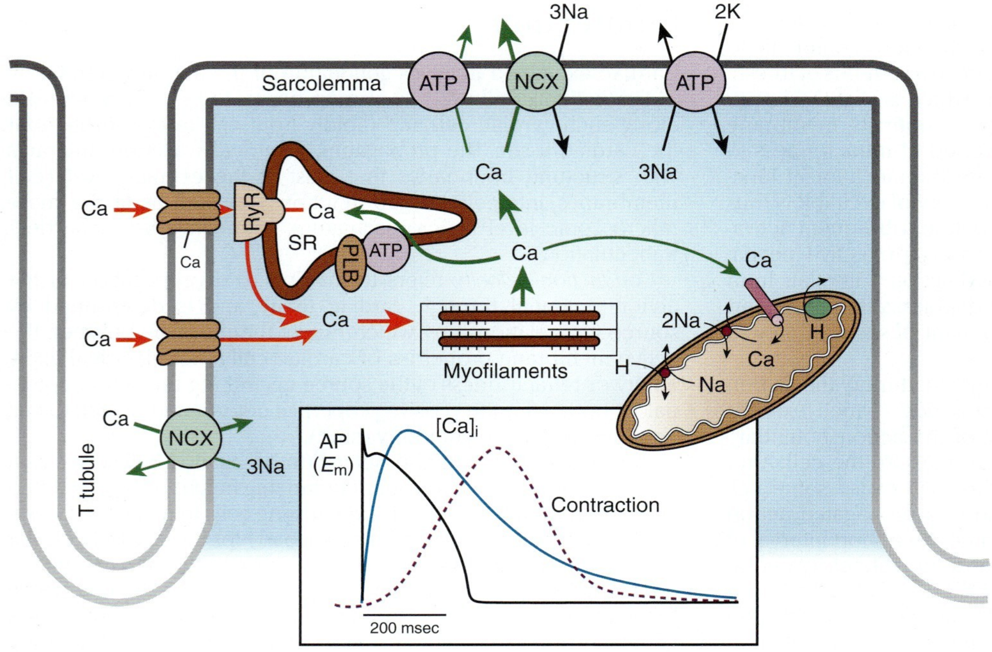

FIGURE 1-3 Ca^{2+} transport in ventricular myocytes. **Inset,** The time course of action potential (AP), Ca^{2+} transient and contraction at 37°C in a rabbit ventricular myocyte. ATP = Ca^{2+} adenosine triphosphatase; NCX = Na^+/Ca^{2+} exchanger; PLB = phospholamban; RyR = ryanodine receptor channel; SR = sarcoplasmic reticulum. *(Modified with permission from Bers DM: Cardiac excitation-contraction coupling. Nature 415:198-205, 2002.)*

or a couplon. When a Ca^{2+} channel opens, local cytosolic Ca^{2+} concentration rises in less than 1 millisecond in the junctional cleft to 10 to 20 μM, and this activates RyR2 to release Ca^{2+} from the sarcoplasmic reticulum. The close proximity of the RyR2 to the T tubule enables each L-type Ca^{2+} channel to activate 4 to 6 RyR2s and generate a Ca^{2+} spark. Ca^{2+} influx via I_{CaL} simultaneously activates approximately 10,000 to 20,000 couplons in each ventricular cardiomyocyte with every action potential.[36-38]

CICR raises cytosolic Ca^{2+} levels from approximately 10^{-7} M to approximately 10^{-5} M. The free Ca^{2+} binds to troponin C, a component of the thin filament regulatory complex, and thus causes a conformational change in the troponin-tropomyosin complex, such that troponin I exposes a site on the actin molecule that is able to bind to the myosin ATPase located on the myosin head. This binding results in ATP hydrolysis that supplies energy for a conformational change to occur in the actin-myosin complex. The result of these changes is a movement (ratcheting) between the myosin heads and the actin, such that the actin and myosin filaments slide past each other and thereby shorten the sarcomere length. Ratcheting cycles occur as long as cytosolic Ca^{2+} levels remain elevated.

CICR typically induces release of only approximately 50% to 60% of sarcoplasmic reticulum Ca^{2+} content. RyR2 channels are inactivated by a feedback mechanism from the rising Ca^{2+} concentration in the cleft and, more importantly, by the decline of sarcoplasmic reticulum Ca^{2+} content (a process referred to as luminal Ca^{2+}-dependent deactivation). This process ensures that the sarcoplasmic reticulum never is fully depleted of Ca^{2+} physiologically.[38,39]

Relaxation requires the removal of Ca^{2+} from the cytosol, a process vital for enabling ventricular chamber relaxation and filling, as well as for prevention of arrhythmias. At the end of phase 2 of the action potential, Ca^{2+} entry into the cell slows, and most of the surplus Ca^{2+} in the cytosol is resequestered into the sarcoplasmic reticulum by the SERCA, the activity of which is controlled by the phosphoprotein phospholamban. Additionally, some of the Ca^{2+} is extruded from the cell by the sarcolemmal Na^{+}-Ca^{2+} exchanger and, to a minor degree, the cell membrane Ca^{2+} ATPase, to balance the Ca^{2+} that enters with I_{CaL}. As the cytosolic Ca^{2+} concentration drops, Ca^{2+} dissociates rapidly from the myofilaments, thus inducing a conformational change in the troponin complex leading to troponin I inhibition of the actin binding site. At the end of the cycle, a new ATP binds to the myosin head and displaces the adenosine diphosphate, and the initial sarcomere length is restored, thus ending contraction. Recurring Ca^{2+} release-uptake cycles provide the basis for periodic elevations of cytosolic Ca^{2+} concentration and contractions of myocytes, hence for the orderly beating of the heart.[38,39]

REFERENCES

1. Zaza A: Control of the cardiac action potential: the role of repolarization dynamics, *J Mol Cell Cardiol* 48:106–111, 2010.
2. Katz AM: The cardiac action potential. In Katz AM, editor: *Physiology of the heart*, ed 5, Philadelphia, 2011, Lippincott Williams & Wilkins, pp 369–400.
3. Grant AO: Cardiac ion channels, *Circ Arrhythm Electrophysiol* 2:185–194, 2009.
4. Katz AM: Cardiac ion channels. In Katz AM, editor: *Physiology of the heart*, ed 5, Philadelphia, 2011, Lippincott Williams & Wilkins, pp 343–368.
5. Bodi I, Mikala G, Koch SE, et al: The L-type calcium channel in the heart: the beat goes on, *J Clin Invest* 115:3306–3317, 2005.
6. Tamargo J, Caballero R, Gomez R, et al: Pharmacology of cardiac potassium channels, *Cardiovasc Res* 62:9–33, 2004.
7. Anumonwo JM, Lopatin AN: Cardiac strong inward rectifier potassium channels, *J Mol Cell Cardiol* 48:45–54, 2010.
8. Oudit GY, Backx PH: Voltage-regulated potassium channels. In Zipes DP, Jalife J, editors: *Cardiac electrophysiology: from cell to bedside*, ed 5, Philadelphia, 2009, Saunders, pp 29–42.
9. Andavan GS, Lemmens-Gruber R: Voltage-gated sodium channels: mutations, channelopathies and targets, *Curr Med Chem* 18:377–397, 2011.
10. Niwa N, Nerbonne JM: Molecular determinants of cardiac transient outward potassium current (I(to)) expression and regulation, *J Mol Cell Cardiol* 48:12–25, 2010.
11. Abriel H: Cardiac sodium channel Na(v)1.5 and interacting proteins: physiology and pathophysiology, *J Mol Cell Cardiol* 48:2–11, 2010.
12. Amin AS, Tan HL, Wilde AA: Cardiac ion channels in health and disease, *Heart Rhythm* 7:117–126, 2010.
13. Charpentier F, Merot J, Loussouarn G, Baro I: Delayed rectifier K(+) currents and cardiac repolarization, *J Mol Cell Cardiol* 48:37–44, 2010.
14. Tristani-Firouzi M, Sanguinetti MC: Structural determinants and biophysical properties of HERG and KCNQ1 channel gating, *J Mol Cell Cardiol* 35:27–35, 2003.
15. Benitah JP, Alvarez JL, Gomez AM: L-type Ca(2+) current in ventricular cardiomyocytes, *J Mol Cell Cardiol* 48:26–36, 2010.
16. van der Heyden MA, Wijnhoven TJ, Opthof T: Molecular aspects of adrenergic modulation of cardiac L-type Ca2+ channels, *Cardiovasc Res* 65:28–39, 2005.
17. Antzelevitch C, Yan GX: J wave syndromes, *Heart Rhythm* 7:549–558, 2010.
18. Wilson LD, Jennings MM, Rosenbaum DS: Point: M cells are present in the ventricular myocardium, *Heart Rhythm* 8:930–933, 2011.
19. Glukhov AV, Fedorov VV, Lou Q, et al: Transmural dispersion of repolarization in failing and nonfailing human ventricle, *Circ Res* 106:981–991, 2010.
20. Janse MJ, Coronel R, Opthof T: Counterpoint: M cells do not have a functional role in the ventricular myocardium of the intact heart, *Heart Rhythm* 8:934–937, 2011.
21. Opthof T, Coronel R, Janse MJ: Is there a significant transmural gradient in repolarization time in the intact heart? Repolarization gradients in the intact heart, *Circ Arrhythm Electrophysiol* 2:89–96, 2009.
22. Mangoni ME, Nargeot J: Genesis and regulation of the heart automaticity, *Physiol Rev* 88:919–982, 2008.
23. Baruscotti M, Barbuti A, Bucchi A: The cardiac pacemaker current, *J Mol Cell Cardiol* 48:55–64, 2010.
24. Lakatta EG: A paradigm shift for the heart's pacemaker, *Heart Rhythm* 7:559–564, 2010.
25. Venetucci LA, Trafford AW, O'Neill SC, Eisner DA: The sarcoplasmic reticulum and arrhythmogenic calcium release, *Cardiovasc Res* 77:285–292, 2008.
26. DiFrancesco D: The role of the funny current in pacemaker activity, *Circ Res* 106:434–446, 2010.
27. Maltsev VA, Lakatta EG: Dynamic interactions of an intracellular Ca2+ clock and membrane ion channel clock underlie robust initiation and regulation of cardiac pacemaker function, *Cardiovasc Res* 77:274–284, 2008.
28. Lakatta EG, Maltsev V: A new functional paradigm for the heart's pacemaker: mutual entrainment of intracellular calcium clocks and surface membrane ion channel clocks. In Zipes DP, Jalife J, editors: *Cardiac electrophysiology: from cell to bedside*, ed 5, Philadelphia, 2009, Saunders, pp 235–247.
29. Ono K, Iijima T: Cardiac T-type Ca(2+) channels in the heart, *J Mol Cell Cardiol* 48:65–70, 2010.
30. Kilborn MF: Electrocardiographic manifestations of supernormal conduction, concealed conduction, and exit block. In Zipes DP, Jalife J, editors: *Cardiac electrophysiology: from cell to bedside*, ed 4, Philadelphia, 2004, Saunders, pp 733–738.
31. Fisch C, Knoebel SB: Supernormal conduction and excitability. In Fisch C, Knoebel SB, editors: *Electrocardiography of clinical arrhythmias*, Armonk, NY, 2000, Futura, pp 237–252.
32. Kleber AG, Rudy Y: Basic mechanisms of cardiac impulse propagation and associated arrhythmias, *Physiol Rev* 84:431–488, 2004.
33. Hund TJ, Rudy Y: Determinants of excitability in cardiac myocytes: mechanistic investigation of memory effect, *Biophys J* 79:3095–3104, 2000.
34. Noorman M, van der Heyden MA, van Veen TA, et al: Cardiac cell-cell junctions in health and disease: electrical versus mechanical coupling, *J Mol Cell Cardiol* 47:23–31, 2009.
35. Amin AS, Asghari-Roodsari A, Tan HL: Cardiac sodium channelopathies, *Pflugers Arch* 460:223–237, 2010.
36. Kushnir A, Marks AR: The ryanodine receptor in cardiac physiology and disease, *Adv Pharmacol* 59:1–30, 2010.
37. Mohamed U, Napolitano C, Priori SG: Molecular and electrophysiological bases of catecholaminergic polymorphic ventricular tachycardia, *J Cardiovasc Electrophysiol* 18:791–797, 2007.
38. Bers DM: Calcium cycling and signaling in cardiac myocytes, *Annu Rev Physiol* 70:23–49, 2008.
39. Gyorke S: Molecular basis of catecholaminergic polymorphic ventricular tachycardia, *Heart Rhythm* 6:123–129, 2009.

CHAPTER 2 Cardiac Ion Channels

Ion channels are pore-forming membrane proteins that regulate the flow of ions passively down their electrochemical gradient across the membrane. Ion channels are present on all membranes of cells (plasma membrane) and intracellular organelles (nucleus, mitochondria, endoplasmic reticulum). There are more than 300 types of ion channels in a living cell. The channels are not randomly distributed in the membrane, but tend to cluster at the intercalated disc in association with modulatory subunits.[1]

Ion channels are distinguished by two important characteristics: ion permeation selectivity and gating kinetics. Ion channels can be classified by the strongest permeant ion (sodium [Na^+], potassium [K^+], calcium [Ca^{2+}], and chloride [Cl^-]), but some channels are less selective or are not selective, as in gap junctional channels. Size, valency, and hydration energy are important determinants of selectivity. Na^+ channels have a selectivity ratio for Na^+ to K^+ of 12:1. Voltage-gated K^+ and Na^+ channels exhibit more than 10-fold discrimination against other monovalent and divalent cations, and voltage-gated Ca^{2+} channels exhibit a more than 1000-fold discrimination against Na^+ and K^+ ions and are impermeable to anions. Ions move through the channel pore at a very high rate (more than 10^6 ions/sec).

Gating is the mechanism of opening and closing of ion channels and represents time-dependent transitions among distinct conformational states of the channel protein resulting from molecular movements, most commonly in response to variations in voltage gradient across the plasma membrane (termed voltage-dependent gating) and, less commonly, in response to specific ligand molecules binding to the extracellular or intracellular side of the channel (ligand-dependent gating) or in response to mechanical stress such as stretch, pressure, shear, or displacement (mechanosensitive gating).

Importantly, channel opening and closing are not instantaneous but usually take time. The transition from the resting (closed) state to the open state is called activation. Once opened, channels do not remain in the open state, but instead they undergo conformational transition in a time-dependent manner to a stable nonconducting (inactivated) state. Inactivated channels are incapable of reopening and must undergo a recovery or reactivation process back to the resting state to regain their ability to open. Inactivation curves of the various voltage-gated ion channel types differ in their slopes and midpoints of inactivation and can overlap, in which case a steady-state or noninactivating current flows.[1]

Ion channels differ with respect to the number of subunits of which they are composed and other aspects of structure. Many ion channels function as part of macromolecular complexes in which many components are assembled at specific sites within the membrane. For most ion channels, the pore-forming subunit is called the α subunit, whereas the auxiliary subunits are denoted β, gamma, and so on. Most ion channels have a single pore; however, some have two.[1]

Sodium Channels

Structure and Physiology

The cardiac Na^+ channel complex is composed of a primary α and multiple ancillary β subunits. The approximately 2000-amino-acid α subunit contains the channel's ion-conducting pore and controls the channel selectivity for Na^+ ions and voltage-dependent gating machinery. This subunit contains all the drug and toxin interaction sites identified to date. The α subunit ($Na_v1.5$), encoded by the *SCN5A* gene, consists of four internally homologous domains (I to IV) that are connected to each other by cytoplasmic linkers (Fig. 2-1). Each domain consists of six membrane-spanning segments (S1 to S6), connected to each other by alternating intracellular and extracellular peptide loops. The four domains are arranged in a fourfold circular symmetry to form the channel. The extracellular loops between S5 and S6 (termed the P segments) have a unique primary structure in each domain (Fig. 2-2). The P segments curve back into the membrane to form an ion-conducting central pore whose structural constituents determine the selectivity and conductance properties of the Na^+ channel.[2]

Four auxiliary β subunits ($Na_v\beta1$ to $Na_v\beta4$, encoded by the genes *SCN1B* to *SCN4B*, respectively) have been identified; each is a glycoprotein with a single membrane-spanning segment. The β_1 subunit likely plays a role in modulation of the gating properties and level of expression of the Na^+ channel.[2]

Na^+ channels are the typical example of voltage-gated ion channels. Na^+ channels switch among three functional states: deactivated (closed), activated (open), and inactivated (closed), depending on the membrane potential (E_m). These channel states control Na^+ ion permeability through the channel into the

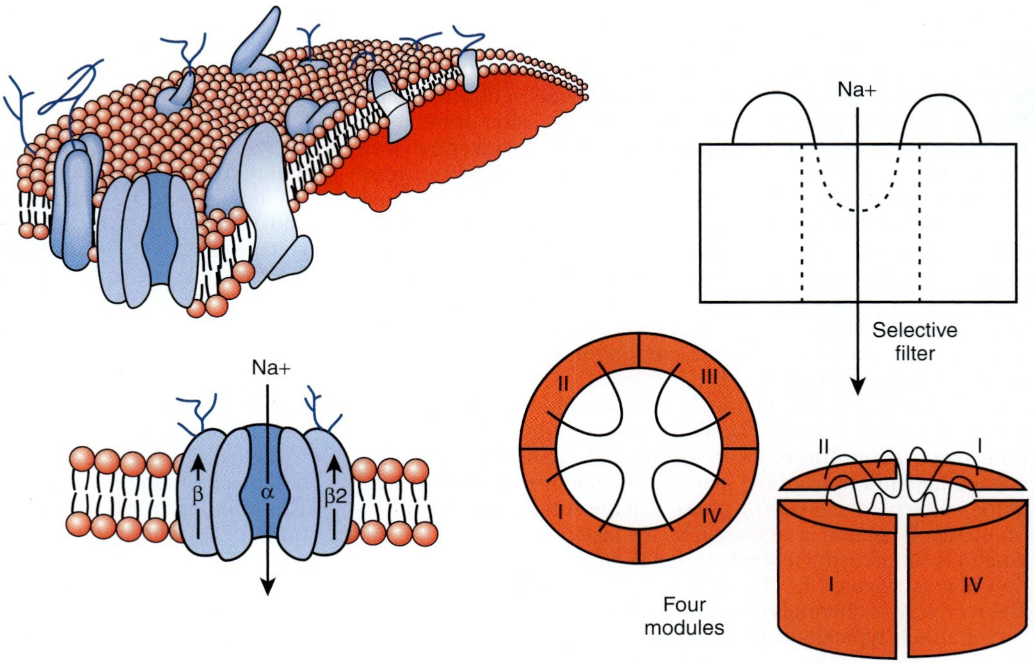

FIGURE 2-1 The sodium channel macromolecular complex. See text for discussion. *(From Boussy T, Paparella G, de Asmundis C, et al: Genetic basis of ventricular arrhythmias. Heart Fail Clin 6:249-266, 2010.)*

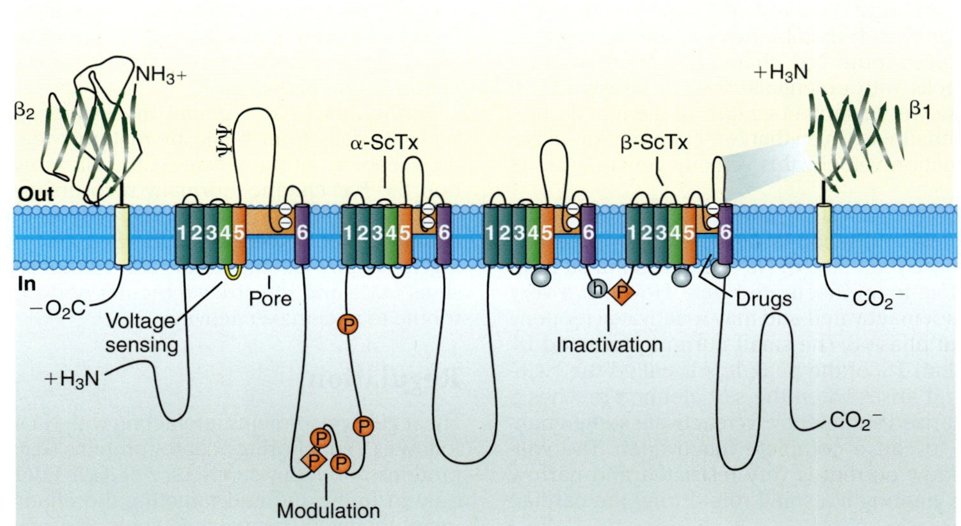

FIGURE 2-2 Transmembrane organization of sodium channel subunits. The primary structures of the subunits of the voltage-gated ion channels are illustrated as transmembrane folding diagrams. Cylinders represent probable α-helical segments: S1 to S3, blue; S4, green; S5, orange; S6, purple; outer pore loop, shaded orange area. Bold lines represent the polypeptide chains of each subunit, with length approximately proportional to the number of amino acid residues in the brain sodium channel subtypes. The extracellular domains of the β_1 and β_2 subunits are shown as immunoglobulin-like folds. Ψ shows sites of probable *N*-linked glycosylation. P represents sites of demonstrated protein phosphorylation by protein kinase A (red circles) and protein kinase C (red diamonds); h in the blue circle signifies an inactivation particle in the inactivation gate loop; the empty blue circles represent sites implicated in forming the inactivation gate receptor. The structure of the extracellular domain of the β subunits is illustrated as an immunoglobulin-like fold based on amino acid sequence homology to the myelin P0 protein. Sites of binding of α and β scorpion toxins (α-ScTx, β-ScTx) and a site of interaction between α and β_1 subunits also are shown. H_3N and NH_3 = ammonia. *(From Caterall WA, Maier SK: Voltage-gated sodium channels and electrical excitability of the heart. In Zipes DP, Jalife J, editors: Cardiac electrophysiology: from cell to bedside, ed 5, Philadelphia, 2009, Saunders, pp 9-17.)*

cardiomyocyte. Na^+ channel activation allows Na^+ ion influx into the cell, and inactivation blocks entry of Na^+ ions.[2]

On excitation of the cardiomyocyte by electrical stimuli from adjacent cells, its resting E_m (approximately −85 mV) depolarizes. The positively charged S4 segment of each domain of the α subunit functions as the sensor of the transmembrane voltage; these segments are believed to undergo rapid structural conformational changes in response to membrane depolarization, thus leading to channel opening (activation) from its resting (closed) state and enabling a large and rapid influx of Na^+ (inward Na^+ current [I_{Na}]) during the rapid upstroke (phase 0) of the action potential in atrial, ventricular, and Purkinje cardiomyocytes.[3]

Normally, activation of Na^+ channels is transient; fast inactivation (closing of the pore) starts simultaneously with activation, but because inactivation is slightly delayed relative to activation, the channels remain transiently open to conduct I_{Na} during phase 0 of the action potential before it closes. Each Na^+ channel opens very briefly (less than 1 millisecond) during phase 0 of the action potential; collectively, activation of the channel lasts a few milliseconds and is followed by fast inactivation.

Na^+ channel inactivation comprises different conformational states, including fast, intermediate, and slow inactivation. Fast inactivation is at least partly mediated by rapid occlusion of the inner mouth of the pore by the cytoplasmic interdomain linker between domains III and IV of the α subunit, which has a triplet of hydrophobic residues that likely functions as a hinged "latch" that limits or restricts Na^+ ion pass through the pore. The carboxyl terminus (C-terminus) also plays an important role in the control of Na^+ channel inactivation and stabilizing the channels in the inactivated state by interacting with the loop linking domains III and IV. Importantly, although most Na^+ channels open before inactivating, some actually inactivate without ever opening (a process known as closed-state inactivation).[1,4]

Once inactivated, Na^+ channels do not conduct any more current and cannot be reactivated (reopened) until after recovery from inactivation. The recovery of the Na^+ channel to reopen is voltage dependent. Channel inactivation is removed when the E_m of the cell repolarizes during phase 4 of the action potential. Membrane repolarization is facilitated by the fast inactivation of the Na^+ channels (limiting the inward current) and is augmented by activation of voltage-gated K^+ channels (allowing the outward current). The recovery of channels from inactivation is also time dependent; Na^+ channels typically activate within 0.2 to 0.3 milliseconds and inactivate completely within 2 to 5 milliseconds.

Following recovery, Na^+ channels enter a closed state that represents a nonconducting conformation, which allows the channels to be activated again during the next action potential. The fraction of channels available for opening varies from almost 100% at −90 mV and 50% at −75 mV to almost 0% at +40 mV. Consequently, highly polarized (−80 to −90 mV) cell membranes can be depolarized rapidly by stimuli because more Na^+ channels reopen, whereas partially depolarized cells with potentials close to threshold −70 mV generate a much slower upstroke because of the inactivation of a proportion of Na^+ channels. Given that Na^+ channels are major determinants of conduction velocity, this velocity generally slows at a reduced E_m.

Na^+ channel activation, inactivation, and recovery from inactivation occur within a few milliseconds. At the end of phase 1 of the action potential, more than 99% of Na^+ channels transit from an open (activated) state to an inactivated state. However, a very few Na^+ channels are not inactivated and may reactivate (reopen) during action potential phase 3. The small current produced by these channels (less than 1% of the peak I_{Na}) is called the "window" current because it arises when the sarcolemma reaches a potential that is depolarized sufficiently to reactivate some channels, but not enough to cause complete inactivation. The voltage range for the window current is very restricted and narrow in healthy hearts, thus granting it a small role during the cardiac action potential.

In addition to these rapid gating transitions, Na^+ channels are also susceptible to slower inactivating processes (slow inactivation) if the membrane remains depolarized for a longer time. These slower events can contribute to the availability of active channels under various physiological conditions. Whereas fast-inactivated Na^+ channels recover rapidly (within 10 milliseconds) during the hyperpolarized interval between stimuli, slow inactivation requires much longer recovery times (ranging from hundreds of milliseconds to many seconds). The molecular movements leading to slow inactivation are less well understood. The P segments seem to play a key role in slow inactivation.[4]

Some Na^+ channels occasionally show alternative gating modes consisting of isolated brief openings occurring after variable and prolonged latencies and bursts of openings during which the channel opens repetitively for hundreds of milliseconds. The isolated brief openings are the result of the occasional return from the inactivated state. The bursts of openings are the result of occasional failure of inactivation.[1] Prolonged opening or reopening of some Na^+ channels during phases 2 and 3 can result in a small late I_{Na} (I_{NaL}). Despite its minor contribution in healthy hearts, I_{NaL} can potentially play an important role in diseased hearts.[3]

Function

Na^+ channels play a pivotal role in the initiation, propagation, and maintenance of the normal cardiac rhythm. The I_{Na} determines excitability and conduction in atrial, His-Purkinje system (HPS), and ventricular myocardium. On membrane depolarization, the voltage-gated Na^+ channels respond within a millisecond by opening, thus leading to the very rapid depolarization of the cardiac cell membrane (phase 0 of the action potential), reflected by the fast (within tenths of a microsecond) subsequent opening of Na^+ channels triggering the excitation-contraction coupling. Na^+ entry during phase 0 of the action potential also modulates intracellular Na^+ levels and, through Na^+-Ca^{2+} exchange, intracellular Ca^{2+} concentration and cell contraction.

The cardiac Na^+ channel also plays a crucial role in the propagation of action potentials throughout the atrium, HPS, and ventricles. The opening of Na^+ channels in the atria underlies the P wave on the ECG, and in the ventricles I_{Na} underlies the QRS complex and enables a synchronous ventricular contraction. Because the upstroke of the electrical potential primarily determines the speed of conduction between adjacent cells, Na^+ channels are present in abundance in tissues where speed is of importance. Cardiac Purkinje cells contain up to 1 million Na^+ channels, a finding that illustrates the importance of rapid conductance in the heart.[2]

Na^+ channels also make a contribution in the plateau phase (phase 2) and help determine the duration of the action potential. After phase 0 of the action potential, I_{Na} decreases to less than 1% of its peak value over the next several milliseconds because of voltage-dependent inactivation. This persistent or "late" inward I_{Na} (I_{NaL}), along with the L-type Ca^{2+} current (I_{CaL}), helps maintain the action potential plateau.[5]

Furthermore, Na^+ channel inactivation is very important as it prevents cells from being prematurely reexcited because of the unavailability of the voltage-gated Na^+ channels. With repolarization, the Na^+ channel normally recovers rapidly from inactivation (within 10 milliseconds) and is ready to open again. Hence, Na^+ channels help to determine the frequency of action potential firing. To a lesser extent, cardiac Na^+ channels are also present in the sinus node and the atrioventricular node (AVN), where they contribute to pacemaker activity.

Regulation

The regulatory proteins interacting with $Na_v1.5$ may be classified as follows: (1) anchoring-adaptor proteins (e.g., ankyrin-G, syntrophin proteins, multicopy suppressor of gsp1 [MOG1]), which play roles only in trafficking and targeting the channel protein in specific membrane compartments; (2) enzymes interacting with and modifying the channel structure (post-translational modifications), such as protein kinases or ubiquitin ligases; and (3) proteins modulating the biophysical properties of $Na_v1.5$ on binding (e.g., caveolin-3, calmodulin, glycerol 3-phosphate dehydrogenase 1–like [G3PD1L], telethonin, Plakophilin-2).[5] Coexpression of $Na_v1.5$ with its β subunits induces acceleration in the recovery from inactivation and enhancement of I_{Na} amplitude.

The cardiac Na^+ channels are subject to phosphorylation and dephosphorylation by kinases or phosphatases. The intracellular linker between domains I and II contains eight consensus sites for cyclic adenosine monophosphate (cAMP)–dependent protein kinase A (PKA) phosphorylation. cAMP-dependent PKA and G protein stimulatory α subunit (Gsα) modulate the function of expressed cardiac Na^+ channels on β-adrenergic stimulation and enhance I_{Na}.[1]

In contrast, activation of α-adrenergic stimulating protein kinase C (PKC) results in the reduction of I_{Na}. The effect of PKC is largely attributable to phosphorylation of a highly conserved serine in the linker between domains III and IV. PKC reduces the maximal conductance of the channels and alters gating. Na^+ channels exhibit a hyperpolarizing shift in the steady-state availability curve, suggesting an enhancement of inactivation from closed states.

All subunits of the Na^+ channel are modified by glycosylation. The β_1 and β_2 subunits are heavily glycosylated, with up to 40% of the mass being carbohydrate. In contrast, the cardiac α subunit is only 5% sugar by weight. Sialic acid is a prominent component of the N-linked carbohydrate of the Na^+ channel. The addition of such a highly charged carbohydrate has predictable effects on the voltage dependence of gating through alteration of the surface charge of the channel protein.[1]

Pharmacology

Na^+ channels are the targets for the action of class I antiarrhythmic drugs. Na^+ channel blockers bind to a specific receptor within the channel's pore. The binding blocks ion movement through the pore and stabilizes the inactivated state of Na^+ channels. Blockade of Na^+ channels tends to decrease tissue excitability and conduction velocity (by attenuating peak I_{Na}) and can shorten action potential duration (by attenuating late I_{Na}).[1,6]

One important component in the action of antiarrhythmic drugs is a voltage-dependent change in the affinity of the drug-binding site (i.e., the channel is a modulated receptor). Additionally, restricted access to binding sites can contribute to drug action, a phenomenon that has been called the guarded receptor model. Open and inactivated channels are more susceptible to block than resting channels, likely because of a difference in binding affinity or state-dependent access to the binding site. Consequently, binding of antiarrhythmic drug occurs primarily during the action potential (known as use-dependent block), and the block dissipates after repolarization (i.e., in the interval between action potentials). When the time interval between depolarizations is insufficient for block to recover before the next depolarization occurs (secondary to either abbreviation of the interval between action potentials during fast heart rates or slow kinetics of the unbinding of the Na^+ channel blocker), block of Na^+ channels accumulates (resulting in an increased number of blocked channels and enhanced blockade).[6] A drug with rapid kinetics produces less channel block with the subsequent depolarization than does a drug with slower recovery. Use-dependent block is important for the action of antiarrhythmic drugs because it allows strong drug effects during fast heart rates associated with tachyarrhythmias but limits Na^+ channel block during normal heart rates. Importantly, drug recovery kinetics can potentially be slowed by pathophysiological conditions such as membrane depolarization, ischemia, and acidosis.[1] This property is known as use-dependence and is seen most frequently with the class IC agents, less frequently with the class IA drugs, and rarely with the class IB agents.

Class I antiarrhythmic drugs can be classified into three groups according to rates of drug binding to and dissociation from the channel receptor. Class IC drugs (flecainide and propafenone) block both the open and inactivated state (which is induced by depolarization) Na^+ channels and have the slowest kinetics of unbinding during diastole. The results are prolongation of conduction at normal heart rates and a further increase in the effect at more rapid rate (use-dependence).

The class IB agents (lidocaine, mexiletine, and tocainide) block both open and inactivated Na^+ channels and dissociate from the channel more rapidly than do other class I drugs. As a consequence, class IB drugs exhibit minimal or no effects on the Na^+ channels in normal tissue but cause significant conduction slowing in depolarized tissue, especially at faster depolarization rates. Furthermore, class IB drugs are less effective in the atrium, where the action potential duration is so short that the Na^+ channel is in the inactivated state only briefly compared with the relatively long diastolic recovery times; thus, accumulation of block is less likely to result from the rapid recovery of block.

Class IA drugs (quinidine, procainamide, and disopyramide) exhibit open state block, have intermediate effects on Na^+ channels, and generally only cause significant prolongation of conduction in cardiac tissue at rapid heart rates. Because the open state block is dominant and recovery from block is slow, these drugs are effective in both the atrium (where action potential duration is short) and the ventricle (where the action potential duration is long).

The late I_{Na} (I_{NaL}) also can be a target for blockade. Several drugs exhibit relative selectivity for block of late I_{NaL} over peak I_{Na}, including mexiletine, flecainide, lidocaine, amiodarone, and ranolazine.

Importantly, class IA drugs also have moderate K^+ channel blocking activity (which tends to slow the rate of repolarization and prolong the action potential duration) and anticholinergic activity, and they tend to depress myocardial contractility. At slower heart rates, when use-dependent blockade of I_{Na} is not significant, K^+ channel blockade becomes predominant (reverse use-dependence), leading to prolongation of the action potential duration and QT interval and increased automaticity. Flecainide and propafenone also have K^+ channel blocking activity and can increase the action potential duration in ventricular myocytes. Propafenone has significant β-adrenergic blocking activity.

Inherited Channelopathies

Mutations in genes that encode various subunits of the cardiac Na^+ channel or proteins involved in regulation of the inward I_{Na} have been linked to several types of electrical disorders (Table 2-1). Depending on the mutation, the consequence is either a gain of channel function (with consequent prolongation of action potential duration because more positive ions accumulate in the cell) or an overall loss of channel function that influences the initial depolarizing phase of the action potential (with consequent decrease in cardiac excitability and electrical conduction velocity). It is noteworthy that a single mutation can cause different phenotypes or combinations thereof.[2]

LONG QT SYNDROME

In contrast to most long QT syndrome (LQTS) phenotypes, which are based on mutations that modify the cardiac K^+ currents, type 3 congenital LQTS (LQT3), which accounts for approximately 8% of congenital LQTS cases, is caused by gain-of-function mutations on the Na^+ channel gene, *SCN5A*. More than 80 mutations have been identified in the *SCN5A* gene, with most being missense mutations mainly clustered in $Na_v1.5$ regions that are involved in fast inactivation (i.e., S4 segment of domain IV, the domain III–domain IV linker, and the cytoplasmic loops between the S4 and S5 segments of domain III and domain IV), or in regions that stabilize fast inactivation (e.g., the C-terminus).[2,4,7]

Several mechanisms have been identified to underlie ionic effects of *SCN5A* mutations in LQT3. Most *SCN5A* mutations cause a gain of function through disruption of fast inactivation, thus allowing repeated reopening during sustained depolarization and resulting in an abnormal, small, but functionally important sustained (or persistent) noninactivating Na^+ current (I_{sus}) during action potential plateau. Because the general membrane conductance is small during the action potential plateau, the presence of a persistent inward I_{Na}, even of small amplitude, can potentially have a major impact on the plateau duration and can be sufficient to prolong repolarization and QT interval. QT prolongation and the risk of developing arrhythmia are more pronounced at slow heart rates, when the action potential duration is longer, thereby allowing more I_{Na} to enter the cell.[2,4,7]

Other less common mechanisms of *SCN5A* mutations to cause LQT3 include increased window current, which results from delayed inactivation of mutant Na^+ channels, occurring at more positive potentials and widening the voltage range during which the Na^+ channel may reactivate without inactivation. Additionally, some mutations cause slower inactivation, which allows longer channel openings and causes a slowly inactivating I_{Na}. This current is I_{NaL} and is to be distinguished from I_{sus} (which does not inactivate). Comparable to I_{sus}, both the window current and I_{NaL} exert

TABLE 2-1 Inherited Cardiac Sodium Channelopathies

CLINICAL PHENOTYPE	GENE	PROTEIN	SODIUM CHANNEL ALTERATION
Long QT syndrome			
LQT3	SCN5A	$Na_v1.5$	Increase in late or sustained I_{Na}
LQT9	CAV3	Caveolin-3	Increase in sustained I_{Na}
LQT10	SCN4B	$Na_v\beta4$	Increase in sustained I_{Na}
LQT12	SNTA1	α_1-syntrophin	Increase in sustained I_{Na}
Brugada syndrome			
Type 1	SCN5A	$Na_v1.5$	Decrease in I_{Na}
Type 2	GPD1L	G3PD1L	Decrease in I_{Na}
Type 5	SCN1B	$Na_v\beta1/\beta1b$	Decrease in I_{Na}
Type 7	SCN3B	$Na_v\beta3$	Decrease in I_{Na}
Progressive cardiac conduction disease	SCN5A SCN1B	$Na_v1.5$ $Na_v\beta3$	Decrease in I_{Na}
Congenital sick sinus syndrome	SCN5A	$Na_v1.5$	Decrease or increase in I_{Na}
Atrial standstill	SCN5A	$Na_v1.5$	Decrease in I_{Na}
Familial atrial fibrillation	SCN5A SCN1B SCN2B	$Na_v1.5$ $Na_v\beta1$ $Na_v\beta2$	Different and discordant molecular phenotypes
Dilated cardiomyopathy	SCN5A	$Na_v1.5$	Different and discordant molecular phenotypes
Sudden infant death syndrome	SCN5A CAV3 GPD1L	$Na_v1.5$ Caveolin-3 G3PD1L	Increase in late I_{Na} or decrease in I_{Na}
SCN5A overlap syndromes			Combination of the molecular phenotypes found in the other clinical entities

I_{Na} = sodium current; LQTS = long QT syndrome.

their effects during phases 2 and 3 of the action potential, in which normally no or very small I_{Na} is present. Other mutations induce prolonged action potential duration by enhancing recovery from inactivation, an effect that leads to larger peak I_{Na} by increasing the fraction of channels available for activation (because of faster recovery) during subsequent depolarizations. Finally, some mutations can cause increased expression of mutant $Na_v1.5$ through enhanced mRNA translation or protein trafficking to the sarcolemma, decreased protein degradation, or altered modulation by β subunits and regulatory proteins. These effects lead to larger I_{Na} density during phase 0 of the action potential. Importantly, one single *SCN5A* mutation can potentially cause several changes in the expression and/or gating properties of the resulting Na^+ channels.[2]

Regardless of the mechanism, increased Na^+ current (I_{sus}, window current, I_{NaL}, or peak I_{Na}) upsets the balance between depolarizing and repolarizing currents in favor of depolarization. The resulting delay in the repolarization process triggers early afterdepolarizations (EADs; i.e., reactivation of the L-type Ca^{2+} channel during phase 2 or 3 of the action potential), especially in Purkinje fiber myocytes, in which action potential durations are intrinsically longer.[2]

LQT9 is caused by gain-of-function mutations on the *CAV3* gene, which encodes caveolin-3, a plasma membrane scaffolding protein that interacts with $Na_v1.5$ and plays a role in compartmentalization and regulation of channel function. Mutations in caveolin-3 induce kinetic alterations of the $Na_v1.5$ current that result in persistent Na^+ current (I_{sus}) and have been reported in cases of sudden infant death syndrome (SIDS).[2,8]

LQT10 is caused by loss-of-function mutations on the *SCN4B* gene, which encodes the β subunit ($Na_v\beta4$) of the $Na_v1.5$ channel. To date, only a single mutation in one patient has been described. This mutation caused a shift in the inactivation of the I_{Na} toward more positive potentials, but it did not change the activation. This resulted in increased window currents at an E_m corresponding to the phase 3 of the action potential.[2,8]

LQT12 is caused by mutations on the *SNTA1* gene, which encodes α_1 syntrophin, a cytoplasmic adaptor protein that enables the interaction among $Na_v1.5$, nitric oxide synthase, and the sarcolemmal Ca^{2+} adenosine triphosphatase (ATPase) complex that appears to regulate ion channel function. By disrupting the interaction between $Na_v1.5$ and the sarcolemmal Ca^{2+} ATPase complex, *SNTA1* mutations cause increased $Na_v1.5$ nitrosylation with consequent reduction of channel inactivation and enhanced I_{sus} densities.[2,9]

BRUGADA SYNDROME

The Brugada syndrome is an autosomal dominant inherited channelopathy characterized by an elevated ST segment or J wave appearing in the right precordial leads. This syndrome is associated with a high incidence of sudden cardiac death (SCD) secondary to a rapid polymorphic ventricular tachycardia (VT) or ventricular fibrillation (VF). Approximately 65% of mutations identified in the *SCN5A* gene are associated with the Brugada syndrome phenotype (Brugada syndrome type 1), and they account for approximately 18% to 30% of cases of Brugada syndrome. So far, more than 200 Brugada syndrome–associated loss-of-function (i.e., reduced peak I_{Na}) mutations have been described in *SCN5A*. Some of these mutations result in loss of function secondary to impaired channel trafficking to the cell membrane (i.e., reduced expression of functional Na^+ channels), disrupted ion conductance (i.e., expression of nonfunctional Na^+ channels), or altered gating function. Altered gating properties comprise delayed activation (i.e., activation at more positive potentials), earlier inactivation (i.e., inactivation at more negative potentials), faster inactivation, and enhanced slow inactivation.[1-3,10]

Most of the mutations are missense mutations, whereby a single amino acid is replaced by a different amino acid. Missense mutations commonly alter the gating properties of mutant channels. Because virtually all reported *SCN5A* mutation carriers are heterozygous, mutant channels with altered gating may cause up to 50% reduction of I_{Na}. Different *SCN5A* mutations can cause different degrees of I_{Na} reduction and therefore different degrees of severity of the clinical phenotype of Brugada syndrome.[10-12]

In addition to *SCN5A* alterations, mutations in the *GPD1L* gene, which encodes the glycerol 3-phosphate dehydrogenase 1–like protein (G3PD1L), affect the trafficking of the cardiac Na^+ channel to the cell surface and result in reduction of I_{Na} and Brugada syndrome type 2.[10] Brugada syndrome associated with *GPD1L* gene mutations is characterized by progressive conduction disease, a low sensitivity to procainamide, and a relatively good prognosis.[2,13]

Furthermore, reduction in I_{Na} can be caused by mutations in the *SCN1B* gene (encoding the β_1 and β_{1b} subunits of the Na^+ channel) and the *SCN3B* gene (encoding the β_3 subunit of the Na^+ channel), resulting in Brugada syndrome type 5 and type 7, respectively.[10,13]

FAMILIAL PROGRESSIVE CARDIAC CONDUCTION DISEASE

Loss-of-function *SCN5A* mutations have been linked to familial forms of progressive cardiac conduction disease (referred to as hereditary Lenègre disease, primary cardiac conduction system disease, and familial atrioventricular [AV] block). This disease is characterized by slowing of electrical conduction through the atria, AVN, His bundle, Purkinje fibers, and ventricles, accompanied by an age-related degenerative process and fibrosis of the cardiac conduction system, in the absence of structural or systemic disease. It is often reflected by varying degrees of AV block and bundle branch block. Whether the age-dependent fibrosis of the conduction system is a primary degenerative process in progressive cardiac conduction disease or a physiological process that is accelerated by I_{Na} reduction remains to be investigated. A single loss-of-function *SCN5A* mutation can cause isolated progressive cardiac conduction disease or can be combined with the Brugada syndrome (overlap syndrome). Loss-of-function mutations in *SCN1B* also have been identified in patients with progressive cardiac conduction disease who carried no mutation in *SCN5A*.[2]

CONGENITAL SICK SINUS SYNDROME

Although I_{Na} does not play a prominent role in sinus node activity, mutations in *SCN5A* have been linked to sick sinus syndrome, manifesting as sinus bradycardia, sinus arrest, sinoatrial block, or a combination of these conditions, which can progress to atrial inexcitability (atrial standstill). Loss-of-function *SCN5A* mutations result in reduced peak I_{Na} density, hyperpolarizing shifts in the voltage dependence of steady-state channel availability, and slow recovery from inactivation. These effects likely cause reduced automaticity, decreased excitability, and conduction slowing or block of impulses generated in the sinus node to the surrounding atrial tissue. Sinus node dysfunction can also manifest concomitantly with other phenotypes that are linked to *SCN5A* loss-of-function mutations such as Brugada syndrome and progressive cardiac conduction disorders.[2,14]

FAMILIAL ATRIAL FIBRILLATION

Loss-of-function mutations, gain-of-function mutations, and common polymorphisms on the *SCN5A* gene have been identified in some cases of atrial fibrillation (AF) occurring in young patients with structurally normal hearts. It is speculated that I_{Na} reduction may predispose to AF by slowing the electrical conduction velocity and thereby facilitating reentry. On the other hand, gain-of-function mutations can potentially predispose to AF by increasing atrial excitability. AF can occur in patients with other phenotypes of Na^+ channelopathies, including LQT3, Brugada syndrome, dilated cardiomyopathy, and sinus node dysfunction. Furthermore, mutations in the *SCN1B* gene (encoding the β_1 subunit of the Na^+ channel) and the *SCN2B* gene (encoding the β_2 subunit of the Na^+ channel) have been identified in patients with AF, many of whom displayed ECG patterns suggestive of the Brugada syndrome.[1,2]

DILATED CARDIOMYOPATHY

Some cases of familial dilated cardiomyopathy have been linked to *SCN5A* mutations. Dilated cardiomyopathy–linked *SCN5A* mutations cause diverse loss-of-function and gain-of-function changes in the gating properties, but how such changes evoke contractile dysfunction is not understood. It is speculated that *SCN5A* mutations disrupt the interactions between the mutant Na^+ channels and intracellular (or extracellular) proteins that are essential for normal cardiomyocyte structure and architecture. Notably, dilated cardiomyopathy with *SCN5A* mutations display atrial or ventricular arrhythmias (including AF, VT, and VF), or both, as well as sinus node dysfunction, AV block, and intraventricular conduction delay.[2]

SUDDEN INFANT DEATH SYNDROME

Gain-of-function mutations in *SCN5A* may be the most prevalent genetic cause of SIDS. *SCN5A* mutations in SIDS commonly increase I_{sus}. Less frequently, loss-of-function mutations in *SCN5A* or *CAV3* and gain-of-function mutations in *GPD1-L* have also been found in infants with SIDS. However, it is possible that in these patients SIDS represents a severe form of the Brugada syndrome or LQTS that manifests during infancy.

Acquired Diseases

In heart failure, peak I_{Na} is reduced (likely secondary to reduced *SCN5A* expression), whereas I_{NaL} is increased (likely because of increased phosphorylation of Na^+ channels). $Na_v1.5$ expression is reduced in the surviving myocytes in the border zone of the myocardial infarct (MI). Importantly, Na^+ channel blockers can increase the risk for SCD in patients with ischemic heart disease, possibly by facilitating the initiation of reentrant excitation waves. Additionally, I_{NaL} increases during myocardial ischemia, explaining why I_{NaL} inhibition may be an effective therapy for chronic stable angina. $Na_v1.5$ expression is reduced in response to persistent atrial tachyarrhythmias as part of the "electrical remodeling" process, leading to attenuation of I_{Na}.[3]

Furthermore, mutations in *SCN5A* can predispose affected individuals to acquired LQTS induced by a variety of drugs such as antihistamines or antibiotics. These mutations result in changes in channel activity that exert a significant impact on action potential duration only when combined with drug-induced alteration of other channels.

Potassium Channels

Structure and Physiology

Cardiac K^+ channels are membrane-spanning proteins that allow the passive movement of K^+ ions across the cell membrane along its electrochemical gradient. The ion-conducting or pore-forming subunit is generally referred to as the α subunit. The tripeptide sequence glycine-tyrosine-glycine GYG is common to the pore of all K^+ channels and constitutes the signature motif for determining K^+ ion selectivity. A gating mechanism controls switching between open-conducting and closed-nonconducting states.[1,15]

K^+ channels represent the most diverse class of cardiac ion channels (Fig. 2-3). Cardiac K^+ currents can be categorized as voltage-gated (K_v) and ligand-gated channels. In K_v channels, pore opening is coupled to the movement of a voltage sensor within the membrane electric field, and they include the rapidly activating and inactivating transient outward current (I_{to}); the ultrarapid (I_{Kur}), rapid (I_{Kr}), and slow (I_{Ks}) components of the delayed rectifier current; and the inward rectifier current (I_{K1}). In contrast, pore opening in ligand-gated channels is coupled to the binding of an organic molecule, including channels activated by a decrease in the intracellular concentration of adenosine triphosphate (K_{ATP}) or activated by acetylcholine (K_{ACh}). Other classes of K^+ channels

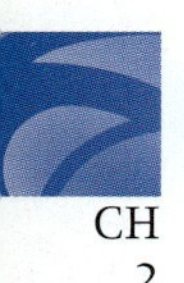

CH 2

K+ Channel α subunits

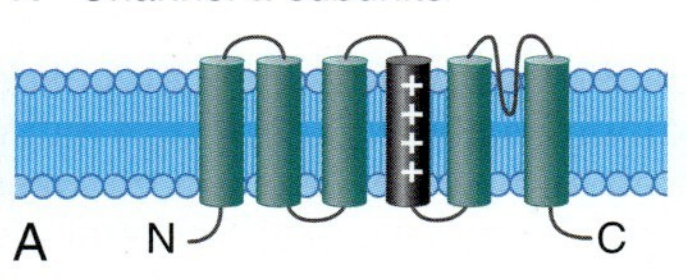

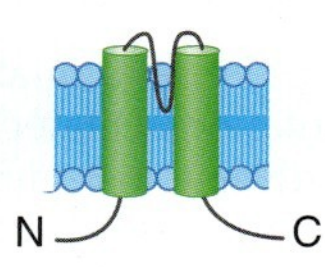

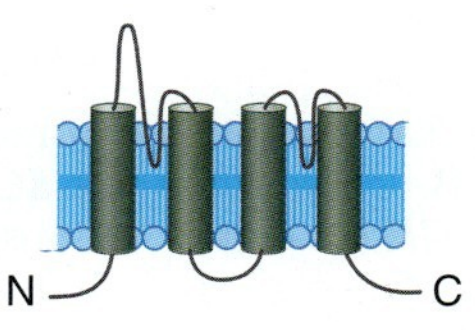

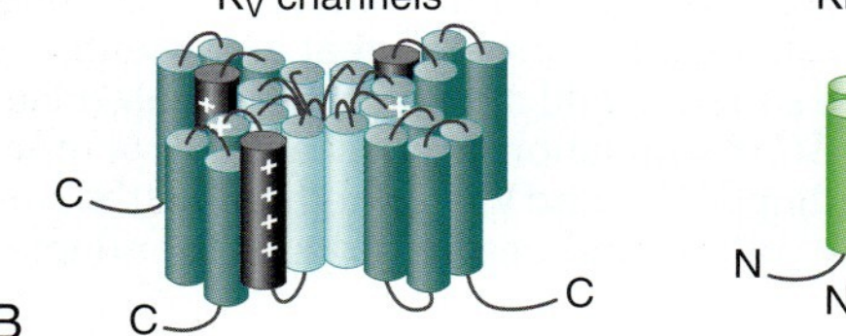

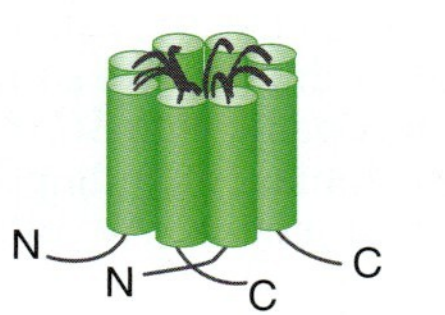

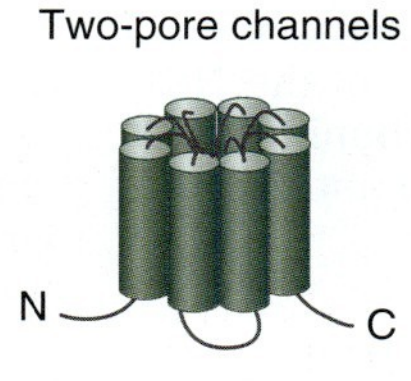

FIGURE 2-3 Molecular compositions of cardiac potassium (K^+) channels. Amino termini (N) and carboxyl termini (C) are indicated. **A,** Voltage-gated (K_v), inward rectifier (Kir), and two-pore α subunits are integral membrane proteins with six, two, and four membrane-spanning domains, respectively. **B,** These α subunits assemble as tetramers or dimers to form K^+-selective pores. *(Modified from Oudit GY, Backx PH: Voltage-regulated potassium channels. In Zipes DP, Jalife J, editors: Cardiac electrophysiology: from cell to bedside, ed 5, Philadelphia, 2009, Saunders, pp 29-42.)*

TABLE 2-2 Genetic and Molecular Basis of Cardiac Ion Currents

CURRENT	α SUBUNIT	α-SUBUNIT GENE	β-SUBUNIT/ ACCESSORY PROTEINS	β-SUBUNIT GENE
$I_{to,f}$	K_v4.2 K_v4.3	KCND2 KCND3	MiRP1 MiRP2 KChIP1 KChIP2 DPP6	KCNE2 KCNE3 KCNIP1 KCNIP2 DPP6
$I_{to,s}$	K_v1.4 K_v1.7 K_v3.4	KCNA4 KCNA7 KCNC4	$K_v\beta1$ $K_v\beta2$ $K_v\beta3$ $K_v\beta4$	KCNB1 KCNB2 KCNB3 KCNB4
I_{Kur}	K_v1.5 (HK2) K_v3.1	KCNA5 KCNC1	$K_v\beta1$ $K_v\beta2$	KCNAB1 KCNAB2
I_{Kr}	K_v10.2 (EAG2) K_v11.1 (HERG)	KCNH2 KCNH2	minK MiRP1	KCNE1 KCNE2
I_{Ks}	K_v7.1 (K_vLQT1)	KCNQ1	minK	KCNE1
I_{K1}	Kir2.1 (IKR1) Kir2.2 (IRK2)	KCNJ2 KCNJ12		
I_{KACh}	Kir3.1 (GIRK1) Kir3.4 (GIRK4)	KCNJ3 KCNJ5		
I_{KATP}	Kir6.2 (BIR)	KCNJ11	SUR2A	ABCC9
K_{2P}	K_{2P}1.1 (TWIK-1) K_{2P}2.1 (TREK1) K_{2P}3.1 (TASK-1) K_{2P}5.1 (TASK-2) K_{2P}6.1 (TWIK-2) K_{2P}9.1 (TASK-3) K_{2P}10.1 (TREK-2) K_{2P}13.1 (THIK-1) K_{2P}17.1 (TASK-4)	KCNK1 KCNK2 KCNK3 KCNK5 KCNK6 KCNK9 KCNK10 KCNK13 KCNK17		

I_f = cardiac pacemaker current; I_{K1} = inward rectifying current; I_{KACh} = acetylcholine-activated potassium current; I_{KATP} = adenosine triphosphate–dependent potassium current; I_{Kr} = rapidly activating delayed outward rectifying current; I_{Ks} = slowly activating delayed outward rectifying current; $I_{to,s}$ = slow transient outward current; K_{2P} = two-pore potassium channel.

respond to different stimuli, including changes in intracellular Ca^{2+} concentration and G proteins.[15]

On the basis of the primary amino acid sequence of the α subunit, K^+ channels have been classified into three major families (Table 2-2):

1. Channels containing six transmembrane segments and a single pore. This architecture is typical of K_v channels.
2. Channels containing two transmembrane segments (M1 and M2) and a pore. This architecture is typical of inward rectifier K^+ (Kir) channels, including K1, K_{ATP}, and K_{ACh} channels. They conduct K^+ currents more in the inward direction than the outward and play an important role in setting the resting potential close to the equilibrium potential for K^+ and in repolarization. Kir channels form either homotetramers or heterotetramers.
3. Channels containing four transmembrane segments and two pores (K_{2P}). These channels exist as homodimers or heterodimers. K_{2P} currents display little time or voltage dependence. There are four classes of cardiac K_{2P}: TASK, TWIK, TREK, and THIK.[15,16]

Each voltage-gated K^+ channel (K_v family) is formed by the coassembly of 4 identical (homotetramers) or a combination of 4 different (from the same subfamily, heterotetramers) α subunits. A total of 38 genes has been cloned and assigned to 12 subfamilies of voltage-gated K channels (K_v1 to K_v12) on the basis of sequence similarities. Each α subunit contains one domain consisting of 6 membrane-spanning segments (S1 to S6), connected to each other by alternating intracellular and extracellular peptide loops (similar to 1 of the 4 domains of voltage-gated Na^+

and Ca^{2+} channels), with both the amino terminus (N-terminus) and the C-terminus located on the intracellular side of the membrane. The central ion-conducting pore region is formed by the S5 and S6 segments and the S5-S6 linker (P segment); the S5-S6 linker is responsible for K^+ ion selectivity. The S4 segment serves as the voltage sensor.[1,15]

The α subunits of K_v channels can generate voltage dependent K^+ current when expressed in heterologous systems. However, the assembly of a functional tetramer can occur only in the presence of multiple auxiliary units (see Table 2-2). In many cases, auxiliary subunits coassociate with the α subunits and likely modulate cell surface expression, gating kinetics, and drug sensitivity of the α subunit complex. Most K^+ channel β subunits assemble with α subunits and give rise to an $\alpha_4\beta_4$ complex. K^+ channel β subunits represent a diverse molecular group, which includes cytoplasmic proteins ($K_v\beta1$ to $K_v\beta3$, KChIP, and KChAP) that interact with the intracellular domains of K_v channels; single transmembrane spanning proteins (e.g., minK and minK-related proteins [MiRPs]) encoded by the *KCNE* gene family; and large ATP-binding cassette (ABC) transport-related proteins (e.g., the sulfonylurea receptors [SURs]).[1,16]

The diversity of K^+ currents in native tissues exceeds the number of K^+ channel genes identified. The explanations for this diversity include alternative splicing of gene products, post-translational modification, and heterologous assembly of β subunits within the same family and assembly with accessory β subunits that modulate channel properties.

As with voltage-dependent Na^+ and Ca^{2+} channels, K_v channels typically fluctuate among distinct conformational states because of molecular movements in response to voltage changes across the cell membrane (voltage-dependent gating). The K_v channel activates (opens) on membrane depolarization, thus allowing the rapid passage of K^+ ions across the sarcolemma. After opening, the channel undergoes conformational transition in a time-dependent manner to a stable nonconducting (inactivated) state. Inactivated channels are incapable of reopening, even if the transmembrane voltage is favorable, unless they "recover" from inactivation (i.e., enter the closed state) on membrane repolarization. Closed channels are nonconducting but can be activated on membrane depolarization.[17]

Three mechanistically distinct types of K_v channel inactivation that are associated with distinct molecular domains have been identified: N-type, C-type, and U-type. N-type ("ball and chain") inactivation involves physical occlusion of the intracellular mouth of the channel pore through binding of a small group of amino acids ("inactivation ball tethered to a chain") at the extreme N-terminus. In contrast, C-type inactivation involves conformational changes in the external mouth of the pore. C-type inactivation exists in almost all K^+ channels and may reflect a slow constriction of the pore. This inactivation process is thought to be voltage independent, coupled to channel opening, and is usually slower than N-type inactivation. Recovery from C-type inactivation is relatively slow and weakly voltage dependent. Importantly, the rate of C-type inactivation and recovery can be strongly influenced by other factors, such as N-type inactivation, drug binding, and changes in extracellular K^+ concentration. These interactions render C-type inactivation an important biophysical process in regulating repetitive electrical activity and determining certain physiological properties such as refractoriness, drug binding, and sensitivity to extracellular K^+.[17]

In addition to N-type and C-type inactivation, some K_v channels also show another type of inactivation (U-type), which exhibits a U-shaped voltage dependence with prolonged stimulation rates. Those channels appear to exhibit preferential inactivation from partially activated closed states, rapid and strongly voltage-dependent recovery from inactivation and, in some channel types, accelerated inactivation with elevation of extracellular K^+. The exact conformational changes underlying U-type inactivation remain unclear. Importantly, there is extreme diversity in the kinetic and potentially molecular properties of K_v channel inactivation, particularly of C-type inactivation.[17]

Function

K^+ channels are a diverse and ubiquitous group of membrane proteins that regulate K^+ ion flow across the cell membrane on the electrochemical gradient and regulate the resting E_m, the frequency of pacemaker cells, and the shape and duration of the cardiac action potential. Because the concentration of K^+ ions outside the cell membrane is approximately 25-fold lower than that in the intracellular fluid, on activation, the opening of K^+ channels generates an outward current resulting from the efflux of positively charged ions that offers a mechanism to counteract, dampen, or restrict the depolarization front (phases 1 through 4 of the action potential) triggered by an influx of cations (Na^+ and Ca^{2+}).[1,3,15,16]

The variation in the level of expression of K^+ channels that participate in the genesis of the cardiac action potential explains the regional differences of the configuration and duration of cardiac action potentials from sinus node and atrial to ventricular myocytes and across the myocardial wall (endocardium, midmyocardium, and epicardium). Moreover, the expression and properties of K^+ channels are not static; heart rate, neurohumoral state, pharmacological agents, cardiovascular diseases (cardiac hypertrophy and failure, MI) and arrhythmias (e.g., AF) can influence those properties, and they underlie the change in action potential configuration in response to variation in heart rate and various physiological and pathological conditions.[1,15,16]

Transient Outward Potassium Current (I_{to})

STRUCTURE AND PHYSIOLOGY

Cardiac I_{to} channels are macromolecular protein complexes, comprising four pore-forming K_v α subunits and a variety of K_v channel accessory (β) subunits (see Fig. 2-3). I_{to} is the sum of a voltage-dependent, Ca^{2+}-independent K^+ current (I_{to1}) and a Ca^{2+}-activated Cl^- or K^+ current (I_{to2}). In human atrial and ventricular myocytes, the presence of I_{to2} has not been clearly demonstrated.

I_{to1} (which is referred to as I_{to}) displays two phenotypes with distinct recovery kinetics: a rapid or fast I_{to} ($I_{to,fast}$ or $I_{to,f}$) phenotype and a slower phenotype ($I_{to,slow}$ or $I_{to,s}$). The transient nature of I_{to} is secondary to its rapid activation (with time constants of less than 10 milliseconds for both $I_{to,f}$ and $I_{to,s}$) and rapid inactivation (25 to 80 milliseconds for $I_{to,f}$ and 80 to 200 milliseconds for $I_{to,s}$). However, whereas $I_{to,f}$ recovers rapidly from inactivation (60 to 100 milliseconds), $I_{to,s}$ recovers slowly (with time constants on the order of seconds).

K_v channels mediating $I_{to,s}$ are formed by the coassembly of four α subunits from the $K_v1.x$ subfamily (primarily $K_v1.4$, and possibly $K_v1.7$ and $K_v3.4$), whereas those mediating $I_{to,f}$ are formed by the coassembly of four α subunits from the $K_v4.x$ subfamily (primarily $K_v4.3$, and possibly $K_v4.2$) (see Table 2-2). Among the various accessory subunits identified, a crucial role has been definitively demonstrated only for KChIP2, and potentially for MiRP2.[1,16,18]

FUNCTION

I_{to} is a prominent repolarizing current; it partially repolarizes the membrane, shapes the rapid (phase 1) repolarization of the action potential, and sets the height of the initial plateau (phase 2). Thus, the activity of I_{to} channels influences the activation of voltage-gated Ca^{2+} channels and the balance of inward and outward currents during the plateau (mainly I_{CaL} and the delayed rectifier K^+ currents), thereby mediating the duration and the amplitude of phase 2.

The density of I_{to} varies across the myocardial wall and in different regions of the heart. In human ventricles, I_{to} densities are much higher in the epicardium and midmyocardium than in the endocardium. Furthermore, $I_{to,f}$ and $I_{to,s}$ are differentially expressed in the myocardium, thus contributing to regional heterogeneities in action potential waveforms. $I_{to,f}$ is the principal subtype expressed

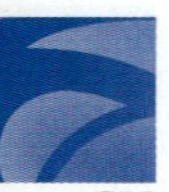

in human atrium. The markedly higher densities of $I_{to,f}$, together with the expression of the ultrarapid delayed rectifier current, accelerate the early phase of repolarization and lead to lower plateau potentials and shorter action potentials in atrial as compared with ventricular cells.[17,18]

Although both $I_{to,f}$ and $I_{to,s}$ are expressed in the ventricle, $I_{to,f}$ is more prominent in the epicardium and midmyocardium (putative M cells) than in the endocardium. These regional differences are responsible for the shorter duration and the prominent phase 1 notch and the "spike-and-dome" morphology of epicardial and midmyocardial compared with endocardial action potentials. A prominent I_{to}-mediated action potential notch in ventricular epicardium but not endocardium produces a transmural voltage gradient during early ventricular repolarization that registers as a J wave or J point elevation on the ECG.[19] I_{to} densities are also reportedly higher in right than in left (midmyocardial and epicardial) ventricular myocytes, consistent with the more pronounced spike-and-dome morphology of right, compared with left, ventricular action potentials.[1,3,17,18]

Furthermore, variations in cardiac repolarization associated with I_{to} regional differences strongly influence intracellular Ca^{2+} transient by modulating Ca^{2+} entry via I_{CaL} and Na^+-Ca^{2+} exchange, thereby regulating excitation-contraction coupling and regional modulation of myocardial contractility and hence synchronizing the timing of force generation between different ventricular regions and enhancing mechanical efficiency.[17]

REGULATION

Transient outward channels are subject to α- and β-adrenergic regulation. α-Adrenergic stimulation reduces I_{to}; concomitant β-adrenergic stimulation appears to counteract the α-adrenergic effect, at least in part. The effects of α- and β-adrenergic stimulation are exerted by phosphorylation of the $K_v1.4$, $K_v4.2$, and $K_v4.3$ α-subunits by PKA as well as PKC. Calmodulin-dependent kinase II, on the other hand, has been shown to be involved in enhancement of I_{to}. Adrenergic stimulation is also an important determinant of transient outward channel downregulation in cardiac disease. Chronic α-adrenergic stimulation and angiotensin II reduce I_{to} channel expression.[20]

KChIP2, when coexpressed with $K_v4.3$, increases surface channel density and current amplitude, slows channel inactivation, and markedly accelerates the recovery from inactivation. In the ventricle, KChIP2 mRNA is 25-fold more abundant in the epicardium than in the endocardium. This gradient parallels the gradient in I_{to} expression, whereas $K_v4.3$ mRNA is expressed at equal levels across the ventricular wall. Thus, transcriptional regulation of the *KChIP2* gene (KChIP2) is the primary determinant of I_{to} expression in the ventricular wall.[1,16]

Observations suggest that MiRP2 is required for the physiological functioning of human $I_{to,f}$ channels and that gain-of-function mutations in MiRP2 predispose to Brugada syndrome through augmentation of $I_{to,f}$.[18]

I_{to} is strongly rate dependent. I_{to} fails to recover from previous inactivation at very fast heart rates, which can be manifest as a decrease in the magnitude of the J wave on the surface ECG. Hence, abrupt changes in rate and pauses have important consequences for the early repolarization of the membrane.[19]

I_{to} can be enhanced by aging, low sympathetic activity, high parasympathetic activity, bradycardia, hypothermia, estrogen reduction, and drugs. Estrogen suppresses the expression of the $K_v4.3$ channel and results in reduced I_{to} and a shallow phase 1 notch.[13]

Phase 1 notch of the action potential modulates the kinetics of slower activating ion currents and consequently the later phases of the action potential. Initial enhancement of phase 1 notch promotes phase 2 dome and delays repolarization, presumably by delaying the peak of I_{CaL}. However, further enhancement of phase 1 notch prevents the rising of phase 2 dome and abbreviates action potential duration, presumably by deactivation or voltage modulation that reduces I_{CaL}. Thus, progressive deepening of phase 1 notch can cause initial enhancement followed by sudden disappearance of phase 2 dome and corresponding prolongation followed by abbreviation of action potential duration. On the other hand, modulators that decrease I_{to} lead to a shift of the plateau phase into the positive range of potentials, thus increasing the activation of the delayed rectifier currents, promoting faster repolarization, and reducing the electrochemical driving force for Ca^{2+} and hence I_{CaL}. Phase 1 notch also affects the function of the Na^+-Ca^{2+} exchanger and subsequently intracellular Ca^{2+} handling and Na^+ channel function.[1,16]

PHARMACOLOGY

Quinidine, 4-aminopyridine, flecainide, and propafenone produce an open channel blockade and accelerate I_{to} inactivation. Quinidine, but not flecainide or propafenone, produces a frequency-dependent block of I_{to} that results from a slow rate of drug dissociation from the channel. Quinidine has relatively strong I_{to} blocking effect, whereas flecainide mildly blocks I_{to}.[18,20]

I_{to} blockers can potentially prolong the action potential duration in the atrial and in ischemic ventricular myocardium. However, because the net effects of I_{to} blockade on repolarization depend on secondary changes in other currents, the reduction of I_{to} density can result in a shortening of the ventricular action potential. Moreover, heterogeneous ventricular distribution of I_{to} can cause marked dispersion of repolarization across the ventricular wall that, when accompanied by prominent conduction delays related to Na^+ channel blockade, results in extrasystolic activity through a phase 2 reentrant mechanisms.[18,20]

Currently, a cardioselective and channel-specific I_{to} opener or blocker is not available for clinical use. Development of an I_{to}-selective drug is expected to be beneficial in patients with primary abnormality in the I_{to} or in other channels, such as the Brugada syndrome, in which heterogeneity in the expression of I_{to} between epicardium and endocardium in the right ventricle (RV) results in the substrate responsible for reentry and ventricular arrhythmias.[18,20]

INHERITED CHANNELOPATHIES

To date, only mutations in *KCNE3* (MiRP2) are linked to inherited arrhythmia. *KCNE3* mutations were identified in five related patients with Brugada syndrome. When expressed with $K_v4.3$, the mutation increased $I_{to,f}$ density.[3]

Another *KCNE3* mutation was identified in one patient with familial AF. The mutation was found to increase $I_{to,f}$ and was postulated to cause AF by shortening action potential duration and facilitating atrial reentrant excitation waves.[3]

A genome wide haplotype-sharing study associated a haplotype on chromosome 7, harboring DPP6, with idiopathic VF in three distantly related families. Overexpression of DPP6, which encodes dipeptidyl-peptidase 6, a putative component of the I_{to} channel complex, was proposed as the likely pathogenetic mechanism. DPP6 significantly alters the inactivation kinetics of both $K_v4.2$ and $K_v4.3$ and promotes expression of these α subunits in the cell membrane.[3,21]

Importantly, the normally functioning I_{to} channels play an important role in the electrophysiological consequences of the ionic current abnormalities in the Brugada and J wave syndromes. Heterogeneity in the distribution of I_{to} channels across the myocardial wall, being more prominent in ventricular epicardium than endocardium, and particularly in the RV, results in the shorter duration and the prominent phase 1 notch and the spike-and-dome morphology of the epicardial action potential as compared with the endocardium. The resultant transmural voltage gradient during the early phases (phases 1 and 2) of the action potential is thought to be responsible for the inscription of the J wave on the surface ECG.[18,19] An increase in net repolarizing current, secondary to either a decrease in the inward currents (I_{Na} and I_{CaL}) or an increase in the outward K^+ currents (I_{to}, I_{Kr}, I_{Ks}, I_{KAch}, I_{KATP}), or both, can accentuate the action potential notch and lead to augmentation of the J wave or the appearance of ST segment elevation on the surface ECG. An outward shift of currents that extends beyond the action potential notch not only can accentuate the J wave but also can lead to partial or complete loss of the dome of the action potential, thus leading to a protracted transmural voltage gradient that manifests as greater ST segment elevation and gives rise to J wave syndromes. The type of the ion current affected and its regional distribution in the ventricles determine the particular phenotype (including the Brugada syndrome, early repolarization syndrome, hypothermia-induced ST segment elevation, and MI-induced ST segment elevation).[18,19,22] The degree of accentuation of the action potential notch leading to loss of the dome depends on the magnitude of I_{to}. These changes are more prominent in regions of the myocardium exhibiting a relatively large I_{to}, such as the RV epicardium; this explains the appearance of coved ST segment elevation, characteristic of Brugada syndrome, in the right precordial ECG leads.[19,20]

In this context, factors that influence the kinetics of I_{to} or the other repolarization currents can modify the manifestation of the J wave on the ECG. Na^+ channel blockers (procainamide, pilsicainide, propafenone, flecainide, and disopyramide), which reduce the inward I_{Na}, can accentuate the J wave and ST segment elevation in patients with concealed J wave syndromes. Quinidine, which inhibits both I_{to} and I_{Na}, reduces the magnitude of the J wave and normalizes ST segment elevation. Additionally, acceleration of the heart rate, which is associated with reduction of I_{to} (because of slow recovery of I_{to} from inactivation), results in a decrease in the magnitude of the J wave. Male predominance can potentially result from larger epicardial I_{to} density versus I_{to} in women.[19,22]

The increased transmural heterogeneity of ventricular repolarization (i.e., dispersion of repolarization between epicardium and endocardium), which is responsible for J point elevation and early repolarization pattern on the surface ECG, is also responsible for the increased vulnerability to ventricular tachyarrhythmias. A significant outward shift in current can cause partial or complete loss of the dome of the action potential in regions where I_{to} is prominent (epicardium), with the consequent loss of activation of I_{CaL}. The dome of the action potential then can propagate from regions where it is preserved (midmyocardium endocardium) to regions where it is lost (epicardium), thus giving rise to phase 2 reentry, which can generate premature ventricular complexes that in turn can initiate polymorphic VT or VF.[19,20,22,23]

ACQUIRED DISEASES

An alteration in the expression and distribution of I_{to} is observed in various pathophysiological conditions. Adrenergic effects seem to be involved in at least some of these I_{to}-regulating processes during heart disease.[20]

In general, myocardial ischemia, MI, dilated cardiomyopathy, and end-stage heart failure cause downregulation of I_{to}. In fact, I_{to} downregulation is the most consistent ionic current change in the failing heart. The reduction in I_{to} results in attenuation of early repolarization (phase 1) and affects the level of plateau (phase 2) of the action potential and other currents involved in delayed repolarization (phase 3), with resulting prolongation and increased heterogeneity of action potential duration. The prominent epicardial I_{to} contributes to the selective electrical depression of the epicardium. This process leads to the development of a marked dispersion of repolarization between normal and abnormal epicardium and between epicardium and endocardium, which provides the substrate for reentrant arrhythmias and may underlie the increased predisposition to ventricular arrhythmias and SCD in patients with heart failure and ischemic heart disease.[18,20,24] Additionally, downregulation of I_{to} in advanced heart failure likely slows the time course of force generation, thereby contributing to reduced myocardial performance.

On the other hand, compensatory ventricular hypertrophy preceding heart failure is associated with an upregulation of I_{to}. The prolongation of the action potential, concomitant with an increase in I_{to}, presumably results from the more negative level of the plateau with less I_{CaL} inactivation and probably less delayed rectifier activation. In contrast, progression of hypertrophy to heart failure is associated with a clear reduction in I_{to}.[20]

Chronic AF reduces I_{to} density and $K_v4.3$ mRNA levels. Hypothyroidism reduces the expression of *KCND2* ($K_v4.2$) genes. Additionally, I_{to} may also be reduced and contribute to QT interval prolongation in diabetes. Importantly, with some delay, insulin therapy partially restores I_{to}, maybe by enhancing $K_v4.3$ expression.[3]

Ultrarapidly Activating Delayed Outward Rectifying Current (I_{Kur})

STRUCTURE AND PHYSIOLOGY

The ion-conducting pore of I_{Kur} channels is formed by four $K_v1.5$ α subunits, whereas the ancillary β subunits $K_v\beta1.2$, $K_v\beta1.3$, and $K_v\beta2.1$ control channel trafficking and plasma membrane integration as well as activation and inactivation kinetics.[3,25]

I_{Kur} activates rapidly on depolarization in the plateau range and displays outward rectification, but it inactivates very slowly during the time course of the action potential. Inactivation accelerates when $K_v1.5$ is coexpressed with its β subunits.[3]

FUNCTION

I_{Kur} is detected only in human atria and not in the ventricles, so that it is the predominant delayed rectifier current responsible for human atrial repolarization and is a basis for the much shorter duration of the action potential in the atrium.[1,3]

REGULATION

β-Adrenergic stimulation enhances I_{Kur}, whereas α-adrenergic stimulation inhibits it, effects likely mediated by PKA and PKC, respectively. Membrane depolarization and elevated extracellular K^+ concentrations reduce $K_v1.5$ expression. Additionally, cAMP, mechanical stretch, hyperthyroidism, and dexamethasone increase $K_v1.5$ expression, whereas extracellular acidosis, phenylephrine, and hypothyroidism decrease it.[1,3]

Coexpression of $K_v\beta1.3$ with $K_v1.5$ induces a fast inactivation and a hyperpolarizing shift in the activation curve (i.e., $K_v\beta1.3$ subunit converts $K_v1.5$ from a delayed rectifier with a modest degree of slow inactivation to a channel with both fast and slow components of inactivation). Data suggest that $K_v\beta1.2$ and $K_v\beta1.3$ subunit modification of $K_v1.5$ currents requires phosphorylation by PKC or a related kinase.

PHARMACOLOGY

I_{Kur} is relatively insensitive to class III antiarrhythmics of the methane-sulfonanilide group, but it is highly sensitive to 4-aminopyridine. Selective inhibition of I_{Kur} by 4-aminopyridine prolongs the human atrial action potential duration.[16]

I_{Kur} is a promising target for the development of new, safer antiarrhythmic drugs to prevent AF or atrial flutter, or both, without a risk of ventricular proarrhythmia. Because I_{Kur} is atrium specific, a drug specifically targeting $K_v1.5$ channels would be expected to terminate AF by preventing reentry through atrial action potential prolongation. The drug vernakalant is an I_{Kur}/I_{Na} channel blocker and is undergoing review by the U.S. Food and Drug Administration for the acute termination of AF. However, because $K_v1.5$ is downregulated in AF, the beneficial effect of I_{Kur} block becomes less certain. Furthermore, because $K_v1.5$ is also expressed in other organs (e.g., brain), discovery of drugs that selectively inhibit atrial $K_v1.5$ channels remains necessary.[1,3,16]

Physiologically, rapid activation of I_{Kur} in the positive potential range following the action potential upstroke can offset depolarizing I_{CaL} and hence lead to the less positive plateau phase in atrial compared with ventricular cardiomyocytes. Conversely, block of I_{Kur} produces a more pronounced spike-and-dome configuration and therefore shifts the potential into a more positive range in which I_{CaL} activation enhances systolic Ca^{2+} influx during a free-running action potential. Such an indirect effect on I_{CaL} should be shared by all I_{Kur} blockers and is expected to result in a positive atrial inotropic effect.[25]

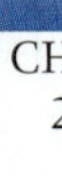
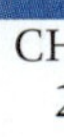
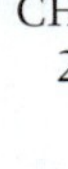

INHERITED CHANNELOPATHIES

KCNA5 nonsense mutations have been reported in individuals with familial AF. Heterologous expression of these mutations revealed complete I_{Kur} loss of function. Absence of I_{Kur} can excessively prolong atrial action potential duration with an enhanced risk of EADs that can trigger or maintain AF.[3,25]

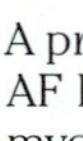
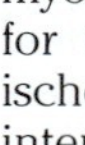
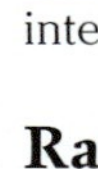

ACQUIRED DISEASES

A prolonged period of rapid activation of the atria as occurs during AF leads to a decrease in I_{Kur}. Additionally, I_{Kur} may be affected in myocardial ischemia. Decreased $K_v1.5$ mRNA levels were reported for the epicardial border zone of infarcted hearts. Moreover, ischemic damage disrupted the normal location of $K_v1.5$ in the intercalated discs.[1,3,26]

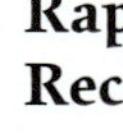
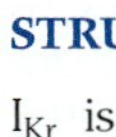
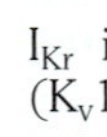

Rapidly Activating Delayed Outward Rectifying Current (I_{Kr})

STRUCTURE AND PHYSIOLOGY

I_{Kr} is formed by coassembly of four pore-forming α subunits ($K_v11.1$, encoded by the *KCNH2* gene, also called the human-ether-a-go-go-related gene, *HERG*, so-named because the mutation in the *Drosophila* fruit fly caused it to shake like a go-go dancer) and β subunits (MiRP1, encoded by the *KCNE2* gene). The current generated by *HERG* channels shows unusual voltage dependence. In contrast to I_{Ks}, I_{Kr} activates relatively rapidly (on the order of 10s of milliseconds) on membrane depolarization. Activation of I_{Kr} occurs with steep voltage dependence and reaches half-maximum activation at membrane voltage of approximately −20 mV. The magnitude of I_{Kr} increases as a function of E_m up to approximately 0 mV, but it declines with stronger depolarization (higher than 0 mV), resulting in a negative slope conductance of the current-voltage relationship. During repolarization of the action potential, I_{Kr} rapidly recovers from inactivation, thus causing the current to peak at −40 mV. The amplitude of the tail current on repolarization exceeds that of the current during the depolarizing pulse.[3,16,27,28]

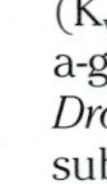
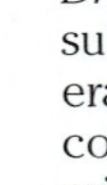
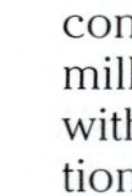
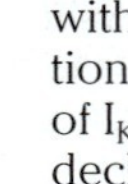
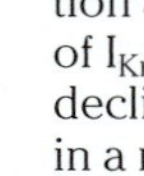
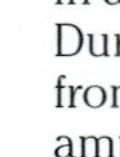
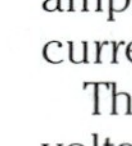

The unusual voltage dependence of I_{Kr} results from a fast, voltage-dependent C-type inactivation process, which limits outward K^+ flow at positive voltages. The large tail current on repolarization from positive voltages results from the rapid recovery of inactivated channels into a conducting state.[27] On repolarization, *HERG* channels deactivate (close) via a slow, voltage-independent process (in contrast to the voltage-dependent inactivation process).[3]

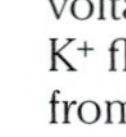
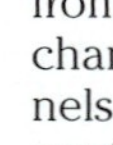
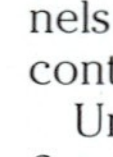
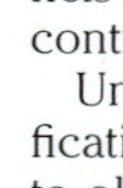
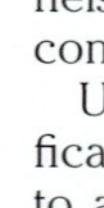
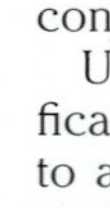
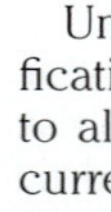
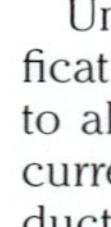

Unlike most K_v channels, *HERG* channels exhibit inward rectification. Rectification describes the property of an ion channel to allow currents preferentially to flow in one direction or limit currents from flowing in the other direction. In other words, conductivity of channels carrying such currents is not constant but is altered at a different E_m. A channel that is inwardly rectifying is one that passes current (positive charge) more easily into the cell. This property is critical for limiting outward K^+ conductance during the plateau phase of the cardiac action potential. Unlike typical Kir channels, in which rectification derives from blockade of the channel pore by intracellular polyamines (see later discussion), the mechanism of *HERG* inward rectification is a very rapid inactivation that develops at far more negative potentials (−85 mV) than channel activation (−20 mV).[28]

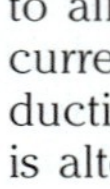
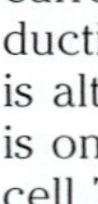
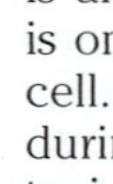
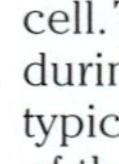
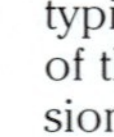

The inactivation of *HERG* channels resembles the C-type inactivation of other K_v channels in its sensitivity to extracellular cations (including K^+ and Na^+) and tetraethyl ammonium (TEA), and to mutations in the P segment. However, the gating behavior is distinctive. First, channel inactivation is much faster than voltage-dependent activation, thus resulting in its characteristic rectification. Second, *HERG* inactivation displays intrinsic voltage dependence. Similar to the classic C-type inactivation, raising the concentration of extracellular K^+ slows *HERG* channel C-type inactivation, an effect that appears to result from occupancy of the pore selectivity filter by K^+.

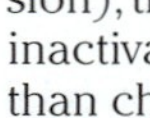
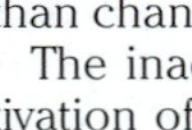
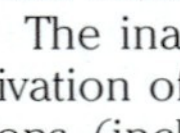
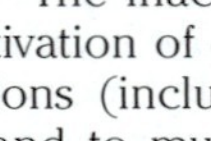
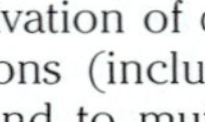
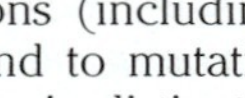
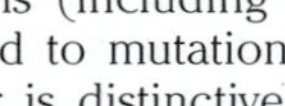
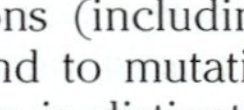
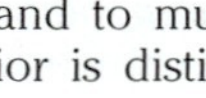
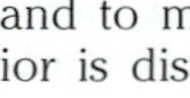
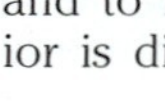
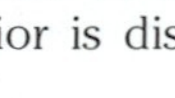
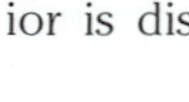
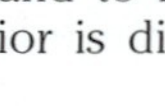
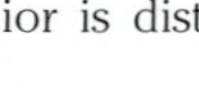
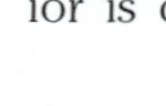
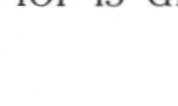

FUNCTION

I_{Kr} presents the principal repolarizing current at the end of the plateau phase in most cardiac cells and plays an important role in governing the cardiac action potential duration and refractoriness. I_{Kr} is differentially expressed, with high levels in left atrial and in ventricular endocardium.

I_{Kr} activates relatively fast on membrane depolarization and allows outward diffusion of K^+ ions in accordance with its electrochemical gradient, but voltage-dependent inactivation thereafter is very fast; hence, only limited numbers of channels remain in the open state, whereas a considerable fraction resides in the nonconducting inactivated state. The fast voltage-dependent inactivation limits outward current through the channel at positive voltages and thus helps maintain the action potential plateau phase that controls contraction and prevents premature excitation. However, as the voltage becomes less positive at the end of the plateau phase of repolarization, the channels recover rapidly from inactivation, thus leading to a progressive increase in I_{Kr} amplitudes during action potential phases 2 and 3, with maximal outward current occurring before the final rapid declining phase of the action potential. Next, the channel deactivates (closes) slowly. The resulting large and transient outward current adds considerably to the ongoing repolarization and makes *HERG* especially suitable for robust control of the repolarization phase.[3,16,27]

REGULATION

β-Adrenergic stimulation and elevation of intracellular cAMP levels enhance I_{Kr} amplitude both through PKA-mediated effects and by direct interaction with the protein. α-Adrenergic stimulation is inhibitory. Coexpression of *HERG* with its β subunit (*KCNE1* or *KCNE2*) accentuates the cAMP-induced voltage shift. The net result of these effects is a reduction in I_{Kr}.[3,16,27]

Extracellular Na^+ potently inhibits I_{Kr} by binding to an outer pore site, and it also speeds recovery from inactivation. The inhibitory effect of Na^+ is potently relieved by physiological levels of extracellular K^+. Competition with external K^+ for a binding site near the external pore explains the finding that elevation of extracellular K^+ concentration paradoxically enhances I_{Kr} despite the decrease in the electrochemical driving force. Hypokalemia causes prolongation of the action potential duration as a result of reduced K^+ conductance. Low extracellular K^+ levels accelerate fast inactivation of the *HERG* channel and further decrease I_{Kr}.[17]

PHARMACOLOGY

I_{Kr} is the target of class III antiarrhythmic drugs of the methanesulfonanilide group (almokalant, dofetilide, D-sotalol, E-4031, ibutilide, and MK-499). These drugs produce a voltage- and use-dependent block, shorten open times in a manner consistent with open channel block, and exhibit low affinity for closed and inactivated states. I_{Kr} blockers prolong atrial and ventricular action potential duration (and the QT interval) and refractoriness in the absence of significant changes in conduction velocity (A-H, H-V, and PR intervals do not prolong). Although selective I_{Kr} blockers exhibit antiarrhythmic properties against reentrant arrhythmias, they are probably not effective against triggered activity or increased automaticity.[16]

Selective I_{Kr} blockers have several disadvantages. These drugs tend to prolong the action potential duration in the Purkinje and midmyocardial cells more than in the subepicardial or subendocardial cells, thus resulting in increased dispersion of repolarization across the ventricular wall and, as a consequence, increased arrhythmogenesis. Moreover, the effects of these drugs increase with decreasing heart rate. This reverse frequency-dependent nature of I_{Kr} blockers can potentially result in excessive prolongation of the QT interval during bradycardia, potentially precipitating torsades de pointes, whereas this prolongation is much less marked or even absent following β-adrenergic stimulation or during sustained tachycardia. This phenomenon limits the efficacy of these drugs in terminating tachyarrhythmias, while maximizing the risk of torsades de pointes during slow heart rates, such as during sinus rhythm after termination of AF. Reverse use-dependence has been attributed, at least in part, to the incomplete deactivation (accumulation) of I_{Ks} during fast heart rates that leads to a progressive increase in current amplitude, which counteracts the action potential prolongation effects of I_{Kr} blockers.[3,16,27]

Azimilide blocks I_{Kr}, I_{Ks}, and I_{Ca}, whereas amiodarone exhibits a complex mechanism of action because it blocks I_{Na}, I_{Ca}, I_{Kr}, I_{Ks}, I_{to}, and I_{KATP}. Quinidine, a class IA agent, also blocks I_{Kr} at concentrations lower than those required to block I_{Ks}, I_{to}, and I_{K1}.

Furthermore, *HERG* channels display an unusual susceptibility to blockade by a variety of drugs compared with other voltage-gated K^+ channels. Increasing numbers of drugs with diverse chemical structures (including some antihistaminics, antipsychotics, and antibiotics) decrease I_{Kr} by depressing *HERG* channel gating, delay ventricular repolarization, prolong the QT interval (acquired LQTS), and induce torsades de pointes. In fact, almost all drugs that cause acquired LQTS target *HERG* channels, likely because of unique structural properties rendering this channel unusually susceptible to a wide range of different drugs. Compared with other cardiac K^+ channels, the *HERG* channel has a large, funnel-like vestibule that allows many small molecules to enter and block the channel. The more spacious inner cavity results from a lack of the S6 helix bending Pro-X-Pro sequence, which presumably facilitates access of drugs to the pore region from the intracellular side of the channel to block the channel current. Additionally, the *HERG* channel contains two aromatic residues located in the S6 domain facing the channel vestibule (not present in most other K^+ channels) that provide high-affinity binding sites for a wide range of structurally diverse compounds. The accessory β subunit (MiRP1, *KCNE2*) also determines the drug sensitivity. Interaction of these compounds with the channel's pore causes functional alteration of its biophysical properties or occlusion of the permeation pathway, or both.[8,16,29]

One novel mechanism for acquired LQTS involves compounds interfering with HERG trafficking (i.e., moving the HERG protein from the endoplasmic reticulum to the cell membrane), rather than direct pore blocking. These compounds include arsenic trioxide, pentamidine, probucol (a cholesterol-lowering therapeutic compound), and cardiac glycosides.[16,29,30]

Some drugs (almokalant, norpropoxyphene, azimilide, candesartan, and E3174, the active metabolite of losartan) can enhance I_{Kr}. Flufenamic acid and niflumic acid also increase I_{Kr} by accelerating channel opening. These observations open the possibility of developing new I_{Kr} openers for the treatment of patients with congenital (LQT2) or drug-induced LQTS.[16]

INHERITED CHANNELOPATHIES

Long QT Syndrome

The LQTS variants in which I_{Kr} is dysfunctional include LQT2 (caused by *KCNH2 [HERG]* loss-of-function mutations) and LQT6 (caused by *KCNE2* [MiRP1] mutations); most are LQT2, which is the second most prevalent type of LQTS. More than 200 putative disease-causing mutations have been identified for *KCNH2;* most appear to disrupt the maturation and trafficking of I_{Kr} α subunit (K_v11.1) to the sarcolemma, thereby reducing the number of functional ion channels at the cell surface membrane. Mutations involving the pore region of the *HERG* channel are associated with a significantly more severe clinical course than nonpore mutations; most pore mutations are missense mutations with a dominant negative effect. Attenuation of I_{Kr} results in prolongation of the action potential and the QT interval and can potentially generate EADs and torsades de pointes.[3,7,27,30]

The trafficking of some mutant channels into the sarcolemma can be restored by *HERG* channel blockers (e.g., cisapride, terfenadine, astemizole, E-4031), even when fexofenadine rescues mutant *HERG* channels at concentrations that do not cause channel block. However, because I_{Kr} blockers failed to rescue other trafficking-defective mutants, it is evident that multiple mechanisms may exist for pharmacological rescue of LQT2 mutations.[7,16]

Proarrhythmia induced by conditions associated with reduction of I_{Kr} (acquired or congenital LQTS) is related to excessive prolongation of action potential duration near plateau voltages, especially those that favor the development of EADs. It is also related to a more marked prolongation of the action potential duration in midmyocardial than in subepicardial or subendocardial ventricular cells possibly because of the relative scarcity of I_{Ks} and hence less "repolarization reserve" in the midmyocardial cells. Thus, triggered focal activity and ventricular reentry associated with an increased heterogeneity of repolarization across the ventricular wall would lead to the development of torsades de pointes.[16]

Short QT Syndrome

Short QT syndrome (SQTS) is a rare disease associated with short QT intervals and increased risk for AF and VF. A gain-of-function mutation in *KCNH2 (HERG)* is linked to SQTS type 1 (SQT1). A gain-of-function mutation on *KCNH2* causes a shift of voltage dependence of inactivation of I_{Kr} by +90 mV out of the range of the action potential leading to a significant increase of I_{Kr} during the action potential plateau. The resulting I_{Kr} increase achieved by altered gating hastens repolarization, thereby shortening action potential duration and facilitating reentrant excitation waves to induce atrial or ventricular arrhythmia, or both. Additionally, gain-of-function mutations in *KCNE2* (MiRP1) have been found in two families with AF.[3,27,30]

ACQUIRED DISEASES

MI can result in reduction in K_v11.1 mRNA levels and I_{Kr} with consequent prolongation of the action potential duration. Conversely, I_{Kr} density increases in subendocardial Purkinje cells in the infarcted heart at 48 hours, which can potentially increase the proarrhythmic effects of I_{Kr} blockers in patients with MI. Additionally, during acute ischemia, I_{Kr} is increased and action potential duration is shortened. Such changes can be arrhythmogenic. I_{Kr} is unchanged in patients with chronic AF and is homogeneously distributed in failing canine hearts.[3,16]

ATP, derived from either glycolysis or oxidative phosphorylation, is critical for *HERG* channel function. Both hyperglycemia and hypoglycemia depress I_{Kr} and can cause QT prolongation and ventricular arrhythmias. In diabetes, K_v11.1 levels are downregulated, leading to reduction in I_{Kr} and contributing to QT interval prolongation. Importantly, insulin therapy restores I_{Kr} function and shortens QT intervals.[3,16]

Unlike with most other K^+ currents, I_{Kr} amplitude increases on elevation of extracellular K^+ concentrations and decreases after removal of extracellular K^+. Elevation of extracellular K^+ concentration reduces C-type inactivation and increases the single channel conductance of *HERG* channels. This explains why the action potential durations are shorter at higher extracellular K^+ concentrations and longer at low concentrations, and it clarifies the associations among hypokalemia, action potential duration prolongation, and induction of torsades de pointes in patients treated with I_{Kr} blockers. In contrast, modest elevations of extracellular K^+ concentrations using K^+ supplements and spironolactone in patients given I_{Kr} blockers or with LQT2 significantly shorten the QT interval and may prevent torsades de pointes. Moreover, the antiarrhythmic actions of I_{Kr} blockers can be reversed during ischemia, which is frequently accompanied by elevations of the extracellular K^+ concentrations in the narrow intercellular spaces and by catecholamine surges that occur with exercise or other activities associated with fast heart rates.[16]

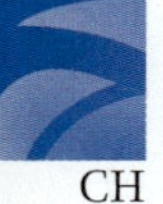

Slowly Activating Delayed Outward Rectifying Current (I_{Ks})

STRUCTURE AND PHYSIOLOGY

I_{Ks} is formed by coassembly of four pore-forming α subunits ($K_v7.1$, encoded by the *KCNQ1* gene, also known as K_vLQT1) and β subunits (minK, encoded by the *KCNE1* gene). I_{Ks} is a K^+-selective current that activates very slowly in response to membrane depolarization to potentials greater than −30 mV and reaches half-maximum activation close to +20 mV. I_{Ks} has a linear current-voltage relationship, its time course of activation is extremely slow, slower than any other known K^+ current, and steady-state amplitude is achieved only with extremely long membrane depolarization.[3,16,27,28]

Inactivation of *KCNQ1* channels is half maximal at −18 mV and, at its maximum, inactivation reduces fully activated current by approximately 35%. In addition, unlike inactivation of other K_v channels, the onset of I_{Ks} inactivation occurs after a delay (a delay of approximately 75 milliseconds at +40 mV). In contrast, when inactivation is induced after transient recovery of channels to open states, the onset of inactivation is 10 times faster. The molecular mechanism of *KCNQ1* channel inactivation is unknown, but in contrast to a classical C-type inactivation, *KCNQ1* inactivation is independent of extracellular K^+ concentration.[28]

FUNCTION

I_{Ks} contributes to human atrial and ventricular repolarization, particularly during action potentials of long duration. I_{Ks} gradually increases during the plateau phase of the action potential because its activation is delayed and very slow. As a consequence, the contribution of I_{Ks} to the net repolarizing current is greatest late in the cardiac action potential plateau phase. I_{Ks} is expressed in all cell types, but it is reduced in midmyocardial cells. The midmyocardial cells have the longest action potential duration across the myocardial wall.[28]

I_{Ks} plays an important role in determining the rate-dependent shortening of the cardiac action potential. As heart rate increases, I_{Ks} increases because channel deactivation is slow and incomplete during the shortened diastole. This allows I_{Ks} channels to accumulate in the open state during rapid heart rates and contribute to the faster rate of repolarization.[16,28]

Importantly, I_{Ks} is functionally upregulated when other repolarizing currents (e.g., I_{Kr}) are reduced, potentially serving as a safeguard against loss of repolarizing power. As such, several redundant mechanisms contribute to repolarization constituting the repolarization reserve, in which I_{Ks} plays an important role.[8,28]

REGULATION

I_{Ks} is markedly enhanced by β-adrenergic stimulation through channel phosphorylation by PKA (requiring A-kinase anchoring protein 9 [AKAP9, also known as Yotiao]) and PKC (requiring minK). This produces a rate-dependent shortening of the action potential duration such as seen during exercise-induced sinus tachycardia. I_{Ks} is also modulated by α-adrenergic receptors through the PKC pathway. Lowering extracellular K^+ and Ca^{2+} concentrations increases I_{Ks}.[16,27]

Coexpression of *KCNQ1* α subunits with minK regulates the α-subunit trafficking and behavior and results in a seven-fold increase in I_{Ks} magnitude, marked slowing of the time course of activation, and removal (or significant slowing) of inactivation of *KCNQ1* channels.[16]

As noted, I_{Kr} and I_{Ks} are functionally linked; when I_{Kr} is reduced, the action potential is prolonged, causing I_{Ks} activation to increase to prevent excess repolarization delay. Hence, the duration of the action potential is very tightly tuned via I_{Ks} and I_{Kr} regulation.[27]

PHARMACOLOGY

I_{Ks} is resistant to methanesulfonanilides (almokalant, dofetilide, D-sotalol, E-4031, ibutilide, and MK-499), but it is selectively blocked by chromanols, indapamide, thiopentone, propofol, and benzodiazepines. I_{Ks} is also blocked, although nonselectively, by amiodarone, dronedarone, and azimilide. *KCNE1* modulates the effects of I_{Ks} blockers and agonists. In fact, *KCNQ1/KCNE1* channels have 6- to 100-fold higher affinity for some I_{Ks} blockers than *KCNQ1* channels.[16]

Selective I_{Ks} blockers prolong the cardiac action potential duration and QT interval and suppress electrically induced ventricular tachyarrhythmias in animals with acute coronary ischemia and exercise superimposed on a healed MI.[16]

I_{Ks} blockade seems to have less proarrhythmic potency as compared with I_{Kr} blockade, likely the result of less drug-induced dispersion in repolarization. Additionally, because I_{Ks} accumulates at fast driving rates because of its slow deactivation, I_{Ks} blockers can be expected to be more effective in prolonging action potential duration and refractoriness at fast rates. Furthermore, because I_{Ks} activation occurs at approximately 0 mV and this voltage is more positive than the Purkinje fiber action potential plateau voltage, I_{Ks} blockade should not be expected to prolong the action potential duration at this level. Conversely, in ventricular muscle, the plateau voltage is more positive (approximately +20 mV), thus allowing I_{Ks} to be substantially more activated, so that I_{Ks} blockade would be expected to markedly increase action potential duration.[16]

β-Adrenergic agonists increase I_{Ks} density and produce a rate-dependent shortening of the action potential duration and can also decrease the antiarrhythmic effects of I_{Ks} blockers. Additionally, in the presence of I_{Ks} blockade, isoproterenol seems to abbreviate the action potential duration of epicardial and endocardial, but not midmyocardial, cells, an effect that can accentuate transmural dispersion of repolarization and precipitate torsades de pointes. These observations may explain the therapeutic actions of β-blockers in patients with LQTS syndromes linked to attenuation of I_{Ks} and the increased risk of fatal cardiac arrhythmias under physical activity or stressful situations that increase sympathetic activity in these patients.[16]

INHERITED CHANNELOPATHIES

KCNQ1 and *KCNE1* mutations can lead to a defective protein and several forms of inherited arrhythmias, including LQTS (comprising the autosomal dominant Romano-Ward syndrome and the autosomal recessive Jervell and Lange-Nielsen syndrome), SQTS, and familial AF.[3,31]

Long QT Syndrome

The most common type of LQTS, LQT1, is caused by autosomal dominant loss-of-function mutations on the *KCNQ1* gene (K_vLQT1). More than 170 mutations of this gene have been reported. They comprise many Romano-Ward (autosomal dominant) syndromes and account for approximately 45% of all genotyped LQTS families.[7] Individuals with the less prevalent LQTS type 5 (LQT5) carry loss-of-function autosomal dominant mutations in *KCNE1* and display a phenotype similar to that seen in patients with LQT1.[8]

Loss-of-function mutations in both alleles of *KCNQ1* or *KCNE1* (i.e., inherited from both parents, autosomal recessive) cause the very rare Jervell and Lange-Nielsen syndrome type 1 or 2, respectively. Jervell and Lange-Nielsen syndrome encompasses 1% to 7% of all genotyped patients with LQTS and is characterized by severe QT interval prolongation, high risk of sudden death, and congenital deafness; the deafness results from deficient endolymph secretion (*KCNQ1* and *KCNE1* are also expressed in the inner ear, where they enable endolymph secretion).[3,8,9,31,32]

LQT11 is caused by loss-of-function mutations on the *AKAP9* gene, which encodes an A-kinase anchoring protein (Yotiao), shown to be an integral part of the I_{Ks} macromolecular complex.

The presence of Yotiao is necessary for the physiological response of the I_{Ks} channel to β-adrenergic stimulation.[9] A mutation in *AKAP9* (Yotiao) in the I_{Ks} channel ($K_v7.1$) binding domain reduces the interaction between the I_{Ks} channel and Yotiao. This, in turn, reduces the cAMP-induced phosphorylation of the channel and prevents the functional response of the I_{Ks} channel to cAMP and adrenergic stimulation (i.e., prevents the increase in magnitude of I_{Ks} and the shortening of action potential duration in response to sympathetic stimulation). The final result is an attenuation of I_{Ks}, resulting in a delay in ventricular repolarization and QT interval prolongation.[3,8]

Mutations in LQT1, LQT5, and LQT11 result in attenuation of I_{Ks}, which causes prolongation of repolarization, action potential duration, and QT interval, which may be especially notable during periods of increased sympathetic activity, such as exercise, when I_{Ks} becomes the predominant repolarization current rather than I_{Kr}. In LQT1, ventricular arrhythmias are usually triggered by emotional or physical stress, probably because mutant I_{Ks} does not increase sufficiently (i.e., has less repolarization reserve) during β-adrenergic stimulation. Accordingly, β-adrenergic blocking drugs suppress arrhythmic events in LQT1.[3,8,33]

Short QT Syndrome

SQT2 is caused by mutations on the *KCNQ1* gene (K_vLQT1). A gain-of-function mutation on *KCNQ1* causes a shift of voltage dependence of activation of I_{Ks} by –20 mV and acceleration of activation kinetics, leading to enhancement of I_{Ks} and shortening of the action potential duration and QT interval. *KCNQ1* gain-of-function mutations likely predispose to AF and VF by shortening refractoriness and facilitating reentry.[3,8]

Familial Atrial Fibrillation

KCNQ1 gain-of-function mutations have been linked to familial AF, with or without the SQTS phenotype.

ACQUIRED DISEASES

Heart failure reduces I_{Ks} in atrial, ventricular, and sinus node myocytes. Given that I_{Kr} is unchanged, I_{Ks} reduction may largely account for the prolonged action potential duration in heart failure.[3]

I_{Ks} density and *KCNQ1/KCNE1* mRNA levels are reduced in myocytes from infarcted border zones 2 days after MI. However, *KCNQ1* expression is restored 5 days after MI, whereas *KCNE1* expression remains decreased.[3]

Inward Rectifying Current (I_{K1})

STRUCTURE AND PHYSIOLOGY

The Kir channels are formed by the coassembly of four α subunits (see Fig. 2-3). The α subunit (Kir2.1) of I_{K1} is encoded by *KCNJ2* and consists of two transmembrane domains (M1 and M2) connected by a pore-forming P loop (H5) along with the cytoplasmic N- and C-termini. The tetrameric Kir channel complex can be formed by identical (homotetramers) or different (heterotetramers) α subunits. Several I_{K1} channels with different conductances are recorded in human atrial myocytes. Similarly, different gene families (Kir2.1 to Kir2.3) have been found in human heart encoding I_{K1}.[16,34]

Kir channels exhibit a strong inward rectification property because conductance to K^+ ions alters at a different E_m. As noted, rectification describes the property of an ion channel to allow currents preferentially to flow in one direction or limit currents from flowing in the other direction. A channel that is inwardly rectifying is one that passes current (positive charge) more easily into the cell. In the case of Kir channels, inward rectification is a strongly voltage-dependent decline of K^+ efflux (i.e., reduction of outward current) on membrane depolarization that produces a characteristic region of so-called negative slope conductance. As such, I_{K1} is a strong rectifier that passes K^+ currents over a limited range of E_m; at a negative E_m, I_{K1} conductance is much larger than that of any other current, and so it clamps the resting E_m close to the reversal potential for K^+ (E_K). On depolarization, I_{K1} channels close almost immediately and thus limit K^+ efflux at potentials more positive than the E_K, remain closed throughout the plateau, and open again at potentials negative to –20 mV. Nevertheless, I_{K1} channels also conduct a substantial outward current at an E_m between –40 and –90 mV. Within this voltage range, outward I_{K1} is larger at more negative potentials. Thus, I_{K1} also contributes to terminal phase 3 of repolarization. Because an E_m negative to E_K is not reached in cardiomyocytes, only the outward I_{K1} plays a role in action potential formation.[16,34]

The phenomenon of inward rectification of I_{K1} channels results from high-affinity and strongly voltage-dependent blockade of the inner channel pore by cytosolic magnesium (Mg^{2+}), Ca^{2+}, and polyamines (spermine, spermidine, putrescine), which plug the channel pore at depolarized potentials, resulting in a decline in outward currents, but are displaced by incoming K^+ ions at hyperpolarized potentials. This voltage-dependent block by polyamines causes currents to be conducted well only in the inward direction. As such, I_{K1} channels are voltage regulated despite the lack of the classic voltage-sensing mechanism of K_v channels.[16,17,34]

FUNCTION

I_{K1} sets and stabilizes the resting E_m and regulates cellular excitability of atrial and ventricular myocytes during phase 4. It also contributes to the terminal portion of phase 3 repolarization. In addition to the contribution of I_{K1} to the T wave on surface ECG, data suggest that the U wave is strongly modulated by I_{K1}.

I_{K1} channels close on depolarization. The strong inward rectification of the I_{K1} limits the outward current during the positive phase of the action potential (phases 0, 1, and 2), thus allowing membrane depolarization following Na^+ channel activation, slowing membrane repolarization, and helping maintain a more prolonged cardiac action potential. This also confers energetic efficiency in the generation of the action potential.[16,34]

I_{K1} density is much higher in ventricular than in atrial myocytes, a finding that explains the steep repolarization phase in the ventricles (where more abundant I_{K1} plays a larger role in accelerating the terminal portion of repolarization) and the more shallow phase in the atria. The higher I_{K1} channel expression in the ventricle protects the ventricular cell from pacemaker activity. By contrast, I_{K1} is almost absent in sinus node and AVN cells, thus allowing for relatively more depolarized resting diastolic potentials compared with atrial and ventricular myocytes.[16,34]

A unique property of Kir currents is the unusual dependence of rectification on extracellular K^+ concentration. Specifically, on increase in extracellular K^+, the I_{K1} current-voltage relationship shifts nearly in parallel with the E_K and leads to a crossover phenomenon. One important consequence of such behavior is that at potentials positive to the crossover, K^+ conductance increases rather than decreases, against an expectation based on a reduced driving force for K^+ ions in response to elevated extracellular K^+ concentration.[34]

Fast heart rates increase the K^+ concentration in the narrow intercellular space to several millimolars and the I_{K1} density, which results in a shortening of the action potential duration that may offset the ability of I_{Kr} blockers to prolong the action potential duration under these conditions.[16,34]

REGULATION

β-Adrenergic stimulation inhibits I_{K1} in ventricular myocytes via PKA-mediated phosphorylation of the channel. In atrial myocytes, α_1-adrenergic stimulation reduces I_{K1} via PKC-dependent pathways.[16,34]

Kir2.1 overexpression increases I_{K1} density, shortens the action potential duration, and hyperpolarizes the resting E_m. In contrast, suppression of I_{K1} prolongs the action potential duration and disrupts effective clamping of the resting E_m, thus precipitating spontaneous pacemaker activity in otherwise nonpacemaking atrial and ventricular cardiomyocytes.[16]

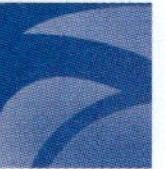

PHARMACOLOGY

Barium (Ba^{2+}) is a potent I_{K1} blocker. Blocking I_{K1} by extracellular Ba^{2+} results in depolarization of the resting potential and mild action potential prolongation.[3,34]

I_{K1} blockers prolong atrial and ventricular action potential duration and are effective against various types of experimental reentrant VTs. Moreover, I_{K1} blockers produce membrane depolarization, an effect that slows conduction velocity as a result of voltage-dependent inactivation of Na^+ channels, and prolongs the QT interval; both actions are proarrhythmic.[16,34]

INHERITED CHANNELOPATHIES

Long QT Syndrome

More than 33 loss-of-function mutations of *KCNJ2* gene encoding Kir2 result in dominant negative effects on the current and have been linked to Andersen-Tawil syndrome (LQT7), a rare autosomal dominant disorder characterized by the triad of skeletal developmental abnormalities, periodic paralysis, and usually ventricular arrhythmias, often associated with prominent U waves and mild QT interval prolongation (Kir2.1 channels are expressed primarily in skeletal muscle, heart, and brain).[3,16,34] The arrhythmias displayed by affected patients are more benign compared with other LQTS and rarely degenerate into hemodynamically compromising rhythms such as torsades de pointes, as ultimately evidenced by the lack of SCD cases so far.[8,35,36]

Disruption of the I_{K1} function can potentially lead to prolongation of the terminal repolarization phase and QT interval, which can predispose to the generation of EADs and delayed afterdepolarizations (DADs) that cause ventricular arrhythmias. However, unlike other types of LQTS in which the afterdepolarizations arise from reactivation of L-type Ca^{2+} channels, the EADs and DADs generated in LQT7 are likely secondary to Na^+-Ca^{2+} exchanger-driven depolarization. It is believed that the differential origin of the triggering beat is responsible for the observed discrepancy in arrhythmogenesis and the clinical features compared with other types of LQTS. Additionally, it is likely that prolongation of the action potential duration in LQT7 is somewhat homogeneous across the ventricular wall (i.e., transmural dispersion of repolarization is less prominent than in other types of LQTS), and this can potentially explain the low frequency of torsades de pointes.[8,35,36]

Catecholaminergic Polymorphic Ventricular Tachycardia

Three novel loss-of-function mutations of *KCNJ2* have been found in patients with catecholaminergic polymorphic VT (CPVT). These patients had prominent U waves, ventricular ectopy, and polymorphic VT, but no dysmorphic features or skeletal muscle abnormalities.[34]

I_{K1} reduction can trigger arrhythmia by allowing inward currents, which are no longer counterbalanced by the strong outward I_{K1}, to depolarize the E_m gradually during phase 4. Membrane depolarization during phase 4 induces arrhythmia by facilitating spontaneous excitability.[3]

Short QT Syndrome

A gain-of-function mutation of *KCNJ2* has been identified and linked to SQTS type 3 (SQT3). The mutation causes a significant increase in the outward I_{K1} at potentials between −75 mV and −45 mV, thus leading to acceleration of the terminal phase of repolarization and, as a consequence, shortening the action potential duration and QT interval and asymmetrical T waves with a rapid terminal phase.[37]

Familial Atrial Fibrillation

A gain-of-function *KCNJ2* mutation has been linked to familial AF. The affected members had normal QT intervals. The mutation was speculated to cause AF by shortening atrial action potential duration and facilitating reentrant excitation waves.[3,34]

ACQUIRED DISEASES

I_{K1} is downregulated in patients with severe heart failure and cardiomyopathy. The downregulation of I_{K1} produces membrane depolarization and prolongation of the action potential duration, and it can facilitate spontaneous excitability and trigger arrhythmia (both EADs and DADs). The ventricular myocytes from patients with idiopathic dilated cardiomyopathy exhibit decreased channel activity, longer action potential duration, and a lower resting E_m than those from patients with ischemic cardiomyopathy. Upregulation of I_{K1} can be observed in ventricular hypertrophy.[3,34]

Atrial I_{K1} is upregulated in patients with chronic AF, resulting in more negative resting potentials and, together with reduced I_{CaL}, accounting for action potential shortening in AF.[3]

Acetylcholine-Activated Potassium Current (I_{KACh})

STRUCTURE AND PHYSIOLOGY

I_{KACh} results from a heterotetrameric complex of two Kir3.1 (encoded by *KCNJ3*) and two Kir3.4 (encoded by *KCNJ5*) α subunits. I_{KACh} is a receptor-activated Kir channel; it has large cytoplasmic domains that harbor specific binding sites for cytosolic effectors (G proteins). The channel conducts I_{KACh} in response to the stimulation of G protein–coupled muscarinic (M_2) and adenosine (A_1) receptors.[16]

Cardiac I_{K1} and I_{KACh} are the major K^+ currents displaying classical strong inward rectification with membrane depolarization, a unique property that is critical for their roles in cardiac excitability.[34]

FUNCTION

I_{KACh} has generally an opposite distribution to that of I_{K1}. I_{KACh} is more prominent in atrial tissue, as well as in the sinus node and AVN, and is largely absent in the ventricles. The regional distribution of I_{KACh} is also heterogeneous within and between the atria.[16,34]

I_{KACh} mediates vagal influences on sinus rate and atrial repolarization, as well as AVN conduction. Activation I_{KACh} by acetylcholine hyperpolarizes the E_m and shortens action potential duration. These effects result in slowing of phase 4 depolarization, reduction in the spontaneous firing rate of the pacemaker cells of the sinus node and AVN, and slowing of AVN conduction. These effects explain why vagal maneuvers or intravenous adenosine can terminate reentrant supraventricular tachycardias using the AVN.[16,34]

REGULATION

Vagal stimulation produces a nonuniform shortening of the atrial action potential duration and refractoriness mediated by activation of I_{KACh}, an effect that can contribute to the perpetuation of AF.[16]

I_{KACh} is also increased by purinergic stimulation. Adrenergic stimulation via β_1-receptor-mediated signaling increases the amplitude of constitutively active current, whereas α_{1a}-stimulation decreases I_{KACh}.

Atrial I_{KACh} is inhibited by membrane stretch, possibly serving as a mechanoelectrical feedback pathway, a property conferred by the Kir3.4 subunit.[16]

PHARMACOLOGY

I_{KACh} activity can be stimulated by intracellular ATP, the phospholipid phosphatidylinositol 4,5-bisphosphate (PIP_2) and ETA endothelin, A opioid, and α_2-adrenergic agonists. α_1-Adenosine receptor agonists stimulate I_{KACh}, whereas methylxanthines, such as theophylline and aminophylline, antagonize the effects of adenosine. Dipyridamole prolongs the action of adenosine by disturbing the action of the cell membrane transporter of adenosine.[1,38]

I_{KACh} is inhibited by several antiarrhythmic drugs, including amiodarone, dronedarone, disopyramide, procainamide, flecainide, and propafenone. Disopyramide and procainamide mainly block the muscarinic receptors, whereas flecainide and propafenone act as open channel blockers. Blockade of I_{KACh} by dronedarone is approximately 100 times more potent than that of amiodarone.[16]

A potent I_{KACh} blocking property is of additional therapeutic value especially for treatment of AF, because I_{KACh} plays a prominent role in vagally induced AF and has been shown to be constitutively active in chronic AF. In fact, I_{KACh} is a promising target for AF therapy, and series of chemical compounds have been tested as antiarrhythmic agents. Inhibition of I_{KACh} in the setting of AF can potentially produce proportionally greater action potential duration prolongation than under control conditions and can even terminate experimental atrial tachyarrhythmias and AF without ventricular side effects.[26]

INHERITED CHANNELOPATHIES

LQT13 is caused by loss-of-function mutations on the *KCNJ5* gene. The *KCNJ5* mutation is the most recently identified LQTS-associated gene, and it exerts dominant-negative effects on Kir3.1-Kir3.4 channel complexes by disrupting membrane targeting and stability of Kir3.4.[39]

ACQUIRED DISEASES

I_{KACh} is downregulated during chronic AF, possibly to counteract the AF-induced nonuniform shortening of the atrial refractoriness.[16] However, I_{KACh} channels can develop constitutive activity during human AF (i.e., these channels become activated despite the absence of stimulating acetylcholine). This increase in functionally uncoupled I_{KACh} in human AF is possibly the result of increased phosphorylation of Kir3 channels by PKC or a reduction in inhibitory $G_{\alpha i\text{-}3}$ subunits. Constitutively active I_{KACh} can hyperpolarize the membrane and, hence, contribute to AF-related electrical remodeling and to the persistence of AF by stabilization of rotors. Therefore, selectively targeting constitutively active I_{KACh} channels only may preserve physiological stimulation by vagal nerves and could serve as a promising remodeling-related drug target.[26,40]

ATP-Dependent Potassium Current (I_{KATP})

STRUCTURE AND PHYSIOLOGY

Cardiac ATP-sensitive K^+ (K_{ATP}) channels (also termed the adenosine diphosphate [ADP]–activated K^+ channel) are formed by the unique combination of two dissimilar proteins: four pore-forming α subunits (Kir6.2, encoded by *KCNJ4*) and four regulatory ATP-binding cassette proteins (sulfonylurea receptor subunits [SUR2A] encoded by *ABCC9*). The Kir6.2 subunits have two transmembrane spans and form the channel's pore and large cytoplasmic domains that provide the binding sites for ATP. The SUR2A subunits have three transmembrane domains and contain two nucleotide-binding domains on the cytoplasmic side. These allow for nucleotide-mediated regulation of K_{ATP} and are critical in its role as a sensor of metabolic status. The SUR2A subunits are also sensitive to sulfonylureas, Mg-ATP, Mg-ADP, and some other pharmacological channel openers. The SUR2A subunit also harbors an ATPase for ATP hydrolysis, which gates the K^+ permeation through the Kir6.2 α subunit.[16,41-43]

K_{ATP} is a receptor-activated weak inward rectifier channel, regulated by intracellular ATP and ADP concentrations. An increase in the ratio of ATP to ADP closes the channel, and a decrease opens it, linking the metabolic state to the cellular E_m.[16,41-43]

FUNCTION

I_{KATP} is inhibited by intracellular ATP and activated by Mg-ADP, so that the channel activity is regulated by the ATP/ADP ratio, coupling cell metabolism to the E_m. In responding to cytoplasmic nucleotide levels, K_{ATP} channel activity provides a unique link between cellular energetics and electrical excitability and hence contractility. Under normal metabolic conditions, sarcolemmal K_{ATP} channels are predominantly closed (inhibited by intracellular ATP), and they do not significantly contribute to the cardiac action potential, resting E_m, or cell excitability. However, when exposed to a severe metabolic stress such as anoxia, metabolic inhibition, or ischemia, K_{ATP} channels become activated (secondary to reduced intracellular ATP levels) and conduct an outward repolarizing K^+ current (I_{KATP}), which results in abbreviation of the action potential duration and reduction of Ca^{2+} influx through L-type Ca^{2+} channels. By reducing Ca^{2+} entry, K_{ATP} channels depress muscle contractility, thereby conserving scarce energy resources, and prevent the damaging effects of intracellular Ca^{2+} overload.[42,43]

Accordingly, cardiac K_{ATP} channels act as membrane-based metabolic sensors that receive energetic signals of cellular distress and provide adaptive response to acute stress capable of controlling cardiac action potential duration and associated cellular functions and adjusting cellular excitability to match demand.[43]

Additionally, activation of I_{KATP} plays an important role in ischemic preconditioning; brief periods of myocardial ischemia confer protection against subsequent prolonged ischemia, reducing MI size, severity of stunning, and incidence of cardiac arrhythmias. However, the role of sarcolemmal K_{ATP} channels in ischemic preconditioning versus that of mitochondrial K_{ATP} channels (which appear to be pharmacologically distinct from sarcolemmal K_{ATP}) has been debated.[42,43]

On the other hand, activation of I_{KATP} also results in shortening of the action potential duration, accumulation of extracellular K^+, membrane depolarization, and slowed conduction velocity, effects that render the ischemic heart vulnerable to reentrant arrhythmias.[42]

K_{ATP} channels have been further implicated in the adaptive cardiac response to chronic pathophysiological hemodynamic load. K_{ATP} channel deficiency affects structural remodeling, renders the heart vulnerable to Ca^{2+}-dependent maladaptation, and predisposes to heart failure.[43]

REGULATION

ATP (with or without Mg^{2+}) inhibits I_{KATP} by stabilizing the closed state of the channel by interacting directly with Kir6.2. In addition, in the presence of Mg^{2+}, ATP and ADP can activate the channel through interaction with the SUR2A subunit. Inhibition by ATP binding to Kir6.2 and activation by Mg nucleotides is the primary physiological regulatory mechanism.[16,41-43]

K_{ATP} channel's sensitivity to ATP is not fixed, and it can be modulated by other cellular factors. Nucleotide diphosphates, lactate, oxygen-derived free radicals, and adenosine α_1 receptor stimulation desensitize K_{ATP} to inhibition by intracellular ATP. Additionally, the phospholipid PIP_2 directly interacts with Kir6.2 subunit stabilizing the open state of the channel and antagonizes ATP inhibition of I_{KATP}.[42]

PHARMACOLOGY

K^+ channel openers (pinacidil, cromakalim, rimakalim, and nicorandil) bind at two distinct regions of SUR2A subunits and can exert cardioprotective effects in patients with acute MI. However, K^+ channel openers also activate vascular K_{ATP} (Kir6.1/SUR2B) and produce hypotensive effects that limit their use in the treatment of myocardial ischemia. Moreover, because I_{KATP} density is larger in the epicardium, K^+ channel openers produce a more marked shortening of action potential duration in epicardial cells, thus leading to a marked dispersion of repolarization and to the development of extrasystolic activity via a mechanism of phase 2 reentry. On the other hand, K^+ channel openers shorten the action potential duration (and QT interval), reduce transmural dispersion of repolarization, and suppress EADs and DADs induced in patients with LQT1.

Thus, K^+ channel openers may prevent spontaneous torsades de pointes when congenital or acquired LQTS is secondary to reduced I_{Kr} or I_{Ks}.[16,42]

I_{KATP} blockers (e.g., sulfonylureas and various antiarrhythmic drugs) prevent the shortening of the action potential duration and can potentially prevent VF during myocardial ischemia. Nonetheless, they can also be arrhythmogenic. Moreover, because K_{ATP} channels are present in pancreatic β cells and vascular smooth muscle, I_{KATP} blockers can produce hypoglycemia and coronary vasoconstriction, effects that may preclude their interest as antiarrhythmic agents.

On the other hand, cardioselective I_{KATP} blockers (clamikalant, HMR 1098) inhibited hypoxia-induced shortening of the action potential duration and prevented VF induced by coronary artery occlusion in postinfarcted conscious dogs at doses that had no effect on insulin release, blood pressure, or coronary blood flow. Thus, these drugs may represent a new therapeutic approach to the treatment of ventricular arrhythmias in patients with coronary heart disease.[16,42]

It is still unclear whether opening of K_{ATP} channels has completely proarrhythmic or antiarrhythmic effects. Increased K^+ conductance should stabilize the E_m during ischemic insults and reduce the extent of infarct and ectopic pacemaker activity. On the other hand, K^+ channel opening accelerates repolarization of the action potential, possibly inducing arrhythmic reentry.[16,42]

INHERITED CHANNELOPATHIES

Mutations in *ABCC9* resulting in reduced intrinsic channel ATPase activity, metabolic sensing deficit, and dysfunctional K_{ATP} channels have been found in patients with idiopathic dilated cardiomyopathy and rhythm disturbances. These mutations confer susceptibility to Ca^{2+}-dependent maladaptive remodeling, progressing to cardiomyopathy and congestive heart failure. Additionally, a loss-of-function *ABCC9* mutation has been linked to predisposition to adrenergic AF. K_{ATP} channel-pore polymorphisms have also been linked to SCD.[43]

Many mutations in the Kir6.2 subunit have now been identified as causal in human neonatal diabetes mellitus, a very severe form of diabetes that typically occurs within the first days or weeks of life. All the identified Kir6.2 mutations result in a reduced channel sensitivity to ATP inhibition, leading to channel activation at elevated glucose, maintained hyperpolarization of pancreatic islet α cells, and electrical inexcitability, with consequent inhibition of insulin secretion. Although cardiac K_{ATP} channels (Kir6.2/SUR2A) have the same Kir6.2 subunit as that in pancreatic K_{ATP} channels (Kir6.2/SUR1), there are no reports of any cardiac abnormalities in patients with neonatal diabetes mellitus; this finding suggests that factors other than nucleotide sensitivity play an important role.[42]

ACQUIRED DISEASES

Metabolic dysregulation of I_{KATP} created by disease-induced structural remodeling appears to contribute to the dysfunction of heart failure.[26,43]

The effects of Kir6.2 modulation in AF have not extensively been studied. However, evidence indicates a reduction of I_{KATP} in patients with chronic AF, a finding suggesting that regulation of this current may not contribute importantly to AF-related ionic remodeling.[26,43]

Two-Pore Potassium Channels (K_{2P})

STRUCTURE AND PHYSIOLOGY

K_{2P} channels are composed of four transmembrane domains and two pore-forming P loops arranged in tandem, one between the first and second transmembrane domains and the other between the third and fourth domains (see Fig. 2-3). The proteins mainly form functional homodimers, although heterodimers combining different K_{2P} subunits have been reported. Several subfamilies of K_{2P} channels have been identified, including the TWIK-related acid-sensitive K^+ (TASK) channels and TWIK-related K^+ (TREK) channels.[44]

TASK channels exhibit sensitivity to variations in extracellular pH over a narrow physiological range. TASK-1 *(KCNK3)* and TASK-3 *(KCNK9)* subunits are functional when associated as homodimers or heterodimers. TASK channels display strong basal currents with very fast activation and inactivation kinetics.

TREK channels, which comprise TREK-1 *(KCNK2)*, TREK-2 *(KCNK10)*, and TRAAK *(KCNK4)*, display low basal activity, but are stimulated by stretch of the cell membrane, lysophospholipids, and arachidonic acid and are inactivated by hypo osmolarity and phosphorylation by PKA and PKC.[44]

Several members of the K_{2P} channel family are expressed in the heart and in the systemic or pulmonary circulations, and some contribute to background K^+ currents and the control of E_m in vascular smooth muscle cells. The K^+ selectivity, voltage-independent gating, and rectification of K_{2P} currents are characteristics that make them strong candidates for mediating background K^+ currents. Importantly, the sensitivity of K_{2P} channels to numerous chemical and physical physiological stimuli (e.g., pH, oxygen, phospholipids, neurotransmitters, G protein–coupled receptors, and stretch) allow these channels to play a role in regulating the E_m and excitability in various cell types under a range of physiological and pathological situations.[44,45]

FUNCTION

There is clear evidence for TREK-1 and TASK-1 in the heart and these channels are likely to regulate cardiac action potential duration through their regulation by stretch, polyunsaturated fatty acids, pH, and neurotransmitters. TREK-1 may also have a critical role in mediating the vasodilator response of resistance arteries to polyunsaturated fatty acids, thus contributing to their protective effect on the cardiovascular system. TASK-1, on the other hand, is a strong candidate for a role in hypoxic vasoconstriction of pulmonary arteries.[44]

In working atrial and ventricular myocytes, background K^+ currents are crucial for stabilizing the E_m at a hyperpolarized value toward the K^+ equilibrium potential and regulating action potential duration in various physiological and pathological conditions. The background current is mainly carried by inward rectifier channels (including I_{K1}, I_{KACh}, and I_{KATP}). Several K_{2P} channels have been proposed to contribute to the cardiac background or "leak" K^+ channels (i.e., channels with properties similar to the steady-state noninactivating K^+ current [I_{ss}] that is well characterized in rodent myocytes). Among them, TREK-1 and TASK-1 have been the most extensively studied.[44]

TREK-1, as an outwardly rectifying current, can potentially participate in balancing the E_m and action potential duration. Indeed, on a beat-to-beat basis, it could be involved in a negative feedback loop, hyperpolarizing the E_m in response to a stretch stimulus following the stretch activation of nonselective cation channels. The expression of TREK-1 appears to be nonuniform in the heart, with stronger TREK-1 mRNA expression in endocardial cells compared with epicardial cells. This finding possibly reflects different amounts of stretch experienced by muscle cells in different parts of the ventricular wall, leading to differential mechanoelectrical feedback and thereby reducing action potential repolarization in areas of the myocardium where conduction velocity is slower. Mechanoelectric feedback following an increase in atrial volume may be arrhythmogenic, changing the shape of the action potential. Physiological evidence of the direct involvement of TREK-1 current in mechanoelectric feedback in the heart has still to be provided.[44]

ACQUIRED DISEASES

TREK-1 activity may have some importance in pathological conditions such as ischemia, when released purinergic agonists such as ADP and ATP lead to arachidonic acid production. Activation of TREK-1 by ATP during ischemia may contribute to electrophysiological disturbances in the ventricular wall. As a stretch-activated K^+ channel in atrial cells, TREK-1 could additionally be involved in regulating the release of atrial natriuretic peptide, which is released by a stretch-induced increase in intracellular Ca^{2+} concentration. Further work will be necessary to clarify the possible role of TREK or other stretch-dependent channels in the pathological heart.[44]

L-Type Calcium Current (I_{CaL})

Structure and Physiology

In cardiac muscle, two types of voltage-dependent Ca^{2+} channels, the L-type and the T-type, transport Ca^{2+} into the cells. The L-type channel (L for long-lasting, because of its slow kinetics of current decay as compared with Na^+ channels) is found in all cardiac cell types. The T-type channel (T for tiny and transient) is found principally in pacemaker, atrial, and Purkinje cells. The term Ca^{2+} channels is used to refer to the L-type channel.[46-48]

Cardiac L-type Ca^{2+} channels are composed of four polypeptide subunits (α_{1C}, β, α_2, delta) and form a heterotetrameric complex. The α_{1C} subunit ($Ca_v1.2$, encoded by the *CACNAIC* gene) has a structure similar to that of the Na^+ channel: four homologous domains (I to IV), each consisting of six transmembrane segments (S1 to S6). The S5 and S6 segments and the membrane-associated pore loop (P loop) between them form the central pore through which ions flow down their electrochemical gradient. The P loop contains four negatively charged glutamate residues (EEEE) that are required for the Ca^{2+} selectivity of the channel. S4 in each homologous domain contains a highly conserved positively charged residue (arginine or lysine) at every third or fourth position. This segment serves as the voltage sensor for gating.[46,47,49]

The α_{1C} subunit is the main and largest subunit, and it determines most of the channel characteristics because it harbors the ion-selective pore, voltage sensor, gating apparatus, and binding sites for channel-modulating drugs and is autoregulatory. To form a functional L-type Ca^{2+} channel, the α_{1C} subunit coassembles with auxiliary subunits in a 1:1:1 ratio: the β subunit, the α_2 subunit, and the delta subunit.[46,47,49]

The β subunit ($Ca_v\beta$, encoded by the *CACNB* gene) is entirely intracellular and is tightly bound to a highly conserved motif in the cytoplasmic linker between domains I and II of the α_{1C} subunit. Coexpression of β subunits modulates the biophysical properties of the α_{1C} subunit. The β subunit has a prominent role in channel expression, trafficking, regulation, and facilitation. Sites possible for phosphorylation by various protein kinases (PKA, PKC, protein kinase G [PKG]) have been identified in these subunits. The β subunits are also involved in channel regulation by β-adrenergic stimulation and in response to the changes of the pH of the cell. In addition, the β subunit increases Ca^{2+} current amplitude, accelerates the kinetics of Ca^{2+} channel activation, and alters pharmacological properties of the channel.[46,47]

The α_2 and delta subunits are encoded by the same gene *(CACNA2D)*; the mature forms of these subunits are derived by posttranslational proteolytic cleavage, but they remain associated through a disulfide bond. The α_2 subunit is completely extracellular, whereas the delta subunit has a single membrane-spanning segment with a very short intracellular part that anchors the α_2-delta subunit complex to the α_{1C} subunit. The α_2-delta subunit complex has less influence on channel function than the β subunit. The α_2-delta subunit slightly increases Ca^{2+} current amplitude and accelerates channel inactivation and can change the properties of Ca^{2+} channel activation. It can also affect channel density trafficking.[46,47]

L-type Ca^{2+} channels are characterized by a large single channel conductance. The channels are closed at the resting potential, but they activate on depolarization to potentials positive to –40 mV. I_{CaL} peaks at 0 to + 10 mV, and tends to reverse at +60 to +70 mV, following a bell-shaped current-voltage relationship.

Although I_{CaL} is normally activated during phase 0 by the regenerative depolarization caused by the fast I_{Na}, I_{CaL} is much smaller than the peak I_{Na}. In addition, the amplitude of I_{CaL} is not maximal near the action potential peak because of the time-dependent nature of I_{CaL} activation, as well as the low driving force (E_m – reversal potential of a cardiac Ca^{2+} channel [E_{Ca}]) for I_{CaL}.[50]

The decay of I_{CaL} during depolarization (i.e., time-dependent inactivation) is very slow and depends on two mechanisms: voltage-dependent inactivation and Ca^{2+}-dependent inactivation. These two mechanisms control Ca^{2+} influx into cardiomyocytes and hence regulate signal transduction to sarcoplasmic reticulum Ca^{2+} channels (ryanodine receptor 2 [RyR2]) and ensure normal contraction and relaxation of the heart.[46-48]

Fast Ca^{2+}-dependent inactivation serves as a negative feedback for Ca^{2+} to limit further Ca^{2+} entry via L-type Ca^{2+} channels. The slow voltage-dependent inactivation (induced by membrane depolarization) prevents a premature rise in I_{CaL} when intracellular Ca^{2+} concentration decreases and Ca^{2+}-dependent inactivation terminates during maintained depolarization. Although still under dispute, the relative contribution of Ca^{2+}-dependent inactivation to total inactivation of I_{CaL} appears to be greater at negative potentials when voltage-dependent inactivation, which typically exhibits a U-shaped availability curve, is weak. After β-adrenergic stimulation, Ca^{2+}-dependent inactivation becomes the main inactivation mechanism as a result of a slowing down of voltage-dependent inactivation.[46-48]

The Ca^{2+}-dependent inactivation mechanism depends primarily on Ca^{2+} released from the sarcoplasmic reticulum. The Ca^{2+}-binding protein calmodulin functions as a critical sensor mediating Ca^{2+}-induced inactivation of L-type Ca^{2+} channels. Calmodulin binds to two α_{1C} subunit amino acid sequences (called domains L and K). When local intracellular Ca^{2+} concentration increases (secondary to influx Ca^{2+} via the L-type Ca^{2+} channel, as well as Ca^{2+}-induced Ca^{2+} release from the sarcoplasmic reticulum), more Ca^{2+} ions bind to calmodulin, which harbors four Ca^{2+}-binding sites. When saturated with Ca^{2+}, conformational change of both calmodulin and α_{1C} subunit leads to blockage of the channel pore.

Voltage steady-state activation and inactivation are sigmoidal, with an activation range over –40 to +10 mV (with a half-activation potential near –15 mV) and a half-inactivation potential near –35 mV. However, a relief of inactivation for voltages positive to 0 mV leads to a U-shaped voltage curve for steady-state inactivation. Overlap of the steady-state voltage-dependent inactivation and activation relations defines a window current near the action potential plateau, within which transitions from closed and open states can occur that may participate in action potential repolarization and may play a major role in the initiation of EADs.[47,48]

After inactivation, the transition of Ca^{2+} channels from the inactivated to the closed resting state (i.e., recovery from inactivation [reactivation, restoration, or repriming]) is also Ca^{2+} and voltage dependent. Reduction of intracellular Ca^{2+} concentration in the immediate vicinity of the channel allows recovery from Ca^{2+}-dependent inactivation. Acceleration of Ca^{2+} channel reactivation, as may occur secondary to reuptake of Ca^{2+} by the sarcoplasmic reticulum during prolonged depolarization, can result in the recovery from Ca^{2+}-dependent inactivation and enable secondary depolarization. This leads to instability of the cell E_m during repolarization and may be the basis for the EADs that are capable of initiating torsades de pointes.[46,48]

Voltage-dependent recovery of I_{CaL} from inactivation between action potentials is slow at a low (depolarized) E_m, and it becomes very fast as the action potential repolarization is nearly complete. As a consequence, I_{CaL} declines in response to repetitive stimulation at a partially depolarized E_m between pulses (resulting from Ca^{2+} channel incomplete recovery from inactivation), and a negative staircase of contractility is observed.

In contrast, at normal resting potentials, recovery of I_{CaL} from inactivation is fast, and I_{CaL} may increase progressively during repetitive stimulation. This positive staircase or rate-dependent potentiation of contractility is Ca^{2+} dependent and likely is the result of diminished Ca^{2+}-dependent inactivation at frequencies with less sarcoplasmic reticulum Ca^{2+} release. Additionally, similar to Ca^{2+}-dependent inactivation, Ca^{2+}-dependent facilitation requires high-affinity binding of calmodulin to the C-terminal tail of the $Ca_v1.2$ channel and may be facilitated by calmodulin kinase II–dependent phosphorylation. Calmodulin kinase II is a Ca^{2+}/calmodulin-dependent serine/threonine kinase that is activated by low intracellular Ca^{2+} concentration. The facilitatory effect of Ca^{2+} entry on subsequent I_{CaL} is distinct from, but coexistent with, Ca^{2+}-dependent inactivation.[46-48]

Function

I_{CaL} is activated by membrane depolarization. It is largely responsible for the action potential plateau and is a major determinant of the duration of the plateau phase and hence of action potential duration and refractoriness. I_{CaL} also links membrane depolarization to myocardial contraction and constitutes the dominant factor in mediating positive inotropy in all types of cardiac tissue. Additionally, I_{CaL} is responsible for the upstroke (phase 0) of slow response action potentials (in pacemaking cardiomyocytes and regions of depressed resting E_m) and contributes to physiological frequency regulation in the sinus node.[46-48]

L-type Ca^{2+} channels are the principal portal of entry of Ca^{2+} into the cells during depolarization. Ca^{2+} influx during the action potential plateau triggers more massive Ca^{2+} release (Ca^{2+} transients) from the sarcoplasmic reticulum into the cytosol via activation of Ca^{2+}-release channels (e.g., RyR2). This amplifying process, termed Ca^{2+}-induced Ca^{2+} release (CICR), causes a rapid increase in intracellular Ca^{2+} concentration (from approximately 100 nM to approximately 1 μM) to a level required for optimal binding of Ca^{2+} to troponin C and induction of contraction. Most of the L-type Ca^{2+} channels in the adult myocyte are localized in the transverse tubules (T tubules) facing the sarcoplasmic reticulum junction and the RyR2, organized as a "complex" that ensures coordinated Ca^{2+} release during excitation-contraction coupling.[46,49]

Cytosolic Ca^{2+} concentration decreases during diastole: contraction is followed by Ca^{2+} release from troponin C and its reuptake by the sarcoplasmic reticulum via activation of the sarcoplasmic reticulum Ca^{2+}-ATPase Ca^{2+} pump, in addition to extrusion across the sarcolemma via the Na^+-Ca^{2+} exchanger. Intracellular Ca^{2+}-dependent inactivation limits Ca^{2+} influx during action potential.[46,47,49]

For maintenance of intracellular Ca^{2+} homeostasis and balanced cardiac activity, Ca^{2+} influx into cytoplasm via L-type Ca^{2+} channels has to be terminated. This is achieved by Ca^{2+}-dependent inactivation of L-type Ca^{2+} channels. This inactivation serves as a negative feedback mechanism for regulating Ca^{2+} entry into the cell and as a physiological safety mechanism against a harmful Ca^{2+} overload in the cell, which can cause both arrhythmias and cell death. Ca^{2+}-dependent inactivation is also a major determinant of action potential duration, and it ensures that contraction and relaxation cycles of the heart muscle fiber are coordinated. A failure to deactivate I_{CaL} completely may possibly be an essential mechanism underlying EADs caused by suppression of the K^+ delayed rectifier currents.[50]

Inhibition of α_{1C} subunit binding to calmodulin eliminates Ca^{2+}-dependent inactivation, thus promoting Ca^{2+}-dependent facilitation, which contributes to a force-frequency relationship in the heart.[46,47,49]

Regulation

Phosphorylation of the pore-forming α_{1C} subunits by different kinases is one of the most important pathways to change the activity of the L-type Ca^{2+} channel. Phosphorylation by PKA is the main mechanism of Ca^{2+} channel activation, because it increases the probability and duration of the open state of the channels and consequently increases I_{CaL}.[46,47,49]

Several different agonists (e.g., catecholamines, glucagon, histamine, serotonin) can activate PKA-mediated phosphorylation and activation of the L-type Ca^{2+} channel via an intracellular signaling cascade. Once one of these agonists binds to its receptor, receptor stimulation activates guanosine triphosphate (GTP)–binding protein (G_s), which activates adenylyl cyclase, which, in turn, mediates the conversion of ATP into cAMP. The increased cAMP levels stimulate cAMP-dependent PKA phosphorylation of the α_{1C} subunit of L-type Ca^{2+} channels and result in an increase in I_{CaL} amplitude and a shift in activation to a more negative E_m. cAMP is degraded by cAMP phosphodiesterases, and the signaling cascade is then suppressed limiting cAMP-dependent phosphorylation; in addition, the signaling cascade is terminated by serine/threonine phosphatases that remove a phosphate group from kinase-phosphorylated proteins.[46,47]

The suppression of adenylyl cyclase activity is one of the most common pathways to interrupt PKA-dependent Ca^{2+} channel stimulation. Adenylyl cyclase is usually suppressed (and cAMP synthesis is blocked) by activation of G_i proteins. Stimulation of various G_i protein–coupled receptors (e.g., M_2 muscarinic receptors, adenosine A_1 receptors, opiates, and atrial natriuretic peptides) does not change basal I_{CaL} in most cases, but reduces I_{CaL} increased via stimulation of β-adrenergic receptors. Activation of phosphodiesterases is another way to reduce PKA-dependent channel phosphorylation. Phosphodiesterases hydrolyze cAMP and cyclic guanosine monophosphate (cGMP) and decrease their intracellular concentrations.[46,47,49]

The physiological functions of cardiac L-type Ca^{2+} channels are under control of catecholamines of circulating and neurohumoral origin. The effects of adrenergic stimulation are exerted by phosphorylation of the L-type Ca^{2+} channel subunits by PKA, PKC, and PKG. β_1-Adrenergic receptors couple exclusively to the G_s protein, thus producing a widespread increase in cAMP levels in the cell, whereas β_2-adrenergic receptors couple to both G_s and G_i, thus producing a more localized activation of L-type Ca^{2+} channels.[46,49]

The effect of PKC-mediated phosphorylation on I_{CaL} can be highly diverse. PKC can either increase or decrease I_{CaL}. Activation of G_q subunits by G_q protein–coupled receptors (e.g., α-adrenergic receptors, endothelin, angiotensin II, and muscarinic receptors) stimulates phospholipase C, which hydrolyzes PIP_2 to inositol 1,4,5-triphosphate ($InsP_3$) and diacylglycerol (DAG). DAG activates PKC, which, in turn, phosphorylates L-type Ca^{2+} channels. The mechanism of the effect of PKC on the activity of cardiac L-type Ca^{2+} channels is not exactly known. PKC phosphorylates the N-terminus of the α_{1C} subunit, and the effect on the channel can be either stimulating or suppressive.[46,47]

Activation of soluble guanylate cyclase (primarily by nitric oxide) results in the conversion of GTP into cGMP. cGMP activates PKG, which phosphorylates the α_{1C} subunit of the L-type Ca^{2+} channel, with a resulting inhibition of I_{CaL}. Besides direct phosphorylation of the L-type Ca^{2+} channel, it is also possible that PKG activates a protein phosphatase, which dephosphorylates the channel, or that cGMP activates phosphodiesterase 2, which reduces cAMP levels. Thus, stimulation of I_{CaL} by PKA is inhibited. However, besides an inhibition of I_{CaL}, stimulatory effects of the PKG pathway have been shown.[46,47,49]

I_{CaL} is blocked by several cations (e.g., Mg^{2+}, nickel [Ni^{2+}], zinc [Zn^{2+}]) and drugs (dihydropyridines, phenylalkylamines, benzothiazepines). In addition, coexpression of the β-subunit increases I_{CaL} amplitude, accelerates the kinetics of Ca^{2+} channel activation, and alters pharmacological properties of the channel.[47,49]

Pharmacology

Cardiac L-type Ca^{2+} channels are the targets for the interaction with class IV antiarrhythmic drugs. The three classes of organic Ca^{2+} channel blockers include dihydropyridines (e.g., nifedipine, nicardipine, amlodipine, felodipine), phenylalkylamines (verapamil), and benzothiazepines (diltiazem). Each drug type binds specifically to separate binding sites on the channel's

α_{1C} subunit. The combined use of Ca^{2+} channel blockers can enhance or weaken the block effect because, at least in part, of the different binding sites for those drugs. It is noteworthy that increased extracellular Ca^{2+} concentrations inhibit the binding of phenylalkylamines and dihydropyridines to their receptors on the Ca^{2+} channel.

Verapamil and diltiazem preferentially block open and inactivated states of the channel. The more frequently the Ca^{2+} channel opens, the better is the penetration of the drug to the binding site; hence, these drugs cause use-dependent block of conduction in cells with Ca^{2+}-dependent action potentials such as those in the sinus node and AVN. This explains their preferential effect on nodal tissue in paroxysmal supraventricular tachycardia.[46,47,49]

The dihydropyridines block open Ca^{2+} channels. However, the lack of use-dependence and the presence of voltage sensitivity of the dihydropyridines with regard to their binding explain their vascular selectivity. The kinetics of recovery from block is sufficiently fast that these drugs produce no significant cardiac effect but effectively block the smooth muscle Ca^{2+} channel because of its low resting potential.[46,47,49]

Inherited Channelopathies

LONG QT SYNDROME

Gain-of-function mutations of the *CACNA1C* gene encoding the α_{1C} subunit ($Ca_v1.2$) result in nearly complete elimination of voltage-dependent inactivation of $Ca_v1.2$ channels, thus leading to inappropriate continuation of the depolarizing I_{CaL} and lengthening the plateau phase. The resultant sustained Ca^{2+} influx, action potential (and QT interval) prolongation, and Ca^{2+} overload promote EADs and DADs. These mutations have been linked to Timothy syndrome, a rare disease with QT interval prolongation (LQT8). Because the Ca^{2+} channel $Ca_v1.2$ is abundant in many tissues, patients with Timothy syndrome have many clinical manifestations including congenital heart disease, autism, syndactyly, and immune deficiency.[3,47,49]

BRUGADA SYNDROME

Approximately 12% of cases of the Brugada syndrome are attributable to loss-of-function mutations in the cardiac Ca^{2+} channel resulting in a reduction of the depolarizing I_{CaL}. Brugada syndrome type 3 is caused by mutations in the *CACNA1C* gene, which encodes the pore-forming α_1 subunit ($Ca_v1.2$). Brugada syndrome type 4 is caused by mutations in the *CACNB2* gene, which encodes for the regulatory β_2 subunit ($Ca_v\beta2$), which modifies gating of I_{CaL}. The mechanism of Brugada syndrome type 3 and type 4 involves a reduction of the depolarizing I_{CaL}. Mutations in the α and β subunits of the Ca^{2+} channel can also lead to a shorter than normal QT interval, creating a new clinical entity consisting of a combined Brugada/short QT syndrome.[10]

SHORT QT SYNDROME

SQT4 is caused by mutations on the *CACNA1C* gene (encoding the α_{1C} subunit, $Ca_v1.2$) and SQT5 is caused by mutations on the *CACNB2* gene (encoding the β_{2b} subunit). Loss-of-function mutations on those genes result in major attenuation in I_{CaL} amplitude, leading to shortening of the action potential duration, and are associated with asymmetrical T waves, an attenuated QT–heart rate relationship, and AF. The three patients reported to harbor these mutations had a Brugada type 1 phenotype.[1,49]

Acquired Diseases

Abnormalities in Ca^{2+} currents or intracellular Ca^{2+} transients, or both, in acquired diseases may induce both arrhythmia and contractile dysfunction. In AF, $Ca_v1.2$ mRNA and protein levels are downregulated, resulting in I_{CaL} reduction, which contributes to action potential shortening.[3]

In heart failure, the membrane density of I_{CaL} channels is reduced. However, channel phosphorylation is increased, leading to reduced response to phosphorylating interventions and causing increased single channel open probability that compensates for the reductions in channel density. Despite unchanged I_{CaL}, sarcoplasmic reticulum Ca^{2+} transients are smaller and slower in heart failure, and they cause contractile dysfunction.[3,24,49]

T-Type Calcium Current (I_{CaT})

Structure and Physiology

The cardiac T-type Ca^{2+} channel (originally called low-voltage–activated channels) is composed of a single α subunit. $Ca_v3.1$ (α_{1G} subunit encoded by *CACNA1G*) and $Ca_v3.2$ (α_{1H} subunit encoded by *CACNA1H*) isoforms are major candidates for the cardiac T-type Ca^{2+} channel. It is not yet clear whether auxiliary subunits exist for native T-type Ca^{2+} channels. The structure of the α_{1H} and α_{1G} subunits is similar to that involved in the L-type Ca^{2+} channels.[46,48]

T-type Ca^{2+} channels can be distinguished from L-type Ca^{2+} channels on the basis of their distinctive gating and conductance properties. Compared with L-type Ca^{2+} channels, T-type Ca^{2+} channels have a smaller conductance and transient openings, and they open at the significantly more negative E_m that overlaps the pacemaker potentials of sinus node cells. The threshold for activation of I_{CaT} is −70 to −60 mV, and I_{CaT} is fully activated at −30 to −10 mV at physiological Ca^{2+} concentration. Membrane depolarization also causes inactivation of I_{CaT}. The inactivation threshold is near −90 mV, with half-maximal inactivation of −60 mV. In contrast to L-type Ca^{2+} channels, T-type Ca^{2+} channels do not inactivate in a Ca^{2+}-dependent manner. The activation and steady-state inactivation overlap near the activation threshold (−60 to −30 mV), thus providing a constant inward current (a window current). This window component may help in facilitating the slow diastolic depolarization in sinus node cells and contribute to automaticity. Unlike L-type channels, T-type Ca^{2+} channels are relatively insensitive to dihydropyridines.[46,48]

Function

Ca_v3 channels conduct the T-type Ca^{2+} current (I_{CaT}), which is important in a wide variety of physiological functions, including neuronal firing, hormone secretion, smooth muscle contraction, cell proliferation of some cardiac tissues, and myoblast fusion. In the heart, T-type channels are abundant in sinus node pacemaker cells and Purkinje fibers of many species and are important for maintenance of pacemaker activity by setting the frequency of action potential firing.[46,48]

T-type Ca^{2+} channels are functionally expressed in embryonic hearts, but they are almost undetectable or markedly reduced in postnatal ventricular myocytes, although some reports described substantial amplitude of I_{CaT}. In the adult heart, the largest I_{CaT} densities are seen in pacemaker cells located in the conduction system.

Because T-type Ca^{2+} channels are most prevalent in the conduction system in the adult heart and the activation range of I_{CaT} overlaps the pacemaker potential, it has been suggested that T-type Ca^{2+} channels play a role in generating pacemaker depolarization and contribute to automaticity. However, experimental evidence indicates that I_{CaT} is not a primary pacemaker current, but it can modify depolarization frequency only slightly. Although organic T-type Ca^{2+} channel blockers (mibefradil) result in marked decrease in firing frequency of sinus node cells in clinical studies, the possibility that these blockers affect other ionic currents, including I_{CaL}, cannot be entirely excluded. In fact, it is has not yet been determined whether I_{CaT} exists functionally in atrial, ventricular, and sinoatrial node cells in the human heart. Further studies are necessary to clarify whether T-type Ca^{2+} channels contribute to the automaticity of the human heart.[48,51]

Acquired Diseases

Interestingly, the T- type Ca^{2+} channels are re-expressed in atrial and ventricular myocytes in animal models under various pathological conditions such as cardiac hypertrophy, MI, and heart failure. These findings reflect a reversion to a fetal or neonatal pattern of gene expression, and I_{CaT} contributes to abnormal electrical activity and excitation-contraction coupling. It is possible that similar remodeling occurs in the hypertrophied human heart; however, to date, T-type Ca^{2+} channels have not been detected in normal or diseased human myocardial cells.[46,48,51]

Furthermore, experimental evidence suggests that T-type Ca^{2+} channels may be of functional importance in arrhythmogenesis in cardiomyocytes in pulmonary veins, which can initiate paroxysmal AF. I_{CaT} may directly and indirectly participate in pacemaker depolarization in sinoatrial and other regions of the heart, and this mechanism may become more important in failing hearts.[46,48]

Cardiac Pacemaker Current (I_f)

Structure and Physiology

Channels responsible for the pacemaker current (I_f; also called the funny current because it displays unusual gating properties) are named hyperpolarization-activated cyclic nucleotide-gated (HCN) channels. HCN channels are members of the voltage-gated cation channel superfamily and, based on sequence homology, are most closely related to the cyclic nucleotide-gated (CNG) channel and ether-a-go-go (EAG) K^+ channel families. Four α-subunit isoforms are described (HCN1 to HCN4, encoded by *HCN1* to *HCN4* genes), which are preferentially expressed in sinus and AVN myocytes and Purkinje fibers. HCN isoforms differ in the extent of voltage-dependent gating and sensitivity to cAMP, and they have different relative rates of activation and deactivation, with HCN1 the fastest, HCN4 the slowest, and HCN2 and HCN3 intermediate. HCN4 is the isoform primarily expressed in the sinus node, AVN, and ventricular conducting system, but low levels of HCN1 and HCN2 have also been reported.

It is likely that the HCN channel is formed by the coassembly of four either identical (homotetramers) or nonidentical (heterotetramers) α subunits that create an ion-conducting pore. Each α subunit comprises six transmembrane segments (S1 to S6), with a voltage sensor domain in the S4 segment and a pore-forming region between S5 and S6 carrying the GYG triplet signature of K^+-permeable channels. Their intracellular C-terminus contains cyclic nucleotide-binding domains, which enable direct cAMP binding. A potential auxiliary subunit of HCN channels is MiRP1 (encoded by *KCNE2*).

I_f is a mixed Na^+-K^+ current, with a threefold higher selectivity for Na^+ than for K^+. Despite the GYG amino acid motif, HCN channels are more permeable Na^+ than K^+ ions. Unlike most voltage-gated channels, which are activated on membrane depolarization, HCN channels are activated on hyperpolarization. The HCN channel activates slowly on hyperpolarization (at voltages lower than approximately –40 to –45 mV) and inactivate slowly in a voltage-independent manner on depolarization. The speed of channel opening is strongly dependent on E_m and is faster at more negative potentials. I_f conducts an inward current during phases 3 and 4 of the action potential and may underlie slow membrane depolarization in cells with pacemaker activity (i.e., cells with I_f and little or no I_{K1}).[52]

Function

I_f is a major player in both generation of spontaneous activity and rate control of cardiac pacemaker cells, and it is sometimes referred to as the pacemaker current.

The I_f channels are deactivated during the action potential upstroke and the initial plateau phase of repolarization, but they begin to activate at the end of the action potential as repolarization brings the E_m to levels more negative than approximately –40 to –50 mV, and they are fully activated at approximately −100 mV. Once activated, I_f depolarizes the membrane back toward a level at which the Ca^{2+} current activates to initiate the action potential.[1] In its range of activation, which quite properly comprises the voltage range of diastolic depolarization in sinus node cells (approximately –40 to –65 mV), the current is inward, and its reversal occurs at approximately −10 to −20 mV. At the end of the repolarization phase of an action potential, because I_f activation occurs in the background of a decaying outward (K^+ time-dependent) current, current flow quickly shifts from outward to inward, giving rise to a sudden reversal of voltage change (from repolarizing to depolarizing) at the maximum diastolic potential. Hence, I_f first opposes and then stops the repolarization process (at the maximum diastolic potential) and finally initiates the diastolic depolarization.[52-55]

The I_f contribution terminates when, in the late part of diastolic depolarization, Ca^{2+}-dependent processes take over, and the threshold for L-type Ca^{2+} current activation and action potential firing is reached. Although deactivation of I_f at depolarized voltages is rapid, complete switch off of the current occurs only during the very early fraction of the action potential, which provides a brief time interval during which I_f carries an outward current at positive voltages.[52]

I_f is not only involved in principal rhythm generation but also plays a key role in heart rate regulation. The degree of activation of I_f determines, at the end of an action potential, the steepness of phase 4 depolarization and hence the frequency of action potential firing. Additionally, I_f represents a basic physiological mechanism mediating autonomic regulation of heart rate. I_f is regulated by intracellular cAMP and is thus activated and inhibited by β-adrenergic and muscarinic M_2 receptor stimulation, respectively.[52,56]

However, given the complexity of the cellular processes involved in rhythmic activity, exact quantification of the extent to which I_f and other mechanisms contribute to pacemaking is still a debated issue.[52]

Regulation

The voltage dependence of I_f activation is regulated by cAMP direct binding to the cyclic nucleotide-binding domain in the HCN channel and not via phosphorylation-dependent activation mechanisms. Direct interaction of cAMP to the channel shifts the activation curve to more depolarized voltages and strongly accelerates channel activation kinetics. Sympathetic stimulation activates I_f and hence accelerates heart rate via β-adrenoceptor-triggered cAMP production, whereas low-level vagal stimulation lowers heart rate via inhibition of cAMP synthesis and an ensuing inhibition of I_f activity. High vagal tone most likely lowers the heart rate mainly via the activation of I_{KACh}.[56]

HCN channels are inhibited by increased intracellular acidity (e.g., during myocardial ischemia). Protons shift the activation of I_f to more hyperpolarized potentials and slow pacemaker activity.

Pharmacology

Given the key role of HCN channels in cardiac pacemaking, I_f has become a pharmacological target for the development of novel and more specific heart rate–reducing agents in patients with ischemic heart disease. Whereas current heart rate–lowering drugs adversely affect cardiac contractility, selective I_f inhibition is believed to lower heart rate without impairing contractility. In the past, several agents inhibiting cardiac I_f were developed. Early drugs identified as pure bradycardic agents include zatebradine and cilobradine, which are derived from the L-type Ca^{2+} channel blocker verapamil. More recently, ivabradine was introduced into clinical use as the first therapeutic I_f blocker for the treatment of chronic stable angina. The principal action of all these substances is to reduce the frequency of pacemaker potentials in the sinus node by inducing a reduction of the diastolic depolarization slope. Ivabradine blocks HCN4 and HCN1 channels by accessing the channels from their intracellular side and by exerting a use- and current-dependent block. Interestingly, ivabradine acts as open channel blocker in HCN4 (as in sinus nodal I_f), whereas block of HCN1 requires channels either to be closed or in a transitional state between an open and closed configuration.[52,56] With the exception of ivabradine, other HCN channel blockers are not specific enough for sinus nodal (mainly HCN4-mediated) I_f; they also block neuronal HCN channels (I_h current) in several regions of the nervous system, and this has prevented their clinical utility.[56]

Clonidine, an α_2-adrenergic agonist, was shown to block sinus nodal I_f. Clonidine produces a shift in the voltage dependence of the channel by 10 to 20 mV to more hyperpolarizing potentials.[56]

Inherited Channelopathies

Heterozygous *HCN4* mutations have been identified in individuals with sinus bradycardia and chronotropic incompetence. Severe bradycardia, QT prolongation, and torsades de pointes have been described in another family. HCN mutations slow channel activation kinetics or, when located in cyclic nucleotide-binding domains, abolish sensitivity of HCN channels to cAMP, thus reducing I_f and the speed of diastolic depolarization.

Acquired Diseases

HCN2/HCN4 expression is upregulated in the atria of patients with AF and in ventricular tissues in cardiac hypertrophy and congestive heart failure. This response may contribute to the arrhythmias observed in these disease states. Enhancement of I_f in these pathological conditions can potentially initiate arrhythmia by triggering spontaneous excitation of nonpacemaker cardiomyocytes.

Sarcoplasmic Reticulum Calcium Release Channels (Ryanodine Receptor 2)

Structure and Physiology

The Ca^{2+} release channel is a macromolecular complex, formed by the cardiac ryanodine receptor isoform (RyR2, encoded by the *RYR2* gene) homotetramer and certain proteins localized on both the cytosolic and the luminal side of the sarcoplasmic reticulum membrane. The cardiac RyR2, by far the largest protein of the complex, operates as a Ca^{2+}-conducting channel. RyR2 channels are approximately 10 times larger than voltage-gated Ca^{2+} and Na^+ channels.[57,58]

Each RyR2 monomer contains a transmembrane domain, the pore-forming region that is composed of an even, but still undetermined number (likely six to eight) of transmembrane segments. This domain encompasses only approximately 10% of the protein clustered at the C-terminus, but it has a critical functional role because it contains sequences that control RyR2 localization and oligomerization and is sufficient to form a functional Ca^{2+} release channel. The remaining 90% of the protein at the N-terminus comprises an enormous cytoplasmic domain that serves as a cytosolic scaffold that interacts with regulatory molecules (including Ca^{2+}, ATP) and proteins (including FKBP12.6, calmodulin). On the luminal (sarcoplasmic reticulum) side, RyR2 forms a part of a large quaternary complex with calsequestrin (CASQ2), triadin, and junctin. Together these four proteins form the core of the Ca^{2+} release channel complex.[57-60]

Cardiac RyR2 functions as a ligand-activated ion channel that activates (opens) on Ca^{2+} binding. However, the exact structural determinants of RyR gating are as yet unknown. RyR2 is normally closed at low cytosolic diastolic Ca^{2+} concentrations (approximately 100 to 200 nM). At submicromolar cytosolic Ca^{2+} concentrations, Ca^{2+} binds to high-affinity binding sites on RyR2 and thus increases the open probability of the channel (two Ca^{2+} ions are required to open the RyR2 channel) and allows Ca^{2+} release from the sarcoplasmic reticulum into the cytosol.[50,59,60]

The precise juxtaposition of the sarcolemmal specialized invaginations (known as T tubules) and sarcoplasmic reticulum forms specific junctional microdomains, creating a 10- to 12-nM gap, known as the dyadic cleft. RyR2s are assembled in a paracrystalline lattice in each dyad, containing 80 to 260 channels, where the RyR2 cytoplasmic region resides, and its transmembrane region spans the sarcoplasmic reticulum membrane to immerse the luminal portion into the sarcoplasmic reticulum Ca^{2+} store. Each array of RyR2s is faced by 10 to 25 L-type Ca^{2+} channels in the sarcolemmal T tubule. Hence, each dyad constitutes a local Ca^{2+} signaling complex, or couplon, whereby these proteins are coordinately regulated via the changing concentrations of Ca^{2+}, Na^+, and K^+ within the dyadic cleft.[50,59,60]

After approximately 10 milliseconds of RyR2 channel opening, Ca^{2+} release from the sarcoplasmic reticulum terminates, and the Ca^{2+} spark signal starts to decay, mostly owing to diffusion of Ca^{2+} away from its source. RyR2 channel activity is maximal at cytosolic Ca^{2+} concentrations of approximately 10 μM. Elevating cytosolic Ca^{2+} concentrations beyond this point leads to a reduction in the open probability of the channel, possibly because of Ca^{2+} binding to low-affinity inhibitory binding sites on the RyR2 channel.[60]

Inactivation of Ca^{2+} release is not well understood. It is likely mediated by Ca^{2+}-induced inactivation of RyR2, thus extinguishing of CICR by stochastic attrition, or by Ca^{2+} depletion of the sarcoplasmic reticulum, or both.

RyR2 open probability increases by elevation of sarcoplasmic reticulum Ca^{2+} concentration. When levels of Ca^{2+} in the sarcoplasmic reticulum reach a critical threshold, spontaneous Ca^{2+} release (spillover) can occur even in the presence of normal channels (store overload–induced Ca^{2+} release [SOICR]). Ca^{2+} concentration in the sarcoplasmic reticulum is physiologically increased as an effect of adrenergic (sympathetic) stimulation.

Function

The RyR2 channels are an essential component of the excitation-contraction coupling and act as sentinels to the large sarcoplasmic reticulum Ca^{2+} store. Excitation-contraction coupling describes the physiological process of converting an electrical stimulus (action potential) to a mechanical response (muscle contraction). The contraction of a cardiac myocyte is governed primarily by intracellular Ca^{2+} concentration (see Fig. 1-3). Ca^{2+} enters the cell during the plateau phase of the action potential through L-type Ca^{2+} channels that line the sarcolemmal T tubules. However, the rise in intracellular Ca^{2+} is small and not sufficient to induce contraction. Nonetheless, the small amount of Ca^{2+} entering the cell via I_{CaL} triggers a rapid mobilization of Ca^{2+} from the sarcoplasmic reticulum into the cytosol by opening the RyR2 channels in the CICR process. Approximately 75% of Ca^{2+} present in the cytoplasm during contraction is released from the sarcoplasmic reticulum. The close proximity of the RyR2 to the T tubule enables each L-type Ca^{2+} channel to activate 4 to 6 RyR2s and generate a Ca^{2+} spark. Ca^{2+} influx via I_{CaL} simultaneously activates approximately 10,000 to 20,000 couplons in each ventricular myocyte with every action potential. Such sophisticated coordination in opening and closing is required to ensure that Ca^{2+} release occurs during the systolic phase of the cardiac cycle and functional silence during diastole.[50,59,60]

Luminal Ca^{2+}-dependent deactivation of RyR2 is a process by which the decline in sarcoplasmic reticulum Ca^{2+} that follows sarcoplasmic reticulum Ca^{2+} release renders RyR2s functionally inactive. This results in termination of CICR and induction of a refractory state that suppresses Ca^{2+} release during the diastolic phase, which is an important determinant of the mechanical refractoriness required for efficient relaxation and refilling of the heart.[50,58]

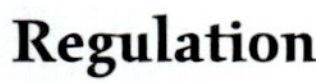

Regulation

Many proteins interact directly and indirectly with the N-terminal cytoplasmic domain of RyR2 including FK506-binding protein (calstabin2 or FKBP12.6), PKA, Ca^{2+}-calmodulin-dependent kinase II (CaMKII), phosphodiesterase 4D3, calmodulin, protein phosphatases 1 and 2A, and sorcin. CASQ2, junctin, and triadin bind with the luminal (sarcoplasmic reticulum) C-terminus of RyR2.[58-60]

CALSEQUESTRIN

CASQ2 is a low-affinity, high-capacity Ca^{2+}-binding protein, which serves as a Ca^{2+} storage reservoir that is able to bind luminal Ca^{2+} (40 to 50 Ca^{2+} ions per molecule) during diastole, thus buffering Ca^{2+} within the sarcoplasmic reticulum (i.e., preventing Ca^{2+} precipitation and lowering luminal free Ca^{2+} concentration) and preventing diastolic Ca^{2+} release via RyR2 to cytosol. CASQ2 presumably serves as a luminal Ca^{2+} sensor that modulates the responsiveness of the RyR2 to luminal Ca^{2+}. At low luminal Ca^{2+} concentrations, CASQ2 interacts with RyR2 via binding to triadin and junctin and inhibits the activity of the RyR2. When sarcoplasmic reticulum Ca^{2+} levels increase, Ca^{2+} binds to CASQ2, resulting in weakened interactions or complete dissociation of CASQ2 from triadin. This process relieves the inhibitory action of CASQ2 on the RyR2 complex, allows Ca^{2+} release to the cytosol, and hence normalizes sarcoplasmic reticulum Ca^{2+} load. Triadin and junctin not only mediate functional interactions of CASQ2 and RyR2 but also modulate RyR2 function by themselves by increasing the activity of the RyR2 channel. This Ca^{2+}-dependent modulation of RyR2s by triadin, junctin, and CASQ2 may contribute to deactivation and refractoriness of RyR2 channels after sarcoplasmic reticulum Ca^{2+} release.[58,60,61]

FK506-BINDING PROTEIN

FKBP12.6 (the 12.6-kDa cytosolic FK506-binding protein), also known as calstabin2 (Ca^{2+} channel-stabilizing binding protein), stabilizes the closed conformational state of the RyR2 channel, thus enabling the channel to close completely during diastole (at low intracellular Ca^{2+} concentrations), preventing aberrant Ca^{2+} leakage from the sarcoplasmic reticulum, and ensuring muscle relaxation. PKA phosphorylation of RyR2 decreases the binding affinity of FKBP12.6 to RyR2 and thereby increases the probability of an open state and amplifies the response to Ca^{2+}-dependent activation.[50,59,60,62]

CALMODULIN

Calmodulin is a Ca^{2+}-binding protein containing four Ca^{2+}-binding sites and four sites that bind to RyR2 monomers. Calmodulin preferentially inhibits RyR2 at Ca^{2+} concentrations lower than 10 μM by binding to a region on RyR2. Calmodulin may function to assist closing RyR2 following sarcoplasmic reticulum Ca^{2+} release in excitation-contraction coupling.[60]

PROTEIN KINASE A

Stimulation of β-adrenergic receptors results in an increase in cAMP and consequent PKA activation. PKA interacts with the RyR2 channel via binding to the muscle A kinase anchoring protein (mAKAP). PKA phosphorylation of RyR2 activates the channel, at least in part by increasing the sensitivity of RyR2 to cytosolic Ca^{2+} and a transient decrease in the binding affinity of calstabin2. This allows for increased sarcoplasmic reticulum Ca^{2+} release on Ca^{2+} influx via I_{CaL} as a part of the fight-or-flight mechanism. By contrast, chronic PKA hyperphosphorylation of RyR2 can result in incomplete channel closure and a Ca^{2+} leak during diastole, which causes depletion of the sarcoplasmic reticulum Ca^{2+} store and reduced Ca^{2+} release on receptor activation.[50,60,62]

CA^{2+}-CALMODULIN-DEPENDENT PROTEIN KINASE II

CaMKII is a dodecameric holoenzyme activated by Ca^{2+}-bound calmodulin, possibly at high cellular Ca^{2+} loads. CaMKII phosphorylation increases RyR2 channel open probability, but to a smaller extent than PKA phosphorylation. CaMKII activity increases at faster heart rates (typically mediated by β-adrenergic stimulation and PKA activation and associated with increased cytosolic Ca^{2+}) and phosphorylates RyR2 to enhance sarcoplasmic reticulum Ca^{2+} release, which helps maintain the positive force-frequency relationship (i.e., cardiac contractility increases as a function of heart rate). Increased CaMKII activity also phosphorylates phospholamban to help accelerate diastolic filling of the ventricles at higher heart rates. Physiologically, sympathetic activation stimulates both PKA and CaMKII, which thus function synergistically. CaMKII is typically considered to be downstream of PKA and elevated Ca^{2+} transients.[50,60,62]

Pharmacology

RyR2s are targets of multiple experimental drugs. However, thus far, no compounds in clinical use are known to target RyR2 directly.

The plant alkaloid ryanodine binds the RyR2 channel with high affinity in a Ca^{2+}-dependent and use-dependent fashion, thus making it an important tool for biochemical characterization of the channel. Two ryanodine-binding sites, a high-affinity site and a low-affinity one, have been described at the C-terminus of RyR2. At the high-affinity site, ryanodine induces long-lasting channel openings at a subconductance state, whereas high concentrations block the channel.

Caffeine, in high concentrations (5 to 20 mM), increases the RyR2 sensitivity to Ca^{2+} and ATP and results in increased RyR2 mean open time and open probability. Caffeine is used experimentally to measure sarcoplasmic reticulum Ca^{2+} content indirectly because its application causes emptying of the sarcoplasmic reticulum Ca^{2+} store.

JTV-519, also known as K201, is a benzothiazepine derivative (an analogue of diltiazem) and an L-type Ca^{2+} channel blocker and stabilizer. JTV-519 can increase the binding affinity of calstabin2 for RyR2, thus stabilizing the closed conformational state of the RyR2 channel and hence preventing diastolic sarcoplasmic reticulum Ca^{2+} leak. JTV-519 can potentially offer an antiarrhythmic benefit in a variety of pathological conditions that lead to destabilization of the RyR2 channel's closed state, such as RyR2 mutations, hyperphosphorylation of the RyR2 during heart failure, and sarcoplasmic reticulum Ca^{2+} overload.

Among class I antiarrhythmic drugs, only flecainide and propafenone were found to inhibit RyR2 channels (by inducing brief closures of open RyR2 to subconductance states), suppress arrhythmogenic Ca^{2+} sparks, and prevent CPVT in experimental studies. The potency of RyR2 channel inhibition rather than Na^{+} channel blockade appears to determine the efficacy of class I agents for the prevention of CPVT. Flecainide has been demonstrated to prevent lethal ventricular arrhythmias in patients with familial CPVT.[63,64]

Several toxins (e.g., the scorpion toxins imperatoxin A and imperatoxin I), some anticancer drugs (e.g., doxorubicin), and some immunosuppressants (e.g., rapamycin) can potentially cause cardiac adverse events likely related to effects on the gating kinetics of RyR2 channels.

Inherited Channelopathies

CPVT is caused by mutations in genes that encode for key Ca^{2+} regulatory proteins. Two genetic variants of CPVT have been described: an autosomal-dominant trait (CPVT1; most common) caused by mutations in the cardiac RyR2 gene, and a recessive form (CPVT2; rare) associated with homozygous mutations in the CASQ2 gene *(CASQ2)*.

Approximately 50% to 70% of patients with CPVT harbor RyR2 mutations. More than 70 RyR2 mutations linked to CPVT have been identified. CPVT mutant RyR2 typically shows gain-of-function defects following channel activation by PKA phosphorylation (in response to β-adrenergic stimulation or caffeine), resulting in uncontrolled Ca^{2+} release from the sarcoplasmic reticulum during electrical diastole. The exaggerated spontaneous Ca^{2+} release from the sarcoplasmic reticulum facilitates the development of DADs and triggered arrhythmias.[58,59]

The molecular mechanisms by which RyR2 mutations alter the physiological properties and function of RyR2 are not completely defined. It has been suggested that CPVT mutations in RyR2 reduce the binding affinity of RyR2 for the regulatory protein FKBP12.6 (calstabin2) that stabilizes the closed conformational state of the RyR2 channel, thus enabling the channel to close completely during diastole (at low intracellular Ca^{2+} concentrations), preventing aberrant Ca^{2+} leakage from the sarcoplasmic reticulum, and ensuring muscle relaxation. PKA phosphorylation (induced by β-adrenergic stimulation) of the mutant channels results in further worsening of the binding affinity of FKBP12.6 to the mutant RyR2 and increases the probability of an open state at diastolic Ca^{2+} concentrations. As a consequence, the mutant RyR2 channel fails to close completely during diastole, with a resulting diastolic Ca^{2+} leak from the sarcoplasmic reticulum during stress or exercise.[58-60]

An alternative hypothesis is that CPVT mutations in RyR2 sensitize the channel to luminal (sarcoplasmic reticulum) Ca^{2+} such that under baseline conditions, when sarcoplasmic reticulum load is normal, there is no Ca^{2+} leak. Under β-adrenergic (sympathetic) stimulation, sarcoplasmic reticulum Ca^{2+} concentration becomes elevated above the reduced threshold, causing Ca^{2+} to leak out of the sarcoplasmic reticulum. A third hypothesis for RyR2-related CPVT is that mutations in RyR2 impair the intermolecular interactions between discrete RyR2 domains necessary for proper folding of the channel and self-regulation of channel gating.[58,60]

So far, seven *CASQ2* mutations linked to CPVT have been reported. Although some of these mutations are thought to compromise CASQ2 synthesis and result in reduced expression or complete absence of CASQ2 in the heart, other mutations seem to cause expression of defective CASQ2 proteins with abnormal regulation of cellular Ca^{2+} homeostasis. *CASQ2* mutations result in disruption of the control of RyR2s by luminal Ca^{2+} required for effective termination of sarcoplasmic reticulum Ca^{2+} release and prevention of spontaneous Ca^{2+} release during diastole, thus leading to diminished Ca^{2+} signaling refractoriness and generation of arrhythmogenic spontaneous Ca^{2+} releases.[58,59,65]

Importantly, in the setting of digitalis poisoning, the abnormal RyR2 behavior leading to spontaneous Ca^{2+} release and DADs is secondary to the elevation of the sarcoplasmic reticulum Ca^{2+} content (SOICR). In CPVT, on the other hand, spontaneous Ca^{2+} release and DADs can occur without Ca^{2+} overload. Mutations in RyR2 or CASQ2 lead to defective Ca^{2+} signaling lowering of the sarcoplasmic reticulum Ca^{2+} threshold for spontaneous Ca^{2+} release to less than the normal baseline level (perceived Ca^{2+} overload).[58]

Missense mutations in RyR2 also been linked to a form of arrhythmogenic cardiomyopathy (ARVD-2) characterized by exercise-induced polymorphic VT that does not appear to have a reentrant mechanism and occurs in the absence of significant structural abnormalities. Patients do not develop characteristic features of ARVD on the 12-lead ECG or signal-averaged ECG, and global RV function remains unaffected. ARVD-2 shows a closer resemblance to familial CPVT in both etiology and phenotype; its inclusion under the umbrella term of ARVD remains controversial.[66-68]

Acquired Diseases

RyR2 dysfunction is a key factor leading to arrhythmias in heart failure. Chronic β-adrenergic stimulation results in PKA hyperphosphorylation of RyR2. This process causes the dissociation of the channel-stabilizing protein calstabin and leads to diastolic Ca^{2+} leak from the sarcoplasmic reticulum and the generation of spontaneous Ca^{2+} waves, which can be maintained despite a reduced Ca^{2+} gradient, thus underlying DAD-induced triggered arrhythmias in heart failure.[24,69,70]

Cardiac Gap Junctions

Structure and Physiology

Cardiomyocytes make contact with each other via multiple intercalated discs, which mediate the transmission of force, electrical continuity, and chemical communication between adjacent cells. Three types of specialized junctions exist in the intercalated disc: (1) the fascia adherens, (2) the macula adherens (desmosome), and (3) the gap junction (nexus). The fascia adherens is an anchoring site for myofibrils, facilitating the transmission of mechanical energy between neighboring cells. The desmosomes link to the cytoskeleton of adjacent cells to provide strong localized adhesion sites that resist shearing forces generated during contraction. Gap junctions are assemblies of intercellular channels that provide electrical continuity and chemical communication between adjacent cells.[71]

In addition to the end-to-end and side-to-side gap junctions localized at the intercalated discs, lateral (side-to-side) gap junctions can exist in nondisc lateral membranes of cardiomyocytes, but they are much less common, occurring more in atrial than ventricular myocardium.[71]

Each gap junction channel is constructed of two hemichannels (connexons) aligned head-to-head in mirror symmetry across a narrow extracellular gap, one provided by each of the adjoining cells. Each connexon is composed of six integral membrane proteins called connexins (Cx) hexagonally arranged around the pore. Each connexin consists of four membrane-spanning domains (M1 to M4), two extracellular loops (E1, E2), one intracellular loop, and cytoplasmic N- and C-termini. The extracellular loops mediate the docking of the two hemichannels.[71,72]

Up to 24 different connexin types have been identified. They are named after their theoretical molecular weight in daltons. In the heart, Cx40, Cx43, and Cx45 are most important for action potential propagation. Although each connexin exhibits a distinct tissue distribution, most cardiomyocytes express more than one connexin isoform. Cx43 is by far the most abundant and is expressed between atrial and ventricular myocytes and distal parts of the Purkinje system. Cx40 is mainly expressed in the atrial myocytes, AVN, and HPS. Cx45 appears to be primarily expressed in nodal tissue (the sinus and compact AVNs), and more weakly in the atrium, His bundle, bundle branches, and Purkinje fibers.[71]

Connexons can be composed by the oligomerization of a single connexin type (homomeric) or of different types (heteromeric). In addition, the gap junction channel as a whole may be formed of two matching hemichannels (homotypic) or nonmatching hemichannels (heterotypic).[71]

Cardiac connexins exhibit distinctive biophysical properties; hence, the connexin composition of a gap junction channel determines its unitary conductance, voltage sensitivity, and ion selectivity. Cx40 gap junctions express the largest conductance, and Cx45 expresses the smallest. Both Cx40 and Cx45 are highly cation selective, and their conductance is voltage dependent. Cx43 has an intermediate conductance and is nonselective.

The individual gap junction channels allow exchange of nutrients, metabolites, ions (e.g., Na^+, Cl^-, K^+, Ca^{2+}) and small molecules (e.g., cAMP, cGMP, inositol triphosphate [IP_3]) with molecular weights up to approximately 1000 Da.[71]

Function

Gap junctions maintain direct cell-to-cell communication in the heart by providing biochemical and low-resistance electrical coupling between adjacent cardiomyocytes. Thus, gap junctions are responsible for myocardial electrical current flow propagation from one cardiac cell to another and are crucial in myocardial synchronization and heart function. Gap junctions also provide biochemical coupling, which allows intercellular movement of second-messenger substances (e.g., ATP, cyclic nucleotides, and IP_3) and hence enables coordinated responses of the myocardial syncytium to physiological stimuli.

The role of gap junction channels in action potential propagation and conduction velocity in cardiac tissue depends primarily on static factors of the channels (e.g., the number of channels, channel conductance, and voltage sensitivity) and dynamic factors (e.g., channel gating kinetics), as well as on properties of the propagated action potential, structural aspects of the cell geometry, and tissue architecture. Tissue-specific connexin expression and gap junction spatial distribution, as well as the variation in the structural composition of gap junction channels, allow for a greater versatility of gap junction physiological features and for disparate conduction properties in cardiac tissue. The myocytes of the sinus and AVNs are equipped with small, sparse, dispersed gap junctions containing Cx45, a connexin that forms low conductance channels; this feature underlies the relatively poor intercellular coupling in nodal tissues, a property that is linked to slowing of conduction. In contrast, ventricular muscle expresses predominantly Cx43 and Cx45, which have larger conductance. Atrial muscle and Purkinje fibers express all three cardiac connexins.

Under physiological conditions, a given cardiomyocyte in the adult working myocardium is electrically coupled to an average of approximately 11 adjacent cells, with gap junctions predominantly localized at the intercalated discs at the ends of the rod-shaped cells. Lateral (side-to-side) gap junctions in nondisc lateral membranes of cardiomyocytes are much less abundant and occur more often in atrial than ventricular tissues.[71] Thus, intercellular current flow occurs primarily at the cell termini, although propagation can occur both longitudinally and transversely. This particular subcellular distribution of gap junctions underlies uniform anisotropic impulse propagation throughout the myocardium, whereby conduction in the direction parallel to the long axis of the myocardial fiber bundles is approximately 3 to 5 times more rapid than that in the transverse direction. This property is attributable principally to the lower resistivity of myocardium provided by the gap junctions in the longitudinal versus the transverse direction.[73-75]

Regulation

Gap junction channels have a voltage-dependent gating mechanism, depending primarily on transjunctional voltage (i.e., the potential difference between the cytoplasm of the two adjacent cells). At rest, when the junctional voltage is zero, the channels usually are open. During the course of a propagated action potential, the channels tend to close in a voltage- and time-dependent manner. Gap junction channel gating can also be altered by specific changes in intracellular ions and by post-translational modifications ("loop" gating). Cytosolic Na^+ and Ca^{2+} overload, acidosis, and reduced ATP levels decrease gap junction channel function. Unlike the voltage gate, which closes rapidly and incompletely, the chemical gate closes slowly and completely.[76]

The regulation of gap junction trafficking, assembly and disassembly, and degradation is likely to be critical in the control of intercellular communication. Phosphorylation also appears to play a key role in channel gating that determines channel conductance and has been implicated in the regulation of the connexin "life cycle" at several stages. Gap junction coupling also is regulated by certain endogenous mediators (e.g., acetylcholine, norepinephrine, and angiotensin), likely via phosphorylation-mediated mechanisms. Importantly, channels composed of different connexins possess different properties and are susceptible to different regulation.[71,76]

Pharmacology

Several agents have been found to decrease gap junction channel coupling, including long-chain alcohols (e.g., heptanol, octanol), fatty acids (myristoleic acid, decanoic acid, palmitoleic acid), general anesthetics (e.g., halothane, isoflurane), carbachol (an acetylcholine analogue), α-adrenergic agonists (phenylephrine), angiotensin, insulin, insulin-like growth factor, and the nonsteroidal agents fenamates (e.g., flufenamic acid, meclofenamic acid). The mechanism of action of those agents remain largely unknown.

Antimalarial drugs, particularly quinine and quinine derivatives such as mefloquine, can reduce gap junction channel conductance, and their effects seem to be connexin subtype specific. In addition, it has been suggested that the cardiac glycosides strophanthidin, ouabain, and digitoxin decrease intercellular coupling.[76]

Experimental evidence suggests that increasing gap junction conductance can potentially confer an antiarrhythmic effect. Some compounds, including antiarrhythmic peptides and their derivatives (e.g., AAP10, ZP123, rotigaptide) can upregulate Cx43 via modulation either synthesis or degradation and enhance gap junctional communication and were found to reduce conduction slowing and prevent AF and ischemic reentrant VT in various cell and animal models. These peptides presumably act by modulating Cx43 phosphorylation.[77,78]

Acquired Diseases

Modification of cell-to-cell coupling occurs in numerous pathophysiological settings (e.g., myocardial ischemia, ventricular hypertrophy, cardiomyopathy) as a consequence of acute changes in the average conductance of gap junctions secondary to ischemia, hypoxia, acidification, or an increase in intracellular $Ca2^+$, or it can be produced by changes in expression or cellular distribution patterns of gap junctions.[74,79-81]

Remodeling includes a decrease in the number of gap junction channels resulting from the interruption of communication between cells by fibrosis and downregulation of Cx43 formation or of trafficking to the intercalated disc. Additionally, gap junctions can become more prominent along lateral membranes of myocytes (so-called structural remodeling). Influences of Cx43 lateralization on impulse propagation have not yet been well defined.[82]

Alterations in distribution and function of cardiac gap junctions are associated with conduction delay or block. Inactivation of gap junctions decreases transverse conduction velocity to a greater degree than longitudinal conduction, thus resulting in exaggeration of anisotropy and providing a substrate for reentrant activity and increased susceptibility to arrhythmias.[74]

AF is associated with abnormal expression and distribution of atrial Cx40, which can potentially lead to inhomogeneous electrical coupling and abnormal impulse formation and conduction and thereby provide the substrate for atrial arrhythmias. Furthermore, a rare single nucleotide polymorphism in the atrial-specific Cx40 gene has been found to increase the risk of idiopathic AF.[83]

Importantly, there is a high redundancy in connexin expression in the heart with regard to conduction of electrical impulse. It has been shown that a 50% reduction in Cx43 does not alter ventricular impulse conduction. Cx43 expression must decrease by 90% to affect conduction, but even then conduction velocity is reduced only by 20%.

REFERENCES

1. Grant AO: Cardiac ion channels, *Circ Arrhythm Electrophysiol* 2:185–194, 2009.
2. Amin AS, Asghari-Roodsari A, Tan HL: Cardiac sodium channelopathies, *Pflugers Arch* 460:223–237, 2010.
3. Amin AS, Tan HL, Wilde AA: Cardiac ion channels in health and disease, *Heart Rhythm* 7:117–126, 2010.
4. Viswanathan PC, Balser JR: Biophysics of normal and abnormal cardiac sodium channel function. In Zipes DP, Jalife J, editors: *Cardiac electrophysiology: from cell to bedside*, ed 5, Philadelphia, 2009, Saunders, pp 93–104.
5. Abriel H: Cardiac sodium channel Na(v)1.5 and interacting proteins: physiology and pathophysiology, *J Mol Cell Cardiol* 48:2–11, 2010.

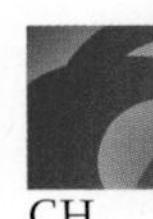

6. January CT, Makielski JC: Pharmacology of the cardiac sodium channel. In Zipes DP, Jalife J, editors: *Cardiac electrophysiology: from cell to bedside*, ed 5, Philadelphia, 2009, Saunders, pp 169–174.
7. Moss AJ, Goldenberg I: Importance of knowing the genotype and the specific mutation when managing patients with long QT syndrome, *Circ Arrhythm Electrophysiol* 1:213–226, 2008.
8. Saenen JB, Vrints CJ: Molecular aspects of the congenital and acquired long QT syndrome: clinical implications, *J Mol Cell Cardiol* 44:633–646, 2008.
9. Lu JT, Kass RS: Recent progress in congenital long QT syndrome, *Curr Opin Cardiol* 25(3):216–221, May 2010.
10. Campuzano O, Brugada R, Iglesias A: Genetics of Brugada syndrome, *Curr Opin Cardiol* 25(3):210–215, May 2010.
11. Gehi AK, Duong TD, Metz LD, et al: Risk stratification of individuals with the Brugada electrocardiogram: a meta-analysis, *J Cardiovasc Electrophysiol* 17:577–583, 2006.
12. Antzelevitch C, Brugada P, Borggrefe M, et al: Brugada syndrome: report of the second consensus conference: endorsed by the Heart Rhythm Society and the European Heart Rhythm Association, *Circulation* 111:659–670, 2005.
13. Morita H, Zipes DP, Wu J: Brugada syndrome: insights of ST elevation, arrhythmogenicity, and risk stratification from experimental observations, *Heart Rhythm* 6(Suppl):S34–S43, 2009.
14. Lei M, Huang CL, Zhang Y: Genetic Na+ channelopathies and sinus node dysfunction, *Prog Biophys Mol Biol* 98:171–178, 2008.
15. Katz AM: Cardiac ion channels. In Katz AM, editor: *Physiology of the heart*, ed 5, Philadelphia, 2011, Lippincott Williams & Wilkins, pp 3433–3468.
16. Tamargo J, Caballero R, Gomez R, et al: Pharmacology of cardiac potassium channels, *Cardiovasc Res* 62:9–33, 2004.
17. Oudit GY, Backx PH: Voltage-regulated potassium channels. In Zipes DP, Jalife J, editors: *Cardiac electrophysiology: from cell to bedside*, ed 5, Philadelphia, 2009, Saunders, pp 29–42.
18. Niwa N, Nerbonne JM: Molecular determinants of cardiac transient outward potassium current (I(to)) expression and regulation, *J Mol Cell Cardiol* 48:12–25, 2010.
19. Antzelevitch C, Yan GX: J wave syndromes, *Heart Rhythm* 7:549–558, 2010.
20. van der Heyden MA, Wijnhoven TJ, Opthof T: Molecular aspects of adrenergic modulation of the transient outward current, *Cardiovasc Res* 71:430–442, 2006.
21. Alders M, Koopmann TT, Christiaans I, et al: Haplotype-sharing analysis implicates chromosome 7q36 harboring DPP6 in familial idiopathic ventricular fibrillation, *Am J Hum Genet* 84:468–476, 2009.
22. Benito B, Guasch E, Rivard L, Nattel S: Clinical and mechanistic issues in early repolarization of normal variants and lethal arrhythmia syndromes, *J Am Coll Cardiol* 56:1177–1186, 2010.
23. Tikkanen JT, Anttonen O, Junttila MJ, et al: Long-term outcome associated with early repolarization on electrocardiography, *N Engl J Med* 361:2529–2537, 2009.
24. Aiba T, Tomaselli GF: Electrical remodeling in the failing heart, *Curr Opin Cardiol* 25:29–36, 2010.
25. Ravens U, Wettwer E: Ultra-rapid delayed rectifier channels: molecular basis and therapeutic implications, *Cardiovasc Res* 89:776–785, 2011.
26. Ehrlich JR: Inward rectifier potassium currents as a target for atrial fibrillation therapy, *J Cardiovasc Pharmacol* 52:129–135, 2008.
27. Charpentier F, Merot J, Loussouarn G, Baro I: Delayed rectifier K(+) currents and cardiac repolarization, *J Mol Cell Cardiol* 48:37–44, 2010.
28. Tristani-Firouzi M, Sanguinetti MC: Structural determinants and biophysical properties of HERG and KCNQ1 channel gating, *J Mol Cell Cardiol* 35:27–35, 2003.
29. Smyth JW, Shaw RM: Forward trafficking of ion channels: what the clinician needs to know, *Heart Rhythm* 7:1135–1140, 2010.
30. Ruan Y, Liu N, Napolitano C, Priori SG: Therapeutic strategies for long QT syndrome: does the molecular substrate matter? *Circ Arrhythm Electrophysiol* 1:290–297, 2008.
31. Roden DM: Clinical practice: long QT syndrome, *N Engl J Med* 358:169–176, 2008.
32. Schwartz PJ, Spazzolini C, Crotti L, et al: The Jervell and Lange-Nielsen syndrome: natural history, molecular basis, and clinical outcome, *Circulation* 113:783–790, 2006.
33. Sy RW, Chattha IS, Klein GJ, et al: Repolarization dynamics during exercise discriminate between LQT1 and LQT2 genotypes, *J Cardiovasc Electrophysiol* 21:1242–1246, 2010.
34. Anumonwo JM, Lopatin AN: Cardiac strong inward rectifier potassium channels, *J Mol Cell Cardiol* 48:45–54, 2010.
35. Lu CW, Lin JH, Rajawat YS, et al: Functional and clinical characterization of a mutation in KCNJ2 associated with Andersen-Tawil syndrome, *J Med Genet* 43:653–659, 2006.
36. Tsuboi M, Antzelevitch C: Cellular basis for electrocardiographic and arrhythmic manifestations of Andersen-Tawil syndrome (LQT7), *Heart Rhythm* 3:328–335, 2006.
37. Schimpf R, Borggrefe M, Wolpert C: Clinical and molecular genetics of the short QT syndrome, *Curr Opin Cardiol* 23:192–198, 2008.
38. Callans DJ: Patients with hemodynamically tolerated ventricular tachycardia require implantable cardioverter defibrillators, *Circulation* 116:1196–1203, 2007.
39. Yang Y, Yang Y, Liang B, et al: Identification of a Kir3.4 mutation in congenital long QT syndrome, *Am J Hum Genet* 86:872–880, 2010.
40. Ravens U, Cerbai E: Role of potassium currents in cardiac arrhythmias, *Europace* 10: 1133–1137, 2008.
41. Nichols CG: KATP channels as molecular sensors of cellular metabolism, *Nature* 440: 470–476, 2006.
42. Zhang H, Flagg TP, Nichols CG: Cardiac sarcolemmal K(ATP) channels: latest twists in a questing tale!, *J Mol Cell Cardiol* 48:71–75, 2010.
43. Kane GC, Liu XK, Yamada S, et al: Cardiac KATP channels in health and disease, *J Mol Cell Cardiol* 38:937–943, 2005.
44. Gurney A, Manoury B: Two-pore potassium channels in the cardiovascular system, *Eur Biophys J* 38:305–318, 2009.
45. Enyedi P, Czirjak G: Molecular background of leak K+ currents: two-pore domain potassium channels, *Physiol Rev* 90:559–605, 2010.
46. Bodi I, Mikala G, Koch SE, et al: The L-type calcium channel in the heart: the beat goes on, *J Clin Invest* 115:3306–3317, 2005.
47. Benitah JP, Alvarez JL, Gomez AM: L-type Ca(2+) current in ventricular cardiomyocytes, *J Mol Cell Cardiol* 48:26–36, 2010.
48. Ono K, Iijima T: Cardiac T-type Ca(2+) channels in the heart, *J Mol Cell Cardiol* 48:65–70, 2010.
49. van der Heyden MA, Wijnhoven TJ, Opthof T: Molecular aspects of adrenergic modulation of cardiac L-type Ca2+ channels, *Cardiovasc Res* 65:28–39, 2005.
50. Bers DM: Calcium cycling and signaling in cardiac myocytes, *Annu Rev Physiol* 70:23–49, 2008.
51. Nerbonne JM, Kass RS: Molecular physiology of cardiac repolarization, *Physiol Rev* 85: 1205–1253, 2005.
52. DiFrancesco D: The role of the funny current in pacemaker activity, *Circ Res* 106:434–446, 2010.
53. Mangoni ME, Nargeot J: Genesis and regulation of the heart automaticity, *Physiol Rev* 88:919–982, 2008.
54. Lakatta EG: A paradigm shift for the heart's pacemaker, *Heart Rhythm* 7:559–564, 2010.
55. Venetucci LA, Trafford AW, O'Neill SC, Eisner DA: The sarcoplasmic reticulum and arrhythmogenic calcium release, *Cardiovasc Res* 77:285–292, 2008 January 15.
56. Biel M, Wahl-Schott C, Michalakis S, Zong X: Hyperpolarization-activated cation channels: from genes to function, *Physiol Rev* 89:847–885, 2009.
57. Zalk R, Lehnart SE, Marks AR: Modulation of the ryanodine receptor and intracellular calcium, *Annu Rev Biochem* 76:367–385, 2007.
58. Gyorke S: Molecular basis of catecholaminergic polymorphic ventricular tachycardia, *Heart Rhythm* 6:123–129, 2009.
59. Mohamed U, Napolitano C, Priori SG: Molecular and electrophysiological bases of catecholaminergic polymorphic ventricular tachycardia, *J Cardiovasc Electrophysiol* 18:791–797, 2007.
60. Kushnir A, Marks AR: The ryanodine receptor in cardiac physiology and disease, *Adv Pharmacol* 59:1–30, 2010.
61. Ter Keurs HE, Boyden PA: Calcium and arrhythmogenesis, *Physiol Rev* 87:457–506, 2007.
62. Blayney LM, Lai FA: Ryanodine receptor-mediated arrhythmias and sudden cardiac death, *Pharmacol Ther* 123:151–177, 2009.
63. Cerrone M, Napolitano C, Priori SG: Catecholaminergic polymorphic ventricular tachycardia: a paradigm to understand mechanisms of arrhythmias associated to impaired Ca(2+) regulation, *Heart Rhythm* 6:1652–1659, 2009.
64. Hwang HS, Hasdemir C, Laver D, et al: Inhibition of cardiac Ca2+ release channels (RyR2) determines efficacy of class I antiarrhythmic drugs in catecholaminergic polymorphic ventricular tachycardia, *Circ Arrhythm Electrophysiol* 4:128–135, 2011.
65. Napolitano C, Priori SG: Diagnosis and treatment of catecholaminergic polymorphic ventricular tachycardia, *Heart Rhythm* 4:675–678, 2007.
66. Otten E, Asimaki A, Maass A, et al: Desmin mutations as a cause of right ventricular heart failure affect the intercalated disks, *Heart Rhythm* 7:1058–1064, 2010.
67. Maass K: Arrhythmogenic right ventricular cardiomyopathy and desmin: another gene fits the shoe, *Heart Rhythm* 7:1065–1066, 2010.
68. Hamilton RM, Fidler L: Right ventricular cardiomyopathy in the young: an emerging challenge, *Heart Rhythm* 6:571–575, 2009.
69. Jin H, Lyon AR, Akar FG: Arrhythmia mechanisms in the failing heart, *Pacing Clin Electrophysiol* 31:1048–1056, 2008.
70. Laurita KR, Rosenbaum DS: Mechanisms and potential therapeutic targets for ventricular arrhythmias associated with impaired cardiac calcium cycling, *J Mol Cell Cardiol* 44:31–43, 2008.
71. Jansen JA, van Veen TA, de Bakker JM, van Rijen HV: Cardiac connexins and impulse propagation, *J Mol Cell Cardiol* 48:76–82, 2010.
72. Yeager M, Harris AL: Gap junction channel structure in the early 21st century: facts and fantasies, *Curr Opin Cell Biol* 19:521–528, 2007.
73. Valderrabano M: Influence of anisotropic conduction properties in the propagation of the cardiac action potential, *Prog Biophys Mol Biol* 94:144–168, 2007.
74. Kleber AG, Rudy Y: Basic mechanisms of cardiac impulse propagation and associated arrhythmias, *Physiol Rev* 84:431–488, 2004.
75. Saffitz JE, Lerner DL: Gap junction distribution and regulation in the heart. In Zipes DP, Jalife J, editors: *Cardiac electrophysiology: from cell to bedside*, ed 4, Philadelphia, 2004, Saunders, pp 181–191.
76. Lewandowski R, Petersen JS, Delmar M: Connexins as potential targets for cardiovascular pharmacology. In Zipes DP, Jalife J, editors: *Cardiac electrophysiology: from cell to bedside*, ed 5, Philadelphia, 2009, Saunders, pp 205–213.
77. Wit AL, Duffy HS: Drug development for treatment of cardiac arrhythmias: targeting the gap junctions, *Am J Physiol* 294:H16–H18, 2008.
78. Lin X, Zemlin C, Hennan JK, et al: Enhancement of ventricular gap-junction coupling by rotigaptide, *Cardiovasc Res* 79:416–426, 2008.
79. van Rijen HV, van Veen TA, Gros D, et al: Connexins and cardiac arrhythmias, *Adv Cardiol* 42:150–160, 2006.
80. Lee PJ, Pogwizd SM: Micropatterns of propagation, *Adv Cardiol* 42:86–106, 2006.
81. Cascio WE, Yang H, Muller-Borer BJ, Johnson TA: Ischemia-induced arrhythmia: the role of connexins, gap junctions, and attendant changes in impulse propagation, *J Electrocardiol* 38(Suppl):55–59, 2005.
82. Cabo C, Yao J, Boyden PA, et al: Heterogeneous gap junction remodeling in reentrant circuits in the epicardial border zone of the healing canine infarct, *Cardiovasc Res* 72:241–249, 2006.
83. Chaldoupi SM, Loh P, Hauer RN, et al: The role of connexin40 in atrial fibrillation, *Cardiovasc Res* 84:15–23, 2009.

CHAPTER 3 Electrophysiological Mechanisms of Cardiac Arrhythmias

The mechanisms responsible for cardiac arrhythmias are generally divided into categories of disorders of impulse formation (automaticity or triggered activity), disorders of impulse conduction (reentry), or combinations of both. Automaticity is the property of cardiac cells to initiate an impulse spontaneously, without need for prior stimulation. Triggered activity is impulse initiation in cardiac fibers caused by depolarizing oscillations in membrane voltage (known as afterdepolarizations) that occur consequent to one or more preceding action potentials.[1] Reentry occurs when a propagating action potential wave fails to extinguish after initial tissue activation; instead, it blocks in circumscribed areas, circulates around the zones of block, and reenters and reactivates the site of original excitation after it recovers excitability. Reentry is the likely mechanism of most recurrent clinical arrhythmias.

Diagnosis of the underlying mechanism of an arrhythmia can be of great importance in guiding appropriate treatment strategies. Spontaneous behavior of the arrhythmia, mode of initiation and termination, and response to premature stimulation and overdrive pacing are the most commonly used tools to distinguish among the different mechanisms responsible for cardiac arrhythmias. Our present diagnostic tools, however, do not always permit unequivocal determination of the electrophysiological (EP) mechanisms responsible for many clinical arrhythmias or their ionic bases. In particular, it can be difficult to distinguish among several mechanisms that appear to have a focal origin with centrifugal spread of activation (automaticity, triggered activity, microreentry). This is further complicated by the fact that some arrhythmias can be started by one mechanism and perpetuated by another.

Automaticity

Automaticity, or spontaneous impulse initiation, is the ability of cardiac cells to depolarize spontaneously, reach threshold potential, and initiate a propagated action potential in the absence of external electrical stimulation. Altered automaticity can be caused by enhanced normal automaticity or abnormal automaticity.[1]

Enhanced normal automaticity refers to the accelerated generation of an action potential by normal pacemaker tissue and is found in the primary pacemaker of the heart, the sinus node, as well as in certain subsidiary or latent pacemakers that can become the functional pacemaker under certain conditions. Impulse initiation is a normal property of these latent pacemakers.

Abnormal automaticity occurs in cardiac cells only when there are major abnormalities in their transmembrane potentials, in particular in steady-state depolarization of the membrane potential. This property of abnormal automaticity is not confined to any specific latent pacemaker cell type but can occur almost anywhere in the heart.

The discharge rate of normal or abnormal pacemakers can be accelerated by drugs, various forms of cardiac disease, reduction in extracellular potassium (K^+), or alterations of autonomic nervous system tone.

Enhanced Normal Automaticity

PACEMAKER MECHANISMS

Normal automaticity involves a spontaneous, slow, progressive decline (less negative) in the transmembrane potential during diastole (spontaneous diastolic depolarization or phase 4 depolarization) (see Chap. 1). Once this spontaneous depolarization reaches threshold (approximately −40 mV), a new action potential is generated.[2]

The ionic mechanisms responsible for normal pacemaker activity in the sinus node are still controversial. The fall in membrane potential during phase 4 seems to arise from a changing balance between positive inward currents, which favor depolarization, and positive outward currents, with a net gain in intracellular positive charges during diastole (i.e., inward depolarizing current; Fig. 3-1).[1-6]

Originally, a major role was attributed to the decay of the delayed K^+ conductance (an outward current) activated during the preceding action potential, (the I_K-decay theory). This model of pacemaker depolarization lost interest on the discovery of the pacemaker current (I_f). Other ionic currents gated by membrane depolarization (i.e., L-type and T-type calcium [Ca^{2+}] currents), nongated and nonspecific background leak currents, and a current generated by the sodium (Na^+)–Ca^{2+} exchanger, were also proposed to be involved in pacemaking.

Evidence suggests that I_f (named the "funny" current because, unlike most voltage-sensitive currents, it is activated by hyperpolarization rather than depolarization) is one of the most important ionic currents involved in the rate regulation of cardiac pacemaker cells, hence its designation as the pacemaker current. I_f is an inward current carried largely by Na^+ and, to a lesser extent, K^+ ions. The I_f channels are deactivated during the action potential upstroke and the initial plateau phase of repolarization. However, they begin to activate at the end of the action potential as repolarization brings the membrane potential to levels more negative than approximately −40 to −50 mV, and I_f is fully activated at approximately −100 mV. Once activated, I_f depolarizes the membrane to a level where the Ca^{2+} current activates to initiate the action potential.[7] In its range of activation, which quite properly comprises the voltage range of diastolic depolarization, the current is inward, and its reversal occurs at approximately −10 to −20 mV because of the mixed Na^+-K^+ permeability of I_f channels. At the end of the repolarization phase of an action potential, because I_f activation occurs in the background of a decaying outward (K^+ time-dependent) current, current flow quickly shifts from outward to inward, thus giving rise to a sudden reversal of voltage change (from repolarizing to depolarizing) at the maximum diastolic potential. The major role of I_f has been reinforced by the findings that drugs such as ivabradine targeted to block I_f slow heart rate and mutations in the I_f channel are associated with slowed heart rate.[2,5,8-10]

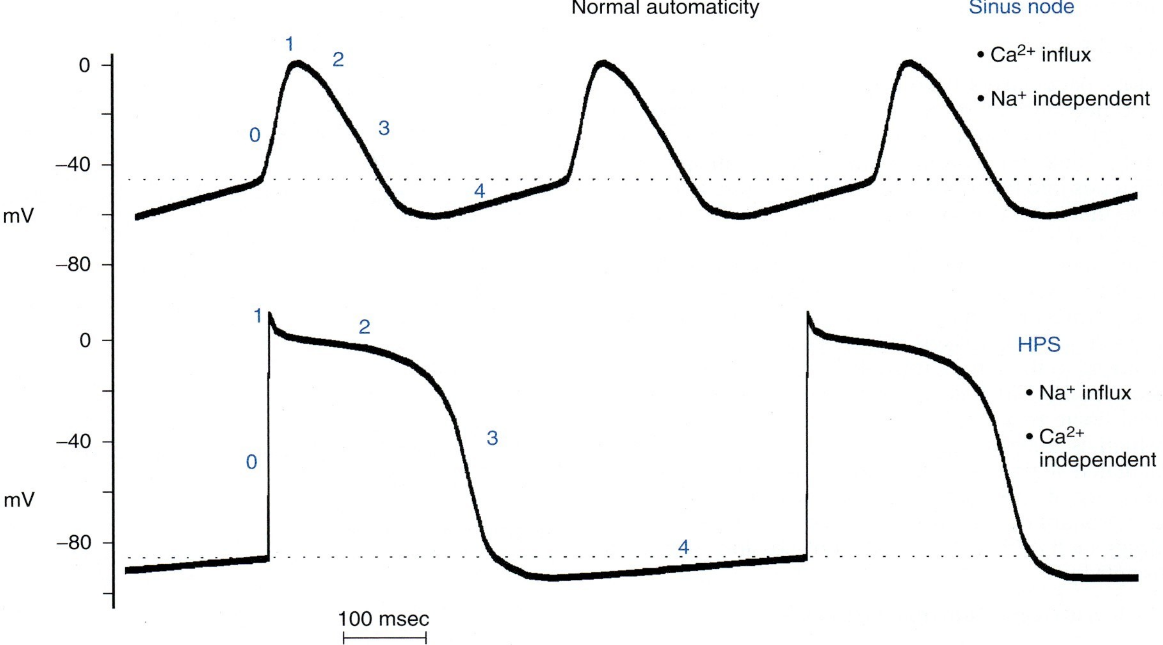

FIGURE 3-1 Normal cardiac automaticity. Action potentials from typical sinus nodal and His-Purkinje cells are shown with the voltage scale on the vertical axes; dashed lines are threshold potential, and numbers on the figure refer to phases of the action potential. Note the qualitative differences between the two types of cells, as well as different rates of spontaneous depolarization. Ca^{2+} = calcium; Na^{+} = sodium.

On the other hand, several studies have shown that I_f is not the only current that can initiate the diastolic depolarization process in the sinus node. In addition to voltage and time, the electrogenic and regulatory molecules on the surface membrane of sinus node cells are strongly modulated by Ca^{2+} and phosphorylation, a finding suggesting that intracellular Ca^{2+} is an important player in controlling pacemaker cell automaticity. Newer evidence points to a substantial impact of another current on the late diastolic depolarization; that is, the Na^+-Ca^{2+} exchanger current activated by submembrane spontaneous rhythmic local Ca^{2+} releases from the sarcoplasmic reticulum, a major Ca^{2+} store within sinus node cells, via ryanodine receptors (RyR2). Activation of the local oscillatory Ca^{2+} releases is independent of membrane depolarization and is driven by a high level of basal state phosphorylation of Ca^{2+} cycling proteins. Critically timed Ca^{2+} releases occur during the later phase of diastolic depolarization and activate the forward mode of the Na^+-Ca^{2+} exchanger (one Ca^{2+} for three Na^+). The result is in an inward membrane current that causes the late diastolic depolarization to increase exponentially, thus driving the membrane potential to the threshold to activate a sufficient number of voltage-gated L-type Ca^{2+} channels and leading to generation of the rapid upstroke of the next action potential (see Fig. 1-3). Although regulated by membrane potential and submembrane Ca^{2+}, the Na^+-Ca^{2+} exchanger does not have time-dependent gating, as do ion channels, but generates an inward current almost instantaneously when submembrane Ca^{2+} concentration increases.[8,9,11]

Such rhythmic, spontaneous intracellular Ca^{2+} cycling has been referred to as an "intracellular Ca^{2+} clock." Phosphorylation-dependent gradation of the speed at which Ca^{2+} clock cycles is the essential regulatory mechanism of normal pacemaker rate and rhythm. The robust regulation of pacemaker function is ensured by tight integration of the Ca^{2+} clock and the classic sarcolemmal "ion channel clock" (formed by voltage-dependent membrane ion channels) to form the overall pacemaker clock. The action potential shape and ion fluxes are tuned by membrane clocks to sustain operation of the Ca^{2+} clock, which produces timely and powerful ignition of the membrane clocks to effect action potentials.

There is some degree of uncertainty about the relative role of I_f versus that of intracellular Ca^{2+} cycling in controlling the normal pacemaker cell automaticity and their individual (or mutual) relevance in mediating the positive-negative chronotropic effect of neurotransmitters. Furthermore, the interactions between the membrane ion channel clock and the intracellular Ca^{2+} clock and the cellular mechanisms underlying this internal Ca^{2+} clock are not completely elucidated.[8,9,11]

Automaticity in subsidiary pacemakers appears to arise via a mechanism similar to that occurring in the sinus node.

HIERARCHY OF PACEMAKER FUNCTION

Automaticity is not limited to the cells within the sinus node. Under physiological conditions, cells in parts of the atria and within the atrioventricular node (AVN) and the His-Purkinje system (HPS) also possess pacemaking capability. However, the occurrence of spontaneous activity in these cells is prevented by the natural hierarchy of pacemaker function that causes these sites to be latent or subsidiary pacemakers.[1] The spontaneous discharge rate of the sinus node normally exceeds that of all other subsidiary pacemakers (see Fig. 3-1). Therefore, the impulse initiated by the sinus node depolarizes subsidiary pacemaker sites and keeps their activity depressed before they can spontaneously reach threshold. However, slowly depolarizing and previously suppressed pacemakers in the atrium, AVN, or ventricle can become active and assume pacemaker control of the cardiac rhythm if the sinus node pacemaker becomes slow or unable to generate an impulse (e.g., secondary to depressed sinus node automaticity) or if impulses generated by the sinus node are unable to activate the subsidiary pacemaker sites (e.g., sinoatrial exit block, or atrioventricular [AV] block). The emergence of subsidiary or latent pacemakers under such circumstances is an appropriate fail-safe mechanism, which ensures that ventricular activation is maintained. Because spontaneous diastolic depolarization is a normal property, the automaticity generated by these cells is classified as normal.

There is also a natural hierarchy of intrinsic rates of subsidiary pacemakers that have normal automaticity, with atrial pacemakers having faster intrinsic rates than AV junctional pacemakers, and AV junctional pacemakers having faster rates than ventricular pacemakers.

CH 3

SUBSIDIARY PACEMAKERS

Subsidiary Atrial Pacemakers

Subsidiary atrial pacemakers have been identified in the atrial myocardium, especially in the crista terminalis, at the junction of the inferior right atrium and inferior vena cava, near or on the eustachian ridge, near the coronary sinus ostium, in the atrial muscle that extends into the tricuspid and mitral valves, and in the muscle sleeves that extend into the cardiac veins (venae cavae and pulmonary veins).[12]

Latent atrial pacemakers can contribute to impulse initiation in the atrium if the discharge rate of the sinus node is reduced temporarily or permanently. In contrast to the normal sinus node, these latent or ectopic pacemakers usually generate a fast action potential (referring to the rate of upstroke of the action potential [dV/dt]) mediated by Na^+ fluxes. However, when severely damaged, the atrial tissue may not be able to generate a fast action potential (which is energy dependent), but rather generates a slow, Ca^{2+}-mediated action potential (which is energy independent). Automaticity of subsidiary atrial pacemakers can also be enhanced by coronary disease and ischemia, chronic pulmonary disease, or drugs such as digitalis and alcohol, possibly overriding normal sinus activity.

Subsidiary Atrioventricular Junctional Pacemakers

Some data suggest that the AVN itself has pacemaker cells, but that concept is controversial. However, it is clear that the AV junction, which is an area that includes atrial tissue, the AVN, and His-Purkinje tissue, does have pacemaker cells and is capable of exhibiting automaticity.

Subsidiary Ventricular Pacemakers

In the ventricles, latent pacemakers are found in the HPS, where Purkinje fibers have the property of spontaneous diastolic depolarization. Isolated cells of the HPS discharge spontaneously at rates of 15 to 60 beats/min, whereas ventricular myocardial cells do not normally exhibit spontaneous diastolic depolarization or automaticity. The relatively slow spontaneous discharge rate of the HPS pacemakers, which further decreases from the His bundle to the distal Purkinje branches, ensures that pacemaker activity in the HPS will be suppressed on a beat-to-beat basis by the more rapid discharge rate of the sinus node and atrial and AV junctional pacemakers. However, enhanced Purkinje fiber automaticity can be induced by certain situations, such as myocardial infarction (MI). In this setting, some Purkinje fibers that survive the infarction develop moderately reduced maximum diastolic membrane potentials and therefore accelerated spontaneous discharge rates.[13]

REGULATION OF PACEMAKER FUNCTION

The intrinsic rate at which the sinus node pacemaker cells generate impulses is determined by the interplay of three factors: the maximum diastolic potential, the threshold potential at which the action potential is initiated, and the rate or slope of phase 4 depolarization (Fig. 3-2). A change in any one of these factors will alter the time required for phase 4 depolarization to carry the membrane potential from its maximum diastolic level to threshold and thus alter the rate of impulse initiation.[1]

The sinus node is innervated by the parasympathetic and sympathetic nervous systems, and the balance between these systems importantly controls the pacemaker rate. The classic concept has been that of a reciprocal relationship between sympathetic and parasympathetic inputs. More recent investigations, however, stress dynamic, demand-oriented interactions, and the anatomical distribution of fibers that allows both autonomic systems to act quite selectively. Muscarinic cholinergic and $beta_1$-adrenergic receptors are nonuniformly distributed in the sinus node, and they modulate both the rate of depolarization and impulse propagation.[1]

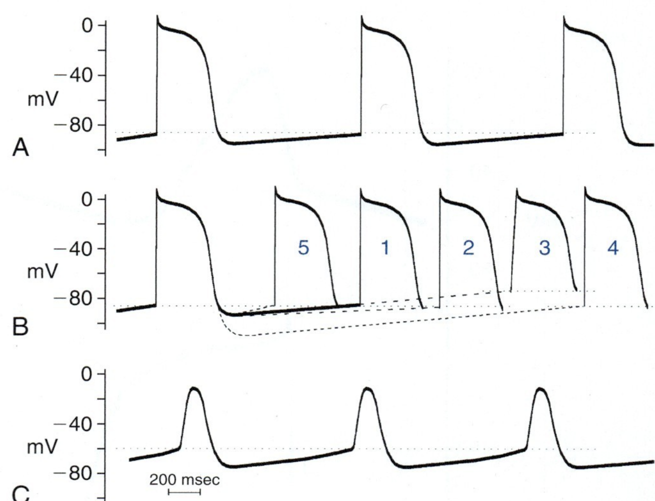

FIGURE 3-2 Abnormalities of automaticity. **A,** Normal His-Purkinje action potential. **B,** Modulation of rate of depolarization from baseline (1) by slowing rate of phase 4 depolarization (2), increasing threshold potential (3), starting from a more negative resting membrane potential (4), all of which slow discharge rate, or by increasing rate of phase 4 depolarization (5), thus yielding a faster discharge rate. **C,** Abnormal automaticity with change in action potential contour (resembling sinus nodal cell) when resting membrane potential is less negative, inactivating most sodium channels.

Parasympathetic Activity

Parasympathetic tone reduces the spontaneous discharge rate of the sinus node, whereas its withdrawal accelerates sinus node automaticity. Acetylcholine, the principal neurotransmitter of the parasympathetic nervous system, inhibits spontaneous impulse generation in the sinus node by increasing K^+ conductance. Acetylcholine acts through M_2 muscarinic receptors to activate the G_i protein, which subsequently results in activation of I_{KACh} (an acetylcholine-activated subtype of inward rectifying current) in tissues of the sinus node and AVN as well as of the atria, Purkinje fibers, and ventricles. The increased outward repolarizing K^+ current (I_K) leads to membrane hyperpolarization (i.e., the resting potential and the maximum diastolic potential become more negative). The resulting hyperpolarization of the membrane potential lengthens the time required for the membrane potential to depolarize to threshold and thereby decreases the automaticity of the sinus node (see Fig. 3-2). In addition, activation of the Gi protein results in inhibition of beta-receptor–stimulated adenylate cyclase activity, thus reducing cyclic adenosine monophosphate (cAMP) and inhibiting protein kinase A, with subsequent inhibition of the inward Ca^{2+} current. This results in reduction of the rate of diastolic depolarization because of less Ca^{2+} entry and subsequent slowing of the pacemaker activity. Inhibition of beta-receptor–stimulated adenylate cyclase activity can also inhibit the inward I_f current.

Sympathetic Activity

Increased sympathetic nerve traffic and the adrenomedullary release of catecholamines increase sinus node discharge rate. Stimulation of $beta_1$-receptors by catecholamines enhances the L-type of inward Ca^{2+} current (I_{CaL}) by increasing cAMP and activating the protein kinase A system; the increment in inward Ca^{2+} current increases the slope of diastolic depolarization and enhances pacemaker activity (see Fig. 3-2). The redistribution of Ca^{2+} can also increase the completeness and the rate of deactivation of the rapid (I_{Kr}) and slow (I_{Ks}) components of the delayed rectifier I_K; the ensuing decline in the opposing outward current results in a further net increase in inward current. Catecholamines can also enhance the inward I_f current by shifting the voltage dependence of I_f to more positive potentials, thus augmenting the slope of phase 4 and increasing the rate of sinus node firing.[10]

In addition to altering ionic conductance, changes in autonomic tone can produce changes in the rate of the sinus node by shifting the primary pacemaker region within the pacemaker complex. Mapping of activation indicates that, at faster rates, the sinus node impulse usually originates in the superior portion of the sinus node, whereas at slower rates, it usually arises from a more inferior portion of the sinus node. The sinus node can be insulated from the surrounding atrial myocytes, except at a limited number of preferential exit sites. Shifting pacemaker sites can select different exit pathways to the atria. As a result, autonomically mediated shifts of pacemaker regions can be accompanied by changes in the sinus rate. Vagal fibers are denser in the cranial portion of the sinus node, and stimulation of the parasympathetic nervous system shifts the pacemaker center to a more caudal region of the sinus node complex, thus resulting in slowing of the heart rate. In contrast, stimulation of the sympathetic nervous system or withdrawal of vagal stimulation shifts the pacemaker center cranially, resulting in an increase in heart rate.

Atrial, AV junctional, and HPS subsidiary pacemakers are also under similar autonomic control, with the sympathetic nervous system enhancing pacemaker activity through beta$_1$-adrenergic stimulation and the parasympathetic nervous system inhibiting pacemaker activity through muscarinic receptor stimulation.[1]

Other Influences

Adenosine binds to A_1-receptors, thus activating I_{KACh} and increasing outward I_K in a manner similar to that of marked parasympathetic stimulation. It also has similar effects on I_f channels.

Digitalis exerts two effects on the sinus rate. It has a direct positive chronotropic effect on the sinus node, resulting from depolarization of the membrane potential caused by inhibition of the Na^+-K^+ exchange pump. The reduction in the maximum diastolic membrane potential decreases the time required for the membrane to depolarize to threshold and thereby accelerates the spontaneous discharge rate. However, digitalis also enhances vagal tone, which decreases spontaneous sinus discharge.

Enhanced subsidiary pacemaker activity may not require sympathetic stimulation. Normal automaticity can be affected by certain other factors associated with heart disease. Inhibition of the electrogenic Na^+-K^+ exchange pump results in a net increase in inward current during diastole because of the decrease in outward current normally generated by the pump, and therefore it can increase automaticity in subsidiary pacemakers sufficiently to cause arrhythmias. This can occur when adenosine triphosphate (ATP) is depleted during prolonged hypoxia or ischemia or in the presence of toxic amounts of digitalis. Hypokalemia can reduce the activity of the Na^+-K^+ exchange pump, thereby reducing the background repolarizing current and enhancing phase 4 diastolic depolarization. The end result would be an increase in the discharge rate of pacemaking cells. Additionally, the flow of current between partially depolarized myocardium and normally polarized latent pacemaker cells can enhance automaticity. This mechanism has been proposed to be a cause of some of the ectopic complexes that arise at the borders of ischemic areas in the ventricle. Slightly increased extracellular K^+ can render the maximum diastolic potential more positive (i.e., reduced or less negative), thereby also increasing the discharge rate of pacemaking cells. A greater increase in extracellular K^+, however, renders the heart inexcitable by depolarizing the membrane potential and inactivating the Na^+ current (I_{Na}).

Evidence indicates that active and passive changes in the mechanical environment of the heart provide feedback to modify cardiac rate and rhythm and are capable of influencing both the initiation and spread of cardiac excitation. This direction of the crosstalk between cardiac electrical and mechanical activity is referred to as mechanoelectric feedback and is thought to be involved in the adjustment of heart rate to changes in mechanical load, which would help explain the precise beat-to-beat regulation of cardiac performance. Acute mechanical stretch enhances automaticity, reversibly depolarizes the cell membrane, and shortens the action potential duration. Feedback from cardiac mechanics to electrical activity involves mechanosensitive ion channels and ATP-sensitive K^+ channels. In addition, Na^+ and Ca^{2+} entering the cells via nonselective ion channels are thought to contribute to the genesis of stretch-induced arrhythmia.[14]

Abnormal Automaticity

In the normal heart, automaticity is confined to the sinus node and other specialized conducting tissues. Working atrial and ventricular myocardial cells do not normally have spontaneous diastolic depolarization and do not initiate spontaneous impulses, even when they are not excited for long periods of time by propagating impulses. Although these cells do have an I_f, the range of activation of this current in these cells is much more negative (–120 to –170 mV) than in Purkinje fibers or in the sinus node. As a result, during physiological resting membrane potentials (–85 to –95 mV), the I_f is not activated, and ventricular cells do not depolarize spontaneously.[1] When the resting potentials of these cells are depolarized sufficiently, to approximately –70 to –30 mV, however, spontaneous diastolic depolarization can occur and cause repetitive impulse initiation, a phenomenon called depolarization-induced automaticity or abnormal automaticity (see Fig. 3-2). Similarly, cells in the Purkinje system, which are normally automatic at high levels of membrane potential, show abnormal automaticity when the membrane potential is reduced to approximately –60 mV or less, as can occur in ischemic regions of the heart. When the steady-state membrane potential of Purkinje fibers is reduced to approximately –60 mV or less, the I_f channels that participate in normal pacemaker activity in Purkinje fibers are closed and nonfunctional, and automaticity is therefore not caused by the normal pacemaker mechanism. It can, however, be caused by an "abnormal" mechanism. In contrast, enhanced automaticity of the sinus node, subsidiary atrial pacemakers, or the AVN caused by a mechanism other than acceleration of normal automaticity has not been demonstrated clinically.[15]

A low level of membrane potential is not the only criterion for defining abnormal automaticity. If this were so, the automaticity of the sinus node would have to be considered abnormal. Therefore, an important distinction between abnormal and normal automaticity is that the membrane potentials of fibers showing the abnormal type of activity are reduced from their own normal level. For this reason, automaticity in the AVN (e.g., where the membrane potential is normally low) is not classified as abnormal automaticity.

Several different mechanisms probably cause abnormal pacemaker activity at low membrane potentials, including activation and deactivation of the delayed rectifier I_K, intracellular Ca^{2+} release from the sarcoplasmic reticulum that causes activation of inward Ca^{2+} currents and the inward I_{Na} (through the Na^+-Ca^{2+} exchanger), and a potential contribution by I_f.[16] It has not been determined which of these mechanisms are operative in the different pathological conditions in which abnormal automaticity can occur.[1]

The upstroke of the spontaneously occurring action potentials generated by abnormal automaticity can be caused by Na^+ or Ca^{2+} inward currents or possibly a combination of the two.[1] In the range of diastolic potentials between approximately –70 and –50 mV, repetitive activity is dependent on extracellular Na^+ concentration and can be decreased or abolished by Na^+ channel blockers. In a diastolic potential range of approximately –50 to –30 mV, Na^+ channels are predominantly inactivated; repetitive activity depends on extracellular Ca^{2+} concentration and is reduced by L-type Ca^{2+} channel blockers.

The intrinsic rate of a focus with abnormal automaticity is a function of the membrane potential. The more positive the membrane potential is, the faster the automatic rate will be (see Fig. 3-2). Abnormal automaticity is less vulnerable to suppression by overdrive pacing (see later). Therefore, even occasional slowing of the sinus node rate can allow an ectopic focus with abnormal automaticity to fire without a preceding long period of quiescence. Catecholamines can increase the rate of discharge caused by abnormal automaticity and therefore can contribute to a shift in the pacemaker site from the sinus node to a region with abnormal automaticity.

The decrease in the membrane potential of cardiac cells required for abnormal automaticity to occur can be induced by a variety of factors related to cardiac disease, such as ischemia and infarction. The circumstance under which membrane depolarization occurs, however, can influence the development of abnormal automaticity. For example, an increase in extracellular K^+ concentration, as occurs in acutely ischemic myocardium, can reduce membrane potential; however, normal or abnormal automaticity in working atrial, ventricular, and Purkinje fibers usually does not occur because of an increase in K^+ conductance (and hence net outward current) that results from the increase in extracellular K^+ concentration.

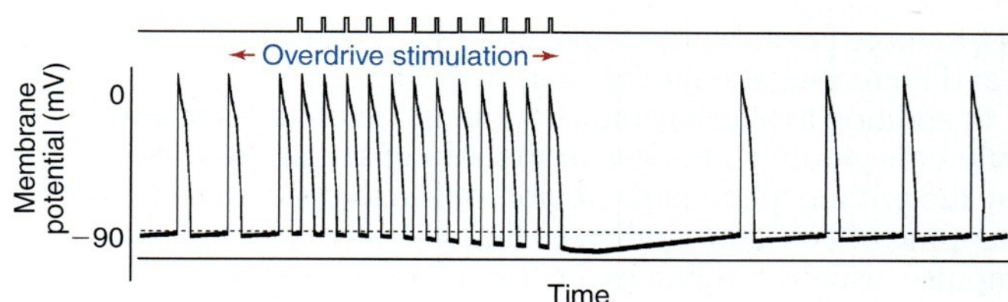

FIGURE 3-3 Overdrive suppression of automaticity. A spontaneously firing cell is paced more rapidly, resulting in depression of resting membrane potential; after pacing is stopped, spontaneous depolarization takes longer than usual and gradually resumes baseline rate. Dashed line = threshold potential.

Overdrive Suppression of Automatic Rhythms

SUPPRESSION OF NORMAL AND ABNORMAL AUTOMATIC SUBSIDIARY PACEMAKERS

The sinus node likely maintains its dominance over subsidiary pacemakers in the AVN and the Purkinje fibers by several mechanisms. During sinus rhythm in a normal heart, the intrinsic automatic rate of the sinus node is faster than that of the other potentially automatic cells. Consequently, the latent pacemakers are excited by propagated impulses from the sinus node before they have a chance to depolarize spontaneously to threshold potential. The higher frequency of sinus node discharge also suppresses the automaticity of other pacemaker sites by a mechanism called overdrive suppression. The diastolic (phase 4) depolarization of the latent pacemaker cells with the property of normal automaticity is actually inhibited because the cells are repeatedly depolarized by the impulses from the sinus node.[1] Electrotonic interaction between the pacemaker cells and the nonpacemaker cells in the surrounding myocardium via intercalated discs and gap junctions can also hyperpolarize the latent pacemakers and contribute to their suppression (Fig. 3-3).

MECHANISM OF OVERDRIVE SUPPRESSION

The mechanism of overdrive suppression is mediated mostly by enhanced activity of the Na^+-K^+ exchange pump that results from driving a pacemaker cell faster than its intrinsic spontaneous rate. During normal sinus rhythm (NSR), latent pacemakers are depolarized at a higher frequency than their intrinsic rate of automaticity. The increased frequency of depolarizations leads to an increase in intracellular Na^+, which enters the cell with every action potential, because more Na^+ enters the cell per unit time.[1] The increased intracellular Na^+ stimulates the Na^+-K^+ exchange pump. Because the Na^+-K^+ exchange pump is electrogenic (i.e., moves more Na^+ outward than K^+ inward), it generates a net outward (hyperpolarizing) current across the cell membrane. This drives the membrane potential more negative, thereby offsetting the depolarizing I_f being carried into the cell and slowing the rate of phase 4 diastolic depolarization. This effectively prevents the I_f from depolarizing the cell to its threshold potential and thereby suppresses spontaneous impulse initiation in these cells.

When the dominant (overdrive) pacemaker is stopped, suppression of subsidiary pacemakers continues because the Na^+-K^+ exchange pump continues to generate the outward current as it reduces the intracellular Na^+ levels toward normal. This continued Na^+-K^+ exchange pump–generated outward current is responsible for the period of quiescence, which lasts until the intracellular Na^+ concentration, and hence the pump current, becomes low enough to allow subsidiary pacemaker cells to depolarize spontaneously to threshold. Intracellular Na^+ concentration decreases during the quiescent period because Na^+ is constantly being pumped out of the cell and little is entering. Additionally, the spontaneous rate of the suppressed cell remains lower than it would be otherwise until the intracellular Na^+ concentration has a chance to decrease. Intracellular Na^+ concentration and pump current continue to decline even after spontaneous discharge begins because of the slow firing rate, thus causing a gradual increase in the discharge rate of the subsidiary pacemaker. At slower rates and shorter overdrive periods, the Na^+ load is of lesser magnitude, as is the activity of the Na^+-K^+ pump, resulting in a progressively rapid diastolic depolarization and warm-up. The higher the overdrive rate or the longer the duration of overdrive, the greater the enhancement of pump activity will be, so that the period of quiescence after the cessation of overdrive is directly related to the rate and duration of overdrive.

The sinus node itself also is vulnerable to overdrive suppression. When overdrive suppression of the normal sinus node occurs, however, it is generally of lesser magnitude than that of subsidiary pacemakers overdriven at comparable rates. The sinus node action potential upstroke is largely dependent on the slow inward current carried by I_{CaL}, and far less Na^+ enters the fiber during the upstroke than occurs in latent pacemaker cells such as the Purkinje fibers. As a result, the accumulation of intracellular Na^+ and enhancement of Na^+-K^+ exchange pump activity occur to a lesser degree in sinus node cells after a period of overdrive; therefore, there is less overdrive suppression caused by enhanced Na^+-K^+ exchange pump current. The relative resistance of the normal sinus node to overdrive suppression can be important in enabling it to remain the dominant pacemaker, even when its rhythm is perturbed transiently by external influences such as transient shifts of the pacemaker to an ectopic site. The diseased sinus node, however, can be much more easily overdrive suppressed, such as in the so-called tachycardia-bradycardia syndrome.

Abnormally automatic cells and tissues at reduced levels of membrane potential are less sensitive to overdrive suppression than cells and tissues that are fully polarized, with enhanced normal automaticity. The amount of overdrive suppression of spontaneous diastolic depolarization that causes abnormal automaticity is directly related to the level of membrane potential at which the automatic rhythm occurs. At low levels of membrane potential, Na^+ channels are inactivated, decreasing the fast inward I_{Na}; therefore, there are reductions in the amount of Na^+ entering the cell during overdrive and the degree of stimulation of the Na^+-K^+ exchange pump. The more polarized the membrane is during phase 4, the larger the amount will be of Na^+ entering the cell with each action potential, and the more overdrive suppression will occur. As a result of the lack of overdrive suppression of abnormally automatic cells, even transient sinus pauses can permit an ectopic focus with a slower rate than the sinus node to capture the heart for one or more beats. However, even in situations in which the cells can be sufficiently depolarized to inactivate the I_{Na} and limit intracellular Na^+ load, overdrive suppression can still be observed because of increased intracellular Ca^{2+} loading. Such Ca^{2+} loading can activate Ca^{2+}-dependent K^+ conductance (favoring repolarization) and promote Ca^{2+} extrusion through the Na^+-Ca^{2+} exchanger and Ca^{2+} channel phosphorylation, thus increasing Na^+ load and thus Na^+-K^+ exchange pump activity. The increase in intracellular Ca^{2+} load can also reduce the depolarizing I_{CaL} by promoting Ca^{2+}-induced inactivation of the Ca^{2+} current.

In addition to overdrive suppression being of paramount importance for maintenance of NSR, the characteristic response of automatic pacemakers to overdrive is often useful to distinguish automaticity from triggered activity and reentry.

Arrhythmias Caused by Automaticity

INAPPROPRIATE SINUS NODE DISCHARGE

Such arrhythmias result simply from an alteration in the rate of impulse initiation by the normal sinus node pacemaker, without a shift of impulse origin to a subsidiary pacemaker at an ectopic site, although there can be shifts of the pacemaker site within the sinus node itself during alterations in sinus rate. These arrhythmias are often a result of the actions of the autonomic nervous system on the sinus node. Examples of these arrhythmias include sinus bradycardia, sinus arrest, inappropriate sinus tachycardia, and respiratory sinus arrhythmia. Respiratory sinus arrhythmia is primarily caused by withdrawal of vagal tone during inhalation and reinstitution of vagal tone during exhalation.

ESCAPE ECTOPIC AUTOMATIC RHYTHMS

Impairment of the sinus node can allow a latent pacemaker to initiate impulse formation. This would be expected to happen when the rate at which the sinus node overdrives subsidiary pacemakers falls considerably below the intrinsic rate of the latent pacemakers or when the inhibitory electrotonic influences between nonpacemaker cells and pacemaker cells are interrupted.

The rate at which the sinus node activates subsidiary pacemakers can be decreased in certain situations, including sinus node dysfunction, with depressed sinus automaticity (secondary to increased vagal tone, drugs, or intrinsic sinus node disease), sinoatrial exit block, AV block, and parasystolic focus. The sinus node and AVN are most sensitive to vagal influence, followed by atrial tissue, with the ventricular conducting system being least sensitive. Moderate vagal stimulation allows the pacemaker to shift to another atrial site, but severe vagal stimulation suppresses the sinus node and blocks conduction at the AVN and therefore can allow a ventricular escape pacemaker to become manifest.

Interruption of the inhibitory electrotonic influences between nonpacemaker cells and pacemaker cells allows those latent pacemakers to fire at their intrinsic rate. Uncoupling can be caused by fibrosis or damage (e.g., infarction) of the tissues surrounding the subsidiary pacemaker cells or by reduction in gap junction conductance secondary to increased intracellular Ca^{2+}, which can be caused by digitalis. Some inhibition of the sinus node is still necessary for the site of impulse initiation to shift to an ectopic site that is no longer inhibited by uncoupling from surrounding cells because the intrinsic firing rate of subsidiary pacemakers is still slower than that of the sinus node.

ACCELERATED ECTOPIC AUTOMATIC RHYTHMS

Accelerated ectopic automatic rhythms are caused by enhanced normal automaticity of subsidiary pacemakers. The rate of discharge of these latent pacemakers is then faster than the expected intrinsic automatic rate. Once the enhanced rate exceeds that of the sinus node, the enhanced ectopic pacemaker prevails and overdrives the sinus node and other subsidiary pacemakers. A premature impulse caused by enhanced automaticity of latent pacemakers comes early in the normal rhythm. In contrast, an escape beat secondary to relief of overdrive suppression occurs late in normal rhythm.

Enhanced automaticity is usually caused by increased sympathetic tone, which steepens the slope of diastolic depolarization of latent pacemaker cells and diminishes the inhibitory effects of overdrive. Such sympathetic effects can be localized to subsidiary pacemakers in the absence of sinus node stimulation. Other causes of enhanced normal automaticity include periods of hypoxemia, ischemia, electrolyte disturbances, and certain drug toxicities. There is evidence that in the subacute phase of myocardial ischemia, increased activity of the sympathetic nervous system can enhance automaticity of Purkinje fibers, thus enabling them to escape from sinus node domination.

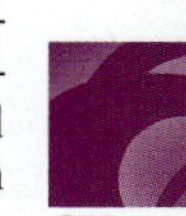

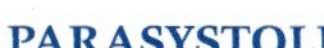

PARASYSTOLE

Parasystole is a result of interaction between two fixed rate pacemakers having different discharge rates. Parasystolic pacemakers can exist in either the atrium or the ventricle. The latent pacemaker is protected from being overdriven by the dominant rhythm (usually NSR) by intermittent or constant entrance block (i.e., impulses of sinus origin fail to depolarize the latent pacemaker secondary to block in the tissue surrounding the latent pacemaker focus). Various mechanisms have been postulated to explain the protected zone surrounding the ectopic focus. It is possible that the depolarized level of membrane potential at which abnormal automaticity occurs can cause entrance block, leading to parasystole. This would be an example of an arrhythmia caused by a combination of an abnormality of impulse conduction and impulse initiation. Such block, however, must be unidirectional, so that activity from the ectopic pacemaker can exit and produce depolarization whenever the surrounding myocardium is excitable. The protected pacemaker is said to be a parasystolic focus. In general, under these conditions, a protected focus of automaticity of this type fires at its own intrinsic frequency, and the intervals between the discharges of each pacemaker are multiples of its intrinsic discharge rate (sometimes described as *fixed parasystole*). Therefore, on the surface ECG, the coupling intervals of the manifest ectopic beats wander through the basic cycle of the sinus rhythm. Accordingly, the traditional ECG criteria used to recognize the fixed form of parasystole are (1) the presence of variable coupling intervals of the manifest ectopic beats, (2) interectopic intervals that are simple multiples of a common denominator, and (3) the presence of fusion beats. Occasionally, the parasystolic focus can exhibit exit block, during which it may fail to depolarize excitable myocardium.[17]

Although the parasystolic focus is protected, it may not be totally immune to the surrounding electrical activity. The effective electrical communication that permits the emergence of the ectopic discharges can also allow the rhythmic activity of the surrounding tissues to electrotonically influence the periodicity of the pacemaker discharge rate (described as *modulated parasystole*). Electrotonic influences arriving during the early stage of diastolic depolarization result in a delay in the firing of the parasystolic focus, whereas those arriving late accelerate the discharge of the parasystolic focus. As a consequence, the dominant pacemaker can entrain the partially protected parasystolic focus and force it to discharge at periods that may be faster or slower than its own intrinsic cycle and give rise to premature discharges whose patterns depend on the degree of modulation and the basic heart rate, occasionally mimic reentry, and occur at fixed coupling intervals. Therefore, appropriate diagnosis of modulated parasystole relies on the construction of a phase response curve as theoretical evidence of modulation of the ectopic pacemaker cycle length (CL) by the electrotonic activity generated by the sinus discharges across the area of protection.[17]

All these features of abnormal automaticity can be found in the Purkinje fibers that survive in regions of transmural MI and cause ventricular arrhythmias during the subacute phase.

ARRHYTHMIAS CAUSED BY ABNORMAL AUTOMATICITY

There appears to be an association between abnormal Purkinje fiber automaticity and the arrhythmias that occur during the acute phase of MI (e.g., an accelerated idioventricular rhythm). However, the role of abnormal automaticity in the development of ventricular arrhythmias associated with chronic ischemic heart disease is less certain. Additionally, isolated myocytes obtained from hypertrophied and failing hearts have been shown to manifest spontaneous diastolic depolarization and enhanced I_f, findings suggesting that abnormal automaticity can contribute to the occurrence of some arrhythmias in heart failure and left ventricular hypertrophy.

Abnormal automaticity can underlie atrial tachycardia, accelerated idioventricular rhythms, and ventricular tachycardia (VT), particularly that associated with ischemia and reperfusion. It has also been suggested that injury currents at the borders of ischemic zones can depolarize adjacent nonischemic tissue, thus predisposing to automatic VT.

Although automaticity is not responsible for most clinical tachyarrhythmias, which are usually caused by reentry, normal or abnormal automaticity can lead to arrhythmias caused by nonautomatic mechanisms. Premature beats, caused by automaticity, can initiate reentry. Rapid automatic activity in sites such as the cardiac veins can cause fibrillatory conduction, reentry, and atrial fibrillation (AF).

Triggered Activity

Triggered activity is impulse initiation in cardiac fibers caused by afterdepolarizations that occur consequent to a preceding impulse or series of impulses.[1] Afterdepolarizations are depolarizing oscillations in membrane potential that follow the upstroke of a preceding action potential. Afterdepolarizations can occur early during the repolarization phase of the action potential (early afterdepolarization [EAD]) or late, after completion of the repolarization phase (delayed afterdepolarization [DAD]; Fig. 3-4). When either type of afterdepolarization is large enough to reach the threshold potential for activation of a regenerative inward current, a new action potential is generated, which is referred to as *triggered*.

Unlike automaticity, triggered activity is not a self-generating rhythm. Instead, triggered activity occurs as a response to a preceding impulse (the trigger). Automatic rhythms, on the other hand, can arise de novo in the absence of any prior electrical activity.

Delayed Afterdepolarizations and Triggered Activity

DADs are oscillations in membrane voltage that occur after completion of repolarization of the action potential (i.e., during phase 4). The transient nature of the DAD distinguishes it from normal spontaneous diastolic (pacemaker) depolarization, during which the membrane potential declines almost monotonically until the next action potential occurs. DADs may or may not reach threshold. Subthreshold DADs do not initiate action potentials or trigger arrhythmias. When a DAD does reach threshold, only one triggered action potential occurs (Fig. 3-5). The triggered action potential can also be followed by a DAD that, again, may or may not reach threshold and may or may not trigger another action potential. The first triggered action potential is often followed by a short or long train of additional triggered action potentials, each arising from the DAD caused by the previous action potential.

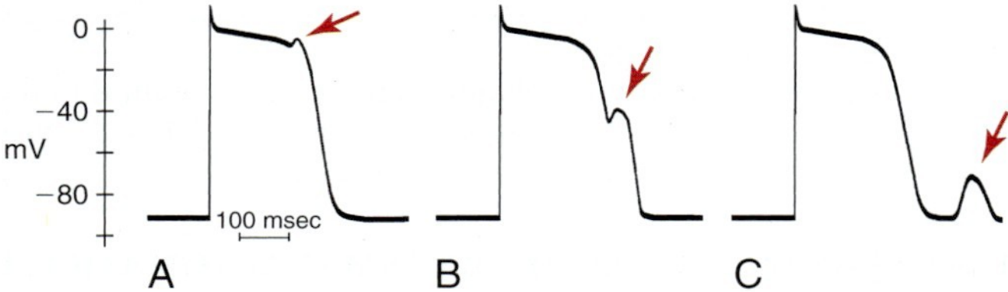

FIGURE 3-4 Types of afterdepolarizations. Afterdepolarizations are indicated by arrows. Purkinje cell action potentials are shown with phase 2 early afterdepolarizations (EADs) **(A)** and phase 3 EADs **(B)**, as well as delayed afterdepolarizations (DADs) **(C)**, which occur after full repolarization.

IONIC BASIS OF DELAYED AFTERDEPOLARIZATIONS

DADs usually occur under a variety of conditions in which Ca^{2+} overload develops in the cytoplasm and sarcoplasmic reticulum. During the plateau phase of the normal action potential, Ca^{2+} flows through voltage-dependent L-type Ca^{2+} channels (I_{CaL}). Although the rise in intracellular Ca^{2+} is small and not sufficient to induce contraction, the small amount of Ca^{2+} entering the cell via I_{CaL} triggers a massive release of Ca^{2+} from the sarcoplasmic reticulum (the major store for Ca^{2+}) into the cytosol by opening the RyR2 channels (present in the membrane of the sarcoplasmic reticulum) in a process known as Ca^{2+}-induced Ca^{2+} release (CICR).[1,6] During repolarization (i.e., diastole), most of the surplus Ca^{2+} in the cytosol is resequestered into the sarcoplasmic reticulum by the sarcoplasmic reticulum Ca^{2+} adenosine triphosphatase (SERCA), the activity of which is controlled by the phosphoprotein phospholamban. Additionally, some of the Ca^{2+} is extruded from the cell by the Na^+-Ca^{2+} exchanger to balance the Ca^{2+} that enters with Ca^{2+} current. Recurring Ca^{2+} release-uptake cycles provide the basis for periodic elevations of the cytosolic Ca^{2+} concentration and contractions of myocytes, hence for the orderly beating of the heart (Fig. 3-6).[18-20]

Under various pathological conditions, Ca^{2+} concentration in the sarcoplasmic reticulum can rise to a critical level during repolarization (i.e., Ca^{2+} overload), at which time a secondary spontaneous release of Ca^{2+} from the sarcoplasmic reticulum occurs after the action potential, rather than as a part of excitation-contraction coupling. This secondary release of Ca^{2+} results in inappropriately timed Ca^{2+} transients and contractions. Spontaneous Ca^{2+} waves are arrhythmogenic; they induce Ca^{2+}-dependent depolarizing membrane currents (transient inward current), mainly by activation of the Na^+-Ca^{2+} exchanger, thereby causing oscillations of the membrane potential known as DADs. After one or several DADs, myoplasmic Ca^{2+} can decrease because the Na^+-Ca^{2+} exchanger extrudes Ca^{2+} from the cell, and the membrane potential stops oscillating.[18-20]

When the DADs are of low amplitude, they usually are not apparent or clinically significant. However, during pathological conditions (e.g., myocardial ischemia, acidosis, hypomagnesemia, digitalis toxicity, and increased catecholamines), the amplitude of the Ca^{2+}-mediated oscillations is increased and can reach the stimulation threshold, and an action potential is triggered. If this process continues, sustained tachycardia will develop. Probably the most important influence that causes subthreshold DADs to reach threshold is a decrease in the initiating CL, because that increases

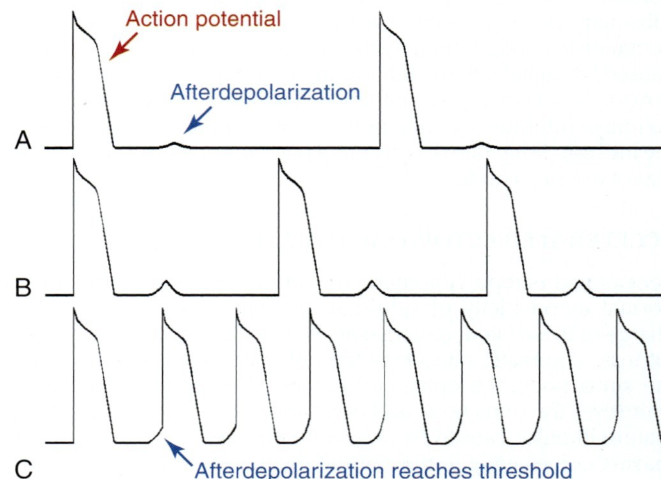

FIGURE 3-5 Behavior of delayed afterdepolarizations (DADs). **A,** The DAD is seen following the action potential at slow rates. **B,** At faster rates, the DAD occurs slightly earlier and increases in amplitude. **C,** At still more rapid rates, the DAD occurs even earlier and eventually reaches threshold, resulting in sustained firing.

both the amplitude and rate of the DADs. Therefore, initiation of arrhythmias triggered by DADs can be facilitated by a spontaneous or pacing-induced increase in the heart rate.

Digitalis causes DAD-dependent triggered arrhythmias by inhibiting the Na^+-K^+ exchange pump. In toxic amounts, this effect results in the accumulation of intracellular Na^+ and, consequentially, an enhancement of the Na^+-Ca^{2+} exchanger in the reverse mode (Na^+ removal, Ca^{2+} entry) and an accumulation of intracellular Ca^{2+}.[16] Spontaneously occurring accelerated ventricular arrhythmias that occur during digitalis toxicity are likely to be caused by DADs. Triggered ventricular arrhythmias caused by digitalis also can be initiated by pacing at rapid rates. As toxicity progresses, the duration of the trains of repetitive responses induced by pacing increases.

Catecholamines can cause DADs by increasing intracellular Ca^{2+} overload secondary to different mechanisms. Catecholamines increase the slow, inward I_{CaL} through stimulation of beta-adrenergic receptors and increasing cAMP, which result in an increase in transsarcolemmal Ca^{2+} influx and intracellular Ca^{2+} overload (see Fig. 3-6). Catecholamines can also enhance the activity of the Na^+-Ca^{2+} exchanger, thus increasing the likelihood of DAD-mediated triggered activity. Additionally, catecholamines enhance the uptake of Ca^{2+} by the sarcoplasmic reticulum and lead to increased Ca^{2+} stored in the sarcoplasmic reticulum and the subsequent release of an increased amount of Ca^{2+} from the sarcoplasmic reticulum during contraction.[16] Sympathetic stimulation can potentially cause triggered atrial and ventricular arrhythmias, possibly some of the ventricular arrhythmias that accompany exercise and those occurring during ischemia and infarction.

Elevations in intracellular Ca^{2+} in the ischemic myocardium are also associated with DADs and triggered arrhythmias. Accumulation of lysophosphoglycerides in the ischemic myocardium, with consequent Na^+ and Ca^{2+} overload, has been suggested as a mechanism for DADs and triggered activity. Cells from damaged areas or surviving the infarction can display spontaneous release of Ca^{2+} from sarcoplasmic reticulum, which can generate waves of intracellular Ca^{2+} elevation and arrhythmias.[19,20]

Abnormal sarcoplasmic reticulum function caused by genetic defects that impair the ability of the sarcoplasmic reticulum to sequester Ca^{2+} during diastole can lead to DADs and be the cause of certain inherited ventricular tachyarrhythmias. Mutations in the cardiac RyR2, the sarcoplasmic reticulum Ca^{2+} release channel in the heart, have been identified in kindreds with the syndrome of catecholaminergic polymorphic VT and ventricular fibrillation (VF) with short QT intervals. It seems likely that perturbed intracellular Ca^{2+}, and perhaps also DADs, underlie arrhythmias in this syndrome (see Fig. 3-6).[18,21]

Several drugs can inhibit DAD-related triggered activity via different mechanisms, including reduction of the inward Ca^{2+} current and intracellular Ca^{2+} overload (Ca^{2+} channel blockers, beta-adrenergic blockers; see Fig. 3-6), reduction of Ca^{2+} release from the sarcoplasmic reticulum (caffeine, ryanodine, thapsigargin, cyclopiazonic acid), and reduction of the inward I_{Na} (tetrodotoxin, lidocaine, phenytoin).

DAD-related triggered activity is thought to be a mechanism for tachyarrhythmia associated with MI, reperfusion injury, some right ventricular outflow tract tachycardia, and some atrial tachyarrhythmias. DADs are more likely to occur with fast spontaneous or paced rates or with increased premature beats.[15,18,20,22]

PROPERTIES OF DELAYED AFTERDEPOLARIZATIONS

The amplitude of DADs and the possibility of triggered activity are influenced by the level of membrane potential at which the action potential occurs. The reduction of the membrane potential during DADs may also result in Na^+ channel inactivation and a slowing of conduction.

The duration of the action potential is a critical determinant of the presence of DADs. Longer action potentials, which are associated with more transsarcolemmal Ca^{2+} influx, are more likely to be associated with DADs. Drugs that prolong action potential duration (e.g., class IA antiarrhythmic agents) can increase DAD amplitude, whereas drugs that shorten action potential duration (e.g., class IB antiarrhythmic agents) can decrease DAD amplitude.

The number of the action potentials preceding the DAD affects the amplitude of the DAD; that is, after a period of quiescence, the initiation of a single action potential can be followed by either no DAD or only a small one. With continued stimulation, the DADs increase in amplitude, and triggered activity can eventually occur.

The amplitude of DADs and the coupling interval between the first triggered impulse and the last stimulated impulse that induced them are directly related to the drive CL at which triggered impulses are initiated. A decrease in the basic drive CL (even a single drive

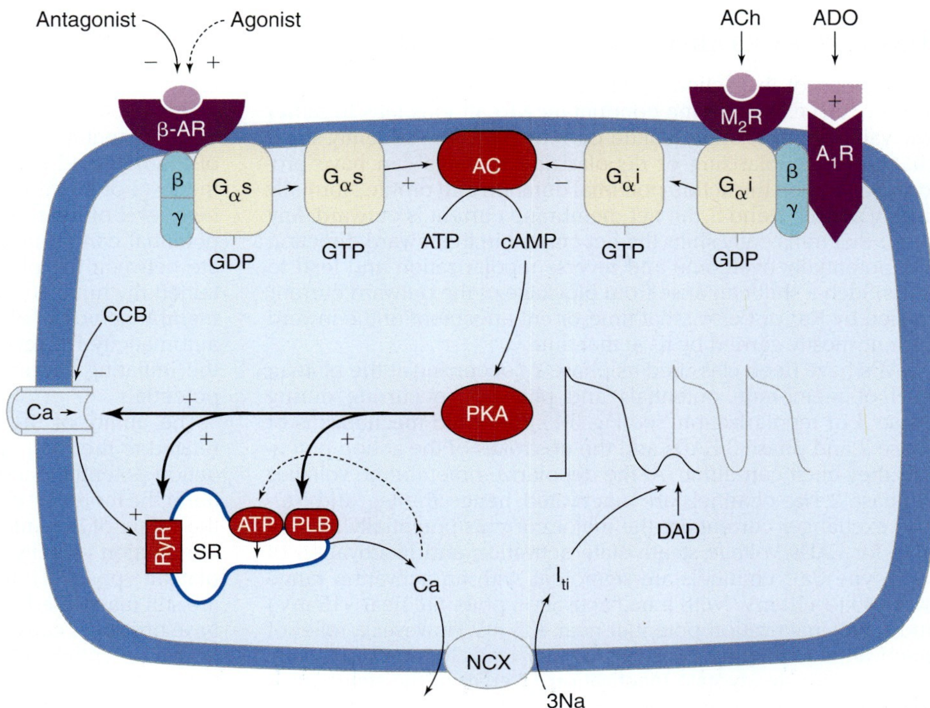

FIGURE 3-6 Signal transduction schema for initiation and termination of cyclic adenosine monophosphate (cAMP)-mediated triggered activity. See text for discussion. AC = adenylyl cyclase; ACh = acetylcholine; ADO = adenosine; A_1R = alpha$_1$-adenosine receptor; ATP = adenosine triphosphate; β-AR = beta-adrenergic receptor; Ca = calcium; CCB = calcium channel blocker; DAD = delayed afterdepolarization; $G_\alpha i$ = inhibitory G protein; $G_\alpha s$ = stimulatory G protein; GDP = guanosine diphosphate; GTP = guanosine triphosphate; I_{ti} = transient inward current; M_2R = muscarinic receptor; Na = sodium; NCX = sodium (Na^+)-calcium (Ca^{2+}) exchanger; PLB = phospholamban; PKA = protein kinase A; RyR = ryanodine receptor; SR = sarcoplasmic reticulum. *(From Lerman BB: Mechanism of outflow tract tachycardia. Heart Rhythm 4:973, 2007.)*

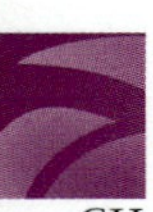

cycle; i.e., premature impulse), in addition to increasing the DAD amplitude, results in a decrease in the coupling interval between the last drive cycle and the first DAD-triggered impulse, with respect to the last driven action potential, and an increase of the rate of DADs. Triggered activity tends to be induced by a critical decrease in the drive CL, either spontaneous, such as in sinus tachycardia, or pacing induced. The increased time during which the membrane is in the depolarized state at shorter stimulation CLs or after premature impulses increases Ca^{2+} in the myoplasm and the sarcoplasmic reticulum, thus increasing the transient inward current responsible for the increased afterdepolarization amplitude, causing the current to reach its maximum amplitude more rapidly, and decreasing the coupling interval of triggered impulses. The repetitive depolarizations can increase intracellular Ca^{2+} because of repeated activation of I_{CaL}. This characteristic property can help distinguish triggered activity from reentrant activity because the relationship for reentry impulses initiated by rapid stimulation is often the opposite; that is, as the drive CL is reduced, the first reentrant impulse occurs later with respect to the last driven action potential because of rate-dependent conduction slowing in the reentrant pathway.

In general, triggered activity is influenced markedly by overdrive pacing. These effects are dependent on both the rate and the duration of overdrive pacing. When overdrive pacing is performed for a critical duration of time and at a critical rate during a catecholamine-dependent triggered rhythm, the rate of triggered activity slows until the triggered rhythm stops, because of enhanced activity of the electrogenic Na^+-K^+ exchange pump induced by the increase in intracellular Na^+ caused by the increased number of action potentials. When overdrive pacing is not rapid enough to terminate the triggered rhythm, it can cause overdrive *acceleration* (in contrast to overdrive suppression observed with automatic rhythms). Single premature stimuli also can terminate triggered rhythms, although termination is much less common than it is by overdrive pacing.

Early Afterdepolarizations and Triggered Activity

EADs are oscillations in membrane potential that occur during the action potential and interrupt the orderly repolarization of the myocyte. EADs manifest as a sudden change in the time course of repolarization of an action potential such that the membrane voltage suddenly shifts in a depolarizing direction.

IONIC BASIS OF EARLY AFTERDEPOLARIZATIONS

The plateau of the action potential is a time of high membrane resistance (i.e., membrane conductance to all ions falls to rather low values), when there is little current flow. Consequently, small changes in repolarizing or depolarizing currents can have profound effects on the action potential duration and profile. Normally, during phases 2 and 3, the net membrane current is outward. Any factor that transiently shifts the net current in the inward direction can potentially overcome and reverse repolarization and lead to EADs. Such a shift can arise from blockage of the outward current, carried by Na^+ or Ca^{2+} at that time, or enhancement of the inward current, mostly carried by K^+ at that time.[1]

EADs have been classified as phase 2 (occurring at the plateau level of membrane potential) and phase 3 (occurring during phase 3 of repolarization; see Fig. 3-4). The ionic mechanisms of phase 2 and phase 3 EADs and the upstrokes of the action potentials they elicit can differ.[1] At the depolarized membrane voltages of phase 2, Na^+ channels are inactivated; hence, the I_{CaL} and Na^+-Ca^{2+} exchanger current are the major currents potentially responsible for EADs. Voltage steady-state activation and inactivation of the L-type Ca^{2+} channels are sigmoidal, with an activation range over −40 to +10 mV (with a half-activation potential near −15 mV) and a half-inactivation potential near −35 mV. However, a relief of inactivation for voltages positive to 0 mV leads to a U-shaped voltage curve for steady-state inactivation. Overlap of the steady-state voltage-dependent inactivation and activation relations defines a "window" current near the action potential plateau, within which transitions from closed and open states can occur. As the action potential repolarizes into the window region, I_{CaL} increases and can potentially be sufficient to reverse repolarization, thus generating the EAD upstroke (Fig. 3-7).[23]

The cardiac Na^+-Ca^{2+} exchanger exchanges three Na^+ ions for one Ca^{2+} ion; the direction is dependent on the Na^+ and Ca^{2+} concentrations on the two sides of the membrane and the transmembrane potential difference. When operating in forward mode, this exchanger generates a net Na^+ influx, thereby resisting repolarization. The increase in the window I_{CaL} further increases the Na^+-Ca^{2+} exchanger, thus possibly facilitating EAD formation and increasing the probability of an EAD-triggered action potential.[23]

EADs occurring late in repolarization develop at membrane potentials more negative than −60 mV in atrial, ventricular, or Purkinje cells that have normal resting potentials. Normally, a net outward membrane current shifts the membrane potential progressively in a negative direction during phase 3 repolarization of the action potential. Despite fewer data, it has been suggested that current through the Na^+-Ca^{2+} exchanger and possibly the I_{Na} can participate in the activation of phase 3 EADs. Nevertheless, this concept was questioned by a study suggesting that phase 2 EADs appear to be responsible for inducing phase 3 EADs through electrotonic interactions and that a large voltage gradient related to heterogeneous repolarization is essential for phase 3 EADs.[23,24]

The upstrokes of the action potentials elicited by phase 2 and phase 3 EADs also differ.[1] Phase 2 EAD-triggered action potential upstrokes are exclusively mediated by Ca^{2+} currents. Even when these triggered action potentials do not propagate, they can substantially exaggerate heterogeneity of the time course of repolarization of the action potential (a key substrate for reentry), because EADs occur more readily in some regions (e.g., Purkinje fibers, mid left ventricular myocardium, right ventricular outflow tract epicardium) than others (e.g., left ventricular epicardium, endocardium). Action potentials triggered by phase 3 EADs arise from more negative membrane voltages. Therefore, the upstrokes can be caused by Na^+ and Ca^{2+} currents and are more likely to propagate.

Under certain conditions, when an EAD is large enough, the decrease in membrane potential leads to an increase in net inward (depolarizing) current, and a second upstroke or an action potential is *triggered* before complete repolarization of the first. The triggered action potential also can be followed by other action potentials, all occurring at the low level of membrane potential characteristic of the plateau or at the higher level of membrane potential of later phase 3 (Fig. 3-8). The sustained rhythmic activity can continue for a variable number of impulses and terminates when repolarization of the initiating action potential returns membrane potential to a high level. As repolarization occurs, the rate of the triggered rhythm slows because the rate is dependent on the level of membrane potential. Sometimes repolarization to the high level of membrane potential may not occur, and membrane potential can remain at the plateau level or at a level intermediate between the plateau level and the resting potential. The sustained rhythmic activity then can continue at the reduced level of membrane potential and assumes the characteristics of abnormal automaticity. However, in contrast to automatic rhythms, without the initiating action potential, there can be no triggered action potentials.

The ability of the triggered action potentials to propagate is related to the level of membrane potential at which the triggered action potential occurs. The more negative the membrane potential is, the more Na^+ channels are available for activation, the greater the influx of Na^+ into the cell during phase 0, and the higher the conduction velocity. At more positive membrane potentials of the plateau (phase 2) and early during phase 3, most Na^+ channels are still inactivated, and the triggered action potentials most likely have upstrokes caused by the inward I_{CaL}. Therefore, those triggered action potentials have slow upstrokes and are less able to propagate. Increased dispersion of repolarization facilitates the ability of phase 2 EADs to trigger propagating ventricular responses.[24]

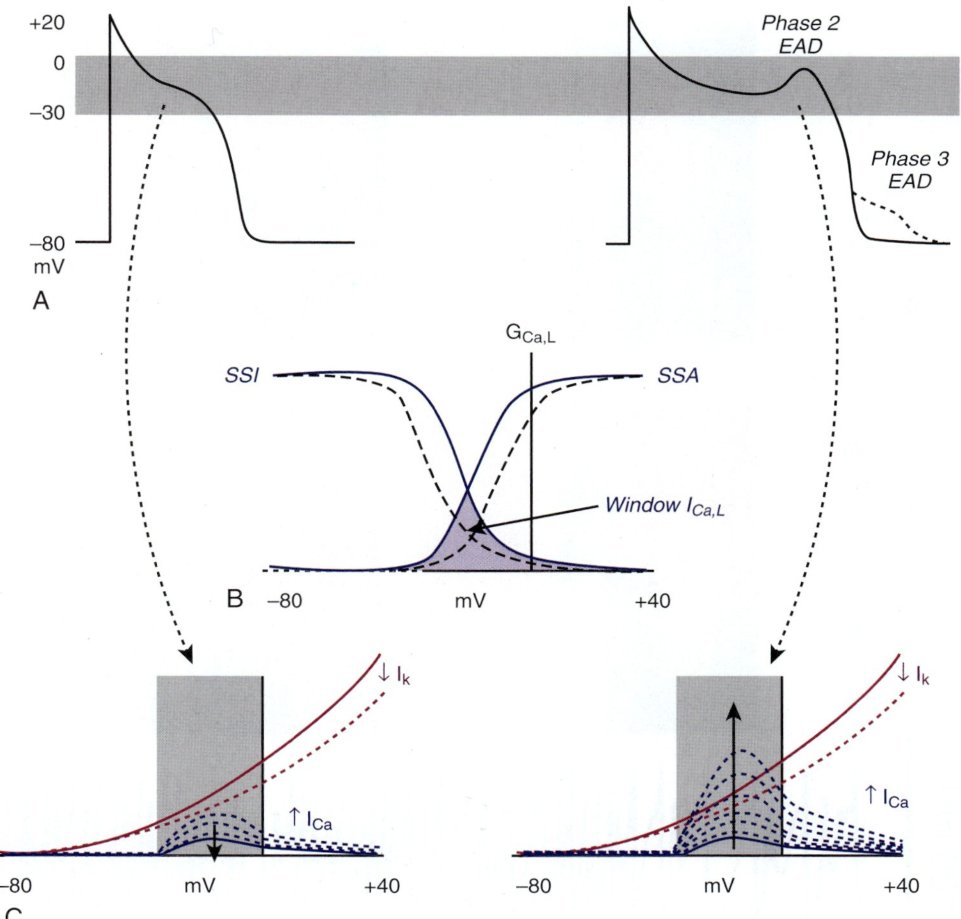

FIGURE 3-7 A, Normal action potential **(left)** and an action potential with phase 2 early afterdepolarization (EAD) (solid line) or phase 3 EAD (dashed line) **(right)**. B, Schematic plot of L-type calcium (Ca^{2+}) channel conductance ($G_{Ca,L}$) versus membrane voltage (mV) showing the window L-type inward Ca^{2+} current ($I_{Ca,L}$) region (purple area) where the steady-state activation (SSA) and steady-state inactivation (SSI) curves overlap and a fraction of Ca channels remain continuously open. Dashed lines show a potential therapeutic intervention that shifts the SSA and SSI curves to reduce the overlapping window current region. C, Schematic diagram illustrating the interaction between time-dependent $I_{Ca,L}$ reactivation (blue dashed lines) and time-dependent deactivation of repolarizing currents (I_K) (dashed red lines) in the window voltage range during action potential repolarization. For the normal action potential **(left)**, the repolarization rate is too fast for $I_{Ca,L}$ to grow larger than I_K. If the repolarization rate is too slow, however, $I_{Ca,L}$ can grow larger than I_K, thereby reversing repolarization to cause an EAD **(right)**. *(From Weiss JN, Garfinkel A, Karagueuzian HS, et al: Early afterdepolarizations and cardiac arrhythmias. Heart Rhythm 7:1891-1899, 2010.)*

A fundamental condition that underlies the development of EADs is action potential prolongation, which is manifest on the surface ECG by QT prolongation. Hypokalemia, hypomagnesemia, bradycardia, and drugs can predispose to the formation of EADs, invariably in the context of prolonging the action potential duration; drugs are the most common cause. Class IA and III antiarrhythmic agents prolong the action potential duration and the QT interval, effects intended to be therapeutic but frequently causing proarrhythmia. Noncardiac drugs such as some phenothiazines, some nonsedating antihistamines, and some antibiotics can also prolong the action potential duration and predispose to EAD-mediated triggered arrhythmias, particularly when there is associated hypokalemia, bradycardia, or both. Decreased extracellular K^+ concentration paradoxically decreases some membrane I_K (particularly the I_{Kr}) in the ventricular myocyte. This finding explains why hypokalemia causes action potential prolongation and EADs. EAD-mediated triggered activity likely underlies initiation of the characteristic polymorphic VT, torsades de pointes, seen in patients with congenital and acquired forms of long QT syndrome (see Chapter 31). Although the genesis of ventricular arrhythmias in these patients is still unclear, marked transmural dispersion of repolarization can create a vulnerable window for development of reentry. EADs arising from these regions can underlie the premature complexes that initiate or perpetuate the tachycardia.[1] Structural heart disease such as cardiac hypertrophy and failure can also delay ventricular repolarization—so-called electrical remodeling—and predispose to arrhythmias related to abnormalities of repolarization. The abnormalities of repolarization in hypertrophy and failure are often magnified by concomitant drug therapy or electrolyte disturbances.

EADs are opposed by ATP-dependent K^+ channel (I_{KATP}) openers (pinacidil, cromakalim, rimakalim, and nicorandil), magnesium, alpha-adrenergic blockade, tetrodotoxin, nitrendipine, and antiarrhythmic drugs that shorten action potential (e.g., lidocaine and mexiletine). Alpha-adrenergic stimulation can exacerbate EADs.

It was traditionally thought that unlike DADs, EADs do not depend on a rise in intracellular Ca^{2+}; instead, action potential prolongation and reactivation of depolarizing currents are fundamental to their production. More recent experimental evidence suggested a previously unappreciated interrelationship between intracellular Ca^{2+} loading and EADs. Cytosolic Ca^{2+} levels can increase when action potentials are prolonged. This situation, in turn, appears to enhance I_{CaL} (possibly via Ca^{2+}-calmodulin kinase activation), thus further prolonging the action potential duration as well as providing the inward current driving EADs. Intracellular Ca^{2+} loading by action potential prolongation can also enhance the likelihood of DADs. The interrelationship among intracellular Ca^{2+}, DADs, and EADs can be one explanation for the susceptibility of hearts that are Ca^{2+} loaded (e.g., in ischemia or congestive heart failure) to develop arrhythmias, particularly on exposure to action potential–prolonging drugs.

PROPERTIES OF EARLY AFTERDEPOLARIZATIONS

EAD-triggered arrhythmias exhibit rate dependence. In general, the amplitude of an EAD is augmented at slow rates when action potentials are longer in duration.[6] Pacing-induced increases in rate shorten the action potential duration and reduce EAD amplitude. Action potential shortening and suppression of EADs with increased stimulation rate are likely the result of augmentation of delayed rectifier I_K and perhaps hastening of Ca^{2+}-induced inactivation of I_{CaL}. Once EADs have achieved a steady-state magnitude at a constant drive CL, any event that shortens the drive CL tends to reduce their amplitude. Hence, the initiation of

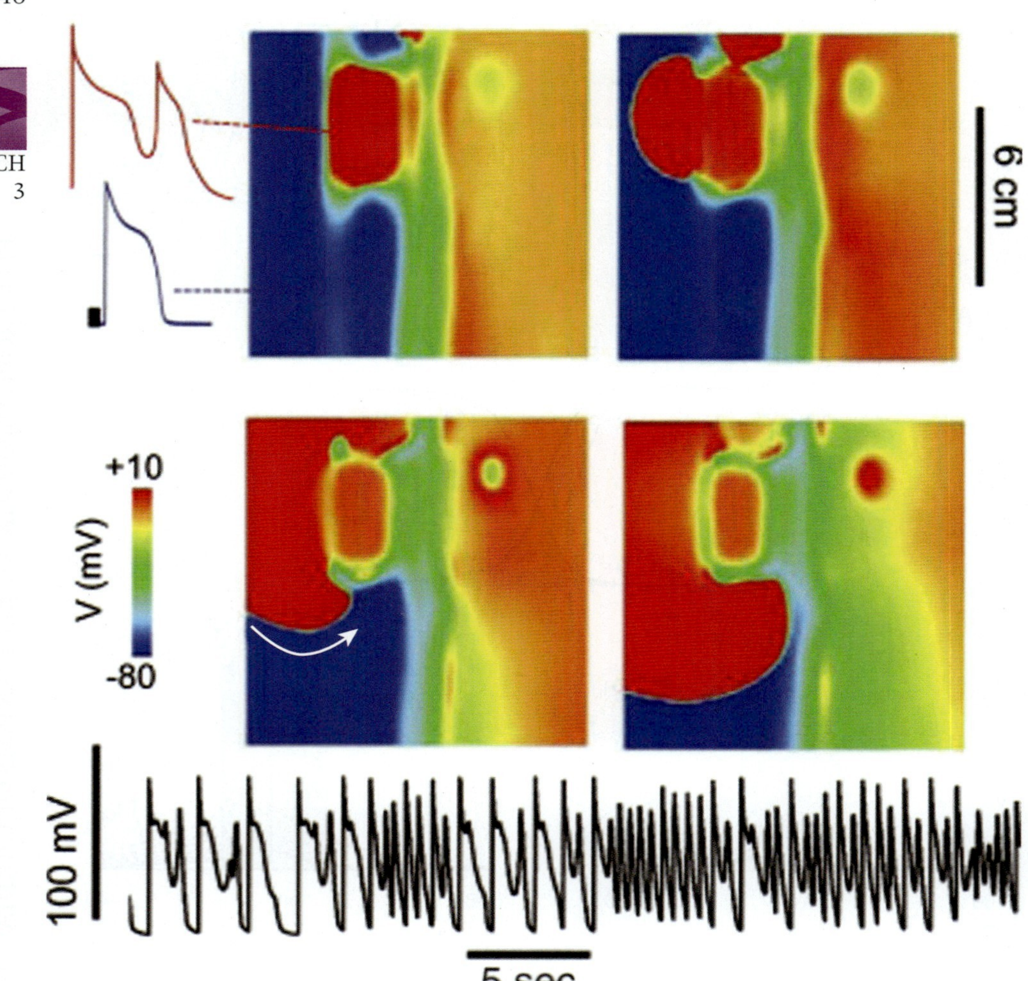

FIGURE 3-8 Mixed focal reentrant polymorphic ventricular tachycardia as a result of early afterdepolarization (EAD)-mediated premature ventricular complexes (PVCs) arising from EAD islands in simulated two-dimensional homogeneous tissue. The tissue was paced from the left edge at a slow rate. Four successive voltage snapshots show an EAD (red in **upper left quadrant**) that generates a PVC (red blob). The PVC then initiates reentry by reentering (white arrow) the receding waveback of the region without EADs (blue blob). The voltage trace below from a representative cell shows multiple EADs followed by rapid tachycardia resulting from a mixture of triggered activity and reentry. *(From Weiss JN, Garfinkel A, Karagueuzian HS, et al: Early afterdepolarizations and cardiac arrhythmias. Heart Rhythm 7:1891-1899, 2010.)*

a single premature depolarization, which is associated with an acceleration of repolarization, will reduce the magnitude of the EADs that accompany the premature action potential; as a result, triggered activity is not expected to follow premature stimulation. The exception is when a long compensatory pause follows a premature ventricular complex. This situation can predispose to the development of an EAD and can be the mechanism of torsades de pointes in some patients with the long QT syndrome. Thus, EADs are more likely to trigger rhythmic activity when the spontaneous heart rate is slow because bradycardia is associated with prolongation of the QT interval and action potential duration (e.g., bradycardia- or pause-induced torsades de pointes). Similarly, catecholamines increase heart rate and decrease action potential duration and EAD amplitude, despite the effect of beta-adrenergic stimulation to increase I_{CaL}.

Reentry

Basic Principles of Reentry

During each normal cardiac cycle, at the completion of normal cardiac excitation, the electrical impulse originating from the sinus node becomes extinct, and the subsequent excitation cycles originate from new pacemaker impulses.[6] Physiological excitation waves vanish spontaneously after the entire heart has been activated because of the long duration of refractoriness in the cardiac tissue compared with the duration of the excitation period; therefore, after its first pass, the impulse, having no place to go, expires. Reentry occurs when a propagating impulse fails to die out after normal activation of the heart and persists to reexcite the heart after expiration of the refractory period. In pathological settings, excitation waves can be blocked in circumscribed areas, rotate around these zones of block, and reenter the site of original excitation in repetitive cycles. The wavefront does not extinguish but rather propagates continuously and thus continues to excite the heart because it always encounters excitable tissue.

Reentrant tachycardia, also called reentrant excitation, reciprocating tachycardia, circus movement, or reciprocal or echo beats, is a continuous repetitive propagation of the activation wave in a circular path, returning to its site of origin to reactivate that site.[1,25,26] Traditionally, reentry has been divided into two types: (1) anatomical reentry, when there is a distinct relationship of the reentry pathway with the underlying tissue structure; and (2) functional reentry, when reentrant circuits occur at random locations without clearly defined anatomical boundaries (Fig. 3-9). Although this distinction has a historical background and is useful for didactic purposes, both the anatomical and functional forms can coexist in a given pathological setting and share many common basic biophysical mechanisms.

The original 3 criteria for reentry proposed by Mines still hold true: (1) unidirectional block is necessary for initiation; (2) the wave of excitation should travel in a single direction around the pathway, returning to its point of origin and then restarting along the same path; and (3) the tachycardia should terminate when one limb of the pathway is cut or temporarily blocked. The 12 conditions that were proposed to prove or identify the existence of reentrant tachycardia in the EP laboratory are listed in Table 3-1.[25,26]

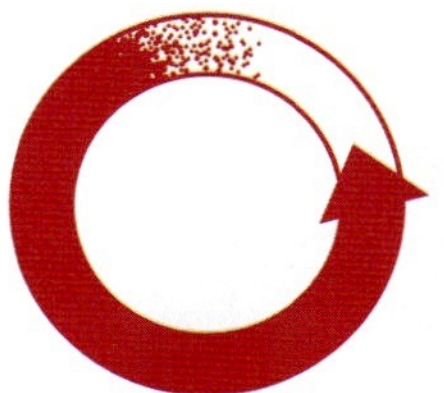

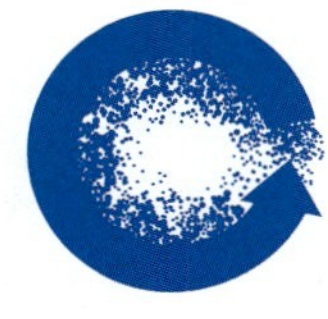

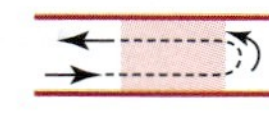

Anatomical reentry Functional reentry Reflected reentry

FIGURE 3-9 Models of reentry; the solid area is completely refractory tissue, and mottled area is partially refractory. In anatomical reentry, the circuit is determined by structures or scar in the heart, and a portion of the circuit that has fully recovered excitability can be stimulated while it awaits the next cycle. In functional reentry, however, the rate is as rapid as it can be and still allow all portions of the circuit to recover.

TABLE 3-1 Criteria for Diagnosis of Reentrant Tachycardia

1. Mapping activation in one direction around the continuous loop
2. Correlation of continuous electrical activity with occurrence of tachycardia
3. Correlation of unidirectional block with initiation of reentry
4. Initiation and termination by premature stimulation
5. Dependence of initiation of the arrhythmia on the site of pacing
6. Inverse relationship between the coupling interval of the initiating premature stimulus and the interval to the first tachycardia beat
7. Resetting of the tachycardia by a premature beat, with an inverse relationship between the coupling interval of the premature beat and the cycle length of the first or return beat of the tachycardia
8. Fusion between a premature beat and the tachycardia beat followed by resetting
9. Transient entrainment (with external overdrive pacing, the ability to enter the reentrant circuit and capture the circuit, resulting in tachycardia at the pacing rate with fused complexes)
10. Abrupt termination by premature stimulation
11. Dependence of initiation on critical slowing of conduction in the circuit
12. Similarity with experimental models in which reentry is proven and is the only mechanism of tachycardia

Requisites of Reentry

SUBSTRATE

The initiation and maintenance of a reentrant arrhythmia require the presence of myocardial tissue with adjacent tissue or pathways having different EP properties, conduction, and refractoriness, and that they be joined proximally and distally, forming a circuit. These circuits can be stationary or can move within the myocardial substrate.

The reentrant circuit can be an anatomical structure, such as a loop of fiber bundles in the Purkinje system or accessory pathways, or a functionally defined pathway, with its existence, size, and shape determined by the EP properties of cardiac tissues in which the reentrant wavefront circulates. The circuit can also be an anatomical-functional combination. The cardiac tissue that constitutes the substrate for reentrant excitation can be located almost anywhere in the heart.[1] The reentrant circuit can be a variety of sizes and shapes and can include different types of myocardial cells (e.g., atrial, ventricular, nodal, Purkinje; Fig. 3-10).

CENTRAL AREA OF BLOCK

A core of inexcitable tissue around which the wavefront circulates is required to sustain reentry. Without this central area of block, the excitation wavefront will not necessarily be conducted around the core of excitable tissue; rather, it could take a shortcut, permitting the circulating excitation wavefront to arrive early at the site where it originated. If it arrives sufficiently early, the tissue at the site of origination will still be refractory, and reentrant excitation will not be possible.

As mentioned earlier, the area of block can be anatomical, functional, or a combination of the two.[6,27] Anatomical block is the result of a nonconductive medium in the center of the circuit, such as the tricuspid annulus in typical atrial flutter (AFL). Functional block at the center of a circuit occurs when there is block of impulses in otherwise excitable cardiac muscle. The central area of functional block develops during the initiation of the reentrant circuit by the formation of a line of block that most likely is caused by refractoriness. When the reentrant circuit forms, the line of block then is sustained by centripetal activation from the circulating wavefront that, by repeatedly bombarding the central area of block, maintains the state of refractoriness of this region. A combination of an anatomical and a functional central area of block in the reentrant circuit has been described in some models of AFL such as the orifice of one or both venae cavae and an area of functional block continuous with or adjacent to either or both caval orifice(s). Additionally, it has now been shown that a functional extension of an anatomical line of block can occur such that it plays a role in creating the necessary or critical substrate for reentry. Thus, a surgical incision in the right atrium made to repair a congenital heart lesion can, under certain circumstances, develop a functional extension to one or both of the venae cavae, such that the substrate to create and sustain AFL develops.

UNIDIRECTIONAL CONDUCTION BLOCK

Transient or permanent unidirectional block is usually a result of heterogeneity of EP properties of the myocardium and is essential for the initiation of reentry. The excitation wavefront propagating in the substrate must encounter unidirectional block; otherwise, the excitation wavefronts traveling down both limbs of the reentrant circuit will collide and extinguish each other.[27]

AREA OF SLOW CONDUCTION

In a successful reentrant circuit, the wavefront of excitation must encounter excitable cells or the tachycardia will terminate. Therefore, a condition necessary for reentry is the maintenance of excitable tissue ahead of the propagating wavefront. In other words, the tissue initially activated by the excitation wavefront should have sufficient time to recover its excitability by the time the reentrant wavefront returns. Thus, conduction of the circulating wavefront must be sufficiently delayed in an alternate pathway to allow for expiration of the refractory period in the tissue proximal to the site of unidirectional block, and there must always be a gap of excitable tissue (fully or partially excitable) ahead of the circulating wavefront (i.e., the length of the reentrant pathway must equal or exceed the reentrant wavelength; see later). This is facilitated by a sufficiently long reentrant pathway (which is especially important when conduction is normal along the reentrant path), sufficiently slow conduction in all or part of the alternative pathway (because sufficiently long pathways are usually not present in the heart), sufficient shortening of the refractory period, or a combination of these factors.[1]

CRITICAL TISSUE MASS

An additional requisite for random reentry is the necessity of a critical mass of tissue to sustain the one or usually more simultaneously circulating reentrant wavefronts. Thus, it is essentially impossible to achieve sustained fibrillation of ventricles of very small, normal, mammalian hearts and equally difficult to achieve sustained fibrillation of the completely normal atria of humans or smaller mammals.

INITIATING TRIGGER

Another prerequisite for reentrant excitation to occur is often, but not always, the presence of an initiating trigger, which invokes the necessary EP milieu for initiation of reentry.[1] Susceptible patients

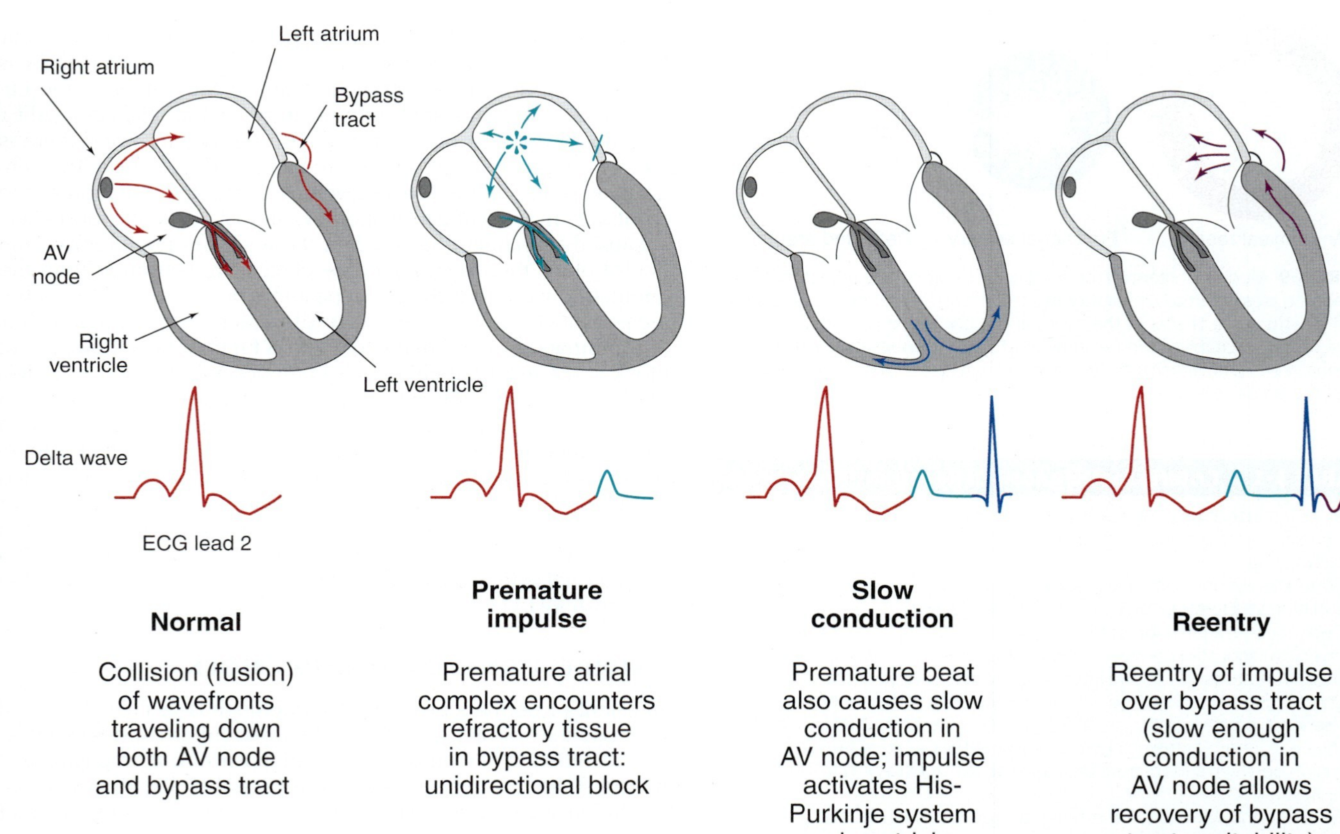

FIGURE 3-10 Reentry in the Wolff-Parkinson-White syndrome. AV = atrioventricular.

with appropriate underlying substrates usually do not suffer from incessant tachycardia because the different EP mechanisms required for the initiation and maintenance of a reentrant tachycardia are infrequently present at exactly the same time. However, changes in heart rate or autonomic tone, ischemia, electrolyte or pH abnormalities, or the occurrence of a premature depolarization can be sufficient to initiate reentrant tachycardia.

The trigger frequently is required because it elicits or brings to a critical state one or more of the conditions necessary to achieve reentrant excitation. In fact, premature depolarizations frequently initiate these tachyarrhythmias because they can cause slow conduction and unidirectional block. Thus, a premature impulse initiating reentry can arrive at one site in the potential reentrant circuit sufficiently early that it encounters unidirectional block, because that tissue has had insufficient time to recover excitability after excitation by the prior impulse. Furthermore, in the other limb of the potential reentrant circuit, the premature arrival of the excitation wavefront causes slow conduction or results in further slowing of conduction of the excitation wavefront through an area of already slow conduction. The resulting increase in conduction time around this limb of the potential reentrant circuit allows the region of unidirectional block in the tissue in the other limb activated initially by the premature beat to recover excitability. It should be noted that the mechanism causing the premature impulse can be different from the reentrant mechanism causing the tachycardia. Thus, the premature impulse can be caused by automaticity or triggered activity.

Types of Reentrant Circuits

ANATOMICAL REENTRY

In anatomically determined circuits, a discrete inexcitable anatomical obstacle creates a surrounding circular pathway, resulting in a fixed length and location of the reentrant circuit. Because the length and location of the reentrant pathway are relatively fixed, the characteristics of the reentrant circuit are determined by the characteristics of the anatomical components of that circuit.

A reentrant tachycardia is initiated when an excitation wavefront splits into two limbs after going around the anatomical obstacle and travels down one pathway and not the other, thus creating a circus movement. Tachycardia rates are determined by the wavelength and by the length of the reentrant pathway (the path length). The initiation and maintenance of anatomical reentry depend on conduction velocity and refractory period. Thus, as long as the extension of the refractory zone behind the excitation wave, the so-called wavelength of excitation, is smaller than the entire length of the anatomically defined reentrant pathway, a zone of excitable tissue, the so-called excitable gap, exists between the tail of the preceding wave and the head of the following wave.[27] In essence, circus movements containing an excitable gap are stable with respect to their frequency of rotation and can persist at a constant rate for hours. In the setting where the wavelength of excitation exceeds the path length, the excitation wavefront becomes extinct when it encounters the not yet recovered inexcitable tissue. A special case is present in the intermediate situation, when the head of the following wavefront meets the partially refractory tail of the preceding wavefront (i.e., the wavelength approximates the path length). This situation is characterized by unstable reentrant CLs and complex dynamics of the reentrant wavefront. There is often a long excitable gap associated with anatomical reentry.

Anatomical circuits therefore are associated with ordered reentry. Examples of this type of reentry are AV reentrant tachycardia associated with an AV bypass tract, AVN reentrant tachycardia, AFL, VT originating within the HPS (bundle branch reentrant VT), and post-MI VT.

FUNCTIONAL REENTRY

In functionally determined circuits, the reentrant pathway depends on the intrinsic heterogeneity of the EP properties of the myocardium, not by a predetermined anatomical circuit (i.e., without involvement of an anatomical obstacle or anatomically defined conducting pathway). Such heterogeneity involves dispersion of excitability or refractoriness and conduction velocity, as well as anisotropic conduction properties of the myocardium.[28]

Functional circuits typically tend to be small and unstable; the reentrant excitation wavefront can fragment, generating other areas of reentry. The location and size of these tachycardias can vary. The circumference of the leading circle around a functional obstacle can be as small as 6 to 8 mm and represents a pathway in which the efficacy of stimulation of the circulating wavefront is just sufficient to excite the tissue ahead, which is still in its relative refractory phase. Therefore, conduction through the functional reentrant circuit is slowed because impulses are propagating in partially refractory tissue. Consequently, this form of functional reentry has a partially excitable gap. The reentry CLs are therefore significantly dependent on the refractory period of the involved tissue.[28]

The mechanisms for functionally determined reentrant circuits include the leading circle type of reentry, anisotropic reentry, and spiral wave reentry. Functional circuits can be associated with ordered reentry (the reentrant circuit remains in the same place) or random reentry (the reentrant circuit changes size and location). Random reentry can occur when leading circle reentry causes fibrillation.

Leading Circle Concept

To explain the properties of a single functional reentrant circuit, Allessie and colleagues formulated the leading circle concept (see Fig. 3-9).[28] It was postulated that during wavefront rotation in tissue without anatomical inexcitable obstacles, the wavefront impinges on its refractory tail and travels through partially refractory tissue. The interaction between the wavefront and the refractory tail determines the properties of functional reentry. In this model, functional reentry involves the propagation of an impulse around a functionally determined region of inexcitable tissue or a refractory core and among neighboring fibers with different EP properties. The tissue within this core is maintained in a state of refractoriness by constant centripetal bombardment from the circulating wavefront. The premature impulse that initiates reentry blocks in fibers with long refractory periods and conducts in fibers with shorter refractory periods and eventually returns to the initial region of block after excitability has recovered there. The impulse then continues to circulate around a central area that is kept refractory because it is bombarded constantly by wavelets propagating toward it from the circulating wavefront. This central area provides a functional obstacle that prevents excitation from propagating across the fulcrum of the circuit.

The leading circle was defined as "the smallest possible pathway in which the impulse can continue to circulate" and "in which the stimulating efficacy of the wavefront is just enough to excite the tissue ahead which is still in its relative refractory phase."[28] Thus, the "head of the circulating wavefront is continuously biting its tail of refractoriness" and the length of the reentrant pathway equals the wavelength of the impulse; as a result, there is usually no fully excitable gap.[28] Because the wavefront propagates through partially refractory tissue, the conduction velocity is reduced.

The velocity value and the length of the circuit depend on the excitability of the partially refractory tissue and on the stimulating efficacy of the wavefront, which is determined by the amplitude and the upstroke velocity of the action potential and by the passive electrical properties of the tissue (e.g., gap junctional conductance). The partially refractory tissue determines the revolution time period. Because of the absence of a fully excitable gap, this form of reentry is less susceptible to resetting, entrainment, and termination by premature stimuli and pacing maneuvers. Leading circle reentry is thought to be the underlying mechanism of AF and VF and of at least some of the ventricular arrhythmias associated with acute ischemia.

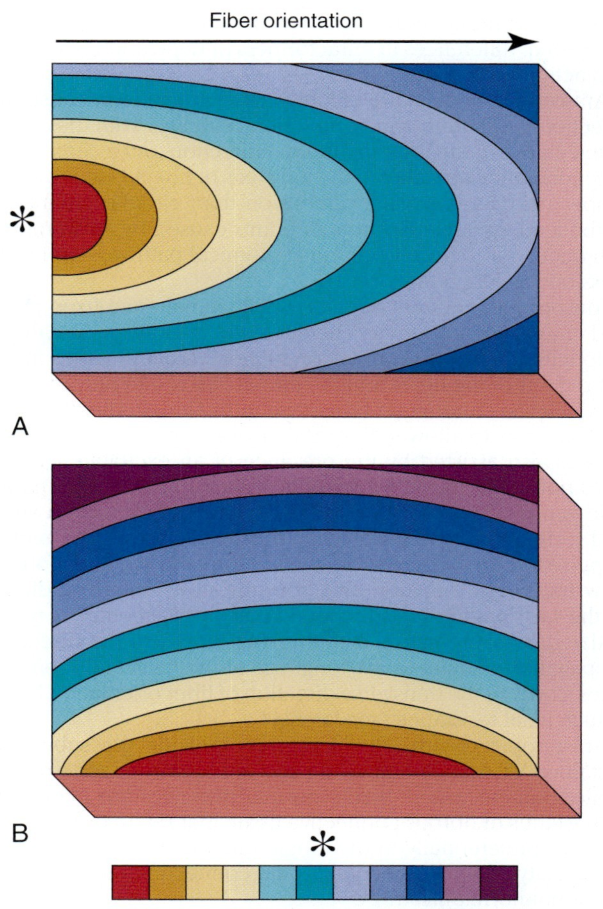

FIGURE 3-11 Anisotropic conduction. Progression of activation wavefronts in blocks of ventricular myocardium with longitudinal fiber orientation are shown. A wavefront stimulated (asterisk) at the left edge progresses more rapidly (wider isochrone spacing, **A**) than one starting perpendicularly (**B**) because of more favorable conduction parameters in the former direction.

Anisotropic Reentry

Isotropic conduction is uniform in all directions; anisotropic conduction is not. Anisotropy is a normal feature of heart muscle and is related to the differences in longitudinal and transverse conduction velocities, which are attributable to the lower resistivity of myocardium in the longitudinal (parallel to the long axis of the myocardial fiber bundles) versus the transverse direction (Fig. 3-11). Anisotropy in myocardium composed of tissue with structural features different from those of adjacent tissue results in heterogeneity in conduction velocities and repolarization properties (see later discussion), which can lead to blocked impulses and slowed conduction, thereby setting the stage for reentry (referred to as anisotropic reentry).

Unlike the functional characteristic that leads to the leading circle type of reentry (differences in refractoriness in adjacent areas caused by local differences in membrane properties), the functional characteristic that is important in functional reentry caused by anisotropy is the difference in effective axial resistance to impulse propagation dependent on fiber direction. In its pure form, the unidirectional conduction block and slow conduction in the reentrant circuit result from anisotropic, discontinuous propagation,

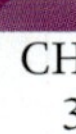

and there is no need for variations in membrane properties, such as regional differences in refractoriness or depression of the resting and action potentials.[29]

Anisotropic circuits are elliptical or rectangular because of the directional differences in conduction velocities, with the long axis of the ellipse in the fast longitudinal direction and a central line of functional block parallel to the long axis of fibers. Circuits with this shape can have a smaller dimension than circular circuits, such as the leading circle. Reentrant circuits caused by anisotropy also can occur without well-defined anatomical pathways and may be classified as functional.

Anisotropic reentrant circuits usually remain in a fixed position and cause ordered reentry. The degree of anisotropy (i.e., the ratio of longitudinal to transverse conduction velocity) varies in different regions of the heart, and the circuit can reside only in a region in which the conduction transverse to the longitudinal axis is sufficiently slow to allow reentry. Stability of anisotropic reentrant circuits is also assisted by the presence of an excitable gap, which does not occur in the leading circle functional circuit. The excitable gap is caused by the sudden slowing of conduction velocity and a decrease in the wavelength of excitation as the reentrant impulse turns the corner from the fast longitudinal direction to the slow transverse direction and from the slow transverse direction to the fast longitudinal direction. Anisotropic reentry is typically initiated by a premature stimulus that blocks in the direction of propagation parallel to the long axis of the cells and then propagates slowly in the transverse direction of fiber orientation because of high axial resistance (see later).[29]

Anisotropic reentry can potentially provide the substrate for sustained VT that occurs in the epicardial border zone region of healed infarcts, where viable normal myocytes are intermingled with islands of fibrous connective tissue that separate muscle-fiber bundles preferentially in the longitudinal direction and decrease the density of side-to-side junctional connections, therefore creating nonuniform anisotropy.

Figure-of-8 Reentry

The model of figure-of-8 or double-loop reentry involves two concomitant excitation wavefronts circulating in opposite directions, clockwise and counterclockwise, around a long line of functional conduction block rejoining on the distal side of the block. The wavefront then breaks through the arc of block to reexcite the tissue proximal to the block. The single arc of block is thus divided into two, and reentrant activation continues as two circulating wavefronts that travel clockwise and counterclockwise around the two arcs in a pretzel-like configuration.[30] This form of reentry has been shown in atrial and ventricular myocardia (Fig. 3-12, Video 1).

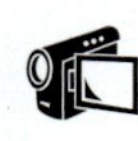

Reflection

Reflection is a special subclass of reentry in which the excitation wavefront does not require a circuit but appears to travel back and forth in a linear segment of tissue (e.g., trabecula or Purkinje fiber) containing an area of conduction block (see Fig. 3-9). In such a situation, an action potential propagates toward, but not through, the inexcitable zone. Subsequently, an electrotonic current conducts passively (i.e., without eliciting an action potential) through the inexcitable zone toward the distal portion of the pathway. If the inexcitable zone is sufficiently small and the magnitude of the electrotonic current is sufficiently large, the segment of tissue distal to the blocked area will be excited (i.e., an action potential is elicited) but with a significant delay. The action potential generated in the distal portion of the pathway will then cause electrotonic current to flow back through the inexcitable zone toward the proximal region. Provided the proximal portion of the conduction pathway recovers quickly enough, this current may be sufficient to elicit a second action potential on the proximal side of the inexcitable zone, which propagates in the opposite direction to the first action potential, thus giving the appearance that the inexcitable zone has reflected the initial action potential. Because reflection can occur within areas of tissue as small as 1 to 2 mm^2, it is likely to appear of focal origin. Its identification as a mechanism of arrhythmia may be difficult even with very high spatial resolution mapping of the electrical activity of discrete sites.

Phase 2 Reentry

As discussed in Chapter 1, substantial differences in the expression levels of ion channels underlie the substantial heterogeneity in action potential duration and configuration between cardiomyocytes across the ventricular wall. Heterogeneity in the distribution of the transient outward I_K (I_{to}) channels across the myocardial wall, being more prominent in ventricular epicardium than endocardium, results in the shorter duration and the prominent phase 1 notch and the "spike and dome" morphology of the epicardial action potential as compared with the endocardium. The resultant transmural voltage gradient during the early phases (phases 1 and 2) of the action potential is thought to be responsible for the inscription of the J wave on the surface ECG (see Fig. 31-6). A significant outward shift of currents, secondary to either a decrease in the inward currents (I_{Na} and I_{CaL}) or an increase in the outward I_K (I_{to}, I_{Kr}, I_{Ks}, I_{KACH}, I_{KATP}), or both, can cause partial or complete loss of the dome of the action potential in the epicardium that leads to exaggeration of transmural voltage gradient and dispersion of repolarization between the epicardium and endocardium. The type of the ion current affected and its regional distribution in the ventricles determine the particular phenotype (including the Brugada syndrome, early repolarization syndrome, hypothermia-induced ST segment elevation, and infarction-induced ST segment elevation).[31]

In this setting, the phase 2 dome (plateau) of the action potential can potentially propagate from regions where it is preserved (midmyocardium and endocardium) to regions where it is abolished (epicardium), thus causing local reexcitation (phase 2 reentry) and the generation of a closely coupled extrasystole that, in turn, can initiate VT or VF (see Fig. 31-7).[32]

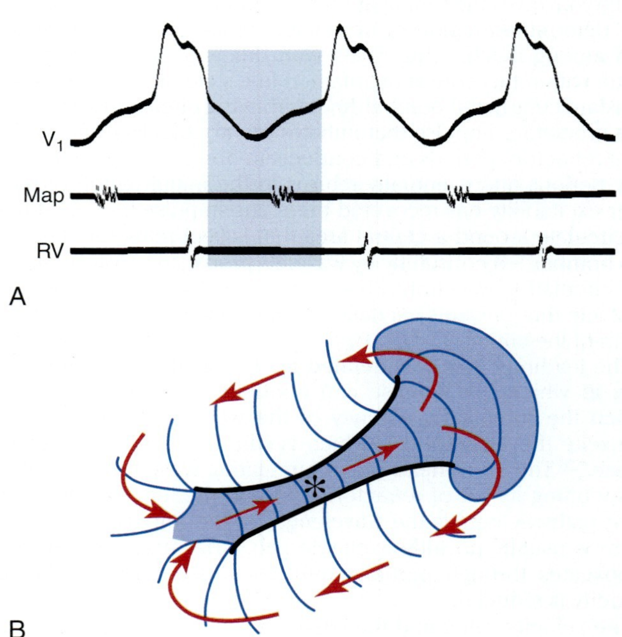

FIGURE 3-12 Figure-of-8 reentry. **A,** ECG and intracardiac recordings from a left ventricular mapping catheter (Map) and the right ventricle (RV) are shown during scar-based ventricular tachycardia. **B,** A stylized tachycardia circuit is shown in which propagation proceeds through a central common pathway (small arrows and asterisk) constrained by scar or other barriers and then around the outside of these same barriers. Activation in the circuit during electrical diastole is shaded (also in **A**).

Spiral Wave (Rotor) Activity

The leading circle concept was based on properties of impulse propagation in a one-dimensional tissue that forms a closed pathway (e.g., a ring). The concept was a major breakthrough in the understanding of the mechanisms of reentrant excitation. However, it became evident that these considerations alone do not fully describe wave rotation in two- and three-dimensional cardiac tissue.[33]

Spiral waves typically describe reentry in two dimensions. The term *rotor* initially described the rotating source, and the spiral wave defined the shape (i.e., curvature) of the wave emerging from the rotating source. In many publications, this difference has been blurred, and terms used in the literature include *rotors, vortices,* and *reverberators*.[27] The center of the spiral wave is called the core, and the distribution of the core in three dimensions is referred to as the filament. The three-dimensional form of the spiral wave is called a scroll wave.[30,33]

Under appropriate circumstances, a pulse in two-dimensional, homogeneous, excitable media can be made to circulate as a rotor. When heterogeneities in recovery exist, the application of a second stimulus over a large geometric area to initiate a second excitation wave only excites a region in which there has been sufficient time for recovery from the previous excitation, not regions that have not yet recovered. An excitation wave is elicited at the excitable site in the form of a rotor because the wave cannot move in the direction of the wake of the previous wave but only in the opposite direction, thus moving into adjacent regions as they in turn recover. The inner tip of the wavefront circulates around an organizing center or core, which includes cells with transmembrane potentials that have a reduced amplitude, duration, and rate of depolarization (i.e., slow upstroke velocity of phase 0); these cells are potentially excitable, but they remain unexcited, instead of a region of conduction block. In the center of the rotating wave, the tip of the wave moves along a complex trajectory and radiates waves into the surrounding medium. In addition, the spiral waves can give rise to daughter spirals that can result in disorganized electrical activity.[34]

The curvature of the spiral wave is the key to the formation of the core and the functional region of block.[27,30] Propagation of two- and three-dimensional waves also depends on wavefront curvature, a property that is not present in one-dimensional preparations.[27] Because the maximal velocity of a convex rotating wavefront can never exceed the velocity of a flat front and the period of rotation remains constant in a stable rotating wave, the velocity has to decrease from the periphery (where the highest value corresponds to linear velocity) to the center of a rotating wave. As a consequence, any freely rotating wave in an excitation-diffusion system has to assume a spiral shape. A prominent curvature of the spiral wave is generally encountered following a wave break, a situation in which a planar wave encounters an obstacle and breaks up into two or more daughter waves. Because it has the greatest curvature, the broken end of the wave moves most slowly. As curvature decreases along the more distal parts of the spiral, propagation speed increases.[30] The rotor, by definition, has a marked curvature, and this curvature slows down its propagation. Slow conduction results from an increased electrical load; that is, not only must a curved wavefront depolarize cells ahead of it in the direction of propagation, but also current flows to cells on its sides.

Because the slow activation by a rotor is not dependent on conduction in relatively refractory myocardium, an excitable gap exists, despite the functional nature of reentry. This type of functional reentrant excitation does not require any inhomogeneities of refractory periods as in leading circle reentry, inhomogeneities in conduction properties as in anisotropic reentry, or a central obstacle, whether functional or anatomical. The heterogeneity that allows initiation can result from a previous excitation wave and the pattern of recovery from that wave. Even though nonuniform dispersions of refractoriness or anisotropy are not necessary for the initiation of reentrant excitation caused by rotors in excitable media, the myocardium, even when normal, is never homogeneous, and anisotropy and anatomical obstacles can modify the characteristics and spatiotemporal behavior of the spiral.

The location of the rotor can occur wherever the second stimulated excitation encounters the wake of the first excitation with the appropriate characteristics. Spirals can be *stationary*, continuously drift or migrate away from their origin, or *anchored*, initially drifting and then becoming stationary by anchoring to a small obstacle.[34,35]

In the heart, spiral waves have been implicated in the generation of cardiac arrhythmias for a long time. Both two-dimensional spiral waves and three-dimensional scroll waves have been implicated in the mechanisms of reentry in atrial and ventricular tachycardia and fibrillation.[27] Monomorphic VT results when the spiral wave is anchored and cannot drift within the ventricular myocardium away from its origin. In contrast, a polymorphic VT, such as the torsades de pointes encountered with long QT syndromes, is thought to be caused by a meandering or drifting spiral wave. VF seems to be the most complex representation of rotating spiral waves in the heart. VF develops when the single spiral wave responsible for VT breaks up, leading to the development of multiple spirals that are continuously extinguished and recreated.[30,34,35]

Excitable Gaps in Reentrant Circuits

WAVELENGTH CONCEPT

The *wavelength* is defined as the product of the conduction velocity of the circulating excitation wavefront and the effective refractory period of the tissue in which the excitation wavefront is propagating.[6] The wavelength quantifies how far the impulse travels relative to the duration of the refractory period. The wavelength of the reentrant excitation wavefront must be shorter than the length of the pathway of the potential reentrant circuit for reentrant excitation to occur; that is, the impulse must travel a distance during the refractory period that is less than the complete reentrant path length to give myocardium ahead of it sufficient time to recover excitability. Slowing of impulse conduction or shortening of refractoriness shortens the wavelength and increases the excitable gap.

For almost all clinically important reentrant arrhythmias resulting from ordered reentry and in the presence of uniform, normal conduction velocity along the potential reentrant pathway, the wavelength would be too long to permit reentrant excitation. Thus, almost all these arrhythmias must have, and do have, one or more areas of slow conduction as a part of the reentrant circuit. The associated changes in conduction velocity, as well as associated changes in refractory periods, actually cause the wavelength to change in different parts of the circuit. However, the presence of one or more areas of slow conduction permits the average wavelength of reentrant activation to be shorter than the path length.

The wavelength concept is a good predictive parameter of arrhythmia inducibility. A decrease in conduction velocity or shortening of refractoriness results in a decrease in the wavelength or lessening of the amount of tissue needed to sustain reentry. This situation favors initiation and maintenance of reentry. In contrast, an increase in conduction velocity or prolongation of refractoriness prolongs the wavelength of excitation and, in this situation, a larger anatomical circuit is necessary to sustain reentry. If a larger circuit is not possible, initiation or maintenance of tachycardia cannot occur.

EXCITABLE GAPS

The excitable gap in a reentrant circuit is the region of excitable myocardium that exists between the head of the reentrant wavefront and the tail of the preceding wavefront and, at any given time, is no longer refractory (i.e., is capable of being excited) if the excitation wavelength is shorter than the length of the reentrant circuit (Fig. 3-13).

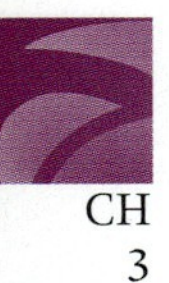

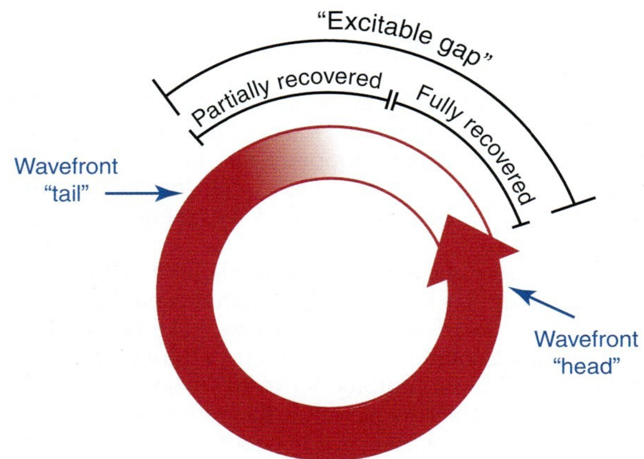

FIGURE 3-13 Excitable gap of recovered tissue in anatomically determined reentry.

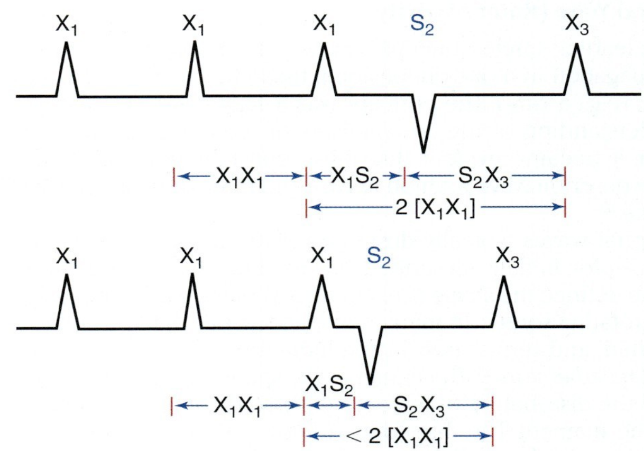

FIGURE 3-14 Response of tachycardia to a single extrastimulus (S_2). The tachycardia cycle length (CL) is [X_1X_1]. The coupling interval of the extrastimulus is [X_1S_2]. The return CL of the first complex of tachycardia after the extrastimulus is [S_2X_3]. In the **top portion** of the figure, the extrastimulus does not affect the tachycardia circuit, and a compensatory pause occurs. Resetting (i.e., advancement) of the tachycardia is shown at the **bottom of the figure**. *(From Frazier DW, Stanton MS: Resetting and transient entrainment of ventricular tachycardia. Pacing Clin Electrophysiol 18:1919, 1995.)*

The occurrence of an excitable gap is dependent on the recovery of excitability of the myocardium from its previous excitation by the reentrant wavefront. A fully excitable gap is defined as the segment of the reentrant circuit in which the tail of the preceding wavefront does not affect the head and velocity of the following wavefront (absence of head-tail interaction). A partially excitable gap is defined as the zone where the rotating wave can be captured by local stimulation in the presence of head-tail interaction. Whereas the excitable gap denotes a length of a segment within the reentrant circuit, the fully or partially excitable period denotes the time period during which a segment within the reentrant circuit is fully or partially excitable, respectively (see Fig. 3-13).

There are two different measurements of the excitable gap. The spatial excitable gap is the distance (in millimeters) of excitability occupied at any moment of time in the circuit ahead of the reentrant wavefront. On the other hand, the temporal excitable gap is the time interval (in milliseconds) of excitability between the head of activation of one impulse and the tail of refractoriness of the prior impulse. Both the spatial and temporal gaps can be composed of partially excitable or fully excitable myocardium, depending on the time interval between successive excitations of the circuit. The size of the spatial gap and the duration of the temporal gap vary in different parts of the circuit as the wavelength of the reentrant impulse changes because of changes in conduction velocity, refractory periods, or both.

The characteristics of the excitable gap can be different in different types of reentrant circuits. Many anatomically determined reentrant circuits have large excitable gaps with a fully excitable component, although, even in anatomically determined circuits, the gap can sometimes be only partially excitable. On the other hand, functional reentrant circuits caused by the leading circle mechanism have very small gaps that are only partially excitable, although parts of some functionally determined reentrant circuits (anisotropic reentrant circuits) can have fully excitable gaps. An excitable gap has been shown to occur during AF, VF, and AFL; these are examples of arrhythmias caused by functional reentrant mechanisms, possibly including spiral waves. The relationship between the excitable gap and the excitable period can be complex if the velocity of propagation changes within the reentry circuit.[27]

The existence and the extent of an excitable gap in a reentrant circuit have important implications.[27] The presence of an excitable gap enables modulation of the frequency of a reentrant tachycardia by a locally applied stimulus or by field stimulation; the longer the excitable gap is, the more likely it will be for an extrastimulus to be able to enter the reentrant circuit and initiate or terminate a reentrant arrhythmia. In addition, resetting and entrainment are more likely to occur when the excitable gap is longer. The excitable gap can be exploited to terminate a reentrant tachycardia. The presence of a significant temporal and spatial excitable gap in some reentrant circuits enables reentry to be terminated by a single premature stimulus or by overdrive stimulation. Termination of arrhythmias by stimulation would be expected to be much more difficult when the reentrant circuit has only a small partially excitable gap. Additionally, the excitable gap can influence the effects of drugs on the reentrant circuit, so that reentry with a partially excitable gap and mainly functional components may respond more readily to drugs that prolong repolarization, without slowing conduction, whereas fixed anatomical reentry with a large excitable gap responds to drugs that decrease conduction velocity, preferentially at pivot points.

The properties of the excitable gap influence the characteristics of arrhythmias caused by reentry. Arrhythmias caused by leading circle reentry, in which the wavefront propagates in the just-recovered myocardium of the refractory tail and in which there is only a small partially excitable gap, are inherently unstable and often terminate after a short period or go on to fibrillation. On the other hand, the reentrant wavefront in anatomical and nonuniform anisotropic reentrant circuits, in general, is not propagating in myocardium that has just recovered excitability, and the excitable gap can be large. This property can contribute to the stability of these reentrant circuits.[27]

The shape of the anatomical obstacle determines the path of a reentrant wave in fixed anatomical reentry. Therefore, instability of anatomical reentry is confined to variations of the rotating interval and wavelength of excitation. This instability is characterized by the wavefront's invading the repolarizing phase of the preceding wave, with resulting oscillations of the rotation period.[27]

Resetting Reentrant Tachycardias

DEFINITION

Resetting is the advancement (acceleration) of a tachycardia impulse by timed premature electrical stimuli. The extrastimulus is followed by a pause that is less than fully compensatory before resumption of the original rhythm. The tachycardia complexes that return first should have the same morphology and CL as the tachycardia before the extrastimulus, regardless of whether single or multiple extrastimuli are used.[36-38]

The introduction of a single extrastimulus (S_2) during a tachycardia yields a return cycle (S_2X_3) if the tachycardia is not terminated (Fig. 3-14). If S_2 does not affect the arrhythmogenic focus, the coupling interval (X_1S_2) plus the return cycle (S_2X_3) will be equal to twice the tachycardia cycle ($2 \times [X_1X_1]$); that is, a fully compensatory pause will occur. Resetting of the tachycardia occurs when a less than fully compensatory pause occurs. In this situation, $X_1S_2 + S_2X_3$ will be less than $2 \times (X_1X_1)$, as measured from the surface ECG. Tachycardia CL stability should be taken into account when the return cycle is measured. To account for any tachycardia CL instability, at least a 20-millisecond shortening of the return cycle is required to demonstrate resetting.[39]

When more than a single extrastimulus is used, the relative prematurity should be corrected by subtracting the coupling interval or intervals from the spontaneous tachycardia cycles when the extrastimuli are delivered.[40]

REENTRANT TACHYCARDIA RESETTING

To reset reentrant tachycardia, the stimulated wavefront must reach the reentrant circuit, encounter excitable tissue within the circuit (i.e., enter the excitable gap of the reentrant circuit), collide in the antidromic (retrograde) direction with the previous tachycardia impulse, and continue in the orthodromic (anterograde) direction to exit at an earlier than expected time and perpetuate the tachycardia (Fig. 3-15).[36-38] If the extrastimulus encounters fully excitable tissue, which commonly occurs in reentrant tachycardias with large excitable gaps, the tachycardia will be advanced by the extent that the stimulated wavefront arrives at the entrance site prematurely. If the tissue is partially excitable, which can occur in reentrant tachycardias with small or partially excitable gaps or even in circuits with large excitable gaps when the extrastimulus is very premature, the stimulated wavefront will encounter some conduction delay in the orthodromic direction within the circuit (see Fig. 3-15). Therefore, the degree of advancement of the next tachycardia beat depends on both the degree of prematurity of the extrastimulus and the degree of slowing of its conduction within the circuit. The reset tachycardia beat consequently can be early, on time, or delayed.

Termination of the tachycardia occurs when the extrastimulus collides with the preceding tachycardia impulse antidromically and blocks in the reentrant circuit orthodromically (see Fig. 3-15). This occurs when the premature impulse enters the reentrant circuit early in the relative refractory period; it fails to propagate in the anterograde direction because it encounters absolutely refractory tissue. In the retrograde direction, it encounters increasingly recovered tissue and can propagate until it encroaches on the circulating wavefront and terminates the arrhythmia.[39,40]

Resetting does not require that the pacing site be located in the reentrant circuit. The closer the pacing site is to the circuit, however, the less premature a single stimulus can be and reach the circuit without being extinguished by collision with a wave emerging from the circuit. The longest coupling interval for an extrastimulus to be able to reset a reentrant tachycardia depends on the tachycardia CL, the duration of the excitable gap of the tachycardia, refractoriness at the pacing site, and the conduction time from the pacing site to the reentrant circuit.[39]

Resetting Zone and Excitable Gap

For an extrastimulus to be able to reset the reentrant circuit, it has to penetrate the circuit during its excitable gap. The difference between the longest and shortest coupling intervals resulting in resetting is defined as the *resetting interval* or *resetting zone*.[37,39] Thus, the coupling intervals over which resetting occurs, the resetting zone, can be considered a measure of the duration of the temporal excitable gap existing in the reentrant circuit. Therefore, the entire extent of the fully excitable gap would be the zone of coupling intervals from the onset of tachycardia resetting until tachycardia termination. The excitable gap, however, can be underestimated by using only a single extrastimulus or by using single or double extrastimuli in the absence of tachycardia termination by the extrastimuli.

All tachycardias reset by a single extrastimulus can be reset by double extrastimuli, unless tachycardia termination occurs. Double extrastimuli produce resetting over a longer range of coupling intervals and should therefore be used to characterize the excitable gap of the reentrant circuit more fully. During EP testing, only the temporal excitable gap of the entire circuit can be evaluated. It is impossible to assess the conduction velocity and refractoriness at any point in the circuit, which certainly must vary, with available technology.

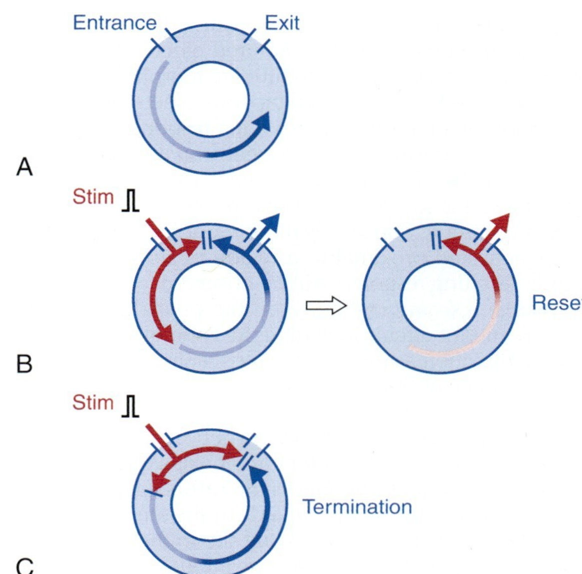

FIGURE 3-15 **A**, Schematic representation of the reentrant circuit is illustrated with separate entrance and exit sites. During tachycardia, a wavefront is shown propagating through the tissue of the reentrant circuit (arrow). The dark portion of the arrow represents fully refractory tissue, and the fading portion represents partially refractory tissue. **B**, A premature stimulus (Stim) introduced during the tachycardia results in a wavefront of depolarization (red arrow), which enters the reentrant circuit and conducts antegradely over fully excitable tissue while it collides retrogradely with the already propagating wavefront (blue arrow). The premature wavefront (red arrow) then propagates around the circuit to the exit site, thus leading to the less than compensatory pause and resetting of the tachycardia. **C**, A more premature extrastimulus (Stim) results in a wavefront of depolarization (red arrow), which enters the circuit at a time when it collides retrogradely with the previously propagating wavefront (blue arrow) and encounters antegrade tissue incapable of sustaining further propagation. As a result, circus movement in the circuit is extinguished, and tachycardia terminates. *(From Rosenthal ME, Stamato NJ, Almendral JM, et al: Coupling intervals of ventricular extrastimuli causing resetting of sustained ventricular tachycardia secondary to coronary artery disease: relation to subsequent termination. Am J Cardiol 61:770, 1988.)*

Return Cycle

The return cycle is the time interval from the resetting stimulus to the next excitation of the pacing site by the new orthodromic wavefront. This corresponds to the time required for the stimulated impulse to reach the reentrant circuit, conduct through the circuit, exit the circuit, and travel back to the pacing site.[37,39] The noncompensatory pause following the extrastimulus and the return cycle are typically measured at the pacing site; however, they may also be measured to the onset of the tachycardia complex on the surface ECG.

When the return cycle is measured from the extrastimulus producing resetting to the onset of the first return tachycardia complex on the surface ECG, conduction time into the tachycardia circuit is incorporated into that measurement. Conduction time between the pacing site and the tachycardia circuit may or may not be equal to that from the circuit to the pacing site. Differences in location of the site of stimulation, as well as the tachycardia circuit entrance and exit, can result in differences in conduction time to and from the pacing site.

Orthodromic and Antidromic Resetting

Antidromic resetting occurs when intracardiac sites are directly captured by the premature stimulus without traversing the reentrant circuit and the zone of slow conduction.[37] Therefore, antidromic resetting of intracardiac sites occurs with a conduction interval from the pacing stimulus to the captured electrogram that is less than the tachycardia CL and with differing morphology of the captured as compared with the spontaneous electrogram. Although demonstration of an antidromic resetting response can indicate a tachycardia mechanism other than reentry, an antidromic resetting pattern can also be observed during reentry with an excitable gap if the pacing site is located distal to a region of slow conduction in the reentry circuit. Conversely, if the recording sites are located in regions activated proximal to a region of slow conduction, an antidromic resetting response will be observed.

Orthodromic resetting occurs when the premature stimulus traverses the reentrant circuit, including the zone of slow conduction, in the same direction as the spontaneous tachycardia impulse and with an identical exit site.[37] Intracardiac areas that are orthodromically reset are advanced by the premature extrastimulus but retain the same morphology because they are activated from the impulse emerging from the same reentrant circuit exit site. The conduction interval from the pacing stimulus to the orthodromically captured electrogram exceeds the tachycardia CL by the time required for the extrastimulus to travel from the pacing site to the reentrant circuit. Thus, an orthodromic resetting response implies that the pacing site is located proximal to a region of slow conduction in the reentry circuit and that the recording site is located distal to this region. The ability to demonstrate orthodromic resetting is critically dependent on the location of pacing and recording electrodes relative to the region of slow conduction in the circuit. Therefore, failure to demonstrate an orthodromic resetting response does not exclude reentry with an excitable gap as a possible tachycardia mechanism.

RESETTING RESPONSE CURVES

Response patterns during resetting are characterized by plotting the coupling interval of the extrastimulus producing resetting versus the return cycle measured at the pacing site. Alternatively, the return cycle is measured to the onset of the first tachycardia complex following stimulation on the surface ECG; then, qualitatively similar but quantitatively different response curves are obtained.[39] Demonstration of a noncompensatory pause following the extrastimulus is required, and the interval encompassing the extrastimulus should be 20 or more milliseconds earlier than the expected compensatory pause following a single extrastimulus and 20 or more milliseconds less than three tachycardia CLs when double extrastimuli are used.[39] As always, it is important to establish the stability of tachycardia CL before assessing any perturbation in tachycardia presumed to be caused by resetting.

Four resetting response patterns are possible (Fig. 3-16)[39]:

1. During the *flat response pattern*, the return cycle is constant (less than a 10-millisecond difference) over a 30-millisecond range of coupling intervals.
2. With the *increasing response* pattern, the return cycle increases as the coupling interval increases.
3. With a *decreasing response pattern*, the return cycle decreases as the coupling interval increases.
4. A *mixed response pattern* meets the criteria for a flat response at long coupling intervals and for an increasing response at shorter coupling intervals.

Occasionally, a response pattern to a single extrastimulus cannot be characterized because resetting occurs over too narrow a range of coupling intervals as a result of significant variability of the baseline tachycardia CL or of variability in the return cycle. Triggered rhythms secondary to DADs usually have a flat or decreasing response. A flat response can be observed in automatic, triggered, or reentrant rhythms.

In all cases in which a single extrastimulus resets the tachycardia, double extrastimuli from the same pacing site produce an identical or expected resetting curve. Thus, if a single extrastimulus produces a flat curve, double extrastimuli will produce a flat or mixed curve. If a single extrastimulus produces an increasing or mixed curve, double extrastimuli will produce the same curve.

The types of resetting curves can vary depending on the site of stimulation. Extrastimuli from different pacing sites likely engage different sites in the reentrant circuit that are in different states of excitability or refractoriness and therefore result in different conduction velocities and resetting patterns.[39]

Flat Response Curves in Reentrant Rhythms

A flat resetting curve implies the presence of a fully excitable gap within the reentrant circuit over a range of coupling intervals. The total duration of the excitable gap should exceed the range of coupling intervals that produce resetting with a flat response. Large excitable gaps are more likely to result in flat response curves, because the increasingly premature extrastimuli are less likely to encroach on the trailing edge of refractoriness and encounter decremental conduction (see Fig. 3-16). The flat return cycle also suggests the presence of fixed sites of entrance and exit from the circuit and fixed conduction time from the stimulation site through the reentrant circuit over a wide range of coupling intervals.

If a single extrastimulus produced resetting with a flat response, the response to double extrastimuli would also be flat. However, because the use of double extrastimuli allows engagement of the reentrant circuit at relatively long coupling intervals with greater prematurity, resetting will begin at longer coupling intervals and will continue over a greater range of coupling intervals than observed with a single extrastimulus. Therefore, double extrastimuli can produce a flat and then increasing response curve.

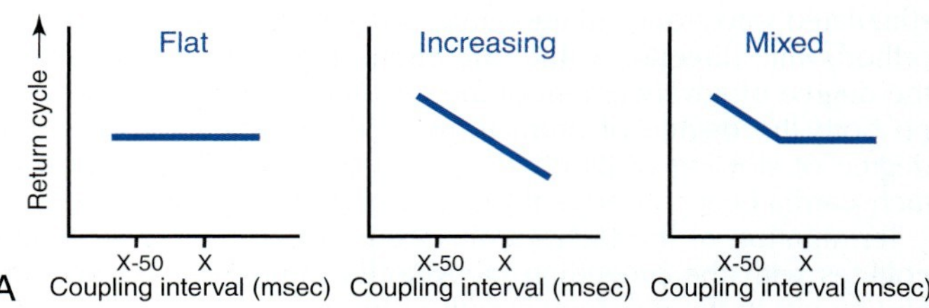

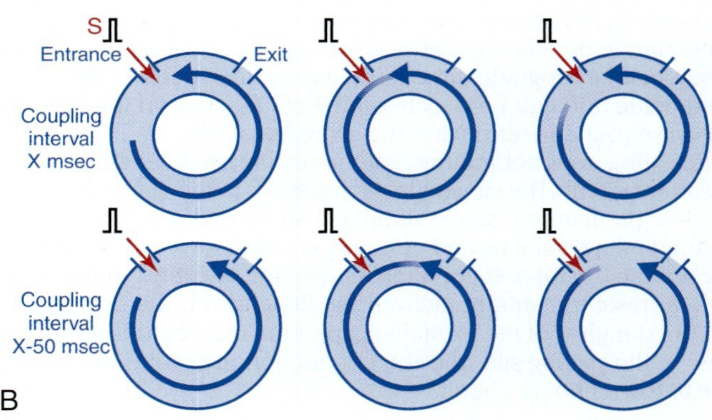

FIGURE 3-16 Mechanisms of various resetting response patterns. **A,** Schemas of three types of resetting response curves. **B,** A theoretical mechanism of resetting patterns in response to extrastimuli at coupling intervals of X and X-50 milliseconds. The reentrant circuit is depicted as having a separate entrance and exit in each pattern. Each tachycardia wavefront is followed by a period of absolute refractoriness (blue arrow), which is then followed by a period of relative refractoriness (fading tail of the arrow) of variable duration. On the **left side,** a flat curve results when the stimulated wavefront reaches the tachycardia circuit and finds a fully excitable gap between the head and tail of the tachycardia wavefront. The gap is still fully excitable at a coupling interval of X-50. Therefore, the conduction time from the entrance to exit is the same. An increasing curve is shown in the **middle;** this results when the initial stimulated wavefront enters the reentrant circuit when the excitable gap is partially refractory. The curve continues to increase at a coupling interval of X-50 because the tissue is still in a relative refractory state. A mixed curve **(right side)** results when the less premature extrastimuli find the reentrant circuit fully excitable, whereas the more premature one (at coupling intervals of X-50) finds it in the relative refractory period. *(From Josephson ME: Recurrent ventricular tachycardia. In Josephson ME, editor: Clinical cardiac electrophysiology, ed 3, Philadelphia, 2004, Lippincott Williams & Wilkins, pp 425-610.)*

Increasing Response Curves in Reentrant Rhythms

Increasing resetting curves result from progressively longer return cycles in response to increasingly premature extrastimuli and indicate a zone of decremental slow conduction, usually located within the reentrant circuit. The most probable mechanism underlying the decremental conduction is encroachment of the advancing wavefront from the premature extrastimuli on an increasingly more refractory tissue within the reentrant circuit, most likely within the zone of slow conduction (see Fig. 3-16).[39] This response pattern is possible only for reentrant arrhythmias and is not observed in triggered or automatic rhythms.

Mixed Response Curves in Reentrant Rhythms

In a mixed response curve, the initial coupling intervals demonstrate a flat portion of the curve of variable duration (but less than 30 milliseconds), followed by a zone during which the return cycle increases (see Fig. 3-16). Occasionally, a flat curve is seen with a single extrastimulus; it is only by using double extrastimuli that an increasing response can be observed.

Decreasing Response Curves in Reentrant Rhythms

Decreasing reset curves are not observed in reentry but can be seen in triggered rhythms, although flat responses are the most common response for triggered activity. The return cycle in triggered activity is typically 100% to 110% of the tachycardia CL.

RESETTING WITH FUSION

Fusion of the stimulated impulse can be observed on surface ECG or intracardiac recordings if the stimulated impulse is intermediate in morphology between a fully paced complex and the tachycardia complex. The ability to recognize ECG fusion requires a significant mass of myocardium to be depolarized by both the extrastimulus and the tachycardia.[37,39,41] With early extrastimuli, the paced antidromic wavefront captures all or most of the myocardium prior to the orthodromic wavefront of the tachycardia impulse exiting from the reentrant circuit. Thus, no ECG fusion is present, although resetting can occur. With later coupled extrastimuli, the orthodromic wavefront exits from the reentrant circuit, thus capturing a certain portion of myocardium before colliding with the paced antidromic wavefront. In this situation, ECG fusion occurs. Resetting with ECG fusion requires wide separation of the entrance and exit of the reentrant circuit, with the stimulus wavefront preferentially engaging the entrance.

If presystolic activity in the reentrant circuit is recorded before delivery of the extrastimulus that resets the tachycardia, one must consider this to represent local fusion (Fig. 3-17).[39] Thus, an extrastimulus that is delivered after the onset of the tachycardia complex and enters and resets the circuit always demonstrates local fusion. Resetting with local fusion and a totally paced complex morphology provides evidence that the reentrant circuit is electrocardiographically small.

The farther the pacing site is from the reentrant circuit, the less likely resetting with ECG fusion will occur because the extrastimulus should be delivered at a shorter coupling interval to reach the circuit with adequate prematurity. Consequently, the stimulated impulse is more likely to capture both the exit and entrance sites and therefore have a purely paced ECG complex morphology without fusion.

Reentrant circuits reset with fusion have a higher incidence of flat resetting curves, longer resetting zones, and significantly shorter return cycles measured from the stimulus to the onset of the tachycardia complex. Resetting with fusion is a potential indication that the pacing site is located proximal to the zone of slow conduction (i.e., prior to the entrance site) within the reentrant circuit, whereas resetting without fusion potentially suggests pacing distal to the zone of slow conduction, because pacing closer to the exit is more likely to capture both the exit and entrance sites and produce resetting without fusion.

RESETTING OF TACHYCARDIAS WITH DIVERSE MECHANISMS

Resetting can be demonstrated for tachycardias based on different mechanisms, including reentry, normal or abnormal automaticity, and triggered activity. Although the ability to reset an arrhythmia is not helpful in distinguishing the underlying mechanism, certain features of the resetting response can be useful for the differential diagnosis.[39]

Site Specificity of Resetting

Triggered activity and automaticity do not demonstrate site specificity for resetting, whereas reentry can. Site specificity for resetting is decreased with the use of multiple extrastimuli.

Resetting Response Curves

Triggered rhythms secondary to DADs usually have a flat or decreasing resetting curve. A flat resetting curve can be seen in automatic, triggered, or reentrant rhythms. Reentrant rhythms never demonstrate a decreasing resetting curve to single or double extrastimuli.

Resetting with Fusion

The ability to reset tachycardia after it has begun activating the myocardium (i.e., resetting with fusion) is diagnostic of reentry and excludes automatic and triggered mechanisms.[37,39,41]

In automaticity or triggered activity, resetting of the arrhythmia by an extrastimulus requires depolarization of the site of origin by

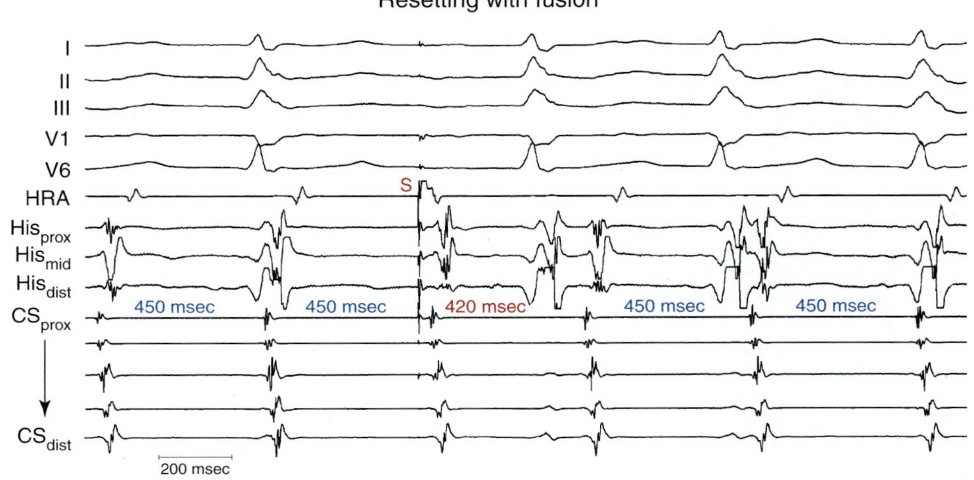

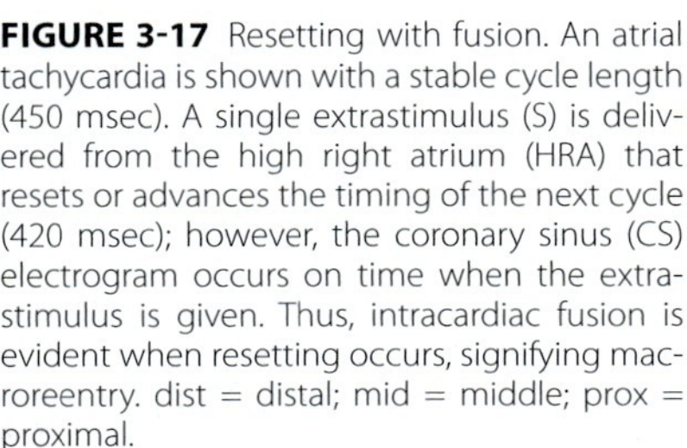
FIGURE 3-17 Resetting with fusion. An atrial tachycardia is shown with a stable cycle length (450 msec). A single extrastimulus (S) is delivered from the high right atrium (HRA) that resets or advances the timing of the next cycle (420 msec); however, the coronary sinus (CS) electrogram occurs on time when the extrastimulus is given. Thus, intracardiac fusion is evident when resetting occurs, signifying macroreentry. dist = distal; mid = middle; prox = proximal.

the paced wavefront. Because the entrance and exit sites of focal rhythms (automatic or triggered) are not separate, a tachycardia wavefront cannot exit the focus once the exit or entrance site has already been depolarized and rendered refractory by the paced wavefront.

During automatic or triggered tachycardias, when an extrastimulus is delivered late in the tachycardia cycle, it can collide with the tachycardia impulse exiting the tachycardia focus and produce fusion of a single beat on the surface ECG or intracardiac recordings. In this case, however, resetting cannot occur because the surrounding myocardium is refractory to the advancing extrastimulus; that is, entrance block occurs. This produces a fully compensatory pause.

Entrainment of Reentrant Tachycardias

BASIC PRINCIPLES OF ENTRAINMENT

Entrainment of reentrant tachycardias by external stimuli was originally defined in the clinical setting as "an increase in the rate of a tachycardia to a faster pacing rate, with resumption of the intrinsic rate of the tachycardia upon either abrupt cessation of pacing or slowing of pacing beyond the intrinsic rate of the tachycardia" and taken to indicate an underlying reentrant mechanism. The ability to entrain a tachycardia also establishes that the reentrant circuit contains an excitable gap.[27,39,42,43]

Orthodromic resetting and transient entrainment are manifestations of the same phenomenon (i.e., premature penetration of a tachycardia circuit by a paced wavefront), and the ability to demonstrate resetting is a strong indication that entrainment can occur from that specific pacing site. Entrainment is the continuous resetting of a reentrant circuit by a train of capturing stimuli. However, following the first stimulus of the pacing train that penetrates and resets the reentrant circuit, the subsequent stimuli interact with the reset circuit, which has an abbreviated excitable gap.[27]

During entrainment, each pacing stimulus creates two activation wavefronts, one in the orthodromic direction and the other in the antidromic direction. The wavefront in the antidromic direction collides with the existing tachycardia wavefront. The wavefront that enters the reentrant circuit in the orthodromic direction (i.e., the same direction as the spontaneous tachycardia wavefront) conducts through the reentrant pathway, resets the tachycardia, and emerges through the exit site to activate the myocardium and collide with the antidromically paced wavefront from the next paced stimulus. This sequence continues until cessation of pacing or block somewhere within the reentrant circuit develops.[37] The first entrained stimulus results in retrograde collision between the stimulated and tachycardia wavefronts, whereas for all subsequent stimuli, the collision occurs between the currently stimulated wavefront and the one stimulated previously. Depending on the degree to which the excitable gap is preexcited (and abbreviated) by the first resetting stimulus, subsequent stimuli fall on fully or partially excitable tissue. Entrainment is said to be present when two consecutive extrastimuli conduct orthodromically through the circuit with the same conduction time while colliding antidromically with the preceding paced wavefront. Because all pacing impulses enter the tachycardia circuit during the excitable gap, each paced wavefront advances and resets the tachycardia. Thus, when pacing is terminated, the last paced impulse will continue to activate the entire tachycardia reentrant circuit orthodromically at the pacing CL and also will activate the entire myocardium orthodromically on exiting the reentrant circuit.[42,43]

Overdrive pacing at long CLs (approximately 10 to 20 milliseconds shorter than the tachycardia CL) can almost always entrain reentrant circuits with large flat resetting curves and a post-pacing interval (PPI) equal to the return cycle observed during the flat part of the resetting curve.[39] During overdrive pacing, once the nth pacing stimulus resets the circuit, the following pacing stimulus $(n + 1)^{th}$ will reach the circuit more prematurely. Depending on how premature it is, this $(n + 1)^{th}$ extrastimulus may produce no change in the return cycle (compared with that in response to the nth extrastimulus), encounter progressive conduction delay (until a fixed, longer return cycle is reached), or terminate the tachycardia. The larger the flat curve observed during resetting or the longer the pacing CL, or both, the more likely the return cycle of the nth and $(n + 1)^{th}$ extrastimuli will be the same. In this case, no matter how many subsequent extrastimuli are delivered, the return cycle will be the same and equal to that observed during the flat portion of the resetting curve. However, if the flat portion of the resetting curve is small, the pacing CL is short, or both, the $(n + 1)^{th}$ extrastimulus will fall on partially refractory tissue and the return cycle will increase. Continued pacing at the same CL will result in a stable but longer return cycle than the nth extrastimulus or termination of the tachycardia. Consequently, circuits with large fully excitable gaps (i.e., large flat resetting curves) can demonstrate prolonged return cycles or even termination at pacing CLs equal to coupling intervals of a single extrastimulus demonstrating a fully excitable gap.

ENTRAINMENT RESPONSE CURVES

During entrainment, the orthodromic wavefront of the last extrastimulus propagates around the circuit to become the first complex of the resumed tachycardia. The conduction time of this impulse to the exit site of the circuit is termed the *last entrained interval*, and it characterizes the properties of the reset circuit during entrainment.[37,39] Measurement of the interval between the last paced extrastimulus to the first nonpaced tachycardia complex (on the surface ECG or presystolic electrogram) during entrainment at progressively shorter pacing CLs characterizes an entrainment response curve, analogous but not identical to resetting response curves with single extrastimuli. In this case, the return cycle depends critically on the number of extrastimuli delivered that reset the circuit before the return cycle is measured, because following the first extrastimulus producing resetting (the nth extrastimulus), subsequent extrastimuli are relatively more premature and can lead to a different return cycle.[42,43]

During entrainment, the return cycle measured at an orthodromically captured presystolic electrogram should equal the pacing CL regardless of the site of pacing, as long as the presystolic electrogram is orthodromically activated at a fixed stimulus-to-electrogram interval (i.e., fixed orthodromic conduction time). This would not be observed if the electrogram were captured antidromically. If the time from the orthodromically activated electrogram to the onset of the return cycle on the surface ECG remains constant, which is a requirement to prove that the electrogram is within or attached to the reentrant circuit proximal to the exit site, then the interval from the stimulus to the surface ECG complex will remain constant. The same is true for the electrogram measured at the stimulation site. In the absence of recording of a presystolic electrogram, other measurements may be used to characterize the last entrained interval at any pacing CL. Therefore, during entrainment, curves relating the pacing CL to the last entrained interval can be measured from the stimulus to the orthodromic presystolic electrogram, to the onset of the surface ECG of the first tachycardia (nonpaced) complex, or to the local activation time at the pacing site of the first tachycardia (nonpaced) complex. These measurements will be qualitatively identical but have different absolute values. As always, it is important to establish the stability of tachycardia CL and document the presence of entrainment before assessing the return cycle and PPI.[42,43]

Termination is the usual response to overdrive pacing of circuits that demonstrate an increasing curve in response to resetting by a single extrastimulus. However, if the number of extrastimuli following the nth extrastimulus is limited to one or two (especially at long pacing CLs), termination may not occur, although the return cycle will be progressively longer following each extrastimulus. Entrainment is not present until two consecutive PPIs are identical. In such cases, when termination does not occur, the return cycle will be longer than that observed if pacing were discontinued following the nth extrastimulus at that pacing CL.[37,39] Thus, if only the return cycle following entrainment is used to analyze the excitable gap, an increasing curve suggesting decremental conduction can result, even though a flat curve is observed with single or double extrastimuli, or both. Therefore, only resetting phenomena describe the characteristics of the reentrant circuit. Entrainment analyzes a reset circuit that has a shorter excitable gap. Flat, mixed (flat and increasing), and increasing curves can be seen during entrainment of macroreentrant circuits. Increasing curves are almost always observed during entrainment of small or microreentrant circuits.

RELATIONSHIP OF PACING SITE AND CYCLE LENGTH TO ENTRAINMENT

As with resetting, entrainment does not require the pacing site be located in the reentrant circuit. The closer the pacing site is to the circuit, however, the less premature a single stimulus can be and reach the circuit and, with pacing trains, the fewer the number of stimuli required before a stimulated wavefront reaches the reentrant circuit without being extinguished by collision with a wave emerging from the circuit.

Overdrive pacing at long CLs (approximately 10 to 20 milliseconds shorter than the tachycardia CL) can almost always entrain reentrant tachycardias. However, the number of pacing stimuli required to entrain the reentrant circuit depends on the tachycardia CL, the duration of the excitable gap of the tachycardia, refractoriness at the pacing site, and the conduction time from the stimulation site to the reentrant circuit.[39,42-45]

DIAGNOSTIC CRITERIA OF ENTRAINMENT

Entrainment is the continuous resetting of a tachycardia circuit. Therefore, during constant rate pacing, entrainment of tachycardia results in the activation of all myocardial tissue responsible for maintaining the tachycardia at the pacing CL, with the resumption of the intrinsic tachycardia morphology and rate after cessation of pacing. Unfortunately, it is almost impossible to document the acceleration of all tissues responsible for maintaining the reentrant circuit to the pacing CL. Therefore, certain surface ECG criteria have been proposed for establishing the presence of entrainment: (1) fixed fusion of the paced complexes at a constant pacing rate; (2) progressive fusion or different degrees of fusion at different pacing rates (i.e., the surface ECG and intracardiac morphology progressively look more like the purely paced configuration and less like the pure tachycardia complex in the course of pacing at progressively shorter pacing CLs); and (3) resumption of the same tachycardia morphology following cessation of pacing, with the first PPI displaying no fusion but occurring at a return cycle equal to the pacing CL.[46] These criteria are discussed in more detail in Chapter 5.[42,43,47]

Mechanism of Slow Conduction in the Reentrant Circuit

As mentioned earlier, a condition necessary for reentry is that the impulse be delayed sufficiently in the alternative pathway or pathways to allow tissues proximal to the site of unidirectional block to recover excitability.[27] All types of reentrant arrhythmias have a basic feature in common—the wavefront must encounter a zone of tissue where local electrical inhomogeneity is present. This inhomogeneity can be related to (1) electrical properties of the individual cardiac myocyte that generates the action potential (inhomogeneity in electrical excitability or refractoriness, or both), (2) passive properties governing the flow of current among cardiac cells (cell-to-cell coupling and tissue geometry), or (3) combinations of those conditions.[48] Such changes can be permanent (e.g., in remodeling after ventricular hypertrophy or infarction), or they can be purely functional (e.g., inhomogeneity of refractoriness in acutely ischemic tissue). Additionally, some of those changes are needed only to set the initial condition for the deviation of the impulse, the so-called unidirectional conduction block. Once the disturbance is initiated, an arrhythmia can develop in a perfectly homogeneous electrical medium.[48]

Slow conduction within the reentrant circuit is also an important determinant of the size of the reentrant circuit. A decrease in conduction velocity results in a reduction in the wavelength and a lessening of the amount of tissue needed to sustain reentry. In contrast, an increase in conduction velocity prolongs the wavelength of excitation, and, hence, a larger anatomical circuit is necessary to sustain reentry. If a larger circuit is not possible, initiation or maintenance of tachycardia cannot occur.[27]

In some cardiac tissues (e.g., the AVN), slow conduction is normal physiology. Slow conduction also can be secondary to pathophysiological settings (e.g., MI) or caused by functional properties that can develop as a result of premature stimulation or evolve during a rapid transitional rhythm.[27]

As discussed in Chapter 1, action potential propagation and conduction velocity in cardiac tissue are determined by source-sink relationships, which reflect the interplay between the active membrane properties of cardiac cells (the source generating the action potential) and the passive properties determined by architectural features of the myocardium (sink), as well as the coupling resistance between source and sink. The current provided by the source must reach the sink. The pathway between the source and sink includes intracellular resistance (provided by the cytoplasm) and intercellular resistance (provided by the gap junctions). Extracellular resistance plays a role, but it can often be neglected. The coupling resistance is mainly determined by resistance of the gap junctions. Therefore, the number and distribution of gap junctions, as well as the conductance of the gap junction proteins (connexins), are important factors for conduction of the action potential.

The safety factor for conduction predicts the success of action potential propagation and is defined as the ratio of the current generated by the depolarizing ion channels of a cell (source) to the current consumed during the excitation cycle of a single cell in the tissue (sink).[39] Thus, the safety factor for propagation is proportional to the excess of source current over the sink needs. By this definition, conduction fails when the safety factor drops to less than 1 and becomes increasingly stable as it rises to more than 1.[49] This concept of propagation safety provides information about the dependence of propagation velocity on the state of the ion channels, cell-to-cell coupling, and tissue geometry. In essence, local source-sink relationships determine the formation of conduction heterogeneities and provide conditions for the development of slow conduction, unidirectional block, and reentry.[27,50,51]

REDUCED MEMBRANE EXCITABILITY

Excitability of a cardiac cell describes the ease with which the cell responds to a stimulus with a regenerative action potential, and it depends on the passive and active properties of the cell membrane.[7] The passive properties include the membrane resistance and capacitance and the intercellular resistance. The more negative the membrane potential is, the more Na^+ channels are available for activation, the greater the influx of Na^+ into the cell during phase 0, and the greater the conduction velocity.

In contrast, membrane depolarization to levels of −60 to −70 mV can inactivate half the Na^+ channels, and depolarization to −50 mV or less can inactivate all the Na^+ channels. Therefore, when stimulation occurs during phase 3 (e.g., during premature stimulation during the relative refractory period), before full recovery and at less negative potentials of the cell membrane, a portion of Na^+ channels will still be refractory and unavailable for activation. As a result, I_{Na} and phase 0 of the next action potential are reduced, and conduction of the premature stimulus is slowed, facilitating reentry.[6,27]

Reduced membrane excitability occurs in numerous physiological and pathophysiological conditions. Genetic mutations that result in loss of Na^+ channel function, as occurs in the Brugada syndrome, can cause reduced membrane excitability.

Reduced membrane excitability is also present in cardiac cells with persistently low levels of resting potential caused by disease (e.g., during acute ischemia, tachycardia, certain electrical remodeling processes, and treatment with class I antiarrhythmic agents).[27,50] At low resting potentials, the availability of excitable Na^+ channels is reduced because of inactivation of a significant proportion of the Na^+ channels and prolonged recovery of Na^+ channels from inactivation. With progressive reduction of excitability, less Na^+ source current is generated, and conduction velocity and the safety factor decrease monotonically. When the safety factor falls to less than 1, conduction can no longer be sustained, and failure (conduction block) occurs. Action potentials with reduced upstroke velocity resulting from partial inactivation of Na^+ channels are called depressed fast responses. These action potential changes are likely to be heterogeneous, with unequal degrees of Na^+ inactivation that create areas with minimally reduced velocity, more severely depressed zones, and areas of complete block. In addition, refractoriness in cells with reduced membrane potentials can outlast voltage recovery of the action potential; that is, the cell can still be refractory or partially refractory after the resting membrane potential returns to its most negative value.[50]

Thus, in a diseased region with partially depolarized fibers, there can be some areas of slow conduction and some areas of conduction block, depending on the level of resting potential and the number of Na^+ channels that are inactivated. This combination can be the substrate for reentry. The chance for reentry in such fibers is even greater during premature activation or during rhythms at a rapid rate, because slow conduction or the possibility of block is increased even further.

REDUCED CELLULAR COUPLING

Intercellular communication is maintained by gap junctional channels that connect neighboring cells and allow biochemical and low-resistance electrical coupling.[52] Although the resistivity of the gap junctional membrane for the passage of ions and small molecules and for electrical propagation is several orders of magnitude higher than the cytoplasmic intracellular resistivity, gap junction coupling provides a resistance pathway that is several orders of magnitude lower compared with uncoupled cell membranes.[53]

In normal adult working myocardium, a given cardiomyocyte is electrically coupled to an average of approximately 11 adjacent cells, with gap junctions being predominantly localized at the intercalated discs at the ends of the rod-shaped cells. Lateral (side-to-side) gap junctions in nondisc lateral membranes of cardiomyocytes are much less abundant and occur more often in atrial than ventricular tissues.[27,53-55] This particular subcellular distribution of gap junctions is a main determinant of anisotropic conduction in the heart; a wavefront must traverse more cells in the transverse direction than over an equivalent distance in the longitudinal direction, because cell diameter is much smaller than cell length. Additionally, less intercellular gap junctional coupling occurs and, hence, greater resistance and slower conduction transversely than longitudinally.[27,52,55]

Modification of intercellular coupling occurs in numerous physiological and pathophysiological conditions.[27] Physiologically, cell-to-cell coupling is reduced in atrial and ventricular myocardium in the transverse direction to the main fiber axis relative to the longitudinal direction. Reduced intercellular coupling also likely contributes to slow impulse conduction in the AVN. In pathophysiological settings (e.g., myocardial ischemia, ventricular hypertrophy, cardiomyopathy),[56] modification of intercellular coupling can occur as a consequence of acute changes in the average conductance of gap junctions secondary to ischemia, hypoxia, acidification, or increase in intracellular Ca^{2+}, or it can be produced by changes in expression or cellular distribution patterns of gap junctions.[57,58] Changes in the distribution and number of gap junctions (gap junction remodeling) have been reported in almost all cardiac diseases predisposing to arrhythmias. Remodeling includes a decrease in some gap junction channels resulting from the interruption of communication between cells by fibrosis and downregulation of connexin-43 (Cx43) formation or trafficking to the intercalated disc. Additionally, gap junctions can become more prominent along lateral membranes of myocytes (so-called structural remodeling).[54,59]

A reduction in the gap junctional conductance increases the intercellular resistance, thus leading to conduction delay or block. Similar to its behavior during reduced membrane excitability, conduction velocity decreases monotonically with reduction in intercellular coupling.[52] However, the resulting reduction of conduction velocities is more than an order of magnitude larger than that observed during a reduction of excitability.[27] Importantly, the changes in the safety factor with uncoupling are opposite to those observed with a reduction in membrane excitability. As cells become less coupled, there is greater confinement of depolarizing current to the depolarizing cell, with less electrotonic load and axial flow of charge to the downstream cells. As a result, individual cells depolarize with a high margin of safety, but conduction proceeds with long intercellular delays. At such low levels of coupling, conduction is very slow but, paradoxically, very robust.[27,57,58]

Importantly, there is a high redundancy in connexin expression in the heart with regard to conduction of electrical impulse, and a large reduction of intercellular coupling is required to cause major slowing of conduction velocity. It has been shown that a 50% reduction in Cx43 does not alter ventricular impulse conduction. Cx43 expression must decrease by 90% to affect conduction, but even then conduction velocity is reduced only by 20%.

TISSUE STRUCTURE AND GEOMETRY

Tissue geometry can influence action potential propagation and conduction velocity. In contrast to an uncoupled cell strand, in which the high resistance junctions alternate with the low cytoplasmic resistance of the cells, a high degree of discontinuity can be produced by large tissue segments (consisting of a segment with side branches) alternating with small tissue segments having a small tissue mass (connecting segments without branches).[27]

When a small mass of cells has to excite the large mass (e.g., an impulse passing abruptly from a fiber of small diameter to one of large diameter or propagating into a region where there is an abrupt increase in branching of the myocardium), transient slowing of the conduction velocity can be observed at the junction. This occurs because of sink-source mismatch, during which the current provided by the excitation wavefront (source) is insufficient to charge the capacity and thus excite the much larger volume of tissue ahead (sink).[27,49,60,61]

In a normal heart, abrupt changes in geometric properties are not of sufficient magnitude to provide sufficient sink-source mismatch and cause conduction block of the normal action potential because the safety factor for conduction is large; that is, there is a large excess of activating current over the amount required for propagation. However, when the action potential is abnormal, the unexcited area has decreased excitability (e.g., in the setting of acute ischemia), or both, anatomical impediments can result in conduction block.

Anisotropy and Reentry

The anisotropic cellular structure of the myocardium is important for the understanding of normal propagation and arrhythmogenesis. Structural anisotropy can relate to cell shape and to the cellular distribution pattern of proteins involved in impulse conduction, such as gap junction connexins and membrane ion channels. The anisotropic architecture of most myocardial regions, consisting of elongated cells forming strands and layers of tissue, leads to a dependence of propagation velocity on the direction of impulse spread.[27,54] In normal ventricular myocardium, conduction in the direction parallel to the long axis of the myocardial fiber bundles is approximately three to five times more rapid than that in the transverse direction. This is attributable principally to the lower resistivity of myocardium in the longitudinal versus the transverse direction; hence, intercellular current flow occurs primarily at the cell termini (although propagation also occurs transversely). As discussed previously, the gap junctions of the intercalated discs form a major source of intercellular resistance to current flow between fiber bundles. Therefore, the structure of the myocardium that governs the extent and distribution of these gap junctions has a profound influence on axial resistance and conduction.[55]

CELLULAR COUPLING: GAP JUNCTIONAL ORGANIZATION

The anisotropic conductive properties of ventricular myocardium are dependent on the geometry of the interconnected cells and the number, size, and location of the gap junction channels between them. Additionally, gap junctions vary in their molecular composition, degree of expression, and distribution pattern, whereby each of these variations can contribute to the specific propagation properties of a given tissue in a given species. Tissue-specific connexin expression and gap junction spatial distribution, as well as the variation in the structural composition of gap junction channels, allow for a greater versatility of gap junction physiological features and enable disparate conduction properties in cardiac tissue. The myocytes of the sinus node and AVN are equipped with small, sparse, dispersed gap junctions containing Cx45, a connexin that forms low conductance channels, thus underlying the relatively poor intercellular coupling in nodal tissues, a property that is linked to slowing of conduction. In contrast, ventricular muscle expresses predominantly Cx43 and Cx45, which have larger conductance. Atrial muscle and Purkinje fibers express all three cardiac connexins.

Alterations in distribution and function of cardiac gap junctions are associated with conduction delay or block. Inactivation of gap junctions decreases transverse conduction velocity to a greater degree than longitudinal conduction, thereby resulting in exaggeration of anisotropy and providing a substrate for reentrant activity and increased susceptibility to arrhythmias.[54,59]

MYOCYTE PACKING AND TISSUE GEOMETRY

Discontinuities in myocardial architecture exist at several levels. In addition to discontinuities imposed by cell borders, microvessels and connective tissue sheets separating bundles of excitable myocytes can act as resistive barriers. A propagating impulse is expected to collide with such barriers and travels around them wherever it encounters excitable tissue.[48]

In some regions of the myocardium (e.g., the papillary muscles), connective tissue septa subdivide the myocardium into unit bundles composed of 2 to 30 cells surrounded by a connective tissue sheath.[6] Within a unit bundle, cells are tightly connected or coupled to each other longitudinally and transversely through intercalated discs that contain the gap junctions and are activated uniformly and synchronously as an impulse propagates along the bundle. Adjacent unit bundles also are connected to each other. Unit bundles are coupled better in the direction of the long axis of its cells and bundles, because of the high frequency of the gap junctions within a unit bundle, than in the direction transverse to the long axis, because of the low frequency of interconnections between the unit bundles. This is reflected as a lower axial resistivity in the longitudinal direction than in the transverse direction in cardiac tissues composed of many unit bundles. Additionally, anisotropy on a macroscopic scale can influence conduction at sites at which a bundle of cardiac fibers branches or separate bundles will coalesce. Marked slowing can occur when there is a sudden change in the fiber direction, causing an abrupt increase in the effective axial resistivity. Conduction block, which sometimes can be unidirectional, can occur at such junction sites, particularly when membrane excitability is reduced.

UNIFORM VERSUS NONUNIFORM ANISOTROPY

Uniform anisotropy is characterized by smooth wavefront propagation in all directions and measured conduction velocity changes monotonically on moving from fast (longitudinal) to slow (transverse) axes, thus indicating relatively tight coupling between groups of fibers in all directions. However, this definition is based on the characteristics of activation at a macroscopic level, where the spatial resolution encompasses numerous myocardial cells and bundles, and therefore it describes the behavior of the myocardial syncytium. In contrast, when the three-dimensional network of cells is broken down into linear single-cell chains, gap junctions can be shown to limit axial current flow and induce saltatory conduction because of the recurrent increases in axial resistance at the sites of gap junctional coupling; that is, conduction is composed of rapid excitation of individual cells followed by a transjunctional conduction delay. In two- and three-dimensional tissue, these discontinuities disappear because of lateral gap junctional coupling, which serves to average local small differences in activation times of individual cardiomyocytes at the excitation wavefront.[49,55]

In multicellular tissue, saltatory conduction reappears only under conditions of critical gap junctional uncoupling, in which it leads to a functional unmasking of the cellular structure and induces ultraslow and meandering conduction, well known to be a key ingredient in arrhythmogenesis.[49] Change in the characteristics of anisotropic propagation at the macroscopic scale from uniform to nonuniform strongly predisposes to reentrant arrhythmias. Nonuniform anisotropy has been defined as tight electrical coupling between cells in the longitudinal direction but uncoupling to the lateral gap junctional connections. Therefore, there is disruption of the smooth transverse pattern of conduction characteristic of uniform anisotropy that results in a markedly irregular sequence or zigzag conduction, producing the fractionated extracellular electrograms characteristic of nonuniform anisotropic conduction (Fig. 3-18). In nonuniformly anisotropic muscle, there also can be an abrupt transition in conduction velocity from the fast longitudinal direction to the slow transverse direction, unlike the case with uniform anisotropic muscle, in which intermediate velocities occur between the two directions.

Nonuniform anisotropic properties can exist in normal cardiac tissues secondary to separation of the fascicles of muscle bundles in the transverse direction by fibrous tissue that proliferates with aging to form longitudinally oriented insulating boundaries (e.g., crista terminalis, interatrial band in adult atria, or ventricular papillary muscle). Similar connective tissue septa cause nonuniform anisotropy in pathological situations such as chronic ischemia or a healing MI, in which fibrosis in the myocardium occurs (see Fig. 3-18).[6,55]

Mechanism of Unidirectional Block in the Reentrant Circuit

Unidirectional block occurs when an impulse cannot conduct in one direction along a bundle of cardiac fibers but can conduct in the opposite direction. As mentioned earlier, this condition is necessary for the occurrence of classic reentrant rhythms. Several mechanisms, involving active and passive electrical properties of cardiac cells, can cause unidirectional block.[29]

INHOMOGENEITY OF MEMBRANE EXCITABILITY AND REFRACTORINESS

Unidirectional block develops when the activation wavefront interacts with the repolarization phase (tail) of a preceding excitation wave. There is a critical or vulnerable window during the relative refractory period of a propagating action potential within which unidirectional block occurs. When a premature stimulus is delivered outside this window, the induced action potential propagates or blocks in both directions; specifically, a stimulus delivered too early fails to induce a propagating action potential in either

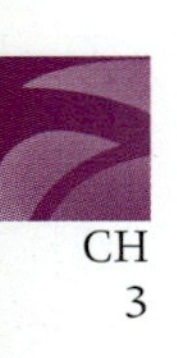

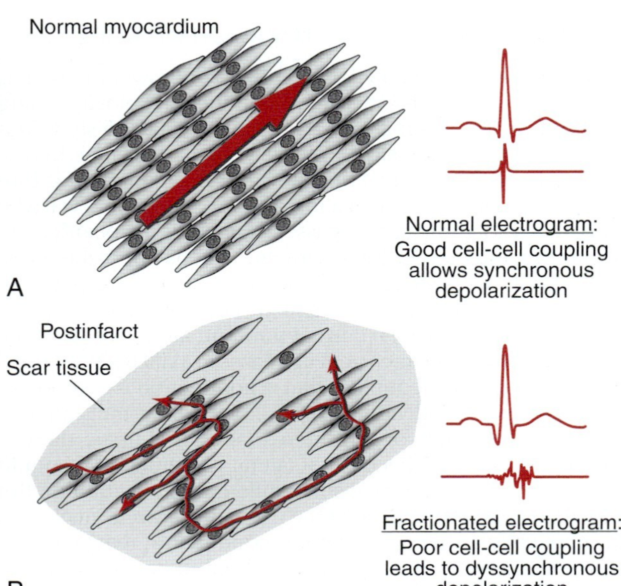

FIGURE 3-18 Effect of scar on electrical propagation. **A,** A homogeneous sheet of myocardium conducts an electrical wavefront rapidly, with synchronous activation of a large number of cells that leads to a sharp electrogram. **B,** Myocardial scarring produces disordered propagation, resulting in a low-amplitude electrogram, with multiple fragmented peaks.

direction (bidirectional block), whereas a late stimulus results in bidirectional conduction (no block). In contrast, when a stimulus is applied within the vulnerable window, the induced action potential propagates incrementally in the retrograde direction because the tissue is progressively more recovered as the distance from the window increases in this direction, but it blocks in the anterograde direction following a short distance of decremental conduction because the tissue is progressively less excitable as the distance from the window increases in this direction.[27]

The size of the vulnerable window provides an index of the vulnerability to the development of reentrant arrhythmias. Therefore, the probability that a premature stimulus will fall inside the window and induce reentry is high when the vulnerable window is large. In contrast, precise timing of a premature stimulus is required to induce reentry in a small window, and the probability of such an event is low. In normal tissue, the vulnerable window is very small, and inducibility of unidirectional block and reentry is negligible. The width of the vulnerable window can be affected by changes in the availability of Na^+ channels for depolarization, cell-to-cell coupling, and repolarizing I_K. Additionally, the size of the vulnerable window can be widened (and reentry facilitated) by factors that increase the spatial inhomogeneity of refractoriness or decrease cellular coupling via gap junctions.

Unidirectional conduction block in a reentrant circuit also can be persistent and independent of premature activation, in which case it often occurs in a region of depressed and heterogeneous excitability (as occurs in acute ischemia); this leads to a widening of the vulnerable window. Asymmetry in excitability, which can occur because of asymmetrical distribution of a pathological event, can lead to an abrupt rise in the threshold for excitation in one direction and to a more gradual rise in the other. Conduction fails when the wavefront encounters the least depressed site first and is successful in the direction in which it encounters the most depressed site first. Additionally, impulses are conducted more easily from a rapidly conducting tissue to a slowly conducting tissue than in the opposite direction.[29]

Local dispersion of refractory periods is a normal feature of ventricular myocardium. Critical increases in the dispersion of refractoriness, the difference between the shortest and longest refractory periods, can result in the local widening of the vulnerability window and an increased probability for the generation of unidirectional block and reentry.[6,27] Increased heterogeneity of repolarization and dispersion of refractoriness can be caused by acute or prolonged ischemia, the long QT syndrome, or electrical remodeling in the setting of ventricular hypertrophy and failure and in the setting of MI. When differences in the duration of the refractory periods occur in adjacent areas, conduction of an appropriately timed premature impulse can be blocked in the region with the longest refractory period, which then becomes a site of unidirectional block, whereas conduction continues through regions with a shorter refractory period.[6]

ANISOTROPY AND UNIDIRECTIONAL BLOCK

The anisotropic properties of cardiac muscle can contribute to the occurrence of unidirectional block.[6] As mentioned earlier, in the anisotropic muscle, the safety factor for conduction is lower in the longitudinal direction of rapid than in the transverse direction of slow conduction. The low safety factor longitudinally is a result of a large current load on the membrane associated with the low axial resistivity and a large membrane capacitance in the longitudinal direction. This low safety factor can result in a preferential conduction block of premature impulses in the longitudinal direction while conduction in the transverse direction continues. The site of block in the longitudinal direction can become a site of unidirectional block that leads to reentry.[6] In contrast to the propensity of premature impulses to block in the longitudinal direction in nonuniformly anisotropic myocardium because of the decreased depolarizing current and low safety factor, when coupling resistance between cells is increased, conduction of all impulses will block first in the transverse direction. Preferential block in this direction occurs because an increase in coupling resistance will reduce the safety factor below the critical level needed to maintain transverse conduction before the safety factor for longitudinal conduction is reduced to this critical level.[6,55]

DISCONTINUITIES IN TISSUE STRUCTURE AND GEOMETRY

Geometric factors related to tissue architecture also can influence impulse conduction and, under certain conditions, lead to unidirectional block.[27] Structural discontinuities exist in the normal heart in the form of trabeculations of the atrial and ventricular walls, sheets interconnected by small trabeculae, or myocardial fibers with different diameters packed in a connective tissue matrix. Structural discontinuities can also be secondary to pathophysiological settings, such as the connective tissue septa characteristic of aging, infarcted, hypertrophic, and failing myocardium. The propagating excitation wave is expected to interact with these normal and abnormal structural discontinuities. These structural features influence conduction by affecting the axial currents that flow ahead of the propagating wavefront.[27] Therefore, an impulse conducting in one direction can encounter a different sequence of changes in fiber diameter, branching, and frequency and distribution of gap junctions than it does when traveling in the opposite direction. The configuration of pathways in each direction is not the same.

REFERENCES

1. Peters NS, Cabo C, Wit AL: Arrhythmogenic mechanisms: automaticity, triggered activity, and reentry. In Zipes DP, Jalife J, editors: *Cardiac electrophysiology: from cell to bedside*, ed 3, Philadelphia, 2000, Saunders, pp 345–355.
2. Mangoni ME, Nargeot J: Genesis and regulation of the heart automaticity, *Physiol Rev* 88:919–982, 2008.
3. Dobrzynski H, Boyett MR, Anderson RH: New insights into pacemaker activity: promoting understanding of sick sinus syndrome, *Circulation* 115:1921–1932, 2007.
4. Couette B, Marger L, Nargeot J, Mangoni ME: Physiological and pharmacological insights into the role of ionic channels in cardiac pacemaker activity, *Cardiovasc Hematol Disord Drug Targets* 6:169–190, 2006.
5. Barbuti A, Baruscotti M, DiFrancesco D: The pacemaker current: from basics to the clinics, *J Cardiovasc Electrophysiol* 18:342–347, 2007.

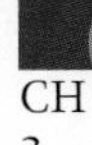

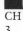

6. Waldo AL, Wit AL: Mechanisms of cardiac arrhythmias and conduction disturbances. In Fuster V, Alexander RW, O'Rourke RA, editors: *Hurst's the heart*, ed 11, Columbus, Ohio, 2004, McGraw-Hill, pp 787–816.
7. Grant AO: Cardiac ion channels, *Circ Arrhythm Electrophysiol* 2:185–194, 2009.
8. Lakatta EG: A paradigm shift for the heart's pacemaker, *Heart Rhythm* 7:559–564, 2010.
9. Venetucci LA, Trafford AW, O'Neill SC, Eisner DA: The sarcoplasmic reticulum and arrhythmogenic calcium release, *Cardiovasc Res* 77:285–292, 2008.
10. DiFrancesco D: The role of the funny current in pacemaker activity, *Circ Res* 106:434–446, 2010.
11. Maltsev VA, Lakatta EG: Dynamic interactions of an intracellular Ca2+ clock and membrane ion channel clock underlie robust initiation and regulation of cardiac pacemaker function, *Cardiovasc Res* 77:274–284, 2008.
12. Haissaguerre M, Jais P, Shah DC, et al: Spontaneous initiation of atrial fibrillation by ectopic beats originating in the pulmonary veins, *N Engl J Med* 339:659–666, 1998.
13. Boyden PA, Hirose M, Dun W: Cardiac Purkinje cells, *Heart Rhythm* 7:127–135, 2010.
14. Kohl P, Bollensdorff C, Garny A: Effects of mechanosensitive ion channels on ventricular electrophysiology: experimental and theoretical models, *Exp Physiol* 91:307–321, 2006.
15. Dun W, Boyden PA: The Purkinje cell: 2008 style, *J Mol Cell Cardiol* 45:617–624, 2008.
16. Venetucci LA, Trafford AW, O'Neill SC, Eisner DA: Na/Ca exchange: regulator of intracellular calcium and source of arrhythmias in the heart, *Ann N Y Acad Sci* 1099:315–325, 2007.
17. Kalbfleisch S, Hart D, Weiss R: Two ventricular tachycardias with cycle length and QRS alternans: insights into the mechanism from mapping and ablation of the tachycardias, *Pacing Clin Electrophysiol* 32:e31–e35, 2009.
18. Gyorke S: Molecular basis of catecholaminergic polymorphic ventricular tachycardia, *Heart Rhythm* 6:123–129, 2009.
19. Laurita KR, Rosenbaum DS: Mechanisms and potential therapeutic targets for ventricular arrhythmias associated with impaired cardiac calcium cycling, *J Mol Cell Cardiol* 44:31–43, 2008.
20. Ter Keurs HE, Boyden PA: Calcium and arrhythmogenesis, *Physiol Rev* 87:457–506, 2007.
21. Kaufman ES: Mechanisms and clinical management of inherited channelopathies: long QT syndrome, Brugada syndrome, catecholaminergic polymorphic ventricular tachycardia, and short QT syndrome, *Heart Rhythm* 6(Suppl):S51–S55, 2009.
22. Scheinman MM: Role of the His-Purkinje system in the genesis of cardiac arrhythmia, *Heart Rhythm* 6:1050–1058, 2009.
23. Weiss JN, Garfinkel A, Karagueuzian HS, et al: Early afterdepolarizations and cardiac arrhythmias, *Heart Rhythm* 7:1891–1899, 2010.
24. Maruyama M, Lin SF, Xie Y, et al: Genesis of phase 3 early afterdepolarizations and triggered activity in acquired long-QT syndrome, *Circ Arrhythm Electrophysiol* 4:103–111, 2011.
25. Mines GR: On circulating excitations in heart muscles and their possible relation to tachycardia and fibrillation, *Trans R Soc Can* 4:43, 1914.
26. Mines GR: On dynamic equilibrium in the heart, *J Physiol* 46:349–383, 1913.
27. Kleber AG, Rudy Y: Basic mechanisms of cardiac impulse propagation and associated arrhythmias, *Physiol Rev* 84:431–488, 2004.
28. Allessie MA, Bonke FI, Schopman FJ: Circus movement in rabbit atrial muscle as a mechanism of tachycardia. III. The "leading circle" concept: a new model of circus movement in cardiac tissue without the involvement of an anatomical obstacle, *Circ Res* 41:9–18, 1977.
29. Segal OR, Chow AW, Peters NS, Davies DW: Mechanisms that initiate ventricular tachycardia in the infarcted human heart, *Heart Rhythm* 7:57–64, 2010.
30. Antzelevitch C: Basic mechanisms of reentrant arrhythmias, *Curr Opin Cardiol* 16:1–7, 2001.
31. Benito B, Guasch E, Rivard L, Nattel S: Clinical and mechanistic issues in early repolarization of normal variants and lethal arrhythmia syndromes, *J Am Coll Cardiol* 56:1177–1186, 2010.
32. Antzelevitch C, Yan GX: J wave syndromes, *Heart Rhythm* 7:549–558, 2010.
33. Lim ZY, Maskara B, Aguel F, et al: Spiral wave attachment to millimeter-sized obstacles, *Circulation* 114:2113–2121, 2006.
34. Tung L, Zhang Y: Optical imaging of arrhythmias in tissue culture, *J Electrocardiol* 39(Suppl): S2–S6, 2006.
35. Chang MG, Zhang Y, Chang CY, et al: Spiral waves and reentry dynamics in an in vitro model of the healed infarct border zone, *Circ Res* 105:1062–1071, 2009.
36. Almendral JM, Rosenthal ME, Stamato NJ, et al: Analysis of the resetting phenomenon in sustained uniform ventricular tachycardia: incidence and relation to termination, *J Am Coll Cardiol* 8:294–300, 1986.
37. Kay GN, Epstein AE, Plumb VJ: Resetting of ventricular tachycardia by single extrastimuli: relation to slow conduction within the reentrant circuit, *Circulation* 81:1507–1519, 1990.
38. Stevenson WG, Weiss JN, Wiener I, et al: Resetting of ventricular tachycardia: implications for localizing the area of slow conduction, *J Am Coll Cardiol* 11:522–529, 1988.
39. Josephson ME: Recurrent ventricular tachycardia. In Josephson M, editor: *Clinical cardiac electrophysiology*, ed 4, Philadelphia, 2002, Lippincott Williams & Wilkins, pp 425–610.
40. Rosman JZ, John RM, Stevenson WG, et al: Resetting criteria during ventricular overdrive pacing successfully differentiate orthodromic reentrant tachycardia from atrioventricular nodal reentrant tachycardia despite interobserver disagreement concerning QRS fusion, *Heart Rhythm* 8:2–7, 2011.
41. Rosenthal ME, Stamato NJ, Almendral JM, et al: Resetting of ventricular tachycardia with electrocardiographic fusion: incidence and significance, *Circulation* 77:581–588, 1988.
42. Deo R, Berger R: The clinical utility of entrainment pacing, *J Cardiovasc Electrophysiol* 20:466–470, 2009.
43. Waldo AL: From bedside to bench: entrainment and other stories, *Heart Rhythm* 1:94–106, 2004.
44. Tritto M, De PR, Zardini M, et al: Comparison of single premature versus continuous overdrive stimulation for identification of a protected isthmus in macro-reentrant atrial tachycardia circuits, *Am J Cardiol* 91:1485–1489, 2003.
45. Morton JB, Sanders P, Deen V, et al: Sensitivity and specificity of concealed entrainment for the identification of a critical isthmus in the atrium: relationship to rate, anatomic location and antidromic penetration, *J Am Coll Cardiol* 39:896–906, 2002.
46. Almendral JM, Gottlieb CD, Rosenthal ME, et al: Entrainment of ventricular tachycardia: explanation for surface electrocardiographic phenomena by analysis of electrograms recorded within the tachycardia circuit, *Circulation* 77:569–580, 1988.
47. Das MK, Scott LR, Miller JM: Focal mechanism of ventricular tachycardia in coronary artery disease, *Heart Rhythm* 7:305–311, 2010.
48. Kleber AG, Fast V: Molecular and cellular aspects of re-entrant arrhythmias, *Basic Res Cardiol* 92(Suppl 1):111–119, 1997.
49. Rohr S: Role of gap junctions in the propagation of the cardiac action potential, *Cardiovasc Res* 62:309–322, 2004.
50. Antzelevitch C: Cellular basis and mechanism underlying normal and abnormal myocardial repolarization and arrhythmogenesis, *Ann Med* 36(Suppl 1):5–14, 2004.
51. Santana LF, Nunez-Duran H, Dilly KW, Lederer WJ: Sodium current and arrhythmogenesis in heart failure, *Heart Fail Clin* 1:193–205, 2005.
52. Sohl G, Willecke K: Gap junctions and the connexin protein family, *Cardiovasc Res* 62: 228–232, 2004.
53. Noorman M, van der Heyden MA, van Veen TA, et al: Cardiac cell-cell junctions in health and disease: electrical versus mechanical coupling, *J Mol Cell Cardiol* 47:23–31, 2009.
54. Saffitz JE, Lerner DL, Yamada KA: Gap junction distribution and regulation in the heart. In Zipes DP, Jalife J, editors: *Cardiac electrophysiology: from cell to bedside*, ed 4, Philadelphia, 2004, Saunders, pp 181–191.
55. Valderrabano M: Influence of anisotropic conduction properties in the propagation of the cardiac action potential, *Prog Biophys Mol Biol* 94:144–168, 2007.
56. Cascio WE, Yang H, Muller-Borer BJ, Johnson TA: Ischemia-induced arrhythmia: the role of connexins, gap junctions, and attendant changes in impulse propagation, *J Electrocardiol* 38(Suppl):55–59, 2005.
57. van Rijen HV, van Veen TA, Gros D, et al: Connexins and cardiac arrhythmias, *Adv Cardiol* 42:150–160, 2006.
58. Lee PJ, Pogwizd SM: Micropatterns of propagation, *Adv Cardiol* 42:86–106, 2006.
59. Dhein S: Cardiac ischemia and uncoupling: gap junctions in ischemia and infarction, *Adv Cardiol* 42:198–212, 2006.
60. Fast VG, Kleber AG: Cardiac tissue geometry as a determinant of unidirectional conduction block: assessment of microscopic excitation spread by optical mapping in patterned cell cultures and in a computer model, *Cardiovasc Res* 29:697–707, 1995.
61. Wang Y, Rudy Y: Action potential propagation in inhomogeneous cardiac tissue: safety factor considerations and ionic mechanism, *Am J Physiol Heart Circ Physiol* 278:H1019–H1029, 2000.

CHAPTER 4 Electrophysiological Testing

Indications

Invasive electrophysiological (EP) testing involves recording a portion of cardiac electrical activity and programmed cardiac electrical stimulation via multipolar catheter electrodes positioned percutaneously strategically at various locations within the cardiac chambers. EP testing is used predominantly in patients with suspected or documented cardiac arrhythmias when the precise EP diagnosis is required for management decisions or when catheter ablation is planned. Additionally, EP testing is of value in selected groups of patients for stratification of risk of life-threatening arrhythmias. The role of EP testing in specific cardiac electrical and structural cardiac diseases is discussed in subsequent chapters.

Periprocedural Management

Preprocedure Evaluation

Heart failure, myocardial ischemia, and electrolyte abnormalities should be treated and adequately controlled before any invasive EP testing is undertaken. Patients with critical aortic stenosis, severe hypertrophic cardiomyopathy, left main or severe three-vessel coronary artery disease, or decompensated heart failure are at higher than average risk of complications. Induction of sustained tachyarrhythmias in these patients can cause severe deterioration. Anticoagulation to achieve an international normalized ratio (INR) in the therapeutic range (2.0 to 3.0) for 4 weeks before the procedure, transesophageal echocardiography (to exclude the presence of intracardiac thrombus), or both, is required before studying patients who have persistent atrial fibrillation (AF) and atrial flutter (AFL) who may have sinus rhythm restored intentionally or inadvertently (i.e., cardioversion of ventricular tachycardia [VT]).

Antiarrhythmic Drugs

Antiarrhythmic drugs are usually, but not always, stopped for at least five half-lives prior to EP testing. In selected cases, antiarrhythmic drugs can be continued if an arrhythmic event occurred while the patient was taking a specific agent.

Consent

Patients generally are not as familiar with EP procedures as they are with other invasive cardiac procedures, such as coronary angiography. Therefore, patient education is an essential part of the procedure. The patient should be informed about the value of the EP study, its risks, and the expected outcome. Patients should also have a realistic idea of the benefit that they can derive from undergoing EP studies, including the possibility that the study result can be negative or equivocal.

Defibrillator Pads

A functioning cardioverter-defibrillator should be available at the patient's side throughout the EP study. Using preapplied adhesive defibrillator pads avoids the need to disrupt the sterile field in the event that electrical defibrillation or cardioversion is needed during the procedure. Biphasic devices are more effective than devices with monophasic waveforms.

Arterial Line

Although accurate monitoring of blood pressure is vital during any invasive procedure, indwelling arterial pressure monitoring lines are not used routinely in most EP laboratories. Automated cuff blood pressure devices are usually adequate. However, invasive blood pressure monitoring is generally used in unstable patients and when transseptal left atrial (LA) access is planned.

Sedation

Many patients benefit from mild sedation. Longer procedures and ablations are now routinely performed using intravenous conscious sedation. The combination of a benzodiazepine (most commonly midazolam) and a narcotic (e.g., fentanyl) is typically used. Propofol is used in some EP laboratories. Bispectral analysis of brain electrical activity is occasionally used for monitoring the depth and safety of sedation. In certain situations, especially when mapping and ablation of an automatic or triggered-activity tachycardia are expected, sedation can suppress the arrhythmic activity and delay or preclude the mapping-ablation procedure. In such cases, avoiding sedation is advisable until inducibility of the tachycardia is ensured.

Urinary Problems

Urinary retention can occur during lengthy EP procedures, particularly in combination with sedation, fluid administration, and tachycardia-related diuresis. When such situations are anticipated, it is useful to insert a urinary drainage catheter before the procedure.

Oxygen and Carbon Dioxide Monitoring

Monitoring of oxygen saturation is used routinely. Exhaled carbon dioxide monitors also can be useful in preventing hypercapnia in patients receiving supplemental oxygen, because oxygen saturation can be misleadingly high.

Anticoagulation

Periprocedural anticoagulation for catheter ablation of persistent AFL or AF is necessary to minimize thromboembolic stroke risk; LA stunning and increased spontaneous echo contrast within the LA can occur following cardioversion or ablation of these arrhythmias. Similarly, patients with mechanical valvular prosthesis require uninterrupted anticoagulation. A perception of increased bleeding risks of invasive procedures in patients taking therapeutic warfarin doses led many operators to adopt a "bridging" strategy of conversion to enoxaparin to allow ablation and subsequent hemostasis to be performed during a pause in anticoagulation.[1] This strategy involves discontinuation of warfarin at least 3 to 5 days prior to ablation, and starting heparin or enoxaparin after cessation of warfarin until the evening prior to the ablation procedure. Both enoxaparin and warfarin are then reinitiated within 4 to 6 hours after ablation and sheath removal, and enoxaparin is maintained until an optimal INR level is achieved.

An alternative strategy of uninterrupted oral anticoagulation during these procedures was found to be safe and feasible and more cost-effective for ablation of typical AFL or AF, without increasing hemorrhagic complications. However, INR testing is required on the day of the procedure to confirm therapeutic anticoagulation. Transesophageal echocardiography is performed in patients with a subtherapeutic INR in the 3 weeks prior to the procedure. Another potential advantage of this strategy is the ability to reverse warfarin effects rapidly in the setting of a bleeding complication (e.g., pericardial bleeding) by using synthetic clotting factor concentrates or fresh frozen plasma infusion, whereas enoxaparin effects remain difficult to reverse; protamine has only a partial effect on its action. This anticoagulation strategy can potentially be used routinely for EP studies and ablation of right-sided arrhythmias for which anticoagulation is required.[2-4]

Catheterization Techniques

Electrode Catheters

Electrode catheters are used during EP testing for recording and pacing. These catheters consist of insulated wires; at the distal tip of the catheter, each wire is attached to an electrode, which is exposed to the intracardiac surface. At the proximal end of the catheter, each wire is attached to a plug, which can be connected to an external recording device. Electrode catheters are generally made of woven Dacron or newer synthetic materials, such as polyurethane. The Dacron catheters have the advantage of stiffness, which helps maintain catheter shape with enough softness at body temperature to allow formation of loops. Catheters made of synthetic materials cannot be easily manipulated and change shape within the body, but they are less expensive and can be made smaller. Some manufacturers use braided metal strands to enhance torque control.

Electrode catheters come in different sizes (3 to 8 Fr). In adults, sizes 5, 6, and 7 Fr catheters are the most commonly used. Recordings derived from electrodes can be unipolar (one pole) or bipolar (two poles). The electrodes are typically 1 to 2 mm in length. The interelectrode distance can range from 1 to 10 mm or more. The greater the interelectrode spacing is on a conventional bipolar electrode, the more the recorded electrogram resembles a unipolar recording. Catheters with a 2- or 5-mm interelectrode distance are most commonly used.[5]

Many multipolar electrode catheters have been developed to facilitate placement of the catheter in the desired place and to fulfill various recording requirements. Bipolar or quadripolar electrode catheters are used to record and pace from specific sites of interest within the atria or ventricles. These catheters come with a variety of preformed distal curve shapes and sizes (Fig. 4-1). Multipolar recording electrode catheters are placed within the coronary sinus (CS) or along the crista terminalis in the right atrium (RA). The Halo catheter is a multipolar catheter used to map atrial electrical activity around the tricuspid annulus during atrial tachycardias, as well as for locating right-sided bypass tracts (BTs) (Fig. 4-2). A decapolar catheter with a distal ring configuration (Lasso catheter) is used to record electrical activity from the pulmonary vein (PV; Fig. 4-3). Basket catheters capable of conforming to the chamber size and shape have also been used for mapping atrial and ventricular arrhythmias (Fig. 4-4). Special catheters are also used to record LA and left ventricular (LV) epicardial activity from the CS branches.[5]

Catheters can have a fixed or deflectable tip. Steerable catheters allow deflection of the tip of the catheter in one or two directions in a single plane; some of these catheters have asymmetrical bidirectional deflectable curves (Fig. 4-5).

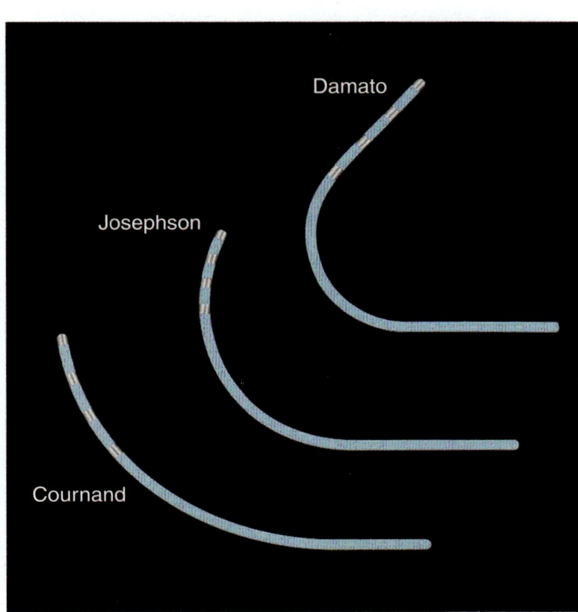

FIGURE 4-1 Multipolar electrode catheters with different preformed curve shapes. *(Courtesy of Boston Scientific, Boston.)*

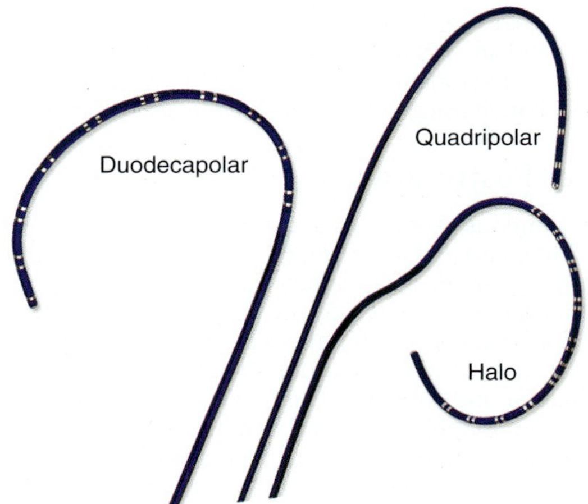

FIGURE 4-2 Multipolar electrode catheters with different electrode numbers and curve shape. **Left to right,** Duodecapolar catheter, quadripolar catheter, and Halo catheter. *(Courtesy of Boston Scientific, Boston.)*

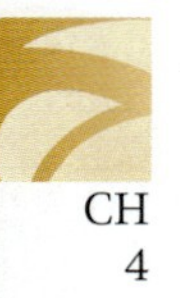

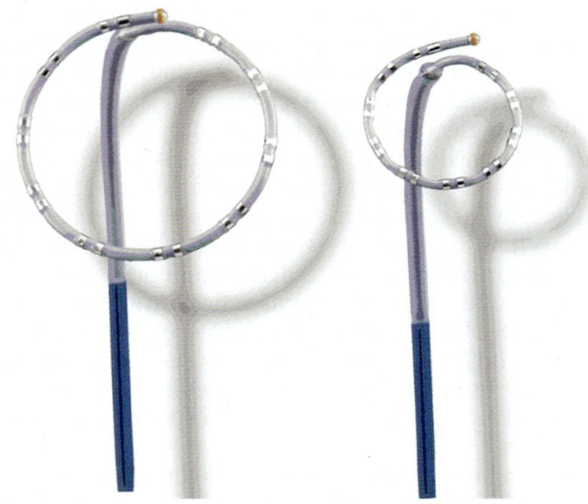

FIGURE 4-3 Lasso catheter with two different loop sizes. *(Courtesy of Biosense Webster, Inc., Diamond Bar, Calif.; www.BiosenseWebster.com.)*

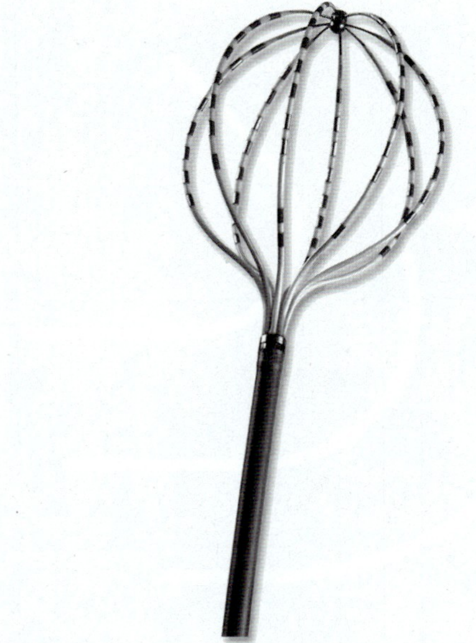

FIGURE 4-4 Basket catheter (Constellation). *(Courtesy of Boston Scientific, Boston.)*

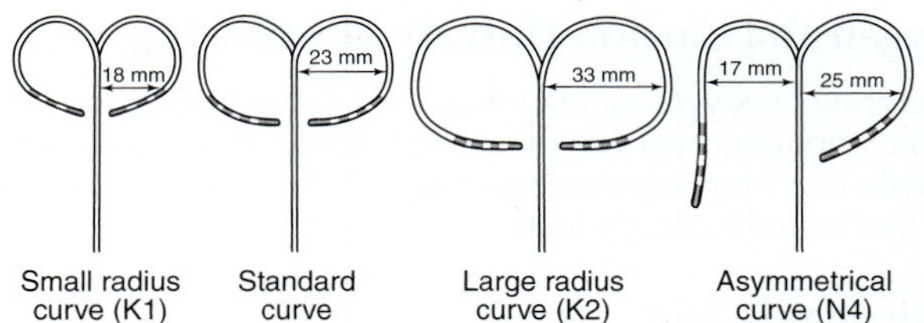

FIGURE 4-5 Deflectable multipolar electrode catheters with different curve sizes and shapes. *(Courtesy of Boston Scientific, Boston.)*

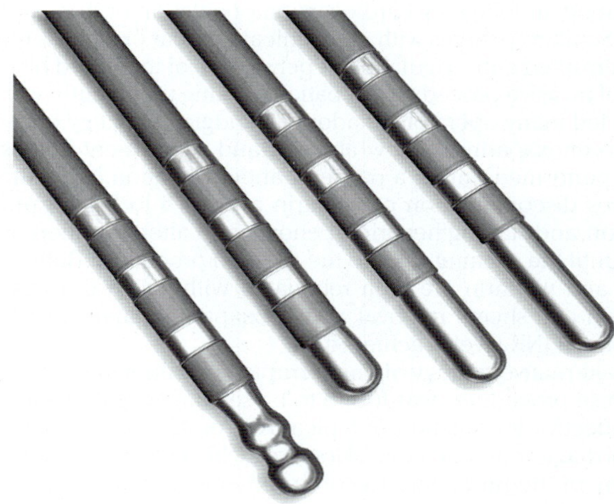

FIGURE 4-6 Ablation catheters with different tip electrode sizes and shapes. **Left to right,** Peanut 8-mm, 2-mm, 4-mm, and 8-mm tip electrodes. *(Courtesy of Boston Scientific, Boston.)*

Ablation catheters have tip electrodes that are conventionally 4 mm long and are available in sizes up to 10 mm in length (Fig. 4-6). The larger tip electrodes on ablation catheters reduce the resolution of a map obtained using recordings from the distal pair of electrodes.

Catheter Positioning

The percutaneous technique is used almost exclusively. RA, His bundle (HB), and right ventricular (RV) electrograms are most commonly recorded using catheters inserted via a femoral vein. Some other areas (e.g., the CS) are more easily reached through the superior vena cava (SVC), although the femoral approach can be adequate in most cases. Insertion sites can also include the antecubital, jugular, and subclavian veins. Femoral arterial access can be required for mapping of the LV or mitral annulus or for invasive blood pressure monitoring. Occasionally, an epicardial approach is required to map and ablate certain VTs and BTs as well as the sinus node. For this purpose, the epicardial surface is accessed via the CS and its branches or percutaneously (subxiphoid puncture).[6]

Fluoroscopy is conventionally used to guide intracardiac positioning of the catheters. It is important to remember that catheters can be withdrawn without fluoroscopy, but they should always be advanced under fluoroscopy guidance. More recently, newer navigation systems have been tested to guide catheter positioning in an effort to limit radiation exposure (see Chap. 6).

Transcaval Approach

The modified Seldinger technique is used to obtain multiple venous accesses. The femoral approach is most common, but the subclavian, internal jugular, or brachial approaches may be used, most often for the placement of a catheter in the CS.[6]

The femoral access should be avoided in patients with any of the following: known or suspected femoral vein or inferior vena cava (IVC) thrombosis, active lower extremity thrombophlebitis or postphlebitic syndrome, groin infection, bilateral leg amputation, extreme obesity, or severe peripheral vascular disease resulting in nonpalpable femoral arterial pulse. IVC umbrella filters are not necessarily a contraindication to the femoral approach.

Typically, the RA, HB, and RV catheters are introduced via the femoral veins. It is advisable to use the left femoral vein for diagnostic EP catheters and to save the right femoral vein for potential ablation or mapping catheter placement, which then would be easier to manipulate because it would be on the side closer to the operator. Multiple venous punctures and single vascular sheaths may be used for the different catheters. Alternatively, a single triport 12 Fr sheath can be used to introduce up to three EP catheters (usually the RA, HB, and RV catheters). The CS catheter is frequently introduced via the right internal jugular or subclavian vein, but also via the femoral approach.

RIGHT ATRIAL CATHETER

A fixed-tip, 5 or 6 Fr quadripolar electrode catheter is typically used. The RA may be entered from the IVC or SVC. The femoral veins are the usual entry sites. Most commonly, stimulation and recording

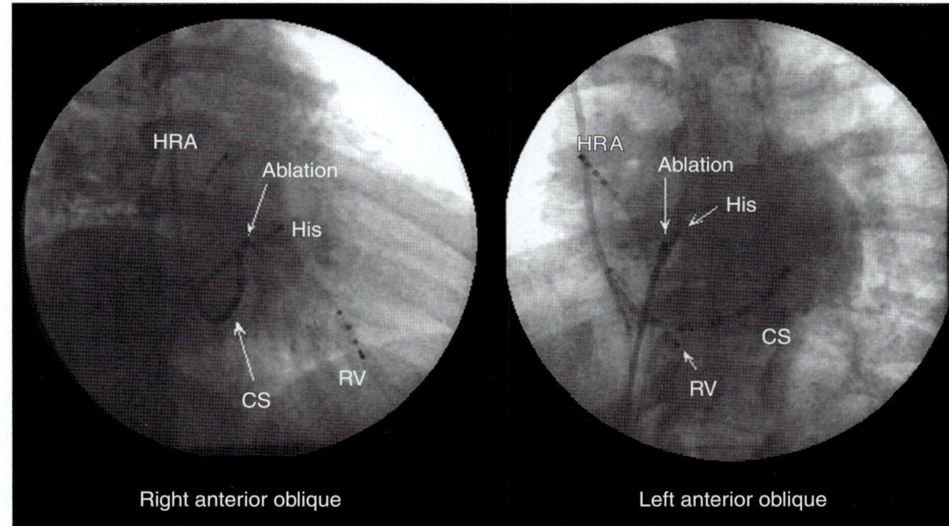

FIGURE 4-7 Fluoroscopic views of catheters in study for supraventricular tachycardia (superoparaseptal bypass tract ablation). Catheters are labeled HRA (high right atrium), right ventricle (RV), and coronary sinus (CS); the CS catheter was inserted from a jugular venous approach.

from the RA is performed by placing the RA catheter tip at the high posterolateral wall at the SVC-RA junction in the region of the sinus node or in the RA appendage (Fig. 4-7).

RIGHT VENTRICULAR CATHETER

A fixed-tip, 5 or 6 Fr quadripolar electrode catheter is typically used. All sites in the RV are accessible from any venous approach. The RV apex is most commonly chosen for stimulation and recording because of stability and reproducibility (see Fig. 4-7).

HIS BUNDLE CATHETER

A fixed- or deflectable-tip, 6 Fr quadripolar electrode catheter is typically used. The catheter is passed via the femoral vein into the RA and across the tricuspid annulus until it is clearly in the RV (under fluoroscopic monitoring, using the right anterior oblique [RAO] view; see Fig. 4-7). It is then withdrawn across the tricuspid orifice while maintaining a slight clockwise torque for good contact with the septum until a His potential is recorded. Initially, a large ventricular electrogram can be observed, then, as the catheter is withdrawn, the right bundle branch (RB) potential can appear (manifesting as a narrow spike less than 30 milliseconds before the ventricular electrogram). When the catheter is further withdrawn, the atrial electrogram appears and grows larger. The His potential usually appears once the atrial and ventricular electrograms are approximately equal in size and is manifest as a biphasic or triphasic deflection interposed between the local atrial and ventricular electrograms. If the first pass was unsuccessful, the catheter should be passed again into the RV and withdrawn with a slightly different rotation. If, after several attempts, a His potential cannot be recorded using a fixed-tip catheter, the catheter should be withdrawn and reshaped, or it may be exchanged with a deflectable-tip catheter. Once the catheter is in place, a stable recording can usually be obtained. Occasionally, continued clockwise torque on the catheter shaft is required to obtain a stable HB recording, which can be accomplished by looping the catheter shaft remaining outside the body and fixing the loop by placing a couple of towels on it, or by twisting the connection cable in the opposite direction so that it maintains a gentle torque on the catheter.

When the access is from the SVC, it is more difficult to record the His potential because the catheter does not lie across the superior margin of the tricuspid annulus. In this case, a deflectable-tip catheter is typically used, advanced into the RV, positioned near the HB region by deflecting the tip superiorly to form a J shape, and then withdrawing the catheter so that it lies across the superior margin of the tricuspid annulus. Alternatively, the catheter can be looped in the RA ("figure-of-6" position); then the body of the loop is advanced into the RV so that the tip of the catheter is pointing toward the RA and lying on the septal aspect of the RA. Gently withdrawing the catheter can increase the size of the loop and allow the catheter tip to rest on the HB location.

Recording of the HB electrogram can also be obtained via the retrograde arterial approach. Using this approach, the catheter tip is positioned in the noncoronary sinus of Valsalva (just above the aortic valve) or in the LV outflow tract (LVOT), along the interventricular septum (just below the aortic valve).

CORONARY SINUS CATHETER

A femoral, internal jugular, or subclavian vein may be used. It is easier to cannulate the CS using the right internal jugular or left subclavian vein versus the femoral vein because the CS valve is oriented anterosuperiorly and, when prominent, can prevent easy access to the CS from the femoral venous approach. A fixed-tip, 6 Fr decapolar electrode catheter is typically used for access from the SVC, whereas a deflectable-tip catheter is preferred for CS access from the femoral veins.

The standardized RAO and left anterior oblique (LAO) fluoroscopic views are used to guide placement of catheters in the CS. Although the CS cannot be directly visualized with standard fluoroscopy, the epicardial fat found in the posteroseptal space just posterior to the CS os can be visualized as a characteristic radiolucency on cine fluoroscopy in the RAO projection, where the cardiac and diaphragmatic silhouettes meet.[7]

When cannulating the CS from the SVC approach, the LAO view is used, the catheter tip is directed to the left of the patient, and the catheter is advanced with some clockwise torque to engage the CS os; electrodes should resemble rectangles rather than ovals when the catheter tip is properly oriented to advance into the CS. Once the CS os is engaged, the catheter is further advanced gently into the CS, so that the most proximal electrodes lie at the CS os (see Fig. 4-7).

During cannulation of the CS from the IVC approach, the tip of the catheter is first placed into the RV, in the RAO fluoroscopy view, and flexed downward toward the RV inferior wall (Video 2). Subsequently, the catheter is withdrawn until it lies at the inferoseptal aspect of the tricuspid annulus. In the LAO or RAO view, the catheter is then withdrawn gently with clockwise rotation until the tip of the catheter drops into the CS os. Afterward, the catheter is advanced into the CS concomitantly with gradual release of the catheter curve (Fig. 4-8). Alternatively, the tip of the catheter is directed toward the posterolateral RA wall and advanced with a tight curve to form a loop in the RA, in the LAO view, with the tip directed toward the

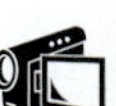

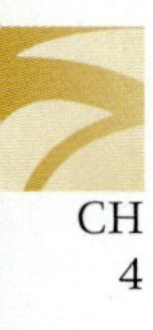

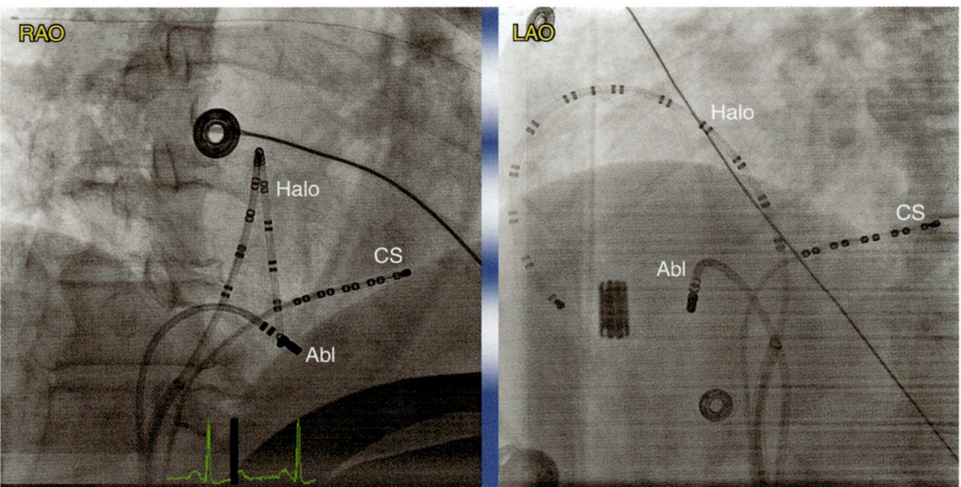

FIGURE 4-8 Right anterior oblique (RAO) and left anterior oblique (LAO) fluoroscopic views of catheters in a study of typical atrial flutter. A 20-pole Halo catheter is positioned along the tricuspid annulus. The coronary sinus (CS) catheter was introduced from a femoral venous approach. The ablation catheter (Abl) is at the cavotricuspid isthmus.

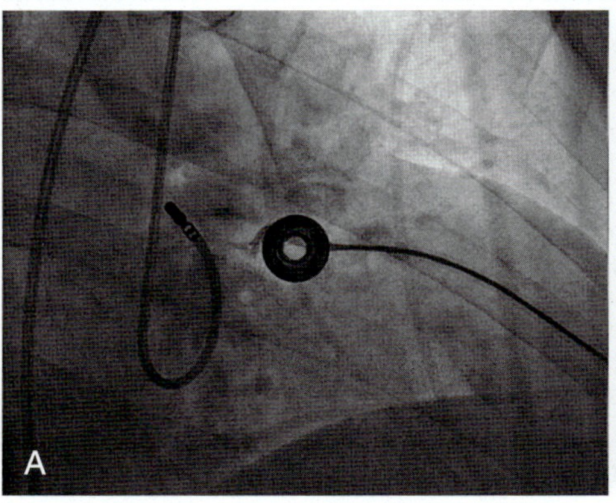

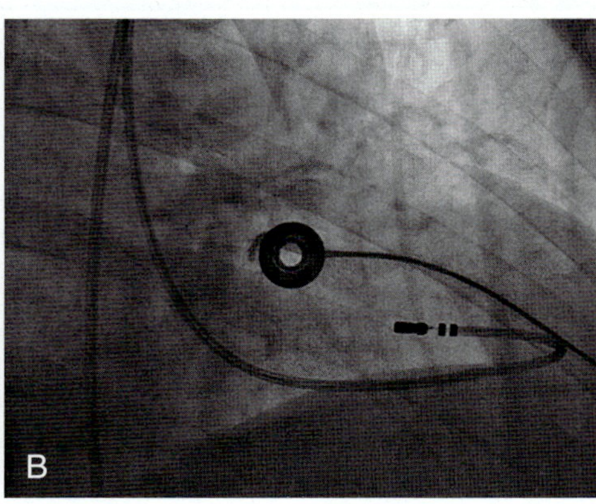

FIGURE 4-9 Right anterior oblique (RAO) fluoroscopic views of a mapping-ablation catheter introduced into the left ventricle (LV) via the retrograde transaortic approach. In a 30-degree RAO view, the curved catheter **(A)** is prolapsed across the aortic valve into the LV **(B)**.

inferomedial RA. The tip is then advanced with gentle up-down, right-left manipulation using the LAO and RAO views to cannulate the CS. In the RAO view, the atrioventricular (AV) fat pad (containing the CS) appears as more radiolucent than surrounding heart tissue.

When attempting CS cannulation, the catheter can enter the RV, and premature ventricular complexes (PVCs) or VT can be observed. Catheter position in the RV outflow tract (RVOT) can be misleading and simulate a CS position. Confirming appropriate catheter positioning in the CS can be achieved by fluoroscopy and recorded electrograms. In the LAO view, further advancement in the CS directs the catheter toward the left heart border, where it curves toward the left shoulder. Conversely, advancement of a catheter lying in the RVOT leads to an upward direction of the catheter toward the pulmonary artery. In the RAO view, the CS catheter is directed posteriorly, posterior to the AV sulcus, whereas the RVOT position is directed anteriorly. Recording from the CS catheter shows simultaneous atrial and ventricular electrograms, with the atrial electrogram falling in the later part of the P wave, whereas a catheter lying in the RVOT records only a ventricular electrogram. The catheter can also pass into the LA via a patent foramen ovale, in which case it takes a straight course toward the left shoulder, and all recordings are atrial.

If used, the CS catheter should be placed first, because its positioning can be impeded by the presence of other catheters. It is also recommended that the CS catheter sheath be sutured to the skin to prevent displacement of the catheter during the course of the EP study.

Transaortic Approach

This approach is generally used for mapping the LV and mitral annulus (for VT and left-sided BTs). The right femoral artery is most commonly used. The mapping-ablation catheter is passed to the descending aorta, and, in this position, a tight J curve is formed with the catheter tip before passage to the aortic root to minimize catheter manipulation in the arch. In a 30-degree RAO view, the curved catheter is advanced through the aortic valve with the J curve opening to the right, so the catheter passes into the LV oriented anterolaterally (Fig. 4-9; Video 3). The straight catheter tip must never be used to cross the aortic valve because of the risk of leaflet damage or perforation and also because the catheter tip can slip into the left or right coronary artery or a coronary bypass graft, thus mimicking entry to the LV and causing damage to these structures.

A long vascular sheath can provide added catheter stability. Anticoagulation should be started once the LV is accessed or before (intravenous heparin, a 5000-unit bolus followed by a 1000-unit infusion is usually used), to maintain the activated clotting time (ACT) between 250 and 300 seconds.

Transseptal Approach

Mapping and ablation in the LA are performed through a transseptal approach. Knowledge of septal anatomy and its relationship with adjacent structures is essential to ensure safe and effective access to the LA. Many apparent septal structures are not truly septal. The true interatrial septum is limited to the floor of the fossa ovalis, the flap valve, and the anteroinferior rim of the fossa. Therefore, the floor of the fossa (with an average diameter of 18.5 ± 6.9 mm [vertically] and 10.0 ± 2.4 mm [horizontally] and 2 mm thickness) is the target for atrial septal crossing. The area between the superior border of the fossa and the mouth of the SVC is an infolding of the atrial wall filled with adipose tissue. Although this area is often referred to as the septum secundum, it is not really a true septum, and puncture in this region would lead to exiting of the heart. The infolded groove ends at the superior margin (superior rim) of the fossa ovalis. Anterior and superior to the fossa ovalis, the RA wall overlies the aortic root. Advancing the transseptal needle in this area can puncture the aorta.

A search for a patent foramen ovale, which is present in 15% to 20% of normal subjects, is initially performed. If one is absent, atrial septal puncture is performed. The challenge for a successful atrial septal puncture is positioning the Brockenbrough needle at the thinnest aspect of the atrial septum, the membranous fossa ovalis, guided by fluoroscopy or intracardiac echocardiography (ICE; Videos 4, 5, and 6).

Although fluoroscopy provides sufficient information to allow safe transseptal puncture in most cases, variations in septal anatomy, atrial or aortic root dilation, the need for multiple punctures, and the desired ability to direct the catheter to specific locations within the LA can make fluoroscopy an inadequate tool for complex LA ablation procedures. Intraoperative transesophageal echocardiography allows identification of the fossa ovalis and its relation to surrounding structures and provides real-time evaluation of the atrial septal puncture procedure, with demonstration of tenting of the fossa prior to entry into the LA and visualization of the sheath advancing across the septum (Video 7). However, the usefulness of transesophageal echocardiography is limited by the fact that the probe obstructs the fluoroscopic field, and it is impractical in the nonanesthetized patient. ICE, which provides similar information on septal anatomy, can be used for the conscious patient and does not impede fluoroscopy.

FLUOROSCOPY-GUIDED TRANSSEPTAL CATHETERIZATION

Equipment required for atrial septal puncture includes the following: a 62-cm, 8 Fr transseptal sheath for LA cannulation (e.g., SR0, SL1, Mullins, or Agilis NxT Steerable sheath, St. Jude Medical, Minnetonka, Minn.), a 0.035-inch J guidewire, a 71-cm Brockenbrough needle (e.g., BRK, St. Jude Medical, Minnetonka, Minn.), and a 190-cm, 0.014-inch guidewire.

Venous access is obtained via the femoral vein, preferably the right femoral vein because it is closer to the operator. The sheath, dilator, and guidewires are flushed with heparinized saline. The transseptal sheath and dilator are advanced over a 0.035-inch J guidewire under fluoroscopy guidance into the SVC. The guidewire is then withdrawn, thus leaving the sheath and its dilator locked in place. The dilator within the sheath is flushed and attached to a syringe to avoid introduction of air into the RA.

Attention is then directed to preparing the transseptal needle. The Brockenbrough needle comes prepackaged with an inner stylet, which may be left in place to protect it as it is advanced within the sheath. Alternatively, the inner stylet may be removed and the needle connected to a pressure transducer line (pressure monitoring through the Brockenbrough needle will be required during the transseptal puncture); continuous flushing through the Brockenbrough needle is used while advancing the needle into the dilator. A third approach, when the use of contrast injection is planned, is to attach the Brockenbrough needle to a standard three-way stopcock via a freely rotating adapter. A 10-mL syringe filled with radiopaque contrast is attached to the other end of the stopcock while a pressure transducer line is attached to the third stopcock valve for continuous pressure monitoring. The entire apparatus should be vigorously flushed to ensure that no air bubbles are present within the circuit.

The Brockenbrough needle is advanced into the dilator until the needle tip is within 1 to 2 cm of the dilator tip. The needle tip must be kept within the dilator at all times, except during actual septal puncture. The curves of the dilator, sheath, and needle should be aligned so that they are all in agreement and not contradicting each other. The sheath, dilator, and needle assembly is then rotated leftward and posteriorly (usually with the Brockenbrough needle arrow pointing at the 3 to 6 o'clock position relative to its shaft) and retracted caudally as a single unit (while maintaining the relative positions of its components) to engage the tip of the dilator into the fossa ovalis. Under fluoroscopy monitoring (30-degree LAO view), the dilator tip moves slightly leftward on entering the RA and then leftward again while descending below the aortic root. A third abrupt leftward movement ("jump") below the aortic root indicates passage over the limbus into the fossa ovalis (Fig. 4-10). This jump generally occurs at the level of the HB region (marked by an EP catheter recording the HB potential). If the sheath and dilator assembly is pulled back farther than intended (i.e., below the level of the fossa and HB region), the needle should be withdrawn and

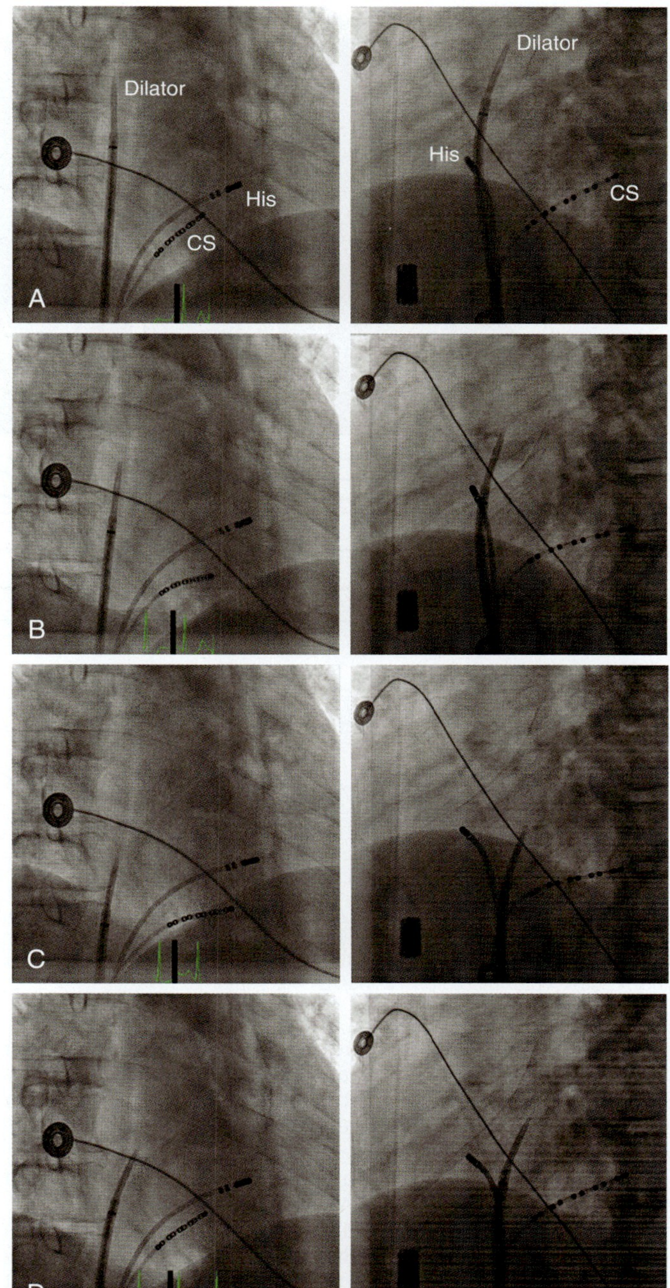

FIGURE 4-10 Right anterior oblique (RAO; **left**) and left anterior oblique (LAO; **right**) fluoroscopic views during transseptal catheterization. **A,** Initially, the transseptal sheath-dilator assembly is advanced into the superior vena cava. **B,** The transseptal assembly is withdrawn into the high right atrium. **C,** With further withdrawal, the dilator tip abruptly moves leftward, indicating passage over the limbus into the fossa ovalis at the level of the His bundle catheter. At the fossa ovalis, the dilator tip has an anteroposterior orientation in the RAO view and a leftward orientation in the LAO view. **D,** The transseptal assembly is advanced across the atrial septum. CS = coronary sinus.

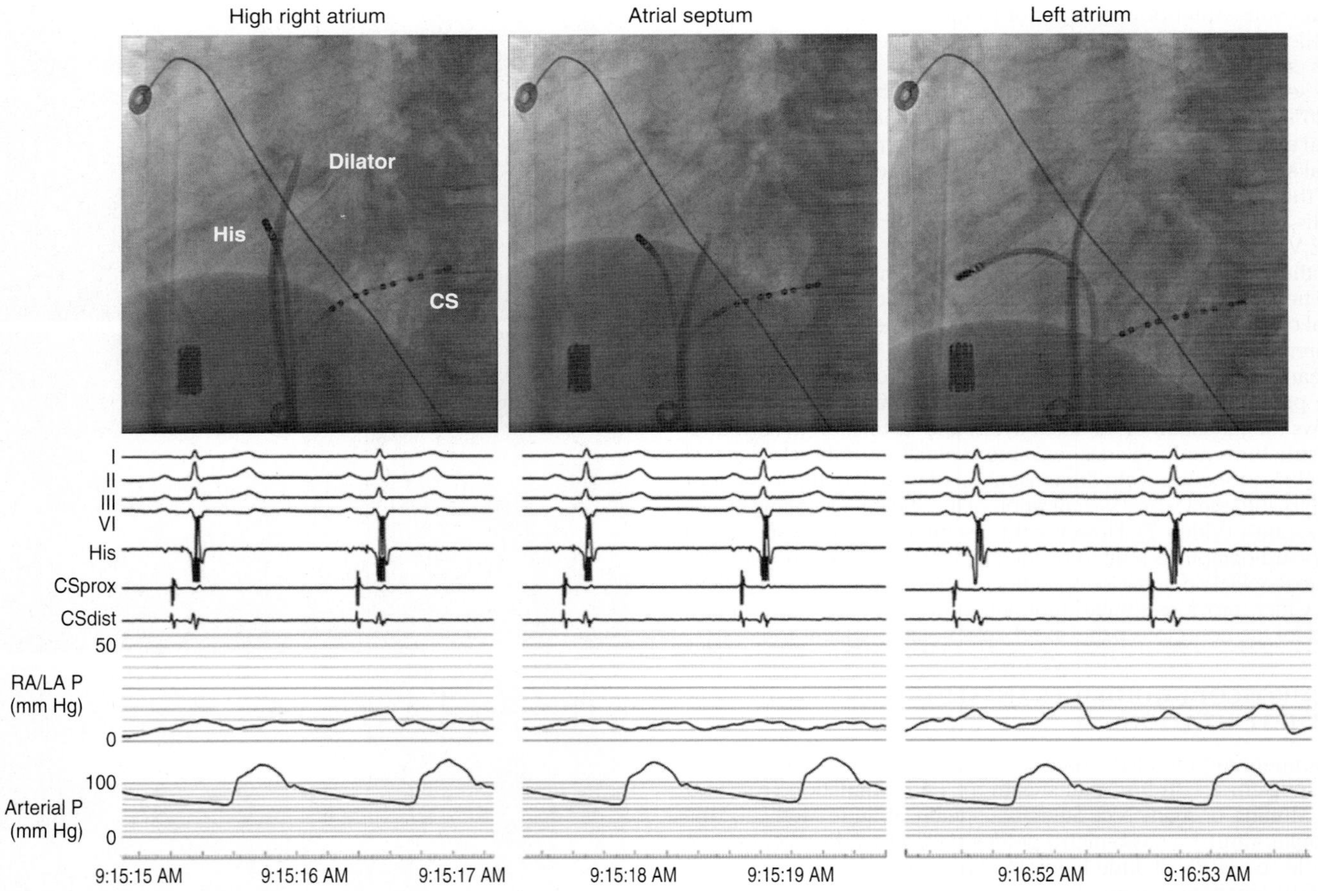

FIGURE 4-11 Left anterior oblique (LAO) fluoroscopic views and simultaneous electrical and pressure (P) recordings during transseptal catheterization. **Left,** The transseptal assembly is in the right atrium (RA), indicated by typical A and V waves of right-heart pressure tracing. **Middle,** The pressure waveform is dampened somewhat as the catheter tip abuts the septum. **Right,** The needle is across the atrial septum, and characteristic waves (V larger than A) are seen. CSdist = distal coronary sinus; CSprox = proximal coronary sinus; LA = left atrium.

the guidewire placed through the dilator into the SVC. The sheath and dilator assembly is then advanced over the guidewire into the SVC and repositioning attempted, as described earlier. The sheath and dilator assembly should never be advanced without the guidewire at any point during the procedure.

Several fluoroscopic markers are used to confirm the position of the dilator tip at the fossa ovalis. As noted, an abrupt leftward movement (jump) of the dilator tip below the aortic knob is observed as the tip passes under the muscular atrial septum onto the fossa ovalis (see Video 4). In addition, the posterior extent of the aortic root can be marked by a pigtail catheter positioned through the femoral artery in the noncoronary cusp or by the HB catheter (recording a stable proximal HB potential), which lies at the level of the fibrous trigone opposite and caudal to the noncoronary aortic cusp. When the dilator tip lies against the fossa ovalis, it is directed posteroinferiorly to the proximal HB electrode (or pigtail catheter) in the RAO view and to the left of the proximal HB electrode (or pigtail catheter) in the LAO view (see Fig. 4-10). Another method that can be used to ensure that the tip is against the fossa ovalis is injection of 3 to 5 mL of radiopaque contrast through the Brockenbrough needle to visualize the interatrial septum. The needle tip then can be seen tenting the fossa ovalis membrane with small movements of the entire transseptal apparatus. Typically, septal staining remains visible after contrast injection, which allows for real-time septal visualization while monitoring the pressure during transseptal puncture.

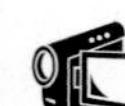

Once the position of the dilator tip is confirmed at the fossa ovalis, the needle, dilator, and sheath assembly is pushed slightly against the interatrial septum, and the needle is then briskly advanced to protrude outside the dilator in the LAO view during continuous pressure monitoring. If excessive force is applied without a palpable "pop" to the fossa, then the Brockenbrough needle likely is not in proper position. After passage through the fossa ovale and before advancing the dilator and sheath, an intraatrial position of the needle tip within the LA, rather than the ascending aorta or posteriorly into the pericardial space, needs to be confirmed. Recording an LA pressure waveform from the needle tip confirms an intraatrial location (Fig. 4-11). An arterial pressure waveform indicates intraaortic position of the needle. Absence of a pressure wave recording can indicate needle passage into the pericardial space or sliding up and not puncturing through the atrial septum. A second method is injection of contrast through the needle to assess the position of the needle tip. Opacification of the LA (rather than the pericardium or the aorta) verifies the successful transseptal access. Alternatively, passing a 0.014-inch floppy guidewire through the Brockenbrough needle into a left-sided PV (beyond the cardiac silhouette in the LAO fluoroscopy view) helps verify that needle tip position is within the LA (see Video 4). If the guidewire cannot be advanced beyond the fluoroscopic border of the heart, pericardial puncture should be suspected. In addition, aortic puncture should be suspected if the guidewire seems to follow the course of the aorta. In these situations, contrast should be injected to assess the position of the Brockenbrough needle before advancing the transseptal dilator. Sometimes, the guidewire enters the LA appendage rather than a PV; in this setting, a clockwise torque of the sheath and dilator assembly can help direct the guidewire posteriorly toward the ostium of the left superior or left inferior PV.

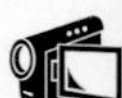

Once the position of the needle tip is confirmed to be in the LA, both the sheath and dilator are advanced as a single unit over the needle by using one hand while fixing the Brockenbrough needle in position with the other hand (to prevent any further advancement of the needle). Preferably, the sheath and dilator assembly is advanced into the LA over a guidewire placed distally into a left-sided PV, which helps direct the path of the assembly as it enters the LA and minimize the risk of inadvertent puncture of the lateral LA wall. Once the dilator tip is advanced into the LA over the needle tip, the needle and dilator are firmly stabilized as a unit—to prevent any further advancement of the needle and dilator—and the sheath is advanced over the dilator into the LA. Once the transseptal sheath tip is within the LA, the dilator and needle are withdrawn slowly during continuous flushing through the needle or while suction is maintained through a syringe placed on the sheath side port to minimize the risk of air embolism and while fixing the sheath with the other hand to prevent dislodgment outside the LA. The sheath should be aspirated until blood appears without further bubbles; this usually requires aspiration of approximately 5 mL. The sheath is then flushed with heparinized saline at a flow rate of 3 mL/min during the entire procedure.

The mapping-ablation catheter is advanced through the sheath into the LA. Flexing the catheter tip and applying clockwise and counterclockwise torque to the sheath help confirm free movement of the catheter tip within the LA, rather than possibly in the pericardium. It is important to recognize that merely recording atrial electrograms does not confirm an LA catheter location because an LA recording can be obtained from the epicardial surface of the LA, from the RA, or even the aortic root.

When two transseptal accesses are required, the second access can be obtained through a separate transseptal puncture performed in a fashion similar to that described for the first puncture. Alternatively, the first transseptal puncture can be used for the second sheath. This technique entails passing a guidewire or thin catheter through the first transseptal sheath into the LA, preferably into the left inferior or superior PV, and then the sheath is pulled back into the RA. Subsequently, a deflectable tip catheter is used through the second long sheath to interrogate the fossa ovalis and to try to access the LA through the initial puncture site. Once this is accomplished, the first sheath is advanced back into the LA, and the guidewire is replaced with the mapping catheter. Alternatively, instead of using a deflectable catheter, the needle, dilator, and sheath assembly is advanced into the SVC and pulled back and positioned at the fossa ovalis (as described earlier for the first transseptal puncture). Once the tip of the dilator falls into the fossa ovalis, gentle manipulation of the assembly under biplane fluoroscopy guidance is performed until the dilator tip passes along the guidewire through the existing transseptal puncture, without advancing the needle through the dilator. The assembly is then advanced as a single unit into the LA.

An intravenous heparin bolus is administered just before or immediately after puncturing the atrial septum, followed by intermittent boluses or continuous heparin infusion to maintain an elevated ACT (more than 250 to 300 seconds).

INTRACARDIAC ECHOCARDIOGRAPHY–GUIDED TRANSSEPTAL CATHETERIZATION

The intent of ICE-guided transseptal catheterization is to image intracardiac anatomy and identify the exact position of the distal aspect of the transseptal dilator along the atrial septum—in particular, to assess for tenting of the fossa ovalis with the dilator tip.

Two types of ICE imaging systems are currently available, the electronic phased-array ultrasound catheter and the mechanical ultrasound catheter.[8] The electronic phased-array ultrasound catheter sector imaging system (AcuNav, Siemens Medical Solutions, Malvern, Pa.) uses an 8 or 10 Fr catheter that has a forward-facing 64-element vector phased-array transducer scanning in the longitudinal plane. The catheter has a four-way steerable tip (160-degree anteroposterior or left-right deflections). The catheter images a sector field oriented in the plane of the catheter. The mechanical ultrasound catheter radial imaging system (Ultra ICE, EP Technologies, Boston Scientific, San Jose, Calif.) uses a 9-MHz catheter-based ultrasound transducer contained within a 9 Fr (110-cm length) catheter shaft. It has a single rotating crystal ultrasound transducer that images circumferentially for 360 degrees in the horizontal plane. The catheter is not freely deflectable.

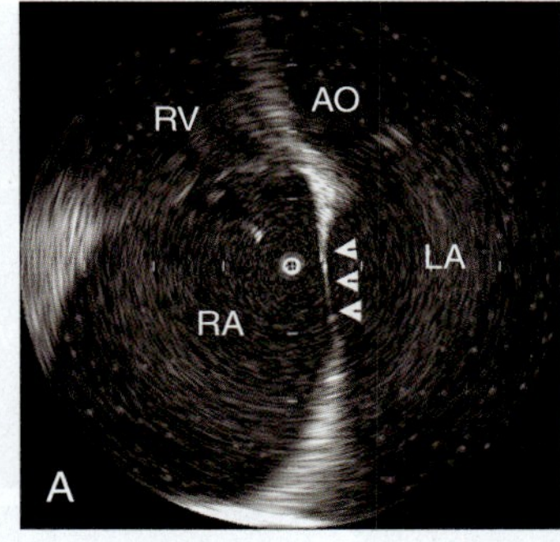

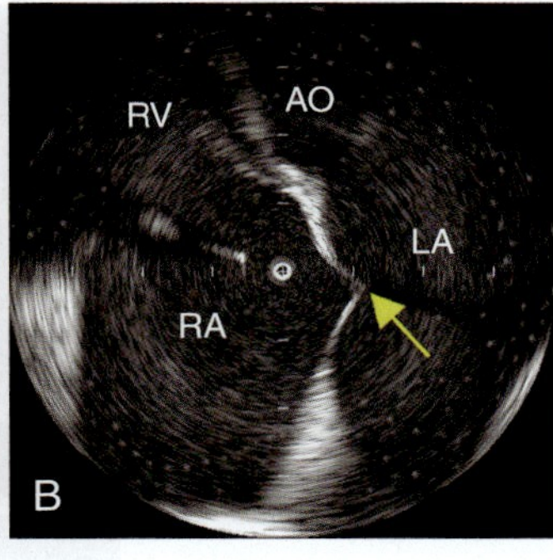

FIGURE 4-12 Intracardiac echocardiography (ICE)-guided transseptal puncture using the Ultra-ICE catheter. These ICE images, with the transducer placed in the right atrium (RA), show **(A)** the RA, fossa ovalis (arrowheads), left atrium (LA), and aorta (AO). **B,** The transseptal needle is properly positioned, with tenting (yellow arrow) against the midinteratrial septum at the fossa ovalis. RV= right ventricle.

When using the mechanical radial ICE imaging system, a 9 Fr sheath, preferably a long, preshaped sheath, for the ICE catheter is advanced via a femoral venous access. To enhance image quality, all air must be eliminated from the distal tip of the ICE catheter by flushing vigorously with 5 to 10 mL of sterile water. The catheter then is connected to the ultrasound console and advanced until the tip of the rotary ICE catheter images the fossa ovalis. Satisfactory imaging of the fossa ovalis for guiding transseptal puncture is viewed from the mid-RA (Fig. 4-12).[8]

The AcuNav ICE catheter is introduced under fluoroscopy guidance through a 23-cm femoral venous sheath. Once the catheter is advanced into the mid-RA with the catheter tension controls in neutral position (the ultrasound transducer oriented anteriorly and to the left), the RA, tricuspid valve, and RV are viewed. This is called the home view (Fig. 4-13A; see Video 5). Gradual clockwise rotation of a straight catheter from the home view allows sequential visualization of the aortic root and the pulmonary artery (see Fig. 4-13B), followed by the CS, the mitral valve, the LA appendage orifice, and a cross-sectional view of the fossa ovalis (see Fig. 4-13C and D). The mitral valve and interatrial septum are usually seen in the same plane as the LA appendage. Posterior deflection or right-left steering of the imaging tip in the RA, or both, is occasionally required to optimize visualization of the fossa ovalis; the tension knob (lock function) can then be used to hold the catheter tip in position. Further clockwise rotation beyond this location demonstrates images of the left PV ostia (see Fig. 4-13E). The optimal ICE image to guide transseptal puncture demonstrates adequate space behind the interatrial septum on the LA side and clearly identify adjacent structures, but it does not include the aortic root because it would be too anterior for the interatrial septum to be punctured safely. In patients with an enlarged LA, a cross-sectional view that includes the LA appendage is also optimal if adequate space exists behind the atrial septum on the LA side.[8]

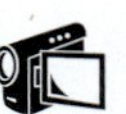

The sheath, dilator, and needle assembly is introduced into the RA, and the dilator tip is positioned against the fossa ovale, as described earlier. Before advancing the Brockenbrough needle, continuous ICE imaging should direct further adjustments in the dilator tip position until ICE confirms that the tip is in intimate contact with the middle of the fossa, confirms proper lateral movement of the dilator toward the fossa, and excludes inadvertent superior displacement toward the muscular septum and aortic valve. With further advancement of the dilator, ICE demonstrates tenting of the fossa (Fig. 4-14 and see Fig. 4-12). If the distance from the tented fossa to the LA free wall is small, minor adjustments in the dilator tip position can be made to maximize the space. The Brockenbrough needle is then advanced. With successful transseptal puncture, a palpable pop is felt, and sudden collapse of the tented

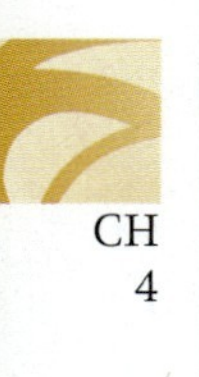

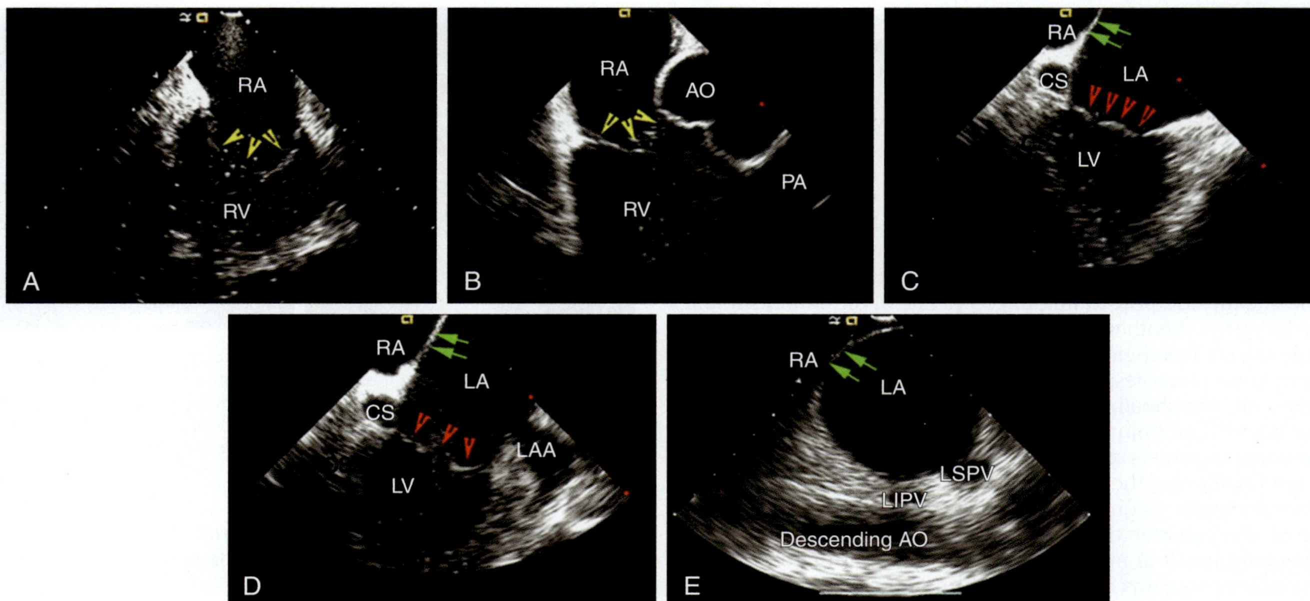

FIGURE 4-13 Phased-array intracardiac echocardiography (ICE) AcuNav serial images with the transducer placed in the middle right atrium (RA) demonstrate serial changes in tomographic imaging views following clockwise rotation of the transducer. Each view displays a left-right (L-R) orientation marker to the operator's left side (i.e., craniocaudal axis projects from image right to left). **A,** Starting from the home view, the RA, tricuspid valve (yellow arrowheads), and right ventricle (RV) are visualized. **B,** Clockwise rotation brings the aorta (AO) into view. PA = pulmonary artery. **C,** Further rotation allows visualization of the interatrial septum (green arrows), left atrium (LA), coronary sinus (CS), left ventricle (LV), and mitral valve (red arrowheads). **D,** Subsequently, the left atrium appendage (LAA) becomes visible. **E,** The ostia of the left superior pulmonary vein (LSPV) and left inferior PV (LIPV) can be visualized with further clockwise rotation. *(Courtesy of AcuNav, Siemens Medical Solutions, Malvern, Pa.)*

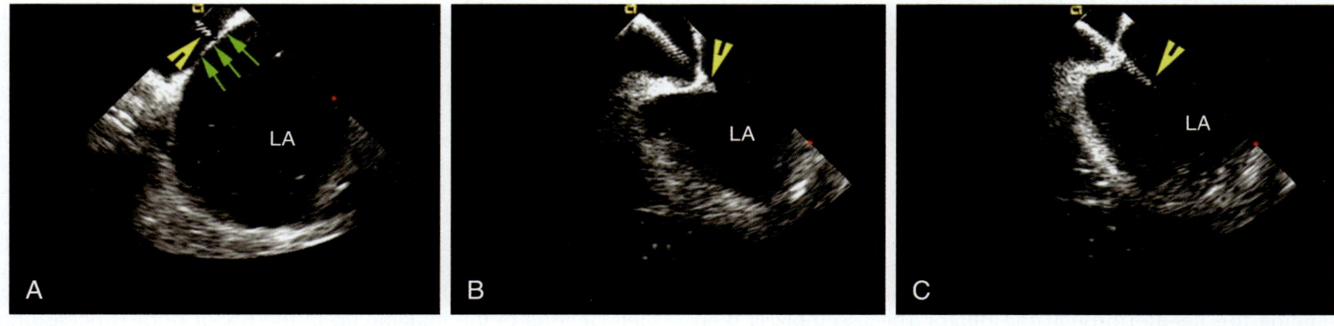

FIGURE 4-14 Phased-array intracardiac echocardiography (ICE)-guided transseptal puncture. **A,** These ICE images, with the transducer placed in the right atrium (RA), show a transseptal dilator tip (yellow arrowhead) lying against the interatrial septum (green arrows). **B,** With further advancement of the dilator, ICE demonstrates tenting of the interatrial septum at the fossa ovalis. **C,** Advancement of the transseptal needle is then performed, with the needle tip visualized in the left atrium (LA), and tenting of the interatrial septum is lost.

fossa is observed (see Fig. 4-14). Advancement of the needle is then immediately stopped. Saline infusion through the needle is visualized on ICE as bubbles in the LA, thus confirming successful septal puncture (see Video 6). With no change in position of the Brockenbrough needle, the transseptal dilator and sheath are advanced over the guidewire into the LA, as described earlier.

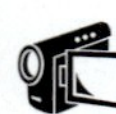

ALTERNATIVE METHODS FOR DIFFICULT TRANSSEPTAL CATHETERIZATION

In some cases, the conventional approach using a Brockenbrough needle sheath fails to pierce the septum because of the presence of a small fossa area, a thick interatrial septum, fibrosis and scarring of the septum from previous interventions, or an aneurysmal septum with excessive laxity. Applying excessive force to the needle, dilator, and sheath assembly against a resistant septum (which can be seen as bending and buckling of the assembly in the RA) can lead to building pressure of the needle tip on the septum, which can potentially lead to an uncontrolled sudden jump of the assembly once across the stiff or fibrotic fossa ovalis, thus perforating the opposing lateral LA wall. Similarly, excessive tenting of the interatrial septum (beyond halfway into the LA) can bring it in close proximity to the lateral LA wall, so that the needle can potentially puncture the lateral LA wall once across the septum. Some of these difficulties can sometimes be overcome by manual reshaping of the curvature of the Brockenbrough needle tip, applying slight rotation on the needle and sheath assembly to puncture a different point on the fossa ovalis, using a sharper transseptal needle type (BRK-1 extra sharp), or utilizing a 0.014-inch, sharp-tipped, J-shaped transseptal guidewire (Safe Sept, Pressure Products, Inc., San Pedro, Calif.).[9-13]

Other techniques to facilitate transseptal puncture include radiofrequency (RF) perforation of the fossa ovalis and the application of pulses of electrosurgical cautery or RF energy to the proximal end of the Brockenbrough needle. Once the position of the dilator tip is confirmed at the fossa ovalis (under ICE guidance), the needle is advanced beyond the tip of the dilator in contact with the septum until resistance is met. RF energy (5 to 30 W for 1 to 11 seconds) can be applied through a conventional ablation catheter electrode brought manually in contact with the proximal hub of the transseptal needle. Typically, the fossa is punctured almost instantaneously (within 1 to 2 seconds) following RF application. Alternatively, electrosurgical cautery (set to 15 to 20 W for a 1- to 2-second pulse of cut-mode cautery) is applied to the proximal hub of the needle as its tip is advanced out of the dilator. Importantly, the cautery should be initiated on the needle handle prior to pushing the needle tip beyond the dilator tip to help minimize the power needed to puncture the septum, and it should be stopped as soon as the needle is pushed out fully.[14-16]

Additionally, a specialized, electrically insulated RF-powered needle (Baylis Medical Company, Inc., Montreal) has been developed to facilitate transseptal puncture. The needle is connected to a proprietary RF generator (RFP-100 RF Puncture Generator, Baylis Medical), which delivers RF energy to the rounded, closed tip of the needle positioned at the interatrial septum. Once septal tenting is visualized on the ICE, RF energy is applied at 10 W for 2 seconds. The RF perforation generators apply a higher voltage for short durations, resulting in a high-energy electric field and an almost instantaneous temperature rise to 100°C, leading to steam popping and septal perforation with minimal collateral tissue damage. In contrast, conventional RF generators deliver a higher power with a lower voltage and impedance range for longer periods of time, with resulting thermal destruction of the local tissue around the needle tip, rather than perforation.[17,18]

These methods help minimize pressure application to the needle as it crosses the septum and tenting of the septum, which can potentially reduce the chances of sudden advancement through the lateral LA as the needle crosses the septum. Nonetheless, the powered needle can potentially be more traumatic at the puncture site than a standard needle, and it is possible that the transseptal puncture site created with a powered needle is less likely to close spontaneously. Similarly, inadvertent cardiac perforation occurring in the setting of powered needles can potentially be associated with greater consequences. Whether RF is more likely to cause a thrombus at the puncture site compared with a standard needle is unknown.[17-19]

COMPLICATIONS OF ATRIAL TRANSSEPTAL PUNCTURE

Injury to cardiac and extracardiac structures is the most feared complication. Because of its stiffness and large caliber, the transseptal dilator should never be advanced until the position of the Brockenbrough needle is confirmed with confidence. Advancing the dilator into an improper position can be fatal. Therefore, many operators recommend the use of ICE-guided transseptal puncture, especially for patients with normal atrial size.[19]

When the aorta is advertently punctured by the Brockenbrough needle—an arterial waveform is recorded from the needle tip and dye injected through the needle is carried away from the heart—the needle should be withdrawn back into the dilator. If the patient remains stable for 15 minutes and echocardiography shows no pericardial effusion, another attempt at LA access can be made. Advancing the dilator and sheath assembly into the aorta can lead to catastrophic consequences.

It is important to recognize that successful atrial septal puncture is a painless procedure for the patient. If the patient experiences significant discomfort, careful assessment should be made of the catheter and sheath locations (pericardial space, aorta).

Another potential complication is embolism of thrombus or air. To avoid air embolism, catheters must be advanced and withdrawn slowly so as not to introduce air into the assembly. Sheaths must be aspirated with a syringe on a stopcock to the amount of their volume (e.g., an 8 Fr sheath contains 5 mL when filled) to remove any retained air. Thromboembolic complications can be avoided by flushing all sheaths and guidewire with heparinized saline and maintaining the ACT at longer than 300 seconds. In addition, a guidewire should not be left in the LA for more than 1 minute, especially if no systemic heparin has been administered. Administration of heparin before, rather than after, the atrial septal puncture can also help reduce thromboembolism.[19]

Occasionally, ST segment elevation in the inferior ECG leads (with or without transient bradycardia or AV block) can occur following transseptal catheterization, potentially secondary to air embolism in coronary arteries, although a Bezold-Jarisch–like reflex mechanism can also be implicated.

Importantly, the presence of an LA thrombus is an absolute contraindication for transseptal catheterization. Additionally, caution should be used in the setting of the presence cardiac or thoracic malformation (e.g., congenital heart disease, kyphoscoliosis).

Transseptal catheterization is feasible and safe in most patients with atrial septal defect or patent foramen ovale repair. Nonetheless, because of the altered anatomical landmarks after repair, fluoroscopic guidance for transseptal puncture can be unreliable, and the procedure can be challenging. In these patients, an understanding of the method of repair and utilization of ICE guidance are essential.

In patients with atrial septal defect closure devices, puncture is preferably performed at the portion of the septum located inferior and posterior to the closure device and not through the device itself. In patients with a septal stitch or pericardial or Dacron patch, puncture can be achieved through the thickened septum or the patch. However, transseptal access is typically not achievable through a Gore-Tex patch (W.L. Gore & Associates, Flagstaff, Ariz.) because of its resistant texture; instead, puncture can be performed directly through neighboring native interatrial tissue. When the patch is wide, sufficient free septal tissue for transseptal puncture may not be available, in which setting transseptal access to the LA may not be feasible.[19,20]

Epicardial Approach

Coronary veins can be used to perform epicardial mapping, but manipulation of the mapping catheter is limited by the anatomical distribution of these vessels. Therefore, the subxiphoid percutaneous approach to the epicardial space is the only technique currently available that allows extensive and unrestricted mapping of the epicardial surface of both ventricles, and it has been used most commonly for VT mapping and ablation. The epicardial approach for mapping and ablation is discussed in Chapter 27.[6]

Baseline Measurements

Intracardiac Electrograms

Whereas the surface ECG records a summation of the electrical activity of the entire heart, intracardiac electrograms recorded by the electrode catheter represent only the electrical activity (phase 0 of the action potential) of the local cardiac tissue in the immediate vicinity of the catheter's electrodes. Cardiac electrograms are generated by the potential (voltage) differences recorded at two recording electrodes during the cardiac cycle. All clinical electrogram recordings are differential recordings from one source that is connected to the anodal (positive) input of the recording amplifier and a second source that is connected to the cathodal (negative) input.[21]

Recorded electrograms can provide three important pieces of information: (1) the local activation time (i.e., the time of activation of myocardium immediately adjacent to the recording electrode relative to a reference), (2) the direction of propagation of electrical activation within the field of view of the recording electrode, and (3) the complexity of myocardial activation within the field of view of the recording electrode.

ANALOG VERSUS DIGITAL RECORDINGS

Intracardiac electrograms are recorded with amplifiers that have high-input impedances (more than 1010 Ω), to decrease unwanted electrical interference and ensure high-quality recordings.[21] Analog recording systems directly amplify the potential from the recording electrodes, plot the potential on a display oscilloscope, and write it to recording paper or store it on magnetic tape, or both. Analog systems have largely been replaced by digital recording systems that use an analog to digital (A/D) converter that converts the amplitude of the potential recorded at each point in time to a number that is stored.

The quality of digital data is influenced by the sampling frequency and precision of the amplitude measurement.[21] The most common digital recording systems sample the signal approximately every 1 millisecond (i.e., 1000 Hz), which is generally adequate for practical purposes of activation mapping. However, higher sampling frequencies can be required for high-quality recording of high-frequency, rapid potentials that can originate from the Purkinje system or areas of infarction. The faster sampling places greater demands on the computer processor and increases the size of the stored data files.

UNIPOLAR RECORDINGS

A unipolar electrogram is the voltage difference recorded between an intracardiac electrode in close association with cardiac tissue and a distant *indifferent* (reference) electrode patch applied to the body surface (so that the indifferent electrode has little or no cardiac signal). The precordial ECG leads, for example, are unipolar recordings that use an indifferent electrode created by connecting the arms and left leg electrodes through high-impedance resistors.[22]

By convention, the exploring electrode in contact with the cardiac tissue is connected to the positive input of the recording amplifier. In this configuration, an approaching wavefront creates a positive deflection that quickly reverses itself as the wavefront passes directly under the electrode, thus generating an RS complex. In normal homogeneous tissue, the maximum negative slope (dV/dt) of the signal coincides with the arrival of the depolarization wavefront directly beneath the electrode, because the maximal negative dV/dt corresponds to the maximum sodium (Na^+) channel conductance; Fig. 4-15). This is true for filtered and unfiltered unipolar electrograms.[21,23]

The unfiltered unipolar recordings provide information about the direction of impulse propagation; positive deflections (R waves) are generated by propagation toward the recording electrode, and negative deflections (QS complexes) are generated by propagation away from the electrode. Therefore, a wavefront of depolarization traveling past a unipolar electrode results in a biphasic electrogram (positive then negative) representing the approach and recession of the activation wavefront.[22]

Unipolar recordings also allow pacing and recording at the same location while eliminating a possible anodal contribution to

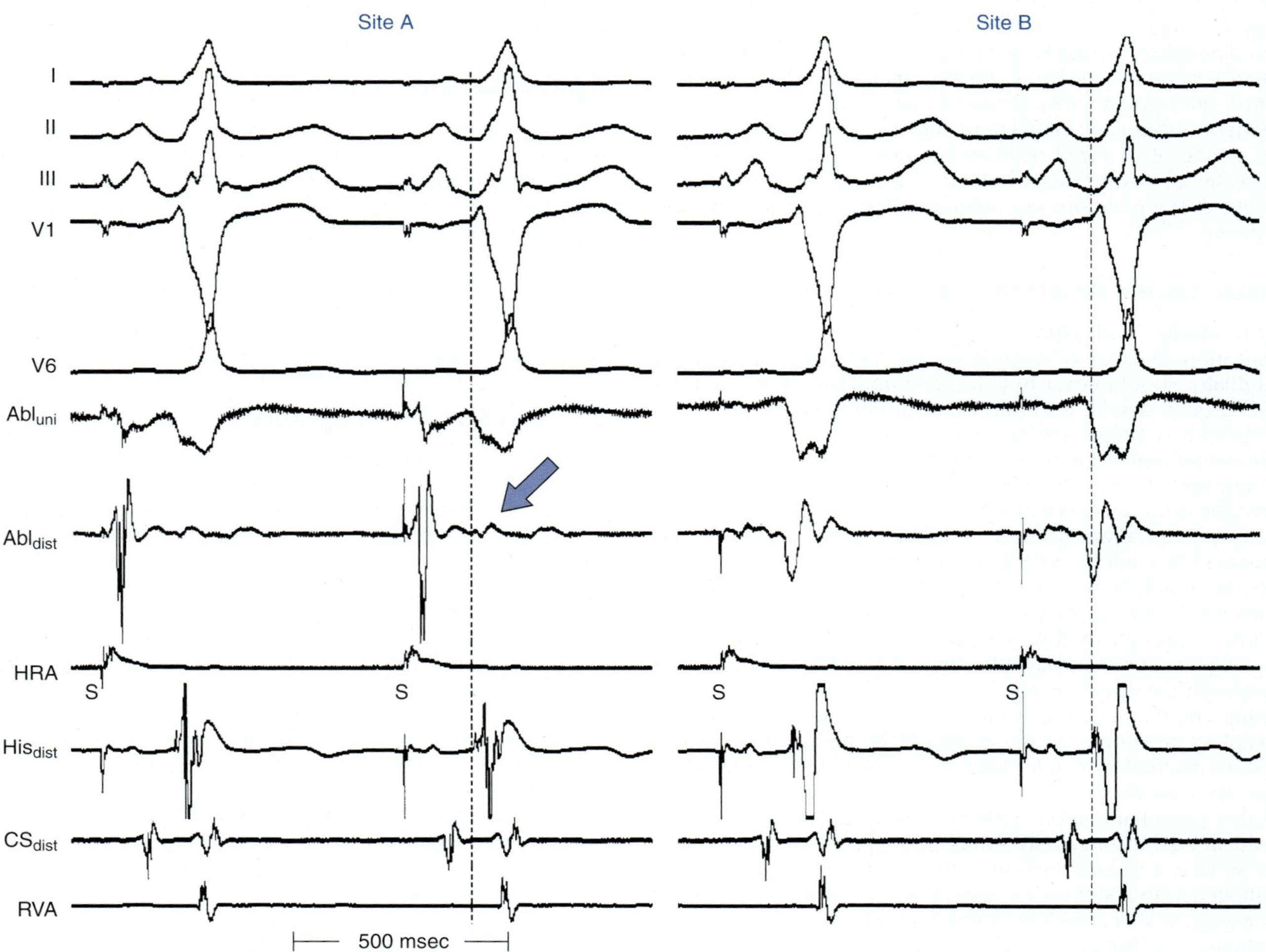

FIGURE 4-15 Unipolar and bipolar recordings. Two complexes from different sites are shown in a patient with Wolff-Parkinson-White syndrome. The dashed line denotes onset of the delta wave. In site A, the unfiltered unipolar recording shows a somewhat blunted "QS" complex and small atrial component, but the filtered (30- to 300-Hz) bipolar signal shows a very large atrial signal and very small ventricular signal (arrow), suggesting a poor choice for ablation site. Site B shows a sharper "QS" in the unipolar signal, with a larger ventricular than atrial electrogram, and the initial nadir of bipolar recording coincides with the maximal negative dV/dt of the unipolar recording. Ablation at this site was successful. Abl_{dist} = distal ablation; Abl_{uni} = unipolar ablation; CS_{dist} = distal coronary sinus; His_{dist} = distal His bundle; HRA = high right atrium; RVA = right ventricular apex.

depolarization that is sometimes seen with bipolar pacing at high output.[21] However, one of the disadvantages of unipolar recording is the inability to record an undisturbed electrogram during or immediately after pacing.

The major disadvantage of unipolar recordings is that they contain substantial far-field signals generated by depolarization of tissue remote from the recording electrode, because the unipolar electrode records a potential difference between widely spaced electrodes.[23] Noise can be reduced by using an indifferent electrode in the IVC. The unipolar electrograms are generally unfiltered (0.05 to 300 Hz or more), but are usually filtered at settings comparable to those of bipolar electrograms (10 to 40 to 300 Hz or more) when an abnormal tissue (scars or infarct areas) is studied, where local electrograms can have very low amplitude and can be masked by larger far-field signals. Filtering the unipolar electrograms can help eliminate far-field signals; however, the filtered unipolar recordings lose the ability to provide directional information.

BIPOLAR RECORDINGS

Bipolar recordings are obtained by connecting two electrodes that are exploring the area of interest to the recording amplifier. At each point in time, the potential generated is the sum of the potential from the positive input and the potential at the negative input. The potential at the negative input is inverted; this is subtracted from the potential at the positive input so that the final recording is the difference between the two.[21]

Unlike unipolar recordings, bipolar electrodes with short interpolar distances are relatively unaffected by far-field events. The bipolar electrogram is simply the difference between the two unipolar electrograms recorded at the two poles. Because the far-field signal is similar at each instant in time, it is largely subtracted out, thus leaving the local signal. Therefore, compared with unipolar recordings, bipolar recordings provide an improved signal-to-noise ratio, and high-frequency components are more accurately seen.[6,23]

Although local activation is less precisely defined, in a homogeneous sheet of tissue the initial peak (or nadir) of a filtered (10 to 40 to 300 Hz or more) bipolar recording coincides with depolarization beneath the recording electrode and corresponds to the maximal negative dV/dt of the unipolar recording (see Fig. 4-15).

Several factors can affect bipolar electrogram amplitude and width, including conduction velocity (the greater the velocity, the higher the peak amplitude of the filtered bipolar electrogram), the mass of the activated tissue, the distance between the electrode and the propagating wavefront, the direction of propagation relative to the bipoles, the interelectrode distance, the amplifier gain, and other signal-processing techniques that can introduce artifacts. To acquire true local electrical activity, a bipolar electrogram with an interelectrode distance of less than 1 cm is desirable.[23]

The direction of wavefront propagation cannot be reliably inferred from the morphology of the bipolar signal. Moreover, bipolar recordings do not allow simultaneous pacing and recording from the same location. To pace and record simultaneously in bipolar fashion at endocardial sites as close together as possible, electrodes 1 and 3 of the quadripolar mapping catheter are used for bipolar pacing, and electrodes 2 and 4 are used for recording.[23]

The differences in unipolar and bipolar recordings can be used to assist in mapping by simultaneously recording bipolar and unipolar signals from the mapping catheter.[21] Although bipolar recordings provide sufficient information for most mapping purposes in clinical EP laboratories, simultaneous unipolar recordings can provide an indication of the direction of wavefront propagation and a more precise measure of the timing of local activation.[23]

SIGNAL FILTERING

The surface ECG is usually filtered at 0.1 to 100.0 Hz. The bulk of the energy is in the 0.1- to 20.0-Hz range. Because of interference from alternating current (AC), muscle twitches, and similar relatively high-frequency interference, it is sometimes necessary to record the surface ECG over a lower frequency range or to use notch filters.[6]

Amplifiers are also used to filter the low- and high-frequency content of the intracardiac electrograms. Intracardiac electrograms are usually filtered to eliminate far-field noise, typically at 30 to 500 Hz. The range of frequencies not filtered out is frequently called the bandpass. The high-pass filter allows frequencies higher than a certain limit to remain in the signal (i.e., it filters out lower frequencies), and the low-pass filter filters out frequencies higher than a certain limit.

High-Pass Filtering

High-pass filtering attenuates frequencies slower than the specified cutoff (corner frequency) of the filter. If intracardiac recordings were not filtered, the signal would wander up and down as this potential fluctuated with respiration, catheter movement, and variable catheter contact.

For bipolar electrograms, high-pass filters with corner frequencies between 10 and 50 Hz are commonly used. Filtering can distort the electrogram morphology and reduce its amplitude. The bipolar signal becomes more complex, and additional peaks are introduced. In general, high-pass filtering can be viewed as differentiating the signal, so that the height of the signal is proportional to the rate of change of the signal, rather than only the amplitude.[22]

Unipolar signals are commonly filtered at 0.05 to 0.5 Hz to remove baseline drift. Filtering at higher corner frequencies (e.g., 30 Hz) alters the morphology of the signal so that the morphology of the unipolar signal is no longer an indication of the direction of wavefront propagation and the presence or absence of a QS complex cannot be used to infer proximity to the site of earliest activation. However, filtering the unipolar signal does not affect its usefulness as a measure of the local activation time.[5] As mentioned earlier, during mapping of areas with infarcts or scars, where local electrograms can have very low amplitude and can be masked by larger far-field signals, high-pass filtering of a unipolar signal (at 30 Hz) can help reduce the far-field signal and improve detection of the lower amplitude local signals.[22]

Low-Pass Filtering

Low-pass filters attenuate frequencies that are faster than the specified corner frequency (usually 250 to 500 Hz). This approach is useful for reducing high-frequency noise without substantially affecting electrograms recorded with clinical systems because most of the signal content is lower than 300 Hz.[22]

Band-Pass Filtering

Defining a band of frequencies to record, such as setting the high-pass filter to 30 Hz and the low-pass filter to 300 Hz, defines a band of frequencies from 30 to 300 Hz that are not attenuated (i.e., bandpass filtering). A notch filter is a special case of bandpass filtering, with specific attenuation of frequencies at 50 or 60 Hz to reduce electrical noise introduced by the frequency of common AC current.

TIMING OF LOCAL EVENTS

As noted, with an unfiltered unipolar electrogram, a wavefront of depolarization that is propagating toward the exploring electrode generates a positive deflection (an R wave). As the wavefront reaches the electrode and propagates away, the deflection sweeps steeply negative. This rapid reversal constitutes the intrinsic deflection of the electrogram and represents the timing of the most local event (i.e., at the site of the electrode). The maximum negative slope (dV/dt) of the signal coincides with the arrival of the depolarization wavefront directly beneath the electrode (see Fig. 4-15).[22]

Filtering the unipolar signal does not affect its usefulness as a measure of the local activation time. The slew rate or dV/dt of the filtered electrogram is so rapid in normal heart tissue that the difference between the peak and the nadir of the deflection is 5 milliseconds or less. Identification of the local event is therefore easy with filtered or unfiltered electrograms in normal tissue. On the other hand, diseased myocardium can conduct very slowly with fractionated electrograms, and this makes local events harder to identify.

To acquire true local electrical activity, a bipolar electrogram with an interelectrode distance of less than 1 cm is preferable. Smaller interelectrode distances record increasingly local events. In normal homogeneous tissue, the initial peak of a filtered (30 to 300 Hz or more) bipolar recording coincides with depolarization beneath the recording electrode and corresponds to the maximal negative dV/dt of the unipolar recording (see Fig. 4-15). However, in the setting of complex multicomponent bipolar electrograms, such as those with marked fractionation and prolonged duration seen in regions with complex conduction patterns, determination of local activation time becomes problematic.[6]

When the intracardiac electrogram of interest is small relative to the size of surrounding electrograms (e.g., His deflection), and the gain must be markedly increased to produce a measurable deflection, clipping the signals can help eliminate the highly amplified surrounding signals to allow concentration on the deflection of interest (Fig. 4-16). It is important to recognize, however, that clippers eliminate the ability to determine the amplitude and timing of the intrinsic deflection (local timing) of the signals being clipped.[5]

CHOICES OF SURFACE AND INTRACARDIAC SIGNALS

Baseline recordings obtained during a typical EP study include several surface ECG leads and several intracardiac electrograms, all of which are recorded simultaneously. Timing of events with respect to onset of the QRS complex or P wave on the surface ECG is often important during the EP study, but it is cumbersome to display all 12 leads of the regular surface ECG. It is more common to use leads I, II, III, V_1, and V_6, which provide most of the information required to determine the frontal plane axis, presence and type of intraventricular conduction abnormalities, and P wave morphology.

Intracardiac leads can be placed strategically at various locations within the cardiac chambers to record local events in the region of the lead. A classic display would include three to five surface ECG leads, high RA recording, HB recording, CS recording, and RV apex recording (Fig. 4-17). Depending on the type of study and information sought, stimulation and recording from other sites can be appropriate and can include RB recording, LV recording, transseptal LA recording, and atrial and ventricular mapping catheter tracings for EP mapping and ablation.[21]

The intracardiac electrograms are generally displayed in the order of normal cardiac activation. The first intracardiac tracing is a recording from the high RA close to the sinus node. The next intracardiac tracing is the HB recording, obtained from a catheter positioned at the HB, which shows low septal RA, HB, and high septal RV depolarizations. One to five recordings may be obtained from the CS, which reflects LA activation, followed by a recording from the RV catheter (see Fig. 4-17).[6]

Right Atrial Electrogram

Depending on the exact location of the RA catheter, the high RA electrogram typically shows a local sharp, large atrial electrogram and a smaller, far-field ventricular electrogram. The catheter is usually positioned in the RA appendage because of stability and reproducibility. The recorded atrial electrogram is earlier in the P wave when the catheter is positioned close to the sinus node. Recordings from this site also help determine the direction of atrial activation (e.g., high-low versus low-high, and right-left versus left-right). Pacing at this position allows evaluation of sinus node function and AV conduction, as well as the induction of supraventricular, and occasionally ventricular, arrhythmias.

Coronary Sinus Electrogram

Because the CS lies in the AV groove, in close contact to both the LA and the LV, the CS catheter records both atrial and ventricular electrograms. However, the CS has a variable relationship with the mitral annulus. The CS lies 2 cm superior to the annulus as it crosses from the RA to the LA. More distally, the CS frequently overrides the LV. Consequently, the most proximal CS electrodes (located at the CS os) are closer to the atrium and typically show a local sharp, large atrial electrogram and a smaller, far-field ventricular

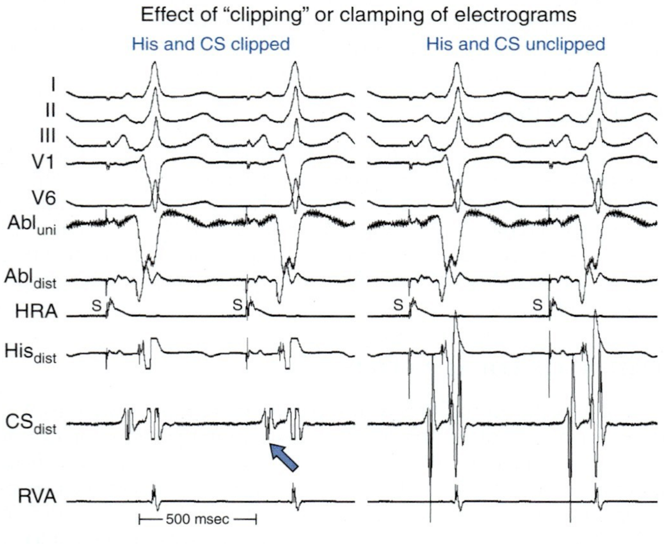

FIGURE 4-16 Effect of electronic clipping on recordings. The same two complexes are shown in both panels. **Left,** Both His and coronary sinus (CS) recordings are electronically attenuated (clipped) to reduce excursions on the display. The CS atrial and ventricular signals appear to have equal amplitude, and the ventricular electrogram in the His recording is small. **Right,** Without clipping, the true signal amplitudes are seen, showing a very large ventricular signal in the His recording and a larger atrial than ventricular signal in the CS recording. Abl_{dist} = distal ablation; Abl_{uni} = unipolar ablation; CS_{dist} = distal coronary sinus; His_{dist} = distal His bundle; HRA = high right atrium; RVA = right ventricular apex.

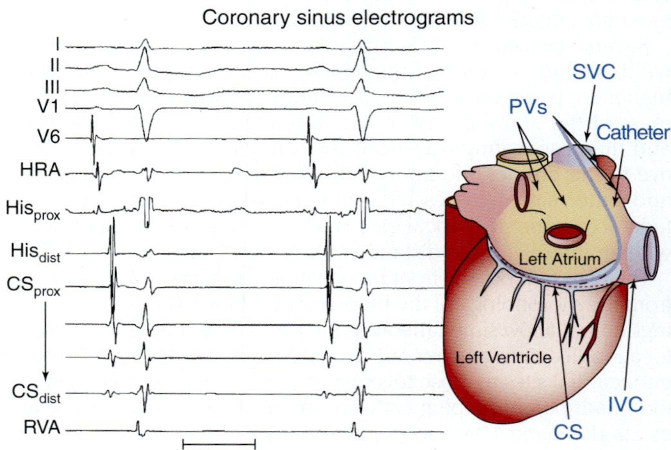

FIGURE 4-17 A classic display of surface ECG and intracardiac recordings during an electrophysiology study of supraventricular tachycardia. Included are four surface ECG leads, high right atrium (HRA) recording, two His bundle recordings (proximal and distal His [His_{prox} and His_{dist}]), five coronary sinus (CS) recordings (in a proximal-to-distal sequence), and a right ventricular apex (RVA) recording. The relative amplitudes of atrial and ventricular electrograms in CS recordings are also shown. **Right,** The back of the heart is shown with a CS catheter in position. The distal portion of the CS (CS_{dist}) is closer to the ventricle (originating as the great cardiac vein on the anterior wall); the CS crosses the atrioventricular groove at the lateral margin and becomes an entirely atrial structure as it empties into the right atrium. **Left,** Thus, proximal CS (CS_{prox}) recordings show large atrial and small ventricular signals, whereas more distal recordings show small atrial, large ventricular signals. IVC = inferior vena cava; PVs = pulmonary veins; SVC = superior vena cava.

electrogram. The more distal CS electrodes, lying closer to the LV than the LA, record progressively smaller, less sharp, far-field atrial electrograms and larger, sharper, near-field ventricular electrograms (see Fig. 4-17).

During normal sinus rhythm (NSR), the atrial activation sequence proceeds from the CS os distally. However, if the CS catheter is deeply seated in the CS, so that the most proximal electrodes are distal to the CS os and the most distal electrodes are anterolateral on the mitral annulus, then both proximal and distal electrodes can be activated at the same time (Fig. 4-18).

His Bundle Electrogram

The HB catheter is positioned at the junction of the RA and RV. Therefore, it records electrograms from local activation of the adjacent atrial, HB, and ventricular tissues (Fig. 4-19). Using a 5- to 10-mm bipolar recording, the His potential appears as a rapid biphasic spike, 15 to 25 milliseconds in duration, interposed between local atrial and ventricular electrograms. The use of a quadripolar catheter allows simultaneous recording of three bipolar pairs.[24]

Before measuring conduction intervals within the HB electrogram, it is important to verify that the spike recorded between the atrial and ventricular electrograms on the HB catheter actually represents activation of the most proximal HB and not the distal HB or RB. The most proximal electrodes displaying the His potential should be chosen, and a large atrial electrogram should accompany the proximal His potential. Anatomically, the proximal portion of the HB originates in the atrial side of the tricuspid annulus; thus, the most proximal HB deflection is the one associated with the largest atrial electrogram. Recording of a His potential associated with a small atrial electrogram can reflect recording of the distal HB or RB and therefore would miss important intra-His conduction abnormalities and falsely shorten the measured HB-ventricular (HV) interval (see Fig. 4-19). Even if a large His potential is recorded in association with a small atrial electrogram, the catheter should be withdrawn to obtain a His potential associated with a larger atrial electrogram. Using a multipolar (three or more) electrode catheter to record simultaneously proximal and distal HB electrograms (e.g., a quadripolar catheter records three bipolar electrograms over a 1.5-cm distance) can help evaluate intra-His conduction.[5]

Validation of the HB recording can be accomplished by assessment of the HV interval and establishing the relationship between the His potential and other electrograms.[24] The HV interval should be 35 milliseconds or longer (in the absence of preexcitation). In contrast, the RB potential invariably occurs within 30 milliseconds before ventricular activation. Atrial pacing can be necessary to distinguish a true His potential from a multicomponent atrial electrogram. With a true His potential, the atrial-HB (AH) interval should increase with incremental pacing rates. HB pacing can also be a valuable means for validating HB recording. The ability to pace the HB through the recording electrode and obtain HB capture (i.e., QRS identical to that during NSR and stimulus-to-QRS interval identical to the HV interval during NSR) provides the strongest evidence validating the His potential. However, this technique is inconsistent in accomplishing HB capture, especially at low current output. Higher output can result in nonselective HB capture. The use of closely spaced electrodes and the reversal of current polarity (i.e., anodal stimulation) can facilitate HB capture. Failure to capture the HB selectively does not necessarily imply that the recorded potential is from the RB.

Other measures that can be used, although rarely required, to validate the HB recording include recording of pressure simultaneously with a luminal electrode catheter (which should reveal atrial pressure wave when the catheter is at the proximal His electrogram position) and simultaneous left and right recording of the His potential. The His potential can be recorded in the noncoronary sinus of Valsalva (just above the aortic valve) or in the LVOT along the interventricular septum (just below the aortic valve). Because these sites are at the level of the central fibrous body, the proximal penetrating portion of the HB is recorded and can be used to time the His potential recorded via the standard venous route. Recording the HB from the noncoronary cusp (versus the LVOT) is preferred because only a true His potential can be recorded from that site.[25]

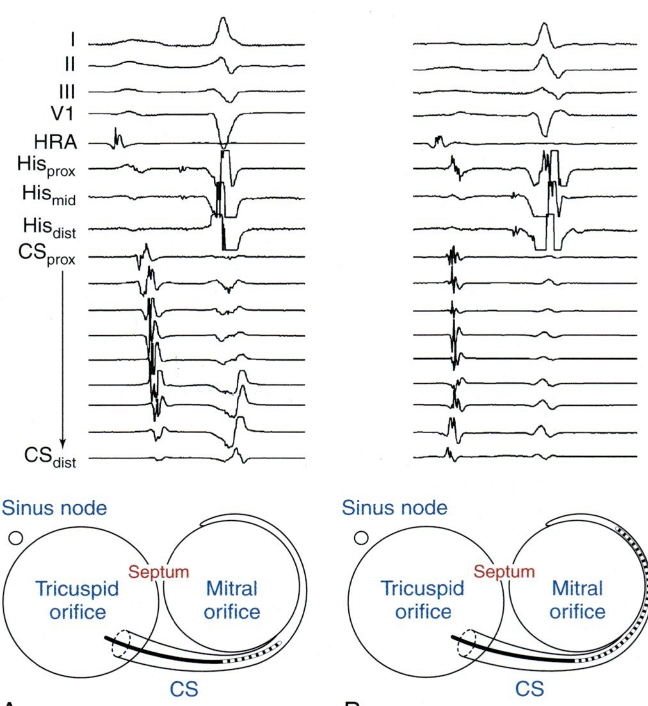

FIGURE 4-18 Influence of catheter position on coronary sinus (CS) atrial electrograms. Two different CS atrial activation sequences are shown from different patients. **A,** A proximal-to-distal sequence is shown. **B,** The latest activation is in the mid-CS electrodes. The diagrams at the bottom show relative positions of the CS catheter in each instance (atrioventricular grooves viewed from above). With more proximal CS position (CS_{prox}), propagation is proximal-distal, indicating relative distance from the sinus node. With a more distal CS position (CS_{dist}), the mid-CS electrodes are farthest from the sinus node. His_{dist} = distal His bundle; His_{mid} = middle His bundle; His_{prox} = proximal His bundle; HRA = high right atrium.

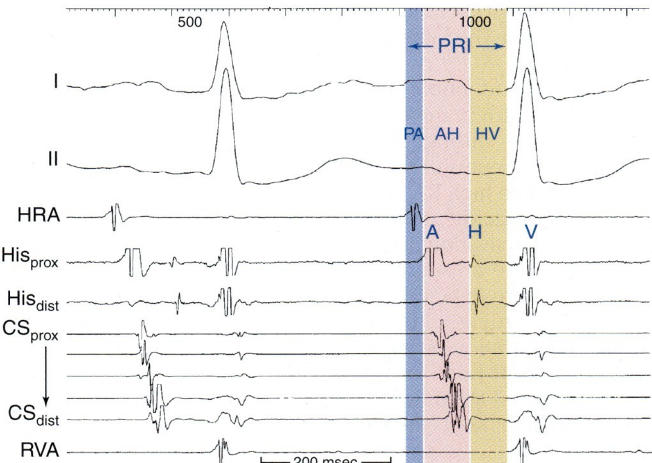

FIGURE 4-19 Intracardiac intervals. Shaded areas represent the P wave–atrial (PA) (blue), atrial–His bundle (AH) (pink), and His bundle–ventricular (HV) (yellow) intervals. It is important that the HV interval be measured from the onset of the His potential in the recording showing the most proximal (rather than the most prominent) His potential (His_{prox}) to the onset of the QRS on the surface ECG (rather than the ventricular electrogram on the His bundle [HB] recording). CS_{dist} = distal coronary sinus; CS_{prox} = proximal coronary sinus; His_{dist} = distal His bundle; HRA = high right atrium; PRI = PR interval; RVA = right ventricular apex. See text for details.

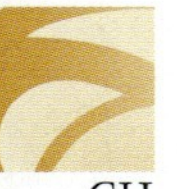

Right Ventricular Electrogram

The RV electrogram typically shows a local sharp and large ventricular electrogram and generally no atrial electrogram. The closer the RV catheter tip position is to the apex, the closer it is to the RB myocardial insertion site and the earlier the ventricular electrogram timing to the onset of the QRS. The catheter is usually positioned in the RV apex because of stability and reproducibility.

Baseline Intervals

The accuracy of measurements made at a screen speed of 100 mm/sec is ±5 milliseconds, and at a speed of 400 mm/sec is ±1 millisecond. In dealing with large intervals (e.g., sinus node function), a speed of 100 mm/sec is adequate. For refractory periods, a speed of 150 to 200 mm/sec is adequate, but for detailed mapping, a speed of 200 to 400 mm/sec is required.

P WAVE–ATRIAL INTERVAL

The P wave–atrial (PA) interval is measured from the first evidence of sinus node depolarization, whether on the intracardiac or surface ECG, to the atrial deflection as recorded in the HB lead. It represents conduction through the RA to the inferoposterior interatrial septum (in the region of the AV node [AVN] and HB; see Fig. 4-19).

The PA interval is a reflection of internodal (sinus node to AVN) conduction; prolonged PA intervals suggest abnormal atrial conduction and can be a clue to the presence of biatrial disease or disease confined to the RA. The normal range of the PA interval is 20 to 60 milliseconds. Rarely, diseased atrial conduction can underlie first-degree AV block, indicated by a prolonged PA interval. A short PA interval suggests an ectopic source of atrial activation.

INTERATRIAL CONDUCTION

Normal atrial activation begins in the high or mid-lateral RA (depending on the sinus rate), spreads from there to the low RA and AV junction, and then spreads to the LA.

Activation of the LA is mediated by three possible routes. Superiorly, activation proceeds through the Bachman bundle; this can be seen in 50% to 70% of patients and can be demonstrated by CS os activation followed by distal CS and then mid-CS activation. Activation also propagates through the mid-atrial septum at the fossa ovalis and at the region of the central fibrous trigone at the apex of the triangle of Koch. The latter provides the most consistent amount of LA activation.

Interatrial conduction is measured by the interval between the atrial electrogram in the high RA lead and that in the CS lead. LA-to-RA activation during LA pacing appears primarily to cross the fossa and low septum and not the Bachman bundle, as reflected by relatively late high RA activation.

Normal retrograde atrial activation proceeds over the AVN. The earliest atrial activation is recorded in the AV junction (HB recording), then in the adjacent RA and CS os, and finally in the high RA and LA. More detailed mapping reveals atrial activation to start at the HB recording, with secondary breakthrough sites in the CS (reflecting activation over the LA extension of the AVN) or the posterior triangle of Koch, or both. At faster ventricular pacing rates, the earliest atrial activation typically shifts to the posterior portion of the triangle of Koch, the CS os, or within the CS itself.

ATRIAL–HIS BUNDLE INTERVAL

The AH interval is measured from the first rapid deflection of the atrial deflection in the HB recording to the first evidence of HB depolarization in the HB recording (see Fig. 4-19). The AH interval is an approximation of the AVN conduction time, because it represents conduction time from the low RA at the interatrial septum through the AVN to the HB.

The AH interval can vary according to the site of atrial pacing. During LA or CS os pacing, the impulse can enter the AVN at a different site that bypasses part of the AVN, or it can just enter the AVN earlier in respect to the atrial deflection in the HB electrogram. Both mechanisms can give rise to a shorter AH interval.

The response of the AH interval to atrial pacing or drugs often provides more meaningful information about AVN function than an isolated measurement of the AH interval. Autonomic blockade with atropine (0.04 mg/kg) and propranolol (0.02 mg/kg) can be used to evaluate AVN function in the absence of autonomic influences. Not enough data, however, are available to define normal responses under these circumstances.[24]

The AH interval has a wide range in normal subjects (50 to 120 milliseconds) and is markedly influenced by the autonomic nervous system. Short AH intervals can be observed in cases of increased sympathetic tone, reduced vagal tone, enhanced AVN conduction, and preferential LA input into the AVN, as well as unusual forms of preexcitation (atrio-His BTs).

Long AH intervals are usually caused by negative dromotropic drugs (such as digoxin, beta blockers, calcium channel blockers, and antiarrhythmic drugs), enhanced vagal tone, and intrinsic disease of the AVN. Artifactually prolonged AH intervals can result from an improperly positioned catheter or the incorrect identification of an RB potential as a His potential. This situation needs to be distinguished from true AH interval prolongation.

HIS POTENTIAL

His potential duration reflects conduction through the short length of the HB that penetrates the fibrous septum. Disturbances of HB conduction can manifest as fractionation, prolongation (longer than 30 milliseconds), or splitting of the His potential.

HIS BUNDLE–VENTRICULAR INTERVAL

The HV interval is measured from the onset of the His potential to the onset of the earliest registered surface or intracardiac ventricular activation. It represents conduction time from the proximal HB through the distal His-Purkinje system (HPS) to the ventricular myocardium (see Fig. 4-19).[24]

The HV interval is not significantly affected by the autonomic tone, and it usually remains stable. The range of HV intervals in normal subjects is narrow, 35 to 55 milliseconds. A prolonged HV interval is consistent with diseased distal conduction in all fascicles or in the HB itself. A validated short HV interval suggests ventricular preexcitation via a BT. A falsely shortened HV interval can occur during sinus rhythm with PVCs or an accelerated idioventricular rhythm that is isorhythmic with the sinus rhythm, or when an RB potential rather than a His potential is inadvertently recorded.

Programmed Electrical Stimulation

Stimulators

Cardiac stimulation is carried out by delivering a pulse of electrical current through the electrode catheter from an external pacemaker (stimulator) to the cardiac surface. Such an electrical impulse depolarizes cardiac tissue near the pacing electrode, which then propagates through the heart. The paced impulses (stimuli) are introduced in predetermined patterns and at precise timed intervals using a programmable stimulator.

A typical stimulator has a constant current source and is capable of pacing at a wide range of CLs and variable current strengths (0.1 to 10 mA) and pulse widths (0.1 to 10 milliseconds). Additionally, current stimulators have at least two different channels of stimulation (preferably four) and allow delivery of multiple extrastimuli (three or more) and synchronization of the pacing stimuli to selected electrograms during intrinsic or paced rhythms.

Pacing Techniques

PACING OUTPUT

Stimulation is usually carried out using an isolated constant current source that delivers a rectangular impulse. Pacing output at twice (2×) diastolic threshold is generally used. *Pacing threshold* is defined as the lowest current required for consistent capture determined in late diastole. The pacing threshold can be influenced by the pacing cycle length (CL); therefore, the threshold should be determined at each pacing CL used. In general, refractory periods are somewhat longer when determined using 2× threshold (as opposed to higher outputs), and this can reduce the incidence of induction of nonclinical tachyarrhythmias.[24] Additionally, diastolic excitability can be influenced by drug administration; re-evaluation of the pacing threshold and adjustment of the pacing output (2× threshold) are therefore required in such situations. A pulse duration of 1 or 2 milliseconds is generally used.

High current strength is generally used for determination of strength-interval curves to overcome drug-induced prolongation of refractoriness, assess the presence and mechanism of antiarrhythmic therapy, and overcome the effect of decreased tissue excitability (e.g., pace mapping in scar-related arrhythmias).

CYCLE LENGTH

During EP testing, CLs often change from beat to beat, so that these measures are more relevant than an overall rate expressed in beats per minute. The use of rates in beats per minute is retained mostly to facilitate communication with physicians who are more comfortable with this terminology. Pacing rate is determined by dividing 60,000 by the CL (in milliseconds).

INCREMENTAL VERSUS DECREMENTAL

The terms *incremental* and *decremental* can have opposite meaning, depending on whether one is considering the pacing rate in beats per minute or the pacing CL in milliseconds. The term *incremental pacing rate* is derived from stimulators controlled by an analog dial. Digitally controlled devices often increase the rate by choosing a sequence of CL decrements, but the term *incremental pacing* may still be used.

OVERDRIVE PACING (STRAIGHT PACING)

Pacing stimuli are delivered at a constant pacing rate (or pacing CL) throughout the duration of the stimulation. The pacing rate is faster than the rate of the baseline rhythm to ensure capture of the spontaneous rhythm.

BURST PACING

Pacing stimuli are delivered at a constant rate for a relatively short duration, but at successively faster rates with each burst until a predetermined maximum rate (or minimum CL) has been reached. This technique is generally used for induction or termination of tachycardias.

STEPWISE RATE-INCREMENTAL PACING

After pacing at a given rate for a predetermined number of stimuli or seconds, the rate is increased (with intervening pauses) in a series of steps until predetermined endpoints are reached. It is important to maintain the pacing at any given rate for at least 15 seconds (period of accommodation) before increasing the pacing rate. Otherwise, the initial stimuli at any given rate can produce effects different from those observed several seconds later, because the ability of a tissue to conduct is affected by the baseline rate or CL of the preceding beats. A disadvantage for this technique is the prolonged pacing required at each rate, which is time-consuming.

RAMP PACING

Ramp pacing implies a smooth change in the interval between successive stimuli, with gradual decrease of the pacing CL every several paced complexes (without intervening pauses). Ramps are often used as an alternative to the stepwise method for assessment of conduction. The pacing rate is slowly increased at 2 to 4 beats/min every several paced beats until block occurs. This method avoids prolonged rapid pacing at each pacing CL and is particularly useful when multiple assessments of conduction are planned (e.g., after therapeutic interventions) and in the assessment of retrograde conduction. Because each successive paced interval differs from its predecessor by only a few milliseconds, the interval at which block occurs can be determined more precisely using the ramp method. However, prolonged episodes of continuous high-rate pacing can provoke significant hypotension, and close monitoring of blood pressure is important while performing these maneuvers.

For tachycardia induction or termination, the ramp is decreased in duration, but the inter-stimulus intervals are decreased more rapidly. Ramp pacing is generally used in antitachycardia pacing algorithms in implantable cardioverter-defibrillators. Programmed rate-incremental ramps are also known as *autodecremental pacing*.

EXTRASTIMULUS TECHNIQUE

S_1-S_1 DRIVE STIMULI. The heart is paced, or driven, at a specified rate and duration (typically eight beats) after which a premature extrastimulus is delivered. The eight drive beats are each termed *S_1 stimulus*. The S_1-S_1 drive stimuli are sometimes called trains. These S_1 drive stimuli can be followed by first, second, third, and n^th^ premature extrastimuli, which are designated as S_2, S_3, S_4, and S_N. When the extrastimuli follow a series of sinus beats, the sinus beats can also be designated as S_1.

S_1, S_2, S_3, . . . SN. S_2 is the first extrastimulus, with the S_1-S_2 interval almost always shorter than the S_1-S_1 interval. S_3, S_4, . . . S_N are the second, third, . . . n^{th} extrastimuli. When stimulation is performed in the atrium, capture of S_1, S_2, S_3, . . . S_N results in atrial depolarizations, termed A_1, A_2, A_3, . . . A_N, respectively, and when stimulation is performed in the ventricle, they are termed V_1, V_2, V_3, . . . V_N, corresponding to the resultant ventricular depolarizations, respectively.

One or more extrastimuli (designated S_2, S_3, and S_N) are introduced at specific coupling intervals based on previous S_1 drive stimuli or spontaneous beats. Thereafter, the S_1-S_2 interval is altered, usually in 10- to 20-millisecond steps, until an endpoint is reached, such as tissue refractoriness or termination or induction of a tachycardia. It is usual to begin late in diastole and successively decrement the S_1-S_2 interval. A second extrastimulus (S_3) can then be introduced, with the S_2-S_3 interval altered similarly to that used for S_1-S_2.

Two methods are in common clinical use for decreasing the coupling intervals during delivery of multiple extrastimuli. In the simple sequential method, the S_1-S_2 coupling interval is decreased until it fails to capture, at which time the coupling interval is increased until it captures (usually within 10 to 20 milliseconds). The S_1-S_2 coupling interval is then held constant while the S_2-S_3 interval is decreased similarly to that used for S_1-S_2, and then the same is done for S_3-S_4. In the tandem method, the S_1-S_2 coupling interval is decreased until S_2 fails to capture, and then the S_1-S_2 coupling interval is increased by 40 to 50 milliseconds and held there. S_3 is then introduced and the S_2-S_3 interval decreased until S_3 fails to capture. At that point, the S_1-S_2 interval is decreased, and S_3 is retested to see whether it captures. From that point on, the S_1-S_2 and S_2-S_3 intervals are decreased in tandem until refractory. As compared with the simple sequential method, the tandem method allows relatively longer intervals and provides a larger number of stimulation runs before moving on to the next extrastimulus. Prospective studies comparing the two methods have shown no differences between the two methods in any of the outcomes assessed.

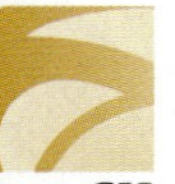

ULTRARAPID TRAIN STIMULATION

Pacing at very short CLs (10 to 50 milliseconds) is rarely performed, mainly for induction of ventricular fibrillation (VF), to test defibrillation threshold during implantation of a cardioverter-defibrillator.

Conduction and Refractoriness

CONDUCTION

During depolarization, the electrical impulse spreads along each cardiac cell, and rapidly from cell to cell, because each myocyte is connected to its neighbors through low resistance gap junctions. As discussed in Chapter 1, conduction velocity refers to the speed of propagation of an electrical impulse through cardiac tissue, which is dependent on both the active membrane properties of the individual cardiac myocyte that generates the action potential (i.e., electrical excitability or refractoriness, or both) and passive properties governing the flow of current between cardiac cells (cell-to-cell coupling and tissue geometry).[26,27]

Conduction can be assessed by observing the propagation of wavefronts during pacing at progressively incremental rates. Rate-incremental pacing is delivered to a selected site in the heart while propagation to a selected distal point is assessed. Conduction velocity is assessed by measuring the time it takes for an impulse to travel from one intracardiac location to another. During tests of conduction, it is usual for capture to be maintained at the site of stimulation and block to occur at a distal point.[6]

REFRACTORINESS

As discussed in Chapter 1, during a cardiac cycle, once an action potential is initiated, the cardiac cell is unexcitable to stimulation (i.e., unable to initiate another action potential in response to a stimulus of threshold intensity) for some duration of time (which is slightly shorter than the "true" action potential duration) until its membrane has repolarized to a certain level.[28-30]

There are different levels of refractoriness during the action potential. During the *absolute refractory period* (which extends over phases 0, 1, 2, and part of phase 3 of the action potential), the tissue is completely unexcitable and a second action potential absolutely cannot be initiated, no matter how large a stimulus is applied, because of inactivation of most Na^+ channels. After the absolute refractory period, a stimulus may cause some cellular depolarization but does not lead to a propagated action potential. The sum of this period (which includes a short interval of phase 3 of the action potential) and the absolute refractory period is termed the *effective refractory period* (ERP). The ERP is followed by the *relative refractory period* (RRP), which extends over the middle and late parts of phase 3 of the action potential. During the RRP, initiation of a second action potential is *inhibited* but not impossible; a larger-than-normal stimulus can result in activation of the cell and lead to a propagating action potential. However, the upstroke of the new action potential is less steep and of lower amplitude and its conduction velocity slower than normal. Of note, there is a brief period in phase 3 of the action potential, the supernormal period, during which excitation is possible in response to an otherwise subthreshold stimulus; that same stimulus fails to elicit a response earlier or later than the supernormal period (see later).

MEASUREMENTS OF REFRACTORY PERIODS

Refractoriness (or, more appropriately, excitability) is defined by the response of a tissue to premature stimulation.[31,32] Refractory periods are analyzed by the extrastimulus technique, with progressively premature extrastimuli delivered after a train of 8 to 10 paced beats at a fixed pacing CL to allow for reasonable (more than 95%) stabilization of refractoriness, which is usually accomplished after 3 or 4 paced beats.

Several variables are considered in the assessment of refractory periods, including the stimulus amplitude and the drive rate or CL. Longer CLs are generally associated with longer refractory periods, but refractory periods of different parts of the conducting system do not respond comparably with changes in the drive CLs.[30]

Additionally, the measured ERP is invariably related to the current used. Thus, standardization of the pacing output is required. In most laboratories, it is arbitrarily standardized at twice the diastolic threshold. A more detailed method of assessing refractoriness is to define the strength-interval curves at these sites. The steep portion of that curve defines the ERP of that tissue. The use of increasing current strengths to 10 mA usually shortens the measured ERP by approximately 30 milliseconds. However, such a method does not offer a useful clinical advantage, except when the effects of antiarrhythmic drugs on ventricular excitability and refractoriness are to be characterized. Moreover, the safety of using high current strengths, especially when multiple extrastimuli are delivered, is questionable, because fibrillation is more likely to occur in such situations.

It is important that measurements of refractory periods be taken at specific sites. Measurements of atrial and ventricular ERP are taken at the site of stimulation. Measurements of AVN ERP and HPS ERP are taken from responses in the HB electrogram.[24]

EFFECTIVE REFRACTORY PERIOD. The ERP is the longest premature coupling interval (S_1-S_2) at a designated stimulus amplitude (usually 2× diastolic threshold) that results in failure of propagation of the premature impulse through a tissue (i.e., fails to capture). ERP therefore must be measured proximal to the refractory tissue.

RELATIVE REFRACTORY PERIOD. The RRP is defined as the longest premature coupling interval (S_1-S_2) that results in prolonged conduction of the premature impulse (an increase in stimulus to distal response time) compared with the conduction of the stimulus delivered during the basic drive train. Conduction is slowed when a wavefront encounters tissue that is not completely repolarized. Thus, the RRP marks the end of the full recovery period, the zone during which conduction of the premature and basic drive impulses is identical. The RRP is generally slightly longer than the ERP by an amount called the *latency period*. During the latency period, the tissue is excitable, but the excitation wavefront conducts with slower or even decremental conduction.

FUNCTIONAL REFRACTORY PERIOD. The functional refractory period (FRP) is the shortest interval between two consecutively conducted impulses out of a cardiac tissue resulting from any two consecutive input impulses into that tissue (i.e., the shortest output interval that can occur in response to *any* input interval in a particular tissue). Because the FRP is a measure of output from a tissue, it is described by measuring points distal to that tissue. It is helpful to think of the FRP as a response-to-response measurement (in contrast, the ERP is a stimulus-to-stimulus measurement). Therefore, the FRP is a measure of refractoriness *and* conduction velocity of a tissue.

The definitions of anterograde ERP and FRP of the AV conduction system are given in Table 4-1.[24]

CYCLE LENGTHS RESPONSIVENESS OF REFRACTORY PERIODS

Normally, refractoriness of the atrial, HPS, and ventricular tissue is directly related to the basic drive CL (i.e., the ERP shortens with decreasing basic drive CL). This phenomenon (termed *peeling of refractoriness*) results from rate-related shortening of the action potential duration and is most marked in the HPS.[32] Abrupt changes in the CL also affect refractoriness of these tissues. A change from a long- to short-drive CL (e.g., with introduction of an extrastimulus [S_2] following a pacing drive [S_1] with a long CL) shortens the ERP of the HPS and atrium, whereas a change from a short to a long drive CL markedly prolongs the HPS ERP but alters the ventricular ERP little, if at all. Refractoriness of the atrial, HPS, and ventricular tissue appears relatively independent of autonomic tone; however,

TABLE 4-1 Definition of Refractory Periods

	ERP	RRP	FRP
Atrium	Longest S_1-S_2 interval that fails to achieve atrial capture	Longest S_1-S_2 interval at which S_2-A_2 is > S_1-A_1	Shortest A_1-A_2 interval (recorded at a designated site, often the HB region) in response to any S_1-S_2
AVN	Longest A_1-A_2 interval (measured at the HB region) that fails to propagate to the HB	Longest A_1-A_2 interval at which A_2-H_2 is > A_1-H_1	Shortest H_1-H_2 interval in response to any A_1-A_2
HPS	Longest H_1-H_2 interval that fails to propagate to the ventricles	Longest H_1-H_2 interval at which H_2-V_2 is > H_1-V_1 or generates an aberrant QRS complex	Shortest V_1-V_2 interval in response to any H_1-H_2
Ventricle	Longest S_1-S_2 interval that fails to achieve ventricular capture	Longest S_1-S_2 interval at which S_2-V_2 is > S_1-V_1	Shortest V_1-V_2 interval (recorded at a designated site or) in response to any S_1-S_2

AVN = atrioventricular node; ERP = effective refractory period; FRP = functional refractory period; HB = His bundle; HPS = His-Purkinje system; RRP = relative refractory period.

TABLE 4-2 Normal Refractory Periods in Adults

STUDY*	ERP ATRIUM (msec)	ERP AVN (msec)	FRP AVN (msec)	ERP HPS (msec)	ERP VENTRICLE (msec)
Denes et al (1974)	150–360	250–365	350–495	—	—
Akhtar et al (1975)	230–330	280–430	320–680	340–430	190–290
Josephson (2002)	170–300	230–425	330–525	330–450	170–290

*Studies performed at 2× threshold.
AVN = atrioventricular node; ERP = effective refractory period; FRP = functional refractory period; HPS = His-Purkinje system.
Data from Denes P, Wu D, Dhingra R, et al: The effects of cycle length on cardiac refractory periods in man. *Circulation* 49:32, 1974; Akhtar M, Damato AN, Batsford WP, et al: A comparative analysis of anterograde and retrograde conduction patterns in man, *Circulation* 52:766, 1975; and Josephson ME: Electrophysiologic investigation: general aspects. In Josephson ME, editor: *Clinical cardiac electrophysiology*, ed 3, Philadelphia, 2002, Lippincott Williams & Wilkins, pp 19-67.

data have shown that increased vagal tone reduces atrial ERP and increases ventricular ERP.[30]

In contrast, the AVN ERP increases with increasing basic drive CL in response to the fatigue phenomenon, which most likely results because AVN refractoriness is time-dependent and exceeds its action potential duration (unlike HPS refractoriness). Additionally, AVN refractory periods are labile and can be markedly affected by the autonomic tone. On the other hand, the response of AVN FRP to changes in pacing CL is variable, but it tends to decrease with decreasing pacing CL.[32] This paradox occurs because the FRP is not a true measure of refractoriness encountered by an atrial extrastimulus (AES; A_2); it is significantly determined by the AVN conduction time of the basic drive beat (A_1-H_1); the longer the A_1-H_1 is, the shorter the calculated FRP will be at any A_2-H_2.[33]

LIMITATIONS OF TESTS OF CONDUCTION AND REFRACTORINESS

It is unusual to be able to collect a complete set of measurements. With refractory period testing, the atrial ERP is often longer than the AVN ERP, so that atrial refractoriness is encountered before AVN refractoriness, thus limiting the ability to assess the latter. Moreover, an AES cannot be used to test the HPS if conduction is blocked at the AVN level. This is a limitation that applies to most patients undergoing conduction or refractory period testing.[31] On the other hand, it is possible to assess anterograde conduction and refractoriness distal to the AVN by direct pacing of the HB. This is not part of the routine EP evaluation, however, and is reserved for cases in which the information is particularly desired.[6]

It is important to recognize that atrial conduction can materially affect the determination of refractory periods. Therefore, refractory periods should not be timed from the site of stimulation, but from the point in the conduction cascade that is being assessed. For example, if the high RA is stimulated in a patient with a left lateral BT, an early AES can encounter the RRP of the atrium, so that intraatrial conduction time is prolonged. Thus, the timing of the S_1-S_2 stimuli in the high RA would be shorter than the timing of the propagated impulse when it arrives at the region of the BT as the local A_1-A_2 interval.

A wide range of normal values has been reported for refractory periods (Table 4-2). However, it is difficult to interpret these so-called normal values because they come from pooled data using different standards (different pacing CLs, stimulus strengths, and pulse widths).[24,31,32]

Atrial Stimulation

Technical Aspects

Atrial stimulation provides a method for evaluation of the functional properties of the sinus node and AV conduction system and of the means of induction of different arrhythmias (supraventricular and, occasionally, ventricular arrhythmias). Atrial stimulation from different atrial sites can result in different patterns of AV conduction. Thus, stimulation should be performed from the same site if the effects of drugs and physiological maneuvers are to be studied. Atrial stimulation is usually performed from the high RA and CS.

Rate-incremental atrial pacing is usually started at a pacing CL just shorter than the sinus CL, with progressive shortening of the pacing CL (by 10- to 20-millisecond decrements) until 1:1 atrial capture is lost, Wenckebach AVN block develops, or a pacing CL of 200 to 250 milliseconds is reached. Ramp atrial pacing is equivalent to rate-incremental pacing if AVN Wenckebach CL is all that is required. Stepwise rate-incremental pacing, however, also allows evaluation of sinus node recovery time at each drive CL. Atrial pacing should always be synchronized because alteration of the coupling interval of the first paced beat of the pacing drive can affect subsequent AV conduction.

During stepwise rate-incremental pacing, pacing should be continued long enough (usually 15 to 60 seconds) at each pacing CL to ensure stability of conduction intervals and to overcome two factors that significantly influence the development of a steady state: the phenomenon of accommodation and the effects of autonomic tone. During rate-incremental pacing, if the coupling interval of the first beat of the drive is not synchronized, it can be shorter, longer, or equal to the subsequent pacing CL. Therefore, one can observe an increasing, decreasing, or stable AH interval pattern for several cycles, and the initial AH interval can be different from the steady-state AH interval. Oscillations of the AH interval, which dampen to a steady level, or AVN Wenckebach can occur under these circumstances. With regard to influence of the autonomic tone on AVN conduction, rapid pacing can produce variations in AVN conduction, depending on the patient's immediate autonomic state. Rapid pacing can also provoke symptoms or hypotension in patients who then produce neurohumoral responses that can alter results. Therefore, for assessment of AV conduction, ramp pacing is often an attractive alternative to the stepwise method. The pacing rate is slowly increased at 2 to 4 beats/min/sec (or the pacing CL is decreased by 10 milliseconds every several paced beats) until block occurs.[24]

AES is used for assessment of atrial and AVN refractory periods and for induction of arrhythmias. During programmed stimulation, a sequence of eight paced stimuli is delivered at a constant rate (the S_1 drive), which allows stable AVN conduction. Following these eight beats, an AES (S_2) is delivered. This stimulation sequence is repeated at progressively shorter S_1-S_2 coupling intervals, thus allowing the response of the sinus node and AVN to be recorded across a range of premature test stimuli.

Normal Response to Rate-Incremental Atrial Pacing

SINUS NODE RESPONSE TO ATRIAL PACING

The sinus node is the prototype of an automatic focus. Automatic rhythms are characterized by spontaneous depolarization, overdrive suppression, and post-overdrive warm-up to baseline CL. Rapid atrial pacing results in overdrive suppression of the sinus rate, with prolongation of the return sinus CL following termination of the pacing train. Longer pacing trains and faster pacing rates further prolong the return cycle. After cessation of pacing, the sinus rate resumes discharge at a slower rate and gradually speeds up (warms up) to return to the prepacing sinus rate.

Sinus node recovery time is the interval between the end of a period of pacing-induced overdrive suppression of sinus node activity and the return of sinus node function, manifested on the surface ECG by a post-pacing sinus P wave.

ATRIOVENTRICULAR NODE RESPONSE TO ATRIAL PACING

The normal AVN response to rate-incremental atrial pacing is for the PR and AH intervals to increase gradually as the pacing CL decreases until AVN Wenckebach block appears (Fig. 4-20). With further decrease in the pacing CL, higher degrees of AV block (2:1 or 3:1) can appear. Infranodal conduction (HV interval) generally remains unaffected.

Wenckebach block is frequently atypical; that is, the AH interval does not increase gradually in decreasing increments but stabilizes for several beats before the block, or it can show its greatest increment in the last conducted beat. The incidence of atypical Wenckebach block is highest during long Wenckebach cycles (longer than 6.5). It is important to distinguish atypical Wenckebach periodicity from Mobitz II AV block. Additionally, it is important to ensure that the ventricular pauses observed during atrial pacing are not secondary to loss of atrial capture or the occurrence of AVN echo beats (pseudoblock; see Fig. 4-20).

AVN Wenckebach CL is the longest pacing CL at which Wenckebach block in the AVN is observed. Normally, Wenckebach CL is 500 to 350 milliseconds, and it is sensitive to the autonomic tone. There is a correlation between the AH interval during NSR and the Wenckebach CL; patients with a long AH interval during NSR tend to develop Wenckebach block at a longer pacing CL, and vice versa.

At short pacing CLs (less than 350 milliseconds), infranodal block can occasionally occur in patients with a normal baseline HV interval and QRS. This occurs especially when atrial pacing is started during NSR with the first or second paced impulses acting as a long-short sequence. The HPS can also show accommodation following the initiation of pacing. Prolongation of the HV interval or infranodal block at a pacing CL longer than 400 milliseconds is abnormal and indicates infranodal conduction abnormalities.

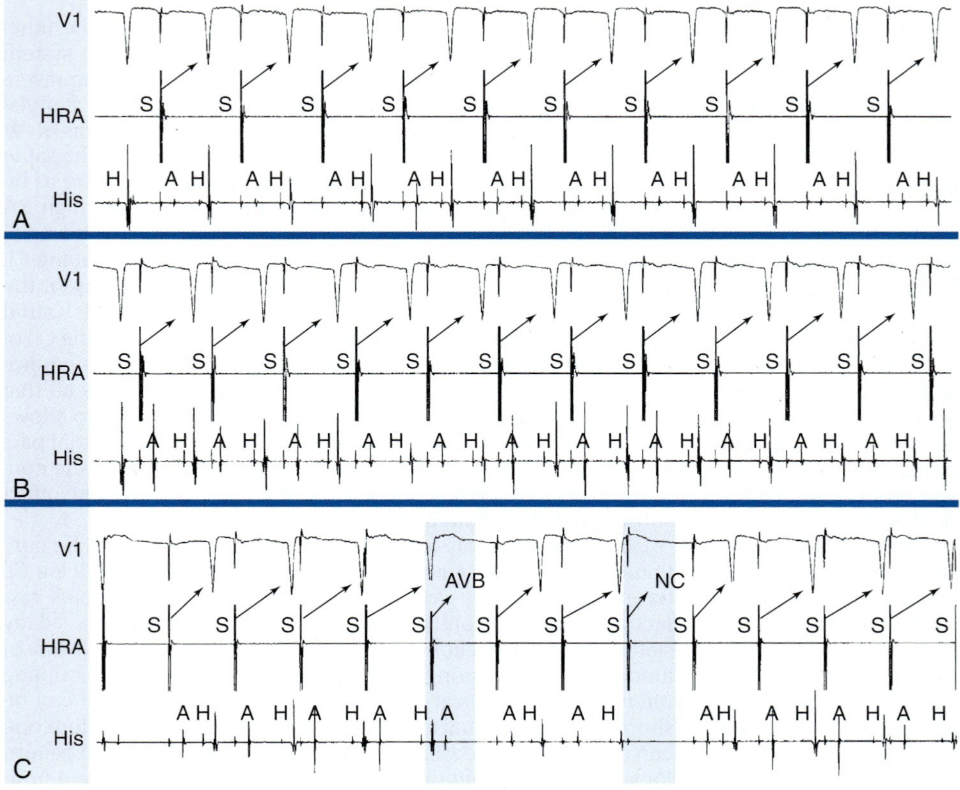

FIGURE 4-20 Normal atrioventricular node (AVN) response to rate-incremental atrial pacing. **A,** Fixed-rate high right atrial (HRA) pacing (S) at a cycle length (CL) of 600 milliseconds. **B,** Decreasing the pacing CL to 500 milliseconds results in prolongation of the atrial–His bundle (AH) interval, as illustrated in the His bundle recording (His). Infranodal conduction (His bundle–ventricular [HV] interval) remains unaffected. **C,** Further decrement of the pacing CL results in progressive prolongation of the AH interval until block occurs in the AVN (AVB), followed by resumption of conduction, indicating Wenckebach CL. The site of block is in the AVN because no His bundle deflection is present after the nonconducted atrial stimulus. Of note, apparent block of another atrial stimulus is observed (pseudoblock) because of failure of the atrial stimulus to capture (NC), which is confirmed by the absence of an atrial electrogram on the His bundle recording after the stimulus artifact.

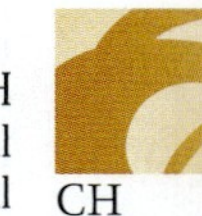

ATRIAL RESPONSE TO ATRIAL PACING

It is usually possible to maintain 1:1 atrial capture with rate-incremental pacing techniques to a pacing CL of 200 to 300 milliseconds. Pacing threshold normally tends to increase at faster rates. Rate-incremental pacing can result in prolongation of the intraatrial (PA interval) and interatrial conduction. At rapid pacing rates, induction of AF is not rare and is not necessarily an abnormal response. Vagal tone and medications such as adenosine and edrophonium can slow the sinus rate, but they tend to shorten the atrial ERP, which makes the atrium more vulnerable to induction of AF.

Normal Response to Atrial Premature Stimulation

SINUS NODE RESPONSE TO ATRIAL EXTRASTIMULATION

Four zones of response of the sinus node to AES have been identified: the zone of collision, the zone of reset, the zone of interpolation, and the zone of reentry (Fig. 4-21).

ZONE I. A late-coupled AES with very long A_1-A_2 intervals (with A_2 falling in the last 20% to 30% of the sinus CL) collides with the impulse already emerging from the sinus node, resulting in fusion of atrial activation (fusion between the AES [A_2] with the spontaneous sinus impulse [A_1]) or paced-only atrial activation sequence; it fails to affect the timing of the next sinus beat, thus producing a fully compensatory pause. This zone, also known as the zone of collision, zone of interference, and nonreset zone, is defined by the range of A_1-A_2 at which A_2-A_3 is fully compensatory (see Fig. 4-21).[24]

ZONE II. An earlier coupled AES results in penetration of the sinus node with resetting so that the resulting pause is less than compensatory (i.e., A_1-A_3 is < 2×[A_1-A_1]), but without changing sinus node automaticity. The range of A_1-A_2 at which resetting of the sinus pacemaker occurs, resulting in a less than compensatory pause, defines zone II, also known as the zone of reset (see Fig. 4-21). This zone is typically of long duration (40% to 50% of the sinus CL). In most patients, A_2-A_3 remains constant throughout zone II, thus producing a plateau in the curve because, although A_2 penetrates and resets the sinus node, it does so without changing the sinus pacemaker automaticity. Hence, A_2-A_3 should equal the spontaneous sinus CL (A_1-A_1) plus the time it takes the AES (A_2) to enter and exit the sinus node. The difference between A_2-A_3 and A_1-A_1 therefore has been taken as an estimate of total sinoatrial conduction time.[24]

ZONE III. A very early coupled AES encounters a refractory sinus node (following the last sinus discharge) and fails to enter or reset the sinus node. The next sinus discharge is on time because the atrium is already fully recovered following that early AES. The range of A_1-A_2 coupling intervals at which A_2-A_3 is less than A_1-A_1, and A_1-A_3 is less than 2× (A_1-A_1), defines zone III, also known as the zone of interpolation (see Fig. 4-21). The A_1-A_2 coupling intervals at which incomplete interpolation is first observed define the RRP of the perinodal tissue. Some refer to this as the sinus node refractory period. In this case, A_3 represents delay of A_1 exiting the sinus node, which has not been affected.[34] The A_1-A_2 coupling interval at which complete interpolation is observed probably defines the ERP of the most peripheral of the perinodal tissue because the sinus impulse does not encounter refractory tissue on its exit from the sinus node. In this case, (A_1-A_2) + (A_2-A_3) = A_1-A_1 and sinus node entrance block is said to exist.[34]

ZONE IV. This zone, also known as the zone of reentry, is defined as the range of A_1-A_2 at which A_2-A_3 is less than A_1-A_1, (A_1-A_2) + (A_2-A_3) is less than A_1-A_1, and the atrial activation sequence and P wave morphology are identical to those of the sinus. The incidence of single beats of sinus node reentry is approximately 11% in the normal population.

ATRIOVENTRICULAR NODAL RESPONSE TO ATRIAL EXTRASIMULATION

Progressively premature AES results in prolongation of PR and AH intervals, with inverse relationship between the AES coupling interval (A_1-A_2) and the AH interval (A_2-H_2). The shorter the coupling interval

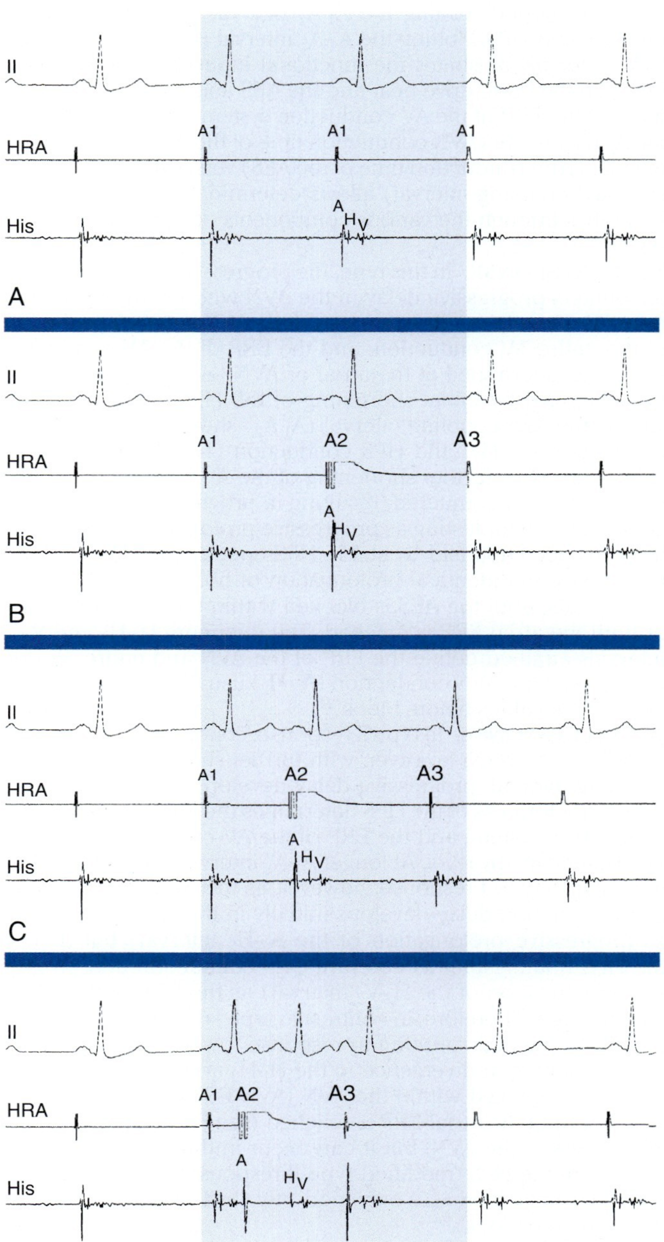

FIGURE 4-21 Normal sinus node and atrioventricular node response to atrial extrastimulation. **A,** Baseline sinus rhythm shown in surface ECG lead II, high right atrium (HRA) recording, and His bundle (His) recording. The shaded area represents two sinus cycle lengths (2× [A_1-A_1]). **B,** A late coupled atrial extrastimulus (AES) (A_2) collides with the exiting sinus impulse and therefore does not affect (or reset) the sinus pacemaker (zone of collision). The next sinus impulse (A_3) occurs at exactly twice the baseline sinus cycle length. **C,** An early coupled AES is able to penetrate and reset the sinus node (zone of resetting). **D,** An even earlier coupled AES reaches refractory tissue around the sinus node and is thus unable to penetrate the sinus node (entrance block); therefore, it does not affect sinus node discharge. The next spontaneous sinus beat (A_3) arrives exactly at the sinus interval (zone of interpolation). The atrial–His bundle (AH) interval progressively prolongs with progressively premature coupling intervals (**B** to **D**). In contrast, the His bundle–ventricular (HV) interval remains constant.

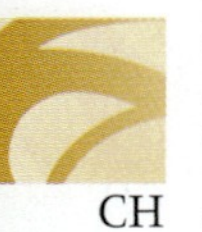

of the AES is, the longer the A_2-H_2 interval will be (see Fig. 4-21). More premature AES can block in the AVN with no conduction to the ventricle (defining AVN ERP). Occasionally, conduction delay and block occur in the HPS, especially when the AES is delivered following long basic drive CLs, because HPS refractoriness frequently exceeds the AVN FRP at long pacing CLs.

The patterns of AV conduction can be expressed by plotting refractory period relating the A_1-A_2 interval to the responses of the AVN and HPS. Plotting the A_1-A_2 interval versus the H_1-H_2 and V_1-V_2 intervals illustrates the functional input-output relationship between the basic drive beat and the AES and provides an assessment of the FRP of the AV conduction system. In contrast, plotting the A_2-H_2 interval (AVN conduction time of the AES) and the H_2-V_2 interval (HPS conduction time of the AES) versus the A_1-A_2 interval (the AES coupling interval) allows determination of the conduction times through the various components of the AV conduction system.[32]

TYPE I RESPONSE. In this type, the progressively premature AES encounters progressive delay in the AVN without any changes in the HPS. Therefore, refractoriness of the AVN determines the FRP of the entire AV conduction, and the ERP of the AV conduction system is determined at the atrial or AVN level. This response is characterized by initial shortening of the H_1-H_2 and V_1-V_2 intervals as the AES coupling interval (A_1-A_2) shortens, whereas AVN conduction (A_2-H_2) and HPS conduction (H_2-V_2) remain stable (Fig. 4-22). With further shortening of the A_1-A_2 interval, the RRP of the AVN is encountered, resulting in progressive delay in AVN conduction (manifesting as progressive prolongation of the A_2-H_2 interval) accompanied by stable HPS conduction (H_2-V_2) and a progressive but identical prolongation of both the H_1-H_2 and V_1-V_2 intervals, until the AES is blocked within the AVN (AVN ERP) or until the atrial ERP is reached. The minimum H_1-H_2 and V_1-V_2 intervals attained define the FRP of the AVN and entire AV conduction system. AVN conduction (A_2-H_2) usually increases by 2 to 3× baseline values before block.[24]

TYPE II RESPONSE. In type II response, conduction delay occurs initially in the AVN; however, with further shortening of the AES coupling interval, progressive delay develops in the HPS. Therefore, refractoriness of the HPS determines the FRP of the entire AV conduction system, and the ERP of the AV conduction system is determined at any level. At longer A_1-A_2 intervals, type II response is similar to type I response; however, as the A_1-A_2 interval shortens, conduction delay develops initially in the AVN (manifesting as progressive prolongation of the A_2-H_2 interval) but then in the HPS (manifesting as aberrant QRS conduction and progressive prolongation of the H_2-V_2 interval) as the RRP of the HPS is encountered. Therefore, in contrast to type I response, both A_2-H_2 and H_2-V_2 intervals prolong in response to progressively shorter A_1-A_2, resulting in divergence in the H_1-H_2 and V_1-V_2 curves until the AES is blocked within the AVN (AVN ERP), in the HPS (HPS ERP), or until the atrial ERP is reached (see Fig. 4-22). Block usually occurs in the AVN, but it can occur in the atrium and occasionally in the HPS (modified type II response). AVN conduction (A_2-H_2) usually increases only modestly (by less than 2× baseline values before block).[24]

TYPE III RESPONSE. In type III response, conduction delay occurs initially in the AVN; however, at a critical AES coupling interval, sudden and marked delay develops in the HPS. Therefore, refractoriness of the HPS determines the FRP of the entire AV conduction system, and the ERP of the AV conduction system is determined at any level. However, in contrast to type II response, the HPS is invariably the first site of block. At longer A_1-A_2 intervals, type II response is similar to type I response; however, as the A_1-A_2 interval shortens, progressive delay is noted initially in the AVN (manifest as progressive prolongation in the A_2-H_2 interval), but then a sudden delay of conduction in the HPS occurs (manifesting as aberrant QRS conduction and a sudden jump in the H_2-V_2 interval). This results in a break in the V_1-V_2 curve, which subsequently descends until, at a critical A_1-A_2 interval, the impulse blocks in the AVN or HPS (see Fig. 4-22). The FRP of the HPS occurs just before the marked jump in H_2-V_2. AVN conduction (A_2-H_2) usually increases by less than 2× baseline values before block.[24]

Type I response is the most common pattern, whereas type III response is the least common. The pattern of AV conduction (type I, II, or III), however, is not fixed in any patient. Drugs (e.g., atropine, isoproterenol) or changes in CL can alter the refractory period relationship among different tissues so that one type of response can be switched to another. For example, atropine can decrease the FRP of the AVN and allow the impulse to reach the HPS during its RRP, changing type I response to type II or III.

The ERP of the atrium is not infrequently reached earlier than that of the AVN, especially when the basic drive is slow (which increases atrial ERP and decreases AVN ERP) or when the patient is agitated, which increases sympathetic tone and decreases AVN ERP. The first site of block is in the AVN in most patients (45%), in the atrium in 40%, and in the HPS in 15%.[31]

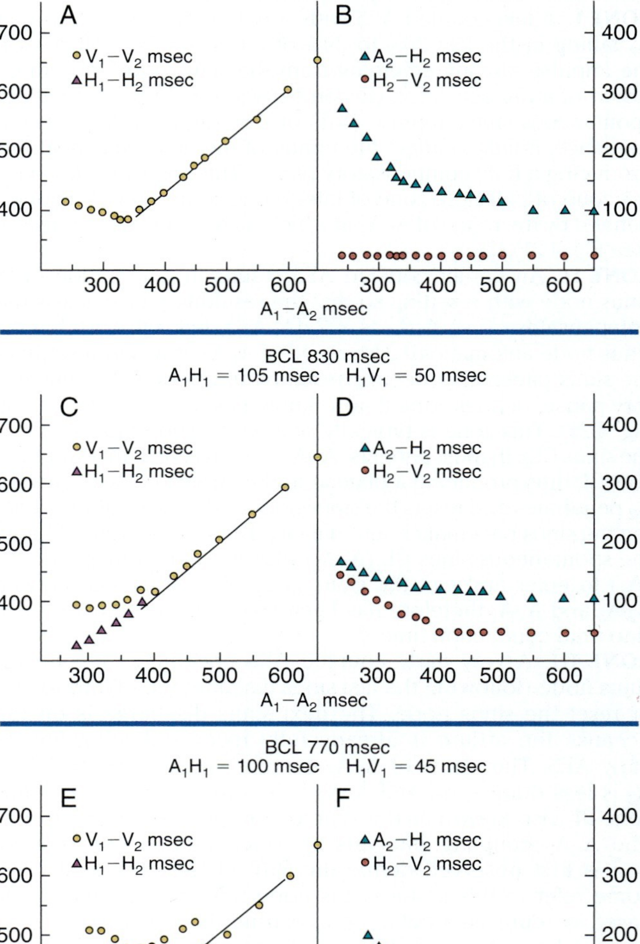

FIGURE 4-22 A and B, Type I pattern of atrioventricular node response to atrial extrastimulation (AES). C and D, Type II pattern of response to AES. E and F, Type III pattern of response to AES. See text for details. BCL = basic cycle length. *(From Josephson ME: Electrophysiologic investigation: general aspects. In Josephson ME, editor: Clinical cardiac electrophysiology, ed 3, Philadelphia, 2002, Lippincott Williams & Wilkins, pp 19-67.)*

ATRIAL RESPONSE TO ATRIAL EXTRASTIMULATION

Early AESs can impinge on the atrial RRP, with resulting local latency (i.e., long interval between the pacing artifact and the atrial electrogram on the pacing electrode).[31] A very early AES delivered during the atrial ERP fails to capture the atrium. The atrial ERP can be longer or shorter than the AVN ERP, especially at long basic drive CLs or in cases of enhanced AVN conduction secondary to autonomic influences.

As with rate-incremental pacing, AES can result in prolongation of intraatrial and interatrial conduction, which is more pronounced in patients with a history of atrial arrhythmias. Development of a fractionated atrial electrogram is more often observed in patients who have a history of AF. Intraatrial block in response to AES is unusual. Occasionally, double or triple AESs induce AF in patients with no history of such arrhythmia. Such episodes usually terminate spontaneously and are not clinically relevant in the absence of a history of known or suspected atrial arrhythmias.

Repetitive Atrial Responses

Atrial stimulation can trigger extra atrial complexes or echo beats. Those complexes can be caused by different mechanisms; the most common are intraatrial reentrant beats and AVN echo beats.

Intraatrial reentrant beats usually occur at short coupling intervals. They can originate anywhere in the atrium, and atrial activation sequence depends on the site of origin of the beat. The incidence of these responses increases with increasing both the number of AESs and the number of drive-pacing CLs and stimulation sites used.

Repetitive atrial responses can also be caused by reentry in the AVN. These patients have anterograde dual AVN physiology, and the last paced beat conducts slowly down the slow AVN pathway and then retrogradely up the fast pathway to produce the echo beat (Fig. 4-23). Atrial activation sequence is consistent with retrograde conduction over the fast AVN pathway, earliest in the HB catheter recording. Atrial and ventricular activations occur simultaneously.

Ventricular Stimulation

Technical Aspects

Ventricular stimulation is used to assess retrograde (ventricular-atrial [VA]) conduction and refractory periods, retrograde atrial activation patterns, including sequences that can indicate the presence of a BT, and vulnerability to inducible ventricular arrhythmias.[31]

Stepwise rate-incremental ventricular pacing or ramp pacing is used in the assessment of VA conduction. It is unusual to provoke ventricular arrhythmias with these tests, even in patients with

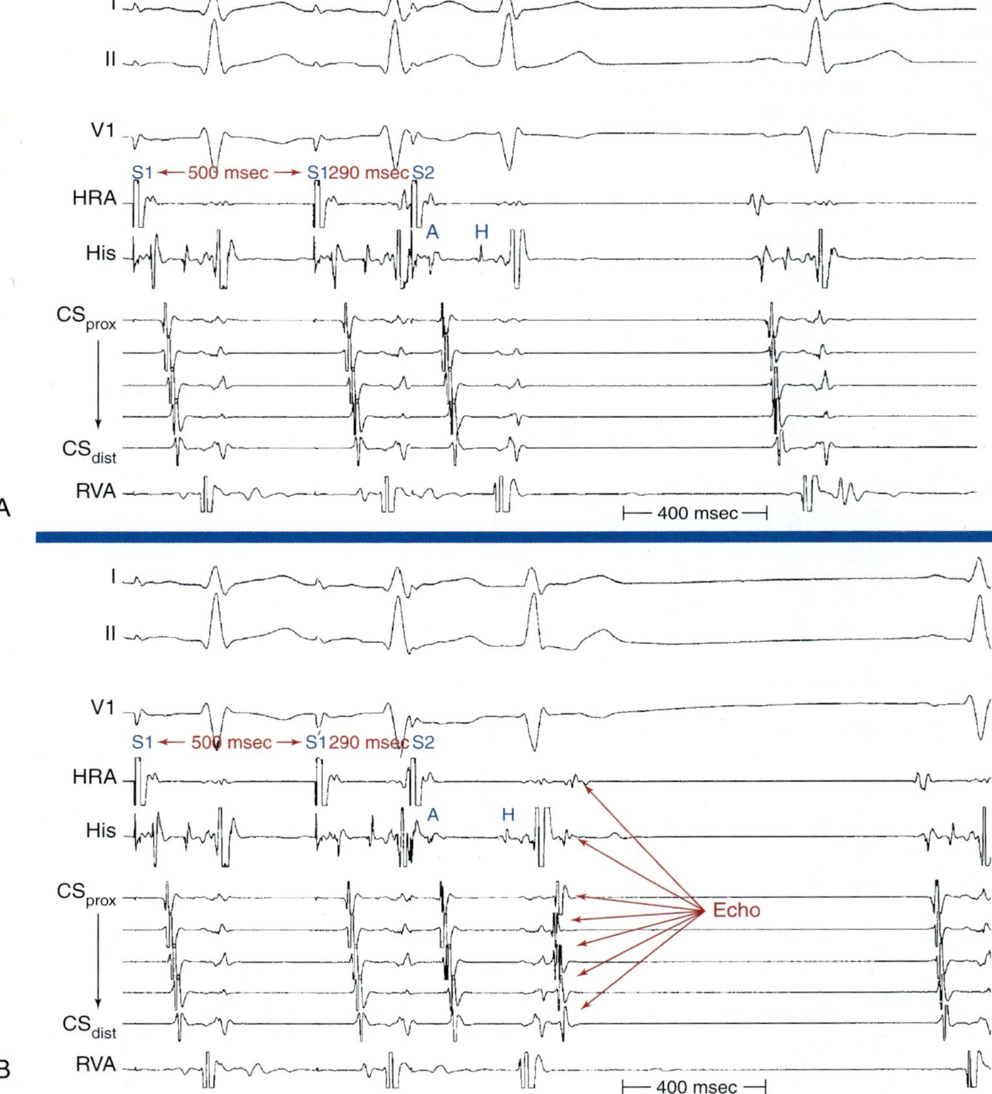

FIGURE 4-23 Anterograde dual atrioventricular nodal pathways. **Top,** A single extrastimulus is introduced from the high right atrium (HRA; S_2) at 290 milliseconds after the last afterdrive stimulus (S_1). This results in an atrial–His bundle (AH) interval of 140 milliseconds. **Bottom,** An extrastimulus is delivered 10 milliseconds earlier than above (280 milliseconds), resulting in marked prolongation of the AH interval to 202 milliseconds and an atrial echo. CS_{dist} = distal coronary sinus; CS_{prox} = proximal coronary sinus; HRA = high right atrium; RVA = right ventricular apex.

known ventricular arrhythmia. Rate-incremental ventricular pacing is usually started at a pacing CL just shorter than the sinus CL, and the pacing CL is then gradually decreased (in 10- to 20-millisecond decrements) down to 300 milliseconds. Shorter pacing CL may be used to assess rapid conduction in patients with supraventricular tachycardia (SVT) or to induce VT. With ramp pacing, the pacing rate is slowly increased at 2 to 4 beats/min/sec (or the pacing CL is decreased by 10 milliseconds every several paced beats) until VA block occurs.

Ventricular extrastimulus (VES) testing is used to assess ventricular, HPS, and AVN refractory periods and to induce arrhythmias.[31] During programmed stimulation, a sequence of eight paced stimuli is delivered at a constant rate (the S_1 drive), which allows stable VA conduction. Following these eight beats, a VES (S_2) is delivered. This stimulation sequence is repeated at progressively shorter S_1-S_2 intervals, thus allowing the response of the HPS and AVN to be recorded across a range of premature test stimuli.

During ventricular stimulation, the HB electrogram shows a retrograde His potential in 85% of patients with a normal QRS during NSR.[24] Ventricular pacing at the base of the heart close to the AV junction facilitates recording a retrograde His potential because it allows the ventricles to be activated much earlier relative to the HB (Fig. 4-24). The ventricular-HB (VH) or stimulus-HB (S-H) interval always exceeds the anterograde HV interval by the time it takes for the impulse to travel from the stimulation site to the ipsilateral bundle branch. In patients with normal HV intervals, a retrograde His potential can usually be seen before the ventricular electrogram in the HB recording during RV apical pacing. In contrast, when ipsilateral bundle branch block (BBB) is present, especially with long HV intervals, a retrograde His potential is less frequently seen; when it is seen, it is usually inscribed after the QRS when pacing from the ipsilateral ventricle (Fig. 4-25).

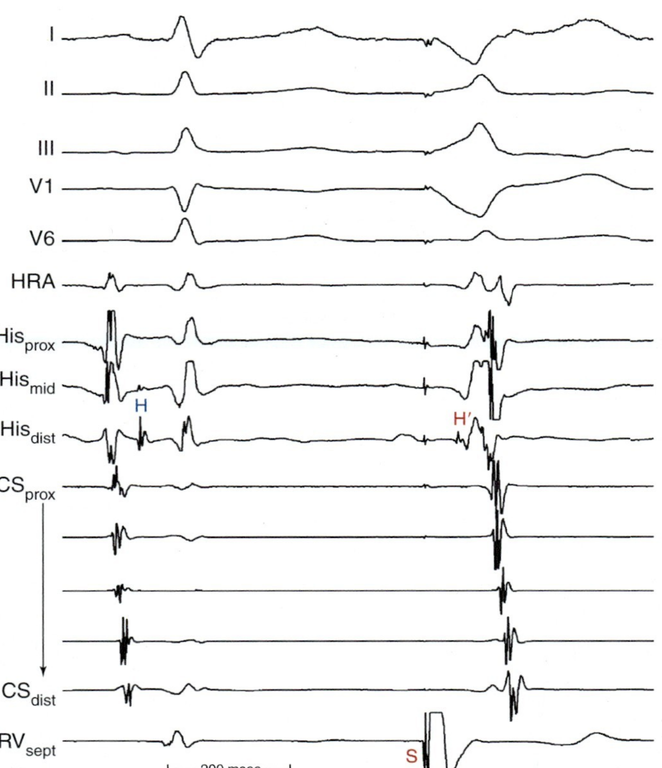

FIGURE 4-24 Retrograde activation with right ventricular (RV) septal (RV_{sept}) stimulation. Sinus and RV septal stimulated complexes (S) are shown. Retrograde atrial activation is concentric, following a retrograde His potential (H′). CS_{dist} = distal coronary sinus; CS_{prox} = proximal coronary sinus; His_{dist} = distal His bundle; HRA = high right atrium.

Ventricular stimulation is relatively safe; however, induction of clinically irrelevant serious arrhythmias, including VF, can occur in patients with normal hearts and those who have not had spontaneous ventricular arrhythmias. The induction of these arrhythmias is directly related to the aggressiveness of the ventricular stimulation protocol. Thus, the stimulation protocol is usually limited to single or double VES in patients without a clinical history consistent with malignant ventricular arrhythmias.[24] The use of high pacing output can also increase the risk of such arrhythmias. Therefore, ventricular stimulation at 2× diastolic threshold and 1-millisecond pulse width is preferable.

Normal Response to Rate-Incremental Ventricular Pacing

Ventricular pacing provides information about VA conduction, which is present in 40% to 90% of patients, depending on the population studied. Absence of VA conduction at any paced rate is common and normal. There is no difference in the capability of VA conduction regarding the site of ventricular stimulation in patients with a normal HPS. When present, normal VA conduction uses the normal AV conduction system, with the earliest atrial activation site usually in the septal region in proximity to the AVN. In some cases, the slow posterior AVN pathway is preferentially engaged so that the earliest atrial activation site is somewhat posterior to the AVN, closer to the CS os.[24]

The normal AVN response to rate-incremental ventricular pacing is a gradual delay of VA conduction (manifest as gradual prolongation of the HA interval) as the pacing CL decreases. Retrograde VA Wenckebach block and a higher degree of block appear at shorter pacing CLs. Occasionally, VA Wenckebach cycles are terminated with ventricular echo beats secondary to retrograde dual AVN physiology. When a retrograde His potential is visible, a relatively constant VH interval at a rapid pacing rate, despite the development of retrograde VA block, localizes the site of block to the AVN (Fig. 4-26). When a retrograde His potential is not visible during ventricular pacing, the site of VA block, when it occurs, must be inferred from the effect of paced impulses on conduction of spontaneous or stimulated atrial beats (i.e., by analyzing the level of retrograde concealment; see Fig. 4-26). If the AH interval of the atrial beat is independent of the time relationship of the paced impulse, the site of block is in the HPS (infranodal). On the other hand, if the AH interval varies according to the coupling interval of the atrial beat to the paced QRS, or if the atrial beat fails to depolarize the HB, the site of block is in the AVN. Moreover, drugs that enhance AVN (but not HPS) conduction (e.g., atropine) improve VA conduction if the site of block is in the AVN, but they do not affect VA conduction if the site of block is in the HPS.

At comparable pacing CLs, anterograde AV conduction is better than retrograde VA conduction in most patients. AVN conduction is the major determinant of retrograde VA conduction. Patients with prolonged PR intervals are much less likely to demonstrate retrograde VA conduction.[31] Furthermore, patients with prolonged AVN conduction are less capable of VA conduction than patients with infranodal conduction delay. Anterograde AV block in the AVN is almost universally associated with retrograde VA block. On the other hand, anterograde AV block in the HPS is associated with some degree of VA conduction in up to 40% of cases. However, the exact comparison between anterograde and retrograde AVN conduction can be limited by the absence of a visible retrograde His potential during ventricular stimulation. Consequently, localization of the exact site of conduction delay or block (AVN versus HPS) may not be feasible. The response to rate-incremental pacing at two different pacing CLs may differ because of the opposite effects of the pacing CL on AVN and HPS refractoriness.[24]

Rapid ventricular pacing can result in ipsilateral retrograde BBB, with subsequent impulse propagation across the septum, retrogradely up the contralateral bundle branch, and then to the HB. Such an event can manifest as sudden prolongation of the HV interval during pacing. This can be followed by resumption

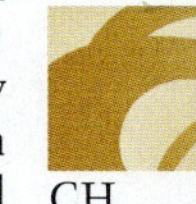

of VA conduction after a period of VA block in the AVN when the VH interval is short, because the delay in the HPS allows recovery of the AVN (the gap phenomenon). This occurrence can permit better visualization of the His potential, and, by comparing the ventricular electrogram in the HB recording when the His potential is clearly delayed with that with normal retrograde ipsilateral bundle branch conduction, a previously unappreciated His potential within that electrogram can then be visualized (see Fig. 4-26).

To exclude the presence of a nondecremental retrogradely conducting BT, the VES technique is usually more effective than rate-incremental ventricular pacing for demonstrating normal

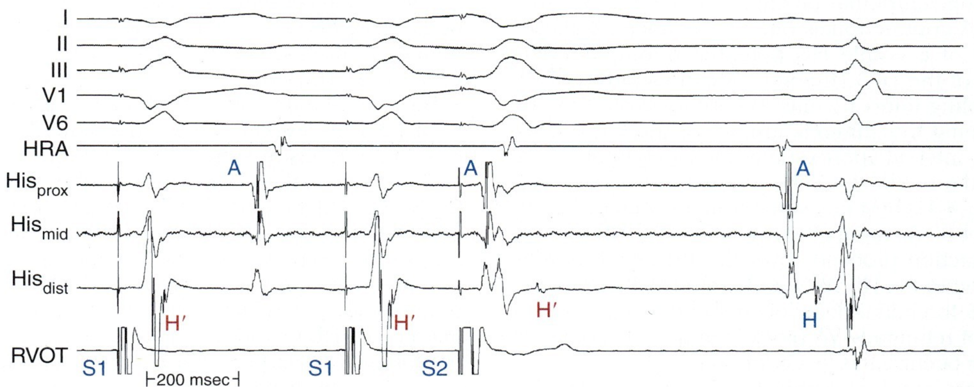

FIGURE 4-25 His recordings in the presence of right bundle branch block (RBBB). Two right ventricular drive complexes (S_1) and an extrastimulus (S_2) are shown, with a subsequent sinus complex with typical RBBB. Retrograde His activation (H′) cannot traverse the blocked right bundle branch and must occur over the left bundle branch following transseptal ventricular activation, resulting in a long S-H′ interval. The S-H′ interval prolongs further following the extrastimulus (S_2). Of note, S_2 is associated with retrograde ventricular-atrial block in the atrioventricular node. His_{dist} = distal His bundle; His_{mid} = middle His bundle; His_{prox} = proximal His bundle; HRA = high right atrium; RVOT = right ventricular outflow tract.

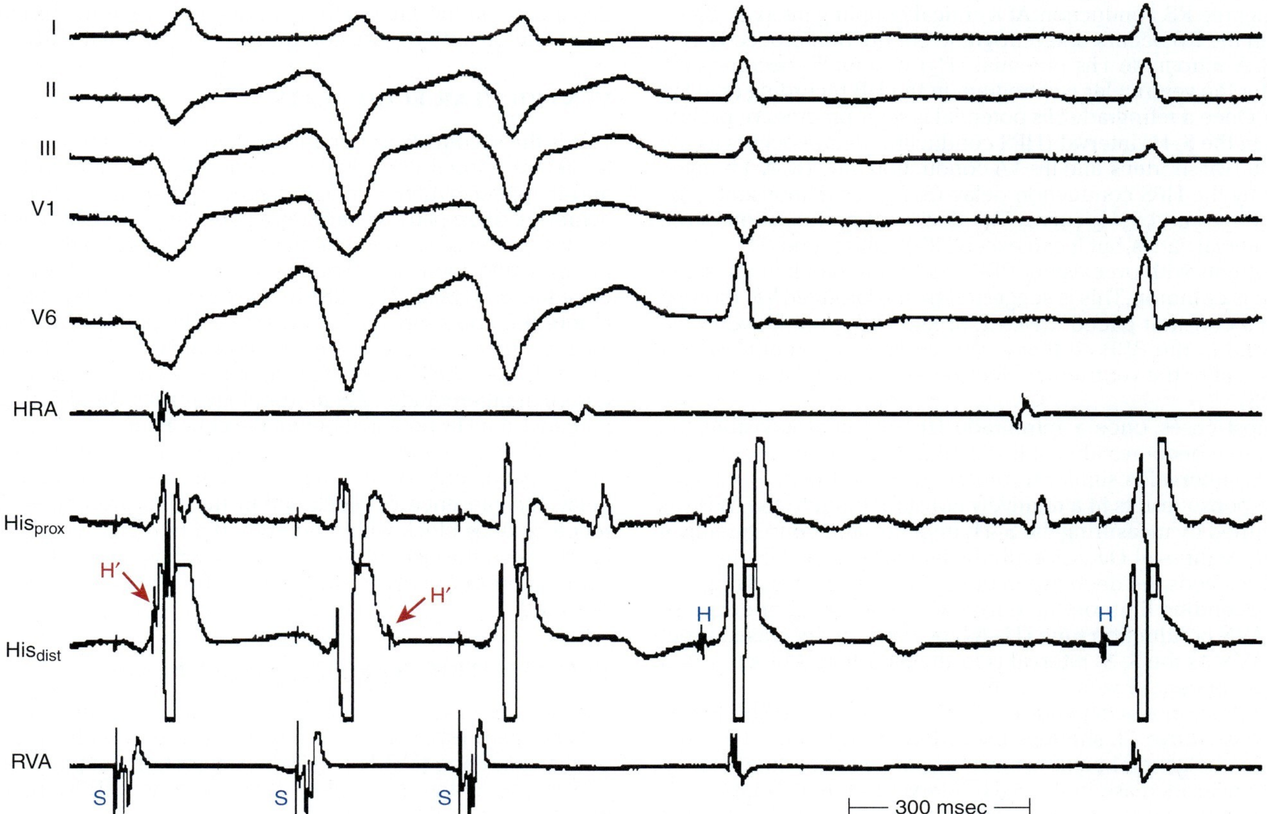

FIGURE 4-26 Complete retrograde ventricular-atrial (VA) block in the atrioventricular node (AVN). Three ventricular paced complexes are shown, the first two of which have a clear retrograde His potential (H′) and no retrograde atrial activation (sinus rhythm in atria), suggesting the AVN as the site of VA block. However, the site of VA block (AVN versus His-Purkinje system) following the third ventricular complex is not obvious because there is no His potential visible following that ventricular stimulus. The site of VA block, however, can be inferred from the effect of paced impulses on conduction of the sinus complex after cessation of pacing. The atrial–His bundle (AH) interval of the conducted sinus complex after the last paced ventricular complex is longer than the baseline AH interval (at right), consistent with retrograde penetration of the AVN by the ventricular stimulus (resulting in concealed conduction) and therefore suggesting the AVN as the site of VA block. His_{dist} = distal His bundle; His_{prox} = proximal His bundle; HRA = high right atrium; RVA = right ventricular apex.

prolongation of the VA interval. If uncertainty continues to exist, adenosine can be extremely helpful, which is much more likely to block AVN conduction than BT.

Normal Response to Ventricular Premature Stimulation

Because a retrograde His potential may not be visible in 15% to 20% of patients during ventricular pacing, evaluation of the HPS, and consequently VA conduction, is often incomplete. Additionally, in the absence of a visible His potential during ventricular pacing, the FRP of the HPS (theoretically, the shortest H_1-H_2 interval at any coupling interval) must be approximated by the S_1-H_2 interval (S_1 being the stimulus artifact of the basic drive CL), so that the S_1-H_2 interval approximates the H_1-H_2 interval, but exceeds it by a fixed amount, the S_1-H_1 interval. Retrograde AVN conduction time (H_2-A_2) is best measured from the end of the His potential to the onset of the atrial electrogram on the HB tracing.

Typically, VA conduction proceeds over the RB or left bundle branch (LB), and then to the HB, AVN, and atrium. With a progressively premature VES, the initial delay occurs in the HPS, and the most common site of retrograde VA block is in the HPS. Delay or block in the AVN can occur but is less common.[31]

The typical response can be graphically displayed by plotting the S_1-S_2 interval versus S_2-H_2, S_2-A_2, and H_2-A_2 intervals, as well as the S_1-S_2 interval versus S_1-H_2 and A_1-A_2 intervals.[31] At long S_1-S_2 intervals, no delay occurs in the retrograde conduction (S_2-A_2). Further shortening of the S_1-S_2 intervals results in prolongation in the S_2-A_2 intervals, and localization of the exact site of S_2-A_2 delay may not be feasible unless a retrograde His potential is visible (Fig. 4-27A and B). During RV pacing, the initial delay usually occurs in retrograde RB conduction. At a critical coupling interval (S_1-S_2), block in the RB occurs, and retrograde conduction proceeds over the LB. A retrograde His potential (H_2) eventually becomes visible after the ventricular electrogram in the HB recording (see Fig. 4-27D). Once a retrograde His potential is seen, progressive prolongation in the S_2-H_2 interval (HPS conduction delay) occurs as the S_1-S_2 interval shortens, and the VA conduction time (S_2-A_2) is determined by the HPS conduction delay (S_2-H_2), as demonstrated by parallel S_2-A_2 and S_2-H_2 curves. The degree of prolongation of the S_2-H_2 interval varies, but it can exceed 300 milliseconds.[24]

In patients with preexistent BBB, retrograde block in the same bundle is common. This is suggested by a prolonged VH interval during a constant paced drive CL or late VES from the ventricle ipsilateral to the BBB, so that a retrograde His potential is usually seen after the ventricular electrogram in the HB tracing (see Fig. 4-25).

In most cases, once a retrograde His potential is visible, the S_1-H_2 curve becomes almost horizontal because the increase in the S_2-H_2 interval is similar to the decrease in the S_1-S_2 interval. This response results in a relatively constant input to the AVN (as determined by measuring the S_1-H_2 interval) and consequently a fixed H_2-A_2 interval. Occasionally, the increase in the S_2-H_2 interval greatly exceeds the decrease in the S_1-S_2 interval, thus giving rise to an ascending limb on the curve, with a subsequent decrease in the AVN conduction time (H_2-A_2) because of decreased input to the AVN. As the S_1-S_2 interval is further shortened, block within the HPS appears, or ventricular ERP is reached.[24]

HPS refractoriness depends markedly on the CL, and shortening of the basic drive CL shortens the FRP and ERP of the HPS and ventricle. The general pattern, however, remains the same, with an almost linear increase in the S_2-H_2 interval as the S_1-S_2 interval is shortened. The curves for S_2-H_2 versus S_1-S_2 are shifted to the left, and the curves for S_1-S_2 versus S_1-H_2 are shifted down.

Repetitive Ventricular Responses

Ventricular stimulation can trigger extra ventricular beats. Those beats can be caused by different mechanisms; the most common are bundle branch reentry (BBR) beats, ventricular echo beats, and intraventricular reentrant beats. Multiple mechanisms may be responsible for repetitive responses in the same patient. Almost always, one of these responses is BBR.

BUNDLE BRANCH REENTRY BEATS

This is the most common response and can occur in up to 50% of normal individuals. In patients with normal hearts, BBR is rarely sustained and is usually self-limiting in one or two complexes. The occurrence of nonsustained BBR in patients with or without structural heart disease is not related to the presence of spontaneous ventricular arrhythmias.

The longest refractory periods in the HPS are found most distally, at or near the Purkinje-myocardial junction. This creates a distal gate that inhibits retrograde conduction of early VES. Thus, when an early VES is delivered to the RV apex, the nearby distal gate of the RB can still be refractory. The results are progressive retrograde conduction delay and block occurring in the distal RB, with subsequent transseptal conduction of the impulse to the LV, leading to retrograde conduction up the LB to the HB (see Fig. 4-27D). At this point, the His potential usually follows the local ventricular electrogram in the HB recording, and retrograde atrial stimulation, if present, follows the His potential. Further decrease in the VES coupling interval produces progressive delay in retrograde HPS conduction. When a critical degree of HPS delay (S_2-H_2) is attained, the impulse can return down the initially blocked RB, thus producing a QRS with a typical LBBB pattern and left-axis deviation, because ventricular activation originates solely from conduction over the RB (see Fig. 4-27E). This beat is called a BBR beat or V_3 phenomenon.[24]

The HV interval of the BBR beat usually approximates that during anterograde conduction. However, it can be shorter or longer, depending on the site of HB recording relative to the turnaround point and on anterograde conduction delay down the RB.

VENTRICULAR ECHO BEATS

This is the second most common response and can occur in 15% to 30% of normal individuals. It is caused by reentry in the AVN, and it appears when a critical degree of retrograde AVN delay is achieved. These patients have retrograde dual AVN physiology, and the last paced beat conducts slowly retrogradely up the slow AVN pathway and then anterogradely down the fast pathway to produce the echo beat (Fig. 4-28). In most cases, this delay is achieved before the appearance of a retrograde His potential beyond the local ventricular electrogram. At a critical H_2-A_2 interval (or V_2-A_2 interval, when the His potential cannot be seen), an extra beat with a normal anterograde QRS morphology results. Atrial activity also precedes the His potential before the echo beat.

This phenomenon can occur at long or short coupling intervals and depends only on the degree of retrograde AVN conduction delay. The presence of block within the HPS prevents its occurrence, as does block within the AVN. If a retrograde His potential can be seen throughout the zone of coupling intervals, a reciprocal relationship between the H_2-A_2 and A_2-H_3 intervals can often be noted.

INTRAVENTRICULAR REENTRANT BEATS

This response usually occurs in the setting of a cardiac pathological condition, especially coronary artery disease with a prior myocardial infarction (MI). It usually occurs at short coupling intervals and can have any morphology, but more often RBBB than LBBB in patients with a prior MI. Such beats occur in fewer than 15% of normal patients with a single VES at 2× diastolic threshold and in 24% with double VESs. In contrast, intraventricular reentrant beats occur following single or double VESs in 70% to 75% of patients with prior VT or VF and cardiac disease. The incidence of this response increases with increasing the number of VESs, basic drive CLs, and stimulation sites used. These responses are usually nonsustained (1 to 30 complexes) and typically polymorphic. In

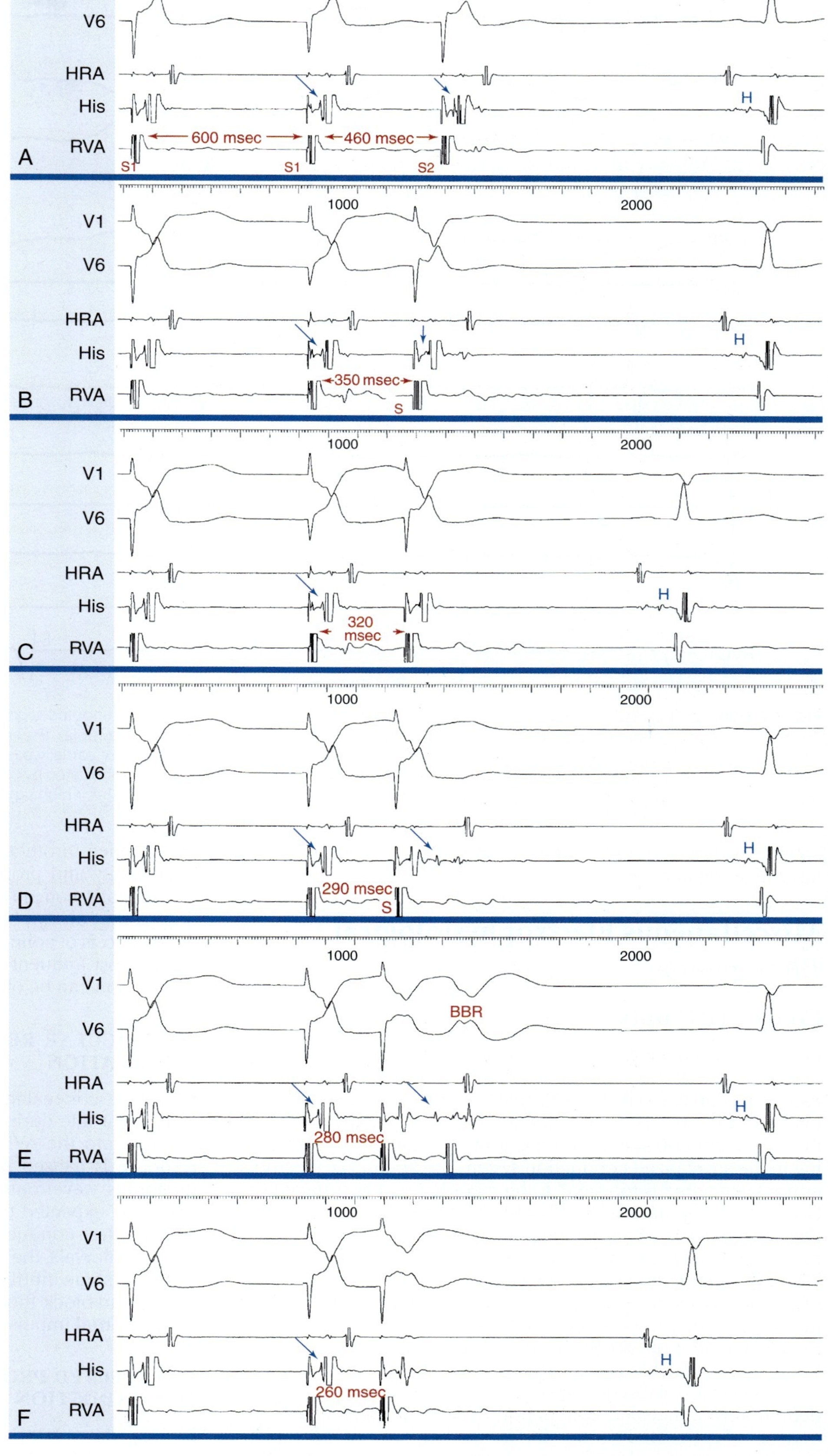

FIGURE 4-27 Normal response to progressively premature ventricular stimulation. Following a drive stimulus (S_1) at a cycle length of 600 milliseconds, a progressively premature ventricular extrastimulus (VES; S_2) is delivered from the right ventricular apex (RVA). **A,** At a VES coupling interval of 460 milliseconds, retrograde His potential (arrows) is visible just before the local ventricular electrogram on the His bundle (HB) tracing, and ventricular-atrial (VA) conduction is intact. **B,** An earlier VES is followed by some delay in VA conduction and prolongation of the His bundle–atrial (HA) interval. **C,** A short coupled VES is followed by VA block. A retrograde His potential is not clearly visible. **D,** An earlier VES is associated with retrograde block in the right bundle branch (RB), followed by transseptal conduction and retrograde conduction up the left bundle branch (LB) to the HB (the retrograde His potential is now visible well after the local ventricular electrogram). VA conduction now resumes because of proximal delay (in the His-Purkinje system [HPS]), allowing distal recovery in the atrioventricular node (AVN; the gap phenomenon). **E,** Further decrement in the VES coupling interval results in progressive delay in retrograde HPS conduction (and further prolongation of the S_2-H_2 interval), allowing for anterograde recovery of the RB, so that the impulse can return down the initially blocked RB, producing a QRS with a typical left bundle branch block pattern (bundle branch reentry beat [BBR]). **F,** A very early VES is followed by ventricular-atrial (VA) block secondary to retrograde block in both the RB and LB; therefore, no His potential is visible. HRA = high right atrium.

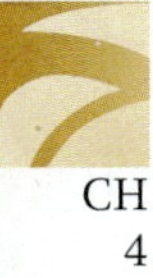

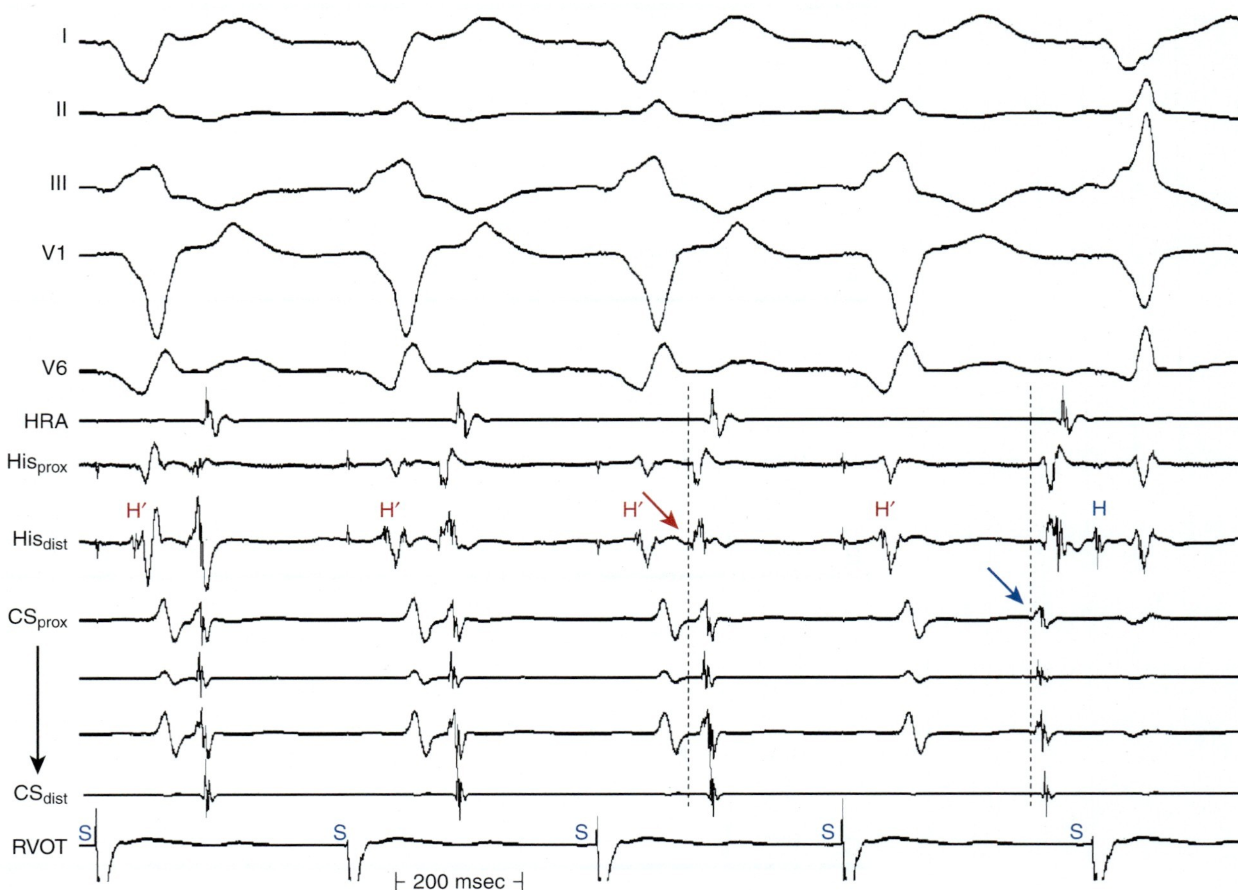

FIGURE 4-28 Retrograde dual atrioventricular pathways. Fixed-rate ventricular pacing results in retrograde conduction; retrograde His potential is labeled H′. The first three complexes are conducted over a fast atrioventricular nodal (AVN) pathway; with the fourth complex, the fast AVN pathway conduction is blocked and retrograde conduction proceeds up the slow pathway (longer VA interval), followed by a fused QRS complex, partially paced and partially conducted to the His bundle anterogradely over the fast pathway. The two AVN pathways have different earliest atrial activation sites, indicated by colored arrows and dashed lines. CS_{dist} = distal coronary sinus; CS_{prox} = proximal coronary sinus; His_{dist} = distal His bundle; His_{prox} = proximal His bundle; HRA = high right atrium; RVOT = right ventricular outflow tract.

patients without prior clinical arrhythmias, such responses are of no clinical significance.

Miscellaneous Electrophysiological Phenomena

Concealed Conduction

Concealed conduction can be defined as the propagation of an impulse within the specialized conduction system of the heart that can be recognized only from its effect on the subsequent impulse, interval, or cycle.[35] This phenomenon can occur in any portion of the AV conduction system. As long as the cardiac impulse is traveling in the specialized conduction system, the amount of electrical current generated is too small to be recorded on the surface ECG. However, if this impulse travels only a limited distance—incomplete anterograde or retrograde penetration—within the system, it can interfere with the formation or propagation of another impulse. When this interference can be recognized in the tracing because of an unexpected behavior of the subsequent impulse, unexpected in the sense that the event cannot be explained on the basis of readily apparent physiological or pathophysiological processes, it is known as concealed conduction.[25,35,36]

The effect on subsequent events is an important part of the definition of concealed conduction because it differentiates the concept of concealed conduction from other forms of incomplete conduction, such as block of conduction at the level of the AVN or HPS. Ideally, a diagnosis of concealed conduction is supported by evidence in other areas of the same tracing where, given the opportunity and proper physiological setting, an impulse that is occasionally concealed can be conducted. However, this condition cannot always be satisfied, nor is it absolutely necessary for the diagnosis of concealed conduction. Following are descriptions of the most frequent clinical circumstances in which concealed conduction can be observed.

VENTRICULAR RESPONSE DURING ATRIAL FIBRILLATION

Repetitive concealed conduction is the mechanism of a slow ventricular rate during AF and AFL, with varying degrees of penetration into the AVN.[25,35,36] During AF, the irregular ventricular response is caused by the varying depth of penetration of the numerous wavefronts approaching the AVN. Although the AVN would be expected to conduct whenever it recovers excitability after the last conducted atrial impulse, which would then be at regular intervals, the ventricular response is irregularly irregular because some fibrillatory impulses penetrate the AVN incompletely and block, thus leaving it refractory in the presence of subsequent atrial impulses.

UNEXPECTED PROLONGATION OR FAILURE OF CONDUCTION

Prolongation of the PR (and AH) interval or AVN block can occur secondary to a nonconducted premature depolarization of any origin (atrium, ventricle, or HB). The premature impulse incompletely penetrates the AVN (anterogradely or retrogradely), resets its refractoriness, and can make it fully or partially refractory in the presence of the next sinus beat, which may then be blocked or may conduct with longer PR interval (see Fig. 4-26). For example, concealed junctional (HB) impulses can manifest as isolated PR interval prolongation, pseudo–type I AV block, or pseudo–type II AV block. ECG clues to concealed junctional extrasystoles causing such unexpected events include abrupt unexplained prolongation of the PR interval, the presence of apparent type II AV block in the presence of a normal QRS, the presence of types I and II AV block in the same tracing, and the presence of manifest junctional extrasystoles elsewhere in the tracing.

UNEXPECTED FACILITATION OF CONDUCTION

When a premature impulse penetrates the AV conduction system, it can result in facilitation of AV conduction and normalization of a previously present AV block or BBB by one of two mechanisms: (1) preexciting parts of the conduction system so that its refractory period ends earlier than expected (i.e., peeling back the refractory period of that tissue, thus allowing more time to recover excitability), or (2) causing CL-dependent shortening of refractoriness of tissues (i.e., atria, HPS, and ventricles) by decreasing the CL preceding the subsequent spontaneous impulse.[25,35,36] Abrupt normalization of the aberration by a PVC, the finding of which proves retrograde concealment as the mechanism for perpetuation of aberration, is based on these principles.

PERPETUATION OF ABERRANT CONDUCTION DURING SUPRAVENTRICULAR TACHYCARDIAS

The most common mechanism (70%) of perpetuation of aberrant conduction during tachyarrhythmias is retrograde penetration of the blocked bundle branch subsequent to transseptal conduction. For example, a PVC from the LV during an SVT can activate the LB early and then conduct transseptally and later penetrate the RB retrogradely. Subsequently, the LB recovers in time for the next SVT impulse, whereas the RB remains refractory. Therefore, the next SVT impulse travels to the LV over the LB (with an RBBB pattern, phase 3 aberration). Conduction subsequently propagates from the LV across the septum to the RV. By this time, the distal RB has recovered, thereby allowing retrograde penetration of the RB by the transseptal wavefront and rendering the RB refractory to each subsequent SVT impulse. This scenario is repeated and RBBB continues until another, well-timed PVC preexcites the RB (and either peels back or shortens its refractoriness), so that the next impulse from above finds the RB fully recovered and conducts without aberration.

Gap Phenomenon

The term *gap* in AVN conduction was originally used to define a zone in the cardiac cycle during which PACs failed to evoke ventricular responses, whereas PACs of greater or lesser prematurity conducted to the ventricles. The physiological basis of the gap phenomenon depends on a distal area with a long refractory period and a proximal site with a shorter refractory period. During the gap phenomenon, initial block occurs distally. With earlier impulses, proximal conduction delay is encountered, which allows the distal site of early block to recover excitability and resume conduction.[35-37]

The gap phenomenon is not an abnormality, but reflects the interplay between conduction velocity and refractory periods at two different levels in the AV conduction system. Demonstration of the gap phenomenon can be enhanced or eliminated by any intervention that alters the relationship between the EP properties of those structures (e.g., changes in the neurohumoral tone created by drugs or changes in the heart rate by pacing).

An example of the most common type of gap phenomenon is an AES (A_2) conducting with modest delay through the AVN that finds

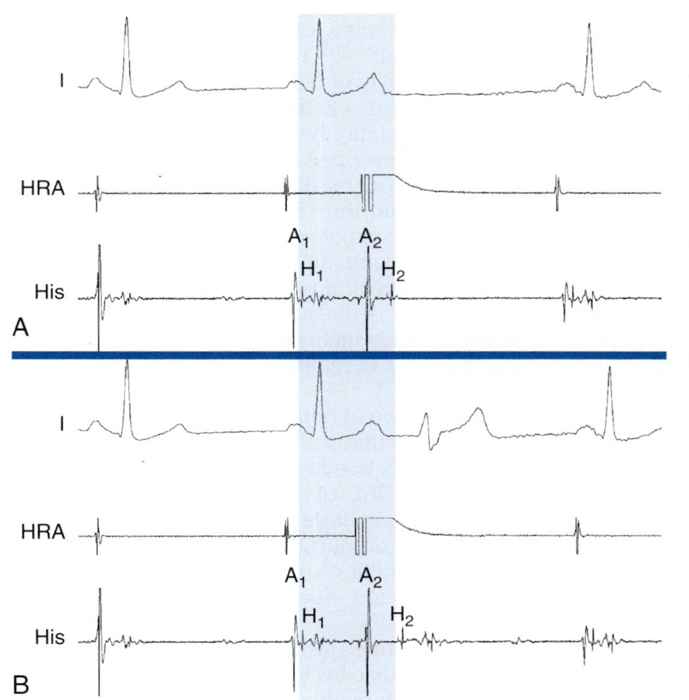

FIGURE 4-29 Anterograde atrioventricular (AV) gap phenomenon. **A,** An atrial extrastimulus (AES; A_2) conducting with modest delay through the AV node (AVN) finds the His bundle (HB) still refractory, causing AV block. **B,** An earlier AES results in further prolongation of the A_2-H_2 interval and the subsequent H_1-H_2 interval (shaded area). The longer H_1-H_2 interval now exceeds the refractory period of the HB, and, by the time the impulse traverses the AVN, the HB has completed its effective refractory period and conduction resumes; however, the conducted QRS has a left bundle branch block morphology and a longer HV interval because the left bundle is still refractory. HRA = high right atrium.

the HB still refractory, thus causing block. With increasing prematurity of the AES, the AES travels more slowly through the AVN (i.e., the A_2-H_2 interval prolongs further), so that the H_1-H_2 interval now exceeds the refractory period of the HB. By the time the impulse traverses the AVN, the HB has completed its ERP and conduction resumes (Fig. 4-29).

Other types of the gap phenomenon are described in which the required conduction delay is in the HB, proximal AVN, or atria. The gap phenomenon depends on the relationship between the EP properties of two sites; any pair of structures in the AV conduction system that has the appropriate physiological relationship can exhibit the gap phenomenon (e.g., AVN-HB, HB-HPS, atrium-AVN, atrium-HPS, proximal AVN–distal AVN, proximal HPS–distal HPS), and gap can occur during anterograde or retrograde stimulation. Therefore, there are almost endless possibilities for gaps, all based on the fundamental precept of "proximal delay allows distal recovery" (see Fig. 4-27C and D).[35,36]

Supernormality

Supernormal conduction implies conduction that is better than anticipated or conduction that occurs when block is expected. Electrocardiographically, however, supernormal conduction is not better than normal conduction, only better than expected. Conduction is better earlier in the cycle than later and occurs when block is expected. When an alteration in conduction can be explained in terms of known physiological events, true supernormal conduction need not be invoked.[35]

Supernormal conduction is dependent on supernormal excitability, a condition that exists during a brief period of repolarization, at the end of phase 3. During the supernormal period, excitation is possible in response to an otherwise subthreshold

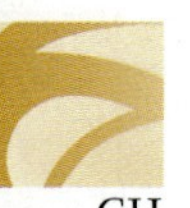

stimulus; that same stimulus fails to elicit a response earlier or later than the supernormal period.[35,36,38] Two factors are responsible for supernormality: the availability of fast Na^+ channels and the proximity of the membrane potential to threshold potential. During the supernormal phase of excitability, the cell has recovered enough to respond to a stimulus. However, because the membrane potential is still reduced, it requires only a little additional depolarization to bring the fiber to threshold; thus, a smaller stimulus than is normally required elicits an action potential. Supernormality has been demonstrated in the HPS, Bachmann bundle in the dog, and working myocardium of the atrium and ventricle, but not in the AVN.

Supernormal excitability is diagnosed when the myocardium responds to a stimulus that is ineffective when applied earlier or later in the cycle. Some ECG manifestations of supernormality include the following:

1. Paradoxical normalization of bundle branch conduction at an R-R interval shorter than that with BBB. This can occur with a premature atrial complex conducting with a normal QRS during baseline NSR with BBB or with acceleration-dependent BBB that normalizes at even faster rates.
2. Intermittent AV conduction during periods of high-degree AV block. Only the P waves falling on or just after the terminal part of the T wave are conducted, whereas other timed P waves fail to conduct.
3. A failing pacemaker captures just at the end of the T wave, but not elsewhere in the cardiac cycle.

Although supernormal conduction is a proven property of the HPS and has been demonstrated in vitro, it is uncertain whether true supernormal conduction is a clinically important phenomenon. Other physiological mechanisms can be invoked to explain almost all reported examples of supernormal conduction in humans. Causes of apparent or pseudosupernormal conduction include the gap phenomenon (the most common mechanism of pseudosupernormal conduction), peeling back of refractoriness, shortening of refractoriness by changing the preceding CL, Wenckebach phenomena in the bundle branches, bradycardia-dependent (phase 4) block, summation, dual AVN physiology, reentry with ventricular echo beats, and concealed junctional extrasystoles.[35,36,38]

Complications

Risks and Complications

The complication rate of EP testing is relatively low (less than that of coronary arteriography) when only right-heart catheterization is performed, with almost negligible mortality. The risk of complications increases significantly in patients with severe or decompensated cardiac disease. Complications of EP testing include vascular injury (hematoma, pseudoaneurysm, and arteriovenous fistula), bleeding requiring transfusion, deep venous thrombosis and pulmonary embolism, systemic thromboembolism, infection at catheter sites, systemic infection, pneumothorax, hemothorax, pericarditis, cardiac perforation and tamponade, MI, worsening heart failure, stroke, complete AV block, and BBB. Although potentially lethal arrhythmias such as rapid VT or VF can occur in the EP laboratory, they are not necessarily regarded as complications, but are often expected and anticipated.

The addition of left-heart access or therapeutic maneuvers (e.g., ablation) to the procedure increases the incidence of complications, especially with the increasing use of extensive ablation to treat AF and ischemic VT. In the 1998 North American Society for Pacing and Electrophysiology (NASPE) Prospective Catheter Ablation Registry, 3357 patients were treated with RF ablation for a variety of cardiac arrhythmias. Major complications were reported in 1% to 4%, with procedure-related deaths in approximately 0.2%. There was no significant difference in the incidence of complications comparing patients older than 60 with those younger than 60 years of age or comparing large-volume centers (more than 100 ablation procedures/year) with lower-volume centers or between teaching and nonteaching hospitals.[2] Complications following specific ablation procedures are discussed in subsequent chapters.

Iatrogenic Problems Encountered during Electrophysiological Testing

Mechanical irritation from catheters during placement inside the heart, even when they are not being manipulated, can cause arrhythmias and conduction disturbances, including induction of atrial, junctional, and ventricular ectopic beats or tachyarrhythmias, BBB, and AV block. AV block can occur especially during RV catheterization in patients with preexisting LBBB, and occasionally secondary to mechanical trauma of the compact AVN. Ventricular stimulation can also occur from physical movement of the ventricular catheter coincident with atrial contraction, thus producing patterns of ventricular preexcitation on the surface ECG. Recognition of all these iatrogenic patterns is important for avoiding misinterpretation of EP phenomena and determining the significance of findings in the laboratory.

AF and VF are to be avoided unless they are the subject of the study. AF obviously does not permit study of any other form of SVT, and VF requires prompt defibrillation. If AF must be initiated for diagnostic purposes (e.g., to assess ventricular response over an AV BT), it is preferably induced at the end of the diagnostic portion of the study. Patients with a prior history of AF are more prone to the occurrence of sustained AF in the EP laboratory. Frequently, this occurs during initial placement of catheters; excessive manipulation of catheters in the atria should therefore be avoided.

Another iatrogenic problem is catheter trauma resulting in abolition of BT conduction or injury to the focus of a tachycardia or to the reentrant pathway, which can make the mapping and curative ablation difficult or impossible.

REFERENCES

1. Calkins H, Brugada J, Packer DL, et al: HRS/EHRA/ECAS expert Consensus Statement on catheter and surgical ablation of atrial fibrillation: recommendations for personnel, policy, procedures and follow-up. A report of the Heart Rhythm Society (HRS) Task Force on catheter and surgical ablation of atrial fibrillation, *Heart Rhythm* 4:816–861, 2007.
2. Finlay M, Sawhney V, Schilling R, et al: Uninterrupted warfarin for periprocedural anticoagulation in catheter ablation of typical atrial flutter: a safe and cost-effective strategy, *J Cardiovasc Electrophysiol* 21:150–154, 2010.
3. Hussein AA, Martin DO, Saliba W, et al: Radiofrequency ablation of atrial fibrillation under therapeutic international normalized ratio: a safe and efficacious periprocedural anticoagulation strategy, *Heart Rhythm* 6:1425–1429, 2009.
4. Kwak JJ, Pak HN, Jang JK, et al: Safety and convenience of continuous warfarin strategy during the periprocedural period in patients who underwent catheter ablation of atrial fibrillation, *J Cardiovasc Electrophysiol* 21:620–625, 2010.
5. Josephson M: Electrophysiologic investigation: technical aspects. In Josephson ME, editor: *Clinical cardiac electrophysiology*, ed 4, Philadelphia, 2008, Lippincott Williams & Wilkins, pp 1–19.
6. Markides V, Koa-Wing M, Peters N: Mapping and imaging. In Zipes DP, Jalife J, editors: *Cardiac electrophysiology: from cell to bedside*, ed 5, Philadelphia, 2009, Saunders, pp 897–904.
7. Habib A, Lachman N, Christensen KN, Asirvatham SJ: The anatomy of the coronary sinus venous system for the cardiac electrophysiologist, *Europace* 11(Suppl 5):v15–v21, 2009.
8. Ren JF, Callans DJ: Utility of intracardiac echocardiographic imaging for catheterization. In Ren JF, Marchlinski FE, Callans DJ, Schwartsman D, editors: *Practical intracardiac echocardiography in electrophysiology*, Malden, Mass., 2006, Wiley-Blackwell, pp 56–73.
9. de Asmundis C, Chierchia GB, Sarkozy A, et al: Novel trans-septal approach using a Safe Sept J-shaped guidewire in difficult left atrial access during atrial fibrillation ablation, *Europace* 11:657–659, 2009.
10. Betensky BP, Park RE, Marchlinski FE, et al: The v(2) transition ratio: a new electrocardiographic criterion for distinguishing left from right ventricular outflow tract tachycardia origin, *J Am Coll Cardiol* 57:2255–2262, 2011.
11. Tomlinson DR, Sabharwal N, Bashir Y, Betts TR: Interatrial septum thickness and difficulty with transseptal puncture during redo catheter ablation of atrial fibrillation, *Pacing Clin Electrophysiol* 31:1606–1611, 2008.
12. De PR, Cappato R, Curnis A, et al: Trans-septal catheterization in the electrophysiology laboratory: data from a multicenter survey spanning 12 years, *J Am Coll Cardiol* 47: 1037–1042, 2006.
13. Hu YF, Tai CT, Lin YJ, et al: The change in the fluoroscopy-guided transseptal puncture site and difficult punctures in catheter ablation of recurrent atrial fibrillation, *Europace* 10:276–279, 2008.
14. McWilliams MJ, Tchou P: The use of a standard radiofrequency energy delivery system to facilitate transseptal puncture, *J Cardiovasc Electrophysiol* 20:238–240, 2009.
15. Bidart C, Vaseghi M, Cesario DA, et al: Radiofrequency current delivery via transseptal needle to facilitate septal puncture, *Heart Rhythm* 4:1573–1576, 2007.
16. Knecht S, Jais P, Nault I, et al: Radiofrequency puncture of the fossa ovalis for resistant transseptal access, *Circ Arrhythm Electrophysiol* 1:169–174, 2008.

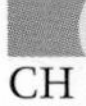

17. Smelley MP, Shah DP, Weisberg I, et al: Initial experience using a radiofrequency powered transseptal needle, *J Cardiovasc Electrophysiol* 21:423–427, 2010.
18. Winkle RA, Mead RH, Engel G, Patrawala RA: The use of a radiofrequency needle improves the safety and efficacy of transseptal puncture for atrial fibrillation ablation, *Heart Rhythm* 8:1411–1415, 2011.
19. Tzeis S, Andrikopoulos G, Deisenhofer I, et al: Transseptal catheterization: considerations and caveats, *Pacing Clin Electrophysiol* 33:231–242, 2010.
20. Lakkireddy D, Rangisetty U, Prasad S, et al: Intracardiac echo-guided radiofrequency catheter ablation of atrial fibrillation in patients with atrial septal defect or patent foramen ovale repair: a feasibility, safety, and efficacy study, *J Cardiovasc Electrophysiol* 19:1137–1142, 2008.
21. Stevenson WG, Soejima K: Recording techniques for clinical electrophysiology, *J Cardiovasc Electrophysiol* 16:1017–1022, 2005.
22. Tedrow UB, Stevenson WG: Recording and interpreting unipolar electrograms to guide catheter ablation, *Heart Rhythm* 8:791–796, 2011.
23. Arora R, Kadish A: Fundamental of intracardiac mapping. In Huang SKS, Wilber DH, editors: *Catheter ablation of cardiac arrhythmias*, Philadelphia, 2006, Saunders, pp 107–134.
24. Josephson M: Electrophysiologic investigation: general aspects. In Josephson ME, editor: *Clinical cardiac electrophysiology*, ed 4, Philadelphia, 2008, Lippincott Williams & Wilkins, pp 20–68.
25. Fisch C, Knoebel SB: Concealed conduction. In Fisch C, Knoebel SB, editors: *Electrocardiography of clinical arrhythmias*, Armonk, NY, 2000, Futura, pp 153–172.
26. Grant AO: Cardiac ion channels, *Circ Arrhythm Electrophysiol* 2:185–194, 2009.
27. Noorman M, van der Heyden MA, van Veen TA, et al: Cardiac cell-cell junctions in health and disease: electrical versus mechanical coupling, *J Mol Cell Cardiol* 47:23–31, 2009.
28. Nerbonne JM, Kass RS: Molecular physiology of cardiac repolarization, *Physiol Rev* 85:1205–1253, 2005.
29. Michael G, Xiao L, Qi XY, et al: Remodelling of cardiac repolarization: how homeostatic responses can lead to arrhythmogenesis, *Cardiovasc Res* 81:491–499, 2009.
30. Hanson B, Sutton P, Elameri N, et al: Interaction of activation-repolarization coupling and restitution properties in humans, *Circ Arrhythm Electrophysiol* 2:162–170, 2009.
31. Akhtar M, Damato AN, Batsford WP, et al: A comparative analysis of antegrade and retrograde conduction patterns in man, *Circulation* 52:766–778, 1975.
32. Denes P, Wu D, Dhingra R, et al: The effects of cycle length on cardiac refractory periods in man, *Circulation* 49:32–41, 1974.
33. Tadros R, Billette J: Rate-dependent AV nodal refractoriness: a new functional framework based on concurrent effects of basic and pretest cycle length, *Am J Physiol Heart Circ Physiol* 297:H2136–H2143, 2009.
34. Chinitz LA, Sethi JS: How to perform noncontact mapping, *Heart Rhythm* 3:120–123, 2006.
35. Josephson ME: Miscellaneous phenomena related to atrioventricular conduction. In Josephson ME, editor: *Clinical cardiac electrophysiology*, ed 4, Philadelphia, 2008, Lippincott Williams & Wilkins, pp 145–159.
36. Kilborn MF: Electrocardiographic manifestations of supernormal conduction, concealed conduction, and exit block. In Zipes DP, Jalife J, editors: *Cardiac electrophysiology: from cell to bedside*, ed 4, Philadelphia, 2004, Saunders, pp 733–738.
37. Fisch C, Knoebel SB: Atrioventricular and ventriculoatrial conduction and blocks, gap, and overdrive suppression. In Fisch C, Knoebel SB, editors: *Electrocardiography of clinical arrhythmias*, Armonk, NY, 2000, Futura, pp 315–344.
38. Fisch C, Knoebel SB: Supernormal conduction and excitability. In Fisch C, Knoebel SB, editors: *Electrocardiography of clinical arrhythmias*, Armonk, NY, 2000, Futura, pp 237–252.

CHAPTER 5 Conventional Intracardiac Mapping Techniques

Cardiac mapping refers to the process of identifying the temporal and spatial distributions of myocardial electrical potentials during a particular heart rhythm. Cardiac mapping is a broad term that covers several modes of mapping such as body surface, endocardial, and epicardial mapping. Mapping during tachycardia aims at elucidation of the mechanism or mechanisms of the tachycardia, description of the propagation of activation from its initiation to its completion within a region of interest, and identification of the site of origin or a critical site of conduction to serve as a target for catheter ablation.

Activation Mapping

Fundamental Concepts

Essential to the effective management of any cardiac arrhythmia is a thorough understanding of the mechanisms of its initiation and maintenance. Conventionally, this has been achieved by careful study of the surface ECG and correlation of the changes therein with data from intracardiac electrograms recorded by catheters at various key locations within the cardiac chambers (i.e., activation mapping). A record of these electrograms documenting multiple sites simultaneously is studied to determine the mechanisms of an arrhythmic event.

The main value of intracardiac and surface ECG tracings consists of the comparative timing of electrical events and the determination of the location and direction of impulse propagation. Additionally, electrogram morphology can be of significant importance during mapping. Interpretation of recorded electrograms is fundamental to the clinical investigation of arrhythmias during electrophysiological (EP) studies. Establishing electrogram criteria, which permit accurate determination of the moment of myocardial activation at the recording electrode, is critical for construction of an area map of the activation sequence. Bipolar recordings are generally used for activation mapping. Unipolar recordings are used to supplement the information obtained from bipolar recordings. The differences in unipolar and bipolar recordings can be used to assist in mapping by simultaneously recording bipolar and unipolar signals from the mapping catheter.[1]

UNIPOLAR RECORDINGS

TIMING OF LOCAL ACTIVATION. The major component of the unipolar electrogram allows determination of the local activation time, although there are exceptions. The point of maximum amplitude, the zero crossing, the point of maximum slope (maximum first derivative), and the minimum second derivative of the electrogram have been proposed as indicators of underlying myocardial activation (Fig. 5-1). The maximum negative slope (i.e., maximum change in potential, dV/dt) of the signal coincides best with the arrival of the depolarization wavefront directly beneath the electrode because the maximal negative dV/dt corresponds to the maximum sodium channel conductance. Using this fiducial point, errors in determining the local activation time as compared with intracellular recordings have typically been less than 1 millisecond. This is true for filtered and unfiltered unipolar electrograms.[1,2]

DIRECTION OF LOCAL ACTIVATION. The morphology of the unfiltered unipolar recording indicates the direction of wavefront propagation. By convention, the mapping electrode that is in contact with the myocardium is connected to the positive input of the recording amplifier. In this configuration, positive deflections (R waves) are generated by propagation *toward* the recording electrode, and negative deflections (QS complexes) are generated by propagation *away* from the electrode (Figs. 5-2 and 5-3). If a recording electrode is at the source from which all wavefronts propagate (at the site of initial activation), depolarization will produce a wavefront that spreads away from the electrode, thus generating a monophasic QS complex. It is also important to recognize that a QS complex can be recorded when the mapping electrode is not in contact with the myocardium, but is floating in the cavity. In that situation, the initial negative slope of the recording is typically slow, suggesting that the electrogram is a far-field signal, generated by tissue some distance from the recording electrode.[1] Filtering at higher corner frequencies (e.g., 30 Hz) alters the morphology of the signal, so that the morphology of the unipolar electrogram is no longer an indication of the direction of wavefront propagation, and the presence or absence of a QS complex cannot be used to infer proximity to the site of earliest activation (Fig. 5-4).[2]

ADVANTAGES OF UNIPOLAR RECORDINGS. One important value of unipolar recordings is that they provide a more precise measure of local activation. This is true for filtered and unfiltered unipolar electrograms. In addition, unfiltered unipolar recordings provide information about the direction of impulse propagation. Using the unipolar configuration also eliminates a possible anodal contribution to depolarization and allows pacing and recording at the same location. This generally facilitates the use of other mapping modalities, namely pace mapping.

DISADVANTAGES OF UNIPOLAR RECORDINGS. The major disadvantage of unipolar recordings is that they have poor signal-to-noise ratio and contain substantial far-field signal generated by depolarization of tissue remote from the recording electrode. Therefore, distant activity can be difficult to separate from local activity. This is especially true when recording from areas of prior myocardial infarction (MI), where the fractionated ventricular potentials are ubiquitous and it is often impossible to select a rapid negative dV/dt when the entire QS potential is slowly inscribed—that is, cavity potential.[2] Another disadvantage is the inability to record an undisturbed electrogram during or immediately after pacing. This is a significant disadvantage when entrainment mapping is to be performed during activation mapping, because recording of the return tachycardia complex on the pacing electrode immediately after cessation of pacing is required to interpret entrainment mapping results.[1]

BIPOLAR RECORDINGS

TIMING OF LOCAL ACTIVATION. Algorithms for detecting local activation time from bipolar electrograms have been more problematic, partly because of generation of the bipolar electrogram

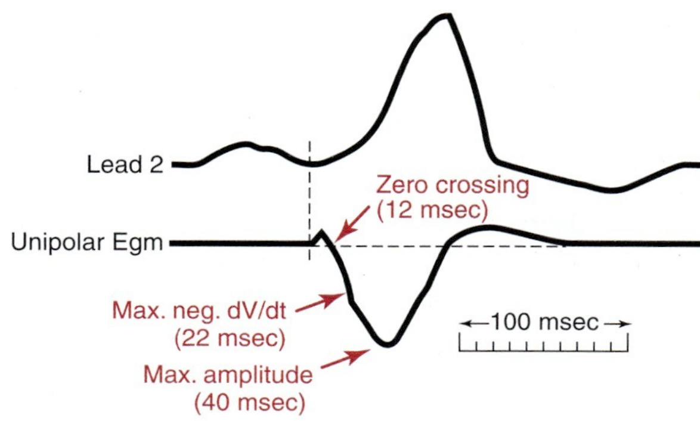

FIGURE 5-1 Unipolar electrogram activation times. A lead II electrocardiogram and a unipolar electrogram (Egm) from the ventricle of a patient with Wolff-Parkinson-White syndrome are shown. The vertical dashed line denotes the onset of the delta wave; the horizontal dotted line is the baseline of the unipolar recording. Several candidates for the timing of unipolar activation are labeled with corresponding activation times relative to delta wave onset.

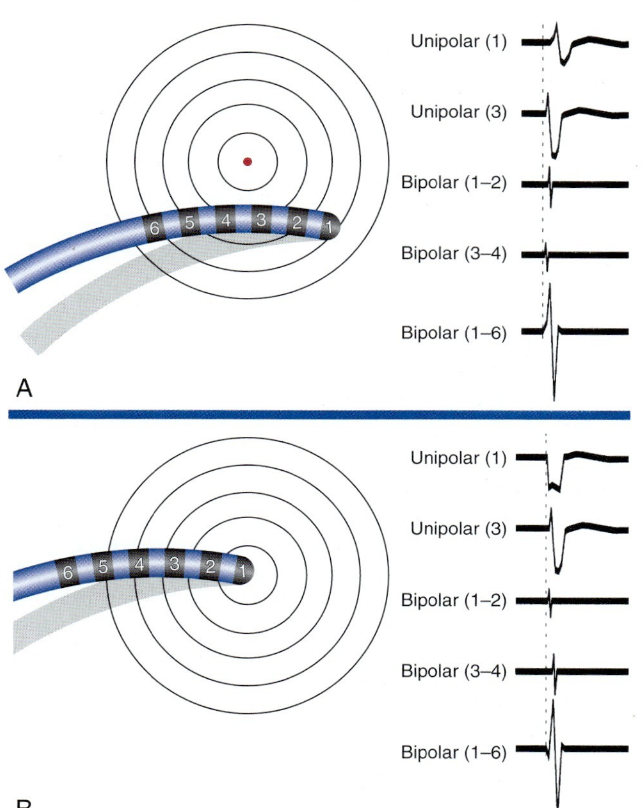

FIGURE 5-2 Hypothetical recordings from a multipolar electrode catheter. **A,** The electrodes are near a point source of activation (red dot in center of concentric rings). Note the timing and shape of the resultant electrogram patterns based on distance from point source, unipolar or bipolar recording, and width of bipole. **B,** The tip electrode (1) is at the point source of activation. Note the differences in timing and shape of the electrograms compared with **A.**

by two spatially separated recording poles. In a homogeneous sheet of tissue, the initial peak of a filtered (30 to 300 Hz) bipolar signal, the absolute maximum electrogram amplitude, coincides with depolarization beneath the recording electrode, appears to correlate most consistently with local activation time, and corresponds to the maximal negative dV/dt of the unipolar recording (see Fig. 5-3).[2] However, in the case of complex multicomponent bipolar electrograms, such as those with marked fractionation and prolonged duration seen in regions with complex conduction patterns (e.g., in regions of slow conduction in macroreentrant

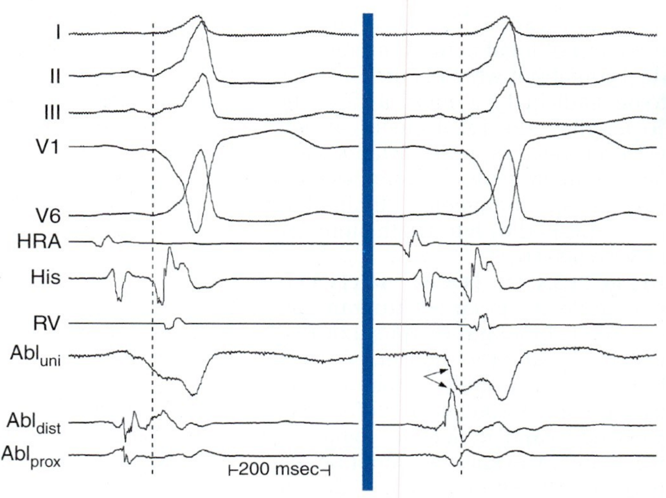

FIGURE 5-3 Unipolar and bipolar recordings from a patient with Wolff-Parkinson-White syndrome. The dashed line denotes the onset of the QRS complex (delta wave). **Right panel,** Recordings at the successful ablation site, characterized by QS in the unipolar recording. The most rapid component precedes the delta wave onset by 22 milliseconds, has the same timing as the peak of the ablation distal electrode recording, and precedes the ablation proximal electrode recording (arrows). **Left panel,** Recordings from a poorer site, with an rS in the unipolar recording; most of the bipolar recordings are atrial. Abl_{dist} = distal ablation; Abl_{prox} = proximal ablation; Abl_{uni} = unipolar ablation; HRA = high right atrium; RV = right ventricle.

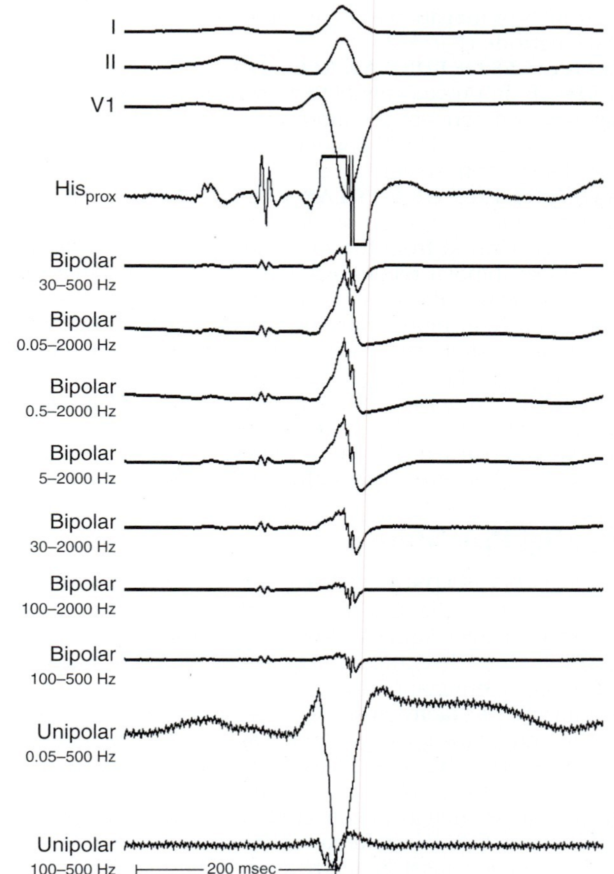

FIGURE 5-4 Effect of filtering on intracardiac recordings. The signal labeled "Bipolar 30-500 Hz" is the same signal as the proximal His bundle signal (His_{prox}) above it, displayed at lower gain. All signals beneath this are of the same gain but different filter bandwidths, and they illustrate progressive loss of signal amplitude as the bandwidth is narrowed. Unipolar signals below are of the same gain.

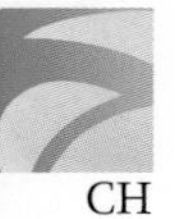

atrial tachycardia [AT] or ventricular tachycardia [VT]), determination of local activation time becomes problematic, and the decision about which activation time is most appropriate needs to be made in the context of the particular rhythm being mapped. To acquire true local electrical activity, a bipolar electrogram with an interelectrode distance of less than 1 cm is desirable. Smaller interelectrode distances record increasingly local events (as opposed to far-field). Elimination of far-field noise is usually accomplished by filtering the intracardiac electrograms, typically at 30 to 500 Hz.[1,2]

DIRECTION OF LOCAL ACTIVATION. The morphology and amplitude of bipolar electrograms are influenced by the orientation of the bipolar recording axis to the direction of propagation of the activation wavefront. A wavefront that is propagating in the direction exactly perpendicular to the axis of the recording dipole produces no difference in potential between the electrodes and hence no signal.[1,2] However, the direction of wavefront propagation cannot be reliably inferred from the morphology of the bipolar signal, although a change in morphology can be a useful finding. For example, when recording from the lateral aspect of the cavotricuspid isthmus during pacing from the coronary sinus (CS), a reversal in the bipolar electrogram polarity from positive to negative at the ablation line indicates complete isthmus block. Similarly, if bipolar recordings are obtained with the same catheter orientation parallel to the atrioventricular (AV) annulus during retrograde bypass tract (BT) conduction, an RS configuration electrogram will be present on one side of the BT, where the wavefront is propagating from the distal electrode toward the proximal electrode, and a QR morphology electrogram will be present on the other side, where the wavefront is propagating from the proximal electrode toward the distal electrode (Fig. 5-5).

ADVANTAGES OF BIPOLAR RECORDINGS. Bipolar recordings provide an improved signal-to-noise ratio. In addition, high-frequency components are more accurately seen, which facilitates identification of local depolarization, especially in abnormal areas of infarction or scar.

DISADVANTAGES OF BIPOLAR RECORDINGS. In contrast to unipolar signals, the direction of wavefront propagation cannot be reliably inferred from the morphology of the bipolar signal. Furthermore, bipolar recordings do not allow simultaneous pacing and recording from the same location. To pace and record simultaneously in bipolar fashion at endocardial sites as close together as possible, electrodes 1 and 3 of the mapping catheter are used for bipolar pacing, and electrodes 2 and 4 are used for recording. The precision of locating the source of a particular electrical signal depends on the distance between the recording electrodes, because the signal of interest can be beneath the distal or proximal electrode (or both) of the recording pair.[1]

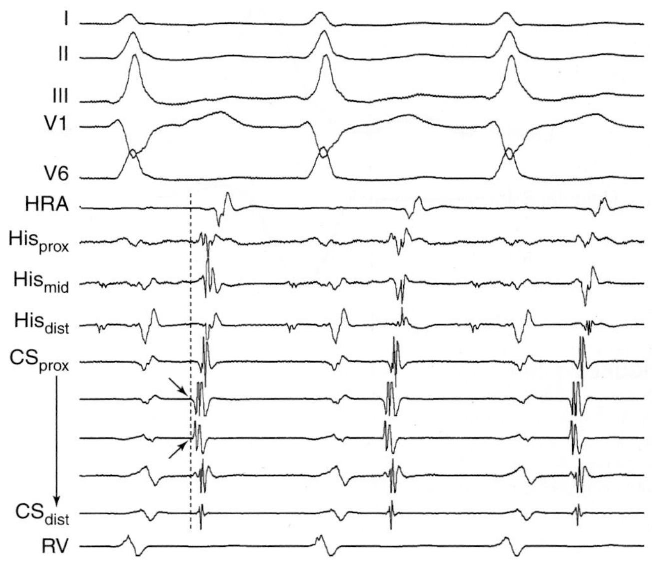

FIGURE 5-5 Recordings from a patient with a left lateral bypass tract during orthodromic atrioventricular reentrant tachycardia showing electrogram inversion at the middle of the coronary sinus (CS) (arrows), where the earliest retrograde atrial activation (over the bypass tract) occurs (dashed line). CS_{dist} = distal coronary sinus; CS_{prox} = proximal coronary sinus; His_{dist} = distal His bundle; His_{mid} = middle His bundle; His_{prox} = proximal His bundle; HRA = high right atrium; RV = right ventricle.

Mapping Procedure

PREREQUISITES FOR ACTIVATION MAPPING. Several factors are important for the success of activation mapping, including inducibility of tachycardia at the time of EP testing, hemodynamic stability of the tachycardia, and stable tachycardia morphology. In addition, determinations of an electrical reference point, of the mechanism of the tachycardia (focal versus macroreentrant), and, subsequently, of the goal of mapping are essential prerequisites.

SELECTION OF THE ELECTRICAL REFERENCE POINT. Local activation times must be relative to some external and consistent fiducial marker, such as the onset of the P wave or QRS complex on the surface ECG or a reference intracardiac electrode. For VT, the QRS complex onset should be assessed using all surface ECG leads to search for the lead with the earliest QRS onset. This lead should then be used for subsequent activation mapping. Similarly, the P wave during AT should be assessed using multiple ECG leads and choosing the one with the earliest P onset. However, determining the onset of the P wave can be impossible if the preceding T wave or QRS is superimposed. To facilitate visualization of the P wave, a ventricular extrastimulus (VES) or a train of ventricular pacing can be delivered to anticipate ventricular activation and repolarization and permit careful distinction of the P wave onset (Fig. 5-6). After determining P wave onset, a surrogate marker, such as a right atrial (RA) or CS electrogram indexed to the P wave onset, where it is clearly seen, can be used rather than the P wave onset.

DEFINING THE GOAL OF MAPPING. Determination of the mechanism of the tachycardia (focal versus macroreentrant) is essential to define the goal of activation mapping. For focal tachycardias, activation mapping entails localizing the site of origin of the tachycardia focus. This is reflected by the earliest presystolic activity that precedes the onset of the P wave (during focal AT) or QRS (during focal VT) by an average of 10 to 40 milliseconds, because only this short amount of time is required after the focus discharges to activate enough myocardium and begin generating a P wave or QRS complex (Fig. 5-7). For mapping macroreentrant tachycardias, the goal of mapping is identification of the critical isthmus of the reentrant circuit, as indicated by finding the site with a continuous activity spanning diastole or with an isolated mid-diastolic potential (see Fig. 5-7).

EPICARDIAL VERSUS ENDOCARDIAL MAPPING. Activation mapping is predominantly performed endocardially. Occasionally, epicardial mapping is required because of an inability to ablate some VTs, ATs, or AV BTs by using the endocardial approach. Limited epicardial mapping can be performed with special recording catheters that can be steered in the branches of the CS. This technique has been used for mapping VTs and AV BTs, but its scope is limited by the anatomy of the coronary venous system.

Another epicardial mapping technique utilizes a subxiphoid percutaneous approach for accessing the epicardial surface. This technique has become an important adjunctive strategy to ablate a diverse range of cardiac arrhythmias including cardiomyopathic VT, BTs, atrial fibrillation, and idiopathic VTs. Transthoracic epicardial mapping and ablation are seeing increasingly wider application, especially in patients with scar-related VT, in whom more reentrant circuits with vulnerable isthmuses are on the epicardial

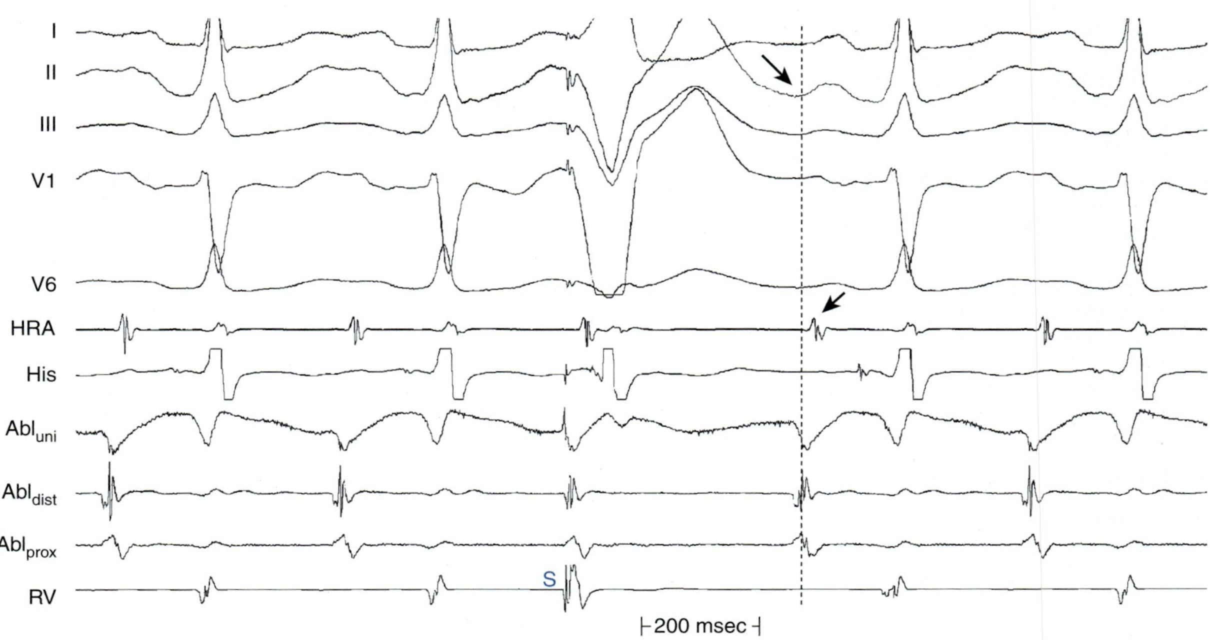

FIGURE 5-6 Use of ventricular extrastimulus (VES) to clarify onset of the P wave during atrial tachycardia (AT). A single VES (S) delivered during AT advances the timing of ventricular activation to show the P wave (long arrow) by itself without the overlying ST segment and T wave, which made it difficult to determine P wave onset during ongoing tachycardia. The dashed line denotes onset of the P wave; timing of the reference electrogram (high right atrium [HRA]; short arrow) can thereafter be used as a surrogate for P wave onset. Abl_{dist} = distal ablation; Abl_{prox} = proximal ablation; Abl_{uni} = unipolar ablation; RV = right ventricle.

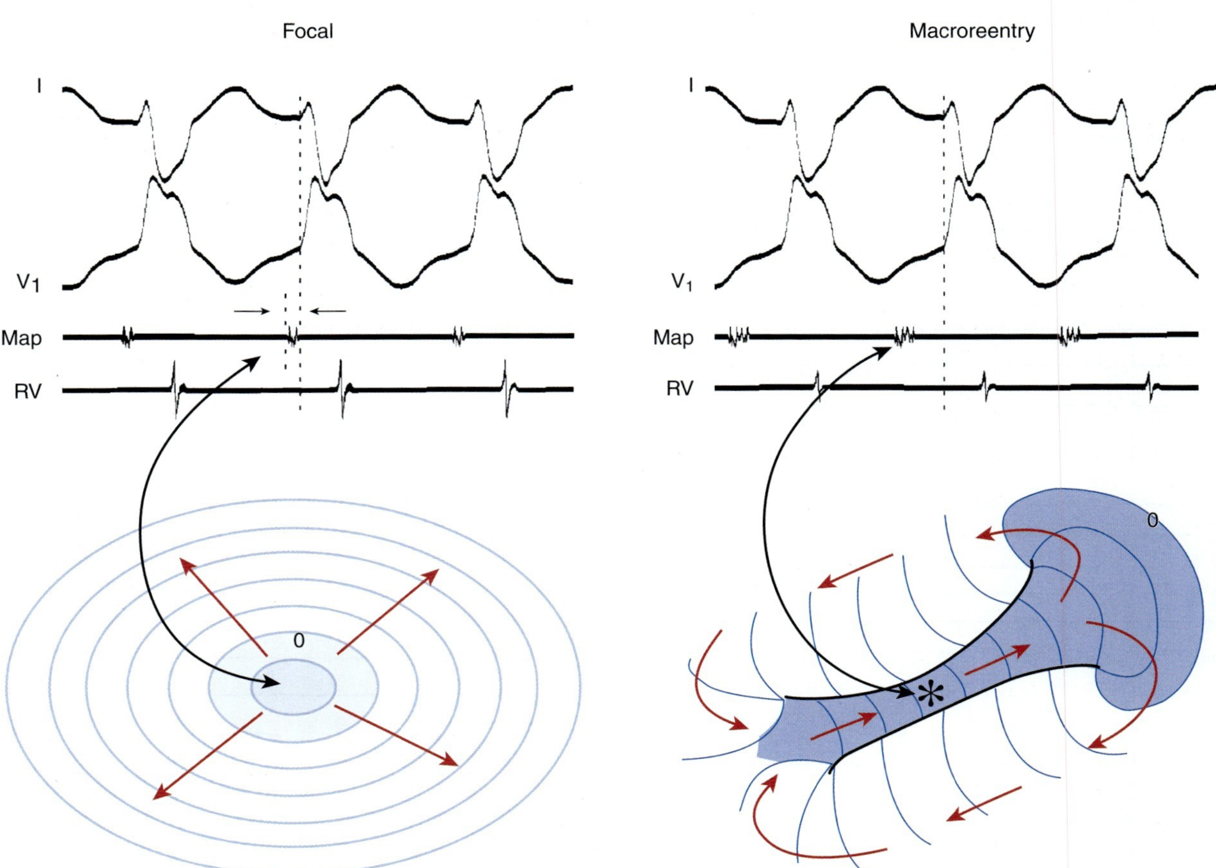

FIGURE 5-7 Focal versus macroreentrant ventricular tachycardia (VT). **Top,** ECG and intracardiac electrograms from the mapping (Map) and right ventricle (RV) catheters. **Bottom,** Depictions of events at sites where mapped electrograms are obtained. **Left,** VT focus fires and activation spreads to normal myocardium within 30 to 40 milliseconds, generating a QRS complex. Thus, the electrogram at the site of the focus is generally 40 milliseconds or less prior to the QRS onset. **Right,** In contrast, in a macroreentrant VT, some myocardium is being activated at each instant in the cardiac cycle. During surface ECG diastole, only a few cells are activating (too few to cause surface ECG deflections). The area of a protected diastolic corridor, often cordoned off by scar, contains mid-diastolic recordings and is an attractive ablation site. The 0 isochrone indicates the time at which the QRS complex begins.

surface. The same fundamental principles of activation mapping are used for both endocardial mapping and epicardial mapping.[3-7]

MAPPING CATHETERS. The simplest form of mapping is achieved by moving the mapping catheter sequentially to sample various points of interest on the endocardium to measure local activation. The precision of locating the source of a particular electrical signal depends on the distance between the recording electrodes on the mapping catheter. For ablation procedures, recordings between adjacent electrode pairs are commonly used (e.g., between electrodes 1 and 2, 2 and 3, and 3 and 4), with 1- to 5-mm interelectrode spacing. In some studies, wider bipolar recordings (e.g., between electrodes 1 and 3 and 2 and 4) have been used to provide an overlapping field of view. For bipolar recordings, the signal of interest can be beneath the distal or proximal electrode (or both) of the recording pair. As noted, this is germane in that ablation energy can be delivered only from the distal (tip) electrode.

MAPPING FOCAL TACHYCARDIAS

The goal of activation mapping of focal tachycardias (automatic, triggered activity, or microreentrant) is identifying the site of origin, defined as the site with the earliest presystolic bipolar recording in which the distal electrode shows the earliest intrinsic deflection and QS unipolar electrogram configuration (Figs. 5-8 and 5-9). Local activation at the site of origin precedes the onset of the tachycardia complex on the surface ECG by an average of 10 to 40 milliseconds. Earlier electrograms occurring in mid-diastole, as in the setting of macroreentrant tachycardias, are not expected and do not constitute a target for mapping.[1]

Endocardial activation mapping of focal tachycardias can trace the origin of activation to a specific area, from which it spreads centrifugally. There is generally an electrically silent period in the tachycardia cycle length (CL) that is reflected on the surface ECG by an isoelectric line between tachycardia complexes. Intracardiac mapping shows significant portions of the tachycardia CL without recorded electrical activity, even when recording from the entire cardiac chamber of tachycardia origin. However, in the presence of complex intramyocardial conduction disturbances, activation during focal tachycardias can extend over a large proportion of the tachycardia CL, and conduction spread can follow circular patterns suggestive of macroreentrant activation.[2,4]

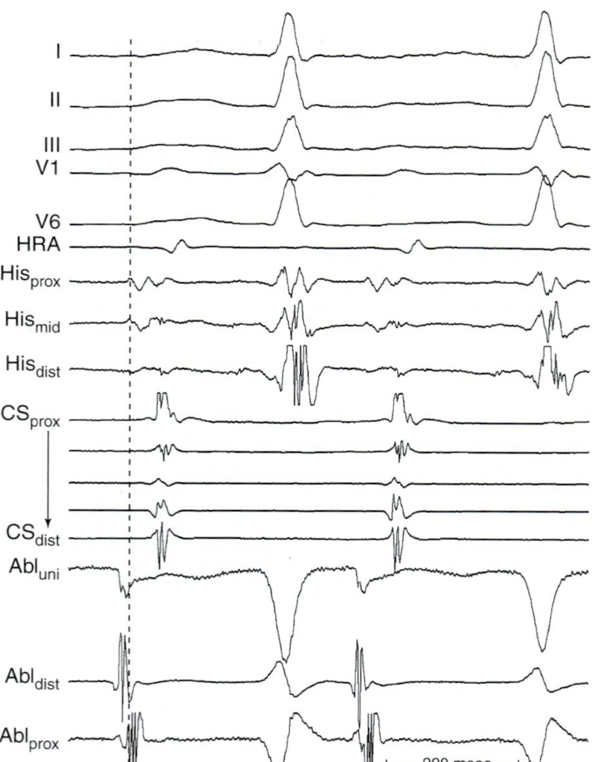

FIGURE 5-8 Focal atrial tachycardia. The unipolar electrogram recorded by the distal ablation electrode (Abl$_{uni}$) shows a QS configuration, and its timing coincides with the distal ablation (Abl$_{dist}$) recording at the site of successful ablation. The dashed line marks the onset of the P wave on the surface ECG. Abl$_{prox}$ = proximal ablation; CS$_{dist}$ = distal coronary sinus; CS$_{prox}$ = proximal coronary sinus; His$_{dist}$ = distal His bundle; His$_{mid}$ = middle His bundle; His$_{prox}$ = proximal His bundle; HRA = high right atrium.

Technique of Activation Mapping of Focal Tachycardias

Initially, one should seek the general region of the origin of the tachycardia as indicated by the surface ECG. In the EP laboratory, additional data can be obtained by placing a limited number of catheters within the heart in addition to the mapping catheter or catheters; these catheters are frequently placed at the right ventricular apex, His bundle region, high RA, and CS. During initial arrhythmia evaluation, recording from this limited number of sites allows a rough estimation of the site of interest. Mapping simultaneously from as many sites as possible greatly enhances the precision, detail, and speed of identifying regions of interest.[1]

Subsequently, a single mapping catheter is moved under the guidance of fluoroscopy over the endocardium of the chamber of interest to sample bipolar signals. Using standard equipment, mapping a tachycardia requires recording and mapping performed at several sites, based on the ability of the investigator to recognize the mapping sites of interest from the morphology of the tachycardia on the surface ECG and baseline intracardiac recordings.

Local activation time is then determined from the filtered (30 to 300 Hz) bipolar signal recorded from the distal electrode pair on the mapping catheter; this time is determined and compared with the timing reference (fiducial point). The distal pole of the mapping catheter should be used for mapping the earliest activation site because it is the pole through which RF energy is delivered. Activation times are generally measured from the onset of the first rapid deflection of the bipolar electrogram to the onset of the tachycardia complex on the surface ECG or surrogate marker (see Fig. 5-6). Using the onset (rather than the peak or nadir) of a local bipolar electrogram is preferable because it is easier to determine reproducibly, especially when measuring heavily fractionated, low-amplitude local electrograms.[4]

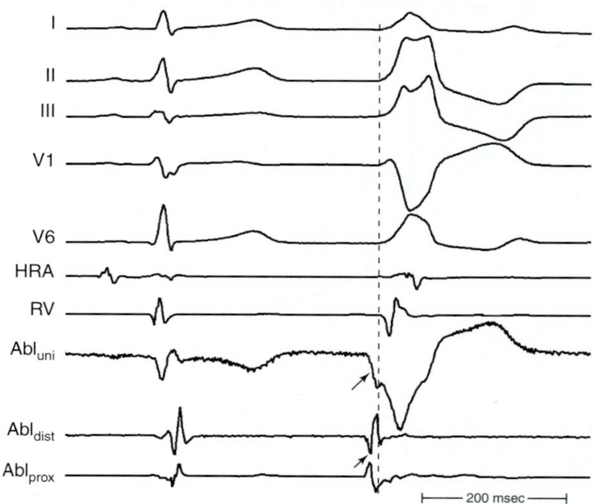

FIGURE 5-9 Sinus rhythm and a single premature ventricular complex from a patient with focal ventricular tachycardia. The unipolar ablation site (Abl$_{uni}$) show a QS configuration, the most rapid slope of which times with the initial peak in the distal ablation (Abl$_{dist}$) recording (arrows) at the site of successful ablation. The dashed line marks the onset of the QRS complex on the surface ECG. Abl$_{prox}$ = proximal ablation; HRA = high right atrium; RV = right ventricle.

Once an area of relatively early local activation is found, small movements of the catheter tip in the general target region are undertaken until the site is identified with the earliest possible local activation relative to the tachycardia complex. Recording from multiple bipolar pairs from a multipolar electrode catheter is helpful in that if the proximal pair has a more attractive electrogram than the distal, the catheter may be withdrawn slightly to achieve the same position with the distal electrode.

Once the site with the earliest bipolar signal is identified, the unipolar signal from the distal ablation electrode should be used to supplement bipolar mapping.[2] The unfiltered (0.05 to 300 Hz) unipolar signal morphology should show a monophasic QS complex with a rapid negative deflection if the site was at the origin of impulse formation (see Figs. 5-8 and 5-9). However, the size of the area with a QS complex can be larger than the tachycardia focus, exceeding 1 cm in diameter. Thus, a QS complex should not be the only mapping finding used to guide ablation. Successful ablation is unusual, however, at sites with an RS complex on the unipolar recording, because these are generally distant from the focus (see Fig. 5-2). Concordance of the timing of the onset of the bipolar electrogram with that of the filtered or unfiltered unipolar electrogram (with the rapid downslope of the S wave of the unipolar QS complex coinciding with the initial peak of the bipolar signal) helps ensure that the tip electrode, which is the ablation electrode, is responsible for the early component of the bipolar electrogram. The presence of ST elevation on the unipolar recording and the ability to capture the site with unipolar pacing are used to indicate good electrode-tissue contact.[4]

MAPPING MACROREENTRANT TACHYCARDIAS

The main goal of activation mapping of macroreentrant tachycardias (e.g., post-MI VT, macroreentrant AT) is identification of the isthmus critical for the macroreentrant circuit.[8] The site of origin of a tachycardia is the source of electrical activity producing the tachycardia complex. Although this is a discrete site of impulse formation in focal rhythms, during macroreentry it represents the exit site from the diastolic pathway (i.e., from the critical isthmus of the reentrant circuit) to the myocardium that gives rise to the ECG deflection. During macroreentry, an isthmus is defined as a corridor of conductive myocardial tissue bounded by nonconductive tissue (barriers) through which the depolarization wavefront must propagate to perpetuate the tachycardia. These barriers can be scar areas or naturally occurring anatomical or functional (present only during tachycardia, but not in sinus rhythm) obstacles. The earliest presystolic electrogram closest to mid-diastole is the most commonly used definition for the site of origin of the reentrant circuit. However, recording continuous diastolic activity or bridging of diastole at adjacent sites, or both, or mapping a discrete diastolic pathway is more specific. Therefore, the goal of activation mapping during macroreentry is finding the site or sites with continuous activity spanning diastole or with an isolated mid-diastolic potential. Unlike focal tachycardias, a presystolic electrogram preceding the tachycardia complex by 10 to 40 milliseconds is not adequate in defining the site of origin of a macroreentrant tachycardia (Figs. 5-10 and 5-11; see also Fig. 5-7).[2,4]

However, identification of critical isthmuses is often challenging. The abnormal area of scarring, where the isthmus is located, is frequently large and contains false isthmuses (bystanders) that confound mapping. Additionally, multiple potential reentry circuits can be present, giving rise to multiple different tachycardias in a single patient. Furthermore, in abnormal regions such as infarct scars, the tissue beneath the recording electrode can be small relative to the surrounding myocardium outside the scar; thus, a large far-field signal can obscure the small local potential. For this reason, despite the limitations of bipolar recordings, these recordings are preferred in scar-related VTs because the noise is removed and high-frequency components are more accurately seen. Unipolar recordings are usually of little help when mapping arrhythmias associated with regions of scar, unless the recordings are filtered to remove far-field signal. Much of the far-field signal in a unipolar recording consists of lower frequencies than the signal generated by local depolarization because the high-frequency content of a signal diminishes more rapidly with distance from the source than the low-frequency content. Therefore, high-pass filtering of unipolar signals (at 30 or 100 Hz) is generally used when mapping scar-related arrhythmias to reduce the far-field signal and improve detection of lower amplitude local signals from abnormal regions.[1]

Although activation mapping alone is usually inadequate for defining the critical isthmus of a macroreentrant tachycardia, it can help guide other mapping modalities (e.g., entrainment or pace mapping, or both) to the approximate region of the isthmus.[4,8]

Continuous Activity

Theoretically, if reentry were the mechanism of the tachycardia, electrical activity should occur throughout the tachycardia cycle. For example, in macroreentrant AT, the recorded electrical activity

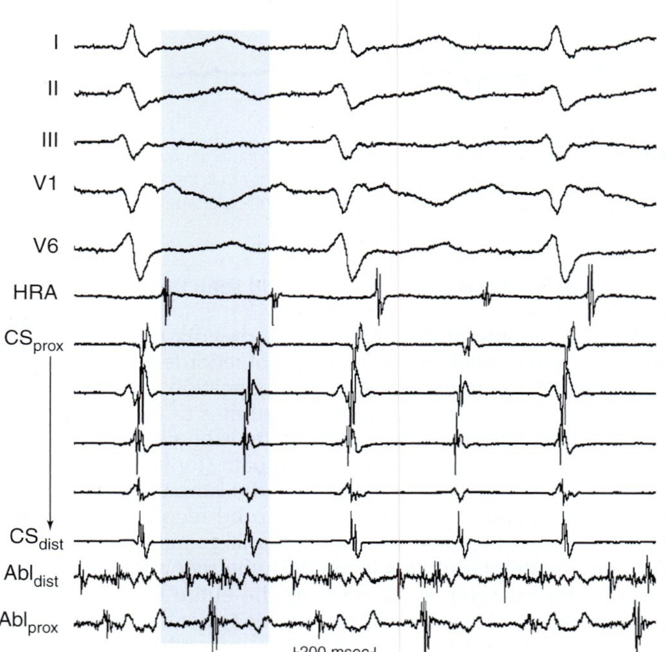

FIGURE 5-10 Macroreentrant atrial tachycardia. Electrical activity spans the tachycardia cycle length (shaded); thus, a merely presystolic electrogram is a poor indicator of optimal ablation site. Abl_{dist} = distal ablation; Abl_{prox} = proximal ablation; CS_{dist} = distal coronary sinus; CS_{prox} = proximal coronary sinus; HRA = high right atrium.

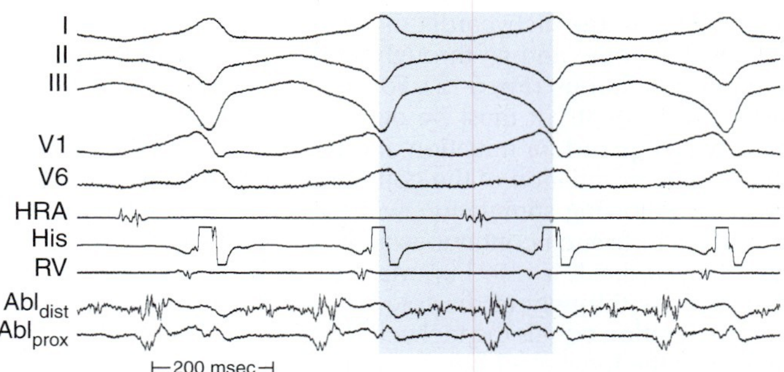

FIGURE 5-11 Macroreentrant post–myocardial infarction ventricular tachycardia. Electrical activity spans diastole and nearly the tachycardia cycle length (shaded); thus, a simply presystolic electrogram is a poor indicator of the optimal ablation site. Abl_{dist} = distal ablation; Abl_{prox} = proximal ablation; HRA = high right atrium; RV = right ventricle.

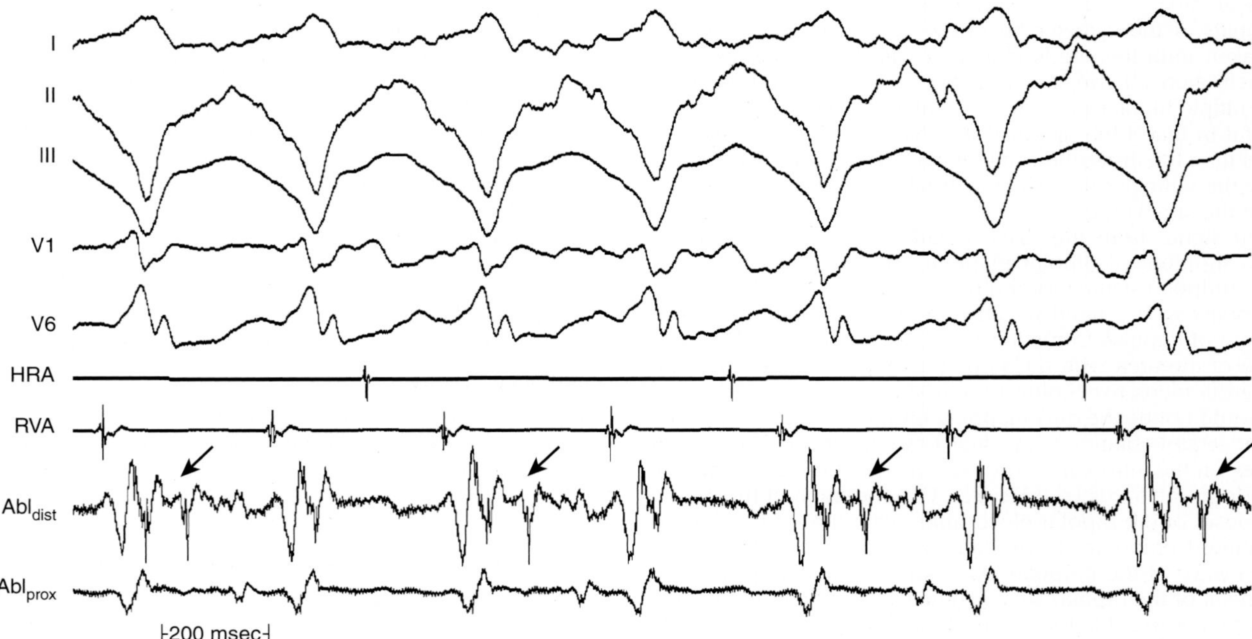

FIGURE 5-12 Diastolic recordings during ventricular tachycardia that have a 2:1 conduction ratio (arrows). Cells causing these recordings are clearly not integrally involved in the ongoing arrhythmia. They are not atrial, because atrial ventricular dissociation is evident in the high right atrium (HRA) recording. Abl_{dist} = distal ablation; Abl_{prox} = proximal ablation; RVA = right ventricular apex.

at different locations in the atrium should span the tachycardia CL (see Fig. 5-10).

For macroreentrant VT, conduction during diastole is extremely slow and is in a small area so that it is not recorded on the surface ECG. The QRS complex is caused by propagation of the wavefront from the exit of the circuit from that isthmus to the surrounding myocardium. After leaving the exit of the isthmus, the circulating wavefront propagates through a broad path (loop) along the border of the scar, back to the entrance of the isthmus (see Fig. 5-7).[8] Continuous diastolic activity is likely to be recorded only if the bipolar pair records a small circuit; if a large circuit is recorded (i.e., the reentrant circuit is larger than the recording area of the catheter, the catheter is not covering the entire circuit, or both), nonholodiastolic activity will be recorded. In such circuits, repositioning of the catheter to other sites may allow visualization of what is termed *bridging of diastole*; electrical activity in these adjacent sites spans diastole.[2,4]

All areas from which diastolic activity is recorded are not necessarily part of the reentrant circuit. Such sites can reflect late activation and may not be related to the tachycardia site of origin. Analysis of the response of these electrograms to spontaneous or induced changes in tachycardia CL is critical in deciding their relationship to the tachycardia mechanism. Additionally, electrical signals that come and go throughout diastole should not be considered continuous (Fig. 5-12). For continuous activity to be consistent with reentry, it must be demonstrated that such electrical activity is required for initiation and maintenance of the tachycardia, so that termination of the continuous activity, either spontaneously or following stimulation, without affecting the tachycardia, would exclude such continuous activity as requisite for sustaining the tachycardia. It is also important to verify that an electrogram that extends throughout diastole is not just a broad electrogram whose duration equals the tachycardia CL. This can be achieved by analyzing the local electrogram during pacing at a CL comparable to tachycardia CL; if pacing produces continuous diastolic activity in the absence of tachycardia, the continuous electrogram has no mechanistic significance. Furthermore, the continuous activity should be recorded from a circumscribed area, and motion artifact should be excluded.[4,8]

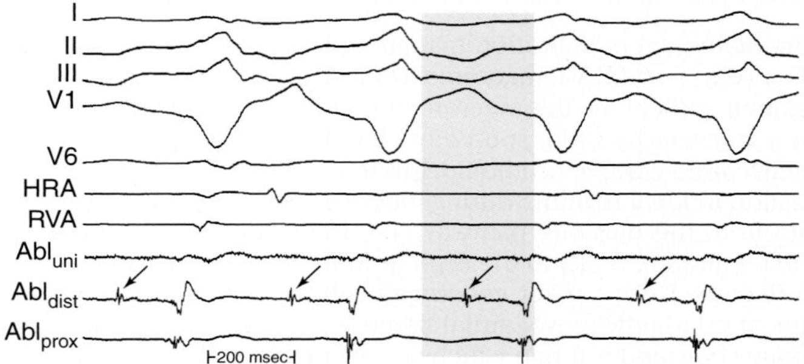

FIGURE 5-13 Mid-diastolic potential during ventricular tachycardia (VT)—duration of diastole (shaded area), with isolated mid-diastolic potential from the site at which ablation eliminated VT (arrows). Abl_{dist} = distal ablation; Abl_{prox} = proximal ablation; Abl_{uni} = unipolar ablation; HRA = high right atrium; RVA = right ventricular apex.

Mid-Diastolic Activity

An isolated mid-diastolic potential is defined as a low-amplitude, high-frequency diastolic potential separated from the preceding and subsequent electrograms by an isoelectric segment (Fig. 5-13). Sometimes, these discrete potentials provide information that defines a diastolic pathway, which is believed to be generated from a narrow isthmus of conduction critical to the reentrant circuit. Localization of this pathway is critical for guiding catheter-based ablation.[8]

Detailed mapping usually reveals more than one site of presystolic activity, and mid-diastolic potentials can be recorded from a bystander site attached to the isthmus. Therefore, regardless of where in diastole the presystolic electrogram occurs (early, middle, or late), its position and appearance on initiation of the tachycardia, although necessary, does not confirm its relevance to the tachycardia mechanism. One must always confirm that the electrogram is required to maintain, and cannot be dissociated from, the tachycardia.[8] Thus, during spontaneous changes in the tachycardia CL or those produced by programmed stimulation, the electrogram, regardless of its position in diastole, should show a fixed relationship with the subsequent tachycardia complex (and

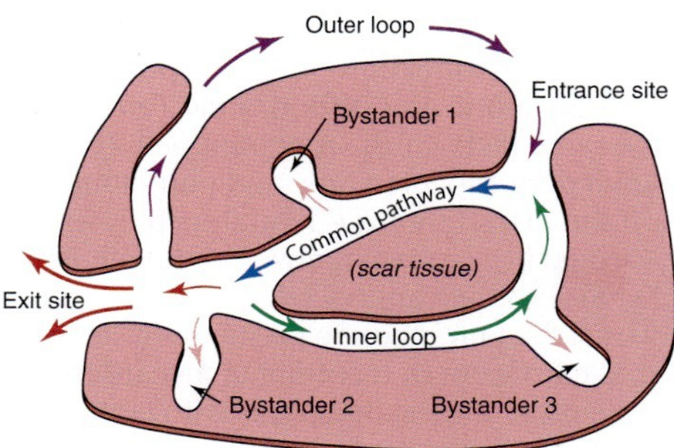

Site	Electrogram timing in VT	Entrainment with concealed fusion	Entrained stimulus-QRS	(S-QRS) VTCL	Post-pacing interval	Sinus rhythm pacemap	
						QRS vs VT	Stimulus-QRS
Common pathway	Diastolic	Present	≈Egm−QRS	<0.7	≈TCL	Same †	≈Egm−QRS †
Inner loop	Systolic	Present	<Egm−QRS	>0.7	≈TCL	Same †	≈Egm−QRS †
Outer loop	Systolic	Absent	<Egm−QRS	>0.7	≈TCL	Different	<Egm−QRS
Entrance site	Early diastolic	Present*	≈Egm−QRS	<0.7	≈TCL	Different	<Egm−QRS
Exit site	Late diastolic	Present	>Egm−QRS	>0.7	>TCL	Same	≈Egm−QRS
Bystander 1	Mid-diastolic*	Present	>Egm−QRS	>0.7	>TCL	Same	>Egm−QRS
Bystander 2	Late diastolic*	Present	>Egm−QRS	>0.7	>TCL	Same	>Egm−QRS
Bystander 3	Early diastolic*	Present*	>Egm−QRS	>0.7	>TCL	Same †	>Egm−QRS

* Variable † Depends on whether captured orthodromically or antidromically

FIGURE 5-14 Representation of a ventricular tachycardia (VT) circuit, showing a common diastolic pathway, entrance and exit sites, inner and outer loops, and bystander dead-end paths in three locations. The accompanying table describes the behavior of each of these locations during VT, as well as pacing during VT and sinus rhythm. Egm = electrogram; S = stimulus; TCL = tachycardia cycle length.

not the preceding one). Very early diastolic potentials, in the first half of diastole, can represent an area of slow conduction at the entrance of a protected isthmus. These potentials remain fixed to the prior tachycardia complex (exit site from the isthmus), and a delay between this complex and the subsequent tachycardia complex would reflect delay in entering or propagating through the protected diastolic pathway.[4]

If, after very detailed mapping, the earliest recorded site is not at least 50 milliseconds presystolic, this suggests that the map is inadequate (most common), the mechanism of tachycardia is not macroreentry, or the diastolic corridor is deeper than the subendocardium (in the midmyocardium or subepicardium).

Limitations

Standard transcatheter endocardial mapping, as performed in the EP laboratory, is limited by the number, size, and type of electrodes that can be placed within the heart. Therefore, these methods do not cover a vast area of the endocardial surface. Time-consuming, point-by-point maneuvering of the catheter is required to trace the origin of an arrhythmic event and its activation sequence in the neighboring areas.

The success of roving point mapping depends on the sequential beat-by-beat stability of the activation sequence being mapped and the ability of the patient to tolerate sustained arrhythmia. Therefore, it can be difficult to perform activation mapping in poorly inducible tachycardias, in hemodynamically unstable tachycardias, and in tachycardias with unstable morphology. Sometimes, poorly tolerated rapid tachycardias can be slowed by antiarrhythmic agents to allow for mapping. Alternatively, mapping can be facilitated by starting and stopping the tachycardia after data acquisition at each site. Additionally, newer techniques (e.g., basket catheter and noncontact mapping) can facilitate activation mapping in these cases by simultaneous multipoint mapping.

Although activation mapping is adequate for defining the site of origin of focal tachycardias, it is deficient by itself in defining the critical isthmus of macroreentrant tachycardias, and adjunctive mapping modalities (e.g., entrainment mapping, pace mapping) are required. Moreover, the laborious process of precise mapping with conventional techniques can expose the electrophysiologist, staff, and patient to undesirable levels of radiation from the extended fluoroscopy time.

Using conventional activation mapping techniques, it is difficult to conceive the three-dimensional orientation of cardiac structures because a limited number of recording electrodes guided by fluoroscopy is used. Although catheters using multiple electrodes to acquire data points are available, the exact location of an acquired unit of EP data is difficult to ascertain because of inaccurate delineation of the location of anatomical structures. The inability to associate the intracardiac electrogram with a specific endocardial site accurately also limits the reliability with which the roving catheter tip can be placed at a site that was previously mapped. This results in limitations when the creation of long linear ablation lesions is required to modify the substrate, as well as when multiple isthmuses or channels are present. The inability to identify, for example, the site of a previous ablation increases the risk of repeated ablation of areas already dealt with and the likelihood that new sites can be missed.

Entrainment Mapping

Fundamental Concepts

To help understand the concept of entrainment, a hypothetical reentrant circuit is shown in Figure 5-14. This reentrant circuit has several components—a common pathway, an exit site, an outer loop, an inner loop, an entry site, and bystander sites. The reentrant wavefront propagates through the common pathway (protected critical isthmus) during electrical diastole. Because this zone is usually composed of a small amount of myocardium and is bordered by anatomical or functional barriers preventing spread of the electrical signal except in the orthodromic direction, propagation of the wavefront in the protected isthmus is electrocardiographically silent. The exit site is the site at which the reentrant wavefront exits the protected isthmus to start activation of the rest of the myocardium, including the outer loop. Activation of the exit site corresponds to the onset of the tachycardia complex on the surface ECG. The outer loop is the path through which the reentrant wavefront propagates while at the same time activating the rest of the myocardium. Activation of the outer loop corresponds to electrical systole (P wave during AT and QRS during VT) on the surface ECG. An inner loop can serve as an integral part of the reentrant circuit or function as a bystander pathway. If conduction through the inner loop is slower than conduction from the exit to entrance sites (through the outer loop), the inner loop will serve as a bystander, and the outer loop will be the dominant. If conduction through the inner loop is faster than conduction through the outer loop, it will form an integral component of the reentrant circuit. The entry site is where the reentrant wavefront enters the critical isthmus. Bystander sites are sites that are activated by the reentrant wavefront but are not an essential part of the reentrant circuit. These sites can be remote, adjacent, or attached to the circuit. Elimination of these sites does not terminate reentry.[4,8]

Understanding the concepts associated with resetting is critical to understanding entrainment. When a premature stimulus is delivered to sites remote from the reentrant circuit, it can interact with the circuit in different ways. When the stimulus is late-coupled, it can reach the circuit after it has just been activated by the reentrant wavefront. Consequently, although the extrastimulus may have resulted in activation of part of the myocardium, it fails to affect the reentrant circuit, and the reentrant wavefront continues to propagate in the critical isthmus and through the exit site to produce the next tachycardia complex on time. To reset reentrant tachycardia, the paced wavefront must reach the reentrant circuit (entry site, critical isthmus, or both), encounter excitable tissue within the circuit (i.e., enter the excitable gap of the reentrant circuit), collide in the antidromic (retrograde) direction with the previous tachycardia complex, and propagate in the orthodromic (anterograde) direction through the same tachycardia reentrant path (critical isthmus) to exit at an earlier than expected time and perpetuate the tachycardia (Fig. 5-15). If the extrastimulus encounters fully excitable tissue, as commonly occurs in reentrant tachycardias with large excitable gaps, the tachycardia is advanced by the extent that the paced wavefront arrives at the entrance site prematurely. If the tissue is partially excitable, as can occur in reentrant tachycardias with small or partially excitable gaps, or even in circuits with large excitable gaps when the extrastimulus is very premature, the paced wavefront will encounter some conduction delay in the orthodromic direction within the circuit. Consequently, the degree of advancement of the next tachycardia complex depends on both the degree of prematurity of the extrastimulus and the degree of slowing of its conduction within the circuit. Therefore, the reset tachycardia complex may be early, on time, or later than expected.[4,8]

Termination of the tachycardia occurs when the extrastimulus collides with the preceding tachycardia impulse antidromically and blocks in the reentrant circuit orthodromically. This occurs when

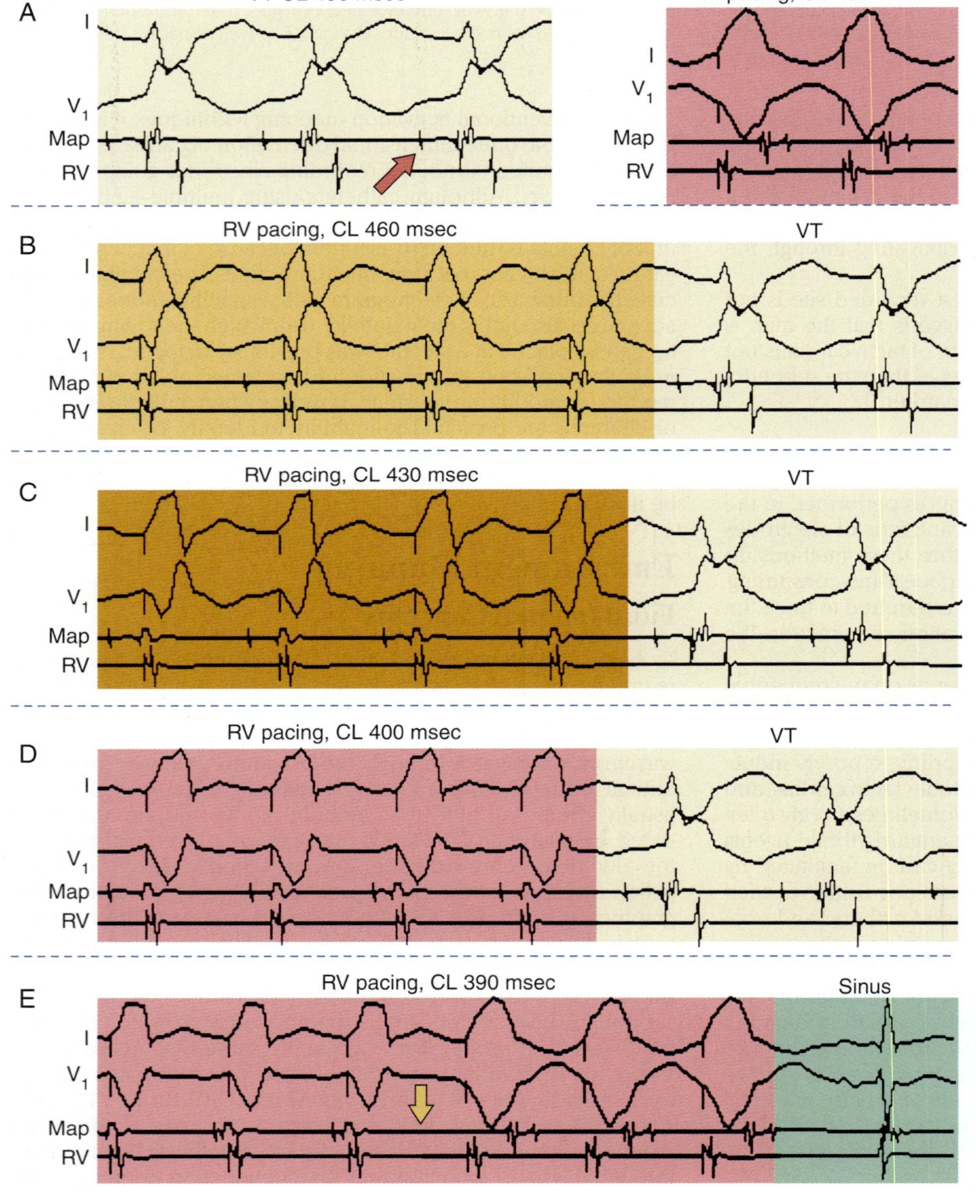

FIGURE 5-15 Entrainment of ventricular tachycardia (VT). **A,** Pure VT is shown in yellow (right bundle branch block, right axis), pure right ventricle (RV) pacing in red (left bundle branch block, left axis). A mid-diastolic potential during VT (arrow) is recorded by the mapping catheter. **B,** Pacing the RV at 460 milliseconds (30 milliseconds faster than VT), each paced complex is a stable blend of pacing and VT (gold). This illustrates fixed fusion. After cessation of pacing, VT resumes. **C,** Pacing the RV faster (430 milliseconds), all complexes are again identical to each other but different than with pacing at 460 milliseconds; they look slightly more like pure RV pacing (deeper gold shading). **D,** Pacing the RV faster still (400 milliseconds), QRS complexes again are identical to each other (fixed fusion) but look progressively more like fully paced (progressive fusion). **E,** Finally, with pacing rapidly enough, an antidromic wavefront captures the diastolic potential, QRS complexes become fully paced, and when pacing ceases, sinus rhythm resumes. This figure demonstrates all established entrainment criteria (fixed fusion at a given paced cycle length [CL], progressive fusion over a range of paced CLs, and antidromic capture of critical circuit elements leading to termination of the tachycardia).

the premature impulse enters the reentrant circuit early enough in the relative refractory period, because it fails to propagate in the anterograde direction, given that it encounters absolutely refractory tissue (see Fig. 5-15). In the retrograde direction, it encounters increasingly recovered tissue and is able to propagate until it meets the circulating wavefront and terminates the arrhythmia.[8]

Entrainment is the continuous resetting of a reentrant circuit by a train of capturing stimuli. However, following the first stimulus of the pacing train that penetrates and resets the reentrant circuit, the subsequent stimuli interact with the reset circuit, which has an abbreviated excitable gap. The first entrained complex results in retrograde collision between the stimulated and tachycardia wavefronts, whereas in all subsequent beats, the collision occurs between the currently stimulated wavefront and that stimulated previously. Depending on the degree that the excitable gap is preexcited by that first resetting stimulus, subsequent stimuli fall on fully or partially excitable tissue. Entrainment is said to be present when two consecutive extrastimuli conduct orthodromically through the circuit with the same conduction time while colliding antidromically with the preceding paced wavefront.[4]

During entrainment, each pacing impulse creates two activation wavefronts, one in the orthodromic direction and the other in the antidromic direction. The wavefront in the antidromic direction collides with the existing tachycardia wavefront. The wavefront that enters the reentrant circuit in the orthodromic direction (i.e., the same direction as the spontaneous tachycardia wavefront) conducts through the critical isthmus, resets the tachycardia, and emerges through the exit site to activate the myocardium and collide with the antidromically paced wavefront from the next paced stimulus. This sequence continues until cessation of pacing or development of block somewhere within the reentrant circuit. Because all pacing impulses enter the tachycardia circuit during the excitable gap, each paced wavefront advances and resets the tachycardia. Thus, when pacing is terminated, the last paced impulse continues to activate the entire tachycardia reentrant circuit orthodromically at the pacing CL and also activates the entire myocardium orthodromically on exiting the reentrant circuit.

Entrainment of reentrant tachycardias by external stimuli was originally defined in the clinical setting as an increase in the rate of a tachycardia to a faster pacing rate, with resumption of the intrinsic rate of the tachycardia on either abrupt cessation of pacing or slowing of pacing beyond the intrinsic rate of the tachycardia, and it was taken to indicate an underlying reentrant mechanism. The ability to entrain a tachycardia also establishes that the reentrant circuit contains an excitable gap.[4,8]

Entrainment does not require that the pacing site be located in the reentrant circuit. The closer the pacing site is to the circuit, however, the less premature a single stimulus needs to be to reach the circuit and, with pacing trains, the fewer stimuli will be required before a stimulated wavefront reaches the reentrant circuit without being extinguished by collision with a wave emerging from the circuit. Overdrive pacing at relatively long CLs (i.e., 10 to 30 milliseconds shorter than the tachycardia CL) can almost always entrain reentrant tachycardias. However, the number of pacing stimuli required to entrain the reentrant circuit depends on the tachycardia CL, the duration of the excitable gap of the tachycardia, refractoriness at the pacing site, and the conduction time from the stimulation site to the reentrant circuit.[8]

During constant-rate pacing, entrainment of a reentrant tachycardia results in the activation of all myocardial tissue responsible for maintaining the tachycardia at the pacing CL, with the resumption of the intrinsic tachycardia morphology and rate after cessation of pacing. Unfortunately, it is almost impossible to document the acceleration of all tissue responsible for maintaining the reentrant circuit to the pacing CL. Therefore, several surface ECG and intracardiac electrogram criteria have been proposed for establishing the presence of entrainment (see Fig. 5-15): (1) fixed fusion of the paced complexes at a constant pacing rate; (2) progressive fusion or different degrees of fusion at different pacing rates (i.e., the surface ECG and intracardiac morphology progressively look more like the purely paced configuration and less like the pure tachycardia beat in the course of pacing at progressively shorter pacing CLs; Fig. 5-16); and (3) resumption of the same tachycardia morphology following cessation of pacing, with the first post-pacing complex

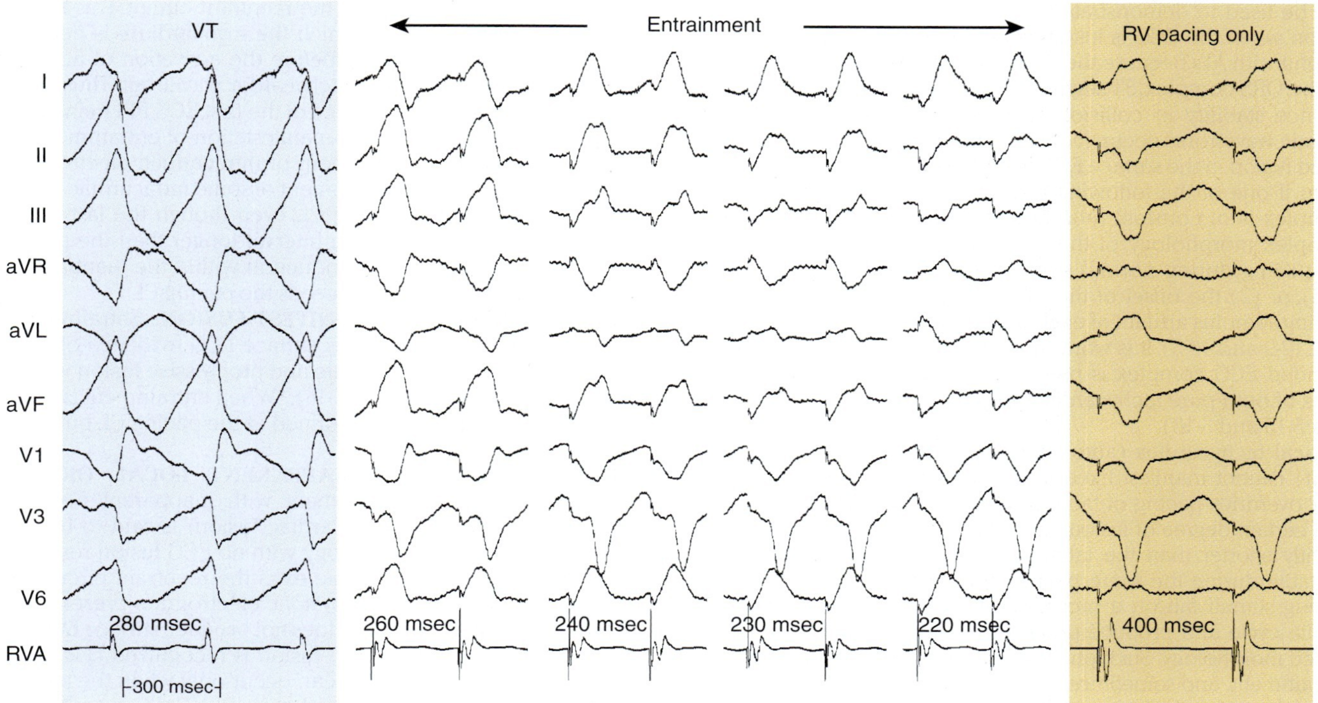

FIGURE 5-16 QRS fusion during entrainment of ventricular tachycardia (VT). Progressive ECG fusion is shown over a range of paced cycle lengths (CLs). Pure tachycardia complexes are shown on the **left**; fully paced complexes are shown on the **right**. As the paced CL shortens, complexes gradually appear more like those that are fully paced. RV = right ventricle.

displaying no fusion but occurring at a return cycle equal to the pacing CL.[8]

FUSION DURING ENTRAINMENT

A stimulated impulse is said to be fused when its morphology is a hybrid between that of a fully paced complex and a tachycardia complex. Fusion can be observed on the surface ECG, intracardiac recordings, or both. For fusion to be observed on the surface ECG, the tachycardia and stimulated wavefronts must collide within the reentrant circuit after the tachycardia wavefront has exited from the isthmus. This requires the paced wavefront to have access to an entrance site of the reentrant circuit that is anatomically distinct from the exit site. If the antidromically stimulated wavefront penetrates the reentrant circuit and collides with the tachycardia wavefront (or the previously stimulated orthodromic wavefront) before the point at which the tachycardia wavefront would be exiting to the mass of the myocardium, then no fusion will be evident on the surface ECG, and the surface ECG will appear entirely paced.[4]

The ability to demonstrate surface ECG fusion requires that a significant mass of myocardium be depolarized by the extrastimulus and the tachycardia. The degree of fusion represents the relative amounts of myocardium depolarized by the two separate wavefronts. The relative degree of myocardium antidromically activated by the paced wavefront depends on the site of pacing relative to the reentrant circuit, the pacing CL, and the degree of conduction delay within the reentrant circuit. With a single extrastimulus, the farther the stimulation site is from the reentrant circuit, the less likely ECG fusion will be to occur, because the extrastimulus must be delivered at a shorter coupling interval, well before the tachycardia wavefront exits the circuit, to reach the circuit with adequate prematurity. Therefore, by the time the tachycardia wavefront exits the circuit, most of the myocardium has already been activated by the paced wavefront. Consequently, the stimulated impulse will have a purely paced morphology with no ECG fusion. Nevertheless, continuous pacing at a slow CL at a site remote from the exit site affords the best opportunity to demonstrate fusion, whereas pacing closer to the presumed exit site shows less fusion. Presystolic electrograms in the reentrant circuit that are activated orthodromically can be used to demonstrate the presence of intracardiac (local) fusion when the ECG is insufficiently sensitive. This is particularly helpful with ATs because the P waves are small and often obscured by the QRS complex, ST segments, and T waves.

Once stability in collision sites of the antidromic and orthodromic wavefronts occurs, constant surface ECG fusion is achieved. Fixed fusion in the surface ECG is said to be present during entrainment if one of the following criteria is met: (1) the surface ECG complex is of constant morphology, representing a hybrid of the complex morphology of the tachycardia and that observed during pacing during normal sinus rhythm (NSR; see Figs. 5-15 and 5-16), or (2) the onset of the surface ECG complex precedes the pacing stimulus artifact of each paced beat by a fixed interval (see Figs. 12-9 and 13-5). It is worth noting that to be certain a hybrid or blended ECG complex is present, one must know the configurations of both pure tachycardia and pure pacing (Fig. 5-17; see also Figs. 5-15 and 5-16).

Focal tachycardias (automatic, triggered activity, or microreentrant) cannot manifest fixed fusion during overdrive pacing. However, overdrive pacing of tachycardia of any mechanism can result in a certain degree of fusion, especially when the pacing CL is only slightly shorter than the tachycardia CL. Such fusion, however, is unstable during the same pacing drive at a constant CL, because pacing stimuli fall on a progressively earlier portion of the tachycardia cycle and produce progressively less fusion and more fully paced morphology. Such phenomena should be distinguished from entrainment, and sometimes this distinction requires pacing for long intervals to demonstrate variable degrees of fusion. Moreover, overdrive pacing frequently results in suppression (automatic) or acceleration (triggered activity) of focal tachycardias, rather than resumption of the original tachycardia with an unchanged tachycardia CL.[4]

Varying degrees of fusion at different pacing rates are caused by a progressive increase in the amount of myocardium activated by the antidromic wavefront at progressively shorter pacing CLs (see Figs. 5-15 and 5-16). At slower pacing CLs, a larger amount of the myocardium is activated by the orthodromic wavefront exiting from the reentrant circuit prior to its intracardiac collision, with the subsequent antidromic wavefront incoming from the pacing site. With a faster pacing rate, more myocardium is antidromically activated because the orthodromic wavefront must continue to traverse the zone of slow conduction within the reentrant circuit, thus creating progressive fusion with changing pacing CLs. In the extreme situation, the antidromic wavefront can capture the exit site of the reentrant circuit and produce a fully paced complex. Once this occurs, pacing at shorter pacing CLs does not cause further progressive fusion, although entrainment is still present. As noted, progressive fusion at decreasing pacing CLs during entrainment of tachycardia excludes the possibility of automaticity or triggered activity as the mechanism of the tachycardia. In those cases, overdrive pacing would yield solely the morphology of the pacing stimulus for a nonprotected focus or would yield varying (not progressive) degrees of fusion for a protected focus with entrance block. Of note, a microreentrant circuit with entrance block could also yield variable fusion during overdrive pacing; thus, this finding would not exclude reentry as the underlying mechanism.[4,8]

On cessation of pacing, the last paced wavefront traverses the protected isthmus and exits the circuit to produce a normal (nonfused) tachycardia complex at the pacing CL, because there is no paced antidromic wavefront with which to fuse. The wavefront continues around the reentrant circuit to maintain the tachycardia. Constant fusion of the surface ECG can occur, however, without the first nonpaced beat occurring at the pacing CL. When surface ECG fusion occurs, the initial portion of the ECG complex usually reflects activation of the myocardium by the paced wavefront, whereas the terminal portion represents the orthodromically activated wavefront exiting from the tachycardia circuit. The point at which this wavefront exits the circuit can be late in the surface ECG complex. The degree to which the first ECG post-pacing interval (PPI) exceeds the pacing CL is primarily a reflection of the time from the onset of the paced surface ECG complex to the exit of the orthodromic wavefront from the reentrant circuit. This represents the period of time during which the myocardium is depolarized by the stimulated wavefront before the activation of any portion of the myocardium by the tachycardia wavefront. Thus, constant fusion occurring in the absence of the first ECG PPI being equal to the pacing CL can be a valid manifestation of entrainment. In this situation, appropriate placement of intracardiac electrodes demonstrates orthodromic entrainment of some intracardiac recording sites occurring at the pacing CL, even though the last entrained ECG complex occurred at an interval longer than the pacing CL. Alternatively, decremental conduction within the reentrant circuit can explain a first PPI that exceeds the pacing CL.[4]

ENTRAINMENT WITH MANIFEST FUSION. Entrainment with manifest fusion demonstrates surface ECG evidence of constant fusion at a constant pacing rate and progressive fusion with incremental-rate pacing (see Fig. 5-16).[8] When entrainment is manifest, the last captured wave is entrained at the pacing CL but does not demonstrate fusion.[9]

ENTRAINMENT WITH INAPPARENT, LOCAL, OR INTRACARDIAC FUSION. Entrainment with inapparent fusion (also referred to as local or intracardiac fusion) is said to be present when a fully paced morphology with no ECG fusion results, even when the tachycardia impulse exits the reentrant circuit (orthodromic activation of the presystolic electrogram present). Fusion is limited to a small area and does not produce surface ECG fusion, and only intracardiac (local) fusion is recognized (Fig. 5-18; see also Fig. 13-5).[8] Local fusion can occur only when the presystolic electrogram is activated orthodromically. Collision with the last paced impulse must occur distal to the presystolic electrogram, either at the exit from the circuit or outside the circuit. In such cases, the return cycle measured at this local electrogram equals

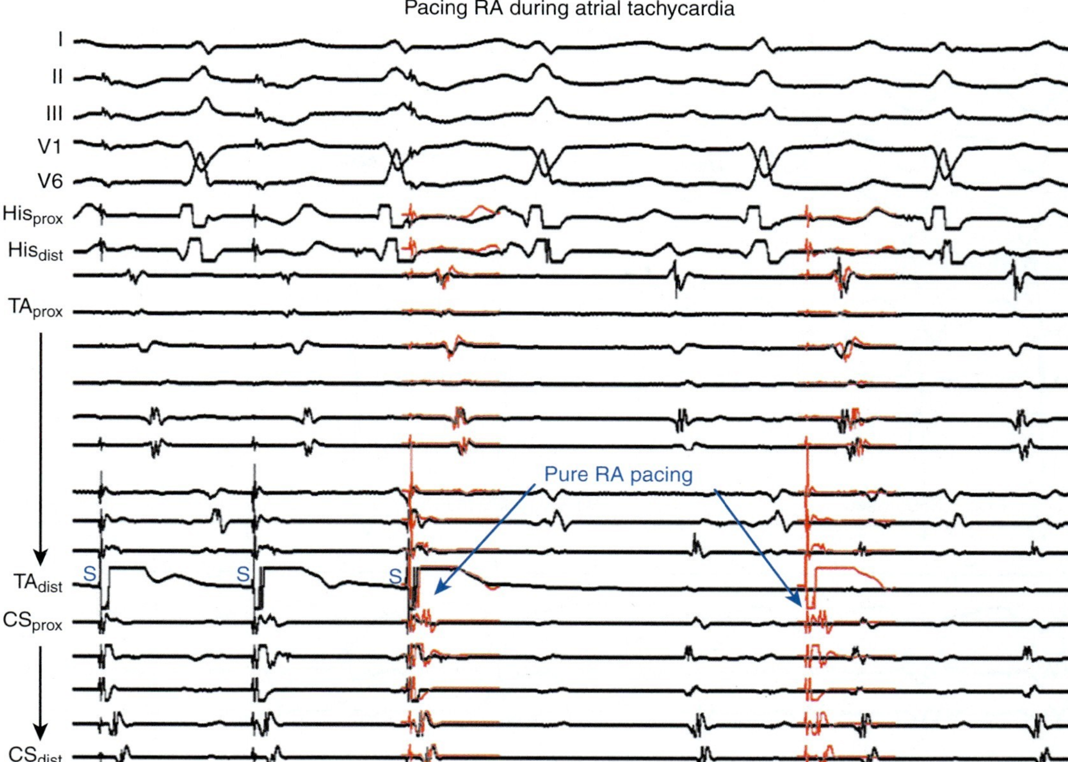

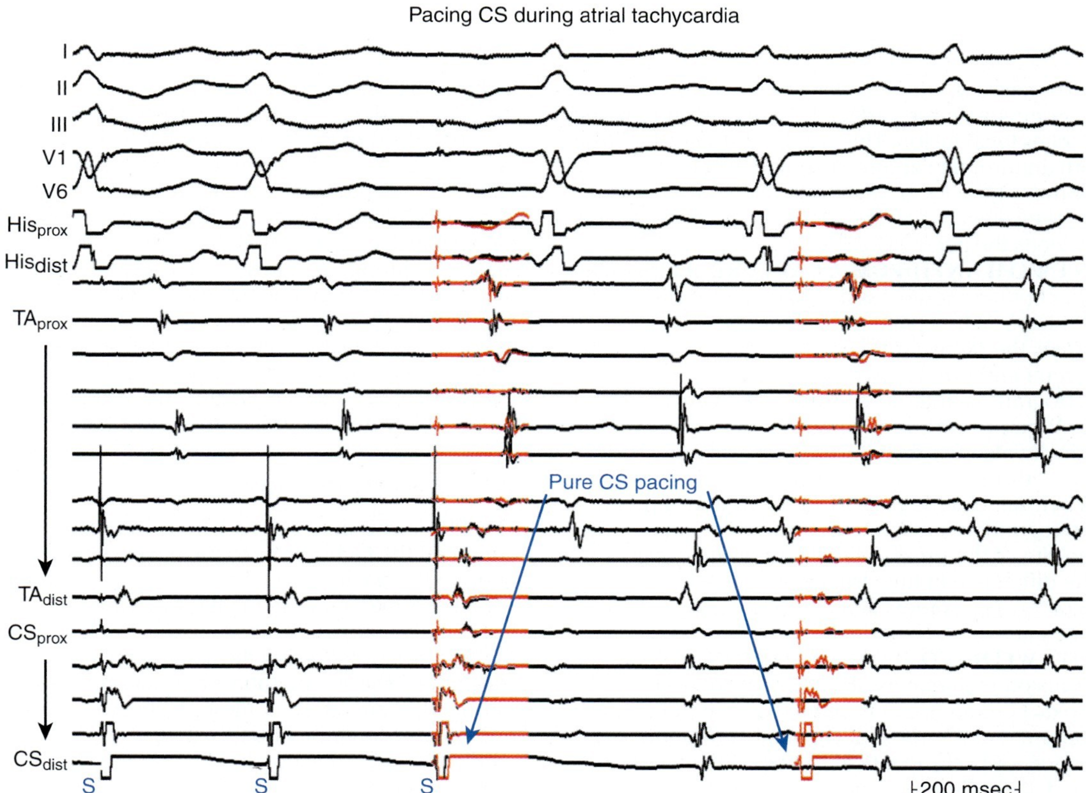

FIGURE 5-17 Overdrive pacing during focal atrial tachycardia (AT). **Top,** The last three complexes of pacing (S) from the high right atrium (RA) are shown, following which AT resumes. The red overlay represents recordings of pure high RA pacing that perfectly match the electrogram sequence of high RA pacing during AT; thus, fusion is absent. **Bottom,** Similar findings with pacing from distal coronary sinus (CS_{dist}). The red overlay of pure CS pacing perfectly matches the electrogram sequence of CS pacing during AT; thus, there is no fusion. CS_{prox} = proximal coronary sinus; His_{dist} = distal His bundle; His_{prox} = proximal His bundle; TA_{dist} = distal tricuspid annulus; TA_{prox} = proximal tricuspid annulus.

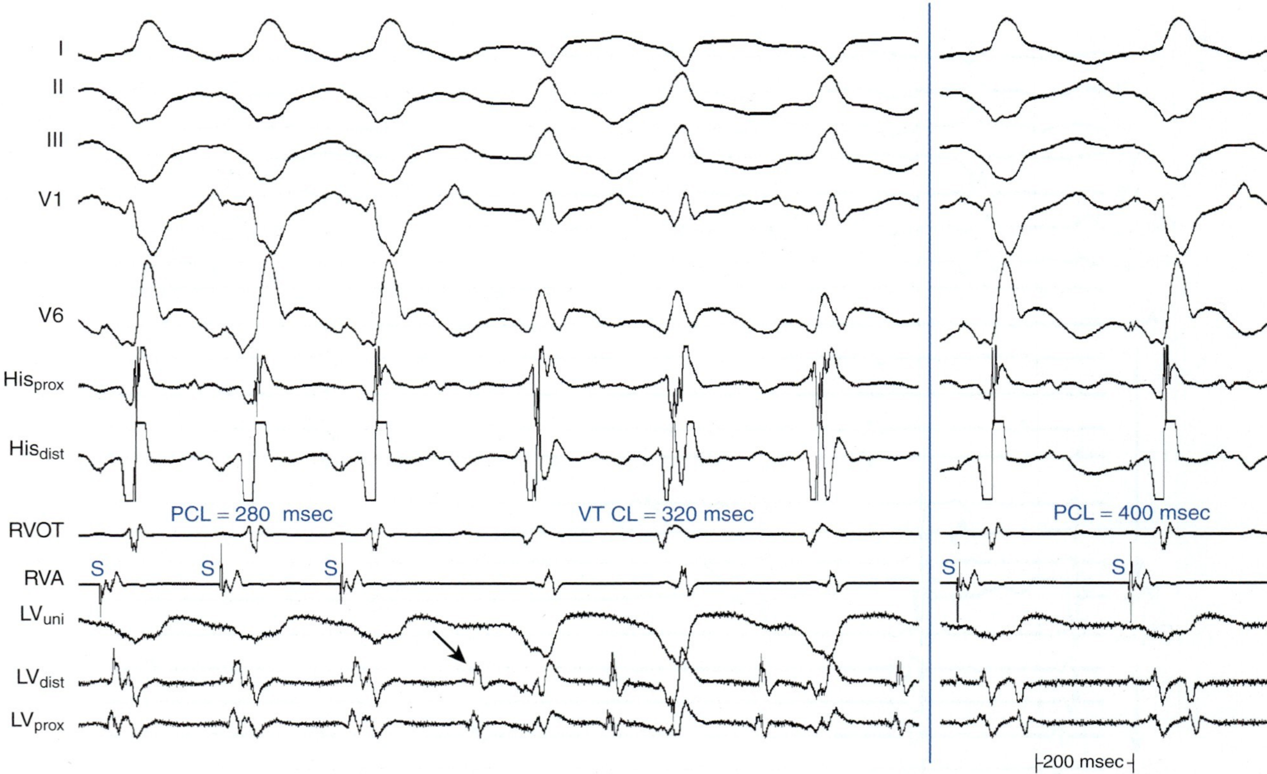

FIGURE 5-18 Inapparent fusion. The last three complexes paced from the right ventricular apex during ventricular tachycardia (VT) are shown; VT resumes on cessation of pacing. Fusion is not evident on the surface ECG because these complexes are identical to fully paced QRS complexes at the **far right**, yet fusion is present on the distal ablation (Abl_{dist}) recording (mid-diastolic potential at arrow seen during pacing as well). CL = cycle length; PCL = pacing cycle length; His_{dist} = distal His bundle; His_{prox} = proximal His bundle; LV_{dist} = distal left ventricle; LV_{prox} = proximal left ventricle; LV_{uni} = unipolar left ventricle; RVA = right ventricular apex; RVOT = right ventricular outflow tract.

the pacing CL. Therefore, a stimulus delivered after the onset of the tachycardia complex on the surface ECG during entrainment always demonstrates local fusion. This is to be distinguished from entrainment with antidromic capture. As noted, when antidromic (retrograde) capture of the local presystolic electrogram occurs, the return cycle, even when measured at the site of the presystolic electrogram, exceeds the pacing CL.[8,9]

ENTRAINMENT WITH ANTIDROMIC CAPTURE. Entrainment with antidromic capture should be distinguished from entrainment with local fusion. When pacing is performed at a CL significantly shorter than the tachycardia CL, the paced impulse can penetrate the circuit antidromically and retrogradely capture the presystolic electrogram so that no exit from the tachycardia circuit is possible. When pacing is stopped, the impulse that conducts antidromically also conducts orthodromically to reset the reentrant circuit with orthodromic activation of the presystolic electrogram. When antidromic (retrograde) capture of the local presystolic electrogram occurs, the return cycle, even when measured at the site of the presystolic electrogram, exceeds the pacing CL by the difference in time from when the electrogram is activated retrogradely (i.e., preexcited antidromically) and when it would have been activated orthodromically.[4,8,9]

ENTRAINMENT WITH CONCEALED FUSION. Entrainment with concealed fusion (sometimes also referred to as concealed entrainment or exact entrainment) is defined as entrainment with orthodromic capture and a surface ECG complex (or intracardiac activation sequence, or both) identical to that of the tachycardia (see Figs. 12-9 and 13-5). Entrainment with concealed fusion suggests that the pacing site is within a protected isthmus inside or outside, but attached to, the reentrant circuit (see Fig. 5-14). In this situation, transient entrainment is achieved when the orthodromically directed stimulated wavefront resets the tachycardia, but the antidromically directed stimulated wavefront collides with the tachycardia wavefront in or near the reentry circuit and fails to exit the slow conduction zone. Only tissue near the pacing site within the critical isthmus is antidromically activated; hence, there is no evidence of fusion. Compared with the intrinsic tachycardia, this antidromic capture may result in earlier intracardiac recordings from sites located adjacent to the pacing region. The morphological appearance of the ECG, however, is the same during entrainment as during the tachycardia. Entrainment with concealed fusion can occur by pacing from bystander pathways, such as a blind alley, alternate pathway, or inner loop, that are not critical to the maintenance of reentry. In this case, activation propagates from the main circuit loop but is constrained by block lines having the shape of a cul-de-sac; ablation there does not terminate reentry (unless it is fortuitously close to a critical portion of the circuit).[4,8,9]

POST-PACING INTERVAL

The PPI is the time interval from the last pacing stimulus that entrained the tachycardia to the next nonpaced recorded electrogram at the pacing site (Fig. 5-19). During entrainment from sites within the reentrant circuit, the orthodromic wavefront from the last stimulus propagates through the reentry circuit and returns to the pacing site, following the same path as the circulating reentry wavefronts. The conduction time required is the revolution time through the circuit. Thus, the PPI (measured from the pacing site recording) should be equal (within 30 milliseconds) to the tachycardia CL (given that conduction velocities and the reentrant path did not change during pacing; see Fig. 5-14). At sites remote from the circuit, stimulated wavefronts propagate to the circuit, then through the circuit, and finally back to the pacing site. Thus, the PPI should equal the tachycardia CL plus the time required for the stimulus to propagate from the pacing site to the tachycardia circuit and back. The greater the difference is between the PPI and

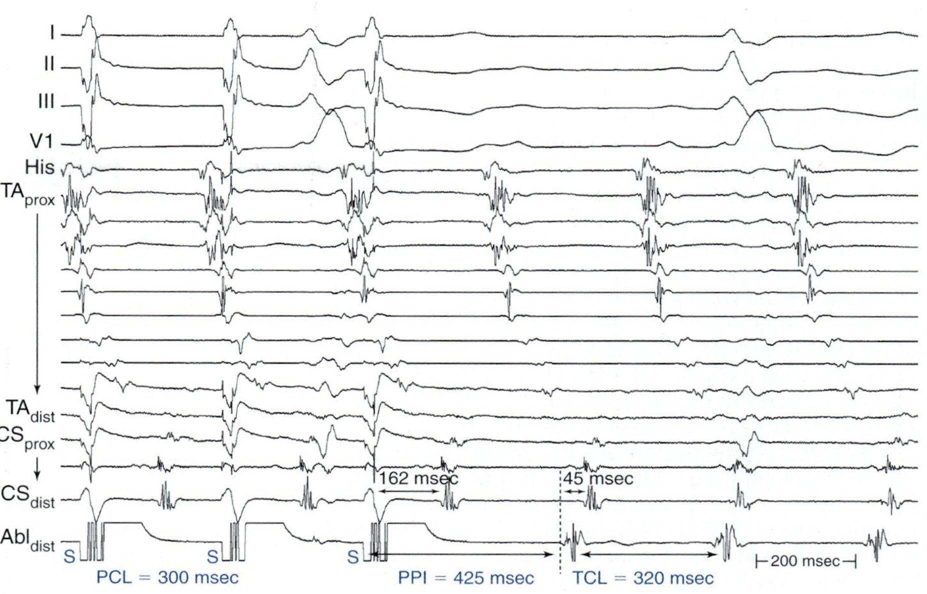

FIGURE 5-19 Bystander site during atypical left atrial (LA) flutter. The last three complexes of pacing from the posterior LA are shown in a patient with LA macroreentry. Although the timing of the electrogram at the pacing site is in early mid-diastole and the paced activation sequence is similar to tachycardia, thereby giving the appearance of an attractive ablation site, the results of entrainment indicate otherwise, with a large difference between the stimulus–coronary sinus (CS) electrogram interval (162 milliseconds) and the ablation recording–CS electrogram interval (45 milliseconds), as well as a large difference between the post-pacing interval (PPI) (425 milliseconds) and tachycardia cycle length (TCL, 320 milliseconds). Abl_{dist} = distal ablation; CS_{dist} = distal coronary sinus; CS_{prox} = proximal coronary sinus; PCL = pacing cycle length; TA_{dist} = distal tricuspid annulus; TA_{prox} = proximal tricuspid annulus.

the tachycardia CL (PPI – tachycardia CL), the longer the conduction time will be between the pacing site and reentry circuit, and the greater the physical distance will be between the pacing site and the circuit (see Figs. 12-9 and 13-5).[9]

Several factors have to be considered when evaluating the PPI. The PPI should be measured to the near-field potential that indicates depolarization of tissue at the pacing site. In regions of scar, electrode catheters often record multiple potentials separated in time, some of which are far-field potentials that result from depolarization of adjacent myocardium. The near-field potential is obscured by capture during pacing, whereas far-field potentials can be undisturbed during pacing. Furthermore, when pacing artifacts obscure recordings from the pacing site and prevent assessment of the PPI, the electrograms from the proximal electrodes of the mapping catheter may be utilized, provided such electrograms are also present in the distal electrode recordings. When the electrograms from the pacing site are not discernible because of stimulus artifact, relating the timing of the near-field potential to a consistent intracardiac electrogram or surface ECG wave can be used to determine the PPI.

CONDUCTION TIME FROM THE PACING SITE TO THE CIRCUIT EXIT SITE

During entrainment of reentrant tachycardia, the interval between the pacing stimulus and the onset of the tachycardia complex on the surface ECG (QRS or P wave) reflects the conduction time from the pacing site to the exit of the reentrant circuit (stimulus-exit interval), regardless of whether the pacing site is inside or outside the reentrant circuit, because activation starts at the pacing site and propagates in sequence to the circuit exit site. On the other hand, during tachycardia, the interval between the local electrogram at a given site and circuit exit (electrogram-exit interval) can reflect the true conduction time between those two sites if they are activated in sequence (as occurs when that particular site is located within the reentrant pathway), or it may be shorter than the true conduction time if those two sites are activated in parallel (which occurs when that particular site is located outside the reentrant circuit) (see Figs. 5-14 and 5-19).[8]

Therefore, at any given pacing site, an electrogram-exit interval that is equal (±20 milliseconds) to the stimulus-exit interval indicates that the pacing site lies within the reentry circuit and excludes the possibility that the site is a dead-end pathway attached to the circuit (i.e., not a bystander). On the other hand, pacing sites outside the reentrant circuit have an electrogram-exit interval significantly (more than 20 milliseconds) shorter than the stimulus-exit interval.

However, the electrogram-exit interval may not be exactly equal to the stimulus-exit interval at sites within the reentrant circuit. Several factors can explain this. One potential factor is decremental conduction properties of the zone of slow conduction that produce lengthening of the stimulus-exit interval during pacing; however, this appears to occur rarely. Therefore, the stimulus-exit interval should be measured during pacing at the slower CL that reliably entrains the tachycardia. Moreover, stimulus latency in an area of diseased tissue can account for a delay in the stimulus-exit interval compared with the electrogram-QRS interval. Additionally, failure of the recording electrodes to detect low-amplitude depolarizations at the pacing site can account for a mismatch of the stimulus-exit and electrogram-exit intervals.[8]

Mapping Procedure

Before attempting to use entrainment methods for mapping, it is necessary to demonstrate that the tachycardia can be entrained, by providing strong evidence that it is caused by reentry rather than by triggered activity or automaticity. Potential ablation sites are sought by pacing at sites thought to be related to the reentrant circuit, based on other mapping modalities, such as activation mapping and pace mapping. The areas of slow conduction can be identified by endocardial mapping revealing fractionated electrograms, mid-diastolic electrograms, or long delays between the pacing stimulus and the captured surface ECG complex (see Fig. 5-14). These sites are then targeted by entrainment mapping. However, proof of entrainment is best obtained by pacing from sites remote from the circuit, which most readily demonstrate fusion.[9]

Entrainment mapping can be reliably carried out only if one can record and stimulate from the same area (e.g., for 2-5-2-mm spacing catheters, record from the second and fourth poles and stimulate from the first and third poles). Pacing is usually started at a CL just shorter (10 to 20 milliseconds) than the tachycardia CL. Pacing should be continued for a long enough duration to allow for entrainment; short pacing trains are usually not helpful. Pacing is then repeated at progressively shorter pacing CLs.[8]

After cessation of each pacing drive, the presence of entrainment should be verified by demonstrating the presence of fixed fusion of the paced complexes at a given pacing CL, progressive fusion at faster pacing CLs, and resumption of the same tachycardia morphology following cessation of pacing with a nonfused complex at a return cycle equal to the pacing CL. The mere acceleration of the tachycardia to the pacing rate and then resumption of the original tachycardia after cessation of pacing do not establish the presence of entrainment. Evaluation of the PPI or other criteria is meaningless when the presence of true entrainment has not been established. Moreover, it is important to verify the absence of termination and reinitiation of the tachycardia during the same pacing drive.[4]

Once the presence of entrainment is verified, several criteria can be used to indicate the relation of the pacing site to the reentrant circuit. The first entrainment criterion to be sought is concealed fusion. Entrainment with concealed fusion indicates that the pacing site is in a protected isthmus located within or attached to the reentrant circuit. Whether this protected isthmus is crucial to the reentrant circuit or is just a bystander site needs to be verified by other criteria, mainly comparing the PPI with the tachycardia CL and comparing the stimulus-exit interval with the electrogram-exit interval. Features of entrainment when pacing from different sites are listed in Table 5-1 (see also Figs. 5-14, 5-18, and 5-19).[9,10]

A graphical representation of entrainment mapping can be constructed by plotting the values of the difference between the PPI and the tachycardia CL [PPI–tachycardia CL] on an electroanatomical mapping system (CARTO, Biosense Webster, Inc., Diamond Bar, Calif.; or NavX, St. Jude Medical, Inc., St. Paul, Minn.) to generate color-coded three-dimensional entrainment maps (see Chap. 6 for discussion).[11,12]

Clinical Implications

Entrainment mapping is the gold standard for ablation of reentrant circuits generating hemodynamically well-tolerated tachycardias. Achievement of entrainment of tachycardia establishes a reentrant mechanism of that tachycardia and excludes triggered activity and abnormal automaticity as potential mechanisms. Entrainment may also be used to estimate how far the reentrant circuit is from the pacing site qualitatively. For example, entrainment of an AT from multiple sites in the RA with a PPI significantly longer than the tachycardia CL can help identify a left atrial origin of the AT before attempting LA access (see Fig. 13-5). In addition, pacing at multiple sites and measuring the difference between the PPI and tachycardia CL provide an indication of how far or near the pacing site is from the circuit (Fig. 5-20).[4,8,9]

Entrainment mapping has been useful to identify the critical isthmus in patients with macroreentrant VT or AT. Focal ablation of all sites defined as within the reentrant circuit may not result in a cure of reentrant tachycardia. Cure requires ablation of an isthmus bordered by barriers on either side, which is critical to the reentrant circuit. Entrainment mapping helps identify this critical part of the reentrant circuit. Sites demonstrating entrainment with concealed fusion are initially sought. Once these sites are identified, their relationship to the reentrant circuit is verified using the PPI or stimulus-exit interval (see earlier). Sites demonstrating concealed fusion, a PPI equal to the tachycardia CL (±30 milliseconds), and a stimulus-exit interval equal to the electrogram-exit interval (±20 milliseconds) have a very high positive predictive value for successful ablation.[4,9,10]

TABLE 5-1 Entrainment Mapping of Reentrant Tachycardias

Pacing from Sites *Outside* the Reentrant Circuit
Manifest fusion on surface ECG or intracardiac recordings, or both
• PPI-tachycardia CL >30 msec
• Stimulus-exit interval > electrogram-exit interval
Pacing from Sites *Inside* the Reentrant Circuit
• Manifest fusion on surface ECG or intracardiac recordings, or both
• PPI-tachycardia CL <30 msec
• Stimulus-exit interval = electrogram-exit interval (±20 msec)
Pacing from a Protected Isthmus Inside the Reentrant Circuit
• Concealed fusion
• PPI-tachycardia CL <30 msec
• Stimulus-exit interval = electrogram-exit interval (±20 msec)

CL = cycle length; PPI = post-pacing interval.

Limitations

One of the limitations of entrainment mapping is the requirement of the presence of sustained, hemodynamically well-tolerated tachycardia of stable morphology and CL. Furthermore, attempts at entrainment can result in termination, acceleration, or transformation of the index tachycardia into a different one, thus making further mapping challenging. Bipolar pacing at relatively high stimulus strengths used during entrainment can result in capture of an area larger than the local area. Additionally, errors can be introduced by the decremental conduction properties of the zone of slow conduction that may cause a rate-dependent lengthening of the PPI. This is more likely to occur at rapid pacing rates.[4,8]

Pacing and recording from the same area are required for entrainment mapping. This requirement is usually satisfied by pacing from electrodes 1 and 3 and recording from electrodes 2 and 4 of the mapping catheter. However, this technique has several limitations:

1. There are differences, albeit slight, of the area from which the second and fourth electrodes record as compared with the first and third. When the local electrogram is not recorded from the same pair of electrodes used for pacing, errors can be introduced when comparing the PPI with the tachycardia CL.
2. The bipolar pacing technique has the potential for anodal contribution to local capture.
3. The total area captured by the pacing stimulus can exceed the local area, especially when high currents (more than 10 mA) are required for stimulation.
4. The pacing artifact can obscure the early part of the captured local electrogram. In such a case, a comparable component of the electrogram can be used to measure the PPI.
5. Far-field electrical signals generated by depolarization of adjacent tissue can cause false-positive entrainment criteria at some sites.[4,8]

Pace Mapping

Fundamental Concepts

Pace mapping is a technique designed to help locate tachycardia sources by pacing at different endocardial sites to reproduce the ECG morphology of the tachycardia. Pace mapping is based on the

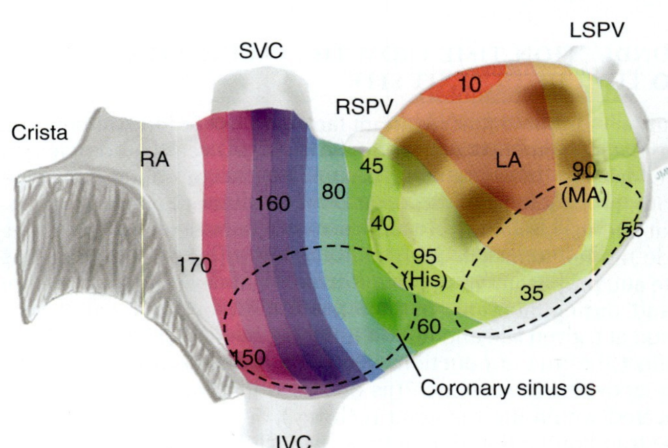

FIGURE 5-20 The post-pacing interval (PPI)–tachycardia cycle length (TCL) interval as an indicator of distance from the pacing site to the reentrant circuit (located in the dome of the left atrium [LA], near 10). In this representation of both atria viewed from the front, colors indicate isochrones of the difference between PPI and TCL in milliseconds at various pacing sites (indicated by numbers). IVC = inferior vena cava; LSPV = left superior pulmonary vein; MA = mitral annulus; os = ostium; RA = right atrium; RSPV = right superior pulmonary vein; SVC = superior vena cava.

principle that pacing from the site of origin of a focal tachycardia at a pacing CL similar to the tachycardia CL results in the same activation sequence as that during the tachycardia.[4]

When myocardial activation originates from a point-like source, such as during focal tachycardia or during pacing from an electrode catheter, ECG configuration of the resultant tachycardia or paced complex (QRS or P wave) is determined by the sequence of myocardial activation, which is largely determined by the initial site of myocardial depolarization, assuming no conduction abnormalities from that site. Analysis of specific surface ECG configurations in multiple leads allows estimation of the pacing site location to within several square centimeters, and comparing the paced complex configuration with that of tachycardia can be used to locate the arrhythmia focus (Fig. 5-21).[13,14]

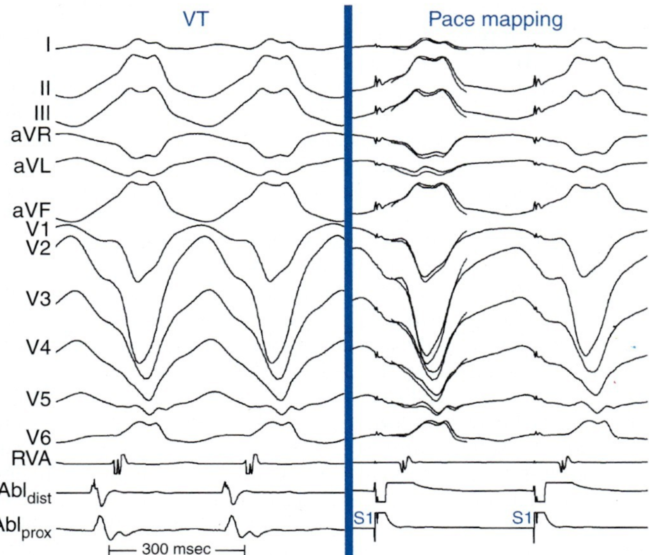

FIGURE 5-21 Pace mapping of ventricular tachycardia (VT). At **left**, 12 ECG leads and intracardiac recordings during idiopathic right ventricular outflow tract VT are shown (cycle length [CL], 280 milliseconds). At **right**, pace mapping from the site of earliest ventricular activation at CL 350 milliseconds produces an identical 12-lead ECG configuration (the VT complex superimposed on the first paced complex). Abl_{dist} = distal ablation; Abl_{prox} = proximal ablation; RVA = right ventricular apex.

On the other hand, reentry circuits in healed infarct scars (e.g., post-MI VT) often extend over several square centimeters and can have various configurations. In many circuits, the excitation wave propagates through surviving myocytes in the scarred region, depolarization of which is not detectable in the standard surface ECG. The QRS complex is then inscribed after the reentry wavefront activates a sufficient amount of muscle outside the dense scar area. At sites at which the reentrant wavefront exits the scar, pace mapping is expected to produce a QRS configuration similar to that of VT. Pace mapping at sites more proximally located in the isthmus of the reentrant circuit should also produce a similar QRS complex, but with a longer stimulus-to-QRS (S-QRS) interval.

INTERPRETATION OF PACE MAPPING

Pace maps with identical or nearly identical matches of tachycardia morphology in all 12 surface ECG leads can be indicative of the site of origin of the tachycardia (Fig. 5-22). Differences in the morphology between pacing and spontaneous tachycardia in a single lead can be critical. For VT, pacing at a site 5 mm from the index pacing site results in minor differences in QRS configuration (e.g., notching, new small component, change in amplitude of individual component, or overall change in QRS shape) in at least one lead in most patients. In contrast, if only major changes in QRS morphology are considered, pacing sites separated by as much as 15 mm can produce similar QRS morphologies.

Although qualitative comparison of the 12-lead ECG morphology between a pace map and clinical tachycardia is frequently performed, there are few objective criteria for quantifying the similarity between 2 12-lead ECG waveform morphologies. Such comparisons are frequently completely subjective or semiquantitative,

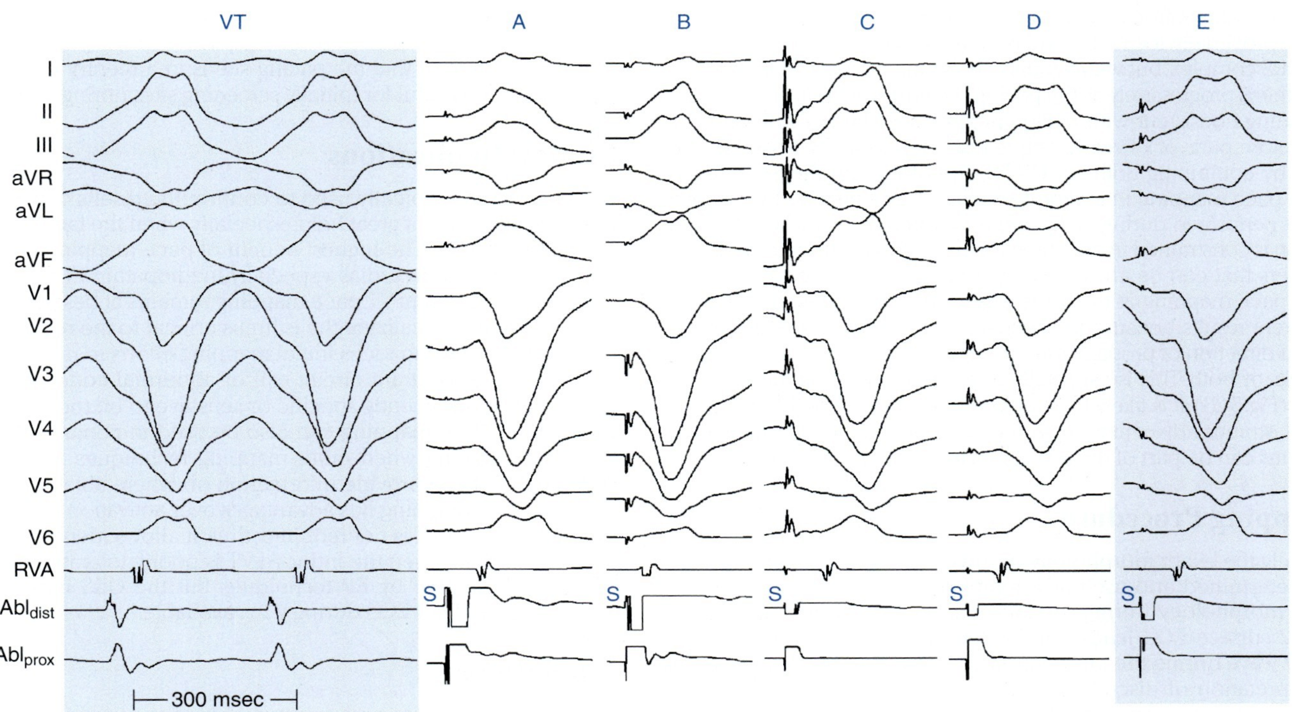

FIGURE 5-22 Pace mapping of ventricular tachycardia (VT). Pace mapping at various sites in the right ventricular outflow tract produces QRS configurations (A to D) with less or more similarity to the VT QRS **(left panel)**; E shows an exact match. Abl_{dist} = distal ablation; Abl_{prox} = proximal ablation; RVA = right ventricular apex.

such as a 10/12 lead match. Unsuccessful ablation can result, in part, from subjective differences in the opinion of a pace map match to the clinical tachycardia. Furthermore, criteria for comparing the similarity in 12-lead ECG waveforms from one laboratory with those of another or for describing such comparisons in the literature are lacking. Two waveform comparison metrics, the correlation coefficient (CORR) and the mean absolute deviation (MAD), have been evaluated to quantify the similarity of 12-lead ECG waveforms during VT and pace mapping objectively. It has been suggested that an automated objective interpretation can have some advantage to qualitative interpretation. Although CORR is more commonly used, MAD is more sensitive to differences in waveform amplitude. The most common human error is not appreciating subtle amplitude or precordial lead transition differences between the ECG patterns. It is important to note that such subtle differences in multiple leads can be reflected in a single quantitative number.

The MAD score grades 12-lead ECG waveform similarity as a single number ranging from 0% (identical) to 100% (completely different). A MAD score of up to 12% was 93% sensitive and 75% specific for a successful ablation site (see Fig. 23-11). It is not surprising that the MAD score is more sensitive than specific; characteristics other than a 12-lead ECG match are necessary for successful ablation, including catheter-tissue contact, catheter orientation, and tissue heating. MAD scores higher than 12%, and certainly higher than 15% (100% negative predictive value), suggest sufficient dissimilarity between the pace map and clinical tachycardia to dissuade ablation at that site. MAD scores of up to 12% should be considered an excellent match, and ablation at these sites is warranted if catheter contact and stability are adequate.

S-QRS INTERVAL DURING PACE MAPPING

Ventricular pacing in normal myocardium is associated with an S-QRS interval shorter than 20 milliseconds. On the other hand, an S-QRS interval longer than 40 milliseconds is consistent with slow conduction from the pacing site and is typically associated with abnormal fractionated electrograms recorded from that site. Thus, pace mapping can provide a measure of slow conduction, as indicated by the S-QRS interval. For post-MI VTs, at sites at which the reentrant wavefront exits the scar, pace mapping is expected to produce a QRS configuration similar to that of the VT. Pace mapping at sites more proximally located in the isthmus should also produce a similar QRS complex, but with a longer S-QRS interval. The S-QRS interval lengthens progressively as the pacing site is moved along the isthmus, a finding consistent with pacing progressively farther from the exit. Therefore, parts of VT reentry circuit isthmuses can be traced during NSR by combining both the QRS morphology and the S-QRS delay from pace mapping in anatomical maps. This works well when pacing is performed during tachycardia, at which time wavefront propagation is constrained in one direction through a corridor bounded by barriers that can be anatomically or functionally determined. However, pace mapping at the same sites during sinus rhythm can yield different results because the barriers may not exist then, the preferential direction of propagation may not be the same as during tachycardia, or both. This is especially true for pacing at circuit entrance sites (Fig. 5-23). It is likely that pacing sites with long S-QRS delays are in an isthmus adjacent to regions of conduction block. However, this isthmus can be part of the reentrant circuit or a bystander.[4]

Mapping Procedure

Initially, the exact morphology of the tachycardia complex should be determined and used as a template for pace mapping. For VT, QRS morphology during the tachycardia should be inspected in all 12 surface ECG leads. For AT, determining the morphology of the P wave during the tachycardia can be challenging, and proper interpretation of discrete changes in P wave shape is limited by its low voltage and distortion or masking by the preceding ST segment and T wave. Therefore, the P wave during AT should be assessed using multiple ECG leads, in addition to the intracardiac electrogram activation sequence. Delivery of a vesicular extrastimulus (or a train of ventricular pacing) to advance ventricular activation and repolarization can allow careful distinction of the P wave onset and morphology. Using multiple intraatrial catheters (e.g., Halo and CS catheters) can provide more intracardiac atrial electrograms that are useful for comparing the paced and tachycardia atrial activation sequence.[4]

Pace mapping during tachycardia (at a pacing CL 20 to 40 milliseconds shorter than the tachycardia CL) is preferable whenever possible, because it facilitates rapid comparison of tachycardia and paced complexes at the end of the pacing train in a simultaneously displayed 12-lead ECG. If sustained tachycardia cannot be induced, mapping is performed during spontaneous nonsustained runs or ectopic beats. In this setting, the pacing CL and coupling intervals of the extrastimuli should match those of spontaneous ectopy. For atrial pace mapping, it is unclear whether the conduction pattern of an atrial stimulus depends on the pacing CL; in fact, some have suggested that it is not mandatory to pace exactly at the same tachycardia CL to reproduce a similar atrial sequence.

Pace mapping is preferably performed with unipolar stimuli (10 mA, 2 milliseconds) from the distal electrode of the mapping catheter (cathode) and an electrode in the inferior vena cava (anode), or with closely spaced bipolar pacing at twice diastolic threshold to eliminate far-field stimulation effects.

The resulting 12-lead ECG morphology is compared with that of the tachycardia. ECG recordings should be reviewed at the same gain and filter settings and at a paper-sweep speed of 100 mm/sec. It is often helpful to display all 12 ECG leads side by side in review windows on screen, as well as a printout of regular 12-lead ECGs for side-by-side comparison on paper. The greater is the degree of concordance between the morphology during pacing and tachycardia, the closer the catheter will be to the site of origin of the tachycardia. Concordance occurring in 12 of 12 leads on the surface ECG is indicative of the site of origin of the tachycardia.

For mapping macroreentrant VT circuits, evaluation of the S-QRS interval, the interval from the pacing stimulus to the onset of the earliest QRS on the 12-lead ECG, is of value. The reentry circuit exit, which is more likely to be at the border of the infarct and close to the normal myocardium, often has a short S-QRS interval during pace mapping during NSR even though it is a desirable target for ablation. A delay between the pacing stimulus and QRS onset is consistent with slow conduction away from the pacing site; this can indicate a greater likelihood that the pacing site is in a reentry circuit. This method can be useful for initially screening sites during NSR.

Clinical Implications

Pace mapping is typically used to confirm the results of activation mapping. It can be of great help, especially when the tachycardia is difficult to induce. The highest benefit of pace mapping has been found in focal tachycardias, especially in idiopathic VT.[13]

For macroreentrant VT, pace mapping remains at best a corroborative method of localizing the isthmus critical to the reentrant circuit. It can be used to focus initial mapping efforts to regions likely to contain the reentrant circuit exit or abnormal conduction, but it may not be sufficiently specific or sensitive to be the sole guide for ablation. Pace mapping can also be used in conjunction with substrate mapping when other mapping techniques are not feasible, so that it can provide information on where ablation can be directed. Pace mapping has advantages over activation mapping in that induction of VT is not required; thus, it allows identification of the site of origin when the induced VT is poorly tolerated or when VT is not inducible by EP techniques but the QRS morphology from a prior 12-lead ECG during VT is available.[4]

Limitations

An optimal spatial pace mapping resolution requires a short maximum distance between two points generating a similar ECG configuration. Usually, the spatial resolution of unipolar stimulation is

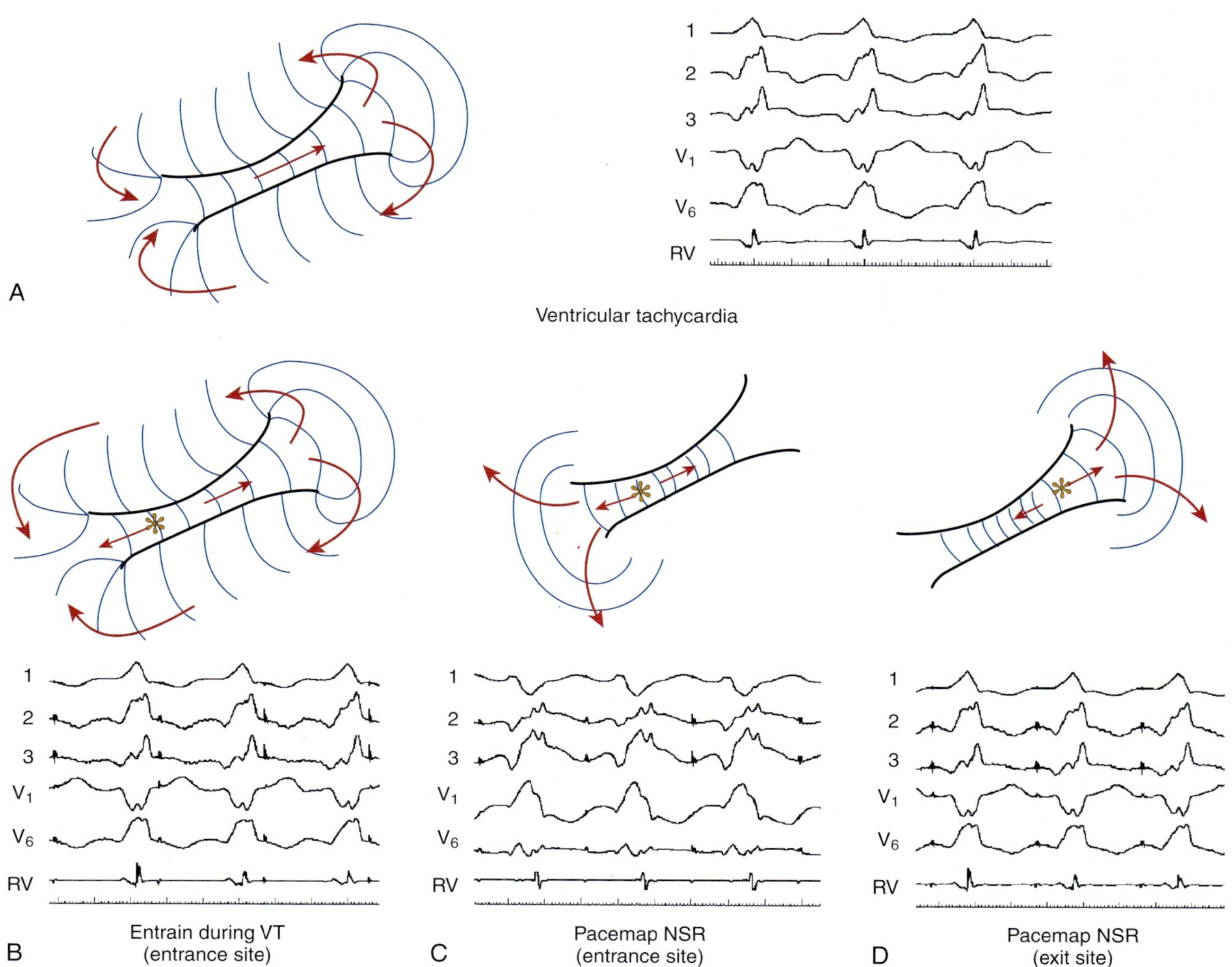

FIGURE 5-23 Pacing to verify ablation sites in reentrant ventricular tachycardia (VT). **A,** Five ECG leads of VT are shown with a figure-of-8 circuit with propagation of the reentrant wavefront (arrows); the protected diastolic corridor is also shown (short straight arrow). **B,** Pacing is performed during VT from a site near the entrance to the diastolic corridor (asterisk); the impulse must traverse a significant slow conduction zone before exiting to generate a QRS complex, resulting in a long S-QRS as shown. **C,** Pacing is performed at the same site as in **B**, but during sinus rhythm; the impulse exits in the opposite direction from **B** because it takes less time to propagate in this direction (short S-QRS). The resulting QRS complex is completely different, despite pacing at the same site. **D,** Pacing is performed during sinus rhythm from a site closer to the exit of the diastolic corridor. The QRS is the same as VT because the path taken is the same as in VT, and the S-QRS is short. NSR = normal sinus rhythm; RV = right ventricle.

5 mm or less. Spatial resolution deteriorates with wide electrodes, bipolar stimulation, and pacing at pathological areas. Spatial resolution worsens with bipolar stimulation by inducing electrical capture at both electrodes with variable contribution of the proximal electrode (generally anode) to depolarization. Such changes in paced ECG morphology that are potentially induced by bipolar pacing can be minimized by low pacing outputs and a small interelectrode distance (5 mm or less).

It is important to understand that morphology of single paced complexes can vary, depending on the coupling interval, and the paced complex morphology during overdrive pacing is affected by the pacing CL. Therefore, the coupling interval or CL of the template arrhythmia should be matched during pace mapping, especially during mapping of VTs. Similarly, spontaneous couplets from the same focus can have slight variations in QRS morphology that must be considered when seeking a pace match.

Pace mapping during post-MI VT has several other limitations. Some areas of conduction block are not anatomically determined but can be functional. Therefore, pacing within the diastolic corridor of the VT circuit during NSR can generate a completely different QRS complex from that of the VT (see Fig. 5-23). Consequently, during pace mapping, a QRS configuration different from VT does not reliably indicate that the pacing site is distant from the reentry circuit. On the other hand, pacing during NSR from sites attached to the reentrant circuit but not part of the circuit can occasionally produce a QRS morphology identical to that of the VT. The reason is that the stimulated wavefront can be physiologically forced to follow the same route of activation as the VT as long as pacing is carried out between the entrance and exit of the protected isthmus. At best, a pace map that matches the VT would identify only the exit site to the normal myocardium, and this site can be distant from the critical sites of the circuit required for ablation.

REFERENCES

1. Josephson M: Electrophysiologic investigation: technical aspects. In Josephson ME, editor: *Clinical cardiac electrophysiology*, ed 4, Philadelphia, 2008, Lippincott Williams & Wilkins, pp 1–19.
2. Stevenson WG, Soejima K: Recording techniques for clinical electrophysiology, *J Cardiovasc Electrophysiol* 16:1017–1022, 2005.
3. Sosa E, Scanavacca M: Epicardial mapping and ablation techniques to control ventricular tachycardia, *J Cardiovasc Electrophysiol* 16:449–452, 2005.
4. Markides V, Koa-Wing M, Peters N: Mapping and imaging. In Zipes DP, Jalife J, editors: *Cardiac electrophysiology: from cell to bedside*, ed 5, Philadelphia, 2009, Saunders, pp 897–904.
5. Tedrow U, Stevenson WG: Strategies for epicardial mapping and ablation of ventricular tachycardia, *J Cardiovasc Electrophysiol* 20:710–713, 2009.

6. d'Avila A: Epicardial catheter ablation of ventricular tachycardia, *Heart Rhythm* 5(Suppl): S73–S75, 2008.
7. Pak HN, Hwang C, Lim HE, et al: Hybrid epicardial and endocardial ablation of persistent or permanent atrial fibrillation: a new approach for difficult cases, *J Cardiovasc Electrophysiol* 18:917–923, 2007.
8. Josephson ME: Recurrent ventricular tachycardia. In Josephson ME, editor: *Clinical cardiac electrophysiology*, ed 4, Philadelphia, 2008, Lippincott Williams & Wilkins, pp 446–642.
9. Deo R, Berger R: The clinical utility of entrainment pacing, *J Cardiovasc Electrophysiol* 20:466–470, 2009.
10. Miyazaki H, Stevenson WG, Stephenson K, et al: Entrainment mapping for rapid distinction of left and right atrial tachycardias, *Heart Rhythm* 3:516–523, 2006.
11. Esato M, Hindricks G, Sommer P, et al: Color-coded three-dimensional entrainment mapping for analysis and treatment of atrial macroreentrant tachycardia, *Heart Rhythm* 6: 349–358, 2009.
12. Santucci PA, Varma N, Cytron J, et al: Electroanatomic mapping of postpacing intervals clarifies the complete active circuit and variants in atrial flutter, *Heart Rhythm* 6:1586–1595, 2009.
13. Azegami K, Wilber DJ, Arruda M, et al: Spatial resolution of pacemapping and activation mapping in patients with idiopathic right ventricular outflow tract tachycardia, *J Cardiovasc Electrophysiol* 16:823–829, 2005.
14. Brunckhorst CB, Delacretaz E, Soejima K, et al: Identification of the ventricular tachycardia isthmus after infarction by pace mapping, *Circulation* 110:652–659, 2004.

CHAPTER 6 Advanced Mapping and Navigation Modalities

Conventional radiofrequency (RF) ablation has revolutionized the treatment of many supraventricular tachycardias (SVTs) as well as ventricular tachycardias (VTs). Success in stable arrhythmias with predictable anatomical locations or characteristics identifying endocardial electrograms, such as idiopathic VT, atrioventricular nodal reentrant tachycardia (AVNRT), atrioventricular reentrant tachycardia (AVRT), or typical atrial flutter (AFL), has approached 90% to 99%. However, as interest has turned to a broad array of more complex arrhythmias, including some atrial tachycardias (ATs), many forms of intraatrial reentry, most VTs, and atrial fibrillation (AF), ablation of such arrhythmias continues to pose a major challenge. This stems in part from the limitations of fluoroscopy and conventional catheter-based mapping techniques to localize arrhythmogenic substrates that are removed from fluoroscopic landmarks and the lack of characteristic electrographic patterns.

Newer mapping systems have transformed the clinical electrophysiology (EP) laboratory, have enabled physicians to overcome some of the limitations of conventional mapping, and have offered new insights into arrhythmia mechanisms. These newer systems are aimed at improving the resolution, three-dimensional (3-D) spatial localization, and rapidity of acquisition of cardiac activation maps. These systems use novel approaches to determine the 3-D location of the mapping catheter accurately, and local electrograms are acquired using conventional, well-established methods. Recorded data of the catheter location and associated intracardiac electrogram at that location are used to reconstruct in real time a representation of the 3-D geometry of the chamber, color-coded with relevant EP information.

The application of these various techniques for mapping of specific arrhythmias is described elsewhere in this text, as are the details of the diagnosis, mapping, and treatment of specific arrhythmias.

Basket Catheter Mapping

Fundamental Concepts

The basket catheter mapping system consists of a basket catheter (Constellation, EPT, Inkster, Mich.), a conventional ablation catheter, the Astronomer (Boston Scientific, Natick, Mass.), and a mapping system.

The basket catheter consists of an open-lumen catheter shaft with a collapsible, basket-shaped, distal end. Currently, baskets are composed of 64 platinum-iridium ring electrodes mounted on eight equidistant, flexible, self-expanding nitinol splines (metallic arms; see Fig. 4-4). Each spline contains eight 1.5-mm electrodes equally spaced at 4 or 5 mm apart, depending on the size of the basket catheter used. Each spline is identified by a letter (from A to H) and each electrode by a number (distal 1 to proximal 8). The basket catheter is constructed of a superelastic material to allow passive deployment of the array catheter and optimize endocardial contact. The size of the basket catheter used depends on the dimensions of the chamber to be mapped, and it requires antecedent evaluation (usually by echocardiogram) to ensure proper size selection.

The Astronomer is used for navigation with the ablation-mapping catheter inside the basket catheter. This system consists of a switching-locating device and a laptop computer with proprietary software. The device and the laptop communicate on a standard RS-232 interface. The device delivers AC current (32 kHz, 320 mA) between the ablation catheter tip electrode and a reference electrode (skin patch), and the resulting electrical potentials are sensed at each basket catheter electrode. On the basis of the sensed voltages at each of the basket catheter electrodes, the Astronomer device determines whether the roving electrode is in close proximity to a basket catheter electrode and lights the corresponding electrodes on a representation of the basket catheter displayed on the laptop.

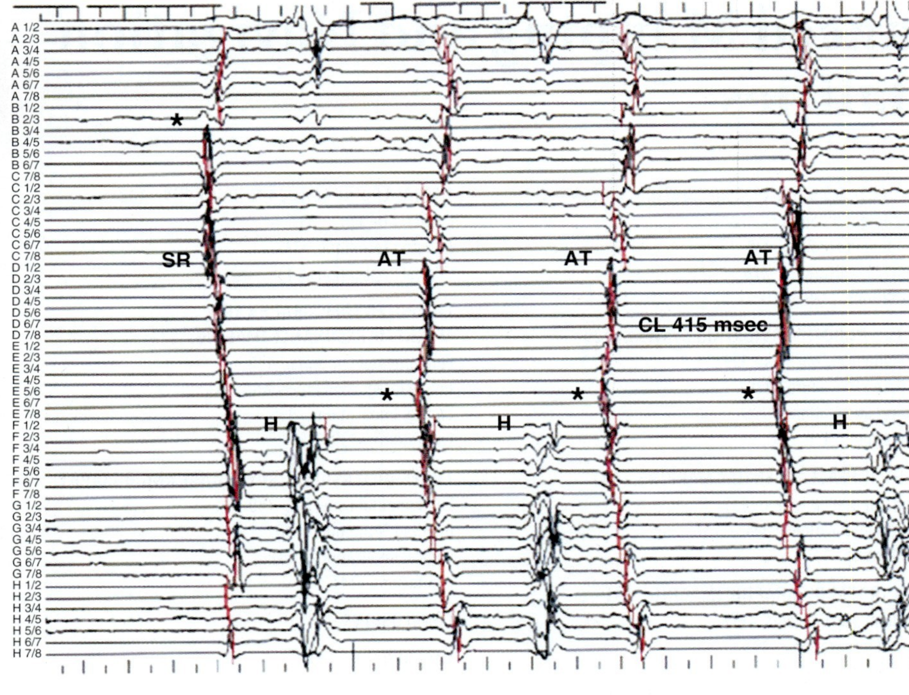

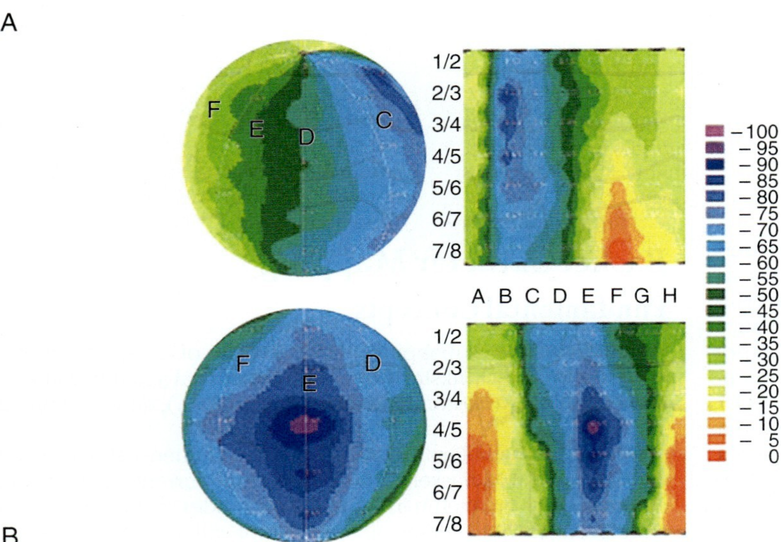

FIGURE 6-1 Basket catheter mapping during focal atrial tachycardia (AT). **A,** Simultaneous recordings of the surface ECG leads I and aVF and 56 bipolar electrograms from the basket catheter in a patient with focal AT. The first beat is a sinus beat. The next three beats are tachycardia beats. His bundle (H) potential is recorded in electrode pairs F2/3 and F3/4. The earliest spot of activation during sinus rhythm (SR) and AT is shown (asterisks). Spline A was located in the anterolateral right atrium (RA), splines B and C in the lateral region, splines D and E in the posterior region, and splines G and H across the tricuspid valve. The activation times are marked with red bars. **B, Upper panel,** Animated map of the SR beats. **Lower panel,** Animated map of the AT beats. Planar and three-dimensional options are shown. During SR, the impulse emerged in the high lateral area (spline B1-2) and propagated rapidly down the lateral wall. The complete activation of the RA took 85 milliseconds. During focal AT, the earliest activity emerged in the midposterior wall (spline E4-5). The activation sequence of the RA was entirely different from that of SR. The complete activation of the RA took 95 milliseconds. CL = cycle length. *(From Zrenner B, Ndrepepa G, Schneider M, et al: Computer-assisted animation of atrial tachyarrhythmias recorded with a 64-electrode basket catheter. J Am Coll Cardiol 34:2051, 1999.)*

The mapping system consists of an acquisition module connected to a computer, which is capable of simultaneously processing bipolar electrograms from the basket catheter, 16 bipolar-unipolar electrogram signals, a 12-lead ECG, and a pressure signal. Color-coded activation maps are reconstructed on-line. The color-coded animation images simplify the analysis of multielectrode recordings and help establish the relation between activation patterns and anatomical structures (Fig. 6-1). The electrograms and activation maps are displayed on a computer monitor, and the acquired signals can be stored on optical disk for off-line analysis. Activation marks are generated automatically with a peak or slope (dV/dt) algorithm, and activation times are then edited manually as needed.

Mapping Procedure

The size of the cardiac chamber of interest is initially evaluated, usually with echocardiography, to help select the appropriate size of the basket catheter. The collapsed basket catheter is advanced under fluoroscopic guidance through a long sheath into the chamber of interest; the catheter is then expanded (Fig. 6-2). Electrical-anatomical relations are determined by fluoroscopically identifiable markers (spline A has one marker and spline B has two markers located near the shaft of the basket catheter) and by the electrical signals recorded from certain electrodes (e.g., ventricular, atrial, or His bundle electrograms), which can help identify the location of those particular splines.

From the 64 electrodes, 64 unipolar signals and 32 to 56 bipolar signals can be recorded (by combining electrodes 1-2, 3-4, 5-6, 7-8, or 1-2, 2-3 until 7-8 electrodes are on each spline). Color-coded activation maps can be reconstructed (see Fig. 6-1). The concepts of activation mapping discussed earlier are then used to determine the site of origin of the tachycardia.

The Astronomer navigation system permits precise and reproducible guidance of the ablation catheter tip electrode to targets identified by the basket catheter. Without the use of this navigation system, it is often difficult to identify the alphabetical order of the splines by fluoroscopic guidance.

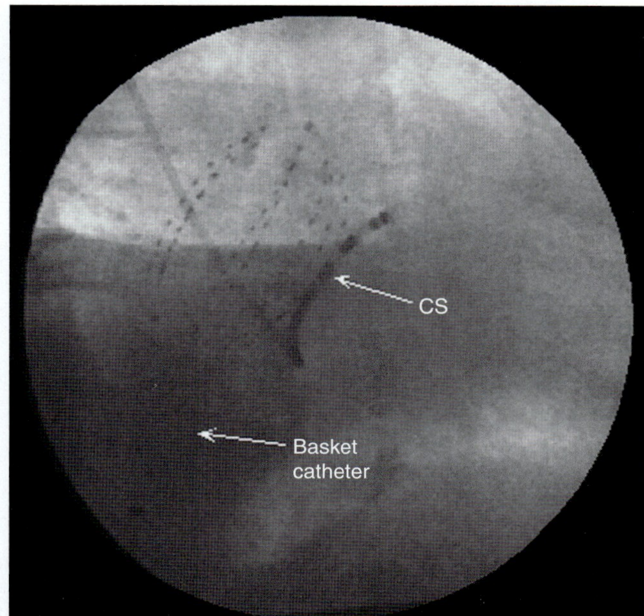

FIGURE 6-2 Fluoroscopic appearance of the basket catheter in the right atrium (right anterior oblique view). Note the radiopaque electrodes on the splines of the basket catheter. CS = coronary sinus.

The electrograms recorded from the basket catheter can be used to monitor changes in the activation sequence in real time and thereby indicate the effects of ablation as lesions are created. The capacity of pacing from most basket electrodes allows the evaluation of activation patterns, pace mapping, and entrainment mapping.

Clinical Implications

The multielectrode endocardial mapping system allows simultaneous recording of electrical activation from multiple sites and fast reconstruction of endocardial activation maps. This can limit the time endured in tachycardia compared with single point mapping techniques without the insertion of multiple electrodes. It also facilitates endocardial mapping of hemodynamically unstable or nonsustained tachycardias. Importantly, the recording of only a single beat can be sufficient to enable analysis of the arrhythmogenic substrate.

Endocardial mapping with a multielectrode basket catheter has been shown to be feasible and safe for various arrhythmias, including AT, AFL, VT, and pulmonary vein (PV) isolation. However, in view of more advanced mapping systems, and because of significant limitations of the current basket catheters, its use has been limited.

Limitations

Because of its poor spatial resolution, the basket catheter in its current iteration has demonstrated only limited clinical usefulness for guiding ablation of reentrant atrial or ventricular arrhythmias. The relatively large interelectrode spacing in available catheters prevents high-resolution reconstruction of the tachycardia and is generally not sufficient for a catheter-based ablation procedure, given the small size and precise localization associated with RF lesions. In addition, the quality of recordings is critically dependent on proper selection of the basket size. Resolution is limited to the proportion of electrodes in contact with the endocardium and by unequal deployment and spacing of the splines. Unfortunately, the electrode array does not expand to provide adequate contact with the entire cardiac chamber; therefore, good electrode contact at all sites on the endocardium is difficult to ensure because of irregularities in the cardiac chamber surface, so that areas crucial to arrhythmia circuit or focus may not be recorded. Moreover, regions such as the right atrial (RA) and left atrial (LA) appendages and cavotricuspid isthmus are incompletely covered by the basket catheter. As a result, arrhythmia substrates involving these structures are not recorded by the basket catheter.

Voltage, duration, and late potential maps are not provided by this mapping approach. Additionally, basket catheter mapping does not permit immediate correlation of activation times to precise anatomical sites, and a second mapping-ablation catheter is still required to be manipulated to the site identified for more precise mapping and localization of the target for ablation, as well as for RF energy delivery. Basket catheters also have limited torque capabilities and limited maneuverability, which hamper correct placement, and they can abrade the endocardium.

Carbonizations occasionally observed after ablation on the splines of the basket catheter can potentially cause embolism. Carbonizations, which appear as dark material attached to the basket catheter electrodes or splines, are thought to be caused by the concentration of RF energy on the thin splines that results in very high local temperatures that induce denaturization of proteins. Carbonization can be greatly diminished with the use of an irrigated tip catheter, as opposed to conventional ablation catheters.

HIGH-DENSITY MAPPING CATHETER

One study evaluated a mapping approach for AT that uses a novel high-density multielectrode mapping catheter (PentaRay, Biosense Webster, Inc., Diamond Bar, Calif.).[1] This 7 Fr steerable catheter (180 degrees of unidirectional flexion) has 20 electrodes distributed over 5 soft, radiating spines (1-mm electrodes separated by 4-4-4 or 2-6-2 mm interelectrode spacing), thus allowing splaying of the catheter to cover a surface diameter of 3.5 cm. The spines have been given alphabetical nomenclature (A to E), and spines A and B are recognized by radiopaque markers (Fig. 6-3).[1]

Localization of the atrial focus can be performed during tachycardia or atrial ectopy.[1] Guided by the ECG appearance, the catheter is sequentially applied to the endocardial surface in various atrial regions to allow rapid activation mapping. By identifying the earliest site of activation around the circumference of the high-density catheter, vector mapping is performed, moving the catheter and applying it to the endocardium in the direction of earliest activation (outer bipoles) to identify the tachycardia origin and bracket activation (i.e., demonstrating later activation in all surrounding regions).

The high-density mapping catheter can offer several potential advantages.[1] In contrast to the basket catheter, which provides a global density of mapping but limited localized resolution, the high-density mapping catheter allows splaying of the spines against the endocardial surface to achieve high-density contact mapping and better localized resolution.[1]

EnSite Noncontact Mapping System

Fundamental Concepts

The noncontact mapping system (EnSite 3000, St. Jude Medical, Inc., St. Paul, Minn.) consists of a catheter-mounted multielectrode array (MEA), which serves as the probe, a custom-designed amplifier system, a computer workstation used to display 3-D maps of cardiac electrical activity, and a conventional ablation catheter.[2,3]

The MEA catheter consists of a 7.5-mL ellipsoid balloon mounted on a 9 Fr catheter around which is woven a braid of 64 insulated 0.003-mm-diameter wires (Fig. 6-4). Each wire has a 0.025-mm break in insulation that serves as a noncontact unipolar electrode.[3] The system acquires more than 3000 noncontact unipolar electrograms from all points in the chamber simultaneously. The unipolar signals are recorded using a ring electrode located on the shaft of the array catheter as a reference. The raw far-field EP data acquired by the array catheter are fed into a multichannel

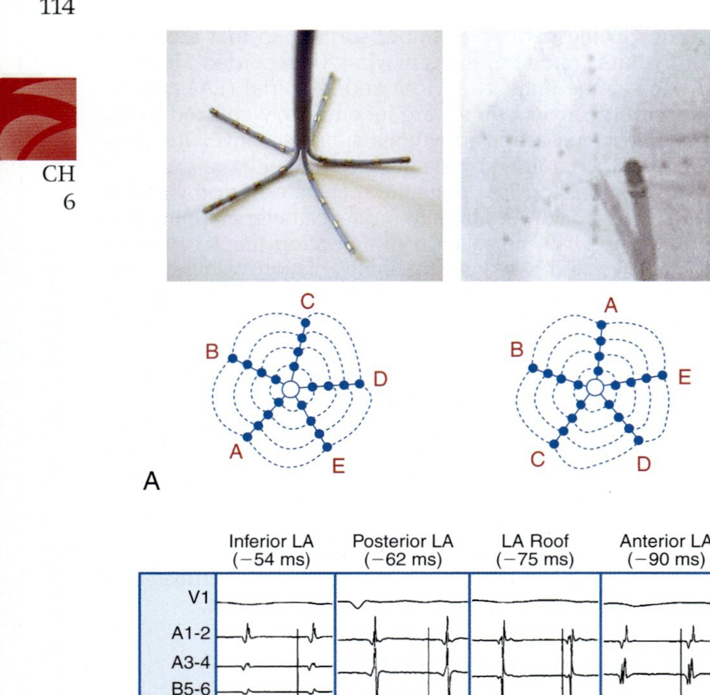

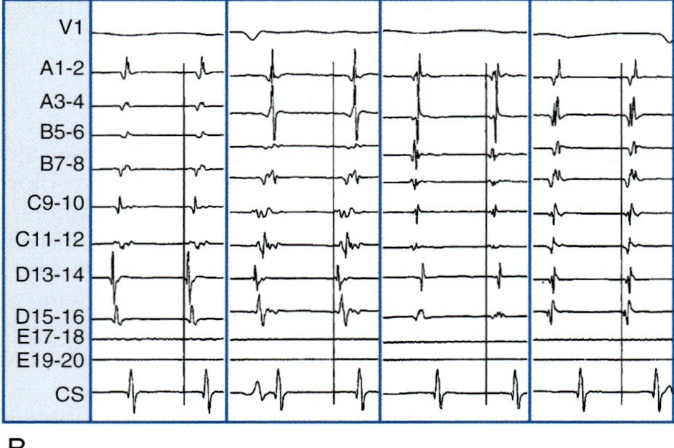

FIGURE 6-3 The high-density mapping catheter. **A,** Picture and a fluoroscopic image of the high-density mapping catheter. Below each figure is a schematic representation indicating the orientation of the catheter spines. Note that the marker band on spine A is between electrodes 1 and 2, and on spine B it is between electrodes 2 and 3. **B,** Vector mapping using the high-density mapping catheter to identify the earliest site of activation of focal atrial tachycardia. Shown is the catheter in four distinct locations within the left atrium (LA). Mapping is commenced along the inferior LA, where the earliest activation is 54 milliseconds ahead of the coronary sinus (CS). The catheter is moved in the direction of the spine demonstrating the earliest activation (spine D). In the midposterior LA, activation precedes the coronary sinus (CS) by 62 milliseconds. Again, the catheter is moved in the earliest direction (spine D) to a more cranial location on the LA roof. At this site, activation precedes the CS by 75 milliseconds. At this site, spine B, which is slightly anterior, is the earliest. Moving the catheter in the direction of spine B to the anterosuperior LA demonstrates the site with the earliest endocardial activation (90 milliseconds ahead of the CS, which was 40 milliseconds ahead of the P wave). *(From Sanders P, Hocini M, Jais P, et al: Characterization of focal atrial tachycardia using high-density mapping, J Am Coll Cardiol. 46:2088, 2005.)*

recorder and amplifier system that also has 16 channels for conventional contact catheters, 12 channels for the surface ECG, and pressure channels. Using data from the 64-electrode array catheter suspended in the heart chamber, the computer uses sophisticated algorithms to compute an inverse solution to determine the activation sequence on the endocardial surface.

The EnSite 3000 mapping system is based on the premise that endocardial activation creates a chamber voltage field that obeys the Laplace's equation. Therefore, when one 3-D surface of known geometry is placed within another of known geometry, if the electrical potential on one surface is known, the potential on the other can be calculated.[3] Because the geometry of the balloon catheter is known, and the geometry of the cardiac chamber can be

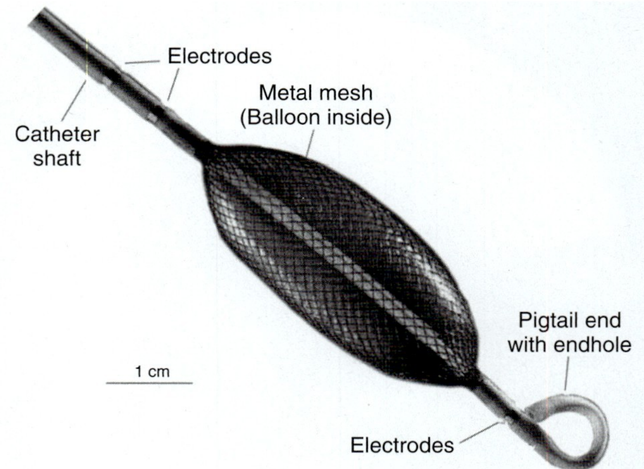

FIGURE 6-4 The multielectrode array for noncontact endocardial mapping.

reconstructed during the procedure (see later), endocardial surface potential can then be determined once the potentials over the balloon catheter are recorded. Using this concept, the raw far-field EP data acquired by the array catheter, which are generally lower in amplitude and frequency than the source potential of the endocardium itself and therefore have limited usefulness, are mathematically enhanced and resolved. The solution to the inverse Laplace's equation using the boundary element method predicts how a remotely detected signal by the MEA would have appeared at its source, the endocardial surface, so that electrograms are reconstructed at endocardial sites in the absence of physical electrode contact at those locations (virtual electrograms). Once the potential field has been established, more than 3000 activation points can be displayed as computed electrograms or as isopotential maps. The activation time at each endocardial site is determined by taking the time instant with maximum negative time derivative (−dV/dt) on the electrogram.

The system can locate any conventional mapping-ablation catheter in space with respect to the array catheter (and thus with respect to the cardiac chamber being mapped).[3] A low-current (5.68 kHz) locator signal is passed between the contact catheter electrode being located and reference electrodes on the noncontact MEA. This creates a potential gradient across the array electrodes, which is then used to position the source. This locator system is also used to construct the 3-D computer model of the endocardium (virtual endocardium) that is required for the reconstruction of endocardial electrograms and isopotential maps. This model is acquired by moving a conventional contact catheter around the endocardial surface of the cardiac chamber; the system collects the location information, thus building up a series of coordinates for the endocardium and generating a patient-specific, anatomically contoured model of its geometry. During geometry creation, only the most distant points visited by the roving catheter are recorded to ignore those detected when the catheter is not in contact with the endocardial wall.

Using mathematical techniques to process potentials recorded from the array, the system is able to reconstruct more than 3000 unipolar electrograms simultaneously and superimpose them onto the virtual endocardium, thus producing isopotential maps with a color range representing voltage amplitudes. Additionally, the locator signal can be used to display and track the position of any catheter on the endocardial model (virtual endocardium) and allows marking of anatomical locations identified using fluoroscopy and electrographic characteristics. During catheter ablation procedures, the locator system is used in real time to navigate the ablation catheter to sites of interest identified from the isopotential color maps, catalog the position of RF energy applications on the virtual endocardium, and facilitate revisitation of sites of interest by the ablation catheter.[2]

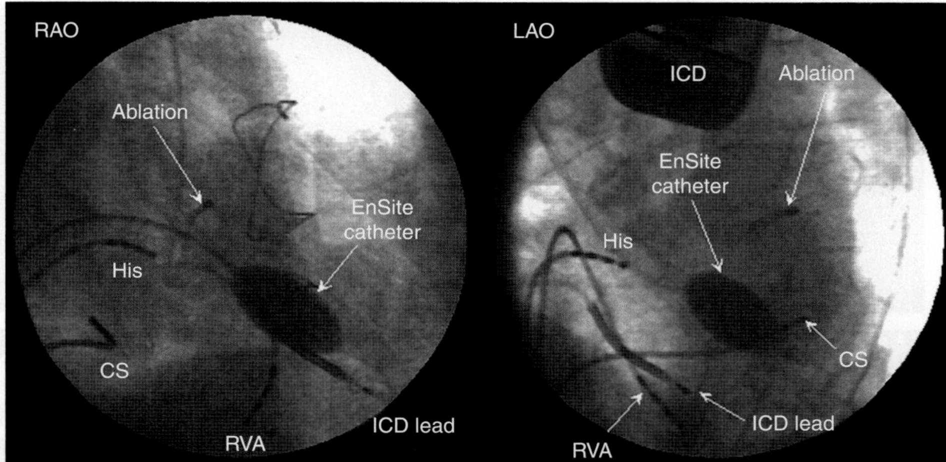

FIGURE 6-5 Fluoroscopic views of noncontact mapping catheter (EnSite, St. Jude Medical, Inc., St. Paul, Minn.) situated in the left ventricle (LV). CS = coronary sinus; ICD = implantable cardioverter-defibrillator; LAO = left anterior oblique; RAO = right anterior oblique; RVA = right ventricular apex.

In addition, the most recent version of the EnSite software provides the capability of point-to-point contact mapping, to allow the creation of activation and voltage maps by acquiring serial contact electrograms and displaying them on the virtual endocardium (see later). This is useful for adding detail, familiarity, and validation of the information obtained by the noncontact method.[4]

Mapping Procedure

The EnSite 3000 system requires placing a 9 Fr MEA and a mapping-ablation catheter.[3] To create a map, the balloon catheter is advanced over a 0.035-inch guidewire under fluoroscopic guidance into the cardiac chamber of interest. For RA arrhythmias, the guidewire is advanced into the SVC and the balloon is deployed in the upper third of the RA for tachycardia originating in the SVC, in the middle third for ectopic AT, and in the lower third for typical AFL. For LA arrhythmias, the guidewire is advanced into the left superior PV, and the balloon is deployed in the middle of the LA. For right ventricular (RV) arrhythmias, the guidewire is advanced into the pulmonary artery, and the balloon is deployed close to the RV outflow tract (RVOT) or in the middle of the RV. The balloon can be filled with contrast dye, thus permitting it to be visualized fluoroscopically (Fig. 6-5). The balloon is positioned in the center of the cardiac chamber of interest and does not come in contact with the walls of the chamber being mapped. In addition, the position of the array in the chamber must be secured to avoid significant movement that would invalidate the electrical and anatomical information. The array must be positioned as closely as possible (and in direct line of sight through the blood pool) to the endocardial surface being mapped, because the accuracy of the map is sensitive to the distance between the center of the balloon and the endocardium being mapped.[2,4,5]

During the use of this mapping modality, systemic anticoagulation is critical to avoid thromboembolic complications. Intravenous heparin is usually given to maintain the activated clotting time longer than 250 seconds for right-sided and longer than 300 seconds for left-sided mapping.

A conventional (roving) deflectable mapping catheter is also positioned in the chamber being mapped and used to collect geometry information. The mapping catheter is initially moved to known anatomical locations, which are tagged. A detailed geometry of the chamber is then reconstructed by moving the mapping catheter and tracing the contour of the endocardium (using the locator technology). To create detailed geometry, attempts must be made to make contact with as much endocardium as possible. This requires maneuvering on all sides of the array, which can be challenging and can require decreasing the profile of the balloon by withdrawing a few milliliters of fluid. This results in the rapid formation of a relatively accurate 3-D geometric model of the cardiac chamber. Creation of chamber geometry can be performed during sinus rhythm or tachycardia.[2,4]

Once the chamber geometry has been delineated, tachycardia is induced and mapping is started. The data acquisition process is performed automatically by the system, and all data for the entire chamber are acquired simultaneously. Following this, the segment must be analyzed by the operator to find the early activation during the tachycardia (Fig. 6-6).

The noncontact mapping system is capable of simultaneously reconstructing more than 3360 unipolar electrograms over the virtual endocardium. From these electrograms, isopotential or isochronal maps can be reconstructed (see Fig. 6-6). Because of the high density of data, color-coded isopotential maps are used to depict graphically regions that are depolarized, and wavefront propagation is displayed as a user-controlled 3-D "movie" (Videos 8 and 9). The color range represents voltage or timing of onset. The highest chamber voltage is at the site of origin of the electrical impulse. Although the electrode closest to the origin of the impulse is influenced the most, all the electrodes on the array catheter are influenced, the degree of influence diminishing with the distance between the electrode and each endocardial point.

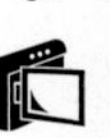

In addition, the system can simultaneously display as many as 32 electrograms as waveforms (see Fig. 6-6). Unipolar or bipolar electrograms (virtual electrograms) can be selected at any given interval of the tachycardia cycle by using the mouse from any part of the created geometry and displayed as waveforms as if from point, array, or plaque electrodes. The reconstructed electrograms are subject to the same electrical principles as contact catheter electrograms, because they contain far-field electrical information from the surrounding endocardium, as well as the underlying myocardium signal vector, and distance from measurement may affect the contribution to the electrogram. These selected unipolar waveforms are used to augment information obtained from the 3-D map by demonstrating the slope of depolarization, the presence of double potentials or fractionation, and differentiation of far-field signals from more relevant endocardial activation.[4]

In the unipolar electrogram, signals associated with high conduction velocity (e.g., the His-Purkinje system) possess a greater slope (–dV/dt), and thus are characterized by high-frequency spectral components (more than 32 Hz). Electrograms recorded in normally conducting atrial or ventricular myocardium possess spectral components in the midrange from 4 Hz to 16 Hz, whereas electrograms in regions of slow conduction are composed of lower frequency spectral components from 1 Hz to 4 Hz. Thus, the high-pass filter must be adjusted between 1 Hz and 32 Hz, helping to modulate the extent to which low-frequency signals are visible on the 3-D display. Identification of true local activation and its differentiation from the far-field signals are essential to successful utilization of noncontact mapping. The true local activation always shows

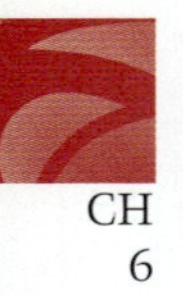

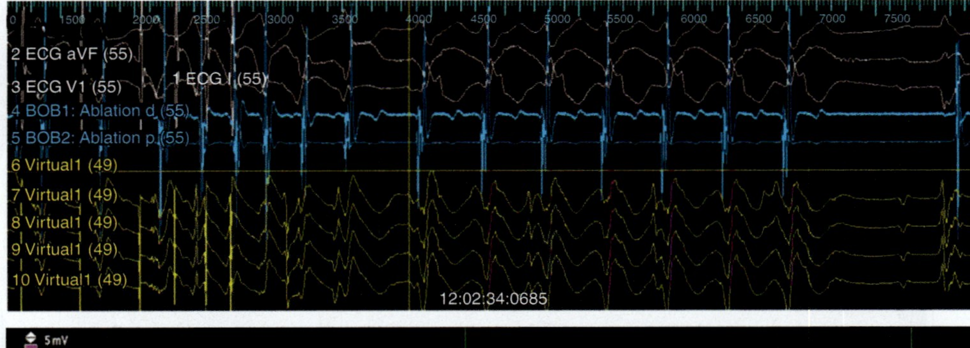

A

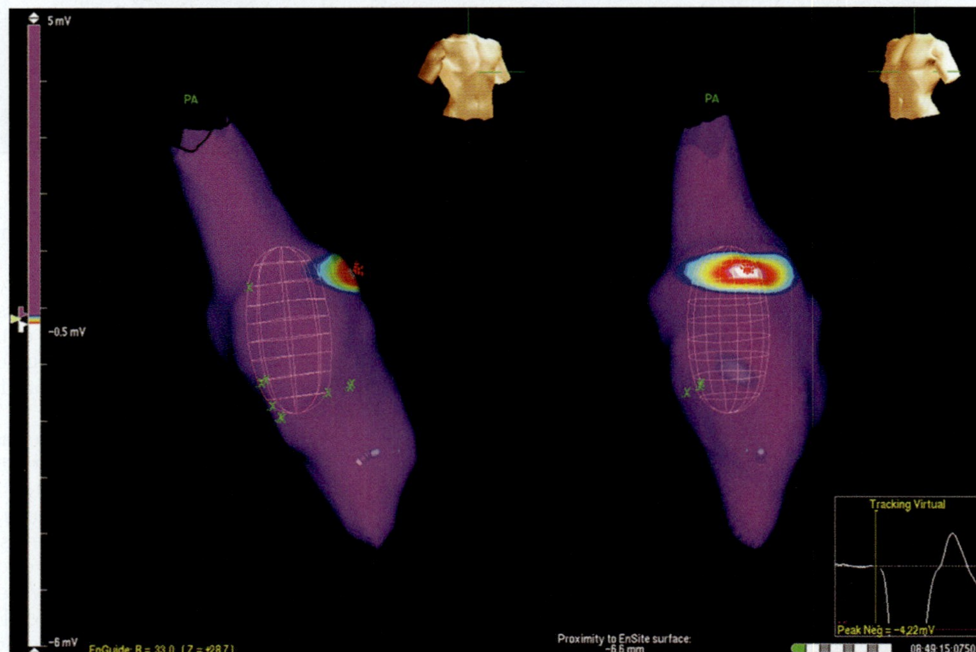

B

FIGURE 6-6 Noncontact mapping of idiopathic right ventricular outflow tract (RVOT) tachycardia. **A,** Right anterior oblique and right lateral views of color-coded isopotential map of RVOT activation during a single premature ventricular complex (PVC). **B,** Surface electrocardiographic (white) and intracardiac contact (blue) and virtual noncontact (yellow, V_{1-1} through V_{1-4}) electrograms are shown during the PVC. **Inset,** Virtual electrograms at the site of earliest activation (note the QS pattern).

advancement of isopotential lines, but far-field signals would show retraction of isopotential lines on the 3-D display when the whole electrograms are traced.[5]

Substrate mapping based on scar or diseased tissue has been introduced to the noncontact mapping technology. High-density voltage mapping of the atrial substrate is performed using the peak negative voltage of the reconstructed unipolar electrograms. Areas with slow conduction are identified along the reentrant circuit of the atypical AFL. An atrial substrate characterized by an abnormally low peak negative voltage can potentially predict areas with slow conduction during macroreentrant tachycardias, which would provide a substrate for reentry.[6]

Clinical Implications

The MEA has been successfully deployed in all four cardiac chambers by using a transvenous, transseptal, or retrograde transaortic approach to map atrial and ventricular tachyarrhythmias.

The biggest advantage of noncontact endocardial mapping is its ability to recreate the endocardial activation sequence from simultaneously acquired multiple data points over a few (theoretically one) tachycardia beats, without requiring sequential point-to-point acquisitions, thus obviating the need for prolonged tachycardia episodes that the patient might tolerate poorly. This technique can be used to map nonsustained arrhythmias, premature atrial complexes (PACs), premature ventricular complexes (PVCs), and irregular rhythms such as AF or polymorphic VT, and rhythms that are not hemodynamically stable, such as very rapid VT (see Fig. 6-6). The system generates isopotential maps of the endocardial surface at successive cross sections of time, and when these are animated, the spread of the depolarization wave can be visualized. These maps are particularly useful for identifying rapid breakthrough points and slowly conducting macroreentrant pathways, such as the critical slow pathways in ischemic VT or reentrant AT in patients with surgically corrected congenital heart disease. In macroreentrant tachycardias such as typical AFL or VT, the reentry circuit can be fully identifiable, along with other aspects, such as the slowing, narrowing, and splitting of activation wavefronts in the isthmus. The system can also map multiple cardiac cycles in real time, a method that discloses changes in the activation sequence from one beat to the next. Because mapping data are acquired without direct contact of conventional electrode catheters with the endocardium, the use of noncontact mapping can help avoid the mechanical induction of ectopic activity that is frequently seen during conventional mapping. An additional advantage of this system is that any catheter from any manufacturer can be used in conjunction with this mapping platform. Other useful features include radiation-free catheter navigation, revisitation of points of interest, and cataloging ablation points on the 3-D model.[2]

In complex substrate-related arrhythmias, the use of activation mapping alone may not be sufficient for rhythm analysis or identifying ablation targets. Substrate mapping based on scar or diseased tissue is of value in these cases. Although substrate mapping used to be relatively limited with the noncontact mapping technology (very low-amplitude signals may not be detected, particularly if the distance between the center of the balloon catheter and endocardial surface exceeds 40 mm), dynamic substrate mapping, which has been introduced, allows the creation of voltage maps from a single cardiac cycle (in contrast to the contact mapping system, in which the mapping catheter is moved point to point over the endocardial surface). Dynamic substrate mapping also provides the capability of identifying low-voltage areas, as well as fixed and functional block, on the virtual endocardium through noncontact methods, provided that points more than 40 mm from the electrode array are excluded from analysis. Combining substrate mapping with the ability of the noncontact system to assess activation over a broad area from a single beat may facilitate ablation of hemodynamically unstable or nonsustained macroreentrant tachycardias.[4,6,7]

Limitations

Because the geometry of the cardiac chamber is contoured at the beginning of the study during sinus rhythm, changes of the chamber size and contraction pattern during tachycardia or administration of medications (e.g., isoproterenol) can adversely affect the accuracy of the location of the endocardial electrograms. Moreover, because isopotential maps are predominantly used, ventricular repolarization must be distinguished from atrial depolarization and diastolic activity. Early diastole can be challenging to map during VT.[8]

The overall accuracy of the reconstructed electrograms decreases with the distance of the area mapped from the array catheter, thus creating problems in mapping large cardiac chambers. Virtual electrogram quality deteriorates at a distance of more than 4 cm from the array catheter and at polar regions. Therefore, the array must be positioned as closely as possible to the endocardial area of interest, and at times it can be necessary to reposition the array catheter to acquire adequate isopotential maps.

Only data segments up to a maximum of 10 seconds in length can be stored retroactively by the EnSite system once the record button has been pushed. Thus, continuous recording and storage of all segments of an arrhythmia are not possible at the time of evaluation of the arrhythmia maps. Therefore, some isolated PACs or PVCs that can be of interest during evaluation and mapping could be missed. In addition, the acquired geometry with the current version of software is somewhat distorted, requiring multiple set points to establish the origin and shape of complicated structures such as the LA appendage or PVs clearly. Otherwise, these structures can be lost in the interpolation among several neighboring points. In addition, synchronized mapping of multiple chambers requires multiple systems. Importantly, maps are highly sensitive to changes in filtering frequencies used in postprocessing analysis.

Sometimes it is difficult to manipulate the ablation catheter around the outside of the balloon, especially during mapping in the LA. Special attention and care also are necessary during placement of the large balloon electrode in a relatively small cardiac chamber. Another disadvantage is that the balloon catheter cannot be moved after completion of geometry creation because it will change the activation localization and result in distortion of isopotential maps.[5]

Although the risk of complications is low, aggressive anticoagulation measures because of balloon deployment in the cardiac chamber expose patients to potential bleeding complications.

CARTO Electroanatomical Mapping System

Fundamental Concepts

The CARTO mapping system (Biosense Webster, Inc.) consists of an ultralow magnetic field emitter, a magnetic field generator locator pad (placed beneath the operating table), an external reference patch (fixed on the patient's back), a deflectable 7 Fr quadripolar mapping-ablation catheter with a 4- or 8-mm tip and proximal 2-mm ring electrodes, location sensors inside the mapping-ablation catheter tip (the three location sensors are located orthogonally to each other and lie just proximal to the tip electrode, totally embedded within the catheter), a reference catheter (placed intracardially), a data processing unit, and a graphic display unit to generate the electroanatomical model of the chamber being mapped.

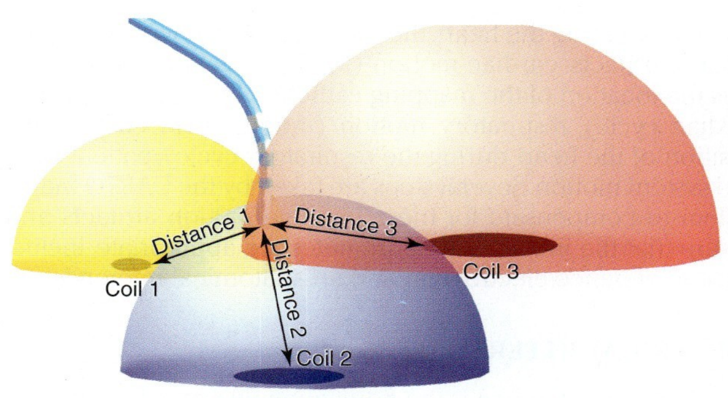

FIGURE 6-7 CARTO (Biosense Webster, Inc., Diamond Bar, Calif.) electroanatomical map setup. The three hemispheres represent fields from three different electromagnets situated beneath the patient. The catheter tip contains an element that is sensed by these fields, and this triangulating information is used to monitor the location and orientation of the catheter tip in the heart.

CARTO is a nonfluoroscopic mapping system that uses a special catheter to generate 3-D electroanatomical maps of the heart chambers. This system uses magnetic technology to determine the location and orientation of the mapping-ablation catheter accurately while simultaneously recording local electrograms from the catheter tip. By sampling electrical and spatial information from different endocardial sites, the 3-D geometry of the mapped chamber is reconstructed in real time and analyzed to assess the mechanism of arrhythmia and the appropriate site for ablation.[2]

Electroanatomical mapping is based on the premise that a metal coil generates an electrical current when it is placed in a magnetic field. The magnitude of the current depends on the strength of the magnetic field and the orientation of the coil in it. The CARTO mapping system uses a triangulation algorithm similar to that used by a global positioning system (GPS). The magnetic field emitter, mounted under the operating table, consists of three coils that generate a low-intensity magnetic field, approximately 0.05 to 0.2 gauss, which is a very small fraction of the magnetic field intensity inside a magnetic resonance imaging (MRI) machine (Fig. 6-7).

The sensor embedded proximal to the tip of a specialized mapping catheter detects the intensity of the magnetic field generated by each coil and allows for determination of its distance from each coil. These distances determine the area of theoretical spheres around each coil, and the intersection of these three spheres determines the location of the tip of the catheter. The accuracy of determination of the location is highest in the center of the magnetic field; therefore, it is important to position the location pad under the patient's chest. In addition to the x, y, and z coordinates of the catheter tip, the CARTO system can determine three orientation determinants—roll, yaw, and pitch—for the electrode at the catheter tip. The position and orientation of the catheter tip can be seen on the screen and monitored in real time as the catheter moves within the electroanatomical model of the chamber mapped. The catheter icon has four color bars (green, red, yellow, and blue), enabling the operator to view the catheter as it turns clockwise or counterclockwise. In addition, because the catheter always deflects in the same direction, each catheter will always deflect toward a single color. Hence, to deflect the catheter to a specific wall, the operator should first turn the catheter so that this color faces the desired wall.[2]

The unipolar and bipolar electrograms recorded by the mapping catheter at each endocardial site are archived within that positional context. Using this approach, local tissue activation at each successive recording site produces activation maps within the framework of the acquired surrogate geometry.

When mapping the heart, the system can deal with four types of motion artifacts: cardiac motion (the heart is in constant motion; thus the location of the mapping catheter changes throughout the cardiac cycle), respiratory motion (intrathoracic change in the position of the heart during the respiratory cycle), patient motion, and system motion. Several steps are taken by the CARTO mapping system to compensate for these possible motion artifacts and to ensure that the initial map coordinates are appropriate, including using a reference electrogram and an anatomical reference.

ELECTRICAL REFERENCE

The electrical reference is the fiducial marker on which the entire mapping procedure is based. The timing of the fiducial point is used to determine the activation timing in the mapping catheter in relation to the acquired points and to ensure collection of data during the same part of the cardiac cycle. It is therefore vital to the performance of the system. All the local activation timing information recorded by the mapping catheter at different anatomical locations during mapping (displayed on the completed 3-D map) is relative to this fiducial point, with the acquisition gated so that each point is acquired during the same part of the cardiac electrical signal (Video 10). It is important that the rhythm being mapped is monomorphic and the fiducial point is reproducible at each sampled site. The fiducial point is defined by the user by assigning a reference channel and an annotation criterion. The system has a great deal of flexibility in terms of choosing the reference electrogram and gating locations. Any surface ECG lead or intracardiac electrogram in bipolar or unipolar mode can serve as a reference electrogram. For the purpose of stability when intracardiac electrograms are selected, coronary sinus (CS) electrograms are usually chosen for mapping supraventricular rhythms, and an RV electrode or a surface ECG lead is commonly chosen as the electrical reference during mapping ventricular rhythms. Care must be taken to ensure that automatic sensing of the reference is reproducible and is not subject to oversensing in the case of annular electrograms (e.g., oversensing of a ventricular electrogram on the CS reference electrode during mapping an atrial rhythm). Any component of the reference electrogram may be chosen for a timing reference, including maximum (peak positive) deflection, minimum (peak negative) deflection, maximum upslope (dV/dt), or maximum downslope.[9,10]

ANATOMICAL REFERENCE

Once the mapping catheter is placed inside the heart, its location in relation to the fixed magnetic field sensors placed under the patient can be determined. However, several of the factors mentioned earlier, including a change in the patient's position during the procedure, can result in loss of orientation of the structures. To overcome the effect of motion artifacts, a reference catheter with a sensor similar to that of the mapping catheter is used. This reference catheter is fixed in its location inside the heart or on the body surface. The anatomical reference (location sensor) is typically placed in an adhesive reference patch secured on the patient's back. The fluoroscopic (anteroposterior view) location of the anatomical reference should be close to the cardiac chamber being mapped. Movement of the anatomical reference indicates movement of the patient's chest, which must be corrected to prevent distortion of the electroanatomical map.

The CARTO mapping system continuously calculates the position of the mapping catheter in relation to the anatomical reference, thus solving the problem of any possible motion artifacts. An intracardiac reference catheter has the advantage of moving with the patient's body and with the heart during the phases of respiration. However, the intracardiac reference catheter can change its position during the course of the procedure, especially during manipulation of the other catheters. It is therefore better to use an externally positioned reference patch strapped to the back of the patient's chest in the interscapular area. The movement of the ablation catheter is then tracked relative to the position of this reference. Should the location reference magnet or patch become displaced during the procedure, the original location is recorded by CARTO to allow proper repositioning.

WINDOW OF INTEREST

Defining an electrical window of interest is a crucial aspect in ensuring the accuracy of the initial map coordinates. The window of interest is defined as the time interval relative to the fiducial point during which the local activation time is determined (Fig. 6-8). Within this window, activation is considered early or late relative to the reference. The total length of the window of interest should not exceed the tachycardia cycle length (CL; usually 90% of the tachycardia CL; Videos 11 and 12). The boundaries are set relative to the reference electrogram. Thus, the window is defined by two intervals, one extending before the reference electrogram and the other after it. For macroreentrant circuits, the sensing window should approximate the tachycardia CL, and designating activation times in a circuit as early or late is arbitrary. In theory, a change in the window or reference would not change a macroreentrant circuit but only result in a phase shift of the map. If the activation window spans two adjacent beats of an arrhythmia, the resulting map can be ambiguous, lack coherency, and give rise to a spurious pattern of adjacent regions of early and late activation (see Fig. 6-8).[9,10]

LOCAL ACTIVATION TIME

Another important concept in CARTO mapping is determination of the local activation time. Once the reference electrogram, anatomical reference, and window of interest have been chosen, the mapping catheter is moved from point to point along the endocardial surface of the cardiac chamber being mapped (Fig. 6-9; see Video 10). These points can be acquired in a unipolar or bipolar configuration. These electrograms are analyzed using the principles of activation mapping discussed in Chapter 5. The local activation time at each sampled site is calculated as the time interval between the fiducial point on the reference electrogram and the corresponding local activation determined from the unipolar or bipolar local electrogram recorded from that site.[2]

CARTOMERGE

The CARTOMerge Module (Biosense Webster, Inc.) allows for images from a preacquired computed tomography (CT) angiogram or MRI scan to be integrated on the electroanatomical image of the cardiac chamber created with the CARTO system (Fig. 6-10).[11] CARTOMerge helps to guide real-time catheter ablation by using the detailed cardiac chamber anatomy acquired from the CT/MRI (see later discussion). These images have also been used in AF catheter ablation procedures to identify correctly the anatomy and location of the PVs, as well as other structures such as the esophagus (Video 13).

CARTOSOUND

The CARTOSound Image Integration Module (Biosense Webster, Inc.) incorporates the electroanatomical map to a map derived from intracardiac echocardiography (ICE) and allows for 3-D reconstruction of the cardiac chambers using real-time ICE. Echocardiographic imaging is performed using a 10 Fr phased-array transducer catheter incorporating a navigation sensor (SoundStar, Biosense Webster, Inc.) that records individual 90-degree sector image planes of the cardiac chamber of interest, including their location and orientation, to the CARTO workspace. A 3-D volume-rendered image is created by obtaining ECG-gated ICE images of the endocardial surface of the cardiac chamber of interest (Fig. 6-11). Following optimizing each image by adjusting frequency (5 to 10 MHz) and contrast, the chamber endocardial surfaces are identified (based on differences in the echo intensity of blood and tissue), and their contours are traced automatically, and

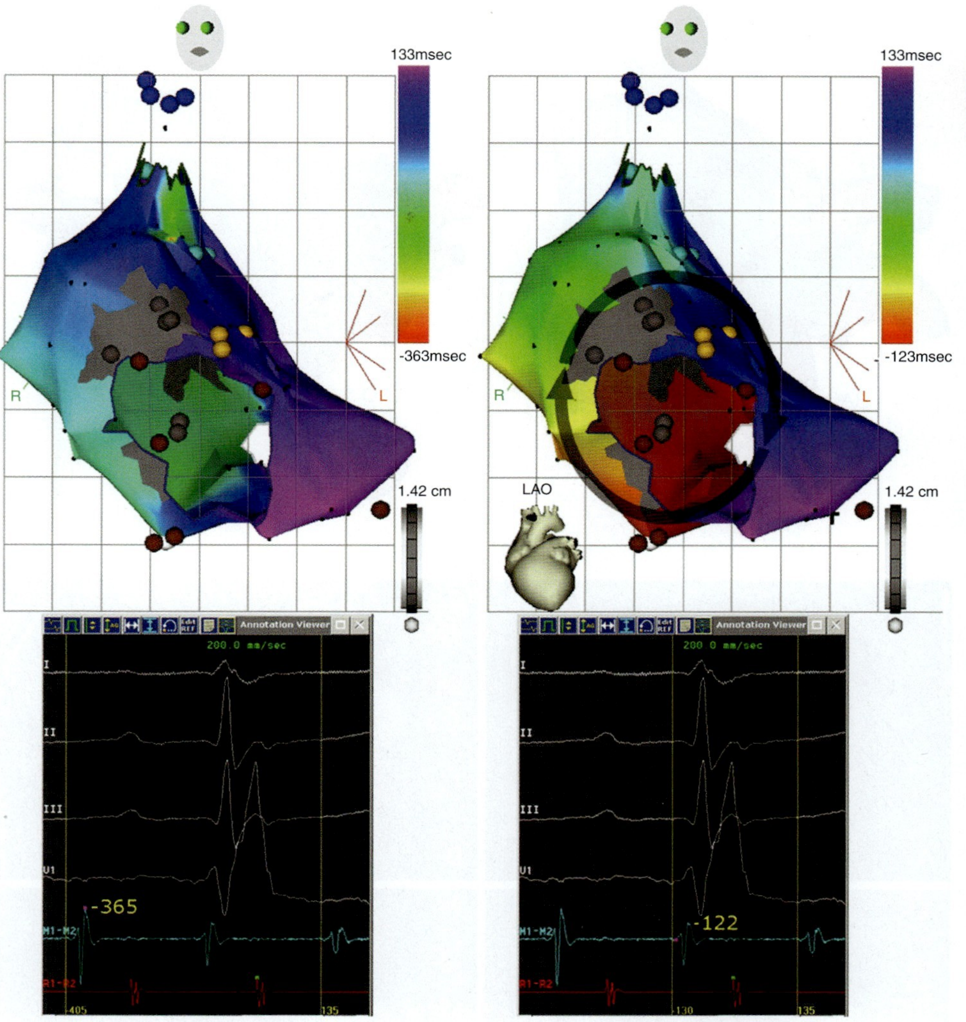

FIGURE 6-8 CARTO (Biosense Webster, Inc., Diamond Bar, Calif.) window of interest and influence on activation map. **Top,** Activation maps of macroreentrant typical atrial flutter (cycle length [CL], 268 milliseconds, with "clockwise" rotation around the tricuspid annulus). **Bottom,** So-called window of interest for the atrial flutter. Figures on **left half** show results of having the window too wide (spanning more than one tachycardia cycle); the computer picks an inappropriately "early" activation time (−365 milliseconds, more than the flutter CL), thus yielding a map (above) that makes little sense. When the same site has correct activation time (−122 milliseconds) assigned by narrowing the window **(lower right),** the color activation map clearly reveals peritricuspid reentry.

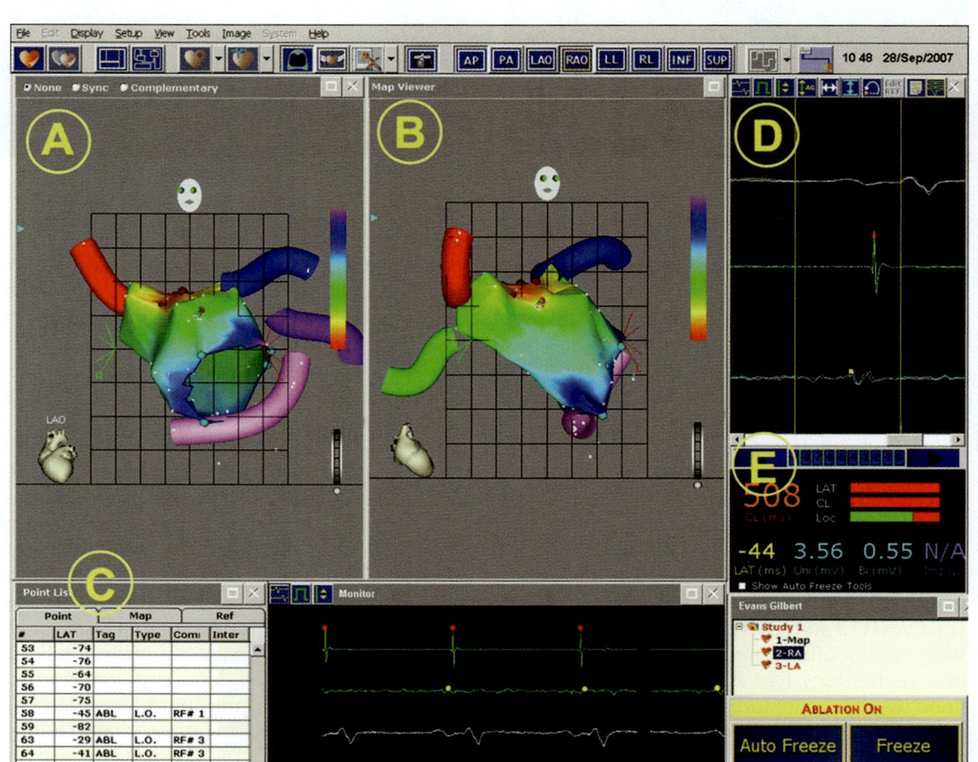

FIGURE 6-9 Screen shot of the CARTO (Biosense Webster, Inc., Diamond Bar, Calif.) electroanatomical mapping system. **A** and **B,** Left anterior oblique and right anterior oblique views of the activation maps of a left atrial tachycardia (AT). **C,** List of saved mapping points selected by the operator. **D,** Selection of surface ECG leads (V1), reference electrogram (R1-R2), and local activation (M1-M2) recorded at the tip of the ablation catheter within the window of interest. **E,** Local electrogram amplitude and local activation time relative to the reference electrogram. Other panels on screen are various controls and indicators for the CARTO system.

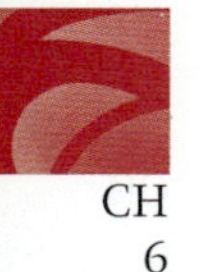

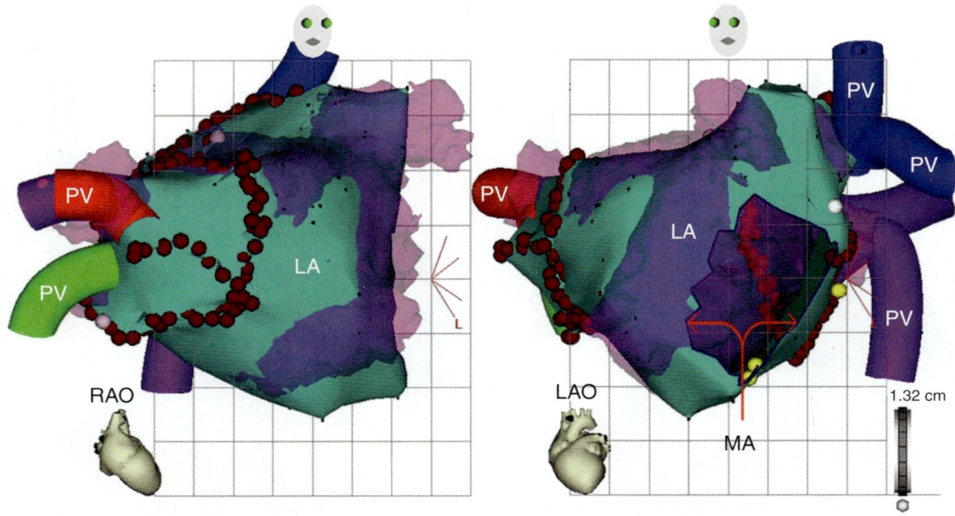

FIGURE 6-10 Integration of CT and electroanatomical mapping data. Right anterior oblique (RAO) and left anterior oblique (LAO) views of the electroanatomical contour acquired with catheter manipulation in the left atrium (LA) during atrial fibrillation ablation are shown overlaid on a CT image of the LA acquired several days earlier. Small red circles are tagged sites at which radiofrequency energy was applied to isolate the pulmonary vein (PV) antra. MA = mitral annulus.

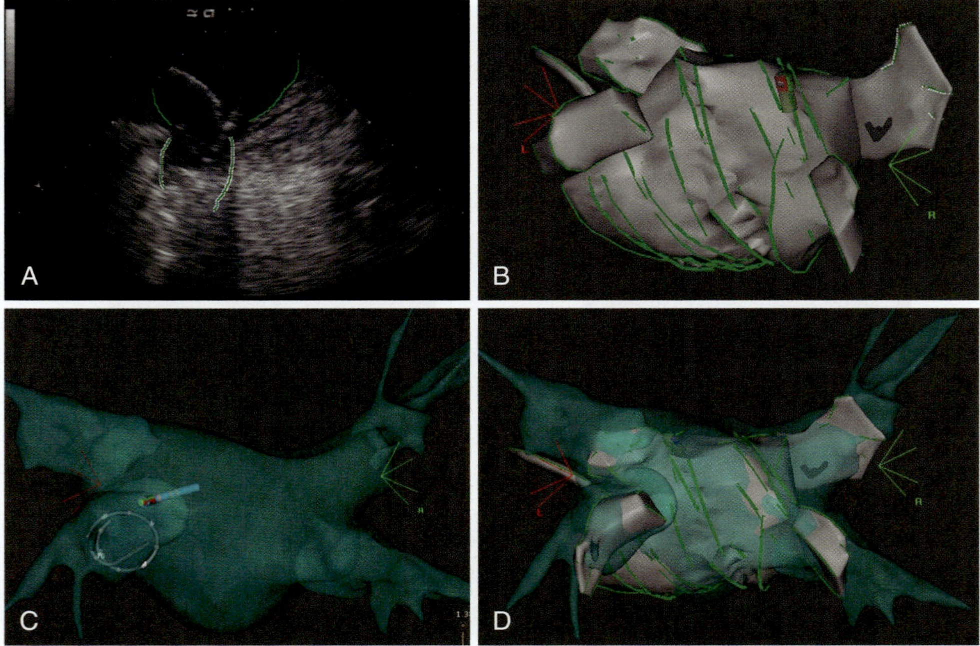

FIGURE 6-11 The CARTOSound Image Integration Module (Biosense Webster, Inc., Diamond Bar, Calif.). **A,** Intracardiac echocardiographic (ICE) image showing the left atrium (LA) and left inferior pulmonary vein (LIPV) obtained using a 10 Fr phased-array transducer catheter. The endocardial surfaces of the LA and LIPV are traced. **B,** Three-dimensional geometry of the LA is reconstructed by interpolation of points on the traced endocardial surface from multiple ICE images. **C,** CARTO 3 anatomical reconstruction of the LA (posterior view). Note that the circular and ablation catheters are visualized in the LIPV. **D,** Integration of the CARTOSound volume and the electroanatomical maps of the LA.

overwritten by hand as necessary, using the CARTOSound software. The software then resolves each contour into a series of discrete spatial points, with an interpoint spacing of up to 3 millimeters (closer spacing on curved contours or at angulations). The CARTO software interpolates these points to create models of the chamber endocardial surface in the CARTO workspace. CARTOSound allows for detailed real-time visualization of the cardiac chamber and of its adjacent structures and elimination of chamber deformity, which often happens with contact mapping (Video 14). The CARTOSound volume map of the cardiac chamber may be used as a stand-alone tool to guide navigation and ablation or as a facilitator of CT/MRI image integration (see later).[12,13]

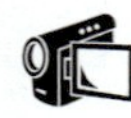

CARTO 3

The CARTO 3 system is the third-generation platform from Biosense Webster that offers three unique features: Advanced Catheter Location Technology, Fast Anatomical Mapping (FAM), and a streamlined workflow feature set referred to as Connection of Choice. Advanced Catheter Location technology is a hybrid technology that combines magnetic location technology and current-based visualization data to provide accurate visualization of multiple catheter tips and curves on the electroanatomical map. It can visualize up to five catheters (with and without the magnetic sensors) simultaneously with clear distinction of all electrodes. Three coils generate a magnetic field, and a location sensor in the catheter measures the strength of the field and the distance from each coil. The location of the sensor in the catheter is determined by the intersection of the three fields. In addition to this magnetic field, CARTO 3 uses an electrical field created by two sets of patches. The magnetic technology calibrates the current-based technology and thereby minimizes distortions at the periphery of the electrical field. The system generates a small current that is sent from the electrodes of the catheters to six patches on the patient's thorax. Each electrode emits current at a unique frequency. The strength of the current emitted by each electrode is measured at each patch and creates a current ratio that is unique to each electrode's location.

Mapping is performed in two steps. Initially, the magnetic mapping permits precise localization of the catheter with the sensor. This is associated with the current ratio of the electrode closest to

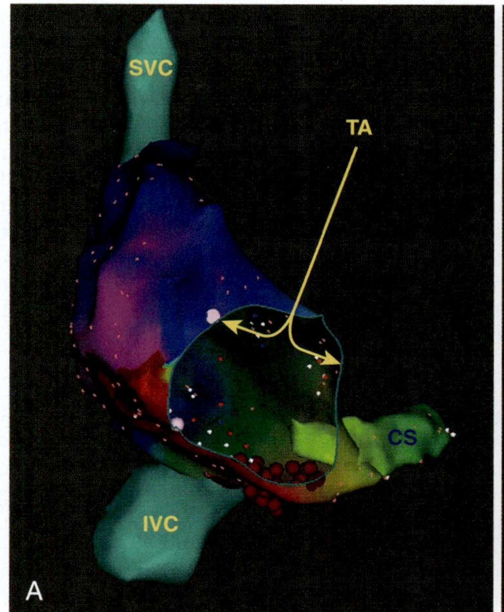

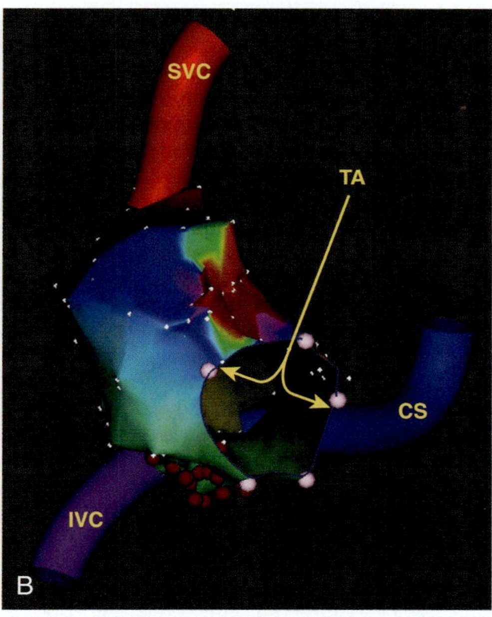

FIGURE 6-12 Electroanatomical CARTO 3 and CARTO XP (Biosense Webster, Inc., Diamond Bar, Calif.) activation maps of the right atrium in the left anterior oblique view constructed during typical atrial flutter. **A**, CARTO 3 activation map during tachycardia. The depolarization wavefront travels counterclockwise around the tricuspid annulus (TA), as indicated by a continuous progression of colors (from red to purple) with close proximity of earliest and latest local activation (red meeting purple). Purple dots denote ablation lesions delivered across the cavotricuspid isthmus. **B**, CARTO XP during clockwise typical tachycardia is shown. Note the difference between the two systems in geometry reconstruction of the cardiac chamber and vascular structures. CS = coronary sinus; IVC = inferior vena cava; SVC = superior vena cava.

the sensor. As the catheter with the sensor moves around a chamber, multiple locations are created and stored by the system. The system integrates the current-based points with their respective magnetic locations, resulting in a calibrated current-based field that permits accurate visualization of catheters and their locations. Each electrode emits a unique frequency that provides clear distinction of the electrodes, especially when they are close to each other. Fast Anatomical Mapping is a feature that permits rapid creation of anatomical maps by movement of a sensor-based catheter throughout the cardiac chamber. Unlike point-by-point electroanatomical mapping, volume data can be collected with Fast Anatomical Mapping (Fig. 6-12; Video 15). Catheters other than the ablation catheter, such as the multipolar Lasso, can further enhance the collection of points and increase the mapping speed. The CARTO 3 system provides highly accurate geometry of a cardiac chamber, which can be visualized in multiple views. Connection of Choice is enabled by a CARTO hardware configuration featuring a central connection point for all catheters and equipment while preserving the signal quality of intracardiac electrograms. Catheter connections have been redesigned for "plug-and-play" functionality and automatic catheter recognition.

Mapping Procedure

Following selection of the reference electrogram, positioning of the anatomical reference, and determination of the window of interest, the mapping catheter is positioned in the cardiac chamber of interest under fluoroscopic guidance. The CARTO system requires the use of a special Biosense Webster catheter with a location sensor embedded in its distal end. The 7 Fr quadripolar catheters come with a deflectable tip in one or two directions in a single plane and various deflectable curve sizes; some of these catheters have asymmetrical bidirectional deflectable curves. The distal tip is capable of RF energy delivery. Catheters with 4- or 8-mm-tip conventional RF ablation electrodes are available, as well as 3.5-mm irrigated tip ablation catheters.

The mapping catheter is initially positioned (using fluoroscopy) at known anatomical points that serve as landmarks for the electroanatomical map. For example, to map the RA, points such as the superior vena cava (SVC), inferior vena cava (IVC), His bundle, tricuspid annulus, and CS ostium (CS os) are marked. The catheter is then advanced slowly around the chamber walls to sample multiple points along the endocardium, thus sequentially acquiring the location of its tip together with the local electrogram.[2]

Points are selected only when the catheter is in stable contact with the wall. The system continuously monitors the quality of catheter-tissue contact and local activation time stability to ensure validity and reproducibility of each local measurement. The stability of the catheter and contact is evaluated at every site by examining the following: (1) local activation time stability, defined as a difference between the local activation calculated from two consecutive beats of less than 2 milliseconds; (2) location stability, defined as a distance between two consecutive gated locations of less than 2 mm; (3) morphological superpositioning of the intracardiac electrogram recorded on two consecutive beats; and (4) CL stability, defined as the difference between the CL of the last beat and the median CL during the procedure. Respiratory excursions that can cause significant shifts in apparent catheter location can be addressed by visually selecting points during the same phase of the respiratory cycle.

Each selected point is tagged on the 3-D map. The local activation time at each site is determined from the intracardiac bipolar electrogram and is measured in relation to the fixed reference electrogram (see Video 10). Lines of block (manifest as double potentials) are tagged for easy identification because they can serve as boundaries for subsequent design of ablation strategies. Electrically silent areas (defined as having an endocardial potential amplitude less than 0.05 mV, which is the baseline noise in the CARTO system and the absence of capture at 20 mA) and surgically related scars are tagged as "scar" and therefore appear in gray on the 3-D maps and are not assigned an activation time (see Figs. 14-1 and 14-2). The map can also be used to catalog sites at which pacing maneuvers are performed during assessment of the tachycardia.

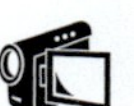

Sampling the location of the catheter together with the local electrogram is performed from a plurality of endocardial sites. The points sampled are connected by lines to form several adjoining triangles in a global model of the chamber. Next, gated electrograms are used to create an activation map, which is superimposed on the anatomical model. The acquired local activation times are then color-coded and superimposed on the anatomical map with red indicating early-activated sites, blue and purple late-activated areas, and yellow and green intermediate activation times (see Figs. 11-17, 11-19, and 12-10). Between these points, colors are interpolated, and the adjoining triangles are colored with these interpolated values. However, if the points are spaced widely apart, no interpolation is done. The degree to which the system interpolates activation times is programmable (as the triangle fill threshold) and can be modified if necessary. As each new site is acquired, the reconstruction is updated in real time to create a 3-D chamber geometry color progressively encoded with activation time.[2]

Sampling an adequate number of homogeneously distributed points is necessary. If a map is incomplete, bystander sites can be mistakenly identified as part of a reentrant circuit. Regions that are poorly sampled have activation interpolated between widely separated points. This can give the appearance of conduction, but critical features such as lines of block can be missed. In addition, low-resolution mapping can obscure other interesting phenomena, such as the second loop of a dual-loop tachycardia. Some arrhythmias, such as complex reentrant circuits, require more than 80 to 100 points to obtain adequate resolution. Other tachycardias can be mapped with fewer points, including focal tachycardias and some less complex reentrant arrhythmias, such as isthmus-dependent AFL.[9,10]

It is also important to identify areas of scar or central obstacles to conduction; failure to do so can confuse an electroanatomical map because interpolation of activation through areas of conduction block can give the appearance of wavefront propagation through, rather than around, those obstacles. This occurrence precludes identification of a critical isthmus in reentrant arrhythmias to target for ablation. A line of conduction block can be inferred if there are adjacent regions with wavefront propagation in opposite directions separated by a line of double potentials or dense isochrones.[9]

The electroanatomical model, which can be seen in a single view or in multiple views simultaneously and freely rotated in any direction, forms a reliable road map for navigation of the ablation catheter. Any portion of the chamber can be seen in relation to the catheter tip in real time, and points of interest can easily be revisited even without fluoroscopy. The electroanatomical maps can be presented in two or three dimensions as activation, isochronal, propagation, or voltage maps.

ACTIVATION MAP

The activation maps display the local activation time color-coded overlaid on the reconstructed 3-D geometry (see Fig. 6-8; also see Figs. 11-17, 11-19, and 12-10). Activation mapping is performed to define the activation sequence. A reasonable number of points homogeneously distributed in the chamber of interest must be recorded. The selected points of local activation time are color-coded—red for the earliest electrical activation areas and orange, yellow, green, blue, and purple for progressively delayed activation areas (see Videos 10 and 11). The electroanatomical maps of focal tachycardias demonstrate radial spreading of activation, from the earliest local activation site (red) in all directions, and, in these cases, activation time is markedly shorter than tachycardia CL (see Figs. 11-17 and 11-19). On the other hand, a continuous progression of colors (from red to purple) around the mapped chamber, with close proximity of earliest and latest local activation, suggests the presence of a macroreentrant tachycardia (see Figs. 12-10, 14-1, and 14-2). It is important to recognize that if an insufficient number of points is obtained in this early meets late zone, it may be falsely concluded through the interpolation of activation times that the wavefront propagates in the wrong direction (Fig. 6-13).[2,9,10]

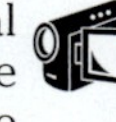

ISOCHRONAL MAP

The system can generate isochrones of electrical activity as color-coded static maps. The isochronal map depicts all the points with an activation time within a specific range (e.g., 10 milliseconds) with the same color. Depending on conduction velocity, each color layer is of variable width; isochrones are narrow in areas of slow conduction and broad in areas of fast conduction. Displaying information as an isochronal map helps demonstrate the direction of wavefront propagation, which is perpendicular to the isochronal lines. Furthermore, isochronal crowding indicating a conduction velocity of 0.033 cm/msec (slower than 0.05 cm/msec) is considered a zone of slow conduction, whereas a collision of two wavefronts traveling in different directions separated temporally by 50 milliseconds is defined as a region of local block. Spontaneous zones of block or slow conduction (less than 0.033 cm/msec) may have a major role in the stabilization of certain arrhythmias.[2]

PROPAGATION MAP

The CARTO system also can generate color-coded animated dynamic maps of activation wavefront (propagation maps). This is a two-colored map, in which the whole chamber is blue and electrical activation waves are seen in red, spreading throughout the chamber as a continuous animated loop (see Figs. 11-19 and 12-10). Propagation of electrical activation is visualized superimposed on the 3-D anatomical reconstruction of the cardiac chamber in relation to the anatomical landmarks and barriers (see Videos 11 and 12). Analysis of the propagation map can allow estimation of the

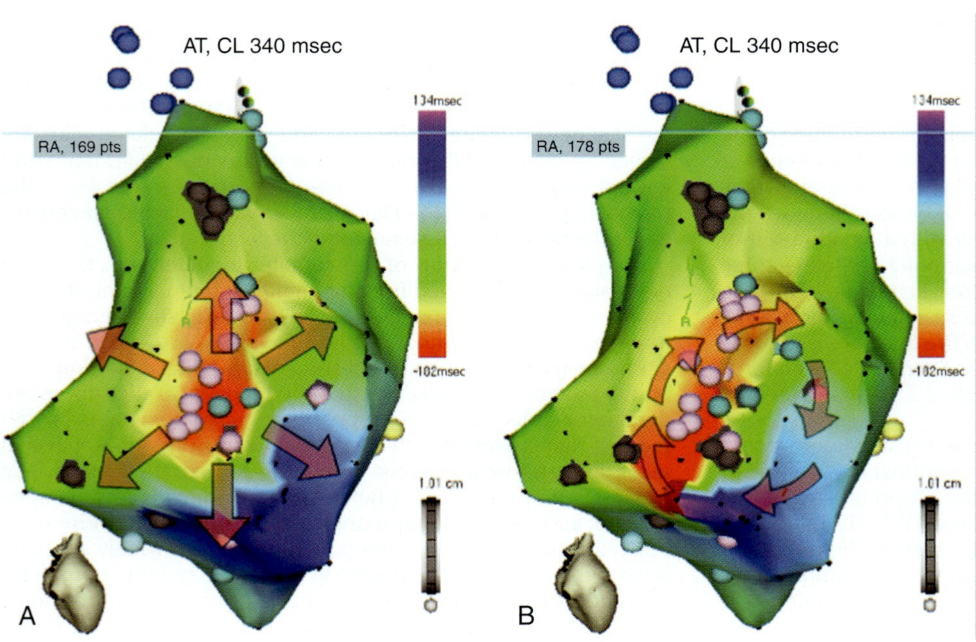

FIGURE 6-13 Right atrial electroanatomical (CARTO, Biosense Webster, Inc., Diamond Bar, Calif.) activation map in a patient with prior atrial tachycardia following atrial septal defect repair years before. The view is from the aspect of the right rib margin (upward toward the lateral right atrium). **A**, The activation pattern suggests a focal process with centrifugal spread of activation from the central red area (169 data points taken). **B**, With additional detailed mapping below the red area, a return path for a reentrant circuit is evident (178 data points). Entrainment data had already diagnosed macroreentry, but the relatively detailed activation map had missed the small area that became clear on more detailed mapping. CL = cycle length.

conduction velocity along the reentrant circuit and identification of areas of slow conduction.

VOLTAGE MAP

The voltage map displays the peak-to-peak amplitude of the electrogram sampled at each site. This value is color-coded and superimposed on the anatomical model, with red as the lowest amplitude and orange, yellow, green, blue, and purple indicating progressively higher amplitudes (Fig. 6-14). The gain on the 3-D color display allows the user to concentrate on a narrow or wide range of potentials. By diminishing the color scale, as may be required to see a fascicular potential or diastolic depolarization during reentry, larger amplitude signals are eliminated. To visualize the broad spectrum of potentials present during a tachycardia cycle, the scale would be opened up to include an array of colors representing a spectrum of voltages. Local electrogram voltage mapping during sinus, paced, or any other rhythm can help define anatomically correct regions of no voltage (presumed scars or electrical scars), low voltage, and normal voltage. The true range of normal is often difficult to define, however, especially with bipolar recordings, and different criteria have been used. Myocardial scars are seen as low voltage, and their delineation can help in understanding the location of the arrhythmia.

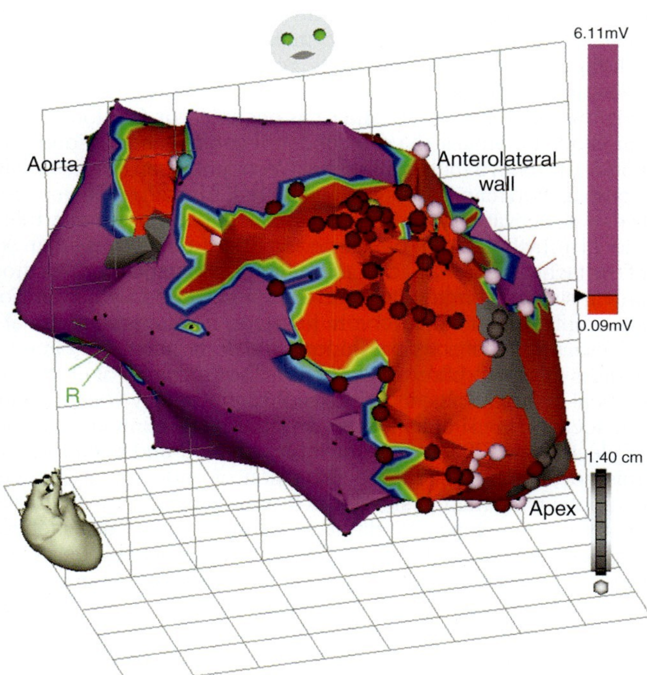

FIGURE 6-14 Electroanatomical (CARTO, Biosense Webster, Inc., Diamond Bar, Calif.) voltage map of the left ventricle in a patient with ventricular tachycardia after anteroapical myocardial infarction. An adjusted voltage scale is shown at right; all sites with voltage lower than 0.5 mV are red on the map, and those with voltage higher than 0.6 mV are purple, with interpolation of color for intermediate amplitudes. The gray area denotes no detectable signal (scar). A large anteroapical infarction is clearly evident. Red circles denote ablation sites.

ENTRAINMENT MAP

A graphical representation of entrainment mapping can be constructed by plotting values of the differences between the postpacing intervals (PPIs) and the tachycardia CLs (PPI–tachycardia CL) on the electroanatomical mapping system to generate color-coded 3-D entrainment maps (Fig. 6-15). This approach can potentially help accurately determine and visualize the 3-D location of the entire reentrant circuit, even though the area of slow conduction of the tachycardia is not specified. Because neither of the electroanatomical mapping systems (CARTO, NavX) contains an algorithm for color-coding of entrainment information, the modus for activation mapping is altered manually. At each 3-D location of the catheter tip stored on the electroanatomical mapping system, entrainment stimulation is performed, and the difference between PPI and tachycardia CL (PPI–tachycardia CL) is calculated and plugged into the electroanatomical mapping system (as if it would be an "activation time"). For that, the local electrogram stored at the 3-D location is completely disregarded. The annotation marker is manually moved into a position where the numeric timing information equals the entrainment information (PPI–tachycardia CL). That timing information then is displayed in a color-coded fashion as if it were activation time, but instead it represents information on the length of the entrainment return cycle. With the color range, red represents points closest to the reentrant circuit (i.e., sites with smaller PPI–tachycardia CL differences, approaching 0, signifying their inclusion in the reentrant circuit) and purple represents points far away from the circuit (i.e., sites with the largest PPI–tachycardia CL differences).[14,15]

Color-coded 3-D entrainment mapping allows determination of the full active reentrant circuit (versus passively activated regions of the chamber) and the obstacle around which the tachycardia is circulating, and it provides very useful information on the location of potential ablation sites (see Fig. 6-15). However, not all these sites will terminate reentry (just as, although the circuit in orthodromic SVT includes the ventricle, ablation at one or two sites in that ventricle will not eliminate reentry); the final choice is determined by location of anatomical barriers and width of putative isthmuses, so that strategic ablation lines, mainly connecting to anatomical barriers, can be applied to transect the circuit and treat the arrhythmia.[14,15]

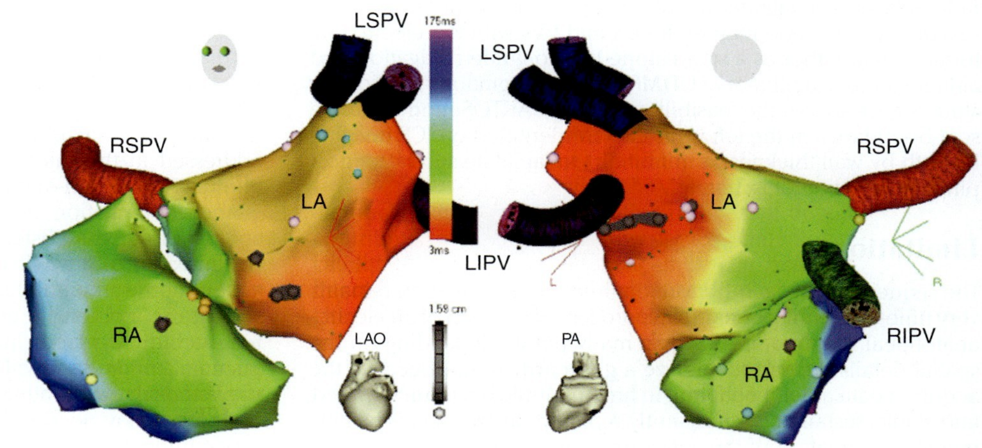

FIGURE 6-15 Right atrial (RA) and left atrial (LA) electroanatomical color-coded entrainment map in a patient with atrial tachycardia following pulmonary vein (PV) isolation for treatment of atrial fibrillation. The colors represent the difference between the postpacing interval at each site following entrainment pacing and the tachycardia cycle length: the less the difference, the closer to the circuit. In this case, the zone of reentry goes around the left inferior PV (LIPV). LAO = left anterior oblique; LSPV = left superior pulmonary vein; PA = posteroanterior; RIPV = right inferior pulmonary vein; RSPV = right superior pulmonary vein.

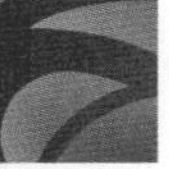

Clinical Implications

The capability of the CARTO system to associate relevant EP information with the appropriate spatial location in the heart and the ability to study activation patterns with high spatial resolution (less than 1 mm) during tachycardia in relation to normal anatomical structures and areas of scar significantly facilitate the mapping and ablation procedure. This mapping system facilitates defining the mechanisms underlying the arrhythmia, making a rapid distinction between a focal origin and macroreentrant tachycardia, precisely describing macroreentrant circuits and the sequence of activation during the tachycardia, understanding the reentrant circuit in relation to native barriers and surgical scars, identifying all slow-conducting pathways, rapidly visualizing the activation wavefront (propagation maps), and identifying appropriate sites for entrainment and pace mapping.

The CARTO system provides a highly accurate geometric rendering of a cardiac chamber with a straightforward geometric display having the capability to determine the 3-D location and orientation of the ablation catheter accurately. The position of the mapping tip at any point in time is readily apparent from a tip icon, provided that the tip is at or beyond the rendered chamber geometry. The catheter can anatomically and accurately revisit a critically important recording site (e.g., sites with double potentials or those with good pace maps) identified previously during the study, even if the tachycardia is no longer present or inducible and map-guided catheter navigation is no longer possible. This accurate repositioning provides significant advantages over conventional techniques and is of great value in ablation procedures. Ablation lesions can be tagged, thus facilitating creation of lines of block with considerable accuracy by serial RF lesion placement and allowing verification of the continuity of the ablation line (see Fig. 6-10). This is of particular value after incomplete ablations caused by catheter dislocation or early coagulum formation, especially if these ablations had caused interruption of the target tachycardia. Extra RF applications can be delivered closely around an apparently successful ablation site to ensure elimination of the arrhythmogenic area.[2]

Voltage maps can help define the arrhythmogenic substrate when the arrhythmia arises in the setting of cardiac structural abnormalities; this is of particular value during mapping of hemodynamically unstable or nonsustained arrhythmias. Additionally, fluoroscopy time can be reduced via electromagnetic catheter navigation, and the catheter can be accurately guided to positions removed from fluoroscopic markers. Although fluoroscopy is always needed for initial orientation, an experienced operator can usually generate an extensive endocardial activation map with substantially reduced radiation exposure for himself or herself and for the patient and laboratory staff.[2]

The CARTOMerge Module has proved very valuable in guiding real-time catheter ablation using the detailed cardiac chamber anatomy acquired from the CT/MRI (see later discussion).[16]

The CARTOSound Image Integration Module has been successfully utilized to facilitate AF catheter ablation by incorporating a real-time ICE volume map of the LA and PVs with the electroanatomical map, either as a stand-alone tool to guide navigation and ablation or as a facilitator of CT/MRI image integration. Additionally, studies have shown the feasibility of using CARTOSound to define scar boundaries in the left ventricle (LV, identified on ICE imaging by both by wall thickness and motion) to facilitate substrate mapping and ablation of ischemic VT.[12,13]

Limitations

The sequential data acquisition required for map creation remains very time-consuming because the process of creation of an electroanatomical map requires tagging many points, depending on the spatial details needed to analyze a given arrhythmia. Because the acquired data are not coherent in time, multiple beats are required, and stable, sustained, or frequently repetitive arrhythmia is usually needed for creation of the activation map. Given that these points do not provide real-time, constantly updated information, more time can be needed for making new maps to see a current endocardial activation sequence, detect a change in arrhythmia, or fully visualize multiple tachycardias. In addition, rapidly changing or transient arrhythmias are not easily recorded and may be mapped only if significant substrate abnormalities are present. For macroreentrant tachycardias, variation of the tachycardia CL by more than 10% can prevent complete understanding of a circuit, and it decreases the confidence in the CARTO map. Single PVCs or PACs or nonsustained events may be mapped, although at the expense of an appreciable amount of time.

One difficulty with current methods is that incorrect assignment of activation for a few electrograms can invalidate the entire activation map, and manual adjustment is often required to achieve the optimal representation. Additionally, data interpolation between mapped points is used to improve the quality of the display; however, areas of unmapped myocardium are then assigned simple estimates of timing and voltage information that may not be accurate.

If highly fractionated and wide potentials are present, it can be difficult to assign an activation time. In some macroreentrant circuits, much of the tachycardia CL is occupied by fractionated low-amplitude potentials. The subjective selection of an individual local potential within a multicomponent electrogram can drastically alter a propagation map. If these potentials are dismissed or assigned relatively late activation times, a macroreentrant tachycardia may mimic a focal arrhythmia, and it will appear as if substantially less than 90% of the tachycardia CL is mapped. Additionally, with current methods, only a single value of timing or voltage can be assigned to those low-amplitude fractionated electrograms, and this is suboptimal in representing their potential importance to the reentrant circuit. To address this issue, one study described a novel form of electroanatomical mapping called "ripple mapping," whereby voltage, timing, and location are simultaneously displayed with continuous display of electrograms that were previously sampled and postprocessed. This novel technique for representation of endocardial activation can potentially help to simplify activation mapping by minimizing operator dependence, to eliminate interpolation of data between mapped points, and to eliminate assignment bias by developing software to register continuous or fractionated electrograms, thereby removing a single, isolated local value as representing an entire coordinate. The extent to which this technology will be incorporated into "real-time" application requires prospective evaluation.[17]

A change in rhythm during the mapping procedure can alter cardiac geometry to the extent that anatomical points acquired during one rhythm cannot be relied on after a change in rhythm. This is relevant during mapping of isolated ectopic beats or nonsustained arrhythmias, because locations assigned to early activation sites during the arrhythmia can potentially be removed from the same locations when they are assigned during normal rhythm (e.g., at the time of RF delivery after tachycardia termination). Therefore, after termination of the arrhythmia, revisiting the site of early activation tagged during PVCs or tachycardia may be unfeasible or even misleading as a target for ablation.

Additionally, significant movement of the patient or the intracardiac reference catheter would necessitate remapping. Older versions of CARTO did not record or display the location of diagnostic/reference catheters; consequently, it was not easy to relocate a displaced intracardiac reference catheter. This issue has been addressed in the third generation of CARTO (CARTO 3), which allows visualization of up to five EP catheters simultaneously.

Another limitation of the CARTO system is the requirement of a special Biosense Webster catheter with a location sensor embedded proximal to its tip. No other catheter types may be used with this system. Furthermore, the magnetic signal necessary for the CARTO system can potentially create interference with other EP laboratory recording systems. Implantable cardioverter-defibrillators and pacemakers are safe with the system, but the magnetic field can prevent device communication with its programmer, and the magnetic field may need to be disabled temporarily to allow device programming.

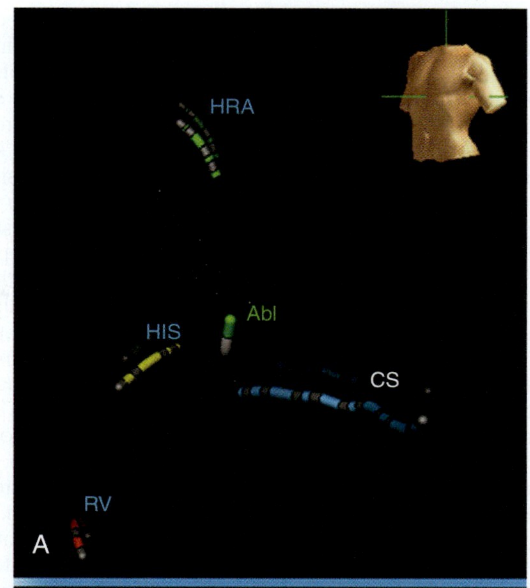

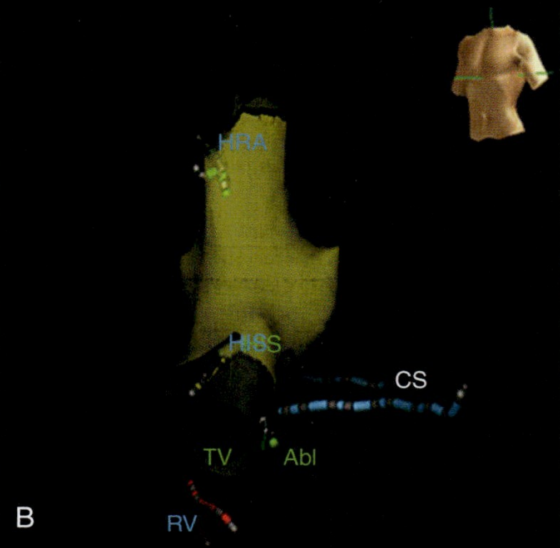

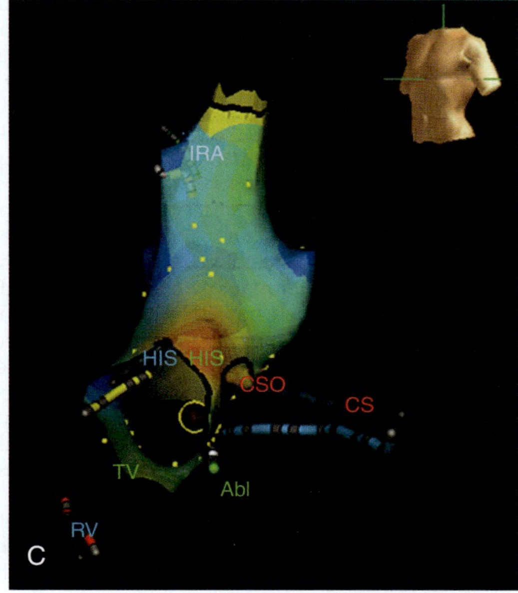

FIGURE 6-16 The NavX system (St. Jude Medical, Austin, Tex.). **A,** Left anterior oblique view of four standard diagnostic catheters (positioned in the high right atrium [HRA], His bundle [HIS], right ventricular [RV] apex, and coronary sinus [CS]) and a standard ablation catheter (Abl) as visualized by the NavX system during mapping of a focal atrial tachycardia. Note the shadows placed over the four diagnostic catheters to record their original position and recognize displacement during the procedure. **B,** Virtual anatomical geometry of the RA is acquired by moving the catheter in all directions throughout the chamber of interest. Any electrode catheter (not just the mapping catheter) can be used to create the three-dimensional (3-D) geometry. **C,** Color-coded activation map superimposed on the RA 3-D geometry localizing the origin of the atrial tachycardia to the triangle of Koch between the His bundle, coronary sinus ostium (CSO), and tricuspid valve (TV).

EnSite NavX Navigation System

Fundamental Concepts

The EnSite NavX system (St. Jude Medical, Austin, Tex.) consists of a set of 3 pairs of skin patches, a system reference patch, 10 ECG electrodes, a display workstation, and a patient interface unit. The reference patch is placed on the patient's abdomen and serves as the electrical reference for the system. The EnSite NavX combines catheter location and tracking features of the LocaLisa system (Medtronic, Minneapolis, Minn.) with the ability to create an anatomical model of the cardiac chamber using only a single conventional EP catheter and skin patches.[8]

This mapping modality is based on currents across the thorax, developed as originally applied in the LocaLisa system. In contrast to the NavX system, LocaLisa does not allow generation of 3-D geometry of the heart cavity because catheters and desired anatomical landmarks are displayed in a cartesian frame of reference.[2] This technology has undergone substantial additional development in the NavX iteration.

For 3-D navigation, 6 electrodes (skin patches) are placed on the skin of the patient to create electrical fields along 3 orthogonal axes (x, y, and z). The patches are placed on both sides of the patient (x-axis), the chest and back of the patient (y-axis), and the back of the neck and inner left thigh (z-axis). Analogous to the Frank lead system, the 3 orthogonal electrode pairs are used to send 3 independent, alternating, low-power currents of 350 mA at a frequency of 5.7 kHz through the patient's chest in 3 orthogonal (x, y, and z) directions, with slightly different frequencies of approximately 30 kHz used for each direction, to form a 3-D transthoracic electrical field with the heart at the center. The absolute range of voltage along each axis varies from each other, depending on the volume and type of tissue subtended between each surface-electrode pair. The voltage gradient is divided by the known applied current to determine the impedance field that has equal unit magnitudes in all 3 axes. Each level of impedance along each axis corresponds to a specific anatomical location within the thorax. As standard catheter electrodes are maneuvered within the chambers, each catheter electrode senses the corresponding levels of impedance, derived from the measured voltage. The mixture of the 30-kHz signals, recorded from each catheter electrode, is digitally separated to measure the amplitude of each of the 3 frequency components. The 3 electrical field strengths are calculated automatically by use of the difference in amplitudes measured from neighboring electrode pairs with a known interelectrode distance for 3 or more different spatial orientations of that dipole. Timed with the current delivery, NavX calculates the x-y-z impedance coordinates at each catheter electrode by dividing each of the 3 amplitudes (V) by the corresponding electrical field strength (V/cm) and expresses them in millimeters to locate the catheters graphically in real time to enable nonfluoroscopic navigation. The NavX system allows real-time visualization of the position and motion of up to 64 electrodes on both ablation and standard catheters positioned elsewhere in the heart (Fig. 6-16).

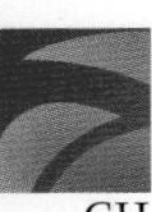

The NavX system also allows for rapid creation of detailed models of cardiac anatomy (see Fig. 6-16). Sequential positioning of a catheter at multiple sites along the endocardial surface of a specific chamber establishes that chamber's geometry. The system automatically acquires points from a nominated electrode at a rate of 96 points/sec. Chamber geometry is created by several thousand points. The algorithm defines the surface by using the most distant points in any given angle from the geometry center, which can be chosen by the operator or defined by the system. In addition, the operator is able to specify fixed points that represent contact points during geometry acquisition; the algorithm that calculates the surface cannot eliminate these points. In addition to mapping at specific points, there is additional interpolation, providing a smooth surface onto which activation voltages and times can be registered. To control for variations related to the cardiac cycle, acquisition can be gated to any electrogram.

Similar to the CARTO system, the voltage or the activation map can be superimposed on the 3-D geometry (see Fig. 6-16). Principles of activation and voltage mapping using the NavX system are similar to those discussed previously for the CARTO system.

Additionally, the NavX Fusion has the capability to integrate images from a preacquired CT/MRI scan on the electroanatomical image the cardiac chamber created with the NavX system to facilitate anatomically based ablation procedures (see later discussion).

Mapping Procedure

NavX-guided procedures are performed using the same catheter setup as conventional approaches. Any electrode can be used to gather data, create static isochronal and voltage maps, and perform ablation procedures. Standard EP catheters of choice are introduced into the heart; up to 12 catheters and 64 electrodes can be viewed simultaneously. The system can locate the position of the catheters from the moment that they are inserted in the vein. Therefore, all catheters can be navigated to the heart under guidance of the EnSite NavX system, and the use of fluoroscopy can be minimized for preliminary catheter positioning. However, interrupted fluoroscopy has to be used repeatedly when an obstacle to catheter advancement is encountered. Once in the heart, one intracardiac catheter is used as reference for geometry reconstruction. A shadow (to record original position) is placed over this catheter to recognize displacement during the procedure, in which case the catheter can be returned easily to its original location under the guidance of NavX. A shadow can also be displayed on each of the other catheters to record the catheter's spatial position (see Fig. 6-16).

Subsequently, 3-D intracardiac geometry is obtained. Respiratory compensation is collected just before mapping to filter low-frequency cardiac shift associated with the breathing cycle. Characteristic anatomical landmarks in the chamber of interest are initially acquired and marked. The system is then allowed to create the geometry automatically. A virtual anatomical geometry is acquired by moving the catheter in all directions throughout the chamber of interest, keeping contact with the endocardial wall.[18] If a CT reconstruction of the mapped cardiac chamber is available, the image can be visualized on a split screen and used to guide finer anatomical definition with the ablation catheter. On completion, maps can be edited to eliminate "false space" (i.e., geometry with sparse geometry points) and erroneous structure definition. Subsequently, a scaling algorithm (Field Scaling) is applied to the completed detailed geometry to compensate for variations in impedance between the heart chambers and venous structures (which can otherwise result in a distortion of the x-y-z coordinates when a "roving" catheter is maneuvered among the differing regions of impedance). Field scaling is based on the measured interelectrode spacing for all locations within the geometry. Adjustments to the local strength of the navigation fields are made so that the computed catheter electrode positions match the known interelectrode spacing of the catheters used to create the geometry.[19]

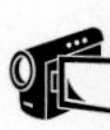

Additional tagging of sites of interest and ablation points can be done during the procedure. Point-to-point activation mapping is carried out to create static isochronal, voltage, and activation maps (Videos 16 and 17; see Fig. 6-16). Standard catheters are used to sample voltage and activation timing at various locations during a sustained rhythm. The system collects and visually organizes activation timing and voltage data and permanently saves 10 beats with every collected point for later review. An unlimited number of maps can be created per procedure. The system works with most manufacturers' ablation catheters, RF generators, or cryogenerators. Ablation lesions can be tagged, thus facilitating creation of lines of block with considerable accuracy by serial RF lesion placement and allowing verification of the continuity of the ablation line.[18]

Clinical Implications

NavX is a novel mapping and navigation system with the ability to visualize and navigate a complete set of intracardiac catheters in any cardiac chamber for diagnostic and therapeutic applications.[8] It enables the electrophysiologist to display in real time up to 64 electrodes simultaneously on 12 catheters with almost every commercially available catheter, including pacemaker leads. Earlier versions of NavX permitted the creation of 3-D cardiac geometry by using all these catheters, without visualization of electrical activity. Thus, they are particularly suitable for ablation of arrhythmias with well-known substrates that can be treated by an anatomical approach, such as AFL and linear LA ablation for AF.[18] A software upgrade allowing point-to-point activation mapping for the NavX system has also been introduced. This is a substantial improvement, permitting the same type of activation mapping and display as are possible with other systems, with the similar advantage of specified voltage mapping as well. This point-to-point mapping, however, is suited only for sustained arrhythmias or frequently recurrent PACs, PVCs, or nonsustained arrhythmias. Unlike with the CARTO system, however, activation times can be acquired simultaneously by the EnSite NavX system from multiple poles on all catheters utilized during the study (and not just the mapping-ablation catheter). This acquisition can be augmented by the addition of noncontact mapping to the procedure.[8]

NavX technology has an important advantage in reducing operator and patient radiation exposure. The ability to position catheters for ablation without the use of fluoroscopy is important because NavX allows the display of catheters from the puncture site to the final destination in the heart. Indeed, this nonfluoroscopic navigation system allows real-time assessment of wall contact and catheter stability, as well as assessment of the anatomical position and the relation between the ablation catheter and other intracardiac catheters. Because of these capabilities, catheter displacement and insufficient wall contact are readily recognized without the use of fluoroscopy, thus resulting in reduction of radiation exposure, procedure duration, and the trend to reduced RF energy delivery.

The ablation procedure is also facilitated by NavX.[8,18] As noted, the system works with most manufacturers' ablation catheters, RF generators, or cryogenerators. The ablation lesions can be tagged, thus facilitating creation of lines of block with considerable accuracy by serial RF lesion placement and allowing verification of the continuity of the ablation line and anatomical visualization of the remaining gaps, where additional RF applications can be delivered. It also helps avoid repeated ablations at the same location. The catheter can anatomically and accurately revisit a critically important recording site identified previously during the study.

As in the CARTO system, the voltage or the activation map can be superimposed on the 3-D geometry. Complex fractionated electrograms can be targeted in persistent AF by using the software to depict the mean electrogram CL map. The NavX system also has the capability to import and integrate 3-D CT or MRI images to facilitate anatomically based ablation procedures. NavX Fusion provides a significant advancement in image integration with the EnSite NavX system and has the ability to mold the created geometry dynamically into the CT/MRI image (see later discussion).

Limitations

The point-to-point activation mapping required while using the NavX system is suited only for sustained arrhythmias or frequently recurrent ectopy or nonsustained arrhythmias. Additionally, in the NavX system, the algorithm defines the surface by using the most distant points in any given angle from the geometric center, and the catheter can protrude out against the wall of the cardiac chamber when acquiring points; thus, chamber geometry of the NavX system is oversized.

Furthermore, with individual interpolation schemes, significant anatomical distortions in complex structures can occur, because there may be interpolations in the region of curvature that do not depict the accurate geometry, especially at areas of exvaginations (e.g., the PVs, LA or RA appendages). One strategy to minimize this is to incorporate a family of fixed points into the geometry to preserve critical junctions between those structures. A second strategy is to create volumes of these structures in separate maps and then combine them to the main chamber.

The position of the intracardiac catheter used as reference for geometry reconstruction needs to be stable throughout the procedure to maintain the accurate position of the electroanatomical map. Any significant shift in its position can frequently lead to remapping. Although a shadow (to record original position) can be placed over the reference catheter to recognize displacement during the procedure, in which case the catheter can be returned to its original location, this may not always be feasible or accurate.

Stereotaxis Magnetic Navigation System

Fundamental Concepts

Catheter navigation by magnetic force was initially introduced in the early 1990s for diagnostic studies in neonates. However, the development of conventional steerable electrodes with integrated pull wires to deflect the catheter tip was pursued, and this constitutes the current technique for catheter ablation. The conventional technique is limited by the fixed maximal catheter deflection and relies mostly on the skill of the operator to ensure stable catheter positioning. A novel magnetic navigation system (MNS; 0.15 T, Telstar, Stereotaxis, St. Louis, Mo.) was introduced to clinical practice. It was proven to be a safe and feasible tool for catheter ablation, although it did not allow remote catheter ablation. The second-generation MNS (Niobe, Stereotaxis) now allows, for the first time, complete, remote RF catheter ablation.[20]

The Niobe MNS consists of two permanent neodymium-iron-boron magnets; their positions, relative to each other, are computer controlled inside a fixed housing and positioned on either side of the single-plane fluoroscopy table.[20] While positioned in the "navigate" position, the magnets create a 360-degree omnidirectional rotation of the device by a uniform magnetic field (0.08 tesla) within an approximately spherical navigation volume 20 cm in diameter (NaviSphere), sufficient to encompass the heart when the patient is properly positioned. The combination of rotation, translation, and tilt movements of the magnets adjusts the magnetic field to any desired orientation within the NaviSphere.[20,21]

The mapping and ablation catheters are extremely flexible distally, especially the distal shaft of the catheter, and have tiny magnets (single or multiple, in various configurations) inserted in their distal portion. The latest catheters have three tiny magnets distributed along the distal shaft and tip of the catheter to increase responsiveness of the catheter to the magnetic field generated (Fig. 6-17). The catheter magnets align themselves with the direction of the externally controlled magnetic field to enable the catheter tip to be steered effectively. By changing the orientation of the outer magnets relative to each other, the orientation of the magnetic field changes, thereby leading to deflection of the catheter.[20]

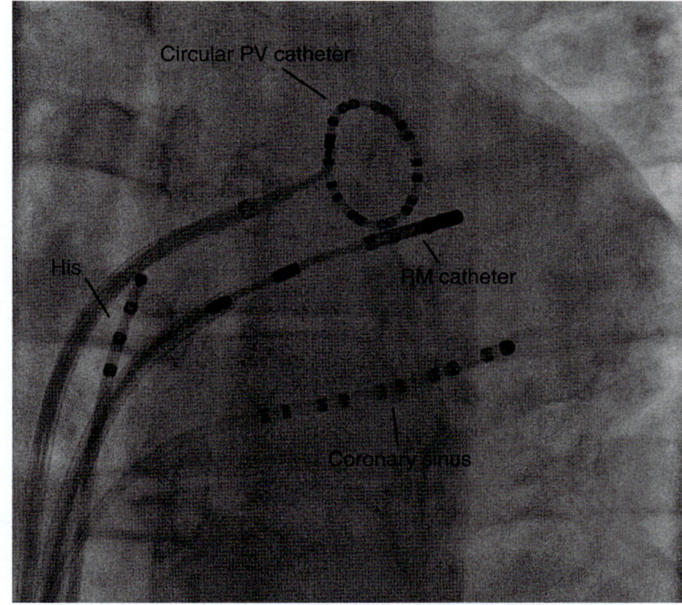

FIGURE 6-17 Stereotaxis catheters (Stereotaxis, St. Louis, Mo.). Anteroposterior fluoroscopic view of the Stereotaxis remote magnetic (RM) catheter in the left atrium. Multipolar circular mapping, coronary sinus, and His bundle catheters are also shown. The RM catheter has a large distal mapping and ablation electrode; this and three other opaque regions more proximally on the catheter shaft contain magnetic elements that conform to changes in direction of an externally applied magnetic field. PV = pulmonary vein.

The system is integrated with a modified C-arm digital x-ray system, mainly a single-plane unit because of the limitations imposed by the magnets, although a biplane system can be installed for use when the magnets are stowed and not in use. Because of the magnets, the rotation of the imaging system is limited to approximately 30 degrees right anterior oblique (RAO) and left anterior oblique (LAO) in Niobe I and almost 45 degrees with Niobe II. In the Niobe I iteration, the magnets can be swung only in (active navigation) or stowed, whereas in the Niobe II the magnets have a different housing and can also be tilted to allow for more angulation of the single-plane C-arm imaging system.[20]

It is important to emphasize that the external magnetic field does not pull or push the tiny magnets and the catheters or guidewires in which they are contained. The position of the magnetic catheter within the heart is controlled by manual advancement or retraction of the catheter through the vascular sheath. A computer-controlled catheter advancer system (Cardiodrive unit, Stereotaxis) is used to allow truly remote catheter navigation without the need for manual manipulation. The operator is positioned in a separate control room, at a distance from the x-ray beam and the patient's body. The graphic workstation (Navigant II, Stereotaxis), in conjunction with the Cardiodrive unit, allows precise orientation of the catheter by 1-degree increments and by 1-mm steps in advancement or retraction. The system is controlled by a joystick or mouse and allows remote control of the ablation catheter from inside the control room. Additionally, the x-ray image data can be transferred from the x-ray system to the user interface of the MNS system to provide an anatomical reference.

Directional catheter navigation is accomplished by drawing a desired magnetic field vector on orthogonal fluoroscopic views with a digitization tablet (Fig. 6-18). A control computer then calculates the appropriate currents to each of the superconducting electromagnets. The resultant composite magnetic field interacts with a permanent magnet in the tip of the magnetic ablation catheter and deflects the catheter to align parallel to the magnetic field. Magnetic field orientations corresponding to specific map points can be stored on the MNS and reapplied to return repeatedly and accurately to previously visited locations on the map. Navigation

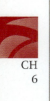

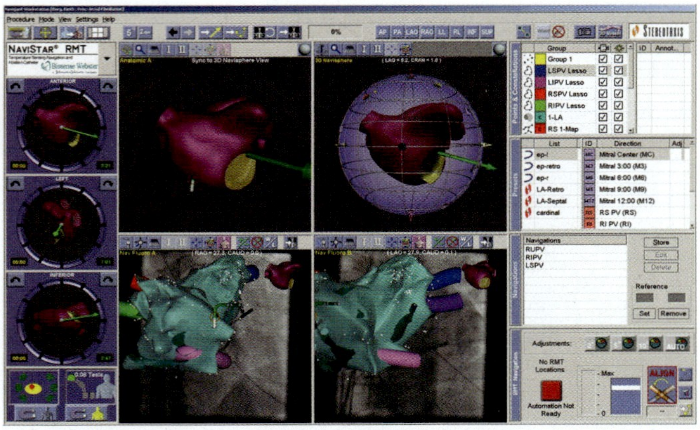

FIGURE 6-18 Stereotaxis monitor—screen shot of the remote magnetic guidance system (Stereotaxis, St. Louis, Mo.). **Top two central panels,** Representation of idealized left atrium shells with a green arrow ("vector") that can be pointed in any direction with a computer mouse, commanding the magnetic steering mechanism to deflect the catheter tip in that direction. **Bottom two central panels,** Shell generated by electroanatomical mapping, integrated with the images on the Stereotaxis unit. These overlie the patient's initial right anterior oblique and left anterior oblique fluoroscopic images. Tubular structures are the pulmonary veins and coronary sinus (pink). Other panels on the screen are various controls and indicators for the Stereotaxis manipulation.

to a particular target often requires two or three manipulations of the magnetic field to refine the catheter position. Each magnetic field manipulation requires less than 20 seconds to activate. By changing the orientation of the outer magnets, the orientation of the magnetic field changes, thereby leading to the deflection of the catheter in parallel.[20]

The MNS has become integrated with CARTO RMT (Biosense Webster, Inc.) electroanatomical mapping system. The CARTO RMT system is similar to the standard CARTO system but is able to localize the ablation catheter without interference from the magnetic field. CARTO RMT is able to send real-time catheter tip location and orientation data to the MNS. It also sends target locations, groups of points, and anatomical surface information from the electroanatomical map to the MNS.

Mapping Procedure

All the components of the MNS, as well as the x-ray, ablator, and stimulator, can be operated from the control room. Therefore, after initial placement of sheaths and catheters, the entire ablation procedure can be performed remotely from the control room. The Navigant system is the computerized graphical user interface system. It includes the software used for image integration and for control of the magnetic fields that orient the catheter within the heart and allow the operator to direct the movement of the tip of the catheter to access the region of interest (see Fig. 6-18).[20]

After synchronizing with respiratory and cardiac cycles, such as inspiration and the end-diastolic period, a pair of best-matched RAO-LAO images is transferred and kept in the Navigant screen as background references for orientation and navigation (see Fig. 6-18). Thus, the real-time catheter location information can be displayed on the Navigant reference x-ray images, thus enabling continuous real-time monitoring of the catheter tip position, even without acquiring a fresh x-ray image.[20]

The operator can access an area of interest by using vector-based or target-based navigation. In vector-based navigation, the operator tells the system, by drawing a vector in virtual 3-D space on the computer, what orientation of the magnetic field is required. In target-based navigation, a target is placed on a specified point using the stored orthogonal fluoroscopic views; the user marks the support or base of the catheter (the distal portion of the sheath) on the pair of x-ray images. This provides Navigant with the data needed to compute field orientations corresponding to particular targets. Each time a vector is selected or a target is marked, the computer sends information to the magnets, which changes their relative orientation, and with it the orientation of the uniform magnetic field in the chest, so that catheter orientation is then changed within a few seconds (see Fig. 6-18). A target can also be defined by selecting a preset magnetic field vector based on a selected study protocol from the list on the Navigant. The software contains several preset vectors selected by the manufacturer, after careful appraisal of multiple CT images and reconstructions, for positioning the catheter at various anatomical landmarks. When a preset vector is applied, it can steer the catheter near the approximate region indicated. In addition, the software can be used to map various chambers of the heart automatically.[20]

The magnetic catheter is advanced to target positions in the cardiac chamber of interest and guided by using the x-ray system, user interface monitors, and catheter advancer (Cardiodrive) system, which allows precise orientation of the catheter in extremely small increments (1-degree increments, by 1-mm steps) within the heart and vessels in advancement or retraction, thus making mapping more accurate. All vectors and targets selected can be saved, as can relative positions of the catheter advancer system, to allow specific areas in the heart or side branches of vessels to be revisited reproducibly.

CARTO RMT has also been integrated with the MNS and has been specifically redesigned to work in the magnetic environment of Stereotaxis. CARTO RMT includes all the latest updates such as CARTOMerge, in which a 3-D reconstruction of a CT or MRI image can be integrated into the electroanatomical map. With the CARTO integration, communication between the two systems allows for real-time catheter orientation and positioning data to be sent from CARTO to the Stereotaxis system and for the catheter tip to be displayed on the saved images stored on the Navigant system. This permits tracking of the ablation catheter without having to update the radiographic image as often. Magnetic vectors can also be applied from the CARTO screen. A feature called "design line" can be used to send a line of points, either for mapping a specific area or potentially as a line of ablation points. "Click and go" is a tool allowing for an area of the map to be clicked on to set a target and have the system guide the catheter to this point. Because Stereotaxis and CARTO have feedback integration, the CARTO system can feed back to the Stereotaxis system if the exact point is not reached, thus allowing for further automatic compensation by the software until the desired point is reached. The combined system has the capability of automatically mapping chambers (anatomy and activation times) by using predetermined scripts. The accuracy of such automaps is highly dependent on the anatomy, as well as where in the heart the operator designates the starting point for mapping. At present, standard 4- and 8-mm-tip and irrigated 3.5-mm-tip RF catheters are available.

Clinical Implications

Precise target localization and catheter stability are prerequisites for successful RF applications and to minimize risks of potential complications. Stiff, manually deflectable catheters, with a unidirectional or bidirectional deflection radius, which deflect in a single plane, have several inherent limitations because stable electrode-tissue contact can be difficult to achieve, particularly in regions of complex cardiac anatomy. In contrast, the promise of the current MNS lies in the precision of catheter movement and the ability to steer the flexible distal portion of the catheter in any direction in 3-D space.[20]

The MNS is increasingly used for ablation of AVNRT, atrioventricular bypass tracts (BTs), AFL, idiopathic outflow tract VT, scar-related VT, and especially AF. Intracardiac electrograms and stimulation thresholds are not significantly different from those recorded with a standard, manually deflected ablation catheter, and the safety of standard EP procedures has not been compromised by use of the MNS.[21-26]

Although the current MNS does not offer a distinct advantage over conventional catheters for navigation to targets that are easily reached, it has potential advantages for complex catheter maneuvers and navigation to sites that are exceptionally difficult to reach with a standard catheter. In addition, catheter mobility and endocardial stability can be superior by virtue of the compliance of the distal catheter and lack of constraints on the magnetic vector used to steer the catheter. Cardiac and respiratory motion can be buffered by the catheter compliance, thereby contributing to endocardial contact stability.

After the diagnostic catheters are positioned, the EP study and ablation process can be performed completely from inside the control room. This offers several potential advantages, including reducing fluoroscopic exposure time for the operator, reducing the strain from standing next to the bed for long periods while wearing a lead apron, and facilitating simultaneous catheter navigation and electrogram analysis.

A unique feature of the current MNS is that the magnetic vector coordinates used to navigate the magnetic catheter to a particular site can be stored and reused later in the study to return to a site of interest. The integration of a stable magnetic catheter with the CARTO electroanatomical mapping system is useful to reconstruct an accurate electroanatomical map by acquiring many more points than are possible manually for successful ablation, even of challenging areas.[20]

The maximum tissue force that can be applied by the flexible catheter used in the MNS is less than the average and significantly less than the maximum that can be applied using a standard catheter. Because of the flexibility of the catheters, cardiac perforation is extremely unlikely.

For certain procedures, notably AF ablation, MNS can decrease fluoroscopy time significantly. Although the use of MNS may increase total procedure duration, procedure times decrease with increasing operator experience.[23-26]

Limitations

A potential limitation of the MNS is the interference induced by the magnetic field in the surface ECG. The origin of the induced potentials is thought to be attributable to blood flow within the magnetic field. Blood is an electrolyte solution that can induce the potential because of motion within the magnetic field. The magnetic field strength used for catheter manipulation is approximately one order of magnitude less than that associated with MRI. The interaction of the magnetic field with the surface ECG is therefore less in magnitude compared with MRI and is restricted to the ST segment, and the temporal distribution of the interfering signal component probably would not compromise cardiac rhythm analysis or analysis of the P wave or QRS morphology. However, interpretation of changes in the ST segment would be predictably compromised by this interference. Whether this distortion will affect arrhythmia analysis is currently being investigated.

Claustrophobia and morbid obesity are contraindications for using the MNS because of the restricted space within the system. The next generation of the MNS features an open design that is more comfortable for obese patients and those with claustrophobia. Patients with pacemakers or defibrillators are also excluded because of electromagnetic interference. Further study is required to determine whether the magnetic field strength is compatible with these devices. Additionally, the MNS requires monitoring instruments that are compatible with magnetic fields.

The angulation of the fluoroscopic system is limited to 30 to 45 degrees for both LAO and RAO projections when the magnets are in the "navigate" position. Although this may not be important in simple ablations, addressing more complex substrates can be more challenging.[20]

The MNS is an evolving technology. Further technical development through the availability of additional catheter designs (e.g., number of recording electrodes) is necessary to address more complex arrhythmias in the future.

The use of the MNS for ablation of AF, atypical AFL, and typical AFL was associated with long procedure times as compared with conventional catheter navigation. The preparation of the devices (registration and positioning of the magnets for MNS; flushing sheaths and gain transseptal access for MNS) is still time-consuming. Furthermore, the use of the MNS for catheter ablation of typical AFL resulted in a lower overall success rate (achievement of cavotricuspid isthmus block and freedom from AFL recurrence during follow-up). A lower success rate of PV electrical isolation was also observed when a standard 4-mm-tip ablation catheter was used. Some reports also expressed concern about a higher incidence of char formation during MNS-guided ablation of AF and AFL.[21,24,25] Irrigated magnetic catheters have become available and may reduce the risk of char formation, and they may also increase lesion efficacy during MNS-guided ablation.[22]

Sensei Robotic Navigation System

Fundamental Concepts

The Sensei robotic navigation system (Hansen Medical, Mountain View, Calif.) is an electromechanical system that realizes catheter navigation by two concentric steerable sheaths (Artisan, Hansen Medical) incorporating an ablation catheter. The outer sheath (14 Fr) and the inner sheath (10.5 Fr) are both manipulated via a pull-wire mechanism by a sheath-carrying robotic arm that is fixed at the foot of the patient's table. The robot arm obeys the commands of the central workstation (master console) positioned in the control room. Catheter navigation is realized using a 3-D joystick (Instinctive Motion Control, Hansen Medical) and allows a broad range of motion in virtually any direction. At the master console, fluoroscopic images, ICE images, and other 3-D representations (electroanatomical maps) are displayed, providing immediate feedback to the operator. Seamless instinctive integration and interpreted motion logic allow the physician to direct catheter movement in 3-D regardless of image orientation or perspective. To provide a representation of tactile feedback, the system continuously monitors the contact force that is exerted by the catheter tip by using a specially designed algorithm (IntelliSense, Hansen Medical). If the contact force exceeds a preset limit, an optical alarm is displayed, and catheter advancement is rendered virtually impossible. In general, all catheters and all electroanatomical mapping systems may be used. Apart from the different navigational approach, the technical aspects of the ablation are identical to the manual ones.[21,27-29]

Mapping Procedure

Both the inner and the outer sheaths should be flushed with heparinized normal saline before insertion and continuously throughout the procedure to prevent clot formation and air embolism. The steerable guide sheath is manually inserted via a 14 Fr sheath in the right femoral vein and advanced manually into the inferior RA under fluoroscopy guidance. To minimize the risk of vascular complications, it is advisable to obtain venous access under ultrasound guidance, initially insert an 8 Fr sheath and upsize to 11 Fr and then 14 Fr, and then insert a long, 30-cm 14 Fr sheath that usually ends at the level of the liver. Through this, the steerable sheath is inserted with the ablation catheter leading by at least 10 cm into the RA. At this level, the ablation catheter is withdrawn into the steerable sheath with only the distal electrodes protruding. Failure to leave the ablation catheter out beyond the end of the Artisan sheath and to observe the catheter system advance up to the RA increases the risk of vascular injury.[29]

Then, the position of the sheath is registered into the robotic catheter remote control system. The registration process involves the use of two orthogonal fluoroscopic views of the heart (anteroposterior and lateral) to allow saving the position of the guide sheath in 3-D space. Following registration, the remote control system is used to steer the tip of the ablation catheter to various targets in all four cardiac chambers.

For ablation of AF, the first transseptal puncture is usually performed manually with a standard transseptal sheath and needle system. The guidewire or a circular catheter placed in the LA through the first transseptal puncture is used as a marker of the second puncture site. Fluoroscopy and ICE images are used for confirmation of robotic navigation system placement in the LA. The second transseptal puncture is performed with the Sensei system by using a transseptal sheath and dilator (Hansen Medical, Inc.); a custom-made transseptal needle (Hansen Medical, Inc.) is advanced through a dilator lumen under fluoroscopy and ICE guidance. After the septum is punctured, the steerable guide sheath and dilator are advanced robotically in the LA, and the dilator is replaced with the ablation catheter, which is then inserted into the guide sheath with approximately 1 cm of the ablation catheter exposed from the tip of the guide sheath. Integration of this robotic system with available mapping systems (CARTO and EnSite NavX) is feasible.

The steerable sheath housing the ablation catheter is remotely controlled by a physician at the master console. Manipulation of other catheters, including the circular mapping catheter, however, is performed manually by a second operator at the procedure tableside.

The amount of energy applied during remote navigation cases is generally lower than that of manual cases, likely because of enhanced catheter contact and stability throughout the cardiac cycle afforded by the robotic sheath. As a result, the rate of steam pop and potential thermal complications may be higher if compensatory energy-lowering strategies are not implemented.[29]

Clinical Implications

Endocardial navigation using conventional manual steerable diagnostic and ablation catheters and transseptal puncture using standard equipment can be challenging and time-consuming, and they require certain skills and experience. The robotic catheter remote control system was designed to facilitate control and allow precise and stable positioning of catheters within the cardiovascular system. It can help overcome the limitations of manual control by combining the ease of navigation with a readily available wide navigational field.

The main advantages of remote navigation are the opportunity to reduce the operator's radiation exposure because of the remote location of the workstation from the fluoroscopy unit. Furthermore, because of better catheter stability and easier navigation with the robotic system, total fluoroscopy time and patient and staff radiation exposure can potentially be reduced; however, this remains to be determined.[21,29,30]

Several studies have shown that robotic navigation and ablation of AF are as safe and effective as manual ablation. Furthermore, the use of the robotic catheter remote control system for transseptal puncture and endocardial navigation is safe and feasible. However, its usefulness in decreasing procedure time and improving procedural efficacy and safety compared with current approaches requires further evaluation in randomized clinical trials. In addition, a comparison between this technology and remote magnetic navigation may be warranted. It is conceivable that, in the future, a completely automated remotely performed procedure could set new and more homogeneous treatment standards for this complex procedure.[21,28]

In contrast to the magnetic guidance system (Niobe, Stereotaxis), which requires specific compatible magnetic-guided catheters, the Sensei robotic navigation system is an open platform system whereby almost any mapping or ablation catheter of appropriate size can be introduced into the remotely steerable catheter or sheath. Additionally, the MNS requires continuous alteration and adjustment of the magnetic field and then advancement of the catheter in that direction. With the use of the Sensei robotic navigation system, a continuous uninterrupted motion of the ablation catheter can be achieved with the use of the instinctive motion controller.[21,29,30] Finally, the Senseirobotic system is, at least in principle, portable and could be transported from one laboratory to another in the facility, whereas the remote MNS requires large magnets permanently installed in one location.

Limitations

Although the remote location of the workstation from the fluoroscopy can significantly reduce radiation exposure to the physician, there is a need for a second physician or operator to manipulate the circular mapping catheter at the bedside during a PV isolation procedure. Radiation exposure is not reduced to this operator or to the patient. With the use of other AF ablation strategies, such as anatomically based ablation, however, there would be no need for a separate mapping catheter. In the future, it is possible that both the ablation and mapping catheters will be controlled in tandem with two coordinated robotic steerable guides.

The steerable robotic sheath is inherently stiff to make it pushable and mechanically steerable, and it has to be advanced through a 14 Fr vascular sheath. The size of the introducer sheath itself increases the likelihood of complications, and advancing the steerable sheath into the vein may cause dissection. The amount of force required to advance the Artisan through the hemostatic valve of the sheath at the groin is significant. Therefore, insertion of the 14 Fr sheath and the Artisan catheter does require special care to avoid retroperitoneal vascular complications.[27,29]

Infrequent cases of cardiac perforations and PV stenosis were reported in several studies using the Sensei robotic navigation system for catheter ablation of AF. Some of those events were thought to be consequent to the use of high power output during RF ablation. Therefore, it is important to recognize that with better catheter contact and stability offered by the robotic sheath, the effectiveness of ablation is increased, and less power is probably needed to achieve adequate attenuation of electrograms. Further studies will be required to evaluate adequate and optimal tissue contact during navigation mapping and ablation, as well as the optimal ablation energy parameters while using a robotic system at different pressure levels, and compare those with the parameters used with conventional manually operated catheters.[27]

During catheter ablation of AF, the major advantage of robotic navigation with respect to stability as compared with manual navigation is along the LA roof. However, at the anterior inferior portion along the lateral circumferential ablation line, catheter stability is suboptimal in almost 50% of the cases despite robotic navigation. This may be explained by the fact that this is the most distant location from the transseptal puncture site. This limitation can be partially compensated for by a "deeper" LA position of the outer sheath and application of a distal bend. Additionally, electrical isolation of the right inferior PV is challenging using this system. Because of the large outer diameter of the sheath, robotic navigation to the distal CS is discouraged. This may limit its use in ablation procedures for long-lasting persistent AF or perimitral LA macroreentrant tachycardias, which frequently require epicardial ablation via the CS.

Certain ablation catheters with flat wire deflection mechanisms, such as the current version of the Cool Path ablation catheter manufactured by St. Jude Medical, are not compatible with the Sensei robotic navigation system, thereby rendering the system truly a semi-open rather than a fully open platform. The flat wire mechanism allows the catheter to only bend along a two-dimensional (2-D) plane described by the flat surface of the wire without causing tension. When the robotic sheath moves in a direction that is not along the 2-D plane of the flat wire, tension is created, resulting in an uncontrolled rebound rapid correction of the system, which can potentially cause cardiac perforation. This rarely happens with manual manipulation of the catheter alone because the operator rotates the catheter appropriately to achieve the desired position.[27,31]

Although the robotic system affords greater stability at ablation targets, complications that occur with the manual approach can also occur with the robotic system. Given the stability of the system and also the stiffness and rigidity of the sheath, it is crucial that the operator understands the anatomy of the LA and adjacent structures. Even more so with the robotic navigation system, it is very important that the operator is cognizant of possible complications and is able to manage such complications effectively.[27]

Body Surface Potential Mapping

Fundamental Concepts

Although the conventional 12-lead ECG is extensively used, its limitations for optimal detection of cardiac abnormalities are widely appreciated. The main deficiency in the 12-lead approach is that only 6 chest electrodes are incorporated, and they cover a relatively constrained area of the precordium. The main reason for the choice of the location of the conventional precordial electrodes, suggested by Wilson in the 1940s, was the need to adopt some standard, which to this day has remained relatively unchallenged. In the years since then, the growing appreciation for the limitations of the conventional precordial electrode positions and the increase in understanding of the localization of various cardiac abnormalities on the body surface have led to the suggestion of various alternatives.[32,33]

One of the most widely studied alternatives to the 12-lead ECG in clinical and experimental electrocardiology has been body surface potential mapping (BSPM). In this approach, 32 to 219 electrodes are used in an attempt to sample all ECG information as projected onto the body's surface. The merits of this enhanced spatial sampling are obvious, in that localized abnormalities that may be difficult to detect using the 12-lead approach can readily be picked up with the additional electrodes.[32]

BSPM is defined as the temporal sequence of potential distributions observed on the thorax throughout one or more electrical cardiac cycles. BSPM is an extension of conventional ECG aimed at refining the noninvasive characterization and use of cardiac-generated potentials. The improved characterization is accomplished by increased spatial sampling of the body surface ECG, recorded as tens or even hundreds of unipolar ECGs, simultaneously or individually, with subsequent time alignment.[33]

BSPMs provide much more electrical and diagnostic information than the 12-lead ECG. They contain all the electrical information that can be obtained from the surface of the body, and they reveal diagnostically significant electrical features in areas that are not sampled by the 12-lead ECG systems. In addition, BSPMs often show distinct electrical manifestations of two or more events simultaneously evolving in the heart; they make it possible to compute any ECG that would be obtained from any pair or combination of body surface electrodes (i.e., from any current or future lead system). In addition, the recorded data can be displayed as a sequence of contour maps, thus allowing isolation of significant ECG events in both space and time.[32]

BSPMs can be used to reconstruct epicardial and, in some cases, endocardial potential distributions, excitation times, and electrograms noninvasively, by means of inverse procedures, which help transform the ECG into an imaging method of electrical activity. This yields 3-D images that depict anatomical features with superimposed activation isochrones or excitation and recovery potentials, isochrones, and electrograms.[33]

In BSPM measurements, unipolar potentials of single heartbeats are acquired simultaneously at more than 60 locations covering the whole thorax. A Wilson central terminal is used as a reference for the unipolar leads. Lead sites in the array are arranged in columns and rows, and the electrodes are attached to flexible plastic strips, attached to dozens of thoracic sites vertically, with the highest electrode density at the left anterior thorax. Recordings are bandpass-filtered at 0.16 to 300 Hz, digitized with a sampling frequency of 1 kHz, and stored on a CD.[33]

BSPMs depict the spatial distribution of heart potentials on the surface of the torso. Initially, all lead tracings are visually screened to reject poor-quality signals. The amplitude of every electrogram is measured at a given time instant during the cardiac cycle and plotted on a chart representing the torso surface. Several analytical procedures are used to convert the grid of data points into map contours. The time interval between successive instantaneous maps (frames) is generally 1 to 2 milliseconds. A sequence of 400 to 800 frames shows the evolution of the potential pattern during the cardiac cycle. Often, 20 to 50 properly selected maps are sufficient to show the essential features of the time-varying surface field.[33]

Localization of the site of origin of focal tachycardia, pacing site, or myocardial insertion site of a BT relates to the thoracic site of greatest negativity in the isointegral map. An activation wavefront moving away from such sites yields a negative body surface identifier because of the dominant effect of activating the remainder of the myocardial mass away from the stimulus site.

Clinical Implications

BSPM has been used for patients with conditions such as pulmonary embolism, aortic dissection, and acute coronary syndromes. It has also been used for diagnosing an old myocardial infarction, localizing the BT in Wolff-Parkinson-White syndrome, recognizing ventricular hypertrophy, and ascertaining the location, size, and severity of myocardial infarction and the effects of different interventions designed to reduce the size of the infarct.[33] From an EP standpoint, BSPM has been studied for the discrimination of clockwise and counterclockwise AFL, localization of the earliest retrograde atrial activation site in dogs with simulated Wolff-Parkinson-White syndrome and orthodromic AVRT, localization of the ventricular insertion site of BTs during preexcitation, localization of sites of origin of ATs and VTs, and localization of endocardial or epicardial pacing sites.

Although ongoing research continues to address the role of BSPM, and how BSPM addresses many of the inadequacies associated with the conventional 12-lead approach, the clinical effectiveness of this procedure has not been established. BSPM is mostly used as a research tool, rather than a routine diagnostic method because of significant limitations.[32]

Limitations

The main limitation of BSPM is the complexity of the recording, which requires many leads from each patient, sophisticated instrumentation, and dedicated personnel.[32] Complexity of the interpretation is another limitation, because it is mostly based on pattern recognition and knowledge of variability in normal subjects and patients, features that are difficult to memorize. Therefore, visual inspection and measurement of BSPMs cannot result, per se, in direct localization of single or multiple electrical events as they occur in the heart. Furthermore, BSPMs do not offer a picture of the heart, but they show an attenuated and distorted projection of epicardial and intracardiac events on the body surface. Additionally, the method of interpolating maps from acquired data is vulnerable to the precision of localization of the electrode sites and to the assurance that each electrode is receiving a true signal.[32]

Electrocardiographic Imaging

Fundamental Concepts

ECGI has three main components: a multielectrode ECG vest, a multichannel mapping system for ECG signal acquisition, and an anatomical imaging modality to determine the heart-torso geometry. ECGI is a cardiac functional imaging modality that noninvasively reconstructs epicardial potentials, electrograms, and isochrones (activation maps) from multichannel body surface potential recordings by using geometrical information from CT and a mathematical algorithm.[34,35]

ECGI has two requirements: ECG unipolar potentials measured over the entire body surface and the heart-torso geometrical relationship relating the epicardial surface to the location of the recording ECG electrodes. The body surface ECG unipolar potentials are

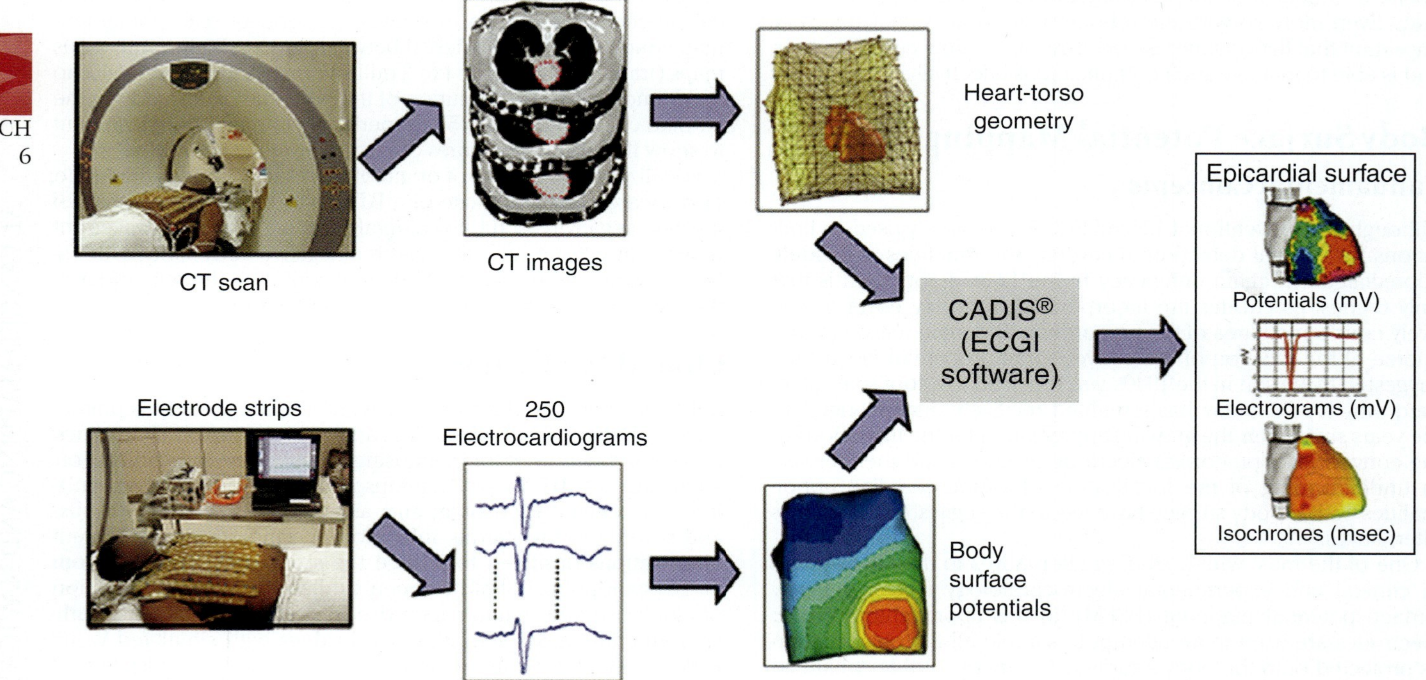

FIGURE 6-19 Electrocardiographic imaging (ECGI) procedure. Body surface potential mapping (BSPM) is recorded using a multichannel (256-electrode) mapping system. Noncontrast CT images with the body surface ECGI electrodes applied simultaneously record the locations of the electrodes (shining dots in CT images) and the geometry of the heart surface. By combining the BSPM and heart-torso geometry information, ECGI reconstructs potential maps, electrograms, and isochrones (activation patterns) on the epicardial surface of the heart. *(From Wang Y, Cuculich PS, Woodard PK, et al: Focal atrial tachycardia after pulmonary vein isolation: noninvasive mapping with electrocardiographic imaging [ECGI]. Heart Rhythm 4:1081, 2007.)*

measured using a multielectrode ECG vest. The prototype ECG vest has 250 electrodes arranged in rows and columns on strips, with Velcro attachments at the sides to secure the vest to the torso (Fig. 6-19). The vest is connected to a multichannel mapping system, which measures ECG unipolar potentials over the entire body surface and facilitates simultaneous signal acquisition and amplification from all channels. Body surface potentials are monitored to ensure proper contact and gain adjustment, and then signals are recorded over several heartbeats.[34-37]

After signal acquisition, the exact geometry of the epicardial and torso surfaces and vest electrode positions is obtained by anatomical imaging modalities, such as thoracic CT or MRI. Scans are usually set to an axial resolution between 0.6 and 1 mm and are typically gated at the R wave of the ECG to obtain diastolic volume (geometry for reconstruction of activation). Systolic volume, gated during the T wave of the ECG, is also measured to obtain suitable geometry for reconstruction during the repolarization phase. The transverse slices are segmented slice by slice to obtain heart geometry (as epicardial contours on each slice) and torso geometry (described by body surface electrode positions, seen as bright dots on the images; see Fig. 6-19). The geometry of the heart and torso surfaces is then assembled in a common x-y-z coordinate system to provide the geometrical heart-torso relationship.[34-37]

ECGI noninvasively computes potentials on the heart surface by solving the Laplace equation within the torso volume, with torso surface potentials and the geometric relationship between the epicardial and torso surfaces as inputs. The potential and geometry data are processed through CADIS, the ECGI software package (see Fig. 6-19). The software has four modules. The pre-processing module pre-processes the acquired ECG signals by noise filtration, baseline correction, elimination of bad signals (poor contact), and interpolation of missing signals. The geometry module includes image segmentation algorithms for heart and body surface segmentation and meshing of heart and torso surfaces. The numerical module includes boundary element algorithms to derive the transfer matrix relating body surface potentials to epicardial potentials and epicardial potential reconstruction algorithms that use regularized inverse solutions such as Tikhonov zero-order or the generalized minimal residual methods to compute unipolar epicardial potentials from the transfer matrix and body surface potentials. Regularization is necessary because of the ill-posed nature of the inverse problem (i.e., large noise fluctuations in the input data [noise on the ECGs or inaccurate electrode locations] may precipitate large errors in the solution). The fourth module is the postprocessing module, which includes tools to analyze reconstructed epicardial data and formats for efficient visualization and analysis.[36,37]

Four modes of display are typically used. Epicardial potential maps depict the spatial distributions of potentials on the epicardium (see Fig. 6-19). Each map depicts one instant of time; maps are computed at 1-millisecond intervals during the entire cardiac cycle. The electrograms depict the variation of potential with respect to time at a single point on the epicardium. The electrograms are computed at many points (typically 400 to 900 sites) around the epicardium. Isochrone maps depict the sequence of epicardial activation based on local activation time, taken as the point of maximum negative derivative ($-dV/dt_{max}$) of the QRS segment in each electrogram (intrinsic deflection). Recovery times are assigned as the point of maximum derivative (dV/dt_{max}) of the T wave segment. Activation times are determined as the time of maximum negative derivative in the epicardial electrograms. Information from neighboring electrograms is used to edit activation times in electrograms with multiple large negative derivatives. Lines of block are drawn to separate sites with activation time differences more than 30 milliseconds.[34,35]

Clinical Implications

A noninvasive imaging modality for cardiac EP is much needed for risk stratification of patients with genetic predisposition or altered myocardial substrate (e.g., after infarction), for specific diagnosis of the arrhythmia mechanism to determine the most suitable intervention, for determination of cardiac location for optimal localized intervention, for evaluation of efficacy and guidance of therapy over time, and for studying the mechanisms and properties of cardiac arrhythmias in humans. Noninvasive diagnosis of arrhythmias is currently based on the standard 12-lead ECG, BSPMs, or paced body surface QRS integral mapping. Standard diagnostic techniques such as the ECG provide only low-resolution projections of cardiac electrical activity on the body surface and cannot provide detailed information on regional electrical activity in the heart, such as the origin of arrhythmogenic activity, sequence of arrhythmic activation, or existence and location of an abnormal EP substrate.

ECGI reconstructs an epicardial electroanatomical map noninvasively by combining a 250-electrode body surface ECG with a CT scan of the heart-torso geometry. The ECGI images can be presented as epicardial potential maps, electrograms, isochrones, or repolarization maps during activation and repolarization. The major strengths of ECGI include the following: characteristics of activation can be analyzed at any point in the cardiac cycle with fine temporal resolution, atrial and ventricular patterns can be displayed, and information about the intramural nature of activation is available.

ECGI has been successfully applied and validated in human subjects, including comparison with intraoperative multielectrode mapping, determination of ECGI accuracy in locating focal sites of initial activation in humans by comparison with known locations of pacing electrodes in various RV and LV positions, comparison with catheter-based localization of focal VT, determination of the origin of human AT, and characterization of reentrant circuits.[34,35,38] ECGI has been applied in humans to reconstruct epicardial activation and repolarization during normal sinus rhythm, right bundle branch block, ventricular pacing, ventricular preexcitation, focal tachycardias, and AFL, in open heart surgery patients, and in patients receiving devices for cardiac resynchronization therapy. Additionally, ECGI can image the reentry pathway and its key components in atrial and ventricular macroreentrant tachycardias, including the critical isthmus, its entry and exit sites, lines of block, and regions of slow and fast conduction. Although clinical reentry usually occurs in the endocardium, the subepicardium plays an important role in the maintenance of reentry in a small proportion of patients undergoing ablation therapy. Interpretation of intramural arrhythmogenic activity can be further enhanced by direct catheter mapping or noncontact catheter reconstruction of EP information on the endocardial surface simultaneously with noninvasive epicardial ECGI. The combination of epicardial and endocardial EP information, with knowledge of the intramural anatomical organization of the myocardium, can provide an unprecedented ability to localize arrhythmogenic activity within the myocardial depth by using only noninvasive or minimally invasive procedures.[36-39]

ECGI's ability to image noninvasively regions of dispersion of repolarization in the form of QRST integral maps (or other metrics of repolarization dispersion) during a single beat provides a feasible and computationally efficient method for evaluating the severity of the substrate in patients at risk of developing arrhythmias. Noninvasive reconstruction of epicardial measures of repolarization dispersion can therefore provide a tool for rapid screening of patients at a high risk of life-threatening arrhythmias. After screening, prophylactic measures (e.g., implantable defibrillators, ablation, drug therapy, or genetic or molecular modification) can be instituted before sudden cardiac death occurs. The significance of applying ECGI for risk stratification is amplified by the lack of sensitivity of body surface measures (e.g., QT dispersion) at reflecting underlying dispersion of repolarization.[36,37,39]

Limitations

ECGI provides EP information about the heart's epicardial surface; it does not directly reconstruct endocardial information in the 3-D myocardium. Computation of endocardial activation is not yet possible because the electrical signal amplitude from the midwall and endocardium is much smaller. Nevertheless, in contrast to BSPMs, epicardial potentials provide high-resolution reflection of underlying intramural activity.[35] In addition, ECGI can have limited success in defining components of arrhythmia pathways that involve small volumes of tissue, such as microreentry. Furthermore, the need to use CT limits the clinical application of ECGI during intervention in the EP laboratory, where CT is not available. To render the ECGI procedure more practical for mainstream adoption, newer methods for obtaining patient-specific geometry using biplane fluoroscopy or pseudo–3-D ultrasound have been developed and successfully tested in the context of ECGI in the EP laboratory.[39]

Intracardiac Echocardiography

Catheter Design

Two types of ICE imaging systems are currently available: the mechanical ultrasound catheter radial imaging system and the electronic phased-array catheter sector imaging system.

MECHANICAL ULTRASOUND CATHETER RADIAL IMAGING SYSTEM

In the mechanical ultrasound catheter (Ultra ICE) radial imaging system (EP Technologies, Boston Scientific), the ultrasound transducer is mounted at the end of a nonsteerable 9 Fr (110-cm length) catheter and has a single, rotating, crystal ultrasound transducer. An external motor drive unit rotates the crystal at 1800 rpm within the catheter to provide an imaging plane that is 360 degrees circumferential and perpendicular to the long axis of the catheter, with the catheter located centrally. Mechanical ICE uses imaging frequencies of 9 to 12 MHz, which provide near-field clarity (within 5 to 7 cm of the transducer) but poor tissue penetration and far-field resolution. As a result, these systems have not allowed clear imaging of the LA and PV, except when they are introduced directly into the LA (transseptally). This technology lacks Doppler capability, and the catheter is not freely deflectable.[40]

ELECTRONIC PHASED-ARRAY CATHETER SECTOR IMAGING SYSTEM

In the electronic phased-array ultrasound catheter (AcuNav) sector imaging system (Acuson Corporation, Siemens Medical Solutions, Malvern, Pa.), the ultrasound transducer is mounted on the distal end of an 8 or 10 Fr (90-cm length) catheter and has a forward-facing 64-element vector phased-array transducer scanning in the longitudinal plane. The catheter has a four-way steerable tip (160 degrees anteroposterior and left-right deflections). The catheter images a sector (wedge-shaped) field in a plane in line with the catheter shaft and oriented in the plane of the catheter. Imaging capabilities include 90-degree sector 2-D, M-mode, and Doppler imaging (pulsed-wave, continuous-wave, color, and tissue Doppler), with tissue penetration up to 16 cm, and variable ultrasound frequency (5.5, 7.5, 8.5, and 10 MHz).[40]

Imaging Technique

USING THE MECHANICAL RADIAL INTRACARDIAC ECHOCARDIOGRAPHIC CATHETER

Initially, all air must be eliminated from the distal tip of the ICE catheter by flushing vigorously with 5 to 10 mL of sterile water to optimize the ultrasound image. The ICE catheter is introduced through a long femoral venous sheath. Because the catheter is not deflectable, preshaped angled long sheaths are preferred to allow some steerability.[40] The mechanical radial ICE catheter generates a panoramic 360-degree image perpendicular to the catheter, with the tip as a central reference point. The catheter is connected to

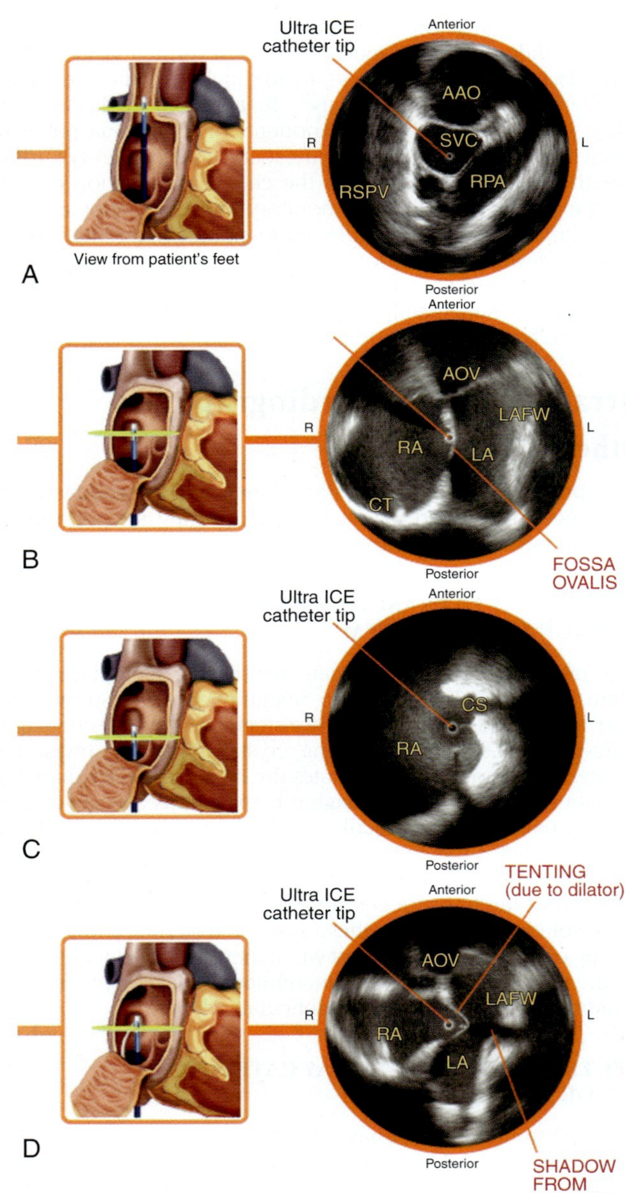

FIGURE 6-20 Mechanical radial intracardiac echocardiographic (ICE) images from different levels in the right atrium (RA) and superior vena cava (SVC). **A,** With the transducer tip in the SVC, typical structures visible in this plane are the ascending aorta (AAO), right pulmonary artery (RPA), and right superior pulmonary vein (RSPV). **B,** Withdrawing the ICE catheter into the mid-RA brings the fossa ovalis into view. Typical structures visible in this plane are the left atrium (LA), LA free wall (LAFW), aortic valve (AOV), and crista terminalis (CT). **C,** Withdrawing the ICE catheter down to the RA floor visualizes the coronary sinus (CS) and inferior vena cava (IVC). **D,** During transseptal puncture, tenting of the fossa is observed on the ICE. *(Courtesy of Boston Scientific, Natick, Mass.)*

the ultrasound console and advanced until the tip of the rotary ICE catheter image is in the RA.

When the transducer is advanced into the SVC, the ascending aorta, the right pulmonary artery, and, occasionally, the right superior PV are viewed.[41] Withdrawing the catheter into the mid-RA brings the fossa ovalis and LA in view; the crista terminalis and aortic valve are usually visible in this view (Fig. 6-20). The LA, left PV orifices, and aortic root are imaged by positioning the transducer at the fossa ovalis. However, visualization of the LA and PV ostia is limited because of limited penetration depth. Withdrawing the catheter to the low RA allows visualization of the eustachian valve, lateral crista terminalis, and CS ostium (see Fig. 6-20).[41] When the transducer is placed in the RV through the tricuspid valve and further advanced into the RVOT, both ventricles and the pulmonary artery can be visualized.

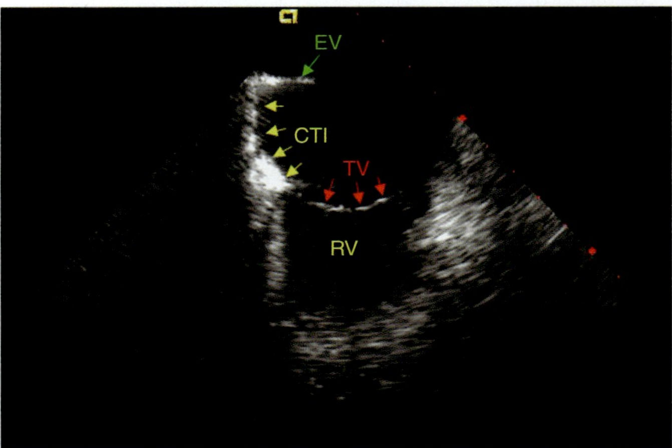

FIGURE 6-21 Intracardiac echocardiographic (ICE) image of the cavotricuspid isthmus (CTI, yellow arrows) between the eustachian valve (EV, green arrow) and the tricuspid valve (TV, red arrows). RV = right ventricle.

USING THE ACUNAV CATHETER

A femoral venous approach is used for the insertion of the ICE catheter. The catheter is advanced to the RA under fluoroscopy guidance. ICE 2-D 90-degree sector scanning demonstrates a cross-sectional anatomical view oriented from the tip to the shaft of the imaging catheter's active face.[40] The left-right (L-R) orientation marker indicates the catheter's shaft side. When the L-R orientation marker is set to the operator's right, the craniocaudal axis projects left to right from the image and the posterior to anterior axis projects from the image top to bottom. Changing the L-R marker to the left side inverts the image but does not change the top-to-bottom image orientation. Image orientation can be adjusted to visualize targeted structures by simple catheter advancement or withdrawal, by tip deflection in four directions (anteroposterior and left-right), or by catheter rotation.

The AcuNav ICE catheter includes variable ultrasound frequency (5.5, 7.5, 8.5, and 10 MHz). Increasing ultrasound frequency improves axial image resolution; however, tissue penetration decreases and reduces imaging depth. An ultrasound frequency of 7.5 MHz is useful for imaging most cardiac structures. Frequency can then be increased (to 8.5 or 10 MHz) for imaging near-field structures, or decreased (to 5.5 MHz) for imaging far-field structures.[40]

RIGHT ATRIAL TARGETS. All RA targets are visualized by advancing or withdrawing the ICE catheter to an appropriate level within the RA and rotating the catheter to bring the target into view. The best resolution of near-field and midfield structures is obtained at an 8.5-MHz frequency. Once the catheter is advanced into the mid-RA with the catheter tension controls in neutral position (the ultrasound transducer oriented anteriorly and to the left), the RA, tricuspid valve, and RV are viewed. This is called the home view (see Fig. 4-13 and Video 5), and it can serve as a starting point; whenever the operator gets lost, he or she can go back to the home view and start over. From the home view, counterclockwise rotation of the catheter brings the RA appendage into view, whereas anterior deflection of the catheter tip toward the RV allows visualization of the tricuspid valve and cavotricuspid isthmus (Fig. 6-21). The superior crista terminalis is visualized when the catheter is advanced to the RA-SVC junction in an anterior direction.[41]

INTERATRIAL SEPTUM. Gradual clockwise rotation of a straight catheter from the home view allows sequential visualization of the aortic root and the pulmonary artery, followed by the CS, mitral valve, the LA appendage orifice, and a cross-sectional

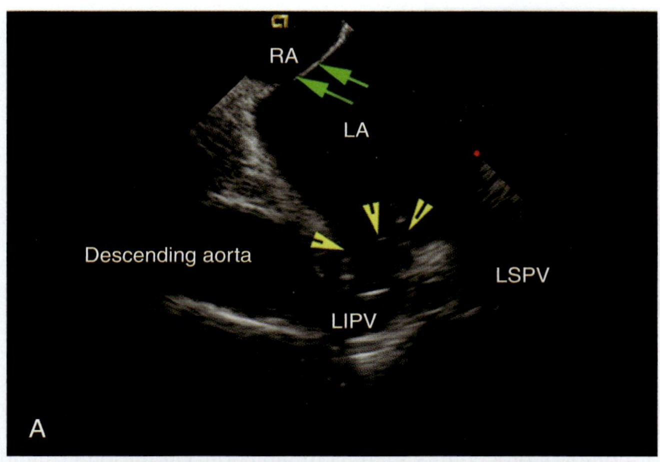

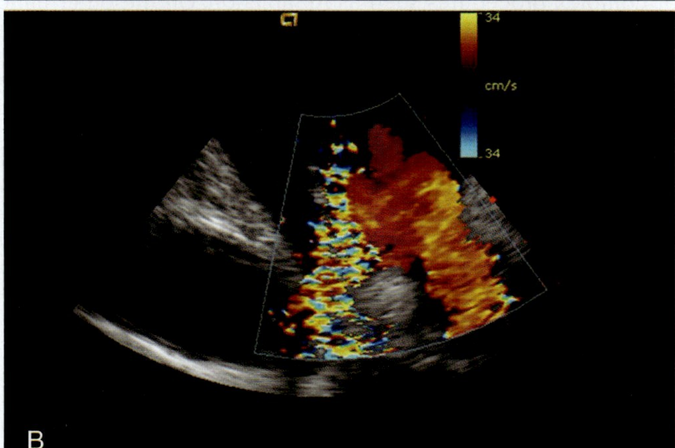

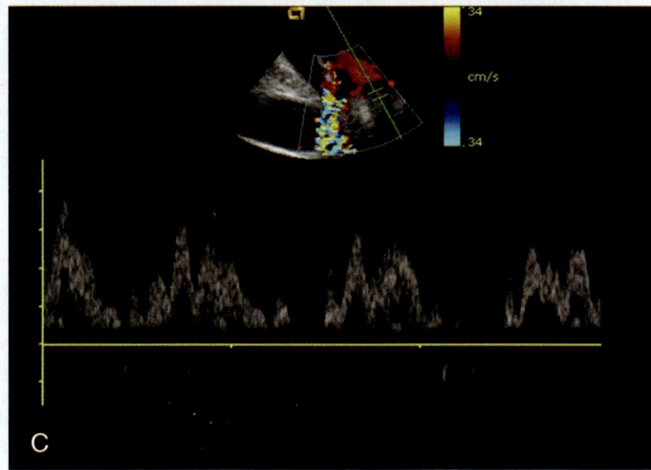

FIGURE 6-22 Intracardiac echocardiographic (ICE) images of the left pulmonary veins with transducer placed in the right atrium (RA). **A,** The RA, interatrial septum (green arrows), left inferior pulmonary vein (LIPV), left superior pulmonary vein (LSPV), and descending aorta are visualized. The Lasso catheter (yellow arrowheads) is visualized at the ostium of the LIPV. Color Doppler images of both LIPV and LSPV **(B)** and a pulsed-wave Doppler tracing **(C)** obtained from the LSPV are shown. LA = left atrium.

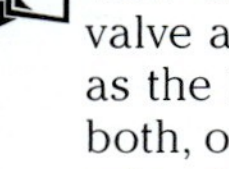

view of the fossa ovalis (see Fig. 4-13 and Video 5). The mitral valve and interatrial septum are usually seen in the same plane as the LA appendage. Posterior deflection, right-left steering, or both, of the imaging tip in the RA is occasionally required to optimize visualization of the fossa ovalis; the tension knob (lock function) can then be used to hold the catheter tip in position. Further clockwise rotation beyond this location demonstrates images of the left PV ostia (see Fig. 4-13). The optimum ICE image to guide

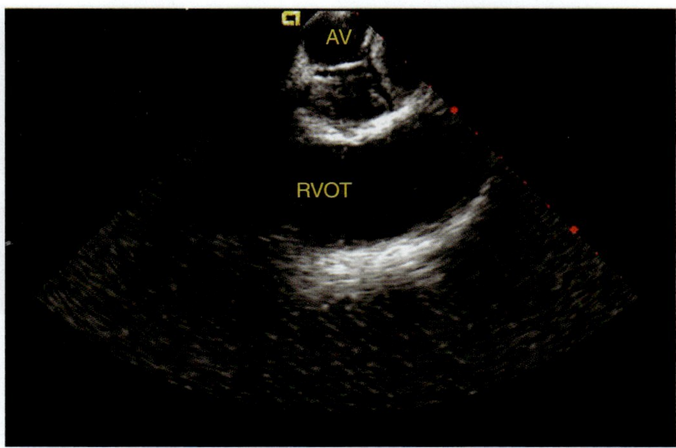

FIGURE 6-23 Short-axis view of the aortic valve (AV) cusps with the intracardiac echocardiographic (ICE) transducer placed in the midright atrium deflected near the posterior wall of the aortic root. RVOT = right ventricular outflow tract.

transseptal puncture demonstrates adequate space behind the interatrial septum on the LA side and clearly identifies adjacent structures (see Fig. 4-14 and Video 6).

LEFT ATRIAL STRUCTURES. A 7.5- or 8.5-MHz imaging frequency optimizes visualization of LA structures and PVs beyond the interatrial septum. PV imaging is possible by first visualizing the membranous fossa from a mid-RA to low-RA catheter tip position. With clockwise catheter rotation, the LA appendage can be visualized, followed by long-axis views of the left superior and inferior PVs (Fig. 6-22; see also Fig. 4-13). Further clockwise rotation of the catheter brings the orifices of the right superior and inferior PVs into view. The ostia of these veins are typically viewed en face, yielding an owl's eyes appearance at the vein's orifice. The LA appendage can also be visualized with the transducer positioned in the CS.

LEFT AND RIGHT VENTRICULAR TARGETS. Imaging of each targeted LV structure at depths of 6 to 15 cm is accomplished with the catheter tip in a low-RA position. When the catheter transducer is placed near the fossa and oriented anteriorly and to the left, the LV outflow tract (LVOT) and truncated LV are imaged. With clockwise rotation and slight adjustment of the transducer level, the mitral valve and LV apex can be viewed. To image the mitral valve in a long-axis, two-chamber view (LA, mitral valve, and LV), a mild degree of apically directed catheter tip deflection can be required. The RVOT, LVOT, and aortic root with coronary artery ostia can be imaged by advancing the catheter in the RA to the level of the outflow tracts (mid-RA), with an appropriate deflection to the right. The aortic valve can also be imaged in its cross section from this region (Fig. 6-23). A long-axis view of the LV can also be visualized by advancing the catheter with its anteriorly deflected tip into the RV with clockwise rotation against the interventricular septum (Fig. 6-24). Further clockwise rotation or right-left steering of the catheter tip allows a short-axis view of the LV, as well as the mitral valve (see Fig. 6-24). Pericardial effusions usually can be readily identified from these views. Withdrawing the catheter back to the base of the RVOT and rotating the shaft allow the RVOT to be visualized in its long axis, with a cross-sectional view of the pulmonic valve.[40]

Clinical Implications

Transesophageal imaging has been used to guide ablation of VT and BTs, as well as transseptal catheterization, and for the closure of atrial septal defects or cardiac biopsy. This approach, however, has been limited in the interventional arena by aspiration risk and patient discomfort accompanying prolonged esophageal intubation, and it requires a second ultrasound operator to complete the study.

Previous human applications of ICE have been limited to those generated by the mechanical rotation of a single piezoelectric

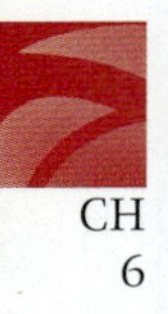

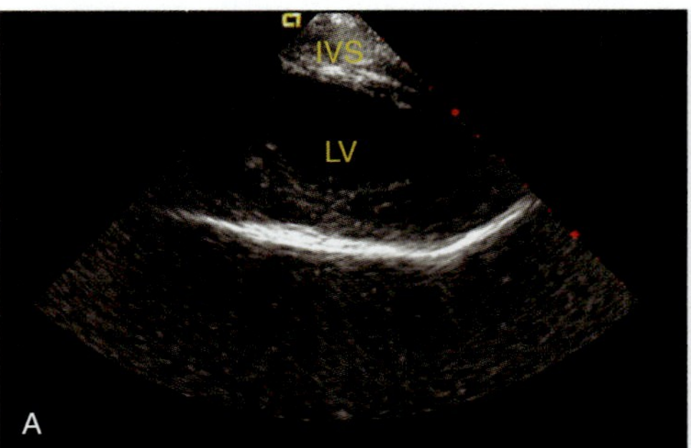

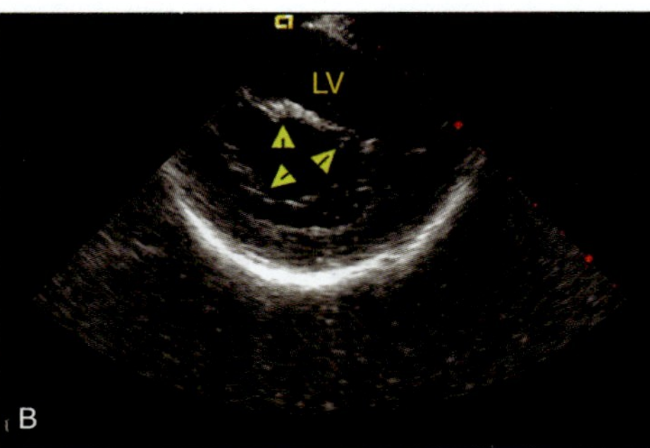

FIGURE 6-24 Intracardiac echocardiographic (ICE) images of the left ventricle (LV), with transducer placed in the right ventricle (RV) against the interventricular septum (IVS). **A,** Long-axis view of the LV. **B,** Short-axis view of the LV at the level of the mitral valve (arrowheads).

element in 6 to 10 Fr catheters. Miniaturization of these elements required the use of higher 10- to 20-MHz transducer frequencies, thus limiting ultrasound penetration to surrounding cardiac tissues. This technology has been applied to the imaging of RA structures in humans and animals, membranous fossa ovalis, crista terminalis, eustachian ridge, tricuspid annulus, and the SVC-RA junction in the region of the sinus node. However, visualization of the LA and PV ostia is limited using this system because of limited penetration depth, except when it is introduced directly into the LA (transseptally).

The electronic phased-array ultrasound system offers deeper field, standard intracardiac visualization of specific right- and left-sided cardiac structures, as well as color flow and pulsed-wave and continuous-wave Doppler imaging by a single operator. These features have been of significant value for PV isolation procedures and LA linear ablation for AF.

Several practical uses for ICE have emerged in the setting of EP procedures, including the following: (1) assessment of catheter contact with cardiac tissues; (2) determination of catheter location relative to cardiac structures (specifically useful in otherwise difficult to localize areas; e.g., the PVs); (3) guidance of transseptal puncture, particularly in the setting of complex or unusual anatomy; (4) facilitation of deployment of mapping or ablation systems (e.g., PV encircling devices, noncontact mapping systems, and basket technologies); (5) visualization of evolving lesions during RF energy delivery; both changing tissue echogenicity and microbubbles reflect tissue heating, with the latter providing a signal for energy termination; (6) evaluation of cardiac structures before and after intervention (e.g., cardiac valves and PVs); (7) assessment of PV anatomy, dimensions, and function via 2-D anatomical imaging and Doppler physiological measurements; (8) assessment of complications (e.g., tamponade, electromechanical dissociation, or thrombus formation; see Fig. 32-1)[42]; (9) identification of the anatomical origin of certain arrhythmias (e.g., ICE can facilitate ablation of inappropriate sinus tachycardia or sinus nodal reentrant tachycardia); and (10) definition of the proximity of the catheter tip and coronary arteries (during mapping and ablation of arrhythmias originating from the aortic cusp).

As mentioned previously, the CARTOSound Image Integration Module (Biosense Webster, Inc.) incorporates the electroanatomical map to an ICE volume map of the cardiac chamber derived from a phased-array transducer catheter incorporating a position sensor (SoundStar, Biosense Webster, Inc.), which may be used as a standalone tool to guide navigation and ablation or as a facilitator of CT/MRI image integration. This navigation approach has been successfully utilized for catheter ablation of AF. Additionally, 3-D ultrasound images can potentially yield anatomically accurate chamber geometries and identify scar in the LV (both by wall thickness and motion) to facilitate substrate mapping and ablation of ischemic VT.[12,13]

Computed Tomography and Magnetic Resonance Imaging

Fundamental Concepts

During catheter ablation procedures, the catheters are usually manipulated under the guidance of fluoroscopy. However, fluoroscopy does not provide adequate depiction of cardiac anatomy because of its poor soft tissue contrast and the 2-D projective nature of the formed image, which hinders its application for complex procedures such as AF ablation. On the other hand, CT and MRI images offer anatomical detail in 3-D. However, these images are presented out of the context of the ablation catheter, thus greatly diminishing their potential value. An optimal strategy would therefore be to integrate the 3-D images generated by CT or MRI with the electrical and navigational information obtained by an interventional system. This can be achieved through the process of integration. Image integration refers to the process of aligning the pre-procedural cardiac CT and MRI images with the real-time 3-D electroanatomical maps reconstructed from multiple endocardial locations. The process of image integration consists of three steps: pre-procedural CT and MRI image acquisition, image segmentation and extraction, and image registration.

IMAGE ACQUISITION

Cross-sectional or axial CT or MRI images are acquired at sufficient resolution to delineate cardiac structures less than 1 to 2 mm in thickness. Images at 0.625-mm thickness can be reconstructed from images obtained at 1.25-mm intervals with currently available multirow helical scanners. A simultaneous ECG is recorded to assign the source images retrospectively to the respective phases of the cardiac cycle. MRI images are similarly obtainable, although at a slightly lower spatial resolution. Reconstructing any cardiac chamber in 3-D from the axial images is performed using any one of various software packages.[43]

IMAGE SEGMENTATION

Image segmentation refers to the process of extracting the 3-D anatomy of individual cardiac structures from its surrounding structures. Methods of image segmentation include thresholding, boundary detection, and region identification. Thresholding involves assigning pixels with intensities lower than a threshold to one class and the remaining pixels to a different class. Connecting adjacent pixels of the same class then forms regions. Boundary differentiation methods use information about intensity differences between adjacent regions to separate the regions from each other. Region identification techniques then form regions by combining pixels of similar properties.[43-45] For cardiac ablation procedures, the volume of cardiac structures is extracted from the whole-volume data set using a computerized algorithm that differentiates the boundary between the blood pool (which is high in contrast) and the endocardium (which is not contrast enhanced). This allows for clear differentiation between the chamber lumen and endocardial wall (Fig. 6-25). Subsequently, the volumes of individual cardiac structures are separated from each other with the use of another algorithm capable of detecting their boundaries. Using a third algorithm, the segmented volumes for individual cardiac structures are extracted as 3-D surface reconstructions. The segmented volumes can be viewed from an external perspective or from within the chamber using virtual endoscopic or cardioscopic displays. These images, in addition to providing a road map for ablation, can also be used for registration (see Fig. 6-25).

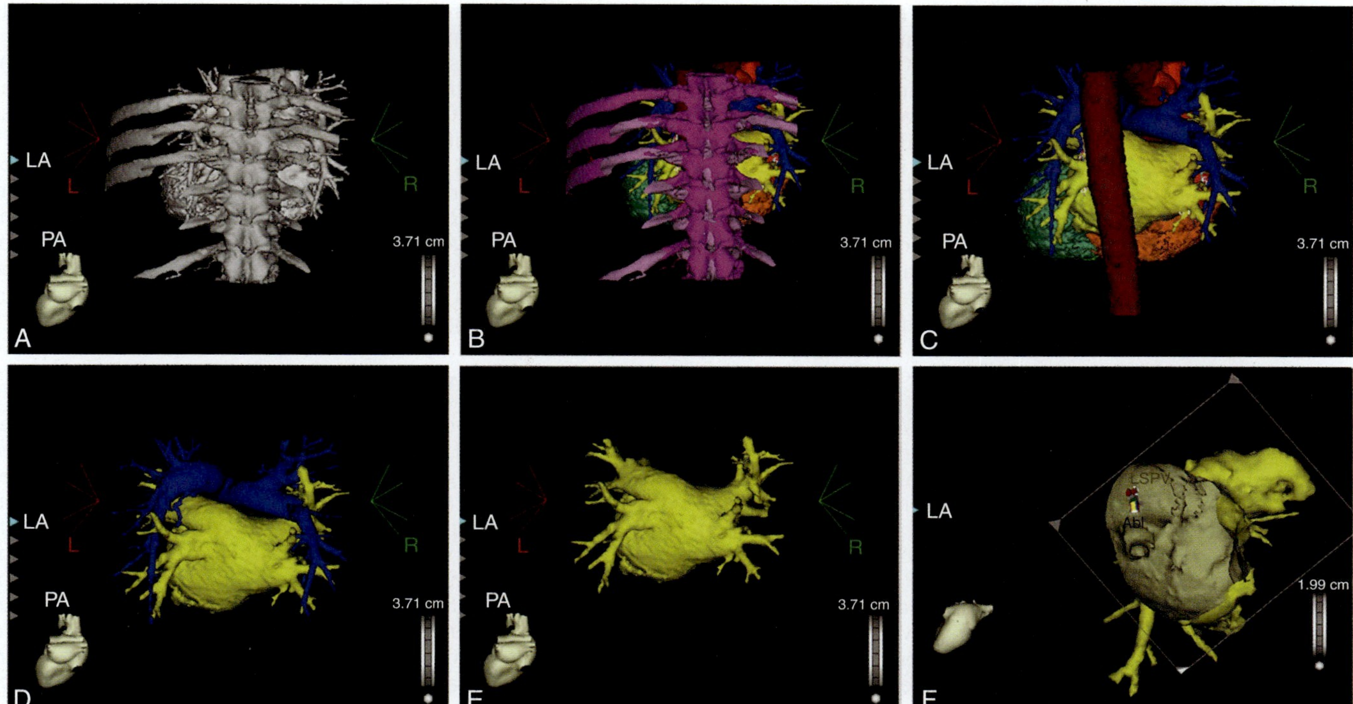

FIGURE 6-25 CT image segmentation and integration with electroanatomical mapping (CARTO) data. **A,** Three-dimensional reconstruction of the heart and part of the spine from the two-dimensional CT image (posteroanterior [PA] view). **B** and **C,** Individual cardiac chambers are segmented from each other using computerized algorithms capable of detecting their boundaries (aorta, red; left atrium [LA], yellow; left ventricle, green; pulmonary artery, blue; right atrium, orange). **D** and **E,** The cardiac chamber is selected (LA in this case), and others are deleted. **F,** Integration of CT and electroanatomical mapping (CARTO) data. Shown is a left lateral cardioscopic view of the ostia of the left pulmonary veins (PVs) during PV electrical isolation. Radiofrequency applications (small red circles) were deployed at the posterior aspect of the ostium of the left superior PV (LSPV). The ablation (Abl) catheter tip is positioned at the inferior aspect of the LSPV.

IMAGE REGISTRATION

Although the segmented structures are highly useful for visualizing the cardiac structures and characteristics of the tissue forming that structure, they do not convey the physiology of an arrhythmia. Integrating that physiology, as captured by electroanatomical or noncontact mapping with the spatial information contained in the CT or MRI images, requires registration of activation or voltage data to an appropriate location on a 3-D representation of a chamber. This is of critical importance in that it establishes the relationship between anatomy and physiology as required for the structure- and activity-based understanding of arrhythmias and for enabling image-guided intervention. Image registration refers to superimposing the 3-D CT/MRI surface reconstruction onto the real-time electroanatomical maps yielded by the 3-D mapping system (see Fig. 6-10).

During registration, the assumption is made that the anatomy of the organ being registered has not changed. Two computerized algorithms are used to accomplish the image registration process: landmark registration and surface registration. Landmark registration aligns the 3-D CT/MRI image reconstruction with corresponding electroanatomical maps through linking two sets of corresponding fiducial points in each set of the images to be registered. Under the guidance of fluoroscopy or ICE, or both, at least three landmark pairs are created by real-time catheter tip locations on the interventional system being used for registration and then placed on their estimated locations on the 3-D CT/MRI image reconstructions. Using more landmark points increases the accuracy of the registration process. Surface registration is an algorithm that attaches the acquired endocardial points to the closest CT/MRI surface to compose the best fit of the two sets of images by minimizing the average distance between the landmarks, and the distance from multiple endocardial locations, to the surface of 3-D CT/MRI image reconstructions. Surface registration complements landmark registration to improve the registration accuracy. However, because of surface indentation and potentially missed areas during mapping, the acquired electroanatomical map does not represent the perfect anatomy of the cardiac chamber.[43-45]

COMPUTED TOMOGRAPHY OVERLAY

A novel application (EP Navigator prototype, Philips Healthcare, Best, The Netherlands) has been developed to superimpose a preacquired segmented 3-D CT image of the LA over real-time fluoroscopy system ("CT overlay") to help in guiding ablation of atrial arrhythmias, particularly AF. This application can be used on monoplane or biplane fluoroscopy. It permits fluoroscopy-directed guiding of an ablation catheter and diagnostic catheters in a virtual 3-D model of the LA, and subsequent tagging of ablation sites on the registered 3-D image without the simultaneous use of an electroanatomical mapping system, thus facilitating the creation of continuous lines and returning to critical ablation sites. Furthermore, it is feasible to identify and segment the esophagus on the CT scan, which can subsequently be overlaid on the fluoroscopic images along with the cardiac structures.[46-48]

Image Integration Procedure

IMAGE REGISTRATION USING CARTOMERGE

The preacquired CT/MRI digital imaging data are imported by a CD into the CARTO XP system equipped with commercially available software (CARTOMerge Image Integration Software Module) that allows structures of interest to be easily and quickly segmented and reconstructed in 3-D. The segmented images are then imported into the real-time mapping system. Once created using the CARTO system (as described previously), the electroanatomical map of the cardiac chamber is "fused" to the CT/MRI. The most frequently used registration technique is a combination of *landmark*

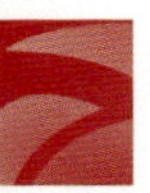

registration and *surface registration*. Landmark registration involves the 3-D orientation of the imported CT/MRI image on the x, y, and z axes and requires the acquisition of at least three noncollinear endocardial landmark points using the mapping-ablation catheter. The precise location of these on the 3-D image is a critical factor in this technique and remains challenging. Biplane fluoroscopy, angiography, and ICE can be used to facilitate identification of the landmark point. Catheter contact is ensured by fluoroscopy visualization of the catheter mobility in relation to the cardiac motion and by a discrete electrogram. The estimated corresponding locations of these endocardial landmark points are then marked on the imported 3-D CT/MRI image, thus creating a landmark pair, with one landmark point on the real-time electroanatomical map and the other on the 3-D CT/MRI image.

Landmark registration approximates the electroanatomical map to the 3-D CT/MRI surface reconstruction by matching the landmark pair. Surface registration fits the 3-D CT/MRI surface reconstruction with the electroanatomical map points by rendering the smallest average distance of the two datasets. Although the registration of surface points should improve alignment of the two images, registering points from the entire surface of the cardiac chamber involves the risk of incorporating errors related to potential indentation of the chamber wall and distortion of chamber geometry resulting from the pressure of the mapping catheter on the most mobile regions. The mapping system then provides an average tip-to-surface distance, which ideally should be less than 2 mm. While manipulating the catheter during ablation, the projected catheter distance to the surface is used as an additional guide to assess catheter contact. This can be complemented by information from electrograms recorded by the catheter, fluoroscopy, and ICE.[16]

IMAGE REGISTRATION USING CARTOSOUND

The CARTOSound utilizes a 10 Fr phased-array ICE catheter with an embedded navigation sensor (SoundStar, Biosense Webster, Inc.), which records individual 90-degree sector image planes of the cardiac chamber of interest, including their location and orientation, to the CARTO workspace. To correct for respiratory phase, all ICE images should be acquired during expiratory breath-hold. Once the CARTOSound volume map of the cardiac chamber is created, registration is performed using CARTOMerge software. First, the CT/MRI image is visually aligned with the ICE-created cardiac chamber anatomical shell. Second, landmark registration is performed whereby three echocardiographically discrete anatomical sites identified with ICE (landmark points) are tagged on the ICE contour and matched to a corresponding location on the CT/MRI image. Finally, the CARTOMerge surface registration algorithm is performed. This algorithm attempts optimally to juxtapose, or integrate, the CT/MRI image spatially with the CARTOSound model to minimize the average distance between each point on the ICE-created anatomical rendering of the cardiac chamber and the corresponding CT/MRI image, thus permitting the CT model to guide navigation.

Registration is based on the best fit between the cardiac chamber surface reconstruction obtained with each ICE contour and the corresponding CT/MRI image, and it is not based on the LA volume obtained with ICE and the corresponding CT/MRI image.[12] ICE-guided focused endocardial surface registration seems to be superior to landmark registration in achieving a better alignment between the CT/MRI image and the electroanatomical map. The 3-D ultrasound images can help create anatomically accurate, real-time chamber geometries and eliminate chamber deformity (as often happens with contact mapping), potentially to yield more accurate CT/MRI registration.[12,13]

IMAGE REGISTRATION USING NAVX FUSION

The cardiac chamber of interest is segmented and reconstructed in 3-D from CT/MRI slices using EnSite Verismo software. The 3-D virtual anatomical geometry of the cardiac chamber is created using NavX Fusion (as described previously). The CT/MRI reconstruction of the mapped cardiac chamber is displayed on a split screen and used to guide finer anatomical definition with the ablation catheter and help edit the virtual 3-D geometry to eliminate "false space." Subsequently, "field scaling" is applied to the geometry to compensate for variations in impedance between the heart chambers and venous structures and render the geometry and navigational space more physiologically relevant and to more closely resemble the CT/MRI image. The field scaled geometry is fused to the CT/MRI in two stages, termed *primary (rigid) fusion* and *secondary (dynamic) fusion*. Primary fusion uses three fiducial (i.e., landmark) corresponding points on the created geometry and the CT/MRI image to superimpose, or lock together, both images (Fig. 6-26). These points are chosen to ensure reasonable 3-D anatomical separation and allow orientation of the CT/MRI, but the registration error is high. Therefore, secondary fusion points or fiducials are applied to the primary fused geometry at sites of local mismatch between the two superimposed geometries.

In this unique component of image fusion, the created geometry surface is molded to the CT/MRI surface while also "bending" the 3-D navigation space within the geometry. This process is continued, adding supplemental (usually more than 15) fiducial point pairs until good correspondence between the NavX geometry and CT/MRI models is achieved. For example, if the anterior wall of the geometry is fused anteriorly to the CT/MRI, the catheter location also will be moved so that, when the catheter is repositioned on the anterior wall after fusion, it should be visualized on the CT/MRI surface and not within the bounds of the original prefusion geometry. Although the principle of CT/MRI image integration is common to both the EnSite NavX Fusion and CARTOMerge systems, there is a significant difference in how registration is achieved.

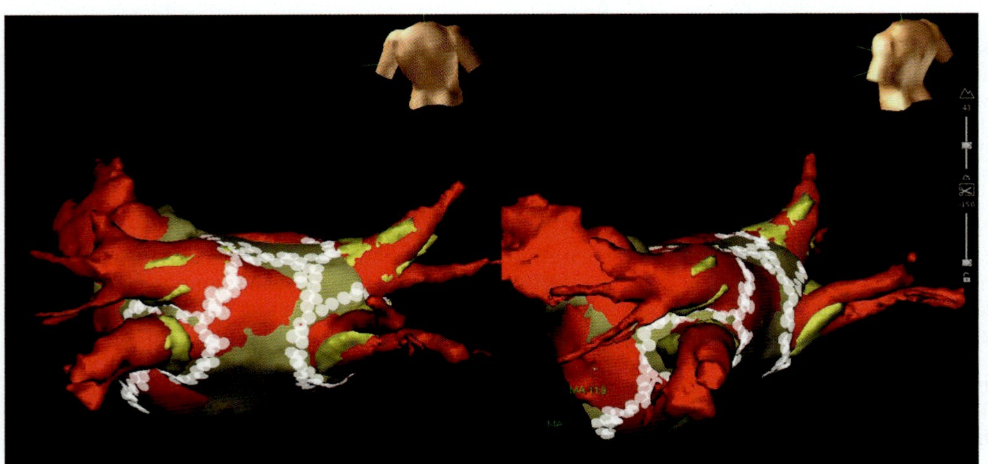

FIGURE 6-26 Integration of CT and ESI-NavX electroanatomical mapping data. Shown are posterior anterior and left lateral views of the electroanatomical contour acquired with catheter manipulation in the left atrium during atrial fibrillation ablation overlaid on a CT image of the left atrium acquired several days earlier. Small white circles are tagged sites at which radiofrequency energy was applied to isolate the pulmonary veins. MA =mitral annulus..

As described previously, the EnSite system uses a dynamic registration process (with four or more fiducials) to optimize both rotation and stretching of the surface of the NavX geometry to match the CT/MRI. With the CARTOMerge system, the whole registration process is rigid with rotation of the CT/MRI to minimize the distance between the surface of the anatomical model generated and that of the CT, but no stretching of the model itself. Despite this difference, the registration error is similar with both techniques (CARTOMerge, 2.3 ± 1.8 mm, versus EnSite NavX Fusion, 3.2 ± 0.9 mm).[19,49]

IMAGE REGISTRATION USING FLUOROSCOPY (CT OVERLAY)

The preacquired CT data set is imported into the software, the cardiac chamber of interest is automatically segmented, and a 3-D volume of the LA and PVs is constructed. Before CT registration is performed, the patient must be properly positioned, and the structure of interest must be isocentered in two orthogonal fluoroscopic projections. Initial registration is based on the heart contour to allow for quick alignment of the CT-rendered volume with the fluoroscopic image. On an anteroposterior fluoroscopic projection (without contrast injection), the CT volume overlay is aligned by first using the right lateral atrial contour. The rest of the cardiac contour then is superimposed on the fluoroscopic image, based on the best visual estimate. Subsequently, fluoroscopic identification of intracardiac landmarks by catheter manipulation within the LA and PVs improves the overlay accuracy (e.g., caudal drop of the catheter when withdrawing from a PV into the LA helps identify the PV ostium; insertion of the ablation catheter into readily identifiable anatomical landmarks such as PV branches immediately connected to PV ostium, accessory PVs; and looping of the ablation catheter in the LA resulting in circumferential catheter-endocardium contact). Finally, angiography of the right and left superior PVs (sequentially or simultaneously) in two orthogonal views is performed to adjust the CT image further and improve registration by matching the superior border of the LA and the superior PV ostia, as well as certain landmarks, such as PV bifurcations, between 3-D image and fluoroscopy.

After registration and locking, the 3-D CT image is always depicted at the same angle as the fluoroscopy (i.e., the CT-generated volume rotates on the screen following the rotation of the C-arm), thus allowing for constant visualization of the CT and fluoroscopic images under the same viewing angle. The transparency of the overlaid CT 3-D volume is adjustable, to allow visualization of the catheters in the fluoroscopic image. In addition, the 3-D image can be clipped with a customizable cutting plane, to permit internal (endoscopic) views. Moreover, tags can be placed on the surface of the registered 3-D image to mark ablation sites and other sites of interest.[46-48]

Clinical Implications

CT and MRI imaging approaches have already been of significant benefit in AF catheter ablation procedures. These approaches provide critical information regarding the number, location, and size of PVs, as needed for planning the ablation and selecting appropriately sized ablation devices.[50] Resulting images also identify branching patterns of potentially arrhythmogenic PVs, disclose the presence of fused superior and inferior veins into antral structures, and clarify the potentially confounding origins of far-field electrograms that masquerade as PV potentials. CT has also been used for postablation evaluation for PV stenosis.

The 21st century has also seen the rapid development of integrated, anatomy-based mapping and ablation. This progress has been driven by a realization of both the critical coupling and dependence of arrhythmias on their underlying anatomy and the limitations of surrogate geometries of contemporary mapping systems for reflecting that anatomy. Over this same time frame, rapid CT and MRI imaging systems have emerged as the mainstays of imaging in the EP laboratory and have been used to plan or guide ablation. Each company is actively working on image incorporation into its system.[11,47,51] Helical 16- to 64-row CT and MRI studies provide a broad anatomy library of an individual patient at one point in time. Segmented CT volumes can be downloaded on the CARTO and NavX platforms. These systems are able to register the surrogate map fully onto actual CT and MRI anatomy; they also enable integration of electroanatomical mapping with preacquired CT and MRI images and allow real-time visualization of the location and orientation of the catheter tip within the registered CT anatomical framework (see Figs. 6-10 and 6-25).[4,16,43-45]

The use of registered CT and MRI images to guide catheter ablation presents a significant advantage over the less detailed surrogate geometry created by previously available 3-D mapping systems. Because it provides detailed anatomical information on the catheter tip location in relation to the true cardiac anatomy, the image integration technique has the potential to facilitate many ablation procedures, especially anatomically based ablation strategies, such as AF ablation (see Video 13), nonidiopathic VT ablation, and ablation of intraatrial reentrant tachycardias following corrective surgery for congenital heart diseases. Initial experience has shown that the registered CT and MRI of LA reconstructions can provide accurate information on the catheter tip location in relation to the important LA structures, such as the PV ostium and LA appendage. The real-time update of the catheter tip location and the marking of ablation lesions on the detailed 3-D image can potentially improve the quality of lesion sets, reduce complications, and shorten procedure and fluoroscopy times.

Registration of a preacquired 3-D CT image on fluoroscopy potentially combines the accuracy of CT with the real-time fluoroscopy to guide catheter ablation of AF. Compared with an established and widely used electroanatomical mapping technique for PV antrum isolation, procedural duration can be shortened significantly without a concomitant increase in radiation burden. An additional advantage to CT overlay is the ability to perform a quick repeat registration in case of major changes in a patient's position. However, unlike the CARTO system, which provides notification for significant patient movements, the operator needs to be alert on discrepancies between catheters and anatomy and must check registration in case of suspected movement. Additionally, with the CARTO system, one can return to the catheter-based LA reconstruction without Merge, which may be more accurate than the CT image.[46-48]

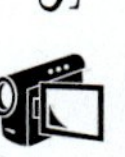

Limitations

Although CT and MRI provide exquisite images of the underlying structures relevant in arrhythmogenesis, they are limited by the requirement of off-line generation of the CT and MRI libraries and the inability to reflect all phases of the cardiac cycle during an arrhythmia. Because CT and MRI is performed prior to the ablation procedure, registration error can arise from interval changes in the heart size because of differences in rhythm, rate, contractility, or fluid status. Performing image registration and ablation procedures within 24 hours after CT and MRI scans and CT and MRI image acquisition and image registration during the same rhythm may help limit interval changes. This situation is confounded by the inevitable imperfection of the created virtual geometry of the cardiac chamber. These factors can impede the clinical utility of image integration in approximately 25% of patients.[52]

Furthermore, the static images of the registered CT and MRI reconstructions provide little information on true catheter-tissue contact. In addition, because the initial landmark points are picked up by the operator using fluoroscopy, the exact location of these points in the 3-D space can be deceptive, and registration errors in the identification of these points are very common, even when angiography and ICE are used for guidance. In addition, because multiple points are needed for surface registration, the accuracy of chamber reconstruction is directly dependent on the number of points taken and the position of the catheter, thus adding a significant amount of time and a manual component to the process.[4,43,47,53]

To overcome some of these limitations, fusion of real-time ICE images with those generated by CT and MRI scans is becoming available and can provide a more real-time interactive display, as well as real-time information on catheter-tissue contact and RF lesion formation. In addition, it is highly likely that subsequent generations of CT or MRI scanners will be sufficiently fast to permit real-time or almost real-time imaging for interventional guidance. Studies have demonstrated the ability to merge the 3-D CT and MRI images with real-time 2-D fluoroscopy images for navigation on virtual anatomy, because the images can be corrected against the background of real-time fluoroscopy as needed.[4,47,54]

The accuracy of registration remains the subject of investigation. 3-D image integration aims at improving the operator's perception of the catheter spatial location in relation to the patient's cardiac structures. However, the success of this approach is primarily dependent on the accuracy of the image integration process. Even if the 3-D cardiac chamber image provides an accurate model of a matched phase of the chamber volume at the time of the procedure, it needs to be accurately registered to the procedural chamber orientation to provide reliable navigation. Current registration algorithms depend on accurate catheter geometry; this requires an accurate update of 3-D coordinates of the catheter tip, as recorded and displayed on the computer image. The exact location of the initial fiducial points picked by the operator using fluoroscopy in the 3-D space may be deceptive. Movement of the catheter tip is complex and is affected by wall motion and respiration. Point collection should therefore be gated to the same phase of the cardiac and respiratory cycle as the CT or MRI scan. Additionally, catheter tip pressure can cause tenting of the chamber wall, thereby distorting the chamber geometry. Stability of catheter contact with the endocardial wall should also be optimized. Catheter contact can vary with the type of ablation catheter and introducer sheath, as well as the degree of regional wall motion; for example, the mitral annulus and appendage are more dynamic than the posterior atrial wall. Ideally, geometry points should be collected from stable catheter positions. The operator can then accept good points or delete bad points. This process can be aided by fluoroscopy, electrogram morphology, and confirmation of the catheter tip location on ICE. However, the process still remains a subjective art.[43,53]

Several studies of AF catheter ablation have reported success using different integration modalities with CT or MRI, by using either noncontact mapping or fluoroscopy as a second integrated image. The registration technique has also varied, including three- or four-point registration or surface registration. Alternatively, a single point and the surface have been used as well (visual alignment). Different techniques for point localization have been reported, including fluoroscopy alone, angiography, or ICE for direct visualization of the catheter at the designated site. The mean error for surface registration in most studies varied between 1.8 and 2.7 mm; one study that compared the landmark registration with and without surface registration found that surface registration increases the accuracy of image integration. On the other hand, a more recent study found that the most accurate landmark registration is achieved when posterior points are acquired at the PV-LA junction, whereas points acquired on the anterior wall, LA appendage, or other structures outside the LA, such as the CS or SVC, afford less accuracy. In addition, surface registration usually results in shifting the landmark points away from the initially acquired position on the corresponding PVs using ICE.[55] Furthermore, accurate surface registration does not guarantee accurate alignment with the important anatomical structures. Another report found that serious inaccuracies of the CARTOMerge image integration algorithms still exist, despite using the precautions discussed earlier.[56] Importantly, registration quality has not yet been shown necessarily to correlate with ablation accuracy.[12,56]

It is important to recognize that the registered CT model still is prone to subjective inaccuracies and should remain only a guide, and a combination of fluoroscopy and the electrogram appearance must also be used in assessing contact with the endocardial surface and the true position of the catheter. Although 3-D mapping systems with image integration have been widely adopted for ablation procedures, many of their theoretical benefits remain unproven; therefore, these systems should remain just one type among the tools facilitating complex catheter ablation procedures and should not distract the electrophysiologist from established EP principles and endpoints.[57]

Three-Dimensional Rotational Angiography

Fundamental Concepts

3-D rotational angiography combines the accuracy of direct angiography with the benefits of computer animation and supplements conventional 2-D fluoroscopy to provide real-time representation of cardiac structures. Its feasibility and clinical utility in the setting of LA imaging and AF ablation have been described. This method provides rapid intraprocedural visualization of LA anatomy and of important nearby structures such as the esophagus. Prior studies have demonstrated that the diagnostic value of 3-D rotational angiography is comparable to that of CT imaging.[58,59]

The principle of 3-D rotational angiography is similar to the CT scan, in which images acquired from different angles are reconstructed to a 3-D image. The C-arc x-ray system is rotated around the patient over 240 degrees to create a circumferential run of many exposure images of the region of interest distributed over the 360-degree (or similar) trajectory. To improve differentiation of the cardiac structures, the cardiac chamber of interest can be opacified with a contrast medium injected either directly into the LA or indirectly into the right side of the heart, in which case rotation of the fluoroscopic system is started after passage of the contrast medium through the lungs. The esophagus can be opacified using a barium paste prior to the image acquisition. The rotational angiographic images of the LA, PVs, esophagus, and other surrounding structures can be segmented and registered with the fluoroscopy on a specialized computer system (EP Navigator, Philips Healthcare or similar system, such as DynaCT Cardiac, Siemens, Forchheim, Germany). The latest version of the software allows registration of the segmented 3-D volume on a live fluoroscopy screen.[60,61]

Imaging Technique

First, the patient must be properly positioned, and the structure of interest must be isocentered. The patient's arms may be extended above the head to reduce mass artifact. Oral contrast (5 mL barium sulfate esophageal cream) is administered immediately prior to initiation of the rotational run, and once it is visualized in the esophagus, intravenous contrast may be injected into the main pulmonary artery, RV, RA, or IVC via a 6 Fr pigtail catheter to obtain adequate levophase opacification of the LA. In general, contrast injection at the IVC-RA junction results in adequate LA and PV opacification in most patients. In addition, this method is technically simpler and potentially safer than more downstream injections. Higher amounts of contrast and longer injection time are generally used with RA and IVC injections than with main pulmonary artery injection. Direct contrast injection into the LA was described and seemed to provide great detail of LA and PV anatomy, but it required a high-dose (30 to 50 mg) adenosine injection immediately prior to the rotational run. Transient cessation of contractions prevents anterograde washout of contrast from the PVs, thus keeping them opacified during the rotational run. Deep sedation, intubation, and RV pacing are usually needed to counteract apnea and asystole produced by adenosine. Additionally, high doses of adenosine are not tolerated by the conscious patient because of the induced flush and dyspnea. Given such complexities, this method may be more difficult to implement in clinical practice.[58-61]

For injection at the RA-IVC junction, 80 to 100 mL of contrast is injected over 4 seconds via a pigtail catheter using a power injector. The C-arm is rotated over a 240-degree arc (120-degree RAO to 120-degree LAO view) in a 4.1-second period. The x-ray acquisition speed is 30 frames per second, which results in a total of 120 frames in the rotational run. Continuous fluoroscopic monitoring for contrast appearance in the LA is used to trigger the rotational run, based on visual guidance rather than on an empirically determined delay. The patient is instructed to stop breathing immediately prior to initiation of the rotational run to prevent respiratory movement of the structure of interest and inadequate reconstruction. Normal breathing can be resumed immediately on the completion of rotation.

The rotational angiogram is judged to be adequate when the LA is filled with contrast during most of the run and antral portions of all PVs are opacified without truncation. A resultant movie file is then transferred to an EP Navigator workstation to be segmented and overlaid on a live fluoroscopy screen. After the catheters are advanced into the LA, the 3-D image is used for navigation. With registration of the 3-D volume, all movements of the C-arm are translated into the appropriate rotation or shift, thus keeping the relationship between the fluoroscopic heart shadow and reconstructed image unchanged.

Image integration of intraprocedural rotational angiography-based 3-D reconstructions of LA and PVs into the electroanatomical mapping system (CARTOMerge) has become feasible. The images of the segmented LA are saved on a compact disc and transferred to the electroanatomical mapping system by using custom-designed software and integrated without further segmentation.

Theoretically, no registration for 3-D rotational angiography image overlay is necessary if the original x-ray table position and the patient's position during the rotational run are maintained. However, moving the x-ray table is often required after 3-D rotational angiography, especially given the fact that intracardiac catheters should be placed only after the rotational run to prevent artifacts. Therefore, registration is often necessary because, in its current iteration, overlay movement is linked only to C-arm rotation and not to x-ray table repositioning. Several registration methods using different primary landmarks, such as catheter placement, heart contour, and PV angiography, have been evaluated. These methods are particularly useful when registering previously obtained CT images on live fluoroscopy (i.e., CT overlay), which is another imaging input available in the EP Navigator (as discussed previously).

The current software version allows for the inner surface of the LA and PVs to be visualized (endoscopic view), further aiding the physician when navigating around the LA. Ablation points can be marked on the overlaid 3-D rotational angiography model to track the completeness of lesions. LA proximity to the esophagus can be evaluated and catheter ablation modified as necessary to avoid ablation near the esophagus.[62-64]

Clinical Implications

One of the advantages of 3-D rotational angiography over conventional 2-D fluoroscopy is the capability of depth perception and volume appreciation. 3-D rotational angiography provides direct visualization of cardiac structures, whereas electroanatomical methods require either operator imagination or confirmation via other imaging modalities, such as CT. Although pre-procedure CT/MRI images provide visualization of the LA and the PVs and facilitate integration with the electroanatomical mapping systems, a significant drawback is the time lag to the actual procedure. Interval changes in volume status, respiratory phase, and cardiac rhythm can result in temporal changes in the size and location of the anatomical structures between the time of image acquisition and the registration process. These limitations may be overcome by intraprocedural acquisition of the LA volume and PV anatomy; 3-D rotational angiography can be performed immediately before ablation using the same fluoroscopic imaging system, thus providing realistic anatomical detail at the time of the intervention.[58-60]

Other advantages of 3-D rotational angiography technology include quick and accurate repeat registration of the 3-D volume in case of patient movement not requiring a new map, as is frequently the case with electroanatomical methods.[61,62]

Despite exclusively fluoroscopic guidance of the ablation catheter using the 3-D rotational angiography technology, total fluoroscopy time and fluoroscopy time for PV isolation have been comparable to reported times for AF ablation procedures performed with different nonfluoroscopic mapping systems. Additionally, 3-D rotational angiography has the potential to eliminate the need for pre-procedural CT/MRI imaging, and the radiation exposure is less than that of CT scanning (estimated at 2.2 ± 0.2 mSv exposure with one rotational angiography run).[63,64]

Imaging by 3-D rotational angiography should not be confined to the LA and PVs. Other cardiac structures (current possibilities include RA and RVOT) can be easily visualized by timing the rotational run with the passage of contrast through the structures. The possibility of "whole heart" imaging has been reported.

Limitations

The use of contrast makes 3-D rotational angiography a less appealing option for patients with heart failure or insufficiency. In addition, the technique is sensitive to patient movements during the study period.

One shortfall of 3-D rotational angiography is the absence of streaming electrogram data. Additionally, because of the lack of respiratory compensation in the 3-D rotational angiography-fluoroscopy fusion, the end-expiratory phase is used as reference for monitoring the position of the ablation catheter tip during RF application.[58,59]

Proper isocentering is important to obtain adequate 3-D rotational angiography. Concerns have been raised about the frequent difficulty in fitting the LA and PVs into one rotational run with the commonly used detector. However, with proper isocentering, even a dilated LA and the PV anatomy can be adequately imaged; truncation may occur more easily if the structures of interest are not at the center of rotation.[58]

3-D rotational angiography is quickly evolving into a true online imaging tool; however, further refinements are needed before it can be widely adopted. These include incorporation of respiratory and cardiac motion compensation and the ability to display electrogram data on the 3-D shell (activation timing, scar and voltage maps, and dominant frequency). Further development is likely to involve several aspects of the method: automation of the workflow, injection protocols, and software; imaging of cardiac structures other than the LA and development of methods to visualize highly mobile structures such as the ventricles; and integration of anatomical 3-D rotational angiography information with electrogram data.[58-60]

Conclusions

Recording and analyzing extracellular electrograms form the basis for cardiac mapping. More commonly, cardiac mapping is performed with catheters introduced percutaneously into the heart chambers that sequentially record the endocardial electrograms with the purpose of correlating local electrogram to cardiac anatomy. These EP catheters are navigated and localized with the use of fluoroscopy.

However, the use of fluoroscopy for these purposes can be problematic for several reasons, including the following: (1) intracardiac electrograms cannot be associated accurately with their precise location within the heart; (2) the endocardial surface is invisible using fluoroscopy, and target sites may be approximated only by their relationship with nearby structures, such as ribs, blood vessels, and the position of other catheters; (3) because of the limitations of 2-D fluoroscopy, navigation is not exact, it is time-consuming, and it requires multiple views to estimate the 3-D location of the catheter; (4) the catheter cannot accurately and precisely be returned to a previously mapped site; and (5) the patient and medical team are exposed to radiation.

The limitations of conventional mapping are being overcome with the introduction of sophisticated mapping systems that integrate 3-D catheter localization with sophisticated complex arrhythmia maps. The choice of a specific mapping system for a particular interventional case is shaped by the importance of a specific characteristic in the mapping process. Advanced mapping systems have a limited role in the ablation of typical AFL, AVNRT, or BTs, given the high success rate of the conventional approach. However, for more complex arrhythmias, such as macroreentrant AT, AF, and unstable VT, advanced mapping modalities offer a clear advantage. Additionally, advanced mapping systems can potentially shorten procedural time, reduce radiation exposure, and enhance the success rate for the ablation of typical AFL, idiopathic outflow tract VT, and sustained, stable macroreentrant VT.

In cases for which an undistorted anatomical rendering with high spatial accuracy is required, the CARTO system is of advantage; it has fewer problems with interstructure delineation and requires fewer fixed or snap points to preserve the anatomy. The CARTO and NavX systems work well for mapping sustained, stable arrhythmias. Mapping nonsustained arrhythmias, PACs, or PVCs can be tedious with each of these three approaches. With these arrhythmias, the noncontact mapping array works well, although the maps can be filter frequency dependent. The noncontact approach provides a quick snapshot of activation during unstable VTs and obviates the need for long periods of tachycardia. Substrate mapping, such as scar or voltage mapping, is a useful alternative to noncontact mapping. CARTO performs very well in this regard. NavX also works reasonably well with its dynamic substrate mapping capabilities.

In some cases, the choice of mapping system depends on the skill and experience of the operator. The user interfaces of the CARTO and NavX systems are acceptably straightforward. The noncontact system requires more steps in the creation of user-friendly working geometry. Each of these systems is currently in the development stage, and their various capabilities can change substantially over the next several years. However, to date, the integration of anatomical, EP, and software information by an experienced physician is an indispensable prerequisite to accomplish a safe and successful procedure. At most, such systems must be used as an adjunctive tool to facilitate mapping and ablation. The operator should understand the advantages and shortcomings of each system and should recognize that these systems can be misleading and confusing and provide inaccurate information as a result of either incorrect data acquisition or inherent limitations of the technology.

REFERENCES

1. Sanders P, Hocini M, Jais P, et al: Characterization of focal atrial tachycardia using high-density mapping, *J Am Coll Cardiol* 46:2088–2099, 2005.
2. Markides V, Koa-Wing M, Peters N: Mapping and imaging. In Zipes DP, Jalife J, editor: *Cardiac electrophysiology: from cell to bedside*, ed 5, Philadelphia, 2009, Saunders, pp 897–904.
3. Schilling R, Friedman P, Stanton M: *Mathematical reconstruction of endocardial potentials with non-contact multielectrode array*, In *Field clinical training manual*, St. Paul, Minn., 2006, Endocardial Solutions.
4. Chinitz LA, Sethi JS: How to perform noncontact mapping, *Heart Rhythm* 3:120–123, 2006.
5. Tai CT, Chen SA: Noncontact mapping of the heart: how and when to use, *J Cardiovasc Electrophysiol* 20:123–126, 2009.
6. Huang JL, Tai CT, Lin YJ, et al: Substrate mapping to detect abnormal atrial endocardium with slow conduction in patients with atypical right atrial flutter, *J Am Coll Cardiol* 48:492–498, 2006.
7. Sivagangabalan G, Pouliopoulos J, Huang K, et al: Comparison of electroanatomic contact and noncontact mapping of ventricular scar in a postinfarct ovine model with intramural needle electrode recording and histological validation, *Circ Arrhythm Electrophysiol* 1:363–369, 2008.
8. Packer DL: Three-dimensional mapping in interventional electrophysiology: techniques and technology, *J Cardiovasc Electrophysiol* 16:1110–1116, 2005.
9. Markowitz SM, Lerman BB: How to interpret electroanatomic maps, *Heart Rhythm* 3:240–246, 2006.
10. Soejima K: How to troubleshoot the electroanatomic map, *Heart Rhythm* 7:999–1003, 2010.
11. Sra J, Krum D, Hare J, et al: Feasibility and validation of registration of three-dimensional left atrial models derived from computed tomography with a noncontact cardiac mapping system, *Heart Rhythm* 2:55–63, 2005.
12. Schwartzman D, Zhong H: On the use of CartoSound for left atrial navigation, *J Cardiovasc Electrophysiol* 21:656–664, 2010.
13. Bunch TJ, Weiss JP, Crandall BG, et al: Image integration using intracardiac ultrasound and 3D reconstruction for scar mapping and ablation of ventricular tachycardia, *J Cardiovasc Electrophysiol* 21:678–684, 2010.
14. Esato M, Hindricks G, Sommer P, et al: Color-coded three-dimensional entrainment mapping for analysis and treatment of atrial macroreentrant tachycardia, *Heart Rhythm* 6:349–358, 2009.
15. Santucci PA, Varma N, Cytron J, et al: Electroanatomic mapping of postpacing intervals clarifies the complete active circuit and variants in atrial flutter, *Heart Rhythm* 6:1586–1595, 2009.
16. Della BP, Fassini G, Cireddu M, et al: Image integration-guided catheter ablation of atrial fibrillation: a prospective randomized study, *J Cardiovasc Electrophysiol* 20:258–265, 2009.
17. Linton NW, Koa-Wing M, Francis DP, et al: Cardiac ripple mapping: a novel three-dimensional visualization method for use with electroanatomic mapping of cardiac arrhythmias, *Heart Rhythm* 6:1754–1762, 2009.
18. Earley MJ, Showkathali R, Alzetani M, et al: Radiofrequency ablation of arrhythmias guided by non-fluoroscopic catheter location: a prospective randomized trial, *Eur Heart J* 27:1223–1229, 2006.
19. Brooks AG, Wilson L, Kuklik P, et al: Image integration using NavX Fusion: initial experience and validation, *Heart Rhythm* 5:526–535, 2008.
20. Pappone C, Vicedomini G, Manguso F, et al: Robotic magnetic navigation for atrial fibrillation ablation, *J Am Coll Cardiol* 47:1390–1400, 2006.
21. Schmidt B, Tilz RR, Neven K, et al: Remote robotic navigation and electroanatomical mapping for ablation of atrial fibrillation: considerations for navigation and impact on procedural outcome, *Circ Arrhythm Electrophysiol* 2:120–128, 2009.
22. Haghjoo M, Hindricks G, Bode K, et al: Initial clinical experience with the new irrigated tip magnetic catheter for ablation of scar-related sustained ventricular tachycardia: a small case series, *J Cardiovasc Electrophysiol* 20:935–939, 2009.
23. Wood MA, Orlov M, Ramaswamy K, et al: Remote magnetic versus manual catheter navigation for ablation of supraventricular tachycardias: a randomized, multicenter trial, *Pacing Clin Electrophysiol* 31:1313–1321, 2008.
24. Vollmann D, Luthje L, Seegers J, et al: Remote magnetic catheter navigation for cavotricuspid isthmus ablation in patients with common-type atrial flutter, *Circ Arrhythm Electrophysiol* 2:603–610, 2009.
25. Di BL, Fahmy TS, Patel D, et al: Remote magnetic navigation: human experience in pulmonary vein ablation, *J Am Coll Cardiol* 50:868–874, 2007.
26. Kim AM, Turakhia M, Lu J, et al: Impact of remote magnetic catheter navigation on ablation fluoroscopy and procedure time, *Pacing Clin Electrophysiol* 31:1399–1404, 2008.
27. Wazni OM, Barrett C, Martin DO, et al: Experience with the Hansen robotic system for atrial fibrillation ablation: lessons learned and techniques modified: Hansen in the real world, *J Cardiovasc Electrophysiol* 20:1193–1196, 2009.
28. Saliba W, Reddy VY, Wazni O, et al: Atrial fibrillation ablation using a robotic catheter remote control system: initial human experience and long-term follow-up results, *J Am Coll Cardiol* 51:2407–2411, 2008.
29. Di BL, Wang Y, Horton R, et al: Ablation of atrial fibrillation utilizing robotic catheter navigation in comparison to manual navigation and ablation: single-center experience, *J Cardiovasc Electrophysiol* 20:1328–1335, 2009.
30. Schmidt B, Chun KR, Tilz RR, et al: Remote navigation systems in electrophysiology, *Europace* 10(Suppl 3):iii57–iii61, 2008.
31. Di BL, Natale A, Barrett C, et al: Relationship between catheter forces, lesion characteristics, "popping," and char formation: experience with robotic navigation system, *J Cardiovasc Electrophysiol* 20:436–440, 2009.
32. Finlay DD, Nugent CD, McCullagh PJ, Black ND: Mining for diagnostic information in body surface potential maps: a comparison of feature selection techniques, *Biomed Eng Online* 4:51, 2005.
33. Taccardi B, Punske B: Body surface potential mapping. In Zipes DP, Jalife J, editors: *Cardiac electrophysiology: from cell to bedside*, ed 5, Philadelphia, 2009, Saunders, pp 803–811.
34. Ghanem RN, Jia P, Ramanathan C, et al: Noninvasive electrocardiographic imaging (ECGI): comparison to intraoperative mapping in patients, *Heart Rhythm* 2:339–354, 2005.
35. Zhang X, Ramachandra I, Liu Z, et al: Noninvasive three-dimensional electrocardiographic imaging of ventricular activation sequence, *Am J Physiol Heart Circ Physiol* 289:H2724–H2732, 2005.
36. Ghosh S, Rhee EK, Avari JN, et al: Cardiac memory in patients with Wolff-Parkinson-White syndrome: noninvasive imaging of activation and repolarization before and after catheter ablation, *Circulation* 118:907–915, 2008.
37. Rudy Y: Cardiac repolarization: insights from mathematical modeling and electrocardiographic imaging (ECGI), *Heart Rhythm* 6(Suppl):S49–S55, 2009.
38. Wang Y, Schuessler RB, Damiano RJ, et al: Noninvasive electrocardiographic imaging (ECGI) of scar-related atypical atrial flutter, *Heart Rhythm* 4:1565–1567, 2007.
39. Ghanem RN: Noninvasive electrocardiographic imaging of arrhythmogenesis: insights from modeling and human studies, *J Electrocardiol* 40(Suppl):S169–S173, 2007.
40. Ren J, Marchlinski F: Intracardiac echocardiography: basic concepts. In Ren JF, Marchlinski FE, Callans DJ, Schwartsman S, editors: *Practical intracardiac echocardiography in electrophysiology*, Malden, Mass., 2006, Blackwell Futura, pp 1–4.
41. Ren J, Weiss J: Imaging technique and cardiac structures. In Ren JF, Marchlinski FE, Callans DJ, Schwartsman S, editors: *Practical intracardiac echocardiography in electrophysiology*, Malden, Mass., 2006, Blackwell Futura, pp 18–40.
42. Ren J, Marchlinski F: Monitoring and early diagnosis of procedural complications. In Ren JF, Marchlinski FE, Callans DJ, Schwartsman S, editors: *Practical intracardiac echocardiography in electrophysiology*, Malden, Mass., 2006, Blackwell Futura, pp 180–207.
43. Sra J, Ratnakumar S: Cardiac image registration of the left atrium and pulmonary veins, *Heart Rhythm* 5:609–617, 2008.
44. Dong J, Calkins H, Solomon SB, et al: Integrated electroanatomic mapping with three-dimensional computed tomographic images for real-time guided ablations, *Circulation* 113:186–194, 2006.
45. Malchano ZJ, Neuzil P, Cury RC, et al: Integration of cardiac CT/MR imaging with three-dimensional electroanatomical mapping to guide catheter manipulation in the left atrium: implications for catheter ablation of atrial fibrillation, *J Cardiovasc Electrophysiol* 17:1221–1229, 2006.

46. Ector J, De BS, Adams J, et al: Cardiac three-dimensional magnetic resonance imaging and fluoroscopy merging: a new approach for electroanatomic mapping to assist catheter ablation, *Circulation* 112:3769–3776, 2005.
47. Sra J, Krum D, Malloy A, et al: Registration of three-dimensional left atrial computed tomographic images with projection images obtained using fluoroscopy, *Circulation* 112:3763–3768, 2005.
48. Stevenhagen J, Van Der Voort PH, Dekker LR, et al: Three-dimensional CT overlay in comparison to CartoMerge for pulmonary vein antrum isolation, *J Cardiovasc Electrophysiol* 21:634–639, 2010.
49. Richmond L, Rajappan K, Voth E, et al: Validation of computed tomography image integration into the EnSite NavX mapping system to perform catheter ablation of atrial fibrillation, *J Cardiovasc Electrophysiol* 19:821–827, 2008.
50. Kato R, Lickfett L, Meininger G, et al: Pulmonary vein anatomy in patients undergoing catheter ablation of atrial fibrillation: lessons learned by use of magnetic resonance imaging, *Circulation* 107:2004–2010, 2003.
51. Triedman J: Virtual reality in interventional electrophysiology, *Circulation* 112:3677–3679, 2005.
52. Bertaglia E, Brandolino G, Zoppo F, et al: Integration of three-dimensional left atrial magnetic resonance images into a real-time electroanatomic mapping system: validation of a registration method, *Pacing Clin Electrophysiol* 31:273–282, 2008.
53. Kistler PM, Earley MJ, Harris S, et al: Validation of three-dimensional cardiac image integration: use of integrated CT image into electroanatomic mapping system to perform catheter ablation of atrial fibrillation, *J Cardiovasc Electrophysiol* 17:341–348, 2006.
54. Sra J, Narayan G, Krum D, et al: Computed tomography-fluoroscopy image integration-guided catheter ablation of atrial fibrillation, *J Cardiovasc Electrophysiol* 18:409–414, 2007.
55. Fahmy TS, Mlcochova H, Wazni OM, et al: Intracardiac echo-guided image integration: optimizing strategies for registration, *J Cardiovasc Electrophysiol* 18:276–282, 2007.
56. Zhong H, Lacomis JM, Schwartzman D: On the accuracy of CartoMerge for guiding posterior left atrial ablation in man, *Heart Rhythm* 4:595–602, 2007.
57. Hsu LF: Image integration for catheter ablation: searching for the perfect match, *Heart Rhythm* 5:536–537, 2008.
58. Orlov MV: How to perform and interpret rotational angiography in the electrophysiology laboratory, *Heart Rhythm* 6:1830–1836, 2009.
59. Li JH, Haim M, Movassaghi B, et al: Segmentation and registration of three-dimensional rotational angiogram on live fluoroscopy to guide atrial fibrillation ablation: a new online imaging tool, *Heart Rhythm* 6:231–237, 2009.
60. Knecht S, Wright M, Akrivakis S, et al: Prospective randomized comparison between the conventional electroanatomical system and three-dimensional rotational angiography during catheter ablation for atrial fibrillation, *Heart Rhythm* 7:459–465, 2010.
61. Kriatselis C, Tang M, Roser M, et al: A new approach for contrast-enhanced X-ray imaging of the left atrium and pulmonary veins for atrial fibrillation ablation: rotational angiography during adenosine-induced asystole, *Europace* 11:35–41, 2009.
62. Knecht S, Skali H, O'Neill MD, et al: Computed tomography-fluoroscopy overlay evaluation during catheter ablation of left atrial arrhythmia, *Europace* 10:931–938, 2008.
63. Nolker G, Gutleben KJ, Marschang H, et al: Three-dimensional left atrial and esophagus reconstruction using cardiac C-arm computed tomography with image integration into fluoroscopic views for ablation of atrial fibrillation: accuracy of a novel modality in comparison with multislice computed tomography, *Heart Rhythm* 5:1651–1657, 2008.
64. Knecht S, Akrivakis S, Wright M, et al: Randomized prospective evaluation of 3D rotational atriography versus CARTO to guide AF ablation, *Heart Rhythm* 2009:PO5–PO17, 2011.

CHAPTER 7 Ablation Energy Sources

Radiofrequency Ablation

Biophysics of Radiofrequency Energy

Radiofrequency (RF) refers to the portion of the electromagnetic spectrum in which electromagnetic waves can be generated by alternating current fed to an antenna.[1] Electrosurgery ablation currently uses hectomeric wavelengths found in band 6 (300 to 3000 kHz), which are similar to those used for broadcast radio. However, the RF energy is electrically conducted, not radiated, during catheter ablation. The RF current is similar to low-frequency alternating current or direct current with regard to its ability to heat tissue and create a lesion, but it oscillates so rapidly that cardiac and skeletal muscles are not stimulated, thereby avoiding induction of arrhythmias and decreasing the pain perceived by the patient. RF current rarely induces rapid polymorphic arrhythmias; such arrhythmias can be observed in response to low-frequency (60-Hz) stimulation. Frequencies higher than 1000 kHz are also effective in generating tissue heating; however, such high frequencies are associated with considerable energy loss along the transmission line. Therefore, frequencies of the RF current commonly used are in the range of 300 to 1000 kHz, a range that combines efficacy and safety.[2,3]

RADIOFREQUENCY ENERGY DELIVERY

Delivery of RF energy depends on the establishment of an electrical circuit involving the human body as one of its in-series elements. The RF current is applied to the tissue via a metal electrode at the tip of the ablation catheter and is generally delivered in a unipolar fashion between the tip electrode and a large dispersive electrode (indifferent electrode, or ground pad) applied to the patient's skin. The polarity of connections from the electrodes to the generator is not important because the RF current is an alternating current. Bipolar RF systems also exist, in which the current flows between two closely apposed small electrodes, thus limiting the current flow to small tissue volumes interposed between the metal conductors. Bipolar systems, partly because of their relative safety, are now the preferred tools in electrosurgery (oncology, plastic surgery, and ophthalmology). Their clinical application for catheter-based ablation has not yet been evaluated.[2,3]

The system impedance comprises the impedance of the generator, transmission lines, catheter, electrode-tissue interface, dispersive electrode-skin interface, and interposed tissues. As electricity flows through a circuit, every point of that circuit represents a drop in voltage, and some energy is dissipated as heat. The point of greatest drop in line voltage represents the area of highest impedance and is where most of that electrical energy becomes dissipated as heat. Therefore, with excessive electrical resistance in the transmission line, the line actually warms up and power is lost. Current electrical conductors from the generator all the way through to the patient and from the dispersive electrode back to the generator have low impedance, to minimize power loss.[2,3]

With normal electrode-tissue contact, only a fraction of all power is effectively applied to the tissue. The rest is dissipated in the blood pool and elsewhere in the patient. With an ablation electrode in contact with the endocardial wall, part of the electrode contacts tissue and the rest contacts blood, and the RF current flows through both the myocardium and the blood pool in contact with the electrode. The distribution between both depends on the impedance of both routes and also on how much electrode surface contacts blood versus endocardial wall. Whereas tissue heating is the target of power delivery, the blood pool is the most attractive route for RF current because blood is a better conductor and has significantly lower impedance than tissue and because the contact between electrode and blood is often better than with tissue. Therefore, with normal electrode-tissue contact, much more power is generally delivered to blood than to cardiac tissue.[2,4]

After leaving the electrode-blood-tissue interface, the current flows through the thorax to the indifferent electrode. Part of the RF power is lost in the patient's body, including the area near the patch. Dissipation of energy can occur at the dispersive electrode site (at the contact point between that ground pad and the skin) to a degree that can limit lesion formation. In fact, if ablation is performed with a high-amplitude current (more than 50 W) and skin contact by the dispersive electrode is poor, it is possible to cause skin burns (Fig. 7-1).[1] Nevertheless, because the surface area of the ablation electrode (approximately 12 mm^2) is much smaller than that of the dispersive electrode (approximately 100 to 250 cm^2), the current density is higher at the ablation site, and heating occurs preferentially at that site, with no significant heating occurring at the dispersive electrode.[5]

The dispersive electrode may be placed on any convenient skin surface. The geometry of the RF current field is defined by the geometry of the ablation electrode and is relatively uniform in the region of volume heating. Thus, the position of the dispersive electrode (on the patient's back or thigh) has little effect on impedance, voltage, current delivery, catheter tip temperature, or geometry of the resulting lesion.[2,3,5]

The size of the dispersive electrode, however, is important. Sometimes it is advantageous to increase the surface area of the dispersive electrode. This increase leads to lower impedance, higher current delivery, increased catheter tip temperatures, and more

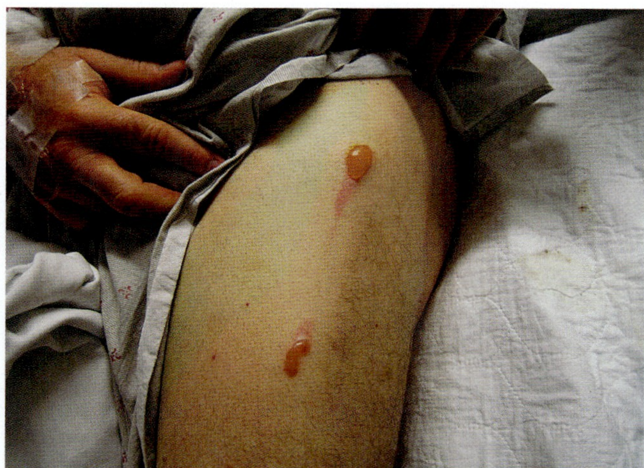

FIGURE 7-1 Second-degree skin burns at the site of ablation ground pad contact to the patient's thigh. Skin burns occurred secondary to poor contact between the skin and the pad during radiofrequency ablation of atrial fibrillation.

effective tissue heating. This is especially true in patients with baseline system impedance greater than 100 Ω. Moreover, when the system is power limited, as with a 50-W generator, heat production at the catheter tip varies with the proportion of the local electrode-tissue interface impedance to the overall system impedance. If the impedance at the skin-dispersive electrode interface is high, then a smaller amount of energy is available for tissue heating at the electrode tip. Therefore, when ablating certain sites, adding a second dispersive electrode or optimizing the contact between the dispersive electrode and skin should result in relatively more power delivery to the target tissue.[5,6]

TISSUE HEATING

During alternating current flow, charged carriers in tissue (ions) attempt to follow the changes in the direction of the alternating current, thus converting electromagnetic (current) energy into molecular mechanical energy or heat. This type of electric current-mediated heating is known as ohmic (resistive) heating. Using Ohm's law, with resistive heating, the amount of power (= heat) per unit volume equals the square of current density times the specific impedance of the tissue. With a spherical electrode, the current flows outward radially, and current density therefore decreases with the square of distance from the center of the electrode. Consequently, power dissipation per unit volume decreases with the fourth power of distance. The thickness of the electrode eliminates the first steepest part of this curve, however, and the decrease in dissipated power with distance is therefore somewhat less dramatic.[2,3]

Approximately 90% of all power that is delivered to the tissue is absorbed within the first 1 to 1.5 mm from the electrode surface. Therefore, only a thin rim of tissue in immediate contact with the RF electrode is directly heated (within the first 2 mm of depth from the electrode). The remainder of tissue heating occurs as a result of heat conduction from this rim to the surrounding tissues. On initiation of fixed-level energy application, the temperature at the electrode-tissue interface rises monoexponentially to reach steady state within 7 to 10 seconds, and the steady state is usually maintained between 80° and 90°C. However, whereas resistive heating starts immediately with the delivery of RF current, conduction of heat to deeper tissue sites is relatively slow and requires 1 to 2 minutes to equilibrate (thermal equilibrium). Therefore, the rate of tissue temperature rise beyond the immediate vicinity of the RF electrode is much slower, resulting in a steep radial temperature gradient as tissue temperature decreases radially in proportion to the distance from the ablation electrode; however, deep tissue temperatures continue to rise for several seconds after interruption of RF delivery (the so-called thermal latency phenomenon).[4] Therefore, RF ablation requires at least 30 to 60 seconds to create full-grown lesions. In addition, when temperature differences between adjacent areas develop because of differences in local current density or local heat capacity, heat conducts from hotter to colder areas, thus causing the temperature of the former to decrease and that of the latter to increase. Furthermore, heat loss to the blood pool at the surface and to intramyocardial vessels determines the temperature profile within the tissue.[2,3]

At steady state, the lesion size is proportional to the temperature measured at the interface between the tissue and the electrode, as well as to the RF power amplitude. By using higher powers and achieving higher tissue temperatures, the lesion size can be increased. However, once the peak tissue temperature exceeds the threshold of 100°C, boiling of the plasma at the electrode-tissue interface can ensue. When boiling occurs, denatured serum proteins and charred tissue form a thin film that adheres to the electrode, thus producing an electrically insulating coagulum, which is accompanied by a sudden increase in electrical impedance that prevents further current flow into the tissue and further heating.[2,3]

The range of tissue temperatures used for RF ablation is 50° to 90°C. Within this range, smooth desiccation of tissue can be expected. If the temperature is lower than 50°C, no or only minimal tissue necrosis results. Because the rate of temperature rise at deeper sites within the myocardium is slow, a continuous energy delivery of at least 60 seconds is often warranted to maximize depth of lesion formation.

CONVECTIVE COOLING

The dominant factor opposing effective heating of myocardium is the convective heat loss into the circulating blood pool. Because the tissue surface is cooled by the blood flow, the highest temperature during RF delivery occurs slightly below the endocardial surface. Consequently, the width of the endocardial lesion matures earlier than the intramural lesion width (20 seconds versus 90 to 120 seconds). Therefore, the maximum lesion width is usually located intramurally, and the resultant lesion is usually teardrop shaped, with less necrosis of the superficial tissue.[3]

As the magnitude of convective cooling increases (e.g., unstable catheter position, poor catheter-tissue contact, or high blood flow in the region of catheter position), there is decreased efficiency of heating as more energy is carried away in the blood and less energy is delivered to the tissue. When RF power is limited, lesion size is reduced by such convective heat loss. On the other hand, when RF power delivery is not limited, convective cooling allows for more power to be delivered into the tissue, and higher tissue temperatures can be achieved (despite low temperatures measured by the catheter tip sensors), resulting in larger lesion size, without the risk of overheating and coagulum formation.[2,3]

The concept of convective cooling can explain why there are few coronary complications with conventional RF ablation. Coronary arteries act as a heat sink; substantive heating of vascular endothelium is prevented by heat dissipation in the high-velocity coronary blood flow, even when the catheter is positioned close to the vessel. Although this is advantageous, because coronary arteries are being protected, it can limit success of the ablation lesion if a large perforating artery is close to the ablation target.[5]

The effects of convective cooling have been exploited to increase the size of catheter ablative lesions. Active electrode cooling by irrigation is currently used to eliminate the risk of overheating at the electrode-tissue contact point and increase the magnitude of power delivery and the depth of volume heating.

CATHETER TIP TEMPERATURE

Ablation catheter tip temperature depends on tissue temperature, convective cooling by the surrounding blood, tissue contact of the ablation electrode, electrode material and its heat capacity, and type and location of the temperature sensor.[2,7]

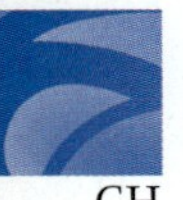

Catheter tip temperature is measured by a sensor located in the ablation electrode. There are two different types of temperature sensors: thermistors and thermocouples. Thermistors require a driving current, and the electrical resistance changes as the temperature of the electrical conductor changes. More frequently used are thermocouples, which consist of copper and constantan wires and are incorporated in the center of the ablation electrode. Thermocouples are based on the so-called Seebeck effect; when two different metals are connected (sensing junction), a voltage can be measured at the reference junction that is proportional to the temperature difference between the two metals.[2,7]

The electrode temperature rise is an indirect process—the ablation electrode is not heated by RF energy, but it heats up because it happens to touch heated tissue. Consequently, the catheter tip temperature is always lower than, or ideally equal to, the superficial tissue temperature. Conventional electrode catheters with temperature monitoring report the temperature only from the center of the electrode mass with one design or from the apex of the tip of the catheter with another design. It is likely that the measured temperature underestimates the peak tissue temperature; it can be significantly lower than tissue temperature.

Several other factors can increase the disparity between catheter tip temperature and tissue temperature, including catheter tip irrigation, large ablation electrode size, and poor electrode-tissue contact. Catheter tip irrigation increases the disparity between tissue temperature and electrode temperature because it results in cooling of the ablation electrode, but not the tissue. With a large electrode tip, a larger area of the electrode tip is exposed to the cooling effects of the blood flow than with standard tip lengths, thus resulting in lower electrode temperatures. Similarly, with poor electrode-tissue contact, less electrode material is in contact with the tissue, and heating of the tip by the tissue occurs at a lower rate, resulting in relatively low tip temperatures.[3,6-8]

Pathophysiology of Lesion Formation by Radiofrequency Ablation

CELLULAR EFFECTS OF RADIOFREQUENCY ABLATION

The primary mechanism of tissue injury by RF ablation is likely to be thermally mediated. Hyperthermic injury to the myocyte is both time- and temperature-dependent, and it can be caused by changes in the cell membrane, protein inactivation, cytoskeletal disruption, nuclear degeneration, or other potential mechanisms.[2,3]

Experimentally, the resting membrane depolarization is related to temperature. In the low hyperthermic range (37° to 45°C), little tissue injury occurs, and a minor change may be observed in the resting membrane potential and action potential amplitude. However, action potential duration shortens significantly, and conduction velocity becomes greater than at baseline. In the intermediate hyperthermic range (45° to 50°C), progressive depolarization of the resting membrane potential occurs, and action potential amplitude decreases. Additionally, abnormal automaticity is observed, reversible loss of excitability occurs, and conduction velocity progressively decreases. In the high temperature ranges (higher than 50°C), marked depolarization of the resting membrane potential occurs, and permanent loss of excitability is observed. Temporary (at temperatures of 49.5° to 51.5°C) and then permanent (at 51.7° to 54.4°C) conduction block develops, and fairly reliable irreversible myocardial injury occurs with a short hyperthermic exposure.[3]

In the clinical setting, the success of ablation is related to the mean temperature measured at the electrode-tissue interface. Block of conduction in an atrioventricular (AV) bypass tract (BT) usually occurs at 62° ± 15°C. During ablation of the AV junction, an accelerated junctional rhythm, which is probably caused by thermally or electrically induced cellular automaticity or triggered activity, is observed at temperatures of 51° ± 4°C, whereas reversible complete AV block occurs at 58° ± 6°C, and irreversible complete AV block occurs at 60° ± 7°C.

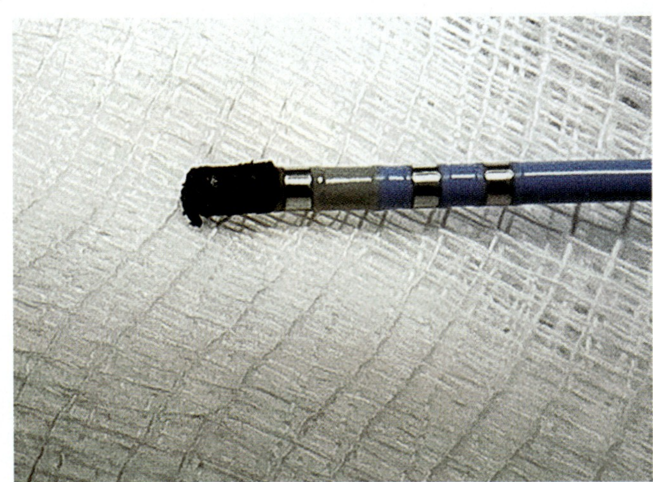

FIGURE 7-2 Standard radiofrequency ablation catheter with char formed on the tip.

RF ablation typically results in high temperatures (70° to 90°C) for a short time (up to 60 seconds) at the electrode-tissue interface, but significantly lower temperatures at deeper tissue sites. This leads to rapid tissue injury within the immediate vicinity of the RF electrode but relatively delayed myocardial injury with increasing distance from the RF electrode. Therefore, although irreversible loss of EP function can usually be demonstrated immediately after successful RF ablation, this finding can be delayed because tissue temperatures continue to rise somewhat after termination of RF energy delivery (thermal latency phenomenon). This effect can account for the observation that patients undergoing AV node (AVN) modification procedures who demonstrate transient heart block during RF energy delivery can progress to persisting complete heart block, even if RF energy delivery is terminated immediately. Reversible loss of conduction can be demonstrated within seconds of initiating the RF application, which can be caused by an acute electrotonic effect. On the other hand, there can be late recovery of electrophysiological (EP) function after an initial successful ablation.[5]

In addition to the dominant thermal effects of RF ablation, some of the cellular injury has been hypothesized to be caused by a direct electrical effect, which can result in dielectric breakdown of the sarcolemmal membrane with creation of transmembrane pores (electroporation), resulting in nonspecific ion transit, cellular depolarization, calcium overload, and cell death. Such an effect has been demonstrated with the use of high-voltage electrical current. However, it is difficult to examine the purely electrical effects in isolation of the dominant thermal injury.

TISSUE EFFECTS OF RADIOFREQUENCY ABLATION

Changes in myocardial tissue are apparent immediately on completion of the RF lesion. Pallor of the central zone of the lesion is attributable to denaturation of myocyte proteins (principally myoglobin) and subsequent loss of the red pigmentation. Slight deformation, indicating volume loss, occurs at the point of catheter contact in the central region of lesion formation. The endocardial surface is usually covered with a thin fibrin layer and, occasionally, if a temperature of 100°C has been exceeded, with char and thrombus (Fig. 7-2). In addition, a coagulum (an accumulation of fibrin, platelets, and other blood and tissue components) can form at the ablation electrode because of the boiling of blood and tissue serum.[2]

On sectioning, the central portion of the RF ablation lesion shows desiccation, with a surrounding region of hemorrhagic tissue and then normal-appearing tissue. Histologic examination of an acute lesion shows typical coagulation necrosis with basophilic stippling consistent with intracellular calcium overload. Immediately surrounding the central lesion is a region of hemorrhage and acute monocellular and neutrophilic inflammation. The progressive changes seen in the evolution of an RF lesion are typical of healing after any acute injury. Within 2 months of the ablation, the lesion shows fibrosis, granulation tissue, chronic inflammatory infiltrates, and significant volume contraction. The lesion border is well demarcated from the surrounding viable myocardium without evidence of a transitional zone. This likely accounts for the absence of proarrhythmic side effects of RF catheter ablation. As noted, because of the high-velocity blood flow within the epicardial coronary arteries, these vessels are continuously cooled and are typically spared from injury, despite nearby delivery of RF energy. However, high RF power delivery in small hearts, such as in pediatric patients, or in direct contact with the vessel can potentially cause coronary arterial injury.[3]

The border zone around the acute pathological RF lesion accounts for several phenomena observed clinically. The border zone is characterized by marked ultrastructural abnormalities of the microvasculature and myocytes acutely, as well as a typical inflammatory response later. The most thermally sensitive structures appear to be the plasma membrane and gap junctions, which show morphological changes as far as 6 mm from the edge of the pathological lesion. The border zone accounts for documented effects of RF lesion formation well beyond the acute pathological lesion. The progression of the EP effects after completion of the ablation procedure can be caused by further inflammatory injury and necrosis in the border zone region that result in late progression of physiological block and a delayed cure in some cases. On the other hand, initial stunning and then early or late recovery of function can be demonstrated in the border zone, thus accounting for the recovery of EP function after successful catheter ablation in the clinical setting, which can be caused by healing of the damaged, but surviving, myocardium.[2]

Determinants of Lesion Size

Lesion size is defined as the total volume or dimensions (width and depth) of the lesion. The size of the lesion created by RF power is determined by the amount of tissue heated to more than the critical temperature for producing irreversible myocardial damage (50°C). As noted, only a thin rim (1 to 2 mm) of tissue immediately under the ablating electrode is directly heated. This heat then radiates to adjacent tissue; however, conduction of heat to deeper tissue sites is relatively slow and very inefficient. The distance at which temperature drops to less than 50°C delimits the depth of lesion formation. The use of higher-power output to achieve higher tissue temperatures results in larger lesions by raising the temperature of the rim of resistively heated tissue to substantially more than 50°C for deeper tissue to reach the 50°C threshold required for tissue necrosis. However, the rim of heated tissue in direct contact with the ablating electrode conducts not only to deeper tissue but also to the electrode tip itself. Higher electrode temperatures either limit further energy delivery (in temperature-controlled power delivery mode) or increase electrode impedance as a result of coagulum formation, or both; these effects potentially limit lesion size. Furthermore, tissue temperatures higher than 100°C are unsafe because they are associated with higher risk of steam "pops." Cooling of the ablating electrode (passively by using a larger electrode length or actively by using catheter irrigation) can help diminish electrode heating, allowing for greater power delivery and creation of larger lesions.[9]

ELECTRODE TIP TEMPERATURE

It is important to understand that it is the amount of RF power delivered effectively into the tissue that determines tissue heating and thus lesion size, and the recorded catheter tip temperature is poorly correlated with lesion size. As noted, catheter tip temperature is always lower than the superficial tissue temperature. With good contact between catheter tip and tissue and low cooling of the catheter tip, the target temperature can be reached with little power, thus resulting in fairly small lesions although a high catheter tip temperature is being measured. In contrast, a low catheter tip temperature can be caused by a high level of convective cooling, which allows a higher amount of RF power to be delivered to the tissue (because it is no longer limited by temperature rise of the ablation electrode) and yields relatively large lesions. This is best illustrated with active cooling of the ablation electrode using irrigation during RF energy delivery; the tip temperature is usually less than 40°C, which allows the application of high-power output for longer durations.

RADIOFREQUENCY DURATION

The RF lesion is predominantly generated within the first 10 seconds of target energy delivery and tissue temperatures, and it reaches a maximum after 30 seconds. Further extension of RF delivery during power-controlled RF delivery does not seem to increase lesion size further.

ELECTRODE-TISSUE CONTACT

The efficiency of energy transfer to the myocardium largely depends on electrode-tissue contact. An improvement in tissue contact leads to a higher amount of RF power that can be effectively delivered to the tissue. Consequently, the same tissue temperatures and lesion size can be reached at a much lower power level. However, at a certain moderate contact force, further increase in contact firmness results in progressively smaller lesions because a lesser amount of RF power is required to reach target temperature.[4]

Additionally, the surface area at the electrode-tissue interface influences the lesion size. When the catheter is wedged (i.e., between ventricular trabeculae or under a valvular leaflet), the electrode surface area exposed to tissue can be much higher. With half the electrode in contact with blood and the other half in contact with (twice) more resistive tissue, the amount of power delivered to blood is two times higher than the amount of power delivered to tissue (as compared with six times with 25% contact). The result is a more than twofold increase in tissue heating. In practice, however, power output rarely reaches 50 W in these situations; a temperature rise of the ablation electrode signals excessive tissue heating and limits power delivery.[4]

Close monitoring of changes in temperature and impedance provides information regarding the degree of electrode-tissue contact. Increased contact results in elevated initial impedance levels (by a mean of 22%) and an increase in the rate and level of impedance reduction, and the plateau is reached later. Additionally, increased electrode-tissue contact results in higher tissue temperatures, and the plateau is achieved later. Beat-to-beat stability of electrograms and pacing threshold also provide some information about tissue contact.

ELECTRODE ORIENTATION

When the catheter tip is perpendicular to the tissue surface, a much smaller surface area is in contact with the tissue (versus that exposed to the cooling effect of blood flow) than when the catheter electrode tip is lying on its side. Clinically, perpendicular electrode orientation yields larger lesion volumes and uses less power than parallel electrode orientation. However, if the RF power level is adjusted to maintain a constant current density, lesion size will increase proportionally to the electrode-tissue contact area, which is larger with parallel tip orientation. Lesion depth is only slightly affected by catheter tip orientation using 4-mm-long tip catheters, but lesions are slightly longer in the parallel orientation as compared with the perpendicular orientation. Moreover, the character of the lesion created with temperature control depends on the placement of the temperature sensors relative to the portion of the electrode in contact with tissue. Thus, the orientation of the electrode and of its temperature sensors determines the appropriate target temperature required to create maximal lesions while avoiding coagulum formation caused by overheating at any location within the electrode-tissue interface.[2,3,10]

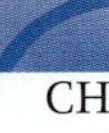

ELECTRODE LENGTH

Ablation catheters have tip electrodes that are conventionally 4 mm long and are available in sizes up to 10 mm long (see Fig. 4-6). An increased electrode size reduces the interface impedance with blood and tissue, but the impedance through the rest of the patient remains the same. The ratio between interface impedance and the impedance through the rest of the patient is thus lower with an 8-mm electrode than with a 4-mm electrode, which reduces the efficiency of power transfer to the tissue. Therefore, with the same total power, lesions created with a larger electrode are always smaller than lesions created with a smaller electrode (Fig. 7-3). A larger electrode size also creates a greater variability in power transfer to the tissue because of greater variability of tissue contact, and tissue contact becomes much more dependent on catheter orientation with longer electrodes. Consequently, an 8-mm electrode may require a 1.5 to 4 times higher power level than a 4-mm electrode to create the same lesion size.[4]

When the power is not limited, however, catheters with large distal electrodes create larger lesions, both by increasing the ablation electrode surface area in contact with the bloodstream, thus resulting in an augmented convective cooling effect, and by increasing the volume of tissue directly heated because of an increased surface area at the electrode-tissue interface (see Fig. 7-3). However, this assumes that the electrode-tissue contact, tissue heat dissipation, and blood flow are uniform throughout the electrode-tissue interface. As the electrode size increases, the likelihood that these assumptions are true diminishes because of variability in cardiac chamber trabeculations and curvature, tissue perfusion, and intracardiac blood flow, which affect the heat dissipation and tissue contact. These factors result in unpredictable lesion size and uniformity for electrodes more than 8 mm long.[2,3]

There is a potential safety concern with the use of long ablation electrodes because of nonuniform heating, with maximal heating occurring at the electrode edges. Thus, large electrode-tipped catheters with only a single thermistor can underestimate maximal temperature and allow char formation and potential thromboembolic complications. Catheter tips with multiple temperature sensors at the electrode edges may be preferable for temperature feedback. In addition, the greater variation in power delivered to the tissue and the greater discrepancy between electrode and tissue temperature make it difficult to avoid intramural gas explosions and blood clot formation. Another point of concern is that the formation of blood clots may only minimally affect electrode impedance by covering a much smaller part of the electrode surface. Therefore, the lower electrode temperature and the absence of any impedance rise may erroneously suggest a safer ablation process.[4]

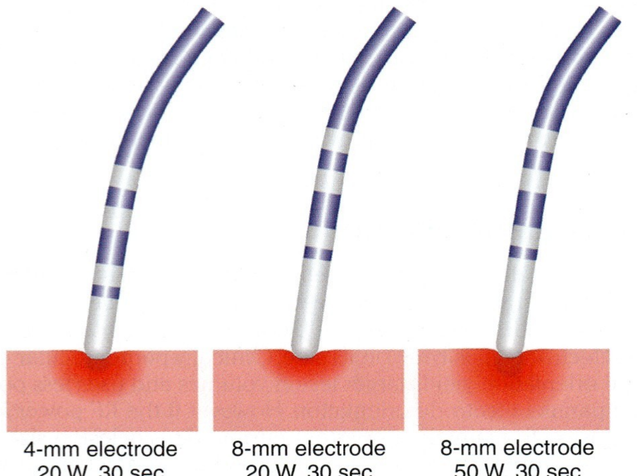

FIGURE 7-3 Effect of electrode size and power delivery on lesion size. Representative blocks of myocardium are shown with lesions (dark shading) resulting from optimal radiofrequency energy delivery for each electrode type. The effect of 20 W delivered for 30 seconds is shown for a 4-mm electrode **(left)** and an 8-mm electrode **(center)**. The larger electrode dissipates more of the energy into the blood pool and thus paradoxically creates a smaller lesion. Because of electrode cooling from its larger surface area, the same 8-mm electrode can deliver more power than the 4-mm electrode and could create a larger lesion **(right)**.

The principal limitations of a large ablation electrode (8 to 10 mm in length) are the reduction in mobility and the flexibility of the catheter, which can impair positioning of the ablation electrode, and a reduction in the resolution of recordings from the ablation electrode, thus making it more difficult to identify the optimal ablation site. A larger electrode dampens the local electrogram, especially that of the distal electrode. With an 8- or 10-mm long distal and a 1-mm short proximal ring electrode, the latter can be the main source for the bipolar electrogram; this then confuses localization of the optimal ablation site. In contrast, a smaller electrode improves mapping accuracy and feedback of tissue heating. Its only drawback is the limited power level that can be applied to the tissue.[4]

ABLATION ELECTRODE MATERIAL

Although platinum-iridium electrodes have been the standard for most RF ablation catheters, gold exhibits excellent electrical conductive properties, as well as a more than four times greater thermal conductivity than platinum (300 versus 70 W/m °K), although both materials have similar heat capacities (130 and 135 J/kg °K). The higher thermal conductivity of gold can potentially lead to a higher mean rate of power because of better heat conduction at the tissue-electrode interface and to enhanced cooling as a result of heat loss to the surrounding blood with this electrode material.[11] Therefore, gold electrodes allow for greater power delivery to create deeper lesions at a given electrode temperature without impedance increases.[12] Enhanced electrode cooling allows for more RF power to be applied at constant temperature, before the temperature limit is reached or before the impedance of the electrode rises.[4] However, the higher thermal conductivity of gold electrodes is no longer an advantage in areas of low blood flow (e.g., among myocardial trabeculae), where convective cooling at the electrode tip is minimal. Under these circumstances, electrode materials with a low thermal conductivity can produce larger lesions.[3,11]

Conflicting results were observed in clinical studies comparing 8-mm gold-tip with platinum-iridium–tip catheters for ablation of the cavotricuspid isthmus.[13] During catheter ablation of the slow AVN pathway in patients with AVN reentrant tachycardia (AVNRT), no significant differences were observed between 4-mm gold-tip and platinum-iridium–tip catheters in the primary endpoint or in the increases of power or temperature at any of the measured time points. However, ablation with gold electrodes seemed to be safe and well tolerated and specifically did not increase the risk of AV block. Interestingly, a significant reduction of charring on gold tips was observed, compared with platinum-iridium material, a finding suggesting a possible advantage of this material beyond its better conduction properties.[11]

REFERENCE PATCH ELECTRODE LOCATION AND SIZE

The RF current path and skin reference electrode interface present significant impedance for the ablation current flow, thereby dissipating part of the power. Increasing patch size (or using two patches) provides for increased heating at the electrode-endocardium interface and thus increases ablation efficiency and increases lesion size. On the other hand, the position of the dispersive electrode (on the patient's back or thigh) has little effect on the size of the resulting lesion.[5]

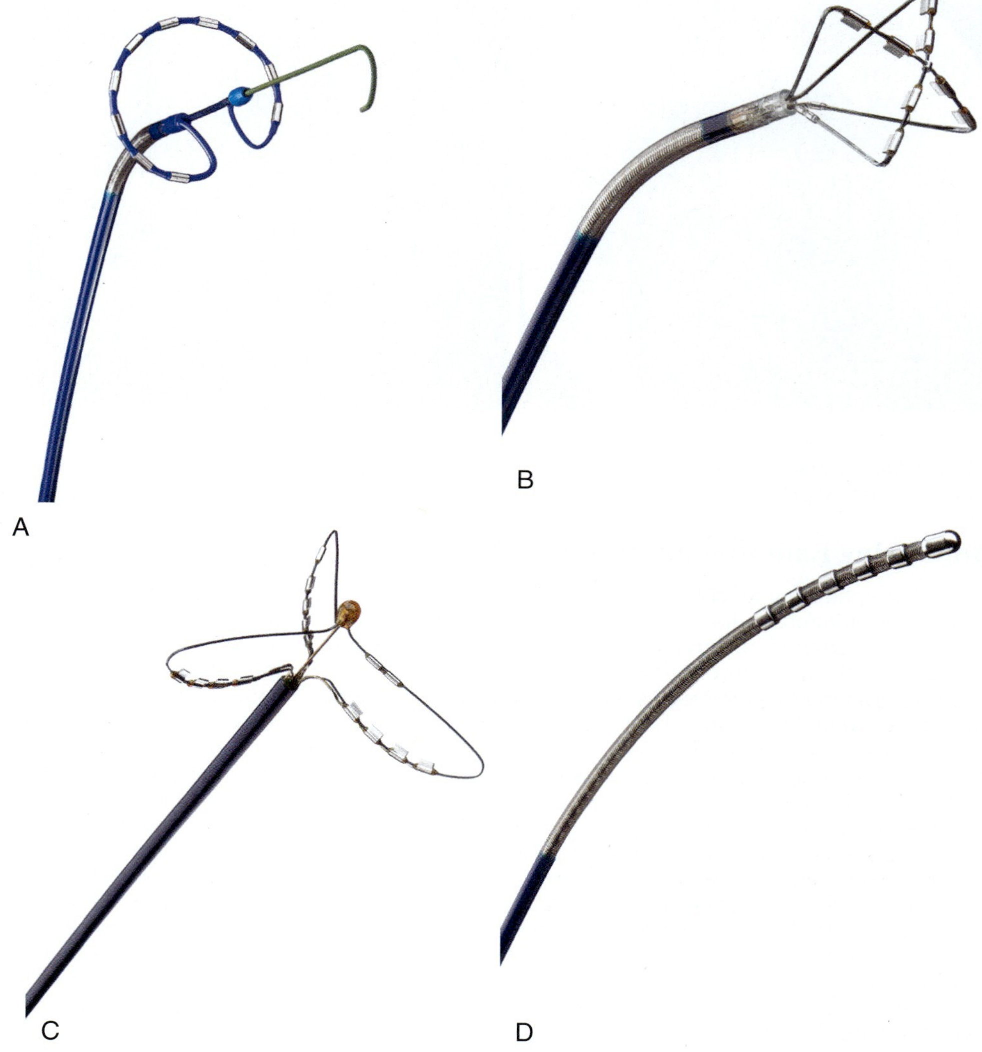

FIGURE 7-4 Novel multipolar electrode catheters (Ablation Frontiers, Inc., Carlsbad, Calif.) using duty-cycled radiofrequency. **A,** The Pulmonary Vein Ablation Catheter (PVAC) is a multielectrode catheter used to map, ablate, and verify isolation of the pulmonary veins. **B,** The Multi-Array Ablation Catheter (MAAC) is a multielectrode catheter designed to map and ablate complex fractionated atrial electrograms in the left atrial body. **C,** The Multi-Array Septal Catheter (MASC) is a multielectrode catheter designed to map and ablate complex fractionated atrial electrograms along the left atrial septum. **D,** The Tip-Versatile Ablation Catheter (TVAC) is a multielectrode catheter for linear ablation. *(Courtesy of Medtronic, Inc., Minneapolis, Minn.)*

BLOOD FLOW

The ablation electrode temperature is dependent on the opposing effects of heating from the tissue and cooling by the blood flowing around the electrode. Because lesion size is primarily dependent on the RF power delivered to the tissue, lesion size varies with the magnitude of local blood flow. At any given electrode temperature, the RF power delivered to the tissue is significantly reduced in areas of low local blood flow (e.g., deep pouch in the cavotricuspid isthmus, dilated and poorly contracting atria, and dilated and poorly contracting ventricles). The reduced cooling associated with low blood flow causes the electrode to reach the target temperature at lower power levels, and if the ablation lesion is temperature-controlled, power delivery will be limited. In these locations, increasing electrode temperature to 65° or 70°C only minimally increases RF power and increases the risk of thrombus formation and impedance rise. In contrast, increasing local blood flow is associated with increased convective cooling of the ablation electrode. Consequently, more power is delivered to the tissue to reach and maintain target temperature, thus resulting in larger lesion volumes.[2,3,7]

RADIOFREQUENCY SYSTEM POLARITY

Most RF lesions are created by applying energy in a unipolar fashion between an ablating electrode touching the myocardium and a grounded reference patch electrode placed externally on the skin. The unipolar configuration creates a highly localized lesion, with the least amount of surface injury. Energy can also be applied in a bipolar mode between two endocardial electrodes. Bipolar energy delivery produces larger lesions than unipolar delivery. A novel ablation system (GENius, Ablation Frontiers, Carlsbad, Calif.) has been developed for ablation of atrial fibrillation (AF), in which duty-cycled and alternating unipolar and bipolar (between adjacent electrodes) energy RF ablation is used to create contiguous lesions in the pulmonary vein (PV) antrum using a ring catheter with 10 electrodes (Pulmonary Vein Ablation Catheter [PVAC], Ablation Frontiers, Medtronic Inc., Minneapolis, Minn.) (Figs. 7-4 and 7-5).[14] Other catheter designs, which use the same multichannel duty-cycled RF generator, also have been developed for left atrial ablation of fractionated electrograms (Multi-Array Ablation Catheter [MAAC], Ablation Frontiers), septal ablation (Multi-Array Septal Catheter [MASC], Ablation Frontiers), and linear ablation (Tip-Versatile Ablation Catheter [TVAC], Ablation Frontiers) (see Fig. 7-4).[15] One advantage of this approach is the simultaneous application of RF energy across an electrode array, intended to create contiguous lesions near an anatomical structure. Additionally, the multielectrode catheters allow selective mapping and ablation through any or all electrodes as required. This system is still undergoing investigation. Another novel ablation catheter system delivers RF energy through a flexible mesh electrode (C.R. Bard, Inc.,

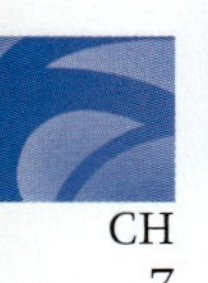

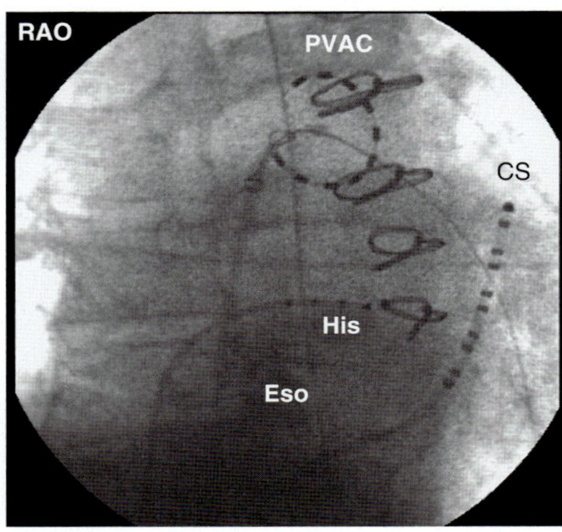

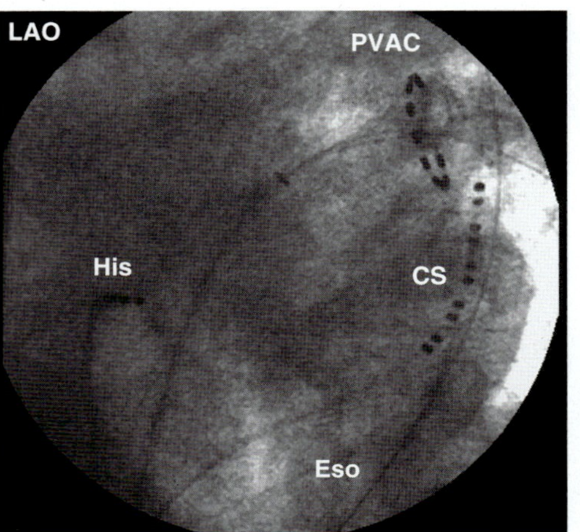

FIGURE 7-5 Ablation Frontiers (Medtronic Inc., Minneapolis, Minn.) Pulmonary Vein Ablation Catheter (PVAC) in the left inferior pulmonary vein. The electrodes of the PVAC catheter, which is deployed over a guidewire into the antrum of a pulmonary vein, can be used for both recording and ablating around the perimeter of the vein. CS = coronary sinus; Eso = esophageal catheter; LAO = left anterior oblique; RAO = right anterior oblique.

Billerica, Mass.) that is deployed in the PV ostium. This system is undergoing investigation for PV isolation.[16]

Monitoring Radiofrequency Energy Delivery

The goal of optimizing RF ablation is to create an adequate-sized lesion while minimizing the chance of an impedance increase because of coagulum formation at the electrode itself, or steam formation within the tissue. As discussed previously, for ablation to be effective, power must be increased sufficiently to achieve temperatures at the tissue directly in contact with the ablating electrode that are substantially higher than 50°C to achieve tissue necrosis. At the same time, for ablation to be safe, the highest tissue temperature must be maintained at less than 100°C to prevent steam pops. Monitoring of RF energy delivery is therefore very important to help achieve successful as well as safe ablation.[9]

Lesion creation is influenced by many factors, some of which can be controlled, whereas others are variable and can be unpredictable. With standard RF, power delivery is titrated to electrode temperature, typically at 55° to 65°C. Higher temperatures can increase the chance of reaching 100°C at edges of the ablation electrode, thus resulting in coagulum formation. An increase in tissue temperature is accompanied by a decrease in impedance, also a reliable marker of tissue heating. Impedance reduction and temperature rise correlate with both lesion width and depth; maximum temperature rise is best correlated with lesion width, and maximum impedance reduction is best correlated with lesion depth.[3,7]

The efficiency of tissue heating (i.e., the temperature per watt of applied power) is dependent on several variables, including catheter stability, electrode-tissue contact pressure, electrode orientation relative to the endocardium, effective electrode contact area, convective heat loss into the blood pool, and target location. Thus, applied energy, power, and current are poor indicators of the extent of lesion formation, and the actual electrode-tissue interface temperature remains the only predictor of the actual lesion size. Currently, although less than ideal, monitoring temperature and impedance are used to help ensure adequate but not excessive heating at the electrode-tissue interface. Newer technologies may be implemented in the future to monitor tissue temperatures during RF delivery, including infrared sensors and ultrasound transducers.

In addition to impedance and catheter tip temperature monitoring, reductions in amplitude and steepness of the local electrogram are important indicators for monitoring lesion growth. These indicators, however, apply only to the unipolar distal electrogram. With a bipolar recording, the signal from the ring electrode may dominate the electrogram, and the bipolar amplitude may theoretically even rise during ablation because of a greater difference between the signals from both electrodes.[4]

Some operators have used visualization of microbubbles on intracardiac ultrasound (ICE) as an indication of excessive tissue heating that is predictive of char and steam pops during ablation and that warrants reduction or termination of RF energy.[6]

IMPEDANCE MONITORING

The magnitude of the current delivered by the RF generator used in ablation is largely determined by the impedance between the ablation catheter and the dispersive electrode. This impedance is influenced by several factors, including intrinsic tissue properties, catheter contact pressure, catheter electrode size, dispersive electrode size, presence of coagulum, and body surface area. Impedance measurement does not require any specific catheter-based sensor circuitry and can be performed with any catheter designed for RF ablation. Larger dispersive electrodes and larger ablation electrodes result in lower impedance.[3,7]

Typically, the impedance associated with firm catheter contact (before tissue heating has occurred) is 90 to 120 Ω. When catheter contact is poor, the initial impedance is 20% to 50% less, because of the lower resistivity of blood. Moreover, larger electrodes have larger contact area and consequently lower impedance.

The impedance drop during RF ablation occurs mainly because of a reversible phenomenon, such as tissue temperature rise, rather than from an irreversible change in tissues secondary to ablation of myocardial tissue. Therefore, impedance provides a useful qualitative assessment of tissue heating; however, it does not correlate well with lesion size.[4] A 5- to 10-Ω reduction in impedance is usually observed in clinically successful RF applications, it correlates with a tissue temperature of 55° to 60°C, and it is rarely associated with coagulum formation. Larger decrements in impedance are noted when coagulum formation is imminent. Once a coagulum is formed, an abrupt rise in impedance to more than 250 Ω is usually observed.[3,7]

To titrate RF energy using impedance monitoring alone, the initial power output is set at 20 to 30 W and is then gradually increased to target a 5- to 10-Ω decrement in impedance. When target impedance is reached, power output should be manually adjusted throughout the RF application, as needed, to maintain the impedance in the target range. A larger decrement of impedance should prompt reduction in power output.

The drop in impedance as a monitoring tool has several limitations. When blood flow rates are low, blood can also be heated, and electrode impedance drops accordingly. Moreover, a large rise in tissue temperature at a small contact area and a smaller rise with better tissue contact can result in a similar drop in impedance. Inversely, similar tissue heating with different tissue contact can result in a different change in impedance. In addition, resistive heating nearby is fast, whereas conductive heating to deeper layers is relatively slow. The former, at close distance, has a much greater effect on impedance than the latter, which occurs at greater distance. Like electrode temperature rise, the drop in impedance during RF application is not a reliable parameter for estimating tissue heating and lesion growth.[3,4,7]

Although coagulum formation is usually accompanied by an abrupt rise in impedance, the absence of impedance rise during ablation does not guarantee the absence of blood clot formation on the tissue contact site, which can unnoticeably be created on the lesion surface. In addition, as noted, with large ablation electrodes, formation of blood clots may only minimally affect electrode impedance by covering a much smaller part of the electrode surface. Any increase in impedance during RF application can, however, indicate the beginning of thrombus formation or unintended catheter movement; in either case, RF application is discontinued.

TEMPERATURE MONITORING

Monitoring of catheter tip temperature and closed-loop control of power output are useful to avoid excessive heating at the tissue surface, which can result in coagulum formation, and to accomplish effective heating at the target area. However, catheter tip temperature is affected by cooling effects and electrode-tissue contact and thus poorly correlates with lesion size. Tissue temperature can be markedly higher than catheter tip temperature; a higher target temperature can increase the incidence of tissue overheating associated with crater formation and coagulum formation. In high-flow areas, the tip is cooled and more RF power is delivered to the tissue to reach target temperature, thus resulting in relatively large lesions and vice versa.[7]

As mentioned earlier, temperature monitoring requires a dedicated sensor within the catheter. Two types of sensors are available: thermistor and thermocouple. No catheter or thermometry technology has been demonstrated to be superior in clinical use; however, closed-loop control of power output is easier to use than manual power titration. Conventional electrode catheters with temperature monitoring report the temperature only from the center of the electrode mass with one design or from the apex of the tip of the catheter with another design, and it is likely that the measured temperature underestimates the peak tissue temperature. Therefore, it is best if target temperatures no higher than 70° to 80°C are selected in the clinical setting.[3,7]

Titration of RF energy using temperature monitoring is usually done automatically by a closed-loop temperature monitoring system. When manual power titration is directed by temperature monitoring, the power initially is set to 20 to 30 W and then is gradually increased until the target temperature is achieved. With both manual and automatic power titration, change in power output is frequently required throughout the RF application to maintain the target temperature. Application of RF energy is continued if the desired clinical effect is observed within 5 to 10 seconds after the target temperature or impedance is achieved. If the desired endpoint does not occur within this time, the failed application is probably because of inadequate mapping. If the target temperature or impedance is not achieved with maximum generator output within 20 seconds, the time it takes to achieve subendocardial steady-state temperature, the RF application can be terminated, and catheter adjustment should be considered to obtain better tissue contact.[7]

The target ablation electrode temperature varies according to the arrhythmia substrate. For AVNRT, target temperature is usually 50° to 55°C. For BT, AV junction, atrial tachycardia (AT), and ventricular tachycardia (VT), a higher temperature (55° to 60°C) is usually targeted.

When using 4-mm-tip catheters, the target temperature should be lower than 80°C. In high-flow areas in the heart, the disparity between tip temperature and tissue temperature is large and a lower target temperature should be considered (e.g., 60°C), whereas in low flow areas tissue temperature is much better reflected by tip temperature and a higher target temperature can be considered (e.g., 70° to 80°C). The duration of RF application can be limited to 30 seconds for nonirrigated 4-mm-tip electrodes. The lesion is predominantly formed within the first 30 seconds. A longer duration does not create larger lesions.

When using 8-mm-tip catheters, a larger portion of the ablation electrode is exposed to the blood and thus cooled by blood flow, and a relatively large difference between catheter tip temperature and tissue temperature can be expected. Consequently, a moderate target temperature (e.g., 60°C) should be chosen; the RF power may be limited to 50 to 60 W to avoid tissue overheating and coagulum formation.[3]

It is important to recognize that prevention of coagulum formation is difficult, even with temperature and impedance monitoring. The clot first adheres to the tissue because that is the site with the highest temperature and may only loosely attach to the cooler electrode. The denaturized proteins probably have higher electrical impedance than blood, but the contact area with the electrode can be small, and RF impedance may not rise noticeably. The absence of flow inside the clot and its presumed higher impedance accelerate local heating and, because of some contact with the electrode, also accelerate heating of the electrode. Desiccation and adherence to the electrode then lead to coagulum formation on the metal electrode and impedance rise. Automatic power reduction by temperature-controlled RF ablation compensates for the reduction of electrode cooling and may prevent desiccation and impedance rise. The clot, however, can still be formed as demonstrated by experimental in vivo studies, and this can remain unnoticeable until it detaches from the tissue. Therefore, the absence of thermal and electrical phenomena does not imply that the ablation has been performed safely.[7]

ULTRASOUND IMAGING

Ultrasound imaging can allow assessment of tissue heating and pops. The presence of microbubbles on intracardiac or transesophageal echocardiography is typically associated with a tissue temperature higher than 60°C and increased lesion size, and continued RF application after the appearance of the bubbles is usually followed by an increase in impedance. Moreover, pops are not always audible but can be seen well on ultrasound, often with a sudden explosion of echocardiographic contrast.[6] Microbubble formation, however, is not a straightforward surrogate for tissue heating. The absence of microbubble formation clearly does not indicate that tissue heating is inadequate or that the power level should be increased, nor does the presence of scattered microbubbles indicate safe tissue heating. This marker is fairly specific for tissue heating as judged by tissue temperatures but is not routinely sensitive. Specifically, scattered microbubbles can occur over the entire spectrum of tissue temperatures, whereas dense showers of microbubbles appear only at tissue temperatures higher than 60°C. Scattered microbubbles can represent an electrolytic phenomenon, whereas dense showers of microbubbles suggest steam formation, with associated tissue disruption and impedance rises.[6]

Clinical Applications of Radiofrequency Ablation

RF is the most frequently used mode of ablation energy and has become a widely accepted treatment for most atrial and ventricular arrhythmias. Studies have demonstrated the effectiveness of RF current in producing precise and effective lesions.

Although RF energy for catheter- and surgical-based treatment of cardiac arrhythmias has been proven to be effective and relatively safe, several limitations exist. Many of these limitations center on how RF creates the tissue lesion. Current flow and energy delivery are critically dependent on a low-impedance electrode-tissue junction, but tissue desiccation, coagulation, and charring around the electrode can result in marked falls in conductivity.

Temporal evolution of ablation lesions can potentially alter the immediate postablation substrate, by producing either lesion expansion (mediated in part by secondary myocyte loss from disrupted microcirculation) or lesion regression (resolution of edema and healing).

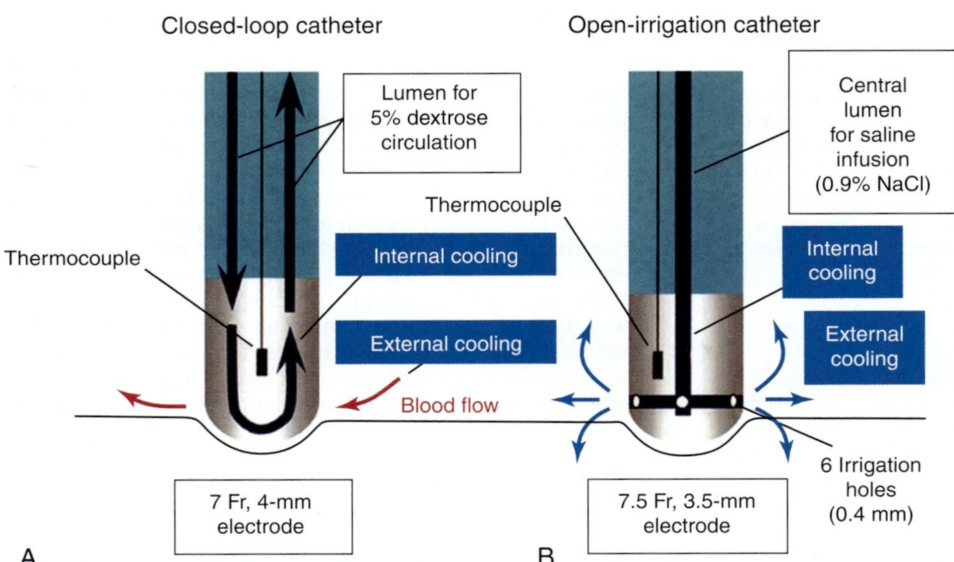

FIGURE 7-6 Schematic representation of irrigated electrode catheters. **A,** The closed-loop irrigation catheter has a 7 Fr, 4-mm-tip electrode with an internal thermocouple. **B,** The open-irrigated catheter has a 7.5 Fr, 3.5-mm-tip electrode with an internal thermocouple and six irrigation holes (0.4-mm diameter) located around the electrode, 1.0 mm from the tip. NaCl = sodium chloride. *(From Yokoyama K, Nakagawa H, Wittkampf FH, et al: Comparison of electrode cooling between internal and open irrigation in radiofrequency ablation lesion depth and incidence of thrombus and steam pop. Circulation 113:11, 2006.)*

A major limitation of RF ablation is the relatively small depth of tissue injury produced by this technique. This can be attributed to the precipitous fall-off of direct tissue heating (volume heating) by the RF energy as the distance from the electrode-tissue interface increases. Deeper tissue layers can be ablated by heat conduction from the volume-heated source, but the maximum lesion depth is limited.

Because the success of RF catheter ablation in the clinical setting is sometimes limited by the relatively small size of the lesion, attempts have been made to increase the size of those lesions reliably and safely. One approach is to increase the size and surface area of the electrode. The RF power needs to be increased comparably to achieve a similar current density and temperature at the electrode-tissue interface, and the results are greater depth of volume heating and a larger lesion. Modifications to the RF energy delivery mechanism, including cooled catheters and pulsed energy, have also helped address some of these limitations. Moreover, investigation into alternative energy sources appears to be more promising, including microwave, ultrasound, laser, and cryoablation.[2]

Delivery of RF energy on the epicardial surface generally requires an irrigated-tip catheter because there is otherwise no passive cooling of the electrode (outside the blood pool) and relatively little power can be delivered without being limited by temperature increases.

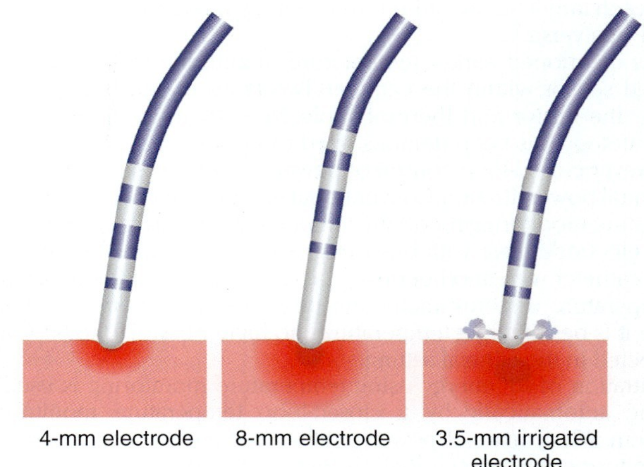

FIGURE 7-7 Effect of electrode type on lesion size. Representative blocks of myocardium are shown with lesions (dark shading) resulting from optimal radiofrequency energy delivery for each electrode type. A 4-mm electrode makes a small shallow lesion **(left)**. An 8-mm electrode makes a larger, deeper lesion **(center)**. The open-irrigated electrode makes a larger, deeper lesion, with a maximum width at some tissue depth **(right)**.

Cooled Radiofrequency Ablation

Biophysics

MECHANISM

Excessive surface heating invites coagulum formation, carbonization, and steam popping. These adverse effects may limit the depth of RF lesions, thus making it difficult to produce lesions of sufficient depth in scar tissue or thickened ventricular walls. Such limitations of conventional RF systems have stimulated the evaluation of modified electrode systems. One important modification involves cooling of the ablation electrode, which was designed to prevent overheating of the endocardium while allowing sufficient energy delivery to achieve a larger lesion size and depth.[17]

There are two methods of active electrode cooling by irrigation: internal and external (Fig. 7-6). With the internal (closed-loop) system (Chilli, Boston Scientific, Natick, Mass.), cooling of the ablation electrode is performed by circulating fluid within the electrode.[18] In contrast, with the external (open-loop) system (Celsius or Navistar ThermoCool, Biosense Webster, Inc., Diamond Bar, Calif.; and Therapy Cool Path, St. Jude Medical, Inc., St. Paul, Minn.), electrode cooling is performed by flushing saline through openings in the porous-tipped electrode (showerhead-type system).[18] Another cooling system is sheath-based open irrigation, which uses a long sheath around the ablation catheter for open irrigation. The latter system was found to provide the best results, but this type of catheter tip cooling is not clinically available.

Active electrode cooling by irrigation can produce higher tissue temperatures and create larger lesions, compared with standard RF ablation catheters, because of a reduction in overheating at the tissue-electrode interface, even at sites with low blood flow. This allows the delivery of higher amounts of RF power for a longer duration to create relatively large lesions with greater depth but without the risk of coagulum and char formation. Unlike with standard RF ablation, the area of maximum temperature with cooled ablation is within the myocardium, rather than at the electrode-myocardial interface. Higher power results in greater depth of volume heating, but if the ablation is power limited, power dissipation into the circulating blood pool can actually result in decreased lesion depth (Fig. 7-7).[18] Compared with large-tip catheters, active cooling has been shown to produce equivalent lesions with energy delivery via smaller electrodes, with less dependence on catheter tip orientation and extrinsic cooling, whereas larger electrodes have significant variability in their electrode-tissue interface, depending on catheter orientation (see Fig. 7-7). For the nonirrigated catheter, greater lesion volumes are observed with a horizontal orientation of the RF electrode compared with a vertical orientation. In contrast, for irrigated catheters, lesion volume increased with a perpendicular electrode orientation compared with the horizontal orientation.[10]

Lesion depth seems to be similar between closed-loop and open-irrigation electrodes. However, open irrigation appears to be more effective in cooling the electrode-tissue interface, as reflected by lower interface temperature, lower incidence of thrombus, and smaller lesion diameter at the surface (with the maximum diameter produced deeper in the tissue). These differences between the two electrodes are greater in low blood flow, presumably because the flow of saline irrigation out of the electrode provides additional cooling of the electrode-tissue interface (external cooling). Ablation with the closed-loop electrode, with irrigation providing only internal cooling, in low blood flow frequently results in high electrode-tissue interface temperature (despite low electrode temperature) and thrombus formation.[18]

When maximum power and temperature parameters that did not result in increased rates of complications and any evidence of excessive heating (including popping, boiling, or impedance rise) for each catheter type were selected, closed-irrigation catheters resulted in slightly larger lesion volumes and greater lesion depths than the open-irrigation catheters. Both cooled catheters fared better than the standard 4-mm-tip and large 10-mm-tip catheters with larger lesions achieved within the range of safe energy delivery.[19]

Monitoring Radiofrequency Energy Delivery

There is a significant discrepancy between monitored electrode temperature and tissue temperature during cooled RF ablation.[6,8] The thermal effects on the electrode temperature are dependent on electrode heating from the tissue, internal cooling by the irrigation fluid, and external cooling from blood flow or open irrigation. With high irrigation flow rates, catheter tip temperature is not representative of tissue temperature, and therefore feedback cannot be used to guide power output. The difference between the electrode temperature and interface temperature is greater with the closed-loop electrode than with the open-irrigation electrode. The discrepancy is likely to be increased in areas of high blood flow, by increasing the irrigation flow rate, or by cooling the irrigant. Saline-irrigated catheters cause peak tissue heating several millimeters from the electrode-tissue interface. Because maximum tissue heating does not occur at the electrode-tissue interface, the value of temperature and impedance monitoring is limited with this type of catheter.

Therefore, it has been challenging to monitor lesion formation and optimize power delivery during cooled RF ablation.[6] Appropriate energy titration is important to allow greater power application and to produce large lesions while avoiding overheating of tissue with steam formation leading to pops. Moreover, the inability to assess tissue heating, and hence to titrate power to an objective endpoint, prevents the operator from determining whether unsuccessful applications are caused by inadequate mapping or inadequate heating.

Electrode-tissue contact and orientation and the cooling effect of blood flow around the electrode and within the tissue are not as easily adjusted, and they also influence tissue heating. However, several other factors can be potentially manipulated to adjust ablation with saline-irrigated catheters, including flow rate, irrigant temperature, and RF power and duration. The most easily controllable factors are the power and duration of RF application. Instead of increasing the power to achieve the desired effect, which increases the likelihood of crater formation, the duration may be increased. A moderate power of 20 to 35 W with a relatively long RF duration of 60 to 300 seconds should be considered to achieve relatively large lesions, with a limited risk of crater formation.[6]

The flow rate of the irrigant determines the degree of cooling. Faster flow rates likely allow greater power application without impedance rises, increase the difference between tissue and electrode temperature, and thereby potentially increase the risk of steam pops if temperature is used to guide ablation. With the internally irrigated ablation system, the approved flow rate is fixed at 36 mL/min and is not currently manipulated.[6] With the externally irrigated ablation system, an irrigation flow rate of 10 to 17 mL/min during RF application (and 2 mL/min during all other times to maintain patency of the pores in the electrode) may be selected in a power-controlled mode with a delivered power of up to 30 W. The irrigation flow rate should be increased to 20 to 30 mL/min with delivery of more than 30 W, to avoid excessive heat development at the superficial tissue layers. Additionally, the temperature of the irrigant can potentially be manipulated. Cooling the irrigant can allow power delivery to be increased without coagulum formation. The cooled irrigant is warmed as it passes through the tubing to reach the catheter and through the length of the catheter. The impact of cooling the irrigant has not been well studied. In most studies, the irrigant that enters the catheter is at room temperature.

Several indicators of tissue heating may be monitored, including catheter tip temperature, EP effects of RF, and the use of ICE. As noted, with cooled RF, the discrepancy between measured electrode temperature and tissue temperature is greater than during standard RF ablation.[8] Identification of microbubbles on ICE has been used as an indication of excessive tissue heating during ablation with nonirrigated and internally irrigated catheters. External irrigation, on the other hand, produces visible bubbles, precluding the use of this method.[17,19]

Evidence of tissue heating from an effect on recorded electrograms or the arrhythmia can be used to guide ablation energy.[6] Interruption of tachycardia (VT, atrial flutter [AFL], supraventricular tachycardia) or block in conduction over a pathway (AVN or BT) during the process of ablation provides immediate feedback about the disruption of tissue integrity. Additionally, an increase in pacing threshold and a decrease in electrogram amplitude can indicate tissue damage. These factors, however, are not easily monitored during the RF application, particularly the change in pacing threshold. Moreover, the decrease in electrogram amplitude is often not visible during RF application because of superimposed electrical artifact.

With the internally irrigated system, the room temperature irrigant flowing at 36 mL/min typically cools the measured electrode temperature to 28° to 30°C. During RF application, the temperature increases; temperatures of 50°C can indicate that cooling is inadequate or has stopped, which warrants termination of RF application. The measured impedance typically decreases during cooled RF ablation by 5 to 10 Ω, in a manner similar to that observed during standard RF ablation.[6]

During open-irrigation RF ablation, initiation of irrigation results in a drop of electrode temperature by several degrees. Failure of electrode temperature to decrease indicates a lack of irrigant flow. When power delivery begins, catheter tip temperature should rise to 36° to 42°C (the presence of rising temperature, not the magnitude, reflects tissue heating). Temperatures higher than 40°C achieved with low power (less than 20 W) can indicate that the electrode is in a location with little or no cooling from the surrounding circulating blood, or that there is a failure of the catheter cooling system that requires attention. In contrast, the absence of any increase in tip temperature should raise the possibility of poor catheter contact.[9]

The optimal method for adjusting power during saline-irrigated RF ablation is not yet clearly defined, but some useful guidelines have emerged. The most commonly recommended approach is to perform ablation in a power-controlled mode, typically starting at 20 to 30 W and gradually increasing power to achieve evidence of tissue heating or damage. An impedance fall likely indicates tissue heating, similar to that observed with conventional RF

When catheter temperature is between 28° and 31°C, power can be ramped up, watching for a 5- to 10-Ω impedance fall. Measured electrode temperature will generally increase. A measured electrode temperature of 37° to 40°C is commonly achieved.

Temperatures exceeding 40° to 42°C with power greater than 30 W during open-irrigation RF ablation can be associated with a greater risk of steam pops and impedance rises, particularly during long RF applications, exceeding 60 seconds. Steam pops are often, but not always, audible. A sudden decrease in temperature, sudden catheter movement (as a consequence of the pop blowing the catheter out of position), and a sudden change in impedance are all potential indications that a pop has occurred. Whether the catheter is maintained in a stable position, as opposed to dragging it across the tissue, also likely influences tissue heating. High power can be applied continuously during dragging with little risk of excessive heating, although the duration of time to spend at each site to create an effective lesion may be difficult to ascertain.[17] As a rule, the lowest effective power setting, shortest duration, and fewest applications should be employed whenever possible.[9]

Clinical Applications of Cooled Radiofrequency Ablation

Cooled tip catheters have several advantages. First, they allow the desired power to be delivered independent of local blood flow, and that results in increased lesion size. Second, they reduce the temperature of the ablation electrode as well as the temperature at the tissue interface, especially with the open-irrigation system, and that helps spare the endocardium and reduce the risk of clots and charring. Third, when compared with standard 8-mm-tip ablation catheters, a 3.5- to 4-mm irrigated electrode offers higher mapping accuracy while providing comparable ablation lesion size.

Cooled tip catheters are preferred (1) for long linear ablations (in the right or left atrium) and complex atrial arrhythmias (AFL or AF), (2) when there is a high probability of encountering thick or trabeculated tissue, (3) for specific areas with low local blood flow (including the coronary sinus [CS], particularly CS aneurysms, and pericardial space), (4) when ablating in the arterial circulation (to minimize the likelihood of arterial thromboembolism), and (5) for targets resistant to previous conventional ablation (focal tachycardias or BTs). Clinical trials have found irrigated tip catheters to be more effective than and as safe as conventional catheters for AFL ablation, thus facilitating the rapid achievement of bidirectional isthmus block. Irrigated tip catheters also were found to be safe and effective in eliminating BT conduction resistant to conventional catheters, irrespective of the location, and they have been successfully used for PV isolation for treatment of AF. Irrigated tip catheters also offer an advantage over conventional RF catheters in the case of scar-related VTs, by facilitating creation of larger and deeper lesions that can help eliminate intramyocardial or subepicardial reentrant pathways necessary for the VT circuit.[9,17,20]

Internally cooled RF ablation is an attractive choice for use in pericardial ablation because no fluid is infused, and one need not worry about monitoring pericardial fluid throughout the ablation procedure, although drainage of irrigant during open-irrigation RF ablation can be managed in this setting.[9]

Power levels typically used during open-irrigation ablation depend on the site of ablation: 25 to 30 W in the left and right atrial free wall, 35 to 40 W for cavotricuspid isthmus and mitral isthmus ablation, 50 W in the left ventricle, and 20 W in the CS. At low power levels, the irrigation flow rate may be set lower than at higher levels; 17 mL/min is used for power output lower than 30 W, whereas 30 mL/min is used for power output of 30 to 50 W. Using a lower irrigation flow rate (10 mL/min) in the left atrium can help maintain some temperature feedback, with a cutoff temperature of 43°C. Lesion formation is monitored via attenuation of the local unipolar electrogram. Because of the very limited or absent temperature feedback, tissue overheating (pops) is a potential risk, especially in thin-walled chambers. The temperature is usually set at 40° to 45°C. If the temperature at the tip is lower than 40°C, the flow rate may be reduced. If the desired power is not met because the target temperature is reached at a lower power, the irrigation flow rate may be increased to a maximum of 60 mL/min.[4] Parameters for epicardial ablation are similar to those used for endocardial ablation.[17]

Potential Risks of Cooled Radiofrequency Ablation

Although creation of larger ablation lesions can improve the efficacy of ablation for some patients, particularly when the targeted arrhythmia originates deep to the endocardium and when large areas require ablation, it is associated with increased risk of damage to tissue outside the target region (Table 7-1).

Higher power can be used with convective cooling, but higher power can cause superheating within the tissue (with subendocardial tissue temperatures exceeding 100°C) that can result in boiling of any liquids under the electrode. Consequently, evaporation and rapid steam expansion can occur intramurally, and a gas bubble can develop in the tissue under the electrode. Continuous application of RF energy causes the bubble to expand and its pressure to increase, which can lead to eruption of the gas bubble (causing a popping sound) through the path with the least mechanical resistance that leaves behind a gaping hole (the so-called pop lesion). This often occurs toward the heat-damaged endocardial surface (crater formation) or, more rarely, across the myocardial wall (myocardial rupture).[18]

Steam pops are often associated with a sudden (although small, less than 10 Ω) impedance rise and a sudden drop in electrode temperature. The consequence of a steam pop depends on the area of the heart being ablated. The risk of cardiac perforation is low in areas of dense ventricular scar. The risk of perforation and cardiac tamponade is likely to be higher for ablation in the thin-walled right ventricular outflow tract and in the atria. Therefore,

TABLE 7-1 Comparison of Features of Ablation Electrodes

FEATURE	4-MM RF	8-MM RF	4-MM COOLED RF (CLOSED)	4-MM COOLED RF (OPEN)	6-MM CRYOABLATION
Electrogram resolution	+++	+	++++	++++	++
Lesion depth	+	+++	+++	+++	++
Lesion surface area	++	++++	++++	++++	+++
Usefulness of temperature monitoring	+++	++	0	0	0
Risk of steam pop	+	++	+++	+++	0
Thrombus risk	++	++++	+++	+	0
Time efficiency of ablation*	++	++++	++++	++++	+

*Inverse function of duration of energy application for effective lesion (higher efficiency = best).

0 = none; + = least, worst; ++ = minimal; +++ = moderate; ++++ = most, best; RF = radiofrequency.

it may be reasonable to take a more conservative approach to power application in these areas. Electrode orientation also seems to affect the significance of pops; pops that occur when the electrode tip is perpendicular to the tissue can be more likely to cause cardiac perforation than those that occur when the electrode is lying horizontally on the tissue. Therefore, one should try to avoid perpendicular (high-pressure) tissue contact, especially at higher power levels.[17] RF applications with steam pops have a greater decrease in impedance and occur at a higher maximum RF power than applications without pops. Because of the considerable overlap of impedance changes in lesions with and without steam pops, it is not possible to advocate a general limit for impedance decrease for all RF lesions. However, when ablation is performed in areas at risk for perforation (i.e., especially in thin-walled structures), reducing power to achieve an impedance decrease of less than 18 Ω is a reasonable strategy to reduce the chance of a pop.[20]

Although increasing power delivery and convective cooling can create large lesions, lesion production is somewhat difficult to control. Surface cooling does reduce the risk of boiling and coagulum formation. However, it does not allow the temperature at the tip to be monitored, and thus some feedback about lesion formation is lost.[18]

These concerns can be more pronounced with internal cooling as compared with open irrigation. Open irrigation cools the electrode and its direct environment, blood, and tissue surface. In contrast, with internal cooling, the main parameter affected by cooling is the temperature of the electrode. There can be minimal cooling of the direct electrode-tissue interface, but only at the true contact site between metal and tissue. Blood flow around the electrode makes it highly unlikely that there will be any noticeable cooling of the tissue surface at a distance of a few millimeters from the contact site. Consequently, one would not expect much effect of internal electrode cooling on the surface area or depth of the lesion. Electrode cooling does, however, enable larger lesions (at higher power levels) because the ablation process is no longer limited by electrode temperature rise. This can also be dangerous; in cases with good tissue contact, power delivery to the tissue can be much higher than average. With standard electrodes, this situation is signaled by an excessive electrode temperature rise, but without this warning, tissue overheating can occur. Blood clots can also be formed, but they do not adhere to a cool electrode and do not cause an impedance rise.[4]

With open-irrigation catheters, extensive ablation often performed for AF and scar-related VT can result in substantial saline administration. Therefore, management of the patient's volume status before, during, and after the procedure is crucial. This is also important during epicardial ablation, in which an obligatory fluid volume enters the pericardial sac and, if not intermittently or continuously evacuated, gradually results in cardiac tamponade. This complication can be prevented by having the side port of the introducer sheath attached to a suction bottle or gravity drain or by intermittent aspiration of accumulated fluid. Internal irrigation, on the other hand, has the advantages that no fluid is infused into the vasculature or pericardial space, and there is no possibility of embolization from the irrigation system.[17]

Cryoablation

Biophysics of Cryothermal Energy

Cryoablation uses a steerable catheter and a dedicated console, which are connected by a coaxial cable used to deliver fluid nitrous oxide to the catheter and to remove the gas from the catheter separately.[21] A tank of fluid nitrous oxide is located inside the console; the gas removed from the catheter to the console is evacuated through a scavenging hose into the vacuum line of the EP laboratory. The system has several sensors to avoid inadvertent leaks of nitrous oxide into the patient body and to check connections of the different cables to the console.

Cryoablation catheters have a terminal segment whose temperature can be lowered to −75°C or less by delivery of precooled compressed liquid refrigerant (nitrous oxide argon) across a sudden luminal widening at the end of the catheters' refrigerant circulation system (Fig. 7-8). Decompression and expansion of the refrigerant (liquid to gas phase change) achieve cooling based on the Joule-Thompson effect.[22]

The effect produced by cryothermal ablation is secondary to tissue freezing, the result of a temperature gradient occurring at the electrode-tissue interface (i.e., local heat absorption by the cooled catheter tip). It greatly depends on the minimum temperature reached, the duration of energy application, and the temperature time constant. The temperature time constant indicates the course of the descent of temperature to the target temperature, and a shorter value (expressed in seconds) identifies a more effective application. Important modulatory variables that can affect tissue damage produced by cryoablation include firmness of the catheter-tissue contact, tip temperature, freeze duration, and blood flow.[22]

At the electrode-tissue interface, the coldest area is the one adjacent to the catheter tip, where functional effects of energy delivery are observed earlier (Fig. 7-9). Conversely, the less cooled area is the one at the periphery of the cryolesion, whose dimensions can also vary according to the duration of freezing. Because of limited cooling of the outer limit of the lesion (both in time and

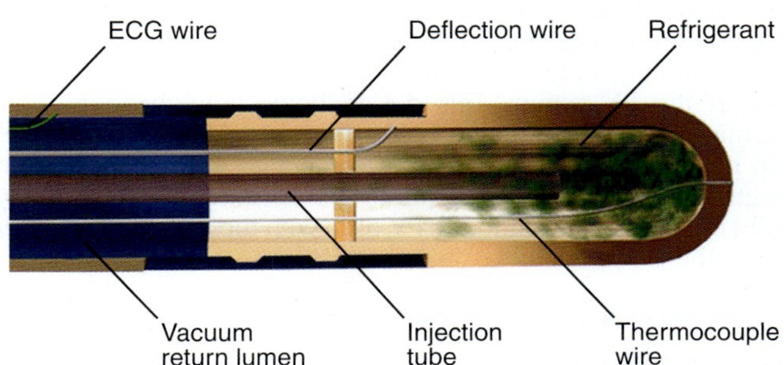

FIGURE 7-8 Schematic diagram demonstrating the CryoCath Freezor cryocatheter internal design. *(Courtesy of CryoCath Technologies, Montreal, Canada.)*

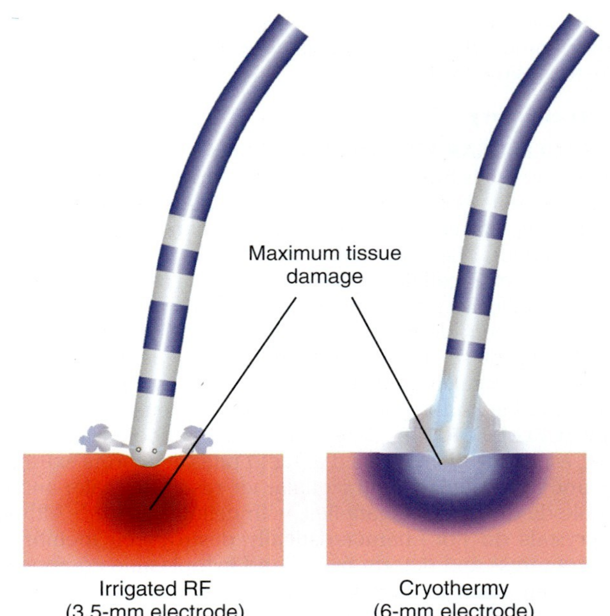

FIGURE 7-9 Depth of maximum tissue injury with irrigated-tip radiofrequency (RF) versus cryothermy. With irrigated RF **(left)**, the maximum tissue heating occurs at some tissue depth because of cooling at the surface. With cryothermy **(right)**, the maximum effect is at the endocardial surface.

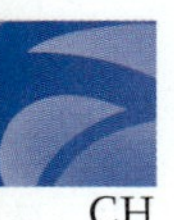

temperature), this region is less likely to suffer irreversible damage. As a consequence, the effects obtained late during cryothermal energy application are likely to be reversible early on rewarming, and, therefore, any expected functional modification induced by cryoenergy should occur early (usually within the first 30 seconds of the application) to obtain a successful and permanent ablation of a given arrhythmogenic substrate.[22]

Currently, two different systems of catheter cryoablation are available for clinical and experimental use: the CryoCath system (CryoCath Technologies, a division of Medtronic, Inc., Minneapolis, Minn.) and the CryoCor system (CryoCor, San Diego, Calif.). CryoCath uses 7 or 9 Fr steerable catheters with 4-, 6-, or 8-mm-long-tip electrodes. The ablation catheter is connected to a dedicated console, which has two algorithms available. The first is for cryomapping with a slow decrease of temperature to –30°C for up to 80 seconds, and the second is for cryoablation with a faster decrease of temperature to –75°C for up to 480 seconds. Additionally, the target temperature can be manually preset on the console at any value between –30° and –75°C. The CryoCor system has 10 Fr steerable catheters with 6.5- or 10-mm-long-tip electrodes. The console has a built-in closed-loop precooler for the fluid nitrous oxide, whose flow at the catheter tip is adjusted during the application to maintain a temperature of –80°C.[22]

An expandable cryoablation balloon catheter (Arctic Front, CryoCath Technologies, Inc.), 18 to 30 mm in diameter, has been specifically designed for PV isolation. The cryoballoon is deployed at the ostium of targeted PVs, and cryoenergy is delivered over the occluding balloon system to create circumferential lesions around the PV ostium. This design helps limit the convective warming effects of the high blood flow at the PV ostium, which can limit lesion size and ablation efficacy, as well as shorten the lengthy procedure times required for circumferential point-by-point cryoablation around the PV ostia with the standard steerable cryocatheters.[23-25]

Pathophysiology of Lesion Formation by Cryoablation

MECHANISM OF TISSUE INJURY

The mechanisms underlying lesion formation by cryoenergy are twofold: direct cell injury and vascular-mediated tissue injury. The mechanisms of cellular death associated with tissue freezing involve immediate cellular effects, as well as late effects that determine the lesion produced.[22]

Direct Cell Injury

EXTRACELLULAR ICE (SOLUTION EFFECT INJURY). Direct cellular injury results from ice formation. Ice forms only extracellularly when the tissue is cooled to mild temperatures (0° to –20°C) and results in hypertonic stress (the extracellular environment becomes hyperosmotic). The consequent shift of water from the intracellular to the extracellular space ultimately causes cell shrinkage and damage to the plasma membrane cellular constituents. These effects are reversible when rewarming is achieved within a short period (30 to 60 seconds). However, extended periods of extracellular freezing result in cellular death, and rewarming then results in cellular swelling sufficient to disrupt cellular membranes.[21]

INTRACELLULAR ICE. When the tissue is cooled to –40°C or lower, especially if it is cooled at rapid rates, ice forms extracellularly and intracellularly. Intracellular ice results in major and irreversible disruption of organelles, with cellular death.[21] Although ice crystals do not characteristically destroy cell membranes, they compress and deform nuclei and cytoplasmic components. Mitochondria are particularly sensitive to ice crystals and are the first structures to suffer irreversible damage. Furthermore, intracellular ice can propagate from one cell to another via intercellular channels, thus potentially resulting in lesion growth. Cellular injury, disruption of membranous organelles in particular, is importantly enhanced on cellular thawing; rewarming causes intracellular crystals to enlarge and fuse into larger masses that extend cellular destruction. Cellular injury can be extended by repeated freeze-thaw cycles. Final rewarming evokes an inflammation response to released cellular constituents and reperfusional hemorrhage, leading to tissue repair and eventual dense scarring.[22] The size of ice crystals and their density depend on the proximity to the cryoenergy source, local tissue temperature achieved, rate of freezing, and surface area in contact with freezing temperatures.[26,27]

Vascular-Mediated Tissue Injury

Tissue freezing results in vasoconstriction, hypoperfusion, and ischemic necrosis.[21] Subsequent tissue rewarming produces a hyperemic response with increased vascular permeability and edema formation. Endothelial disruption within the frozen tissue is also observed and results in platelet aggregation, microthrombi, and microcirculatory stagnation within the lesion. Cryolesions, however, are associated with substantially less degree of endothelial damage and overlying thrombus formation than standard RF lesions. Extensive surgical experience has shown that cryolesions result in dense homogeneous fibrosis, with a well-demarcated border zone. They are nonarrhythmogenic and preserve the underlying extracellular matrix and tensile strength.[22]

In the final phase of cryoinjury, replacement fibrosis and apoptosis of cells near the periphery of frozen tissue give rise to a mature lesion within weeks. Typically, these lesions are well circumscribed, with distinct borders, dense areas of fibrotic tissue, contraction band necrosis, and a conserved tissue matrix, including endothelial cell layers.[26]

DETERMINANTS OF LESION SIZE

During cryoablation, lesion size and tissue temperature are related to convective warming, electrode orientation, electrode contact pressure, electrode size, refrigerant flow rate, and electrode temperature.[28] Lesion sizes during catheter cryoablation can be maximized by use of larger ablation electrodes with higher refrigerant delivery rates. A horizontal electrode orientation to the tissue and firm contact pressure also enhance lesion size. For a given electrode size, electrode temperature may be a poor predictor of tissue cooling and lesion size. In contrast to RF ablation, cryoablation in areas of high blood flow can result in limited tissue cooling and smaller lesion sizes because of convective warming. Conversely, cryoablation lesion size can be maximized in areas of low blood flow.[22,28] The time to reach –80°C can predict cryoablation lesion size; cryoablation lesion volume increases as the time to reach –80°C decreases.[29] The 6- and 8-mm electrode-tip cryocatheters produce ablation lesions of similar depth that are more than two- and threefold larger than 4-mm catheters, respectively. Despite larger lesions, endothelial cell layers remain intact and devoid of thrombosis. Surface areas and volumes may be particularly sensitive to catheter tip-to-tissue contact angles with larger electrodes. As such, particular attention in catheter orientation is required with 8-mm electrode-tip cryocatheters to produce desired lesions.[27]

Technical Aspects of Cryoablation

The intervention is often performed in two steps. First, "cryomaps" are obtained by moderate reversible cooling of tissue (electrode-tissue interface temperature approximately –28° to –32°C). Second, cryoablation cools the selected cryomapped pathways to much lower temperatures (electrode-tissue interface temperature lower than –68°C) and produces ice formation inside and outside of cells, a mechanism of irreversible cellular injury.[22]

CRYOMAPPING

Cryomapping is designed to verify that ablation at the chosen site will have the desired effect and to ensure the absence of complications (i.e., to localize electric pathways to be destroyed or spared).

This procedure is generally performed using various pacing protocols that can be performed during cryomapping (or ice mapping) at −32°C. At this temperature, the lesion is reversible (for up to 60 seconds), and the catheter is stuck to the adjacent frozen tissue because of the presence of an ice ball that includes the tip of the catheter (cryoadherence). This permits programmed electrical stimulation to test the functionality of a potential ablation target during ongoing ablation and prior to permanent destruction. It also allows ablation to be performed during tachycardia without the risk of catheter dislodgment on termination of the tachycardia.

In the cryomapping mode, the temperature is not allowed to drop to less than −30°C, and the time of application is limited to 60 seconds. Formation of an ice ball at the catheter tip and adherence to the underlying myocardium are signaled by the appearance of electrical noise recorded from the ablation catheter's distal bipole. Once an ice ball is formed, programmed stimulation is repeated to verify achievement of the desired effect. If cryomapping does not yield the desired result within 20 to 30 seconds or results in unintended effect (e.g., AV conduction delay or block), cryomapping is interrupted, to allow the catheter to thaw and become dislodged from the tissue. After a few seconds, the catheter may be moved to a different site and cryomapping repeated.[22]

CRYOABLATION

When sites of successful cryomapping are identified by demonstrating the desired effect with no adverse effects, the cryoablation mode is activated, in which a target temperature lower than −75°C is sought (a temperature of −75° to −80°C is generally achieved). The application is then continued for 4 to 8 minutes, thus creating an irreversible lesion. If the catheter tip is in close contact with the endocardium, a prompt drop in catheter tip temperature should be observed as soon as the cryoablation mode is activated. A slow decline in catheter tip temperature or a very high flow rate of refrigerant during ablation suggests poor electrode-tissue contact. In such cases, cryoablation is interrupted, and the catheter is repositioned.[22]

Advantages of Cryoablation

The use of cryoablation in the EP laboratory provides some distinct advantages not seen with conventional RF ablation. The slow development of the cryolesion (approximately 240 seconds), although time-consuming, enables the creation of reversible lesions and modulation of lesion formation in critical areas. As noted, cryomapping allows functional assessment of a putative ablation site during ongoing ablation and prior to permanent destruction. This offers a safety advantage when ablation is performed close to critical structures such as the AVN or His bundle (HB).[30]

Compared with standard RF lesions, cryolesions are associated with a substantially lower degree of endothelial disruption, less platelet activation, and lower thrombogenic tendency. Therefore, the risk of coagulum formation, charring, and steam popping is less than with RF ablation (see Table 7-1). Furthermore, cryoablation results in dense homogeneous fibrotic lesions with a well-demarcated border zone and does not cause collagen denaturation or contracture related to hyperthermic effects. Therefore, cryothermal energy application in close proximity to the coronary arteries (e.g., during epicardial ablation) or in venous vessels (CS, middle cardiac vein, and PVs) does not result in damage, perforation, or chronic stenosis of their lumen.[22,30]

The cryoadherence effect results in the formation of a very focal lesion because of fixed and stable tip electrode contact to adjacent frozen tissue throughout the whole application. This has a particular safety advantage, especially for ablation in the proximity of critical areas, such as the AVN and HB. In addition, cryoadherence augments catheter stability throughout the energy application, even when sudden changes in heart rhythm that can potentially displace the ablation catheter (e.g., tachycardia termination) occur. At the same time, cryoadherence does not compromise safety. On discontinuation of cryothermal application, the defrost phase is fast (within 3 seconds), and the catheter can be immediately disengaged from the ablation position.

Cryothermal energy application is characterized by the absence of pain perception in nonsedated patients. In fact, cryoablation can be performed without analgesia. Occasionally, a light sense of cold or headache is perceived as minor discomfort. This characteristic can be particularly useful in younger and pediatric patients.[22]

Clinical Applications of Cryoablation

As noted, catheter-based cryoablation can have specific advantages over RF catheter ablation, including greater safety as a result of greater catheter stability, reduced risk of systemic embolization, low propensity for thrombus formation and endothelial disruption, and preservation of ultrastructural tissue integrity. As a result, cryoablation has quickly been adapted for specific arrhythmogenic substrates in which RF has specific limitations that can potentially be overcome by cryothermy.[30]

It is unlikely that cryoablation will replace standard RF ablation in unselected cases. Nevertheless, for the previously mentioned peculiarities, cryothermal ablation has proven effective and safe for the ablation of arrhythmogenic substrates close to the normal conduction pathways. It has become the first-choice method to ablate superoparaseptal and midseptal BTs and difficult cases of AVNRT because of its widely demonstrated safety profile. As the technology evolves and further iterations of the catheter proceed, the role for this technology is likely to grow.[31]

ATRIOVENTRICULAR NODAL REENTRANT TACHYCARDIA

So far, slow pathway ablation for AVNRT by cryothermal energy represents the larger experience in the clinical application of this technology.[21,32] Previously published reports with cryoablation of AVNRT in pediatric patients demonstrated procedural success rates of 83% to 97% and recurrence rates ranging from 0% to 20%. Although the use of bonus cryoapplications to consolidate the acutely successful cryoablation and the availability of larger tip cryocatheters (6 to 8 mm and 6 mm versus 4 mm) to create larger lesions have been associated with fewer recurrences on long-term follow-up without compromising safety, the overall procedural success rates have remained consistently lower than those (95% to 99%) with RF ablation.[31,33-36]

According to current data, cryothermal energy is a valuable and useful alternative to RF energy to treat patients with AVNRT. The absence of permanent inadvertent damage of AV conduction makes this new technology particularly useful for patients with difficult anatomy, after an unsuccessful prior standard ablation procedure, in pediatric patients, and in patients in whom even the small risk of AV block associated with RF ablation is considered unacceptable. Cryoablation can be of particular advantage in several situations, including posterior displacement of the fast pathway or AVN, a small space in the triangle of Koch between the HB and the CS ostium, and the need for ablation to be performed in the midseptum. However, given the high success rate and low risk of RF slow pathway ablation, it can be difficult to demonstrate a clinical advantage of cryoablation over RF ablation in unselected AVNRT cases.[22]

BYPASS TRACTS

Cryothermal ablation of BTs in the superoparaseptal and midseptal areas, both at high risk of complete permanent AV block when standard RF energy is applied, is highly safe and successful (Fig. 7-10).[32] Cryoablation can also be successfully and safely used to ablate selected cases of epicardial left-sided BTs within the CS, well beyond the middle cardiac vein, once attempts using the transseptal and transaortic approaches have failed.[21] However, the experience with cryoablation in unselected BTs is more limited

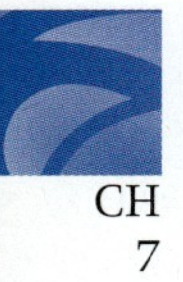

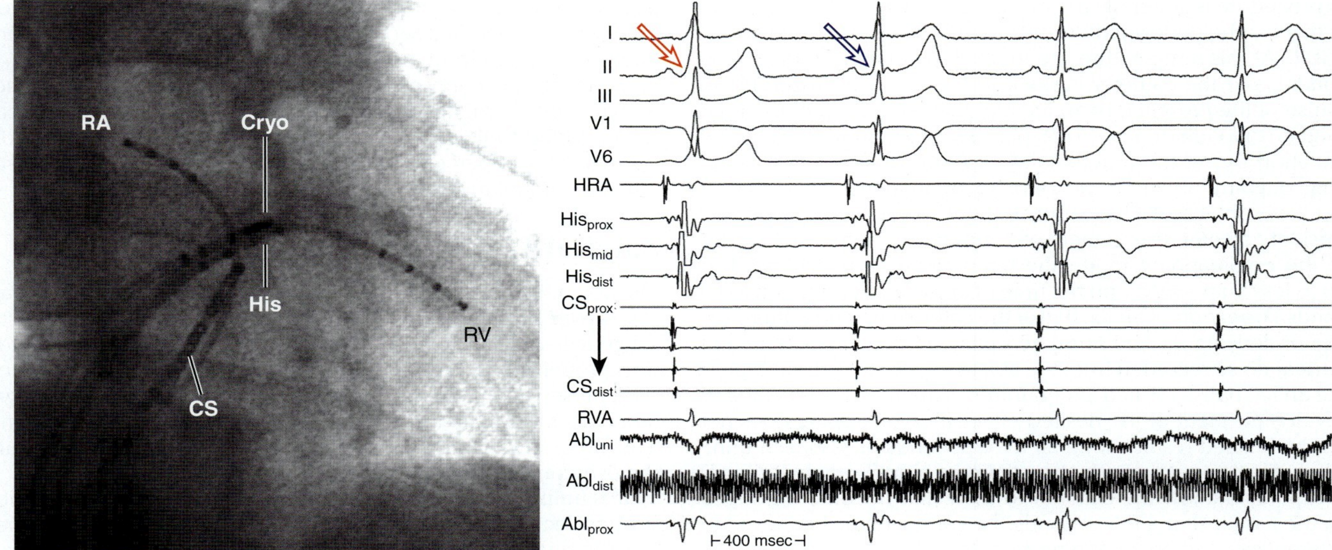

FIGURE 7-10 Cryoablation of a para-Hisian bypass tract (BT). Right anterior oblique fluoroscopic view of cryoablation catheter (Cryo) position and ECG and intracardiac recordings during cryoablation of para-Hisian BT. The first two QRS complexes at left are preexcited, with the second QRS complex (blue arrow) less so than the first (red arrow), as cryoablation begins to affect pathway conduction. Preexcitation disappears afterward. The ablation recordings at bottom are severely disrupted by the delivery of cryoenergy. Abl_{dist} = distal ablation site; Abl_{prox} = proximal ablation site; Abl_{uni} = unipolar ablation site; CS = coronary sinus; CS_{dist} = distal coronary sinus; CS_{prox} = proximal coronary sinus; His_{dist} = distal His bundle; His_{mid} = middle His bundle; His_{prox} = proximal His bundle; HRA = high right atrium; RA = right atrium; RV = right ventricle; RVA = right ventricular apex.

and less satisfactory; this can be related to multiple factors, including the learning curve and the smaller size of the lesion produced by cryoablation. In addition, all the peculiarities of cryothermal energy, which are optimal for septal ablation, are less important or even useless for ablation of BTs located elsewhere.[21]

In more recent series, the short-term success rate of cryoablation of BTs in the superoparaseptal and midseptal regions exceeded 90%; however, resumption of BT conduction with recurrence of symptoms can occur in up to 20% of patients, and overall success rates have been lower than those of AVNRT cryoablation. It is, however, important to note that alternatives for elimination of some of those BTs are limited by a prohibitive risk of AV block with RF ablation. Although transient modifications of the normal AVN conduction pathways can be observed during cooling and right bundle branch block has occurred on occasion, no permanent modifications have been observed, and inadvertent AV block has yet to be reported. In fact, immediate discontinuation of cryothermal energy application at any temperature on observation of modification of conduction over normal pathways results in return to baseline condition soon after discontinuation.[30]

FOCAL ATRIAL TACHYCARDIA

Occasionally, successful cryoablation of focal AT has been reported. Its safety has also been confirmed for ablation of atrial foci located close to the AVN. Cryoenergy can also be particularly valuable in ablating focal sources within venous structures.[30]

TYPICAL ATRIAL FLUTTER

Complete cavotricuspid isthmus block can be achieved by cryothermal ablation. In addition to the safety advantages of cryoenergy discussed earlier, cryolesions are limited by convective warming effects of blood flow, which reduces the risk of damage to nearby coronary arteries. Another advantage of using cryothermal energy for the ablation of typical AFL is the absence of pain perception related to energy application.[30,37] Previous studies reported cryoablation of the cavotricuspid isthmus for typical AFL with short-term and long-term success comparable to results with RF ablation. However, a more recent prospective randomized study comparing RF and cryothermal energy for ablation of typical AFL suggested that lesion durability from cryoablation was significantly inferior to that of RF ablation. Although acutely successful ablation rates in the cryoablation group were comparable to those for RF ablation (89% versus 91%), persistence of bidirectional isthmus block in patients treated with cryoablation reinvestigated 3 months following ablation was inferior to that in patients treated with RF ablation, as evidenced by the higher recurrence rate of symptomatic, ECG-documented AFL (10.9% versus 0%), and higher asymptomatic conduction recurrence rates (23.4% versus 15%). Additionally, compared with RF ablation, cryoablation is associated with significantly longer procedure times. This is driven mainly by differences in ablation duration, which can be attributed to the longer duration of each cryoablation (4 minutes) compared with RF ablation (up to 60 seconds).[22,38]

PULMONARY VEIN ISOLATION

For the characteristics mentioned earlier, cryothermal energy ablation can be considered an ideal and safer energy source for PV isolation, and the incidence of PV stenosis and thromboembolic events is expected to be dramatically reduced compared with RF ablation. Additionally, cryoablation has never been associated with atrioesophageal fistula.[39,40] On the other hand, cryothermal injury is sensitive to surrounding thermal conditions. The high flow of the PVs can present a considerable heat load to cryothermal technologies, which can limit the size and depth of the lesion produced by cryothermal energy at the ostium of the PV. Furthermore, cryoablation of PVs by standard steerable catheters is very time-consuming, considering that one single ablation point takes about 4 minutes.

A new catheter design for circumferential ostial ablation of the PVs has been developed, with the option of deploying an inflatable balloon in the PVs to reduce the heat load related to blood flow (Fig. 7-11).[21,39] The cryoballoon is deployed at the ostium of targeted PVs, and cryoenergy is delivered over the occluding balloon system to create circumferential lesions around the PV ostium. The clinical short-term and long-term success rates of this approach are acceptable; however, the risk of phrenic nerve injury is relatively high because of ablation in the region of the right superior PV. To date, thromboembolism or PV stenosis has yet to be reported.[23-25,41-45]

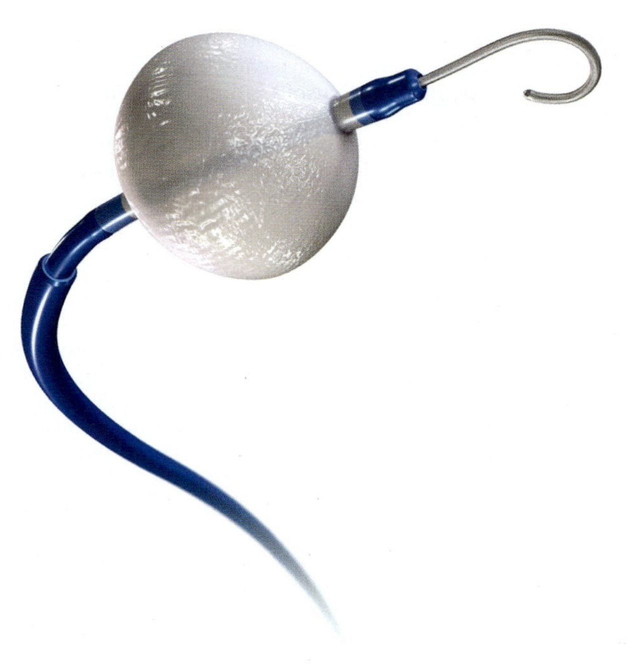

FIGURE 7-11 Cryothermal balloon catheter. *(Courtesy of Medtronic, Inc., Minneapolis, Minn.)*

VENTRICULAR TACHYCARDIA

Data regarding cryoablation for VT remain scant. Small reports described feasibility and success of cryoenergy for ablation of outflow tract VT. Additionally, cryothermal energy can be of potential advantage in percutaneous subxiphoid epicardial ablation of VT because of less potential damage to the epicardial coronary arteries. The reduced heat load in the pericardial space related to the absence of blood flow limits RF energy delivery but can be to the advantage of cryoablation, with the possibility of producing larger transmural lesions.[22]

Microwave Ablation

Biophysics of Microwave Energy

Microwaves are the portion of the electromagnetic spectrum between 0.3 and 300 GHz. For the ablation of cardiac arrhythmias, microwave energy has been used at frequencies of 0.915 and 2.450 GHz. Similar to RF, microwave energy produces thermal cell necrosis. However, in contrast to heating by electrical resistance as observed during RF ablation, the mechanism of heating from a high-frequency microwave energy source is dielectrics. Dielectric heating occurs when high-frequency electromagnetic radiation stimulates the oscillation of dipolar molecules (e.g., water molecules) in the surrounding medium at a very high speed, thereby converting electromagnetic energy into kinetic energy. This high-speed vibration favors friction between water molecules within the myocardial wall that results in an increase of myocardial tissue heat.[1] This mode of heating lends microwave ablation the potential for a greater depth of volume heating than RF ablation and should theoretically result in a larger lesion size.[46]

Microwave energy is not absorbed by blood and can propagate through blood, desiccated tissue, or scar. It also can be deposited directly into the myocardial tissue at a distance, regardless of the intervening medium. The microwave energy field generated around the ablation catheter antenna can create myocardial lesions up to 6 to 8 mm in depth without overheating the endocardial surface, a feature that can potentially limit the risk of charring, coagulum formation, and intramyocardial steam explosions. Penetration depth achieved with microwave energy depends on several factors—dielectric properties of the tissue, frequency of the microwave energy, antenna design, and composition and thickness of the cardiac layers.

The effectiveness of microwave ablation depends on the radiating ability of the microwave antenna that directs the electric field and determines the amount transmitted into the myocardium, which is critical for heating. An end-firing monopolar antenna has been used to produce lesions at depths of 1 cm without disruption of the endocardium in porcine ventricles. The depth of these lesions increased exponentially over time as compared with standard nonirrigated RF energy, which had minimal lesion expansion after 60 seconds of ablation.[1] To concentrate more of the energy distribution near the electrode tip, circularly polarized coil antennas have been developed. Other configurations of the microwave antenna include helical, dipole, and whip designs; these have a large effect on the magnetic field created. However, many of these catheters are still under clinical investigation.

Pathophysiology of Lesion Formation by Microwave Ablation

Microwave energy produces thermal cell necrosis and transmural damage, with foci of coagulation necrosis of myocytes in the central part of the lesion. Hyperthermia (more than 56°C) causes protein denaturation and changes in myocardial cellular EP properties resulting from movement of mobile ions within the aqueous biological medium and altering membrane permeability. The acute myocyte changes include architectural disarray, loss of contractile filaments, and focal interruption of the plasma membrane, which are signs of irreversible injury. Additionally, occlusion of the lumen of the small intramyocardial vessels and severe disruption of endothelial and adventitial layers are observed.[46] Carbonization does not occur on tissue surfaces because of the good penetration of microwave energy. Fibrotic tissue eventually replaces the necrotic muscle, which typically becomes sharply demarcated from normal myocardium.[46]

In vitro and in vivo experiments have demonstrated good uniformity in the distribution of the electromagnetic energy throughout the tissue and excellent penetration depth, with no areas of discontinuity over the length of the ablating probe. Energy distribution is maximal near the center of the ablating element, a finding indicating that depth of ablation is relatively deeper at the midpoint of a lesion. There is no indication of edge effect along the ablating tip, which can potentially produce overheating of the tissue surface and induce charring. The temperature at the tissue surface typically remains at less than 100°C over the time required to produce a 6-mm-deep lesion. This is a critical finding because the ability to raise the tissue temperature to 50°C while maintaining it at less than 100°C is paramount to effective and safe hyperthermic ablation.

In addition to the frequency of the microwave energy and length of antenna used, penetration of microwave into the tissue and lesion dimensions is proportional to the power and duration of energy application.

Although microwave ablation in theory should be less likely than RF to induce surface overheating, in vivo studies found that a higher targeted temperature of 90°C resulted in a surface temperature of more than 70°C and was associated with some tissue surface charring when compared with lower temperatures. Therefore, the use of the temperature-controlled mode of microwave energy delivery to limit the targeted temperature to 80°C may prevent tissue overheating and reduce the risk of tissue charring. It should be noted that no coagulation formation and no popping were observed during any of the microwave ablations performed.[47,48]

In contrast to RF energy, in which lesion expansion is maximal after 60 seconds, microwave lesion size continues to increase after 300 seconds of energy application. As compared with conventional 4-mm-tip RF ablation, microwave ablation creates a similar lesion depth and width. Lesion length created by a 10-mm antenna is comparable to that created by 8-mm-tip RF ablation. However, because of the lack of physical limitations on the length of the microwave antenna that can be made, microwave ablation may be more advantageous in creating long linear lesions by using longer antenna. Nevertheless, a parallel antenna orientation is needed for optimal energy delivery because the growth in lesion sizes is limited beyond the energy field as a result of the finite radial energy distribution of the microwave ablation antenna. Furthermore, the lesion depth created with an 8-mm-tip or saline-irrigated electrode catheter appears to be larger than the lesion depth created by microwave ablation. However, direct comparisons among these different ablation technologies are not available.[47,48]

Clinical Applications of Microwave Ablation

Microwave ablation can be a promising technique that is potentially capable of treating a wide range of ventricular and supraventricular arrhythmias. The physics of the microwave energy source can be particularly useful for transmural ablation lesions of atrial tissue, as well as the treatment of tachyarrhythmias arising from deep foci of ventricular myocardium.[46]

Microwave can potentially overcome several limitations of RF energy for linear ablation. In contrast to resistive heating produced by RF, microwave generates frictional heat by inducing oscillation of dipoles in a medium such as water. Tissue with higher water content, such as cardiac tissue, allows better energy transfer during the propagation of microwave energy deep into the tissue. Therefore, microwave energy is capable of creating deeper lesions, to penetrate scar tissue and to reduce surface heating with less endocardial disruption or coagulation formation. Furthermore, delivery of microwave energy is not limited by electrode size as in RF, and microwave ablation can be applied over a larger surface by modifying antenna size and shape. Another hypothetical advantage of microwave energy is that it provides sufficient lesions, independent of contact. However, experimental data have shown that penetration of electromagnetic fields into tissue declines exponentially, and the decline is steep when using frequencies in the microwave range; therefore, distance is still an important consideration. Nevertheless, this theoretical advantage can potentially improve the versatility of microwave ablation, especially in areas where muscular ridges and valleys may pose problems for conventional RF ablation.[1,49]

Currently, microwave ablation has been increasingly used intraoperatively (epicardially or endocardially) during surgical maze procedures. The ability to make microwave antennas into flexible linear applicators and place them parallel to the endocardium by means of clamps has increased the effectiveness of microwave as a tool in open-chest surgery and in minimally invasive surgery.[50,51]

The development and manufacture of antennae for delivery of microwave energy is technically more complex than for RF electrodes because the efficacy of microwave energy transmission depends mainly on its delivery apparatus. As a result, microwave antennae were previously bulky and were limited to surgical use. Developments in the catheter-based microwave system may allow the transvenous delivery of microwave energy for endocardial ablation. Only a few case reports have described the successful use of transvenous catheter microwave ablation of the AV junction and cavotricuspid isthmus.[47,52,53]

Currently, only one transvenous microwave catheter system (MedWaves, San Diego, Calif.) is available for investigational use. This system includes a deflectable, 10 Fr catheter with 10-mm or 20-mm helical coil antenna with temperature monitoring, bipolar electrode recording, and a generator delivering microwave at 900 to 930 MHz. Microwave energy is delivered by using a temperature-controlled mode in which the generator automatically adjusts the power output to maintain the targeted temperature of the temperature sensor inside the antenna. For ablation of typical AFL, linear lesions are created with a point-by-point technique with gradual pullback of the microwave catheter across the cavotricuspid isthmus. Interestingly, microwave causes no perception of pain during ablation of the cavotricuspid isthmus with energy delivery in the inferior vena cava region.[49,53]

Clinical studies on the use of transvenous catheter microwave ablation for AF and AFL ablation are currently under way to investigate the safety and feasibility of this technique.[52,53]

Ultrasound Energy

Biophysics of Ultrasound Energy

Sound is a propagation of cyclical (oscillatory) displacements of atoms and molecules around their average position in the direction of propagation. When the cyclical events occur at frequencies of more than 20,000 Hz (i.e., higher than the average threshold of the human hearing), the sound is defined as ultrasound.[1,52]

Ultrasound beams can be treated in a manner analogous to light beams, including focusing (ultrasonic lens) and minimization of convergence and divergence (collimation). These optical geometric manipulations allow for ultrasound to be directed toward confined distant (deep) tissue volumes. This is a pivotal capability of therapeutic ultrasound.

Ultrasound energy transmission is subject to attenuation with distance and medium, especially with air. The amount of ultrasound energy transferred to tissue is proportional to the intensity of the wave and the absorption coefficient of the tissue. Because of this property, ultrasound ablation does not require direct contact with the myocardium, in contrast to RF ablation. Ultrasound energy decreases proportionally with the distance ($1/r$), whereas RF ablation electrical conduction decreases with the square of the distance ($1/r^2$). This feature allows ultrasound energy to create deeper and transmural lesions. The duration of application and acoustic power used have a direct relationship with the lesion depth.[52]

Pathophysiology of Lesion Formation by Ultrasound Energy

Tissue injury caused by ultrasound is mediated by two mechanisms: thermal and mechanical energy. Ultrasound waves can propagate through living tissue and fluids without causing any harm to the cells. However, by focusing highly energetic ultrasound waves (high-intensity focused ultrasound [HIFU]) to a well-defined volume, local heating (achieving a tissue temperature of 65° to 100°C) occurs and causes rapid tissue necrosis by coagulative necrosis. Thermal energy results when the energy transported by an ultrasound beam becomes attenuated as it propagates through viscous (viscoelastic) media, such as human soft tissue. The attenuation partly represents conversion of ultrasound energy into heat. Another mechanism by which HIFU destroys tissue is mechanical energy, which results from pressure waves (sound waves) propagating in gas-containing tissues as they cyclically expand (explode) and shrink (implode) microbubbles in the tissue (i.e., oscillation and collapse of gas microbubbles), a process known as microcavitation. This process of vibration of cellular structures causes local hyperthermia and mechanical stress by bubble formation because of rapid changes in local pressure, thus leading to cell death.[1]

Previous studies showed that rapid, focused absorption of HIFU energy in noncardiac tissue produced a steep tissue temperature gradient (2° to 5°C/sec) between the focus and the surrounding tissue, thus allowing for the production of sharply demarcated lesions and reducing collateral damage. However, a more recent study using HIFU for PV isolation in canine hearts found that HIFU produced a dual temperature profile, probably because of immediate direct acoustic heating and subsequent conductive heating. Additionally, the region of direct acoustic heating with HIFU energy in vivo was largely predictable from the distance of the target tissue to the HIFU balloon surface; actual tissue temperatures exceeding 50°C (the temperature at which permanent tissue damage is supposed to occur) were focused within a 7-mm width and 7.5-mm depth around the HIFU exit site (significantly larger than the 2- to 3-mm area of resistive heating observed with RF energy). However, the actual distribution of tissue temperatures during lesion generation may be affected by other factors, such as the following: blood circulation; location of different tissue thicknesses within the atrium, venoatrial junction, or PV; or energy attenuation at various interfaces between the target tissue and the energy source.[54]

HIFU lesion depth increases with longer duration of energy delivery from 15 to 60 seconds, and there is a linear relationship between increasing power and depth of lesions.[1] HIFU applications were found to achieve transmural lesions and PV isolation. However, although this can translate into increased effectiveness of ablation, it also can potentially lead to collateral damage, namely to the phrenic nerve and esophagus. HIFU ablation can produce damage to the phrenic nerve when it is located within 4 to 7 mm of HIFU exit.[54]

Clinical Applications of Ultrasound Energy

HIFU is an attractive alternative energy source. Because it can be focused at specific depths, ultrasound can be advantageous when considering epicardial ablation. The presence of epicardial fat makes the use of standard RF current difficult, both with catheter-based epicardial ablation and minimally invasive surgical ablation.[1,55] Furthermore, the ability of ultrasound to be collimated through echolucent fluid medium (e.g., water, blood) makes it ideal for a balloon delivery system, which can potentially facilitate circumferential ablation at the PV orifice with a single energy delivery.[1] Another potential advantage of ultrasound is that it does not rely on extensive heating on the vein surface. This can be of value in PV isolation procedures, to help prevent PV stenosis seen with RF ablation. Because HIFU is delivered at the beam convergence site rather than at the tissue surface, successful ablation is less dependent on absolute balloon-tissue contact than other balloon-based technologies. Furthermore, unlike other energy sources, HIFU can be deflected within the balloon to create a wide, focused zone of energy delivery outside the PV orifice, thereby mimicking current wide area circumferential ablative approaches. Currently, no HIFU catheters are available that can be used for linear (instead of circular) ablation.[54,56-58]

An 8-MHz cylindrical transducer mounted within a saline-filled balloon has been designed for PV isolation. The ablation system (Atrionix, Palo Alto, Calif.) consists of a 0.035-inch-diameter luminal catheter with a distal balloon (maximum diameter, 2.2 cm) housing a centrally located ultrasound transducer. The system is advanced over a guidewire into the target PV. Tissue surface temperature monitoring is achieved by thermocouples on the balloon and the ultrasound transducer. Despite initial enthusiasm, the long-term report including 33 patients was disappointing, with a long-term cure rate of approximately 30%, although short-term electrical isolation was achieved in all but 1 of the PVs targeted. Surprisingly, several applications were required to achieve PV isolation. The variability of the PV anatomy was the main culprit for the system failure. In larger PV orifices, it was difficult to achieve adequate heating. The system delivered a narrow band of ultrasound energy radially from a centrally located transducer, and it was at times challenging to place the catheter in all PVs at the proximal portion. Therefore, foci at the most proximal lip of a PV may not be ablated successfully.

More recently, a forward-projecting HIFU balloon catheter (ProRhythm, Inc., Ronkonkoma, N.Y.) was developed for circumferential PV isolation outside the PV ostia (to limit the risk of PV stenosis). Radially emitted ultrasound is reflected from the back of the balloon, thus resulting in forward projection of ultrasound energy, with a focal point at the balloon-endocardial interface (Fig. 7-12). This system has two noncompliant balloons. A 9-MHz ultrasound crystal is located in the distal balloon filled with contrast and water. The proximal balloon, filled with carbon dioxide, forms a parabolic interface with the distal balloon to reflect the ultrasound energy in the forward direction, by focusing a 360-degree ring (sonicating ring) of ultrasound energy 2 to 6 mm in front of the distal balloon surface. The distal balloon has three sizes—24, 28, or 32 mm in diameter—producing sonicating rings of 20, 25, or 30 mm in diameter. The acoustic power of the system is 45 W for all three balloons, with negligible loss of power in the balloon. The distal balloon is irrigated with contrast and water at 20 mL/min during ablation to keep the balloon cool (lower than 42°C). The catheter has a central lumen used for insertion of a hexapolar, spiral mapping catheter (ProMap, ProRhythm, Inc.) for real-time assessment of PV potentials.[59-61]

Clinical application of this system for PV isolation was evaluated and was shown to be feasible, but fatal esophageal injury was also observed.[56-58] A study of 28 patients using an esophageal

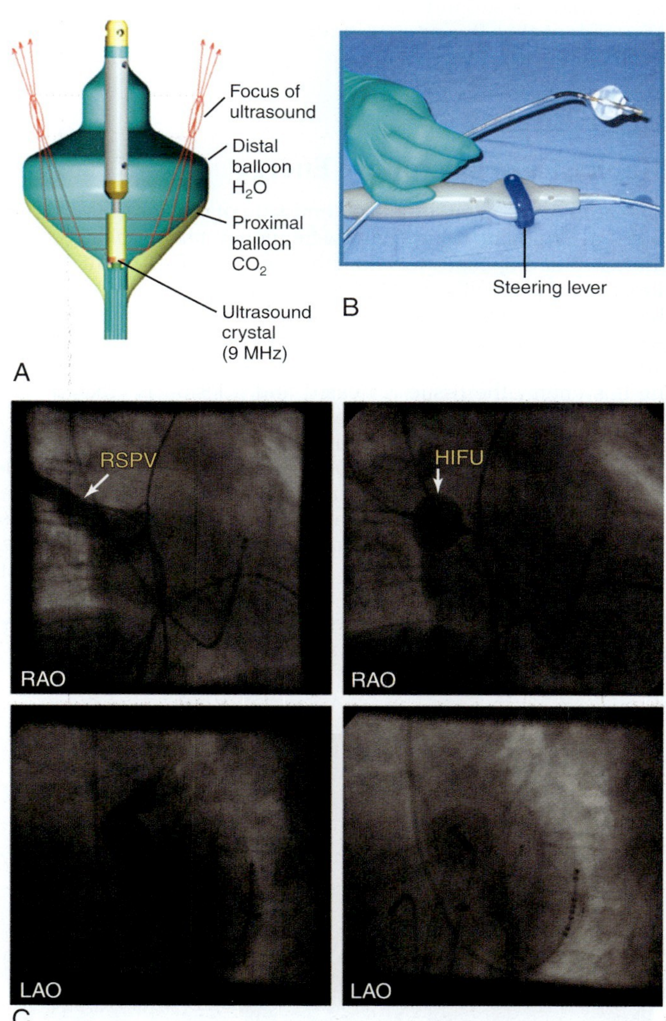

FIGURE 7-12 Circumferential antral pulmonary vein (PV) isolation using the high-intensity focused ultrasound (HIFU) balloon catheter. **A,** Schematic representation of the HIFU balloon catheter designed to focus ultrasound energy circumferentially outside the PV (PV antrum). **B,** HIFU balloon. **C,** Right anterior oblique (RAO) and left anterior oblique (LAO) fluoroscopic views of the angiograms **(right)** and HIFU balloon positioning **(left)** in the right superior PV (RSPV). *(From Schmidt B, Antz M, Ernst S, et al: Pulmonary vein isolation by high-intensity focused ultrasound: first-in-man study with a steerable balloon catheter. Heart Rhythm 4:575, 2007.)*

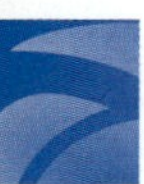

temperature–guided safety algorithm demonstrated that acute PV electrical isolation with HIFU ablation could be achieved in only 77% of PVs. Eight percent of PVs could not be isolated with HIFU as a result of excessive esophageal heating or balloon catheter dislodgment. In only 32% of patients, all PVs could be isolated using HIFU ablation only. Although power modulation did not negatively influence short-term success rates of PV electrical isolation, it also did not prevent esophageal temperature from exceeding levels higher than 40.0°C at the end of the ablation; elevated esophageal temperature prompting cessation of energy delivery occurred in 9% of PVs. Despite use of the safety algorithm and continuous phrenic nerve pacing, transient and persistent phrenic nerve palsy occurred in 14% and 7% of patients, respectively. Even worse, use of the safety algorithm could not prevent occurrence of esophageal thermal damage and lethal atrioesophageal fistula. PV isolation with HIFU has proven to be successful but is not yet safe for everyday clinical use. The problems of phrenic nerve palsy and atrioesophageal fistula occurrence remain unresolved. Still, the concept of the energy source and mode of energy delivery may be very interesting for future treatment of AF. With mean PV isolation times of less than 15 seconds and a high number of complications, it is evident that the present energy source is too powerful in some patients.[59]

Laser Energy

Biophysics of Microwave Energy

Light amplification by stimulated emission of radiation (laser) produces a monochromatic (narrow-frequency range) phase-coherent beam at a specific wavelength (Fig. 7-13). This beam can be directed for a specific duration and intensity, and as it penetrates the tissue, it is absorbed and scattered. The photothermal effect occurs with the absorption of photon energy, thus producing a vibrational excited state in molecules (chromophores). By absorbing this energy, the tissue is heated and a lesion is created (i.e., tissue injury is thermally mediated).[1]

Laser energy can be delivered in a continuous or a pulsed mode. Laser energy is selectively absorbed by the tissues over several millimeters, and it decays exponentially as it passes through the tissue secondary to absorption and scatter, the extent of which depends on laser beam diameter and the optical properties of the tissue. Lesion size is determined by the extent of light diffusion and heat transport.[1]

Three major laser systems are used: argon laser, neodymium:yttrium-aluminum-garnet (Nd:YAG) laser, and diode laser.

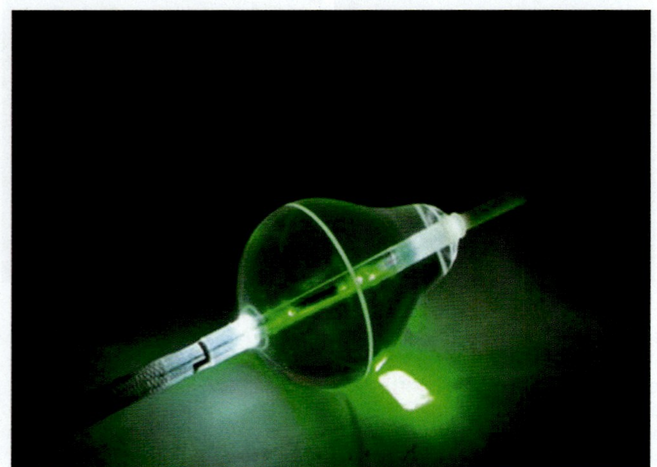

FIGURE 7-13 Laser balloon aiming beam. *(Courtesy of CardioFocus, Inc., Marlborough, Mass.)*

ARGON LASER. This system uses a gaseous lasing medium (argon), which emits light at a wavelength of 500 nM. With this system, the light energy is absorbed rapidly in the first few millimeters of tissue, with resulting surface vaporization with crater formation.

NEODYMIUM:YTTRIUM-ALUMINUM-GARNET LASER. This system uses a solid lasing medium (Nd:YAG), which emits energy at a wavelength of 1060 to 2000 nM in the infrared spectrum. This system is associated with significant scatter in tissue. It causes more diffuse and deeper tissue injury and results in photocoagulation necrosis.

DIODE LASER. This system uses semiconductors and emits energy at a wavelength of 700 to 1500 nM (near-infrared).

Clinical Applications of Laser Energy

Early studies of laser ablation used a high-energy laser that carried a high risk of crater formation and endothelial damage. These studies focused on the intraoperative use of lasers in the ultraviolet and visible range (308- to 755-nm wavelength), and they appeared to show effectiveness of the lesions placed. Laser energy can also be delivered along the entire length of a linear diffuser, which provides uniform linear laser ablation and a superior transmural lesion when compared with previous end-firing optical delivery systems. The use of the linear diffuser in combination with lasers in the infrared or near-infrared wavelength (800 to 1100 nm) is currently under investigation.[1,62]

Laser energy is absorbed by blood; as a consequence, its application directly into blood results in thrombus formation. This limitation is obviated by application of laser energy through a fluid-filled balloon positioned against the tissue to provide a bloodless interface for ablation. Laser energy has been used with balloon technology for PV isolation. The most recent generation of this balloon catheter is a nonsteerable, variable-diameter, compliant balloon (CardioFocus, Inc., Marlborough, Mass.). The laser balloon is inserted at the PV antrum through a 12 Fr deflectable sheath. Varying balloon inflation pressure allows for adjustment to the individual PV anatomy to optimize PV occlusion and maximize balloon-tissue contact. The balloon is filled with a mixture of contrast and deuterium dioxide and irrigated internally at 20 mL/min to minimize absorption of laser energy.

The efficacy of the laser balloon ablation depends on good contact around the balloon circumference. The laser ablation catheter system incorporates an endoscopic visualization capability using a 2 Fr fiberoptic endoscope positioned at the proximal end of the balloon. Once the balloon is deployed, the endoscope enables real-time visualization of the face of the balloon at the targeted PV antrum and monitoring for the intrusion of blood into the space between the balloon and the tissue.[62,63]

The arc generator consists of an optical fiber located within the central shaft that projects a 30-degree arc of light onto regions of balloon-tissue contact guided by an endoscopic view of the PV antrum (areas of balloon-tissue contact are visualized as blanched white, whereas contact with blood is visualized as red). This arc serves as an aiming beam for laser delivery and can be steered along the balloon face with endoscopic visualization, to facilitate individual lesion application in an anatomically flexible lesion design that adapts to the highly variable PV anatomy. Once the proper location is identified, a diode laser is used to deliver laser energy at 980 nm. The laser fiber can be advanced or withdrawn to shift the site of lasing along the longitudinal axis of the catheter. Lesions are deployed in a point-by-point fashion; each individual ablation lesion covers 30 degrees of a circle. Laser energy is delivered at power output of 5.5 to 18 W for 20 to 30 seconds, depending on the thickness of tissue or the proximity of the esophagus, or both.

The laser ablation catheter technology is still in clinical trials. The initial clinical experience with this technology suggests the ability to achieve reliable and lasting PV electrical isolation in patients with highly variable PV shapes and sizes.[62-65]

REFERENCES

1. Cummings JE, Pacifico A, Drago JL, et al: Alternative energy sources for the ablation of arrhythmias, *Pacing Clin Electrophysiol* 28:434–443, 2005.
2. Haines DE: Biophysics of radiofrequency lesion formation. In Huang SKS, Wood MA, editors: *Catheter ablation of cardiac arrhythmias*, Philadelphia, 2006, Saunders, pp 3–20.
3. Cesario D, Boyle N, Shivumar K: Lesion forming technologies for catheter ablation. In Zipes DP, Jalife J, editors: *Cardiac electrophysiology: from cell to bedside*, ed 5, Philadelphia, 2009, Saunders, pp 1051–1058.
4. Wittkampf FH, Nakagawa H: RF catheter ablation: lessons on lesions, *Pacing Clin Electrophysiol* 29:1285–1297, 2006.
5. Haines D: Biophysics of ablation: application to technology, *J Cardiovasc Electrophysiol* 15(Suppl):S2–S11, 2004.
6. Stevenson WG, Cooper J, Sapp J: Optimizing RF output for cooled RF ablation, *J Cardiovasc Electrophysiol* 15(Suppl):S24–S27, 2004.
7. Demazumder D, Schwartzman D: Titration of radiofrequency energy during endocardial catheter ablation. In Huang SKS, Wood MA, editors: *Catheter ablation of cardiac arrhythmias*, Philadelphia, 2006, Saunders, pp 21–34.
8. Bruce GK, Bunch TJ, Milton MA, et al: Discrepancies between catheter tip and tissue temperature in cooled-tip ablation: relevance to guiding left atrial ablation, *Circulation* 112:954–960, 2005.
9. Lustgarten DL, Spector PS: Ablation using irrigated radiofrequency: a hands-on guide, *Heart Rhythm* 5:899–902, 2008.
10. Wood MA, Goldberg SM, Parvez B, et al: Effect of electrode orientation on lesion sizes produced by irrigated radiofrequency ablation catheters, *J Cardiovasc Electrophysiol* 20:1262–1268, 2009.
11. Stuhlinger M, Steinwender C, Schnoll F, et al: GOLDART: gold alloy versus platinum-iridium electrode for ablation of AVNRT, *J Cardiovasc Electrophysiol* 19:242–246, 2008.
12. Lewalter T, Bitzen A, Wurtz S, et al: Gold-tip electrodes: a new "deep lesion" technology for catheter ablation? In vitro comparison of a gold alloy versus platinum-iridium tip electrode ablation catheter, *J Cardiovasc Electrophysiol* 16:770–772, 2005.
13. Kardos A, Foldesi C, Mihalcz A, Szili-Torok T: Cavotricuspid isthmus ablation with large-tip gold alloy versus platinum-iridium-tip electrode catheters, *Pacing Clin Electrophysiol* 32(Suppl 1):S138–S140, 2009.
14. Wieczorek M, Hoeltgen R, Akin E, et al: Results of short-term and long-term pulmonary vein isolation for paroxysmal atrial fibrillation using duty-cycled bipolar and unipolar radiofrequency energy, *J Cardiovasc Electrophysiol* 21:399–405, 2010.
15. Boll S, Dang L, Scharf C: Linear ablation with duty-cycled radiofrequency energy at the cavotricuspid isthmus, *Pacing Clin Electrophysiol* 33:444–450, 2010.
16. Steinwender C, Honig S, Leisch F, Hofmann R: One-year follow-up after pulmonary vein isolation using a single mesh catheter in patients with paroxysmal atrial fibrillation, *Heart Rhythm* 7:333–339, 2010.
17. Vest JA, Seiler J, Stevenson WG: Clinical use of cooled radiofrequency ablation, *J Cardiovasc Electrophysiol* 19:769–773, 2008.
18. Yokoyama K, Nakagawa H, Wittkampf FH, et al: Comparison of electrode cooling between internal and open irrigation in radiofrequency ablation lesion depth and incidence of thrombus and steam pop, *Circulation* 113:11–19, 2006.
19. Everett TH, Lee KW, Wilson EE, et al: Safety profiles and lesion size of different radiofrequency ablation technologies: a comparison of large tip, open and closed irrigation catheters, *J Cardiovasc Electrophysiol* 20:325–335, 2009.
20. Seiler J, Roberts-Thomson KC, Raymond JM, et al: Steam pops during irrigated radiofrequency ablation: feasibility of impedance monitoring for prevention, *Heart Rhythm* 5:1411–1416, 2008.
21. Skanes AC, Klein G, Krahn A, Yee R: Cryoablation: potentials and pitfalls, *J Cardiovasc Electrophysiol* 15(Suppl):S28–S34, 2004.
22. Novak P, Dubuc M: Catheter cryoablation: biophysics and applications. In Huang SKS, Wood MA, editors: *Catheter ablation of cardiac arrhythmias*, Philadelphia, 2006, Saunders, pp 49–68.
23. Neumann T, Vogt J, Schumacher B, et al: Circumferential pulmonary vein isolation with the cryoballoon technique results from a prospective 3-center study, *J Am Coll Cardiol* 52:273–278, 2008.
24. Tang M, Kriatselis C, Nedios S, et al: A novel cryoballoon technique for mapping and isolating pulmonary veins: a feasibility and efficacy study, *J Cardiovasc Electrophysiol* 21:626–631, 2010.
25. Ahmed H, Neuzil P, Skoda J, et al: The permanency of pulmonary vein isolation using a balloon cryoablation catheter, *J Cardiovasc Electrophysiol* 21:731–737, 2010.
26. Khairy P, Dubuc M: Transcatheter cryoablation part I: preclinical experience, *Pacing Clin Electrophysiol* 31:112–120, 2008.
27. Khairy P, Rivard L, Guerra PG, et al: Morphometric ablation lesion characteristics comparing 4, 6, and 8 mm electrode-tip cryocatheters, *J Cardiovasc Electrophysiol* 19:1203–1207, 2008.
28. Wood MA, Parvez B, Ellenbogen AL, et al: Determinants of lesion sizes and tissue temperatures during catheter cryoablation, *Pacing Clin Electrophysiol* 30:644–654, 2007.
29. Pilcher TA, Saul JP, Hlavacek AM, Haemmerich D: Contrasting effects of convective flow on catheter ablation lesion size: cryo versus radiofrequency energy, *Pacing Clin Electrophysiol* 31:300–307, 2008.
30. Lemola K, Dubuc M, Khairy P: Transcatheter cryoablation part II: clinical utility, *Pacing Clin Electrophysiol* 31:235–244, 2008.
31. Chanani NK, Chiesa NA, Dubin AM, et al: Cryoablation for atrioventricular nodal reentrant tachycardia in young patients: predictors of recurrence, *Pacing Clin Electrophysiol* 31:1152–1159, 2008.
32. Friedman PL, Dubuc M, Green MS, et al: Catheter cryoablation of supraventricular tachycardia: results of the multicenter prospective "frosty" trial, *Heart Rhythm* 1:129–138, 2004.
33. Opel A, Murray S, Kamath N, et al: Cryoablation versus radiofrequency ablation for treatment of atrioventricular nodal reentrant tachycardia: cryoablation with 6-mm-tip catheters is still less effective than radiofrequency ablation, *Heart Rhythm* 7:340–343, 2010.
34. Silver ES, Silva JN, Ceresnak SR, et al: Cryoablation with an 8-mm tip catheter for pediatric atrioventricular nodal reentrant tachycardia is safe and efficacious with a low incidence of recurrence, *Pacing Clin Electrophysiol* 33:681–686, 2010.
35. Rivard L, Dubuc M, Guerra PG, et al: Cryoablation outcomes for AV nodal reentrant tachycardia comparing 4-mm versus 6-mm electrode-tip catheters, *Heart Rhythm* 5:230–234, 2008.
36. Drago F, Russo MS, Silvetti MS, et al: Cryoablation of typical atrioventricular nodal reentrant tachycardia in children: six years' experience and follow-up in a single center, *Pacing Clin Electrophysiol* 33:475–481, 2010.
37. Feld GK, Daubert JP, Weiss R, et al: Acute and long-term efficacy and safety of catheter cryoablation of the cavotricuspid isthmus for treatment of type 1 atrial flutter, *Heart Rhythm* 5:1009–1014, 2008.
38. Kuniss M, Vogtmann T, Ventura R, et al: Prospective randomized comparison of durability of bidirectional conduction block in the cavotricuspid isthmus in patients after ablation of common atrial flutter using cryothermy and radiofrequency energy: the CRYOTIP study, *Heart Rhythm* 6:1699–1705, 2009.
39. Hoyt RH, Wood M, Daoud E, et al: Transvenous catheter cryoablation for treatment of atrial fibrillation: results of a feasibility study, *Pacing Clin Electrophysiol* 28(Suppl 1):S78–S82, 2005.
40. Skanes AC, Jensen SM, Papp R, et al: Isolation of pulmonary veins using a transvenous curvilinear cryoablation catheter: feasibility, initial experience, and analysis of recurrences, *J Cardiovasc Electrophysiol* 16:1304–1308, 2005.
41. Chun KR, Furnkranz A, Metzner A, et al: Cryoballoon pulmonary vein isolation with real-time recordings from the pulmonary veins, *J Cardiovasc Electrophysiol* 20:1203–1210, 2009.
42. Siklody CH, Minners J, Allgeier M, et al: Pressure-guided cryoballoon isolation of the pulmonary veins for the treatment of paroxysmal atrial fibrillation, *J Cardiovasc Electrophysiol* 21:120–125, 2010.
43. Klein G, Oswald H, Gardiwal A, et al: Efficacy of pulmonary vein isolation by cryoballoon ablation in patients with paroxysmal atrial fibrillation, *Heart Rhythm* 5:802–806, 2008.
44. Linhart M, Bellmann B, Mittmann-Braun E, et al: Comparison of cryoballoon and radiofrequency ablation of pulmonary veins in 40 patients with paroxysmal atrial fibrillation: a case-control study, *J Cardiovasc Electrophysiol* 20:1343–1348, 2009.
45. Chun KR, Schmidt B, Metzner A, et al: The "single big cryoballoon" technique for acute pulmonary vein isolation in patients with paroxysmal atrial fibrillation: a prospective observational single centre study, *Eur Heart J* 30:699–709, 2009.
46. Climent V, Hurle A, Ho SY, et al: Early morphologic changes following microwave endocardial ablation for treatment of chronic atrial fibrillation during mitral valve surgery, *J Cardiovasc Electrophysiol* 15:1277–1283, 2004.
47. Tse HF, Liao S, Siu CW, et al: Determinants of lesion dimensions during transcatheter microwave ablation, *Pacing Clin Electrophysiol* 32:201–208, 2009.
48. de Gouveia RH, Melo J, Santiago T, Martins AP: Comparison of the healing mechanisms of myocardial lesions induced by dry radiofrequency and microwave epicardial ablation, *Pacing Clin Electrophysiol* 29:278–282, 2006.
49. Yiu KH, Siu CW, Lau CP, et al: Transvenous catheter-based microwave ablation for atrial flutter, *Heart Rhythm* 4:221–223, 2007.
50. Hurle A, Ibanez A, Parra JM, Martinez JG: Preliminary results with the microwave-modified Maze III procedure for the treatment of chronic atrial fibrillation, *Pacing Clin Electrophysiol* 27:1644–1646, 2004.
51. Khargi K, Hutten BA, Lemke B, Deneke T: Surgical treatment of atrial fibrillation; a systematic review, *Eur J Cardiothorac Surg* 27:258–265, 2005.
52. Yiu K, Lau C, Lee KL, Tse H: Emerging energy sources for catheter ablation of atrial fibrillation, *J Cardiovasc Electrophysiol* 17(Suppl 3):S56, 2006.
53. Chan JY, Fung JW, Yu CM, Feld GK: Preliminary results with percutaneous transcatheter microwave ablation of typical atrial flutter, *J Cardiovasc Electrophysiol* 18:286–289, 2007.
54. Okumura Y, Kolasa MW, Johnson SB, et al: Mechanism of tissue heating during high intensity focused ultrasound pulmonary vein isolation: implications for atrial fibrillation ablation efficacy and phrenic nerve protection, *J Cardiovasc Electrophysiol* 19:945–951, 2008.
55. Soejima K, Stevenson WG, Sapp JL, et al: Endocardial and epicardial radiofrequency ablation of ventricular tachycardia associated with dilated cardiomyopathy: the importance of low-voltage scars, *J Am Coll Cardiol* 43:1834–1842, 2004.
56. Nakagawa H, Antz M, Wong T, et al: Initial experience using a forward directed, high-intensity focused ultrasound balloon catheter for pulmonary vein antrum isolation in patients with atrial fibrillation, *J Cardiovasc Electrophysiol* 18:136–144, 2007.
57. Schmidt B, Chun KR, Kuck KH, Antz M: Pulmonary vein isolation by high intensity focused ultrasound, *Indian Pacing Electrophysiol J* 7:126–133, 2007.
58. Schmidt B, Antz M, Ernst S, et al: Pulmonary vein isolation by high-intensity focused ultrasound: first-in-man study with a steerable balloon catheter, *Heart Rhythm* 4:575–584, 2007.
59. Neven K, Schmidt B, Metzner A, et al: Fatal end of a safety algorithm for pulmonary vein isolation with use of high-intensity focused ultrasound, *Circ Arrhythm Electrophysiol* 3:260–265, 2010.
60. Schmidt B, Chun KR, Metzner A, et al: Pulmonary vein isolation with high-intensity focused ultrasound: results from the HIFU 12F study, *Europace* 11:1281–1288, 2009.
61. Borchert B, Lawrenz T, Hansky B, Stellbrink C: Lethal atrioesophageal fistula after pulmonary vein isolation using high-intensity focused ultrasound (HIFU), *Heart Rhythm* 5:145–148, 2008.
62. Metzner A, Schmidt B, Fuernkranz A, et al: One-year clinical outcome after pulmonary vein isolation using the novel endoscopic ablation system in patients with paroxysmal atrial fibrillation, *Heart Rhythm* 8:988–993, 2011.
63. Schmidt B, Metzner A, Chun KR, et al: Feasibility of circumferential pulmonary vein isolation using a novel endoscopic ablation system, *Circ Arrhythm Electrophysiol* 3:481–488, 2010.
64. Reddy VY, Neuzil P, Themistoclakis S, et al: Visually-guided balloon catheter ablation of atrial fibrillation: experimental feasibility and first-in-human multicenter clinical outcome, *Circulation* 120:12–20, 2009.
65. Reddy VY, Neuzil P, d'Avila A, et al: Balloon catheter ablation to treat paroxysmal atrial fibrillation: what is the level of pulmonary venous isolation? *Heart Rhythm* 5:353–360, 2008.

CHAPTER 8 Sinus Node Dysfunction

General Considerations

Anatomy and Physiology of the Sinus Node

The sinus node is the dominant pacemaker of the heart. Its pacemaker function is determined by its low maximum diastolic membrane potential and steep phase 4 spontaneous depolarization. The molecular mechanisms of pacemaker function of the sinus node are discussed in detail in Chapters 1 and 3.[1]

The sinus node is a subepicardial specialized muscular structure located laterally within the epicardial groove of the sulcus terminalis of the right atrium (RA) at the junction of the anterior trabeculated appendage with the posterior smooth-walled venous component. The endocardial aspect of the sulcus terminalis is marked by the crista terminalis. Starting epicardially at the junction of the superior vena cava (SVC) and the RA appendage, it courses downward and to the left along the sulcus terminalis, to end subendocardially almost to the inferior vena cava (IVC). The sinus node is a spindle-shaped structure with a central body and tapering ends; the head extends toward the interatrial groove, and the tail extends toward the orifice of IVC. In adults, the sinus node measures 10 to 20 mm long and 2 to 3 mm wide and thick.[1-5]

The sinus node consists of densely packed specialized myocytes of no definite orientation within a background of extracellular connective tissue matrix.[4] The nodal margins can be discrete with fibrous separation from the surrounding atrial myocardium or interdigitate though a transitional zone. Commonly, prongs of nodal (P) cells and transitional (T) cells extend from the nodal body into the atrial myocardium, but actual cell-to-cell interaction is uncertain.[6]

The sinus node is in reality a region, which is functionally larger and less well defined than initially believed. It is composed of nests of principal pacemaker cells (referred to as P cells because of their relatively pale appearance on electron micrography), which spontaneously depolarize. In addition to this principal nest of cells, other nests contain cells with slower intrinsic depolarization rates and serve as backup pacemakers in response to changing physiological and pathological conditions. Normal conduction velocities within the sinus node are slow (2 to 5 cm/sec), thus increasing the likelihood of intranodal conduction block.

The pacemaker activity is not confined to a single cell in the sinus node; rather, sinus node cells function as electrically coupled oscillators that discharge synchronously because of mutual entrainment. In fact, it is likely that sinus rhythm results from impulse origin at widely separated sites, with two or three individual wavefronts created that merge to form a single, widely disseminated wavefront. The sinus node is insulated electrically from the surrounding atrial myocytes, except at a limited number of preferential exit sites. Neural and hormonal factors influence both the site of pacemaker activation, likely via shifting points of initial activity, and the point of exit from the sinus node complex. At faster rates, the sinus impulse originates in the superior portion of the sinus node, whereas at slower rates, it arises from a more inferior portion.[7] High-density simultaneous endocardial unipolar mapping studies demonstrated the frequent occurrence of spontaneous variations in the P wave and sinus activation sequence in normal individuals. These findings suggested that the sinus node complex in normal hearts displays a dynamic range of activation sites along the posterolateral RA. Furthermore, preferential pathways of conduction were also found to exist between the sinus node and the atrial exit sites, thus potentially contributing to the multicentricity of the sinus node complex.[1,5,8]

The blood supply to the sinus node region is variable and is therefore vulnerable to damage during operative procedures. The blood supply predominantly comes from a large central artery, the sinus nodal artery, which is a branch of the right coronary artery in 55% to 60% of patients, and from the circumflex artery in 40% to 45%. The sinus nodal artery typically passes centrally through the length of the sinus body, and it is disproportionately large, which is considered physiologically important in that its perfusion pressure can affect the sinus rate. Distention of the artery slows the sinus rate, whereas collapse causes an increase in rate.[1,3]

The sinus node is densely innervated with postganglionic adrenergic and cholinergic nerve terminals (threefold greater density of beta-adrenergic and muscarinic cholinergic receptors than adjacent atrial tissue), both of which influence the rate of spontaneous depolarization in pacemaker cells and can cause a shift in the principal pacemaker site within the sinus node region, which is often associated with subtle changes in P wave morphology. Enhanced vagal activity can produce sinus bradycardia, sinus arrest, and sinoatrial exit block, whereas increased sympathetic activity can increase the sinus rate and reverse sinus arrest and sinoatrial exit block. Sinus node responses to brief vagal bursts begin after a short latency and dissipate quickly; in contrast, responses to sympathetic stimulation begin and dissipate slowly. The rapid onset and offset of responses to vagal stimulation allow dynamic beat-to-beat vagal modulation of the heart rate, whereas the slow temporal response to sympathetic stimulation precludes any beat-to-beat regulation by sympathetic activity.[1]

Periodic vagal bursting (as may occur each time a systolic pressure wave arrives at the baroreceptor regions in the aortic and carotid sinuses) induces phasic changes in the sinus cycle length (CL) and can entrain the sinus node to discharge faster or slower at periods identical to those of the vagal burst.[3] Because the peak vagal effects on sinus rate and atrioventricular node (AVN) conduction occur at different times in the cardiac cycle, a brief vagal burst can slow the sinus rate without affecting AVN conduction or can prolong AVN conduction time and not slow the sinus rate.[1]

Pathophysiology of Sinus Node Dysfunction

The cause of sinus node dysfunction (SND) can be classified as intrinsic (secondary to a pathological condition involving the sinus node proper) or extrinsic (caused by depression of sinus node function by external factors such as drugs or autonomic influences).

INTRINSIC SINUS NODE DYSFUNCTION

Idiopathic degenerative disease is probably the most common cause of intrinsic SND.[2] Ischemic heart disease can be responsible for one third of cases of SND. Transient slowing of the sinus rate or sinus arrest can complicate acute myocardial infarction, which is usually seen with acute inferior wall infarction and is caused by autonomic influences. Possible mechanisms for sinus bradycardia after an acute myocardial infarction include neurological reflexes (Bezold-Jarisch reflex), coronary chemoreflexes (vagally mediated), humoral reflexes (enzymes, adenosine, potassium [K^+]), oxygen-conserving reflex ("diving" reflex), and infarction or ischemia of the sinus node or the surrounding atrium (e. g., secondary to proximal occlusion of the right or the circumflex coronary artery).

Cardiomyopathy, long-standing hypertension, infiltrative disorders (e.g., amyloidosis and sarcoidosis), collagen vascular diseases, and surgical trauma can also result in SND.[9,10] Orthotropic cardiac transplantation with atrial-atrial anastomosis is associated with a high incidence of SND in the donor heart (likely because of sinus nodal artery damage). Musculoskeletal disorders such as myotonic dystrophy or Friedreich ataxia are rare causes of SND. Congenital heart disease, such as sinus venosus and secundum atrial septal defects, can be associated with SND, even though no surgery has been performed.[11] Surgical trauma is responsible for most cases of SND in the pediatric population. Most commonly associated with this complication is the Mustard procedure for transposition of the great arteries and repair of atrial septal defects, especially of the sinus venosus type.[11]

Furthermore, atrial tachyarrhythmias can precipitate SND, likely secondary to remodeling of sinus node function. Although early studies implicated anatomical structural abnormalities in the sinus node, which suggested a fixed SND substrate, more recent evidence implicated a functional, and potentially reversible, component involving remodeling of sinus node ion channel expression and function. This finding was supported clinically by the observation that successful catheter ablation of atrial fibrillation (AF) and atrial flutter can be followed by significant improvements in sinus node function. In particular, downregulation of the funny current (I_f) and malfunction of the calcium (Ca^{2+}) clock (characterized by reduced sarcoplasmic reticulum Ca^{2+} release and downregulated ryanodine receptors in the sinus node) seem to account largely for atrial tachycardia–induced remodeling of sinus node. The remodeled atria are associated with more caudal activation of the sinus node complex, slower conduction time along preferential pathways, and only modest shifts within the functional pacemaker complex.[5,12,13]

On the other hand, SND has been associated with an increased propensity of atrial tachyarrhythmias, AF in particular. The mechanism leading to AF in patients with SND is unlikely to be bradycardia-dependent because AF was found to develop despite pacing in these patients. Importantly, patients with SND appear to have more widespread atrial changes beyond the sinus node, a finding indicating atrial myopathy, as evidenced by increased atrial refractoriness, prolonged P wave duration, delayed conduction, slowing electrogram fractionation, regions of low voltage and scar, and caudal shift of the pacemaker complex with loss of normal multicentric pattern of activation. Furthermore, abnormal atrial electromechanical properties, chronic atrial stretch, and neurohormonal activation are likely contributors to SND and its related atrial myopathy. The diffuse atrial myopathy potentially underlies the increased propensity to AF. The cause of these diffuse atrial abnormalities remains unknown, but there appears to be a relationship between atrial remodeling that predisposes to AF and sinus node remodeling that results in SND.[5,14]

Genetic defects in ion channels and structural proteins have been shown to contribute to SND, manifesting as sinus bradycardia, sinus arrest, sinoatrial block, or a combination. Mutations in the *SCN5A* gene (which encodes the alpha subunit of the cardiac sodium [Na^+] channel [I_{Na}]), the *HCN4* gene (which encodes the protein that contributes to formation of I_f channels), the *KCNQ1* gene (which encodes the alpha subunit of the voltage-gated slowly activating delayed rectifier K^+ channel responsible for I_{Ks}), the *GJA5* gene (which encodes for connexin 40, a gap junction protein), the *ANK2* gene (which encodes for ankyrin, which links the integral membrane proteins to the underlying cytoskeleton), and the *EMD* gene (which encodes the nuclear membrane protein emerin) have been associated with familial forms of SND, many of which also exhibit an increased propensity to AF.[15-18]

EXTRINSIC SINUS NODE DYSFUNCTION

In the absence of structural abnormalities, the predominant causes of SND are drug effects and autonomic influences. Drugs can alter sinus node function by direct pharmacological effects on nodal tissue or indirectly by neurally mediated effects.[19] Drugs known to depress sinus node function include beta blockers, calcium channel blockers (verapamil and diltiazem), digoxin, sympatholytic antihypertensive agents (e.g., clonidine), and antiarrhythmic agents (classes IA, IC, and III).

SND can sometimes result from excessive vagal tone in individuals without intrinsic sinus node disease. Hypervagotonia can be seen in hypersensitive carotid sinus syndrome and neurocardiogenic syncope. Well-trained athletes with increased vagal tone occasionally may require some deconditioning to help prevent symptomatic bradyarrhythmias.[20] Surges in vagal tone also can occur during Valsalva maneuvers, endotracheal intubation, vomiting, and suctioning. Sinus slowing in this setting is characteristically paroxysmal and may be associated with evidence of AV conduction delay, secondary to effects of the enhanced vagal tone on both the sinus node and AVN. Less common extrinsic causes of SND include electrolyte abnormalities such as hyperkalemia, hypothermia, increased intracranial pressure (the Cushing response), sleep apnea, hypoxia, hypercapnia, hypothyroidism, advanced liver disease, typhoid fever, brucellosis, and sepsis.

Clinical Presentation

More than 50% of the patients with SND are older than 50 years. Patients often are asymptomatic or have symptoms that are mild and nonspecific, and the intermittent nature of these symptoms makes documentation of the associated arrhythmia difficult at times. Symptoms, which may have been present for months or years, include paroxysmal dizziness, presyncope, or syncope, which are predominantly related to prolonged sinus pauses. Episodes of syncope are often unheralded and can manifest in older patients as repeated falls. The highest incidence of syncope associated with SND probably occurs in patients with tachycardia-bradycardia syndrome, in whom syncope typically occurs secondary to a long sinus pause following cessation of the supraventricular tachycardia (usually AF). Occasionally, a stroke can be the first manifestation of SND in patients presenting with paroxysmal AF and thromboembolism.[3,19,21]

Patients with sinus bradycardia or chronotropic incompetence can present with decreased exercise capacity or fatigue (Fig. 8-1). Chronotropic incompetence is estimated to be present in 20% to 60% of patients with SND.[22,23] Other symptoms include irritability, nocturnal wakefulness, memory loss, lightheadedness, and lethargy. More subtle symptoms include mild digestive disturbances, periodic oliguria or edema, and mild intermittent dyspnea. Additionally, symptoms caused by the worsening of conditions such as congestive heart failure and angina pectoris can be precipitated by SND.

Natural History

The natural history of SND can be variable, but slow progression (over 10 to 30 years) is expected. The prognosis largely depends on the type of dysfunction and the presence and severity of the

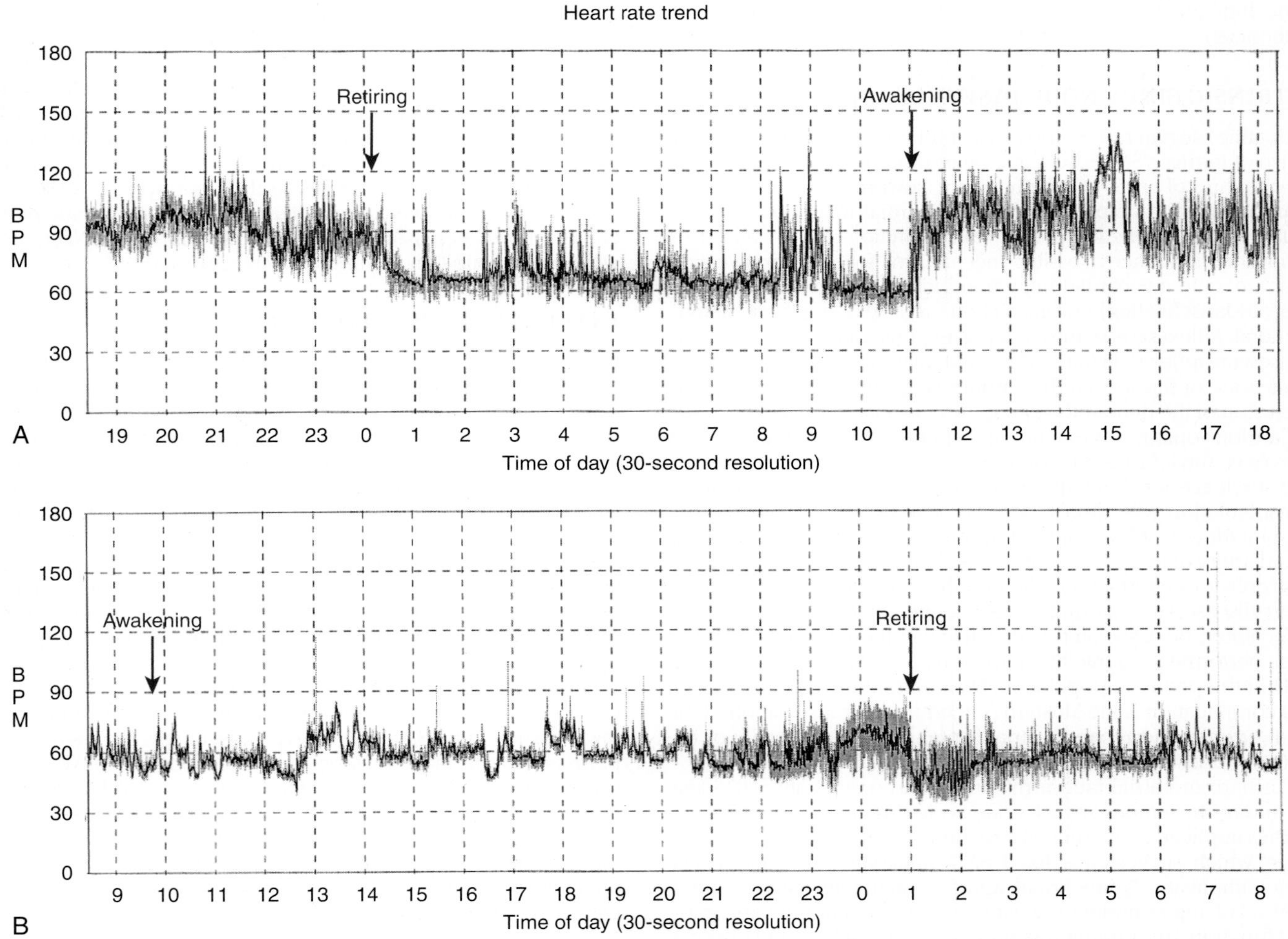

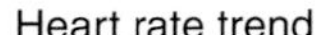

FIGURE 8-1 Chronotropic incompetence. **A,** A 24-hour Holter recording in a normal subject showing normal sinus rate diurnal variation and response to activity. **B,** A 24-hour Holter recording in a different patient with chronotropic incompetence and activity intolerance. Note the blunted response of the sinus rate to activity during waking hours and the slow average heart rate.

underlying heart disease. The worst prognosis is associated with the tachycardia-bradycardia syndrome (mostly because of the risk for thromboembolic complications), whereas sinus bradycardia is much more benign. The incidence of new-onset AF in patients with SND is about 5.2% per year. New atrial tachyarrhythmias occur with less frequency in patients who are treated with atrial pacing (3.9%) compared with a greatly increased incidence of similar arrhythmias in patients with only ventricular pacing (22.3%).[24] Furthermore, thromboembolism occurs in 15.2% among unpaced patients with SND versus 13% among patients treated with only ventricular pacing versus 1.6% among those treated with atrial pacing.[19,21,25]

The incidence of advanced AV conduction system disease in patients with SND is low (5% to 10%), and, when present, its progression is slow. At the time of diagnosis of SND, approximately 17% of the patients have some degree of AV conduction system disease (PR interval longer than 240 milliseconds, bundle branch block, His bundle–ventricular (HV) interval prolongation, AV Wenckebach rate less than 120 beats/min, or second- or third-degree AV block). New AV conduction abnormalities develop at a rate of approximately 2.7% per year. The incidence of advanced AV block during long-term follow-up is low (approximately 1% per year).[21]

Diagnostic Evaluation

Generally, the noninvasive methods of ECG monitoring, exercise testing, and autonomic testing are used first. However, if symptoms are infrequent and noninvasive evaluation is unrevealing, invasive electrophysiological (EP) testing may be pursued.[26]

ELECTROCARDIOGRAM AND AMBULATORY MONITORING. A 12-lead electrocardiogram (ECG) needs to be obtained in symptomatic patients. However, the diagnosis of SND as the cause of the symptoms is rarely made from the ECG. In patients with frequent symptoms, 24- or 48-hour ambulatory Holter monitoring can be useful. Cardiac event monitoring or implantable loop recorders may be necessary in patients with less frequent symptoms.[27] Documentation of symptoms in a diary by the patient while wearing the cardiac monitor is essential for correlation of symptoms with the heart rhythm at the time. In some cases, ambulatory monitoring can exclude SND as the cause of symptoms if normal sinus rhythm (NSR) is documented at the time of symptom occurrence. In contrast, recorded sinus pauses may not be associated with symptoms.

AUTONOMIC MODULATION. An abnormal response to carotid sinus massage (pause longer than 3 seconds) can indicate SND, but this response can also occur in asymptomatic older individuals. Heart rate response to the Valsalva maneuver (normally decreased) or upright tilt (normally increased) can also be used to verify that the autonomic nervous system itself is intact. Complete pharmacological autonomic blockade is used to determine the intrinsic heart rate (see later).[3]

EXERCISE TESTING. Exercise testing to assess chronotropic incompetence is of value in patients with exertional symptoms (see later).

ELECTROPHYSIOLOGICAL TESTING. Noninvasive testing is usually adequate in establishing the diagnosis of SND and guiding subsequent therapy. However, invasive EP testing can be of value in symptomatic patients in whom SND is suspected but cannot be documented in association with symptoms. In addition to assessing SND, EP testing can be useful in evaluating other potential causes for symptoms of syncope and palpitations (e.g., AV block, supraventricular tachycardia, and ventricular tachycardia).[19,21]

Electrocardiographic Features

SINUS BRADYCARDIA. Sinus bradycardia (less than 60 beats/min) is considered abnormal when it is persistent, unexplained, and inappropriate for physiological circumstances. Sinus bradycardia slower than 40 beats/min (not associated with sleep or physical conditioning) is generally considered abnormal.[3]

SINUS PAUSES. Sinus arrest and sinoatrial exit block can result in sinus pauses, and they are definite evidence of SND.

SINUS ARREST. The terms sinus arrest and sinus pause are often used interchangeably; sinus arrest is a result of total cessation of impulse formation within the sinus node. The pause is not an exact multiple of the preceding P-P interval but is random in duration (Fig. 8-2). Although asymptomatic pauses of 2 to 3 seconds can be seen in up to 11% of normal individuals and in one third of trained athletes, pauses longer than 3 seconds are rare in normal individuals and may or may not be associated with symptoms, but they are usually caused by SND.[3]

SINOATRIAL EXIT BLOCK. Sinoatrial exit block results when a normally generated sinus impulse fails to conduct to the atria because of delay in conduction or block within the sinus node itself or perinodal tissue. Sinoatrial exit block produces a pause that is eventually terminated by a delayed sinus beat or an atrial or junctional escape beat.[28] In theory, sinoatrial exit block can be distinguished from sinus arrest because the exit block pause is an exact multiple of the baseline P-P interval. However, sinus arrhythmia causing normal beat-to-beat variations in the sinus rate often makes the distinction impossible. Furthermore, establishing the diagnosis of sinoatrial exit block versus sinus arrest is often of academic interest only.[3]

Exit block is classified into three types, analogous to those of AV block: first-degree, second-degree, and third-degree exit block.[28] First-degree sinoatrial exit block is caused by abnormal prolongation of the sinoatrial conduction time (SACT). It occurs every time a sinus impulse reaches the atrium, but it is conducted with a delay at a fixed interval. This type of sinoatrial exit block is concealed on the surface ECG and can be diagnosed only by direct sinus node recording or indirect measurement of SACT during an EP study. Second-degree sinoatrial exit block is marked by intermittent failure of the sinus impulse to exit the sinus node. Type I block is viewed as Wenckebach periodicity of the P wave on the surface ECG, and it manifests as progressive delay in conduction of the sinus-generated impulse through the sinus node to the atrium, finally resulting in a nonconducted sinus impulse and absence of a P wave on the surface ECG. Because the sinus discharge is a silent event on the surface ECG, this arrhythmia can be inferred only, because of a missing P wave and the signs of Wenckebach periodicity seen with this type of arrhythmia. The increment in delay in impulse conduction through the sinus node tissue is progressively less; thus, the P-P intervals become progressively shorter until a P wave fails to occur. The pauses associated with this type of sinoatrial exit block are less than twice the shortest sinus cycle. Type II block manifests as an abrupt absence of one or more P waves because of failure of the atrial impulse to exit the sinus node, without previous progressive prolongation of SACT (and without progressive shortening of the P-P intervals). Sometimes, two or more consecutive sinus impulses are blocked within the sinus node, thus creating considerably long pauses. The sinus pause should be an exact multiple of the immediately preceding P-P interval. However, normal variations in the sinus rate caused by sinus arrhythmia can obscure this measurement. Third-degree or complete sinoatrial exit block manifests as absence of P waves, with long pauses resulting in lower pacemaker escape rhythm. This type of block is impossible to distinguish from sinus arrest with certainty without invasive sinus node recordings.[21,29,30]

TACHYCARDIA-BRADYCARDIA SYNDROME. Tachycardia-bradycardia syndrome, frequently referred to as sick sinus syndrome, is a common manifestation of SND, and it refers to the presence of intermittent sinus or junctional bradycardia alternating with atrial tachyarrhythmias (Fig. 8-3). The atrial tachyarrhythmia is most commonly paroxysmal AF, but atrial tachycardia, atrial flutter, and occasionally AVN reentrant tachycardia or AV reentrant tachycardia can also occur.[3]

Apart from underlying sinus bradycardia of varying severity, these patients often experience prolonged sinus arrest and asystole on termination of the atrial tachyarrhythmia, resulting from overdrive suppression of the sinus node and secondary pacemakers by the tachycardia. Long sinus pauses that occur following electrical cardioversion of AF constitute another manifestation of SND.

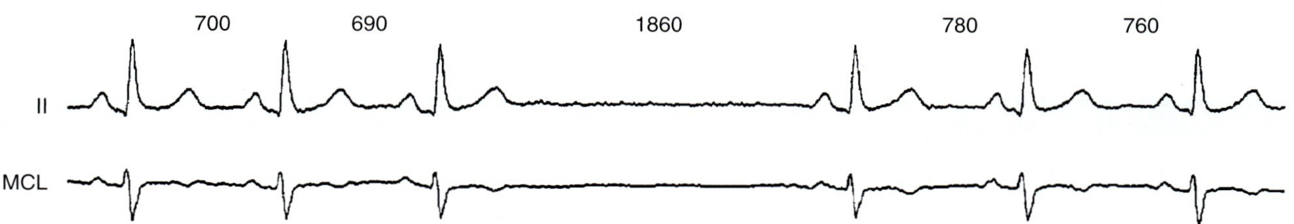

FIGURE 8-2 Sinus pause is shown in two monitor leads. Although the sinus rate is slightly irregular, the pause significantly exceeds any two P-P intervals (excluding sinus exit block). MCL = modified chest-lead.

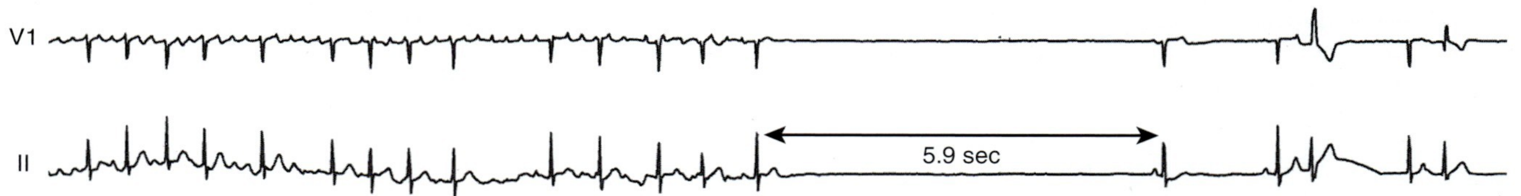

FIGURE 8-3 Tachycardia-bradycardia syndrome. Two surface ECG leads showing atrial fibrillation that spontaneously terminates followed by a 5.9-second pause before sinus rhythm resumes. The patient became lightheaded during this period.

Therapeutic strategies to control the tachyarrhythmias often result in the need for pacemaker therapy (Fig. 8-4). On the other hand, atrial tachyarrhythmias can be precipitated by prolonged sinus pauses.[2,3,31,32] SND is often caused by functional remodeling from the tachycardia and can be reversible in some patients, thus obviating the need for pacing.

ATRIAL FIBRILLATION WITH SLOW VENTRICULAR RESPONSE. Persistent AF with a slow ventricular response in the absence of AVN blocking drugs is often present in patients with SND. These patients can demonstrate very slow ventricular rates at rest or during sleep and occasionally have long pauses. Occasionally, they can develop complete AV block with a junctional or ventricular escape rhythm. They can also conduct rapidly and develop symptoms caused by tachycardia during exercise. In some cases, cardioversion results in a long sinus pause or junctional escape rhythm before the appearance of sinus rhythm. Although a combination of sinus node and AV conduction disease can be present in many cases, examples of rapid ventricular responses during atrial tachyarrhythmias are frequently found.[2]

PERSISTENT ATRIAL STANDSTILL. Atrial standstill is a rare clinical syndrome in which there is no spontaneous atrial activity and the atria cannot be electrically stimulated. The surface ECG usually reveals junctional bradycardia without atrial activity. The atria are generally fibrotic and without any functional myocardium. Lack of mechanical atrial contraction poses a high risk for thromboembolism in these patients.[33,34]

CHRONOTROPIC INCOMPETENCE. Treadmill exercise testing can be of substantial value in assessing the chronotropic response ("competence") to increases in metabolic demands in patients with sinus bradycardia who are suspected of having SND. Although the resting heart rate can be normal, these patients may be unable to increase their heart rate during exercise or may have unpredictable fluctuations in the heart rate during activity. Some patients can initially experience a normal increase in the heart rate with exercise, which then plateaus or decreases inappropriately.[22,23,29,30]

The definition of chronotropic incompetence is not agreed on, but it is reasonable to designate it as an abnormally slow heart rate response to exercise manifesting as a less than normal increase in the sinus rate at each stage of exercise, with a plateau at less than 70% to 75% of the age-predicted maximum heart rate (220 – age) or an inability to achieve a sinus rate of 100 to 120 beats/min at maximum effort. Irregular (and nonreproducible) increases, and even decreases, in the sinus rate during exercise, can also occur but are rare. Other patients with SND can achieve an appropriate peak heart rate during exercise but may have slow sinus rate acceleration in the initial stage or rapid deceleration of heart rate in the recovery stage.[22,23]

CAROTID SINUS HYPERSENSITIVITY. An abnormal response to carotid sinus massage (pause longer than 3 seconds) can indicate SND, but this response may also occur in asymptomatic older individuals (Fig. 8-5).[1,28-30]

SINUS ARRHYTHMIA. Respiratory sinus arrhythmia, in which the sinus rate increases with inspiration and decreases with expiration, is not an abnormal rhythm and is most commonly seen in young healthy subjects. Sinus arrhythmia is present when the P wave morphology is normal and consistent and the P-P intervals vary by more than 120 milliseconds. Nonrespiratory sinus arrhythmia, in which phasic changes in sinus rate are not related to the respiratory cycle, can be accentuated by the use of vagal agents such as digitalis and morphine; its mechanism is unknown. Patients with nonrespiratory sinus arrhythmia are likely to be older and to have underlying cardiac disease, although the arrhythmia is not a marker for structural heart disease. None of the sinus arrhythmias (respiratory or nonrespiratory) indicate SND. Additionally, respiratory variation in the sinus P wave contour

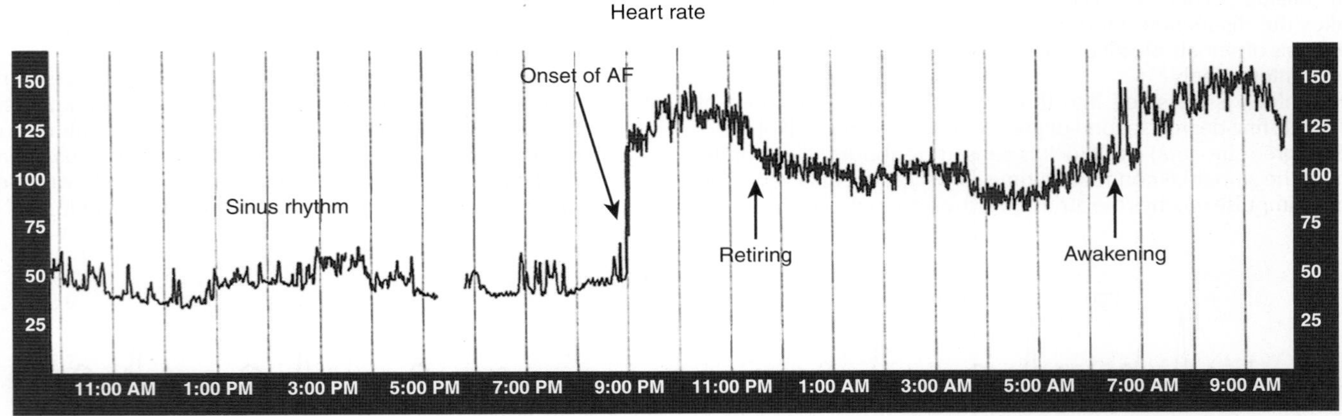

FIGURE 8-4 A 24-hour Holter heart rate trend showing slow sinus rhythm rates during waking hours. Onset of atrial fibrillation (AF) is associated with rapid ventricular response, even during sleep hours. Pacing was required in this patient to prevent symptomatic bradycardia and allow the use of drug therapy to control the tachycardia.

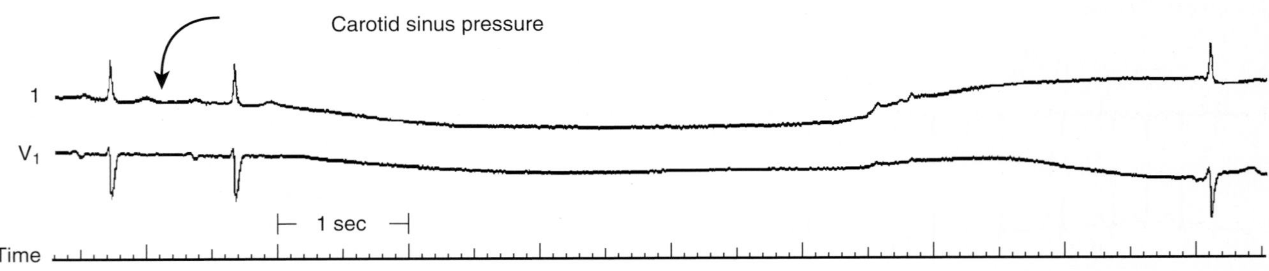

FIGURE 8-5 Carotid sinus hypersensitivity. Two surface ECG leads are shown during carotid sinus pressure, as indicated. The PR interval is prolonged, followed by a 7.5-second sinus pause ended by a P wave and probable junctional escape complex. The patient was nearly syncopal during this period.

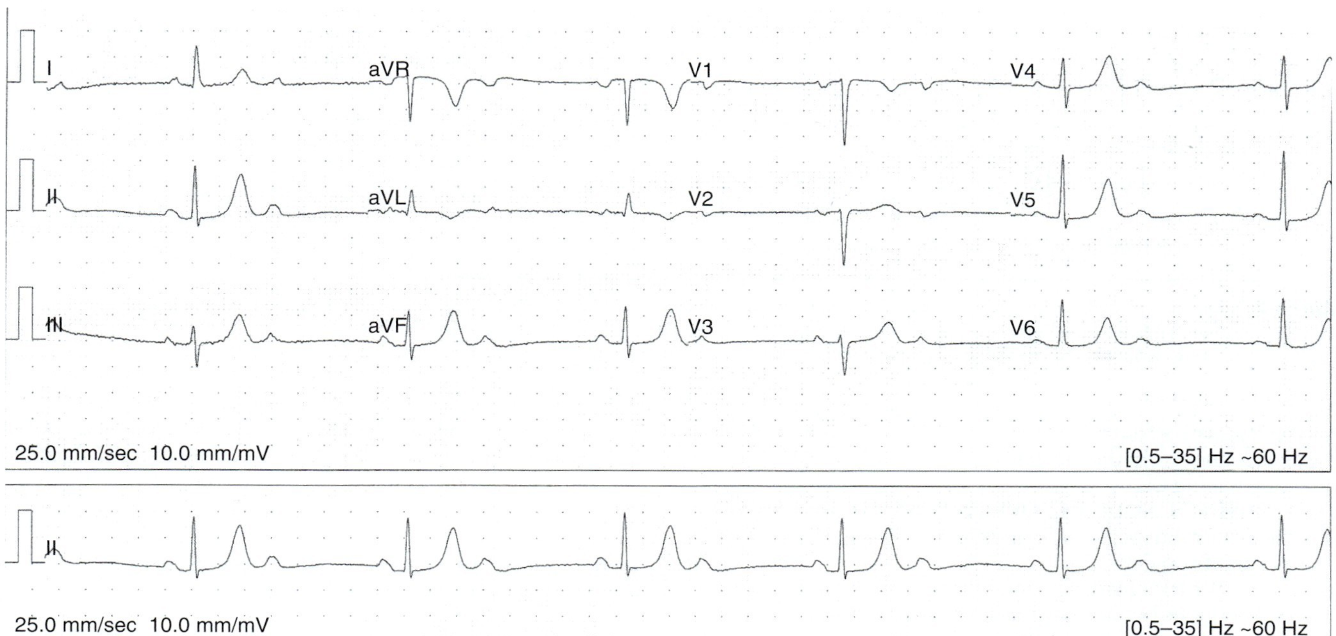

FIGURE 8-6 Ventriculophasic sinus arrhythmia. Surface ECG during sinus rhythm with second-degree 2:1 atrioventricular block. Consecutive sinus P waves enclosing a QRS occur at shorter intervals than that of consecutive P waves without a QRS in between (ventriculophasic arrhythmia).

can be seen in the inferior leads and should not be confused with wandering atrial pacemaker, which is unrelated to breathing and therefore is not phasic.[29,30]

Ventriculophasic sinus arrhythmia is an unusual rhythm that occurs when sinus rhythm and high-grade or complete AV block coexist; it is characterized by shorter P-P intervals when they enclose QRS complexes and longer P-P intervals when no QRS complexes are enclosed (Fig. 8-6). The mechanism is uncertain but may be related to the effects of the mechanical ventricular systole itself: ventricular contraction increases the blood supply to the sinus node, thereby transiently increasing its firing rate. Ventriculophasic sinus arrhythmia is not a pathological arrhythmia and should not be confused with premature atrial complexes or sinoatrial block.

Electrophysiological Testing

Role of Electrophysiological Testing

The diagnosis of SND usually can be made based on clinical and ECG findings, which are typically adequate for deciding subsequent treatment. Once symptoms and SND are correlated with ECG findings, further documentation by invasive studies is not required. Similarly, asymptomatic patients with evidence of SND need not be tested because no therapy is indicated. However, EP testing can be important to assess sinus node function in patients who have had symptoms compatible with SND and in whom no documentation of the arrhythmia responsible for these symptoms has been obtained by prolonged monitoring. In these cases, EP testing can yield information that may be used to guide appropriate therapy. The most useful measures of the overall sinus node function are a combination of the responses to atropine and exercise and the sinus node recovery time (SNRT).[28]

Sinus Node Recovery Time

The sinus node is the archetype of an automatic focus. Automatic rhythms are characterized by spontaneous depolarization, overdrive suppression, and post-overdrive warm-up or a gradual return to baseline CL. SNRT is the interval between the end of a period of pacing-induced overdrive suppression of sinus node activity and the return of sinus node function, manifest on the surface ECG by a post-pacing sinus P wave. Clinically, SNRT is used to test sinus node automaticity.[29,30,35]

TECHNIQUE

PACING SITE. Pacing is performed in the high RA at a site near the sinus node, to decrease the conduction time to and from the sinus node.[28]

PACING CYCLE LENGTH. SNRT is preferably measured after pacing at multiple CLs. Pacing is started at a CL just shorter than the sinus CL. After a 1-minute rest, pacing is repeated at progressively shorter CLs (with 50- to 100-millisecond decrements) down to a pacing CL of 300 milliseconds.[28]

PACING DURATION. Pacing is continued for 30 or 60 seconds at a time. Although pacing durations beyond 15 seconds usually have little effect on the SNRT in healthy subjects, patients with SND can have marked suppression after longer pacing durations. It is also preferable to perform pacing at each CL for different durations (30, 60, or 120 seconds), to ensure that sinus entrance block has not obscured the true SNRT.[28]

MEASUREMENTS

Several intervals have been used as a measure of SNRT.

SINUS NODE RECOVERY TIME. SNRT is the longest pause from the last paced beat to the first sinus return beat at a particular pacing CL. Normally, the SNRT is less than 1500 milliseconds, with a scatter on multiple tests of less than 250 milliseconds (Fig. 8-7). SNRT tends to be shorter with shorter baseline sinus CLs, and therefore various corrections have been introduced.[29,30,35]

CORRECTED SINUS NODE RECOVERY TIME. Corrected SNRT equals SNRT minus the baseline sinus CL. Normal values of corrected SNRT have been reported from 350 to 550 milliseconds, with 500 milliseconds most commonly used (see Fig. 8-7). However, the use of corrections at slow sinus rates can produce odd results. For example, in a patient with symptomatic bradycardia at a 1500-millisecond CL and an SNRT of 2000 milliseconds, the corrected SNRT is 500 milliseconds. For cases of severe bradycardia, an abnormal uncorrected SNRT of 2000 milliseconds is more accurate; in fact, one does not need SNRT to make the clinical diagnosis.

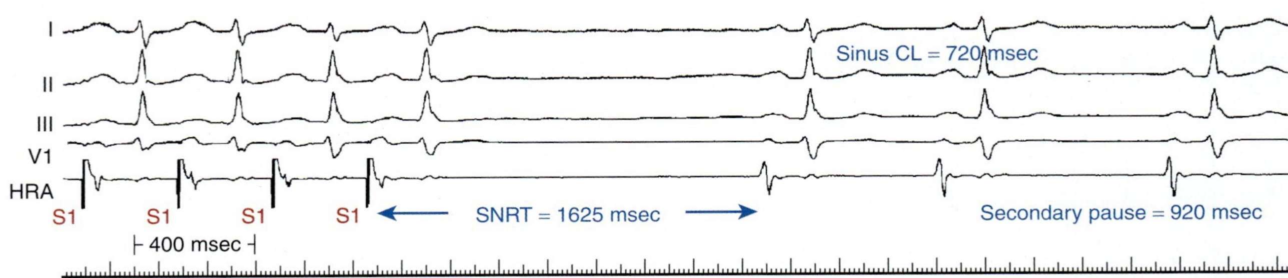

FIGURE 8-7 Sinus node recovery time (SNRT). Surface ECG leads and high right atrial (HRA) recordings are shown at the end of a burst of atrial pacing, suppressing sinus node automaticity. The interval at which the first sinus complex returns (SNRT) is abnormally long at 1625 milliseconds. With a baseline sinus cycle (CL) of 720 milliseconds, the corrected SNRT (1625 − 720 = 905 milliseconds) is also prolonged. In addition, there is a secondary pause after the first two sinus complexes.

MAXIMUM SINUS NODE RECOVERY TIME. Maximum SNRT is the longest pause from the last paced beat to the first sinus return beat at any pacing CL.

RATIO OF SINUS NODE RECOVERY TIME TO SINUS CYCLE LENGTH. The ratio of [(SNRT/sinus CL) × 100%] is lower than 160% in normal subjects.

TOTAL RECOVERY TIME. On cessation of atrial pacing, the pattern of subsequent beats returning to the basic sinus CL should be analyzed. Various patterns exist.[28] Total recovery time equals the time to return to basic sinus CL (normal total recovery time is less than 5 seconds, usually by the fourth to sixth recovery beat).

SECONDARY PAUSES. Normally, following cessation of overdrive pacing, a gradual shortening of the sinus CL is observed until the baseline sinus CL is reached, typically within a few beats. Limited oscillations of recovery CLs before full recovery can be observed, especially at faster pacing rates.[28] Secondary pauses are identified when there is an initial shortening of the sinus CL after the SNRT, followed by an unexpected lengthening of the CL (see Fig. 8-7). Sudden and marked secondary pauses occurring during sinus recovery are abnormal. Sinoatrial exit block of variable duration is the primary mechanism of prolonged pauses, with a lesser component of depression of automaticity. Both may, and often do, coexist. However, secondary pauses can be a normal reflex following hypotension induced by pacing at rapid rates or in response to pressure overshoot in the first recovery beat resulting from the prolonged filling time. Because these secondary pauses represent SND and because they occur more frequently following rapid atrial pacing, pacing should be performed at rates up to 200 beats/min.[28,29,35,36]

LIMITATIONS OF SINUS NODE RECOVERY TIME

Many factors in addition to automaticity are involved in the measurement of SNRT, including proximity of the pacing site to the sinus node and conduction time from the pacing site to the sinus node and vice versa, as well as conduction time in and out of the sinus node. Sinus node entrance block during rapid atrial pacing can lead to a shorter SNRT, whereas sinus node exit block after cessation of pacing can result in marked prolongation of the SNRT.[28] Moreover, sometimes SNRT cannot be measured because of atrial ectopic or junctional escape beats that preempt the sinus beat.[29,30]

Despite these limitations, SNRT is probably the best and most widely used test for sinus node automaticity. Pacing at rates near the baseline sinus CL causes no overdrive suppression, so that the interval between the last paced beat and the next sinus beat is comparable with the baseline CL. If the SNRT after pacing at 500 milliseconds is shorter than after 600 milliseconds, or if there is marked variation (more than 250 milliseconds) in the SNRTs when multiple tests are performed after pacing at 500 milliseconds, this finding can imply that some impulses have not penetrated the sinus node (i.e., some degree of atrial-nodal block exists). At pacing CLs shorter than 500 milliseconds, there is usually little further prolongation of the SNRT; on the contrary, changes in neurohumoral tone may result in shorter SNRTs.[29,35]

The durations of the maximum SNRT and corrected SNRT are independent of age. Evaluation of the corrected SNRT following pharmacological denervation (see later) can increase the sensitivity of the test.[36]

SINUS NODE RECOVERY TIME IN PATIENTS WITH SINUS NODE DYSFUNCTION

The sensitivity of a single SNRT measurement is approximately 35% in patients with SND. This rises to more than 85% when multiple SNRTs at different rates are recorded, along with scatter and total recovery time, with a specificity of more than 90%. A prolonged SNRT or corrected SNRT is found in 35% to 93% of patients suspected of having SND (depending on the population studied). The incidence is lowest in patients with sinus bradycardia. Marked abnormalities in the corrected SNRT usually occur in symptomatic patients with clinical evidence of sinoatrial block or bradycardia-tachycardia syndrome.[28,36]

The pacing CL at which maximum suppression occurs in patients with SND is unpredictable and, unlike in healthy subjects, tends to be affected by the rate and duration of pacing. However, if sinus entrance block is present, the greatest suppression is likely to occur at relatively long pacing CLs. If the longest SNRT occurs at pacing CLs longer than 600 milliseconds, a normal value can reflect the presence of entrance block. In such cases, a normal SNRT is an unreliable assessment of sinus node automaticity. The fact that the longest SNRT occurs at pacing CLs longer than 600 milliseconds is in itself a marker of SND.[28]

Marked secondary pauses are another manifestation of SND and can occasionally occur in the absence of prolongation of SNRT, in which case sinoatrial block is the mechanism. Approximately 69% of patients with secondary pauses have clinical evidence of sinoatrial exit block, and 92% of patients with sinoatrial exit block demonstrate marked secondary pauses.[28]

Sinoatrial Conduction Time

Although the sinus node is the dominant cardiac pacemaker, neither sinus node impulse initiation nor conduction is visible on the surface ECG or on the standard intracardiac recordings because depolarization within the sinus node is of very low amplitude. Sinus node function therefore has usually been assessed indirectly. Normal sinus node function is assumed when the atrial musculature is depolarized at a normal rate and in a normal temporal sequence—so-called *normal sinus rhythm.* In NSR, the atrial rate is assumed to correspond to the rate of impulse formation within the sinus node; however, the time of impulse conduction from the sinus node to the atrium cannot be ascertained. Several methods have been developed for the assessment of SACT, either indirectly (the Strauss and Narula methods) or by directly recording the sinus node electrogram. Signal-averaging techniques have also been used to measure SACT noninvasively.[29,30,36]

DIRECT RECORDINGS

Sinus node depolarization can be recorded directly using high-gain unfiltered electrograms in approximately 50% of patients.[28] A catheter with a 0.5- to 1.5-mm interelectrode distance is used. The catheter is placed directly at the SVC-RA junction, or a loop is formed in the RA and the tip of the catheter is then placed at the SVC-RA junction. Optimizing the filter setting can help reduce baseline drift (0.1 to 0.6 Hz to 20 to 50 Hz), with signal gain at 50 to 100 mV/cm.[36]

SACT is measured as the interval between the pacemaker prepotential on the local electrogram and the onset of the rapid atrial deflection (Fig. 8-8). When SACT is normal, a smooth upstroke slope merges into the atrial electrogram. When SACT is prolonged, an increasing amount of sinus node potential becomes visible before the rapid atrial deflection. Sinoatrial block is said to occur when the entire sinus node electrogram is seen in the absence of a propagated response to the atrium.[28]

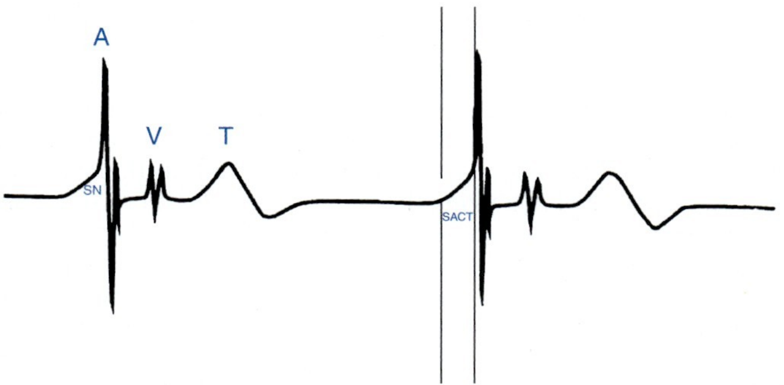

FIGURE 8-8 Schematic illustration showing the direct measurement of sinoatrial conduction time (SACT). A schematic copy of a sinus node electrogram is shown. On the sinus node electrogram, high right atrial depolarization (A), ventricular depolarization (V), T wave (T), and the sinus node potential (SN) are identified. In the second beat, reference lines are drawn through the point at which the SN potential first becomes evident and the point at which atrial activation begins. SACT is the interval between these two reference lines. *(From Reiffel JA: The human sinus node electrogram: a transvenous catheter technique and a comparison of directly measured and indirectly estimated sinoatrial conduction time in adults. Circulation 62:1324, 1980.)*

The sinus node electrogram can be validated by the ability to record the electrogram in only a local area, with loss of the upstroke potential during overdrive atrial pacing. Additionally, persistence of the sinus node electrogram following carotid sinus massage, following induced pauses, or during pauses following overdrive suppression is an important method for validation.

STRAUSS TECHNIQUE

The Strauss technique uses atrial premature stimulation to assess SACT. Baseline sinus beats are designated A_1. Progressively premature atrial extrastimuli (AESs; A_2) are delivered after every eighth to tenth A_1, and the timing of the recovery beat (A_3) is measured.[28] The Strauss method is useful as part of an overall EP study when information is also sought on conduction system refractoriness or possible dual AVN physiology or bypass tracts during sinus rhythm. Four zones of response of the sinus node to AES have been identified. SACT can be measured only in the zone of reset (Fig. 8-9).[29,30,35]

1. ZONE I: ZONE OF COLLISION, ZONE OF INTERFERENCE, NONRESET ZONE. This zone is defined by the range of A_1-A_2 intervals at which the A_2-A_3 interval is fully compensatory (see Fig. 8-9). Very long A_1-A_2 intervals (with A_2 falling in the last 20% to 30% of the sinus CL) generally result in collision of the AES (A_2) with the spontaneous sinus impulse (A_1). The sinus pacemaker and the timing of the subsequent sinus beat (A_3) are therefore unaffected by A_2, and a complete compensatory pause occurs—that is, A_1-$A_3 = 2 \times (A_1$-$A_1)$.

2. ZONE II: ZONE OF RESET. The range of A_1-A_2 intervals at which reset of the sinus pacemaker occurs, resulting in a less than compensatory pause, defines the zone of reset (see Fig. 8-9). Shorter A_1-A_2 intervals result in penetration of the sinus node with

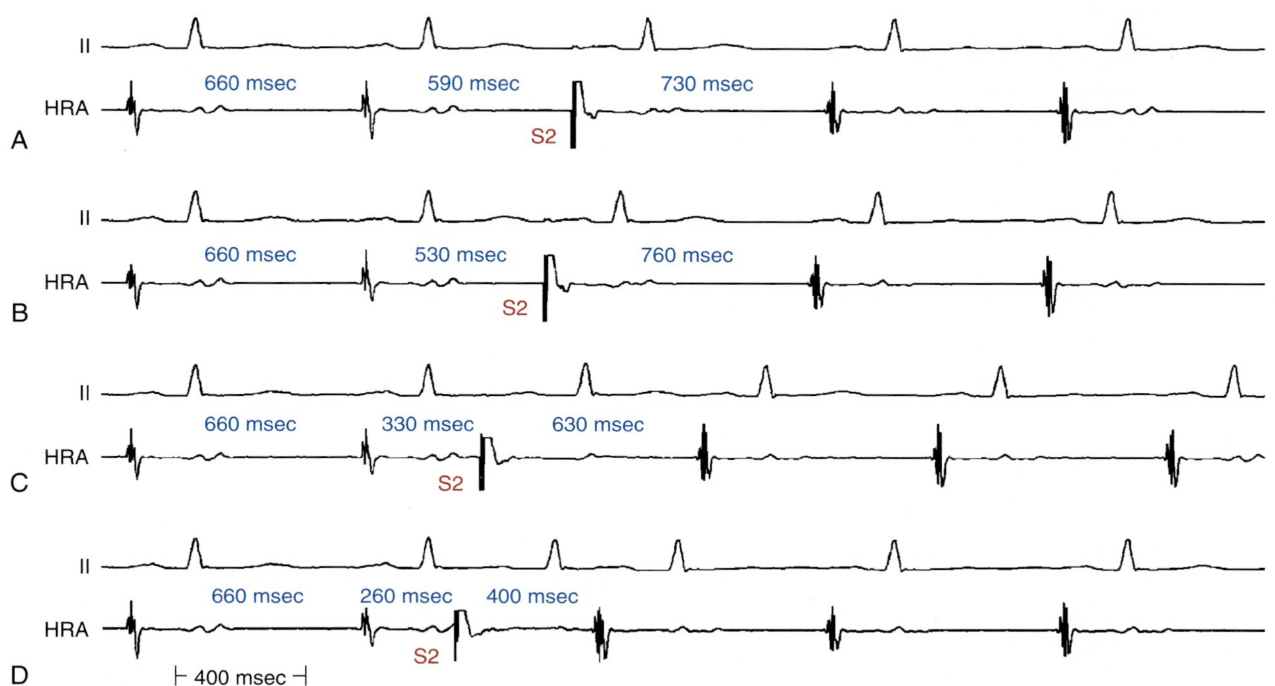

FIGURE 8-9 Strauss sinoatrial conduction time zones. Leads 2 and recording from the high right atrium (HRA) are shown, with a single extrastimulus (S) delivered during sinus rhythm (cycle length, 660 milliseconds) at progressively shorter coupling intervals as indicated relative to the preceding sinus complex. The timing of the subsequent sinus P wave relative to when it would be expected if there were no extrastimulus determines the zone of effect: **A,** collision; **B,** reset; **C,** interpolation; and **D,** reentry. See text for details.

resetting so that the resulting pause is less than compensatory—A_1-A_3 < 2 × (A_1-A_1)—but without changing sinus node automaticity. This zone typically occupies a long duration (40% to 50% of the sinus CL). In most patients, the A_2-A_3 interval remains constant throughout zone II, thus producing a plateau in the curve because A_2 penetrates and resets the sinus node, but it does so without changing the sinus pacemaker automaticity. Hence, the A_2-A_3 interval should equal the spontaneous sinus CL (A_1-A_1) plus the time it takes the AES (A_2) to enter and exit the sinus node. The difference between the A_2-A_3 and A_1-A_1 intervals therefore has been taken as an estimate of total SACT (Fig. 8-10).[36]

Conventionally, it is assumed that conduction times into and out of the sinus node are equal (i.e., SACT = [A_2-A_3 − A_1-A_1]/2). Data, however, suggest that conduction time into the sinus node is shorter than that out of the sinus node (see Fig. 8-10). The Strauss method for assessment of SACT can be affected by the site of stimulation; the farther the site of stimulation is from the sinus node, the greater the overestimation of SACT will be (because conduction through more intervening atrial and perinodal tissue will be incorporated in the measurement). The value of SACT can also be affected by the prematurity of the AES (A_2); the more premature is an A_2, the more likely it will be to encroach on perinodal or atrial refractoriness and slow conduction into the sinus node. In addition, an early AES commonly causes pacemaker shift to a peripheral latent pacemaker, which can exit the atrium earlier because of its proximity to the tissue, thus shortening conduction time out of the sinus node.[28,29,36]

Despite those limitations, for practical purposes, the Strauss method is a reasonable estimate of functional SACT, provided that stimulation is performed as closely as possible to the sinus node and the measurement is taken when a true plateau is present in zone II.[28] SACT appears to be independent of the spontaneous sinus CL. However, marked sinus arrhythmia invalidates the calculation of SACT because it is impossible to know whether the return cycle is a result of spontaneous oscillation or is a result of the AES. To eliminate the effects of sinus arrhythmia, multiple tests need to be performed at each coupling interval. Alternatively, atrial pacing drive at a rate just faster than the sinus rate is used instead of delivery of AES during NSR (Narula method; see later). However, this latter method can result in depression of sinus node automaticity, pacemaker shifts, sinus entrance block, sinus acceleration (if the drive pacing CL is within 50 milliseconds of sinus CL), and shortening of sinus action potential and can lead to an earlier onset of phase IV; each of these actions can yield misleading results.[35,36]

In an occasional patient, in response to progressively premature AESs, the A_2-A_3 interval prolongs either continuously or after a brief plateau (in both cases, the pause remains less than compensatory). This progressive prolongation of the A_2-A_3 interval during zone II can be caused by suppression of sinus node automaticity, a shift to a slower latent pacemaker, or an increase in conduction time into the sinus node because of encroachment of A_2 on perinodal tissue refractoriness. Thus, it is recommended to use the first third of zone II to measure SACT because it is less likely to introduce such errors.[28] Analysis of the A_3-A_4 interval may provide insights into changes in sinus node automaticity or pacemaker shift. If the A_3-A_4 interval is longer than the A_1-A_1 interval, depression of sinus node automaticity is suggested. Therefore, the calculated SACT overestimates the true SACT, and correction of SACT is necessary (in which case the A_3-A_4 interval is used as the basic sinus CL to which the A_2-A_3 interval is compared).[28]

3. ZONE III: ZONE OF INTERPOLATION. This zone is defined as the range of A_1-A_2 intervals at which the A_2-A_3 interval is less than the A_1-A_1 interval and the A_1-A_3 interval is less than twice the A_1-A_1 interval (see Fig. 8-9).[28] The A_1-A_2 coupling intervals at which incomplete interpolation is first observed define the relative refractory period of the perinodal tissue. Some investigators refer to this as the sinus node refractory period. In this case, A_3 represents delay of A_1 exiting the sinus node, which has not been affected.[28] The A_1-A_2 coupling interval at which complete interpolation is observed probably defines the effective refractory period of the most peripheral of the perinodal tissue because the sinus impulse does not encounter refractory tissue on its exit from the sinus node. In this case, (A_1-A_2) + (A_2-A_3) = A_1-A_1, and sinus node entrance block is said to exist.

4. ZONE IV: ZONE OF REENTRY. This zone is defined as the range of A_1-A_2 intervals at which the A_2-A_3 interval is less than the A_1-A_1 interval and (A_1-A_2) + (A_2-A_3) is less than A_1-A_1, and the atrial activation sequence and P wave morphology are identical to sinus beats. The incidence of single beats of sinus node reentry is approximately 11% in the normal population.[29,30,35]

NARULA METHOD

The Narula method for measuring SACT is simpler than the Strauss technique. Instead of atrial premature stimulation, atrial pacing at a rate slightly faster (10 beats/min or more) than the sinus rate is used as A_2. It is assumed that such atrial pacing will depolarize the sinus node without significant overdrive suppression. The SACT is then calculated using the same formula as for the Strauss method. The Narula method is the quickest and easiest to perform, but it gives only SACT and does not provide information about the AV conduction system.[29,30,35]

KIRKORIAN-TOUBOUL METHOD

In contrast to the Strauss method, which uses progressively premature AESs delivered during NSR to evaluate SACT, the Kirkorian-Touboul method uses progressively premature AESs delivered following an eight-beat pacing train at a fixed rate. This method was designed to determine SACT independently of baseline sinus CL, which can normally be somewhat variable. It can have several advantages, especially for the study of drug effects at identical basic rates, but it is less widely used than the other methods.

SINOATRIAL CONDUCTION TIME IN PATIENTS WITH SINUS NODE DYSFUNCTION

The normal SACT is 45 to 125 milliseconds. There is a good correlation between direct and indirect measurements of SACT in a patient with or without SND. However, SACT is an insensitive indicator of SND, especially in patients with isolated sinus bradycardia. SACT is prolonged in only 40% of patients with SND, and more frequently (78%) in patients with sinoatrial exit block or bradycardia-tachycardia syndrome, or both.[28] In patients with sinus pauses, corrected SNRT is more commonly abnormal than SACT (80% versus 53%). SACT appears to be directly related to the baseline

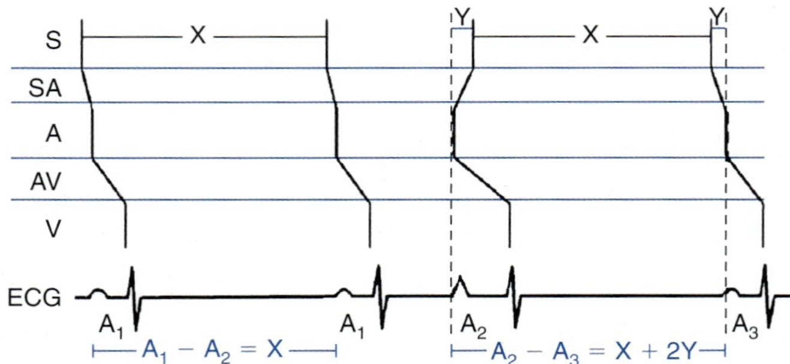

FIGURE 8-10 Calculation of sinoatrial conduction time (SACT) using the Strauss method. The baseline sinus cycle length (A_1-A_2) equals X. The third P wave represents an atrial extrastimulus (A_2) that reaches and discharges the sinoatrial (SA) node, which causes the next sinus cycle to begin at that time. Therefore, the A_2-A_3 interval = X + 2Y milliseconds, assuming no depression of sinus node automaticity. Consequently, SACT = Y = ([A_2-A_3] − [X])/2. AV = atrioventricular. *(From Olgin JE, Zipes DP: Specific arrhythmias: diagnosis and treatment. In Libby P, Bonow RO, Mann DL, Zipes DP, editors: Braunwald's heart disease: a textbook of cardiovascular medicine, ed 8, Philadelphia, 2008, Saunders, pp 869.)*

sinus CL, and the sinus node refractory period is directly related to the drive CL.[36]

Effects of Drugs

AUTONOMIC BLOCKADE (INTRINSIC HEART RATE). Autonomic blockade is the most commonly used pharmacological intervention for evaluation of SND, and it is used to determine the intrinsic heart rate (i.e., the rate independent of autonomic influences). Autonomic blockade is accomplished by administering atropine, 0.04 mg/kg, and propranolol, 0.2 mg/kg (or atenolol, 0.22 mg/kg). The resulting intrinsic heart rate represents sinus node rate without autonomic influences. The normal intrinsic heart rate is age-dependent and can be calculated using the following equation: intrinsic heart rate (beats/min) = 118.1 − (0.57 × age); normal values are ±14% for age younger than 45 years and ±18% for age older than 45 years. A low intrinsic heart rate is consistent with intrinsic SND. A normal intrinsic heart rate in a patient with known SND suggests extrinsic SND caused by abnormal autonomic regulation. Autonomic blockade with atropine and propranolol also results in shortening of corrected SNRT, as well as sinus CL and SACT.[36]

ATROPINE. The normal sinus node responses to atropine are an acceleration of heart rate to more than 90 beats/min and an increase over the baseline rate by 20% to 50%. Atropine-induced sinus rate acceleration is usually blunted in patients with intrinsic SND. Failure to increase the sinus rate to more than the predicted intrinsic heart rate following 0.04 mg/kg of atropine is diagnostic of impaired sinus node automaticity. Atropine (1 to 3 mg) markedly shortens SNRT and, in most cases, corrected SNRT. Atropine also abolishes the marked oscillations frequently observed following cessation of rapid pacing. Atropine occasionally results in the appearance of a junctional escape rhythm on cessation of pacing before sinus escape beats in normal subjects (especially in young men with borderline slow sinus rate) and, more commonly, in patients with SND. When this occurs, the junctional escape rhythm is usually transient (lasting only a few beats). Persistence of junctional rhythm and failure of the sinus rate to increase are indicative of SND.[28] Atropine, with or without propranolol, shortens SACT (unrelated to its effects on the sinus rate).[35,36]

PROPRANOLOL. Propranolol (0.1 mg/kg) produces a 12% to 22.5% increase in sinus CL in normal subjects. Patients with SND have a similar chronotropic response to propranolol, a finding suggesting that sympathetic tone or responsiveness, or both, is intact in most patients with SND. Propranolol increases SNRT by 160% in approximately 40% of patients with SND and increases SACT in most patients with SND. The mechanism of these effects is unclear. Effects are minimal in normal subjects.[28]

ISOPROTERENOL. Isoproterenol (1 to 3 mg/min) produces sinus acceleration of at least 25% in normal subjects. An impaired response to isoproterenol correlates well with a blunted chronotropic response to exercise observed in some patients with SND.[28]

DIGOXIN. Digoxin shortens SNRT or corrected SNRT, or both, in some patients with clinical SND, probably because of increased perinodal tissue refractoriness with consequent sinus node entrance block.[28]

VERAPAMIL AND DILTIAZEM. Verapamil and diltiazem have minimal effects on SNRT and SACT in normal persons. Effects in patients with SND have not been studied, but worsening of the SND is expected.[28]

ANTIARRHYTHMIC AGENTS. Procainamide, quinidine, mexiletine, dronedarone, and amiodarone can adversely affect sinus node function in patients with SND. Severe sinus bradycardia and sinus pauses are the most common problems encountered. Amiodarone is the worst offender and has even caused severe SND in patients without prior evidence of SND. In general, other drugs have minimal effects on sinus node function in normal persons.[29,36]

Principles of Management

Although pacing is the mainstay of treatment for symptomatic SND, identifying transient or reversible causes for SND is the first step in management. Withdrawal of any offending drugs, correction of any electrolyte abnormalities, and treatment of any extrinsic causes for SND (e.g., obstructive sleep apnea, hypothyroidism, hypoxemia) should be considered prior to permanent pacing therapy. Additionally, the specific clinical circumstance in which SND occurred should be analyzed to document potential heightened vagal tone as a cause of sinus bradycardia or pauses. Hypervagotonia as a cause of SND is often suspected by its transient nature and by the symptoms associated with specific clinical circumstances associated with surges in vagal tone, such as vomiting, coughing, gagging, endotracheal intubation, nasogastric tube placement, airway suctioning, and neurocardiogenic syncope. Vagally induced SND may respond to atropine, but it needs to be treated only if the patient is symptomatic.

Pharmacological therapy (atropine, isoproterenol) is effective only as a short-term emergency measure until pacing can be accomplished. Temporary percutaneous or transvenous pacing is necessary in patients with hemodynamically significant SND and bradycardia, to provide immediate stabilization prior to permanent pacemaker placement or to provide pacemaker support when the bradycardia is precipitated by what is presumed to be a transient event, such as electrolyte abnormality or drug toxicity.

Once all reversible causes are excluded or treated, correlation of symptoms with ECG evidence of SND is an essential part of the management strategy. Because of the episodic nature of symptomatic arrhythmias, ambulatory monitoring is often required. For the patient with asymptomatic bradycardia or sinus pauses, the long-term prognosis is generally benign, and no treatment is necessary. For symptomatic patients with SND, pacing is the mainstay of treatment (Table 8-1). SND is currently the most common reported diagnosis for pacemaker implantation, and it accounts for 40% to 60% of new pacemaker implants. For symptomatic

TABLE 8-1 Guidelines for Permanent Pacing in Sinus Node Dysfunction

Class I

- Sinus node dysfunction with documented symptomatic bradycardia, including frequent sinus pauses that produce symptoms
- Symptomatic chronotropic incompetence
- Symptomatic sinus bradycardia that results from required drug therapy for medical conditions

Class IIa

- Sinus node dysfunction with heart rate <40 beats/min when a clear association between significant symptoms consistent with bradycardia and the actual presence of bradycardia has not been documented
- Syncope of unexplained origin when clinically significant abnormalities of sinus node function are discovered or provoked in electrophysiological studies

Class IIb

- Minimally symptomatic patients with chronic heart rate <40 beats/min while awake

Class III

- Sinus node dysfunction in asymptomatic patients
- Sinus node dysfunction in patients whose symptoms suggestive of bradycardia have been clearly documented to occur in the absence of bradycardia
- Sinus node dysfunction with symptomatic bradycardia caused by nonessential drug therapy

From Epstein AE, DiMarco JP, Ellenbogen KA, et al: ACC/AHA/HRS 2008 guidelines for device-based therapy of cardiac rhythm abnormalities: a report of the American College of Cardiology/American Heart Association Task Force on Practice Guidelines (writing committee to revise the ACC/AHA/NASPE 2002 guideline update for implantation of cardiac pacemakers and antiarrhythmia devices). Developed in collaboration with the American Association for Thoracic Surgery and Society of Thoracic Surgeons. *Circulation* 117:e350-e408, 2008.

patients with tachycardia-bradycardia syndrome, pacing may be required to prevent symptomatic bradycardia and allow the use of drug therapy for control of the tachycardia (see Fig. 8-4). These patients are at increased risk for thromboembolism, and the issue of long-term anticoagulation for stroke prevention should be addressed.[25,26,29,30,37-39]

Once the decision to pace is made, choosing the optimal pacemaker prescription is essential. For those patients with SND who have normal AV conduction, a single-chamber atrial pacemaker is a reasonable consideration, although in the United States, a dual-chamber pacemaker is usually implanted, largely because of the 1% to 3% annual risk of developing AV block.[40] The use of rate-adaptive pacing is important for patients with chronotropic incompetence. For patients with intermittent atrial tachyarrhythmias, atrial pacing has been shown to decrease the incidence of AF and thromboembolism greatly, whereas patients who have only ventricular pacing have not seen a similar benefit.[24] Current pacemakers used to treat the tachycardia-bradycardia syndrome follow a special algorithm to switch from a DDD or DDDR mode of operation to a VVI, VVIR, DDI, or DDIR mode on sensing an atrial tachyarrhythmia, and back again to DDD or DDDR mode when a normal atrial rate is sensed. For patients with permanent AF, implantation of a single-chamber ventricular pacemaker is appropriate.[3,25,29,30]

REFERENCES

1. Rubart M, Zipes DP: Genesis of cardiac arrhythmias: electrophysiological considerations. In Zipes DP, Libby P, Bonow R, Braunwald E, editors: *Braunwald's heart disease: a textbook of cardiovascular medicine*, ed 7, Philadelphia, 2004, Saunders, pp 653–688.
2. Dobrzynski H, Boyett MR, Anderson RH: New insights into pacemaker activity: promoting understanding of sick sinus syndrome, *Circulation* 115:1921–1932, 2007.
3. Line D, Callans D: Sinus rhythm abnormalities. In Zipes DP, Jalife J, editors: *Cardiac electrophysiology: from cell to bedside*, ed 4, Philadelphia, 2004, Saunders, pp 479–484.
4. Sanchez-Quintana D, Cabrera JA, Farre J, et al: Sinus node revisited in the era of electroanatomical mapping and catheter ablation, *Heart* 91:189–194, 2005.
5. Lau D, Roberts-Thomson K, Sanders P: Sinus node revisited, *Curr Opin Cardiol*, 2010 November 22 [Epub ahead of print].
6. Basso C, Ho SY, Thiene G: Anatomical and histopathological characteristics of the conductive tissues of the heart. In Gussak I, Antzelevitch C, editors: *Electrical diseases of the heart: genetics, mechanisms, treatment, prevention*, London, 2008, Springer, pp 37–51.
7. Boullin J, Morgan JM: The development of cardiac rhythm, *Heart* 91:874–875, 2005.
8. Stiles MK, Brooks AG, Roberts-Thomson KC, et al: High-density mapping of the sinus node in humans: role of preferential pathways and the effect of remodeling, *J Cardiovasc Electrophysiol* 21:532–539, 2010.
9. Sanders P, Kistler PM, Morton JB, et al: Remodeling of sinus node function in patients with congestive heart failure: reduction in sinus node reserve, *Circulation* 110:897–903, 2004.
10. Kistler PM, Sanders P, Fynn SP, et al: Electrophysiologic and electroanatomic changes in the human atrium associated with age, *J Am Coll Cardiol* 44:109–116, 2004.
11. Walsh EP: Interventional electrophysiology in patients with congenital heart disease, *Circulation* 115:3224–3234, 2007.
12. Yeh YH, Burstein B, Qi XY, et al: Funny current downregulation and sinus node dysfunction associated with atrial tachyarrhythmia: a molecular basis for tachycardia-bradycardia syndrome, *Circulation* 119:1576–1585, 2009.
13. Joung B, Lin SF, Chen Z, et al: Mechanisms of sinoatrial node dysfunction in a canine model of pacing-induced atrial fibrillation, *Heart Rhythm* 7:88–95, 2010.
14. Sweeney MO, Bank AJ, Nsah E, et al: Minimizing ventricular pacing to reduce atrial fibrillation in sinus-node disease, *N Engl J Med* 357:1000–1008, 2007.
15. Mohler PJ, Anderson ME: New insights into genetic causes of sinus node disease and atrial fibrillation, *J Cardiovasc Electrophysiol* 19:516–518, 2008.
16. Lei M, Huang CL, Zhang Y: Genetic Na^+ channelopathies and sinus node dysfunction, *Prog Biophys Mol Biol* 98:171–178, 2008.
17. Lei M, Zhang H, Grace AA, Huang CL: SCN5A and sinoatrial node pacemaker function, *Cardiovasc Res* 74:356–365, 2007.
18. Nof E, Glikson M, Antzelevitch C: Genetics and sinus node dysfunction, *J Atr Fibrillation* 1:328–336, 2009.
19. Wolbrette D, Naccarelli G: Bradycardias: sinus nodal dysfunction and atrioventricular conduction disturbances. In Topol E, editor: *Textbook of cardiovascular medicine*, ed 3, Philadelphia, 2007, Lippincott Williams & Wilkins, pp 1038–1049.
20. Schuchert A, Wagner SM, Frost G, Meinertz T: Moderate exercise induces different autonomic modulations of sinus and AV node, *Pacing Clin Electrophysiol* 28:196–199, 2005.
21. Sakai Y, Imai S, Sato Y, et al: Clinical and electrophysiological characteristics of binodal disease, *Circ J* 70:1580–1584, 2006.
22. Brubaker PH, Kitzman DW: Prevalence and management of chronotropic incompetence in heart failure, *Curr Cardiol Rep* 9:229–235, 2007.
23. Kitzman DW: Exercise intolerance, *Prog Cardiovasc Dis* 47:367–379, 2005.
24. Ellenbogen KA: Pacing therapy for prevention of atrial fibrillation, *Heart Rhythm* 4(Suppl):S84–S87, 2007.
25. Sweeney M: Sinus node dysfunction. In Zipes D, Jalife J, editors: *Cardiac electrophysiology: from cell to bedside*, ed 4, Philadelphia, 2004, Saunders, pp 879–883.
26. Mangrum JM, DiMarco JP: The evaluation and management of bradycardia, *N Engl J Med* 342:703–709, 2000.
27. Maggi R, Menozzi C, Brignole M, et al: Cardioinhibitory carotid sinus hypersensitivity predicts an asystolic mechanism of spontaneous neurally mediated syncope, *Europace* 9:563–567, 2007.
28. Josephson ME: Sinus node function. In Josephson ME, editor: *Clinical cardiac electrophysiology*, ed 4, Philadelphia, 2008, Lippincott Williams & Wilkins, pp 69–92.
29. Miller JM, Zipes DP: Diagnosis of cardiac arrhythmias. In Zipes D, Libby P, Bonow R, Braunwald E, editors: *Braunwald's heart disease: a textbook of cardiovascular medicine*, ed 7, Philadelphia, 2004, Saunders, pp 697–712.
30. Benditt DG, Sakaguchi S, Lurie K, Lu F: Sinus node dysfunction. In Willerson J, Cohn J, Wellens HJ, Holmes D, editors: *Cardiovascular medicine*, New York, 2007, Springer, pp 1925–1941.
31. Hocini M, Sanders P, Deisenhofer I, et al: Reverse remodeling of sinus node function after catheter ablation of atrial fibrillation in patients with prolonged sinus pauses, *Circulation* 108:1172–1175, 2003.
32. Hadian D, Zipes DP, Olgin JE, Miller JM: Short-term rapid atrial pacing produces electrical remodeling of sinus node function in humans, *J Cardiovasc Electrophysiol* 13:584–586, 2002.
33. Disertori M, Marini M, Cristoforetti A, et al: Enormous bi-atrial enlargement in a persistent idiopathic atrial standstill, *Eur Heart J* 26:2276, 2005.
34. Fazelifar AF, Arya A, Haghjoo M, Sadr-Ameli MA: Familial atrial standstill in association with dilated cardiomyopathy, *Pacing Clin Electrophysiol* 28:1005–1008, 2005.
35. Krumerman A, Fisher JD: Electrophysiological testing. In Topol E, editor: *Textbook of cardiovascular medicine*, ed 3, Philadelphia, 2007, Lippincott Williams & Wilkins, pp 1012–1037.
36. Masood A: Techniques of electrophysiological evaluation. In Fuster V, Alexander R, O'Rourke R, editors: *Hurst's the heart*, ed 11, Columbus, Ohio, 2011, McGraw-Hill, pp 935–948.
37. Alboni P, Gianfranchi L, Brignole M: Treatment of persistent sinus bradycardia with intermittent symptoms: are guidelines clear? *Europace* 11:562–564, 2009.
38. Vardas PE, Auricchio A, Blanc JJ, et al: Guidelines for cardiac pacing and cardiac resynchronization therapy: the Task Force for Cardiac Pacing and Cardiac Resynchronization Therapy of the European Society of Cardiology. Developed in collaboration with the European Heart Rhythm Association, *Europace* 9:959–998, 2007.
39. Epstein AE, DiMarco JP, Ellenbogen KA, et al: ACC/AHA/HRS 2008 guidelines for device-based therapy of cardiac rhythm abnormalities: a report of the American College of Cardiology/American Heart Association Task Force on Practice Guidelines (writing committee to revise the ACC/AHA/NASPE 2002 guideline update for implantation of cardiac pacemakers and antiarrhythmia devices). Developed in collaboration with the American Association for Thoracic Surgery and Society of Thoracic Surgeons, *Circulation* 117:e350–e408, 2008.
40. Lamas GA, Lee KL, Sweeney MO, et al: Ventricular pacing or dual-chamber pacing for sinus-node dysfunction, *N Engl J Med* 346:1854–1862, 2002.

CHAPTER 9 Atrioventricular Conduction Abnormalities

General Considerations

Anatomy and Physiology of the Atrioventricular Junction

INTERNODAL AND INTRAATRIAL CONDUCTION

Evidence indicates the presence of preferential impulse propagation from the sinus node to the atrioventricular node (AVN)—that is, higher conduction velocity between the nodes in some parts of the atrium than in other parts. However, whether preferential internodal conduction is caused by fiber orientation, size, or geometry or by the presence of specialized preferentially conducting pathways located between the nodes has been controversial.[1-3]

Anatomical evidence suggests the presence of three intraatrial pathways. The anterior internodal pathway begins at the anterior margin of the sinus node and curves anteriorly around the superior vena cava (SVC) to enter the anterior interatrial band, called the Bachmann bundle. This band continues to the left atrium (LA), with the anterior internodal pathway entering the superior margin of the AVN. The Bachmann bundle is a large muscle bundle that appears to conduct the cardiac impulse preferentially from the right atrium (RA) to the LA. The middle internodal tract begins at the superior and posterior margins of the sinus node, travels behind the SVC to the crest of the interatrial septum, and descends in the interatrial septum to the superior margin of the AVN. The posterior internodal tract starts at the posterior margin of the sinus node and travels posteriorly around the SVC and along the crista terminalis to the eustachian ridge, and then into the interatrial septum above the coronary sinus (CS), where it joins the posterior portion of the AVN. Some fibers from all three pathways bypass the crest of the AVN and enter its more distal segment. These groups of internodal tissue are best referred to as *internodal atrial myocardium*, not tracts, because they do not appear to be histologically recognizable specialized tracts, only plain atrial myocardium. Detailed electroanatomical activation maps do not reveal more rapidly conducting tracts.

ATRIOVENTRICULAR NODE

The AVN is an interatrial structure, measuring approximately 5 mm long, 5 mm wide, and 0.8 mm thick in adults. The AVN is located beneath the RA endocardium at the apex of the triangle of Koch. The triangle of Koch is septal and constitutes the RA endocardial surface of the muscular AV septum. It is bordered anteriorly by the annulus of the septal leaflet of the tricuspid valve, posteriorly by the tendon of Todaro, and inferiorly by the orifice of the CS ostium (CS os) (see Fig. 17-1). The central fibrous body is composed of a thickened area of fibrous continuity between the leaflets of the mitral and aortic valves, termed the right fibrous trigone, together with the membranous component of the cardiac septum. The tendon of Todaro runs within the eustachian ridge and inserts into the central fibrous body; the annulus of the septal leaflet of the tricuspid valve crosses the membranous septum.[4-6]

The compact AVN lies anterior to the CS os and directly above the insertion of the septal leaflet of the tricuspid valve, where the tendon of Todaro merges with the central fibrous body. Slightly more anteriorly and superiorly is where the His bundle (HB) penetrates the AV junction through the central fibrous body and the posterior aspect of the membranous AV septum.[7] The compact node is adjacent to the central fibrous body on the right side but is uninsulated by fibrous tissue on its other sides, thus allowing contiguity with the atrial myocardium. Because the AV valves are not isoplanar (the attachment of the tricuspid valve into the most anterior part of the central body is a few millimeters apically relative to the mitral valve), the AVN lies just beneath the RA endocardium. When traced inferiorly, toward the base of the triangle of Koch, the compact AVN area separates into two extensions, usually with the artery supplying the AVN running between them. The prongs bifurcate toward the tricuspid and mitral annuli, respectively. The rightward posterior extensions have been implicated in the so-called slow pathway in AVN reentrant tachycardia (AVNRT) circuit.[4-6]

The normal AV junctional area can be divided into distinct regions: the transitional cell zone (which represents the approaches from the working atrial myocardium to the AVN), the compact AVN, and the penetrating part of the HB.[8] The AVN and perinodal area are composed of at least three electrophysiologically distinct cells: the atrionodal (AN), nodal (N), and nodal-His (NH) cells. The AN region corresponds to the cells in the transitional region that are activated shortly after the atrial cells. Transitional cells are histologically distinct from both the cells of the compact AVN and the working atrial myocytes, and they are not insulated from the surrounding myocardium, but tend to be separated from one another by thin fibrous strands. Transitional cells do not represent conducting tracts but a bridge funneling atrial depolarization into the compact AVN via discrete AVN inputs (approaches). Transitional cells approaches connect the working atrial myocardium from the left and right sides of the atrial septum to the left and right margins of the compact node, with wider extensions inferiorly and posteriorly between the compact node and the CS os and into the eustachian ridge. In humans and animals, two such inputs are commonly recognized in the right septal region: the anterior (superior) approaches, which travel from the anterior limbus of the fossa ovalis and merge with the AVN closer to the apex of the triangle of Koch; and the posterior (inferior) approaches, which are located in the inferoseptal RA and serve as a bridge with the atrial myocardium at the CS os. Although both inputs have traditionally been assumed to be RA structures, growing evidence supports the AV conduction apparatus as a transseptal structure that reaches both atria. A third, middle group of transitional cells has also been identified to account for the nodal connections with the septum and LA.[4-6]

The N region corresponds to the region where the transitional cells merge with midnodal cells. The N cells represent the most typical of the nodal cells, which are smaller than atrial myocytes, are closely grouped, and frequently are arranged in an interweaving fashion. The N cells in the compact AVN appear to be responsible for the major part of AV conduction delay and exhibit decremental properties in response to premature stimulation because of their slow rising and longer action potentials. Fast pathway conduction through the AVN apparently bypasses many of the N cells by transitional cells, whereas slow pathway conduction traverses the entire compact AVN. Importantly, the recovery of excitability after conduction of an impulse is faster for the slow pathway than for the fast pathway, for reasons that are unclear.[4]

The NH region corresponds to the lower nodal cells, connecting to the insulated penetrating portion of the HB. Sodium (Na^+) channel density is lower in the midnodal zone of the AVN than in the AN and NH cell zones, and the inward L-type calcium (Ca^{2+}) current is the basis of the upstroke of the N cell action potential. Therefore, conduction is slower through the compact AVN than the AN and NH cell zones.[9,10]

The AVN is the only normal electrical connection between the atria and the ventricles; the fibrous skeleton acts as an insulator to prevent electrical impulses from entering the ventricles by any other route. The main function of the AVN is modulation of atrial impulse transmission to the ventricles, thereby coordinating atrial and ventricular contractions. The AVN receives, slows down, and conveys atrial impulses to the ventricles. A primary function of the AVN is to limit the number of impulses conducted from the atria to the ventricles. This function is particularly important during fast atrial rates (e.g., during atrial fibrillation [AF] or atrial flutter), in which only a few impulses are conducted to the ventricles, and the remaining impulses are blocked in the AVN. Additionally, fibers in the lower part of the AVN can exhibit automatic impulse formation, and the AVN may serve as a subsidiary pacemaker.[5,6,9]

The AVN region is innervated by a rich supply of cholinergic and adrenergic fibers. Sympathetic stimulation shortens AVN conduction time and refractoriness, whereas vagal stimulation prolongs AVN conduction time and refractoriness. The negative dromotropic response of the AVN to vagal stimulation is mediated by activation of the inwardly rectifying potassium (K^+) current I_{KACh}, which results in hyperpolarization and action potential shortening of AVN cells, increased threshold of excitation, depression of action potential amplitude, and prolonged conduction time. The positive dromotropic effect of sympathetic stimulation arises as a consequence of activation of the L-type Ca^{2+} current.[7]

The blood supply to the AVN predominantly comes from a branch of the right coronary artery in 85% to 90% of patients and from the circumflex artery in 10% to 15%.

HIS BUNDLE

The HB connects with the distal part of the compact AVN and passes through the fibrous core of the central fibrous body in a leftward direction (away from the RA endocardium and toward the ventricular septum). The HB then continues through the annulus fibrosis (where it is called the nonbranching portion) as it penetrates the membranous septum, along the crest of the left side of the interventricular septum, for 1 to 2 cm and then divides into the right and left bundle branches.[4]

Proximal cells of the penetrating portion are heterogeneous and resemble those of the compact AVN; distal cells are larger, similar to cells in the proximal bundle branches and ventricular myocytes. The HB is insulated from the atrial myocardium by the membranous septum and from the ventricular myocardium by connective tissue of the central fibrous body, thus preventing atrial impulses from bypassing the AVN. The area of fibrous continuity between the aortic and mitral valves adjacent to the membranous septum marks the HB as viewed from the left ventricle (LV). Viewed from the aorta, the HB passes beneath the part of the membranous septum that adjoins the interleaflet fibrous triangle between the right and the noncoronary sinuses.[4]

The HB has a dual blood supply from branches of the anterior and posterior descending coronary arteries that makes the conduction system at this site less vulnerable to ischemic damage unless the ischemia is extensive.

The AVN and the HB region are innervated by a rich supply of cholinergic and adrenergic fibers, with a density exceeding that found in the ventricular myocardium. Although neither sympathetic stimulation nor vagal stimulation affects normal conduction in the HB, either can affect abnormal AV conduction.

Pathophysiology of Atrioventricular Block

Block or delay of a cardiac impulse can take place anywhere in the heart, or even within a single cell. AV block can be defined as a delay or interruption in the transmission of an impulse from the atria to the ventricles caused by an anatomical or functional impairment in the conduction system. The conduction disturbance can be transient or permanent.

CONGENITAL ATRIOVENTRICULAR BLOCK

Congenital complete AV block is thought to result from embryonic maldevelopment of the AVN (and, much less frequently, the His-Purkinje system [HPS]), mainly secondary to a lack of connection between the atria and the peripheral conduction system, with fatty replacement of the AVN and nodal approaches.[4] The incidence of congenital complete AV block varies from 1 in 15,000 to 1 in 22,000 live births. The defect usually occurs proximal to the HB, and QRS duration is shorter than 120 milliseconds.[11] Maternal lupus, caused by antibodies targeting intracellular ribonucleoproteins that cross the placenta to affect the fetal heart but not the maternal heart, is responsible for 60% to 90% of cases of congenital complete AV block.[12]

Approximately 50% of patients with congenital AV block have concurrent congenital heart disease (e.g., congenitally corrected transposition of the great vessels, AV discordance, ventricular septal defects, AV canal defect, tricuspid atresia, and Ebstein anomaly of the tricuspid valve).[13] The AV conduction system may be displaced if atrial and ventricular septa are malaligned, AV arrangements are discordant, or the heart is univentricular. Generally, if the AV conduction system is displaced, it will also tend to be more fragile and susceptible to degeneration, thus placing patients at greater risk for AV block.[14]

HEREDITARY PROGRESSIVE CARDIAC CONDUCTION DISEASE

Cardiac ion channelopathies have been described as a rare cause of familial forms of AV block. Mutations in the *SCN5A* gene (encoding the alpha-subunit of the cardiac Na^+ channel) and the *KCNJ2* gene (encoding the inward rectifier Kir2.1, a critical component of the cardiac inward K^+ rectifier current, I_{K1}) have been associated with AV block. Additionally, mutations in the *PRKAG2* gene (encoding the gamma$_2$ regulatory subunit of adenosine monophosphate–activated protein kinase) have been described in patients with Wolff-Parkinson-White syndrome and AV conduction block.[15,16]

ACQUIRED ATRIOVENTRICULAR BLOCK

DRUGS. Various drugs can impair conduction and cause AV block. Digoxin and beta blockers act indirectly on the AVN through their effects on the autonomic nervous system. Calcium channel blockers and other antiarrhythmic drugs, such as amiodarone and dronedarone, act directly to slow conduction in the AVN. Class I and III antiarrhythmic drugs can also affect conduction in the HPS that results in infranodal block. These effects, however, typically occur in patients with preexisting conduction abnormalities. Patients with a normal conduction system function rarely develop complete heart block as a result of using antiarrhythmic agents.[17]

ACUTE MYOCARDIAL INFARCTION. AV block occurs in 12% to 25% of all patients with acute myocardial infarction (MI);

first-degree AV block occurs in 2% to 12% second-degree AV block occurs in 3% to 10%, and third-degree AV block occurs in 3% to 7%. First-degree AV block and type 1 second-degree (Wenckebach) AV block occur more commonly in inferior MI, usually caused by increased vagal tone and generally associated with other signs of vagotonia, such as sinus bradycardia and responsiveness to atropine and catecholamine stimulation. Wenckebach AV block in the setting of acute inferior MI is usually transient (resolving within 48 to 72 hours of MI) and asymptomatic, and it rarely progresses to high-grade or complete AV block. Wenckebach AV block occurring later in the course of acute inferior MI is less responsive to atropine and probably is associated with ischemia of the AVN or the release of adenosine during acute MI. In this setting, Wenckebach AV block rarely progresses to more advanced block and commonly resolves within 2 to 3 days of onset. The site of conduction block is usually in the AVN.

Type 2 second-degree (Mobitz type II) AV block occurs in only 1% of patients with acute MI (more commonly in anterior than inferior MI) and has a worse prognosis than type 1 second-degree block. Type 2 second-degree AV block occurring during acute anterior MI is typically associated with HB or bundle branch ischemia or infarction and frequently progresses to complete heart block.

Complete AV block occurs in 8% to 13% of patients with acute MI. It can occur with anterior or inferior acute MI. In the setting of acute inferior MI, the site of the block is usually at the level of the AVN, and it results in a junctional escape rhythm with a narrow QRS complex and a rate of 40 to 60 beats/min. The block tends to be reversed by vagolytic drugs or catecholamines and usually resolves within several days. Development of complete AV block in the setting of acute anterior MI, however, is associated with a higher risk of ventricular tachycardia (VT) and ventricular fibrillation, hypotension, pulmonary edema, and in-hospital mortality. In this setting, the block is usually associated with ischemia or infarction of the HB or bundle branches and is less likely to be reversible. Complete AV block during acute anterior MI is often preceded by bundle branch block (BBB), fascicular block, or type 2 second-degree AV block. The escape rhythm usually originates from the bundle branch and Purkinje system, with a rate less than 40 beats/min and a wide QRS complex. In general, patients who develop transient or irreversible AV block are older and have a larger area of damage associated with their acute MI.[11,18]

CHRONIC ISCHEMIC HEART DISEASE. Chronic ischemic heart disease, with or without infarction, can result in persistent AV block secondary to fibrotic changes in the bifurcating HB and bundle branches. Transient AV block can occur during angina pectoris and Prinzmetal angina.

DEGENERATIVE DISEASES. Fibrosis and sclerosis of the conduction system are the most common causes of acquired conduction system disease. These disorders account for approximately half the cases of AV block and can be induced by several different conditions, which often cannot be distinguished clinically.

Progressive cardiac conduction disease (including Lev disease or Lenègre disease) manifests as progressive slowing of electrical conduction through the atria, AVN, HB, Purkinje fibers, and ventricles, accompanied by an age-related degenerative process, in which fibrosis affects only the cardiac conduction system. Complete AV block can develop and cause syncope or sudden death. Lev disease is a result of proximal bundle branch calcification or fibrosis and is often described as senile degeneration of the conduction system. It is postulated as a hastening of the aging process by hypertension and arteriosclerosis of the blood vessels supplying the conduction system. Lenègre disease is a sclerodegenerative process that occurs in a younger population and involves the more distal portions of the bundle branches. As noted, in heritable progressive cardiac conduction disease (referred to as hereditary Lenègre disease, progressive cardiac conduction disease, and familial AV block), conduction slowing may be attributed to loss-of-function mutations in *SCN5A*. Whether age-dependent fibrosis of the conduction system is a primary degenerative process in progressive cardiac conduction disease or a physiological process that is accelerated by Na^+ current (I_{Na}) reduction is still unknown.[16]

Calcification of the aortic or (less commonly) mitral valve annulus can extend to the nearby conduction system and produce AV block. As noted, the HB penetrates the central fibrous body adjacent to the fibrous continuity between the aortic and mitral valves that is the usual site of dystrophic calcification, and extension of calcification can directly involve the HB or the origin of the left bundle branch, or both.[4,11,18]

RHEUMATIC DISEASES. AV block can occur in association with collagen vascular diseases such as scleroderma, rheumatoid arthritis, Reiter syndrome, systemic lupus erythematosus, ankylosing spondylitis, and polymyositis. Polyarteritis nodosa and Wegener granulomatosis also can cause AV block.

INFILTRATIVE PROCESSES. Infiltrative cardiomyopathies such as amyloidosis, sarcoidosis, hemochromatosis, and tumors can be associated with AV block.

NEUROMYOPATHIES. AV conduction disturbance is usually the major cardiac manifestation of neuromuscular diseases, including Becker muscular dystrophy, peroneal muscular dystrophy, Kearns-Sayre syndrome, Erb dystrophy, and myotonic muscular dystrophy. AV block can be an important cause of mortality in such cases.[19]

INFECTIOUS DISEASES. Infective endocarditis (especially of the aortic valve) and myocarditis of various viral, bacterial, and parasitic causes (including Lyme disease, rheumatic fever, Chagas disease, tuberculosis, measles, and mumps) result in varying degrees of AV block. Complete AV block occurs in 3% of cases.[17] Lyme carditis is of particular importance because in most cases, AV block resolves completely within weeks.

IATROGENIC. Cardiac surgery can be complicated by varying degrees of AV block caused by trauma and ischemic damage to the conduction system. AV block is most frequently associated with aortic valve replacement; less commonly, it occurs following coronary artery bypass grafting.[20] Repair of congenital heart defects in the region of the conduction system, such as endocardial cushion malformations, ventricular septal defects, and tricuspid valve abnormalities, can lead to transient or persistent AV block.[13,21,22] The block is usually temporary and is thought to be secondary to postoperative local inflammation. However, AV block can appear years later, usually in patients who had transient block just after the operation.[23,24] Intracardiac catheter manipulation can inadvertently produce varying degrees of heart block, which is usually temporary. Alcohol septal ablation in patients with obstructive hypertrophic cardiomyopathy also can be complicated by AV block. Complete heart block can occur during right-sided heart catheterization in a patient with preexisting left BBB (LBBB) or during LV catheterization (LV angiography or ablation procedures) in a patient with preexisting right BBB (RBBB).[25] AV block can also complicate catheter ablation of AVNRT, bypass tracts and atrial tachycardias in the AVN vicinity, as well as VTs originating in the interventricular septum adjacent to the HB.[26]

VAGALLY MEDIATED ATRIOVENTRICULAR BLOCK. Vagally induced AV block can occur in otherwise normal patients, in those with cough or hiccups, and during swallowing or micturition when vagal discharge is enhanced.[27] Vagally mediated AV block occurs in the AVN, is associated with a narrow QRS complex, and is generally benign. The block is characteristically paroxysmal and is often associated with clearly visible sinus slowing on the ECG because the vagal surge can cause simultaneous sinus slowing and AVN block. Additionally, transient AV block can occur secondary to enhanced vagal tone caused by carotid sinus massage, hypersensitive carotid sinus syndrome, or neurocardiogenic syncope. AV block in athletes is typically type 1 second-degree block, probably an expression of hypervagotonia related to physical training, and it resolves after physical deconditioning. This form of AV block may or may not be associated with sinus bradycardia because the relative effects of sympathetic and parasympathetic systems on the AVN and sinus node can differ.

LONG QT SYNDROME. In long QT syndrome (LQTS) with a very long QT interval (e.g., in LQT2, LQT3, LQT8, and LQT9), functional block between the HB and ventricular muscle caused by prolonged ventricular refractoriness can lead to 2:1 AV block and severe bradycardia. Conduction abnormalities of the HPS, including PQ prolongation and RBBB or LBBB, occur in some patients with LQTS.

Clinical Presentation

Symptoms in patients with AV conduction abnormalities are generally caused by bradycardia and loss of AV synchrony. Individuals with first-degree AV block are usually asymptomatic; however, patients with marked prolongation of the PR interval (longer than 300 milliseconds) can experience symptoms similar to those with pacemaker syndrome caused by loss of AV synchrony and atrial contraction against closed AV valves. Additionally, in patients with LV dysfunction, severe first-degree AV block can cause worsening of heart failure symptoms.[28] Symptoms caused by more advanced AV block can range from exercise intolerance, easy fatigability, dyspnea on exertion, angina, mental status changes, dizziness, and near syncope to frank syncope.[11,18] In patients with paroxysmal or intermittent complete heart block, symptoms are episodic, and routine ECGs may not be diagnostic.

Congenital AV block can be apparent in utero or at birth; however, many individuals have few or no symptoms and reach their teens or young adulthood before the diagnosis is made. Because of the presence of reliable subsidiary HB pacemakers with adequate rates (especially in the presence of catecholamines), syncope is rare with congenital complete AVN block. Some patients become symptomatic only when aging produces chronotropic incompetence of the HB rhythm.[11,18]

Natural History of Atrioventricular Block

The natural history of patients with AV block depends on the underlying cardiac condition; however, the site of the block and the resulting rhythm disturbances themselves contribute to the prognosis. Patients with first-degree AV block have an excellent prognosis, even when the condition is associated with chronic bifascicular block, because the rate of progression to third-degree AV block is low.[28] Type 1 second-degree AV block is generally benign; however, when type 1 AV block occurs in association with bifascicular block, the risk of progression to complete heart block is significantly increased because of probable infranodal disease. Type 2 second-degree AV block, usually seen with BBB, carries a high risk of progression to advanced or complete AV block. The prognosis of 2:1 AV block depends on whether the site of block is within or below the AVN.[11]

The prognosis for patients with symptomatic acquired complete heart block is very poor in the absence of pacing, regardless of the extent of underlying heart disease. Once appropriate pacing therapy has been established, however, the prognosis depends on the underlying disease process.[17] Complete heart block secondary to anterior MI carries a poor prognosis because of the coexisting extensive infarction and pump failure. In contrast, complete heart block secondary to idiopathic fibrosis of the conduction system in the absence of additional cardiac disease carries a more benign prognosis.[11] AV block after valve surgery can recover; however, if conduction has not recovered by 48 hours after surgery, permanent pacing will likely be necessary.[29]

Congenital complete heart block generally carries a more favorable prognosis than the acquired form when it is not associated with underlying heart disease. Patients with concomitant structural heart disease, a wide QRS complex, LQTS, or complete heart block discovered at an early age are more likely to develop symptoms early and are at an increased risk for sudden death.

Diagnostic Evaluation of Atrioventricular Block

Because the prognosis and, in some cases, the treatment of AV block differ depending on whether the block is within the AVN or is infranodal, determining the site of block is important. In most cases, this can be achieved noninvasively.

ELECTROCARDIOGRAPHY

The QRS duration, PR interval, and ventricular rate on the surface ECG can provide important clues for localizing the level of AV block (see later).

AUTONOMIC MODULATION

Whereas the AVN is richly innervated and highly responsive to both sympathetic and vagal stimuli, the HPS is influenced minimally by the autonomic nervous system. Carotid sinus massage increases vagal tone and worsens second-degree AVN block, whereas exercise and atropine improve AVN conduction because of sympathetic stimulation or parasympatholysis, or both. In contrast, carotid sinus massage can improve second-degree infranodal block by slowing the sinus rate and allowing HPS refractoriness to recover. Also, exercise and atropine worsen infranodal block because of the enhanced function of the sinus node and AVN and, as a consequence, the increased rate of impulses conducted to the HPS without changing HPS refractoriness.[11,18]

EXERCISE TESTING

Vagolysis and increased sympathetic drive that occur with exercise enhance AVN conduction. Thus, patients with first-degree AV block can have shorter PR intervals during exercise, and patients with type 1 second-degree AV block can develop higher AV conduction ratios (e.g., 3:2 at rest becoming 6:5 during exercise).

Exercise testing can be a useful tool to help confirm the level of block in second- or third-degree AV block associated with a narrow or wide QRS complex. Patients with presumed type 1 block or congenital complete heart block and a normal QRS complex usually have an increased ventricular rate with exercise. On the other hand, patients with acquired complete heart block and a wide QRS complex usually show minimal or no increase in ventricular rate. Additionally, patients with 2:1 AV block in whom the site of conduction block is uncertain can benefit from exercise testing by observing whether the AV conduction ratio increases in a Wenckebach-like manner (e.g., to 3:2 or 4:3) or decreases (e.g., to 3:1 or 4:1). In the latter case, the increase in the sinus rate finds the HPS refractory, thus causing the higher degrees of block. This response is always abnormal, and it indicates intra-Hisian or infra-Hisian block, which requires permanent cardiac pacing.

ELECTROPHYSIOLOGICAL TESTING

Electrophysiological (EP) testing is usually not required for the diagnosis or treatment of AV block, because the previously described noninvasive measures are usually adequate. Nevertheless, EP testing can be of value in symptomatic patients in whom AV conduction abnormalities are suspected but cannot be documented or in patients with equivocal ECG findings.

Electrocardiographic Features

First-Degree Atrioventricular Block (Delay)

First-degree AV block manifests on the surface ECG as a PR interval longer than 200 milliseconds following a normally timed (nonpremature) P wave. All P waves are conducted, but with delay; each P wave is followed by a QRS complex with a constant, prolonged PR interval.

SITE OF BLOCK

The degree of PR interval prolongation and QRS duration can help predict the site of conduction delay. Very long (more than

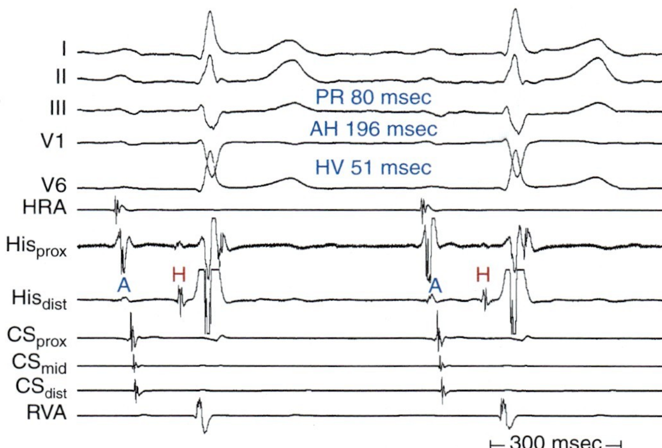

FIGURE 9-1 First-degree atrioventricular block caused by intranodal conduction delay, as indicated by the prolonged atrial–His bundle (AH) and normal PA and His bundle–ventricular (HV) intervals. CS_{dist} = distal coronary sinus; CS_{mid} = middle coronary sinus; CS_{prox} = proximal coronary sinus; His_{dist} = distal His bundle; His_{prox} = proximal His bundle; HRA = high right atrium; RVA = right ventricular apex.

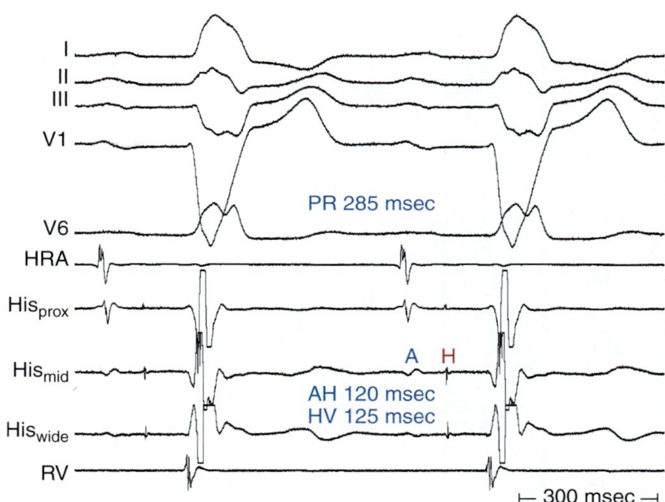

FIGURE 9-2 First-degree atrioventricular block secondary to His-Purkinje system disease. The atrial–His bundle (AH) interval is normal but the His bundle–ventricular (HV) interval is markedly prolonged and associated with complete left bundle branch block. His_{mid} = middle His bundle; His_{prox} = proximal His bundle; His_{wide} = wide His bundle; HRA = high right atrium; RV = right ventricle.

300 milliseconds) or highly variable PR intervals suggest involvement of the AVN. Normal QRS duration also suggests involvement of the AVN.[17,30]

ATRIOVENTRICULAR NODE. Although conduction delay can be anywhere along the AVN-HPS, the AVN is the most common site of delay (87% when the QRS complex is narrow, and more than 90% when the PR interval is longer than 300 milliseconds; Fig. 9-1).

HIS-PURKINJE SYSTEM. Intra-Hisian conduction delay or HPS disease can cause first-degree AV block. First-degree AV block in the presence of BBB is caused by infranodal conduction delay in 45% of cases. A combination of delay within the AVN and in the HPS must also be considered (Fig. 9-2).

ATRIUM. First-degree AV block caused by intraatrial or interatrial conduction delay is not uncommon. An LA enlargement pattern on the ECG (i.e., prolonged P wave duration) reflects the presence of interatrial conduction delay. RA enlargement can prolong the PR interval (Fig. 9-3). In certain cases of congenital structural heart disease, such as Ebstein anomaly of the tricuspid valve or endocardial cushion defects, intraatrial conduction delay can cause first-degree AV block.[31]

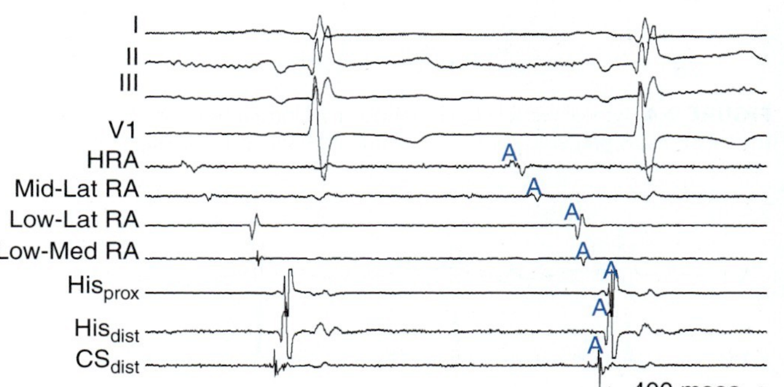

FIGURE 9-3 First-degree atrioventricular block caused by intraatrial conduction delay. The long PR interval (240 milliseconds) is caused by prolonged conduction in the right atrium (prolonged PA interval) in a patient who has undergone Fontan repair for complex congenital heart disease. CS_{dist} = distal coronary sinus; His_{dist} = distal His bundle; His_{prox} = proximal His bundle; HRA = high right atrium; Low-Lat RA = low lateral right atrium; Low-Med RA = low medial right atrium; Mid-Lat RA = middle lateral right atrium.

Second-Degree Atrioventricular Block

The term *second-degree AV block* is applied when intermittent failure of AV conduction is present (i.e., one or more atrial impulses that should be conducted fail to reach the ventricles). This term encompasses several conduction patterns. Types 1 and 2 AV block are ECG patterns that describe the behavior of the PR intervals (in sinus rhythm) in sequences (with at least two consecutively conducted PR intervals) in which a *single* P wave fails to conduct to the ventricles. The anatomical site of block should not be characterized as either type 1 or type 2 because type 1 and type 2 designations refer only to ECG patterns.[11]

TYPE 1 SECOND-DEGREE ATRIOVENTRICULAR BLOCK

Type 1 second-degree AV block (Wenckebach or Mobitz type I block) manifests on the surface ECG as progressive prolongation of the PR interval before failure of an atrial impulse to conduct to the ventricles. The PR interval immediately after the nonconducted P wave returns to its baseline value, and the sequence begins again.

The behavior of Wenckebach block can be simplified by relating it to an abnormally long relative refractory period of the AVN. In this setting, the rate of AVN conduction depends on the time that the impulse arrives at the AVN. The earlier it arrives at the AVN, the longer it takes to propagate through the AVN, and the longer the PR interval will be; the later it arrives, the shorter the conduction time, and the shorter the PR interval. Thus, Wenckebach periodicity develops because each successive atrial impulse arrives earlier and earlier in the relative refractory period of the AVN, thus resulting in longer and longer conduction delay and PR interval, until one impulse arrives during the absolute refractory period and fails to conduct, with a consequent ventricular pause. In other words, the shorter the RP interval is, the longer the PR interval will be; and the longer the RP interval is, the shorter the PR interval will be. This is referred to as RP-PR reciprocity or RP-dependent PR interval. Using this concept, it is easy to explain the behavior of the PR interval during the Wenckebach periodicity. The first atrial impulse conducting after the pause has an unusually long RP interval, whereas with the following atrial impulse, the RP interval dramatically shortens, thus resulting in prolongation of the PR interval. Although the following atrial impulses have shorter RP intervals, such shortening is not as dramatic, and consequently the progressive prolongation of the PR interval is of lesser degree. In other words, although each successive PR interval prolongs, it does so at a decreasing increment. So, for example, if the PR interval following the first conducted P wave

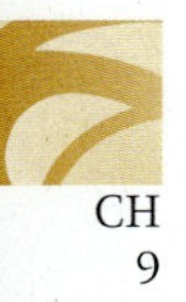

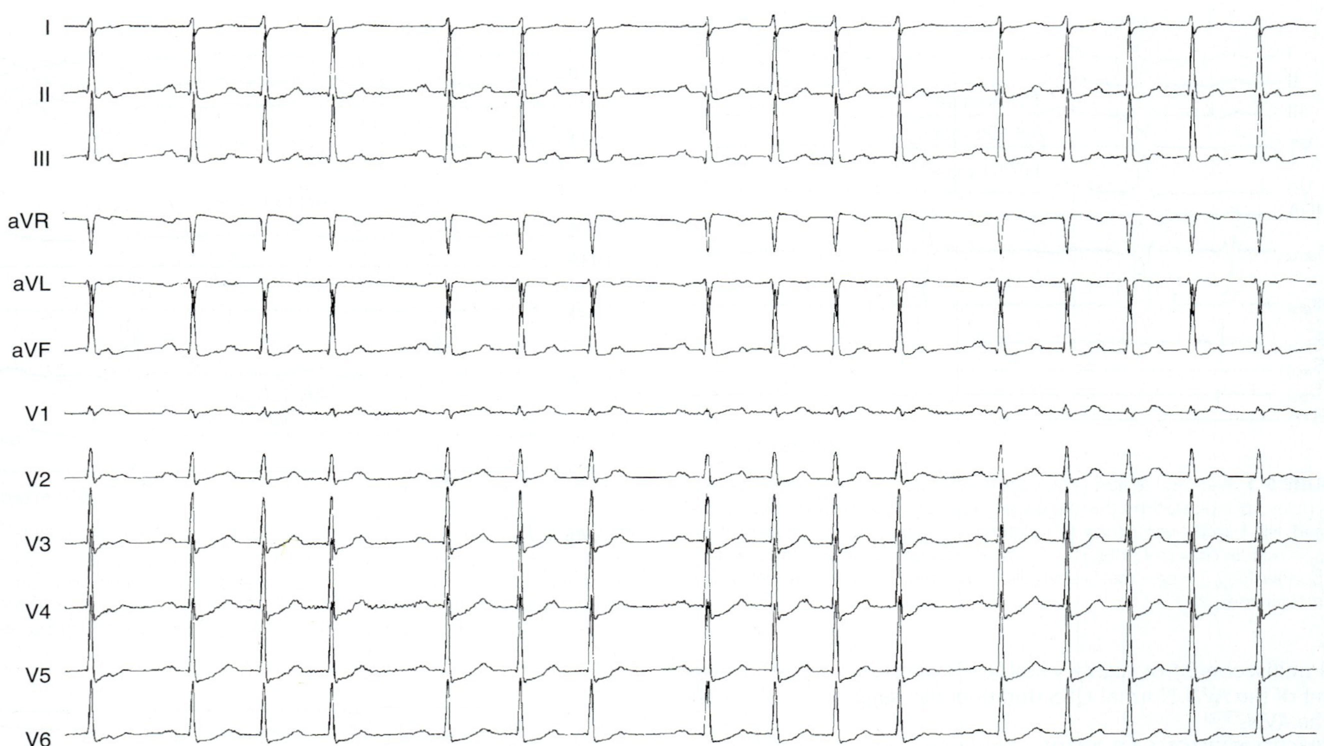

FIGURE 9-4 Typical Wenckebach periodicity. Normal sinus rhythm with type 1 second-degree atrioventricular block is characterized by progressive prolongation of the PR intervals preceding the nonconducted P wave and group beating.

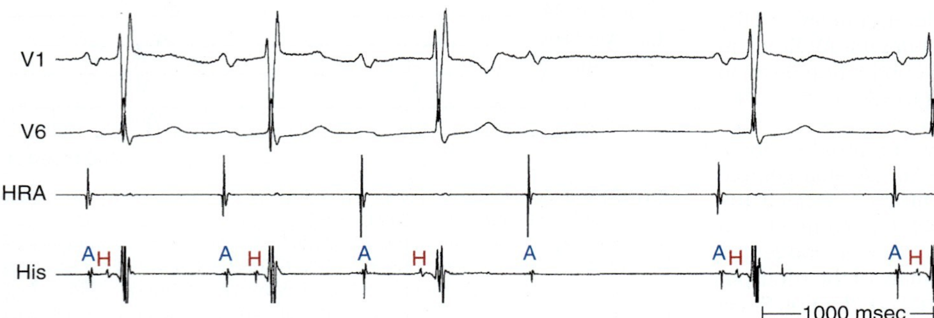

FIGURE 9-5 Atypical Wenckebach periodicity (type 1 second-degree atrioventricular [AV] block) caused by heightened vagal tone. Note the greatest increment occurs in the PR interval of the last conducted beat in the cycle and not in the second PR interval after the pause. Also note the slowing in the sinus rate coinciding with significant prolongation in the PR interval and then AV block, a finding suggesting that increased vagal tone is responsible for both slowing of the sinus rate and atrioventricular nodal block. HRA = high right atrium.

in the cycle increased by 100 milliseconds, the PR interval of the next beat would increase by 50 milliseconds, and so forth.

Features of typical Wenckebach periodicity include the following: (1) progressive lengthening of the PR interval throughout the Wenckebach cycle; (2) lengthening of the PR interval occurring at progressively decreasing increments and resulting in progressively shorter R-R intervals; (3) a pause between QRS complexes encompassing the nonconducted P wave that is less than the sum of R-R intervals of any two consecutively conducted beats; (4) shortening of the PR interval after block, compared with the PR interval just preceding the blocked cycle; and (5) group beating, which offers a footprint that identifies Wenckebach periodicity (Fig. 9-4). It is important to recognize that, during Wenckebach periodicity, the atrial impulse conducted to the ventricles is not always represented by the P wave that immediately precedes the QRS complex; the PR interval can be very long and exceed the P-P interval.[11,18]

Less than 50% of type 1 AV block cases follow this typical pattern. Typical Wenckebach periodicity is more frequently observed during pacing-induced AV block. Atypical patterns are more likely found with longer Wenckebach periods (more than 6:5). In patients with dual AVN physiology, Wenckebach cycles are almost always atypical; the greatest increment in the AH interval occurs when block occurs in the fast pathway, whichever beat this may be. Differentiating atypical from typical patterns is of little clinical significance. However, an atypical pattern can be misdiagnosed as type 2 second-degree AV block. Some possible atypical features of Wenckebach periodicity include the following: (1) the second (conducted) PR interval (after the pause) often fails to show the greatest increment, and the increment may actually increase for the PR interval of the last conducted beat in the cycle (Fig. 9-5); (2) very little incremental conduction delay and no discernible change in the duration of the PR intervals for a few beats just before termination of a sequence (this is seen most often during long Wenckebach cycles and in association with increased vagal tone, and is usually accompanied by slowing of the sinus rate; Fig. 9-6); (3) the PR interval can actually shorten and then lengthen in the middle of a Wenckebach sequence; and (4) a junctional escape beat can end the pause following a nonconducted P wave, resulting in an apparent shortening of the PR interval.[30,32]

AVN block usually can be reversed completely or partially by altering the autonomic tone (e.g., with atropine). However, these measures fail occasionally, especially in the presence of structural damage (congenital heart disease or inferior wall MI) to the AVN. In such cases, progression to complete AV block can occur, although such an event is more likely to occur with block in the HPS.

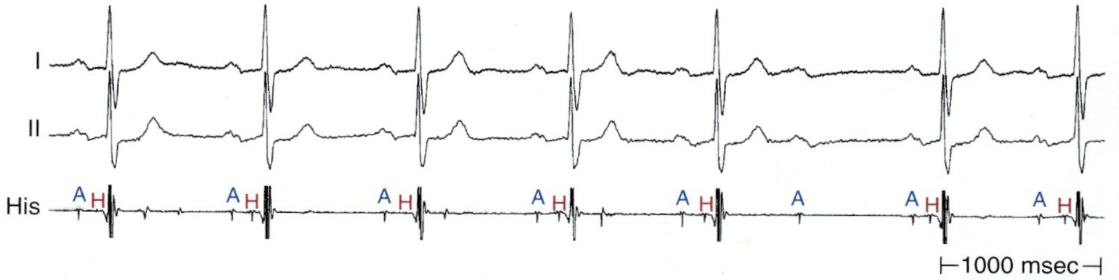

FIGURE 9-6 Atypical Wenckebach periodicity (type 1 second-degree atrioventricular block). Note the very small increments in the duration of the PR intervals for a few beats just before termination of a sequence. The first conducted P wave after the pause, however, is associated with obvious shortening of the PR interval.

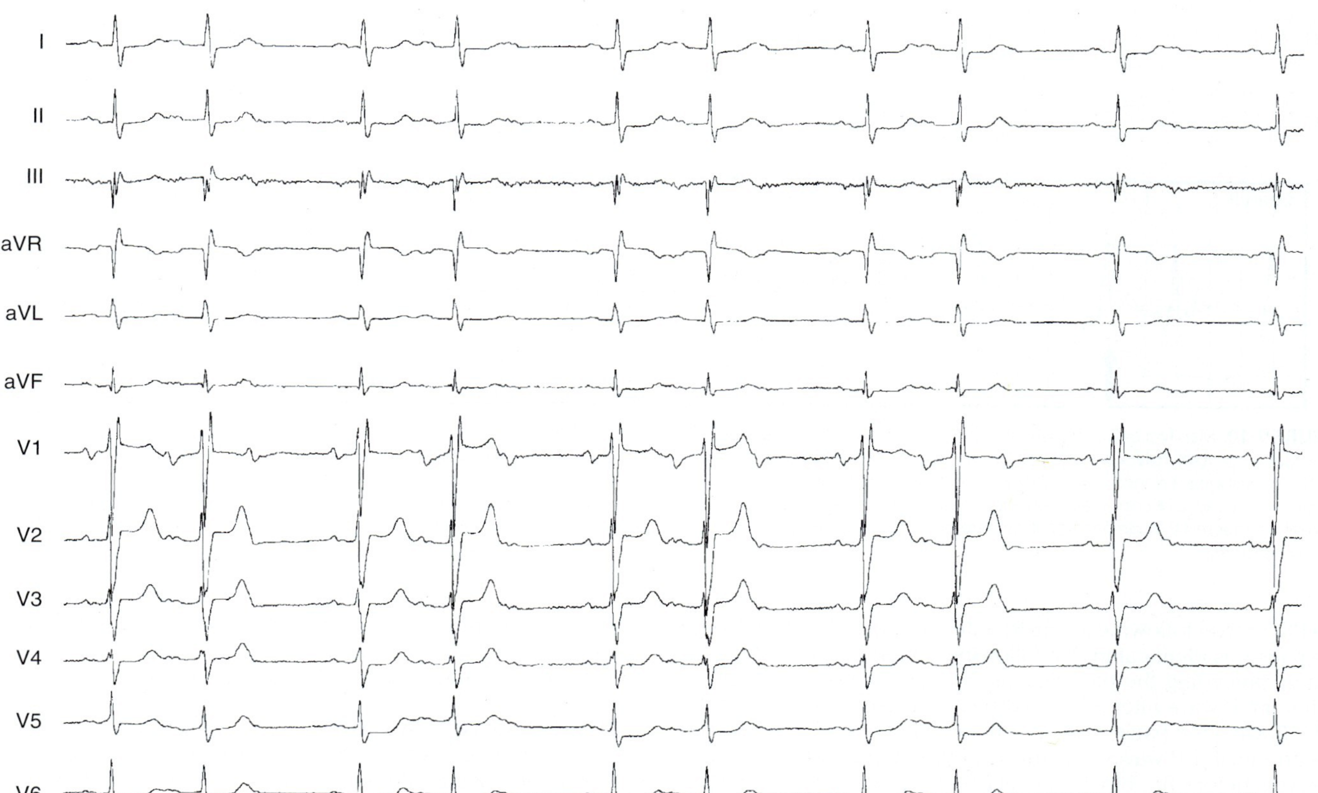

FIGURE 9-7 Typical Wenckebach periodicity. Normal sinus rhythm with type 1 second-degree atrioventricular (AV) block is characterized by progressive prolongation of the PR intervals preceding the nonconducted P wave and group beating. Despite the presence of His-Purkinje system disease (as indicated by incomplete right bundle branch block), Wenckebach AV block is more common in the atrioventricular node. At right, the last four P waves encountered 2:1 AV block.

Site of Block

The degree of PR interval prolongation and QRS duration can help predict the site of block. A normal QRS duration usually suggests AVN involvement, whereas the presence of BBB suggests (but does not prove) HPS involvement. Furthermore, short baseline PR interval and small PR interval increments preceding the block suggest HPS involvement.[30,32]

ATRIOVENTRICULAR NODE. Wenckebach block is almost always within the AVN (and rarely intra-Hisian) when a narrow QRS complex is present.

HIS-PURKINJE SYSTEM. When type 1 block is seen with the presence of BBB, the block is still more likely to be in the AVN (Fig. 9-7), but it can also be localized within or below the HPS (Fig. 9-8). In this setting, a very long PR interval is more consistent with AVN block.[30,32]

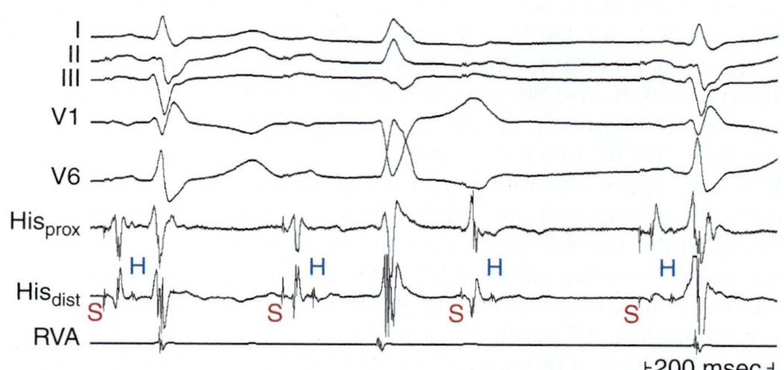

FIGURE 9-8 Infra-Hisian second-degree Wenckebach atrioventricular (AV) block. Atrial pacing in a patient with a normal prolonged atrial–His bundle (AH) interval but prolonged His bundle–ventricular (HV) interval and right bundle branch block (RBBB). On the second complex, the HV is dramatically prolonged and left bundle branch block is present, suggesting very slow conduction over the right bundle branch. With the third paced complex, AV block occurs below the His bundle recording, and on the fourth complex, conduction with RBBB resumes, suggesting a Wenckebach cycle in the His-Purkinje system. His_{dist} = distal His bundle; His_{prox} = proximal His bundle; RVA = right ventricular apex.

TYPE 2 SECOND-DEGREE ATRIOVENTRICULAR BLOCK

Type 2 second-degree (Mobitz type II) AV block is characterized on the surface ECG by a constant (normal or prolonged) PR interval of *all* conducted P waves, followed by sudden failure of a P wave to be conducted to the ventricles (Fig. 9-9). RP-PR reciprocity, the hallmark of type 1 block, is absent in type 2 block. Consequently,

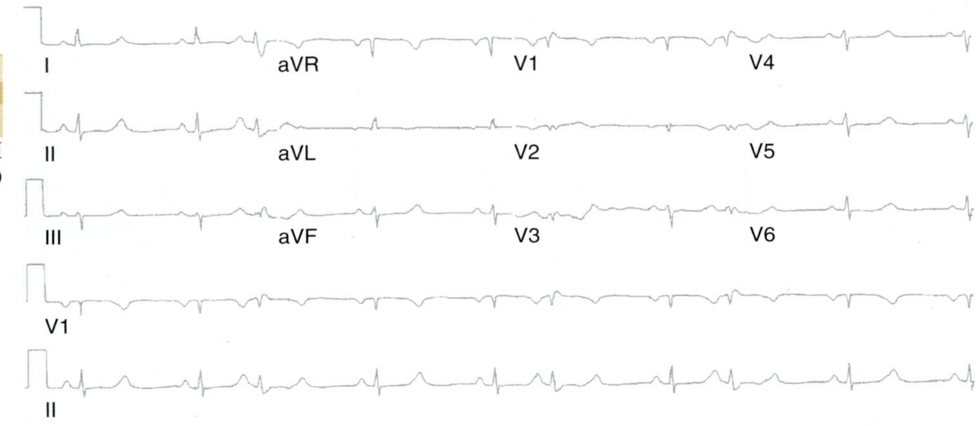

FIGURE 9-9 Second-degree atrioventricular block. Despite the presence of narrow QRS complexes, the site of block is likely intra-Hisian, as suggested by the short PR intervals on conducted beats and no increment in the PR intervals on 3:2 cycles. The P waves frequently are partially concealed within the preceding T waves (especially in view of the presence of long QT intervals) and are more obvious in lead V_3. Note slight QRS aberrancy resulting from the long-short RR intervals.

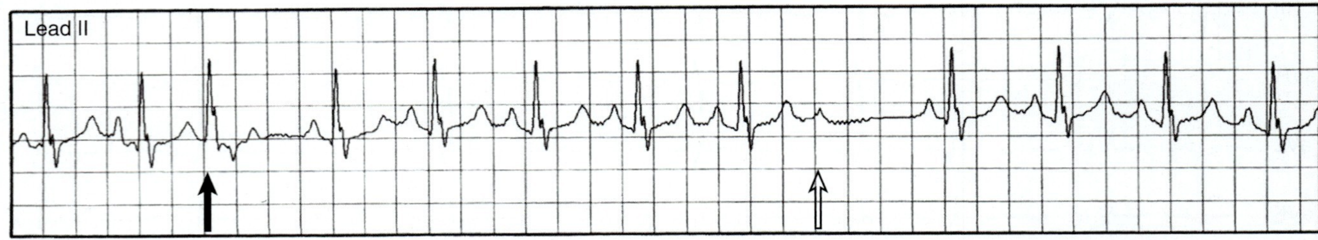

FIGURE 9-10 Manifest and concealed His bundle (junctional) extrasystoles. The lead II rhythm strip shows sinus rhythm with normal atrioventricular conduction, but the second complex (black arrow) is a normal QRS not preceded by a P wave (thus His extrasystole) with retrograde conduction (inverted P wave following QRS). The white arrow shows a nonconducted P wave that would ordinarily indicate Mobitz II block, but in this patient with known His extrasystoles, the P wave more likely fails to conduct because of concealed conduction into the atrioventricular node following a concealed His extrasystole (no resultant QRS or retrograde P wave). Note that the nonconducted P wave has a slightly different contour, perhaps as a result of fusion between the sinus P wave and retrograde atrial capture from the concealed His extrasystole.

the PR interval following a long RP interval (immediately following the pause) is identical to that following a short RP interval (immediately preceding the pause). Type 2 block cannot be diagnosed if the first P wave after a blocked beat is absent or if the PR interval following the pause is shorter than all the other PR intervals of the conducted P waves, regardless of the number of constant PR intervals before the block (see Fig. 9-6). The P-P intervals remain constant, and the pause encompassing the nonconducted P wave equals twice the P-P interval.

A true Mobitz type II AV block in conjunction with a narrow QRS complex is relatively rare and occurs without sinus slowing and without the characteristic Wenckebach sequences. Atypical forms of Wenckebach block with only minimal PR interval variation should be excluded (see Fig. 9-6). Apparent type 2 second-degree AV block can be observed under the influence of increased vagal tone during sleep, in which case Wenckebach block without discernible or measurable increments in the PR intervals is the actual diagnosis; sinus slowing with AV block essentially excludes Mobitz type II block.[30] When an apparent Mobitz type II–like pattern with a narrow QRS complex occurs with intermittent Wenckebach AV block sequences (as in Holter recordings), a true Mobitz type II block can be safely excluded because narrow QRS type 1 and type 2 second-degree AV blocks almost never coexist within the HB. Sustained advanced second-degree AV block is far more common in association with true Mobitz type II block than with Wenckebach block or its variant.

Apparent Mobitz type II AV block can also be caused by concealed junctional extrasystoles (confined to the specialized conduction system and not propagated to the myocardium) and junctional parasystole (Fig. 9-10). Exercise-induced second-degree AV block is most commonly infranodal and rarely is secondary to AVN disease or cardiac ischemia.

Site of Block

HIS-PURKINJE SYSTEM. Type 2 second-degree AV block is almost always below the AVN, occurring in the HB in approximately 30% of cases and in the bundle branches in the remainder. Infrequently, type 2 second-degree AV block is found with a narrow QRS complex and is caused by intra-Hisian block (Fig. 9-11; see Fig. 9-9).

ATRIOVENTRICULAR NODE. Type 2 second-degree AV block has not yet been convincingly demonstrated in the body of the AVN or the N zone. Although multiple reports have described the occurrence of type 2 second-degree AV block in the AVN, in each case either the block could have been localized to the HPS, rather than the AVN, or the block probably was atypical Wenckebach block.

2:1 ATRIOVENTRICULAR BLOCK

When only alternate beats are conducted, resulting in a 2:1 ratio, the PR interval is constant for the conducted beats, provided that the atrial rhythm is regular (Fig. 9-12). A 2:1 AV block cannot be classified as type 1 or type 2; using the term *type 1* to describe 2:1 AV block when the lesion is in the AVN or when there is evidence of decremental conduction and using the term *type 2* to describe 2:1 AV block when it is infranodal or when there is evidence of all-or-none conduction should be discouraged because this practice violates the well-accepted traditional definitions of types 1 and 2 block based on ECG patterns, not on the anatomical site of block. Both types 1 and 2 block can progress to a 2:1 AV block, and a 2:1 AV block can regress to type 1 or 2 block.

Site of Block

Fixed 2:1 AV block poses a diagnostic dilemma because it can be difficult to localize the site of block by the surface ECG alone. Several ECG features can help in the differential diagnosis:

1. 2:1 AV block associated with a narrow QRS complex is likely to be intranodal, whereas that associated with a wide QRS complex is likely to be infranodal, but it could still be at the level of the AVN (Fig. 9-13; see Fig. 9-12).

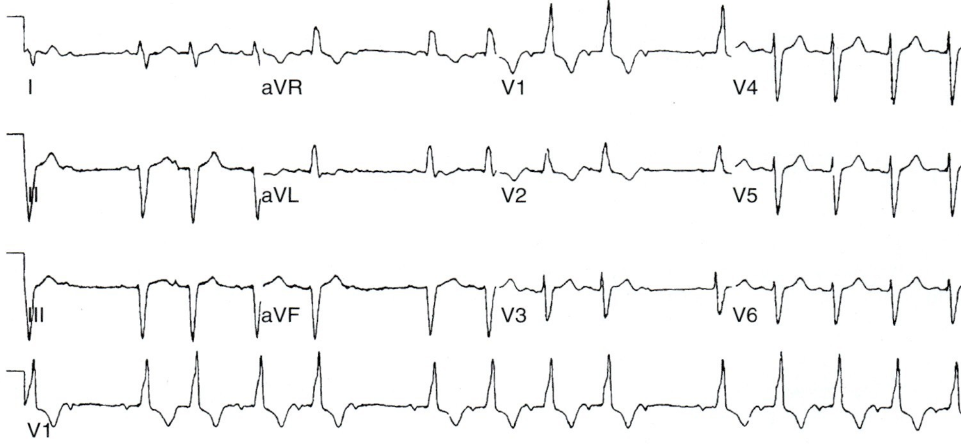

FIGURE 9-11 Second-degree infranodal atrioventricular block. Bifascicular block (right bundle branch block and left anterior fascicular block) and normal, constant PR intervals (196 milliseconds) are observed during conducted beats, consistent with infranodal block.

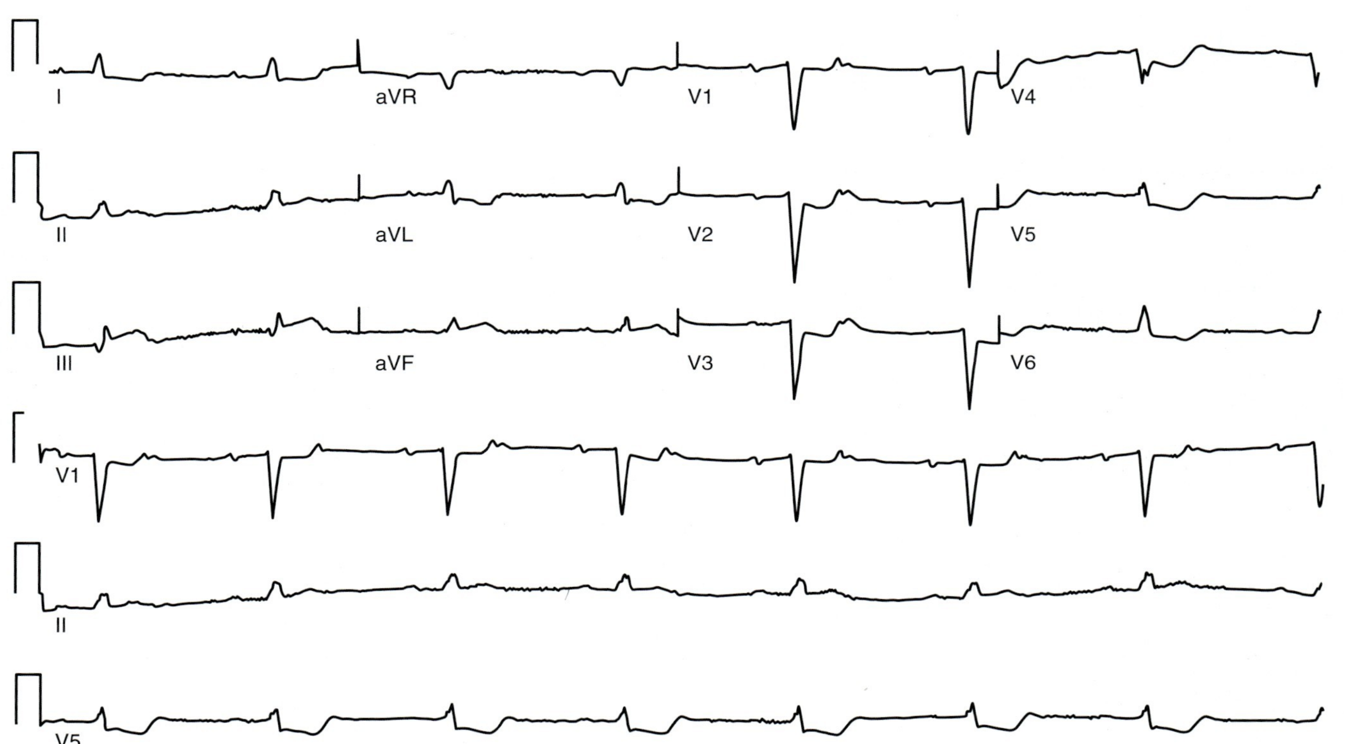

FIGURE 9-12 Second-degree 2:1 atrioventricular block. Note the long PR interval during conducted complexes and the narrow QRS complexes, suggesting intranodal block. The acute current of injury in the inferior leads is consistent with an acute inferior wall myocardial infarction and an intranodal site of AV conduction block.

2. Fixed 2:1 AV block with PR intervals shorter than 160 milliseconds suggests intra-Hisian or infra-Hisian block, whereas very long PR intervals (more than 300 milliseconds) suggest AVN block.
3. If the PR interval of all the conducted complexes is constant despite a varying RP interval, infranodal block is likely.
4. The presence of Wenckebach block before or after episodes of 2:1 AV block is highly suggestive of block at the AVN level (see Fig. 9-7).
5. Improvement of block with atropine or exercise suggests AVN block; however, the absence of such response does not exclude intranodal block.[30]

HIGH-GRADE ATRIOVENTRICULAR BLOCK

Failure of conduction of two or more consecutive P waves when AV synchrony is otherwise maintained is sometimes termed *high-grade AV block* or *advanced second-degree AV block* (Fig. 9-14).[17] This block must happen because of the existing block itself, and not because of retrograde concealment in the AVN or HPS resulting from junctional or ventricular escape complexes that prevent conduction.

Site of Block

The level of block can be at the AVN or the HPS. When high-degree AV block is caused by block in the AVN, QRS complexes of the conducted beats are usually narrow. Wenckebach periodicity can also be seen, and atropine administration produces lesser degrees of AV block. Features suggesting block in the HPS are conducted beats with BBB and no improvement in block with atropine.

Third-Degree (Complete) Atrioventricular Block

AV block is termed *complete* when all P waves fail to conduct, despite having ample opportunity for conduction. Therefore, if there is less than optimal opportunity for the AVN-HPS to conduct, it

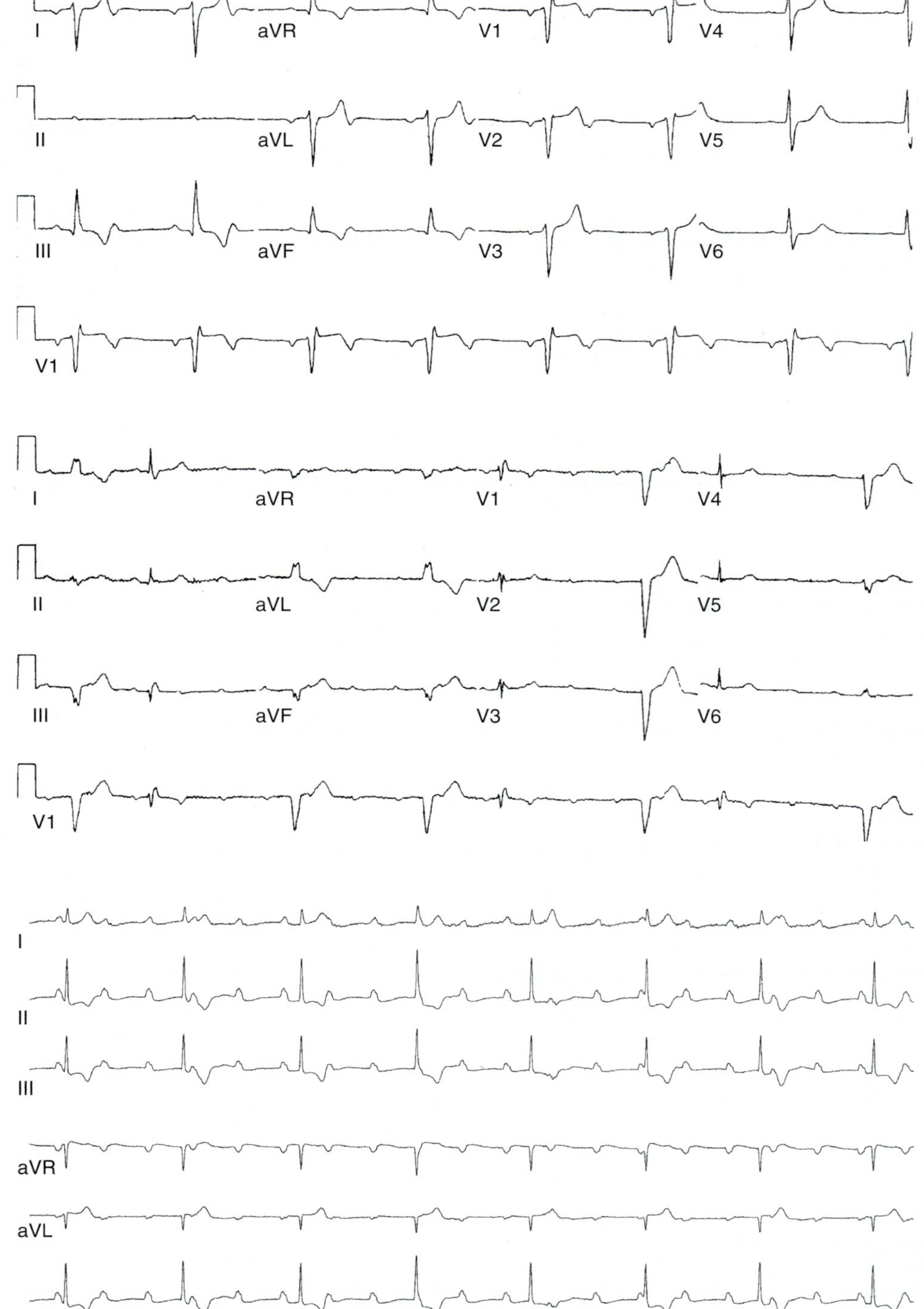

FIGURE 9-13 Second-degree 2:1 atrioventricular block. Note the short PR interval during conducted complexes and the wide QRS complexes, suggesting block in the His-Purkinje system.

FIGURE 9-14 High-grade atrioventricular block. Note that only three P waves conducted to the ventricle in the whole tracing. Conducted P waves were associated with normal PR intervals and right bundle branch block, a finding suggesting infranodal block. All other P waves were blocked, and ventricular escape rhythm with a left bundle branch block pattern is observed. Note that the block is not caused by retrograde concealment in the atrioventricular node or His-Purkinje system from the ventricular escape complexes because the conducted P waves occurred at a short cycle following the escape complexes.

FIGURE 9-15 Congenital third-degree atrioventricular (AV) block. Sinus rhythm with complete AV block and junctional escape rhythm with a narrow QRS are seen, consistent with intranodal block.

cannot be regarded as a failure if it does not conduct. Third-degree AV block is seen on the surface ECG as completely dissociated P waves and QRS complexes, each firing at its own pacemaker rate, with a continuously changing P-R relationship as the P waves march through all phases of the ventricular cycle in the presence of a regular ventricular rhythm (Fig. 9-15). Every possible chance for conduction is afforded, with the P waves occurring at every conceivable RP interval, but the atrial impulse is never conducted to the ventricles. The atrial rate is always faster than the ventricular rate (Fig. 9-16).[30,32]

SITE OF BLOCK

ATRIOVENTRICULAR NODE. Most cases of congenital third-degree AV block are localized to the AVN (see Fig. 9-15), as is transient AV block associated with acute inferior wall MI, beta blockers, calcium channel blockers, and digitalis toxicity. Complete AVN block is characterized by a junctional escape rhythm with a narrow QRS complex and a rate of 40 to 60 beats/min, which tends to increase with exercise or atropine. However, in 20% to 50% of patients with chronic AV block, a wide QRS escape rhythm may occur. Rhythms originating in the distal HB may have a wide QRS. Those rhythms are usually slower and nonresponsive to atropine.[30]

HIS-PURKINJE SYSTEM. Acquired complete heart block is usually associated with block in the HPS that results in an escape rhythm with a wide QRS complex with a rate of 20 to 40 beats/min (Fig. 9-17).

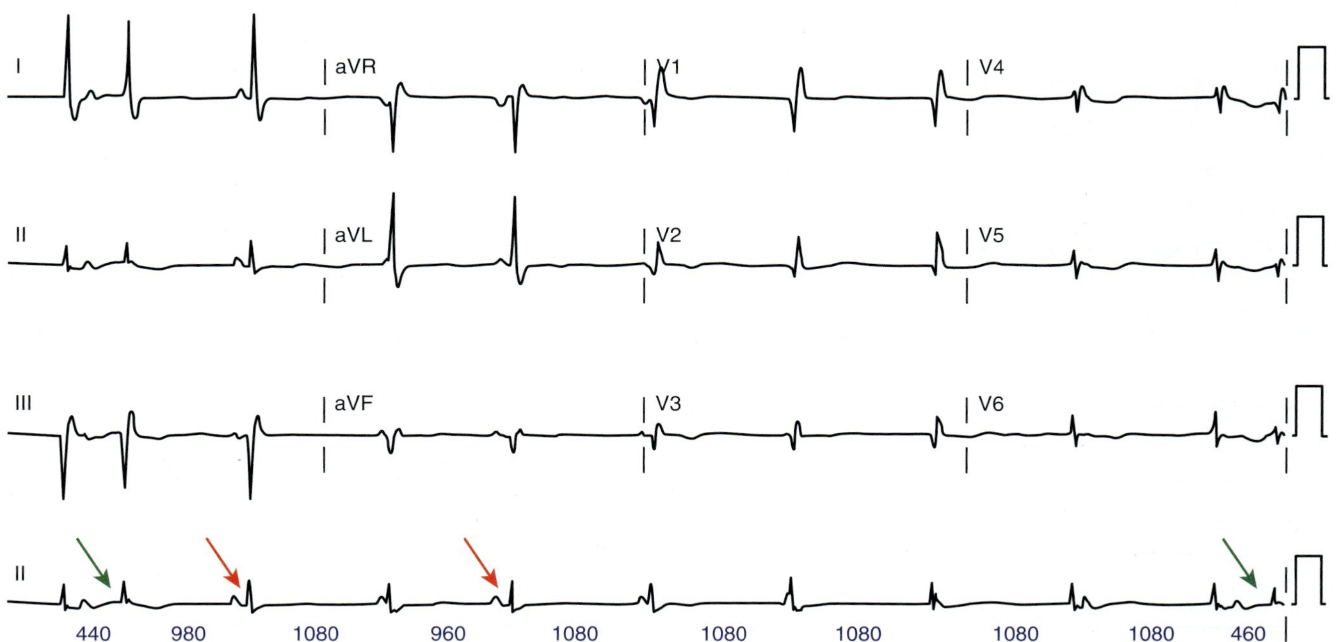

FIGURE 9-16 Surface ECG of sinus bradycardia at a cycle length (CL) of 1180 milliseconds and junctional escape rhythm at a shorter CL (1080 milliseconds). Junctional impulses fail to conduct retrogradely to the atrium, thus setting the stage for atrioventricular (AV) dissociation, which is observed during most of the recording. Note that no pathological AV block is present; failure of AV conduction of several sinus impulses occurred secondary to the physiological refractoriness of the atrioventricular node (AVN) and His bundle (HB) caused by retrograde concealment by the escape junctional impulses. However, whenever sinus P waves occurred at appropriate timings, they did conduct to the ventricle (red and green arrows) and elicited QRS complexes at CLs shorter than the expected junctional rhythm CL. Note that retrograde concealment of the junctional impulses occurred in the AVN and not just the HB, evident by the prolonged PR intervals of conducted sinus P waves when they closely follow the preceding QRS complex (green arrows). Numbers denote R-R intervals in milliseconds.

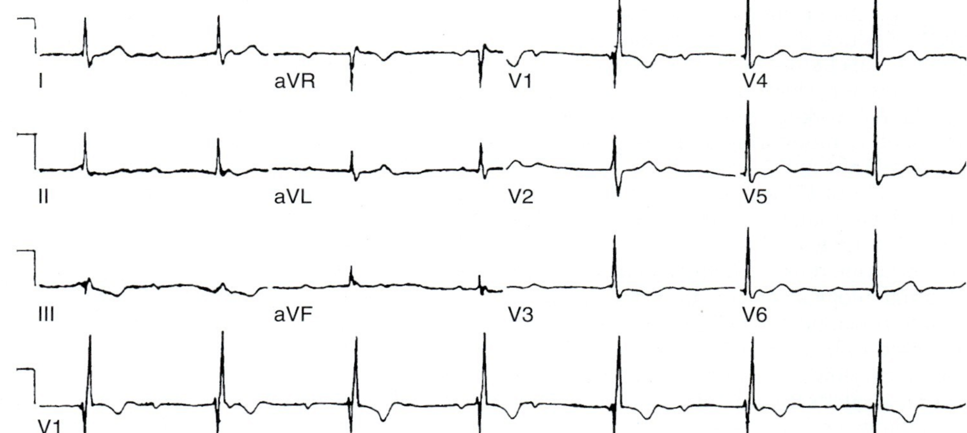

FIGURE 9-17 Complete infranodal atrioventricular (AV) block. Complete AV dissociation is observed, and all the P waves fail to conduct despite having ample opportunity for conduction. Note the slow ventricular escape rhythm with a wide QRS complex and a rate of 40 beats/min, consistent with block in the His-Purkinje system.

Paroxysmal Atrioventricular Block

CLINICAL PRESENTATION

Paroxysmal AV block is characterized by abrupt and sustained AV block in the absence of structural heart disease.[32] The block usually starts following a conducted or nonconducted premature atrial complex (PAC) or premature ventricular complex (PVC), and it persists until another PAC or PVC terminates it (Fig. 9-18). Episodes of AV block are commonly associated with prolonged periods of ventricular asystole (of unpredictable duration) precipitating presyncope or syncope or even sudden death. The natural history of paroxysmal AV block is unknown, and it is unclear whether paroxysmal AV block is reversible.[33]

MECHANISM

Paroxysmal AV block is a unique disorder of the HPS and is believed to be caused by local phase 4 block in the HB or in the bundle branches after a critical change in the H-H interval (see Chap. 10). During a long pause (prolonged diastolic period), the fibers of the often-diseased HPS spontaneously depolarize (membrane potential becomes less negative) and become less responsive to subsequent impulses as a result of Na^+ channel inactivation. Once such critical diastolic membrane potential is reached, conduction may no longer resume without an appropriately timed escape beat or premature beat (sinus or ectopic) that can reset the transmembrane potential to its maximal resting value. Nonetheless, this explanation is controversial because experimental data indicate that partial membrane depolarization can actually *improve* conduction, given that the voltage is closer to threshold. Prolongation of the H-H interval can result from spontaneous sinus rate slowing or post-extrasystolic pauses following atrial, ventricular, or His extrasystoles or tachycardia.[33]

DIAGNOSTIC EVALUATION

No specific or optimal tests exist to diagnose paroxysmal AV block. Patients with paroxysmal AV block may not have structural heart

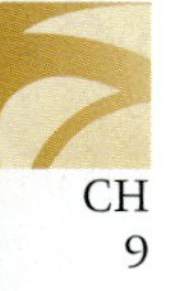

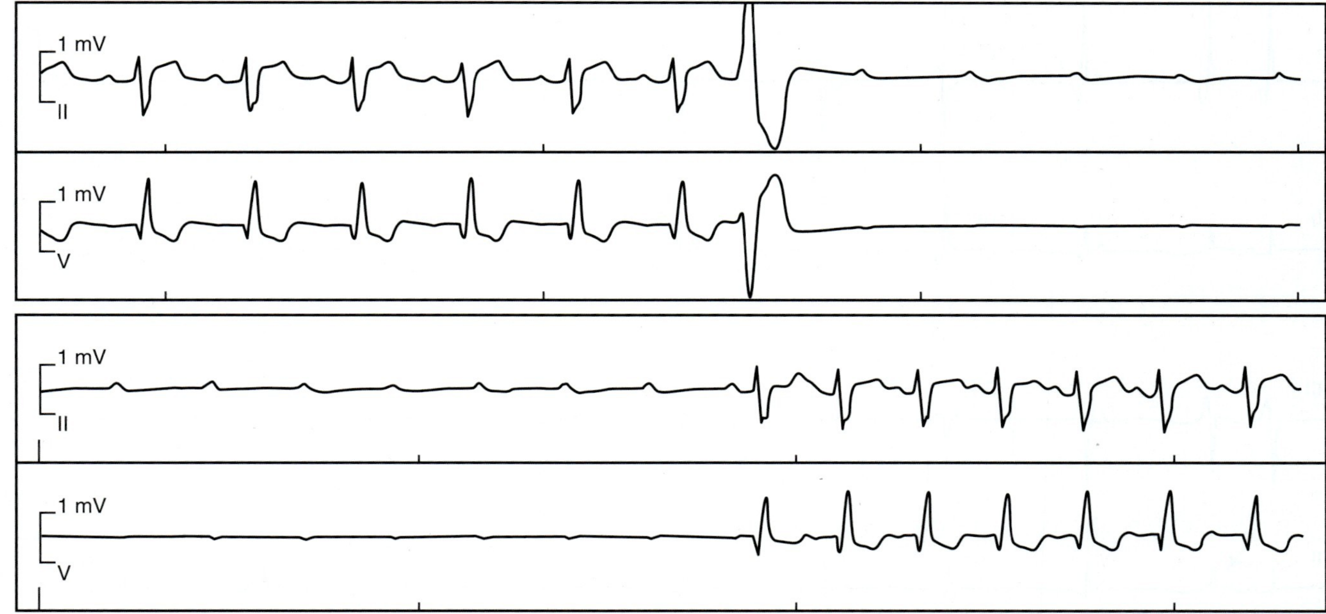

FIGURE 9-18 Paroxysmal atrioventricular block. Shown are two-channel rhythm strips during sinus rhythm with prolonged but stable PR interval and right bundle branch block. A premature ventricular complex (middle, top panel) occurs and is followed by a string of nonconducted P waves for almost 10 seconds until conduction resumes (at a faster sinus rate and with slightly shorter PR intervals, likely because of sympathetic discharge during the asystole).

disease at baseline, and conduction abnormalities may not be evident on resting ECGs. Although no established predictors for paroxysmal AV block exist, evidence of distal conduction disease at baseline is often present, with RBBB the most common finding. A positive response to carotid sinus massage for paroxysmal AV block includes P-P lengthening without changes in preceding PR intervals before heart block (in contrast to a vagally mediated AV block, for which the PR interval lengthens before the block). Additional workup for arrhythmogenic causes including long-term ambulatory monitoring or an implantable loop recorder can also be of value.[33,34]

The role of EP testing remains uncertain because there is no predictable marker for identifying patients at risk for paroxysmal AV block. EP testing is recommended when suspicion for arrhythmic syncope remains high despite a negative noninvasive workup. Pharmacological provocation (using ajmaline or procainamide) of infranodal block or HV lengthening (via stressing the HPS) was reported to be a potentially useful tool in diagnosing infra-Hisian AV block. However, a positive ajmaline or procainamide response simply suggests infranodal conduction disorder and is not specific for identifying patients at risk of developing paroxysmal AV block over other types of acquired AV block. Paroxysmal AV block may also be reproduced in an EP laboratory via critically timed atrial or ventricular extrastimulus and during rapid ventricular pacing. However, a negative EP study result does not exclude the diagnosis of paroxysmal AV block; at least 10% of patients with baseline BBB and syncope developed paroxysmal AV block during a 3-year follow-up despite a negative EP study result. Furthermore, a normal HV interval cannot rule out a risk for paroxysmal AV block. EP testing is therefore a specific test with low sensitivity, and it should be used in conjunction with supplementary clinical data obtained from personal history and ambulatory and implantable loop recordings.[33]

PAROXYSMAL VERSUS VAGAL ATRIOVENTRICULAR BLOCK

Distinction between paroxysmal AV block and the often benign and reversible vagal AV block (whereby an abrupt complete AV block can be precipitated by heightened vagal tone) has important prognostic and therapeutic implications. Unlike vagal AV block, paroxysmal AV block is often initiated by a PAC or PVC or by tachycardia, with sinus acceleration occurring during ventricular asystole without affecting the block (see Fig. 9-18). In contrast, a classic vagal effect on the conduction system includes gradual slowing of the sinus rate and AV conduction (first-degree or Wenckebach block), occasionally followed by sinus arrest or complete AV block (although a more prominent AV response with sudden block can also occur with heightened vagal tone). Subsequently, the sinus rate continues to slow down during ventricular asystole, followed by gradual resumption of AV conduction and sinus acceleration. Additionally, the clinical history, such as during micturition and phlebotomy, among others, can be highly suggestive of heightened vagal tone.[33,34]

Electrophysiological Testing

Role of Electrophysiological Testing

ECG diagnosis of AV block is usually adequate for deciding subsequent treatment. Once symptoms and AV block are correlated with ECG findings, further documentation by invasive studies is not required unless additional information is needed. Similarly, asymptomatic patients with transient Wenckebach block associated with increased vagal tone should not undergo EP testing.

Nevertheless, EP testing can help diagnose an equivocal ECG pattern or delineate the site of conduction abnormality, if that is required for decision making. EP testing is indicated in a patient with suspected high-grade AV block as the cause of syncope or presyncope when documentation cannot be obtained noninvasively. Similarly, in patients with coronary artery disease, it can be unclear whether symptoms are secondary to AV block or VT; therefore, EP testing can be useful in establishing the diagnosis. Some patients with known second- or third-degree block can benefit from an invasive study to localize the site of AV block to help determine therapy or assess prognosis.[30,32]

Normal Atrioventricular Conduction

The normal PR interval is 120 to 200 milliseconds. This interval reflects the conduction time from the high RA to the point of ventricular activation (i.e., QRS onset), and it includes activation of the

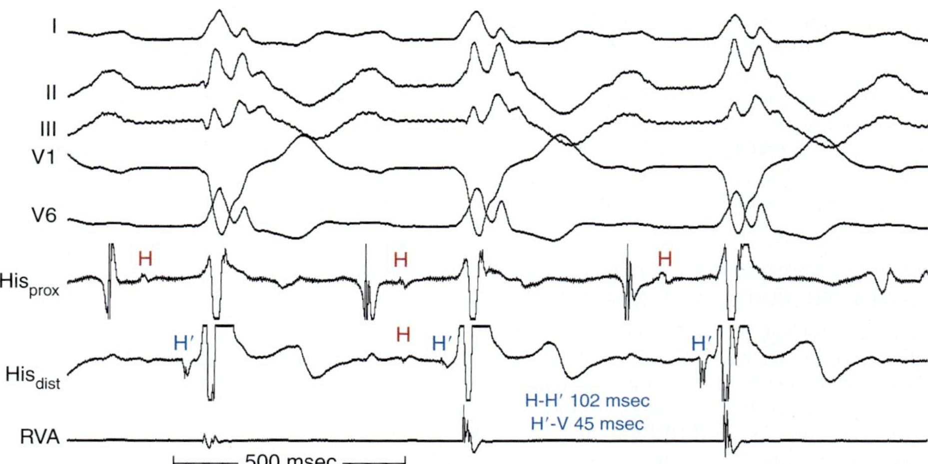

FIGURE 9-19 Split His potentials in a patient with cardiomyopathy and left bundle branch block. Recording only the distal His signal (H′) would give the false impression of normal infranodal conduction (H′V = 42 milliseconds). His_{dist} = distal His bundle; His_{prox} = proximal His bundle; RVA = right ventricular apex.

atrium, AVN, HB, bundle branches and fascicles, and terminal Purkinje fibers. To measure the different components of the conduction system contained in the PR interval, intracardiac tracings from the high RA and HB region are required (see Fig. 4-19).

The PA interval, measured from the high RA electrogram to the low RA deflection in the HB recording, gives an indirect approximation of the intraatrial conduction time. The normal PA interval is 20 to 60 milliseconds.

The atrial-HB (AH) interval is measured from the first rapid deflection of the atrial deflection in the HB recording to the first evidence of HB depolarization in the HB recording. The AH interval is an approximation of AVN conduction time because it represents conduction time from the low RA at the interatrial septum through the AVN to the HB. The AH interval has a wide range in normal subjects (50 to 120 milliseconds) and is markedly influenced by the autonomic tone.

His potential duration reflects conduction through the short length of the HB that penetrates the fibrous septum. Disturbances of the HB conduction can manifest as fractionation, prolongation (more than 30 milliseconds), or splitting of the His potential.

The HB-ventricular (HV) interval is measured from the onset of the His potential to the onset of the earliest registered surface or intracardiac ventricular activation, and it represents conduction time from the proximal HB through the distal HPS to the ventricular myocardium. The most proximal electrodes displaying the His potential should be chosen, and a large atrial electrogram should accompany the proximal His potential. The HV interval is not significantly affected by the autonomic tone, and it usually remains stable. The range of HV intervals in normal subjects is narrow, 35 to 55 milliseconds.

Localization of the Site of Atrioventricular Block

EP testing allows analysis of the HB electrogram, as well as providing atrial and ventricular pacing to uncover conduction abnormalities. A markedly prolonged HV interval (100 milliseconds or longer) is associated with a high incidence of progression to complete heart block. In addition, a His potential 30 milliseconds or longer in duration or that is frankly split into two deflections is indicative of intra-Hisian conduction delay.

When the His potential is recorded during atrial pacing at progressively shorter cycle lengths (CLs), the AH interval normally gradually lengthens until Wenckebach block develops. The HV interval normally remains constant despite different pacing rates. Abnormal AVN conduction produces Wenckebach block at slower atrial pacing rates than what is normally seen (i.e., at a pacing CL longer than 500 milliseconds). To determine whether AVN disease is truly present or whether AVN conduction is just under the influence of excessive vagal tone, atropine or isoproterenol can be administered to evaluate for improvement in conduction. Infranodal block is present when the atrial deflection is followed by the His potential but no ventricular depolarization is seen. Block below the HB is abnormal unless it is associated with short pacing CLs (350 milliseconds or less). Block in the HB can be masked by prolonged AVN conduction time or refractoriness. When block in the AVN develops at slow pacing rate, atropine can be administered to improve AVN conduction and allow evaluation of the HPS at faster pacing rates.

SITE OF FIRST-DEGREE ATRIOVENTRICULAR BLOCK

ATRIOVENTRICULAR NODE. An AH interval longer than 130 milliseconds with a normal HV interval indicates intranodal conduction delay (see Fig. 9-1). Dual AVN physiology can produce transient, abrupt, or alternating first-degree block caused by block in the fast AVN pathway and conduction down the slow pathway. The change in the PR interval seen on the surface ECG corresponds to a jump in the AH interval viewed on the HB electrogram.[30]

HIS-PURKINJE SYSTEM. As long as at least one fascicle conducts normally, the HV interval should not exceed 55 milliseconds (or 60 milliseconds in the presence of LBBB). A prolonged HV interval (more than 55 to 60 milliseconds) with or without prolonged His potential duration (more than 30 milliseconds) or a split His potential is diagnostic for HPS disease, even in the presence of a normal PR interval (Fig. 9-19; see Fig. 9-2). A prolonged HV interval is almost always associated with an abnormal QRS because the impairment of intra-Hisian conduction is not homogeneous. Most patients have an HV interval of 60 to 100 milliseconds, and occasionally more than 100 milliseconds. With pure intra-Hisian conduction delay, the atrial-to-proximal His (AH) interval and the distal His-to-ventricular (H′-V) interval are normal, whereas the duration of the His potential is longer than 30 milliseconds, with a notched, fragmented, or split His potential. In this case, verification of the origin of the "split H" from the HB (and not part of the atrial or ventricular electrograms) is critical. This can be achieved by dissociation of the His potential from atrial activation with atrial pacing, adenosine, or vagal stimulation and dissociation of the His potential from ventricular activation by documenting that the HV interval is longer than 30 milliseconds.[30]

ATRIUM. A prolonged PA interval with normal AH and HV intervals indicates intraatrial conduction delay (see Fig. 9-3).

SITE OF TYPE 1 SECOND-DEGREE ATRIOVENTRICULAR BLOCK

ATRIOVENTRICULAR NODE. Wenckebach block in the AVN is characterized by progressive prolongation of the AH interval, until an atrial deflection is not followed by His and ventricular deflections (see Figs. 9-5 and 9-6).

HIS BUNDLE. A prolonged His potential duration or a split His potential is indicative of intra-Hisian disease. Intra-Hisian Wenckebach block can occur between the two His deflections, characterized by progressive conduction delay until the first His deflection is not followed by the second one.

BUNDLE BRANCHES. In Wenckebach AV block secondary to block below the HB, progressive prolongation of the HV interval is followed by a His deflection without an associated ventricular activation (see Fig. 9-8).

SITE OF TYPE 2 SECOND-DEGREE ATRIOVENTRICULAR BLOCK (MOBITZ TYPE II BLOCK)

HIS-PURKINJE SYSTEM. The blocked cycle features atrial and HB deflections without ventricular depolarization (Fig. 9-20). The conducted beats usually show evidence of infranodal conduction system disease, with a prolonged HV interval, or even a split His potential, and BBB. Multilevel AV block (intranodal and infranodal) can also occur, especially during rapid atrial tachycardias or atrial pacing. Typically, infranodal AV block occurs in the presence of prolonged HPS refractoriness caused by antiarrhythmic agents or during Wenckebach cycles in the AVN (Fig. 9-21).

SITE OF THIRD-DEGREE (COMPLETE) ATRIOVENTRICULAR BLOCK

ATRIOVENTRICULAR NODE. Complete heart block at the AVN level is usually seen on the intracardiac tracings as His potentials consistently preceding each ventricular electrogram. The atrial electrograms are dissociated from the HV complexes (Fig. 9-22). Most often, the escape rhythm originates in the HB (with normal QRS preceded by a His potential and normal HV interval); however, in 20% to 50% of patients with chronic AV block, a wide QRS escape rhythm can occur. Rhythms originating in the distal HB can have a QRS preceded by a retrograde His potential or no His potential at all. Those rhythms are usually slower and nonresponsive to atropine. The stability of the HB rhythm can be assessed by noting the effects of overdrive suppression produced by ventricular pacing (in a manner analogous to testing sinus node function); prolonged pauses (i.e., the lack of HB escapes) herald failure of the escape rhythm.[30]

HIS-PURKINJE SYSTEM. The intracardiac electrogram shows HB deflections consistently following atrial electrograms, but ventricular depolarizations are completely dissociated from the AH complexes. Block below the HB is thus demonstrated.[17,32]

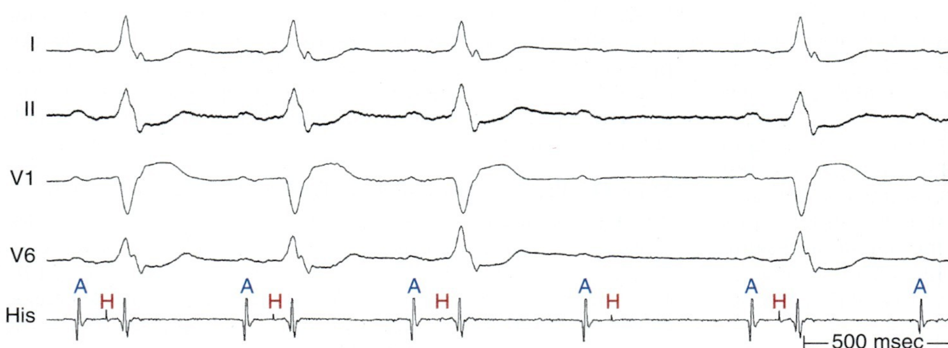

FIGURE 9-20 Type 2 second-degree (Mobitz type II) atrioventricular (AV) block. Sinus rhythm is observed with a wide QRS complex. The PR interval of all conducted P waves is constant and slightly prolonged (224 milliseconds). The fourth P wave fails to conduct to the ventricle but is followed by a His potential, suggesting that the level of AV block is infra-Hisian.

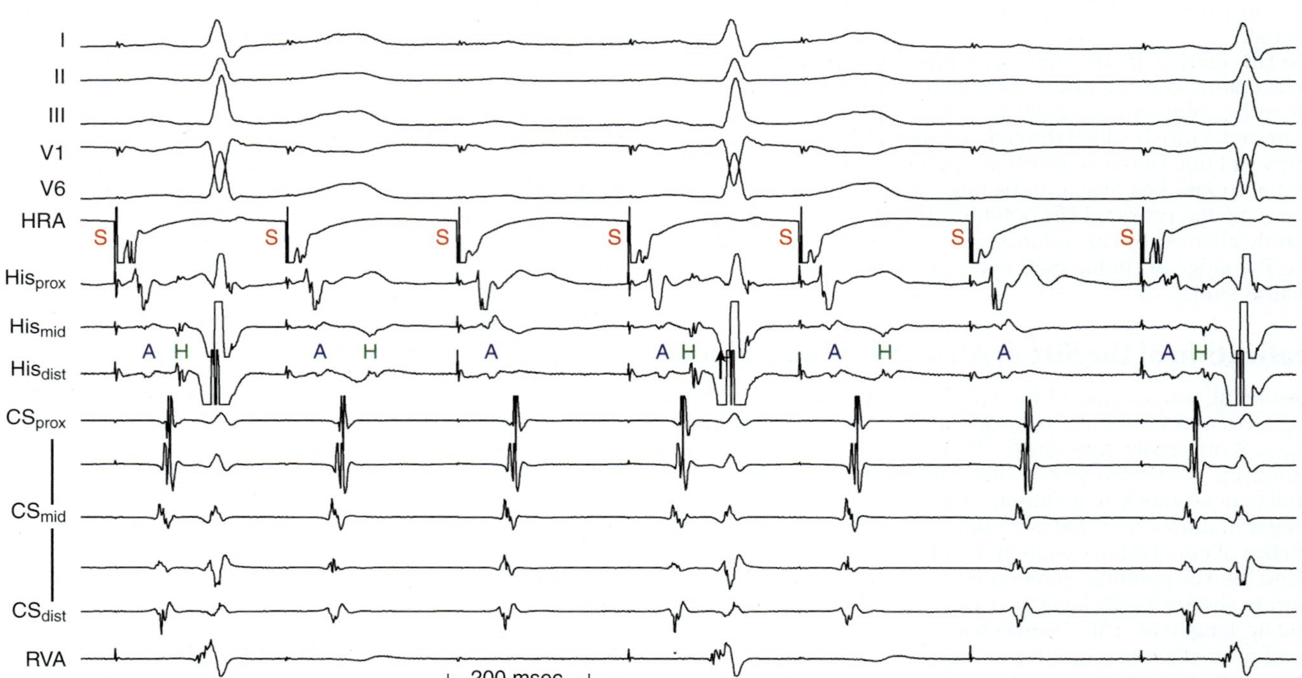

FIGURE 9-21 Multiple levels of atrioventricular block. Rapid atrial pacing (at a cycle length of 330 milliseconds) from the high right atrium (HRA) shows repeating pattern of atrial impulses with normal atrio-His (AH) intervals conducted to the ventricle, atrial impulses associated with AH interval prolongation with block below the His bundle, and atrial impulses associated with atrioventricular nodal block (no His potential). CS_{dist} = distal coronary sinus; CS_{mid} = middle coronary sinus; CS_{prox} = proximal coronary sinus; His_{dist} = distal His bundle; His_{mid} = middle His bundle; His_{prox} = proximal His bundle; RVA = right ventricular apex.

Exclusion of Other Phenomena

NONCONDUCTED PREMATURE ATRIAL COMPLEXES

Early PACs can arrive at the AVN during the absolute refractory period and fail to conduct to the ventricle. This condition can be misdiagnosed as type 1 or type 2 second-degree AV block. Similarly, atrial bigeminy, with failure of conduction of the PACs, can be misinterpreted as 2:1 AV block (Fig. 9-23). In type 2 second-degree AV block, the atrial rhythm is regular, the P-P interval is constant, the nonconducted P wave occurs on time as expected, and P wave morphology is constant. On the other hand, in the setting of nonconducted PACs, the P wave occurs prematurely and usually has a different morphology from that of the baseline atrial rhythm. Nonconducted PACs can often be hidden in the preceding T wave (Fig. 9-24). Additionally, the mere occurrence of PACs in a trigeminal or quadrigeminal pattern can produce a periodicity mimicking Wenckebach periodicity (Fig. 9-25).

CONCEALED JUNCTIONAL ECTOPY

Ectopic beats arising from the HB that fail to conduct to both the atria and ventricles, with retrograde concealment in the AVN, slowing or blocking conduction of the following sinus P wave, can manifest as type 2 second-degree AV block. Such a phenomenon can be difficult to differentiate from actual block without EP testing. ECG clues to concealed junctional extrasystoles causing such unexpected events include the following: (1) abrupt, unexplained prolongation of the PR interval; (2) the presence of apparent Mobitz type II block in the presence of a normal QRS; (3) the presence of types 1 and 2 AV block in the same tracing; and (4) the presence of manifest junctional extrasystoles elsewhere in the tracing (see Fig. 9-10).

ATRIOVENTRICULAR DISSOCIATION

The distinction between AV dissociation and complete AV block is important. AV dissociation is present when the atria and ventricles

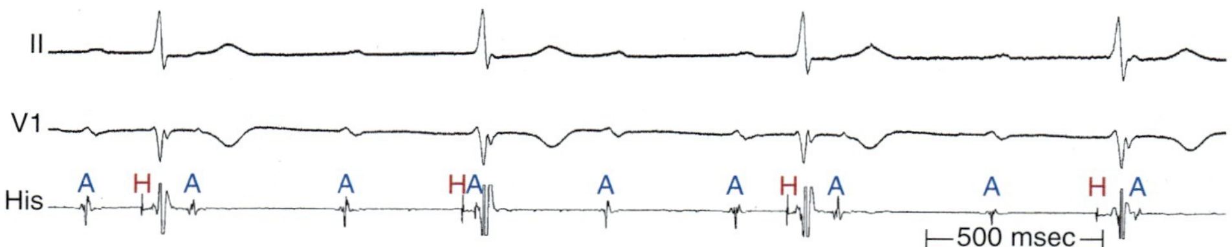

FIGURE 9-22 Complete atrioventricular (AV) block. Complete AV dissociation is observed, and all the P waves fail to conduct despite having ample opportunity for conduction. Note the junctional escape rhythm with a narrow QRS complex and a rate of 45 beats/min, consistent with block in the AVN. Note that the P waves surrounding a QRS complex occur at a faster rate when compared with the P waves that occur sequentially without an intervening QRS complex (ventriculophasic arrhythmia).

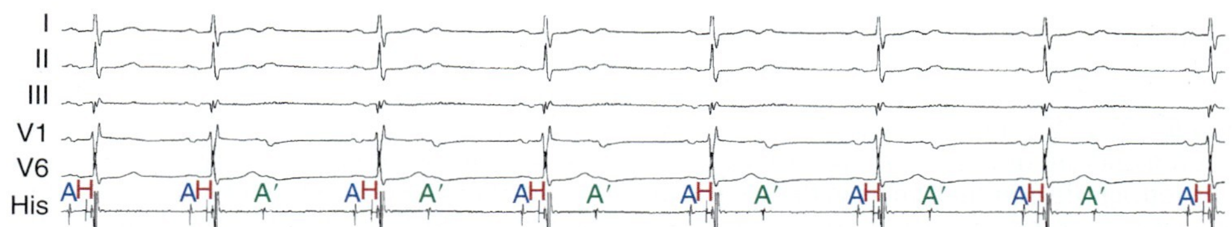

FIGURE 9-23 Sinus rhythm atrial bigeminy mimicking 2:1 atrioventricular block. Frequent premature atrial complexes (PACs; A′) are observed in a bigeminal pattern. The PACs arrive at the atrioventricular node during the absolute refractory period and fail to conduct to the ventricle, thus mimicking 2:1 AV block. In contrast to 2:1 AV block, the nonconducted P waves are premature (compare with the first A-A interval, which is not interrupted by a PAC) and have different morphology than the conducted sinus P waves.

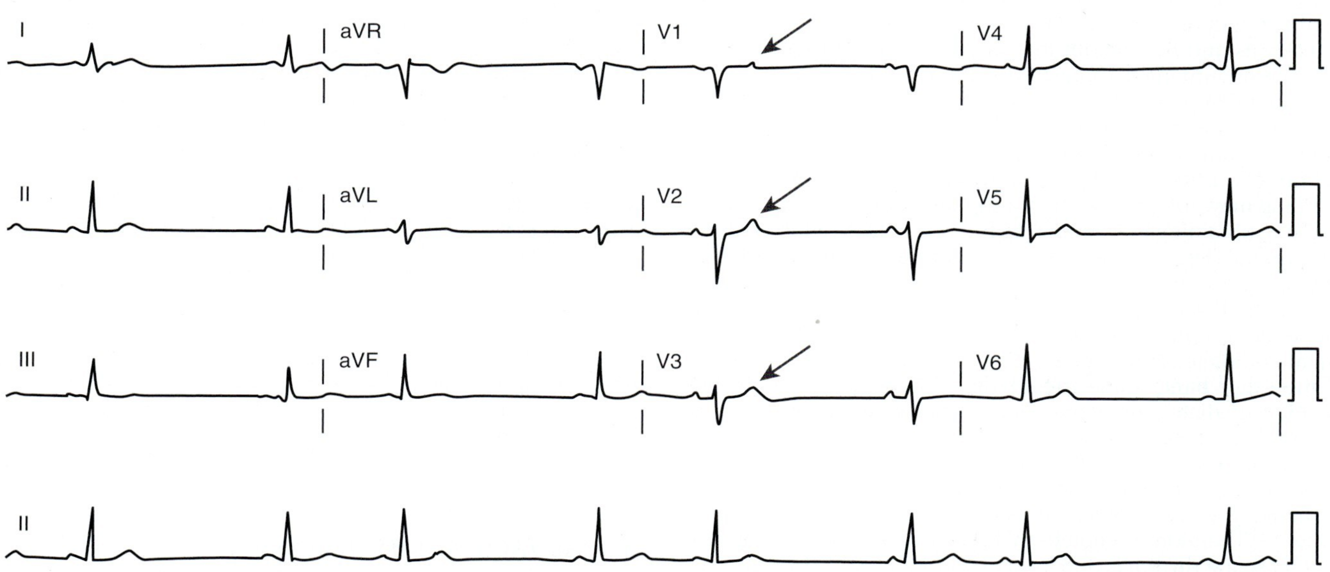

FIGURE 9-24 Sinus rhythm with atrial trigeminy resulting from blocked premature atrial complexes mimicking Mobitz type II atrioventricular block. Note the nonconducted P waves occur early (premature) and lie within the preceding T wave (arrows). All sinus P waves are conducted with a normal, constant PR interval.

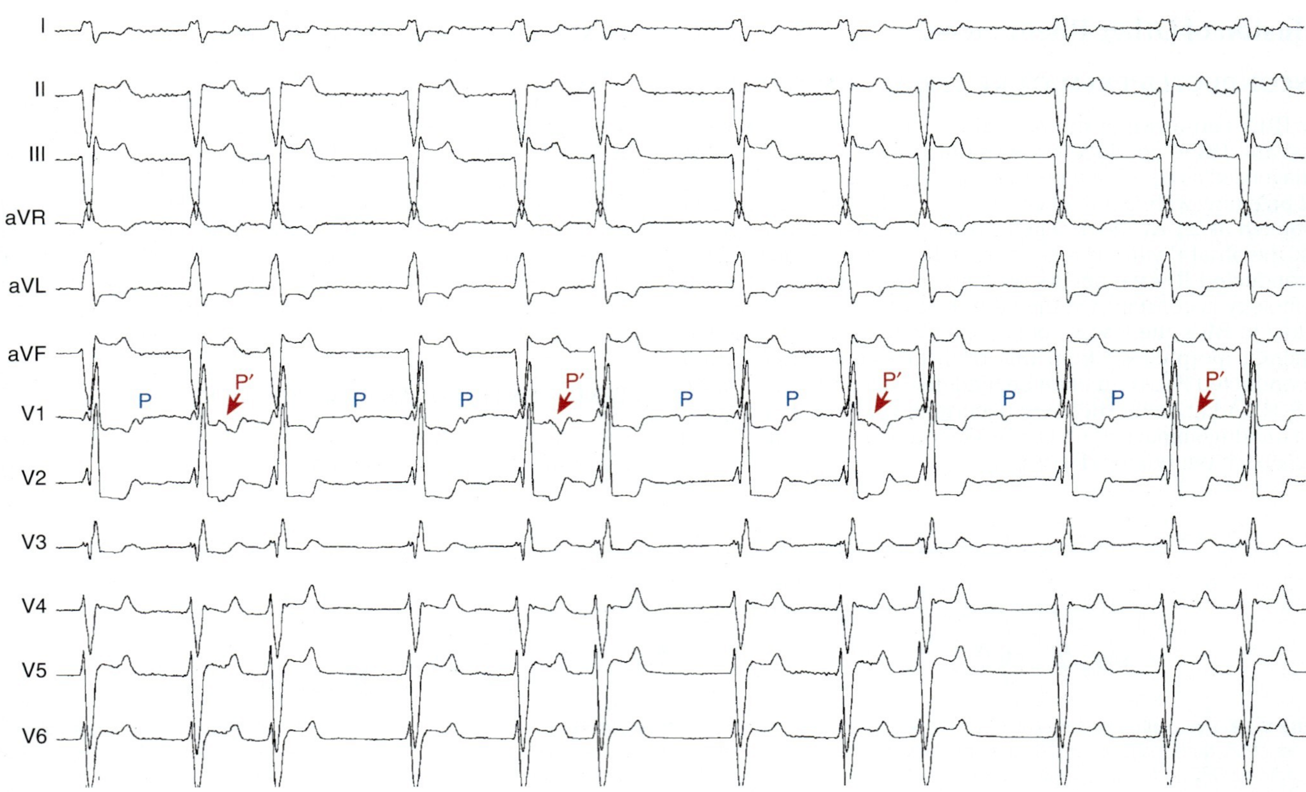

FIGURE 9-25 Sinus rhythm with marked first-degree atrioventricular (AV) block and bifascicular block (right bundle branch block and left anterior fascicular block). Frequent premature atrial complexes (PACs; P′) are observed in a trigeminal pattern. The PACs are conducted to the ventricles; however, they produce a periodicity, thus mimicking Wenckebach AV block. Note that no P waves fail to conduct to the ventricle. Despite the presence of marked His-Purkinje system disease, the marked prolongation of the PR intervals (420 milliseconds) suggests the atrioventricular node as the site of AV conduction delay.

depolarize independently of each other. The ventricles are activated by a nonatrial source and are uninfluenced by atrial activity. By definition, there is no retrograde conduction from the ventricles to the atria.[17] AV dissociation can occur secondary to complete AV block, atrial bradycardia with a faster independent junctional-ventricular escape rhythm, or increased discharge rate of a subsidiary pacemaker that takes control of the ventricular rhythm.[11,35]

In complete AV block, the atrial rate is faster than the ventricular rate. For AV block to be diagnosed, the P waves must fail to conduct, given every opportunity for optimal conduction. Thus, failure of conduction of all the P waves, even those occurring at long RP intervals and throughout the phases of the ventricular cycle, has to be documented. Occasionally, the rate of the junctional or ventricular rhythm during AV dissociation is only slightly different from that of the atrial rhythm. In this case, the standard ECG may not provide a recording opportunity long enough to verify failure of conduction, because all the P waves recorded on a single ECG recording may not occur at an appropriate time to allow conduction. Thus, obtaining ECG recording for an adequate length of time is important (Fig. 9-26). Regularity of both atrial and ventricular rhythms with constantly changing P-R relationships, despite the fact that the P wave falls at every conceivable RP interval, and an independent ventricular rate of 40 beats/min or less (faster in congenital complete AV block) are diagnostic of complete AV block. On the other hand, some irregularity of the ventricular rhythm should immediately draw attention to the possibility of intermittent conduction of P waves, which may reflect lesser degrees of AV block or incomplete AV dissociation. Moreover, with complete AV block, the ventricular rate is almost always slower than the atrial rate, whereas in other forms of AV dissociation, the reverse is true.[11,35] Therefore, complete AV block with a junctional or ventricular escape rhythm is one form of AV dissociation. However, AV dissociation (complete or incomplete) can occur in the absence of AV block.

In the setting of atrial bradycardia, the atrial rate can become slower than a subsidiary escape focus from the AV junction or ventricle. When the faster junctional or ventricular escape rhythm is associated with VA block, it results in failure of the atrial impulses to conduct anterogradely secondary to retrograde concealment by the escape rhythm impulses (see Fig. 9-16).

An increase in the discharge rate of a subsidiary pacemaker, such as accelerated junctional rhythm, accelerated idioventricular rhythm, or VT, which then exceeds the normal sinus rate, can result in a competing junctional or ventricular rhythm, in which case the atrial rate is always slower than the ventricular rate (see Fig. 9-26).

AV dissociation can be complete or incomplete. In the setting of complete AV dissociation, both the atrial and ventricular rates remain constant and, therefore, the PR interval varies, with none of the atrial complexes conducted to the ventricles. In incomplete AV dissociation, ventricular capture beats occur because some of the atrial impulses arrive at the AV junction when the AV junction is no longer refractory. This phenomenon is common in advanced AV block with periodic capture beats.

ECHO BEATS

AVN echo beats can manifest as "group beating" and be misdiagnosed as Wenckebach block. Verification of constant P-P intervals and P wave morphology during the Wenckebach cycle can avoid such misinterpretation. On the other hand, in the presence of dual AVN physiology, not infrequently Wenckebach AV block can result in AVN echo beats.

ATRIAL TACHYARRHYTHMIAS

Failure of the AVN to conduct during fast atrial tachyarrhythmias (atrial tachycardia or flutter) should not be considered

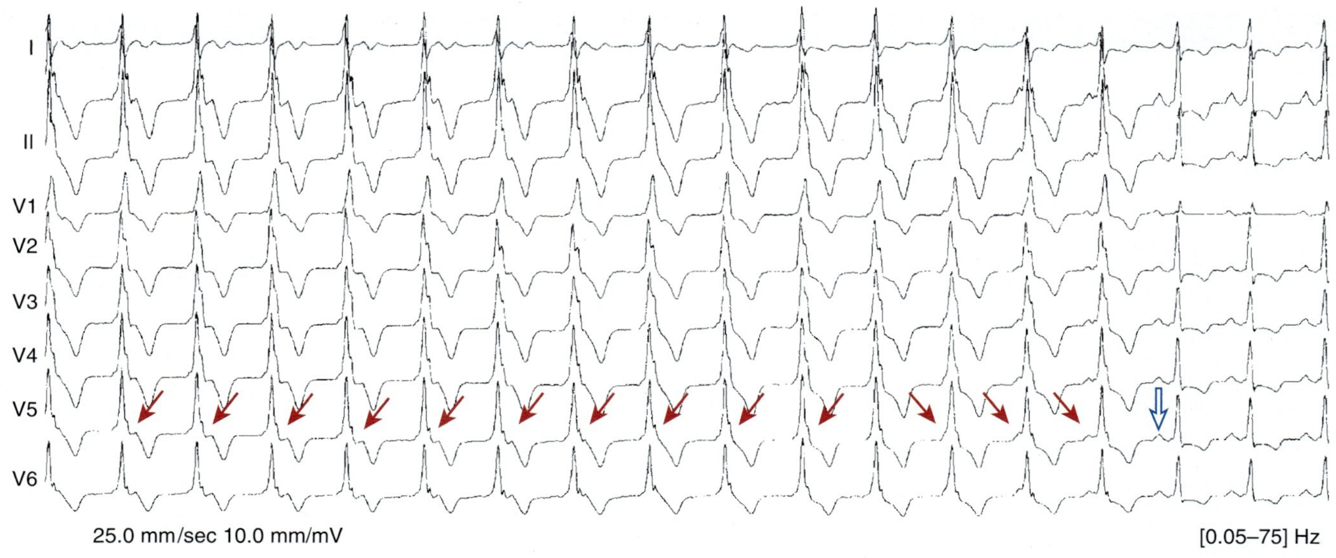

FIGURE 9-26 Atrioventricular (AV) dissociation. Slow ventricular tachycardia and normal sinus rhythm coexist with slightly different rates and ventricular-atrial dissociation. Sinus P waves are marked by red arrows. Note that no AV block is present, and that once the sinus P wave had the chance to conduct, it did (blue arrow).

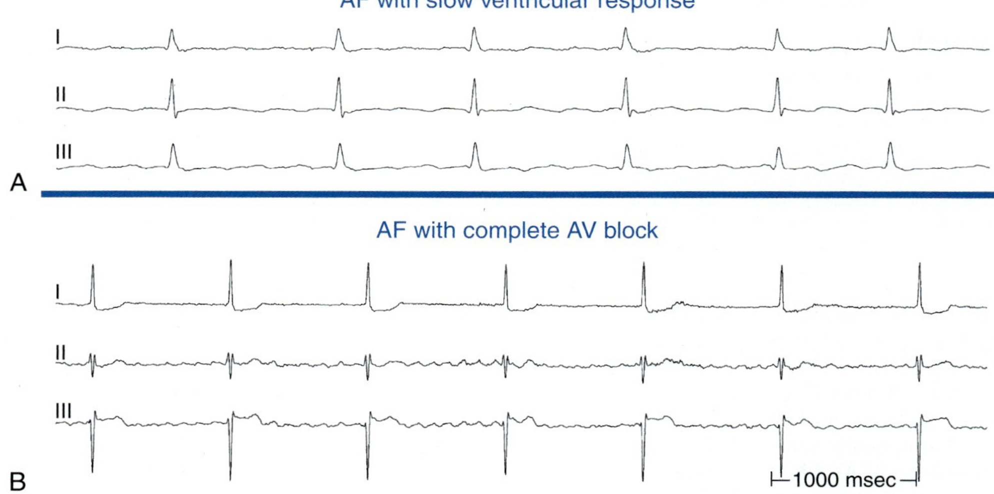

FIGURE 9-27 Atrial fibrillation (AF) with slow ventricular rate. **A,** The ventricular rhythm is irregular, indicating that it is the result of conducted atrial beats. **B,** The ventricular rhythm is regular, consistent with the presence of complete atrioventricular (AV) block and a regular junctional escape rhythm.

pathological AV block. One of the main physiological roles of the AVN is to safeguard the ventricles from rapid atrial rates. Therefore, failure of the AVN to conduct every atrial impulse occurring at a fast rate should be considered a normal physiological finding caused by normal refractoriness. In such situations, terms such as *3:2* and *2:1 AV conduction* are more appropriate than *3:2* or *2:1 AV block*.

ATRIAL FIBRILLATION WITH SLOW VENTRICULAR RATE

AF with slow ventricular response can be misinterpreted as complete AV block. Verification of the regularity of the slow ventricular rhythm is critical. When AV block is present, the escape rhythm is regular, whereas in AF associated with very slow ventricular response, the ventricular rhythm is a result of conducted atrial beats and is irregular (Fig. 9-27).

VENTRICULOPHASIC SINUS ARRHYTHMIA

Ventriculophasic sinus arrhythmia can be observed whenever there is second- or third-degree AV block, and it is manifest as intermittent differences in the P-P intervals based on their relationship with the QRS complex. The two P waves surrounding a QRS complex have a shortened interval or occur at a faster rate when compared with two P waves that occur sequentially without an intervening QRS complex (see Fig. 9-22). The mechanism of this phenomenon is not certain. However, it has been suggested that ventricular contractions enhance sinus node automaticity by increasing the pulsatile blood flow through the sinus nodal artery and by mechanical stretch on the sinus node.

Principles of Management

Pacing is the mainstay of treatment for symptomatic AV block (Table 9-1). Identifying transient or reversible causes for AV conduction disturbances is the first step in management. Withdrawal of any offending drugs, correction of any electrolyte abnormalities, or treatment of any infectious processes or myocardial ischemia should be considered prior to permanent pacing therapy. Pharmacological therapy (atropine, isoproterenol) can be effective in intranodal AV block but only as a short-term emergency measure until pacing can be accomplished. Temporary percutaneous or transvenous pacing is necessary in patients with hemodynamically significant AV block and bradycardia to provide immediate stabilization

TABLE 9-1 Indications for Permanent Pacing in Acquired Atrioventricular Block in Adults

Class I

Third-degree and advanced second-degree AV block at any level, associated with any one of the following:
- Symptomatic bradycardia (including heart failure)
- Ventricular arrhythmias presumed to result from AV block
- Arrhythmias and other conditions that require drugs that result in symptomatic bradycardia
- Asymptomatic awake patients with documented periods of asystole ≥3.0 seconds or any escape rate <40 beats/min, or with an escape rhythm that is below the AVN
- After catheter ablation of the AV junction
- Postoperative AV block that is not expected to resolve
- Neuromuscular diseases, such as myotonic muscular dystrophy, Kearns-Sayre syndrome, Erb dystrophy (limb-girdle muscular dystrophy), and peroneal muscular atrophy, with or without symptoms
- Awake, symptom-free patients with atrial fibrillation and bradycardia with one or more pauses of at least 5 seconds
- Average awake ventricular rates of 40 beats/min or faster if cardiomegaly or left ventricular dysfunction is present or if the site of block is below the AVN

Second-degree AV block with associated symptomatic bradycardia regardless of type or site of block
Second- or third-degree AV block during exercise in the absence of myocardial ischemia

Class IIa

Persistent third-degree AV block with an escape rate >40 beats/min in asymptomatic adult patients without cardiomegaly
Asymptomatic second-degree AV block at intra-Hisian or infra-Hisian levels found at electrophysiological study
First- or second-degree AV block with symptoms similar to those of pacemaker syndrome or hemodynamic compromise
Asymptomatic type II second-degree AV block with a narrow QRS; when type II second-degree AV block occurs with a wide QRS, including isolated right bundle branch block, pacing becomes a class I recommendation

Class IIb

Neuromuscular diseases such as myotonic muscular dystrophy, Erb dystrophy (limb-girdle muscular dystrophy), and peroneal muscular atrophy with any degree of AV block (including first-degree AV block), with or without symptoms, because there may be unpredictable progression of AV conduction disease
AV block in the setting of drug use and/or drug toxicity when the block is expected to recur even after the drug is withdrawn

Class III

Asymptomatic first-degree AV block
Asymptomatic type I second-degree AV block at the AVN level or that which is not known to be intra-Hisian or infra-Hisian
AV block that is expected to resolve and is unlikely to recur (e.g., drug toxicity, Lyme disease, or transient increases in vagal tone, or during hypoxia in sleep apnea syndrome in the absence of symptoms)

AV = atrioventricular; AVN = atrioventricular node.
From Epstein AE, DiMarco JP, Ellenbogen KA, et al: ACC/AHA/HRS 2008 guidelines for device-based therapy of cardiac rhythm abnormalities: a report of the American College of Cardiology/American Heart Association Task Force on Practice Guidelines (writing committee to revise the ACC/AHA/NASPE 2002 guideline update for implantation of cardiac pacemakers and antiarrhythmia devices). Developed in collaboration with the American Association for Thoracic Surgery and Society of Thoracic Surgeons. *Circulation* 117:e350-408, 2008.

prior to permanent pacemaker placement or to provide pacemaker support when the block is precipitated by what is presumed to be a transient event, such as ischemia or drug toxicity.[36]

Once all reversible causes are excluded or treated, correlation of symptoms with ECG evidence of AV block is an essential part of the diagnostic strategy. In the setting of intermittent AV block or Wenckebach AV block, ambulatory monitoring often is required to correlate symptoms with the presence and severity of AV conduction abnormalities. As discussed previously, exercise testing can be a useful tool to help confirm the level of block in second- or third-degree AV block associated with a narrow or wide QRS complex. Additionally, EP testing can be required in a patient with suspected high-grade AV block as the cause of syncope or presyncope when documentation cannot be obtained noninvasively. Similarly, in patients with coronary artery disease, in whom symptoms can be secondary to AV block or VT, EP testing can be useful in establishing the diagnosis. Some patients with known second- or third-degree block also can benefit from an invasive study to localize the site of AV block to help determine therapy or assess prognosis.

Permanent pacemaker implantation is indicated in most patients with symptomatic advanced heart block, regardless of the site of block. Permanent pacemakers are also indicated in asymptomatic patients with complete heart block or infra-Hisian second-degree AV block, especially those with documented ventricular pauses longer than 3 seconds or a ventricular escape rhythm of less than 40 beats/min.[36]

In children with congenital heart block, permanent pacing is recommended in those with exercise intolerance, abrupt pauses in the intrinsic rate (longer than two to three times the basic CL), or inappropriately slow average ventricular rate (less than 50 beats/min). Furthermore, prophylactic pacing can considerably reduce the incidence of syncope and sudden death in asymptomatic patients with congenital heart block with severe bradycardia (resting heart rate less than 40 beats/min), ventricular pauses longer than 3 seconds, wide QRS escape rhythm, complex congenital heart disease, ventricular dysfunction, complex ventricular ectopy, or a long QT interval.[22,36]

Dual-chamber pacing can be beneficial in some patients with marked first-degree AV block (more than 300 milliseconds) and symptoms similar to pacemaker syndrome, as well as in patients with LV dysfunction and heart failure symptoms in whom a shorter AV interval results in hemodynamic improvement, presumably by decreasing LA filling pressure. The latter recommendation, however, is now questionable because a conventional DDD(R) pacemaker with an optimized AV delay would have to pace the ventricle almost 100% of the time. The benefit of pacing with optimized AV synchrony (with a shorter AV delay) should be weighed against the impairment of LV function produced by right ventricular pacing with resultant LV dyssynchrony. However, such a determination can be difficult or impossible.[28]

Temporary pacing is sometimes required in patients with acute MI (more often in anterior than inferior wall MI). Patients with asymptomatic first-degree or type 1 second-degree AV block do not require pacing. However, patients with type 2 second-degree or complete AV block should be temporarily paced, even if they are asymptomatic. In the setting of MI, the criteria for permanent pacing depends less on the presence of symptoms (Table 9-2). If type 2 second-degree or complete AV block persists once past the peri-infarct period, permanent pacing is indicated. Even if the type 2 or third-degree AV block was transient but associated with BBB that persists following resolution of the AV block, permanent pacing of the post-MI patient improves long-term survival.[36]

TABLE 9-2 Indications for Permanent Pacing in Atrioventricular Block with Acute Myocardial Infarction

Class I
Persistent second-degree AV block in the His-Purkinje system with bilateral bundle branch block or third-degree AV block within or below the His-Purkinje system after acute MI
Transient advanced (second- or third-degree) infranodal AV block and associated bundle branch block; if the site of block is uncertain, an electrophysiology study may be necessary
Persistent and symptomatic second- or third-degree AV block
Class IIb
Persistent second- or third-degree AV block at the AV node level, even in the absence of symptoms
Class III
Transient AV block in the absence of intraventricular conduction defects
Transient AV block in the presence of isolated left anterior fascicular block
Acquired left anterior fascicular block in the absence of AV block
Persistent first-degree AV block in the presence of bundle branch block that is old or age indeterminate

AV = atrioventricular; MI = myocardial infarction.

Most patients with AV block require dual-chamber pacemakers to maintain AV synchrony, prevent development of pacemaker syndrome, and, possibly, prevent subsequent development of AF. In patients with normal sinus node function and AV block, VDD pacing using a single lead with a series of electrodes for atrial sensing and ventricular pacing and sensing is appropriate. In patients with permanent AF and bradycardia, rate-responsive single-chamber ventricular pacing (VVIR) is adequate.

REFERENCES

1. Cosio FG, Anderson RH, Kuck KH, et al: Living anatomy of the atrioventricular junctions: a guide to electrophysiologic mapping. A Consensus Statement from the Cardiac Nomenclature Study Group, Working Group of Arrhythmias, European Society of Cardiology, and the Task Force on Cardiac Nomenclature from NASPE, *Circulation* 100:e31–e37, 1999.
2. Lockwood D, Nakagawa H, Jackman W: Electrophysiological characteristics of atrioventricular nodal reentrant tachycardia: implications for the reentrant circuit. In Zipes DP, Jalife J, editors: *Cardiac electrophysiology: from cell to bedside*, ed 5, Philadelphia, 2009, Saunders, pp 615–646.
3. Valderrabano M: Atypical atrioventricular nodal reentry with eccentric atrial activation: is the right target on the left? *Heart Rhythm* 4:433–434, 2007.
4. Basso C, Ho SY, Thiene G: Anatomical and histopathological characteristics of the conductive tissues of the heart. In Gussak I, Antzelevitch C, editors: *Electrical diseases of the heart: genetics, mechanisms, treatment, prevention*, London, 2008, Springer, pp 37–51.
5. Kurian T, Ambrosi C, Hucker W, et al: Anatomy and electrophysiology of the human AV node, *Pacing Clin Electrophysiol* 33:754–762, 2010.
6. Lee PC, Chen SA, Hwang B: Atrioventricular node anatomy and physiology: implications for ablation of atrioventricular nodal reentrant tachycardia, *Curr Opin Cardiol* 24:105–112, 2009.
7. Anderson R, Ho S: *The anatomy of the atrioventricular node. Heart Rhythm Society*, 2008, http://www.hrsonline.org/ Education/SelfStudy/Articles/Anderson_ho1.cfm.
8. Luc PJ: Common form of atrioventricular nodal reentrant tachycardia: do we really know the circuit we try to ablate? *Heart Rhythm* 4:711–712, 2007.
9. Mazgalev T: *AV nodal physiology. Heart Rhythm Society*, 2008, http://www.hrsonline.org/Education/SelfStudy/Articles/mazgalev.cfm.
10. Shryock J, Belardinelli L: *Pharmacology of the AV node. Heart Rhythm Society*, 2008, http://www.hrsonline.org/Education/SelfStudy/Articles/shrbel.cfm.
11. Schwartzman D: Atrioventricular block and atrioventricular dissociation. In Zipes DP, Jalife J, editors: *Cardiac electrophysiology: from cell to bedside*, ed 4, Philadelphia, 2004, Saunders, pp 485–489.
12. Friedman DM, Rupel A, Buyon JP: Epidemiology, etiology, detection, and treatment of autoantibody-associated congenital heart block in neonatal lupus, *Curr Rheumatol Rep* 9:101–108, 2007.
13. Walsh EP: Interventional electrophysiology in patients with congenital heart disease, *Circulation* 115:3224–3234, 2007.
14. Khairy P, Balaji S: Cardiac arrhythmias in congenital heart diseases, *Indian Pacing Electrophysiol J* 9:299–317, 2009.
15. Smits JP, Veldkamp MW, Wilde AA: Mechanisms of inherited cardiac conduction disease, *Europace* 7:122–137, 2005.
16. Amin AS, Asghari-Roodsari A, Tan HL: Cardiac sodium channelopathies, *Pflugers Arch* 460: 223–237, 2010.
17. Wolbrette D, Naccarelli G: Bradycardias: sinus nodal dysfunction and atrioventricular conduction disturbances. In Topol E, editor: *Textbook of cardiovascular medicine*, ed 2, Philadelphia, 2002, Lippincott Williams & Wilkins, pp 1385–1402.
18. Wellens HJ: Atrioventricular nodal and subnodal ventricular disturbances. In Willerson J, Cohn J, Wellens HJ, Holmes D, editors: *Cardiovascular medicine*, New York, 2007, Springer, pp 1991–1998.
19. Sovari AA, Bodine CK, Farokhi F: Cardiovascular manifestations of myotonic dystrophy-1, *Cardiol Rev* 15:191–194, 2007.
20. Huynh H, Dalloul G, Ghanbari H, et al: Permanent pacemaker implantation following aortic valve replacement: current prevalence and clinical predictors, *Pacing Clin Electrophysiol* 32:1520–1525, 2009.
21. Gross GJ, Chiu CC, Hamilton RM, et al: Natural history of postoperative heart block in congenital heart disease: implications for pacing intervention, *Heart Rhythm* 3:601–604, 2006.
22. Villain E: Indications for pacing in patients with congenital heart disease, *Pacing Clin Electrophysiol* 31(Suppl 1):S17–S20, 2008.
23. Tucker EM, Pyles LA, Bass JL, Moller JH: Permanent pacemaker for atrioventricular conduction block after operative repair of perimembranous ventricular septal defect, *J Am Coll Cardiol* 50:1196–1200, 2007.
24. Liberman L, Pass RH, Hordof AJ, Spotnitz HM: Late onset of heart block after open heart surgery for congenital heart disease, *Pediatr Cardiol* 29:56–59, 2008.
25. Padanilam BJ, Morris KE, Olson JA, et al: The surface electrocardiogram predicts risk of heart block during right heart catheterization in patients with preexisting left bundle branch block: implications for the definition of complete left bundle branch block, *J Cardiovasc Electrophysiol* 21:781–785, 2010.
26. Topilski I, Rogowski O, Glick A, et al: Catheter-induced mechanical trauma to fast and slow pathways during radiofrequency ablation of atrioventricular nodal reentry tachycardia: incidence, predictors, and clinical implications, *Pacing Clin Electrophysiol* 30:1233–1241, 2007.
27. Shirayama T, Hadase M, Sakamoto T, et al: Swallowing syncope: complex mechanisms of the reflex, *Intern Med* 41:207–210, 2002.
28. Barold SS, Ilercil A, Leonelli F, Herweg B: First-degree atrioventricular block: clinical manifestations, indications for pacing, pacemaker management and consequences during cardiac resynchronization, *J Interv Card Electrophysiol* 17:139–152, 2006.
29. Kim MH, Deeb GM, Eagle KA, et al: Complete atrioventricular block after valvular heart surgery and the timing of pacemaker implantation, *Am J Cardiol* 87:649–651, A10, 2001.
30. Josephson ME: Atrioventricular conduction. In Josephson ME, editor: *Clinical cardiac electrophysiology*, ed 4, Philadelphia, 2008, Lippincott Williams & Wilkins, pp 93–113.
31. Spodick DH, Ariyarajah V: Interatrial block: the pandemic remains poorly perceived, *Pacing Clin Electrophysiol* 32:667–672, 2009.
32. Fisch C, Knoebel S: Atrioventricular and ventriculoatrial conduction and blocks, gap, and overdrive suppression. In Fisch C, Knoebel S, editors: *Electrocardiography of clinical arrhythmias*, Armonk, NY, 2000, Futura, pp 315–344.
33. Lee S, Wellens HJ, Josephson ME: Paroxysmal atrioventricular block, *Heart Rhythm* 6: 1229–1234, 2009.
34. Silver ES, Pass RH, Hordof AJ, Liberman L: Paroxysmal AV block in children with normal cardiac anatomy as a cause of syncope, *Pacing Clin Electrophysiol* 31:322–326, 2008.
35. Fisch C, Knoebel S: Atrioventricular conduction abnormalities. In Fisch C, Knoebel S, editors: *Electrocardiography of clinical arrhythmias*, Armonk, NY, 2000, Futura, pp 129–149.
36. Epstein AE, DiMarco JP, Ellenbogen KA, et al: ACC/AHA/HRS 2008 guidelines for device-based therapy of cardiac rhythm abnormalities: a report of the American College of Cardiology/American Heart Association Task Force on Practice Guidelines (writing committee to revise the ACC/AHA/NASPE 2002 guideline update for implantation of cardiac pacemakers and antiarrhythmia devices). Developed in collaboration with the American Association for Thoracic Surgery and Society of Thoracic Surgeons, *Circulation* 117:e350–e408, 2008.

CHAPTER 10 Intraventricular Conduction Abnormalities

General Considerations

A narrow QRS complex requires highly synchronous electrical activation of the ventricular myocardium, which can be achieved only through the rapidly conducting His-Purkinje system (HPS). The term *intraventricular conduction disturbances* (IVCDs) refers to abnormalities in the intraventricular propagation of supraventricular impulses resulting in changes in the morphology or duration, or both, of the QRS complex. These changes in intraventricular conduction can be fixed and present at all heart rates, or they can be intermittent (transient) and tachycardia- or bradycardia-dependent. They can be caused by structural abnormalities in the HPS or ventricular myocardium, functional refractoriness in a portion of the conduction system (i.e., aberrant ventricular conduction), or ventricular preexcitation over a bypass tract.[1]

Transient Bundle Branch Block

The term aberration is used to describe transient bundle branch block (BBB) and does not include QRS abnormalities caused by preexisting BBB, preexcitation, or the effect of drugs. Transient BBB can have several mechanisms, including phase 3 block, phase 4 block, and concealed conduction. These mechanisms of aberration can occur anywhere in the HPS, and, unlike in chronic BBB, the site of block during aberration can shift. Right BBB (RBBB) is the most common pattern of aberration, occurring in 80% of patients with aberration and in up to 100% of cases of aberration in normal hearts.[2-7]

PHASE 3 BLOCK

Conduction velocity depends, in part, on the rate of rise of phase 0 of the action potential (dV/dt) and the height to which it rises (V_{max}). These factors, in turn, depend on the membrane potential at the time of stimulation. The more negative the membrane potential is, the more sodium (Na^+) channels are available for activation, the greater the influx of Na^+ into the cell during phase 0, and the greater the conduction velocity. Therefore, when stimulation occurs during phase 3 of the action potential, before full recovery and at less negative potentials of the cell membrane, a portion of Na^+ channels remains refractory and unavailable for activation. Consequently, the Na^+ current and phase 0 of the next action potential are reduced, and conduction is then slower.[6,8-10]

Phase 3 block, also called tachycardia-dependent block, occurs when an impulse arrives at tissues that are still refractory caused by incomplete repolarization. Manifestations of phase 3 block include BBB and fascicular block, as well as complete atrioventricular (AV) block.[3,11]

Functional or physiological phase 3 aberration can occur in normal fibers if the impulse is sufficiently premature to encroach on the physiological refractory period of the preceding beat, when the membrane potential is still reduced. This is commonly seen with very early premature atrial complexes (PACs) that conduct aberrantly. Phase 3 aberration can also occur pathologically if electrical systole and the refractory period are abnormally prolonged (with refractoriness extending beyond the action potential duration or the QT interval) and the involved fascicle is stimulated at a relatively rapid rate.[3,11] Transient left BBB (LBBB) is less common than RBBB (only 25% of phase 3 aberration is of the LBBB type). The block usually occurs in the very proximal portion of the bundle branch.[6,9,10]

Phase 3 block constitutes the physiological explanation of several phenomena, including aberration caused by premature excitation, Ashman phenomenon, and acceleration-dependent aberration.

Aberration Caused by Premature Excitation

Premature excitation can cause aberration (BBB) by encroaching on the refractory period of the bundle branch prior to full recovery of the action potential, namely during so-called voltage-dependent refractoriness (see Fig. 4-29).[11] In normal hearts, this type of aberration is almost always in the form of RBBB (Fig. 10-1), whereas such aberration in the abnormal heart can be that of RBBB or LBBB.

At normal heart rates, the effective refractory period (ERP) of the right bundle branch (RB) exceeds the ERP of the AV node (AVN), HB, and left bundle branch (LB). At faster heart rates, the ERP of both bundle branches shortens. However, RB ERP shortens to a greater degree than LB ERP, so that the duration of the refractory periods of the two bundles crosses over, and LB ERP becomes longer than that of the RB. This explains the tendency of aberration to be in the form of RBBB when premature excitation occurs during normal heart rates and in the form of LBBB when it occurs during fast heart rates.[2,3,6,8-10,12]

Ashman Phenomenon

The Ashman phenomenon refers to aberration occurring when a short cycle follows a long one (long-short cycle sequence) (see Fig. 10-1).[11,13] Aberrancy is caused by the physiological changes of the conduction system refractory periods associated with the R-R interval. Normally, the refractory period of the HPS lengthens as the heart rate slows and shortens as the heart rate increases, even when heart rate changes are abrupt. Thus, aberrant conduction can result when a short cycle follows a long R-R interval. In this scenario, the QRS complex that ends the long pause is conducted normally but creates a prolonged ERP of the bundle branches. If the next QRS complex occurs after a short coupling interval, it may be conducted aberrantly because one of the bundles is still refractory as a result of a lengthening of the refractory period (phase 3 block; Fig. 10-2).[6,7]

RBBB aberration is more common than LBBB in this setting because the RB has a longer ERP than the LB. The Ashman phenomenon can occur during second-degree AV block (see Fig. 9-9), but it is most common during atrial fibrillation (AF), whereby the irregularity of the ventricular response results in frequently occurring long-short cycle sequences.

The aberrancy can be present for one beat and have a morphology resembling a premature ventricular complex (PVC), or it can involve several sequential complexes, a finding suggesting ventricular tachycardia (VT). In the setting of aberrancy during AF, the long-short cycle sequence characteristic of the Ashman phenomenon may not be helpful in differentiating aberration from ventricular ectopy. Although a long cycle (pause) sets the stage for the Ashman phenomenon, it also tends to precipitate ventricular ectopy. Furthermore, concealed conduction occurs frequently

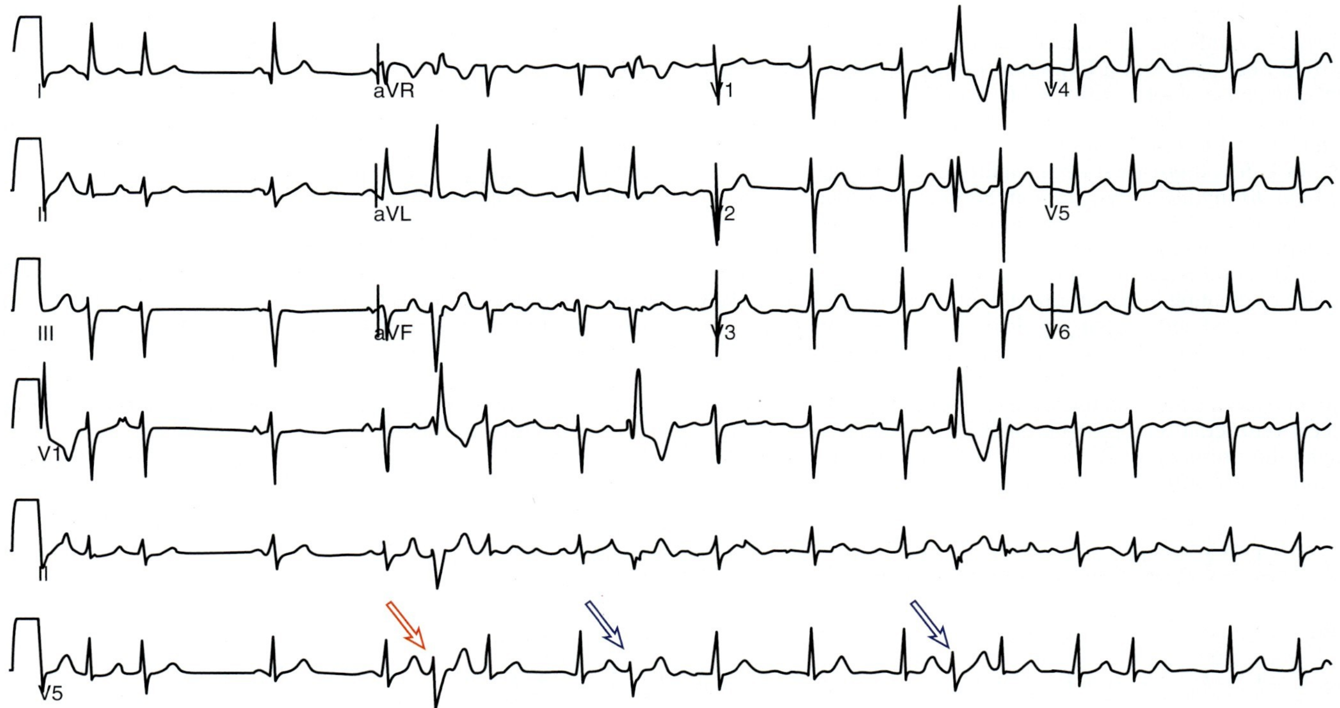

FIGURE 10-1 Ashman phenomenon. A premature atrial complex (PAC, red arrow) during sinus rhythm induces atrial fibrillation (AF). Note that the PAC is conducted with right bundle branch block (RBBB) aberrancy (phase 3 block). During AF, long-short cycle sequences occur repeatedly and are associated with RBBB aberrancy (Ashman phenomenon, phase 3 block). Note that the aberrantly conducted complex (blue arrows) during AF occur at variable coupling intervals to the preceding beats. See text for discussion.

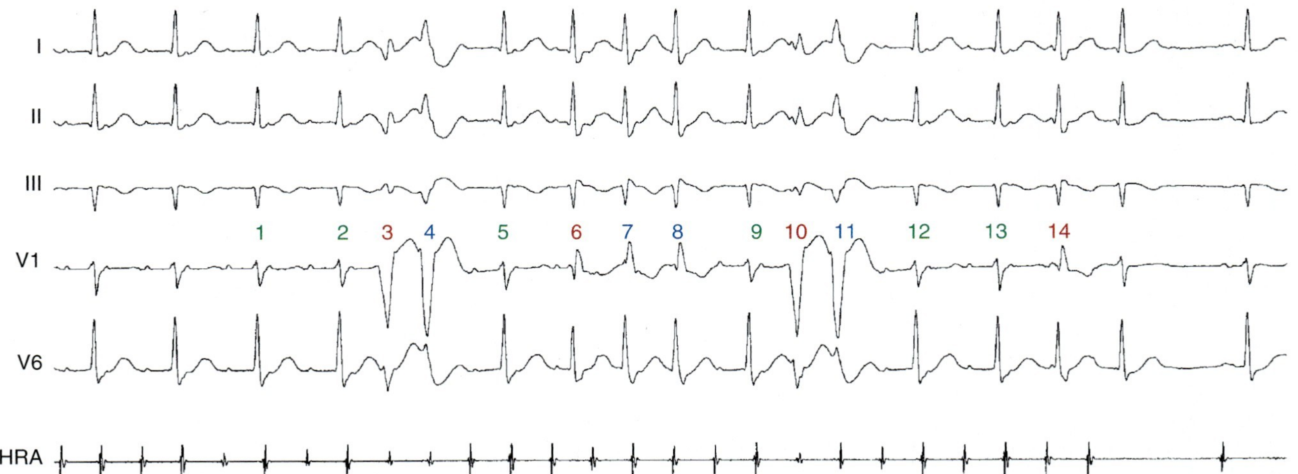

FIGURE 10-2 Atrial tachycardia (AT) with variable atrioventricular (AV) conduction and intermittent aberrancy. **Left,** AT with 2:1 AV conduction and normal QRS morphology is observed. Once 1:1 AV conduction occurs (QRS 3), left bundle branch block (LBBB) aberration develops (caused by long-short cycle sequence, phase 3 block). LBBB aberration is also observed during QRS 4, likely secondary to concealed transseptal conduction causing perpetuation of aberration. After a pause, both bundle branches recover from refractoriness producing a normal QRS 5. Ashman phenomenon (long-short cycle sequence) explains phase 3 block during QRS 6, but this time it manifests as a right bundle branch block (RBBB) pattern. This is because activation during QRS 4 propagated down the right bundle branch (RB) and across the septum, thus activating the left bundle branch (LB) retrogradely after some delay (concealed transseptal conduction), so that the LB-LB interval (between QRS 4 and QRS 5) resulted in a shorter effective refractory period (ERP) of the LB following QRS 5. Conversely, the RB-RB interval (between QRS 4 and QRS 5) was longer and, consequently, the ERP of the RB was still prolonged following QRS 5, thereby setting the stage for a long-short cycle sequence of the RB but not the LB. Therefore, RBBB (rather than LBBB) aberration develops. RBBB aberration during QRS complexes 7 and 8 is secondary to either concealed transseptal conduction or rate-dependent aberration. However, because LBBB (rather than RBBB) was observed during QRS 4 (although QRS 4 occurred following a similar cycle length to that of QRS 8), concealed transseptal conduction is more likely to be the mechanism of aberration. After a pause, both bundle branches recover from refractoriness to produce a normal QRS 9. Long-short cycle sequence explains phase 3 block during QRS 10, but this time it manifests as LBBB. This is because activation during QRS 8 propagated down the LB and across the septum, thus activating the RB after some delay (concealed transseptal conduction). The result is that the RB-RB interval (following QRS 8) and ERP of the RB became shorter, whereas the LB-LB interval (following QRS 8) was longer. Consequently, the ERP of the LB was still prolonged following QRS 9, thereby setting the stage for a long-short cycle sequence and LBBB aberration. LBBB aberration during QRS 11 is caused by concealed transseptal conduction. The Ashman phenomenon (long-short cycle sequence) underlies RBBB aberration during QRS 14. HRA = high right atrium.

during AF, and, therefore, it is never possible to know from the surface ECG exactly when a bundle branch is activated. Thus, if an aberrant beat does end a long-short cycle sequence during AF, it can be because of refractoriness of a bundle branch secondary to concealed conduction into it, rather than because of changes in the length of the ventricular cycle.[8-10,12]

Nevertheless, there are several features of ventricular ectopy that can help distinguish a PVC from an aberrantly conducted or Ashman beat during AF. PVCs are usually followed by a longer R-R cycle, indicating the occurrence of a compensatory pause, the result of retrograde conduction into the AVN and anterograde block of the impulse originating in the atrium. A ventricular origin is also likely when there is a fixed coupling cycle between the normal and aberrant QRS complexes. The presence of long and identical R-R cycles after the aberrated beats and the absence of a long-short cycle sequence associated with the wide or aberrant QRS complex also suggest ventricular ectopy. Additionally, the absence of aberrancy, despite the presence of R-R cycle length (CL) combinations that are longer and shorter than those associated with the wide QRS complex, suggests ventricular ectopy. QRS morphology inconsistent with LBBB or RBBB aberrancy argues against aberration (Fig. 10-3).[6,8-10,12]

Aberration caused by the Ashman phenomenon can persist for several cycles. The persistence of aberration can reflect a time-dependent adjustment of refractoriness of the bundle branch to the abrupt change in CL, or it can be the result of concealed transseptal activation (see later).

Aberration Caused by Heart Rate Acceleration

As the heart rate accelerates, the HPS refractory period shortens; normal conduction tends to be preserved because of this response. However, refractoriness of the HPS eventually reaches a critical value beyond which an increase in heart rate no longer abbreviates it; at this point, AV block may occur. Conversely, the refractory period lengthens as the heart rate slows. Acceleration-dependent BBB is a result of failure of the action potential of the bundle branches to shorten, or, paradoxically, the action potential lengthens in response to acceleration of the heart rate (Fig. 10-4).[3,11] As

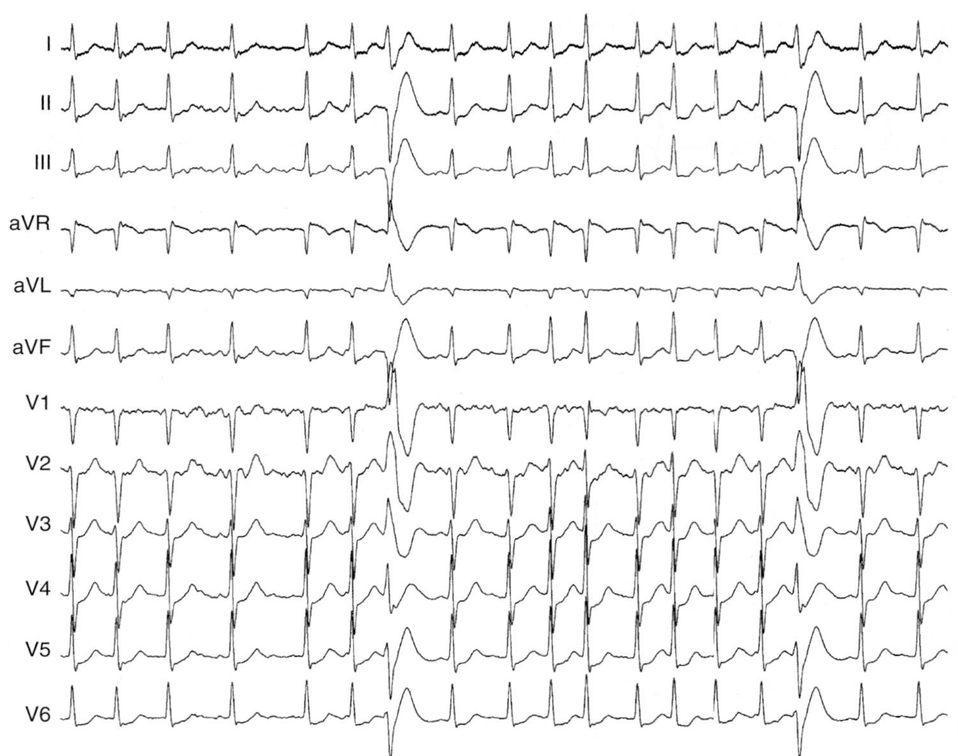

FIGURE 10-3 Premature ventricular complexes during atrial fibrillation. Several features suggest that the wide QRS complexes are caused by ventricular ectopy rather than aberration. QRS morphology is inconsistent with LBBB or RBBB aberrancy. Additionally, there is a fixed coupling cycle between the normal and aberrant QRS complex. The absence of a long-short cycle sequence associated with the wide QRS complex and the absence of aberrancy despite the presence of R-R cycle length combinations that are longer and shorter than those associated with the wide QRS complex also suggest ventricular ectopy.

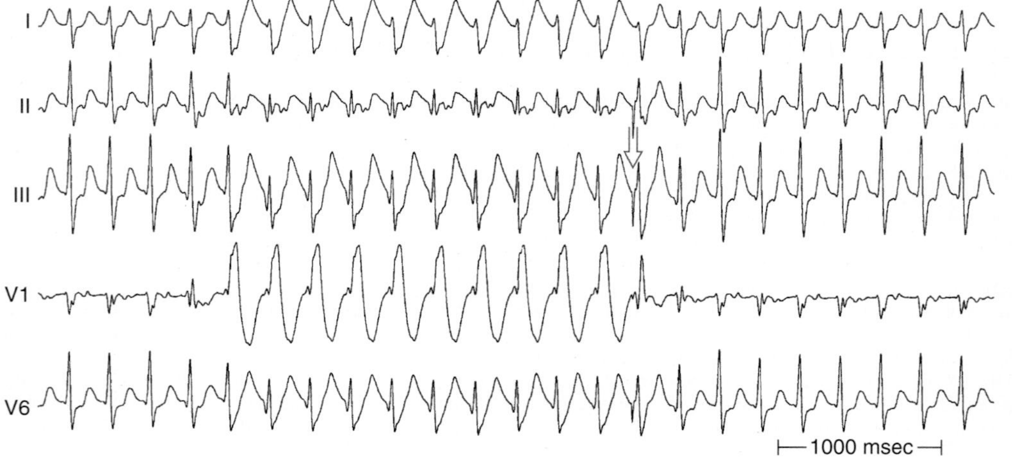

FIGURE 10-4 Supraventricular tachycardia (SVT) with tachycardia-dependent (phase 3) right bundle branch block. Delivery of a late ventricular extrastimulus (arrow) during the SVT preexcites the right bundle branch (and either peels back or shortens its refractoriness) and restores normal conduction.

noted, the ERP of the RB normally shortens at faster heart rates to a greater degree than that of the LB; this finding explains the more frequent RBBB aberration at longer CLs and LBBB aberration at shorter CLs.[4,8,10]

This form of aberration is a marker of some type of cardiac abnormality when it appears at relatively slow heart rates (less than 70 beats/min), displays LBBB (Fig. 10-5), appears after several cycles of accelerated but regular rate, or appears with gradual rather than abrupt acceleration of the heart rate and at CL shortening by less than 5 milliseconds. Because of the small changes in the duration of the CL that may initiate aberration (critical cycle), recognition of acceleration-dependent aberration may require a long record to document the gradual, and at times minimal, shortening of the R-R interval.[8-10]

With increasing heart rate or persistence of fast heart rate, acceleration-dependent aberration can occasionally disappear. The normalization of a previously aberrant QRS complex can be explained by a greater shortening of the ERP of the bundle branches than that of the AVN or by a time-dependent gradual shortening of the refractory period of the affected bundle branch (a phenomenon occasionally referred to as *restitution*).[6]

During slowing of the heart rate, intraventricular conduction often fails to normalize at the critical CL, and aberration persists at cycles longer than the critical cycle that initiated the aberration. Once acceleration-dependent BBB is established, the actual cycle for the blocked bundle does not begin until approximately halfway through the QRS complex because of concealed transseptal conduction (see later); thus, it is necessary for the heart rate to slow down more than would be expected to reestablish normal conduction.[8-10]

PHASE 4 BLOCK

Phase 4 block occurs when conduction of an impulse is blocked in tissues well after their normal refractory periods have ended.[3,11] Phase 4 block is governed by the same physiological principles as those for phase 3 block. Membrane responsiveness is determined by the relationship of the membrane potential at excitation with the maximum height of phase 0. The availability of the Na^+ channels is reduced at less negative membrane potentials, and activation at a reduced membrane potential is likely to cause aberration or block.[6]

The cause of membrane depolarization (i.e., reduction of membrane potential) in the setting of phase 4 block, however, is different from that in phase 3 block. Enhanced phase 4 depolarization within the bundle branches can be caused by enhanced automaticity or partial depolarization of injured myocardial tissue, or both. In this setting, the maximum diastolic potential immediately follows repolarization, from which point the membrane potential is steadily reduced (by the pacemaker current). This reduction, in turn, results in inactivation of some Na^+ channels. Thus, an action potential initiated early in the cycle (immediately after repolarization) would have a steeper and higher phase 0 and consequently better conduction than would an action potential initiated later in the cycle when the membrane potential at the time of the stimulus is reduced, with resulting reductions in the velocity and height of phase 0 and slower conduction.[8,10,12]

Phase 4 aberration is one explanation for the development of aberration at the end of a long cycle. As a result of a gradual spontaneous depolarization made possible by a prolonged cycle, the cell is activated from a less negative potential, and the result is impaired

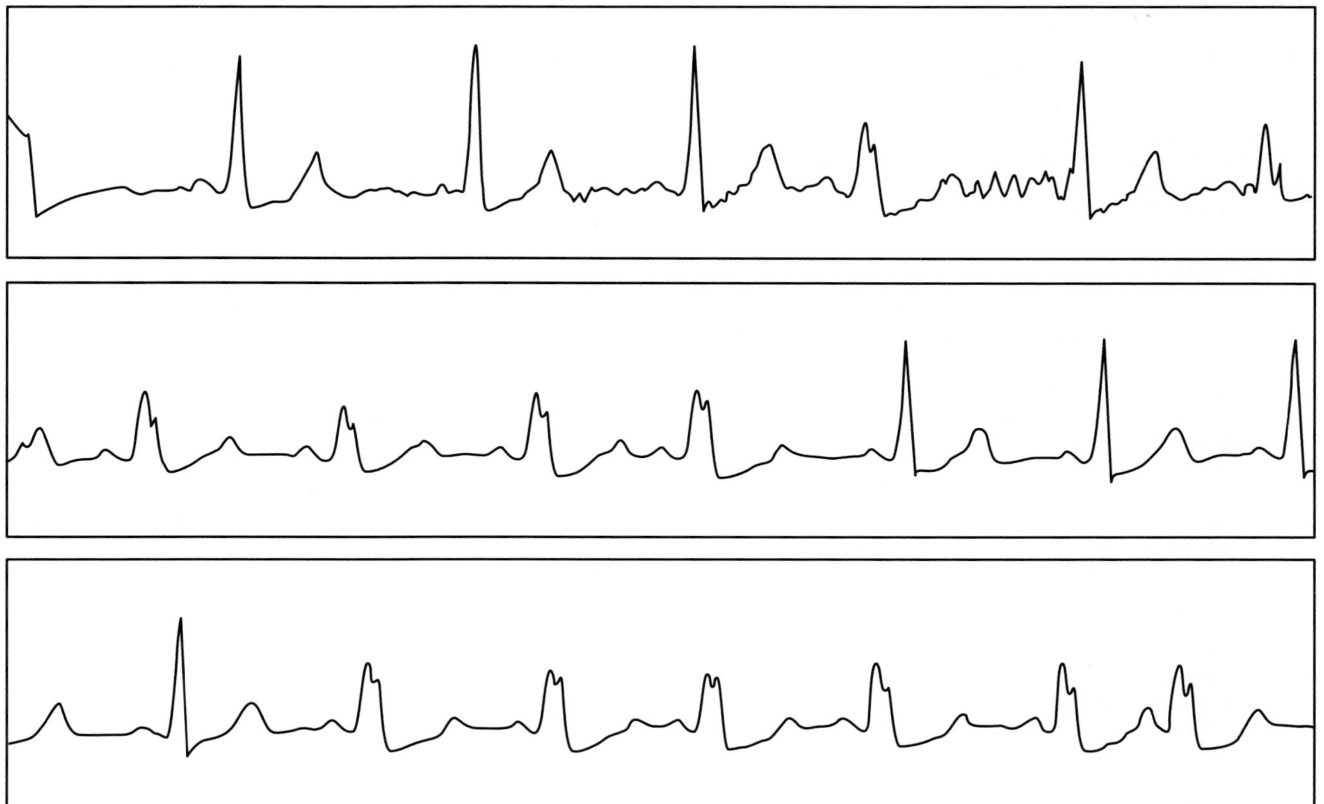

FIGURE 10-5 Acceleration-dependent aberration. The lead II continuous rhythm strip demonstrates sinus rhythm with rate-related left bundle branch block (LBBB). Note that small changes in rate can result in acceleration-dependent aberration. LBBB develops at a sinus rate faster than 70 beats/min, and normal QRS complexes are observed at slower sinus rates. The LBBB and the slow rate at which aberration develops strongly suggest an abnormality in the left bundle branch (LB), rather than physiological aberration, often associated with underlying structural heart disease such as cardiomyopathy. Interestingly, the onset and offset of the LBBB demonstrate hysteresis in that the cycle length (CL) required to initiate the LBBB is shorter than the CL required to maintain it, probably because of retrograde concealed penetration of the LB.

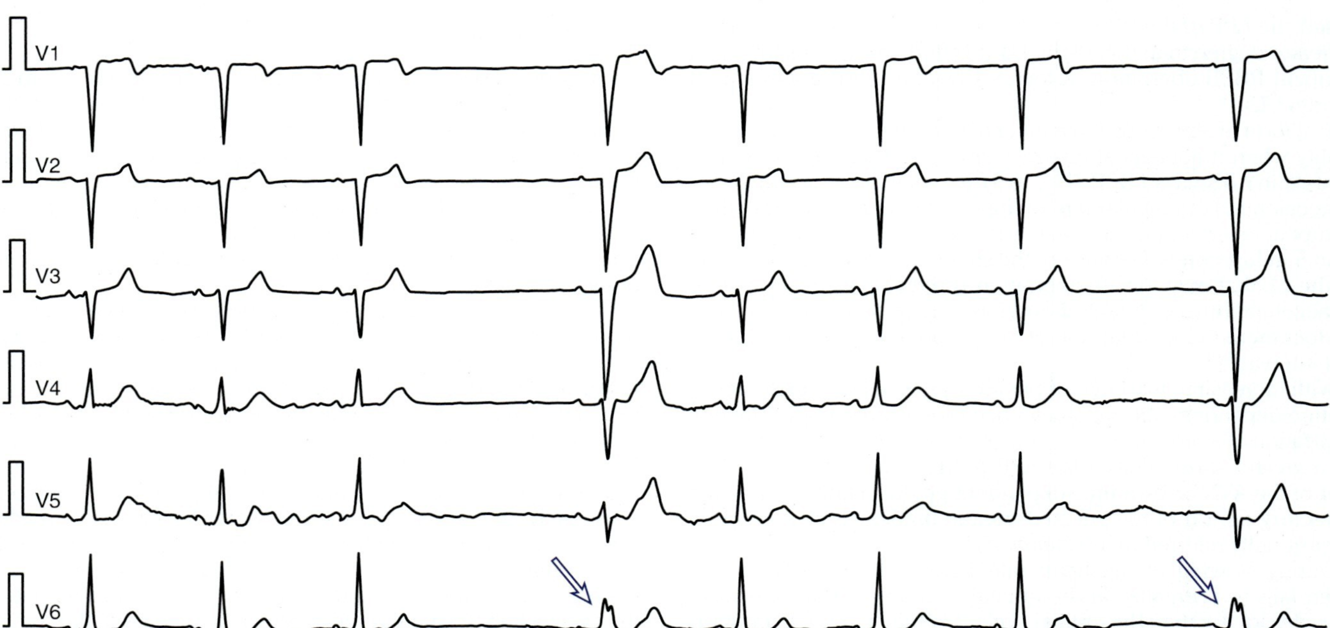

FIGURE 10-6 Bradycardia-dependent left bundle branch block (LBBB). Normal intraventricular conduction is observed during sinus rhythm. Premature atrial complexes (hidden within the T waves) are not conducted to the ventricles, resulting in pauses. The sinus complex following the pause is conducted with LBBB pattern (arrows) presumably secondary to phase 4 block. See text for discussion.

conduction. This type of aberration is sometimes referred to as bradycardia-dependent BBB (Fig. 10-6).[6] Importantly, the membrane potential has to depolarize significantly before conduction becomes impaired. Mild depolarization can actually improve conduction because the voltage is closer to threshold.

Phase 4 aberration would be expected in the setting of bradycardia or enhanced normal automaticity. However, despite the fact that bradycardia is common and cells with phase 4 depolarization are abundant, phase 4 block is not commonly seen; most reported cases are associated with structural heart disease. One explanation for this phenomenon is that in normal fibers, conduction is well maintained at membrane potentials more negative than −70 to −75 mV. Significant conduction disturbances are first manifested when the membrane potential is less negative than −70 mV at the time of stimulation; local block appears at −65 to −60 mV. Because the threshold potential for normal His-Purkinje fibers is −70 mV, spontaneous firing occurs before the membrane can actually be reduced to the potential necessary for conduction impairment or block. Phase 4 block is therefore pathological when it does occur, and it requires one or more of the following: (1) the presence of slow diastolic depolarization, which needs to be enhanced; (2) a decrease in excitability (a shift in threshold potential toward zero) so that, in the presence of significant bradycardia, sufficient time elapses before the impulse arrives, thus enabling the bundle branch fibers to reach a potential at which conduction is impaired; and (3) a deterioration in membrane responsiveness so that significant conduction impairment develops at −75 mV instead of −65 mV; this occurrence would also negate the necessity for such a long cycle before conduction fails.[8,10,12]

Bradycardia-dependent or phase 4 block almost always manifests an LBBB pattern, likely because the left ventricular (LV) conduction system is more susceptible to ischemic damage and has a higher rate of spontaneous phase 4 depolarization than the right ventricle (RV).[12]

Both tachycardia-dependent and bradycardia-dependent BBB can be seen in the same patient with an intermediate range of CLs associated with normal conduction. The prognosis of rate-dependent BBB largely depends on the presence and severity of the underlying heart disease. Its clinical implications are not clear, and it usually occurs in diseased tissue and in the setting of myocardial infarction (MI), especially inferior wall MI.[6]

ABERRATION CAUSED BY CONCEALED TRANSSEPTAL CONDUCTION

Concealed transseptal conduction is the underlying mechanism of aberration occurring in several situations, including perpetuation of aberrant conduction during tachyarrhythmias, unexpected persistence of acceleration-dependent aberration, and alternation of aberration during atrial bigeminal rhythm.[8-10,12,14,15]

Perpetuation of Aberrant Conduction during Tachyarrhythmias

During a supraventricular tachycardia (SVT) with normal ventricular activation, a PVC originating from the RV can retrogradely activate the RB early, whereas retrograde activation of the LB occurs later, following transseptal conduction of the PVC. Consequently, although the RB ERP expires in time for the next SVT impulse, the LB remains refractory because its actual cycle began later than the RB. Therefore, the next SVT impulse traveling down the His bundle (HB) encounters an excitable RB and a refractory LB; thus, it propagates to the RV over the RB (with an LBBB pattern, phase 3 aberration). Conduction subsequently propagates from the RV across the septum to the LV. By this time, the distal LB has recovered, allowing for retrograde penetration of the LB by the SVT impulse propagating transseptally, thereby rendering the LB refractory to each subsequent SVT impulse (Fig. 10-7). This process is repeated, and the LBBB pattern continues until another well-timed PVC preexcites the LB (and either peels back or shortens its refractoriness), so that the next impulse from above finds the LB fully recovered (see Fig. 10-4).[4,14,15]

Unexpected Persistence of Acceleration-Dependent Aberration

Acceleration-dependent BBB develops at a critical rate faster than the rate at which it disappears (Fig. 10-8). This paradox is most commonly ascribed to concealed conduction from the contralateral conducting bundle branch across the septum with delayed activation of the blocked bundle. Such concealed transseptal activation results in a bundle branch–to–bundle branch (RB-RB or LB-LB) interval shorter than the manifest R-R cycle. The reason is that the actual cycle for the blocked bundle does not begin until approximately halfway through the QRS complex, because it takes 60 to 100 milliseconds for the impulse to propagate down the RB and transseptally reach the blocked LB. Consequently, for normal

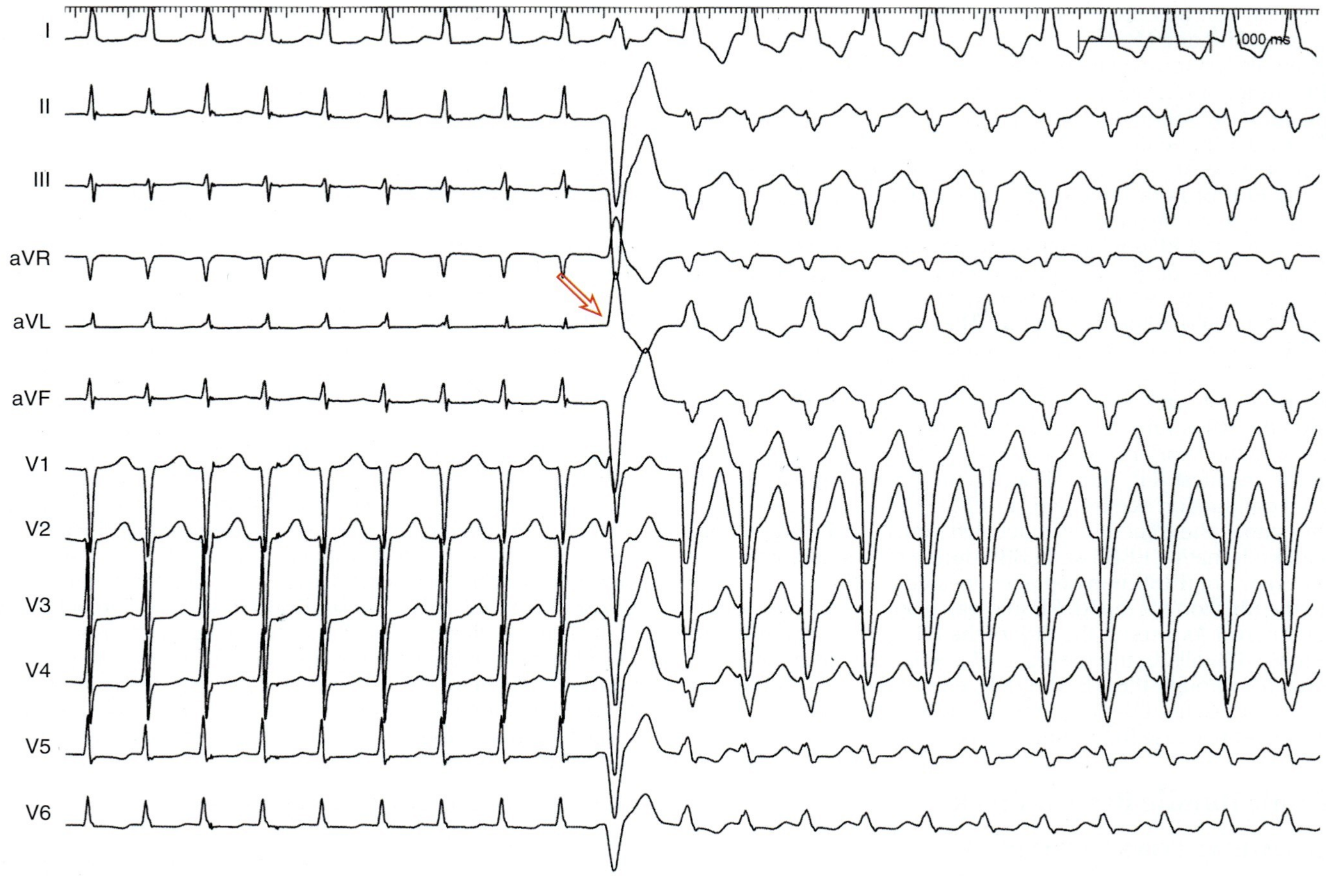

FIGURE 10-7 Perpetuation of aberrant conduction during supraventricular tachycardia (SVT) secondary to concealed transseptal conduction. At **left,** SVT is associated with normal ventricular activation and narrow QRS complexes. Critically timed ventricular extrastimulus delivered from the right ventricle (arrow) precipitates left bundle branch block aberrancy during the SVT. See text for discussion.

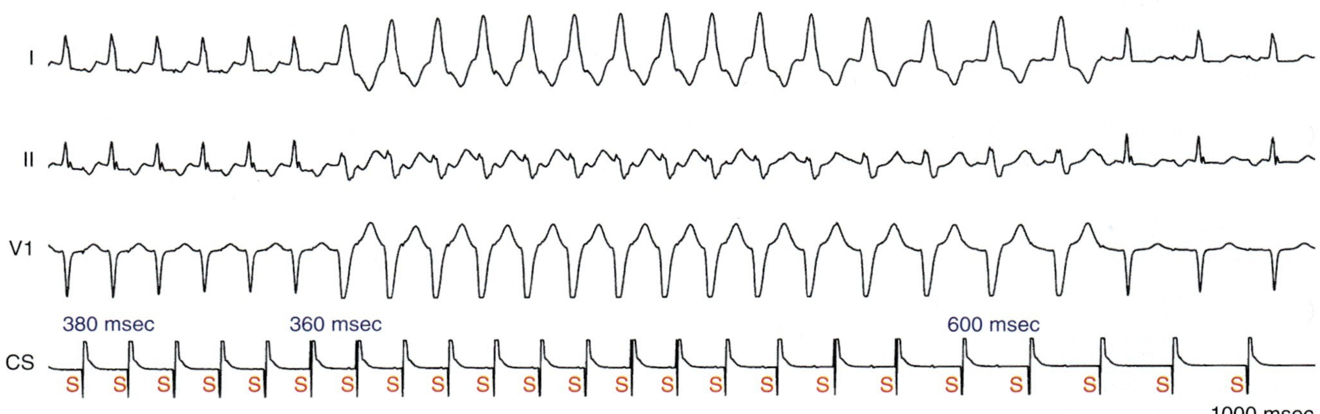

FIGURE 10-8 Unexpected persistence of acceleration-dependent aberration. During incremental-rate atrial pacing from the coronary sinus (CS), acceleration-dependent bundle branch block develops at a cycle length (CL) of up to 370 milliseconds. Aberrancy continues despite progressively increasing the pacing CL and disappears only when pacing at a CL of more than 600 milliseconds. See text for discussion.

conduction to resume, the cycle (R-R interval) during deceleration must be longer than the critical cycle during acceleration by at least 60 to 100 milliseconds.[8-10,12,14,15]

However, unexpected delay of normalization of conduction cannot always be explained by concealed conduction. Conduction sometimes normalizes with slowing of the heart rate, only to recur at cycles that are still longer than the critical cycle. Such a sequence excludes transseptal concealment as the mechanism of recurrence of the aberration. Similarly, when the discrepancy between the critical cycle and the cycle at which normalization finally occurs is longer than the expected transseptal activation time (approximately 60 milliseconds in the normal heart and 100 milliseconds in the diseased states), transseptal concealment alone cannot explain the delay (see Fig. 10-8). Fatigue and overdrive suppression have been suggested as possible mechanisms of the delayed normalization of conduction.[8-10]

Alternation of Aberration during Atrial Bigeminal Rhythm

A bigeminal rhythm can be caused by atrial bigeminy, 3:2 AV block, or atrial flutter with alternating 2:1 and 4:1 AV conduction. The alternation can be between a normal QRS complex and BBB or between RBBB and LBBB.

When alternation occurs between a normal QRS complex and RBBB during atrial bigeminy, the ERP of both RB and LB starts simultaneously following the normally conducted PAC, and the ERP of both branches is relatively short because of the preceding short cycle. After the pause, the sinus beat conducts normally, and the ERP of both bundle branches starts simultaneously but is relatively long because of the preceding long cycle. However, because the RB ERP is relatively longer than that of the LB, the next PAC encroaches on the RB refractoriness and conducts with an RBBB pattern (phase 3 block). Subsequently, that PAC is conducted down the LB and across the septum. The PAC activates the RB retrogradely after some delay (concealed transseptal conduction), so that the RB-RB interval (during the following pause) and the RB ERP become shorter. As a result, by the time the next PAC reaches the RB, the RB is fully recovered because of its abbreviated ERP (reflecting the shorter preceding RB-RB interval, which is shorter than the manifest R-R interval during the preceding pause), and normal conduction occurs (see Fig. 10-2).[14,15]

The same phenomenon (concealed transseptal conduction) explains alternating RBBB and LBBB during bigeminal rhythms. In the presence of RBBB, transseptal concealed conduction from the LB to the RB shortens the RB-RB interval relative to the now longer LB-LB interval. As a result, the ERP of the LB is longer and conduction in the LB fails. In the presence of a refractory LB, conduction propagates through the RB. The delayed transseptal activation of the LB shortens the LB-LB interval. The ERP of the RB is now relatively longer, because RB conduction is blocked.[9,10,12]

Chronic Bundle Branch Block

ANATOMICAL CONSIDERATIONS

Normal ventricular activation requires the synchronized participation of the distal components of the specialized conduction system (i.e., the main bundle branches and their ramifications). An IVCD is the result of abnormal activation of the ventricles caused by conduction delay or block in one or more parts of the specialized conduction system. Abnormalities of local myocardial activation can further alter the specific pattern of venticular activation.[1,6]

Traditionally, three major fascicles are considered to be operative in normal persons: the RB, the left anterior fascicle (LAF), and the left posterior fascicle (LPF). An estimated 65% of individuals have a third fascicle of the LB, the left median fascicle (LMF). The HB divides at the junction of the fibrous and muscular boundaries of the intraventricular septum into the RB and LB. The RB is an anatomically compact unit that travels as the extension of the HB after the origin of the LB. The LB and its divisions are, unlike the RB, diffuse structures that fan out just beyond their origin. The LAF represents the superior (anterior) division of the LB, the LPF represents the inferior (posterior) division of the LB, and the LMF represents the septal (median) division of the LB.[6]

The bundle branches and fascicles consist of bundles of Purkinje cells covered by a dense sheath of connective tissue. The terminal Purkinje fibers connect the ends of the bundle branches to the ventricular myocardium. Purkinje fibers form interweaving networks on the endocardial surface of both ventricles and penetrate only the inner third of the endocardium, and they tend to be less concentrated at the base of the ventricle and at the papillary muscle tips. Purkinje cells are specialized to conduct rapidly, at 1 to 3 m/sec, because phase 0 of the action potential is dependent on the rapid inward Na^+ current (I_{Na}). This characteristic results in almost simultaneous depolarization of the terminal HPS and propagation of the cardiac impulse to the entire RV and LV endocardium.[6]

Characteristics of the Right Bundle

The RB courses down the right side of interventricular septum near the endocardium in its upper third, deeper in the muscular portion of the septum in the middle third, and then again near the endocardium in its lower third. The RB is a long, thin, discrete structure. It does not divide throughout most of its course, and it begins to ramify as it approaches the base of the right anterior papillary muscle, with fascicles going to the septal and free walls of the RV.

The RB is vulnerable to stretch and trauma for two thirds of its course when it travels subendocardially. Chronic RBBB pattern can result from three levels of conduction delay in the RV: proximal, distal, or terminal.[3] Proximal RBBB is the most common site of conduction delay. Distal RBBB occurs at the level of the moderator band, and it is an unusual site of conduction delay unless there has been transection of the moderator band during surgery. Terminal RBBB involves the distal conduction system of the RB or, more likely, the ventricular muscle itself, and it can be produced by ventriculotomy or transatrial resection of parietal bands in repair of tetralogy of Fallot. In addition, RBBB can be induced by events in the HB, because certain fibers of the HB are organized longitudinally and predestined to activate only one fascicle or bundle branch. Disease in these areas can result in activation that is asynchronous from that in the rest of the infranodal conducting system, possibly with resulting bundle branch or fascicular block.

The development of RBBB after a normal pattern can suggest the presence of structural heart disease, although less often than the development of LBBB; however, RBBB in younger individuals generally is not indicative of serious underlying heart disease. Causes of RBBB include increased RV pressure, RV hypertrophy or dilatation, ischemic heart disease, myocarditis, cor pulmonale, acute and chronic pulmonary embolism, hypertension, cardiomyopathies, congenital heart disease, and mechanical damage, as well as Lev and Lenègre diseases.

Characteristics of the Left Bundle and Its Fascicles

The predivisional portion of the LB penetrates the membranous portion of the interventricular septum under the aortic ring and then divides into three discrete branches: the LAF, the LPF, and the LMF.[3] The LAF crosses the anterobasal LV region toward the anterior papillary muscle and terminates in the Purkinje system of the anterolateral wall of the LV. The LPF appears as an extension of the main LB and is large in its initial course. It then fans out extensively toward the posterior papillary muscle and terminates in the Purkinje system of the posteroinferior wall of the LV. The LMF runs to the interventricular septum; it arises in most cases from the LPF, less frequently from the LAF, or from both, and in a few cases it has an independent origin from the central part of the main LB at the site of its bifurcation.[16]

The clinical presentation of conduction disturbances, in order of decreasing incidence, is LAF block, RBBB, LBBB, and LPF block. This rank depends not only on the intrinsic, anatomical, and genetically determined differences among branches and fascicles but also on the manner in which the intraventricular conduction system is exposed to the various pathological processes of the surrounding cardiac structures. LBBB is usually caused by ischemic or mechanical factors, and the site of block is typically in the predivisional segment at the junction of the LB and HB. LBBB is encountered usually in patients with structural heart disease involving dilation, hypertrophy, or fibrosis of the LV such as ischemic heart disease, valvular heart disease, and various cardiomyopathies. LBBB can also be caused by Lev and Lenègre diseases. The location of conduction delay in LBBB can be proximal (particularly in diffuse myocardial disease), distal, or a combination of both.

The LAF can be injured by diseases that involve primarily the LV basal septum, the anterior half of the ventricular septum, and the anterolateral LV wall. In fact, isolated LAF block is the most common type of IVCD seen in acute anterior MI. Other disorders and situations that can also cause LAF block include hypertension, cardiomyopathies, aortic valve disease, Lev and Lenègre diseases, spontaneous and surgical closure of a ventricular septal defect, and other surgical procedures.[16-18]

In contrast, the LPF is the least vulnerable segment of the whole system because it is short and wide and is located in the inflow tract of the LV, which is a less turbulent region than the outflow tract. Additionally, the LPF has a dual blood supply, from the anterior and posterior descending coronary arteries, and it is not related to structures that are so potentially dangerous.[16] LPF block is a rare finding, and rather nonspecific for cardiac disease. LPF block is almost always associated with RBBB.

SITE OF BLOCK

Interest in the site of block stems from the fact that bifascicular block (especially RBBB and LAF block) is the most common ECG pattern preceding the development of AV block. Determining the site of block therefore can help predict the risk of AV block.

Despite ECG anatomical correlates, the site of block producing BBB patterns is not certain in all cases. Data suggest that fibers to the RV and LV are already predestined within the HB and that lesions in the HB can produce characteristic BBB patterns. Longitudinal dissociation with asynchronous conduction in the HB can give rise to abnormal patterns of ventricular activation; hence, the conduction problem may not necessarily lie in the individual bundle branch. Moreover, it is not uncommon for intra-Hisian disease to be accompanied by BBB (especially LBBB).[3] Pacing distal to the site of block can normalize the QRS. Furthermore, the problem may not be actual block, because conduction *delay* within the bundle in the range of 10 milliseconds can give rise to an ECG pattern of BBB.

CLINICAL RELEVANCE

The prognosis of BBB is related largely to the type and severity of the underlying heart disease and to the possible presence of other conduction disturbances. Isolated BBB in the absence of apparent structural heart disease and not associated with block in the other fascicles is usually benign.

Bifascicular block (especially RBBB and LAF block) is the most common ECG pattern preceding complete heart block in adults. Other forms of IVCD precede the bulk of the remaining cases of complete intra-Hisian and infra-Hisian AV block. The incidence of progression to complete AV block is approximately 2% in asymptomatic patients with an IVCD and approximately 6% in patients with an IVCD and neurological symptoms (e.g., syncope).[19,20]

Patients with BBB have an unusually high incidence of cardiac disease and sudden cardiac death. The highest incidence of sudden cardiac death is among patients with LBBB and cardiac disease.[19-22] However, most sudden cardiac deaths are caused by VT or ventricular fibrillation, do not seem to be related to AV block, and are not prevented by pacemakers (although pacing can potentially relieve symptoms such as syncope). Complete electrophysiological (EP) testing and ventricular stimulation are therefore necessary in patients with syncope and BBB because VT can be found in up to 30% to 50%. Although the poor prognosis associated with BBB is related to myocardial dysfunction, heart failure, and ventricular fibrillation rather than heart block, symptoms such as syncope are often related to heart block.[23-25]

RBBB is a common finding in the general population. In patients without evidence of structural heart disease, RBBB has no prognostic significance. However, new-onset RBBB does predict a higher rate of coronary artery disease, heart failure, and cardiovascular mortality. When cardiac disease is present, the coexistence of RBBB suggests advanced disease. RBBB is an independent predictor of all-cause mortality in patients with known or suspected coronary heart disease, and in the setting of an acute MI, RBBB is associated with a significant increase in mortality.[26]

The prevalence of LBBB in the general population has been reported to vary considerably according to population size and sampling criteria; it ranges from 0.1% to 0.8%. The presence of isolated LBBB has no adverse prognostic significance. In patients with LBBB associated with ischemic heart disease, hypertension, or cardiomyopathy, the prognosis depends on the severity of the underlying heart disease. Nevertheless, among patients with acute MI, cardiomyopathy, and heart failure, the presence of LBBB is associated with a worse prognosis. Because the presence of LBBB can represent the clinical onset of LV structural disease such as dilated cardiomyopathy or an infective, hypertensive, or valvular heart disease, the finding of LBBB on resting ECG requires further evaluation with echocardiogram and Holter monitoring for assessment of LV function, as well as identifying both advanced degrees of AV block and heart disease-related tachyarrhythmias. Evaluation for ischemic heart disease can be necessary based on the presence of risk factors and typical symptoms.[26]

The prevalence of LAF block in the general population ranges from 0.9% to 6.2%. Isolated LAF block does not itself imply a risk factor for cardiac mortality or morbidity, and in a healthy population it should be regarded as an incidental ECG finding.[16] The prognosis of LAF block is primarily related to the underlying heart disease. LAF block in the setting of acute MI is probably associated with increased mortality.

As noted, LPF block is a rare finding and rather nonspecific for cardiac disease. LPF block is almost always associated with RBBB, in that LPF block and RBBB share cause, pathogenesis, and prognosis. The combination of LPF block and RBBB in acute MI is associated with a high mortality rate (80% to 87%) during the first weeks after the coronary event. Similarly, the risk of progression toward complete AV block (a form of trifascicular block) is also considerable (42%), and approximately 75% of these patients die of pump failure.[16]

Electrocardiographic Features

Bundle Branch Block

The ECG criteria for different types of fascicular blocks and BBB are listed in Table 10-1. The ECG pattern of BBB can represent complete block or conduction delay (relative to the other fascicles) that produces asynchronous ventricular activation without necessarily implying complete failure of conduction in the diseased fascicle. Therefore, an ECG pattern of complete BBB can have varying degrees or alternate with contralateral complete BBB pattern, phenomena explained by delay, rather than complete block, as the underlying pathophysiologic feature of the ECG pattern.[3,20,27]

BBB leads to prolongation of the QRS duration and sometimes to alterations in the QRS vector. The degree of prolongation of the QRS duration depends on the severity of the impairment. With complete BBB, the QRS is 120 milliseconds or longer in duration; with incomplete BBB, the QRS duration is 100 to 120 milliseconds. The QRS vector in BBB is generally oriented in the direction of the myocardial region in which depolarization is delayed.[1]

BBB is characteristically associated with secondary repolarization (ST-T) abnormalities. The T wave is typically opposite in polarity to the last deflection of the QRS, a discordance that is caused by the altered sequence of repolarization that occurs secondary to altered depolarization.

RIGHT BUNDLE BRANCH BLOCK

Development of RBBB alters the activation sequence of the RV but not the LV. Because the LB is not affected, the initial septal activation (the initial 30 milliseconds of the QRS complex), which depends on the LB, remains normal, occurring from left to right, and results in septal q waves in leads I, aVL, and V_6 and r waves in leads V_1, V_2, and aVR.[26] Thus, the Q wave of a prior MI remains unchanged. Septal activation is followed by LV activation (within the subsequent 40 to 60 milliseconds), occurring over the LB in a leftward and posterior vector and resulting in R waves in the leftward leads (I, aVL, and V_6), as well as s (or S) waves in the anterior precordial leads (V_1 and V_2). This appearance is usually similar to that in normal subjects.

The asynchronous depolarization caused by RBBB is primarily manifested in the later portion of the QRS, at 80 milliseconds and beyond. During this time, RV activation spreads slowly by conduction through working muscle fibers rather than the specialized Purkinje system, and it occurs predominantly after activation of the LV has completed. The forces generated by the late, unopposed RV free wall activation result in a terminal rightward and anterior positivity, manifesting as a second positive deflection that can be small (r′) or large (R′) in the anterior precordial leads (V_1 and V_2) and S waves in the leftward leads (I, aVL, and V_6; Fig. 10-9).[3,26] The QRS axis is unaffected by RBBB; left or right axis deviation can indicate concurrent LAF or LPF block, respectively (see Fig. 10-9).

TABLE 10-1 ECG Criteria for Fascicular and Bundle Branch Block

Complete Right Bundle Branch Block

- QRS duration ≥120 msec in adults
- Broad, notched secondary R waves (rsr′, rsR′, or rSR′ patterns) in right precordial leads (V_1 and V_2); R′ or r′ deflection usually wider than the initial R wave; in a minority of patients, a wide and often notched R wave pattern may be seen in lead V_1 and/or V_2
- Wide, deep S waves (qRS pattern) of greater duration than R wave or greater than 40 msec in leads I and V_6
- Normal R wave peak time in leads V_5 and V_6 but >50 msec in lead V_1
- Of the foregoing criteria, the first three should be present to make the diagnosis; when a pure dominant R wave with or without a notch is present in V_1, criterion 4 should be satisfied

Complete Left Bundle Branch Block

- QRS duration ≥120 msec in adults
- Broad notched or slurred R wave in leads I, aVL, V_5, and V_6 and an occasional RS pattern in V_5 and V_6 attributed to displaced transition of QRS complex
- Absent q waves in leads I, V_5, and V_6, but in the lead aVL, a narrow q wave may be present in the absence of myocardial disease
- R wave peak time >60 msec in leads V_5 and V_6 but normal in leads V_1, V_2, and V_3, when small initial r waves can be discerned in the above leads
- ST and T waves usually opposite in direction to QRS
- Positive T wave in leads with upright QRS may be normal (positive concordance)
- Depressed ST segment and/or negative T wave in leads with negative QRS (negative concordance) are abnormal
- Appearance of LBBB may change the mean QRS axis in the frontal plane to the right, to the left, or superiorly, in some cases in a rate-dependent manner

Left Anterior Fascicular Block

- Frontal plane axis between −45 and −90 degrees
- qR pattern in lead aVL
- R wave peak time in lead aVL ≥45 msec
- QRS duration <120 msec

Left Posterior Fascicular Block

- Frontal plane axis between 90 and 180 degrees in adults
- rS pattern in leads I and aVL
- qR pattern in leads III and aVF
- QRS duration <120 msec

RBBB also results in an abnormality of ventricular repolarization of the RV myocardium. Thus, there are often secondary ST segment and T wave changes present in the right precordial leads. The ST segment change is usually small and, when present, is discordant (i.e., has an axis in the opposite direction) to the terminal mean QRS spatial vector. The T wave also tends to be discordant to the terminal conduction disturbance, resulting in inverted T waves in the right precordial leads (where there is a terminal R′ wave) and upright T waves in the left precordial leads (where there is a terminal S wave).

The time interval necessary for full depolarization of the ventricular free wall (from the endocardium to the epicardium) beneath any given ECG electrode corresponds to the interval from the beginning of the QRS complex to the time of initial downstroke of the R wave after it has peaked (or to the time of initial upstroke of the S wave after it has reached its nadir). This interval is termed *R wave peak time* (in preference to the term *intrinsicoid deflection*). In the right precordial leads, the upper limit of normal for R wave peak time is 35 milliseconds, whereas in the left precordial leads, it is 45 milliseconds. In RBBB, the R wave peak time is delayed in the right precordial leads (more than 50 milliseconds).[1]

Atypical Right Bundle Branch Block

Atypical RBBB can be caused by attenuation or loss of posterior deflections in the anteroposterior leads, resulting in an rsR′, qR, or M-shaped QRS pattern in V_1. This pattern can be a normal variant, a consequence of a gain of midtemporal anterior forces secondary to RV enlargement or concurrent LAF block, or the result of a loss of posterior forces caused by a posterior wall MI.

Incomplete Right Bundle Branch Block

An incomplete RBBB can result from lesser degrees of conduction delay in the RB. The ECG pattern of incomplete RBBB is similar to that of complete RBBB, except that the QRS duration is between 110 and 120 milliseconds (see Fig. 10-9). An RBBB pattern with a QRS duration shorter than 100 milliseconds can be a normal variant, presumably reflecting a slight delay in the terminal posterobasal forces in some individuals.[1]

The ECG pattern of incomplete or complete RBBB in association with a distinct ST segment elevation in the right precordial leads can be observed in the Brugada syndrome. The Brugada ECG pattern, however, is characterized by the absence of a wide terminal S wave in the left lateral leads (I, aVL, V_5, V_6) and no broad terminal R wave in aVR, findings indicating that true RBBB is not present

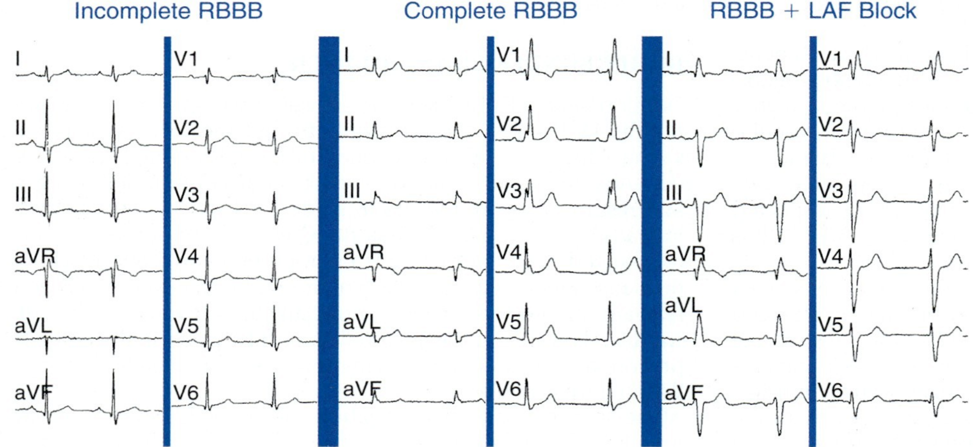

FIGURE 10-9 Surface ECG of incomplete and complete right bundle branch block (RBBB) and bifascicular block. LAF = left anterior fascicle.

(see Fig. 31-5). Additionally, the ECG manifestations of the Brugada syndrome are often dynamic or concealed and can be unmasked or modulated primarily by sodium channel blockers but also during a febrile state or with vagotonic agents.[28]

LEFT BUNDLE BRANCH BLOCK

The normal sequence of ventricular activation is altered dramatically in LBBB. Complete LBBB results in delayed and abnormal activation and diffuse slowing of conduction throughout the LV. Activation of the LV originates from the RB in a right to left direction, in contrast to the normal situation in which the first part of the LV myocardium to be activated is the septum in a left to right direction via a small septal branch of the LB. Thus, LBBB results in reversal of the direction of the initial septal activation sequence (within the initial 30 milliseconds of the QRS complex), with the activation traveling from right to left and from apex to base and to the RV apex and free wall. RV activation is typically completed within the first 45 milliseconds of the onset of the QRS, before the onset of LV activation. However, because the septum is a larger structure than the RV free wall, septal activation predominates, eliciting a leftward and usually anterior vector and resulting in loss of the normal small q waves and initiation of a wide, slurred R wave in leads I, aVL, and V_6 and an rS or QS pattern in lead V_1 (Fig. 10-10). Thus, Q waves of a prior MI may disappear, and new Q waves can emerge.

Following septal activation, LV activation (starting as late as 44 to 58 milliseconds into the QRS) spreads slowly by conduction through working muscle fibers rather than the specialized conduction system, with spatial vectors oriented to the left and posteriorly because the LV is a leftward and posterior structure. As a consequence, the delayed LV activation (unopposed by the now completed RV activation) produces large, broad, and notched or slurred R waves (without q or s waves) in the leftward leads (I, aVL, and V_6), with delayed R wave peak time in the left precordial leads (more than 60 milliseconds). The slowing and notching of the mid-QRS portion are caused by slow transseptal conduction. The terminal activation vector results from depolarization of the anterolateral LV wall that produces a small vector that is also directed to the left and posteriorly.[1,3,25]

The altered activation sequence also changes the sequence of repolarization. Both the ST segment and T wave vectors are discordant from the QRS complex.

Incomplete Left Bundle Branch Block

Incomplete LBBB can result from lesser degrees of conduction delay in the LB. Although LV activation begins abnormally on the right side of the septum (as in complete LBBB), much of the subsequent LV activation occurs via the normal conduction system. Incomplete LBBB is characterized by the following: (1) QRS duration of 110 to 119 milliseconds; (2) presence of an LV hypertrophy pattern; (3) R wave peak time longer than 60 milliseconds in leads V_4, V_5, and V_6; and (4) absence of q wave in leads I, V_5, and V_6 and frequent replacement by a slurred initial upstroke (pseudo-delta wave) (see Fig. 10-10). This entity can bear an ECG resemblance to a Wolff-Parkinson-White ECG pattern secondary to the delayed upstroke of the R wave, although the PR interval is usually short in Wolff-Parkinson-White syndrome, whereas it should be normal in cases of incomplete LBBB.[1]

Fascicular Block

Hemiblocks in the LB system affect the LAF, LPF, or LMF. Fascicular block generally does not substantially prolong QRS duration, but alters only the sequence of LV activation. The primary ECG change is a shift in the frontal plane QRS axis because the conduction disturbance primarily involves the early phases of activation. The QRS duration is usually less than 100 milliseconds (unless complicated by BBB or hypertrophy), although some investigators allow a QRS duration of up to 120 milliseconds, or 20 milliseconds higher than the previous baseline.[16-18]

LEFT ANTERIOR FASCICULAR BLOCK

The LAF normally initiates activation in the upper part of the septum, the anterolateral LV free wall, and the left anterior papillary muscle. Delayed activation of these regions secondary to damage to the LAF causes unopposed activation wavefronts by the LPF and LMF early during the QRS complex and unopposed anterosuperior forces late during ventricular activation. All these changes occur with a QRS that widens no more than 20 milliseconds in pure and uncomplicated LAF block.[16]

As a consequence, the initial (first 20 milliseconds) QRS vector is normal in time, but it has an abnormal direction. Rather than proceeding superiorly and to the left, the QRS vector depicts an inferior and rightward shift in the frontal plane (frontal plane axis more than +120 degrees) that produces a small, sharp r wave in the

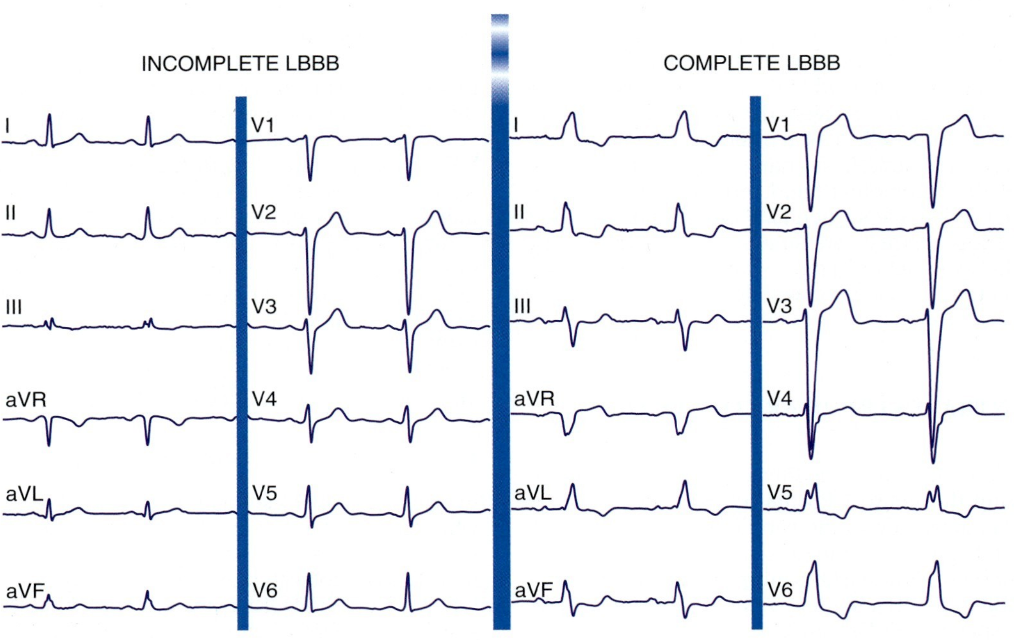

FIGURE 10-10 Surface ECG of incomplete and complete left bundle branch block (LBBB).

inferior leads (II, III, and aVF) and a small q wave in leads I, aVL, V_5, and V_6. Additionally, the inferior and rightward shift in the initial QRS forces can occasionally result in a small, sharp q wave in leads V_2 and V_3 (mimicking old anteroseptal infarction patterns) when the electrodes are placed at the normal level and, in almost all cases, when they are placed in a higher position.[16]

During the midportion of the QRS, the main forces of LV activation are oriented superiorly and to the left (frontal plane axis more than −45 or −60 degrees), with a wide-open counterclockwise-rotated loop in the frontal plane caused by the delayed activation of the high lateral wall, which is normally activated by the LAF. This results in deep S waves in leads II, III, and aVF (S wave deeper in lead III than in lead II), and R waves in aVR and aVL. The net effect is an rS pattern in leads II, III, and aVF and a qR or R pattern in leads I, aVL, V_5, and V_6. Additionally, as a result of the superiorly directed forces, deeper S waves are recorded in leads V_5 and V_6; these waves tend to disappear when the electrodes are placed above the normal level and are deeper when the electrodes are placed below the normal level.[1,16-18]

The ECG pattern of LAF block can simulate LV hypertrophy in limb leads I and aVL. Conversely, it can conceal signs of LV hypertrophy in the left precordial leads, and it can also hide signs of inferior ischemia.

LEFT POSTERIOR FASCICULAR BLOCK

The early unopposed activation of the anterolateral wall of the LV by the normally conducting LAF and LMF causes the initial forces to be oriented superiorly and to the left, producing initial small r waves in leads I, aVL, V_1, and V_6 and small q waves in leads II, III, and aVF. However, the main and terminal forces of the QRS are directed posteriorly, inferiorly, and to the right with a wide-open clockwise-rotated loop, because of the late unopposed activation of the areas normally activated by the LPF (the inferoposterior LV free wall). This is responsible for the characteristic rightward frontal plane axis of +120 to +180 degrees. As a result, there is a qR morphology in leads II, III, and aVF and an rS morphology in leads I and aVL. In fact, the ECG pattern of LPF block is the exact mirror image of LAF block in the standard and unipolar leads. LPF block is almost always associated with RBBB. Isolated LPF block is extremely rare, and a firm diagnosis requires that other causes of right axis deviation have been excluded.[1,16]

LEFT MEDIAN FASCICULAR BLOCK

The ECG pattern seen with LMF block is probably determined by the differences in the sites of insertion of the LMF, LAF, and LPF. Functional block in the LMF can lead to the apparent loss of anterior forces and can result in the transient development of q waves in leads V_1 and V_2, which normally have a positive initial deflection caused by septal depolarization. These changes are similar to those that occur in septal MI. On the other hand, prominent R waves are seen in the right precordial leads when LMF block leads to a gain of anterior forces. These changes are similar to those caused by true posterior MI. The prominence of the R waves may be increased when LMF block occurs in association with RBBB.

Other Types

NONSPECIFIC INTRAVENTRICULAR CONDUCTION DEFECTS

A nonspecific IVCD is the result of diffuse slowing of impulse conduction involving the entire HPS that causes a generalized and uniform delay in activation of the ventricular myocardium. A nonspecific IVCD is diagnosed in the presence of a QRS duration longer than 120 milliseconds and a QRS morphology that does not resemble either LBBB or RBBB and may even resemble the normal QRS complex. Nonspecific IVCDs can be classified as LV or RV IVCD, depending on the site of delayed R wave peak time and the direction of the terminal forces.

BIFASCICULAR BLOCKS

Bifascicular block refers to different combinations of fascicular block and BBB. Examples of bifascicular block include RBBB with LAF block (most common; see Fig. 10-9), RBBB with LPF block, and LAF block plus LPF block (which manifests as LBBB).

TRIFASCICULAR BLOCKS

Trifascicular block involves conduction delay in the RB and either the main LB or both the LAF and LPF. The resulting ECG pattern depends on the relative degree of conduction delay in the affected fascicles. Ventricular activation starts at the insertion site of the fastest conducting fascicle, with subsequent spread of activation from that site to the remainder of the ventricles. ECG documentation of trifascicular block during 1:1 AV conduction is rare. ECG manifestations of trifascicular block include the following: (1) complete AV block with a slow ventricular escape rhythm with a wide, bizarre QRS; (2) alternating RBBB and LBBB; and (3) fixed RBBB with alternating LAF and LPF block.

The combination of bifascicular block (RBBB plus LAF block, RBBB plus LPF block, or LBBB) with first-degree AV block on the surface ECG (Fig. 10-11) cannot be considered as trifascicular block because the site of AV block can be in the AVN or HPS, and such a pattern can reflect slow conduction in the AVN with concomitant bifascicular block. In such circumstances, the PR interval on the ECG does not appear to be helpful in selecting those individuals with a prolonged His bundle–ventricular (HV) interval because a normal PR interval can easily conceal a significantly prolonged HV interval and a prolonged PR interval can be caused by a prolonged atrial–His bundle (AH) interval. However, two criteria can be of value: (1) a short PR interval (less than 160 milliseconds) makes a markedly prolonged HV interval (i.e., more than 100 milliseconds) unlikely, and (2) a markedly prolonged PR interval (more than 300 milliseconds) almost always indicates that at least some of the abnormality, if not all, is caused by AVN conduction.

ALTERNATING BUNDLE BRANCH BLOCK

Alternating RBBB and LBBB is manifested by QRS complexes with LBBB morphology coexisting with complexes with RBBB morphology (Fig. 10-12). Often, every other complex is an RBBB or LBBB. Spontaneous alternating BBB, especially when associated with a change in the PR interval, represents the most common ominous sign for progression to AV block (Fig. 10-13). Beat-to-beat alternation is the most concerning, whereas a change in BBB noted on different days is less ominous.

This phenomenon implies instability of the HPS and a disease process involving the HB or bundle branches. In most patients with diffuse HPS disease, delay or block in one of the bundle branches consistently predominates, and alternating BBB is uncommon. The HV interval in alternating BBB is almost universally prolonged and typically varies with the change in BBB. This group has the highest incidence of HV interval exceeding 100 milliseconds.[3]

Alternating BBB is infrequent but is associated with the most predictable progression to complete AV block (70% of patients develop high-grade AV block within weeks of diagnosis). As a rule, AV conduction delay or block can be assumed to be caused by BBB only in the presence of an alternating or intermittent RBBB and LBBB with a changing PR interval. Not infrequently, the bilateral BBB is caused by acceleration-dependent aberration.

INTERMITTENT BUNDLE BRANCH BLOCK

Intermittent BBB, either right or left, is diagnosed on the surface ECG when there are occasional QRS complexes with RBBB or LBBB morphology, interspersed with QRS complexes that have a normal morphology. Most often, the intermittent BBB is rate-related; thus, the R-R intervals of the QRS complexes manifesting the BBB are shorter when compared with the intervals of the normal QRS complexes. In other cases, there is no rate-related change in the QRS intervals, but the occurrence of the BBB is a random or sporadic event.

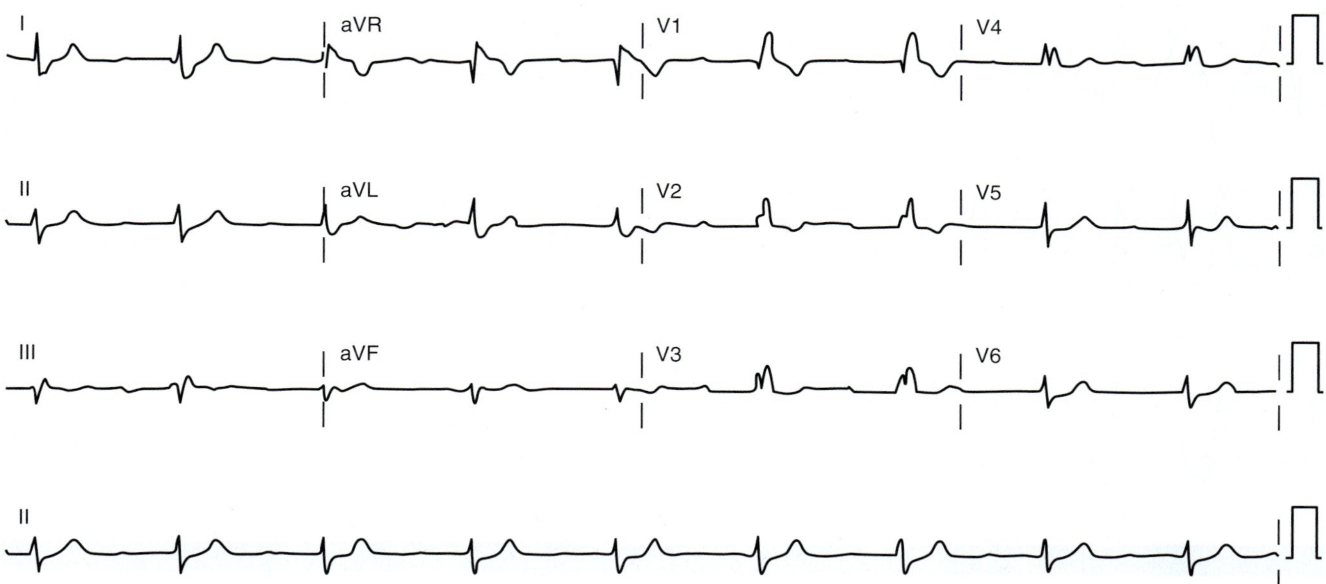

FIGURE 10-11 Surface ECG of sinus rhythm with first-degree atrioventricular (AV) block and bifascicular block (right bundle branch block and left anterior fascicular block). The PR interval is markedly prolonged (480 msec), which suggests that at least some of the AV conduction delay, if not all, occurs in the atrioventricular node and is not exclusively in the His-Purkinje system. A diagnosis of trifascicular block cannot be made solely based on this ECG.

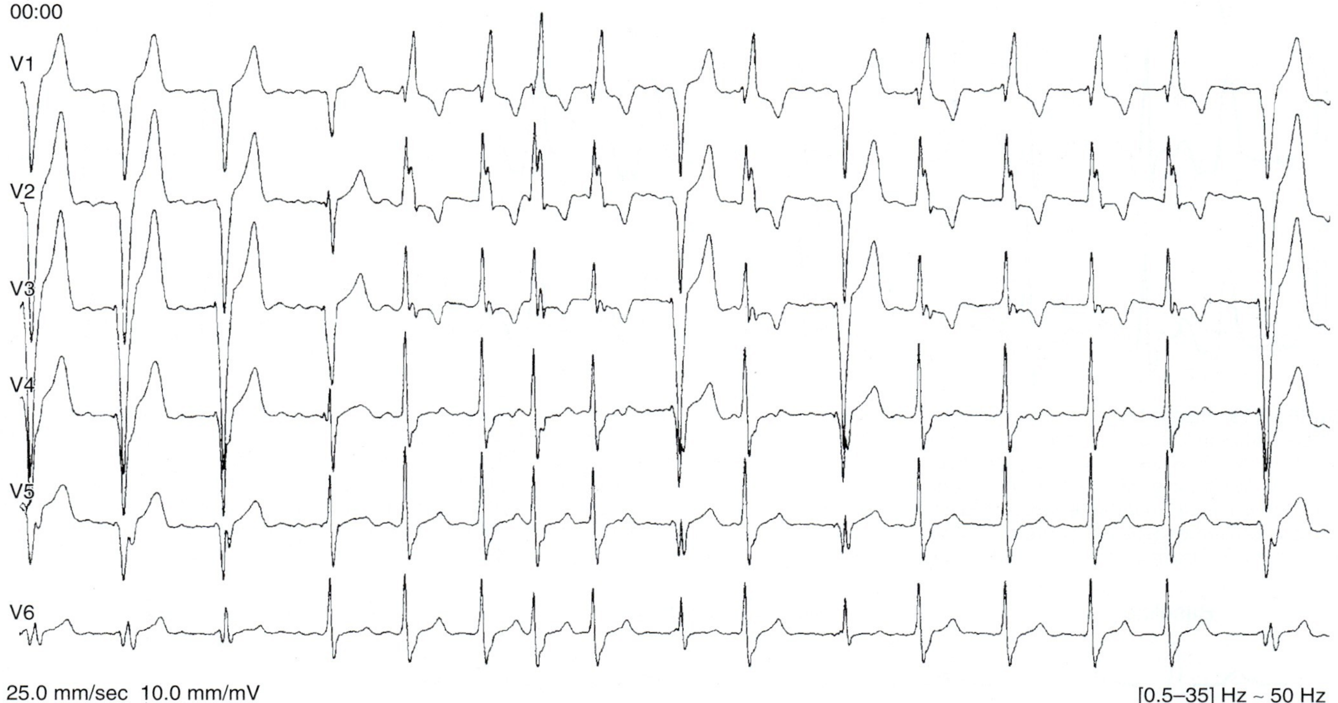

FIGURE 10-12 Alternating bundle branch block: surface ECG precordial leads during atrial fibrillation. QRS complexes with left bundle branch block configuration are observed mostly at long cycle lengths, and complexes with right bundle branch block configuration are observed mostly at shorter cycle lengths.

Electrophysiological Testing

Baseline Intervals

HIS BUNDLE–VENTRICULAR INTERVAL

The use of multipolar catheters to record distal, middle, and proximal HB potentials can help localize the site of conduction delay or block within the HB. The value of prolonged HV interval in predicting the risk of AV block is controversial. Studies have shown that an HV interval longer than 70 milliseconds predicts a higher risk of AV block, especially in symptomatic patients. The risk of AV block, however, even in the high-risk group, approaches at most only 6% per year. An HV interval exceeding 100 milliseconds identifies a group of patients at a very high risk of AV block (25% over 22 months).[3]

In the presence of RBBB with or without additional fascicular block, the HV interval should be normal as long as conduction is unimpaired in the remaining fascicle (Fig. 10-14). However, 50% of patients with RBBB plus LAF block and 75% of those with LBBB have a prolonged HV interval; thus, a prolonged HV interval itself is nonspecific as a predictor of AV block.

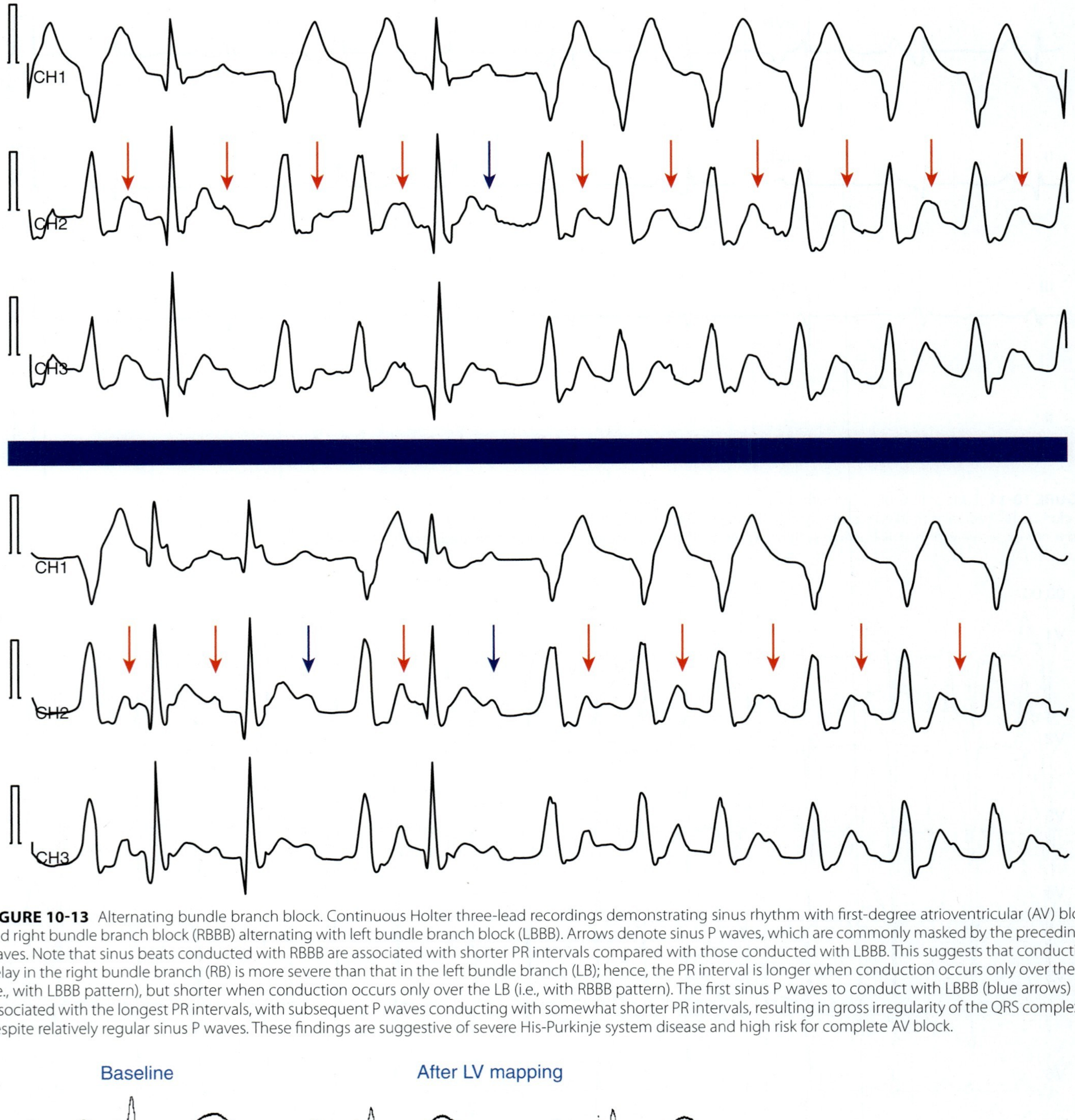

FIGURE 10-13 Alternating bundle branch block. Continuous Holter three-lead recordings demonstrating sinus rhythm with first-degree atrioventricular (AV) block and right bundle branch block (RBBB) alternating with left bundle branch block (LBBB). Arrows denote sinus P waves, which are commonly masked by the preceding T waves. Note that sinus beats conducted with RBBB are associated with shorter PR intervals compared with those conducted with LBBB. This suggests that conduction delay in the right bundle branch (RB) is more severe than that in the left bundle branch (LB); hence, the PR interval is longer when conduction occurs only over the RB (i.e., with LBBB pattern), but shorter when conduction occurs only over the LB (i.e., with RBBB pattern). The first sinus P waves to conduct with LBBB (blue arrows) are associated with the longest PR intervals, with subsequent P waves conducting with somewhat shorter PR intervals, resulting in gross irregularity of the QRS complexes despite relatively regular sinus P waves. These findings are suggestive of severe His-Purkinje system disease and high risk for complete AV block.

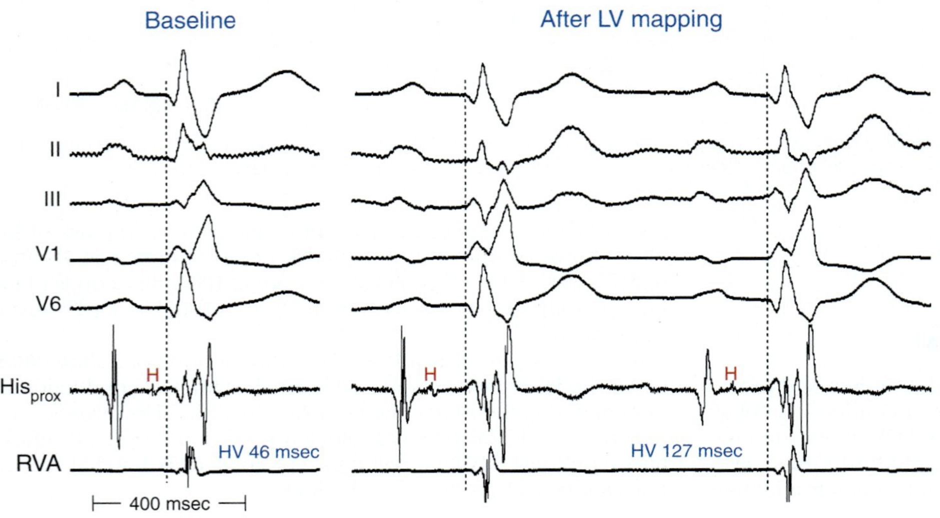

FIGURE 10-14 Catheter-induced His bundle–ventricular (HV) interval prolongation. Right bundle branch block with a normal HV is present at baseline (at **left**). Prolongation of the HV interval is observed after introducing a mapping catheter into the left ventricle that traumatized a portion of the His-Purkinje system. The QRS is also slightly different from baseline. His$_{prox}$ = proximal His bundle; RVA = right ventricular apex.

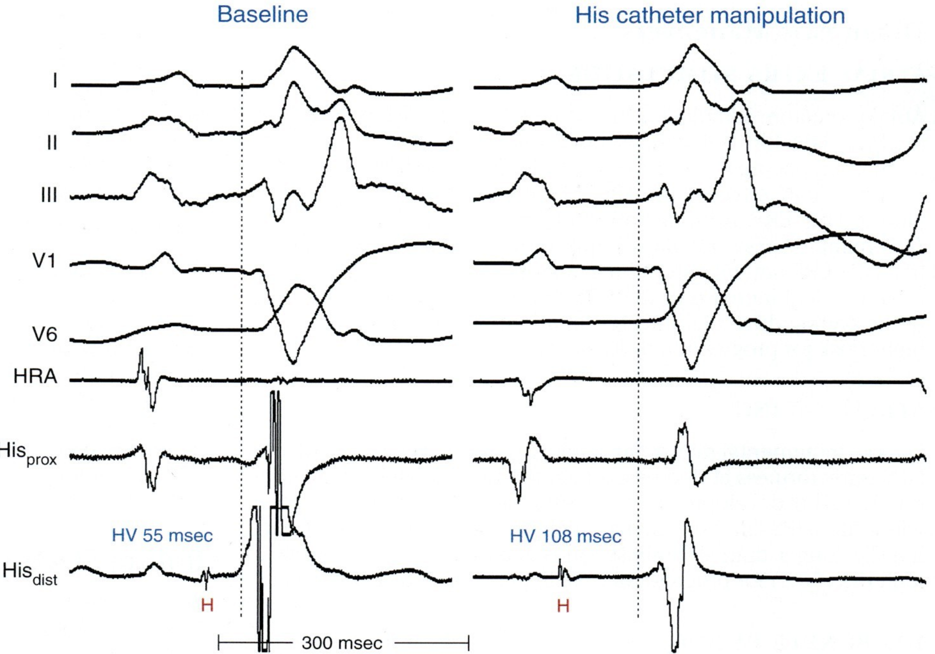

FIGURE 10-15 Catheter-induced His bundle–ventricular (HV) interval prolongation. Left bundle branch block (LBBB) and HV interval at the upper limit of normal are observed at baseline (at left). Manipulation of the His bundle recording catheter results in prolongation of the HV interval. This is not an artifact of the location of His recording, because the PR interval is also prolonged. There is no change in the QRS complex (LBBB pattern), suggesting trauma to the right bundle (RB) or His fibers destined to the RB. His_{dist} = distal His bundle; His_{prox} = proximal His bundle; HRA = high right atrium.

In the presence of LBBB, and in the absence of a change in the HB-RB and HB-RV intervals, the HV interval may be slightly prolonged because the earliest site of depolarization on the left side of the septum via the LB precedes activation of the RB by 5 to 15 milliseconds. Therefore, an HV interval of up to 60 milliseconds in the presence of LBBB should be considered normal and does not by itself indicate associated RB or HB disease (Fig. 10-15).[3]

Catheter manipulation in the LV or RV can inadvertently produce prolongation of the HV interval and varying degrees of AV block or BBB, or both, usually temporarily (see Figs. 10-14 and 10-15). Complete heart block can occur during right-sided heart catheterization in a patient with preexisting LBBB or during LV catheterization (LV angiography or ablation procedures) in a patient with preexisting RBBB. Among patients with chronic LBBB, the presence of an r wave of more than 1 mm in lead V_1 appears to identify a subgroup at lower risk for complete AV block in response to catheter trauma to the RB. This ECG sign likely suggests intact conduction over the septal fibers of the LBB.[29]

LOCALIZATION OF THE SITE OF BLOCK IN RIGHT BUNDLE BRANCH BLOCK

As noted, a chronic RBBB pattern can result from three levels of conduction delay in the RV: proximal RBBB, distal RBBB at the level of the moderator band, and terminal RBBB involving the distal conduction system of the RB or, more likely, the muscle itself.

With proximal RBBB, loss of RB potential occurs where it is typically recorded. Activation at these RV septal sites is via transseptal spread following LV activation. The transseptal activation begins at the apex and then sequentially activates the midanterior wall and base of the RV. The midseptum and apical septum are activated at least 30 milliseconds after the onset of the QRS.

In the setting of distal RBBB, activation of the HB and proximal RB is normal. RB potentials persist at the base of the moderator band and are absent at the midanterior wall (where the moderator band normally inserts). The apical and midseptum are normally activated, but activation of the free wall at the level of the moderator band is delayed, as is the subsequent activation of the RV outflow tract (RVOT) and the remaining RV.

With terminal RBBB, activation along the HB and RB remains normal up the Purkinje-myocardium junction. Activation of the midanterior wall also remains normal, and only the RVOT shows delayed activation.

Measurement of activation times at different areas of the RV has been used to assess conduction properties of the RB indirectly. In the presence of RBBB, measuring the HV interval, HB–proximal RB interval, ventricular-RV (V-RV) apex interval (from onset of the surface QRS to RV apical local activation), and V-RVOT interval can help localize the site of block (Fig. 10-16). In the presence of RBBB, a normal HV interval and a V-RV apex interval of less than 30 milliseconds suggest terminal RBBB. On the other hand, a normal HV interval and a V-RV apex interval of less than 30 milliseconds, with delayed activation in the anterior wall (prolonged V-RVOT interval), suggest distal RBBB. With proximal RBBB, the V-RV apex interval is longer than 30 milliseconds.

LOCALIZATION OF THE SITE OF BLOCK IN LEFT BUNDLE BRANCH BLOCK

Measurement of activation times at different areas of the LV to assess conduction properties of the LB, LAF, and LPF indirectly has many limitations. It is not as feasible as that used for evaluation of the RB, mainly because the LB does not divide into two discrete fascicles, but it rapidly fans out over the entire LV. Therefore, for practical reasons, clinical evaluation has primarily focused on the surface ECG pattern and the HV interval.

In chronic LBBB, RV activation occurs relatively earlier in the QRS. A discrete LV breakthrough site is absent, in contrast to normal findings, in which two or three breakthrough sites may be seen. Moreover, transseptal conduction is slow. In LBBB with normal axis, the latest LV site activated is the AV sulcus, as it is with normal conduction.

A common observation in patients with LBBB is a delay in transseptal activation. The pattern in which the LV is activated initially (i.e., the site of breakthrough), as well as the remainder of the LV endocardium and transmural activation, depends critically on the nature of the underlying heart disease; the bizarreness of the QRS width and morphology is more a reflection of the underlying LV disease than of the primary conduction disturbance.[3] Patients with normal hearts and those with cardiomyopathy appear to have an intact distal conducting system and, hence, early engagement and rapid spread throughout the rest of the intramural myocardium. In patients with large infarcts, the bulk of their distal specialized conducting system has been destroyed; consequently, endocardial activation occurs via muscle-to-muscle conduction and thus is much slower.

Diagnostic Maneuvers

ATRIAL EXTRA STIMULATION

Atrial premature stimulation helps determine the ERP of HPS. Normally, the HPS ERP is 450 milliseconds or less and it decreases with decreasing pacing drive CL. Because the AVN functional refractory period usually exceeds the HPS ERP, it can be difficult to evaluate the HPS ERP. Administration of atropine can help decrease AVN refractoriness and allow impulses to reach the HPS earlier so that HPS ERP can be determined. A grossly prolonged HPS ERP or a paradoxical increase in the HPS ERP in response to shortening of the pacing drive CL indicates an abnormal HPS and predicts a higher risk for progression to AV block.

ATRIAL PACING

During incremental-rate atrial pacing, normal shortening of the HPS refractoriness at decreased pacing CLs facilitates 1:1 AV conduction. The development of second- or third-degree AV block within the HPS (in the absence of changing AH intervals) at pacing CLs longer than 400 milliseconds is abnormal and suggests a high risk (50%) for progression to high-grade AV block (Fig. 10-17).

HIS BUNDLE PACING

Normalization of the QRS during HB pacing is suggestive of HB disease proximal to the pacing site (Fig. 10-18).

VENTRICULAR PACING

Assessment of retrograde VH (or VA) conduction is not useful as an indicator of anterograde HPS reserve. Anterograde RBBB is usually proximal, whereas during RV stimulation, block usually occurs at the gate, which is at the distal HPS–myocardial junction. Bidirectional RBBB is characterized by His activation following local ventricular activation in the HB recording, caused by propagation from the RV pacing site across the interventricular septum to the LB and then to the HB, rather than the more direct retrograde route up the RB (Fig. 10-19).

PROCAINAMIDE CHALLENGE

The administration of drugs known to impair the HPS (e.g., procainamide) can unmask extraordinary sensitivity to the usual therapeutic doses of the drug, which can itself indicate poor HPS reserve. In normal persons and in most patients with a moderately increased HV interval (55 to 80 milliseconds), procainamide typically produces a 10% to 20% increase in the HV interval. Abnormal HV interval responses to procainamide representing evidence of a higher risk for infra-Hisian AV block include any of the following: (1) doubling of the HV interval, (2) prolongation of the HV interval to more than 100 milliseconds, or (3) second- or third-degree infra-Hisian block.

Role of Electrophysiological Testing

The guidelines for pacing in chronic BBB are listed in Table 10-2. EP testing is used to obtain information that could predict which patients are at risk for syncope, AV block, or sudden cardiac death (Table 10-3).[3,18] Complete EP testing with programmed atrial and ventricular stimulation is necessary in patients with syncope and BBB because VT can be induced in 30% to 50% of such patients. Pacemaker therapy clearly can help prevent syncope in those patients in whom that event most likely was caused by transient bradyarrhythmia, but it has not been shown to prevent sudden cardiac death or reduce cardiac mortality.[3,18,30]

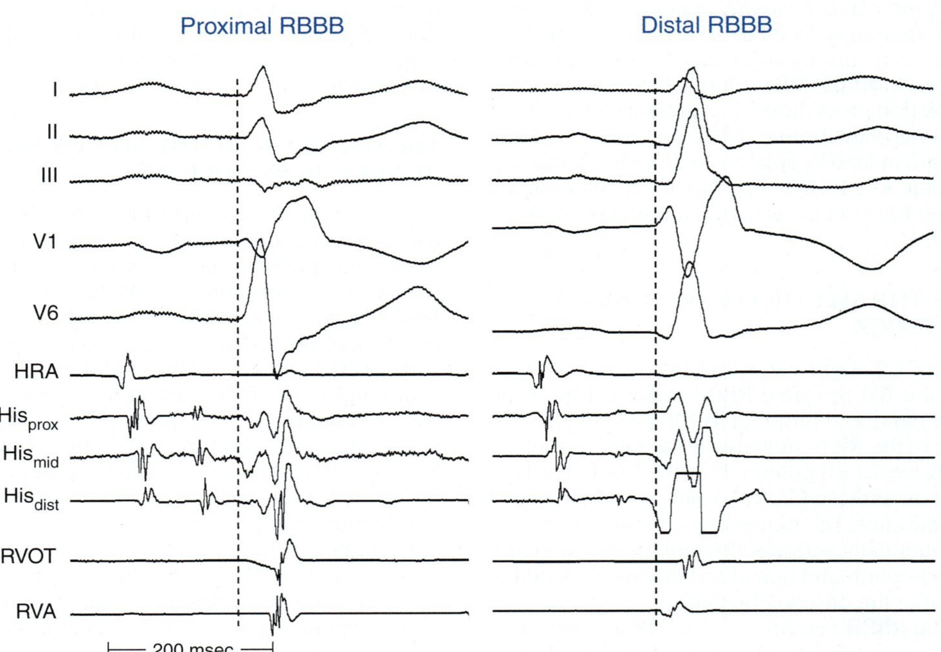

FIGURE 10-16 Localization of the site of block in right bundle branch block (RBBB). Two complexes from different patients are shown, with proximal (left panel) and distal (right panel) RBBB, distinguished by the interval from QRS onset to right ventricle apical (RVA) recording. His_{dist} = distal His bundle; His_{mid} = middle His bundle; His_{prox} = proximal His bundle; RVA = right ventricular apex; RVOT = right ventricular outflow tract.

I
II
III
V1
V6
HRA
PCL 330 msec
S
S
S
S
His$_{prox}$
HV 75 msec
His$_{dist}$
H
H
H
H
H
RVA
HV 108 msec
300 msec

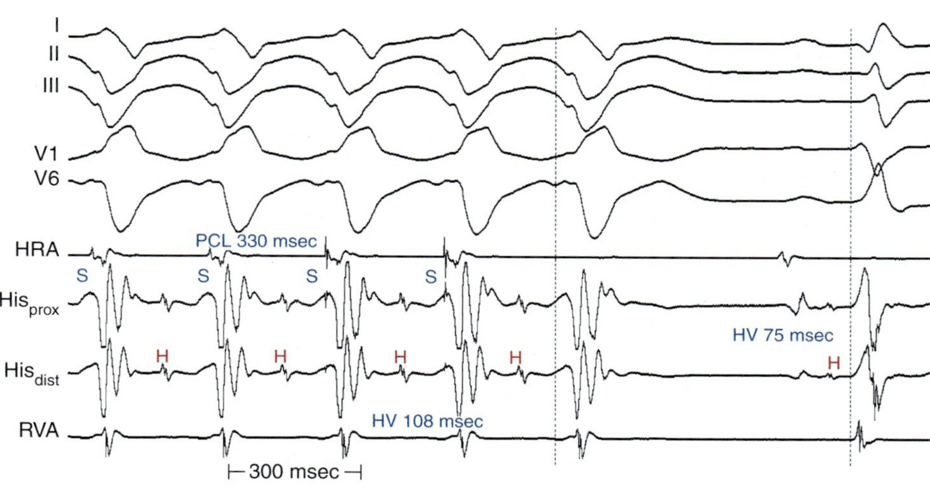

FIGURE 10-17 His-Purkinje system (HPS) disease. The PR interval is borderline (210 milliseconds), and the His bundle–ventricular (HV) interval is prolonged (75 milliseconds) during normal sinus rhythm (at **right**). Atrial pacing at a cycle length of 330 milliseconds results in stressing the HPS and further prolonging the HV interval (108 milliseconds). Right bundle branch block also develops during atrial pacing, a finding suggesting slower conduction over the right bundle than the left bundle. His$_{dist}$ = distal His bundle; His$_{prox}$ = proximal His bundle; HRA = high right atrium; PCL = pacing cycle length.

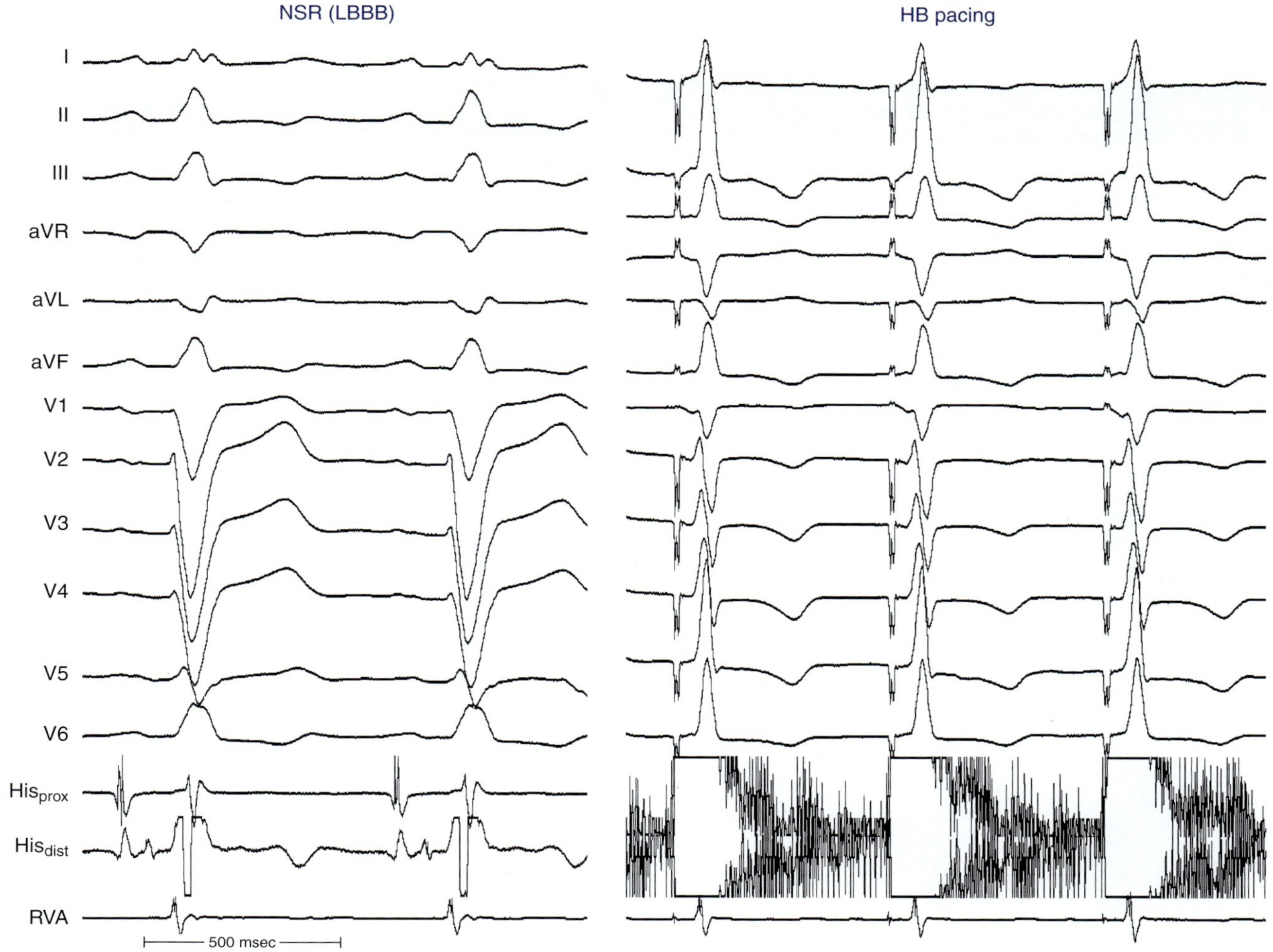

NSR (LBBB)
HB pacing
I
II
III
aVR
aVL
aVF
V1
V2
V3
V4
V5
V6
His$_{prox}$
His$_{dist}$
RVA
500 msec

FIGURE 10-18 Left bundle branch block (LBBB) secondary to intra-Hisian disease. **Left,** ECG leads and intracardiac recordings in a patient with complete LBBB. **Right,** Pacing from the His bundle (HB) pacing normalizes the QRS complex, a finding suggesting that the LBBB is caused by HB disease proximal to the pacing site. His$_{dist}$ = distal His bundle; His$_{prox}$ = proximal His bundle; NSR = normal sinus rhythm; RVA = right ventricular apex.

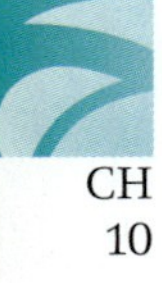

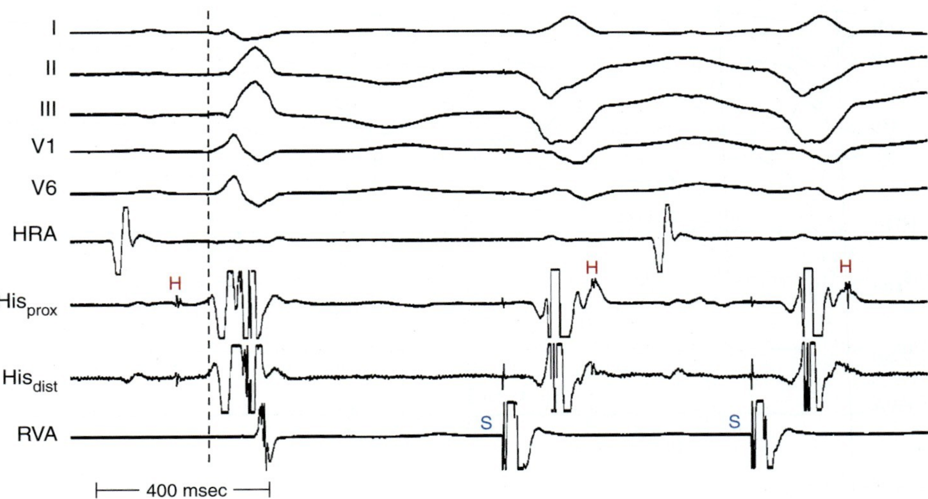

FIGURE 10-19 Bidirectional right bundle branch block (RBBB). The sinus complex at left has proximal RBBB, indicated by a very prolonged ventricular–right ventricular apical (V-RVA) time (more than 100 milliseconds). RV pacing with the next two complexes show His activation following local ventricular activation in the His bundle (HB) recording, caused by propagation from the RV pacing site across the interventricular septum to the left bundle and then to the HB, rather than the more direct route retrogradely up the right bundle. This is consistent with both anterograde and retrograde proximal RBBB. His$_{dist}$ = distal His bundle; His$_{prox}$ = proximal His bundle; HRA = high right atrium; RVA = right ventricular apex.

TABLE 10-2 Guidelines for Permanent Pacing in Chronic Bifascicular and Trifascicular Block

Class I

- Advanced second-degree AV block or intermittent third-degree AV block
- Type 2 second-degree AV block
- Alternating bundle branch block

Class IIa

- Syncope not demonstrated to result from AV block, when other likely causes have been excluded, especially ventricular tachycardia
- Incidental finding at EP study of HV interval ≥100 msec
- Incidental finding at EP study of pacing-induced block below the bundle of His that is not physiological

Class IIb

- Neuromuscular diseases, with or without symptoms

Class III

- Fascicular block without AV block or symptoms
- Fascicular block with first-degree AV block without symptoms

AV = atrioventricular; EP = electrophysiological; HV = His bundle–ventricular.

TABLE 10-3 Role of Electrophysiological Testing in Patients with Bundle Branch Block

EP Indicators of HPS Disease

- HV interval >55 msec
- Infra-Hisian block at atrial pacing CL ≥400 msec
- HPS ERP ≥450 msec
- HPS ERPs inversely related to pacing CLs
- Abnormal response to procainamide: prolongation of the HV interval by 100% or to >100 msec, or second- or third-degree infra-Hisian AV block

EP Indicators of High Risk for AV Block in Patients with IVCD

- HV interval >100 msec
- Infra-Hisian AV block or HV interval prolongation at atrial pacing CL >400 msec
- HPS-ERPs inversely related to pacing CLs
- Infra-Hisian AV block or doubling of the HV interval following procainamide in patients with neurological symptoms compatible with bradyarrhythmia

Recommendations for Pacing in Patients with IVCD

- LBBB, RBBB, IVCD, RBBB + LAF block, or RBBB + LPF block associated with the following: HV interval >100 msec or HV interval = 60-99 msec in the presence of unexplained syncope or presyncope
- Infra-Hisian block at atrial pacing CL ≥400 msec (regardless of HV interval or presence of symptoms)
- Alternating BBB (regardless of HV interval or presence of symptoms)

AV = atrioventricular; BBB = bundle branch block; CL = cycle length; EP = electrophysiological; ERP = effective refractory period; HPS = His-Purkinje system; HV = His bundle–ventricular; IVCD = intraventricular conduction defect; LAF = left anterior fascicle; LBBB = left bundle branch block; LPF = left posterior fascicle; RBBB = right bundle branch block.

REFERENCES

1. Surawicz B, Childers R, Deal BJ, et al: AHA/ACCF/HRS recommendations for the standardization and interpretation of the electrocardiogram. Part III. Intraventricular conduction disturbances: a scientific statement from the American Heart Association Electrocardiography and Arrhythmias Committee, Council on Clinical Cardiology; the American College of Cardiology Foundation; and the Heart Rhythm Society. Endorsed by the International Society for Computerized Electrocardiology, *J Am Coll Cardiol* 53:976–981, 2009.
2. Chilson DA, Zipes DP, Heger JJ, et al: Functional bundle branch block: discordant response of right and left bundle branches to changes in heart rate, *Am J Cardiol* 54:313–316, 1984.
3. Josephson ME: Intraventricular conduction disturbances. In Josephson ME, editor: *Clinical cardiac electrophysiology*, ed 4, Philadelphia, 2008, Lippincott Williams & Wilkins, pp 114–144.
4. Eckardt L, Breithardt G, Kirchhof P: Approach to wide complex tachycardias in patients without structural heart disease, *Heart* 92:704–711, 2006.
5. Pavri BB, Kocovic DZ, Hanna M: Long-short RR intervals and the right bundle branch, *J Cardiovasc Electrophysiol* 10:121–123, 1999.
6. Rubart M, Zipes DP: Genesis of cardiac arrhythmias: electrophysiological considerations. In Zipes DP, Libby P, Bonow R, Braunwald E, editors: *Braunwald's heart disease: a textbook of cardiovascular medicine*, ed 7, Philadelphia, 2004, Saunders, pp 653–688.
7. Suyama AC, Sunagawa K, Sugimachi M, et al: Differentiation between aberrant ventricular conduction and ventricular ectopy in atrial fibrillation using RR interval scattergram, *Circulation* 88:2307–2314, 1993.
8. Josephson ME: Miscellaneous phenomena related to atrioventricular conduction. In Josephson ME, editor: *Clinical cardiac electrophysiology*, ed 4, Philadelphia, 2008, Lippincott Williams & Wilkins, pp 145–159.
9. Kilborn MF: Electrocardiographic manifestations of supernormal conduction, concealed conduction, and exit block. In Zipes DP, Jalife J, editors: *Cardiac electrophysiology: from cell to bedside*, ed 4, Philadelphia, 2004, Saunders, pp 733–738.
10. Wellens HJ, Boss DL, Farre J, Brugada P: Functional bundle branch block during supraventricular tachycardia in man: observations on mechanisms and their incidence. In Zipes DP, Jalife J, editors: *Cardiac electrophysiology and arrhythmias*, New York, 1995, Grune & Stratton, pp 435–441.
11. Fisch C, Knoebel S: Wolff-Parkinson-White syndrome. In Fisch C, Knoebel S, editors: *Electrocardiography of clinical arrhythmias*, Armonk, NY, 2000, Futura, pp 293–314.
12. Fisch C, Knoebel S: Atrioventricular and ventriculoatrial conduction and blocks, gap, and overdrive suppression. In Fisch C, Knoebel S, editors: *Electrocardiography of clinical arrhythmias*, Armonk, NY, 2000, Futura, pp 315–344.
13. Gouaux JL, Ashman R: Auricular fibrillation with aberration simulating ventricular paroxysmal tachycardia, *Am Heart J* 34:366–373, 1947.
14. Fisch C, Zipes DP, McHenry PL: Electrocardiographic manifestations of concealed junctional ectopic impulses, *Circulation* 53:217–223, 1976.
15. Fisch C, Knoebel SB: Concealed conduction. In Fisch C, Knoebel S, editors: *Electrocardiography of clinical arrhythmias*, Armonk, NY, 2000, Futura, pp 153–172.
16. Elizari MV, Acunzo RS, Ferreiro M: Hemiblocks revisited, *Circulation* 115:1154–1163, 2007.
17. Biagini E, Elhendy A, Schinkel AF, et al: Prognostic significance of left anterior hemiblock in patients with suspected coronary artery disease, *J Am Coll Cardiol* 46:858–863, 2005.
18. MacAlpin RN: In search of left septal fascicular block, *Am Heart J* 144:948–956, 2002.
19. Imanishi R, Seto S, Ichimaru S, et al: Prognostic significance of incident complete left bundle branch block observed over a 40-year period, *Am J Cardiol* 98:644–648, 2006.
20. McCullough PA, Hassan SA, Pallekonda V, et al: Bundle branch block patterns, age, renal dysfunction, and heart failure mortality, *Int J Cardiol* 102:303–308, 2005.
21. Baldasseroni S, Opasich C, Gorini M, et al: Left bundle-branch block is associated with increased 1-year sudden and total mortality rate in 5517 outpatients with congestive heart failure: a report from the Italian network on congestive heart failure, *Am Heart J* 143:398–405, 2002.
22. Auricchio A, Fantoni C, Regoli F, et al: Characterization of left ventricular activation in patients with heart failure and left bundle-branch block, *Circulation* 109:1133–1139, 2004.
23. Stenestrand U, Tabrizi F, Lindback J, et al: Comorbidity and myocardial dysfunction are the main explanations for the higher 1-year mortality in acute myocardial infarction with left bundle-branch block, *Circulation* 110:1896–1902, 2004.
24. Wong CK, Stewart RA, Gao W, et al: Prognostic differences between different types of bundle branch block during the early phase of acute myocardial infarction: insights from the Hirulog and Early Reperfusion or Occlusion (HERO)-2 trial, *Eur Heart J* 27:21–28, 2006.
25. Francia P, Balla C, Paneni F, Volpe M: Left bundle-branch block: pathophysiology, prognosis, and clinical management, *Clin Cardiol* 30:110–115, 2007.
26. Agarwal AK, Venugopalan P: Right bundle branch block: varying electrocardiographic patterns. Aetiological correlation, mechanisms and electrophysiology, *Int J Cardiol* 71:33–39, 1999.
27. Rogers RL, Mitarai M, Mattu A: Intraventricular conduction abnormalities, *Emerg Med Clin North Am* 24:41–51, vi, 2006.
28. Kamakura S, Ohe T, Nakazawa K, et al: Long-term prognosis of probands with Brugada-pattern ST-elevation in leads V1-V3, *Circ Arrhythm Electrophysiol* 2:495–503, 2009.
29. Padanilam BJ, Morris KE, Olson JA, et al: The surface electrocardiogram predicts risk of heart block during right heart catheterization in patients with preexisting left bundle branch block: implications for the definition of complete left bundle branch block, *J Cardiovasc Electrophysiol* 21:781–785, 2010.
30. Epstein AE, DiMarco JP, Ellenbogen KA, et al: ACC/AHA/HRS 2008 guidelines for device-based therapy of cardiac rhythm abnormalities: executive summary, *Heart Rhythm* 5:934–955, 2008.

CHAPTER 11 Focal Atrial Tachycardia

Classification of Atrial Tachycardias

Previous classification of regular atrial tachycardias (ATs) had been based exclusively on the surface electrocardiogram (ECG). According to this classification, AT is defined as a regular atrial rhythm at a constant rate greater than 100 beats/min originating outside the sinus node region. The mechanism can be caused by focal pacemaker activity (automaticity or triggered activity) or reentry (microreentry or macroreentry). Atrial flutter (AFL) refers to a pattern of regular tachycardia with a rate of 240 beats/min or more (tachycardia cycle length [CL] 250 milliseconds or less) lacking an isoelectric baseline between deflections. Differentiation between AFL and AT depends on a rate cutoff of approximately 240 to 250 beats/min and the presence of an isoelectric baseline between atrial deflections in AT, but not in AFL. Atypical AFL is only a descriptive term for an AT with an ECG pattern of continuous undulation of the atrial complex, different from typical clockwise or counterclockwise isthmus-dependent AFL, at an atrial rate of 240 beats/min or more.

This ECG classification, however, has several major limitations. Neither rate nor lack of isoelectric baseline is specific for any tachycardia mechanism. Rapid ATs in a diseased atrium can mimic AFL. On the other hand, true AFL may show distinct isoelectric intervals between flutter waves. This dilemma is not solvable in terms of analyses of routine ECGs. Moreover, AT mechanisms, defined by electrophysiological (EP) studies and radiofrequency (RF) catheter ablation, do not correlate with ECG patterns as defined currently.

Therefore, ECG-based classifications are obsolete for this purpose, and a mechanistic classification of ATs has been proposed (Table 11-1).[1,2] If the mechanism of AT or AFL can be elucidated, either through conventional mapping and entrainment or with special multipoint mapping techniques, description of the mechanism should be stated. However, even when using this classification, there are other tachycardias described in the literature that cannot be well classified because of inadequate understanding of their mechanisms, including "type II" AFL, inappropriate sinus tachycardia, and fibrillatory conduction from a focal source with rapid, regular discharge.

This chapter discusses focal AT. Typical AFL and macroreentrant AT are discussed in subsequent chapters.

Pathophysiology

Focal AT is characterized by atrial activation starting rhythmically at a small area (focus), from which it spreads out centrifugally.[1] "Focal" implies that the site of origin cannot be mapped spatially beyond a single point or a few adjacent points with the resolution of a standard 4-mm-tip catheter. In contrast, macroreentrant AT is defined by activation that can be recorded over the entire tachycardia CL around a large central obstacle, which is generally several centimeters in diameter.[1] Relatively small reentry circuits may resemble focal AT, especially if limited numbers of endocardial recordings are collected. The term *localized reentry* has been used to refer to reentry in which the circuit is localized to a small area (covering a surface diameter of less than 3 cm) and does not have a central obstacle. Focal AT CL is usually longer than 250 milliseconds; however, it can be as short as 200 milliseconds. Over a prolonged period of observation (minutes to hours), the AT CL can exhibit significant variations.

Most focal ATs arise from the right atrium (RA), approximately two thirds of which are distributed along the long axis of the crista terminalis (cristal tachycardias) from the sinus node to the coronary sinus (CS) and atrioventricular (AV) junction (called the "ring of fire"), with an apparent gradation in frequency from superior to inferior.[3,4] This particular anatomical distribution of ATs may be related to the marked anisotropy characterizing the region of the crista terminalis. Such anisotropy, which is related to the poor transverse cell-to-cell coupling, favors the development of microreentry by creating regions of slow conduction. Fractionated electrograms often seen at a successful AT ablation site may be markers of the requisite nonuniformly anisotropic substrate. In addition, the normal sinus pacemaker complex is distributed along the long axis of the crista terminalis. The presence of automatic tissue, together with relative cellular uncoupling, may be a requirement for abnormal automaticity such that a normal atrium is prevented from electrotonically inhibiting abnormal phase 4 depolarization. The presence of structural heart disease increases the probability of RA location of the AT, but from sites outside the crista terminalis.

The pulmonary vein (PV) ostia are the most common sites of origin of focal tachycardias within the left atrium (LA), and they account for between 3% and 29% of all focal ATs and approximately 67% of LA ATs.[5-7] Other sites of AT clustering include the CS ostium (CS os),[4,8-11] mitral and tricuspid annuli,[3,5,12,13] bases of RA and LA appendages, para-Hisian region, and atrial septum. Experience gained during catheter ablation of atrial fibrillation (AF) has indicated that focal ATs also can arise within the vein of Marshall, superior vena cava (SVC),[14] or inferior vena cava (IVC). ATs have been described originating from the noncoronary cusp of the aortic valve. The distribution of AT foci may differ, depending on the patient population.[15,16]

Available information suggests that focal activity can be caused by automaticity, triggered activity, or microreentry. There is some overlap based on the pharmacological characterization of these different AT mechanisms. Delineating the mechanism of focal AT, however, can be difficult, and the means of distinguishing focal

TABLE 11-1 Classification of Atrial Tachycardias

Focal Atrial Tachycardia	• Automatic atrial tachycardia • Triggered-activity atrial tachycardia • Microreentrant atrial tachycardia	
Macroreentrant Atrial Tachycardia	Cavotricuspid isthmus-dependent atrial flutters	• Clockwise and counterclockwise typical atrial flutter • Double-loop reentry • Lower-loop reentry • Intraisthmus reentry
	Noncavotricuspid isthmus-dependent right atrial macroreentry (atypical atrial flutter)	• Upper-loop reentry • Lesional or scar-related right atrial macroreentry
	Left atrial macroreentry (atypical atrial flutter)	• Perimitral macroreentry • Pulmonary vein macroreentry • Scar-related macroreentry • Left septal macroreentry • Postsurgical/postablation macroreentry

AT mechanisms are fraught with exceptions.[17] The major limiting factor in the analysis of mechanisms is the absence of a gold standard for determining the tachycardia mechanism, so these remain largely descriptive. In addition, there is a significant overlap in the EP characteristics of tachycardias with differing mechanisms.[18] It is especially difficult to discriminate definitively between triggered activity and microreentry as a mechanism of focal AT; therefore, some investigators have classified focal ATs as automatic or nonautomatic.[1] Furthermore, it is not clear that making such mechanistic distinctions among various types of focal ATs carries any clinical significance, although it is possible that such information could be useful in guiding drug therapy. In contrast, determination of the likely focal versus macroreentrant mechanism is critical for planning mapping and ablation strategy.

The term "incessant" is applied to an AT that is present for at least 50% of the time that a patient is monitored.[19] Incessant AT frequently is automatic, but it can also be secondary to reentry or triggered activity. Incessant tachycardias occur in approximately 25% of patients with focal AT. Foci arising from the atrial appendages and PVs are frequently incessant.[20]

Arrhythmias originating from the PVs can have a critical role in the development of AF in susceptible individuals. Focal ATs arising from the PVs, however, appear to be a distinct clinical entity from the PV arrhythmias associated with AF. Patients with focal PV ATs do not seem to be at risk of AF in the long term; they resemble patients with focal ATs originating elsewhere with a localized isolated substrate that is successfully addressed with a focal ablative approach. Several potential explanations have been suggested for the different behavior. The underlying pathophysiological process in patients with AF is probably fundamentally different. It is a generalized process diffusely affecting the muscular sleeves in all four PVs, with frequently multiple PV foci originating distally (up to 2 to 4 cm) within the vein, compared with the focal nature of the process in patients with isolated PV tachycardia. Additionally, the CLs of the PV ATs are longer (mean CL 340 milliseconds) than the reported CLs of PV tachycardia in AF patients (130 milliseconds). The CL of AT also tends to be irregular in patients with AF but not in patients with PV AT. It is possible that foci with shorter CL and irregular activity may not conduct in a 1:1 fashion from the PV to the LA, with resulting fibrillatory conduction and AF. Furthermore, patients with AF tend to be older than those with PV AT and consequently more prone to more widespread atrial remodeling associated with age, hypertension, or other pathologic processes.[6,7,21,22]

Up to 10% of patients with focal AT have ATs with more than one focus. In these patients, the AT appears to have different EP characteristics from focal AT with a single focus, because it tends to involve the LA and has greater cardiovascular comorbidity, shorter CL, longer total activation time, and lower acute and long-term success rates of catheter ablation.[23]

Other forms of AT in which EP testing and catheter ablation are not indicated are beyond the scope of this chapter and are discussed briefly. Multifocal AT is usually caused by enhanced automaticity and is characterized by varying morphology of the P waves and the PR interval (Fig. 11-1). This finding suggests that the pacemaker arises in different atrial locations, but a single focus with different exit pathways or abnormalities in intraatrial conduction can produce identical electrocardiographic manifestations. Nonparoxysmal AT typically occurs in patients with significant heart disease or digitalis toxicity, or both. The latter may be caused by triggered activity. Repetitive automatic AT, also called repetitive focal AT, is thought to be caused in most cases by enhanced automaticity. It frequently occurs in patients with structural heart disease and is often related to some acute event, such as a myocardial infarction, pulmonary decompensation, infection, alcohol excess, hypokalemia, hypoxia, or use of stimulants, cocaine, or theophylline.

Early studies of sinus node function described the response to a single atrial extrastimulus (AES). The curve produced by plotting return cycles against the coupling interval could be divided into several phases, including compensatory pause, reset, interpolation, and reentry. Sinus node reentrant tachycardia was described on the basis of these findings as a tachycardia that could be induced and terminated by programmed electrical stimulation with a P wave morphology identical or similar to sinus P waves and tachycardia CLs of 350 to 550 milliseconds (see Fig. 16-3).[24] There have been some reports of endocardial ablation of sinus node reentrant tachycardias identified by these criteria. However, the precise identification of sinus node reentrant tachycardia remains elusive. The mechanism of focal AT can be reentrant, and the CL of such ATs completely overlaps that described for sinus node reentrant tachycardia. The location of AT foci is often along the crista terminalis, very close to the supposed location of the sinus node. An added problem is that the origin of the sinus activation can be variable, according to epicardial mapping studies. Furthermore, endocardial origin of sinus activation during normal sinus rhythm (NSR) has not been systematically studied in humans, and specific criteria do not exist to pinpoint a specific sinus node area. Finally, reentry strictly limited to the sinus node area has never been demonstrated and has even been questioned.[24]

Clinical Considerations

Epidemiology

Nonsustained AT is frequently found on Holter recordings and is seldom associated with symptoms. Sustained focal ATs are relatively infrequent; they are diagnosed in approximately 5% to 15% of patients referred for catheter ablation of supraventricular tachycardia (SVT).[25] However, ATs comprise a progressively greater proportion of paroxysmal SVTs with increasing age and account for 23% in patients older than 70 years. Age-related changes in the atrial EP substrate, including cellular coupling and autonomic influences, can contribute to the increased incidence of AT in older individuals.[25]

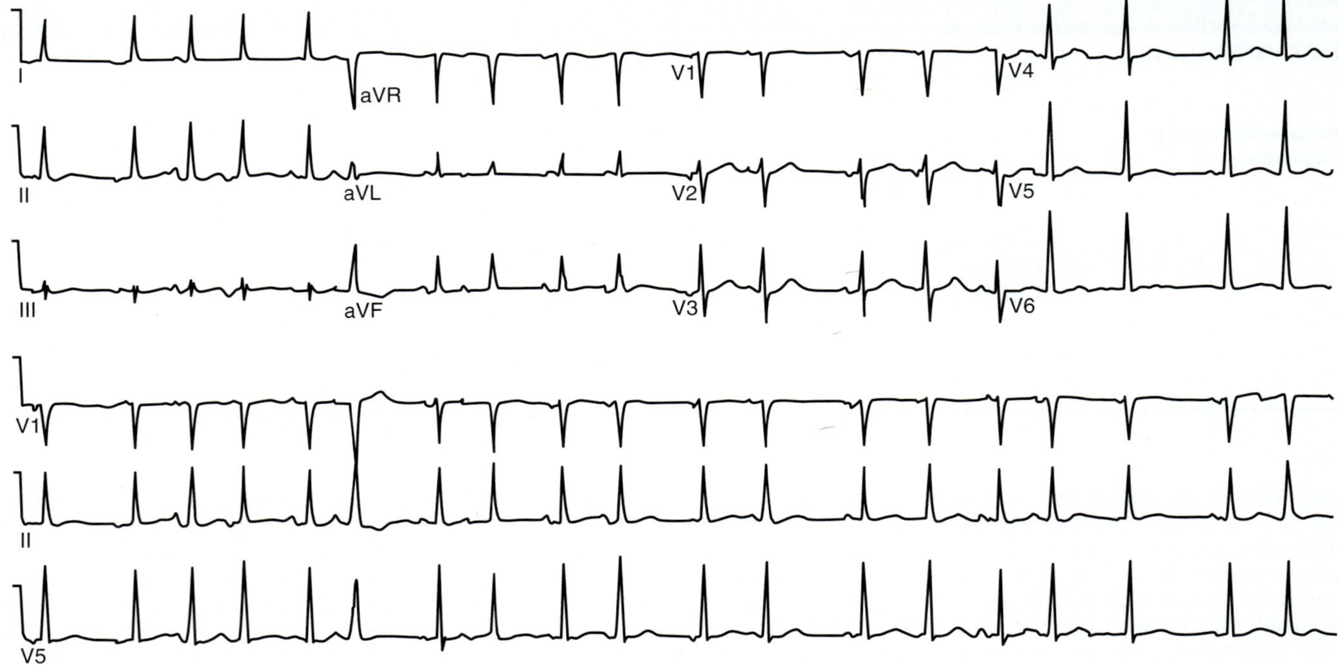

FIGURE 11-1 Surface ECG of multifocal atrial tachycardia. Note the varying morphology of the P waves and the PR intervals.

In adults, focal AT can occur in the absence of cardiac disease, but it is often associated with underlying cardiac abnormalities. Not infrequently, two or more foci of AT can be found in the same patient.[26]

Clinical Presentation

Focal ATs can manifest as paroxysmal or incessant tachycardias. When paroxysmal, AT manifests with the clinical syndrome of paroxysmal SVT (discussed in Chap. 20). Symptoms, however, may be more severe or associated with cardiac decompensation caused by the higher prevalence of structural heart disease in this group of patients. Incessant tachycardia can result in tachycardia-induced cardiomyopathy and manifest with symptoms of congestive heart failure. AT can also manifest as a frequently repetitive tachycardia, with frequent episodes of AT interrupted by short periods of NSR. The repetitive type may be tolerated well for years. It may cause symptoms only in cases of fast heart rates during phases of tachycardia, and it infrequently induces dilated cardiomyopathy.

In one study, tachycardia-induced ventricular cardiomyopathy occurred in 10% of the total population of patients with focal AT. Incessant tachycardia was necessary for the development of cardiomyopathy, and cardiomyopathy was observed in approximately one third of patients with incessant AT. Incessant tachycardias precipitating cardiomyopathy characteristically tend to have slower atrial rates as compared with ATs not associated with cardiomyopathy. In contrast to patients with rapid paroxysmal AT, incessant tachycardia may produce negligible symptoms and may go unrecognized by the patient until symptoms related to cardiomyopathy develop.[20]

Initial Evaluation

History, physical examination, 12-lead ECG, and echocardiography constitute an appropriate initial evaluation. Differentiation of paroxysmal AT from other mechanisms of SVT can be challenging and may require invasive EP testing. However, diagnosis of the incessant and frequently repetitive forms of AT usually can be readily made based on P wave morphology and the frequent presence of AV block during the tachycardia on ECG recordings. An ECG pattern of AT with discrete P waves and isoelectric intervals is suggestive of a focal mechanism of the AT, but it does not rule out macroreentrant AT, especially if complex structural heart disease is present or there has been prior surgery for congenital heart disease, or both. The diagnosis of focal AT can be established with certainty only by an EP study. ATs often occur in older patients and in the context of structural heart disease; therefore, coronary artery disease and left ventricular (LV) dysfunction should be excluded.

Principles of Management

SHORT-TERM MANAGEMENT

On rare occasions, ATs can be terminated with vagal maneuvers. Conversely, a significant proportion of focal ATs will terminate with administration of adenosine. Persistence of the tachycardia with AV block is also a common response to adenosine. In addition, ATs responsive to intravenous verapamil or beta blockers have been reported. It is conceivable that the mechanism of AT in these patients relates to microreentry, involving tissue with slow conduction, or to triggered activity. Class IA or IC drugs can suppress automaticity or prolong action potential duration and hence can be effective in some patients with AT.

For patients with automatic AT, atrial pacing (or adenosine) can result in transient slowing but no tachycardia termination. Similarly, DC cardioversion seldom terminates automatic ATs, but DC cardioversion can be successful for those in whom the tachycardia mechanism is microreentry or triggered activity. An attempt at DC cardioversion should therefore be considered for symptomatic patients with drug-resistant arrhythmia.

The usual acute therapy for AT consists of intravenous beta blockers or calcium channel blockers either to terminate the arrhythmia, which is rare, or to achieve rate control through AV block, which is often difficult.[19] Direct suppression of the tachycardia focus may be achieved by the use of intravenous class IA and IC or class III agents. Intravenous class IA or IC agents may be taken by patients without heart failure, whereas intravenous amiodarone is preferred for those with poor LV function.[19]

LONG-TERM MANAGEMENT

As with other forms of SVT, AT is usually benign and associated with only mild to moderate symptoms. Thus, most patients with AT are treated initially with medical therapy. Patient preference and refractoriness to pharmacological therapy are reasonable indications for catheter ablation.[19]

The efficacy of antiarrhythmic drugs is poorly defined because the clinical definition of focal ATs is often not rigorous. No large studies have been conducted to assess the effect of pharmacological treatment in patients with focal ATs, but both paroxysmal and, especially, incessant ATs are reported to be difficult to treat medically. Available data support a recommendation for initial therapy with calcium channel blockers or beta blockers because these agents may prove to be effective and have minimal side effects. If these drugs are unsuccessful, then class IA agents, class IC (flecainide and propafenone) agents in combination with an AV node (AVN) blocking agent, or class III agents (sotalol and amiodarone) may be tried; however, the potential benefit should be balanced by the potential risks of proarrhythmia and toxicity. Because ATs often occur in older patients and in the context of structural heart disease, class IC agents should be used only after cardiomyopathy and coronary artery disease are excluded.[19]

For patients with drug-refractory AT or incessant AT, especially when tachycardia-induced cardiomyopathy has developed, the best therapy appears to be catheter ablation of the AT focus. In case reports and small series, patients with tachycardia-induced cardiomyopathy frequently have complete resolution of LV dysfunction with successful RF catheter ablation of the atrial focus.[19,20] Regardless of whether the arrhythmia is caused by abnormal automaticity, triggered activity, or microreentry, focal AT is ablated by targeting the site of origin of the AT. Catheter ablation for focal AT carries a success rate of more than 90%, with a recurrence rate of 9%. The incidence of significant complications is relatively low (1% to 3%) in experienced centers.

Electrocardiographic Features

P Wave Morphology

During AT, typically there are discrete P waves at rates of 130 to 240 beats/min, but possibly as slow as 100 beats/min or as fast as 300 beats/min. Antiarrhythmic drugs can slow the tachycardia rate without abolishing the AT. Classically, there are clearly defined isoelectric intervals between the P waves in all leads (Fig. 11-2). However, in the presence of rapid rates, intraatrial conduction disturbances, or both, the P waves can be broad, and there may be no isoelectric baseline. In these cases, the ECG shows an AFL pattern (continuous undulation without isoelectric baseline; Fig. 11-3).[1] Nevertheless, one report demonstrated a high sensitivity (90%) and specificity (90%) of *quantitative* ECG indexes of shorter atrial activation and longer diastolic intervals in distinguishing focal from macroreentrant AT. This approach was effective in cases with and without 1:1 AV conduction and when the P or flutter waves overlay T waves.[27]

P wave morphology depends on the location of the atrial focus, and it can be used to localize the site of origin of the AT approximately. However, the P wave can be partially masked by the preceding ST segment or T wave, or both. Vagal maneuvers and adenosine infusion to provide transient AV block can be used to obtain a clear view of the P wave, assuming that the tachycardia does not terminate with AV block. The compensatory pause following a premature ventricular complex during the AT can also be used to delineate P wave morphology (Fig. 11-4). It has been suggested that the multilead body surface potential recording can be used to help localize the site of origin of the tachycardia.

One report described a clinical application of ECG imaging (ECGI) as an adjunctive noninvasive technology to identify the site of origin of a focal AT accurately prior to catheter ablation (Fig. 11-5).[28]

Focal automatic ATs start with a P wave identical to the P wave during the arrhythmia, and the rate generally increases gradually (warms up) over the first few seconds. In comparison, intraatrial reentry or triggered-activity AT is usually initiated by a P wave from a premature atrial complex (PAC) that generally differs in morphology from the P wave during the established arrhythmia (Fig. 11-6).

QRS Morphology

QRS morphology during AT is usually the same as during NSR. However, functional aberration can occur at rapid atrial rates.

P/QRS Relationship

The atrial to ventricular relationship is usually 1:1 during ATs, but Wenckebach (Fig. 11-7) or 2:1 AV block (see Figs. 11-3 and 11-4) can occur at rapid rates, in the presence of AVN disease, or in the presence of drugs that slow AVN conduction. The presence of AV block during an SVT strongly suggests AT, excludes AV reentrant tachycardia (AVRT), and renders AVN reentrant tachycardia (AVNRT) unlikely.

ATs usually have a long RP interval, but the RP interval can also be short, depending on the degree of AV conduction delay (i.e., PR interval prolongation) during the tachycardia.

Localization of the Atrial Tachycardia Site of Origin Using P Wave Morphology

GENERAL OBSERVATIONS RELATING P WAVE MORPHOLOGY TO SITE OF ORIGIN OF ATRIAL TACHYCARDIA

P wave morphology provides a useful guide to the localization of focal AT in patients without structural heart disease. In patients with prior surgery or extensive atrial ablation or in those with significant structural heart disease, activation patterns can be altered, significantly rendering P wave morphology less helpful.[29]

ECG lead V_1 is the most useful in identifying the likely anatomical site of origin for focal AT. Lead V_1 is located to the right and anteriorly in relation to the atria, which should be considered anatomically as right anterior and left posterior structures. Thus, for example, tachycardias originating from the tricuspid annulus have negative P waves in lead V_1 because of the anterior and rightward location of this structure (i.e., activation travels *away* from lead V_1). The P wave in lead V_1 is universally positive for tachycardias originating from the PVs because of the posterior location of these structures (i.e., the impulse travels *toward* lead V_1).[6,30,31]

Several features of P wave morphology can help predict whether an AT is arising from the RA or the LA. In one report, a negative or biphasic (positive-negative) P wave in lead V_1 was associated with 100% specificity, 100% positive predictive value, 69% sensitivity, and 66% negative predictive value for a tachycardia arising from the RA. Conversely, a positive or negative-positive biphasic P wave in lead V_1 had 100% sensitivity, 81% specificity, 76% positive predictive value, and 100% negative predictive value for an LA origin. A positive or biphasic P wave in lead aVL predicted an RA focus; however, some patients with right superior PV foci had positive P waves in lead aVL. An isoelectric or negative P wave in lead I was 100% specific (but only 50% sensitive) for LA foci.[6]

The predictive value of P wave morphology for localizing the atrium of origin is more limited when the tachycardia foci arise from the interatrial septum. Those ATs are associated with variable P wave morphology and considerable overlap for tachycardias located on the left and right sides of the septum. Of note, P waves during ATs arising near the septum are generally narrower than those arising in the RA or LA free wall.

P waves identical to the sinus P wave are suggestive of sinus node reentrant tachycardia or perinodal AT. Negative P waves in the anterior precordial leads suggest an anterior RA or LA free wall location. Negative P waves in the inferior leads suggest a low (inferior) atrial origin.

Several algorithms have been proposed for ECG localization of focal AT using P wave morphology. Figure 11-8 summarizes some of those algorithms.[6]

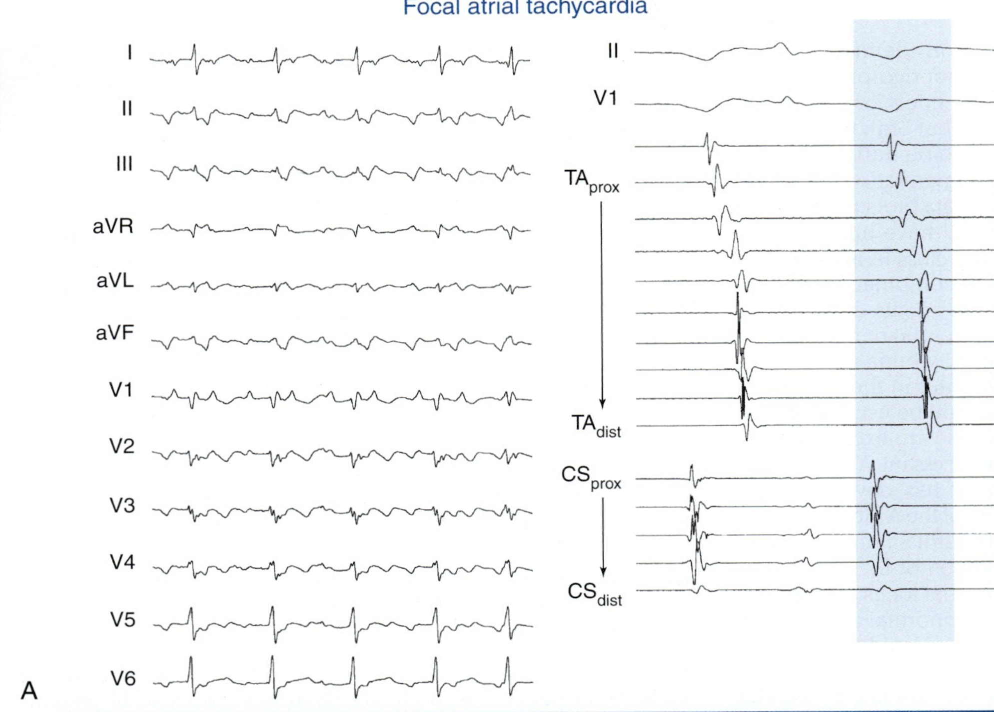

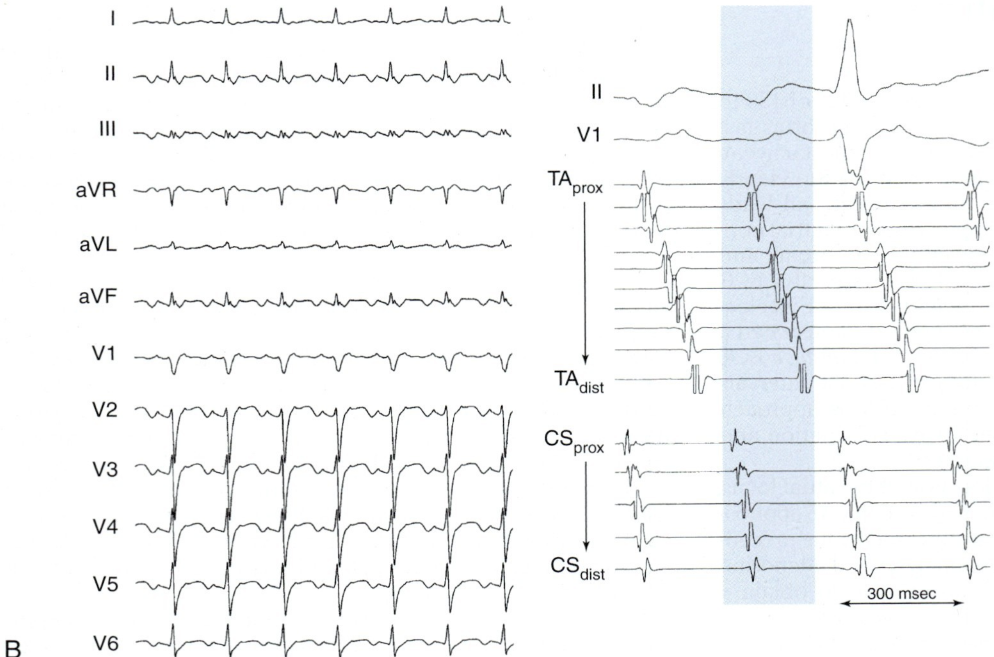

FIGURE 11-2 Comparison of focal and macroreentrant atrial tachycardia (AT). **A,** Surface ECG and endocardial activation sequence of focal AT originating from inferior aspect of the mitral annulus with 2:1 atrioventricular (AV) conduction. **B,** Endocardial activation macroreentrant AT around the tricuspid annulus (counterclockwise, typical atrial flutter) with 2:1 AV conduction. As illustrated in this case, discrimination between focal and macroreentry as the mechanism of AT based on the presence of distinct isoelectric intervals between the tachycardia P waves can be challenging caused by superimposition of the QRS and ST-T waves. Endocardial activation (shaded area), however, clearly demonstrates that biatrial activation from all electrodes of the 20-pole ("Halo") catheter (around the tricuspid annulus [TA]) and the coronary sinus (CS) catheter occupies only a small fraction (less than 50%) of the tachycardia cycle length (CL) during focal AT with over half of the tachycardia CL without recorded activity. In contrast, biatrial activation occupies most (~90%) of the tachycardia CL during macroreentrant AT. dist = distal; prox = proximal.

RIGHT ATRIAL TACHYCARDIAS

Cristal ATs (i.e., ATs arising from the crista terminalis) are characterized by right-to-left activation sequence resulting in P waves that are positive and broad in leads I and II, positive in lead aVL, and biphasic in lead V_1 (Fig. 11-9). A negative P wave in lead aVR predicts a cristal origin compared with anterior RA foci with a sensitivity of 100% and specificity of 93%. Biphasic P waves (positive-negative) in lead V_1 (or positive V_1 during both tachycardia and sinus rhythm), positive P waves in leads I and II, and negative P waves in lead aVR predict a cristal origin with 93% sensitivity, 95% specificity, 84% positive predictive value, and 98% negative predictive value. Although there can be overlap in P wave morphology between the superior crista and the right superior PV as a result of the anatomical proximity of the two sites, these can be distinguishable on the basis of changes to the P wave morphology in lead V_1 during tachycardia as compared with sinus P waves. In right superior PV AT, P waves in lead V_1 are invariably upright during tachycardia and biphasic (positive-negative) in sinus rhythm. When cristal AT has an upright P wave in lead V_1 (approximately 10%), it is invariably also upright

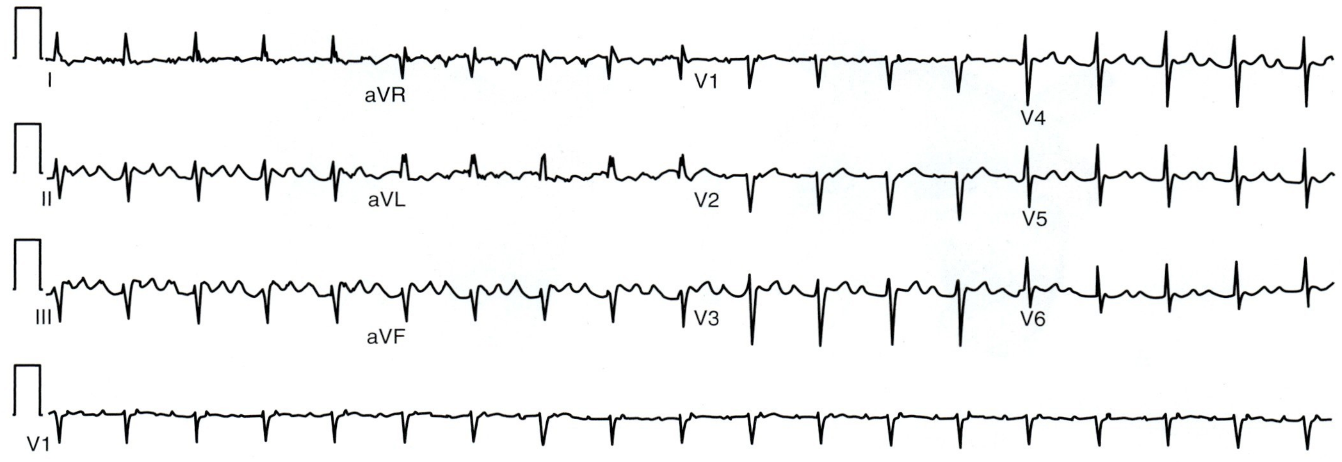

FIGURE 11-3 Surface ECG of focal atrial tachycardia originating from the right superior pulmonary vein. Second-degree 2:1 atrioventricular block is observed during the tachycardia. Note that the tachycardia in the inferior leads mimics atrial flutter as a result of intraatrial conduction abnormalities as well as overlapping T waves.

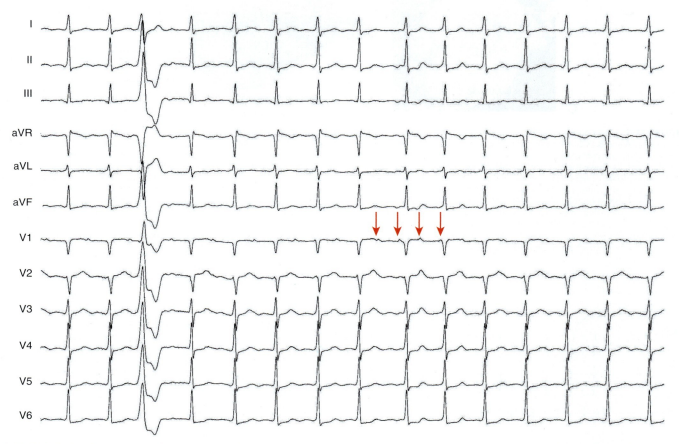

FIGURE 11-4 Surface ECG of focal atrial tachycardia with 2:1 atrioventricular (AV) block. Note that every other P wave lies within the QRS, a pattern mimicking supraventricular tachycardia with 1:1 AV conduction. Careful inspection of the whole recording reveals the hidden P waves sometimes occurring at varying timings within the QRS, as indicated by the arrows.

during sinus rhythm. High, middle, or low cristal locations can be identified by P wave polarity in the inferior leads.[29]

In anteroseptal ATs (originating above the membranous septum), the P wave is biphasic or negative in lead V_1 and positive in the inferior leads. Because of relatively simultaneous biatrial activation, P wave duration is approximately 20 milliseconds narrower than the sinus P wave. Those ATs can mimic slow-fast AVNRT or orthodromic AVRT with superoparaseptal bypass tracts (BTs).

Midseptal ATs (originating below the membranous septum and above the CS os) are associated with P waves that are biphasic or negative in lead V_1 and negative in the inferior leads. Those ATs can mimic fast-intermediate AVNRT or orthodromic AVRT with midseptal BTs.

In the setting of posteroseptal ATs (originating below and around the CS os), the P wave is positive in lead V_1, negative in the inferior leads, and positive in leads aVL and aVR. Those ATs can mimic fast-slow AVNRT or orthodromic AVRT using a posteroseptal BT.

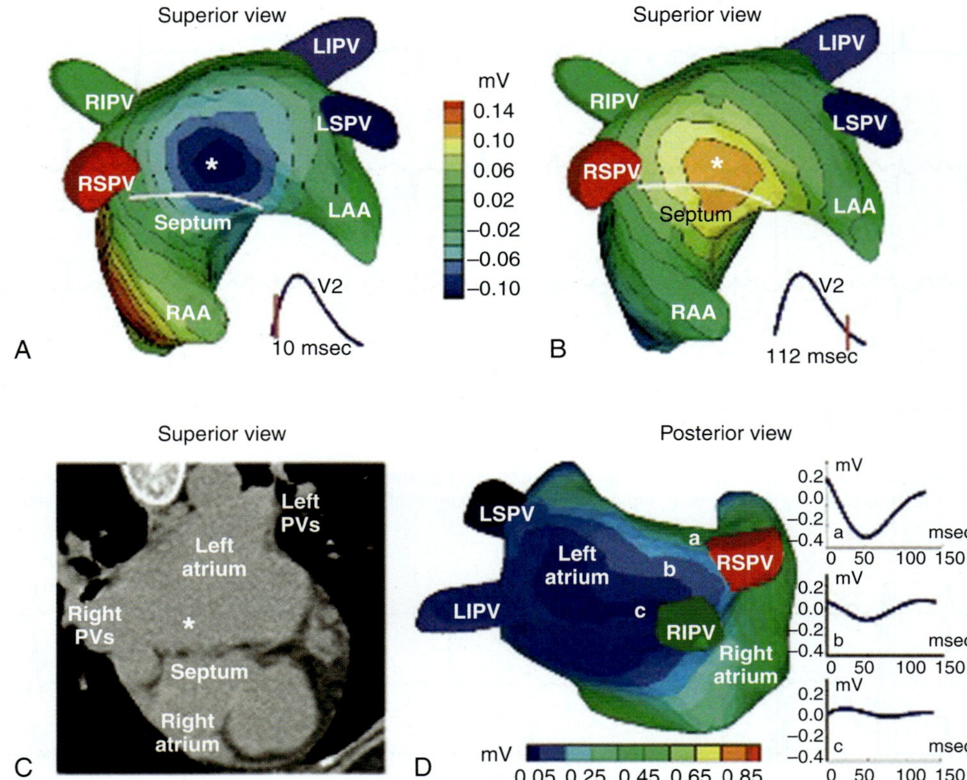

FIGURE 11-5 ECG imaging (ECGI) three-dimensional voltage and electrogram maps during focal atrial tachycardia in a patient with prior pulmonary vein (PV) electrical isolation. **A** and **B**, ECGI-reconstructed atrial epicardial surface voltage maps were produced for a single P wave extracted during the tachycardia at 10 and 112 milliseconds after the onset of the surface P wave. At the onset of the surface P wave, an epicardial breakthrough (local potential minimum, white asterisk) was imaged on the left atrium (LA), near the atrial septum **(A)**. During the end of the surface P wave, a repolarization pattern with reverse polarity (local potential maximum) appeared at the same site (**B**, white asterisk). These observations strongly suggested the existence of an activation source at the breakthrough site. **C** superimposes the site of the breakthrough (white asterisk) on a computed tomography image of the atria. As shown, the earliest site of activation determined by ECGI was located on the roof of the LA, between the right superior PV and the atrial septum **(C)**. **D** is an electrogram magnitude map (peak-to-peak) reconstructed by ECGI (posterior view). The dark blue represents a region of low-magnitude electrograms that indicates a scar region. Three electrograms selected from a nonscar region (a) and from the scar region (b, c) are shown. Location of low-magnitude electrograms is consistent with prior PV isolations and LA substrate modification. LAA = LA appendage; LIPV = left inferior PV; LSPV = left superior PV; RAA = right atrial appendage; RIPV = right inferior PV; RSPV = right superior PV. *(From Wang Y, Cuculich PS, Woodard PK, et al: Focal atrial tachycardia after pulmonary vein isolation: noninvasive mapping with electrocardiographic imaging (ECGI), Heart Rhythm 4:1081-1084, 2008; with permission.)*

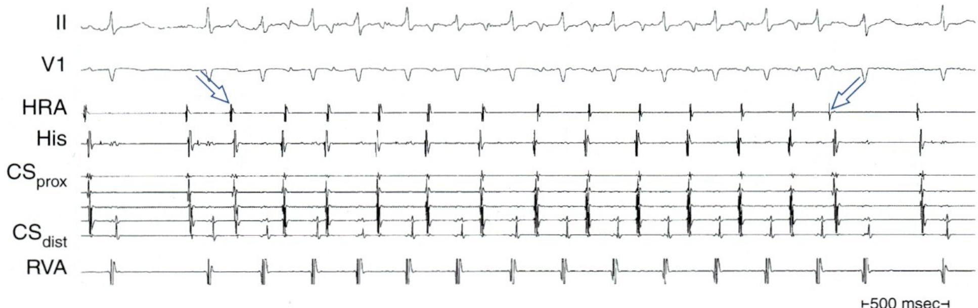

FIGURE 11-6 Spontaneous initiation and termination of a midseptal focal atrial tachycardia (AT; arrows). The tachycardia is initiated and terminated by a premature atrial complex of different morphology from that of the AT, a finding suggesting a nonautomatic mechanism. Note the narrow P wave during AT, consistent with a septal origin. CS_{dist} = distal coronary sinus; CS_{prox} = proximal coronary sinus; HRA = high right atrium; RVA = right ventricular apex.

The circumference of the tricuspid annulus is the second most common site of origin for RA tachycardias. A common feature of tricuspid annular ATs is the presence of an inverted P wave in leads V_1 and V_2 with late precordial transition to an upright appearance. The nonseptal sites demonstrate negative P waves in lead V_1, whereas anteroinferior sites tend to have inverted P waves across the precordial leads, and superior sites closer to the septum show transition from negative in lead V_1 through biphasic to upright in the lateral precordial leads.[3] In general, the polarity of leads II and III is deeply negative for an inferoanterior location and low amplitude, positive, or biphasic for a superior location. Additionally, tricuspid annular ATs typically have positive P waves in lead aVL and positive or isoelectric P waves in lead I.[29]

Focal ATs originating from the RA appendage typically originate from the lateral base of the appendage but are also well described from an apical location. Because of their close anatomical proximity, these tachycardias are generally indistinguishable from superior tricuspid annular foci; they exhibit negative P waves in leads V_1 and V_2 and variable precordial transition to positive in lead V_6. P waves in the inferior leads characteristically have low positive amplitudes.[29,32]

LEFT ATRIAL TACHYCARDIAS

ATs arising from the PVs are characterized by entirely positive P waves in lead V_1 (in 100% of cases) and across the precordial leads, isoelectric or negative waves in lead aVL in 86%, and negative

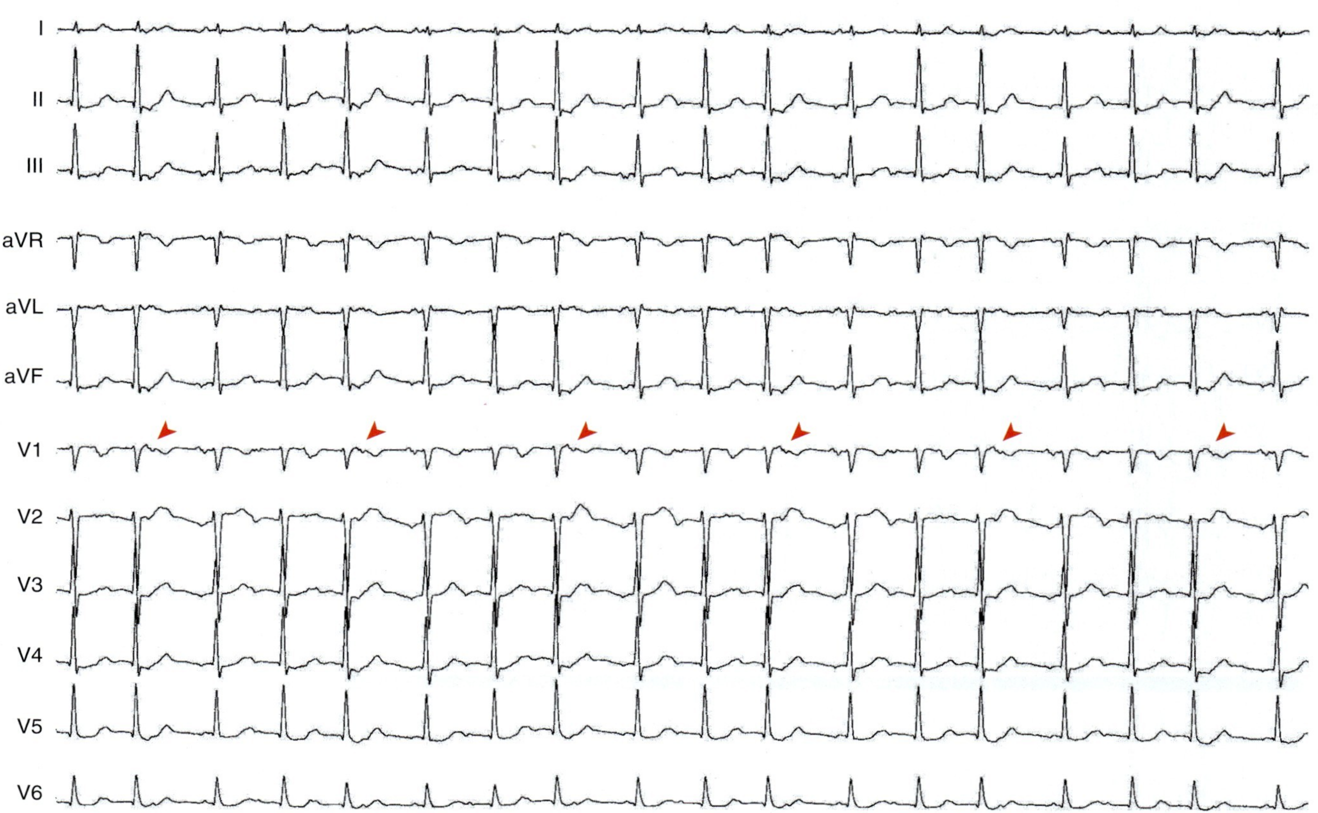

FIGURE 11-7 Surface ECG of focal atrial tachycardia originating from the inferior portion of the right atrial septum. Wenckebach atrioventricular block is observed. Arrowheads indicate blocked P waves.

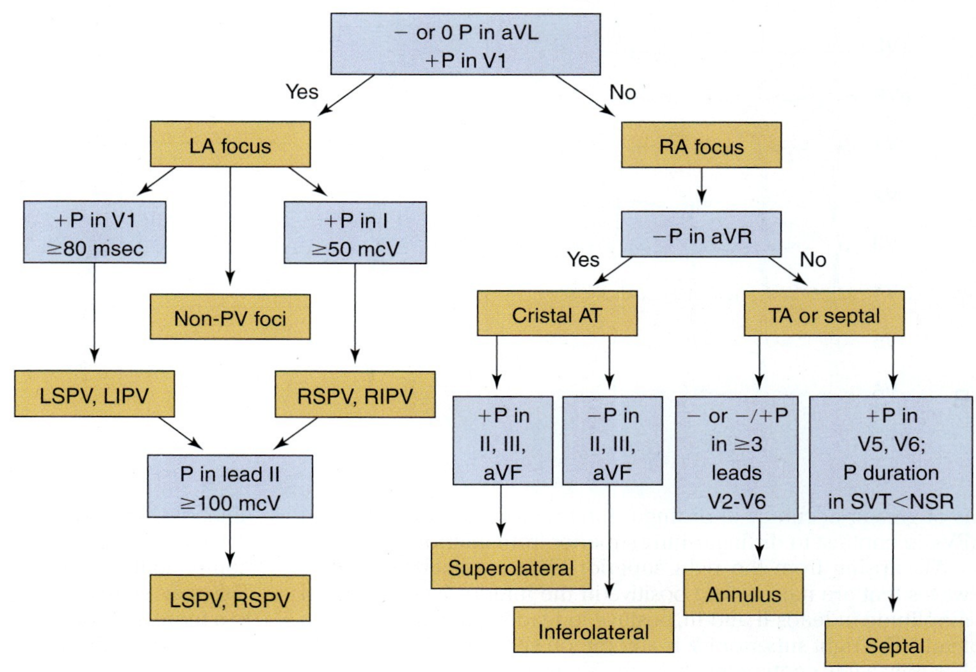

FIGURE 11-8 Algorithm for localization of atrial tachycardia (AT) origin based on P wave morphology on the surface ECG. – /+ = biphasic P wave; LA = left atrial; LIPV = left inferior pulmonary vein; LSPV = left superior pulmonary vein; mcV = microvolt; NSR = normal sinus rhythm; 0 = isoelectric P wave; +P = positive P wave; –P = negative P wave; RA = right atrial; RIPV = right inferior pulmonary vein; RSPV = right superior pulmonary vein; TA = tricuspid annulus. *(From Ellenbogen KA, Wood MA: Atrial tachycardia. In Zipes DP, Jalife J, editors: Cardiac electrophysiology: from cell to bedside, ed 4, Philadelphia, 2002, Saunders, pp 500-511.)*

waves in lead aVR in 96%. Lead aVL can be biphasic or positive in right-sided PV ATs.[7] Compared with the right-sided PVs, the left-sided PV foci have several characteristics: positive notching in the P waves in two or more surface leads, an isoelectric or negative P wave in lead I, P wave amplitude in lead III/II ratio greater than 0.8, and broad P waves in lead V_1 (Fig. 11-10). Right-sided PV foci usually have positive P waves in lead I. ATs arising from the superior PVs invariably have a positive P wave in the inferior leads. In contrast, ATs arising from the inferior PVs can have inverted, low-amplitude positive or isoelectric inferior P waves. However, because of the close proximity of the superior and inferior veins and marked anatomical variation, P wave morphology generally

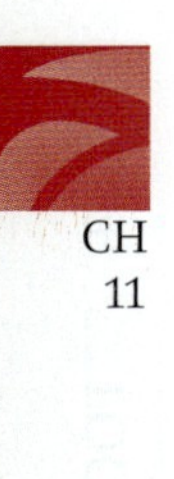

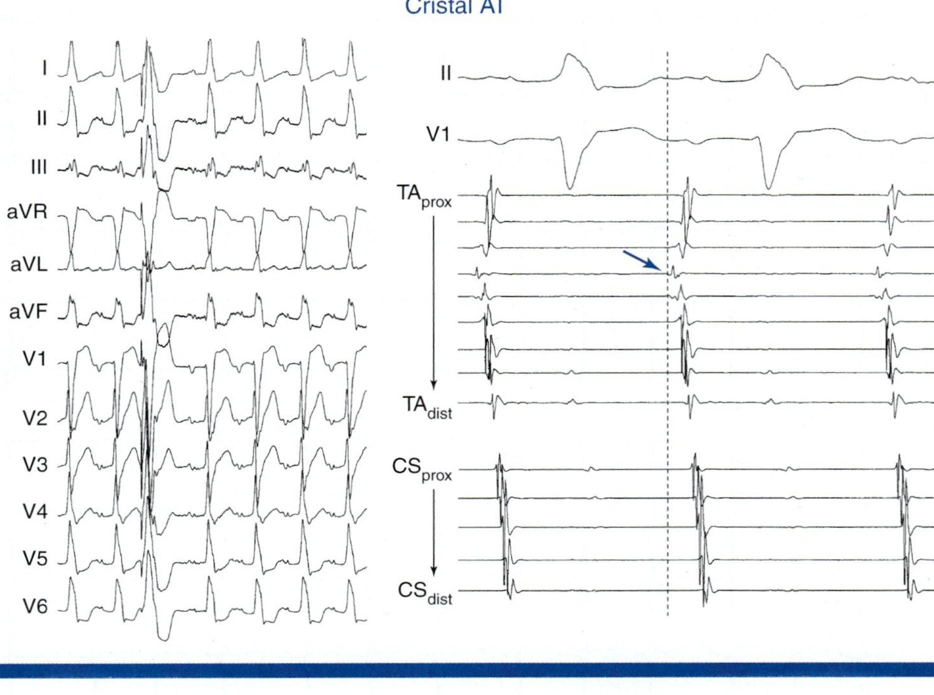

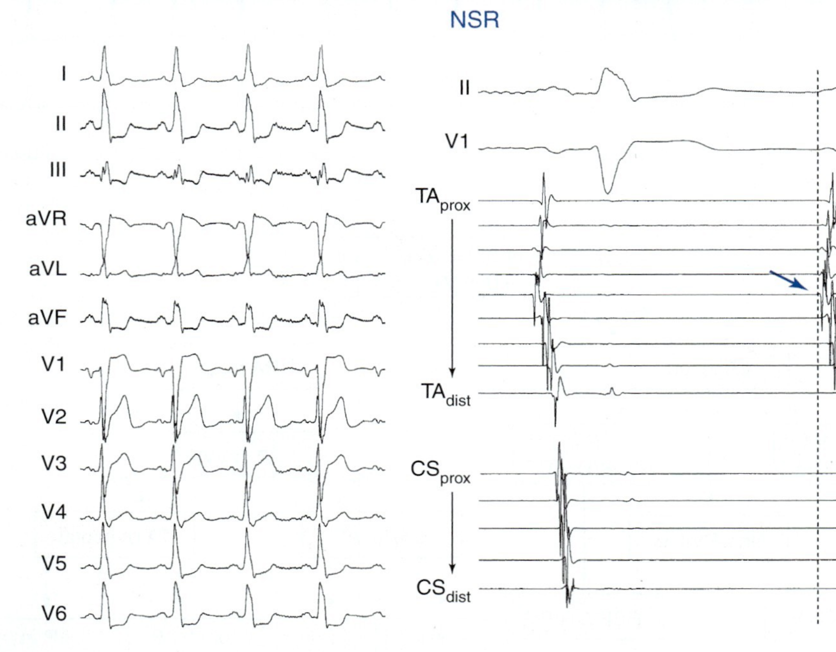

FIGURE 11-9 Comparison of P wave morphology and endocardial atrial activation sequence between focal atrial tachycardia (AT) originating from the crista terminalis **(A)** and normal sinus rhythm (NSR) **(B)** in the same patient. A Halo catheter is positioned around the tricuspid annulus (TA). CS_{dist} = distal coronary sinus; CS_{prox} = proximal coronary sinus.

is of greater accuracy in distinguishing right-sided from left-sided PVs, in contrast to distinguishing superior from inferior PVs.

ATs arising from the right superior PV are associated with P waves that are narrow and positive in the inferior leads, of equal amplitude in leads II and III, positive in lead V_1, and isoelectric in lead I. The right superior PV is a common site of origin for LA ATs. It is only a few centimeters from the sinus node. Activation rapidly crosses the septum via Bachmann's bundle to activate the RA in a fashion similar to NSR, a feature explaining the similarities in P wave morphology. However, whereas the P wave is biphasic in lead V_1 during NSR, it is positive in that lead during right superior PV AT (Fig. 11-11).[7]

Despite prior posterior LA ablation, the surface ECG morphology of ATs originating from the PV ostia in patients with prior AF ablation procedures is similar to those in patients without prior ablation. However, ATs originating from the bottom of the right or left PVs after prior PV isolation can have a significant negative component or can be completely negative in the inferior leads. This may be related to prior ablation in the superoposterior LA or to a more inferior origin of the tachycardia after prior ablation outside the PV ostium.[33]

In the setting of LA appendage ATs, the P wave is positive in the inferior leads (more positive in lead III than in II), positive in lead V_1, and negative in leads I and aVL. The LA appendage is closely approximated to the left superior PV, and, as such, ATs arising from those locations tend to have similar P wave morphologies. When P wave morphology suggestive of a left superior PV focus (broad upright and notched in lead V_1 and in the inferior leads) exhibits a deeply inverted P wave in lead I, an origin from the LA appendage should be strongly suspected. P waves are typically more positive

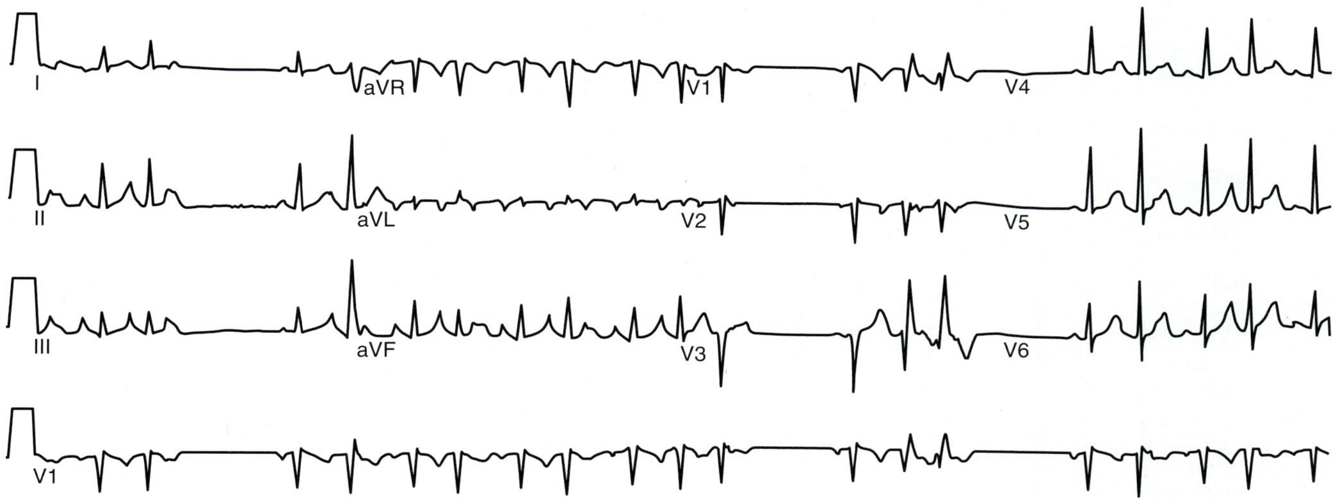

FIGURE 11-10 Surface ECG of nonsustained focal atrial tachycardia originating from the ostium of the left superior pulmonary vein.

in lead III than in lead II. A negative P wave in leads I and aVL predicts an LA appendage focus with a sensitivity and specificity of 92% and 97%, respectively.[29]

Mitral annular ATs typically cluster at the superior aspect of the mitral annulus in close proximity to the aortomitral continuity. ATs originating in this circumscribed area are characterized by P waves with an initial narrow negative deflection in lead V_1 followed by a positive deflection. The positivity of the P wave becomes progressively less from V_1 through V_6. The P wave is negative in leads I and aVL and isoelectric or slightly positive in the inferior leads.[34]

ATs arising from the CS musculature typically demonstrate deeply inverted P waves in the inferior leads. Lead V_1 usually exhibits isoelectric-positive or biphasic (negative-positive) P waves, with variable precordial transition. P waves are invariably positive in leads aVL and aVR.[4] Compared with AT originating from the CS os, AT originating from 3 to 4 cm into the body of the CS have broad and upright P waves in lead V_1.[29]

ATs have been described originating from the noncoronary cusp of the aortic valve. Because of the close anatomical proximity, the P wave morphology is similar to that of ATs arising from the aortomitral continuity. The P waves in leads V_1 and V_2 are also characteristically negative. However, unlike aortomitral ATs, those arising from the noncoronary cusp demonstrate upright P waves in leads I and aVL. In the inferior leads, the P waves are biphasic negative-positive but of low amplitude.[15,16,29]

Electrophysiological Testing

Baseline Observations during Normal Sinus Rhythm

Preexcitation, when present, suggests AVRT but does not exclude AT. In addition, the presence of dual AVN physiology suggests AVNRT but does not exclude AT. On the other hand, broad sinus P wave and intraatrial conduction delay suggest macroreentrant AT.

Induction of Tachycardia

Frequently, AT foci can become inactive in the EP laboratory environment because of sedative medications, changes in autonomic tone that can be caused by prolonged supine position, patient anxiety, deviation from normal diet, or other changes in daily activities that can have an impact on the circadian variation of AT activity. Thus, in preparation for an AT ablation procedure, several measures should be undertaken. Antiarrhythmic drugs should be discontinued for at least five half-lives before the EP study. Sedation should be minimized throughout the procedure. It may be an appropriate policy to monitor the patient in the EP laboratory initially without sedation. If no spontaneous tachycardia is induced, isoproterenol is administered. If no AT can be induced, a single quadripolar catheter is placed in the RA, and programmed electrical stimulation is performed without and, if no AT is induced, with isoproterenol infusion. If AT remains quiescent, the procedure is aborted and retried at a future date. If AT is inducible at any step, the full EP catheter arrangement and EP study are undertaken (Table 11-2).[17,24,31]

INITIATION BY ATRIAL EXTRASTIMULATION OR ATRIAL PACING

Microreentrant AT is usually easy to initiate with a wide range of AES coupling intervals (A_1-A_2 intervals). The initiating AES coupling interval and the interval between the initiating AES and first beat of AT are inversely related. Triggered ATs also can be initiated by AES or (more commonly) atrial pacing. However, initiation frequently requires catecholamines (isoproterenol), and, in contrast to microreentrant AT, there is usually a direct relationship between the coupling interval or pacing CL initiating the AT and the interval to the onset of the AT and the early CL of the AT. On the other hand, automatic ATs cannot be reproducibly initiated by AES or atrial pacing.

In the setting of microreentry and triggered activity, the first tachycardia P wave is different from subsequent P waves; the first P wave is usually a PAC or an AES that is necessary to start the AT (see Fig. 11-6). In contrast, the first tachycardia P wave and subsequent P waves during automatic AT are identical; the AT does not require a PAC to start (Fig. 11-12). Furthermore, the automatic AT CL tends to shorten progressively (warm up) for several beats until its ultimate rate is achieved.

No delay in the atrial–His bundle (HB) interval (AH interval) or PR interval is required for initiation of AT, although it can occur. AV block can also occur at initiation.[24]

INITIATION BY VENTRICULAR EXTRASTIMULATION OR VENTRICULAR PACING

It is uncommon to initiate AT with ventricular extrastimulation (VES) or ventricular pacing because decremental retrograde conduction over the AVN prevents adequate prematurity of atrial activation. However, in the presence of an AV BT, fast retrograde atrial activation mediates adequate prematurity of the conducted ventricular stimulus to the atrium, and AT may be induced.[24]

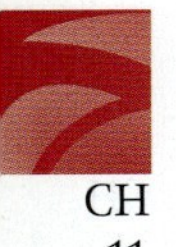

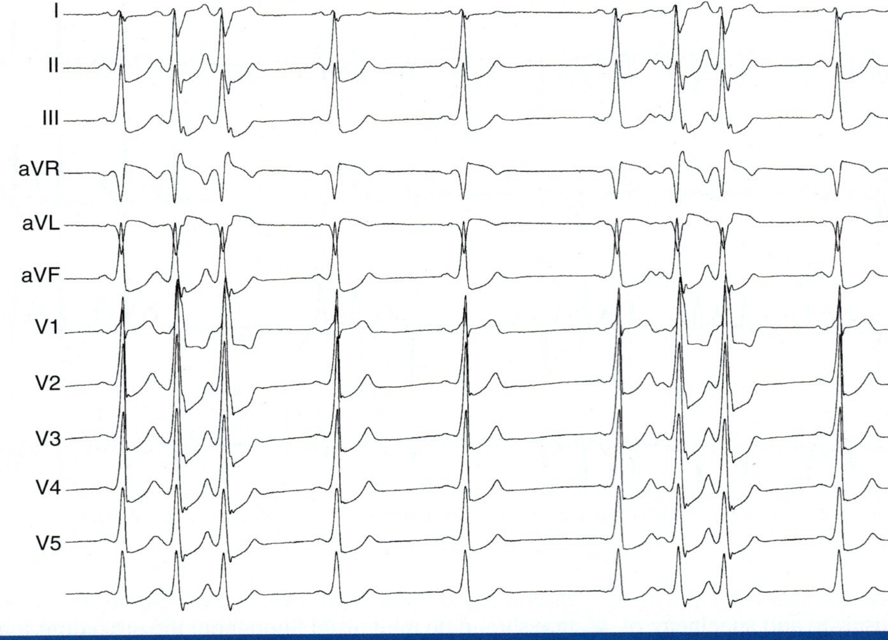

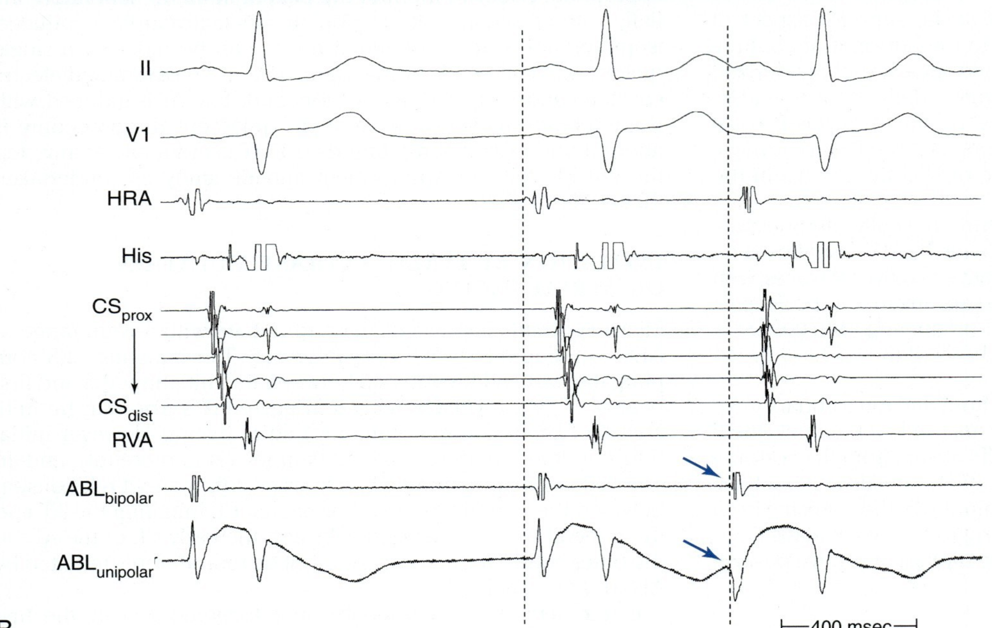

FIGURE 11-11 Premature atrial complexes (PACs) originating from the right superior pulmonary vein (PV). **A,** 12-lead surface ECG illustrating atrial couplets during normal sinus rhythm (NSR). Note the similarities in P wave morphology during PACs versus NSR. **B,** Intracardiac recordings from the same patient. Detailed mapping localized the origin of the PACs to the ostium of the right superior PV (as illustrated by bipolar and unipolar recordings from the ablation catheter [ABL]). Note the concordance of timing of the bipolar and unipolar recordings and the QS unipolar electrogram morphology (blue arrows), suggesting the site of origin of activation and a good ablation site. CS_{dist} = distal coronary sinus; CS_{prox} = proximal coronary sinus; HRA = high right atrium; RVA = right ventricular apex.

TABLE 11-2 Programmed Electrical Stimulation Protocol for Electrophysiological Testing of Atrial Tachycardia

- Atrial burst pacing from the RA and CS (down to a pacing CL at which 2:1 atrial capture occurs)
- Single and double AES at multiple CLs (600–400 msec) from the RA and CS (down to atrial ERP)
- Ventricular burst pacing from the RV apex (down to VA Wenckebach CL)
- Single and double VES at multiple CLs (600–400 msec) from the RV apex (down to ventricular ERP)

AES = atrial extrastimulation; CL = cycle length; CS = coronary sinus; ERP = effective refractory period; RA = right atrium; RV = right ventricle; VA = ventricular-atrial; VES = ventricular extrastimulation.

Tachycardia Features

ATRIAL ACTIVATION SEQUENCE

P wave morphology and atrial activation sequence depend on the site of origin of the AT. Intracardiac mapping shows significant portions of the tachycardia CL without recorded atrial activity, and atrial activation time is markedly less than the tachycardia CL (see Fig. 11-2).[24] However, in the presence of extensive atrial scarring or prior ablation, depolarization from the AT focus can occasionally be followed by very disordered and prolonged conduction so that activation of the entire chamber can extend over (or even exceed) the entire tachycardia CL, thus mimicking macroreentrant AT.[12] Conversely, long isoelectric intervals can occur between the P waves during macroreentrant ATs and can incorrectly suggest a focal mechanism. This pattern is particularly observed for LA

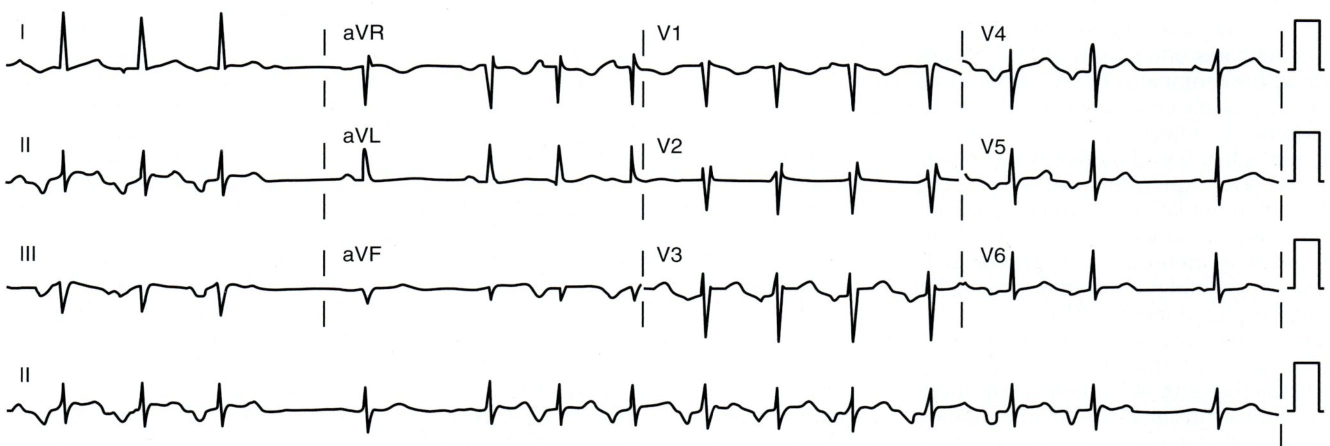

FIGURE 11-12 Surface ECG of repetitive nonsustained atrial tachycardia (AT). Note that the first P wave of the tachycardia is similar in morphology to the subsequent P waves, consistent with abnormal automaticity as the mechanism of the AT.

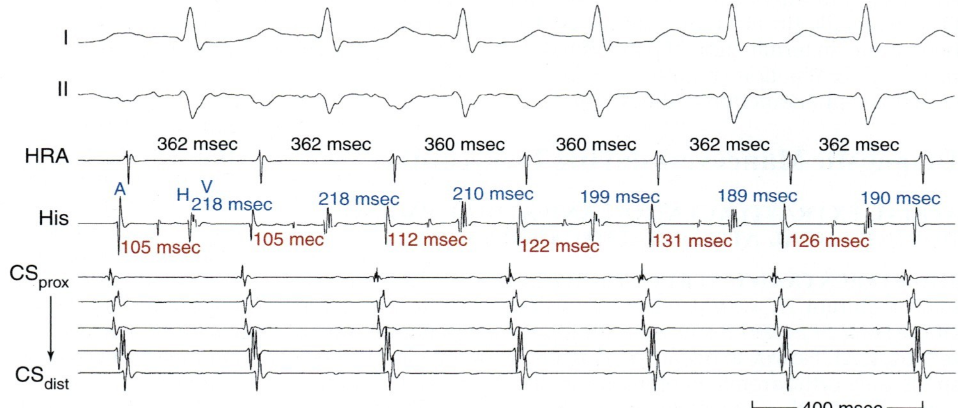

FIGURE 11-13 Supraventricular tachycardia (SVT) with concentric atrial activation sequence. Note the constant atrial cycle length (numbers in black) but variable atrial–His bundle (AH) interval (numbers in red) and ventricular-atrial (VA) interval (numbers in blue). This observation favors atrial tachycardia (originating from the posteroseptal region) as the mechanism of the tachycardia over other types of SVTs. CS_{dist} = distal coronary sinus; CS_{prox} = proximal coronary sinus; HRA = high right atrium.

flutters in the presence of large areas of electrical scar. However, a *thorough* intracardiac activation map reveals atrial activation spanning the tachycardia CL. When mapping is limited to only the atrium contralateral to the origin of the macroreentrant circuit or to only parts of the ipsilateral atrium, a focal mechanism can be falsely implied.

ATRIAL-VENTRICULAR RELATIONSHIP

The AH and PR intervals during AT are appropriate for the AT rate and are usually longer than those during NSR. The faster the AT rate is, the longer the AH and PR intervals will be. Thus, the PR interval may be shorter than, longer than, or equal to the RP interval. The PR interval may also be equal to the RR, and the P wave may fall inside the preceding QRS, thereby mimicking typical AVNRT.[24]

AV block can be observed during AT because neither the AVN nor the ventricle is part of the AT circuit. Most incessant SVTs with AV block are probably automatic ATs.

OSCILLATION IN THE TACHYCARDIA CYCLE LENGTH

Oscillation of the ventricular CL occurs frequently during AT and is the result of changes either in the AT CL or in AVN conduction. When CL variability results from oscillation of the AT CL, changes in the atrial CL are expected to precede and predict similar changes in the ventricular CL. On the other hand, ventricular CL variability can be caused by changes in AV conduction instead of changes in the CL of the AT, in which setting ventricular CL variability is not predicted by a prior change in atrial CL. Because there is no VA conduction during AT, ventricular CL variability by itself is not expected to result in atrial CL variability during AT.[35] Additionally, spontaneous changes in the PR and RP intervals with fixed A-A intervals favor AT over other types of SVT (Fig. 11-13).

In contrast to AT, typical AVNRT and orthodromic AVRT generally have CL variability caused by changes in anterograde AVN conduction. Because retrograde conduction through a fast AVN pathway or a BT generally is much less variable than the anterograde conduction through the AVN, the changes in ventricular CL that result from variability in anterograde AVN conduction are expected to precede the subsequent changes in atrial CL.[35]

Variation in the AT CL of more than 15% has been suggested as a reliable marker of a focal AT. In contrast, it is rare for macroreentrant ATs to display considerable variation in the CL. However, a regular AT can be either focal or macroreentrant.[36]

EFFECTS OF BUNDLE BRANCH BLOCK

Bundle branch block may occur during AT but does not affect the tachycardia CL because the ventricles are not participants in AT.[24]

TERMINATION AND RESPONSE TO PHYSIOLOGICAL AND PHARMACOLOGICAL MANEUVERS

In the setting of spontaneous termination, ATs terminate with a QRS complex following the last P wave of the tachycardia. Most ATs (50% to 80%) are terminated by adenosine; therefore, termination of an SVT in response to adenosine is not helpful in differentiating AT from other SVTs.[24,37] Usually (in 80% of cases), termination of AT in response to adenosine occurs prior to the onset of AV block (i.e., termination occurs with a tachycardia P wave followed by a

QRS). Reproducible termination with a P wave not followed by a QRS indicates other types of SVT because it occurs in AT only if adenosine terminates the AT at the same moment it causes AV block, an unlikely coincidence. In the atrium, adenosine produces antiadrenergic effects (presumably responsible for terminating triggered activity) and increases the acetylcholine- or adenosine-activated potassium (K^+) current (I_{KACh}). The results are shortening of the action potential duration and reduction of the resting membrane potential, which may be responsible for terminating atrial microreentry. Adenosine can also help identify automatic ATs, which are generally transiently slowed but not terminated, with gradual resumption of the AT rate.[1]

Carotid sinus massage, vagal maneuvers, and adenosine reproducibly slow or terminate sinus node reentrant tachycardia and 25% of microreentrant ATs (especially those with long tachycardia CLs and those arising in the RA). Spontaneous termination of AT is usually accompanied by progressive prolongation of the A-A interval, with or without changes in AV conduction. Triggered activity AT also can terminate in response to carotid sinus massage, vagal maneuvers, adenosine, verapamil, beta blockers, and sodium channel blockers. In contrast, although carotid sinus massage can cause AV block and adenosine can slow automatic AT, these interventions generally do not terminate the AT. Only beta blockers have been useful in termination of paroxysmal (but not incessant) automatic AT. Termination of automatic AT is usually preceded by a cool-down phenomenon of the AT rate.[1]

Diagnostic Maneuvers during Tachycardia

ATRIAL EXTRASTIMULATION AND ATRIAL PACING DURING FOCAL ATRIAL TACHYCARDIA

MICROREENTRANT ATRIAL TACHYCARDIA. AES can reset microreentrant AT with a resetting response classic for reentry (increasing or mixed response). Atrial pacing can entrain microreentrant AT. However, because the microreentrant circuit is very small, only orthodromic capture is usually observed. In addition, entrainment with constant fusion (at a fixed pacing CL) or progressive fusion (at progressively shorter pacing CLs), as demonstrated by intermediate P wave morphologies on the surface ECG, or partial activation change recorded by multiple endocardial electrodes, or both, cannot be demonstrated in microreentrant AT.

Fusion during resetting or entrainment (a hallmark of macroreentrant tachycardias) cannot be demonstrated in microreentrant AT. For atrial fusion (i.e., fusion of atrial activation from both the tachycardia wavefront and the atrial stimulus) to occur during resetting or entrainment, the atrial paced impulse should be able to enter the reentrant circuit while at the same time the tachycardia wavefront should be able to exit the circuit. This requires spatial separation between the entry and exit sites to the reentrant circuit, a condition that is lacking in the setting of focal AT. Once the tachycardia wavefront exits the reentry circuit to activate the atrium, any atrial stimulus delivered beyond that time and that results in atrial fusion would not be capable of reaching the reentry circuit because the entry-exit site is already refractory as a result of activation by the exiting tachycardia wavefront, and the atrial stimulus has no alternative way for reaching the circuit. Similarly, once an atrial stimulus is capable of reaching the reentry circuit, the shared entry-exit site is made refractory and incapable of allowing a simultaneous exit of the tachycardia wavefront. Therefore, during entrainment of microreentrant AT by atrial pacing, the atrial activation sequence and P wave morphology are always that of pure paced morphology.

However, it is important to understand that overdrive pacing of a tachycardia of any mechanism (automatic, triggered activity, or microreentrant) can result in a certain degree of fusion, especially when the pacing CL is only slightly shorter than the tachycardia CL. Such fusion, however, is unstable during the same pacing drive at a constant CL because pacing stimuli fall on a progressively earlier portion of the tachycardia cycle, thus producing progressively less fusion and more fully paced morphology. Such phenomena should be distinguished from entrainment, and sometimes this requires pacing for many cycles to demonstrate variable degrees of fusion.

During entrainment of microreentrant AT, the return CL and post-pacing interval (PPI) are fixed regardless of the number of beats in the pacing train. AES and atrial pacing can almost always terminate microreentrant AT (especially sinus node reentrant tachycardia).[24]

TRIGGERED-ACTIVITY ATRIAL TACHYCARDIA. AES can reset triggered-activity AT (with a decreasing resetting response). However, triggered-activity AT cannot be entrained by atrial pacing. Following the delivery of an AES or atrial overdrive pacing during triggered-activity AT, the return CL tends to shorten with shortening of the AES coupling interval or pacing CL. AES and, more effectively, atrial pacing can usually terminate triggered-activity AT.[24]

AUTOMATIC ATRIAL TACHYCARDIA. The response of automatic AT to AES is similar to that of the sinus node. A late-coupled AES collides with the tachycardia impulse already exiting the AT focus (zone of collision), resulting in fusion of atrial activation (fusion between the paced and the tachycardia wavefronts) or paced-only atrial activation sequence, and it does not affect the timing of the next AT complex (producing a full compensatory pause). An earlier coupled AES enters the AT focus before the time of the next tachycardia wavefront and therefore resets the AT focus (zone of reset), with a return CL that is not fully compensatory. The return cycle usually remains constant over a range of coupling intervals during the zone of reset. A very early coupled AES encounters a refractory AT focus (following the last tachycardia complex) and would not be able to enter or reset the AT focus. Therefore, the next AT complex is on time because the atrium is already fully recovered following that early AES (zone of interpolation).

Automatic AT cannot be entrained by atrial pacing. Rapid atrial pacing results in overdrive suppression of the AT rate. The AT resumes after cessation of atrial pacing but at a slower rate and gradually speeds up (warms up) to return back to prepacing tachycardia CL. The tachycardia return CL following cessation progressively prolongs with increasing the duration of overdrive pacing. Occasionally, overdrive pacing produces no effect at all on automatic AT.[24]

VENTRICULOATRIAL LINKING. Following cessation of overdrive atrial pacing (with 1:1 AV conduction) during focal AT, the VA interval (the interval between the last captured QRS complex and the first AT complex) can vary significantly from the VA interval during AT, because the timing of the AT return cycle is not related to the preceding QRS. In contrast, in the setting of typical AVNRT and orthodromic AVRT, the post-pacing VA interval remains fixed and similar to that during tachycardia (with a less than 10-millisecond variation) after different attempts at SVT entrainment. VA linking occurs in the setting of typical AVNRT and orthodromic AVRT because the timing of atrial activation is related to or dependent on ventricular activation and is the result of retrograde VA conduction over the AVN fast pathway (during typical AVNRT) or the BT (during orthodromic AVRT).[38,39]

DIFFERENTIAL-SITE ATRIAL PACING. Differential-site atrial pacing can help distinguish AT from other mechanisms of SVT. Overdrive pacing is performed during tachycardia from different atrial sites (high RA [HRA] and proximal CS) at the same pacing CL. Once the presence of 1:1 AV conduction during atrial pacing is verified and the SVT resumes following cessation of pacing, the maximal difference in the post-pacing VA intervals (the interval from the last captured ventricular electrogram to the earliest atrial electrogram of the initial tachycardia beat after pacing) among the different pacing sites is calculated (ΔVA interval). In one report, a ΔVA interval of more than 14 milliseconds was diagnostic of AT, whereas a ΔVA interval of less than 14 milliseconds favored AVNRT or orthodromic AVRT (with the sensitivity, specificity, and positive and negative predictive values all equal to 100%). In orthodromic AVRT and AVNRT, the initial atrial complex following cessation of atrial pacing entraining the SVT is *linked* to, and cannot be dissociated from, the last captured ventricular complex. In contrast, in the setting of AT, the first atrial return cycle following cessation of pacing is dependent on the distance between the AT origin and pacing site, atrial conduction properties, and mode of the resetting response of the AT, and it is not related to the preceding ventricular activation. Hence, the post-pacing VA intervals vary among the pacing sites, and the ΔVA interval is relatively large (more than 14 milliseconds).[39]

VARIABILITY IN POST-PACING INTERVALS. The global pattern of activation of an atrial arrhythmia can be rapidly determined by comparing the differences in PPIs obtained with overdrive pacing from a single site (proximal CS) at CLs 10, 20, and 30 milliseconds shorter than the tachycardia CL. Relative stability of the PPI, regardless of its relation to the tachycardia CL, is highly suggestive of circuitous activation of the atrium. High variability of the PPI, on the other hand, is nearly diagnostic of a centrifugal activation pattern. In fact, in one report, PPI variability was significantly shorter for macroreentrant ATs (6.0 ± 2.5 milliseconds) than for focal ATs (56.5 ± 20.6 milliseconds). A clinical prediction rule was derived wherein low PPI variability (less than 10 milliseconds) identified macroreentrant ATs with a sensitivity of 94% and a specificity of 100%, whereas high PPI variability (more than 30 milliseconds) identified focal ATs with a sensitivity of 93% and a specificity of 100%.[40]

In macroreentry, the PPI reflects the time required for the stimulated wavefront to travel to a reentrant circuit, revolve once around the circuit, and travel back to the pacing site. Because this distance remains unchanged, pacing at faster rates should theoretically not change the distance traveled, and thus the PPI remains stable (PPI variability should approach zero). Faster pacing rates, however, can decrease conduction velocity because of decremental tissue conduction leading to prolongation of the PPI. Nevertheless, this is less likely to occur when overdrive pacing CLs are limited to within 30 milliseconds of the tachycardia CL. In contrast, variability in the PPI is expected in the setting of automatic ATs; by virtue of the phenomenon of overdrive suppression, automatic foci tend to require more time for recovery as pacing rate or duration increases. Unexpectedly, however, large PPI variability was exhibited by all centrifugal tachycardias regardless of mechanism (including microreentry). By virtue of their small circuits, the microreentrant ATs have a short excitable gap; it is likely that the paced wavefront will penetrate the circuit during relative refractoriness, with decremental conduction resulting in progressive PPI prolongation.[40]

VENTRICULAR EXTRASTIMULATION AND VENTRICULAR PACING DURING FOCAL ATRIAL TACHYCARDIA

It is uncommon for VES or ventricular pacing to affect an AT unless rapid 1:1 VA conduction is present (especially in the presence of an AV BT) and the tachycardia CL is relatively long. Cessation of overdrive ventricular pacing during AT (with 1:1 VA conduction without terminating the tachycardia) results in an A-A-V pattern, which is suggestive of AT as the mechanism of the SVT and practically excludes AVNRT and orthodromic AVRT, whereas an A-V pattern is consistent with AVNRT or orthodromic AVRT and makes AT less likely.[24]

ATRIAL AND VENTRICULAR ELECTROGRAM SEQUENCE FOLLOWING CESSATION OF VENTRICULAR PACING

TECHNIQUE. During SVT, ventricular pacing is initiated at a pacing CL 10 to 60 milliseconds shorter than the tachycardia CL until 1:1 VA conduction occurs, at which point pacing is discontinued. If pacing results in termination of the tachycardia, SVT is reinduced, and the maneuver is repeated. If ventricular pacing does not terminate the tachycardia and the presence of stable 1:1 VA conduction is verified, the electrogram sequence immediately after the last paced ventricular complex is categorized as atrial-ventricular (A-V) or atrial-atrial-ventricular (A-A-V) (Fig. 11-14).

INTERPRETATION. During AVNRT or orthodromic AVRT, when the ventricle is paced at a CL shorter than the tachycardia CL and all electrograms are accelerated to the pacing rate without terminating the tachycardia (i.e., entrainment of the tachycardia is achieved), VA conduction occurs through the retrograde limb of the circuit. Therefore, after the last paced ventricular complex, the anterograde limb of the tachycardia circuit is not refractory, and the last entrained retrograde atrial complex can conduct to the ventricle. This results in an A-V response following cessation of pacing. However, when the ventricle is paced during AT and 1:1 VA conduction is produced, retrograde conduction occurs through the AVN. In this setting, the last retrograde atrial complex resulting from ventricular pacing is unable to conduct to the ventricle because the AVN is refractory to anterograde conduction, and the result is an A-A-V response.

PITFALLS. This pacing maneuver is not useful when 1:1 VA conduction during ventricular pacing is absent. Thus, when determining the response after ventricular pacing during SVT, the presence of 1:1 VA conduction must be confirmed. Isorhythmic VA dissociation can mimic 1:1 VA conduction, especially when the pacing train is not long enough or the pacing CL is too slow (see Fig. 11-14).

A pseudo–A-A-V response can occur during atypical AVNRT. Because retrograde conduction during ventricular pacing occurs through the slow pathway, the VA interval is long and can be longer than the pacing CL (V-V interval), so that the last paced QRS is followed first by the atrial complex resulting from slow VA conduction of the preceding paced QRS and then by the atrial complex resulting from the last paced QRS. Careful examination of the last atrial electrogram that resulted from VA conduction during ventricular pacing avoids this potential pitfall; the last retrograde atrial complex characteristically occurs at an A-A interval equal to the ventricular pacing CL, whereas the first tachycardia atrial complex usually occurs at a different return CL. A pseudo–A-A-V response may also occur when 1:1 VA conduction is absent during overdrive ventricular pacing, during typical AVNRT with long HB-ventricular (HV) intervals or short HA intervals whereby atrial activation may precede ventricular activation, and in patients with a bystander BT. Replacing ventricular activation with HB activation (i.e., characterizing the response as A-A-H or A-H instead of A-A-V or A-V, respectively) can be more accurate and can help eliminate the pseudo–A-A-V response in patients with AVNRT and long HV intervals, short HA intervals, or both.[41]

On the other hand, a pseudo–A-V response can occur with automatic AT when the maneuver is performed during isoproterenol infusion. Ventricular pacing with 1:1 VA conduction can result in overdrive suppression of the atrial focus, and isoproterenol may cause an increase in junctional automaticity, so that an apparent A-V response occurs. Therefore, when ventricular pacing is performed during an isoproterenol infusion, it is important to determine that the response after cessation of ventricular pacing is reproducible.[39]

A pseudo–A-V response can theoretically occur when AT coexists with retrograde dual AVN pathways or bystander BT. In such cases, the last retrograde atrial complex would have an alternative route for anterograde conduction to the ventricle, other than the one used for retrograde VA conduction during ventricular pacing, thus resulting in an A-V response. However, clinical occurrence of these theoretical scenarios has not been observed, probably because of retrograde penetration of both AVN pathways or of the AVN and the BT during ventricular pacing, so that both pathways are refractory to anterograde conduction on cessation of pacing.[39]

Exclusion of Other Arrhythmia Mechanisms

Focal AT should be differentiated from other SVTs, including AVNRT, orthodromic AVRT, and macroreentrant AT. Programmed electrical stimulation is usually adequate in excluding AVNRT and AVRT as the mechanism of SVT (Tables 11-3 and 11-4).[24] Macroreentry, however, can be more difficult to exclude, and electroanatomical mapping is of value in some cases (Table 11-5).

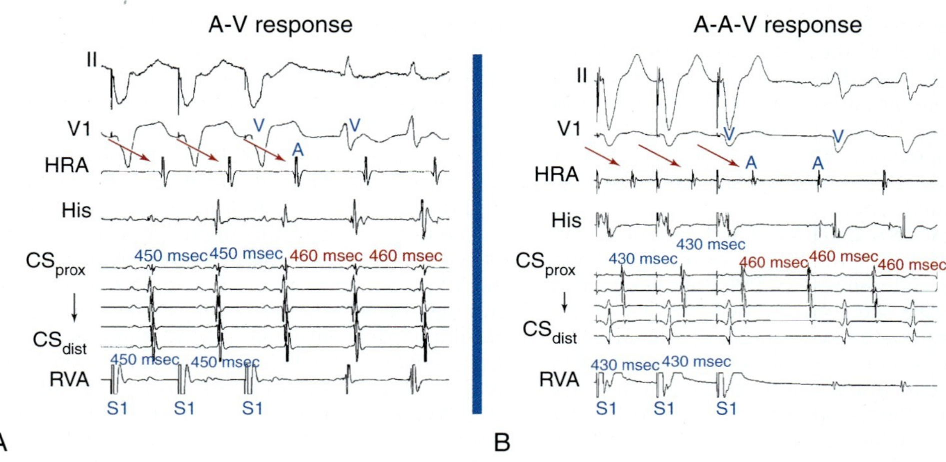

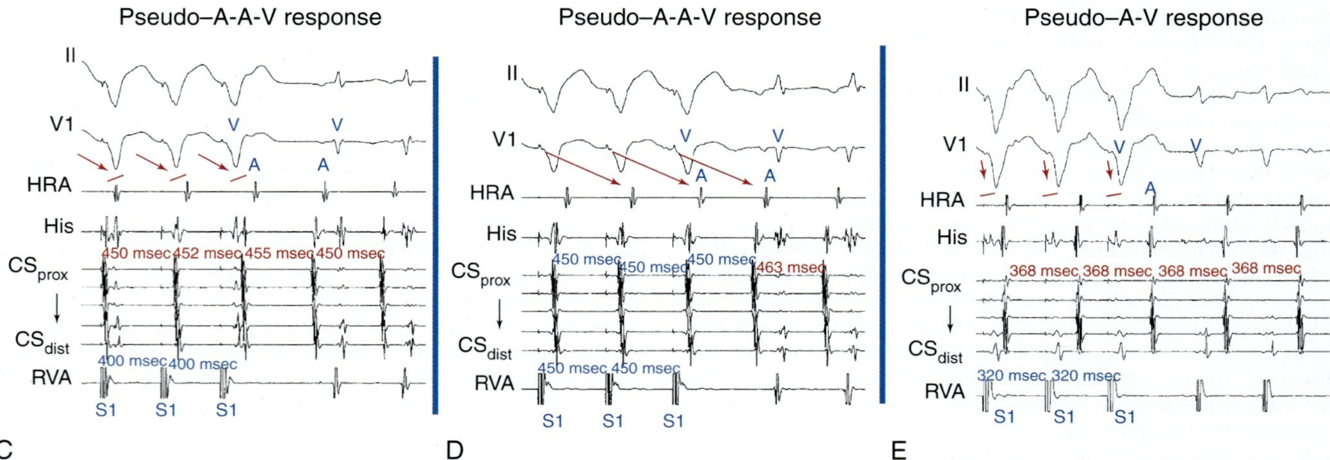

FIGURE 11-14 A-V versus A-A-V response after ventricular pacing during supraventricular tachycardia (SVT). Overdrive ventricular pacing is performed during five SVTs with concentric atrial activation sequence. Red arrows track ventricular-atrial (VA) conduction during ventricular pacing. Numbers indicate ventricular pacing cycle lengths (CLs) and atrial CLs during and after pacing. **A,** A-V response is observed following cessation of pacing during typical atrioventricular nodal reentrant tachycardia (AVNRT), which is inconsistent with atrial tachycardia (AT). **B,** A-A-V response is observed, consistent with AT originating in the posteroseptal region. **C,** Pseudo–A-A-V response is observed during atypical AVNRT secondary to VA dissociation (i.e., absence of VA conduction) during ventricular pacing. **D,** Pseudo–A-A-V response is observed during atypical AVNRT despite the presence of 1:1 VA conduction during ventricular pacing. Retrograde conduction during ventricular pacing, however, occurs through the slow atrioventricular node pathway with a long VA interval (red arrows) that is longer than the pacing CL; hence, the last ventricular paced impulse will be followed first by the P wave conducted slowly from the previous paced QRS, and then by the P wave resulting from the last paced QRS, thus mimicking an A-A-V response. This is verified by observing that the last retrograde atrial complex characteristically occurs at an A-A interval equal to the ventricular pacing CL, whereas the first tachycardia atrial complex usually occurs at a different return CL. **E,** Pseudo–A-V response is observed during focal AT secondary to VA dissociation (i.e., absence of VA conduction) during ventricular pacing. CS_{dist} = distal coronary sinus; CS_{prox} = proximal coronary sinus; HRA = high right atrium; RVA = right ventricular apex.

Mapping

Activation Mapping

Activation mapping entails localizing the site of earliest presystolic activity to the onset of the P wave during AT. Endocardial activation mapping can trace the origin of activation to a specific area, from which it spreads to both atria. However, spread of activation from the focus or origin may not be uniformly radial; anatomical or functional pathways and barriers can influence conduction and force the tachycardia wavefront to travel away from the focal source into noncentrifugal patterns.

There is generally an electrically silent period in the atrial CL reflected by an isoelectric line between atrial deflections on the surface ECG. Intracardiac mapping typically shows significant portions of the tachycardia CL without recorded activity, even when recording from the entire RA, LA, or CS (see Fig. 11-2). However, in the presence of complex intraatrial conduction disturbances, intraatrial activation may extend over a large proportion of the tachycardia CL, and conduction spread may follow circular patterns suggestive of macroreentrant activation.[17,24,31,42]

As noted, the term localized reentry has been used to refer to reentry in which the circuit is localized to a small area and does not have a central obstacle. Thus, if activity accounting for more than 85% of the tachycardia CL is present in an area with a diameter of up to 3 cm, localized reentry is considered (Fig. 11-15).

Determining the onset of the tachycardia P wave is important in activation mapping, but it may be impossible if the preceding T wave or QRS is superimposed. Thus, the P wave during AT should be assessed using multiple surface ECG leads and choosing the one with the earliest P onset. To facilitate visualization of the P wave, a VES (or a train of ventricular pacing) is delivered to accelerate ventricular activation and repolarization and permit careful distinction of the P wave onset. After determining P wave onset, a surrogate marker that is easier to track during mapping, such as an HRA or CS electrogram indexed to P wave onset where it is clearly seen, may be used, rather than the P wave onset on the surface ECG (Fig. 11-16).

TABLE 11-3 Exclusion of Atrioventricular Nodal Reentrant Tachycardia

PARAMETER	FEATURES
Atrial activation sequence	• Eccentric atrial activation sequence generally excludes AVNRT (with the exception of left variant of AVNRT).
AV block	• Spontaneous or induced AV block with continuation of the tachycardia is uncommon in AVNRT.
Oscillations in SVT CL	• Spontaneous changes in PR and RP intervals with fixed A-A interval excludes AVNRT.
Overdrive ventricular pacing during SVT	• If overdrive pacing entrains the SVT with an atrial activation sequence different from that during the SVT, AVNRT is unlikely. • The presence of an A-A-V electrogram sequence following cessation of overdrive ventricular pacing practically excludes AVNRT.
Overdrive atrial pacing during SVT	• ΔAH ($AH_{pacing} - AH_{SVT}$) <20 msec excludes AVNRT. • If entrainment cannot be achieved or overdrive suppression is demonstrated, AVNRT is excluded.
Atrial pacing during NSR at the tachycardia CL	• ΔAH ($AH_{pacing} - AH_{SVT}$) <20 msec excludes AVNRT.

AH = atrial–His bundle interval; AV = atrioventricular; AVNRT = atrioventricular nodal reentrant tachycardia; CL = cycle length; NSR = normal sinus rhythm; SVT = supraventricular tachycardia.

A single roving catheter is used to find the site, with the earliest atrial electrogram using unipolar and bipolar recordings. Small movements of the catheter tip in the general target region are undertaken under the guidance of fluoroscopy until the site with the earliest possible atrial activation relative to the P wave is identified.[17,24,31,42] Activation times are generally measured from the onset or the first rapid deflection of the atrial bipolar electrogram to the onset of the P wave or (preferably) surrogate marker during AT. Using the onset of the local bipolar electrogram is preferable, because it is easier to determine reproducibly when measuring heavily fractionated, low-amplitude atrial electrograms. On the recording system display, placing the intracardiac channel with the earliest local activation timing adjacent to the mapping catheter channel allows the operator to recognize early activation times immediately at sites sequentially visited by the mapping catheter by visual inspection, rather than having to pause and manually measure local activation times. A triggered sweep mode (constant temporal alignment of the display to a reference electrogram) can also be useful for rapid visual assessment of relative timing of mapped sites. The distal pole of the mapping catheter should be the one used for mapping for the earliest atrial activation site because it is the pole through which RF energy is delivered.

Unipolar recordings from the distal ablation electrode are used to supplement conventional bipolar activation mapping. Unipolar signals can be filtered or unfiltered, but unfiltered signals offer more directional information. Unipolar recordings are helpful by showing negative (QS) patterns with sharp initial deflections at the location of the focus (see Fig. 11-11). Timing of the unipolar electrograms can help ensure that the tip electrode, which is the ablation electrode, is responsible for the early component of the bipolar electrograms. The site of origin of the AT is defined as the site with the earliest presystolic (i.e., preceding the onset of the P wave on the surface ECG) bipolar recording in which the distal tip shows the earliest intrinsic deflection and QS unipolar electrogram configuration (see Fig. 11-11).

Low-amplitude early signals followed by a sharper discrete signal may represent early components of a fragmented electrogram or far-field signal associated with a second discrete local signal.

TABLE 11-4 Exclusion of Orthodromic Atrioventricular Reentrant Tachycardia

PARAMETER	FEATURES
Atrial activation sequence	• Initial atrial activation site away from the AV groove excludes orthodromic AVRT.
VA interval	• VA interval <70 msec or V-high RA interval <95 msec during SVT excludes orthodromic AVRT.
AV block	• Spontaneous or induced AV block with continuation of the SVT excludes orthodromic AVRT.
Oscillations in SVT CL	• Spontaneous changes in PR and RP intervals with a fixed A-A interval excludes orthodromic AVRT.
VES delivered during the SVT	• With failure to reset (advance or delay) atrial activation with early VES on multiple occasions and at different VES coupling intervals, despite advancement of the local ventricular activation at all sites (including the site of the suspected BT) by >30 msec, orthodromic AVRT and presence of AV BT are excluded.
Overdrive ventricular pacing during SVT	• Ventriculoatrial dissociation during overdrive pacing excludes AVRT. • If overdrive pacing entrains the SVT with an atrial activation sequence different from that during the SVT, orthodromic AVRT is unlikely. • The presence of an A-A-V electrogram sequence following cessation of overdrive ventricular pacing practically excludes orthodromic AVRT. • Lack of VA linking (i.e., the VA interval following the last entrained QRS varies [>14 msec] depending on site, CL, or duration of pacing) argues against orthodromic AVRT.
Overdrive ventricular pacing during SVT	• If entrainment cannot be achieved or overdrive suppression is demonstrated, orthodromic AVRT is excluded. • If the VA interval of the return cycle after cessation of atrial pacing is variable, orthodromic AVRT is excluded.
Ventricular pacing during NSR at the tachycardia CL	• VA block during pacing excludes orthodromic AVRT.

AV = atrioventricular; AVRT = atrioventricular reentrant tachycardia; BT = bypass tract; CL = cycle length; NSR = normal sinus rhythm; RA = right atrium; SVT = supraventricular tachycardia; VA = ventriculoatrial; VES = ventricular extrastimulation.

This is most likely to happen in the superior posterior RA, where it can actually represent electrical activity generated from the right superior PV. In this situation, the unipolar electrogram demonstrates a sharp negative deflection timing with the later, high-frequency potential on the bipolar electrogram.

Transient catheter-induced interruption of AT by pressure of the catheter may suggest an appropriate site for ablation. This sign is more useful when it is a reproducible phenomenon. Often, however, the tachycardia terminates as the catheter is passing the area, and where the catheter comes to rest may not be the same site as where transient AT termination occurred.

Assessment of simultaneous RA and CS activation sequences by using a multipolar catheter (e.g., duodecapolar or Halo catheters) in the RA around the tricuspid annulus and a decapolar catheter in the CS can facilitate mapping of ATs. In addition to predicting the likely origin of AT, it may facilitate recognition of transformation of the index tachycardia to a different morphology induced by catheter manipulation or by pacing maneuvers. This can be especially important when mapping nonsustained AT or PACs.

TABLE 11-5 Exclusion of Macroreentrant Atrial Tachycardia

PARAMETER	FEATURES
ECG	• Focal AT usually has a clearly defined isoelectric baseline between P waves in all leads. • Macroreentrant AT usually lacks an isoelectric baseline between deflections.
Atrial activation sequence	• Focal AT is characterized by atrial activation starting rhythmically at a small area (focus), and intracardiac mapping shows significant portions of the CL without recorded atrial activity. • Macroreentrant AT endocardial recordings typically show activation spanning the whole tachycardia CL.
Programmed electrical stimulation	• Focal AT is defined on the basis of dissociation of almost the entire atria from the tachycardia with AES. • Macroreentrant AT circuit usually incorporates large portions of the RA or LA, which would be identified with resetting and entrainment mapping.
Tachycardia CL variability	• Variation in the AT CL of >15% favors focal AT.
Entrainment mapping	• Focal AT cannot be entrained, except for microreentrant AT; in this case, because the microreentrant circuit is very small, only orthodromic capture is usually observed. In addition, constant or progressive fusion, as demonstrated by intermediate P wave morphologies on the ECG, cannot be demonstrated. • Macroreentrant AT is defined by demonstration of concealed or manifest entrainment of the tachycardia with atrial pacing.
PPI variability	• PPI variability of >30 msec favors focal ATs. • PPI variability of <10 msec favors macroreentrant ATs.
Electroanatomical three-dimensional mapping	• Focal AT is suggested by electroanatomical maps demonstrating radial spreading of activation, from the earliest local activation site in all directions. • Macroreentrant AT is suggested by electroanatomical maps demonstrating continuous progression of colors around the RA with close proximity of earliest and latest local activation.
Response to adenosine	• Focal AT usually responds to adenosine by slowing or termination. • Macroreentrant AT usually is not influenced by adenosine and may actually accelerate (when the tachycardia CL is refractoriness-dependent) secondary to shortening of atrial refractoriness by adenosine.

AES = atrial extrastimulation; AT = atrial tachycardia; CL = cycle length; LA = left atrium; RA = right atrium.

Occasionally, multiple unstable focal ATs or PACs can be encountered during mapping. In this setting, the goal should be to focus mapping on the most frequently encountered AT or PAC. Ablation of the most frequent AT often results in organization of the atria and allows for mapping and ablation of other successive ATs. Importantly, care has to be taken to ensure that the correct AT is being mapped and to avoid incorrect sampling of activation times during beats originating from the different foci, which can result in erroneous and confusing activation maps. This can be facilitated by careful attention to changes in P wave morphology or shifting of atrial activation sequences (in the RA or CS) or CLs, or both, during the mapping procedure.[43]

Occasionally, several areas may show equivalently early activation, sometimes even with a central area of early local activation time surrounded with areas having later local activation times. This finding may indicate a deeper focus (e.g., in the crista terminalis) or multiple breakthrough sites from a single focus. This can obviously cause confusion during mapping and ablation attempts, with little apparent effect of ablation at a site with very good electrogram characteristics or successful ablation at a site with less optimal parameters.

Special attention should be given to ATs mapped to the midseptum and the right anteroseptal region. For ATs mapped to the midseptum, especially if presystolic activity is not particularly early (i.e., less than 30 milliseconds presystolic), the electrogram is not fractionated, and multiple sites have similar activation times, exclusion of LA ATs using transseptal access to the LA is important (Fig. 11-17). For ATs arising from the PVs, CS activation times may not clearly indicate an LA site of origin. For ATs mapped to the right anteroseptal region (HB region), great care must be given to the anteromedial LA septum, right superior PV, and LA free wall because sites in these regions break through early to the right anteroseptal region, where ablation not only is unsuccessful but also can result in AV block.

Endocardial atrial activation sequences from the RA, HB, and CS catheters can help predict the location of PAC or AT foci in the SVC versus the right superior PV before atrial transseptal puncture. In one report, the difference in *interatrial* conduction time (between the HRA and distal CS [CS_{dist}] recording electrodes) during NSR versus PAC ($[HRA - CS_{dist}]_{NSR\text{-}PAC}$) was significantly larger for right superior PV tachycardias compared with SVC tachycardias, and a cutoff value of 20 milliseconds or more of the interatrial conduction time $[HRA - CS_{dist}]_{NSR\text{-}PAC}$ was able to differentiate 100% between both locations. During SVC tachycardia, after exiting the SVC and entering the RA, the tachycardia wavefront activates the RA in a high-low sequence and at the same time propagates through the interatrial connection to the LA similar to the activation pathway in NSR. As a consequence, there is little change in the interatrial conduction time compared with that during NSR. Conversely, during right superior PV tachycardias, after leaving the vein and entering the LA, the tachycardia wavefront travels to the rest of the LA and simultaneously crosses the interatrial septum to activate the RA. Thus, the interatrial conduction time would be much shorter than that during NSR. As a consequence, the difference of interatrial conduction time $[HRA - CS_{dist}]_{NSR\text{-}PAC}$ between the two groups of tachycardias can be a useful prospective method to define the sources of tachycardia before atrial transseptal puncture.[44]

Similarly, analyzing *intraatrial* conduction times can facilitate the distinction between PACs or ATs originating from the SVC and high crista terminalis from PV foci. The time interval between HRA and HB atrial activation during PACs originating from the SVC and crista terminalis is significantly longer than that of the sinus beats. A difference in intraatrial conduction time ($[HRA - HB]_{NSR\text{-}PAC}$) of less than 0 milliseconds favors SVC or crista terminalis origin. The increased intraatrial conduction delay between HRA and HB recording electrodes is a physiological response to the PACs from the SVC and crista terminalis in the human atrium. In contrast, intraatrial conduction time between the HRA and HB electrodes is shortened in the setting of PV tachycardias because both locations are activated in parallel during PV tachycardias, but in sequence during NSR.[45]

Pace Mapping

When atrial activation originates from a point-like source, such as during focal AT or during pacing from an electrode catheter, the resultant P wave recorded on the surface ECG is determined by the sequence of atrial activation, which depends to a large extent on the initial site of myocardial depolarization. Additionally, analysis of specific P wave configurations in multiple leads allows estimation of the pacing site location to within several square centimeters. Therefore, comparing the paced P wave configuration with that of

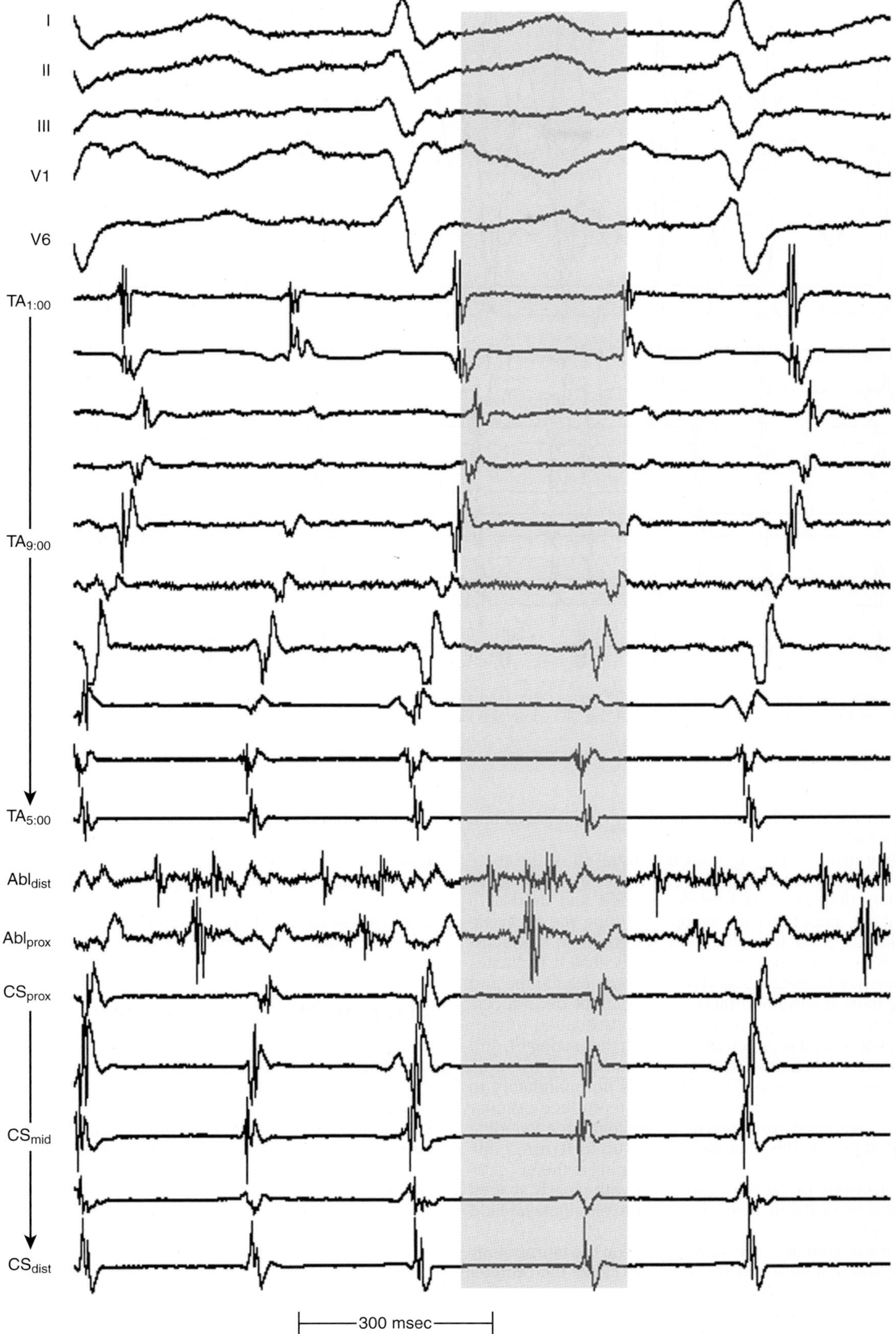

FIGURE 11-15 Localized atrial reentry. Atrial tachycardia had a pattern of activation consistent with emanation from a focus yet could be entrained from multiple sites without evidence of ECG or intracardiac fusion. Electrogram at ablation site is very prolonged and fractionated, occupying more than 80 milliseconds of tachycardia CL (shaded), consistent with microreentry or localized reentry. Abl_{dist} = distal ablation site; Abl_{prox} = proximal ablation site; CS_{dist} = distal coronary sinus; CS_{mid} = middle coronary sinus; CS_{prox} = proximal coronary sinus; TA = tricuspid annulus.

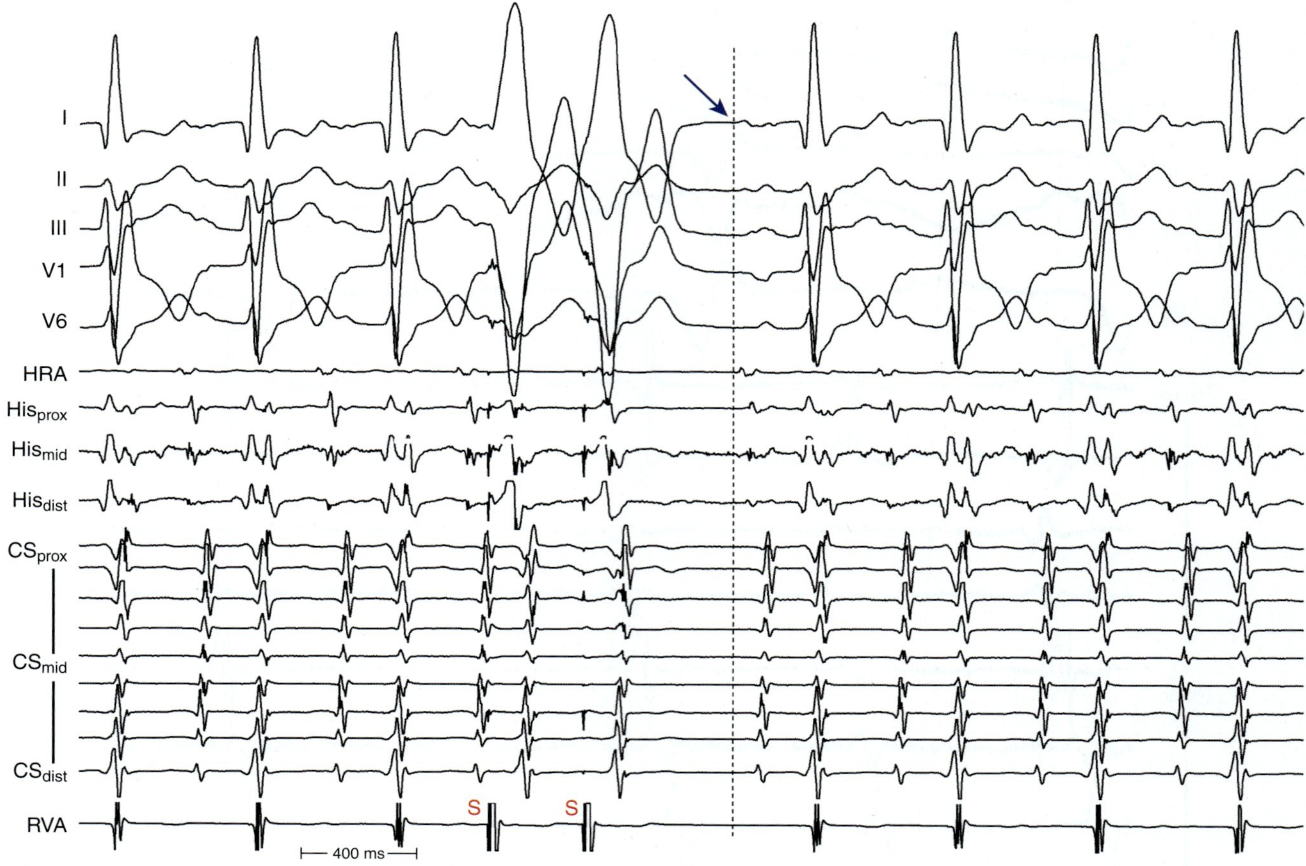

FIGURE 11-16 P wave onset during atrial tachycardia (AT) revealed by premature ventricular stimulation. During AT, P wave onset is difficult to discern (buried in T wave). Double ventricular extrastimuli (S) during AT pull the QRS complexes earlier and allow the P wave to be seen clearly (dark arrow, dashed line). Thereafter, a stable atrial electrogram (e.g., high right atrium [HRA] or proximal coronary sinus [CS_{prox}]) can be used as a surrogate marker for the P wave onset during mapping. CS_{dist} = distal coronary sinus; His_{dist} = distal His bundle; His_{mid} = middle His bundle; His_{prox} = proximal His bundle; HRA = high right atrium; RVA = right ventricular apex.

AT is particularly useful for locating a small arrhythmia focus in a structurally normal heart.[5,17,24]

Pace mapping involves pacing from the distal tip of the mapping catheter at sites of interest. Initially, the exact morphology of the tachycardia complex should be determined and used as a template for pace mapping. Pace mapping during the tachycardia (at a pacing CL 20 to 40 milliseconds shorter than the tachycardia CL) is preferable whenever possible because it facilitates rapid comparison of tachycardia and paced complexes at the end of the pacing train. If sustained tachycardia cannot be induced, mapping is performed during spontaneous nonsustained runs or ectopic beats. Although it is preferable to match the pacing CL and coupling intervals of AESs to those of spontaneous tachycardia or PACs, some reports have suggested that it is not mandatory to stimulate exactly at the same tachycardia CL to reproduce a similar atrial activation sequence and P wave morphology. Pace mapping is preferably performed with unipolar stimuli (up to 10 mA, 2 milliseconds) from the distal electrode of the mapping catheter (cathode) and an electrode in the IVC (anode), or with closely spaced bipolar pacing at twice the diastolic threshold, to eliminate far-field stimulation effects.[17]

The greater the degree of concordance between the morphology during pacing and that during tachycardia, the closer the catheter will be to the site of origin of the tachycardia. Pace maps with identical or nearly identical matches of the tachycardia morphology in all 12 surface ECG leads and intracardiac atrial electrograms can be indicative of the site of origin of the tachycardia (Fig. 11-18).

Pace mapping is used as an adjunct to other methods of mapping to corroborate putative ablation sites. It can be of great help, especially when the AT is difficult to induce. Although there are some limitations to this technique, many studies have demonstrated efficacy using pace mapping to choose ablation target sites; concordance of P wave morphology during pace mapping and AT has a sensitivity of 86% and a specificity of 37%. However, difficulties in precisely comparing P wave morphologies and intracardiac activation sequences limit the applicability of pace mapping. Moreover, the spatial resolution of atrial pace mapping is up to 2 cm, which is too imprecise.

Mapping Post-Pacing Intervals

Following overdrive atrial pacing from a given site during a relatively regular and stable focal AT, the PPI represents the sum of the conduction time to reach the perifocal tissue, the time required to penetrate the perifocal tissue and reset the focus, the tachycardia CL, and the conduction back to the pacing site. Consequently, if the pacing site is directly at the AT focus, the PPI should be equivalent to the AT CL as a result of the minimal perifocal conduction time between the pacing site and the AT focus. Conversely, pacing at sites distant from the AT focus results in a PPI that is greater than the AT CL as a result of conduction delay between the pacing site and the focus. In fact, the difference between the PPI and tachycardia CL ([PPI – AT CL] difference) after atrial overdrive pacing of a focal AT was found to have a direct relationship with proximity to the focus, regardless of whether or not the tachycardia was actually entrained. The [PPI – AT CL] difference approaches zero (and is no more than 20 milliseconds) when pacing directly at the focus of the tachycardia. There appears to be no significant overdrive suppression or acceleration of the AT when pacing at a rate just faster than the AT rate, regardless of the underlying AT mechanism.

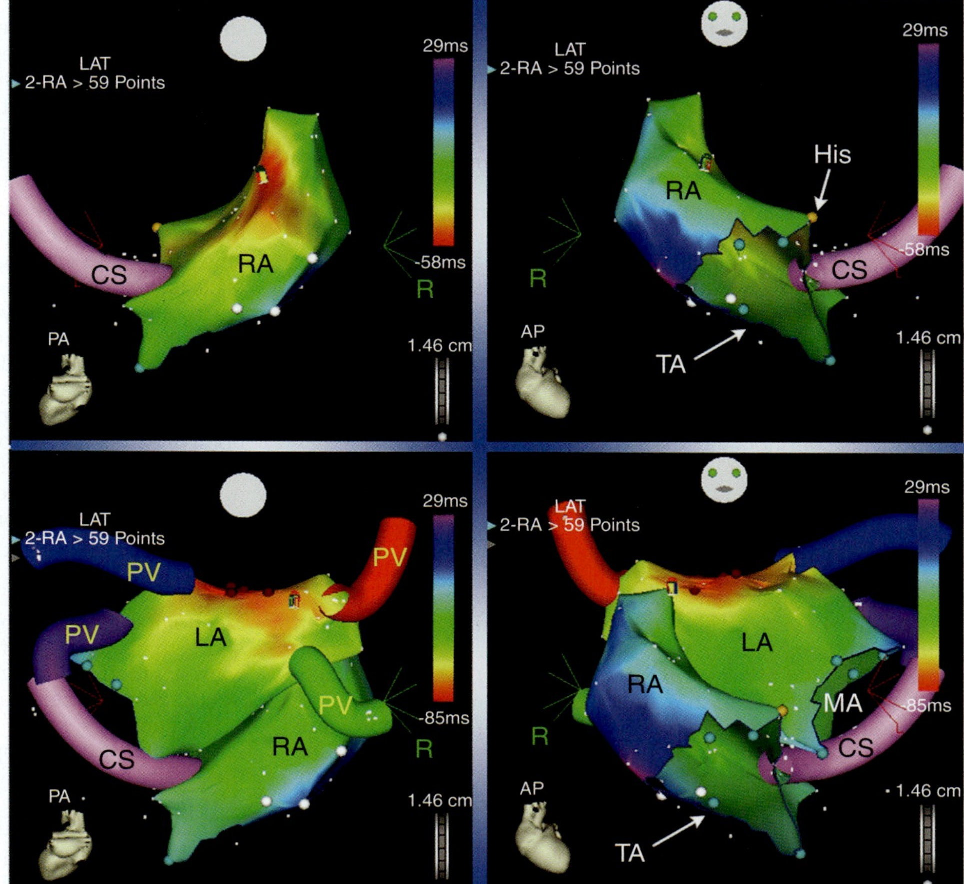

FIGURE 11-17 Three-dimensional electroanatomical (CARTO, Biosense Webster, Diamond Bar, Calif.) activation map of focal atrial tachycardia (AT) originating from the left atrial (LA) roof. **Upper panels,** Posteroanterior (PA) and anteroposterior (AP) projections of the CARTO activation map of the right atrium (RA). **Lower panels,** PA and AP projections of the CARTO activation map of both the RA and left atrium (LA). When mapping is limited to the RA **(upper panels),** the site of earliest atrial activation was localized to the interatrial septum, with local activation preceding the reference electrogram by 58 milliseconds. When activation mapping is extended to the LA **(lower panels),** a site with earlier local activation (preceding the reference electrogram by 85 milliseconds) was localized to the LA roof. Radiofrequency ablation (red dots) at that site eliminated the tachycardia. LAT = local activation time; MA = mitral annulus; PV = pulmonary vein; TA = tricuspid annulus.

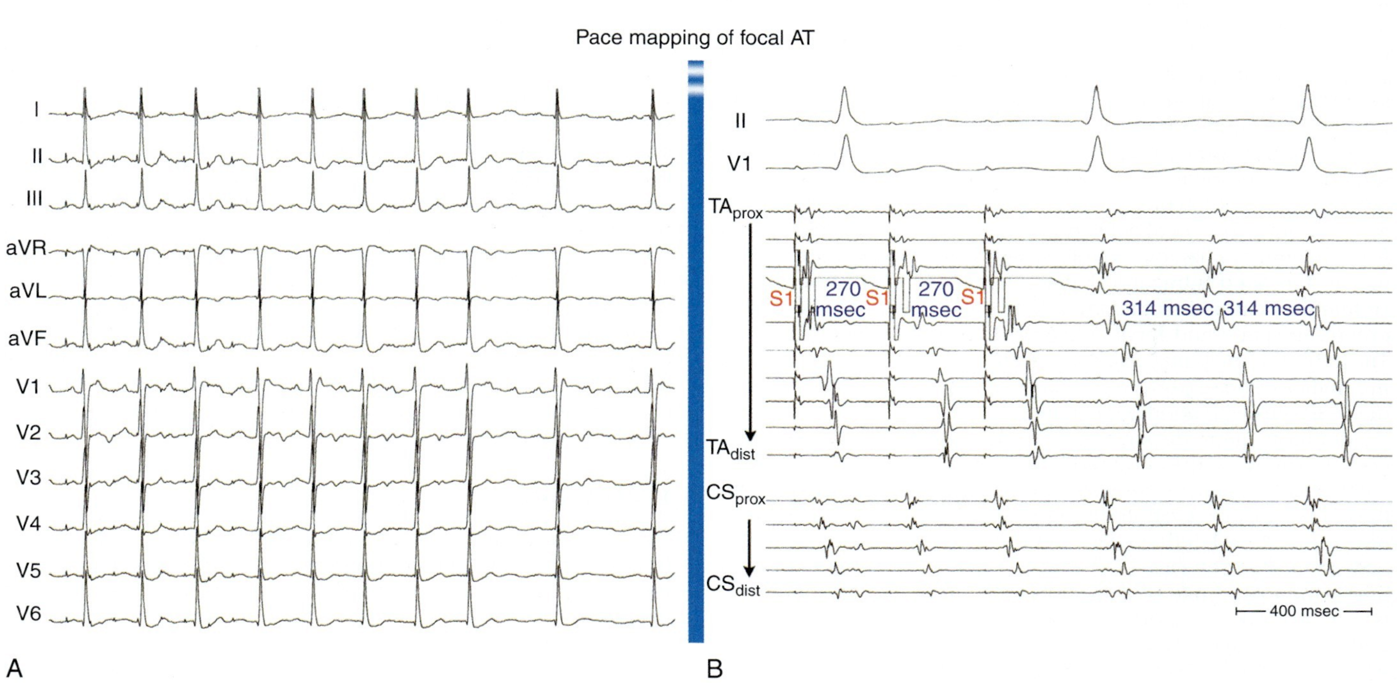

FIGURE 11-18 Surface ECG (**A**) and intracardiac recordings (**B**) demonstrating pace mapping performed during sustained focal atrial tachycardia (AT) originating from the interatrial septum. Atrial pacing (left aspect of the ECG and intracardiac recordings) is performed during the tachycardia at a cycle length (CL) of 270 milliseconds from the site of earliest activation (recorded by the Halo catheter positioned around the tricuspid annulus [TA]). Concordance between paced (at the left aspect of the ECG and intracardiac recordings) and tachycardia (at the right aspect of the ECG and intracardiac recordings) P wave morphology on the surface ECG **(A)**, as well as an endocardial atrial activation sequence **(right panel)**, suggests proximity of the pacing site to the AT focus. CS_{dist} = distal coronary sinus; CS_{prox} = proximal coronary sinus.

Therefore, the [PPI – AT CL] difference can be a useful adjunct to localize the AT focus and guide successful ablation sites.[46]

Additionally, the [PPI – AT CL] difference can be valuable in distinguishing AT in close proximity to the sinus node from sinus tachycardia. It appears that AT foci, unlike the sinus node, have a very short perifocal conduction time, a finding suggesting that there was little "perifocal tissue" as compared with the sinus node. As a consequence, the [PPI – AT CL] difference in the setting of focal AT is determined predominantly by the distance from the focus with minimal contribution of the time required to traverse any perifocal tissue, thus explaining the finding that the [PPI – AT CL] difference approaches zero when pacing is performed directly at the AT focus. In contrast, overdrive pacing during sinus tachycardia is associated with a PPI that always exceeds (by more than 80 milliseconds) the sinus CL, even when pacing is performed directly at the origin of the sinus impulse. This finding suggests significant perinodal conduction delay. The [PPI – AT CL] difference can therefore be used to distinguish perinodal focal AT from sinus tachycardia.[46]

Electroanatomical Mapping

MAPPING TECHNIQUE

Electromagnetic three-dimensional (3-D) mapping (CARTO mapping system [Biosense Webster, Diamond Bar, Calif.] or EnSite NavX system [St. Jude Medical, St. Paul, Minn.] uses a single mapping catheter attached to a system that can precisely localize the catheter tip in 3-D space and store activation time on a 3-D anatomical reconstruction.[5,47] Initially, selection of the reference electrogram, positioning of the anatomical reference, and determination of the window of interest are undertaken. The reference catheter is usually placed in the CS (because of its stability) by using an electrode recording a prominent atrial electrogram and ensuring that the ventricular electrogram is not the one picked up by the system.

A 4-mm-tip mapping-ablation catheter is initially positioned, using fluoroscopy, at known anatomical points that serve as landmarks for the electroanatomical map. Anatomical and EP landmarks (IVC, SVC, CS, HB, and tricuspid annulus for RA mapping and the mitral annulus and PVs for LA mapping) are tagged. The catheter is then advanced slowly around the chamber walls to sample multiple points along the endocardium, thus sequentially acquiring the location of its tip together with the local electrogram (see Fig. 11-17 and Video 10).

Activation mapping is performed to define the atrial activation sequence. A reasonable number of points homogeneously distributed in the RA or LA, or both, must be recorded (approximately 80 to 100 points). The local activation time at each site is determined from the intracardiac bipolar electrogram and is measured in relation to the fixed intracardiac electrogram obtained from the CS (reference) catheter. Points are added to the map only if stability criteria in space and local activation time requirements are met. The activation map may also be used to catalog sites at which pacing maneuvers are performed during assessment of the tachycardia (e.g., sites with good pace maps).

Activation maps display the local activation time by a color-coded overlay on the acquired 3-D geometry. The electroanatomical maps of focal ATs demonstrate radial spread of activation, from the earliest local activation site (red in CARTO, white in NavX) in all directions (a well-defined early activation site surrounded by later activation sites; see Figs. 11-17 and 6-16). In these cases, activation time—the total range of activation times, from earliest to latest—is usually markedly shorter than the tachycardia CL. Conversely, a continuous progression of colors (from red to purple in CARTO, white to purple in NavX), with close proximity of earliest and latest local activation, suggests the presence of a macroreentrant tachycardia. In these cases, total activation time is in a similar range to tachycardia CL (see Fig. 12-10).

A stepwise strategy for mapping of RA and LA focal tachycardias was described in a study using CARTO to avoid time-consuming whole-chamber maps.[47] Using this approach, mapping is started with the acquisition of four or five anatomically defined sites at the superior and septal aspects of the tricuspid annulus, and the mapping procedure is strategically continued according to this initial activation sequence. If the initial four-point activation map shows the earliest atrial activation to be at the superior aspect of the tricuspid annulus, mapping is continued toward the free wall of the RA, including the crista terminalis. When the earliest atrial activation within the four-point area is found at the septal aspect of the tricuspid annulus, the map is expanded to the triangle of Koch and the paraseptal space. This strategy was found to differentiate reliably between ATs arising from the free wall of the RA, including the crista terminalis and RA appendage, from those arising from the triangle of Koch and paraseptal space, as well as from left-sided ATs. Once the general area of interest is identified, high-density mapping of this area is undertaken, together with conventional electrographic analysis (see earlier), to identify the site of the earliest activation within this target area. If the unipolar electrogram at the point of earliest activation at the RA septum or at the high posterior wall still shows a significant R wave, or if RF ablation at that site is unsuccessful, a left-sided AT origin is assumed, and the procedure is extended to the LA for dual-chamber maps.

ADVANTAGES

Electroanatomical mapping systems provide a highly accurate geometric rendering of the cardiac chamber with a straightforward geometric display that has the capability to determine the 3-D location and orientation of the ablation catheter accurately.

The capability of the mapping system to associate relevant EP information with the appropriate spatial location in the heart and the ability to study activation patterns (with high spatial resolution [less than 1 mm]) during tachycardia in relation to normal anatomical structures and areas of scar significantly facilitate the mapping and ablation procedure. It can suggest the mechanisms underlying the arrhythmia (distinguishing between a focal origin and macroreentrant tachycardia) and allows rapid visualization of the activation wavefront (propagation maps; Fig. 11-19), thus facilitating the identification of appropriate sites for entrainment mapping and pace mapping.

Both electroanatomical mapping systems (CARTO and NavX) provide the capability to create and tag several potential points of interest during the mapping process (e.g., double potentials and sites with good pace maps) and return to them with great precision. These features provide significant advantages over conventional techniques. The catheter can anatomically and accurately revisit a critically important recording site identified previously during the study, even if the tachycardia is no longer present or inducible and map-guided catheter navigation is no longer possible. This accurate repositioning can allow pace mapping from, or further application of, RF energy current to critically important sites that otherwise cannot be performed with a high degree of accuracy and reproducibility. Additionally, fluoroscopy time can be reduced via electromagnetic catheter navigation, and the catheter can be accurately guided to positions removed from fluoroscopic markers (see Fig. 11-17).

LIMITATIONS

The sequential data acquisition required for creation of the electroanatomical map remains time-consuming, because the process requires tagging many points, depending on the spatial details needed to analyze a given arrhythmia. Furthermore, because the acquired data are not coherent in time, multiple beats are required, and stable, sustained, or frequently repetitive arrhythmia is usually needed for creation of the activation map. Single PACs or nonsustained AT can be mapped, although at the expense of an appreciable amount of time. Unlike with the CARTO system, activation times can be acquired simultaneously by the EnSite NavX system from multiple poles on all catheters used during the study (and not just the mapping-ablation catheter).

One difficulty with current methods is that incorrect assignment of activation for a small number of electrograms can invalidate the entire activation map; manual adjustment is often required to achieve the optimal representation. Additionally, data interpolation between mapped points is used to improve the quality of the display; however, areas of unmapped myocardium are then assigned simple estimates of timing and voltage information that may not be accurate.

Additionally, the patient or intracardiac reference catheter may move, thus necessitating remapping. Although a shadow (to record original position) can be placed over this catheter to recognize displacement during the procedure, in which case the catheter can be returned to its original location, this may not always be feasible or accurate. Another limitation specific to the CARTO system is the requirement of a proprietary mapping catheter; no other catheter types can be used with this system. In contrast, the EnSite NavX system can work with most manufacturers' ablation catheters and RF or cryogenerators.

Mapping Nonsustained Focal Atrial Tachycardia

Several alternative mapping modalities can be used when AT is short-lived or cannot be reproducibly initiated, including simultaneous multisite data acquisition systems (noncontact mapping system, basket catheter, or localized high-density mapping). Moreover, the electroanatomical mapping and pace mapping techniques discussed can be used in these situations.

ENSITE NONCONTACT MAPPING SYSTEM

The EnSite 3000 noncontact mapping system (St. Jude Medical, St. Paul, Minn.) consists of a noncontact catheter with a multielectrode array surrounding a 7.5-mL balloon mounted at the distal end. Raw data detected by the multielectrode are transferred to a silicon graphics workstation via a digitalized amplifier system. The multielectrode array is used to construct a 3-D computer model of the virtual endocardium. The system is able to reconstruct more than 3000 unipolar electrograms simultaneously and superimpose them onto the virtual endocardium, thus producing isopotential maps with a color range representing voltage amplitude. Electrical potentials at the endocardial surface some distance away are calculated. Sites of early endocardial activity, which are likely adjacent to the origin of the AT, are usually identifiable. Noncontact mapping can rapidly identify AT foci and thus delineate starting points for conventional mapping.[48,49]

The main advantage of noncontact endocardial mapping is its ability to recreate the endocardial activation sequence from simultaneously acquired multiple data points over a few (theoretically one) tachycardia beats, without requiring sequential point-to-point acquisitions. Therefore, it can be of great value in mapping nonsustained arrhythmias, PACs, irregular ATs, and rhythms that are not hemodynamically stable.[48,49]

TECHNIQUE. The EnSite 3000 system requires placing a 9 Fr multielectrode array and a 7 Fr conventional (roving) deflectable mapping-ablation catheter in the cardiac chamber of interest. The balloon catheter is advanced over a 0.035-inch guidewire under fluoroscopy guidance and positioned in the atrium and deployed. The balloon is positioned in the center of the atrium and does not come in contact with the atrial walls being mapped. Activated clotting time is kept at 250 to 300 seconds for right-sided and 300 to 400 seconds for left-sided mapping.

The mapping-ablation catheter is positioned in the atrium and used to collect geometry information. The mapping catheter is initially moved to known anatomical locations (IVC, SVC, CS, HB, and tricuspid annulus for RA mapping and mitral annulus and PVs for LA mapping), which are tagged. A detailed geometry of the chamber is then reconstructed by moving the mapping catheter around the atrium. Using this information, the computer creates a model of the atrium.

After the chamber geometry is determined, mapping of the arrhythmia can begin. The data acquisition process is performed automatically by the system, and all data for the entire chamber are acquired simultaneously. The system then reconstructs unipolar electrograms simultaneously and superimposes them onto the virtual endocardium, thus producing isopotential maps with a color range representing voltage amplitude. A default high-pass filter setting of 2 Hz is used to preserve components of slow conduction on the isopotential map. Color settings are adjusted so that

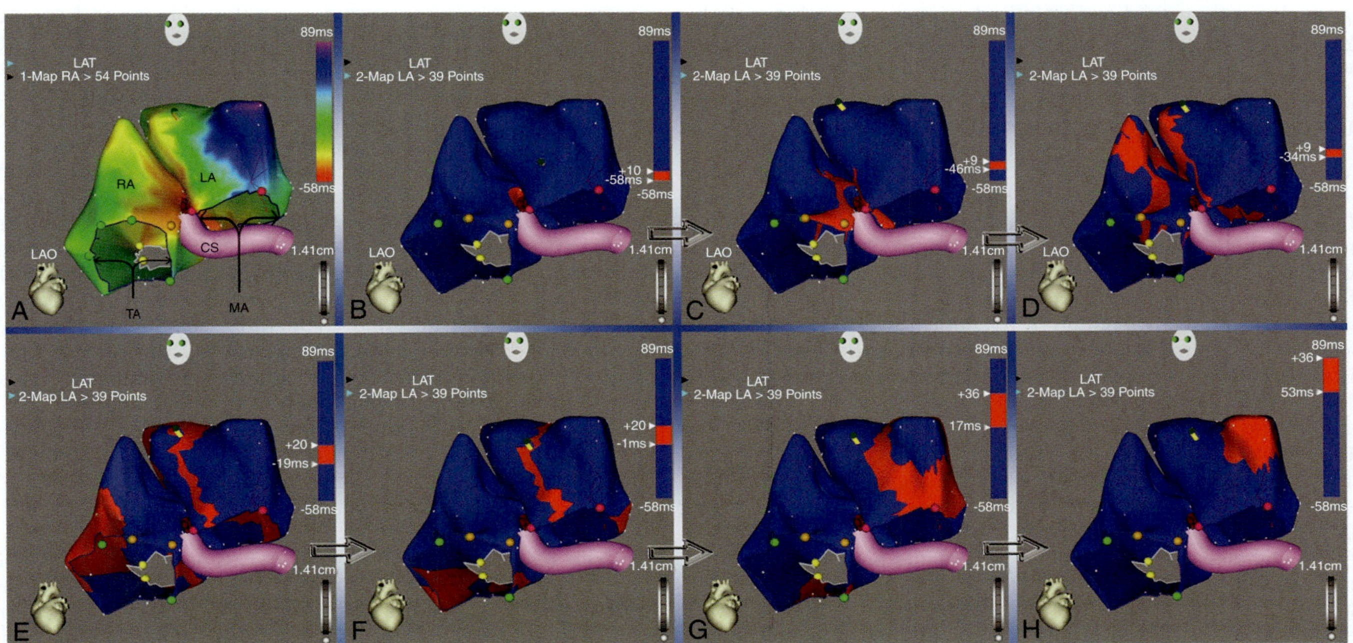

FIGURE 11-19 A, Three-dimensional electroanatomical (CARTO, Biosense Webster, Diamond Bar, Calif.) biatrial activation map in the left anterior oblique (LAO) view constructed during focal atrial tachycardia (AT) originating posterosuperior to the coronary sinus (CS) ostium. During tachycardia, the activation wavefront propagates from the earliest local activation site (red) in all directions. **B** to **H**, Biatrial propagation map during the focal AT. LAT = local activation time; MA = mitral annulus; TA = tricuspid annulus.

the color range matches 1 to 1 with the millivolt range of the electrogram deflection of interest. The color scale for each isopotential map is set so that white indicates most negative potential and blue indicates least negative potential. Activation can be tracked on the isopotential map throughout the cycle to the onset of the tachycardia beat. Virtual electrograms are then reconstructed at sites of earliest activation on the isopotential maps to look for a unipolar QS pattern. If the atrial electrograms overlap with the T wave, a VES may be delivered to accelerate ventricular depolarization and repolarization and may reveal the following atrial complex without far-field interference.

Isochronal maps can also be created. These maps represent progression of activation throughout the chamber relative to a user-defined electrical reference timing point. Contact mapping using the conventional ablation catheter may also be performed at sites of interest to supplement noncontact mapping findings, and color-coded contact activation maps can be displayed on the same 3-D geometry. Once earliest activation is identified, the site is labeled on the 3-D map, and the locator signal is used to navigate the ablation catheter to it in real time during tachycardia or during normal rhythm when sustained tachycardia is not inducible.[49]

The origin of AT is defined as the earliest site showing a single spot on the isopotential map and a QS pattern on the noncontact unipolar electrogram. Early sites with an rS pattern can represent foci that are epicardial in origin or early activation sites in an adjacent structure. The earliest site that shows an rS pattern with a sudden increase of peak negative potential on the noncontact unipolar electrogram after the AT depolarizes is considered to represent the "break-out point" or "exit" from the tachycardia focus, and the path between the origin and the break-out point likely represents the preferential pathway of conduction from the origin of the AT. As such, the traditionally defined origin of focal AT (by contact mapping techniques), whereby centrifugal activation occurs, potentially represents the break-out point, rather than the real origin of the tachycardia. Ablation at the origin of tachycardia or along the proximal path to the break-out point typically eliminates the arrhythmia.[49]

LIMITATIONS. Very-low-amplitude signals may not be detected, particularly if the distance between the center of the balloon catheter and the endocardial surface exceeds 40 mm, thus limiting the accurate identification of diastolic signals. Furthermore, a second catheter is still required for additional mapping and for ablation. Aggressive anticoagulation is required using this mapping modality, and special attention and care are necessary during placement of the large balloon electrode in a nondilated atrium.

MULTIELECTRODE BASKET CATHETER MAPPING

The basket catheter consists of an open-lumen catheter shaft with a collapsible, basket-shaped, distal end. The catheter is composed of 64 electrodes mounted on 8 flexible, self-expanding, equidistant metallic splines (each spline carrying 8 ring electrodes). The electrodes are equally spaced 4 or 5 mm apart, depending on the size of the basket catheter used (with diameters of 48 or 60 mm, respectively). Each spline is identified by a letter (from A to H) and each electrode by a number (from 1 to 8, with electrode 1 having the distal position on the splines). The basket catheter is constructed of a superelastic material to allow passive deployment of the array catheter and optimization of endocardial contact.

TECHNIQUE. The size of the atrium is initially evaluated (usually with echocardiography) to help select the appropriate size of the basket catheter. The collapsed basket catheter is advanced under fluoroscopy guidance through an 11 Fr long sheath into the RA or LA; the catheter is then expanded (Fig. 11-20). Electroanatomical relations are determined by fluoroscopically identifiable markers (spline A has one marker and spline B has two markers located near the shaft of the basket catheter). Additionally, the electrical signals recorded from certain electrodes (e.g., annular or HB electrograms) can help identify the location of those particular splines.

From the 64 electrodes, 64 unipolar signals and 32 to 56 bipolar signals can be recorded (by combining 1-2, 3-4, 5-6, 7-8 or 1-2, 2-3 until 7-8 electrodes are on each spline). Color-coded activation maps are reconstructed. The concepts of activation mapping discussed earlier are then used to determine the site of origin of the tachycardia. The capacity of pacing from the majority of basket electrodes allows the evaluation of activation patterns, pace mapping, and entrainment mapping. The electrograms recorded from the basket catheter can be used to monitor changes in the activation sequence in real time and thereby indicate the effects of ablation as lesions are created.

After basket catheter deployment, the conventional catheters are introduced and placed in standard positions. The ablation catheter is placed in the region of earliest activity and is used for more detailed mapping of the site of origin of the AT (see Fig. 11-20). The Astronomer (Boston Scientific, Natick, Mass.) navigation system permits precise and reproducible guidance of the ablation catheter tip electrode to targets identified by the basket catheter.

LIMITATIONS. The electrode array does not expand to provide adequate contact with the entire atrium. In addition, the system does not permit immediate correlation of activation times to precise anatomical sites. Furthermore, a second catheter is still required for additional mapping and for ablation.

LOCALIZED HIGH-DENSITY MAPPING CATHETER

The PentaRay (Biosense Webster, Diamond Bar, Calif.) is a high-density, multielectrode mapping catheter that may be used for mapping of focal AT. This 7 Fr steerable catheter (180 degrees of unidirectional flexion) has 20 electrodes distributed over 5 soft radiating spines (1-mm electrodes separated by 4-4-4 or 2-6-2 mm interelectrode spacing), allowing splaying of the catheter to cover a surface diameter of 3.5 cm. The spines have alphabetical nomenclature (A to E), with spines A and B recognized by radiopaque markers (see Fig. 6-3).[50]

Localization of the atrial focus can be performed during tachycardia or atrial ectopy. Guided by the ECG appearance and previous mapping information, the catheter is sequentially applied to the endocardial surface in various atrial regions to allow rapid activation mapping. Mapping is performed to identify the earliest endocardial activity relative to the P wave or to a fixed catheter positioned within the CS, or both. By identifying the earliest site of activation around the circumference of the high-density catheter, vector mapping is performed, moving the catheter and applying it to the endocardium in the direction of earliest activation (outer bipoles) to identify the tachycardia origin and bracket activation (i.e., demonstrating later activation in all surrounding regions). Ablation is performed at the site of earliest endocardial activation relative to the P wave when tachycardia is bracketed.

The high-density mapping catheter may offer several potential advantages. Whereas basket catheter mapping has the ability to perform rapid simultaneous contact mapping of the chamber and provides a global density of mapping, its localized resolution is limited. In contrast, this newer mapping modality allows splaying of the spines against the endocardial surface to achieve high-density contact mapping to localize and characterize the origin of focal ATs accurately. Additionally, the ability to position multiple electrodes in a circumscribed part of the endocardium is particularly advantageous for use within the LA and for mapping complex focal AT.

Ablation

Target of Ablation

The site of origin (or focus) of focal AT is the target of ablation.[31,42] Bipolar electrograms at the site of successful ablation are typically fractionated and demonstrate moderate to marked presystolic timing. Average presystolic intervals at sites of successful ablation are generally longer than 30 milliseconds (but not mid-diastolic, as in the case of macroreentrant AT). However, the key to successful mapping is finding the earliest site, because there is great variability in the presystolic interval that will be obtained at successful ablation sites (10 to 80 milliseconds). QS unipolar electrogram morphology is highly predictive of the successful ablation site and supplements findings of bipolar mapping. Timings of the earliest bipolar and unipolar electrogram should be in agreement (see Fig. 11-11).

Focal ATs arising from the PVs can be targeted by either focal ablation or electrical isolation of the culprit PV. The latter approach can potentially limit the risk of PV stenosis, especially when targeting more distal foci within the PV.[21,22]

Ablation Technique

RF power delivery should be adjusted to achieve a tip temperature of 55° to 65°C.[31,42] The response of the AT focus to a successful RF application should be rapid, typically within a few seconds of RF energy delivery. The most common response to successful ablations is abrupt termination. However, in some patients, transient acceleration precedes termination; in others, gradual slowing precedes termination (Fig. 11-21). If the tachycardia is not affected within 10 to 20 seconds, RF energy application is terminated, and the catheter is repositioned slightly for a repeat attempt. Prolonged RF applications beyond 10 to 20 seconds without accompanying changes in AT rate are usually nonproductive.

Extensive ablation in one area that does not terminate AT may cause enough damage to block the spread of activation partially in the region, thus causing a change in P wave morphology (although the actual focus may not have changed), as well as slow propagation of the tachycardia impulse away from the focus of the tachycardia to activate atrial myocardium. The latter effect can result in an increase in the interval between the presystolic electrogram at the focus and P wave onset (Fig. 11-22).

If the AT terminates or changes rate noticeably during the 10-second application, the RF application is continued for 30 to 60 seconds. However, in some patients, applications that may be just slightly off target can cause acceleration of the AT without terminating it. In these cases, the tachycardia rate usually remains accelerated as long as the RF application is in progress, and it returns immediately to the baseline rate when the RF delivery is discontinued. If adequate catheter tip temperature is achieved and good contact is ensured (which can be assessed by observing ST elevation on the unipolar recording), this probably suggests that the catheter is close to, but not exactly at, the proper target area. Continued RF application at a site that produces only acceleration (but not termination) after 15 seconds invites the possibility of transient injury to the AT focus that impedes further ablation and can result in later AT recurrence.

Ablation of focal ATs near the AVN or HB (in the triangle of Koch) requires special precautions. Titrated RF energy output should be used, starting with 5 W and increasing by 5 W every 10 seconds of energy application, up to a maximum of 40 W. Additionally, it is preferable to deliver RF energy during AT; if AT terminates during RF delivery, the RF application is continued at the same power output

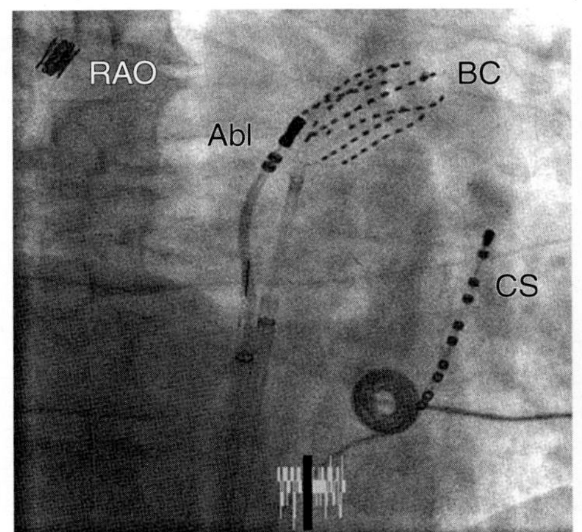

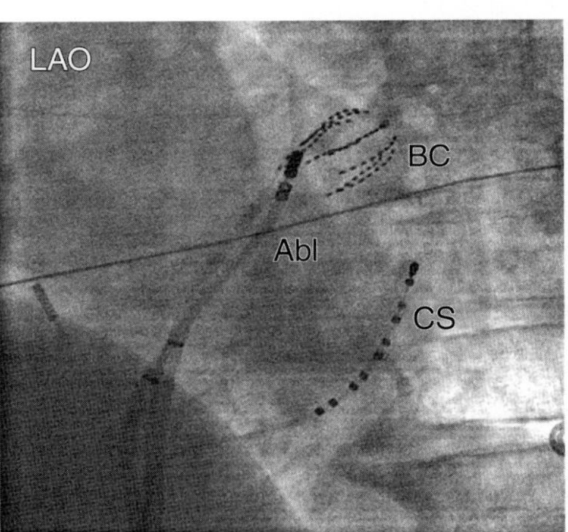

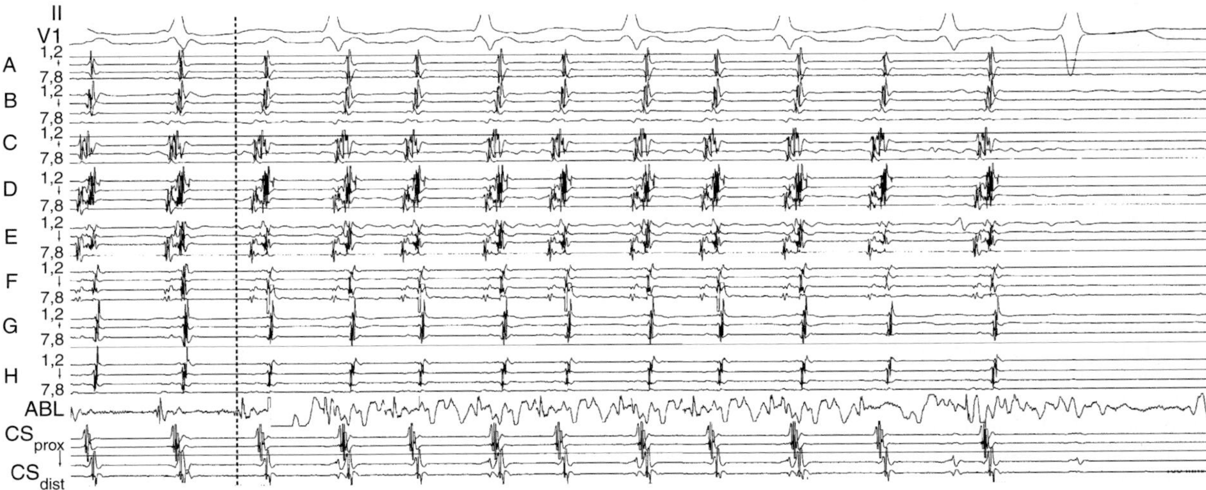

FIGURE 11-20 Basket catheter (BC) mapping of atrial tachycardia (AT). **Upper panels,** Fluoroscopic views (right anterior oblique [RAO], 30 degrees; left anterior oblique [LAO], 60 degrees) of the BC positioned at the ostium of the left superior pulmonary vein (PV). **Lower panel,** BC bipolar electrograms (1-2, 3-4, 5-6, 7-8) from the eight splines (A to H) are displayed. The earliest atrial activation during AT is recorded by the proximal electrodes of the E spline of the basket catheter. Detailed mapping obtained by the ablation catheter (Abl) recorded an even earlier activation (dashed line) at a site in the left atrial roof just outside the PV ostium. Radiofrequency energy delivery at that site resulted in termination of the tachycardia within a few seconds. CS_{dist} = distal coronary sinus; CS_{prox} = proximal coronary sinus.

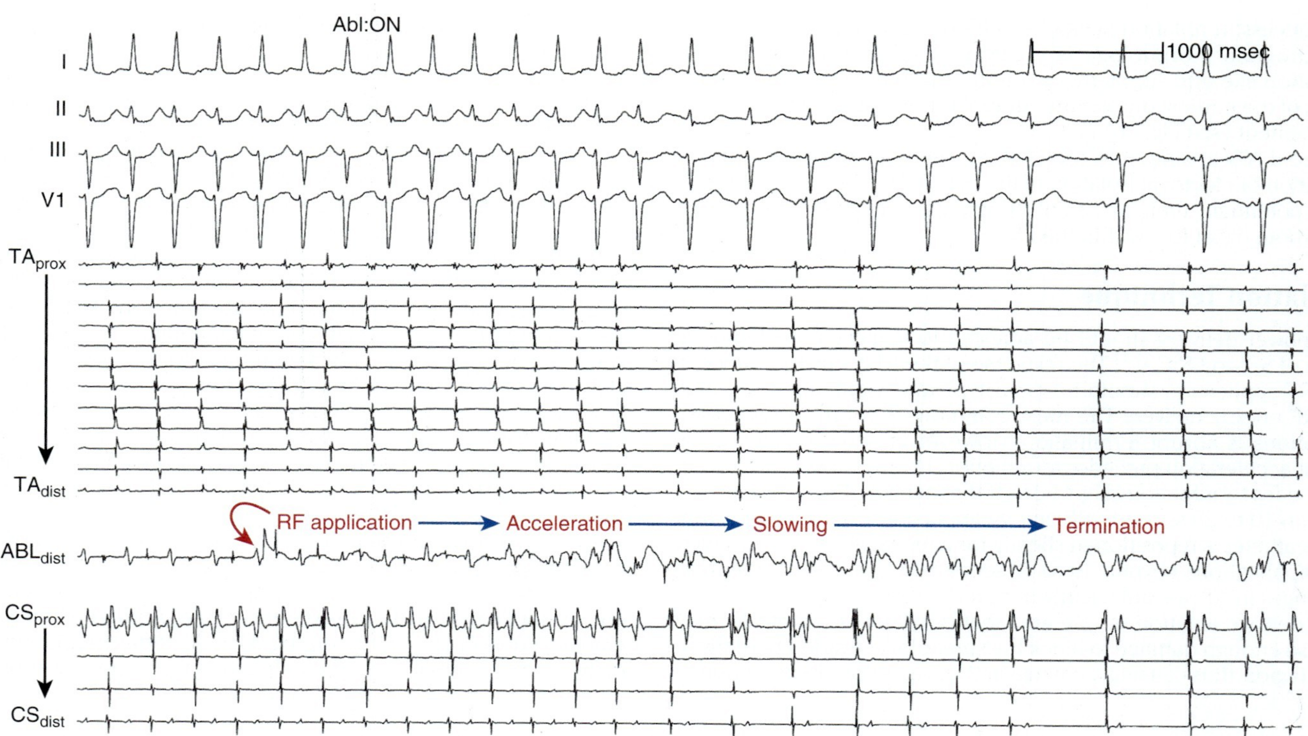

FIGURE 11-21 Catheter ablation of focal atrial tachycardia (AT) originating from the superoanterior aspect of the mitral annulus. Four surface ECG leads and intracardiac recordings from a catheter in the coronary sinus (CS) and a 20-pole Halo catheter positioned around the tricuspid annulus (TA) are shown. Radiofrequency (RF) energy delivery at the successful ablation site resulted within a few seconds in acceleration then slowing of the tachycardia rate followed by termination of the AT and restoration of sinus rhythm. ABL$_{dist}$ = distal ablation site; dist = distal; prox = proximal.

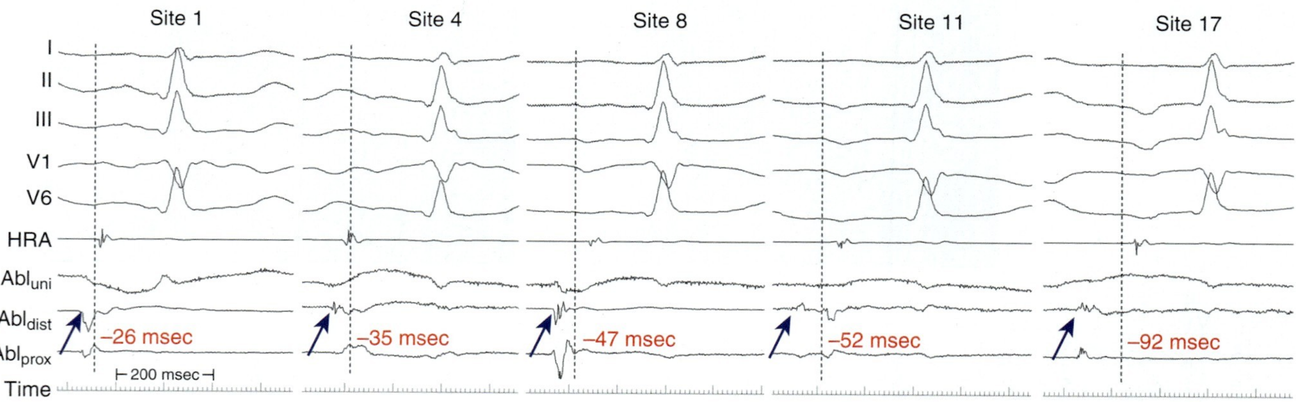

FIGURE 11-22 Recordings from focal right atrial (RA) tachycardia during progressive ablation. Examples are shown from selected ablation sites. Site 2 shows tachycardia from high RA with a site 26 milliseconds prior to the P wave onset. Ablation here changed the P wave morphology as shown in subsequent examples, and progressive ablation at sites in the lateral RA resulted in lengthening of the interval from electrogram to P wave onset (up to 92 milliseconds). Note also progressive fragmentation of the bipolar ablation recording and degradation of the unipolar recording. Abl$_{dist}$ = distal ablation site; Abl$_{prox}$ = proximal ablation site; Abl$_{uni}$ = unipolar ablation site; HRA = high right atrium.

for 30 seconds and then repeated for 30 seconds or more. If the AT does not terminate with an RF output of 40 W for 30 seconds, then another site should be sought. If accelerated junctional rhythm develops after AT termination, overdrive atrial pacing should be performed to monitor AV conduction, or RF application should be stopped and other sites sought. To reduce the risk of AV block, RF delivery should be immediately discontinued when (1) impedance rises suddenly (more than 10 Ω), (2) the PR interval (during NSR, atrial pacing, or AT) prolongs, (3) AV block develops, (4) retrograde conduction block is observed during junctional ectopy, or (5) fast junctional tachycardia (CL shorter than 350 milliseconds) occurs because it may herald imminent heart block.

USE OF INTRACARDIAC ECHOCARDIOGRAPHY TO GUIDE MAPPING AND ABLATION

Intracardiac echocardiography (ICE) can be useful to provide focused real-time images of the endocardial surfaces critical for positioning of catheters, establish catheter tip–tissue contact, and monitor energy delivery in the beating heart. In particular, ICE has been used in cristal ATs. In view of the variability in the anatomical course of the crista terminalis, ICE can assist in accurate positioning of the multipolar mapping catheter and guide precise mapping along this structure with the mapping-ablation catheter (Fig. 11-23).

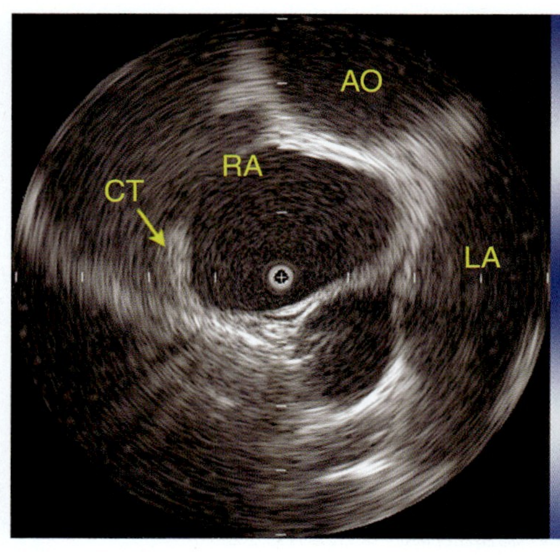

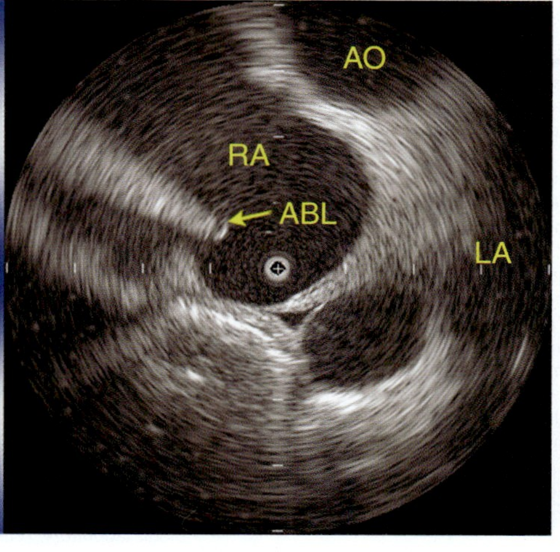

FIGURE 11-23 Intracardiac echocardiographic view (using the mechanical radial imaging system) of the high crista terminalis (CT) showing the anatomical structures and location of the ablation catheter (ABL) at the site of radiofrequency application **(right panel).** The ablation catheter is located on the high lateral CT. AO = aorta; LA = left atrium; RA = right atrium.

ICE can also help demonstrate the close anatomical relation between the superior crista terminalis and right upper PV and can facilitate careful and subtle mapping to determine whether a tachycardia is high cristal or in the right upper PV. This is important when making a decision about the necessity to proceed with a transseptal puncture, in which case ICE can also be helpful. Echocardiographic lesion characteristics defined by ICE can provide a guide for directing additional RF lesions. The effective RF lesion has an increased or changed echo density completely extending to the epicardium, with the development of a trivial linear low-echo density or echo-free interstitial space, a finding suggesting a transmural RF lesion.

Endpoints of Ablation

TACHYCARDIA TERMINATION DURING RADIOFREQUENCY ENERGY APPLICATION. Sudden termination of a sustained AT during RF application suggests a successful ablation. However, reliance on AT termination during RF application as the sole criterion of successful ablation may be misleading because AT may terminate spontaneously or in response to PACs induced by the RF application, and AT termination may not be a result of ablation of the AT focus. Furthermore, sudden termination of the AT can be associated with catheter dislodgment from the critical site to another site, thus making it difficult to deliver additional lesions at the critical site.

NONINDUCIBILITY OF TACHYCARDIA. To use this criterion as a reliable endpoint, careful assessment of inducibility should be performed prior to ablation; the feasibility and best method of reproducible induction of the AT should be documented at baseline before ablation. In the setting of easy inducibility prior to ablation, one may consider the lack of inducibility as an indicator of successful ablation. Noninducibility of the arrhythmia is inapplicable if the original arrhythmia is noninducible at baseline or was inadvertently terminated mechanically. Inducibility should be reassessed 30 minutes after the last successful RF application.

Outcome

The short-term success rate is variable (range, 69% to 100%; mean, 91%). Complication rates range from 0% to 8% (mean, 3%). Recurrence rates range from 0% to 25% (mean, 9%). The mechanism of AT can influence outcome.

Phrenic nerve injury can occur during ablation of ATs in the right or left free wall, SVC, right superior PV, or left PVs. The ability to pace the phrenic nerve at a candidate ablation site should prompt attempting to find a slightly different site or, if this is not possible, applying RF energy at low power or for a short duration. Even when the phrenic nerve cannot be paced, intermittent fluoroscopic visualization of the ipsilateral diaphragm movement should be performed during RF application at high-risk sites, and RF delivery should be terminated if diaphragmatic excursion decreases. An alternative approach is to position a catheter in the SVC at a site at which the phrenic nerve can be consistently captured and pace the phrenic nerve during ablation. RF energy delivery should be stopped immediately if diaphragmatic contraction becomes less vigorous or ceases.

Sinus node dysfunction can develop during ablation of ATs originating near the sinus node. The risk is usually low because of the diffuse distribution of the sinus node complex, except in older patients or in those with preexisting sinus node dysfunction.

AV block can complicate ablation of ATs originating in the anteroseptal region. When the HB potential is detectable at the ablation catheter location, titrated RF energy output and RF application for short duration should be used, coupled with overdrive atrial pacing to monitor AV conduction in case accelerated junctional rhythm occurs. Alternatively, cryoablation may be used in this region with its slightly better safety margin for AV conduction. Moreover, detailed mapping in the right and left anteroseptal regions is required, because ATs arising along the anterior and anteroseptal LA and even the right superior PV frequently have earliest RA activation at the HB region, with a normal activation pattern along the posterior LA, as recorded by the CS electrodes.

REFERENCES

1. Saoudi N, Cosio F, Waldo A, et al: Classification of atrial flutter and regular atrial tachycardia according to electrophysiologic mechanism and anatomic bases: a statement from a joint expert group from the Working Group of Arrhythmias of the European Society of Cardiology and the North American Society of Pacing and Electrophysiology, *J Cardiovasc Electrophysiol* 12:852–866, 2001.
2. Scheinman MM, Yang Y, Cheng J: Atrial flutter: part II. Nomenclature, *Pacing Clin Electrophysiol* 27:504–506, 2004.
3. Morton JB, Sanders P, Das A, et al: Focal atrial tachycardia arising from the tricuspid annulus: electrophysiologic and electrocardiographic characteristics, *J Cardiovasc Electrophysiol* 12:653–659, 2001.
4. Badhwar N, Kalman JM, Sparks PB, et al: Atrial tachycardia arising from the coronary sinus musculature: electrophysiological characteristics and long-term outcomes of radiofrequency ablation, *J Am Coll Cardiol* 46:1921–1930, 2005.
5. Hoffmann E, Reithmann C, Nimmermann P, et al: Clinical experience with electroanatomic mapping of ectopic atrial tachycardia, *Pacing Clin Electrophysiol* 25:49–56, 2002.
6. Kistler PM, Roberts-Thomson KC, Haqqani HM, et al: P-wave morphology in focal atrial tachycardia: development of an algorithm to predict the anatomic site of origin, *J Am Coll Cardiol* 48:1010–1017, 2006.
7. Kistler PM, Sanders P, Fynn SP, et al: Electrophysiological and electrocardiographic characteristics of focal atrial tachycardia originating from the pulmonary veins: acute and long-term outcomes of radiofrequency ablation, *Circulation* 108:1968–1975, 2003.
8. Tritto M, Zardini M, De Ponti R, Salerno-Uriarte JA: Iterative atrial tachycardia originating from the coronary sinus musculature, *J Cardiovasc Electrophysiol* 12:1187–1189, 2001.
9. Volkmer M, Antz M, Hebe J, Kuck KH: Focal atrial tachycardia originating from the musculature of the coronary sinus, *J Cardiovasc Electrophysiol* 13:68–71, 2002.
10. Pavin D, Boulmier D, Daubert JC, Mabo P: Permanent left atrial tachycardia: radiofrequency catheter ablation through the coronary sinus, *J Cardiovasc Electrophysiol* 13:395–398, 2002.
11. Navarrete AJ, Arora R, Hubbard JE, Miller JM: Magnetic electroanatomic mapping of an atrial tachycardia requiring ablation within the coronary sinus, *J Cardiovasc Electrophysiol* 14:1361–1364, 2003.

12. Medi C, Kalman JM: Prediction of the atrial flutter circuit location from the surface electrocardiogram, *Europace* 10:786–796, 2008.
13. Matsuoka K, Kasai A, Fujii E, et al: Electrophysiological features of atrial tachycardia arising from the atrioventricular annulus, *Pacing Clin Electrophysiol* 25:440–445, 2002.
14. Tsai CF, Tai CT, Hsieh MH, et al: Initiation of atrial fibrillation by ectopic beats originating from the superior vena cava: electrophysiological characteristics and results of radiofrequency ablation, *Circulation* 102:67–74, 2000.
15. Das S, Neuzil P, Albert CM, et al: Catheter ablation of peri-AV nodal atrial tachycardia from the noncoronary cusp of the aortic valve, *J Cardiovasc Electrophysiol* 19:231–237, 2008.
16. Shehata M, Liu T, Joshi N, et al: Atrial tachycardia originating from the left coronary cusp near the aorto-mitral junction: anatomic considerations, *Heart Rhythm* 7:987–991, 2010.
17. Wharton M, Shenasa H, Barold H, et al: Ablation of atrial tachycardia in adults. In Huang SKS, Wilber DJ, editors: *Radiofrequency catheter ablation of cardiac arrhythmias: basic concepts and clinical applications*, ed 2, Armonk, NY, 2000, Futura, pp 139–164.
18. Roberts-Thomson KC, Kistler PM, Kalman JM: Focal atrial tachycardia I: clinical features, diagnosis, mechanisms, and anatomic location, *Pacing Clin Electrophysiol* 29:643–652, 2006.
19. Blomstrom-Lundqvist C, Scheinman MM, Aliot EM, et al: ACC/AHA/ESC guidelines for the management of patients with supraventricular arrhythmias—executive summary: a report of the American College of Cardiology/American Heart Association Task Force on Practice Guidelines and the European Society of Cardiology Committee for Practice Guidelines (writing committee to develop guidelines for the management of patients with supraventricular arrhythmias), *Circulation* 108:1871–1909, 2003.
20. Medi C, Kalman JM, Haqqani H, et al: Tachycardia-mediated cardiomyopathy secondary to focal atrial tachycardia: long-term outcome after catheter ablation, *J Am Coll Cardiol* 53:1791–1797, 2009.
21. Teh AW, Kalman JM, Medi C, et al: Long-term outcome following successful catheter ablation of atrial tachycardia originating from the pulmonary veins: absence of late atrial fibrillation, *J Cardiovasc Electrophysiol* 21:747–750, 2010.
22. Baranowski B, Wazni O, Lindsay B, et al: Focal ablation versus single vein isolation for atrial tachycardia originating from a pulmonary vein, *Pacing Clin Electrophysiol* 33:776–783, 2010.
23. Hu YF, Higa S, Huang JL, et al: Electrophysiologic characteristics and catheter ablation of focal atrial tachycardia with more than one focus, *Heart Rhythm* 6:198–203, 2009.
24. Josephson ME: Supraventricular tachycardias. In Josephson ME, editor: *Clinical cardiac electrophysiology*, ed 4, Philadelphia, 2008, Lippincott Williams & Wilkins, pp 175–284.
25. Porter MJ, Morton JB, Denman R, et al: Influence of age and gender on the mechanism of supraventricular tachycardia, *Heart Rhythm* 1:393–396, 2004.
26. Hillock RJ, Kalman JM, Roberts-Thomson KC, et al: Multiple focal atrial tachycardias in a healthy adult population: characterization and description of successful radiofrequency ablation, *Heart Rhythm* 4:435–438, 2007.
27. Brown JP, Krummen DE, Feld GK, Narayan SM: Using electrocardiographic activation time and diastolic intervals to separate focal from macro-re-entrant atrial tachycardias, *J Am Coll Cardiol* 49:1965–1973, 2007.
28. Wang Y, Cuculich PS, Woodard PK, et al: Focal atrial tachycardia after pulmonary vein isolation: noninvasive mapping with electrocardiographic imaging (ECGI), *Heart Rhythm* 4:1081–1084, 2007.
29. Teh AW, Kistler PM, Kalman JM: Using the 12-lead ECG to localize the origin of ventricular and atrial tachycardias: part 1. Focal atrial tachycardia, *J Cardiovasc Electrophysiol* 20:706–709, 2009.
30. Ellenbogen KA, Stambler BS, Wood MA: Atrial tachycardia. In Zipes DP, Jalife J, editors: *Cardiac electrophysiology: from cell to bedside*, ed 5, Philadelphia, 2009, Saunders, pp 589–604.
31. Hsieh M, Chen S: Catheter ablation of focal atrial tachycardia. In Zipes DP, Haissaguerre M, editors: *Catheter ablation of arrhythmias*, Armonk, NY, 2002, Futura, pp 185–204.
32. Roberts-Thomson KC, Kistler PM, Haqqani HM, et al: Focal atrial tachycardias arising from the right atrial appendage: electrocardiographic and electrophysiologic characteristics and radiofrequency ablation, *J Cardiovasc Electrophysiol* 18:367–372, 2007.
33. Gerstenfeld EP, Dixit S, Bala R, et al: Surface electrocardiogram characteristics of atrial tachycardias occurring after pulmonary vein isolation, *Heart Rhythm* 4:1136–1143, 2007.
34. Kistler PM, Sanders P, Hussin A, et al: Focal atrial tachycardia arising from the mitral annulus: electrocardiographic and electrophysiologic characterization, *J Am Coll Cardiol* 41:2212–2219, 2003.
35. Crawford TC, Mukerji S, Good E, et al: Utility of atrial and ventricular cycle length variability in determining the mechanism of paroxysmal supraventricular tachycardia, *J Cardiovasc Electrophysiol* 18:698–703, 2007.
36. Knecht S, Matsuo S, Lim K-T, et al: Focal vs. macroreentrant atrial tachycardia after prior ablation: value of cycle length variability, *Heart Rhythm* 4(Suppl S):S238, 2007.
37. Iwai S, Markowitz SM, Stein KM, et al: Response to adenosine differentiates focal from macroreentrant atrial tachycardia: validation using three-dimensional electroanatomic mapping, *Circulation* 106:2793–2799, 2002.
38. Knight BP, Ebinger M, Oral H, et al: Diagnostic value of tachycardia features and pacing maneuvers during paroxysmal supraventricular tachycardia, *J Am Coll Cardiol* 36:574–582, 2000.
39. Maruyama M, Kobayashi Y, Miyauchi Y, et al: The VA relationship after differential atrial overdrive pacing: a novel tool for the diagnosis of atrial tachycardia in the electrophysiologic laboratory, *J Cardiovasc Electrophysiol* 18:1127–1133, 2007.
40. Colombowala IK, Massumi A, Rasekh A, et al: Variability in post-pacing intervals predicts global atrial activation pattern during tachycardia, *J Cardiovasc Electrophysiol* 19:142–147, 2008.
41. Vijayaraman P, Lee BP, Kalahasty G, et al: Reanalysis of the "pseudo A-A-V" response to ventricular entrainment of supraventricular tachycardia: importance of His-bundle timing, *J Cardiovasc Electrophysiol* 17:25–28, 2006.
42. Josephson ME: Catheter and surgical ablation in the therapy of arrhythmias. In Josephson ME, editor: *Clinical cardiac electrophysiology*, ed 4, Philadelphia, 2008, Lippincott Williams & Wilkins, pp 746–888.
43. Morady F: Catheter ablation of supraventricular arrhythmias: state of the art, *J Cardiovasc Electrophysiol* 15:124–139, 2004.
44. Chang KC, Chen JY, Lin YC, Huang SK: Usefulness of interatrial conduction time to distinguish between focal atrial tachyarrhythmias originating from the superior vena cava and the right superior pulmonary vein, *J Cardiovasc Electrophysiol* 19:1231–1235, 2008.
45. Lee SH, Tai CT, Lin WS, et al: Predicting the arrhythmogenic foci of atrial fibrillation before atrial transseptal procedure: implication for catheter ablation, *J Cardiovasc Electrophysiol* 11:750–757, 2000.
46. Mohamed U, Skanes AC, Gula LJ, et al: A novel pacing maneuver to localize focal atrial tachycardia, *J Cardiovasc Electrophysiol* 18:1–6, 2007.
47. Wetzel U, Hindricks G, Schirdewahn P, et al: A stepwise mapping approach for localization and ablation of ectopic right, left, and septal atrial foci using electroanatomic mapping, *Eur Heart J* 23:1387–1393, 2002.
48. Seidl K, Schwacke H, Rameken M, et al: Noncontact mapping of ectopic atrial tachycardias: different characteristics of isopotential maps and unipolar electrogram, *Pacing Clin Electrophysiol* 26:16–25, 2003.
49. Higa S, Tai CT, Lin YJ, et al: Focal atrial tachycardia: new insight from noncontact mapping and catheter ablation, *Circulation* 109:84–91, 2004.
50. Sanders P, Hocini M, Jais P, et al: Characterization of focal atrial tachycardia using high-density mapping, *J Am Coll Cardiol* 46:2088–2099, 2005.

CHAPTER 12 Typical Atrial Flutter

Pathophysiology

Right Atrial Anatomy

The right atrial (RA) endocardial surface is composed of many orifices and embryonic remnants, accounting for an irregular, complex surface. The RA endocardium is architecturally divided into three anatomically distinct regions; each is a remnant of embryological development. The posterior smooth-walled RA, derived from the embryonic sinus venosus, receives the superior vena cava (SVC), the inferior vena cava (IVC), and the coronary sinus (CS). It also contains the fossa ovalis, the sinus node, and the atrioventricular (AV) node (AVN). The anterolateral trabeculated "true" RA, derived from the true embryonic RA, is lined by horizontal, parallel ridges of muscle bundles that resemble the teeth of a comb (the pectinate muscle). It contains the RA appendage and free wall. The atrial septum is primarily derived from the embryonic septum primum and septum secundum.

The posterior smooth-walled RA and the anterolateral trabeculated RA are separated by the crista terminalis on the lateral wall and the eustachian ridge in the inferior aspect. The sulcus terminalis, where the sinus node is located, is a subtle groove on the epicardial surface of the heart corresponding to the crista terminalis. The crista terminalis is a C-shaped, convex, thick muscular ridge that runs from the high septum, anterior to the orifice of the SVC superiorly, and courses caudally along the posterolateral aspect of the RA. In its inferior extent, it courses anteriorly to the orifice of the IVC. As the crista reaches the region of the IVC, it is extended by the eustachian valve ridge. The eustachian valve is the remnant of the embryonic sinus venosus valve, which manifests as a flap of variable thickness and mobility along the orifice of the IVC; this valve can continue as a ridge superiorly along the floor of the RA to the ostium of the CS (CS os), to join the valve of the CS, form the tendon of Todaro, and then continue onto the interatrial septum as the inferior limbus of the fossa ovalis.[1]

The SVC enters the roof of the RA between the base of the RA appendage and the superior margin of the interatrial septum. The IVC enters the posterolateral portion of the floor of the RA along the inferior margin of the interatrial septum. The CS enters the inferior aspect of the RA adjacent to the inferior margin of the interatrial septum, slightly more anterior and medial relative to the orifice of the IVC, and closer to the tricuspid annulus. On the lower third of the interatrial septum lies the fossa ovalis.

The tricuspid annulus lies anterior to the body of the RA, and its inferior portion lies a short distance (approximately 1 to 4 cm) anterior to the eustachian ridge, although its course varies among individuals.[2] The cavotricuspid isthmus (CTI) is the part of the RA between the ostium of the IVC and the eustachian ridge (posteriorly) and the tricuspid annulus (anteriorly). The CTI runs in an anterolateral-to-posteromedial direction, from the low anterior RA to the low septal RA (see Fig. 17-1). Its width and muscle thickness are variable, from a few millimeters to more than 3 cm in width and more than 1 cm in depth. The CTI becomes wider in a medial-to-lateral direction, and it is thinnest in its central portion. A thick eustachian ridge (greater than 4 mm) is seen in 24% of patients. At mid-diastole, the central isthmus is straight in 8% of patients, concave in 47% of patients, and pouch-like (more than 5 mm) in 45% of patients.[3,4] The eustachian ridge (often composed of partly or largely fibrous tissue) occurs as an elevation on the CTI. The area between the tricuspid annulus and the eustachian ridge is referred to as the subeustachian isthmus, whereas the downslope of the eustachian ridge leads to the junction of the RA and IVC. The pectinates, as they fan out from the crista terminalis or other muscle bundles on the CTI, typically spare the myocardium just atrial to the tricuspid valve. This smooth portion of the cavotricuspid annulus is referred to as the vestibular portion.[1] In the normal heart, CTI anatomy can be flat, "hilly" (from prominent eustachian ridge or pectinate muscles, or both), concave, or have a pouch-like recess.

Typical Atrial Flutter Circuit

Typical atrial flutter (AFL) is a type of macroreentrant atrial tachycardia (AT) that uses the CTI as an essential part of its circuit. The circuit boundaries are the tricuspid annulus, crista terminalis, IVC orifice, eustachian ridge, CS os, and probably fossa ovalis. These barriers (lines of conduction block) can be functional or anatomical and are necessary to provide adequate path length for the flutter reentry circuit. Whereas the anterior boundary of the tachycardia circuit has been well established as being the tricuspid ring, the posterior boundaries are more complex and not as well defined, and they occur at a variable distance from the anterior border; the posterior borders are narrowest in the region of the eustachian ridge and widest in the anterior part of the RA.[2,5-8]

The CTI provides the protected zone of slow conduction necessary for the flutter reentry circuit. The area of slowest conduction is probably localized in the lateral aspect of the CTI in younger patients and in the medial aspect in older patients.[9] Conduction velocity in the CTI during pacing in sinus rhythm is slower in patients with typical AFL compared with those without any history of AFL.[3,10] The mechanism of the slower conduction velocity in the CTI, relative to the interatrial septum and RA free wall, is uncertain but can be related to the anisotropic fiber orientation. With aging or atrial dilation, intercellular fibrosis can change the density of gap junctions and produce nonuniform anisotropic conduction through the trabeculations of the CTI. Additionally, the CTI and RA in patients with typical AFL are significantly larger than those in a control population.[6]

The crista terminalis plays an important role as a functional barrier during typical AFL. Conduction delay and rate-related transverse block across the crista terminalis has been consistently observed in sinus rhythm and during pacing in humans. A line of transverse conduction block along the crista terminalis serving as a lateral boundary can be determined by the presence of double and split potentials recorded during AFL or rapid pacing from either side of the crista terminalis during electrophysiological (EP) testing. Structural characteristics of the crista terminalis influence transverse conduction; steep slope and arborization of the crista terminalis have been implicated as geometric factors in its transverse conduction block. Typical AFL is more likely to occur in the setting of a thicker and continuous crista terminalis, and these patients are more likely to exhibit transverse crista terminalis conduction block at longer cycle lengths (CLs) as opposed to controls. Similarly, the region posterior to the crista terminalis (the posterior smooth-walled RA) also has been shown to demonstrate functional transverse conduction block during AFL or rapid pacing.[11,12]

Typical AFL is of two types: counterclockwise and clockwise.[5] In counterclockwise AFL, the activation wavefront propagates caudocephalically up the septal side of the tricuspid annulus toward the crista terminalis and advances cephalocaudally along the lateral wall of the RA to reach the lateral tricuspid annulus, after which it propagates through the CTI ("counterclockwise" as viewed in the left anterior oblique [LAO] view from the ventricular side of the tricuspid annulus). The width of the activation wavefront in typical AFL varies considerably, determined by the distance between the anterior and posterior boundaries at any given part of the circuit. It is very narrow inferiorly at the CTI and substantially wider moving upward. The substantial distance between anterior and posterior borders as well as the anatomical barriers superiorly, combined with variability in the completeness of the posterior border, creates conditions for substantial variability in the upper part of the circuit. Despite a relatively similar activation sequence, the active circuit (as determined by entrainment mapping) is variable. Most commonly, the reentrant wavefront courses not around the tricuspid annulus but obliquely between anterior and posterior borders away from the tricuspid annulus along any available, more rapidly conducting segments. Consequently, significant portions of the RA, including areas around the tricuspid annulus, can often be passively activated. In many subjects, the upper portions of the circuit pass behind the RA appendage and lie near or at the posterior circuit border, or they bifurcate around the SVC or RA appendage, or both. The posterior border can extend completely or partially between the IVC and the SVC.[7,8]

The flutter circuit is entirely confined within the RA. Left atrial (LA) activation occurs as a bystander and follows transseptal conduction across the inferior CS-LA connection, Bachmann bundle, or fossa ovalis.[2,6]

In clockwise (reverse typical) AFL, activation propagates in the direction opposite to that in counterclockwise typical AFL (Fig. 12-1). Clockwise AFL is observed in only 10% of clinical cases, despite the fact that it is easily inducible in the EP laboratory with programmed electrical stimulation. Clockwise AFL can be induced in the EP laboratory in approximately 50% of patients who clinically present with only counterclockwise AFL. The 9:1 clinical predominance of counterclockwise AFL can be related to the localization of

Counterclockwise typical AFL

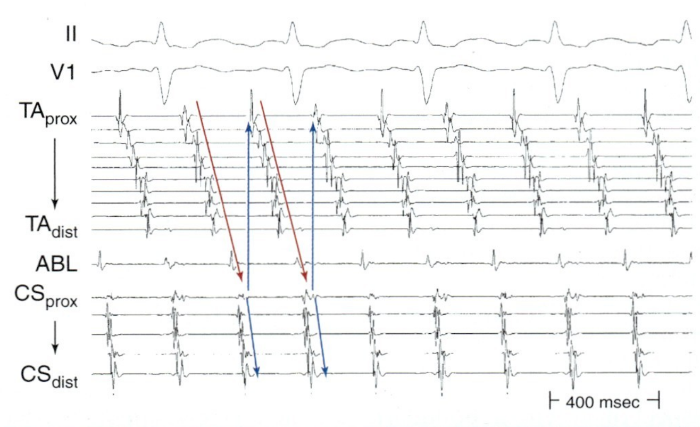

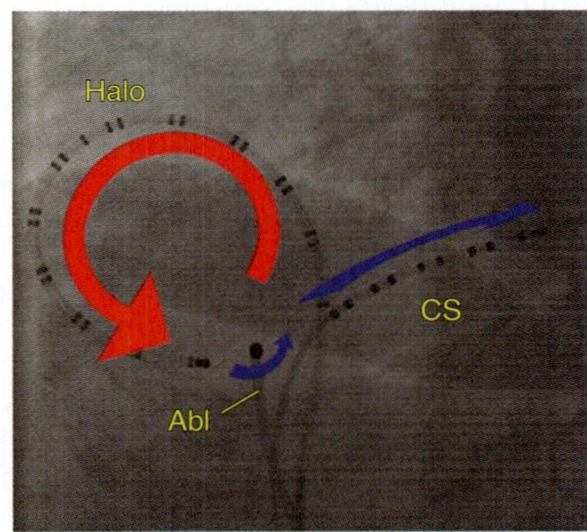

Clockwise typical AFL

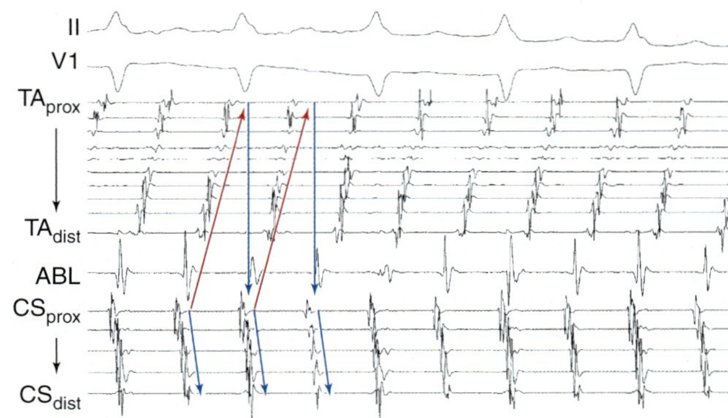

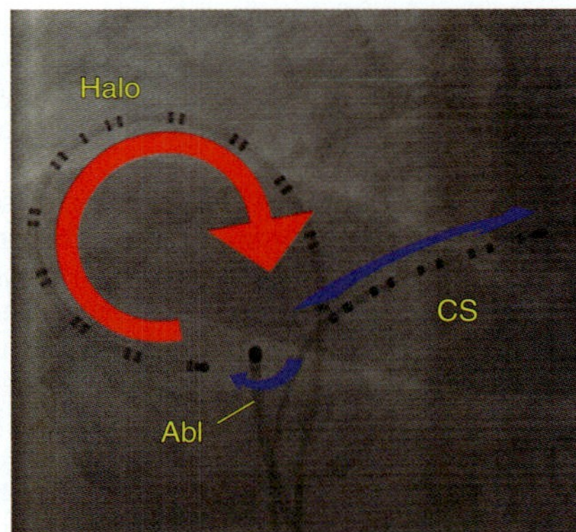

FIGURE 12-1 Endocardial activation during counterclockwise **(upper panel)** and clockwise **(lower panel)** typical atrial flutter (AFL) in the same patient. Catheter position and wavefront activation during the tachycardia are illustrated in a left anterior oblique fluoroscopic view **(right side).** The ablation catheter (Abl) is positioned at the cavotricuspid isthmus (CTI), and the Halo catheter is positioned around the tricuspid annulus, with the distal end at the lateral aspect of the CTI. ABL = ablation site; CS = coronary sinus; CS_{dist} = distal coronary sinus; CS_{prox} = proximal coronary sinus; TA_{dist} = distal tricuspid annulus; TA_{prox} = proximal tricuspid annulus.

an area with a low safety factor for conduction in the CTI, close to the atrial septum. Additionally, counterclockwise AFL is more likely to be induced with rapid atrial pacing from the CS os. Conversely, clockwise AFL is more likely to be induced with pacing from the low lateral RA pacing. These observations may be related to the anisotropic properties of the CTI and the development of rate-dependent conduction delays and unidirectional block necessary for tachycardia induction, which may be affected by the site of stimulation.[2,6] Spontaneous AFL initiation may be related to rapid bursts of pulmonary vein discharges (atrial fibrillation [AF]).

Double-Wave Reentry

A typical AFL circuit with a large excitable gap may allow a second excitation wave to be introduced into the flutter circuit by a critically timed atrial extrastimulus (AES), so that two wavefronts occupy the same circuit simultaneously. This type of AFL is designated double-wave reentry.

Double-wave reentry is manifest by acceleration of the tachycardia rate but with identical surface and intracardiac electrogram morphology. It can be recognized by the simultaneous activation of the superior and inferior regions of the tricuspid annulus, with all activation being sequential. This rhythm rarely lasts for more than a few beats and can serve as a trigger for AF. Because the CTI is still a necessary part of the circuit, double-wave reentry is amenable to CTI ablation.[2,6]

Clinical Considerations

Epidemiology

It is estimated that the overall incidence of AFL in the United States is 88 per 100,000 person-years. AFL accounts for approximately 15% of supraventricular arrhythmias and frequently coexists with or precedes AF. Although in clinical practice AFL appears to be less common than paroxysmal supraventricular tachycardia, population-based data show that in the general population, AFL is diagnosed for the first time more than twice as often. Adjusted for age, the incidence of AFL in men is more than 2.5 times that of women. Paroxysmal AFL can occur in patients with no apparent structural heart disease, whereas chronic AFL is usually associated with underlying heart disease, such as valvular or ischemic heart disease or cardiomyopathy. At highest risk of developing AFL are men, older adults, and individuals with preexisting heart failure or chronic obstructive lung disease. In approximately 60% of patients, AFL occurs as part of an acute disease process, such as exacerbation of pulmonary disease, following cardiac or pulmonary surgery, or during acute myocardial infarction.[13]

Clinical Presentation

Patients with AFL may be completely asymptomatic, or they may present with a spectrum of symptoms ranging from palpitations, lightheadedness, fatigue, reduced activity tolerance, or dyspnea to acute pulmonary edema or acute coronary syndrome in susceptible patients. The severity of symptoms usually depends on the ventricular rate during the AFL, the presence of structural heart disease, and baseline left ventricular function. Some patients remain asymptomatic until they present with a thromboembolic event or with decompensated heart failure secondary to tachycardia-induced cardiomyopathy. AFL occurs in approximately 25% to 35% of patients with AF, in which case AFL may be associated with more intense symptoms because of more rapid ventricular rates.

Initial Evaluation

ECG diagnosis of typical AFL is frequently accurate, but it can occasionally be misleading (see later). Cardiac evaluation with echocardiography is required to assess for structural heart disease. Other tests may be required to evaluate for potential substrates or triggers of AFL.

Principles of Management

ACUTE MANAGEMENT

Acute therapy for patients with AFL depends on the clinical presentation and may include cardioversion and the use of AVN blockers to slow the ventricular rate during the AFL. Cardioversion (electrical or chemical) is commonly the initial treatment of choice. Electrical cardioversion is almost always successful in terminating AFL, and it often requires relatively low energies (less than 50 J). Chemical cardioversion can be achieved with intravenous ibutilide in 38% to 76% of cases, and this agent is more effective than intravenous amiodarone, sotalol, and class IC agents. Overdrive atrial pacing (via a catheter in the esophagus or the RA) can effectively terminate typical AFL, but it can also induce conversion of AFL into AF. Anticoagulation in the pericardioversion period should be considered and is guided by the duration of the AFL and the patient's stroke risk factors, by using the same criteria as for AF (see Chap. 15).[14]

Rate control is typically achieved with oral or intravenous AVN blockers such as verapamil, diltiazem, beta blockers, and digoxin. Rate control tends to be more difficult to achieve during AFL than AF because of the slower and more regular atrial rate.

CHRONIC MANAGEMENT

When AFL occurs as part of an acute disease process, long-term therapy of the arrhythmia is usually not required after sinus rhythm is restored and the underlying disease process is treated. The long-term success rate of antiarrhythmic drugs to prevent AFL recurrence appears to be limited, and complete suppression of AFL can be difficult to achieve. On the other hand, ablation is highly successful at the conclusion of a relatively short and low-risk procedure. Therefore, catheter ablation of the CTI is the treatment of choice for typical AFL, whether paroxysmal or persistent, and long-term drug therapy is rarely indicated and should be reserved for unusual circumstances.[2]

Several antiarrhythmic drugs have demonstrated efficacy in suppression of AFL, including class IA (quinidine, procainamide, and disopyramide), class IC (flecainide and propafenone), and class III (sotalol, amiodarone, dofetilide, and dronedarone) agents. In the absence of structural heart disease, class IC agents are the drugs of choice. The use of antiarrhythmic agents should be instituted in conjunction with AVN blockers to avoid the risk of rapid ventricular rates secondary to the vagolytic effects of class I drugs and slowing of the flutter rate.[14]

Ablation of the AV junction and pacemaker implantation may be indicated for patients in whom curative ablation of the AFL, antiarrhythmic therapy, and rate control strategies have failed. Stroke prevention is recommended and is usually achieved with aspirin or an oral anticoagulant depending on the patient's stroke risk factors, by using the same criteria as for AF.

Electrocardiographic Features

P Waves

Flutter waves appear as atrial complexes of constant morphology, polarity, and CL. Typically, flutter waves are most prominent in the inferior leads (II, III, aVF) and lead V_1. In the inferior leads, they resemble a picket fence (sawtooth) because the leads are primarily negative. This consists of a downsloping segment, followed by a sharper negative deflection, and then a sharp positive deflection, with a positive overshoot leading to the next downsloping plateau. The relative size of each component can vary markedly.[2]

Counterclockwise AFL (Fig. 12-2) can be characterized by pure negative deflections in the inferior leads, negative and then positive deflections that are equal in size, or a small negative and then a larger positive deflection. Those three varieties coexist with tall positive, small positive, or biphasic P waves in lead V_1, respectively. With progression across the precordium, the initial component rapidly becomes inverted and the second component isoelectric usually by lead V_2 to V_3. This produces the overall impression of an upright flutter wave in lead V_1, which becomes inverted by lead V_6. A negative deflection always precedes the positive deflection in the inferior leads in counterclockwise AFL, and the degree of positivity in the inferior leads appears to be related to the coexistence of heart disease and LA enlargement. Lead I is low-amplitude isoelectric, and lead aVL is usually upright.[15]

The surface ECG appearance of clockwise typical AFL is more variable than that of counterclockwise typical AFL, but in many respects, clockwise AFL presents an inversion of the appearance in counterclockwise AFL. Clockwise AFL generally has broad positive deflections in the inferior leads, with characteristic notching (see Fig. 12-2).[2] However, there is an inverted component preceding the upright notched component. Depending on the amplitude of this component, the appearance can be of continuous undulation without an obviously predominant upright or inverted component. On other occasions, it may appear that the inverted component is dominant, thus superficially mimicking counterclockwise AFL. Lead V_1 is characterized by a wide negative and usually notched deflection. There is transition across the precordium to an upright deflection in lead V_6. Lead I is usually upright, and lead aVL is low-amplitude negative and notched.[15]

Typical AFL usually has an atrial rate of 240 to 340 beats/min. However, AFL can be slower in patients receiving antiarrhythmic agents or after incomplete CTI ablation (Fig. 12-3), whereby flutter CLs as long as 450 milliseconds have been observed. If the ventricular response is half the atrial rate, it can be difficult to identify flutter waves "buried" within the QRS or T waves (Fig. 12-4). Close inspection of the QRS and T waves, and comparisons with ECGs obtained in normal sinus rhythm, can help identify buried flutter waves. Furthermore, vagal maneuvers and AVN blockers can slow AV conduction and unmask the flutter waves.

In patients who have undergone extensive LA ablation for treatment of AF, the P wave morphology during CTI-dependent AFL can be very different from the foregoing discussion because of alteration of intraatrial and interatrial wavefront propagation. Similarly, non–CTI-dependent macroreentrant ATs can mimic typical CTI-dependent AFL on the surface ECG. Thus, arrhythmias that appear to be typical AFL may not be, whereas others that are actually typical AFL may not appear to be.

Atrioventricular Conduction

Most commonly, 2:1 AV conduction is present during AFL. Variable AV conduction and larger multiples (e.g., 4:1 or 6:1) are not uncommon. Slowing the atrial rate during AFL caused by antiarrhythmic drugs or following a prior incomplete CTI ablation can result in a paradoxical increase in the ventricular rate caused by better AVN conduction of the slower flutter beats (Fig. 12-5). Rapid 1:1 AV conduction is most commonly seen in patients with anterogradely conducting bypass tracts (Fig. 12-6), but it may also be present in cases of enhanced AVN conduction secondary to high sympathetic tone (e.g., exercise, sympathomimetic drugs).[2]

QRS Morphology

The QRS complex during AFL is often identical to that during sinus rhythm. However, flutter beats can be aberrantly conducted because of functional bundle branch block, most frequently right bundle branch block (see Fig. 12-5). Even with normal ventricular conduction, the QRS complex may be slightly distorted by temporal superimposition of flutter waves on the QRS complex. Thus, the QRS complex can appear to acquire a new or larger R, S, or Q wave.[2]

Electrophysiological Testing

Typically, a decapolar catheter (positioned into the CS with the proximal electrodes bracketing the CS os) and a multipolar (20 or 24 pole) Halo catheter (positioned at the tricuspid annulus) are used to map typical AFL. The distal tip of the Halo catheter is positioned at 6 to 7 o'clock in the LAO view, so that the distal electrodes will record the middle and lateral aspects of the CTI, the middle electrodes will record the anterolateral RA, and the proximal electrodes may record the RA septum (depending on the catheter used and RA size). Instead of the Halo and CS catheters, some laboratories use a single duodecapolar catheter around the tricuspid annulus, thus extending the catheter tip inside the CS. Such a catheter can straddle the CTI and provide recording and pacing from the medial and lateral aspects of the isthmus, assuming good catheter-tissue contact at these locations. In the latter arrangement, however, the body of the duodecapolar catheter crossing over the CTI can potentially hinder manipulation and

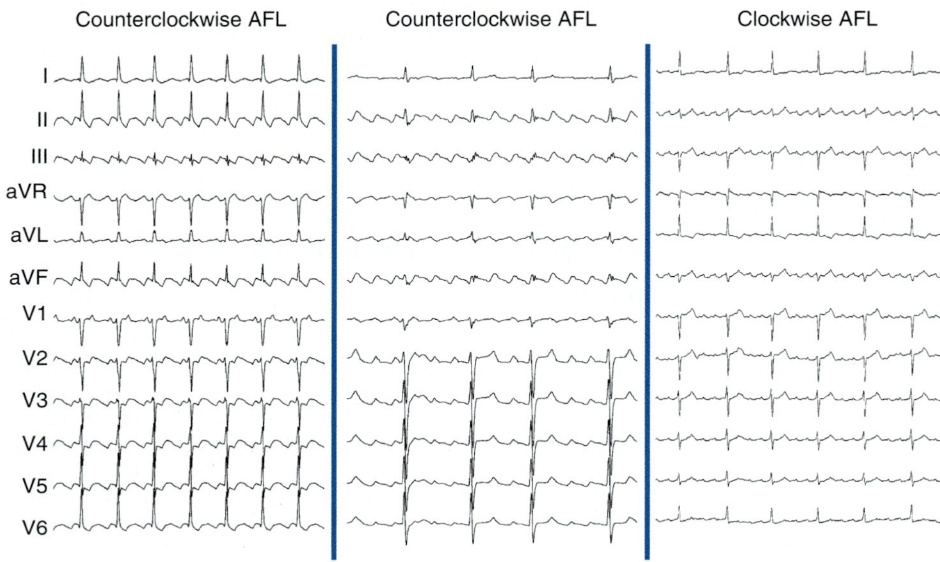

FIGURE 12-2 Surface 12-lead ECG of counterclockwise typical atrial flutter (AFL) with 2:1 atrioventricular (AV) conduction **(left)**, counterclockwise typical AFL with variable AV conduction **(middle)**, and clockwise typical AFL with 4:1 AV conduction **(right)**.

positioning of the ablation catheter tip to achieve adequate tissue contact for effective ablation.

Induction of Tachycardia

Programmed electrical stimulation protocol typically involves atrial burst pacing from the high RA and CS (down to the pacing CL at which 2:1 atrial capture occurs) and single and double AESs (down to the atrial effective refractory period [ERP]) at multiple CLs (600 to 200 milliseconds) from the high RA and CS. Administration of an isoproterenol infusion (0.5 to 4 μg/min) may be required to facilitate tachycardia induction.

AFL can be induced readily with programmed electrical stimulation in most patients with a clinical history of AFL. Reproducible initiation of counterclockwise AFL is possible in more than 95% of patients.[16] Rapid atrial pacing is more likely to induce AFL than a single AES, but as likely as introducing two AESs. On the other hand, the frequency of single or double AESs initiating AFL is low in patients without a history of AFL (less than 10%). Counterclockwise AFL is more likely to be induced by stimulation from the CS os; conversely, clockwise AFL is more likely to be induced with low lateral RA pacing. Induction of AFL usually occurs once unidirectional CTI block develops during pacing (Fig. 12-7). The faster the pacing rate and the shorter the AES coupling intervals, the more likely it will be that AF is induced, which is usually self-terminating but can be sustained in less than 10% of patients with no clinical history of AF. The significance of induction of AF in these patients is uncertain.

Tachycardia Features

Typical AFL is characterized by a constant CL, polarity, morphology, and amplitude of the recorded bipolar electrograms and by the presence of a single constant macroreentrant circuit with a constant atrial activation sequence. The atrial rate is very regular, with cycle-to-cycle variation of less than 2%; it is rare for AFL to display considerable variation in the CL. The atrial CL is usually between 190 and 250 milliseconds, although the atrial rate can be slower in patients receiving antiarrhythmic agents or following a prior unsuccessful ablation of the CTI. It is not uncommon for clockwise and counterclockwise AFLs to occur in the same patient, and they often have similar rates, although clockwise AFL can have a slower rate.

As noted, AFL is usually associated with 2:1 AV conduction, but variable AV conduction and larger multiples are not uncommon. Variable AV block is the result of multilevel block; for example, proximal 2:1 AV block and more distal 3:2 Wenckebach block result in 5:2 AV Wenckebach block. It is likely that the proximal 2:1 block occurs in the upper part of the AVN, whereas Wenckebach block occurs in the lower part of the AVN. Distal Wenckebach behavior in the His bundle (HB) would result in a similar AV conduction pattern but is unlikely to occur. In most cases, the nonconducted flutter impulses block in the AVN. However, infranodal AV block can occur, especially in the presence of prolonged His-Purkinje system refractoriness caused by antiarrhythmic agents or during Wenckebach cycles in the AVN that leads to long-short cycle activation of the His-Purkinje system.

The presence of anterogradely conducting bypass tracts with a short refractory period can result in preexcited AFL with rapid 1:1 AV conduction. Infusion of isoproterenol can enhance AVN function and occasionally facilitate 1:1 AV conduction, especially when the atrial rate is relatively slow.[2] Adenosine increases the degree of AV block, but it also shortens atrial refractoriness and can result in the degeneration of AFL into AF.

Diagnostic Maneuvers during Tachycardia

ATRIAL EXTRASTIMULATION DURING ATRIAL FLUTTER

An AES from the high RA or CS or along the Halo catheter is introduced at a coupling CL 10 milliseconds shorter than the flutter CL, with progressive shortening of the coupling CL by 10 to 30 milliseconds.

An AES commonly results in resetting of the AFL circuit.[16] The closer the site of atrial stimulation is, the easier the resetting of the AFL circuit at longer coupling intervals will be. AFL has a resetting response pattern typical of reentrant circuits with fully excitable

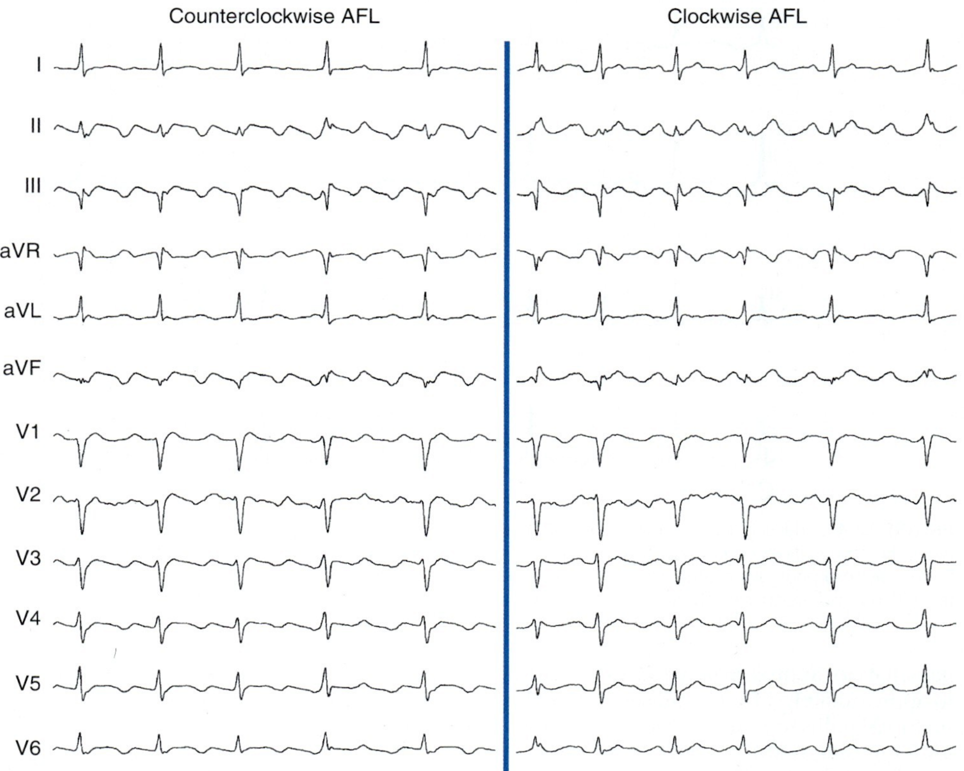

FIGURE 12-3 Surface 12-lead ECGs during counterclockwise **(left)** and clockwise **(right)** typical atrial flutter (AFL) in a patient on flecainide therapy. Note the slow flutter cycle length (approximately 350 milliseconds) secondary to the effects of flecainide.

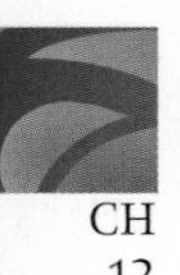

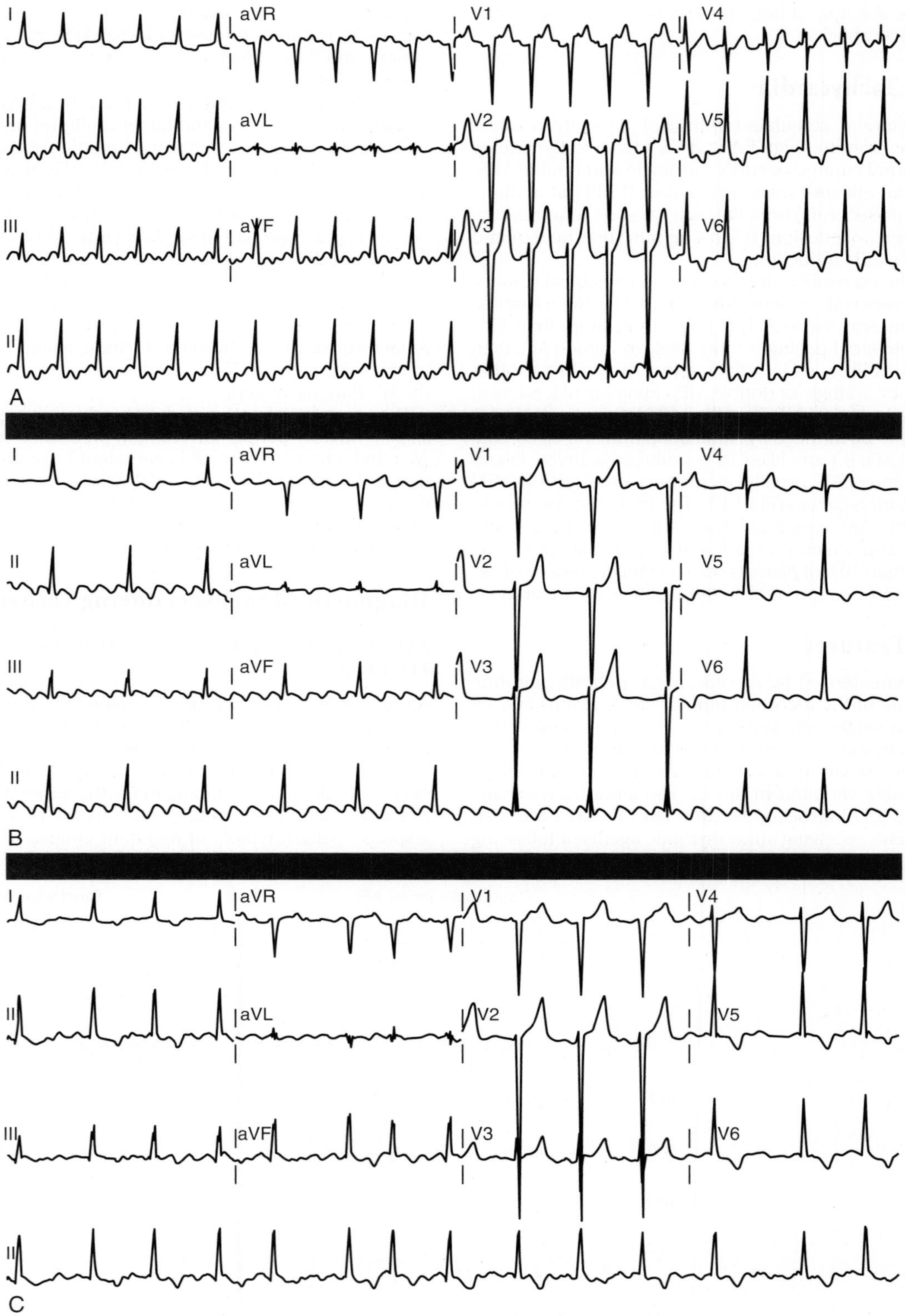

FIGURE 12-4 Surface 12-lead ECG of counterclockwise typical atrial flutter (AFL) with 2:1 atrioventricular (AV) conduction **(A)** and with 4:1 AV conduction **(B).** Note that when the ventricular response is half the atrial rate, it is difficult to identify flutter waves "buried" within the QRS or T waves **(A).** However, when the ventricular rate is slowed, flutter wave morphology becomes more easily visualized. **C** shows atrial fibrillation that developed in the same patient after ablation of the cavotricuspid isthmus. Note that fibrillation waves are coarse and can mimic flutter waves; however, close inspection reveals changes in rate and morphology of atrial activity that are inconsistent with AFL.

gaps: flat (for approximately 15% to 30% of the tachycardia CL, equal to approximately 30 to 63 milliseconds in the absence of drugs, and up to 100 milliseconds with class I antiarrhythmic agents) and then an increasing return CL with progressively shorter coupling intervals. The ability to capture the atrium without affecting (resetting) the AFL circuit timing indicates that the pacing site is outside the AFL circuit (e.g., RA appendage or distal CS).

It is usually difficult for a single AES to terminate AFL because AFL has a sizable fully excitable gap (15% to 30% of the tachycardia CL) that makes it difficult for a single AES to penetrate the AFL

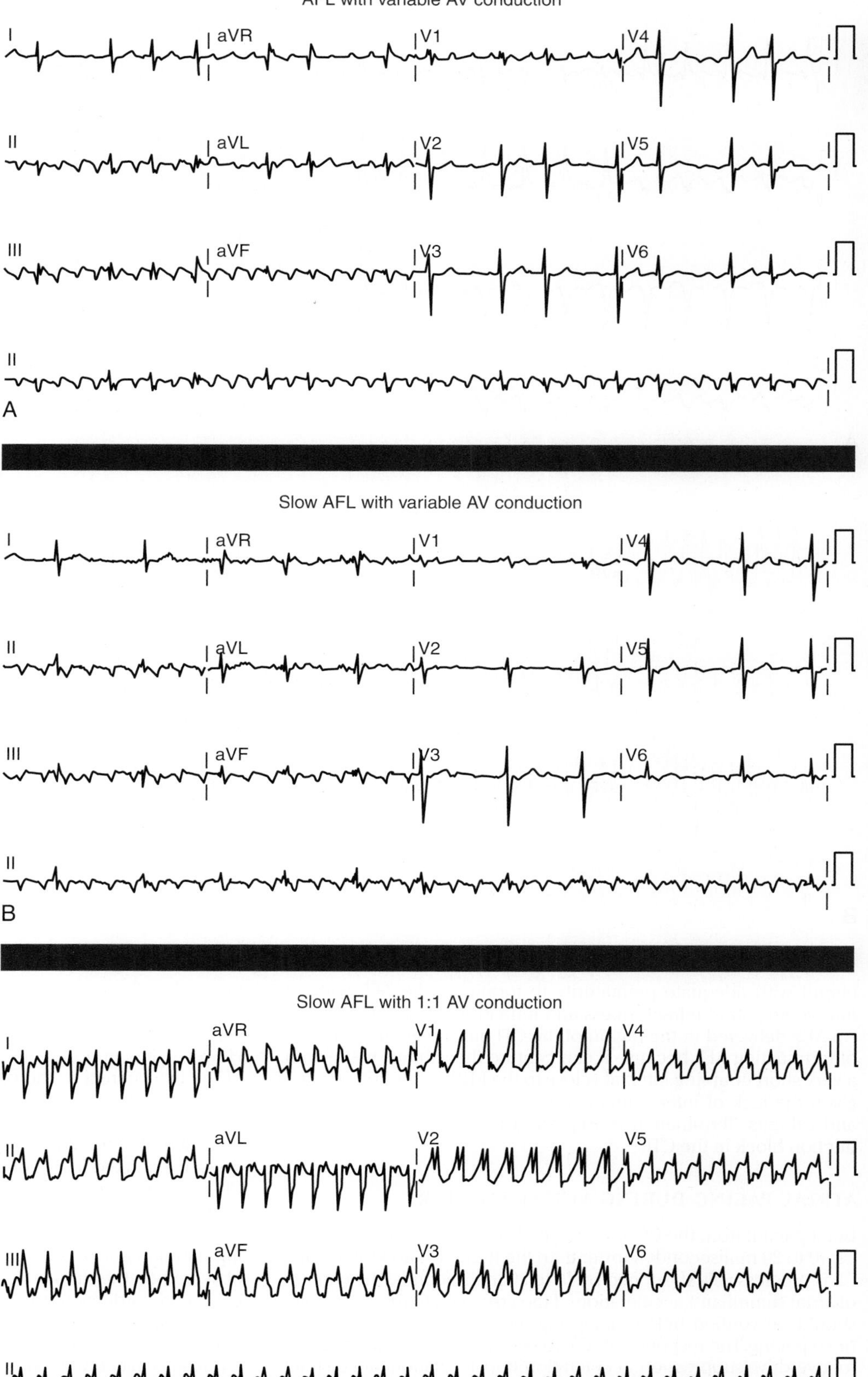

FIGURE 12-5 Effects of antiarrhythmic drugs on typical atrial flutter (AFL). Baseline surface ECG in a patient with AFL and variable atrioventricular (AV) conduction **(A)**. Treatment with propafenone results in slowing of the atrial rate during AFL **(B)** and a paradoxical increase in the ventricular rate caused by better AV nodal conduction of the slower flutter beats **(C)**. Right bundle branch block aberrancy is observed during 1:1 AV conduction.

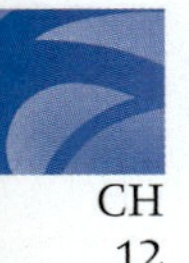

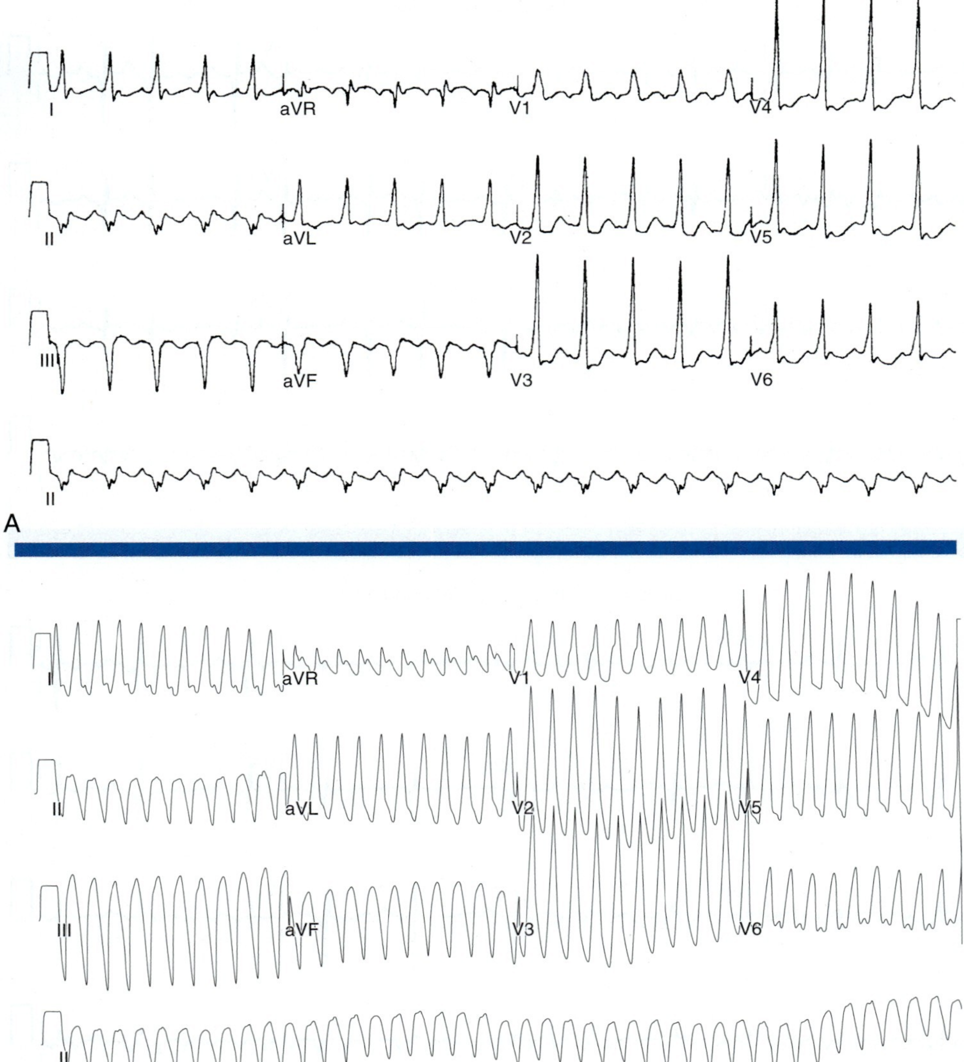

FIGURE 12-6 Surface 12-lead ECGs during clockwise typical atrial flutter in a patient with a left posteroseptal bypass tract (BT). **A,** 2:1 atrioventricular (AV) conduction with QRS fusion (secondary to conduction over both the BT and the AV node). **B,** 1:1 AV conduction over the BT with fully preexcited QRS morphology.

circuit with adequate prematurity to terminate the AFL without intervening atrial refractoriness and intraatrial conduction delays. An AES delivered in the region of the CTI has the greatest chance of terminating AFL because it can capture the isthmus tissue with a very short coupling interval (close to the ERP of this critical site), given the lack of intervening tissue between the stimulation site and isthmus. Termination of AFL always occurs because of conduction block in the CTI.

ATRIAL PACING DURING ATRIAL FLUTTER

Burst pacing from the CS or along the Halo catheter is started at a CL 10 to 20 milliseconds shorter than the flutter CL, and the pacing CL is progressively shortened by 10 to 20 milliseconds. The capture of atrial stimuli and acceleration of the atrial rate to the paced rate should be verified before analyzing the flutter response to overdrive pacing. The response of AFL to overdrive pacing is evaluated for overdrive suppression, acceleration, transformation into distinct uniform AFL morphologies or AF, entrainment, and ability and pattern of termination.

ENTRAINMENT. Overdrive atrial pacing at long CLs (i.e., 10 to 30 milliseconds shorter than the tachycardia CL) can almost always entrain typical AFL. The slower the pacing rate and the farther the pacing site from the reentrant circuit, the longer the pacing drive will need to be to penetrate and entrain the tachycardia. As discussed in detail in Chapter 13, achievement of entrainment of the AT establishes a reentrant mechanism of the tachycardia and excludes triggered activity and abnormal automaticity as potential mechanisms. However, it is important to understand that the mere acceleration of the tachycardia to the pacing rate and then resumption of the original tachycardia after cessation of pacing do not establish the presence of entrainment. After cessation of each pacing drive, the presence of entrainment should be verified by demonstrating the presence of fixed fusion of the paced complexes at a given pacing CL, progressive fusion at faster pacing CLs, and resumption of the same tachycardia morphology following cessation of pacing with a nonfused complex at a return cycle equal to the pacing CL. During entrainment of AFL, fusion of the stimulated impulse can be observed on the surface ECG, but it is easier to recognize on intracardiac recordings from the Halo and CS catheters. Entrainment with manifest fusion can be demonstrated with pacing from sites outside the CTI, such as lateral RA and CS. Conversely, pacing at the CTI results in entrainment with concealed fusion, whereby P waves (on the surface ECG and intracardiac recordings) during pacing are identical to those during the tachycardia.[17,18]

TERMINATION. More rapid atrial burst pacing (pacing CL 20 to 50 milliseconds shorter than the AFL CL) results in termination of AFL in most cases.[16] Termination of AFL during rapid pacing can be indicated by a sudden change of P wave morphology on the surface ECG and by a change of atrial activation sequence in the

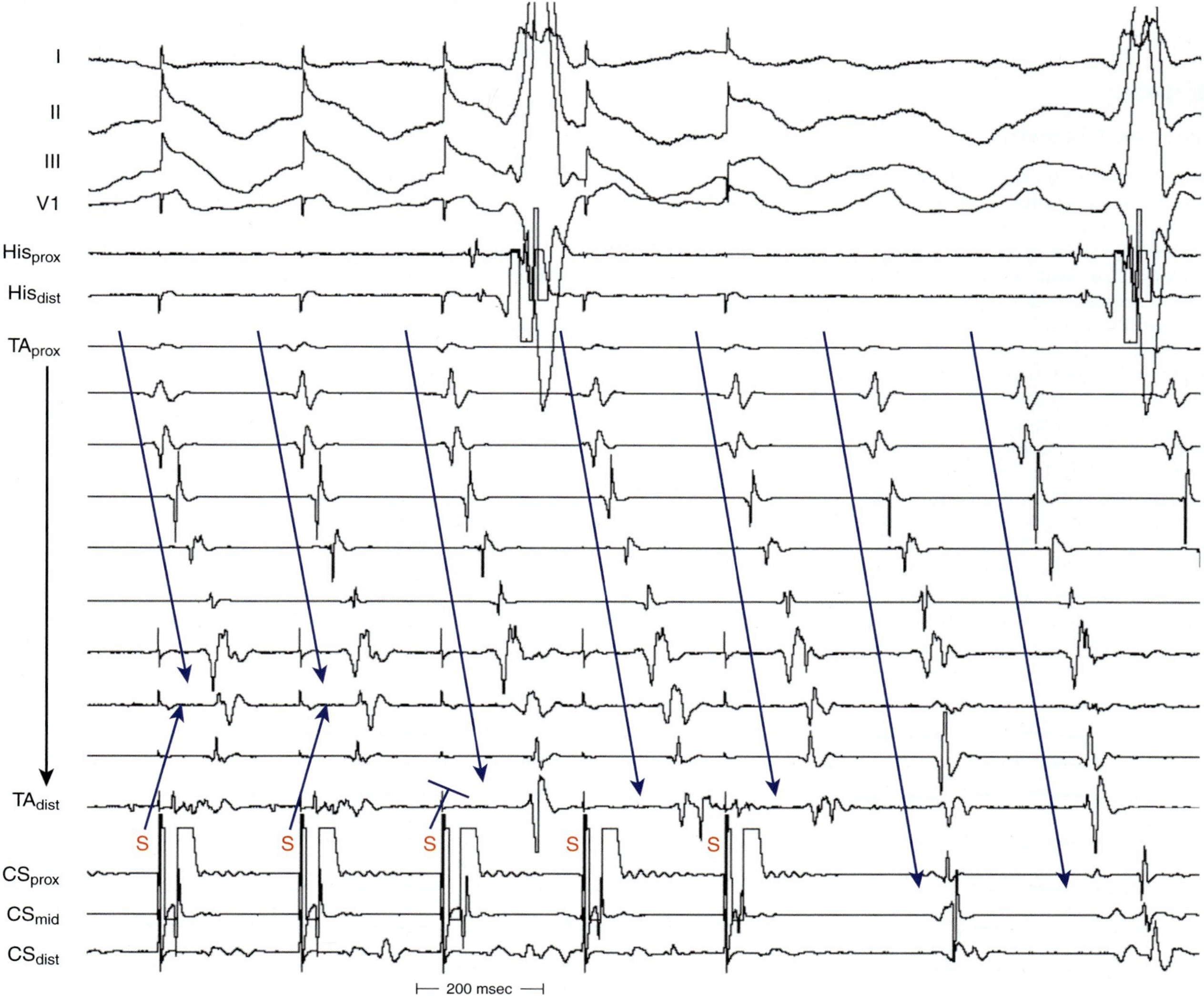

FIGURE 12-7 Surface ECG and intracardiac recordings of initiation of counterclockwise typical AFL. Burst pacing from the coronary sinus (CS) results in wavefronts proceeding in both directions around the tricuspid annulus (TA), colliding around TA 5-6 (arrows); on the third cycle, one wavefront blocks before arriving at TA 1-2 but proceeds around the TA in the opposite direction. When pacing stops, this unopposed wavefront continues around the TA as counterclockwise AFL. dist = distal; prox = proximal.

HB and CS os recordings. This is seen particularly with high RA pacing during counterclockwise AFL, whereby on termination of AFL, the negative flutter waves in the inferior leads change suddenly into upright P waves, thus reflecting a change in the atrial activation sequence to one of high RA pacing (i.e., simultaneous RA lateral and septal activation in a craniocaudal direction).[5] However, if the pacing site is distant from the AFL circuit (e.g., distal CS), a large mass of the atrial tissue can be captured by the pacing stimulus, to produce a marked change in P wave morphology (i.e., manifest fusion) without terminating the AFL. Failure to terminate AFL with rapid pacing can be caused by any of the following: (1) a short period of pacing or pacing at a relatively long CL—the closer the pacing CL is to the tachycardia CL, the longer the pacing duration will need to be to terminate the tachycardia; (2) a pacing site distant from the AFL circuit, with the intervening atrial tissue preventing penetration of the AFL circuit; or (3) the possibility that an apparent AFL on the ECG may actually be AF with streaming of the RA activation wavefront or may be a focal nonreentrant AT.[5,16]

OVERDRIVE SUPPRESSION. Overdrive suppression analogous to that seen with automatic AT is not expected in AFL. The post-pacing interval (PPI, measured from the last pacing stimulus that entrained the tachycardia to the next near-field recorded electrogram at the pacing site) remains relatively stable when entrainment of AFL is performed at the same site, regardless of the length of the pacing drive. This is in contrast to overdrive suppression seen in automatic ATs, which would be associated with progressive delay of the first tachycardia beat return cycle with progressively longer overdrive pacing drives.

ACCELERATION. Acceleration by overdrive pacing refers to sustained shortening of the tachycardia CL following cessation of pacing. Atrial pacing rarely can accelerate AFL into one of two different tachycardias: double-wave reentry or lower loop reentry.[16] Double-wave reentry is manifest by acceleration of the tachycardia rate but with identical surface and intracardiac electrogram morphology, and it can be recognized by having simultaneous activation of the superior and inferior regions of the tricuspid annulus, with all activation being sequential. This rhythm rarely lasts for more than a few beats and may serve as a trigger for AF. Lower loop reentry is a form of CTI-dependent AFL with a reentrant circuit around the IVC. This arrhythmia is usually transient and terminates by itself or converts spontaneously into AFL or AF (see Chap. 13).[19-21]

TRANSFORMATION. Rapid atrial burst pacing may convert AFL into AF. This is less likely with a slower pacing CL or pacing from sites within the AFL circuit. Induction of other forms of atrial macroreentry can also be observed, especially with faster pacing rates.[5]

Mapping

Activation Mapping

The simultaneous recording from endocardial sites around the tricuspid annulus (which encompasses most of the flutter macroreentrant circuit) by the Halo and CS catheters significantly facilitates activation mapping during typical AFL, and sequential point-by-point activation mapping is usually not required. The RA activation sequence during counterclockwise AFL occurs sequentially down the lateral RA wall and adjacent to the crista terminalis, across the CTI (with some delay because of slow conduction across the CTI), past the CS os, up the atrial septum, over the roof of the RA, and back to the lateral free wall of the RA (in a proximal-to-distal direction along the Halo electrodes; see Fig. 12-1). This sequence is reversed during clockwise AFL (see Fig. 12-1).

During AFL, double potentials are seen on the crista terminalis and along the eustachian ridge and indicate lines of block (fixed or functional) along those structures. Activation of the CS propagates in a proximal-to-distal direction.[12]

The atrial activation sequence in AFL is different from that during sinus rhythm or focal AT originating from the upper RA or LA, in which the activation wavefront propagates from the upper RA (middle or proximal Halo electrodes) down both the RA septum and lateral wall in a craniocaudal direction, toward the distal and proximal-most Halo electrodes.

Occasionally, P wave morphology on the surface ECG resembles typical AFL, but intracardiac recordings show that parts of the atria (commonly the LA) have disorganized atrial activity (Fig. 12-8). Such rhythms behave more like AF than AFL, but they may be converted to true typical AFL with antiarrhythmic drugs.[16]

As noted, double-wave reentry is characterized by an activation sequence identical to that of typical AFL, but at a faster atrial rate and with simultaneous activation of the superior and inferior regions of the tricuspid annulus, with all activation being sequential.

Entrainment Mapping

Entrainment mapping provides information about sites of the RA or LA that are part of the reentrant circuit, those that are outside the circuit, and the critical isthmus in the macroreentrant circuit. Entrainment also qualitatively estimates how far the reentrant circuit is from the pacing site. However, before attempting to use entrainment methods for mapping, it is necessary first to demonstrate that the tachycardia can be entrained, thus providing strong evidence that it is caused by reentry rather than by triggered activity or automaticity. At sites of entrainment, there should be confirmation of consistent capture of the atrium at the pacing CL for several beats with minimal or no change in the surface

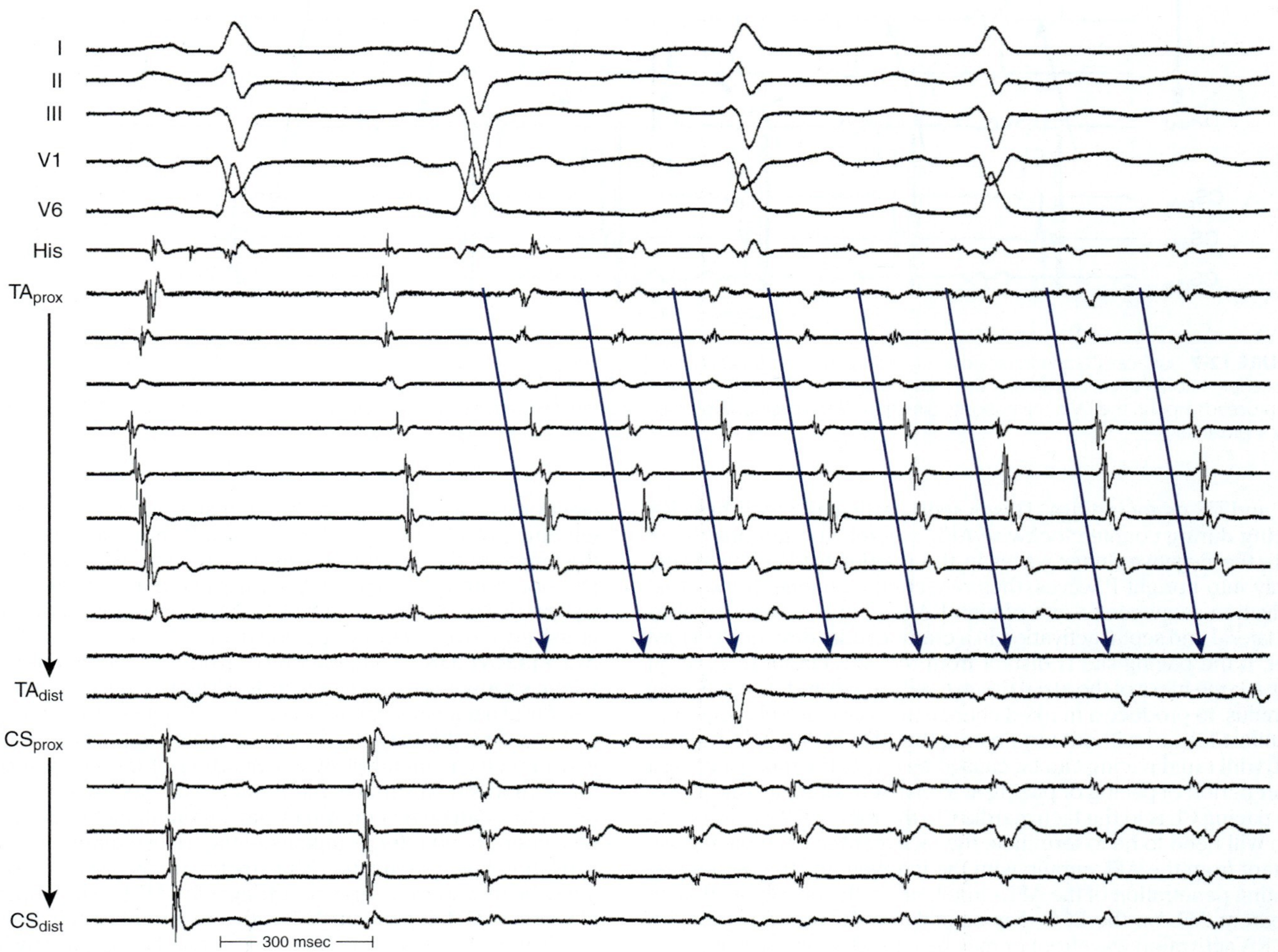

FIGURE 12-8 Surface ECG and intracardiac recordings of the onset of an episode of atrial fibrillation following cavotricuspid isthmus ablation. Activation around the tricuspid annulus (TA) follows a pattern like that in counterclockwise flutter (arrows) because of "streaming" of the wavefront between the crista terminalis and the TA. CS_{dist} = distal coronary sinus; CS_{prox} = proximal coronary sinus; TA_{dist} = distal tricuspid annulus; TA_{prox} = proximal tricuspid annulus.

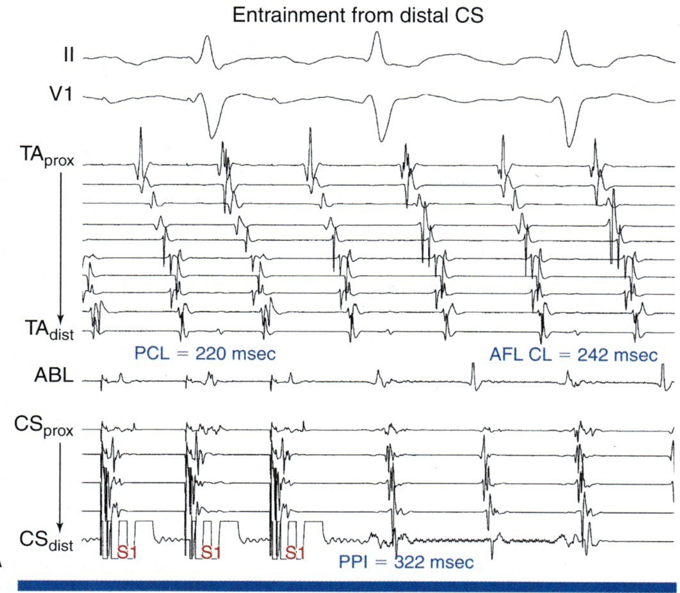

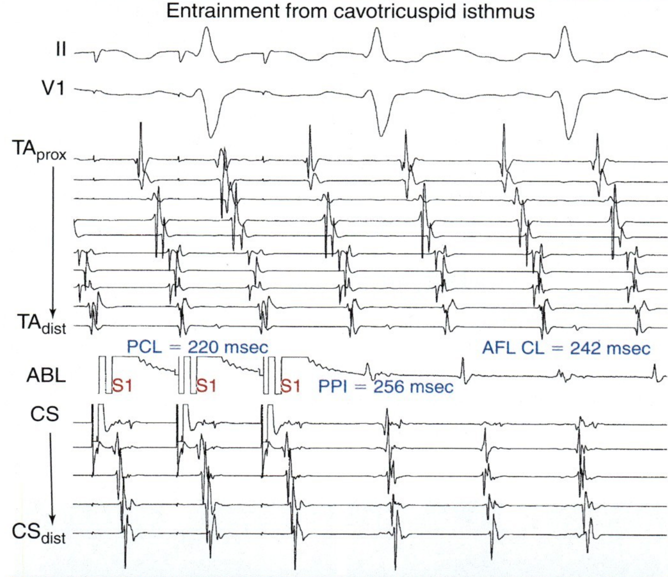

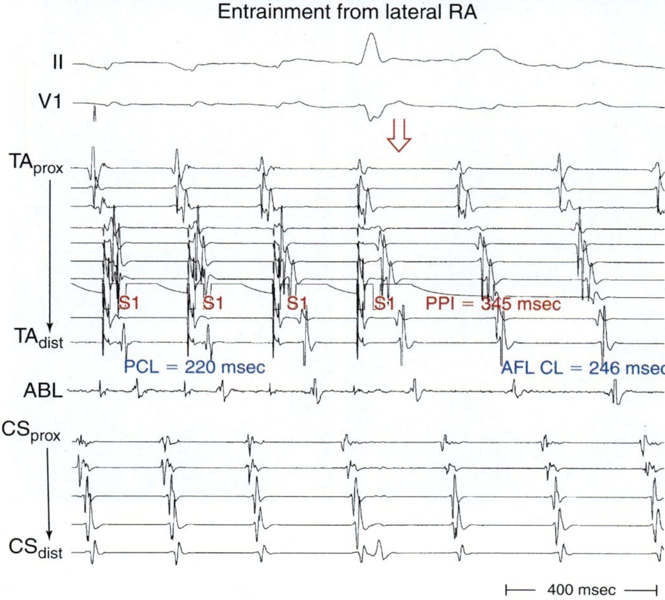

FIGURE 12-9 Entrainment of counterclockwise typical atrial flutter (AFL). **A,** Entrainment from the distal coronary sinus (CS) results in manifest atrial fusion and a long post-pacing interval (PPI; PPI – AFL cycle length [CL] = 80 milliseconds) because the distal CS is far from the reentrant circuit. **B,** Entrainment from ablation catheter positioned at the cavotricuspid isthmus (CTI) results in concealed atrial fusion with a short PPI (PPI – AFL CL = 14 milliseconds), a finding indicating that the CTI is part of the reentrant circuit. **C,** Entrainment from the lateral RA wall is attempted; however, the last paced stimulus fails to capture the atrium (open arrow); therefore, calculation of the PPI in this case is invalid and produces erroneous results. ABL = ablation site; CS_{dist} = distal coronary sinus; CS_{prox} = proximal coronary sinus; PCL = pacing cycle length; TA_{dist} = distal tricuspid annulus; TA_{prox} = proximal tricuspid annulus.

morphology or intracardiac electrograms and continuation of the identical tachycardia after pacing. Evaluation of the PPI or other criteria is meaningless when the presence of true entrainment has not been established. Additionally, it is important to verify the absence of termination and reinitiation of the tachycardia during the same pacing drive.[7]

Pacing is performed from the CTI, high RA, mid-lateral RA, and proximal and distal CS, but not on the septum, to avoid the possibility of capturing the LA, which could be confusing in distinguishing RA from LA flutters.

Once the presence of entrainment is verified, several criteria can be used to indicate the relation of the pacing site to the reentrant circuit. As discussed in detail in Chapter 13, the first entrainment criterion to be sought is concealed fusion. Entrainment with concealed fusion indicates that the pacing site is in a protected isthmus located within or attached to the reentrant circuit. Whether this protected isthmus is crucial to the reentrant circuit or just a bystander site needs to be verified by other criteria, mainly comparing the PPI with the tachycardia CL and the stimulus-exit interval with the electrogram-exit interval (Fig. 12-9). The diagnosis of CTI-dependent AFL is established when pacing from the CTI results in entrainment with concealed fusion and a PPI that is equal (within 20 milliseconds) to the flutter CL and an electrogram-exit interval that is equal (within 20 milliseconds) to the stimulus-exit interval. During counterclockwise AFL, a site medial to the CTI, such as the CS os, may be used to represent the exit of the reentrant wavefront. Conversely, in clockwise AFL, a site lateral to the tricuspid annulus, such as the distal Halo electrode, may be used (Table 12-1).[17,18]

Electroanatomical Mapping

Although atrial activation sequences in the Halo and CS catheters combined with entrainment mapping techniques are usually adequate for the diagnosis of CTI-dependent typical AFL and facilitation of ablation of the CTI, electromagnetic three-dimensional (3-D) mapping (CARTO mapping system [Biosense Webster, Diamond Bar, Calif.] or EnSite NavX system [St. Jude Medical, St. Paul, Minn.]) can help distinguish between a focal origin and macroreentrant tachycardia by providing precise description of the macroreentrant circuit and sequence of atrial activation during the tachycardia and rapid visualization of the activation wavefront.

Initially, selection of the reference electrogram, positioning of the anatomical reference, and determination of the window of interest are undertaken. The reference catheter is usually placed in the CS (because of its stability), and an electrode recording a prominent atrial electrogram is selected, thus ensuring that the ventricular electrogram is not the one detected by the system.

The mapping-ablation catheter is initially positioned, using fluoroscopy, at known anatomical points that serve as landmarks for the electroanatomical map. Anatomical and EP landmarks (IVC, SVC, CS, HB, and tricuspid annulus) are tagged. A set of six specific points (three at the tricuspid annulus and three at the mouth of the IVC) is acquired to delineate the individual isthmus anatomy. The catheter is then advanced slowly around the chamber walls to sample multiple points along the endocardium, thereby sequentially acquiring the location of its tip together with the local electrogram. Activation mapping is performed to define the atrial activation sequence. Reasonable numbers of points are homogeneously distributed in the RA, with careful mapping of endocardial sites around the tricuspid annulus and CTI. The local activation time at each site is determined from the intracardiac bipolar electrogram and is measured in relation to the fixed intracardiac electrogram obtained from the CS (reference) catheter. The activation map may also be used to catalog sites at which pacing maneuvers are performed during assessment of the tachycardia (e.g., sites with good pace maps). Activation maps display the local activation time by a color-coded overlay on the reconstructed 3-D geometry (see Videos 11 and 16). The selected points of local activation time are color-coded.

TABLE 12-1 Entrainment Mapping of Typical Atrial Flutter

Pacing from sites *outside* the AFL circuit (e.g., from RA appendage or middle or distal CS) results in the following:
• Manifest atrial fusion on the surface ECG or intracardiac recordings (fixed fusion at a single pacing CL, or both, and progressive fusion on progressively shorter pacing CLs). During entrainment, any difference in atrial activation sequence compared with that during tachycardia (as determined by analysis of all available surface ECG and intracardiac recordings) is considered to represent manifest fusion. • PPI – tachycardia CL > 20 msec • The interval between the stimulus artifact to the onset of the flutter wave on the surface ECG is longer than the interval between the local electrogram on the pacing site to the onset of the flutter wave on the surface ECG.
Pacing from sites inside the AFL circuit (e.g., from the CS os or around the tricuspid annulus) results in the following:
• Manifest atrial fusion on surface ECG or intracardiac recordings (fixed fusion at a single pacing CL, or both, and progressive fusion on progressively shorter pacing CL) • PPI – tachycardia CL < 20 msec • The interval between the stimulus artifact to the onset of the flutter wave on the surface ECG is equal to the interval between the local electrogram on the pacing site to the onset of the flutter wave on the surface ECG.
Pacing from a protected isthmus inside the circuit (cavotricuspid isthmus) results in the following:
• Concealed atrial fusion (i.e., paced atrial waveform on the surface ECG and intracardiac recordings is identical to the AFL waveform) • PPI – tachycardia CL < 20 msec • The interval between the stimulus artifact to the onset of the flutter wave on the surface ECG is equal to the interval between the local electrogram on the pacing site to the onset of the flutter wave on the surface ECG.

AFL = atrial flutter; CL = cycle length; CS = coronary sinus; CS os = coronary sinus ostium; PPI = post-pacing interval; RA = right atrium.

High-density 3-D electroanatomical maps during AFL can be useful in delineating the specific features of the AFL circuit and global RA activation during AFL. The activation map typically demonstrates a continuous progression of colors (from red to purple in the CARTO system and from white to purple in the NavX system) around the tricuspid annulus with close proximity of earliest and latest local activation and an activation time in a similar range to tachycardia CL, consistent with macroreentry (Figs. 12-10 and 12-11). The activation wavefront exits the CTI as a broad wavefront, spreading anterosuperiorly around the tricuspid annulus and posterosuperiorly. Lateral spread of the posterior wavefront is blocked along the vertical line in the posterolateral RA, a region marked by double potentials that coincides with the crista terminalis. The posterior wavefront propagates cranially around the SVC to merge with the activation wavefront circulating around the tricuspid annulus. The anterolateral wall of the RA is the last to activate as the wavefront reenters the lateral aspect of the CTI.

The 3-D electroanatomical maps can also provide information about the voltage characteristics of the tissues involved in the CTI. The lower the voltage, the easier it is to achieve block in the tissue. Thus, 3-D electroanatomical mapping may help choose a path in the CTI that is easier to ablate, a path that may not necessarily be the shortest across the isthmus.

Noncontact Mapping

The EnSite 3000 noncontact mapping system (St. Jude Medical, St. Paul, Minn.) consists of a noncontact catheter with a multielectrode array surrounding a 7.5-mL balloon mounted at the distal end. The 9 Fr balloon catheter is advanced over a 0.035-inch guidewire under fluoroscopy guidance and is positioned in the middle

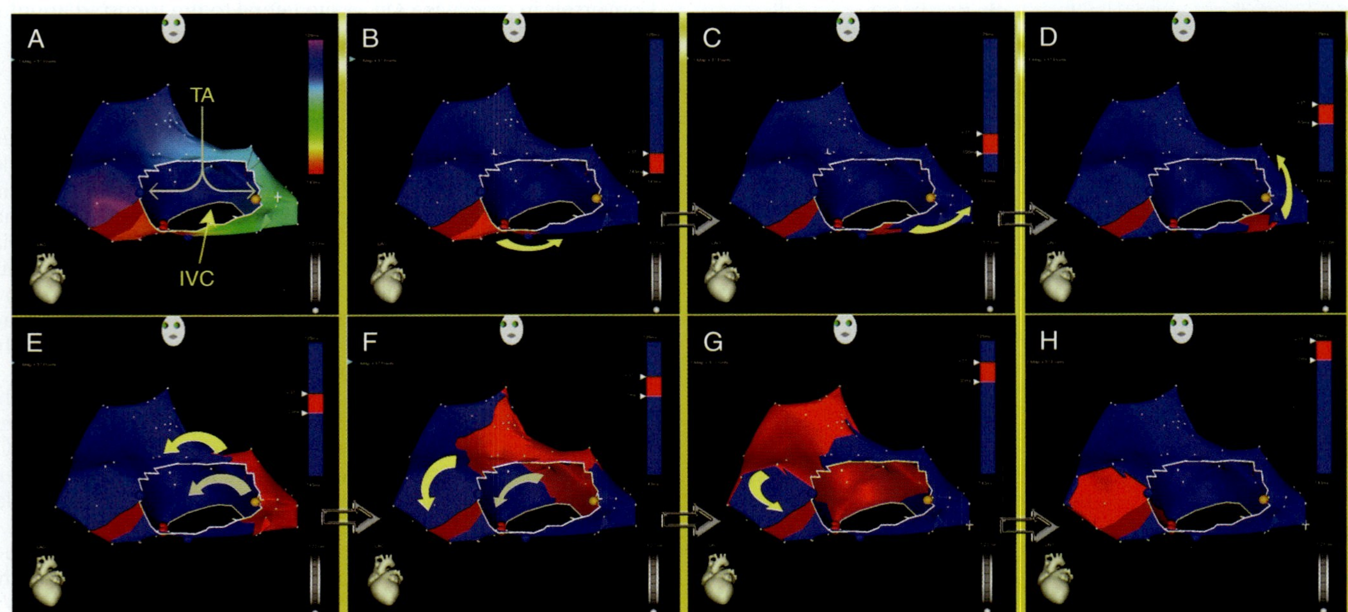

FIGURE 12-10 **A,** Three-dimensional electroanatomical (CARTO, Biosense Webster, Diamond Bar, Calif.) activation map of the right atrium (RA) in the left anterior oblique view constructed during counterclockwise typical atrial flutter (AFL). During tachycardia, the depolarization wavefront travels counterclockwise around the tricuspid annulus (TA), as indicated by a continuous progression of colors (from red to purple) with close proximity of earliest and latest local activation (red meeting purple). **B** to **H,** Propagation map of the RA during counterclockwise typical AFL (arrows). IVC = inferior vena cava.

and lower portion of the RA. The balloon is positioned in the center of the atrium and does not come in contact with the atrial walls being mapped. Intravenous heparin is administered before balloon deployment to keep the activated clotting time at 250 to 300 seconds. A conventional mapping-ablation catheter is used to collect geometry information. The mapping catheter is initially moved to known anatomical locations (IVC, SVC, CS, HB, and tricuspid annulus), which are tagged. Detailed geometry of the chamber is then reconstructed by moving the mapping catheter around the atrium.

After the chamber geometry is determined, mapping of the arrhythmia can begin. The data acquisition process is performed automatically by the system, and all data for the entire chamber are acquired simultaneously. The system then reconstructs unipolar electrograms simultaneously and superimposes them onto the virtual endocardium, to produce isopotential maps with a color range representing voltage amplitude (Fig. 12-12; see Video 9). A default high-pass filter setting of 2 Hz is used to preserve components of slow conduction on the isopotential map. Color settings are adjusted so that the color range matches 1 to 1 with the millivolt range of the electrogram deflection of interest. Activation can be tracked on the isopotential map throughout the tachycardia cycle. Isochronal maps can also be created that represent progression of activation throughout the chamber relative to a user-defined electrical reference timing point (see Fig. 12-12).[22]

Although typical AFL is usually readily treated using standard ablation techniques, noncontact mapping can be used to confirm the anatomical location of the flutter circuit, reduce fluoroscopy time, and confirm CTI block after ablation. Noncontact mapping

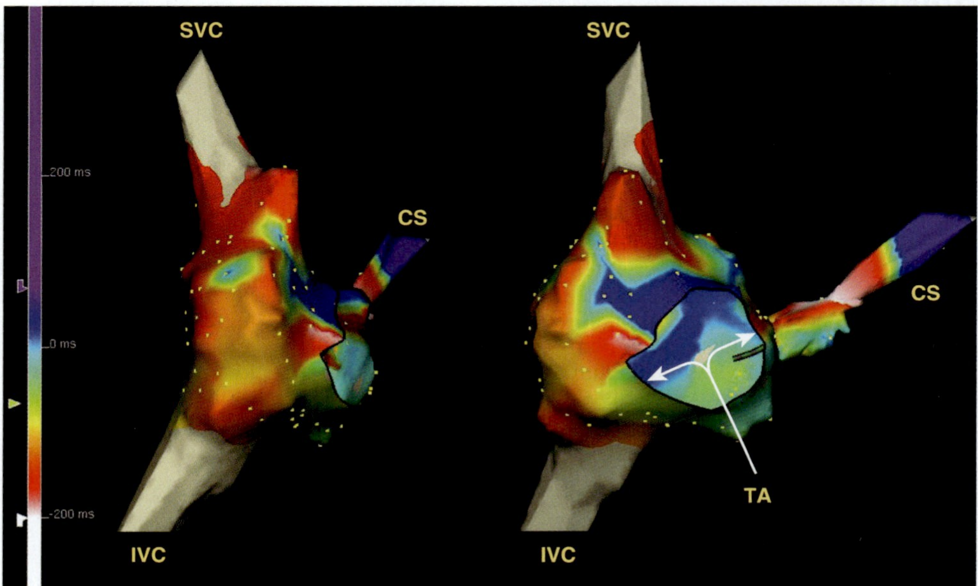

FIGURE 12-11 EnSite-NavX (St. Jude Medical, St. Paul, Minn.) three-dimensional electroanatomical activation map of the right atrium in the left anterior oblique **(left)** and anteroposterior **(right)** views constructed during counterclockwise typical atrial flutter. During tachycardia, the depolarization wavefront travels counterclockwise around the tricuspid annulus (TA), as indicated by a continuous progression of colors (from white to purple) with close proximity of earliest and latest local activation. CS = coronary sinus; IVC = inferior vena cava; SVC = superior vena cava.

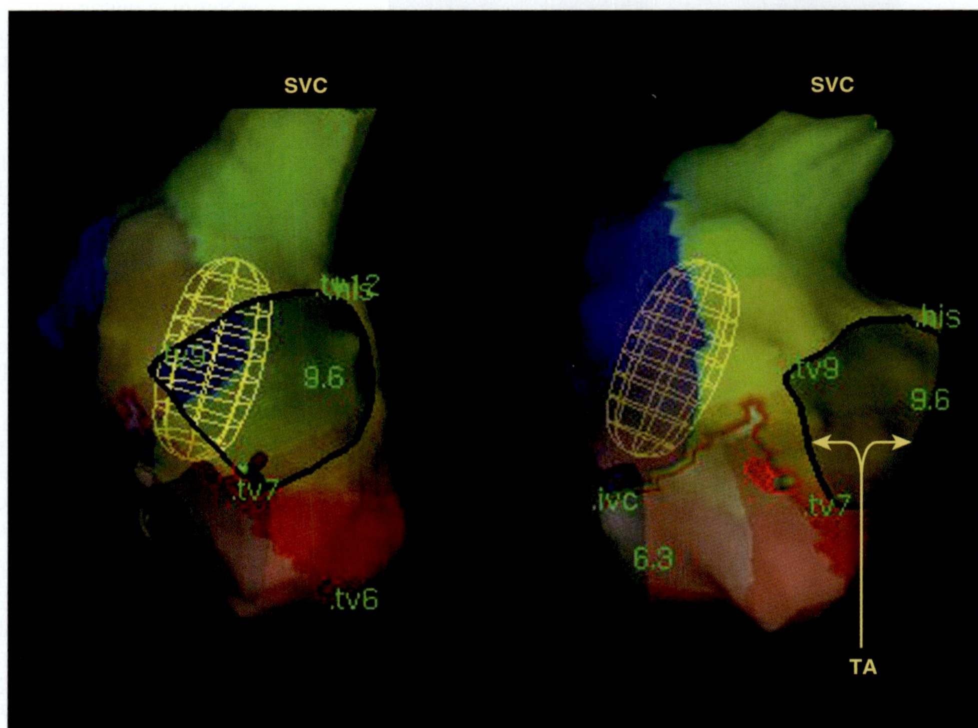

FIGURE 12-12 Noncontact mapping of typical atrial flutter (AFL). Shown are left anterior oblique and posteroanterior views of a color-coded isopotential map of right atrial activation during counterclockwise typical AFL. SVC = superior vena cava; TA = tricuspid annulus.

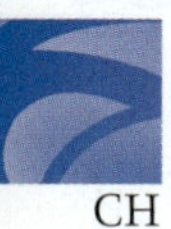

has also been used to identify and guide radiofrequency (RF) ablation of the site of residual conduction following incomplete linear ablation lesions at the isthmus. Because of its ability to record from multiple sites simultaneously, noncontact mapping can rapidly identify gaps in linear lesions. This is accomplished by analysis of one or more paced complexes originating adjacent to the line being assessed. This capability can be particularly helpful in patients who have recurrent AFL following a previous ablation. Because any number of maps can be superimposed on the initial geometry, bidirectional block at the ablation site can be rapidly identified during pacing following ablation. Tagging ablation areas during delivery of each RF impulse and a constantly visible ablation line offer another advantage—they ensure that no area is overlooked or ablated repeatedly.

Ablation

Target of Ablation

The CTI is the ideal target of AFL ablation because it is accessible, relatively narrow, short, safe to ablate, and essential for the AFL circuit (and not because it is the diseased area or the structure causing the AFL).[23] The central part of the isthmus (the 6 o'clock region in a fluoroscopic LAO view) appears to be the optimal target site because it is the thinner part of the isthmus (19 ± 4 mm; range, 13 to 26 mm) and therefore is less likely to resist RF ablation. Other advantages of the central isthmus are the increased distance from the paraseptal isthmus, which contains, in 10% of cases, extensions of the AVN or AVN artery, and the increased distance from the inferolateral isthmus, where the right coronary artery is in close proximity to the endocardium (less than 4 mm).[1,24]

Alternatively, the tricuspid annulus–CS or IVC-CS isthmuses may be targeted (Fig. 12-13). However, for this approach to be successful, ablation within the CS is probably necessary. Such approaches are less successful in curing AFL.[16] The paraseptal isthmus (tricuspid annulus–CS isthmus) has the thickest wall, compared with other parts of the inferior RA isthmus, although there is significant interindividual variability, and this structure is close to the arterial branch supplying the AVN and, in some cases, can contain the inferior extensions of the AVN. The inferolateral isthmus is the longest and is in closest proximity to the right coronary artery.[24]

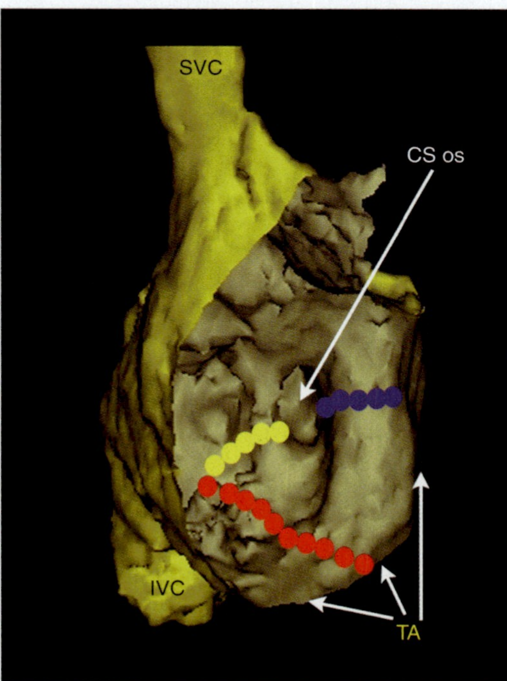

FIGURE 12-13 Computed tomography scan of the right atrium (RA; cardioscopic view) illustrating the typical location for linear ablation of the cavotricuspid isthmus (red dots), the tricuspid valve–coronary sinus (CS) isthmus (blue dots), and the CS–inferior vena cava (IVC) isthmus (yellow dots). CS os = coronary sinus ostium.

Ablation Technique

Periprocedural anticoagulation for catheter ablation of persistent AFL is necessary to minimize thromboembolic stroke risk. LA stunning and increased spontaneous echo contrast within the LA can occur following cardioversion or ablation of these arrhythmias. A perception of increased bleeding risks of invasive procedures undertaken while a patient is receiving therapeutic warfarin doses led many operators to adopt a "bridging" strategy of conversion to enoxaparin, to allow ablation and subsequent hemostasis to be performed during a pause in anticoagulation (a strategy also recommended by the Heart Rhythm Society/European Heart Rhythm Association/European Cardiac Arrhythmia Society expert consensus statement).[25] This strategy involves discontinuation of warfarin at least 3 to 5 days prior to ablation and starting heparin or enoxaparin after cessation of warfarin until the evening prior to the ablation procedure. Both enoxaparin and warfarin are then reinitiated within 4 to 6 hours after ablation and sheath removal, and enoxaparin is maintained until an optimal international normalized ratio (INR) level is achieved. However, an alternative strategy of uninterrupted periprocedure oral anticoagulation was found to be safer and more cost-effective for ablation of typical AFL. Bleeding complications were less frequent. Using this strategy, INR testing is required on the day of the procedure to confirm therapeutic anticoagulation, and transesophageal echocardiography is performed in patients with a subtherapeutic INR in the 3 weeks prior to the procedure. Another potential advantage of this strategy is the ability to reverse the effects of warfarin rapidly in the setting of a bleeding complication (e.g., pericardial bleeding) by using synthetic clotting factor concentrates or fresh frozen plasma infusion, whereas the effects of enoxaparin remain difficult to reverse; protamine has only a partial effect on its action.[26]

CATHETER POSITIONING

A steerable ablation catheter with a distal ablation electrode of 4 or 8 mm is generally used.[27] The catheter's curve size and shape can affect the ability to position the catheter on the CTI, and the use of preshaped guiding sheaths (e.g., SR0, SL1, or ramp sheath; Daig, Minnetonka, Minn.) can help stabilize the catheter position and prevent the catheter from sliding off the CTI and in and out of the right ventricle (RV).

The CTI can be localized electroanatomically. The ablation catheter is advanced to the RV under fluoroscopy (right anterior oblique [RAO] view); the tip is deflected to achieve contact with the RV inferior wall and is withdrawn progressively until the electrogram shows small atrial and large ventricular electrograms. The distal tip of the ablation catheter is then adjusted under fluoroscopy on the CTI in the LAO view until it is midway between the atrial septum and RA lateral wall (pointing toward 6 o'clock in a 45-degree LAO view; Fig. 12-14; Video 18).

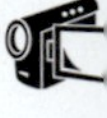

The ratio of the atrial and ventricular electrogram amplitude (A/V ratio) can help localize the position of the ablation catheter; the A/V ratio is typically 1:4 or less at the tricuspid annulus, 1:2 to 1:1 at the CTI, and 2:1 to 4:1 near the IVC. The location of the catheter at the CTI can also be confirmed by demonstrating entrainment with concealed fusion during AFL.

RADIOFREQUENCY ABLATION

After positioning of the ablation catheter on or near the tricuspid annulus, the catheter is gradually withdrawn either toward the IVC during continuous energy application (50 to 70 W, 60 to 120 seconds, targeting a temperature of 55°C to 60°C), or in a stepwise manner with sequentially interrupted point-by-point application of

RF energy (50 to 70 W, 30 to 60 seconds, targeting a temperature of 55°C to 60°C). The first RF lesion is initiated from the tricuspid annulus edge with large ventricular and small atrial electrograms, and the last lesion is completed at the IVC edge. It is important that linear lesions span completely from the tricuspid annulus to the IVC (Fig. 12-15). After each RF application, the electrogram loses voltage and may become fragmented; the catheter is then withdrawn (2 to 4 mm at a time) toward the IVC until a new area of sharp atrial electrogram is reached, and the next RF application is delivered. This is repeated until the lack of atrial electrograms indicates that the catheter has reached the IVC. Before each RF application, the position of the ablation catheter is confirmed fluoroscopically, as described, or by using a 3-D mapping-navigation system.

During delivery of RF energy, AFL can terminate or its CL can increase transiently or permanently, and a gradual delay in activation of the low lateral RA wall can occur. This indicates that the ablation lesions have affected the circuit and should lead to continuation of RF delivery or extension of the lesion to ensure the achievement of complete conduction block across the CTI.

Ablation of the CTI may require more than one pass of RF delivery across the isthmus. It may be necessary to rotate the ablation catheter away from the initial line of energy application, medially or laterally in the isthmus, to create new or additional lines of block. At the time of the second pass-over, the ablation line isthmus electrograms will be fragmented, of low voltage, and often double.

A complete line of block is identified by a continuous corridor of double potentials separated by an isoelectric interval (Fig. 12-16). Further ablation is usually not needed at sites that exhibit double potentials because this finding generally indicates that local conduction block is already present. Gaps in the ablation line (i.e., sites of persistent conduction) are characterized by single- or triple-fractionated potentials centered on or occupying the isoelectric interval of the adjacent double potential (see Fig. 12-16). These gaps should be ablated until complete CTI block is achieved. In 15% to 20% of cases, it can be extremely difficult to produce CTI block, which can be secondary to one or more of the following: (1) a very prominent eustachian ridge; (2) a thick isthmus, preventing transmural ablation; and (3) local edema, clot, or superficial damage forming a barrier for deeper penetration of subsequent RF applications.[23]

MAXIMUM VOLTAGE-GUIDED TECHNIQUE

The maximum voltage-guided technique is based on the hypothesis that discrete muscle bundles in the CTI participate in the flutter circuit. Large atrial electrogram voltages identify the location of these muscle bundles along the isthmus and are selectively targeted for ablation. In effect, bidirectional CTI block is produced by the summation of a series of discrete focal ablations, rather than a continuous ablation line across the CTI.[28]

Using this technique, the CTI is mapped in the 6 o'clock position, and bipolar atrial electrograms (during AFL or, preferably, during sinus rhythm or CS pacing) are measured from peak to peak during a continuous pull-back along the isthmus. The site of maximum voltage is noted and used as a marker for a presumed muscle bundle. The ablation catheter is positioned at this site, regardless of the location along the line, and RF ablation is performed for 40 to 60 seconds until an amplitude reduction of 50% or more is achieved. If the ablation lesion does not result in bidirectional CTI block, the line is remapped, and the next largest atrial electrogram is sequentially targeted for ablation. This is repeated until bidirectional CTI block is achieved. This technique therefore targets the signals with

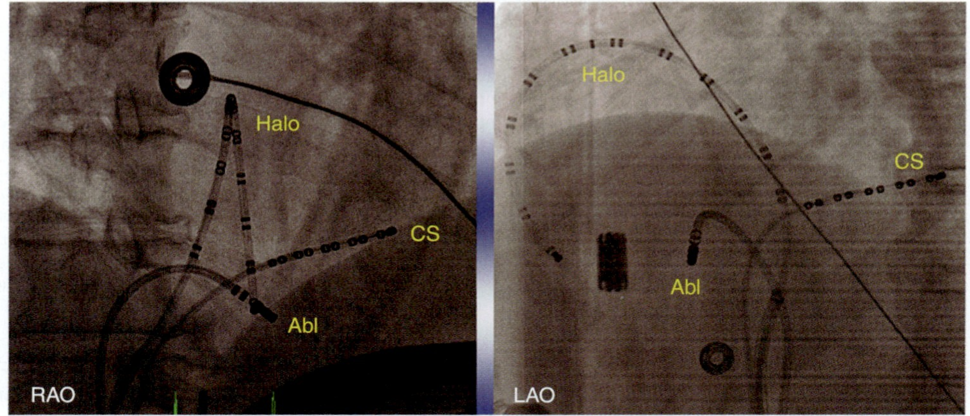

FIGURE 12-14 Fluoroscopic views (right anterior oblique [RAO] and left anterior oblique [LAO]) illustrating catheter location during ablation (Abl) of the cavotricuspid isthmus. CS = coronary sinus.

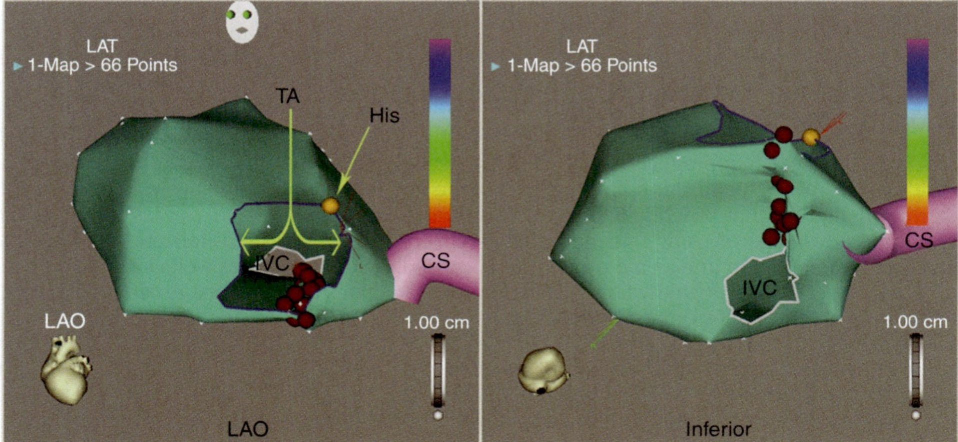

FIGURE 12-15 Ablation of the cavotricuspid isthmus (CTI) guided by CARTO (Biosense Webster, Diamond Bar, Calif.). The left anterior oblique (LAO) and inferior views of the reconstructed right atrium geometry are shown. Linear ablation (red dots) is performed across the CTI between the tricuspid annulus (TA) and inferior vena cava (IVC). CS = coronary sinus.

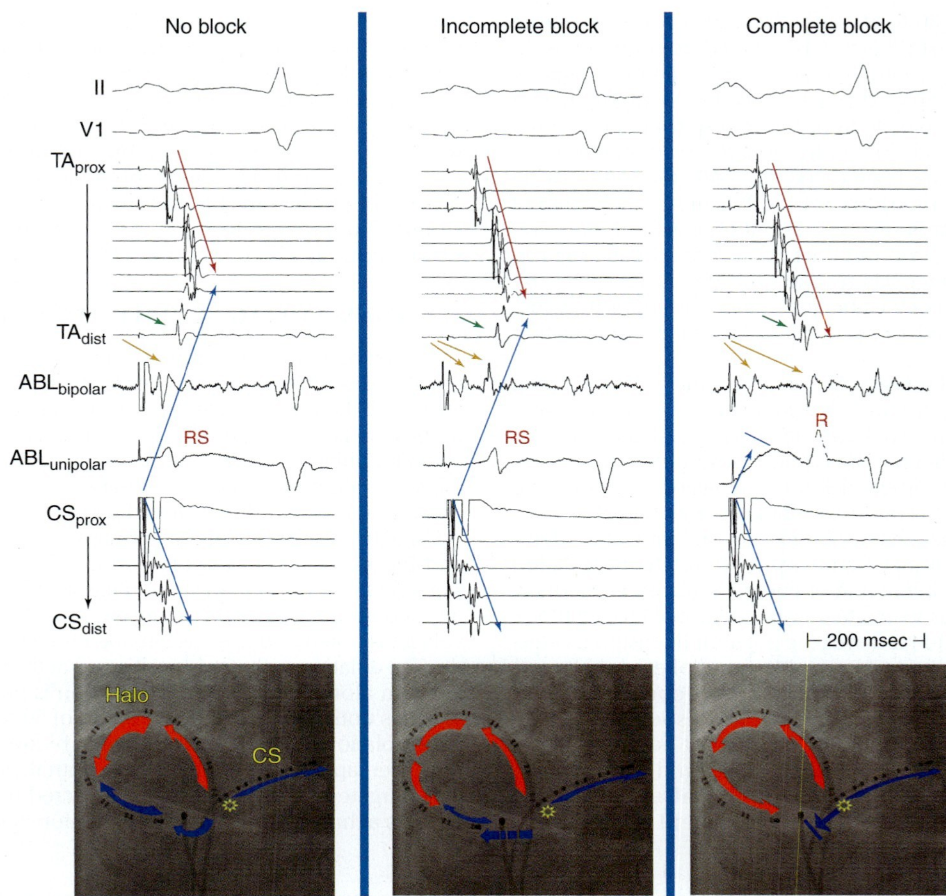

FIGURE 12-16 The use of coronary sinus (CS) pacing to verify the presence of clockwise cavotricuspid isthmus (CTI) block. **Upper panels,** Intracardiac recordings from the right atrium (RA), CS, and CTI. **Lower panels,** Left anterior oblique fluoroscopic view illustrating the position of the ablation catheter at the CTI, and the Halo catheter around the tricuspid annulus (TA), with the distal end at the lateral end of the CTI. When CTI conduction is intact (**left panel),** pacing from the coronary sinus ostium results in the collision of activation wavefronts in the lateral RA wall (red and blue arrows). **Middle panel,** The collision point moves toward the low lateral RA wall when incomplete block is present. **Right panel,** Complete clockwise CTI block is indicated by the observation of a purely descending wavefront at the lateral wall down to the CTI (proximal-to-distal Halo sequence). The bipolar electrogram recording from the CTI initially shows a single atrial potential (**left panel,** gold arrow). With partial CTI ablation, the atrial electrogram splits into two closely adjacent potentials (**middle panel,** gold arrows). Complete CTI block is indicated by the observation of double potentials separated by an isoelectric interval (**right panel,** gold arrows). Additionally, bipolar electrogram polarity reversal (**left panel**) is observed in the distal Halo and the distal ablation electrode recordings when complete block is achieved (as compared with before complete CTI block is achieved in the **right** and **middle panels**), thus indicating reversal of the direction of the activation wavefront lateral to the line of block (green and gold arrows). Positive (R wave) morphology of the unipolar recording lateral to the line of block also indicates complete CTI block (in contrast to biphasic [RS] electrogram morphology when intact conduction or only incomplete block is present). ABL = ablation site; CS_{dist} = distal coronary sinus; CS_{prox} = proximal coronary sinus; TA_{dist} = distal tricuspid annulus; TA_{prox} = proximal tricuspid annulus.

highest amplitude along the CTI and does not necessitate a contiguous line of ablation. This technique was found to reduce ablation times significantly compared with a purely anatomical approach; however, this did not translate into a reduction in fluoroscopy or overall procedure time.[28-31]

ROLE OF THREE-DIMENSIONAL ELECTROANATOMICAL MAPPING NAVIGATION SYSTEMS

Electroanatomical mapping systems (CARTO or NavX) can provide precise spatial localization and tracking of the ablation catheter along the CTI that potentially help shorten fluoroscopy time. The main advantage of using this mapping system for AFL is the visibility of an ablation line as the procedure is carried out so that no area is left out or repeatedly ablated. Therefore, it facilitates the creation of ablation lines devoid of gaps across the entire isthmus (see Fig. 12-15).[32]

After the usual anatomical landmarks are taken, detailed CTI mapping is performed by withdrawing the catheter at 2- to 3-mm intervals and taking several points along the line. Additionally, multiple points at the tricuspid annulus and at the mouth of the IVC are acquired to delineate isthmus anatomy. One specific point is acquired at the most inferior point of the tricuspid annulus, whereby a small atrial electrogram and a larger ventricular electrogram are recorded. The catheter is then slightly rotated to two additional points at the tricuspid annulus, 1.5 to 2 cm septally and laterally. Three points are then acquired at the mouth of the IVC: one directly opposite to the inferior point of the tricuspid annulus and the other two points slightly lateral and medial to this point. In this way, the myocardial isthmus extension can be clearly defined and can be depicted in the 3-D space. The isthmus region forms a relatively flat rectangular surface in a caudal projection, and a side-on view is provided by the RAO projection.[33] These views allow visualization of lateral and septal displacement of the catheter tip, as well as the distance from the tricuspid annulus and the IVC. The ablation line can be planned by a trial run across the isthmus. During RF application, the line is placed to connect the most anterior and posterior points in the CTI. Each tag is approximately 4 mm in diameter, thus permitting visual estimation of the density of applications needed to produce a linear lesion during the drag. This helps avoid redundant lesion application and can identify potential gaps in the ablation line.[32]

Furthermore, electroanatomical mapping also provides information about the voltage characteristics of the tissues involved in the CTI. This information can be of value in selecting ablation targets and choosing a path across the isthmus that is easier to ablate, which may not necessarily be the shortest path. Voltage mapping of the isthmus is particularly helpful in patients with recurrent AFL following previous ablation attempts; high-voltage and breakthrough sites identified during activation and voltage mapping may then be chosen as ablation targets.

Verification of CTI conduction block following ablation can also be carried out using electroanatomical mapping systems. The activation wavefront during AFL halts at the previously completed line but continues through the breakthrough site (see later).

The benefits of electroanatomical mapping compared with conventional mapping for catheter ablation have been clearly demonstrated in various arrhythmia entities, such as focal AT, macroreentrant AT ("atypical AFL"), AF, and ventricular tachycardia. These benefits include the ability of the technology for exact anatomical reconstruction, renavigation of the catheter accurately to positions removed from fluoroscopic markers, and precise electroanatomical identification of an arrhythmia origin or reentrant circuit. In the setting of typical AFL, however, the reentrant circuit and critical isthmus can be identified in most cases by using conventional mapping and fluoroscopic methods. Therefore, it is not surprising that the use of electroanatomical mapping and ablation in one report did not improve on the efficacy and the duration of the procedure as compared with the conventional technique. Nevertheless, fluoroscopy exposure time in that study was significantly reduced in the electroanatomical ablation group by almost 50%. However, this achievement was associated with an increase in the cost of the procedure.[33]

APPROACH TO THE DIFFICULT CAVOTRICUSPID ISTHMUS ABLATION

Although ablation of typical AFL is successful in more than 90% of cases, occasionally inordinate difficulties can be encountered when attempting to terminate the flutter and create bidirectional conduction block across the CTI. The first step in these instances is to reconfirm the diagnosis of CTI-dependent AFL by entrainment mapping on the septal, lateral, and middle portion of the isthmus. Once the diagnosis of typical AFL is verified, other potential contributors to failure of CTI ablation should be considered, including poor catheter contact, inadequate power delivery, thick myocardium, and discontinuous ablation line, typically caused by the presence of pouches, recesses, ridges, and trabeculations within the CTI. These factors can also be responsible for recovery of CTI conduction and recurrent AFL in the follow-up after an acutely successful ablation.[1,34,35]

RF ablation catheters with a large (8-mm) distal electrode and irrigated-tip catheters allow the creation of larger lesions in high- and low-flow regions. These catheters can facilitate ablation of the CTI by achieving a high success rate with a smaller number of RF lesions, shorter procedure times, and less fluoroscopy exposure, as compared with a standard 4-mm electrode.[27,36,37]

When present, deep subeustachian pouches tend to be most prominent in the vestibular portion close to the septum and are typically associated with a prominent thebesian valve (which guards the CS os). The presence of a prominent subeustachian pouch can be suggested by a characteristic inferior dip of the catheter tip when the ablation catheter is dragged back across the isthmus toward the IVC. Catheter stability and power delivery for ablation within these pouches are suboptimal, and it is difficult to create a contiguous ablation line. Performing ablation relatively more laterally, particularly over the vestibular portion of the isthmus, may circumvent the problems with power delivery and potential perforation when ablating within a pouch. If linear ablation more laterally is unsuccessful because of poor catheter stability or thick myocardium, internal or external irrigation catheters may be used, with careful titration of energy delivery to avoid steam pops. When ablation is still unsuccessful, adequate visualization of the pouch (using RA angiography or phased-array intracardiac echocardiography) can be necessary to guide ablation within or around the pouch.[1,34,35]

Prominent pectinate muscles encroaching on the CTI can be suggested by the presence of sites with unusually high-voltage electrograms (from pectinate muscle ridges) surrounded by areas where abrupt impedance rises and minimal power delivery (likely from poor blood flow in the crevices between pectinate muscles) occurs. The thickness of prominent pectinates can prevent transmural ablation lesions and hamper adequate catheter stability. Additionally, the catheter tip can become wedged between the pectinate muscles with consequent inadequate power delivery with impedance rise, and coagulum formation may occur because of poor blood circulation. In these situations, performing ablation closer to the septum, where the pectinate muscle is less prominent, and using large-tip or irrigated-tip catheters can help achieve successful ablation.[1,34,35]

A prominent eustachian ridge can hinder catheter manipulation to the septal aspect of the isthmus because the crest of the ridge can act as a fulcrum, directing the catheter tip laterally (instead of the expected medial rotation) when clockwise torque is applied. Additionally, when the eustachian ridge is prominent, electrode contact may be difficult to maintain on the upslope of the ridge (the portion between the crest of the eustachian ridge and the tricuspid annulus). In these situations, the use of preshaped guiding sheaths (e.g., SR0, SL1, or ramp sheath) often solves the problem.[1,34]

DUTY-CYCLED, BIPOLAR-UNIPOLAR RADIOFREQUENCY ABLATION

A novel ablation system (GENius, Ablation Frontiers, Inc., Carlsbad, Calif.) has been developed, in which duty-cycled and alternating unipolar and bipolar RF energy is delivered using a multielectrode ablation catheter (the Tip-Versatile Ablation Catheter [T-VAC], Ablation Frontiers) to create contiguous linear ablation lesions across the CTI.[38]

The T-VAC is a 9 Fr hexapolar catheter with a 4-mm tip electrode and five 2-mm band electrodes (all on 3-mm interelectrode spacing, see Fig. 7-4). The catheter has bidirectional asymmetric steering. All six electrodes contain two thermocouples, on opposite sides of the ring face, each directed toward the endocardial surface when the device is steered, to allow optimal sensing of endocardial surface temperature.

The multichannel generator delivers RF energy in a temperature-controlled, power-limited manner, but only up to a maximum of 45 W at the tip electrode and 20 W for each ring electrode. As a result of this configuration, a 30-mm-long contiguous linear lesion can be created with one RF application. The entire catheter is laid flat across the isthmus and then is pressed on the isthmus by pulling the entire catheter caudally to avoid the gaps in the ablation line. Additionally, the multielectrode catheter allows selective mapping and ablation through any or all electrodes as required.[39]

This system is still undergoing investigation. Preliminary clinical experience has been promising. Bidirectional block across the CTI could be achieved with fewer than three RF applications, thus leading to significant decreases in procedure time, RF time, and fluoroscopy exposure.[39]

CRYOABLATION

Complete CTI block can also be achieved by cryothermal ablation. Although there is no reason to believe that cryothermal ablation will be more effective than RF ablation of the CTI, cryothermal ablation has the advantage of being less painful. Acute success rates are comparable to those for RF ablation.[40] A prospective randomized trial comparing RF and cryothermal energy for ablation of typical AFL suggested that lesion durability from cryoablation (using an 8-mm-tip catheter [Freezor MAX, Medtronic CryoCath, Montreal]) was significantly inferior to that of RF ablation. Although acutely successful ablation rates in the cryoablation group were comparable to those for RF ablation (89% versus 91%), persistence of bidirectional CTI block in patients treated with cryoablation reinvestigated 3 months following ablation was inferior to that in patients treated with RF ablation, as evidenced by the higher recurrence rate of symptomatic, ECG-documented AFL (10.9% versus 0%) and higher asymptomatic conduction recurrence rates (23.4% versus 15%). Additionally, compared with RF ablation, cryoablation is associated with significantly longer procedure times. This is driven mainly by differences in ablation duration, which can be attributed to the longer duration of each cryoablation (4 minutes) compared with RF ablation (up to 60 seconds).[41,42]

Endpoints of Ablation

Ablation can be performed during AFL or CS pacing.[43] If ablation is carried out during AFL, the first endpoint is to terminate AFL during RF energy delivery. If AFL is terminated, programmed electrical stimulation and burst atrial pacing should be performed immediately to determine whether AFL is still reinducible. If AFL is not terminated or is reinducible, ablation should be repeated. If AFL is terminated and is not reinducible, pacing maneuvers should be performed to determine whether there is bidirectional block in the CTI. Termination of AFL during RF delivery is often not associated with complete bidirectional CTI block and should not be considered a reliable ablation endpoint by itself. Once complete bidirectional CTI block has been achieved, reconfirmation should be repeated 30 minutes after the last RF application.[2,6]

If ablation is performed during sinus rhythm, it is usually performed during CS pacing to help monitor the activation sequence in the lateral RA wall. During ablation of the CTI, gradual delay in activation of the low lateral RA can be observed prior to achieving complete bidirectional CTI block.

CONFIRMATION OF BIDIRECTIONAL CAVOTRICUSPID ISTHMUS BLOCK

1. ATRIAL ACTIVATION SEQUENCE DURING ATRIAL PACING. Complete bidirectional CTI block is demonstrated by pacing from the CS os and RA lateral wall and observing that sequential atrial activation terminates at the ablation line, on the contralateral side from the pacing site.

Normally, during atrial pacing at a CL of 600 milliseconds from the CS os, one wavefront propagates from the CS pacing site in a clockwise direction through the CTI to the low lateral RA. The other wavefront from the CS os ascends up the atrial septum to the high RA in a counterclockwise direction, with resulting collision of wavefronts at the upper part of the lateral RA (the exact location of wavefront collision depends on the relative conduction velocities of the RA and the CTI) and generating an atrial activation sequence with a chevron pattern (see Fig. 12-16). Clockwise CTI block is indicated by the observation of a purely descending wavefront at the lateral wall down to the CTI (proximal-to-distal activation sequence on the Halo catheter positioned around the tricuspid annulus) when pacing from the CS os (i.e., pacing of the septal side of the ablation line; see Video 9). This block is associated with marked prolongation of the CTI conduction duration (i.e., the interval from the CS os to the low lateral RA; see Fig. 12-16). Incomplete clockwise CTI block is said to occur when a descending wavefront at the lateral RA wall still allows the lateral part of the CTI to be activated from the CS os in a clockwise direction across the CTI but at a slower conduction velocity, resulting in displacement of collision of the clockwise and counterclockwise wavefronts to the lower part of lateral RA. The distal bipole of the Halo catheter (Halo 1-2) at the lateral part of the CTI is activated slightly before or at the same time as bipole Halo 3-4, situated more laterally (see Fig. 12-16).[2,6]

It is important to recognize that monitoring only the atrial activation sequence of the RA lateral wall recorded by the Halo catheter during CS pacing can lead to diagnostic errors in a large percentage of patients. This is because of the inability to detect very slow residual isthmus conduction that allows the wavefront propagating in an opposite direction to reach the ablation line earlier than the transisthmus conduction. Theoretically, slow but persistent isthmus conduction that can be confined within the ablation line or part of the isthmus distant from an area mapped by the multipolar catheter can therefore be misdiagnosed, no matter how closely the distal tip of the Halo catheter is placed to the ablation line, or even if the Halo catheter is positioned across the ablation line.[2,6]

During low lateral RA pacing prior to ablation, the RA activation sequence (with intact counterclockwise CTI conduction) exhibits two ascending wavefronts (septal and lateral) leading to impulse collision at the high lateral wall. The caudocranial activation of the RA septum following counterclockwise propagation of the paced wavefront through the CTI results in atrial activation in the CS os preceding that in the HB region (Fig. 12-17). Furthermore, intact conduction through the CTI permits the paced wavefront to proceed rapidly to activate the LA from below (and CS activation propagates in a proximal-to-distal direction), thus giving rise to an inverted P wave in the inferior leads. Counterclockwise CTI block is indicated by the observation of a single ascending wavefront at the lateral wall (distal-to-proximal Halo sequence) followed by a completely descending wavefront at the septum to reach the CS os.

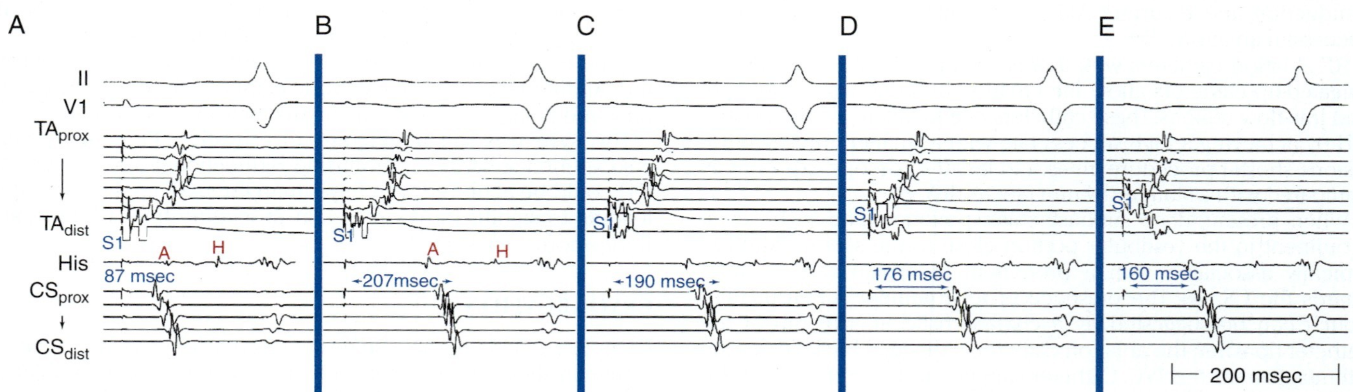

FIGURE 12-17 The use of differential pacing from the lateral right atrial (RA) wall to verify the presence of counterclockwise cavotricuspid isthmus (CTI) block. **A,** Pacing from the lateral aspect of the CTI (Halo 1,2) before CTI ablation. **B** to **E,** Pacing from different lateral RA sites along the Halo catheter after CTI ablation (**B,** pacing from Halo 3,4; **C,** pacing from Halo 5,6; **D,** pacing from Halo 7,8; **E,** pacing from Halo 9,10). When CTI conduction is intact, coronary sinus ostium (CS os) activation occurs via a counterclockwise wavefront across the CTI, and because the CS os is anatomically closer to the pacing site than the His bundle (HB), atrial activation in the CS os electrode precedes that in the HB electrode. In the presence of counterclockwise CTI block, CS os activation occurs via the wavefront propagating in a clockwise direction up the RA lateral wall, over the RA roof, and then down the septum. Consequently, CS os activation (as measured by the stimulus-to–local electrogram interval) occurs progressively earlier during pacing from more cephalic sites along the lateral RA wall (**B** to **E**). Additionally, activation of the CS os occurs after the high RA and the HB region. CS_{dist} = distal coronary sinus; CS_{prox} = proximal coronary sinus; TA_{dist} = distal tricuspid annulus; TA_{prox} = proximal tricuspid annulus.

Therefore, compared with baseline, counterclockwise CTI block is associated with inversion of the direction of the septal activation from ascending to descending. Furthermore, the CS os electrogram is activated after the high RA and the HB region (see Fig. 12-17). Additionally, counterclockwise conduction block in the CTI forces the wavefront to activate the LA from above via the Bachmann bundle—and CS activation propagates in a distal-to-proximal direction—and gives rise to a different P wave morphology, with the terminal portion positive in the inferior leads.[2,6]

2. TRANSISTHMUS CONDUCTION INTERVAL. The transisthmus conduction interval is measured during CS os or low lateral RA pacing; it is equal to the interval from the stimulus artifact from one side of the isthmus to the atrial electrogram recorded on the contralateral side. Prolongation of this interval by more than 50% (or to an absolute value of 150 milliseconds or more) suggests CTI block (see Fig. 12-16). This criterion has sensitivity and negative predictive values of 100%. However, the specificity and positive predictive values are less than 90%.

3. DOUBLE POTENTIALS. Double potentials, separated by an isoelectric interval of 30 milliseconds or longer, straddle a line of block. Double potentials along the ablation line across the CTI are generally considered the gold standard for determining complete bidirectional block (see Fig. 12-16). When there is a gap in a line of block, the isoelectric period between the double potentials shortens the closer the electrograms are to the gap. At the gap, in the line of block, double potentials are no longer present, and the electrogram is typically long and fractionated but can also be discrete. When the interval between the double potentials is more than 110 milliseconds, CTI block is present. When that interval is less than 90 milliseconds, complete bidirectional block is absent.

This technique is probably more difficult to perform than the classic activation mapping technique, mainly because of the ambiguity of electrogram interpretation along the ablation line, especially after extensive ablation attempts. When double potentials cannot be visualized, the interval between the pair of electrograms immediately on either side of the line of block (the [DP + 1] interval) when pacing immediately septal and lateral to the line of block can be used as an alternative method for verifying complete bidirectional CTI block. This technique requires positioning of a duodecapolar catheter around the tricuspid annulus while extending the catheter tip inside the CS, so that the catheter straddles the CTI and provides recording and pacing from the medial and lateral aspects of the isthmus. The [DP + 1] interval cutoff of 140 milliseconds seems to have better or equal sensitivity, specificity, and positive predictive values than other criteria. Nevertheless, it is still very difficult to distinguish incomplete block with very slow conduction from complete block. Additionally, gaps along the ablation line remote from the duodecapolar catheter would result in a [DP + 1] interval that is long in the absence of complete CTI block.[44]

4. UNIPOLAR ELECTROGRAM CONFIGURATION. The morphology of the unfiltered unipolar recording indicates the direction of wavefront propagation. Positive deflections (R waves) are generated by propagation toward the recording electrode; negative deflections (QS complexes) are generated by propagation away from the electrode. During proximal CS pacing, the unfiltered unipolar signals recorded from the CTI typically demonstrate an RS configuration as the paced impulse propagates clockwise across the isthmus. In addition, because atrial depolarization along the CTI occurs sequentially in the clockwise direction, the polarity of the initial depolarization is the same from each pair of recording electrodes when using unfiltered unipolar recording on the CTI. When complete clockwise CTI block is achieved, depolarization of the electrode just medial to the line of block retains its original polarity, but its morphology changes to a single positive deflection (monophasic R wave) because the recording site becomes a dead end for impulse conduction. Conversely, atrial tissue lateral to the line of block is depolarized from the counterclockwise direction, which is opposite to the original direction of depolarization. Accordingly, the polarity of the atrial electrograms on the CTI lateral to the line of block reverses (see Fig. 12-16). The same maneuver can be performed with pacing from the low lateral RA to evaluate counterclockwise CTI block.

Some studies have suggested that bipolar electrogram morphology could also be used for verification of the presence of CTI block. However, it is important to emphasize that bipolar recordings predominantly reflect local activation time; signal subtraction used to create a bipolar signal largely eliminates morphology information at either electrode. Nevertheless, bipolar electrogram polarity reversal can indicate a reversed wavefront direction that has been used in addition to the activation sequence for verifying bidirectional CTI block (see Fig. 12-16).

5. DIFFERENTIAL PACING. During unidirectional activation of the CTI (e.g., during low lateral RA pacing), the double electrograms recorded along the ablation line reflect activation in its immediate vicinity. The initial component reflects activation at the border ipsilateral to the pacing site, and the terminal component reflects that at the contralateral border. Pacing from another site farther away from the ablation line (e.g., midlateral RA) would obviously delay the stimulus to initial component timing, whereas the response of the terminal component would depend on the presence or absence of conduction through the ablation line. If the two components of the electrogram represent slow conduction across the isthmus ablation line, the terminal component will be delayed similar to the initial component because both components are activated by the same wavefront penetrating through the ablation line. In contrast, when complete CTI block is achieved, the two components represent two opposing activation wavefronts; the second component is advanced because it is activated by the wavefront going around, instead of through, the ablation line, given that the length of the detour is shortened by withdrawal of the pacing site.

Using the same principle, the local activation time at the CS os electrode during fixed-rate pacing performed from the low lateral and midlateral RA can be used for evaluation of counterclockwise CTI block. Normally (with intact isthmus conduction), CS os activation occurs via propagation of the paced wavefront across the CTI in a counterclockwise direction. Therefore, CS os activation occurs earlier during pacing from the low lateral RA compared with the midlateral RA because the low lateral RA is anatomically closer to the CS os. In contrast, when counterclockwise CTI block is present, CS os activation occurs via the wavefront propagating in a clockwise direction up the RA lateral wall, over the RA roof, and then down the septum (see Fig. 12-17). Consequently, CS os activation occurs earlier during pacing from the midlateral compared with the low lateral RA because the length of the detour is shortened by pacing from the midlateral RA.

6. RATE-DEPENDENT ISTHMUS BLOCK. Incomplete CTI block can mimic the activation pattern related to complete block and can produce intraatrial conduction delay at the low lateral RA. Residual CTI conduction is usually decremental and is worsened at faster pacing rates. Rate-dependent CTI block (during CS os or low lateral RA pacing) is associated with a change of the direction of impulse propagation and an increase of conduction time when the pacing rate is increased.

This maneuver helps distinguish isthmus block from long local conduction delay across the isthmus. With incomplete CTI block, activation of the low lateral RA during CS os pacing can be delayed, but activation can still occur via the CTI at the same time or just earlier than the wavefront coming to the low lateral RA from the counterclockwise direction. Increasing the pacing rate results in decremental conduction across the now diseased isthmus and causes further delay in activation of the low lateral RA (Fig. 12-18). In contrast, when complete CTI block is present, the lateral RA is activated in a counterclockwise direction across the atrial septum and RA roof. Because these atrial regions conduct nondecrementally, pacing at faster rates should not change the timing of low lateral RA activation significantly, as long as the pacing CL is longer than atrial refractoriness. The same maneuver can be performed with pacing from the low lateral RA to evaluate counterclockwise CTI block.

7. ELECTROANATOMICAL MAPPING. Electroanatomical 3-D activation mapping can be used to verify CTI block. When clockwise block in the CTI is achieved, proximal CS pacing results in an activation wavefront propagating in a counterclockwise fashion, with the latest activation in the CTI immediately lateral to the ablation line (Fig. 12-19). When conduction across the CTI is still intact, CS pacing produces an activation wavefront that propagates rapidly through the CTI, with the anterolateral RA wall activated last. Similar maps can be generated during low lateral RA pacing to confirm counterclockwise block in the CTI. Activation maps can also be evaluated for the presence of gaps in the ablation lines, as indicated by the early breakthroughs from the ablation line. However, following CTI ablation, the local electrograms at the ablation line can be complex—with double, triple, or fragmented potentials and unclear local activation time—and electroanatomical activation mapping can be challenging.

Outcome

With the availability of precise catheter locator systems, more effective ablation tools, and accurate endpoints for ablation, the inability to create complete CTI block and to eliminate recurrences of CTI-dependent AFL successfully is unusual in contemporary practice. Acute success rate of ablation of typical AFL is higher than 90% when large-tip or irrigated RF catheters are used.[45,46] A repeat ablation procedure is performed in 5% to 15% of patients, and the long-term success rate in preventing recurrent AFL is 97%.[45] Advances in AFL ablation technologies have had less effect on short-term success rates than

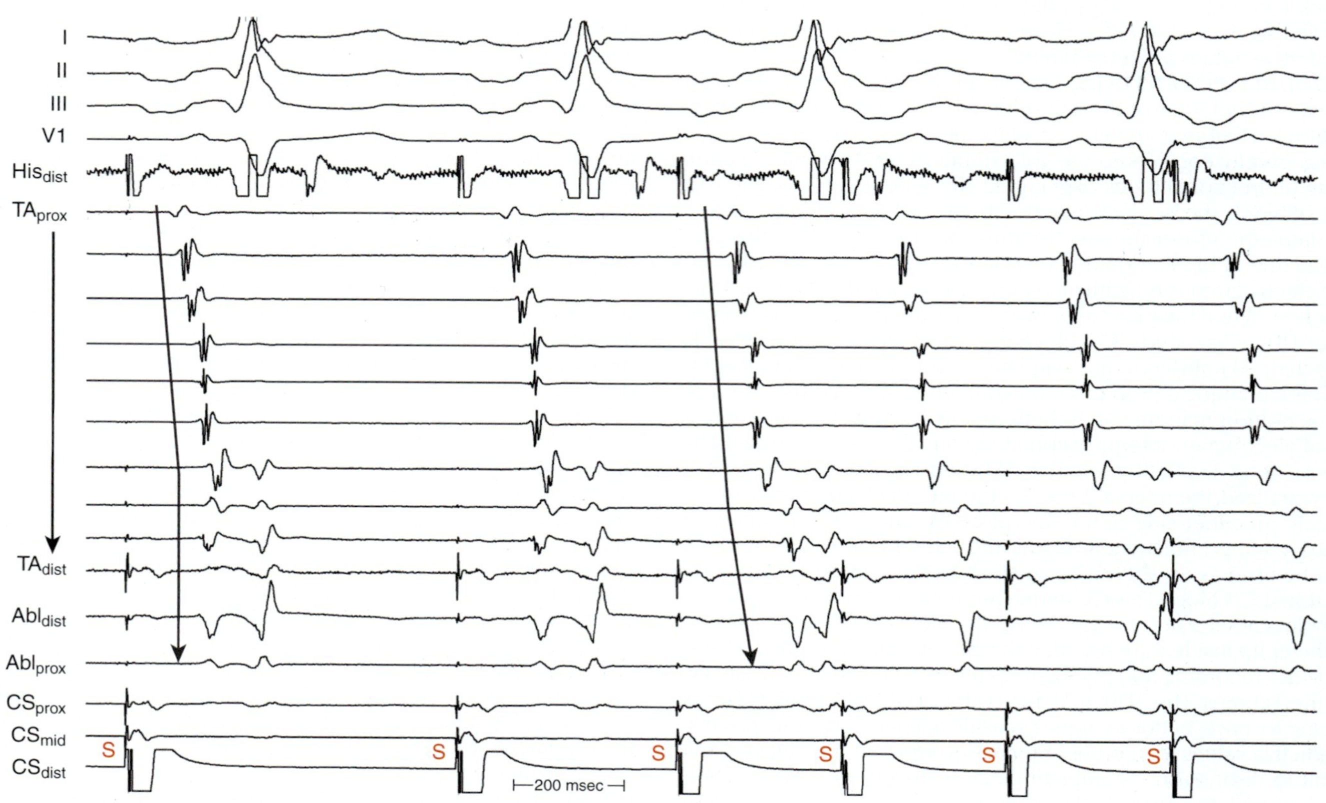

FIGURE 12-18 Surface ECG and intracardiac recordings following incomplete ablation of the cavotricuspid isthmus (CTI). The activation sequence around the tricuspid annulus (TA) during coronary sinus (CS) pacing suggests block in the CTI (continuous line, arrow); however, pacing at a faster rate at right shows a "straighter" line of activation along the TA and thus reveals that conduction had been present in the CTI at the slower paced rate. Abl = ablation site; dist = distal; mid = middle; prox = proximal.

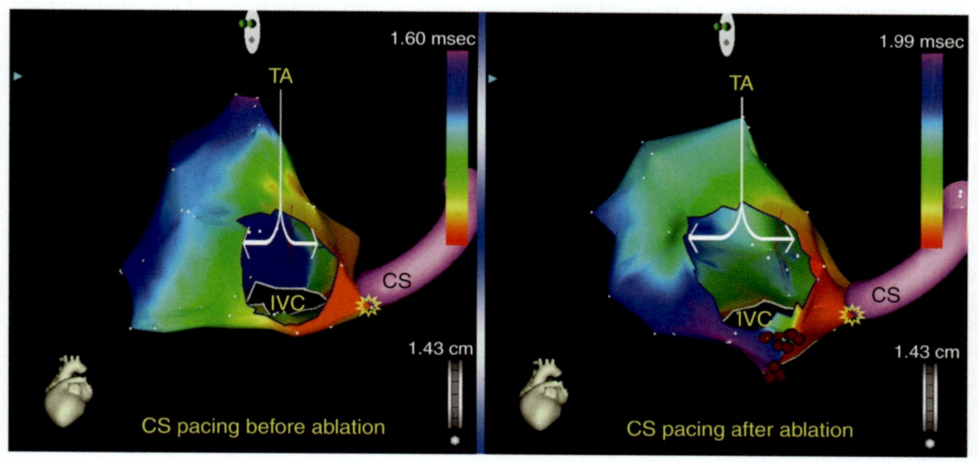

FIGURE 12-19 CARTO (Biosense Webster, Diamond Bar, Calif.) activation map of coronary sinus (CS) pacing before **(left)** and after **(right)** cavotricuspid isthmus (CTI) ablation. During CS ostium pacing (yellow star), complete CTI block in the clockwise direction is indicated by the absence of activation proceeding through the ablation line (red dots); activation of the entire tricuspid annulus (TA) remains counterclockwise, except for the small portion that is situated between the pacing site and the line of block. IVC = inferior vena cava.

on reducing AFL recurrences. On the other hand, the use of the more stringent endpoint of bidirectional block significantly reduces the AFL recurrence rate. For patients in whom typical AFL recurs after ablation, conduction through the CTI is usually responsible. Presumably, such recurrences reflect a failure to achieve bidirectional CTI block during the initial procedure, incorrect initial assessment of bidirectional block, or resumption of conduction across an initially blocked isthmus. The incidence of AFL recurrence does not increase beyond 1 to 6 months of follow-up, a finding suggesting that if recovery of isthmus conduction is going to occur, it will have done so by 6 months.[46]

Serious complications associated with AFL ablation are rare (0.4%) and include AV block (most common, 0.2%), cardiac tamponade, groin hematoma, transient inferior ST segment elevation or acute occlusion of the right coronary artery,[47] thromboembolic complications, and ventricular tachycardia.[45]

Following AFL ablation, AF can develop in approximately 20% to 30% (with short-term follow-up, approximately 1 year) and in up to 82% (with long-term follow-up, approximately 4 years) of patients with or without a prior history of AF.[2,6,48] It appears that AFL is often an early marker of atrial electrical disease that frequently progresses to AF even after curative treatment for AFL. This has led some investigators to advocate ablation of AF at the same time of AFL ablation.[49] In a meta-analysis, over an average follow-up of 16 months, AF occurred in 23.1% of patients with no preablation history of AF and in 52.7% of patients with a history of AF, despite successful AFL ablation. The occurrence of AF was not influenced by the ablation technology or procedural endpoints. This finding has serious implications for patient selection, long-term arrhythmia-free success rates, postprocedure antiarrhythmic drug use, and postprocedure anticoagulation. Because AF predating ablation of AFL is very likely to recur, thus limiting the ability to discontinue antiarrhythmic medications or anticoagulation in many patients, the potential benefits of ablation of only AFL should be seriously scrutinized.[46]

REFERENCES

1. Asirvatham SJ: Correlative anatomy and electrophysiology for the interventional electrophysiologist: right atrial flutter, *J Cardiovasc Electrophysiol* 20:113–122, 2009.
2. Waldo AL, Atiezna F: Atrial flutter: mechanisms, features, and management. In Zipes DP, Jalife J, editors: *Cardiac electrophysiology: from cell to bedside*, ed 5, Philadelphia, 2009, Saunders, pp 567–576.
3. Tai CT, Chen SA: Cavotricuspid isthmus: anatomy, electrophysiology, and long-term outcome of radiofrequency ablation, *Pacing Clin Electrophysiol* 32:1591–1595, 2009.
4. Saremi F, Pourzand L, Krishnan S, et al: Right atrial cavotricuspid isthmus: anatomic characterization with multi-detector row CT, *Radiology* 247:658–668, 2008.
5. Waldo AL: Atrial flutter: from mechanism to treatment. In Camm AJ, editor: *Clinical approaches to tachyarrhythmias*, Armonk, NY, 2001, Futura, pp 1–56.
6. Feld G, Srivatsa U, Hoppe B: Ablation of isthmus-dependent atrial flutters. In Huang SKS, Wood M, editors: *Catheter ablation of cardiac arrhythmias*, Philadelphia, 2006, Saunders, pp 195–218.
7. Santucci PA, Varma N, Cytron J, et al: Electroanatomic mapping of postpacing intervals clarifies the complete active circuit and variants in atrial flutter, *Heart Rhythm* 6:1586–1595, 2009.
8. Anselme F: Macroreentrant atrial tachycardia: pathophysiological concepts, *Heart Rhythm* 5(Suppl):S18–S21, 2008.
9. Huang JL, Tai CT, Lin YJ, et al: Right atrial substrate properties associated with age in patients with typical atrial flutter, *Heart Rhythm* 5:1144–1151, 2008.
10. Feld GK, Mollerus M, Birgersdotter-Green U, et al: Conduction velocity in the tricuspid valve-inferior vena cava isthmus is slower in patients with type I atrial flutter compared to those without a history of atrial flutter, *J Cardiovasc Electrophysiol* 8:1338–1348, 1997.
11. Morita N, Kobayashi Y, Horie T, et al: The undetermined geometrical factors contributing to the transverse conduction block of the crista terminalis, *Pacing Clin Electrophysiol* 32:868–878, 2009.
12. Tai CT, Chen SA: Conduction barriers of atrial flutter: relation to the anatomy, *Pacing Clin Electrophysiol* 31:1335–1342, 2008.
13. Granada J, Uribe W, Chyou PH, et al: Incidence and predictors of atrial flutter in the general population, *J Am Coll Cardiol* 36:2242–2246, 2000.
14. Blomstrom-Lundqvist C, Scheinman MM, Aliot EM, et al: ACC/AHA/ESC guidelines for the management of patients with supraventricular arrhythmias—executive summary: a report of the American College of Cardiology/American Heart Association Task Force on Practice Guidelines and the European Society of Cardiology Committee for Practice Guidelines (writing committee to develop guidelines for the management of patients with supraventricular arrhythmias), *Circulation* 108:1871–1909, 2003.
15. Medi C, Kalman JM: Prediction of the atrial flutter circuit location from the surface electrocardiogram, *Europace* 10:786–796, 2008.
16. Josephson ME: Atrial flutter and fibrillation. In Josephson ME, editor: *Clinical cardiac electrophysiology*, ed 4, Philadelphia, 2008, Lippincott Williams & Wilkins, pp 285–338.
17. Miyazaki H, Stevenson WG, Stephenson K, et al: Entrainment mapping for rapid distinction of left and right atrial tachycardias, *Heart Rhythm* 3:516–523, 2006.
18. Deo R, Berger R: The clinical utility of entrainment pacing, *J Cardiovasc Electrophysiol* 20:466–470, 2009.
19. Zhang S, Younis G, Hariharan R, et al: Lower loop reentry as a mechanism of clockwise right atrial flutter, *Circulation* 109:1630–1635, 2004.
20. Bochoeyer A, Yang Y, Cheng J, et al: Surface electrocardiographic characteristics of right and left atrial flutter, *Circulation* 108:60–66, 2003.
21. Garan H: Atypical atrial flutter, *Heart Rhythm* 5:618–621, 2008.
22. Higa S, Tai CT, Lin YJ, et al: Focal atrial tachycardia: new insight from noncontact mapping and catheter ablation, *Circulation* 109:84–91, 2004.
23. Cosio FG, Pastor A, Nunez A, Giocolea A: Catheter ablation of typical atrial flutter. In Zipes DP, Haissaguerre M, editors: *Catheter ablation of arrhythmias*, Armonk, NY, 2002, Futura, pp 131–152.
24. Nakao M, Saoudi N: More on isthmus anatomy for safety and efficacy, *J Cardiovasc Electrophysiol* 16:409–410, 2005.
25. Calkins H, Brugada J, Packer DL, et al: HRS/EHRA/ECAS expert consensus statement on catheter and surgical ablation of atrial fibrillation: recommendations for personnel, policy, procedures and follow-up. A report of the Heart Rhythm Society (HRS) Task Force on Catheter and Surgical Ablation of Atrial Fibrillation, *Heart Rhythm* 4:816–861, 2007.
26. Finlay M, Sawhney V, Schilling R, et al: Uninterrupted warfarin for periprocedural anticoagulation in catheter ablation of typical atrial flutter: a safe and cost-effective strategy, *J Cardiovasc Electrophysiol* 21:150–154, 2010.
27. Marrouche NF, Schweikert R, Saliba W, et al: Use of different catheter ablation technologies for treatment of typical atrial flutter: acute results and long-term follow-up, *Pacing Clin Electrophysiol* 26:743–746, 2003.
28. Gula LJ, Redfearn DP, Veenhuyzen GD, et al: Reduction in atrial flutter ablation time by targeting maximum voltage: results of a prospective randomized clinical trial, *J Cardiovasc Electrophysiol* 20:1108–1112, 2009.
29. Ozaydin M, Tada H, Chugh A, et al: Atrial electrogram amplitude and efficacy of cavotricuspid isthmus ablation for atrial flutter, *Pacing Clin Electrophysiol* 26:1859–1863, 2003.
30. Redfearn DP, Skanes AC, Gula LJ, et al: Cavotricuspid isthmus conduction is dependent on underlying anatomic bundle architecture: observations using a maximum voltage-guided ablation technique, *J Cardiovasc Electrophysiol* 17:832–838, 2006.
31. Subbiah RN, Gula LJ, Krahn AD, et al: Rapid ablation for atrial flutter by targeting maximum voltage-factors associated with short ablation times, *J Cardiovasc Electrophysiol* 18:612–616, 2007.
32. Ventura R, Rostock T, Klemm HU, et al: Catheter ablation of common-type atrial flutter guided by three-dimensional right atrial geometry reconstruction and catheter tracking using cutaneous patches: a randomized prospective study, *J Cardiovasc Electrophysiol* 15:1157–1161, 2004.
33. Hindricks G, Willems S, Kautzner J, et al: Effect of electroanatomically guided versus conventional catheter ablation of typical atrial flutter on the fluoroscopy time and resource use: a prospective randomized multicenter study, *J Cardiovasc Electrophysiol* 20:734–740, 2009.
34. Gami AS, Edwards WD, Lachman N, et al: Electrophysiological anatomy of typical atrial flutter: the posterior boundary and causes for difficulty with ablation, *J Cardiovasc Electrophysiol* 21:144–149, 2010.
35. Lo LW, Tai CT, Lin YJ, et al: Characteristics of the cavotricuspid isthmus in predicting recurrent conduction in the long-term follow-up, *J Cardiovasc Electrophysiol* 20:39–43, 2009.
36. Atiga WL, Worley SJ, Hummel J, et al: Prospective randomized comparison of cooled radiofrequency versus standard radiofrequency energy for ablation of typical atrial flutter, *Pacing Clin Electrophysiol* 25:1172–1178, 2002.
37. Schreieck J, Zrenner B, Kumpmann J, et al: Prospective randomized comparison of closed cooled-tip versus 8-mm-tip catheters for radiofrequency ablation of typical atrial flutter, *J Cardiovasc Electrophysiol* 13:980–985, 2002.
38. Boll S, Dang L, Scharf C: Linear ablation with duty-cycled radiofrequency energy at the cavotricuspid isthmus, *Pacing Clin Electrophysiol* 33:444–450, 2010.
39. Erdogan A, Guettler N, Doerr O, et al: Randomized comparison of multipolar, duty-cycled, bipolar-unipolar radiofrequency versus conventional catheter ablation for treatment of common atrial flutter, *J Cardiovasc Electrophysiol* 21:1109–1113, 2010.
40. Timmermans C, Ayers GM, Crijns HJ, Rodriguez LM: Randomized study comparing radiofrequency ablation with cryoablation for the treatment of atrial flutter with emphasis on pain perception, *Circulation* 107:1250–1252, 2003.
41. Collins NJ, Barlow M, Varghese P, Leitch J: Cryoablation versus radiofrequency ablation in the treatment of atrial flutter trial (CRAAFT), *J Interv Card Electrophysiol* 16:1–5, 2006.
42. Kuniss M, Vogtmann T, Ventura R, et al: Prospective randomized comparison of durability of bidirectional conduction block in the cavotricuspid isthmus in patients after ablation of common atrial flutter using cryothermy and radiofrequency energy: the CRYOTIP study, *Heart Rhythm* 6:1699–1705, 2009.
43. Tada H, Oral H, Ozaydin M, et al: Randomized comparison of anatomic and electrogram mapping approaches to ablation of typical atrial flutter, *J Cardiovasc Electrophysiol* 13:662–666, 2002.
44. Zambito PE, Palma EC: DP+1: another simple endpoint for atrial flutter ablation, *J Cardiovasc Electrophysiol* 19:10–13, 2008.
45. Morady F: Catheter ablation of supraventricular arrhythmias: state of the art, *J Cardiovasc Electrophysiol* 15:124–139, 2004.
46. Perez FJ, Schubert CM, Parvez B, et al: Long-term outcomes after catheter ablation of cavotricuspid isthmus dependent atrial flutter: a meta-analysis, *Circ Arrhythm Electrophysiol* 2:393–401, 2009.
47. Mykytsey A, Kehoe R, Bharati S, et al: Right coronary artery occlusion during RF ablation of typical atrial flutter, *J Cardiovasc Electrophysiol* 21:818–821, 2010.
48. Ellis K, Wazni O, Marrouche N, et al: Incidence of atrial fibrillation post-cavotricuspid isthmus ablation in patients with typical atrial flutter: left-atrial size as an independent predictor of atrial fibrillation recurrence, *J Cardiovasc Electrophysiol* 18:799–802, 2007.
49. Navarrete A, Conte F, Moran M, et al: Ablation of atrial fibrillation at the time of cavotricuspid isthmus ablation in patients with atrial flutter without documented atrial fibrillation derives a better long-term benefit, *J Cardiovasc Electrophysiol* 22:34–38, 2011.

CHAPTER 13 Macroreentrant Atrial Tachycardia ("Atypical Atrial Flutter")

Pathophysiology

The term *typical atrial flutter* (AFL) is reserved for an atrial macroreentrant arrhythmia rotating clockwise or counterclockwise around the tricuspid annulus and using the cavotricuspid isthmus (CTI) as an essential part of the reentrant circuit. *Atypical AFL* is a term commonly used to describe all other *macroreentrant* atrial tachycardias (MRATs), regardless of the atrial cycle length (CL), but the former term introduces unnecessary confusion, and a mechanistic description of the tachycardia circuit is preferred.

The mechanism of MRAT is reentrant activation around a large central obstacle, generally several centimeters in diameter, at least in one of its dimensions. The central obstacle can consist of normal or abnormal structures. Additionally, the obstacle can be fixed, functional, or a combination of both. There is no single point of origin of activation, and atrial tissues outside the circuit are activated from various parts of the circuit.

A description of MRAT mechanisms must be made in relation to atrial anatomy, including a detailed description of the obstacles or boundaries of the circuit and the critical isthmuses that may be targets for therapeutic action. Typically, chronic or long-lasting atrial tachycardias (ATs) are macroreentrant. Focal ATs are more frequently responsible for irregular ATs with frequent spontaneous interruption and reinitiation than are ATs observed with macroreentry. Microreentrant ATs, by definition, use a smaller circuit and in many regards behave more like other forms of focal ATs.

Atypical Isthmus-Dependent Right Atrial Macroreentry

Lower loop reentry and intraisthmus reentry are macroreentrant circuits that are confined to the right atrium (RA) and incorporate the CTI as a critical part of the circuit. However, in contrast to typical AFL, the circuit is not peritricuspid (Fig. 13-1). Nevertheless, because the CTI is still a necessary part of the circuit, these arrhythmias are amenable to CTI ablation, as is true for patients with typical AFL.[1]

LOWER LOOP REENTRY

Lower loop reentry is a form of CTI-dependent AFL with a reentrant circuit around the inferior vena cava (IVC); therefore, it is confined to the lower part of the RA (see Fig. 13-1). It often coexists with counterclockwise or clockwise typical AFL and involves posterior breakthrough across the crista terminalis. Lower loop reentry can rotate around the IVC in a counterclockwise (i.e., the impulse within the CTI travels from the septum to the lateral wall) or clockwise fashion. A breakdown in the inferoposterior boundaries of the CTI produced by the eustachian ridge and lower crista terminalis causes the circuit to revolve around the IVC (instead of around the tricuspid annulus), across the eustachian ridge, and through the crista terminalis, with slow conduction because of transverse activation through that structure. Alternatively, the circuit can exit at the apex of Koch triangle and come behind the eustachian ridge to break through across the crista terminalis behind the IVC and then return to the CTI. This arrhythmia is usually transient and terminates by itself or converts spontaneously into AFL or atrial fibrillation (AF).[1]

INTRAISTHMUS REENTRY

Intraisthmus reentry is a reentrant circuit usually occurring within the region bounded by the medial CTI and coronary sinus ostium (CS os; see Fig. 13-1). Circuits in the lateral portion of the CTI can also occur but are less common. This arrhythmia can be sustained and usually occurs in patients who have undergone prior, and often extensive, ablation at the CTI. Intracardiac recordings usually resemble typical AFL. However, in this form of CTI-dependent AFL, entrainment pacing from the lateral CTI demonstrates a post-pacing interval (PPI) longer than the tachycardia CL, a finding indicating that the lateral CTI is not part of the reentrant circuit. On the other hand, pacing from the region of medial CTI or CS os demonstrates concealed entrainment with PPI equal to the tachycardia CL. Fractionated or double potentials usually can be recorded in this area and can be entrained. Although the anatomical basis of this arrhythmia remains unknown, a linear lesion across the medial CTI, usually at the site of a very prolonged electrogram, can cure the tachycardia.

Non–Isthmus-Dependent Right Atrial Macroreentry

LESIONAL RIGHT ATRIAL MACROREENTRANT TACHYCARDIA

Atrial macroreentry in the right free wall is the most common form of non–CTI-dependent RA MRAT. These circuits can propagate around a central obstacle of a low-voltage area or scar in the lateral or posterolateral RA wall, arising spontaneously or as a consequence of prior atrial surgery. The central obstacle of the macroreentrant circuit can be an atriotomy scar (in patients who have undergone surgery for congenital or valvular heart disease), a septal prosthetic patch, a suture line, or a line of fixed block secondary to

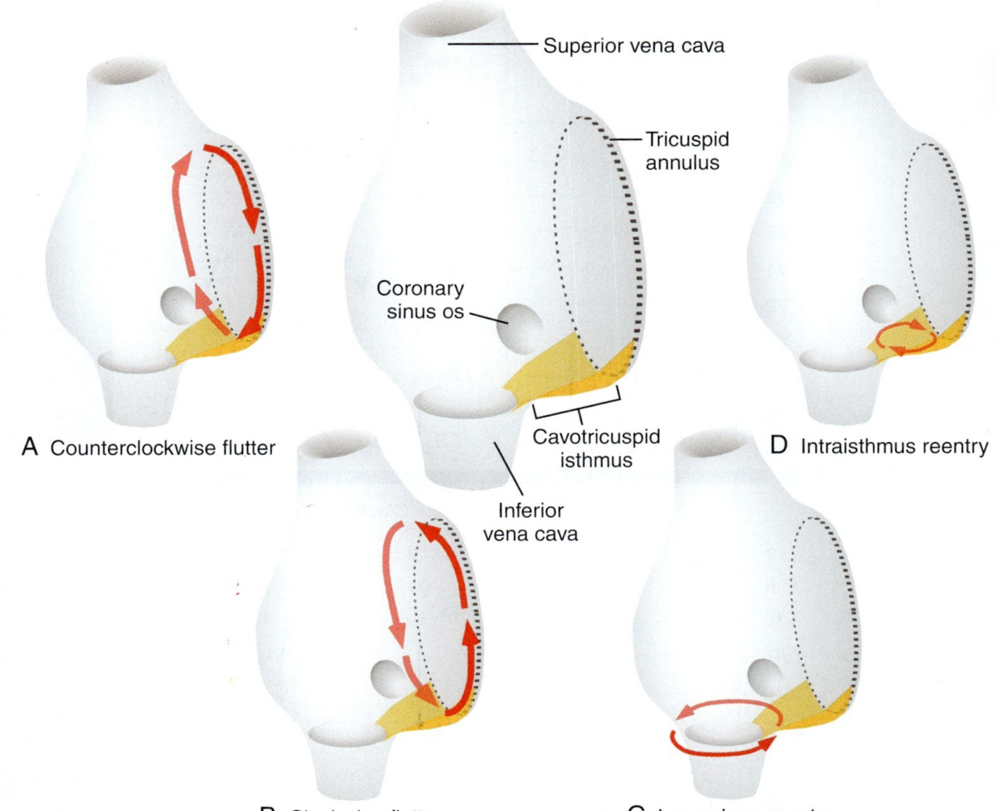

FIGURE 13-1 Anatomy of cavotricuspid-dependent atrial flutter circuits. **Top, center,** The right atrium is viewed from the right lateral aspect, with the lateral wall semitransparent. The cavotricuspid isthmus is shaded orange. **A,** Counterclockwise flutter circuit. **B,** Clockwise flutter circuit. **C,** Lower loop reentry circuit. **D,** Intraisthmus reentry circuit. See text for discussion. Os = ostium.

radiofrequency (RF) ablation. Other obstacles can also include anatomical structures located in the vicinity of the scar (superior vena cava [SVC], IVC). Occasionally, these ATs are associated with areas of electrical silence, a finding suggesting atrial scarring in patients who have not undergone prior atrial surgery. These patients have a characteristic posterolateral and lateral distribution of RA scarring and frequently have more than one tachycardia mechanism. Low-voltage electrograms characterizing areas of scar and double potentials characterizing a line of block can be observed during both normal sinus rhythm (NSR) and AT. In one study, electroanatomical mapping revealed that RA electrically silent areas (electrogram amplitude 0.03 mV or lower) were involved in the tachycardia mechanism in two thirds of the patients with non–CTI-dependent RA MRAT.[2,3]

Patients with congenital heart disease have a high prevalence of AT, particularly after they have undergone reparative or palliative surgical procedures. For MRATs in adults with repaired congenital heart disease, three RA circuits are generally identified: lateral wall circuits with reentry around or related to the lateral atriotomy scar, septal circuits with reentry around an atrial septal patch, and typical AFL circuits using the CTI. These arrhythmias are discussed separately in Chapter 14.[1,4]

UPPER LOOP REENTRY

This type of MRAT involves the upper portion of the RA, with transverse conduction over the crista terminalis and wavefront collision occurring at a lower part of the RA or within the CTI. When upper loop reentry was first reported, it was thought to be a reentrant circuit using the channel between the SVC, fossa ovalis, and crista terminalis. Noncontact mapping studies have shown that this form of MRAT employs the crista terminalis as its functional central obstacle. The impulse rotating in the circuit can be in a counterclockwise or clockwise direction. The CTI is not an intrinsic part of the reentrant circuit. Upper loop reentry can be abolished by linear ablation of the gap in the crista terminalis.[5,6]

DUAL-LOOP REENTRY

Although RA MRAT (lesional RA macroreentry or upper loop reentry) can manifest as an isolated arrhythmia (single-loop reentry), it can occur in conjunction with typical clockwise or counterclockwise AFL, or both, as well as lower loop reentry. When two atrial macroreentrant circuits coexist and use neighboring anatomical structures, they create the so-called *dual-loop reentry*. Not uncommonly, ablation of one tachycardia results in transition to the other, and ablation of both circuits is necessary for clinical success. Detection of this change requires careful attention to the atrial activation sequence and ECG pattern after each RF application. The recording of multiple simultaneous electrograms, as continuous endocardial references, facilitates detection of these activation changes. Fusion between two simultaneous left atrial (LA) macroreentrant circuits is possible after prior AF ablation.[7]

Left Atrial Macroreentry

LA MRATs are less common than typical AFL and are frequently related to or coexist with AF. LA MRAT is a known complication of surgical and catheter-based therapies of AF, and it can occur in up to 50% of patients following extensive catheter ablation strategies (see Chap. 15).[8] Additionally, cardiac surgery involving the LA or atrial septum can produce different LA macroreentrant circuits. However, LA circuits also can be found in patients without a history of atriotomy or prior ablation. Electroanatomical maps in the latter group often show low-voltage or areas of scar in the LA, which act as a central obstacle or barrier in the circuit. These areas are typically located at the posterior wall (45%), superior region (roof, 28%), or anteroseptal region (27%) of the LA. The pathogenesis of these areas

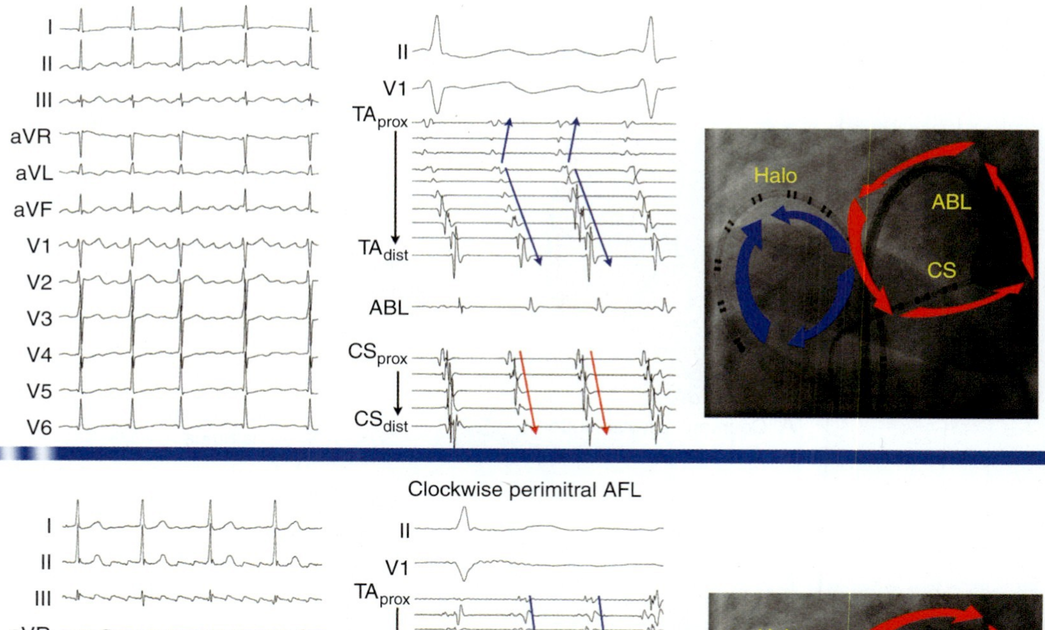

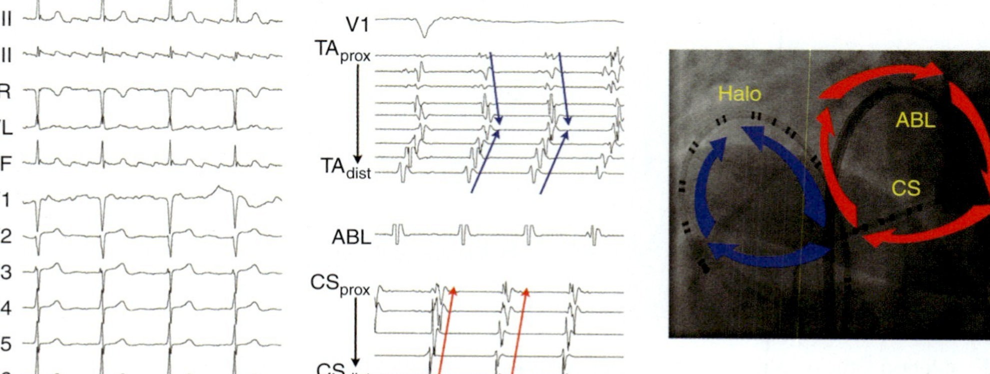

FIGURE 13-2 Surface ECGs and intracardiac recordings during clockwise **(lower panel)** and counterclockwise **(upper panel)** perimitral macroreentrant atrial tachycardia. Catheter position and wavefront activation during the tachycardia are illustrated in a left anterior oblique fluoroscopic view **(right side).** The ablation catheter (ABL) is positioned at the mitral isthmus, and the Halo catheter is positioned around the tricuspid annulus (TA), with the distal end at the lateral end of the cavotricuspid isthmus. AFL = atrial flutter; CS = coronary sinus; CS_{dist} = distal coronary sinus; CS_{prox} = proximal coronary sinus; TA_{dist} = distal tricuspid annulus; TA_{prox} = proximal tricuspid annulus.

with no electrical signals is not well established. Potential causes include volume and pressure overload (mitral valve disease, hypertension, heart failure), ischemia (atrial branch occlusion), postinflammation scarring (after myocarditis), atrial amyloidosis, atrial dysplasia, and tachycardia-related structural remodeling. These macroreentrant circuits show considerable anatomical variability and frequently involve multiple simultaneous loops.[1,2]

PERIMITRAL ATRIAL FLUTTER

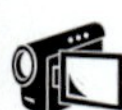

This circuit involves reentry around the mitral annulus in a counterclockwise or clockwise fashion (Fig. 13-2, see Video 12). This arrhythmia is more common in patients with structural heart disease; however, it has been described in patients without obvious structural heart disease, but, in these patients, electroanatomical voltage mapping often shows scar or low-voltage areas on the posterior wall of the LA as a posterior boundary of this circuit. Perimitral MRAT is the most common MRAT in patients with prior LA ablation procedures for AF.

CIRCUITS INVOLVING THE PULMONARY VEINS WITH OR WITHOUT LEFT ATRIAL SCAR

Various reentrant circuits involve the pulmonary veins (PVs), especially in patients with AF or mitral valve disease and those with prior catheter ablation of AF (particularly with linear LA ablation lesions), including reentrant circuits around two or more PVs (it is unusual for a circuit to involve one PV) and posterior scar or low-voltage areas (see Video 17).

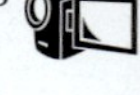

LEFT SEPTAL CIRCUITS

Left septal circuits represent a rare form of MRAT occurring in the absence of prior cardiac surgery. These circuits involve the LA septum primum, which acts as a central obstacle for the reentrant circuit. The right PV ostia serve as its posterior boundary, whereas the mitral annulus serves as its anterior boundary. Atrial dilation and concomitant antiarrhythmic drug therapy also seem to play a role by the prolongation of left intraatrial conduction, which then allows stable macroreentry circuits to persist.[2] In patients with a history of surgery for atrial septal defects, scars or the patch on the septum can serve as the anatomical substrate of left septal circuits.

Clinical Considerations

Epidemiology

MRAT comprises a heterogeneous group of RA or LA macroreentrant circuits related to different anatomical and electrophysiological (EP) substrates. These arrhythmias are frequently associated with structural heart disease, congenital cardiac defects, previous cardiac surgical procedures, or surgical or catheter ablation procedures for AF. Often, these arrhythmias coexist with AF. However, MRAT occasionally occurs in a patient with no apparent structural heart disease.[4]

Although its exact prevalence among cardiac arrhythmias is difficult to establish clinically, MRAT is not a rare arrhythmia. It seems that the incidence of MRAT is increasing. This may be related to aging of the general population, which implies progressive alteration of the atrial electrical properties with development of an arrhythmogenic substrate, as well as to the increased numbers of surgical and catheter based procedures in the atria for treatment of AF.[4,9]

Clinical Presentation

Macroreentrant ATs are typically chronic or long lasting. As with AF and typical AFL, patients can present with symptoms related to rapid ventricular response, loss of atrioventricular (AV) synchrony, tachycardia-induced cardiomyopathy, or deterioration of preexisting cardiac disease. Additionally, typical AFL and MRAT can contribute to systemic thromboembolic complications and stroke.

Initial Evaluation

Outside typical AFL, the clinician is faced with a wide spectrum of ATs for which therapy and prognosis cannot be defined with routine noninvasive testing, and definitive diagnosis typically requires intracardiac mapping. ECG alone is frequently inadequate to distinguish MRAT from focal AT or typical AFL. Detailed evaluation of cardiac function and anatomy is typically required, especially in patients with congenital heart disease and those with previous cardiac procedures (surgical or catheter-based). Additionally, detailed knowledge of the congenital anomaly and previous surgical or ablative procedures is very important, such as location of surgical incisions and the presence and location of prosthetic patch material.

Principles of Management

Medical management of MRAT is practically similar to that for AF. Antiarrhythmic drugs (class IA, IC, and III) have been first-line therapy. Long-term anticoagulation for stroke prevention is typically recommended. Rate control versus rhythm control strategies are evaluated, depending on several factors, including severity of symptoms, response to rate-controlling medications, cardiac function, and associated noncardiac diseases.

With recent advances in the technology to visualize and modify the arrhythmia substrate, ablation of non–CTI-dependent MRAT has become increasingly successful, but it can be substantially more difficult than ablation of typical AFL. MRAT can have complex circuits that demand a thorough knowledge of atrial anatomy and a great deal of experience to correlate activation patterns with anatomical landmarks. When this type of AT is suspected, such as in patients with congenital heart disease who have had surgery, referral to an experienced center should be considered.[4]

Catheter ablation of the AV junction and pacemaker insertion should be considered if catheter ablative cure is not possible and the patient has a rapid ventricular response that is not responding to drug therapy.

Electrocardiographic Features

P wave morphology on the surface ECG is usually of limited value for precise anatomical localization of macroreentrant circuits. Analysis of the P wave can be impeded by partial or complete concealment of the P wave within the QRS complexes or T waves when the AT is associated with 1:1 or 2:1 AV conduction. Additionally, P wave morphology of a spectrum of RA and LA MRATs is highly variable. The presence of complex anatomy secondary to congenital abnormalities, prior atrial surgery, or a large low-voltage zone (secondary to underlying atrial substrate or extensive catheter or surgical atrial ablation) can modify atrial wavefront propagation in a nonuniform manner, resulting in deviated atrial activation vectors or low amplitude P waves. Furthermore, P waves produced by different underlying substrates may appear similar if the direction of activation of the atrial septum and LA is similar. The surface ECG morphology is most characteristic (and hence predictive) for establishing a diagnosis of counterclockwise typical AFL. Nevertheless, atypical ECG patterns have been described for typical AFL after AF ablation. Although clockwise typical AFL also has a characteristic appearance, this is more variable, and it can be mimicked by various other MRATs.[5,10] On the other hand, AFL may show distinct isoelectric intervals between P waves, especially in the presence of extensive atrial scarring or a localized macroreentrant circuit, similar to focal AT.

UPPER LOOP REENTRY. The surface ECG of upper loop reentry closely mimics that of clockwise typical AFL, with positive P waves in the inferior leads, because in most cases, both arrhythmias share a similar activation sequence of the LA, the septum, and caudocranial activation of the lateral RA. However, negative or isoelectric or flat P waves in lead I favor upper loop reentry over clockwise typical AFL. Conversely, positive P waves in lead I with an amplitude of more than 0.07 mV favor clockwise typical AFL. Additionally, the CL of upper loop reentry is usually shorter in comparison with typical AFL.[5,6]

LOWER LOOP REENTRY. The surface morphology of lower loop reentry is highly variable and can be similar to that of counterclockwise or clockwise typical AFL, but lower loop reentry associated with higher crista terminalis breaks can produce unusual ECG patterns. Sometimes, the changes are manifested by decreased amplitude of the late positive waves in the inferior leads, probably as a result of wavefront collision over the lateral RA wall.

INCISIONAL RIGHT ATRIAL MACROREENTRANT TACHYCARDIA. The surface ECG morphology of free wall MRAT in a patient with a previous atriotomy is highly variable, depending on factors including the location of the scars and low-voltage areas, the direction of rotation, the presence of coexisting conduction block in the atrium, and the presence of a simultaneous typical AFL. The morphology of the atrial complex on the surface ECG can range from that similar to typical AFL to that characteristic of focal AT (see Fig. 14-5). Often, inverted P waves can be observed in lead V_1. Depending on the predominant direction of septal activation, RA free wall MRAT can mimic either clockwise or counterclockwise typical AFL.[5]

LEFT ATRIAL MACROREENTRANT TACHYCARDIA. The surface ECG morphology of LA MRAT caused by the different reentrant circuits is variable, and ECG findings are often similar for different underlying substrates, thus making the localization within the LA based on the ECG difficult. LA MRATs are usually associated with prominent positive P waves in lead V_1 and upright (but frequently of low amplitude) deflections in leads II, III, and aVF. However, LA MRAT can result in ECG patterns of focal AT (discrete P waves and isoelectric baseline) because of a high prevalence of generalized atrial disease and slower conduction. Infrequently, LA MRAT can mimic typical AFL on the surface ECG.[5]

PERIMITRAL ATRIAL MACROREENTRY. Most of these tachycardias show prominent forces in leads V_1 and V_2, with diminished amplitude in the inferior leads (see Fig. 13-2). It has been suggested that a posterior LA scar allows for domination by anterior LA forces. This constellation of findings may mimic counterclockwise or clockwise CTI-dependent AFL, but the decreased amplitude of frontal plane forces suggests an LA circuit. In patients with prior PV isolation procedures, the surface ECG morphology of counterclockwise perimitral MRAT can be different from that in patients without prior ablation, possibly related to varying degrees of prior LA ablation or scar. In these patients, counterclockwise perimitral MRAT demonstrates positive P waves in the inferior and precordial leads and a significant negative component in leads I and aVL. Furthermore, counterclockwise perimitral MRAT in these patients can have a morphology similar to that of left PV ATs. However, counterclockwise perimitral MRAT is suggested by

a more negative component in lead I, an initial negative component in lead V_2, and a lack of any isoelectric interval between P waves. Clockwise perimitral MRAT has limb lead morphology that is the converse of that of counterclockwise perimitral MRAT and an initial negative component in the lateral precordial leads. The positive P wave in leads I and aVL differentiates clockwise perimitral MRAT from counterclockwise CTI-dependent AFL and left PV AT.

PULMONARY VEIN CIRCUITS. Because these circuits are related to low-voltage or scar areas, the surface ECG usually shows low-amplitude or flat P waves. These tachycardias have the most variable surface ECG patterns.

LEFT SEPTAL CIRCUITS. Because the reentry circuit is on the septum, the surface ECG shows prominent, usually positive, P waves only in lead V_1 or V_2 and almost flat waves in most other leads (Fig. 13-3). This pattern can be caused by a septal circuit with anteroposterior forces projecting in lead V_1 and the cancellation of caudocranial forces. This pattern was 100% sensitive for an LA septal circuit, but the specificity of this pattern for any type of LA MRAT was only 64%.

Electrophysiological Testing

Typically, a decapolar catheter (positioned into the CS with the proximal electrodes bracketing the CS os) and a multipolar (20- or 24-pole) Halo catheter (positioned at the tricuspid annulus) are used to map typical AFL. The distal tip of the Halo catheter is positioned at 6 to 7 o'clock in left anterior oblique (LAO) view, so that the distal electrodes will record the middle and lateral aspects of the CTI, the middle electrodes will record the anterolateral RA, and the proximal electrodes may record the RA septum (depending on the catheter used). Instead of the Halo and CS catheters described, some laboratories use a single duodecapolar catheter around the tricuspid annulus while extending the catheter tip inside the CS. Such a catheter would straddle the CTI and provide recording and pacing from the medial and lateral aspects of the isthmus.

Induction of Tachycardia

The programmed electrical stimulation protocol should include atrial burst pacing from the high RA and CS—down to a pacing CL at which 2:1 atrial capture occurs—and atrial extrastimulation (AES), single and double, at multiple CLs (600 to 300 milliseconds) from the high RA and CS (down to the atrial effective refractory period). Isoproterenol infusion (0.5 to 4 μg/min) is administered as needed to facilitate tachycardia induction. The goals of EP testing in patients with MRAT are listed in Table 13-1.

Tachycardia Features

MRAT is characterized by a constant CL, P wave polarity, morphology, and amplitude of the recorded bipolar electrograms and by the presence of a single constant macroreentrant circuit with a constant atrial activation sequence. The atrial activation sequence and atrial CL depend on the origin and type of the macroreentrant circuit. However, considerable variation in the atrial CL for a single macroreentry circuit is unusual, although it can be observed in the atrium contralateral to atrium of origin of the tachycardia. In contrast, focal ATs classically exhibit alterations in CL with speeding (warm-up) and slowing (cool-down) at the onset and termination of tachycardia. Variation in the AT CL of greater than 15% has been suggested as a reliable marker of a focal AT. However, a regular AT can be either focal or macroreentrant.[11] Additionally, focal ATs often manifest as bursts of tachycardia with spontaneous onset and termination, although they can be incessant, and they may accelerate in response to sympathetic stimulus.[5] Several criteria can help distinguish focal AT from MRAT (see Table 11-5).

Atrial activation during MRATs spans the whole tachycardia CL. In contrast, intracardiac mapping in the setting of focal ATs shows significant portions of the tachycardia CL without recorded atrial activity, and atrial activation time is markedly less than the tachycardia CL, even when recording from the entire

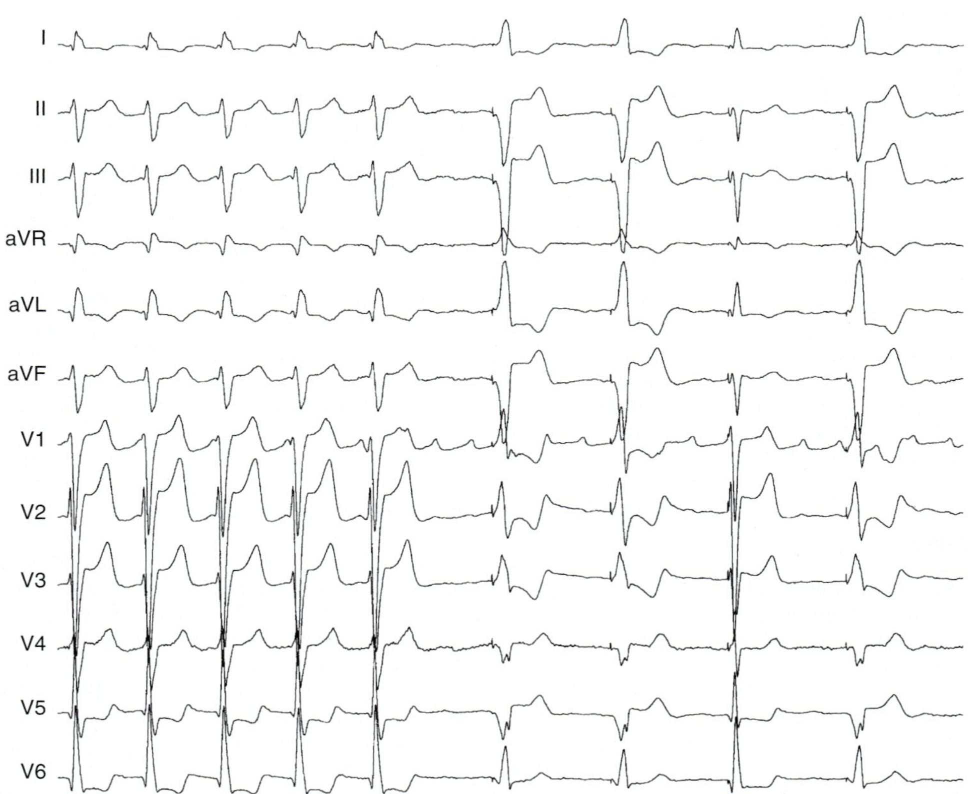

FIGURE 13-3 Surface ECG of left septal macroreentrant atrial tachycardia in a patient with tachycardia-bradycardia syndrome and permanent pacemaker implantation. The P waves are masked by the QRS and T waves during 2:1 atrioventricular (AV) conduction. Administration of adenosine results in AV block and reveals P wave morphology. Note the prominent positive P waves only in lead V1 and almost flat waves in most of the other leads.

cardiac chamber of tachycardia origin (see Fig. 11-2). However, in the presence of complex intramyocardial conduction disturbances, activation during focal tachycardias can extend over a large proportion of the tachycardia CL, and conduction spread can follow circular patterns suggestive of macroreentrant activation.[5] On the other hand, long isoelectric intervals can occur between P waves during MRATs, especially when mapping is limited to only the atrium contralateral to the origin of the macroreentrant circuit or to only parts of the ipsilateral atrium; a focal activation can be observed, incorrectly suggesting a focal mechanism. This is particularly observed for LA MRATs in the presence of large areas of electrical silence. However, a *thorough* intracardiac activation mapping reveals atrial activation spanning the tachycardia CL.

TABLE 13-1 Goals of Programmed Stimulation during Macroreentrant Atrial Tachycardia

1. To confirm that the tachycardia is an AT
2. To confirm that the AT is a macroreentrant circuit • Atrial activation spanning the tachycardia CL • Resetting response consistent with reentry • Entrainment mapping consistent with reentry
3. To exclude cavotricuspid isthmus-dependent atrial flutter • Entrainment mapping at the cavotricuspid isthmus
4. Localization of the circuit in the RA versus LA • ECG morphology of the atrial complex • Isolated variation of the RA CL • RA activation time <50% of the tachycardia CL • Entrainment pacing from different RA sites
5. To define the tachycardia circuit • Activation mapping • Electroanatomical mapping • Entrainment mapping
6. To define the critical isthmus in the tachycardia circuit • Entrainment mapping

AT = atrial tachycardia; CL = cycle length; LA = left atrium; RA = right atrium.

Occasionally, P wave morphology on the surface ECG resembles AFL, but intracardiac recordings show that parts of the atria (commonly the LA) have disorganized atrial activity (Fig. 13-4). Such rhythms behave more like AF than AT, but they may be converted to true typical AFL with antiarrhythmic drugs.

MRAT is usually associated with 2:1 AV conduction, although variable AV conduction and larger multiples are not uncommon. Variable AV block is the result of multilevel block; for example, proximal 2:1 AV block and more distal 3:2 Wenckebach block result in 5:2 AV Wenckebach block. Macroreentrant circuits can have long CLs in the presence of extensive atrial disease and antiarrhythmic agents, in which case fast ventricular response and 1:1 AV conduction may occur.

Diagnostic Maneuvers during Tachycardia

ATRIAL EXTRASTIMULATION

A focal mechanism is defined on the basis of dissociation of almost the entire atria from the tachycardia with AES. In contrast, the MRAT circuit usually incorporates large portions of the RA

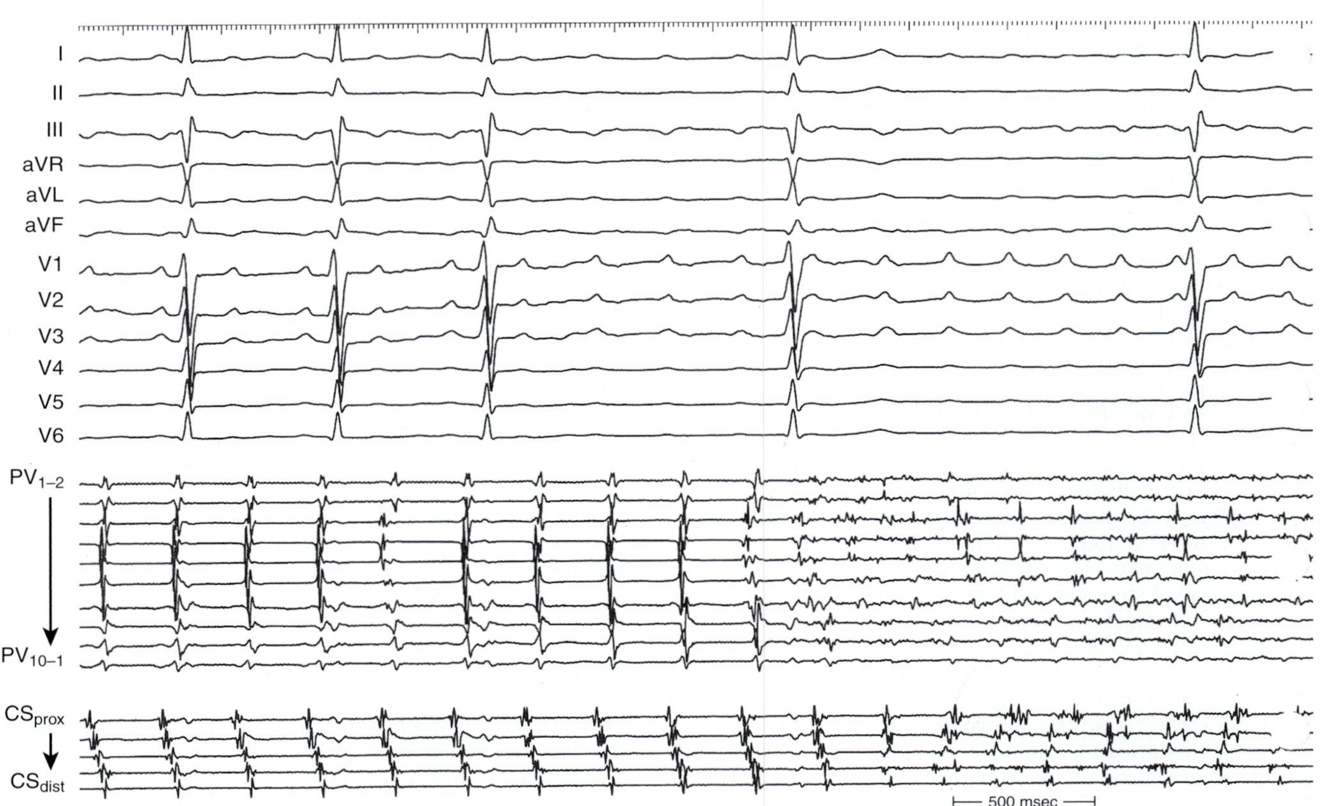

FIGURE 13-4 Surface 12-lead ECG and intracardiac recordings during left atrial tachycardia (AT) that use a small macroreentrant circuit near the ostium of the right superior pulmonary vein (PV) in a patient with prior extensive wide area circumferential PV ablation and linear ablation for atrial fibrillation (AF). On the **left,** P waves are separated by isoelectric intervals, mimicking focal AT, as a result of extensive scarring in the left atrium. In the middle of the recording, the AT converts spontaneously to AF. Note the intracardiac recordings demonstrate grossly irregular atrial activity during AF as compared with AT; however, on the surface ECG, atrial activity remained relatively organized, and conversion from AT into AF was manifest on the surface ECG by a change in rate and minor changes in morphology of atrial complexes. CS_{dist} = distal coronary sinus; CS_{prox} = proximal coronary sinus.

or LA, as demonstrated by resetting. In response to AES, MRATs typically demonstrate an increasing or mixed (flat, then increasing) resetting response. AES usually fails in terminating the AT. AES at short coupling intervals may result in transformation of the tachycardia into a different AT or AF. To minimize the risk to transform or interrupt tachycardia, atrial stimulation maneuvers during the tachycardia should be used sparingly and only when needed to confirm the diagnosis or more precisely localize the critical portion of the AT circuit as guided by the initial activation mapping.[12]

ATRIAL PACING

Burst pacing from the CS or along the Halo catheter is started at a CL 10 to 20 milliseconds shorter than the atrial CL, and then the pacing CL is progressively shortened by 10 to 20 milliseconds. The capture of atrial stimuli and acceleration of the atrial rate to the paced rate should be verified before analyzing the tachycardia response to overdrive pacing. The response of AT to overdrive pacing is evaluated for entrainment, overdrive suppression, transformation into distinct uniform AT morphologies or AF entrainment, and ability and pattern of termination.

Entrainment

Overdrive atrial pacing at long CLs (i.e., 10 to 30 milliseconds shorter than the tachycardia CL) usually can entrain MRAT. The slower the pacing rate and the farther the pacing site from the reentrant circuit, the longer the pacing drive required to penetrate and entrain the tachycardia. Achievement of entrainment of the AT establishes a reentrant mechanism of the tachycardia and excludes triggered activity and abnormal automaticity as potential mechanisms (Fig. 13-5). Entrainment can also be used to estimate qualitatively how far the reentrant circuit is from the pacing site (see later).

ENTRAINMENT CRITERIA. During constant-rate pacing, entrainment of a reentrant tachycardia results in the activation of all myocardial tissue responsible for maintaining the tachycardia at the pacing CL, with resumption of the intrinsic tachycardia morphology and rate after cessation of pacing. However, the mere acceleration of the tachycardia to the pacing rate and the subsequent resumption of the original tachycardia after cessation of pacing do not establish the presence of entrainment. After cessation of each pacing drive, the presence of entrainment should be verified by demonstrating (1) the presence of fixed fusion of the paced complexes at a given pacing CL, (2) progressive fusion at faster pacing CLs, and (3) resumption of the same tachycardia morphology following cessation of pacing with a nonfused complex at a return cycle equal to the pacing CL.

ENTRAINMENT WITH FUSION. During entrainment of MRAT, fusion of the stimulated impulse can be observed on the surface ECG, but it is easier to recognize on intracardiac recordings from the Halo and CS catheters. The stimulated impulse has hybrid morphology between the fully paced atrial impulse and the tachycardia impulse. The ability to demonstrate surface ECG fusion requires a significant mass of atrial myocardium to be depolarized by both the paced stimulus and the tachycardia. The farther the stimulation site from the reentrant circuit, the less likely entrainment will manifest ECG fusion. It is important to understand that overdrive pacing of a tachycardia of any mechanism can result in a certain degree of fusion, especially when the pacing CL is only slightly shorter than the tachycardia CL. Such fusion, however, is unstable during the same pacing drive at the same pacing CL because pacing stimuli fall on a progressively earlier portion of the tachycardia cycle, thus producing progressively less fusion and more fully paced morphology. Such phenomena should be distinguished from entrainment, and sometimes this requires pacing for long intervals to demonstrate variable degrees of fusion. Focal ATs (automatic, triggered activity, or microreentrant) cannot manifest fixed or progressive fusion during overdrive pacing. Moreover, overdrive pacing frequently results in suppression (automatic) or acceleration (triggered activity) of focal ATs, rather than resumption of the original tachycardia with an unchanged tachycardia CL.

ENTRAINMENT WITH MANIFEST FUSION. Entrainment of MRATs commonly produces manifest fusion that is stable (fixed) during the pacing drive at a given pacing CL. Repeated entrainment at pacing CLs progressively shorter than the tachycardia CL results in different degrees of fusion, with the resultant P wave configuration looking more like a fully paced configuration.

ENTRAINMENT WITH INAPPARENT FUSION. Entrainment with inapparent fusion (also referred to as local or intracardiac fusion) is said to be present when a fully paced P morphology (with no ECG fusion) results, even when the tachycardia impulse exits the reentrant circuit (orthodromic activation of the presystolic electrogram is present). Fusion is limited to a small area and does not produce surface ECG fusion, and only intracardiac (local) fusion can be recognized.

ENTRAINMENT WITH CONCEALED FUSION. Entrainment with concealed fusion (sometimes also referred to as concealed entrainment or exact entrainment) is defined as entrainment with orthodromic capture and a surface ECG complex identical to that of the tachycardia. Entrainment with concealed fusion suggests that the pacing site is within a protected isthmus, either inside or outside but attached to the reentrant circuit (i.e., the pacing site can be in, attached to, or at the entrance to a protected isthmus that forms the diastolic pathway of the circuit).

POST-PACING INTERVAL. The PPI is the interval from the last pacing stimulus that entrained the tachycardia to the next recorded electrogram at the pacing site. The PPI should be measured to the near-field potential that indicates depolarization of tissue at the pacing site. The PPI remains relatively stable when entrainment of MRAT is performed at the same site, regardless of the length of the pacing drive.

Termination

Rapid atrial burst pacing can usually terminate MRAT. However, termination is less likely when the pacing drive is short or the pacing site is distant from the reentrant circuit.

Overdrive Suppression

Overdrive suppression analogous to that seen with automatic AT is not expected in MRAT. As noted, the PPI remains relatively stable when entrainment of MRAT is performed at the same site, regardless of the length of the pacing drive. This is in contrast to overdrive suppression seen in automatic ATs, which would be associated with progressive delay of the first tachycardia beat return cycle with progressively longer overdrive pacing drives.

Transformation

Rapid atrial burst pacing may convert an MRAT into AF, clockwise or counterclockwise typical AFL, or another type of MRAT. Detection of this change requires careful attention to the atrial activation sequence and the ECG pattern after cessation of pacing. The recording of multiple simultaneous electrograms, as continuous endocardial references, facilitates detection of these activation changes.

Mapping

Because the reentrant circuit can involve any of multiple barriers, the usual anatomically guided ablation, as performed for typical CTI-dependent AFL, is not possible. Mapping is required to determine the precise circuit and define its vulnerable segment (critical isthmus) to provide a specifically tailored ablation solution. The goals of mapping of macroreentrant circuits include localization of the tachycardia circuit (RA versus LA), identification of possible lines of block, identification of an isthmus of tissue bounded between two long barriers, and determination of whether the line of block is a critical part of the circuit.

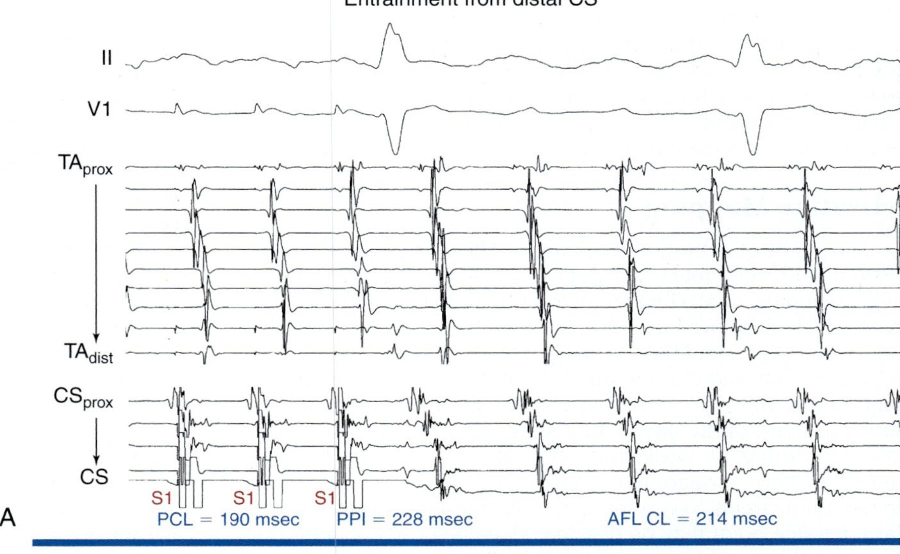

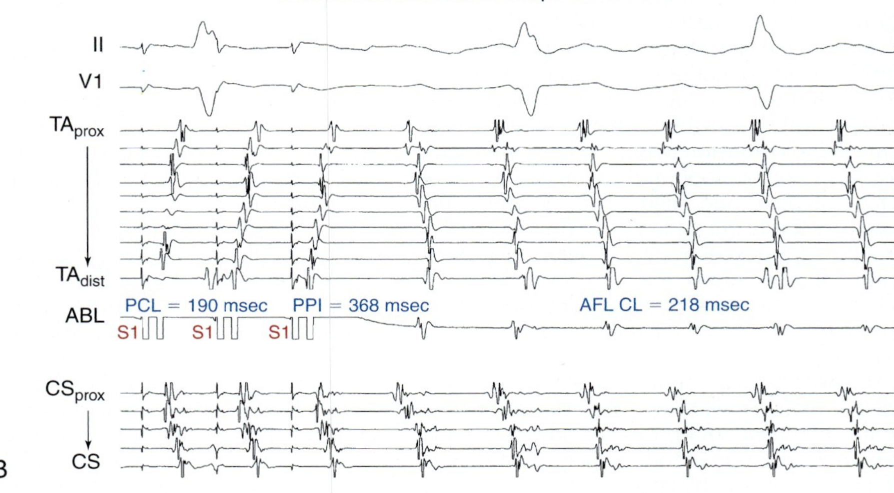

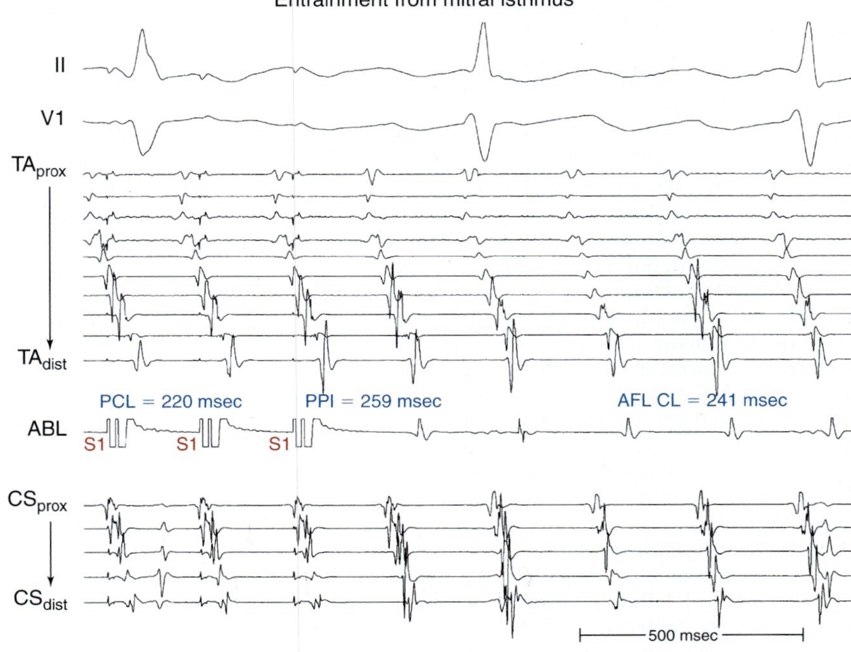

FIGURE 13-5 Entrainment of counterclockwise perimitral macroreentrant atrial tachycardia (AT). **A,** Entrainment from the distal coronary sinus (CS) results in intracardiac atrial fusion (as demonstrated in CS activation sequence) and a short post-pacing interval (PPI) [PPI – AT CL = 14 msec] because the distal CS is close to the reentrant circuit. **B,** Entrainment from the ablation catheter (ABL) positioned at the cavotricuspid isthmus (CTI) results in manifest atrial fusion with a long PPI (PPI – AT CL = 150 msec), suggesting that the CTI is not part of the reentrant circuit. **C,** Entrainment from the ablation catheter positioned at the mitral isthmus, concealed atrial fusion, and a short PPI (PPI – AT CL = 18 msec), suggesting that the mitral isthmus is the critical isthmus of the reentrant circuit. CL = cycle length; CS_{dist} = distal coronary sinus; CS_{prox} = proximal coronary sinus; PCL = pacing CL; TA_{dist} = distal tricuspid annulus; TA_{prox} = proximal tricuspid annulus.

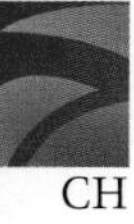

Detailed knowledge of the congenital anomaly and the surgical procedure, if present, is important in interpreting the results of mapping, in knowing how to access the RA, in assessing the feasibility of the transseptal puncture, and in determining whether fluoroscopy is helpful in localizing the catheters or whether intracardiac echocardiography or transesophageal echocardiography is needed.

Activation Mapping

The main goal of activation mapping of MRAT is identification of the complete reentrant circuit and its mid-diastolic critical isthmus. Unlike mapping focal AT, whereby tracking the site with the earliest presystolic local activation timing is the goal of mapping, there is no early or late region for MRAT because the wavefront is continuously propagating around the circuit. Activation can be continuously mapped, and an earlier activation time can always be found for any particular point of the circuit. Endocardial recordings often show activation during the isoelectric intervals on the surface ECG. The concept of early activation is not applicable to any particular site in the reentrant circuit. Nevertheless, for illustrative purposes, a particular reference point may be designated as the origin of activation (time 0), but it should be understood that this is always arbitrary.

The complete reentrant circuit can be defined as the spatially shortest route of unidirectional activation encompassing the complete CL of the tachycardia in terms of activation timing and returning to the site of earliest activation. Activation wavefronts that do not fulfill these conditions are bystander wavefronts and are not critical to the arrhythmia circuit. However, incomplete mapping can lead to confusion about the bystander status of a given activation wavefront or loop, and an incomplete loop can be mistaken for a complete one. High-density mapping or entrainment mapping can clarify this situation by documenting wavefront collision or a long PPI, respectively (see later). If activation recorded at different atrial locations does not cover most of the tachycardia CL, two possibilities must be considered: focal AT and small, localized reentrant circuits, which require much more detailed activation mapping to be identified.

Sometimes, it can be impossible to map the entire circuit, especially in patients with repaired congenital heart disease, because of the complex suture lines, baffles, or both. Entrainment then becomes an essential tool in these cases to confirm participation of specific areas in the circuit and to try to locate a suitable isthmus area (see later).

Identification of the tachycardia circuit barriers is very important to help understand propagation of the reentrant activation wavefront in relation to these barriers, identify the tachycardia critical isthmus, and, equally important, plan an ablation strategy to abolish the tachycardia. For RA MRAT, the tricuspid annulus often provides one important barrier. Other naturally fixed barriers (i.e., independent of the precise form of activation and present also in NSR) include the IVC, SVC, and CS os. For LA MRAT, the mitral annulus and PVs often provide important barriers. Acquired barriers include surgical incisions or patches and electrically silent regions devoid of electrical activity (of uncertain origin). A line of block can be identified by the presence of double potentials, thus reflecting conduction up one side of the barrier and down the other side, with the bipolar electrogram recording both waves of activation. Significant large areas devoid of electrical activity can be easily recognized as electrical scars, provided that catheter contact is verified. Narrow lines of block can easily be missed unless the conduction delay across them is maximized by the appropriate choice of pacing sites and CLs. Therefore, to avoid overlooking any such scar, it may be necessary to perform mapping during more than one form of activation (e.g., during both proximal CS and low lateral RA pacing).

During macroreentry, an isthmus is defined as a corridor of conductive myocardial tissue bounded by nonconductive tissue (barriers) through which the depolarization wavefront must propagate to perpetuate the tachycardia. These barriers can be scar areas or naturally occurring anatomical or functional (present only during tachycardia, but not in sinus rhythm) obstacles. The earliest presystolic electrogram closest to mid-diastole is the most commonly used definition for the center of the isthmus of the reentrant circuit.

It is very important to ensure that the correct AT is being mapped at all points of time, and to remain vigilant to identify any change in CL or activation sequence that can result from catheter manipulation, pacing maneuvers, or ablation. Such changes can indicate transition to another tachycardia requiring reassessment. The transition may be obvious, but it is often quite subtle and sometimes imperceptible if only the CS activation is analyzed. Simultaneous recording RA activation (using a Halo catheter around the tricuspid annulus) and CS activation (using a decapolar catheter) can help rapid identification of tachycardia transformation.[7]

Variations in the tachycardia CL during MRAT can suggest variations in activation pathways resulting from circuit transformation or simply changes in conduction time; the latter is usually manifest as CL alternans. The absence of ECG alterations accompanying changes in activation sequences can occur because of an insufficient change in electromotive force, either because of distance from the recording electrodes or because of insufficient electrically active tissue. At all points of time, it is necessary to ensure that the change of activation sequence is not secondary to unintentional movement of the recording catheters. A single-loop tachycardia with a fixed barrier as its core typically remains stable and unchanged during catheter manipulation, and it may even be difficult to pace-terminate, although mechanical bump termination rendering the tachycardia noninducible suggests mechanical stimulation close to a restricted and relatively fragile isthmus.

A change in ECG morphology without a change in the tachycardia CL can occur secondary to transformation of a multiple loop tachycardia by interruption of one loop, a change in bystander activation sufficient to be visible on the surface ECG (typified by the change in CS and LA activation observed during incomplete ablation of the CTI in counterclockwise typical AFL), a change from tachycardia in one atrium to that in the other (Fig. 13-6), or activation of the same circuit in the opposite direction (the last possible only if the first AT stops at least transiently).

In addition to analyzing the RA and LA activation sequences during the tachycardia as recorded by the peritricuspid Halo catheter and CS catheter, activation mapping is started in the RA by using a roving catheter. Local activation time at each site is measured relative to a reference intracardiac electrogram (e.g., middle CS). Placing the intracardiac reference channel adjacent to the mapping catheter channel on the display allows the operator immediately to know which parts (early, middle, or late) of the cycle are being mapped by visual inspection and sequential electronic caliper measured delay. When activation from 10 evenly distributed sites in the RA (including 3 or 4 points at the tricuspid annulus) occupies less than 50% of the tachycardia CL, the arrhythmia is probably not located in the RA. The only exception is the presence of a small reentrant circuit in the RA.

During LA MRATs, in the absence of LA mapping through transseptal catheterization, long segments of the tachycardia CL may not be covered by recorded electrograms. RA mapping typically shows nonreentrant activation patterns, clearly different from typical clockwise and counterclockwise AFL. Early RA septal activation relative to other parts of the RA can suggest a focal septal origin in some cases when LA recordings are not obtained (Fig. 13-7; see Fig. 13-2). Local RA conduction disturbances, such as CTI block (from prior isthmus ablation), transverse block at the crista terminalis, or both, can result in activation of the anterior and septal RA in opposite directions that mimics reentrant RA activation of typical AFL. In these cases, entrainment mapping clarifies the location of the reentrant circuit.[13]

The CS activation sequence has frequently been suggested as a useful way to determine the chamber of interest; however, this is not without limitations. Whereas in RA MRAT the CS is frequently activated from proximal to distal, this is not always true, particularly with MRAT localized to the superior RA. Similarly, although most circuits with distal to proximal activation of the CS are caused by

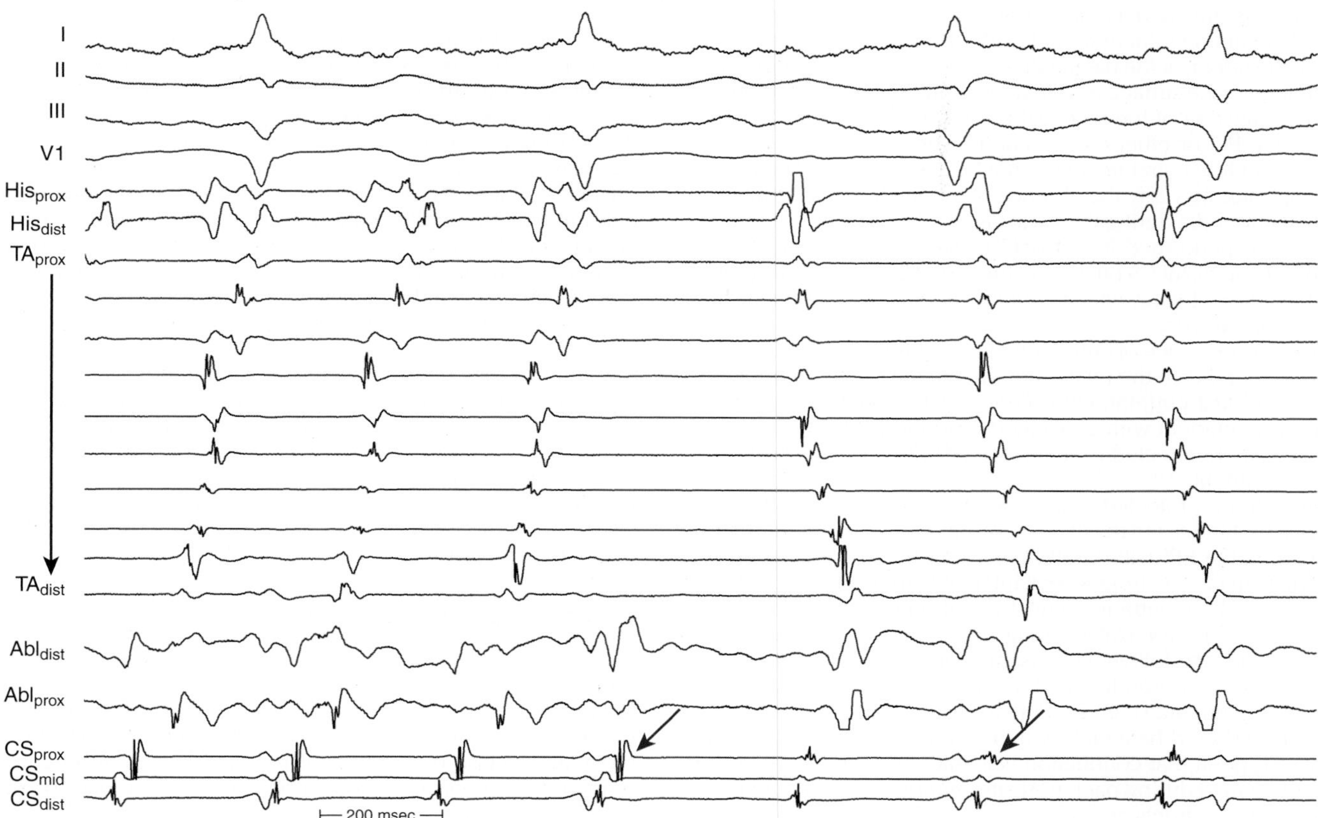

FIGURE 13-6 A change in atrial activation sequence is observed during right atrial ablation during macroreentrant atrial tachycardia that interrupts one circuit while another (left atrial) circuit persists (note coronary sinus [CS] activation from distal to proximal throughout [arrows]). Abl_{dist} = distal ablation site; Abl_{prox} = proximal ablation site; CS_{dist} = distal coronary sinus; CS_{mid} = middle coronary sinus; CS_{prox} = proximal coronary sinus; His_{dist} = distal His bundle; His_{prox} = proximal His bundle; TA_{dist} = distal tricuspid annulus; TA_{prox} = proximal tricuspid annulus.

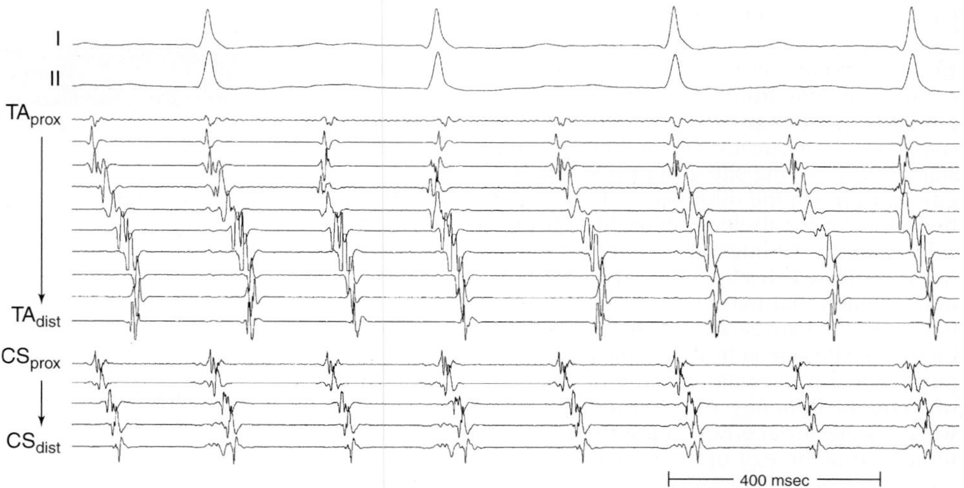

FIGURE 13-7 Surface ECG leads I and II and intracardiac recording during left atrial (LA) macroreentry. Note the large spontaneous variations in the right atrial cycle length (CL) and activation sequence (as recorded by a Halo catheter around the tricuspid annulus, TA), with a constant LA CL and activation sequence (as recorded by the coronary sinus [CS] catheter). CS_{dist} = distal coronary sinus; CS_{prox} = proximal coronary sinus; TA_{dist} = distal tricuspid annulus; TA_{prox} = proximal tricuspid annulus.

LA MRAT, this sequence may also be seen in some cases of RA MRAT (see Fig. 13-2), and some LA MRATs (e.g., counterclockwise perimitral MRAT) can activate the CS proximally to distally.

For LA macroreentry, identification of the complete reentrant circuit can be challenging. The initial step is activation mapping to determine whether activation of the entire tachycardia CL can be recorded within the LA. In particular, mapping should be carefully carried out around the mitral annulus because this maneuver is easy to perform and identifies a common form of LA MRAT, perimitral MRAT.

Entrainment Mapping

Entrainment mapping provides information about sites of the RA or LA that are part of the reentrant circuit, those that are outside the circuit, and the critical isthmus in the macroreentrant circuit. Entrainment also qualitatively estimates how far the reentrant circuit is from the pacing site. However, before attempting to use entrainment methods for mapping, it is necessary first to demonstrate that the tachycardia can, in fact, be entrained, thus providing strong evidence that it is

caused by reentry rather than by triggered activity or automaticity. At sites of entrainment, there should be confirmation of consistent capture of the atrium at the pacing CL for several beats, with minimal or no change in the surface morphology or intracardiac electrograms, and continuation of the identical tachycardia after pacing. Evaluation of the PPI or other criteria can be very misleading when the presence of true entrainment has not been established. Additionally, it is important to verify the absence of termination and reinitiation of the tachycardia during the same pacing drive.[14]

Pacing is performed from the CTI, high RA, midlateral RA, and proximal and distal CS, but not on the septum, to avoid the possibility of capturing the LA, which could be confusing in distinguishing RA from LA MRATs.

Once the presence of entrainment is verified, several criteria can be used to indicate the relation of the pacing site to the reentrant circuit. The first entrainment criterion to be sought is concealed fusion. Entrainment with concealed fusion indicates that the pacing site is in a protected isthmus located within or attached to the reentrant circuit.[15,16]

Whether this protected isthmus is crucial to the reentrant circuit or just a bystander site needs to be verified by other criteria, mainly comparing the PPI with the tachycardia CL and the stimulus-exit interval with the electrogram-exit interval. During entrainment from sites within the reentrant circuit, the orthodromic wavefront from the last stimulus propagates through the reentry circuit and returns to the pacing site, following the same path as the circulating reentry wavefronts. The conduction time required is the revolution time through the circuit. Thus, the PPI (measured from the pacing site recording) should be equal (within 20 milliseconds) to the tachycardia CL, given that conduction velocities and the reentrant path did not change during pacing. At sites remote from the circuit, the stimulated wavefronts propagate to the circuit, then through the circuit, and finally back to the pacing site. Thus, the PPI should equal the tachycardia CL plus the time required for the stimulus to propagate from the pacing site to the tachycardia circuit and back. The greater the difference is between the PPI and the tachycardia CL (PPI – AT CL), the longer the conduction time is between the pacing site and reentry circuit, and the greater the physical distance is between the pacing site and circuit. Features of entrainment when pacing from different sites are listed in Table 13-2.[15,16]

During entrainment of MRAT, the interval between the pacing stimulus and the onset of the P wave on the surface ECG reflects conduction time from the pacing site to the exit of the reentrant circuit (stimulus-exit interval), regardless of whether the pacing site is inside or outside the reentrant circuit, because activation starts at the pacing site and propagates in sequence to the circuit exit site. On the other hand, during tachycardia, the interval between the local electrogram at a given site and circuit exit (electrogram-exit interval) can reflect the true conduction time between those two sites if they are activated in sequence (which occurs when that particular site is located within the reentrant pathway), or can be shorter than the true conduction time if those two sites are activated in parallel (which occurs when that particular site is located outside the reentrant circuit). Because of frequent difficulty of determination of the onset of the P wave on the surface ECG, a reference intracardiac electrogram representing the exit of the circuit is usually used. Therefore, at any given pacing site, an electrogram-exit interval that is equal (± 20 milliseconds) to the stimulus-exit interval indicates that the pacing site lies within the reentry circuit and excludes the possibility that the site is a dead-end pathway attached to the circuit (i.e., not a bystander). On the other hand, pacing sites outside the reentrant circuit have an electrogram-exit interval significantly (more than 20 milliseconds) shorter than the stimulus-exit interval (see Table 13-2).

LIMITATION OF ENTRAINMENT MAPPING

Entrainment techniques can be difficult in patients with incisional AT caused by low-amplitude or absent atrial potentials in the area of surgical incisions. Fusion is difficult to assess on the surface ECG because the pacing artifact and QRS complex frequently obscure the surface P waves, which often have low amplitude in these patients. Furthermore, methodological problems can affect the validity of the PPI. Decremental conduction during pacing increases the PPI and causes false-negative assessment results at some reentry circuit sites. The occasional presence of far-field potentials can also impair the accuracy of entrainment mapping. Additionally, it is difficult to identify exact catheter positions in relation to anatomical barriers because visualization of these barriers is not possible fluoroscopically. Spontaneous changes in the tachycardia CL in some MRATs can also make interpretation of the PPI impossible. Combining entrainment mapping with electroanatomical mapping can reduce the difficulties created by some of these limitations. Finally, reconstruction of the complete circuit can be extremely difficult to achieve, and the risk of transformation of the clinical tachycardia to another morphology or to AF is high. Therefore, it is advisable to begin with electroanatomical mapping, while pacing maneuvers are used sparingly, just to confirm the participation of precise areas in the reentry circuit and to improve understanding of the tachycardia further.

Electroanatomical Mapping

Electromagnetic three-dimensional (3-D) mapping (CARTO mapping system [Biosense Webster, Inc., Diamond Bar, Calif.] or EnSite NavX system [St. Jude Medical, St. Paul, Minn.]) can help distinguish between a focal origin and macroreentrant tachycardia by providing precise description of the macroreentrant circuit and sequence of atrial activation during the tachycardia and rapid visualization of the activation wavefront (see Videos 12 and 17). This can contribute to the understanding of the reentrant circuit in relation to native barriers and surgical scars, identification of all slow-conducting pathways and appropriate sites for entrainment mapping, planning of ablation lines, navigation of the ablation catheter, and verification of conduction block produced by RF ablation.

TABLE 13-2 Entrainment Mapping of Macroreentrant Atrial Tachycardia

Pacing from sites *outside* the AT circuit results in manifest entrainment:
1. Manifest atrial fusion on surface ECG and intracardiac recordings (fixed fusion at a single pacing CL and progressive fusion on progressively shorter pacing CLs). Any change in atrial activation sequence, compared with baseline tachycardia and that of pure pacing, as determined by analysis of all available surface and intracardiac ECG recordings, is considered to represent manifest fusion.
2. PPI – AT CL > 20 msec
3. The interval between the stimulus artifact and the onset of the P wave on the surface ECG is longer than the interval between the local electrogram on the pacing site and the onset of the P wave on the surface ECG.

Pacing from sites *inside* the AT circuit results in manifest entrainment:
1. Manifest atrial fusion on the surface ECG and intracardiac recordings (fixed fusion at a single pacing CL and progressive fusion on progressively shorter pacing CLs)
2. PPI – AT CL < 20 msec
3. The interval between the stimulus artifact and the onset of the P wave on the surface ECG equals the interval between the local electrogram on the pacing site and the onset of the P wave on the surface ECG.

Pacing from *a protected isthmus* inside the circuit results in concealed entrainment:
1. Concealed atrial fusion (i.e., paced atrial waveform on the surface ECG and intracardiac recordings is identical to the tachycardia waveform)
2. PPI – AT CL < 20 msec
3. The interval between the stimulus artifact and the onset the P wave on the surface ECG equals the interval between the local electrogram on the pacing site and the onset of the P wave on the surface ECG.

AT = atrial tachycardia; CL = cycle length; PPI = post-pacing interval.

MAPPING TECHNIQUE

Initially, selection of the reference electrogram, positioning of the anatomical reference, and determination of the window of interest are undertaken. The reference catheter is usually placed in the CS (because of its stability), by using a recording with a prominent atrial electrogram and ensuring that the ventricular electrogram is not the one detected by the system. The onset of the window of interest is usually set at the mid-diastole between two consecutive P waves with a window duration spanning 95% of the tachycardia CL. Anatomical and EP landmarks (IVC, SVC, CS, His bundle, and tricuspid annulus for RA mapping, and mitral annulus and PVs for LA mapping) are marked.

Activation mapping is performed to define the atrial activation sequence. Reasonable numbers of points homogeneously distributed in the RA or LA, or both, must be recorded (80 to 100). Each point is tagged on the 3-D map as follows: The local activation time at each site is determined from the intracardiac bipolar electrogram and is measured in relation to the fixed intracardiac electrogram obtained from the CS (reference) catheter. Points are added to the map only if stability criteria in space and local activation time are met. The end-diastolic location stability criterion is a variation of less than 2 mm, and the local activation time stability criterion is less than 2 milliseconds. Lines of block (manifest as double potentials) are tagged for easy identification because they can serve as boundaries for a subsequent design of ablation strategies. Silent areas are defined as having an atrial potential amplitude lower than 0.05 mV and the absence of atrial capture at 20 mA. Such areas and surgically related scars, such as atriotomy scars in the lateral RA or atrial septal defect closure patches, are tagged as "scar" (see Figs. 14-1 and 14-2). At sites with double potential, entrainment of the tachycardia can help evaluate which potentials are captured by the pacing stimulus. Local activation times are then reviewed, and the apparent far-field signal is excluded from the activation maps. The activation map can also be used to catalog sites at which pacing maneuvers are performed during assessment of the tachycardia.

ACTIVATION MAP

A continuous progression of colors (from red to purple in the CARTO system and from white to purple in the NavX system) around the RA (or LA), with close proximity of earliest and latest local activation, suggests the presence of an RA (or LA) macroreentrant tachycardia. In these cases, RA (or LA) activation time is in a similar range as the tachycardia CL (Fig. 13-8). Conversely, the electroanatomical maps of focal ATs demonstrate radial spreading of activation, from the earliest local activation site in all directions. In these cases, atrial activation time is markedly shorter than the tachycardia CL. When the onset of the window of interest is set at the mid-diastole between two consecutive P waves, the mid-diastolic isthmus of the reentrant circuit can be identified by the interface of early and late activation (i.e., the region where "early meets late" on the color-coded activation map). High-density mapping is then performed in and around the isthmus to define its limits and width precisely. It is important to recognize that if an insufficient number of points is obtained in the isthmus region, it may be falsely concluded through the interpolation of activation times that the wavefront propagates from a focal source (Fig. 13-9).[9]

VOLTAGE MAP

Voltage mapping is performed to define areas of electrical scars, which can be involved in the reentrant circuit and/or can potentially serve as boundaries for the subsequent design of ablation strategies. Silent areas are defined as having an atrial potential amplitude of less than 0.05 mV and the absence of atrial capture at 20 mA.

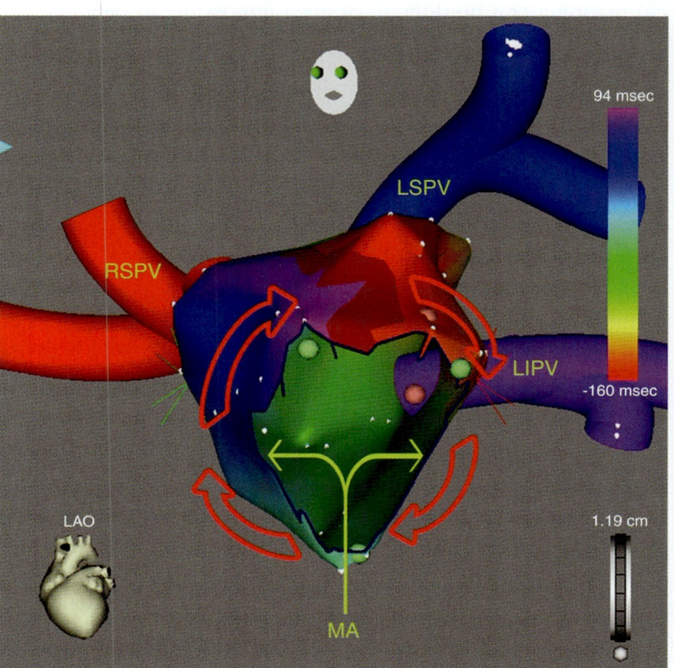

FIGURE 13-8 Three-dimensional electroanatomical (CARTO, Biosense Webster, Inc., Diamond Bar, Calif.) activation map of the left atrium in the left anterior oblique (LAO) view constructed during clockwise perimitral macroreentrant atrial tachycardia. During tachycardia, the activation wavefront travels clockwise around the mitral annulus (MA), as indicated by a continuous progression of colors (from red to purple) with close proximity of earliest and latest local activation (red meeting purple). LIPV = left inferior pulmonary vein; LSPV = left superior pulmonary vein; RSPV = right superior pulmonary vein.

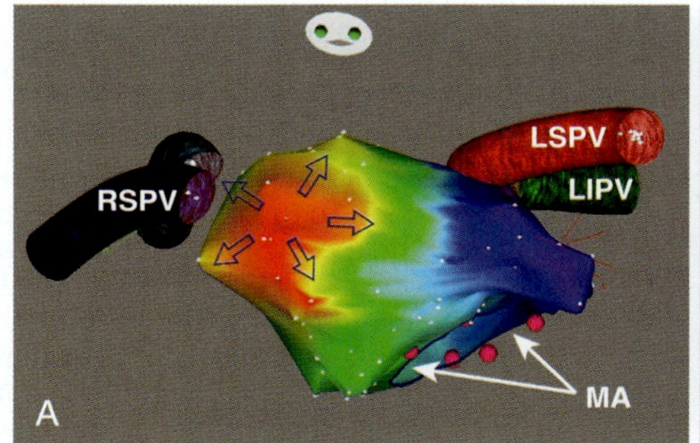

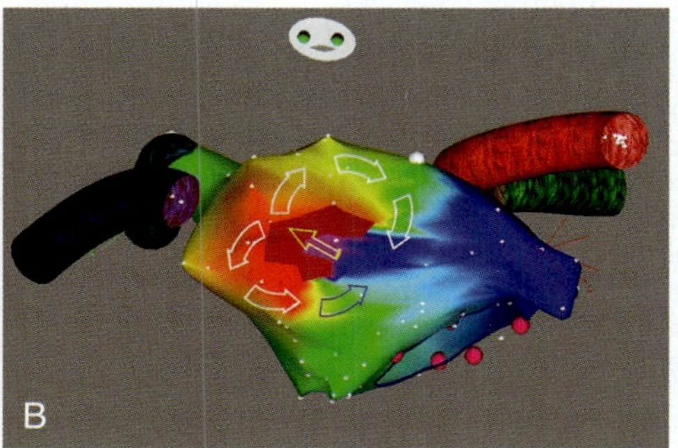

FIGURE 13-9 Left atrial electroanatomical (CARTO, Biosense Webster, Inc., Diamond Bar, Calif.) activation map in a patient with atrial tachycardia following pulmonary vein (PV) isolation for treatment of atrial fibrillation. The view is from the aspect of the right shoulder. **A,** The activation pattern suggests a focal process in the left atrium roof close with centrifugal spread of activation from the central red area. **B,** With additional detailed mapping below the red area, a small figure-of-8 macroreentrant circuit is evident. Entrainment data had already diagnosed macroreentry, but the relatively detailed activation map had missed the small area that became clear on more detailed mapping. LIPV = left inferior pulmonary vein; LSPV = left superior pulmonary vein; MA = mitral annulus; RSPV = right superior pulmonary vein .

PROPAGATION MAP

Propagation of electrical activation can be superimposed on the 3-D anatomical reconstruction of the RA or LA, thereby allowing visualization of the reentrant circuit of AT in relation to the anatomical and EP landmarks and barriers. Analysis of the propagation map may allow estimation of the conduction velocity along the reentrant circuit and identification of areas of slow conduction and may thus help locate appropriate sites for entrainment mapping and catheter ablation.

LIMITATION OF THE USE OF ELECTROANATOMICAL MAPPING

Variation of the tachycardia CL by more than 10% may prevent complete understanding of the circuit and decreases the confidence in the electroanatomical map. Similarly, electroanatomical mapping can be difficult or even impossible in patients with nonsustained AT. In these cases, 3-D mapping systems based on a single-beat analysis, such as the multielectrode basket catheter or the noncontact mapping system, may be an alternative to electroanatomical mapping technology. For unstable tachycardia with changes in morphology or CL, amiodarone infusion can help stabilize the arrhythmia.

Electroanatomical Mapping of Post-Pacing Intervals

A graphical representation of entrainment mapping can be constructed by plotting the values of the [PPI – AT CL] differences on an electroanatomical mapping system (CARTO or NavX) to generate color-coded 3-D entrainment maps (see Fig. 13-1). This approach can potentially help accurately determine and visualize the 3-D location of the entire reentrant circuit, even though the area of slow conduction of the tachycardia is not described. Because neither of the electroanatomical mapping systems (CARTO, NavX) contains an algorithm for color-coding of entrainment information, the modus for activation mapping is altered manually. At each 3-D location of the catheter tip stored on the electroanatomical mapping system, entrainment stimulation is performed, and the difference between PPI and tachycardia CL (PPI – AT CL) is calculated and entered into the electroanatomical mapping system (as if it would be an "activation time"). For that, the local electrogram stored at the 3-D location is completely disregarded. The annotation marker is manually moved into a position where the numerical timing information equaled the entrainment information (PPI – tachycardia CL). That timing information then is displayed in a color-coded fashion as if it were activation time, but, in fact, it represents information on the length of the entrainment return cycle (see Fig. 13-1). With the color range, red (in CARTO) or white (in NavX) represents points closest to the reentrant circuit (i.e., sites with smaller [PPI – AT CL] differences, approaching 0, signifying their inclusion in the reentrant circuit), and purple represents points far away from the circuit (i.e., sites with the largest [PPI – AT CL] differences).[14,17]

Color-coded 3-D entrainment mapping allows determination of the full active reentrant circuit (versus passively activated regions of the chamber) and the obstacle around which the tachycardia is circulating, and it provides very useful information on the location of potential ablation sites. However, not all these sites terminate reentry; the final choice is determined by location of anatomical barriers and width of putative isthmuses, so that strategic ablation lines, mainly connecting to anatomical barriers, can be applied to transect the circuit and eliminate the arrhythmia.[14,17]

Noncontact Mapping

When AT is short-lived or cannot be reproducibly initiated, simultaneous multisite data acquisition using the noncontact mapping system (EnSite 3000, St. Jude Medical, Inc., St. Paul, Minn.) can help localize the AT origin. This system can recreate the endocardial activation sequence from simultaneously acquired multiple data points over a few tachycardia beats without requiring sequential point-to-point acquisitions.

The EnSite 3000 system requires a 9 Fr multielectrode array and a 7 Fr mapping-ablation catheter. To create a map, the balloon catheter is positioned over a 0.035-inch guidewire under fluoroscopic guidance in the cardiac chamber of interest. The balloon is then deployed, and it can be filled with a mixture of contrast and saline to be visualized fluoroscopically. The balloon is positioned in the center of the atrium and does not come into physical contact with the atrial walls being mapped. The position of the array in the chamber must be secured to avoid significant movement that would invalidate the electrical and anatomical information. The array must be positioned as closely as possible (and in direct line of sight through the blood pool) to the endocardial surface being mapped, because the accuracy of the map is sensitive to the distance between the center of the balloon and the endocardium being mapped.[18]

Systemic anticoagulation is critical to avoid thromboembolic complications. Intravenous heparin is usually given to maintain the activated clotting time at 250 to 300 seconds and 300 to 350 seconds for right-sided and left-sided mapping, respectively.

A conventional deflectable mapping-ablation catheter is also positioned in the chamber and used to collect geometry information. The mapping catheter is initially moved to known anatomical locations (IVC, SVC, CS, His bundle, and tricuspid annulus for RA mapping and mitral annulus and PVs for LA mapping), which are tagged. Subsequently, detailed geometry of the chamber is reconstructed by moving the mapping catheter around the atrium. Using this information, the computer creates a model, called a convex hull, of the chamber during diastole.

Once chamber geometry has been delineated, tachycardia is induced, and mapping can begin. The data acquisition process is performed automatically by the system, and all data for the entire chamber are acquired simultaneously. The system then reconstructs more than 3000 unipolar electrograms simultaneously and superimposes them onto the virtual endocardium, to produce color-coded isopotential maps that graphically depict depolarized regions. Activation can be tracked on the isopotential map throughout the tachycardia cycle, and wavefront propagation can be displayed as a user-controlled 3-D "movie." The color range represents voltage or timing of onset. A default high-pass filter setting of 2 Hz is used to preserve components of slow conduction on the isopotential map. When conduction through gaps in a line of block is very slow, the high-pass filter may be set at 1.0 to 0.5 Hz. Color settings are adjusted so that the color range matches 1 to 1 with the millivolt range of the electrogram deflection of interest. Isochronal maps can also be created that represent progression of activation throughout the chamber relative to user-defined electrical reference timing point. If the atrial electrograms overlap with the T wave, a ventricular extrastimulus may be delivered to accelerate ventricular depolarization and repolarization and reveal the following atrial complex without far-field interference.[19]

In addition, the system can simultaneously display as many as 32 electrograms as waveforms. Unipolar or bipolar electrograms (virtual electrograms) can be selected (at any given interval of the tachycardia cycle) by using the mouse from any part of the created geometry and displayed as waveforms as if from point, array, or plaque electrodes. The reconstructed electrograms are subject to the same electrical principles as contact catheter electrograms because they contain far-field electrical information from the surrounding endocardium, as well as the underlying myocardial signal vector, and distance from the point where the signal is generated to the array can affect the contribution to the electrogram. The maps are particularly useful for identifying slowly conducting pathways, such as the critical slow pathways and rapid breakthrough points of MRAT. The reentry circuit can be fully identified, along with other aspects such as the slowing, narrowing, and splitting of activation wavefronts in the isthmus. The locator technology used to collect the geometry information for the convex hull can then be used to guide an ablation catheter to the proper location in the heart. Ablation lesions can be tagged, thus facilitating performing linear ablation devoid of gaps across the tachycardia critical isthmus.[19]

Substrate mapping based on scar or diseased tissue, which has been introduced into noncontact mapping technology, can be of value in mapping and ablation of MRAT. Dynamic substrate mapping allows the creation of voltage maps from a single cardiac cycle and can identify low-voltage areas, as well as fixed and functional block, on the virtual endocardium through noncontact methodology. High-density voltage mapping of the atrial substrate is performed using the peak negative voltage of the reconstructed unipolar electrograms. An atrial substrate characterized by an abnormally low peak negative voltage (less than 30% of the maximal peak negative voltage) can potentially predict the slow conduction path within the protected isthmus of the MRAT. When combined with the activation sequence, substrate mapping provides essential information for guiding ablation, even when the arrhythmia is nonsustained.[20]

LIMITATIONS OF NONCONTACT MAPPING

Very low-amplitude signals may not be detected, particularly if the distance between the center of the balloon catheter and the endocardial surface exceeds 40 mm or regions near its poles, thus limiting the accurate identification of diastolic signals. In addition, the acquired geometry with the current version of software is somewhat distorted, and multiple set points are required to establish the origin and shape of complicated structures clearly, such as the LA appendage or PVs. Otherwise, these structures may be lost in the interpolation among several neighboring points. A second catheter is still required for more detailed mapping to find the precise site to ablate, and sometimes it is difficult to manipulate an ablation catheter around the outside of the balloon, especially during mapping in the LA. Moreover, aggressive anticoagulation is required when using this system, and special attention and care are necessary during placement of the large balloon electrode in a nondilated atrium.

Practical Approach to Mapping Macroreentrant Atrial Tachycardia

EXCLUSION OF CAVOTRICUSPID ISTHMUS DEPENDENCE

Because CTI-dependent typical AFL is the most common MRAT, exclusion of the CTI as part of the reentrant circuit is an important initial step, even when the ECG pattern is not classically typical counterclockwise or clockwise AFL. In fact, typical AFL frequently manifests with an atypical 12-lead ECG appearance (so-called pseudoatypical flutter) in the setting of markedly abnormal atrial substrate. CTI-dependent AFL can be rapidly diagnosed or excluded by mapping of the tricuspid annulus and by entrainment maneuvers at the CTI. Exclusion of the CTI as part of the reentrant circuit can be established by any of the following: (1) demonstration of bidirectional activation of the CTI during AT, with resulting collision or fusion within the isthmus by activation from opposing directions (the low lateral RA and CS; see Fig. 13-2); (2) recording of double potentials separated by an isoelectric and constant interval throughout the full extent of the CTI during tachycardia; or (3) entrainment mapping from the CTI that demonstrates manifest atrial fusion with a long PPI (see Fig. 13-5).[7]

LOCALIZATION OF THE REENTRANT CIRCUIT CHAMBER (RIGHT ATRIUM VERSUS LEFT ATRIUM)

PATIENT HISTORY. A history of prior surgery or ablation within a particular atrial chamber should focus the intensity of the search for the arrhythmia substrate in that chamber. Such macroreentrant arrhythmias can occur in isolation or involve anatomical structures to create dual- or multiple-loop or circuit reentry. In the setting of previous cardiac surgery, a right-sided location of the arrhythmia is more likely and is often seen years later in patients who had a right lateral atriotomy and who underwent surgical closure of an atrial or ventricular septal defect or valve repair. These arrhythmias can also be seen after more complex surgical correction of congenital heart disease, such as the Mustard or Senning correction of transposition of the great vessels, and also after tricuspid valve surgery. LA macroreentry is more likely in the presence of left heart disease, such as hypertrophic cardiomyopathy or mitral valve disease, and following catheter or surgical ablation of AF. In these patients, spontaneous conduction abnormalities and areas of electrical silence forming the substrate for arrhythmia have been observed.

ELECTROCARDIOGRAPHIC FINDINGS. Lead V_1 is the most useful lead for distinguishing LA from RA origin, but much overlap exists. In the absence of previous cardiac surgery or catheter ablation (particularly involving linear lesions in the LA), P waves that are completely negative or have an initial isoelectric (or inverted) component followed by an upright component in lead V_1 is more frequently associated with RA free wall circuits. Conversely, in the absence of counterclockwise typical AFL, broad-based upright (or biphasic positive-negative) P waves in lead V_1 are more frequently associated with LA circuits. LA circuits have also been reported to generate low-amplitude P waves frequently, with some of them having visible waves only in lead V_1.[5]

TACHYCARDIA CYCLE LENGTH VARIATIONS. Large spontaneous variations (30 to 125 milliseconds) or even 2:1 conduction in the RA CL with concomitant variations of less than 20 milliseconds in CS recordings suggest an LA origin of the macroreentrant circuit (see Fig. 13-7).

ACTIVATION MAPPING. As noted, when activation timing from 10 roughly evenly distributed sites in the RA, including 3 or 4 points at the tricuspid annulus, spans less than 50% of the tachycardia CL (in the absence of extensive RA scarring or prior CTI ablation), the arrhythmia is probably not located in the RA. In the setting of LA MRATs, RA mapping typically shows a nonreentrant activation pattern with early RA septal activation relative to other parts of the RA when LA recordings are not obtained (see Figs. 13-2 and 13-7). CS activation usually propagates in a proximal-to-distal direction in the setting of RA MRATs and in a distal-to-proximal direction in the setting of LA MRATs. However, this is not always true; MRATs localized to the superior RA can result in distal-to-proximal CS activation, and some LA MRATs (e.g., counterclockwise perimitral MRAT) can activate the CS in a proximal-to-distal direction (see Fig. 13-2).[13]

ENTRAINMENT MAPPING. If macroreentry has been demonstrated, a difference between the PPI and tachycardia CL of more than 40 milliseconds at three or more different points in the RA (including the CTI and RA free wall, but excluding the septum and CS) denotes an LA circuit (see Fig. 5-20).

IDENTIFICATION OF BARRIERS AND POTENTIAL LINES OF BLOCK

Identification of the tachycardia circuit barriers is very important to help understand propagation of the reentrant activation wavefront in relation to these barriers, to identify the tachycardia critical isthmus, and to plan an ablation strategy to abolish the tachycardia. For RA macroreentry, the tricuspid annulus often provides one important barrier. Other naturally fixed barriers include the IVC, SVC, and CS os. For LA macroreentry, the mitral annulus and PVs often provide important barriers. Acquired barriers include surgical incisions or patches, surgical or catheter ablation lines, and atrial regions devoid of electrical activity (electrical scars). A line of block can be identified by the presence of double potentials, thus reflecting conduction up one side of the barrier and down the other side, with the bipolar electrogram recording both waves of activation. The use of an electroanatomical mapping system (CARTO or NavX) can facilitate tagging these anatomical and EP

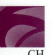

landmarks and understanding potential circuit routes, as well as performing voltage mapping to define areas of electrical scars.

IDENTIFICATION OF THE COMPLETE REENTRANT CIRCUIT

Activation mapping is performed to define the atrial activation sequence. Reasonable numbers of points homogeneously distributed in the atrium of origin of the tachycardia must be recorded. Use of an electroanatomical mapping system (CARTO or NavX) can facilitate tagging each point on the 3-D map. The complete reentrant circuit is the spatially shortest route of unidirectional activation encompassing the complete CL of the tachycardia in terms of activation timing and returning to the site of earliest activation. Using electroanatomical mapping, this translates into continuous progression of colors (from red to purple in the CARTO system and from white to purple in the NavX system) around the atrium, with close proximity of earliest and latest local activation. Additionally, propagation of electrical activation superimposed on the 3-D anatomical reconstruction of the atrium can be visualized as a propagation map in relation to the anatomical and EP landmarks and barriers. For LA MRAT, activation mapping should be carefully carried out around the mitral annulus because this maneuver is easy to perform and identifies a common form of LA macroreentry, perimitral MRAT. If activation recorded at different atrial locations does not cover most of the tachycardia CL, two possibilities must be considered: focal AT and small, localized reentrant circuits (i.e., electrical activity accounting for more than 85% of the tachycardia CL is present within an area with a diameter of 3 cm or less). Identification of small circuits requires much more detailed activation mapping (see Fig. 13-9).

Additionally, entrainment mapping can be used to indicate the relation of pacing sites to the reentrant circuit, and it qualitatively estimates how far the reentrant circuit is from the pacing site. For RA MRAT, a [PPI – AT CL] difference of less than 50 milliseconds at the proximal CS distinguishes typical AFL from a lateral RA MRAT. With LA MRAT, a [PPI – AT CL] difference of less than 50 milliseconds at the proximal and distal CS distinguished perimitral MRAT from macroreentrant circuits involving the right PVs and septum.[15] When entrainment does not localize the circuit in the LA or RA, a focal or small reentrant arrhythmia should be considered. Color-coded 3-D entrainment mapping can facilitate determination of the full active reentrant circuit (versus passively activated regions of the chamber) and the obstacle around which the tachycardia is circulating, and it provides very useful information on the location of potential ablation sites.

Noncontact mapping may also be used to define the atrial substrate and reentrant circuit, and it can be of significant value when the tachycardia is short-lived or cannot be reproducibly initiated.

IDENTIFICATION OF THE CRITICAL ISTHMUS

Once a scar or fixed barrier is localized, its role in supporting reentry is important in determining whether the isthmuses formed around it need ablation. Whether an isthmus is a critical part of the reentrant circuit can be determined by activation mapping during sustained stable reentry and entrainment mapping. The critical isthmus may lie between two anatomical landmarks (e.g., the mitral annulus and the left inferior PV), or it may be a relatively narrow channel bounded by sites of scar or double potentials. During electroanatomical activation mapping, when the onset of the window of interest is set at mid-diastole between two consecutive P waves, mid-diastolic isthmus of the reentrant circuit can be identified by the interface of early and late activation (i.e., the region where "early meets late" on the color-coded activation map). High-density mapping is then performed in and around the isthmus to define its limits and width precisely.[9]

For identification of the critical isthmus of the reentrant circuit, entrainment mapping is performed at selected atrial sites identified during activation mapping and propagation mapping in relation to atrial scars, barriers, and lines of block. Entrainment with concealed fusion should be sought, to indicate that the pacing site is in a protected isthmus located within or attached to the reentrant circuit. Whether this protected isthmus is crucial to the reentrant circuit or is just a bystander site needs to be verified by comparing the PPI with the tachycardia CL and the stimulus-exit interval with the electrogram-exit interval, as outlined in Table 10-2.[15,16]

Ablation

Target of Ablation

The choice of ablation sites should be among those segments of the reentry circuit that offer the most convenient and safest opportunity for creating conduction block. Among other factors are the isthmus size, anticipated catheter stability, and risk of damage to adjacent structures (e.g., phrenic nerve, sinus node, and AV node).

Ablation is performed by targeting the narrowest identifiable isthmus of conduction accessible within the circuit (allowing the best electrode-tissue contact along the desired line). The ablation line is chosen to transect an area critical for the circuit and, at the same time, to connect two anatomical areas of block, an electrically silent area to an anatomical zone of block (e.g., IVC, SVC, tricuspid annulus, PV, or mitral annulus), or two electrically silent areas.

In patients with incomplete maps, the ablation is guided by activation, entrainment, and voltage mapping targeting a critical isthmus or a zone of slow conduction shown to be part of the circuit by pacing maneuvers.[9,20]

When double potentials separated by an isoelectric interval can be traced in a convergent configuration, with a progressively decreasing interpotential interval, and culminate in a fractionated continuous electrogram, this finding indicates one end of a line of block and activation through the resulting isthmus or around a pivot point at the end of the line of block. If the fractionated low-amplitude electrogram is of longer duration, this suggests a protected corridor of slow conduction, whereas single high-amplitude electrograms suggest a wider and relatively large ablation target. An electrophysiologically defined isthmus may therefore be smaller than the anatomically defined isthmus. EP guidance for determining the target site probably offers greater certitude of RF delivery at a desired location because the same tip electrodes are used for both localization and RF delivery.

Contact or noncontact voltage maps can be used to guide the choice of the ablation site. The likelihood of achieving a complete and transmural ablation line is probably greater in low-amplitude areas.[9,20]

RIGHT ATRIAL MACROREENTRY

RA MRATs are frequently localized to the free wall of the RA, because of either previous atriotomy or a spontaneous area of conduction block. In the latter setting, the area with slow conduction (mid-diastolic isthmus, as defined by activation, entrainment, and voltage mapping) is the target of choice.

LEFT ATRIAL MACROREENTRY

IN SETTING OF PREVIOUS SURGERY OR SPONTANEOUS REGIONS OF SCAR. The goal is to localize the area with scar and extend this line of conduction block to an anatomical obstacle, or to transect the circuit by joining anatomical structures. Although this strategy is achievable in most of the atria, it is advisable to avoid attempting to connect the anterior septal region to the mitral annulus in the region of the low left septum because the thickness of the tissue prohibits complete lesions in approximately 40% of patients despite the use of irrigated-tip catheters. The exception to this is the presence of a narrow mid-diastolic isthmus (defined by activation, entrainment, and voltage mapping); this target is then preferable and usually much easier than longer linear lesions.

MACROREENTRANT ATRIAL TACHYCARDIAS FOLLOWING ABLATION OF ATRIAL FIBRILLATION. Knowledge of the type of the initial ablation procedure is critical before embarking on LA AT ablation. ATs following PV isolation procedures can often be focal, typically originating from the vicinity of a reconnected PV.[7] Most of the ATs complicating circumferential and linear LA ablations are macroreentrant, most commonly with circuits around the mitral annulus or involving the LA roof or septum. These circuits are most often related to gaps in ablation lines or to isthmuses created between the ablation lines and other obstacles in the LA. Multiple macroreentrant circuits and multiple-loop reentrant circuits are not infrequently encountered. Additionally, localized reentrant circuits are not uncommon, and they usually arise from the vicinity of the isolated PVs or linear lesions (see Video 17).[21]

Mapping and ablation of LA MRATs following circumferential LA ablation or circumferential PV isolation are frequently challenging. Detailed mapping with a high density of points is necessary to elucidate a more complete understanding of the activation pattern during the AT. In addition, mapping of the previously performed ablation lesions is critical to determine whether the ablation lines, PV isolation, or both, are complete. When the macroreentrant circuit can be mapped, ablation lesions should be tailored to interrupt the path of the reentrant circuit (see Fig. 15-59). In the absence of complete block across the old ablation lines, the gaps must be reablated. Empirical treatment of unmappable ATs primarily involves electrical isolation of all reconnected PVs and, if needed, empirical linear lesions within the tachycardia circuit, often including a line between the mitral annulus and left inferior PV and a line between the superior PVs.[22]

LEFT ATRIAL MACROREENTRY IN THE ABSENCE OF PREVIOUS SURGERY OR ATRIAL FIBRILLATION ABLATION. Spontaneous LA circuits have been observed. The circuits can propagate around spontaneous scars, frequently located in the posterior LA, but also around the mitral annulus or PVs. More recently, LA circuits have been reported to rotate around the fossa ovalis, and they are amenable to RF ablation using a linear lesion connecting the fossa ovalis to the mitral annulus.

PERIMITRAL ATRIAL MACROREENTRY. An ablation lesion connecting the mitral annulus and one other anatomical barrier (usually the left inferior PV; Fig. 13-10) or the posterior scar can eliminate this arrhythmia. Another option is to use an anterior line from the anterior mitral annulus to the ostium of the left superior PV or to a region of scar through the anterior LA.

ATRIAL MACROREENTRY AROUND THE RIGHT PULMONARY VEINS. Circuits propagating around the right PVs demonstrate colliding wavefronts along the mitral annulus and a PPI during entrainment that is much longer at the mitral isthmus than at the roof or posterior LA. This arrhythmia is observed more frequently in the current approach of wide-area atrial ablation to isolate the PVs, because the lesions performed to isolate right and left PVs may create a narrow isthmus in the posterior LA that then forms the substrate for MRAT. A linear lesion connecting both superior PVs through the roof is the best option. This procedure is best performed along the roof, rather than the posterior wall, to avoid the potential risk of atrioesophageal fistulas.

ATRIAL MACROREENTRY AROUND THE LEFT PULMONARY VEINS. Circuits around the left PVs seem rare. They can be abolished with a linear lesion joining the left inferior PV to the mitral annulus or with a roofline connecting both superior PVs.

LEFT SEPTAL CIRCUITS. A linear lesion from right PVs to the fossa ovalis or from the mitral annulus to the fossa ovalis usually terminates the tachycardia.

UNMAPPABLE LEFT ATRIAL MACROREENTRANT TACHYCARDIAS. Some LA MRATs can show some degree of variation in their CL during mapping, in which case conventional and electroanatomical mapping is less useful. An empirical strategy that commences with ablation at the mitral isthmus and the LA roof is then justified because such ablation lines interrupt the most dominant circuits in the LA. CL variation can in some cases facilitate activation mapping by revealing when electrograms "lead" versus "follow," but it severely compromises use of entrainment mapping, which assumes that the [PPI – AT CL] differences result only from proximity of the pacing site to the circuit and not from variable conduction velocity to, from, or within the circuit.

Ablation Technique

Once the ablation target is identified, ablation involves placing a series of RF lesions to sever the critical isthmus to connect two anatomical or surgical barriers. RF energy can be delivered sequentially point by point to span the targeted isthmus or by dragging the ablation catheter tip during continuous energy administration. RF energy is maintained for up to 60 to 120 seconds until the bipolar atrial potential recorded from the ablation electrode is decreased by 80% or split into double potentials, thus indicating local conduction block. Lesion contiguity and continuity depend on ensuring the coalescence of multiple transmural lesions; this is best ensured by documenting the breakdown of the target electrogram (at each site) into double potentials and continuing RF delivery at this point for 30 to 40 seconds more to ensure a stable lesion. The documentation of electrogram breakdown into double potentials depends on the direction of activation relative to the ablation lesion and its size relative to that of the recording bipole and is maximized by activation orthogonal to the lesion's largest dimension.

During delivery of RF energy, the tachycardia can terminate, or its CL can increase transiently or permanently. These findings indicate that the lesions have affected the circuit and should lead to continuation of RF delivery or extension of the lesion to ensure the achievement of complete conduction block across the isthmus.

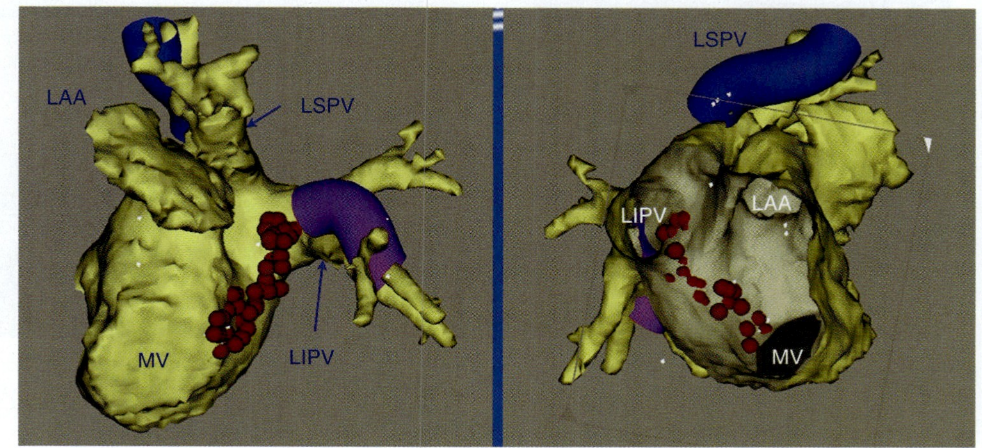

FIGURE 13-10 Integrated computed tomography (CT) and electroanatomical (CARTO, Biosense Webster, Inc., Diamond Bar, Calif.) map of the left atrium acquired during catheter ablation of the mitral isthmus. Left anterior oblique and endoscopic views of the CT scan are shown. Tubular-appearing structures are pulmonary veins; small red circles are tagged sites at which radiofrequency energy was applied across the isthmus between the annulus of the mitral valve (MV) and left inferior pulmonary vein (LIPV). LAA = LA appendage; LSPV = left superior pulmonary vein.

The coalescence of multiple RF lesions can be facilitated by any 3-D localization system (e.g., CARTO, NavX). Ablation sites may be tagged to permit visualization of the ablation line on the electroanatomical map. CARTO is also invaluable in localizing the gaps in the scar line through which the impulse can propagate. Focal ablation of these gaps can abolish the tachycardia.[9,20]

It is not uncommon for the arrhythmia mechanism to switch rather than terminate following successful ablation. A change in atrial activation sequence or P wave morphology or a sudden change in the atrial CL may indicate that the tachycardia that was being ablated has changed to a different loop or to a different tachycardia. In this setting, it is very important to reevaluate the mechanism and location of the new arrhythmia systematically by using activation and entrainment mapping and to move to the new target if necessary.[12,23] However, the transition to a different loop of a tachycardia or to a different tachycardia may occur with no discernible change in the activation sequence among the atrial electrograms that are being recorded, P wave morphology, or CL. It is important to keep this in mind when ablation across an isthmus appears not to affect the tachycardia. The isthmus may have already been blocked and may no longer be participating in the tachycardia. This should be suspected if double potentials are present along the ablation line, and it is easily confirmed by entrainment mapping near the ablation line. If that site was confirmed previously to be part of the reentrant circuit (PPI – AT CL difference less than 20 milliseconds) and now it is outside the tachycardia circuit (PPI – AT CL difference more than 30 milliseconds), this finding indicates that the tachycardia circuit has changed.[7]

ABLATION OF THE MITRAL ISTHMUS

The mitral isthmus is short (2 to 4 cm), anatomically bounded by the mitral annulus, left inferior PV ostium, and superiorly by the LA appendage (see Fig. 13-10). The average thickness of the atrium along the mitral isthmus is 3.8 mm, with maximum thickness up to 7.7 mm. The CS muscle sleeve, present in up to 75% of patients, inserts into the LA inferior to the mitral isthmus and occasionally extends onto the mitral valve.[24,25] Mitral isthmus ablation is performed by linear ablation to join the lateral mitral isthmus to the left inferior PV.

If possible, the CS catheter is positioned to bracket the planned linear lesion between its proximal and distal bipoles. The ablation catheter, bent with a 90- to 180-degree curve and introduced through a long sheath to achieve good contact and stability, is first positioned at the ventricular edge of the lateral mitral annulus, where the A:V electrogram shows a 1:1 to 2:1 ratio, to begin ablation. The sheath and catheter are then rotated clockwise to extend the lesion posteriorly, ending at the left inferior PV ostium (Fig. 13-11). In general, ablation is commenced at about the 3- or 4-o'clock position on the mitral isthmus and reaches the 2- to 3-o'clock position at the upper end of the line. A more anterior extension to the posterior root of the LA appendage occasionally is required.

RF energy is delivered with an 8-mm-tip catheter with a target temperature of 50° to 55°C and a power of 50 to 60 W. Externally irrigated catheters are preferably used with a power of 25 to 35 W and continuous titration of flow from 5 to 60 mL/min to achieve a target temperature of 40° to 42°C. Higher-power delivery in this region carries a significant risk of cardiac perforation with tamponade because of the particular regional anatomy, as well as the catheter-tissue geometry. The stability of the catheter is monitored during RF applications by using electrogram recordings and intermittent fluoroscopy to exclude inadvertent displacement, which could result in high-energy delivery in the left inferior PV ostium or LA appendage.[12,23]

When ablation is performed during NSR, the effect of each RF application is assessed on the local electrogram during pacing from the proximal bipole of the CS catheter located immediately posteromedial of the line, to maximize conduction delay. Splitting of the local potentials, with a resulting increase in the delay from the pacing artifact, is considered evidence of an effective local lesion. After the initial attempt to create this line, mapping is performed along the line to identify and ablate endocardial gaps, defined as sites showing the shortest delay between the pacing artifact and the local atrial potential, which can be single, narrow double, or fractionated.

Persisting epicardial conduction is suspected when the linear lesion results in adequate voltage abatement on the endocardial

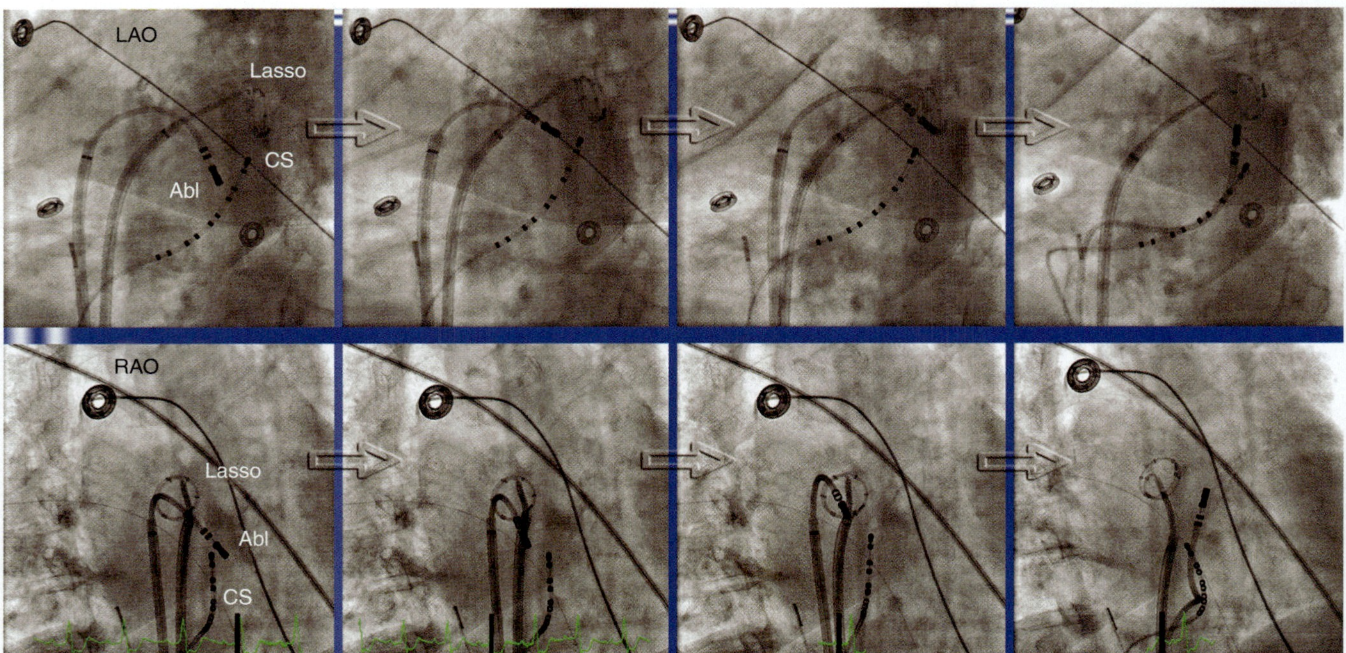

FIGURE 13-11 Right anterior oblique (RAO; **upper panels**) and left anterior oblique (LAO; **lower panels**) fluoroscopy views of catheter placement during mitral isthmus ablation. A ring catheter (Lasso) is positioned at the ostium of the left inferior pulmonary vein (PV). Ablation is started with the ablation catheter (Abl) at the ventricular edge of the mitral annulus **(left panel).** The catheter is then moved gradually to the midisthmus and subsequently to the junction with the ostium of the left inferior PV **(middle panels).** When the endocardial approach fails, epicardial ablation of the mitral isthmus is attempted through the coronary sinus (CS; **right panel**).

aspect and endocardial conduction delay recorded on the ablation catheter but not on the adjacent distal bipole of the CS catheter (anterolateral to the ablation line). Epicardial ablation within the CS is required to achieve block in approximately 70% of cases. The relatively low success rate of mitral isthmus block can be explained by several mechanisms. The shape and depth of the atrial myocardium vary greatly around the mitral isthmus, and the depth of the tissue (resulting from the double muscular layers of LA and CS) may be the limiting factor in achieving transmural lesion by endocardial ablation alone. Additionally, local cooling effects of blood flow in the circumflex coronary artery and the great cardiac vein (both pass in close proximity to the mitral isthmus) may act as a heat sink, preventing adequate tissue heating by RF delivery and making isthmus block difficult. Temporary displacement of the venous blood pool by using an air-filled CS balloon can potentially facilitate transmural mitral isthmus lesions during endocardial catheter ablation.[24,26,27]

When epicardial ablation is required, the ablation catheter is withdrawn from the LA and is introduced into the CS to map the epicardial side of the isthmus and identify fractionated or early potentials suggestive of an epicardial gap. Ablation within the CS is performed using an externally irrigated-tip catheter with a power limit of 20 to 25 W, and usually maximal flow (60 mL/min) is necessary (see Fig. 13-11).[12,23] RF application should be discontinued if there is a rapid rise or fall in impedance or a rapid rise in temperature. Sometimes a power setting of 30 to 35 W is required for successful ablation. A higher power setting should be considered when a tachycardia fails to respond to ablation with 20 to 25 W and when entrainment mapping or activation mapping indicates that the CS is still an appropriate target site.[7]

One report described an alternative approach to ablation of perimitral MRAT. Linear ablation between the anterior-anterolateral mitral annulus and the ostium of the left superior PV (modified anterior line) was found to be safe, feasible, and successful in the short term in terminating perimitral MRAT in more than 96% of cases, and in achieving bidirectional block across the ablation line in 86% of cases, without the need for RF ablation within the CS. The ablation catheter is advanced through the transseptal sheath to the anterior-anterolateral mitral annulus, and delivery of RF lesions is started when the A/V ratio is 1:2. Linear ablation is then performed with clockwise (posterior) rotation of the transseptal sheath and progressive release of the ablation catheter curve. The ablation line is extended just medial to the orifice of the LA appendage, and it ends at the ostium of the left superior PV.[28]

Endpoints of Ablation

TACHYCARDIA TERMINATION DURING RADIOFREQUENCY ENERGY APPLICATION

Sudden termination of an incessant AT during RF application suggests that the lesion has severed a critical isthmus and that site should be targeted for additional lesions. However, reliance on AT termination during RF application as the sole criterion of a successful ablation is hazardous because such an AT can terminate spontaneously, in which case termination can be misleading. RF application itself can induce premature atrial complexes that can then terminate AT without eliminating the substrate. Moreover, the sudden termination of AT can be accompanied by catheter displacement from the critical site to another site, thus making it difficult to deliver additional energy applications at the critical site. Additionally, RF application can cause a transient but not permanent block in the critical isthmus. Such a block can last long enough to terminate the tachycardia, but it can resolve after seconds or minutes.

NONINDUCIBILITY OF TACHYCARDIA

To use the criterion of noninducibility of tachycardia as a reliable endpoint, careful assessment of inducibility should be performed prior to ablation, and the feasibility and best method of reproducible induction of the AT should be documented at baseline before ablation. In the setting of easy inducibility prior to ablation, one can consider the lack of inducibility as an indicator of successful ablation. Noninducibility of the arrhythmia is inapplicable if the original arrhythmia is either noninducible at baseline or was inadvertently terminated mechanically. Noninducibility may also reflect conduction delay in the critical isthmus, and not stable block, or it may be secondary to changes in autonomic tone.

DOCUMENTATION OF A LINE OF BLOCK

Complete stable conduction block within the reentry path is the most useful and objective endpoint. However, achieving this endpoint can be challenging and is not as feasible as in typical AFL ablation. To confirm complete conduction block following ablation, the mapping catheter is used to retrace the same ablation line (during NSR or atrial pacing), thus showing the absence of electrograms or a complete line of block demonstrated by parallel double potentials recorded all along the line. Pacing close to the ablation line (at a site within 30 milliseconds of conduction time to the ablation lesion) and demonstration of marked delay and reversal in the direction of activation on the opposite side of the linear lesion across the isthmus indicate isthmus block, although very slow conduction can be difficult to exclude.

CONFIRMATION OF MITRAL ISTHMUS BLOCK

For perimitral MRAT, the mitral isthmus is the target of ablation. Mitral isthmus ablation has a well-defined demonstrable procedural endpoint of bidirectional conduction block analogous to CTI ablation. Validation of mitral isthmus conduction block is greatly facilitated by its proximity to the CS that allows pacing and recording on either side of the ablation line to confirm bidirectional block. Differential pacing can also be performed to exclude slow conduction through an incomplete line.

Several criteria are used to confirm the presence of bidirectional mitral isthmus block:

1. The presence of widely separated (by 150- to 300-millisecond intervals) local double potentials along the length of the ablation line during CS pacing septal of the ablation line.
2. Mapping the activation detour during pacing from either side of the ablation line. Pacing on the septal side of the line through the CS demonstrates activation toward the line both septally and laterally. Pacing lateral to the line through the ablation catheter placed endocardially demonstrates a proximal-to-distal activation sequence along the CS septal side of the line, thus confirming bidirectional conduction block (Fig. 13-12). Such an activation detour can also be determined using 3-D electroanatomical mapping.
3. Differential pacing to distinguish slow conduction across the mitral isthmus from complete block. With the distal bipole of the CS catheter placed just septal to the linear lesion, the pacing site is changed from the distal to the proximal bipole of the CS catheter without moving any of the catheters. The stimulus-to-electrogram timing at a site lateral to the ablation line is measured before and after changing the pacing site. With complete block, the stimulus-to-electrogram interval is shortened after shifting the pacing site from the distal to proximal CS bipole (Fig. 13-13; see Fig. 13-12).

CONFIRMATION OF MODIFIED ANTERIOR LINE BLOCK

The achievement of a complete block along the modified anterior line can be verified by (1) mapping of the line during pacing from the distal CS or LA appendage and verification of the presence of double potentials along its entire length, (2) electroanatomical activation mapping during LA appendage pacing with earliest LA activation lateral to the ablation line and an early-meets-late zone along the entire length of the ablation line, or (3) evaluation of the CS activation pattern during pacing just laterally and medially to

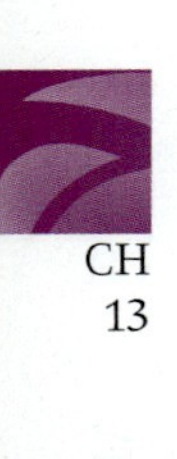

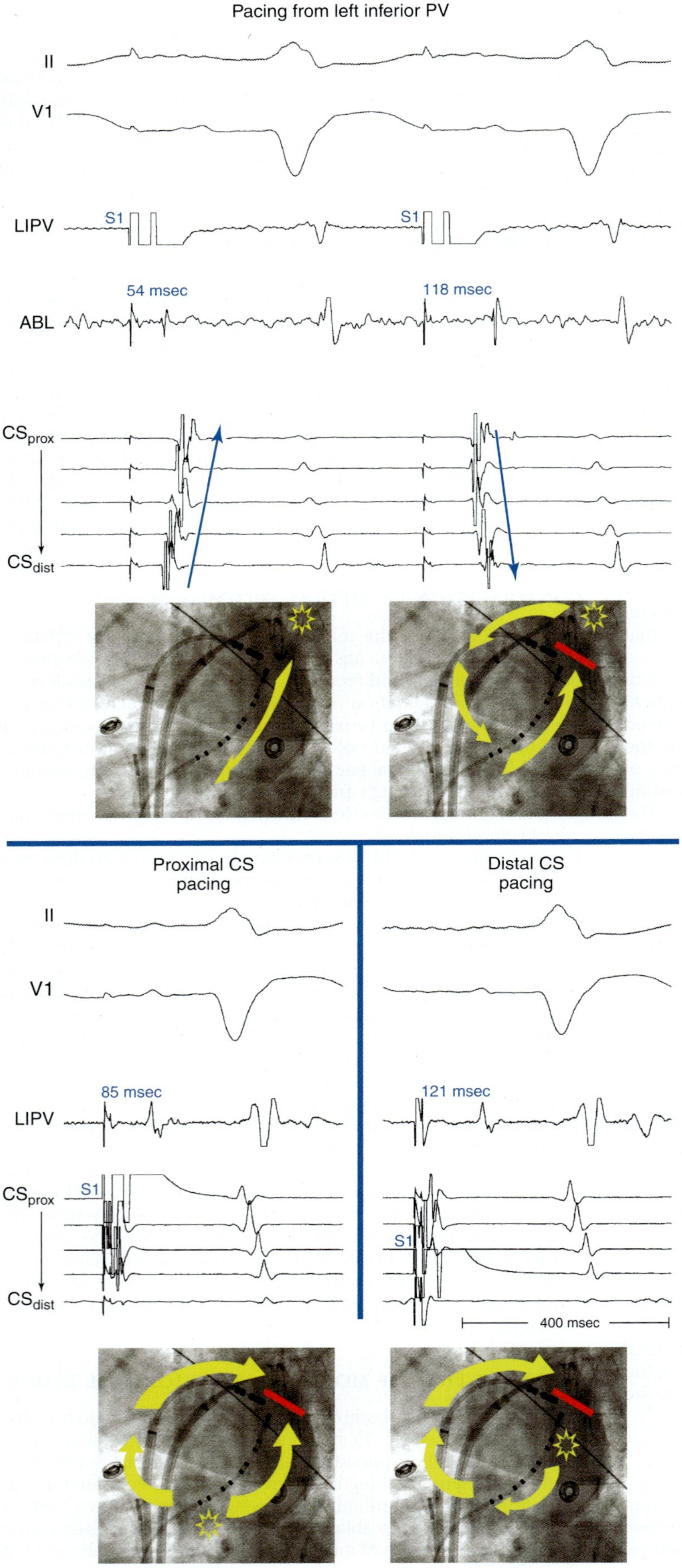

FIGURE 13-12 Verification of bidirectional mitral isthmus block. **Upper panel,** Ablation of the mitral isthmus is performed during pacing lateral to the ablation line (a Lasso catheter positioned at the ostium of the left inferior pulmonary vein [LIPV] is used in this case). With intact isthmus conduction, coronary sinus (CS) activation occurs through the wavefront propagating in the counterclockwise direction; thus, a distal-to-proximal CS activation sequence is observed. When clockwise isthmus block is achieved, CS activation occurs through the wavefront propagating in the clockwise direction; thus, reversal of the CS activation sequence is observed. The ablation catheter (ABL) is positioned at the septal aspect of the line of block. The stimulus-to-electrogram interval recorded by the ablation catheter prolongs suddenly on development of clockwise isthmus block. **Lower panels,** Differential pacing is performed from the proximal and distal CS (CS_{prox}, CS_{dist}) bipoles (both positioned at the septal aspect of the ablation line) to verify the presence of counterclockwise isthmus block. In the presence of counterclockwise block, activation lateral to the ablation line (as recorded by the Lasso catheter in the LIPV) occurs through the wavefront propagating in a clockwise direction up the left atrial (LA) septal wall and over the LA roof. Consequently, LIPV activation occurs earlier during pacing from the proximal CS **(left panel)** compared with the distal CS **(right panel).** A yellow star marks the pacing site.

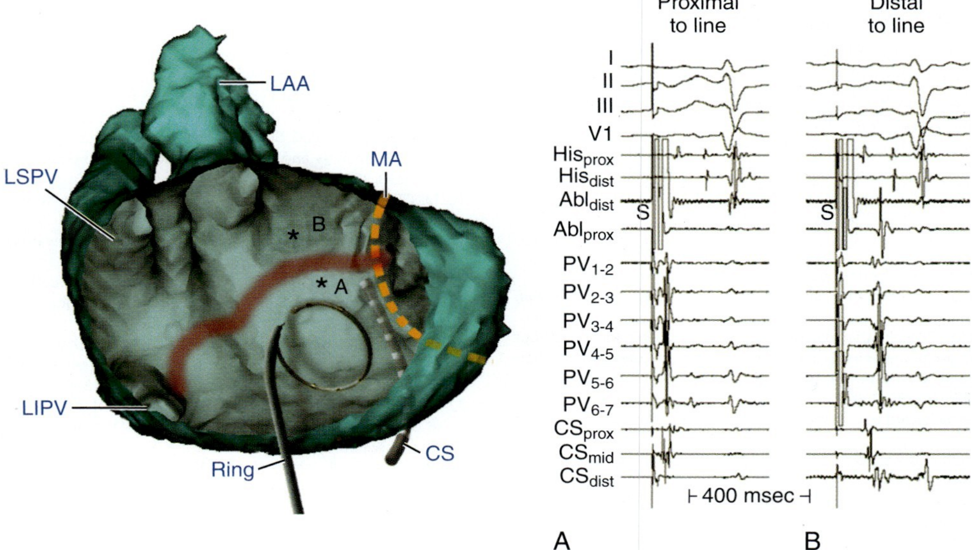

FIGURE 13-13 Endoscopic view of a CT scan of the left side of the left atrium (LA). The orifices of the left superior pulmonary vein (LSPV) and left inferior PV (LIPV) and LA appendage (LAA) are shown. An ablation line (red shading) has been made between mitral annulus (MA, orange dashes) and the LIPV orifice to transect the mitral isthmus. A multipolar ring catheter is situated on the LA endocardium as shown; the tip of the coronary sinus (CS) catheter (situated epicardial to the LA) is proximal to the ablation line. During pacing from A (asterisk), proximal to the ablation line, the ring catheter recordings appear soon after the stimulus artifact and CS electrodes are activated from distal to proximal. Pacing from B (asterisk), distal to the ablation line, shows the ring electrodes are activated much later than before, and the CS is now activated from proximal to distal, thus indicating bidirectional block at the mitral isthmus. Abl_{dist} = distal ablation site; Abl_{prox} = proximal ablation site; CS_{dist} = distal coronary sinus; CS_{mid} = middle coronary sinus; CS_{prox} = proximal coronary sinus; His_{dist} = distal His bundle; His_{prox} = proximal His bundle; PV = pulmonary vein.

the line with the ablation catheter (translinear pacing maneuver). Complete linear block is confirmed if pacing laterally to the line results in a distal to proximal CS activation pattern, whereas after moving the catheter to the septal side of the line, the CS is activated from proximal to distal.[28]

FAILURE OF RADIOFREQUENCY ABLATION

Atrial enlargement can interfere with RF energy delivery secondary to difficulty in achieving stable, firm catheter contact and to the probable high convective heat loss associated with the large chamber volume. In addition, targets for ablation can have low surrounding blood flow; thus, target temperature can be achieved at very low energy outputs because of inadequate cooling of the tip of a standard ablation catheter, with consequent limited energy delivery. Furthermore, some surgical repairs are associated with myocardial hypertrophy, which makes achievement of a transmural lesion difficult or impossible.

Outcome

SUCCESS

Short-term success rates are reasonably good (approximately 90%). However, recurrence rates of the same or other tachycardias are high; up to 54% of cases required repeat ablation in some studies. The long-term success rate is approximately 72%.

Despite frequent underlying structural heart disease, the incidence of AF after ablation is relatively low (9% to 21%) in patients without prior history of AF. This may be related to the presence of silent areas and lines of block (spontaneous and created by RF), which could reduce the electrically active atrial mass to less than the critical threshold for AF. In the context of MRATs propagating through incomplete lines of block delivered for AF ablation, the long-term follow-up is even better, at least in patients for whom complete block is achieved.

In patients with perimitral MRAT, block at the mitral isthmus can be achieved in 76% to 92% of patients with 20 ± 10 minutes of endocardial RF application; an additional 5 ± 4 minutes of epicardial RF application from within the CS is required in 68% of patients.

SAFETY OF ABLATION OF LEFT ATRIAL MACROREENTRANT TACHYCARDIA

Thromboembolic risk during LA ablation can be reduced by the following: (1) anticoagulation for 4 weeks prior to the procedure; (2) preprocedural transesophageal echocardiography, to exclude the presence of atrial clots; (3) perfusion of the LA sheath under pressure, to achieve a flow of approximately 2 to 4 mL/min; (4) intravenous heparin administration immediately before or immediately after transseptal puncture and throughout the LA procedure, to maintain an activated clotting time between 250 and 350 seconds; and (5) the use of irrigated-tip catheters.

Free wall perforation can occur during atrial septal puncture or during the rest of the procedure. The LA appendage is the site of the highest risk of perforation because of the very thin tissue encountered between the pectinate muscles. To prevent perforation caused by steam popping during RF delivery, it is important to limit the delivered power, especially around the PVs, posterior LA, and LA dome.

PV stenosis is another potential complication, and limiting RF power output and duration can reduce this risk. Left phrenic palsy is uncommon and is usually associated with RF delivery at the anterior LA or base of the LA appendage, or both. Right phrenic nerve injury can be observed during ablation at the anterior aspect of the right PVs.

SAFETY OF RIGHT ATRIAL MACROREENTRY ABLATION

Right phrenic nerve injury can be observed during ablation at the anterior aspect of the SVC and lateral RA. Pacing at a high output of 10 mA from the ablation catheter at the site without capture of the phrenic nerve and continuous pacing in the SVC to capture the

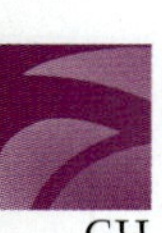

phrenic nerve during RA ablation are reassuring, but their efficacy has never been assessed. Early recognition of phrenic nerve injury during RF delivery, based on cough, hiccup, or reduced diaphragmatic respiratory motion, allows the immediate interruption of the application prior to the onset of permanent injury and is associated with the rapid recovery of phrenic nerve function. Furthermore, limiting the power delivered to 20 to 25 W further minimizes the risk of this complication.

REFERENCES

1. Garan H: Atypical atrial flutter, *Heart Rhythm* 5:618–621, 2008.
2. Anselme F: Macroreentrant atrial tachycardia: pathophysiological concepts, *Heart Rhythm* 5(Suppl):S18–S21, 2008.
3. Fiala M, Chovancik J, Neuwirth R, et al: Atrial macroreentry tachycardia in patients without obvious structural heart disease or previous cardiac surgical or catheter intervention: characterization of arrhythmogenic substrates, reentry circuits, and results of catheter ablation, *J Cardiovasc Electrophysiol* 18:824–832, 2007.
4. Triedman JK: Atypical atrial tachycardias in patients with congenital heart disease, *Heart Rhythm* 5:315–317, 2008.
5. Medi C, Kalman JM: Prediction of the atrial flutter circuit location from the surface electrocardiogram, *Europace* 10:786–796, 2008.
6. Yuniadi Y, Tai CT, Lee KT, et al: A new electrocardiographic algorithm to differentiate upper loop re-entry from reverse typical atrial flutter, *J Am Coll Cardiol* 46:524–528, 2005.
7. Morady F, Oral H, Chugh A: Diagnosis and ablation of atypical atrial tachycardia and flutter complicating atrial fibrillation ablation, *Heart Rhythm* 6(Suppl):S29–S32, 2009.
8. Kron J, Kasirajan V, Wood MA, et al: Management of recurrent atrial arrhythmias after minimally invasive surgical pulmonary vein isolation and ganglionic plexi ablation for atrial fibrillation, *Heart Rhythm* 7:445–451, 2010.
9. De PR, Marazzi R, Zoli L, et al: Electroanatomic mapping and ablation of macroreentrant atrial tachycardia: comparison between successfully and unsuccessfully treated cases, *J Cardiovasc Electrophysiol* 21:155–162, 2010.
10. Chugh A, Latchamsetty R, Oral H, et al: Characteristics of cavotricuspid isthmus-dependent atrial flutter after left atrial ablation of atrial fibrillation, *Circulation* 113:609–615, 2006.
11. Knecht S, Matsuo S, Lim K-T, et al: Focal vs. macroreentrant atrial tachycardia after prior ablation: value of cycle length variability, *Heart Rhythm* 4(Suppl):S238, 2007.
12. Jais P, Matsuo S, Knecht S, et al: A deductive mapping strategy for atrial tachycardia following atrial fibrillation ablation: importance of localized reentry, *J Cardiovasc Electrophysiol* 20:480–491, 2009.
13. Steven D, Seiler J, Roberts-Thomson KC, et al: Mapping of atrial tachycardias after catheter ablation for atrial fibrillation: use of bi-atrial activation patterns to facilitate recognition of origin, *Heart Rhythm* 7:664–672, 2010.
14. Santucci PA, Varma N, Cytron J, et al: Electroanatomic mapping of postpacing intervals clarifies the complete active circuit and variants in atrial flutter, *Heart Rhythm* 6:1586–1595, 2009.
15. Miyazaki H, Stevenson WG, Stephenson K, et al: Entrainment mapping for rapid distinction of left and right atrial tachycardias, *Heart Rhythm* 3:516–523, 2006.
16. Deo R, Berger R: The clinical utility of entrainment pacing, *J Cardiovasc Electrophysiol* 20:466–470, 2009.
17. Esato M, Hindricks G, Sommer P, et al: Color-coded three-dimensional entrainment mapping for analysis and treatment of atrial macroreentrant tachycardia, *Heart Rhythm* 6: 349–358, 2009.
18. Tai CT, Chen SA: Noncontact mapping of the heart: how and when to use, *J Cardiovasc Electrophysiol* 20:123–126, 2009.
19. Higa S, Tai CT, Lin YJ, et al: Focal atrial tachycardia: new insight from noncontact mapping and catheter ablation, *Circulation* 109:84–91, 2004.
20. Huang JL, Tai CT, Lin YJ, et al: Substrate mapping to detect abnormal atrial endocardium with slow conduction in patients with atypical right atrial flutter, *J Am Coll Cardiol* 48: 492–498, 2006.
21. Takahashi Y, Takahashi A, Miyazaki S, et al: Electrophysiological characteristics of localized reentrant atrial tachycardia occurring after catheter ablation of long-lasting persistent atrial fibrillation, *J Cardiovasc Electrophysiol* 20:623–629, 2009.
22. Knecht S, Veenhuyzen G, O'Neill MD, et al: Atrial tachycardias encountered in the context of catheter ablation for atrial fibrillation part II: mapping and ablation, *Pacing Clin Electrophysiol* 32:528–538, 2009.
23. Weerasooriya R, Jais P, Wright M, et al: Catheter ablation of atrial tachycardia following atrial fibrillation ablation, *J Cardiovasc Electrophysiol* 20:833–838, 2009.
24. Matsuo S, Wright M, Knecht S, et al: Peri-mitral atrial flutter in patients with atrial fibrillation ablation, *Heart Rhythm* 7:2–8, 2010.
25. Anousheh R, Sawhney NS, Panutich M, et al: Effect of mitral isthmus block on development of atrial tachycardia following ablation for atrial fibrillation, *Pacing Clin Electrophysiol* 33:460–468, 2010.
26. Choi JI, Pak HN, Park JH, et al: Clinical significance of complete conduction block of the left lateral isthmus and its relationship with anatomical variation of the vein of Marshall in patients with nonparoxysmal atrial fibrillation, *J Cardiovasc Electrophysiol* 20:616–622, 2009.
27. d'Avila A, Thiagalingam A, Foley L, et al: Temporary occlusion of the great cardiac vein and coronary sinus to facilitate radiofrequency catheter ablation of the mitral isthmus, *J Cardiovasc Electrophysiol* 19:645–650, 2008.
28. Sivagangabalan G, Pouliopoulos J, Huang K, et al: Comparison of electroanatomic contact and noncontact mapping of ventricular scar in a postinfarct ovine model with intramural needle electrode recording and histological validation, *Circ Arrhythm Electrophysiol* 1: 363–369, 2008.

CHAPTER 14 Atrial Tachyarrhythmias in Congenital Heart Disease

Pathophysiology

Patients with congenital heart disease have a high prevalence of atrial tachycardias (ATs), particularly after they have undergone reparative or palliative surgical procedures. For macroreentrant ATs in adults with repaired congenital heart disease, three right atrial (RA) circuits are generally identified: lateral wall circuits with reentry around or related to the lateral atriotomy scar, septal circuits with reentry around an atrial septal patch, and typical atrial flutter (AFL) circuits using the cavotricuspid isthmus (CTI). Typical clockwise or counterclockwise isthmus-dependent AFL is the most common macroreentrant tachycardia in this patient population. Left atrial (LA) macroreentrant circuits are infrequent in this group of patients. Atrial macroreentry in the right free wall is the most common form of non–isthmus-dependent RA macroreentry (atypical flutter). Very complex or multiple reentry circuits can be seen after placement of an intraatrial baffle (Mustard or Senning correction for transposition of the great vessels) in an extremely dilated RA, after a Fontan procedure, and in patients with a univentricular heart.[1,2]

Anatomical factors promoting macroreentry in patients with congenital heart disease include abnormalities of the underlying cardiac anatomy, surgically created anastomoses, and atriotomy scars, resulting in anatomical barriers to impulse propagation. Additionally, extensive cardiac surgery and hemodynamic overload result in myocardial hypertrophy and diffuse areas of atrial scarring with surviving myocardial fibers embedded within scar areas, which provide the substrate for potential reentry circuits.[3,4]

The best characterization of macroreentrant AT caused by atriotomy is activation around an incision scar in the lateral RA wall, with a main superoinferior axis (Fig. 14-1). This is a common problem in patients who have undergone surgery for congenital or valvular heart disease. The length, location, and orientation of the atriotomy incisions, as well as potential electrical conduction gaps across the atriotomy, are important determinants of arrhythmogenicity.[5] Typically, the reentry circuit is located in the lateral RA wall. Not only does the central obstacle include the scar, but also functional block can magnify this obstacle to include the superior vena cava (SVC). The anterior RA wall is commonly activated superoinferiorly (descending activation pattern), as in counterclockwise typical AFL. However, the septal wall frequently lacks a clear-cut inferosuperior (ascending) activation pattern. Participation of the anterior RA wall in the circuit can be confirmed with entrainment mapping. A line of double potentials can be recorded in the lateral RA, extending superoinferiorly. Double potential separation can be more marked and demonstrate a voltage lower than in typical AFL. Narrow passages (isthmuses) in the circuit can be found between the SVC and the superior end of the atriotomy scar, between the inferior vena cava (IVC) and the inferior end of the atriotomy, between the atriotomy scar and the tricuspid annulus, between the atriotomy and the crista terminalis, or even within the scar itself (Fig. 14-2). These isthmuses can be areas of slow conduction. Stable pacing of the critical isthmus can be difficult or impossible in RA atriotomy tachycardia because of tachycardia interruption. Isthmus participation in the circuit is often proven by tachycardia interruption with catheter pressure (Fig. 14-3), as well as by tachycardia interruption and noninducibility after radiofrequency (RF) application in the area. A single, wide, fractionated electrogram can be recorded from the lower pivot point of the circuit (Fig. 14-4) in the low lateral RA, close to the IVC, and perhaps also from other isthmuses of the circuit. The line of double potentials or fractionated, low-voltage electrograms can also often be recorded in normal sinus rhythm, to allow tentative localization of the scar and the associated anatomical isthmuses.[2]

Typical AFL is also often associated with RA atriotomy. In fact, the single most common form of AT among patients with congenital heart disease appears to be isthmus-dependent AFL, particularly in patients with simpler anatomical lesions (e.g., tetralogy of Fallot, atrial and ventricular septal defects) (Fig. 14-5). Moreover, the CTI was found to be part of the reentrant circuit in approximately 70% of patients with postoperative intraatrial reentrant tachycardia. In one report, ablation of this isthmus alone resulted in elimination of the tachycardia in 27% of these patients. Factors such as an atriotomy or atrial fibrosis and hypertrophy serve as promoters for early development of the typical form of AFL.

Reentry circuits can also occur in the sinus node region, possibly as a result of injury related to the superior atrial cannulation site for the bypass pump. These circuits can be quite small, often manifesting as focal tachycardia in the sinus node region, and they frequently can be ablated in a single location without establishing a particular line of block.[4]

Focal mechanisms underlying postoperative AT have been rarely reported in this patient population. Nonautomatic focal ATs are predominantly found in adults, with most foci in the RA. The reasons behind this laterality are unknown. The mechanism underlying focal AT is unknown. Both triggered and microreentrant mechanisms have been suggested.[6] Viable myocardial fibers embedded within areas of scar tissue, which play a pivotal role in the initiation and perpetuation of macroreentrant tachycardias, can also be the site of origin of a focal AT and thus play an important role in the pathogenesis of these ATs.[3]

Arrhythmias are also frequently observed in the early postoperative period after corrective surgery in children, occurring in 14% to 48% in the first few days after surgery. The most common arrhythmia in this period is junctional tachycardia, occurring in 5% to 10% of the operated children and usually self-limiting. Other supraventricular arrhythmias are also seen in 4%. The occurrence of early postoperative arrhythmias seems to be related to procedural factors of cardiac surgery, which are, in turn, related to the complexity of the congenital malformation. Early postoperative arrhythmias influence the long-term outcome of patients with congenital heart disease and have been found to be a predictor of late complications, such as ventricular dysfunction, late arrhythmias, and late mortality. Whether

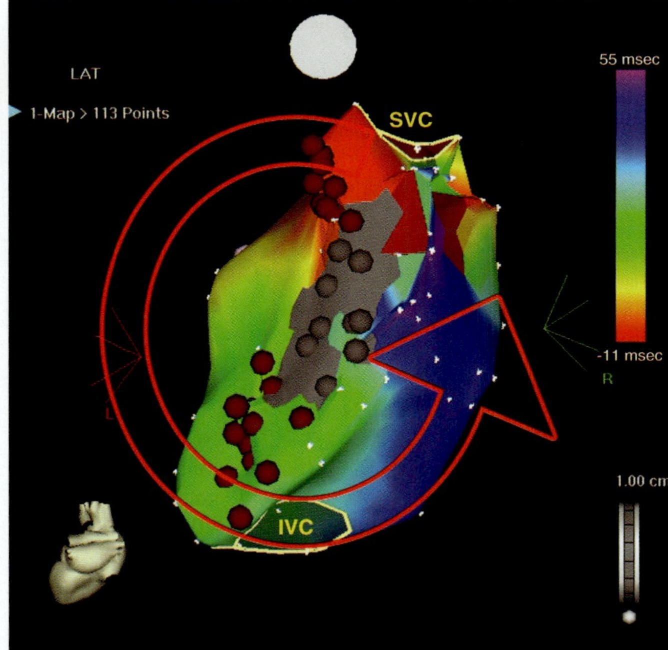

FIGURE 14-1 Three-dimensional electroanatomical (CARTO, Biosense Webster, Inc., Diamond Bar, Calif.) activation map of macroreentrant atrial tachycardia in a patient with previous surgical repair of an atrial septal defect. Gray areas in the posterolateral right atrium represent areas of unexcitable scar related to previous atriotomy, characterized by very low-voltage electrograms. During tachycardia, the activation wavefront travels in a macroreentrant circuit around the atriotomy scar. Ablation lines (red dots) connecting the atriotomy scar to the inferior vena cava (IVC) and superior vena cava (SVC) successfully eliminated the tachycardia.

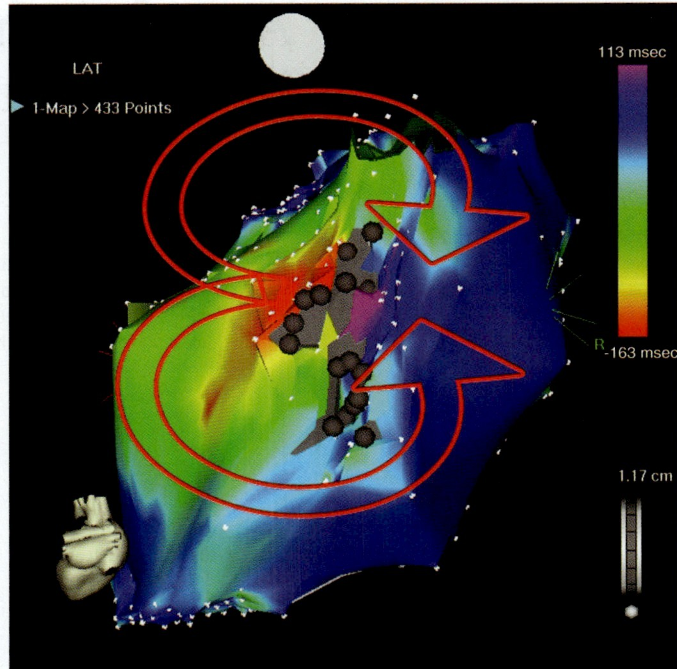

FIGURE 14-2 Three-dimensional electroanatomical (CARTO, Biosense Webster, Inc., Diamond Bar, Calif.) activation map of macroreentrant atrial tachycardia in a patient with previous surgical repair of an atrial septal defect. Gray areas in the posterolateral right atrium (RA) represent areas of unexcitable scar related to previous atriotomy, characterized by very low-voltage electrograms. During tachycardia, the activation wavefront travels from the midposterior RA superiorly and inferiorly, and both counterclockwise and clockwise wavefronts return to the region proximal to the exit site (purple) to complete the circuit by propagating through a narrow isthmus bounded by two areas of unexcitable scar (figure-of-8 reentry). Radiofrequency ablation targeting the gap in the atriotomy scar successfully eliminated the tachycardia. IVC = inferior vena cava; SVC = superior vena cava.

preventing these arrhythmias will influence the long-term survival of patients with congenital heart disease is unknown.[7]

Clinical Considerations

Epidemiology

Macroreentrant AT is the most common mechanism for symptomatic tachycardia in the adult population with congenital heart disease. Surgical incisions in the RA for repair of atrial septal defects are probably the most common causes of lesion-related reentry in adults. Usually, macroreentrant AT appears many years after operations that involved an atriotomy or other surgical manipulation. This arrhythmia can infrequently follow simple procedures, such as closure of an atrial septal defect, but the incidence is highest among patients with advanced dilation, thickening, and scarring of their RA. Other risk factors for macroreentrant AT include the severity of myocardial dysfunction, poor hemodynamic status, concomitant sinus node dysfunction, and older age at the time of heart surgery. It should be recognized, however, that typical AFL is more common than non–isthmus-dependent AFL even in this population, and typical and atypical flutter circuits often coexist in a single patient.

Interestingly, compared with patients with structurally normal hearts, the incidence of atrial fibrillation (AF) in patients with congenital heart disease is relatively low. AF is less common than one would anticipate, especially considering the often extremely dilated RA in this patient population.[8] AF is typically associated predominantly with markers of left-sided heart disease (i.e., lower left ventricular ejection fraction and LA dilation) and is most commonly seen in patients with congenital aortic stenosis, mitral valve disease, palliated single ventricles, or end-stage heart disease.[1,9]

The occurrence of frequent sustained tachycardia is associated with poorer clinical outcome and probably represents a specific risk factor for thrombosis and thromboembolism. It is important to consider the possibility that new-onset atrial arrhythmias may herald worsening ventricular function or tricuspid regurgitation, or both.

ATRIAL SEPTAL DEFECT

Macroreentrant ATs are the most frequent arrhythmias encountered in patients with secundum and sinus venosus atrial septal defects. In the absence of surgical repair, the prevalence of supraventricular arrhythmias increases with age. These arrhythmias have been reported in 20% of these patients at the age of 40 years, and typical AFL is the most common circuit. In the presence of atriotomy incisions, sutures, or patches, non–isthmus-dependent macroreentrant circuits can occur or coexist with typical AFL. Common substrates include macroreentry along the lateral RA wall and double-loop or figure-of-8 circuits. The septal patch itself is rarely a critical conduction obstacle. Surgical closure of an atrial septal defect during childhood provides a substantially lower incidence of arrhythmias. In contrast, surgical closure at adult age is far less effective; approximately 60% of these patients continue to have atrial arrhythmias during follow-up after surgery. The impact of transcatheter atrial septal defect closure on atrial arrhythmias is less clear. In one series, all patients with persistent arrhythmias remained in AF or AFL after closure.[7,8,10]

UNIVENTRICULAR HEARTS WITH FONTAN PALLIATION

Among patients with congenital heart disease, the incidence of macroreentrant AT is highest (16% to 56%) among older patients who have undergone older-style Fontan (atriopulmonary anastomosis) operations, in which extensive suture lines and long-term hemodynamic stress result in marked atrial hypertrophy and fibrosis.[4] The incidence of atrial tachyarrhythmias appears lower

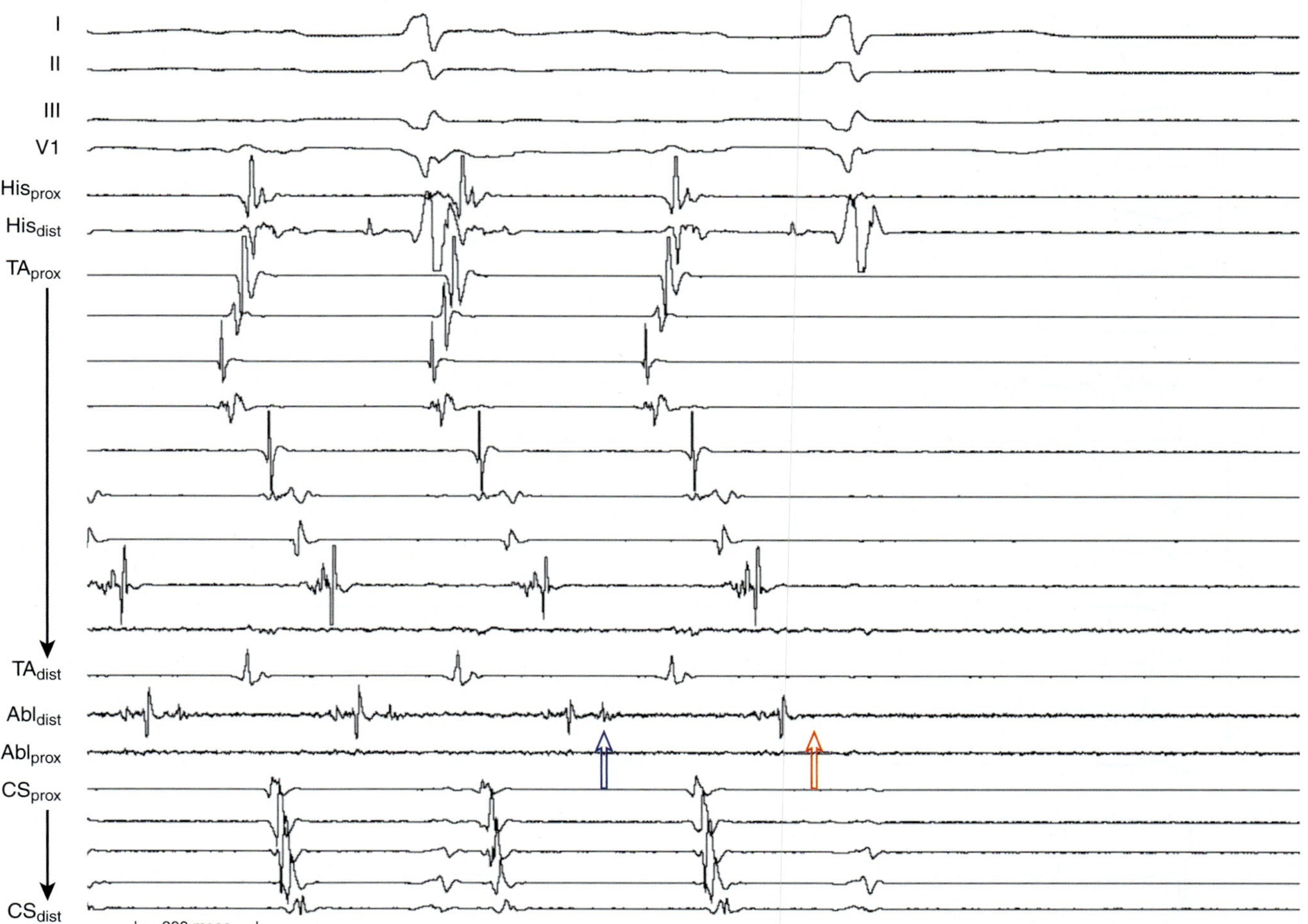

FIGURE 14-3 Catheter-induced termination of macroreentrant atrial tachycardia (AT). ECG leads and intracardiac recordings are shown during an episode of non–isthmus-dependent atrial macroreentrant AT in a patient with prior atriotomy. The episode had lasted 3 months at the time of the study, yet catheter pressure at the site from which the distal ablation site (Abl_{dist}) recording was made terminated AT twice. Note the multicomponent electrogram (blue arrow), the last portion of which is missing when AT terminates (red arrow). Abl_{prox} = proximal ablation site; CS_{dist} = distal coronary sinus; CS_{prox} = proximal coronary sinus; His_{dist} = distal His bundle; His_{prox} = proximal His bundle; TA_{dist} = distal tricuspid annulus; TA_{prox} = proximal tricuspid annulus.

in patients with total cavopulmonary connections in comparison with classical atriopulmonary connections. Overall, the most common arrhythmia is atrial macroreentry. Tachycardia circuits may be complex or multiple. Single circuits that are quite amenable to catheter ablation can occasionally be encountered.[11]

TETRALOGY OF FALLOT

ATs occur commonly (12% to 34%) during extended follow-up after tetralogy of Fallot repair. The observed prevalence of atrial arrhythmias (20.1%) is modestly higher than that of ventricular arrhythmias (14.6%).[12] The most common atrial circuit is typical clockwise or counterclockwise AFL. Other circuits often involve the lateral RA wall and may be multiple, often with a double-loop type of reentry. Nonautomatic focal ATs most commonly arise adjacent to suture points, with radial spread of activation.

The prevalence of AF increases with advancing age. In the first few decades of life, AF is far less common than macroreentrant AT, but it becomes more common (more than 30%) than macroreentrant AT after 55 years of age.[12]

D-TRANSPOSITION OF THE GREAT ARTERIES

The Mustard or Senning atrial switch procedures were performed from the early 1960s until approximately 1985 as the major long-term surgical palliation procedures for young children having D-transposition of the great arteries. Hence, there is a population of patients in their late 20s to early 50s who have undergone these operations and who are at great risk of having supraventricular arrhythmias (15% to 48%), with similar rates in patients with Mustard and Senning baffles.[4,11] Most ATs in this patient group are typical AFL, but non–isthmus-dependent macroreentrant ATs with critical zones of slow conduction between a suture line and the SVC orifice, mitral valve annulus, and pulmonary vein orifice have all been described. Focal ATs adjacent to suture lines are also not uncommon. Currently, arterial switch surgery has supplanted atrial redirection as the procedure of choice for D-transposition of the great arteries, and it has been associated with a lower risk of arrhythmias.[8,10]

Reports suggest that atrial tachyarrhythmias are important contributors to sudden death. Contributing factors may include longer cycle lengths (CLs) than in typical AFL (favoring 1:1 conduction), impaired atrioventricular (AV) transport with failure to augment right ventricular filling rates during tachycardia, systemic ventricular dysfunction, and subendocardial ischemia resulting from right coronary circulation irrigation of a systemic ventricle.[8]

Clinical Presentation

Macroreentrant ATs are typically chronic or long-lasting. As with AF and typical AFL, patients can present with symptoms related to rapid ventricular response, tachycardia-induced cardiomyopathy, or deterioration of preexisting cardiac disease.

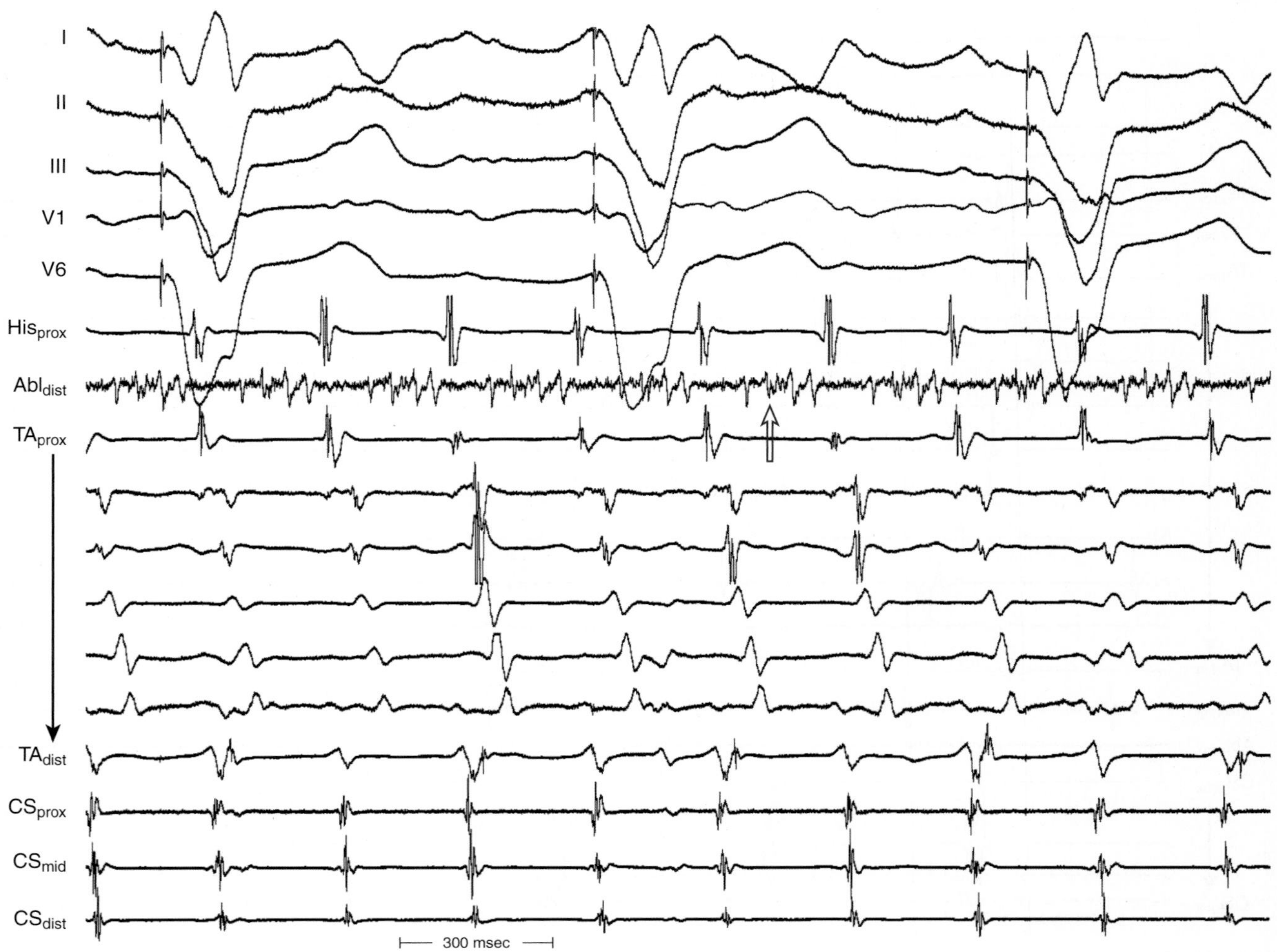

FIGURE 14-4 Postatriotomy right atrial macroreentry (atypical atrial flutter). ECG leads and intracardiac recordings are shown during non–isthmus-dependent macroreentrant atrial tachycardia (AT) in a patient with a repaired atrial septal defect. A prolonged, fractionated diastolic electrogram is observed at the ablation site. Note the repetitive recording (arrow) that nearly spans the cardiac cycle. The patient had a right atriotomy as the basis of AT and incurred complete heart block during surgery (hence the ventricular pacemaker). Abl$_{dist}$ = distal ablation site; CS$_{dist}$ = distal coronary sinus; CS$_{mid}$ = middle coronary sinus; CS$_{prox}$ = proximal coronary sinus; His$_{prox}$ = proximal His bundle; TA$_{dist}$ = distal tricuspid annulus; TA$_{prox}$ = proximal tricuspid annulus.

Generally, in the adult population with congenital heart disease, macroreentrant ATs tend to be slower than typical AFL, with atrial rates in the range of 150 to 250 per minute. In the setting of a healthy AV node (AVN), such rates frequently conduct in a rapid 1:1 AV pattern and can potentially result in hypotension, syncope, or possibly circulatory collapse in patients with limited myocardial reserve. This phenomenon can potentially be compounded by ineffective atrial transport and ventricular dysfunction. Even if the ventricular response rate is well controlled, sustained macroreentrant AT can cause debilitating symptoms in some patients because of the loss of AV synchrony and can contribute to thromboembolic complications when the duration is protracted.[9]

Late-onset supraventricular arrhythmias can potentially have a major impact notably not only on morbidity but also on mortality in patients with congenital heart disease. Not only can arrhythmias be the cause of rapid hemodynamic deterioration, but also they have been linked to an increased risk of sudden death. A multicenter study of defibrillator recipients suggested that supraventricular arrhythmias can trigger ventricular arrhythmias (tachycardia-induced tachycardia). It is likely that the rapid ventricular response is not well tolerated by the impaired ventricle, thus resulting in ventricular tachycardia or fibrillation.[7,11]

Initial Evaluation

In patients with congenital heart disease, arrhythmia onset can herald a changing hemodynamic profile and can be the first sign of deterioration. Therefore, if arrhythmias occur, a thorough evaluation of the hemodynamic status is warranted.[7,13]

Additionally, detailed evaluation of cardiac function and anatomy and knowledge of the congenital anomaly and previous surgical procedures are very important. This evaluation can require transthoracic or transesophageal echocardiography, right or left heart catheterization, angiography of the desired cardiac chamber, and cardiac magnetic resonance imaging (MRI).

Principles of Management

Generally, short-term termination of the tachycardia can be successfully achieved with electrical cardioversion, overdrive pacing, or administration of certain class I or class III antiarrhythmic drugs. However, long-term control of the arrhythmia is far more challenging. Chronic anticoagulation for stroke prevention is typically recommended.

Although the use of antiarrhythmic agents from every class has been reported, none of these drugs have demonstrated clear long-term efficacy. Furthermore, most antiarrhythmic agents carry

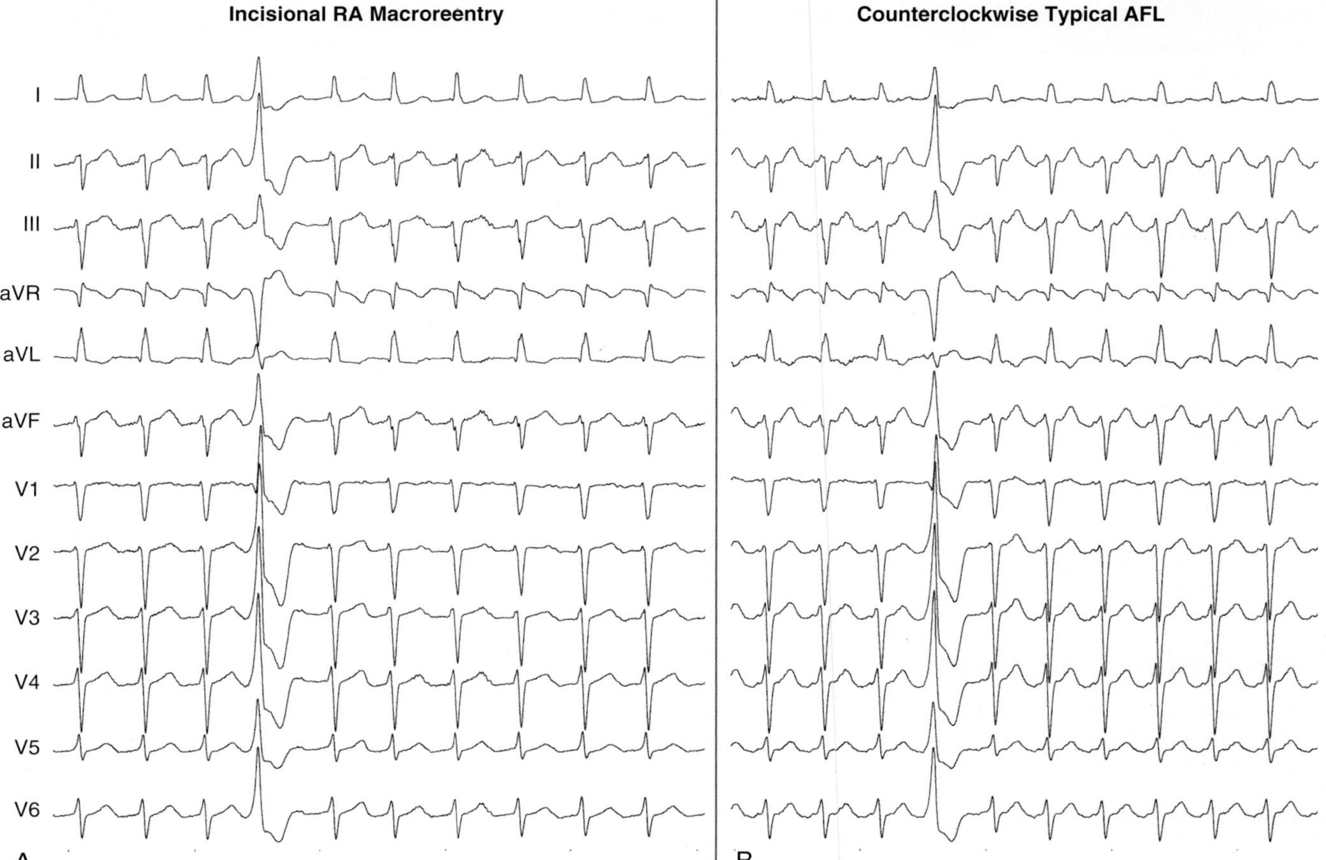

FIGURE 14-5 Surface ECGs of two types of atrial macroreentrant atrial tachycardia in a patient with previous surgical repair of atrial septal defect. **A,** A macroreentrant circuit around the atriotomy scar. **B,** Counterclockwise typical atrial flutter that developed following successful ablation of the scar-related macroreentry. Spontaneous premature ventricular complexes allow better visualization of the P wave (flutter wave) morphology. RA = right atrial; AFL = atrial flutter.

the risk of proarrhythmia, and many agents aggravate sinus node dysfunction and compromise ventricular function, thus diminishing their utility in these patients, particularly in the absence of pacemaker therapy.[9]

Because the general experience with long-term pharmacological therapy has been discouraging, catheter ablation has been adopted as an early intervention for recurrent macroreentrant AT. Catheter ablation carries short-term success rates of nearly 90%, although later tachycardia recurrence is still disappointingly common. The recurrence risk appears to be particularly high in the population of patients who have undergone Fontan procedures. These patients tend to have multiple AT circuits and the thickest and largest atrial dimensions. Nonetheless, ablation results are far superior to the extent of control obtained with medications alone.[9] It is important to recognize that macroreentrant ATs in patients with congenital heart disease can have complex reentrant circuits, the ablation of which can be far more difficult than ablation of typical AFL. This complexity requires that the electrophysiologist be well acquainted with the details of congenital heart lesions and the types of surgical repairs. Therefore, referral to an experienced center should be considered.

Pacemaker implantation can be useful for those patients who have concomitant sinus node dysfunction as a prominent component of their clinical picture. In these patients, prevention of severe sinus bradycardia not only allows for the use of drugs necessary for rate and rhythm control but also can potentially improve the hemodynamic status and often result in marked reduction in AT frequency. Pacemakers with advanced programming features that incorporate AT detection and automatic burst pacing can also be beneficial in select cases, but they carry the risk of accelerating the atrial rate and must thus be used cautiously in patients with rapid AV conduction.[9]

Surgical ablation (RA maze procedure) can be considered in patients with AT refractory to medical therapy and catheter ablation or in those requiring reoperation for hemodynamic reasons. This procedure is used most commonly for patients with failing Fontan procedures and the most refractory variety of macroreentrant AT and is usually combined with a revision of the Fontan connection or conversion from an older atriopulmonary anastomosis to a cavopulmonary connection. This typically includes debulking the RA, removing thrombus, excising RA scar tissue, implanting an epicardial pacemaker, performing a modified RA maze procedure, and, in patients with prior documented AF, performing a left-sided maze procedure as well.[9] Case series with short-term follow-up report promising results, with arrhythmia recurrence rates of 13% to 30%.[11]

It is also important to understand that although effective tachycardia therapy appears to reduce symptoms and the need for cardioversion and improves quality of life in patients with congenital heart disease, it is unclear at present that it improves survival free of major events. If the target arrhythmia is a marker, rather than a cause of poor outcome, therapy should be directed toward the suppression of symptoms while exposing the patient to minimal risk of procedure-related adverse events. Therefore, depending on the expected complexity of the arrhythmia substrate and the underlying structural heart disease, ablation may be reserved for symptomatic patients who are not responding to, or intolerant of, antiarrhythmic medications. Therapeutic decisions are made case by case.[1]

TABLE 14-1 Conditions Associated with Challenges for Vascular and Cardiac Chamber Access

OCCLUSION OR ACCESS CHALLENGE	ASSOCIATED CONDITIONS	ALTERNATE STRATEGIES
Iliofemoral venous occlusion	• D-TGA undergoing BAS as newborn prior to 1985 • Any complex patient with history of multiple catheterizations	• Internal jugular, subclavian veins • Transhepatic venous (especially for transseptal access)
Interrupted inferior vena cava (above renal veins)	• Heterotaxy (left atrial isomerism)	• Internal jugular, subclavian veins • Transhepatic venous (especially for transseptal access) • Femoral vein to azygous vein
Access to pulmonary venous atrium	• "Lateral tunnel," TCPC types of Fontan procedures	• Transbaffle puncture (consult interventionalist?) • Through baffle fenestration, if present • Hybrid procedure (cardiothoracic surgeon performs limited thoracotomy, atrial pursestring)
Access to supra-annular rim of systemic venous atrium	• Fontan procedure–treated patients with supra-annular patch (especially in double inlet ventricle)	• Retrograde from aorta
Access to pulmonary venous atrium	• D-TGA after Mustard or Senning procedure	• Transbaffle puncture (consult interventionalist?) • Retrograde from aorta
Access to atrial mass	• Fontan procedure–treated patients with extracardiac conduit	• Transthoracic puncture (consult cardiothoracic surgeon) • Hybrid procedure (cardiothoracic surgeon performs limited thoracotomy, atrial purse string) • Retrograde from aorta

BAS = balloon atrial septostomy; D-TGA = D-transposition of the great arteries; TCPC = total cavopulmonary connection.
Adapted with permission from Kanter RJ: Pearls for ablation in congenital heart disease, *J Cardiovasc Electrophysiol* 21:223-230, 2010.

Electrocardiographic Features

As noted, macroreentrant ATs in the adult population with congenital heart disease tend have relatively slow atrial rates (in the range of 150 to 250 per minute), and can be associated with 1:1 AV conduction.

The surface ECG morphology of RA free wall macroreentry in a patient with a previous atriotomy is highly variable. The presence of complex anatomy secondary to congenital abnormalities, prior atrial surgery, or large low-voltage zones can modify P wave propagation in nonuniform manner, with resulting altered atrial activation vectors or low-amplitude P waves.[14]

P wave morphology on the surface ECG is usually of limited value for precise anatomical localization of macroreentrant circuits. Even typical isthmus-dependent AFL frequently manifests with an atypical 12-lead ECG appearance (so-called pseudoatypical flutter) in the setting of markedly complex congenital malformation or surgical correction, or both.

Variation in the direction of wavefront rotation, the presence of coexisting conduction block in the atrium, and the presence of simultaneous typical AFL can add to the variability of P wave morphology. Additionally, analysis of the flutter wave can be impeded by partial or complete concealment of the P wave within the QRS complexes or T waves when the AT is associated with 1:1 or 2:1 AV conduction.

The morphology of the atrial complex on the surface ECG can range from that similar to typical AFL to that characteristic of focal AT (see Fig. 14-5). Often, inverted flutter waves can be observed in lead V_1. Depending on the predominant direction of septal activation, RA free wall macroreentrant AT can mimic either clockwise or counterclockwise typical AFL.[14]

Mapping

Detailed knowledge of the of the patient's congenital and operative anatomy is important in the interpretation of the results of mapping, in ascertaining how to access the RA, in determining the feasibility of the transseptal puncture, and in deciding whether fluoroscopy is helpful in localizing the catheters or whether intracardiac or transesophageal echocardiography is needed. Careful preprocedural planning includes a detailed review of prior operative notes, hemodynamic catheterization reports, angiography, and other imaging studies (echocardiography, cardiac computed tomography [CT], or MRI).[13] Table 14-1 includes those conditions that are expected to pose vascular or cardiac chamber access challenges and methods that have been reported to allow catheter access. There is often limited opportunity to place the standard number of diagnostic electrode catheters; alternative approaches to pacing and recording may include the esophagus and hepatic veins and a retrograde approach to the atria from the ventricles.[10]

Exclusion of Cavotricuspid Isthmus Dependence

Exclusion of the CTI as part of the AT circuit is an important initial step because typical clockwise or counterclockwise AFL is the most common macroreentrant AT in patients with congenital heart disease (particularly in patients with simpler anatomical lesions such as the tetralogy of Fallot and atrial and ventricular septal defects), even if the P wave morphology is not characteristic for these arrhythmias. Isthmus-dependent AFL can be rapidly diagnosed or excluded by mapping of the tricuspid annulus and by entrainment maneuvers at the CTI. Exclusion of the CTI as part of the reentrant circuit can be established by any of the following: (1) demonstration of bidirectional activation of the CTI during AT, with resulting collision or fusion within the isthmus by activation from opposing directions (the low lateral RA and coronary sinus [CS]); (2) recording of double potentials separated by an isoelectric and constant interval throughout the full extent of the CTI during tachycardia; or (3) entrainment mapping from the CTI demonstrating manifest atrial fusion with a long post-pacing interval.[4]

Identification of Barriers and Potential Lines of Block

If typical AFL is excluded, attention should be directed to potential reentrant circuits anchored by a right lateral atriotomy scar or a surgical patch. Subsequently, more complex or dual- or multiple-loop reentrant circuits (especially in patients with complex congenital malformations) should be considered; these require a more comprehensive and detailed mapping approach.

Mapping of macroreentrant ATs in patients with congenital heart disease follows the same principles discussed for mapping of other types of macroreentrant ATs (see Chap. 13 for detailed discussion). Electromagnetic three-dimensional (3-D) mapping (CARTO mapping system [Biosense Webster, Inc., Diamond Bar, Calif.] or EnSite NavX system [St. Jude Medical, St. Paul, Minn.]) is typically used to help facilitate identification of the macroreentrant circuit and the sequence of atrial activation during tachycardia and rapid visualization of the activation wavefront in the context of the relevant anatomy. Integration of preacquired cardiac CT or MRI images on the 3-D shell of the cardiac chamber created with the electroanatomical system can further facilitate the procedure. Angiography of the desired chamber may be considered.[4,13] Noncontact mapping may also be used to define the atrial substrate and reentrant circuit, and it can be of significant value when the flutter is short-lived or cannot be reproducibly initiated.

Initially, potential tachycardia circuit barriers are identified (during sinus rhythm or tachycardia) and marked on the electroanatomical map to help understand propagation of the reentrant activation wavefront in relation to these barriers, identify potential slow-conducting pathways critical to the reentrant circuit, identify sites to target by entrainment mapping, and plan subsequent ablation strategy to abolish the tachycardia. The tricuspid annulus often provides one important barrier. Other naturally fixed barriers (i.e., independent of the precise form of activation and present also in sinus rhythm) include the IVC, SVC, and CS ostium. Acquired barriers include surgical incisions or patches, lines of block, and electrical scars. Silent areas are defined as having an atrial potential amplitude of less than 0.05 mV and the absence of atrial capture at 20 mA. Such areas and surgically related scars, such as atriotomy scars in the lateral RA or atrial septal defect closure patches, are tagged as "scar" (see Figs. 14-1 and 14-2).[3,4,13]

Identification of the Complete Reentrant Circuit

Activation electroanatomical mapping during AT is performed to define the atrial activation sequence and identify the complete reentrant circuit and its mid-diastolic critical isthmus. Reasonable numbers of points homogeneously distributed in the atrium must be recorded. The local activation time at each site is determined from the intracardiac bipolar electrogram and is measured in relation to the fixed intracardiac electric reference (usually an electrogram obtained from the CS catheter). The complete reentrant circuit is the spatially shortest route of unidirectional activation encompassing the complete CL of the tachycardia in terms of activation timing and returning to the site of earliest activation. Using electroanatomical mapping, this translates into continuous progression of colors (from red to purple in the CARTO system and from white to purple in the NavX system) around the atrium, with close proximity of earliest and latest local activation. Additionally, propagation of electrical activation superimposed on the 3-D anatomical reconstruction of the atrium can be visualized as a propagation map in relation to the anatomical and EP landmarks and barriers.

Unlike in mapping focal AT, in which tracking the site with the earliest presystolic local activation timing is the goal of mapping, there is no early or late region for macroreentrant AT because the wavefront is continuously propagating around the circuit.

It is very important to remain vigilant during the mapping process and identify any change in CL or activation sequence, or both, that can result from catheter manipulation, pacing maneuvers, or ablation. Such changes can indicate transformation of a multiple loop tachycardia by interruption of one loop, change in bystander activation, or transition to another tachycardia, which requires reassessment. The transition may be obvious but also is often quite subtle and sometimes imperceptible if only the CS activation is analyzed. Simultaneous recording RA activation (using a Halo catheter around the tricuspid annulus) and CS activation (using a decapolar catheter) can help rapid identification of tachycardia transformation.[15]

Sometimes, it can be impossible to map the entire circuit, especially in patients with repaired congenital heart disease, because of the complex suture lines, baffles, or both. In this setting, a combination of activation, entrainment, and voltage mapping data is used to identify the potential isthmus or zone of slow conduction critical to the reentrant circuit, which is then targeted by catheter ablation.[4]

Identification of the Critical Isthmus

Once one or more potential isthmuses are identified during activation mapping and propagation mapping in relation to atrial scars, barriers, and lines of block, entrainment is performed to determine their role for supporting the reentrant circuit. Entrainment with concealed fusion should be sought; this indicates that the pacing site is in a protected isthmus located within or attached to the reentrant circuit. It is important to understand, however, that in patients with complex anatomy and surgical repairs, critical corridors of slow conduction can exist anywhere in the RA mass, and multiple circuits are the rule. As a consequence, entrainment with concealed fusion is highly nonspecific for most circuits in these patients. Therefore, whether the protected isthmus is crucial to the reentrant circuit or just a bystander site needs to be verified by comparing the post-pacing interval with the tachycardia CL and the stimulus-exit interval with the electrogram-exit interval. Features of entrainment when pacing from different sites are listed in Table 13-2.[10,16,17]

Ablation

Target of Ablation

The choice of ablation sites should be among those segments of the reentry circuit that offer the most convenient and safest opportunity for creating conduction block. Among other factors are the isthmus size, anticipated catheter stability, and risk of damage to adjacent structures (e.g., phrenic nerve, sinus node, and AVN).

Ablation is performed by targeting the narrowest identifiable isthmus of conduction accessible within the circuit (allowing the best electrode-tissue contact along the desired line). The ablation line is chosen to transect an area critical for the circuit and, at the same time, connect two anatomical areas of block, an electrically silent area to an anatomical zone of block (e.g., IVC, SVC, or tricuspid annulus), or two electrically silent areas.

Although success in most of these studies has been achieved by targeting the "slow zone" of atrial conduction presumed necessary for maintenance of the reentry, some investigators have emphasized the need for considering both the anatomy and electrophysiology simultaneously to identify a susceptible bridge of tissue, which connects two areas of electrical block. Such an approach requires careful review of the details of the atrial surgery, in addition to detailed mapping of the atria in its "usual" rhythm and during reentry.[4]

Because typical isthmus-dependent AFL is the most common mechanism underlying macroreentrant AT in the patient population with congenital heart disease, determination of the role of the CTI in supporting reentry is evaluated first, and this isthmus is targeted by ablation if it is proved to be critical to the AT circuit (see Chap. 12 for detailed discussion). Ablation of the CTI may also be reasonable in every patient with congenital heart disease, even patients presenting with non–isthmus-dependent RA macroreentry, because the CTI can support reentry in most patients with prior right atriotomy.

Successful CTI ablation can result in termination of the tachycardia and restoration of sinus rhythm, thus confirming participation of the CTI in the circuit. Alternatively, the tachycardia may transform to a different arrhythmia, as indicated by a change in activation sequence or CL, or both. Additionally, after extensive ablation and even appearance of dissociated electrograms in the CTI, AT may persist with little discernible change in CL or activation sequence. This usually indicates multiple circuits, often with a double-loop type of reentry that uses the lateral wall as well as the CTI, and is now dependent on a different isthmus (e.g., the lateral RA around or within the atriotomy scar).[18]

If participation of the CTI in the reentrant circuit is excluded, or if the tachycardia persists or transforms into a different tachycardia after ablation of the CTI, the participation of the lateral RA wall in the AT circuit should be assessed. Non–isthmus-dependent RA macroreentry is frequently localized to the free wall of the RA, anchored by the atriotomy scar, in which setting the ablation strategy includes any of the following: (1) to target the slow conduction area (critical isthmus of the reentrant circuit) as identified by detailed activation and entrainment mapping; (2) to extend the atriotomy (double potential or scar) to the IVC (see Fig. 14-1); or (3) to extend the scar area to the SVC. The last approach can result in injury of the sinus node or phrenic nerve. Therefore, when possible, extending the atriotomy to the IVC is preferable. As noted, additional ablation of the CTI may be considered in these patients because these circuits are often combined with a circuit around the tricuspid annulus in a figure-of-8 reentry, such that ablation of both the CTI and one of the lateral wall options must be performed to eliminate and prevent reentrant AT.[4,18]

Rarely, more complex circuits, such as around the right septal patch, as seen in patients with Mustard or Senning repairs, are observed. However, the approach to ablation is the same: the area with slow conduction or scar is extended to an anatomical obstacle.

Another focus for reentry circuits is the sinus node region, possibly because of injury related to the superior atrial cannulation site for the bypass pump. These circuits may be quite small, often manifesting as focal tachycardia in the sinus node region, and they can often be ablated in a single location without establishing a particular line of block.[4]

In patients with incomplete maps, a combination of activation, entrainment, and voltage mapping data is used to identify the potential isthmus or zone of slow conduction critical to the reentrant circuit, which is then targeted by catheter ablation. When limitations to this approach still exist (from poor inducibility or frequent change in morphology of the tachycardia), a stepwise ablation strategy may be employed. Because the reentrant circuit in most patients is anchored to the CTI or the atriotomy scar, or both, ablation of the CTI is initially performed. Then, if the tachycardia persists, linear ablation is carried out by targeting the isthmuses related to the lateral atriotomy scar (i.e., connecting the atriotomy to either the IVC or SVC). Additional ablation lines connecting other areas of conduction block (scar, surgical incision, septal patch, baffle, or natural barriers) may be considered based on substrate mapping findings.[4]

Ablation Technique

Once the ablation target is identified, ablation involves placing a series of RF lesions to sever the critical isthmus to connect two anatomical or surgical barriers. Because some congenital malformations and surgical repairs are associated with myocardial hypertrophy and extensive fibrotic regions, thus making the achievement of a transmural lesion difficult, ablation is performed with an irrigated (25 to 50 W) or 8-mm (target temperature, 60° to 70°C; 50 to 60 W) electrode-tip RF catheter.[18]

RF application is maintained for up to 60 to 120 seconds until the bipolar atrial potential recorded from the ablation electrode is decreased by 80% or split into double potentials, indicating local conduction block. The coalescence of multiple RF lesions can be facilitated by the use of an electroanatomical mapping system.

During delivery of RF energy, the tachycardia can terminate, or its CL can increase transiently or permanently. These findings indicate that the lesions have affected the circuit and should lead to continuation of RF delivery or extension of the lesion to ensure the achievement of complete conduction block across the isthmus. Alternatively, the tachycardia may transform to a different loop or to a different tachycardia (rather than terminate), as indicated by a change in activation sequence or CL, or both, in which setting reassessment of the new tachycardia mechanism and location is necessary before continued RF ablation. However, if ablation across an isthmus that was initially found to be critical to the tachycardia circuit (by entrainment mapping techniques) appears to be not affecting the tachycardia, it is important to verify whether the isthmus is still critical to the reentrant circuit by repeating entrainment mapping. Sometimes, complete isthmus block is already achieved (as suggested by the presence of double potentials along the ablation line), and the isthmus is no longer participating in the tachycardia circuit (as suggested by entrainment mapping findings), as a result of a change in the tachycardia circuit that occurred during ablation.[15,19,20]

Ablation near the region of the superior crista terminalis and SVC can result in right phrenic nerve injury and diaphragmatic paralysis. Pacing with a high output (10 mA at 2 milliseconds) from the ablation catheter at the target site can help identify the location of the right phrenic nerve. Additionally, suspicion of phrenic nerve injury should be considered in the case of hiccup, cough, or decrease in diaphragmatic excursion during energy delivery. Early recognition of phrenic nerve injury during RF delivery allows the immediate interruption of the application prior to the onset of permanent injury and is associated with the rapid recovery of phrenic nerve function.[4]

Endpoints of Ablation

TACHYCARDIA TERMINATION DURING RADIOFREQUENCY ENERGY APPLICATION

Sudden termination of AT during RF application suggests that the lesion has affected a critical isthmus, and that site should be targeted for additional lesions. However, AT termination during RF application as the sole criterion of a successful ablation is hazardous because such an AT can also terminate spontaneously, secondary to premature atrial complexes induced by RF energy delivery, and by partial, rather than complete, isthmus block. Therefore, termination of AT during RF application is insufficient by itself as an endpoint.[4,18]

NONINDUCIBILITY OF TACHYCARDIA

To use this criterion as a reliable endpoint, careful assessment of inducibility should be performed prior to ablation, and the feasibility and best method of reproducible induction of the AT should be documented at baseline before ablation. In the setting of easy inducibility prior to ablation, one can consider the lack of inducibility as an indicator of successful ablation. Noninducibility of the arrhythmia is inapplicable if the original arrhythmia either is noninducible at baseline or was inadvertently terminated mechanically. Noninducibility may also reflect conduction delay in the critical isthmus, and not stable block, or it may be secondary to changes in autonomic tone.[4,18]

DOCUMENTATION OF A LINE OF BLOCK

Complete stable conduction block within the reentry path is the most useful and objective endpoint for ablation of macroreentrant AT. Complete conduction block following linear ablation across the isthmus can be confirmed by atrial pacing on one side of the ablation line and mapping along the line demonstrating absence of electrograms or the presence of widely separated parallel double potentials recorded all along the line with marked delay and reversal in the direction of activation on the opposite side of the linear lesion. For a vertically oriented RA free wall atriotomy, assessment of conduction block can be facilitated by the use of a multielectrode Halo-type catheter, which can document activation sequences anterior and posterior to the scar, so that when pacing close to the contiguously ablated isthmus, the absence of a wavefront penetrating the scar and isthmus is used to indicate conduction block. Additionally, assessment of electrical block across the ablation line can be facilitated by the use of the noncontact mapping system (EnSite, St. Jude Medical, St. Paul, Minn.), which allows for simultaneous mapping of the entire chamber of interest (versus sequential point-by-point mapping) during pacing on either side of the ablation line.[4,18]

Outcome

Atrial enlargement and myocardial hypertrophy and extensive scarring in patients with congenital heart disease can interfere with RF energy delivery and limit RF lesion depth. Additionally, the complexity of anatomy, vascular access issues, and the multiplicity of circuits in some patients can render the mapping and ablation procedure very challenging. Nonetheless, the combined use of 3-D mapping and tip cooling techniques has improved acute success rates to nearly 90%. However, high recurrence rates and the onset of new arrhythmias remain problematic (up to 30% to 45% within the first year), which may be related, at least in part, to ongoing changes in the arrhythmia substrate.[8]

Importantly, in some congenital heart malformations (e.g., AV canal defects), the AVN is displaced just anterior to the mouth of the CS. Consequently, ablating in the right inferior paraseptal region can cause AV block. Therefore, for patients with CTI-dependent macroreentry, lateral ablation lines are generally preferred, to prevent AV block.[10]

REFERENCES

1. Triedman JK: Atypical atrial tachycardias in patients with congenital heart disease, *Heart Rhythm* 5:315–317, 2008.
2. Garan H: Atypical atrial flutter, *Heart Rhythm* 5:618–621, 2008.
3. de Groot NM, Zeppenfeld K, Wijffels MC, et al: Ablation of focal atrial arrhythmia in patients with congenital heart defects after surgery: role of circumscribed areas with heterogeneous conduction, *Heart Rhythm* 3:526–535, 2006.
4. Saul JP: Role of catheter ablation in postoperative arrhythmias, *Pacing Clin Electrophysiol* 31(Suppl 1):S7–S12, 2008.
5. Anselme F: Macroreentrant atrial tachycardia: pathophysiological concepts, *Heart Rhythm* 5(Suppl):S18–S21, 2008.
6. Seslar SP, Alexander ME, Berul CI, et al: Ablation of nonautomatic focal atrial tachycardia in children and adults with congenital heart disease, *J Cardiovasc Electrophysiol* 17:359–365, 2006.
7. Roos-Hesselink JW, Karamermer Y: Significance of postoperative arrhythmias in congenital heart disease, *Pacing Clin Electrophysiol* 31(Suppl 1):S2–S6, 2008.
8. Khairy P, Balaji S: Cardiac arrhythmias in congenital heart diseases, *Indian Pacing Electrophysiol J* 9:299–317, 2009.
9. Warnes CA, Williams RG, Bashore TM, et al: ACC/AHA 2008 guidelines for the management of adults with congenital heart disease: a report of the American College of Cardiology/American Heart Association Task Force on Practice Guidelines (writing committee to develop guidelines on the management of adults with congenital heart disease), *Circulation* 118:e714–e833, 2008.
10. Kanter RJ: Pearls for ablation in congenital heart disease, *J Cardiovasc Electrophysiol* 21:223–230, 2010.
11. Khairy P, Van Hare GF: Catheter ablation in transposition of the great arteries with Mustard or Senning baffles, *Heart Rhythm* 6:283–289, 2009.
12. Khairy P, Aboulhosn J, Gurvitz MZ, et al: Arrhythmia burden in adults with surgically repaired tetralogy of Fallot: a multi-institutional study, *Circulation* 31(122):868–875, 2010.
13. Khairy P: EP challenges in adult congenital heart disease, *Heart Rhythm* 5:1464–1472, 2008.
14. Medi C, Kalman JM: Prediction of the atrial flutter circuit location from the surface electrocardiogram, *Europace* 10:786–796, 2008.
15. Morady F, Oral H, Chugh A: Diagnosis and ablation of atypical atrial tachycardia and flutter complicating atrial fibrillation ablation, *Heart Rhythm* 6(Suppl):S29–S32, 2009.
16. Miyazaki H, Stevenson WG, Stephenson K, et al: Entrainment mapping for rapid distinction of left and right atrial tachycardias, *Heart Rhythm* 3:516–523, 2006.
17. Deo R, Berger R: The clinical utility of entrainment pacing, *J Cardiovasc Electrophysiol* 20:466–470, 2009.
18. Khairy P, Stevenson WG: Catheter ablation in tetralogy of Fallot, *Heart Rhythm* 6:1069–1074, 2009.
19. Weerasooriya R, Jais P, Wright M, et al: Catheter ablation of atrial tachycardia following atrial fibrillation ablation, *J Cardiovasc Electrophysiol* 20:833–838, 2009.
20. Jais P, Matsuo S, Knecht S, et al: A deductive mapping strategy for atrial tachycardia following atrial fibrillation ablation: importance of localized reentry, *J Cardiovasc Electrophysiol* 20:480–491, 2009.

CHAPTER 15 Atrial Fibrillation

Pathophysiology

Classification of Atrial Fibrillation

Atrial fibrillation (AF) has been described in various ways, such as paroxysmal or persistent, lone, idiopathic, nonvalvular, valvular, or self-terminating. Each of these classifications has implications regarding mechanisms, as well as response to therapy. At the initial detection of AF, it may be difficult to be certain of the subsequent pattern of duration and frequency of recurrences. Thus, a designation of first-detected episode of AF is made on the initial diagnosis, irrespective of the duration of the arrhythmia. When the patient has experienced two or more episodes, AF is classified as recurrent. After the termination of an episode of AF, the rhythm can be classified as paroxysmal or persistent. *Paroxysmal AF* is characterized by self-terminating episodes that generally last less than 7 days. *Persistent AF* generally lasts longer than 7 days and often requires electrical or pharmacological cardioversion. *Permanent AF* refers to AF in which cardioversion has failed or AF that has been sustained for more than 1 year, or when further attempts to terminate the arrhythmia are deemed futile. With the advent of catheter ablation interventions for AF, patients with persistent AF for longer than 1 year who are considered for ablation have been referred to as having *longstanding persistent AF*, to distinguish them from patients with permanent AF in whom attempts to restore normal sinus rhythm (NSR) were unsuccessful or have been abandoned.[1,2]

Although useful, this arbitrary classification does not account for all presentations of AF. Paroxysmal AF often progresses to longer, non–self-terminating episodes. Additionally, the pattern of AF can change in response to treatment. AF that has been persistent can become paroxysmal with antiarrhythmic drug therapy, and AF that had been permanent may be cured or made paroxysmal by surgical or catheter-based ablation. Furthermore, the distinction between persistent and permanent AF is not only a function of the underlying arrhythmia but also a reflection of the clinical pragmatism of the patient and physician. The severity of symptoms associated with AF, anticoagulation status, and patient preference all affect the decision of whether and when cardioversion will be attempted. This decision would then affect the duration of sustained AF and could lead to a diagnosis of persistent or permanent AF.[3]

Mechanism of Atrial Fibrillation

The pathogenesis of AF remains incompletely understood and is believed to be multifactorial. Two concepts of the underlying mechanism of AF have received considerable attention: factors that trigger and factors that perpetuate the arrhythmia. In general, patients with frequent, self-terminating episodes of AF are likely to have a predominance of factors that trigger AF, whereas patients with AF that does not terminate spontaneously are more likely to have a predominance of perpetuating factors. Although such a gross generalization has clinical usefulness, there is often considerable overlap of these mechanisms. The typical patient with paroxysmal AF has identifiable ectopic foci initiating the arrhythmia, but these triggers cannot be recorded in all patients. Conversely, occasional patients with persistent or permanent AF may be cured of their arrhythmia by ablation of a single triggering focus, a finding suggesting that perpetual firing of the focus may be the mechanism sustaining this arrhythmia in some cases.

Advanced mapping technologies, along with studies in animal models, have suggested the potential for complex pathophysiological substrates and modifiers responsible for AF, including the following: (1) continuous aging or degeneration of atrial tissue and the cardiac conduction system; (2) progression of structural heart disease (e.g., valvular heart disease and cardiomyopathy); (3) myocardial ischemia, local hypoxia, electrolyte derangement, and metabolic disorders (e.g., atherosclerotic heart disease, chronic lung disease, hypokalemia, and hyperthyroidism); (4) inflammation related to pericarditis or myocarditis, with or without cardiac surgery; (5) genetic predisposition; (6) drugs; and (7) autonomic effects.[2]

MECHANISM OF INITIATION OF ATRIAL FIBRILLATION

The factors responsible for the onset of AF include triggers that induce the arrhythmia and the substrate that sustains it. The triggers are diverse yet may not cause AF in the absence of other contributors. There are two different types of arrhythmias that can potentially play a role in generating AF: premature atrial complexes (PACs) that initiate AF (focal triggers) and focal tachycardia that either induces fibrillation in the atria or mimics AF by creating a pattern of rapid and irregular depolarization wavefronts in the atria for as long as the focus continues to discharge.[2,4]

The mechanism of initiation of AF is not certain in most cases and likely is multifactorial. Triggers propagating into the atrial myocardium can initiate multiple reentering wavelets and AF. In some patients with paroxysmal AF, impulses initiated by ectopic focal activity propagate into the left atrium (LA) and encounter heterogeneously recovered tissue. If reentry were assumed to be the mechanism of AF, initiation would require an area of conduction block and a wavelength of activation short enough to allow the reentrant circuits to persist in the myocardium.[2,4]

Once triggered, AF can be self-sustained, in which case the continued firing of the focus may not be required for maintenance of the arrhythmia, and ablation of the focus may not terminate AF, but rather may prevent the reinitiation of AF. Conversely, initiation and maintenance of AF can depend on uninterrupted periodic activity of a few discrete reentrant or triggered sources localized to the LA (i.e., focal driver), emanating from such sources to propagate through both atria and interact with anatomical or functional obstacles, or both, thus leading to fragmentation and multiple wavelet formation. Factors such as wavefront curvature, sink-source relationships, and spatial and temporal organization all are relevant to the understanding of the initiation of AF by the interaction of the propagating wavefronts with such anatomical or functional obstacles. Indeed, all these factors, which differ from triggers, importantly affect the initiators of AF.

AF triggering factors include sympathetic or parasympathetic stimulation, bradycardia, PACs (which are the most common cause; Fig. 15-1), atrial flutter (AFL), supraventricular tachycardias (SVTs; especially those mediated by atrioventricular [AV] bypass tracts [BTs]; Fig. 15-2), and acute atrial stretch. Identification of these triggers has clinical importance because treatment approaches directed at elimination of the triggers (e.g., radiofrequency [RF] ablation of the initiating PACs or SVT) can be curative in selected patients.

PULMONARY VEIN TRIGGERS. Triggering foci of rapidly firing cells within the sleeves of atrial myocytes extending into the pulmonary veins (PVs) have been clearly shown to be the underlying mechanism in most cases of paroxysmal AF.[4] Supporting this idea are clinical studies of impulses generated by single foci propagating from individual PVs or other atrial regions to the remainder of the atria as fibrillatory waves and abolition of AF by RF ablation to eliminate or isolate the venous foci.

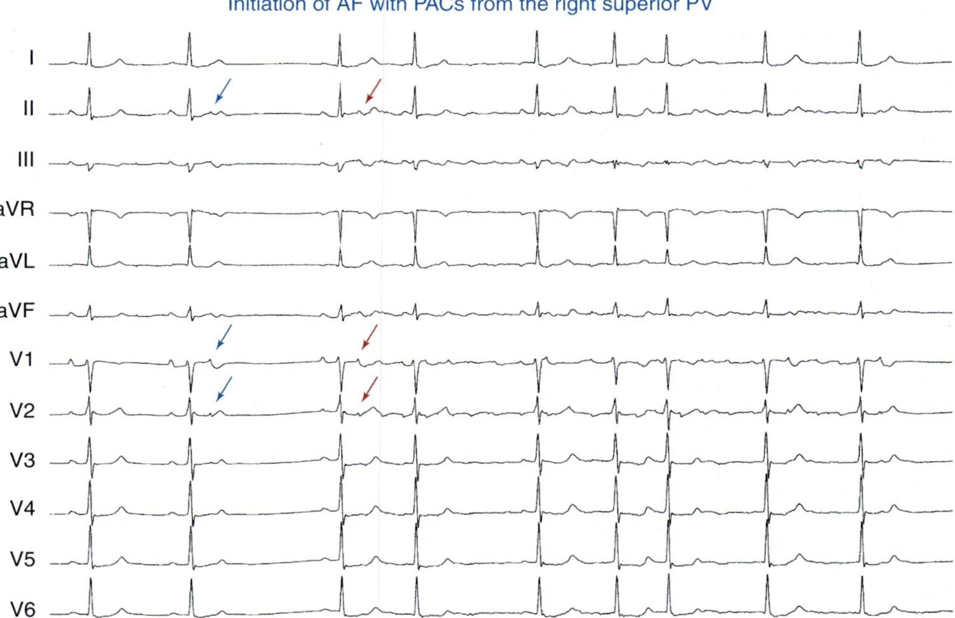

FIGURE 15-1 Atrial fibrillation (AF) induction by premature atrial complexes (PACs) originating from the right superior pulmonary vein (PV). Two monomorphic PACs (arrows) occur at short coupling intervals and are inscribed within the T wave. The second PAC (red arrows) triggers AF.

Based on several features, the thoracic veins are highly arrhythmogenic. The PV-LA junction has discontinuous myocardial fibers separated by fibrotic tissues and hence is highly anisotropic. Insulated muscle fibers can promote reentrant excitation, automaticity, and triggered activity. These regions likely resemble the juxtaposed islets of atrial myocardium and vascular smooth muscle in the coronary sinus (CS) and AV valves that, under normal circumstances, manifest synchronous electrical activity but develop delayed afterdepolarizations and triggered activity in response to catecholamine stimulation, rapid atrial pacing, or acute stretch.[5]

Furthermore, the PVs of patients with paroxysmal AF demonstrate abnormal properties of conduction so that there can be markedly reduced refractoriness within the PVs, progressive conduction delay within the PV in response to rapid pacing or programmed stimulation, and often conduction block between the PV and the LA. Such findings are much more common in patients with paroxysmal AF than in normal subjects.[2,6] Rapidly firing foci can often be recorded within the PVs with conduction block to the LA. Administration of catecholamines such as isoproterenol can lead to shortening of the LA refractory period, thereby allowing these foci to propagate to the LA with the induction of AF.[6] These discontinuous properties of conduction within the PV can also provide a substrate for reentry within the PV itself, although this remains to be proven.[5]

NON–PULMONARY VEIN TRIGGERS. Although more than 90% of triggering foci that are mapped during electrophysiological (EP) studies in patients with paroxysmal AF occur in the PVs, foci within the superior vena cava (SVC), small muscle bundles in the ligament of Marshall, and the musculature of the CS have been identified. Although these latter locations of triggering foci are uncommon in patients with paroxysmal AF, the common factor is that the site of origin is often within a venous structure that connects to the atrium. Other sites of initiating foci can be recorded in the LA wall or along the crista terminalis in the right atrium (RA).[5]

MECHANISM OF MAINTENANCE OF ATRIAL FIBRILLATION

Having been initiated, AF can be brief; however, various factors can act as perpetuators, thus ensuring the maintenance of AF.[2] One factor is the persistence of the triggers and initiators that induced the AF, which then act as an engine driving the continuation of AF. In this setting, maintenance of AF is dependent on the continued firing of the focus (the so-called focal driver). However, AF can persist even in the absence of the focal drivers. Without focal drivers, persistence of AF results from a combination of electrical and structural remodeling processes characterized by atrial dilation and shortening of atrial refractoriness (see later). These factors can be present at baseline or, alternatively, induced by the AF itself.

Several theories have been proposed to explain the EP mechanisms underlying AF, including the multiple wavelet theory, the single circuit reentry theory, and rapidly discharging atrial focus with fibrillatory conduction.

MULTIPLE WAVELET THEORY. For many years, the most widely held theory on the maintenance of AF was the multiple wavelet hypothesis, which was a key development in our understanding of the mechanism of AF. Moe and associates noted that, "The grossly irregular wavefront becomes fractionated as it divides about islets or strands of refractory tissue, and each of the daughter wavelets may now be considered as independent offspring. Such a wavelet may accelerate or decelerate as it encounters tissue in a more or less advanced state of recovery."[7] Moe and associates subsequently hypothesized that AF is sustained by multiple randomly wandering wavelets that collided with each other and were extinguished, or divided into daughter wavelets that continually reexcited the atria.[7] Those functional reentrant circuits are therefore unstable; some disappear, whereas others reform. These circuits have variable, but short, cycle lengths (CLs), resulting in multiple circuits to which atrial tissue cannot respond in a 1:1 fashion. As a result, functional block, slow conduction, and multiple wavefronts develop. It has been suggested that at least four to six independent wavelets are required to maintain AF. These wavelets rarely reenter themselves but can reexcite portions of the myocardium recently activated by another wavefront, a process called random reentry. As a result, there are multiple wavefronts of activation that can collide with each other and extinguish themselves or create new wavelets and wavefronts, thereby perpetuating the arrhythmia.

The persistence of multiple-circuit reentry depends on the ability of a tissue to maintain enough simultaneously reentering wavefronts so that electrical activity is unlikely to extinguish simultaneously in all parts of the atria. Therefore, the more wavelets are present, the more likely it is that the arrhythmia will be sustained. The number of wavelets on the heart at any moment depends on the atrial mass, refractory period, conduction velocity, and anatomical obstacles in different portions of the atria. In essence, a large atrial mass with short refractory periods and conduction delay would yield increased wavelets and would present the most favorable situation for AF to be sustained.[2,8]

SINGLE CIRCUIT REENTRY THEORY. Studies in isolated human atrial preparations questioned the randomness of atrial activity and suggested the presence of a single source of stable reentrant activity ("mother rotor") that serves as a periodic background focus, with break-up of emanating waves in atrial tissue of variable electrical properties and anatomical obstacles into multiple wavelets spreading in various directions. Although well represented in animal studies, rotors have not been observed in whole human atria studied at the time of thoracic surgery. More recent data using different techniques have shown that functional reentry (or anatomical reentry with a functional component), in the form of spiral waves rotating around microreentrant circuits approximately 1 cm in diameter, was suggested to be the most likely cause of AF. Other studies have shown that these dominant

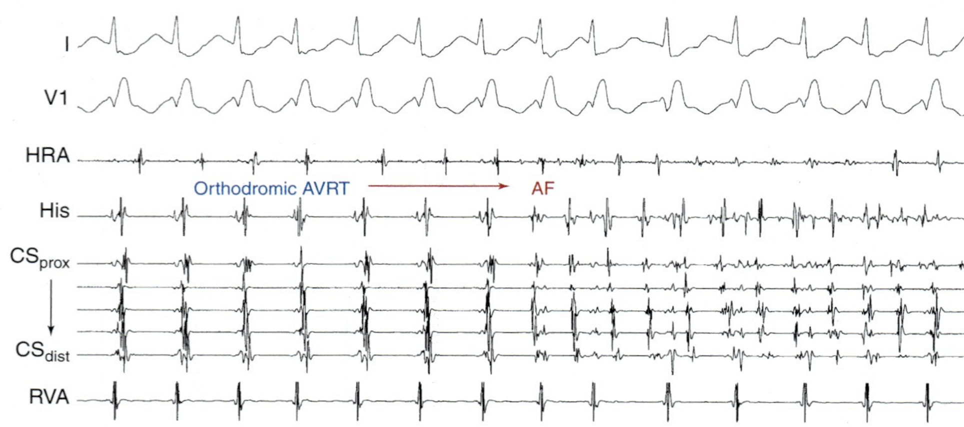

FIGURE 15-2 Atrial fibrillation (AF) induction by orthodromic atrioventricular reentrant tachycardia (AVRT). CS_{dist} = distal coronary sinus; CS_{prox} = proximal coronary sinus; HRA = high right atrium; RVA = right ventricular apex.

rotors that drive AF invariably originate and anchor in the LA, with the RA activated passively.[8,9]

FOCAL DRIVERS WITH FIBRILLATORY CONDUCTION. Although multiple wandering wavelets probably account for most cases of AF, occasionally a single, rapidly firing focus can be identified with EP mapping. Impulses initiated by ectopic focal activity propagate into the atria to encounter heterogeneously recovered tissue. When cardiac impulses are continuously generated at a rapid rate from any source or any mechanism, they activate the tissue of that cardiac chamber in a 1:1 manner, up to a critical rate. However, when this critical rate is exceeded, so that not all the tissue of that cardiac chamber can respond in a 1:1 fashion (e.g., because the CL of the driver is shorter than the refractory periods of those tissues), fibrillatory conduction develops. Fibrillatory conduction can be caused by spatially varying refractory periods or by the structural properties of atrial tissue, with source-sink mismatches providing spatial gradients in the response.[2] Thus, fibrillatory conduction is characterized by activation of tissues at variable CLs, all longer than the CL of the driver, because of variable conduction block. In that manner, activation is fragmented.[2] This is the mechanism of AF in several animal models in which the driver consists of a stable, abnormally automatic focus of a very short CL, a stable reentrant circuit with a very short CL, or an unstable reentrant circuit with a very short CL. It also appears to be the mechanism of AF in patients in whom activation of the atria at very short CLs originates in one or more PVs. The impulses from the PVs seem to precipitate and maintain AF. Autonomic influences (parasympathetic or sympathetic) can cause some of these rapid discharges. Of note, it has also been suggested that fibrillatory conduction caused by a reentrant driver can potentially be the cause of ventricular fibrillation (VF).

Substrate for Atrial Fibrillation

AF results from the interplay between a trigger for initiation and a vulnerable EP substrate for maintenance. The fact that most potential triggers do not initiate AF suggests some role for functional and structural substrates in most patients. However, the relative contribution of triggers versus substrate can vary with the clinical context, and the exact nature of the interaction between triggers and substrate remains to be elucidated.[8]

AF commonly occurs in the context of other cardiac or noncardiac pathological conditions, such as valvular disease, hypertension, ischemic heart disease, heart failure, or hyperthyroidism. Depending on the type, extent, and duration of such external stressors, a cascade of time-dependent adaptive, as well as maladaptive, atrial responses develops in order to maintain homeostasis (so-called atrial remodeling), including changes at the ionic channel level, cellular level, or extracellular matrix level, or a combination of these, thus resulting in structural, functional, and electrical consequences. A hallmark of atrial structural remodeling is atrial dilation, often accompanied by a progressive increase in interstitial fibrosis. Atrial arrhythmias, especially AF, are the most common manifestations of electrical remodeling.[10]

Increased dispersion in atrial refractoriness and inhomogeneous dispersion of conduction abnormalities, including block, slow conduction, and dissociation of neighboring atrial muscle bundles, are key elements in the development of the substrate of AF. Importantly, different pathological conditions can be associated with a different set of remodeling responses in the atria.[11]

Even in the setting of lone AF, whereby no structural heart disease is apparent, there is accumulating evidence that occult abnormalities (e.g., patchy fibrosis, inflammatory infiltrates, loss of myocardial voltage, conduction slowing, altered sinus node function, and vascular dysfunction) can be observed and likely represent an early stage of atrial remodeling contributing to the substrate of AF.[12]

ATRIAL ELECTROPHYSIOLOGICAL PROPERTIES

The normal atrial myocardium consists of so-called fast response tissues that depend on the rapidly activating sodium (Na^+) current for phase 0 of the action potential. As a result, the atrium has several properties that permit the development of very complex patterns of conduction and an extremely rapid atrial rate, as seen in AF. The action potential duration is relatively short, reactivation can occur partially during phase 3 and usually completely within 10 to 50 milliseconds after return to the diastolic potential, the refractory period shortens with increasing rate, and very rapid conduction can occur.

Patients with lone AF appear to have increased dispersion of atrial refractoriness, which correlates with enhanced inducibility of AF and spontaneous episodes. Some patients have site-specific dispersion of atrial refractoriness and intraatrial conduction delays resulting from nonuniform atrial anisotropy. This appears to be a common property of normal atrial tissue, but there are further conduction delays to and within the posterior triangle of Koch in patients with induced AF, a finding suggesting an important role for the low RA in the genesis of some forms of AF.

ATRIAL FIBROSIS

Atrial fibrosis plays an important role in the pathophysiology of AF. Atrial fibrosis results from various cardiac insults that share common fibroproliferative signaling pathways. Fibrotic myocardium exhibits slow and inhomogeneous conduction, likely secondary to reduced intercellular coupling, discontinuous branching architecture, and zigzagging circuits. When combined with inhomogeneous dispersion of refractoriness within the atria, conduction block provides an ideal substrate for reentry. The greater the slowing of conduction velocity is in scarred myocardium, the shorter the anatomical circuit will need to be to sustain a reentrant wavelet. In fact, reentrant circuits need be only a few millimeters in length in discontinuously conducting tissue. Thus, atrial regions with advanced fibrosis can be local sources for AF. Such a hypothesis would not preclude the remainder of the atria from showing fibrillatory conduction or intact, functional reentrant waves, or both.[10,13]

The normal aging process results in anatomical changes likely to yield inhomogeneous conduction that can potentially create the milieu necessary for the development of reentry. These changes are probably magnified by the presence of certain disease processes, such as hypertension, coronary artery disease, and heart failure. The strong association of sinus node dysfunction and AF (the bradycardia-tachycardia syndrome) also suggests that replacement of atrial myocytes by interstitial fibrosis likely plays an important part in the pathogenesis of AF in older adults, although in some instances the bradycardia component is a functional response to the tachycardia. Furthermore, AF itself seems to produce various alterations of atrial architecture that further contribute to atrial remodeling, mechanical dysfunction, and perpetuation of fibrillation. Longstanding AF results in loss of myofibrils, accumulation of glycogen granules, disruption in cell-to-cell coupling at gap junctions, and organelle aggregates.[10]

Changes in AF characteristics during evolving fibrosis also have a direct impact on why electrical or drug treatment, or both, ultimately fails to achieve conversion to NSR. In the markedly fibrotic and discontinuous atrial tissue, characterized by discontinuous anisotropy, a marked degree of gap junctional uncoupling, and fiber branching, the safety factor for propagation is higher than in normal tissue. As a consequence, blocking of the Na^+ current to the same degree as is necessary for the termination of functional reentry may not terminate reentry caused by slow and fractionated conduction in fibrotic scars of remodeled atria. Conduction in discontinuous tissue is mostly structurally determined and leads to excitable gaps behind the wavefronts. If a gap is of critical size, the effectiveness of drugs that prolong atrial refractoriness will be limited. Furthermore, scar tissue is likely to exhibit multiple entry and exit points and multiple sites at which unidirectional block occurs. This can potentially lead to activity whose appearance in local extracellular electrograms changes from beat to beat, as well as beat-to-beat CL variability. Although such regions can be expected to respond to defibrillation, AF may resume after extrasystoles or normal sinus beats immediately after conversion, with unidirectional block recurring as a result of the presence of scar.

ATRIAL STRETCH

Atrial stretch and dilation can play a role in the development and persistence of AF. Clinically, AF episodes occur more frequently in association with conditions known to cause elevated LA pressure and atrial stretch, such as acutely decompensated systolic or diastolic heart failure. Additionally, the echocardiographic LA volume index and restrictive transmitral Doppler flow patterns are strong predictors of the development of AF.[8,14]

The structure of the dilated atria can potentially have important EP effects related to stretch of the atrial myocardium (so-called electromechanical feedback). Acute atrial stretch reduces the atrial refractory period and action potential duration and depresses atrial conduction velocity, potentially through a reduction of cellular excitability by the opening of stretch-activated channels or changes in cable properties (membrane resistance, capacitance, core resistance), or both. Regional stretch for less than 30 minutes turns on the immediate early gene program, thus initiating hypertrophy and altering action potential duration in affected areas. Moreover, acutely altered stress and strain patterns augment the synthesis of angiotensin II, which induces myocyte hypertrophy. By regionally increasing L-type calcium (Ca^{2+}) current (I_{CaL}) and decreasing the transient outward potassium (K^+) current (I_{to}), angiotensin II can contribute to arrhythmogenic electrical dispersion. Altered stretch of atrial myocytes also results in opening of stretch-activated channels, increasing G protein–coupled pathways. This leads to increased protein kinase A and C activity, and enhanced I_{CaL} through the cell membrane, and increased release of Ca^{2+} from the sarcoplasmic reticulum, thus promoting afterdepolarizations and triggered activity.[10] Furthermore, acute stretch can promote an increase in dispersion of refractoriness and spatial heterogeneity by causing conduction block and potentially contributing to the development of AF.[8,14,15]

INFLAMMATION AND ATRIAL FIBRILLATION

There is increasing evidence that implicates inflammation in the pathogenesis of AF. Clinically, AF occurs frequently in the setting of inflammatory states such as cardiac surgery and acute pericarditis. Additionally, the levels of inflammatory biomarkers (C-reactive protein [CRP] and interleukin-6 [IL-6]) are significantly increased in patients with AF, findings suggesting the presence of systemic inflammation in these patients. Elevation of the levels of CRP and IL-6 has been shown to predict future development, recurrence, and burden of AF.[16-18] There is also evidence suggesting that inflammation is involved in electrical and structural atrial remodeling. Furthermore, inflammation appears to increase the inhomogeneity of atrial conduction directly, potentially via disruption of expression of connexin proteins, leading to impaired intercellular coupling.[16]

It is also likely that inflammation can be a consequence of AF. CRP levels decrease following restoration of sinus rhythm. Rapid atrial activation in AF results in Ca^{+2} overload in atrial myocytes that can potentially result in cell death, which induces a low-grade inflammatory response. The inflammation, in turn, can induce healing and repair that likely enhance remodeling and promote perpetuation of the arrhythmia.[16]

Currently, the exact role of inflammation in AF is poorly defined, and it remains unclear whether inflammation is actually involved in the mechanisms underlying AF or whether it is simply an epiphenomenon. Therapies directed at attenuating the inflammatory burden (e.g., glucocorticoids, statins, and angiotensin II inhibitors) appear promising, although early clinical trials do not support a significant benefit.[19]

Atrial Remodeling in Atrial Fibrillation

It is well known from clinical practice that AF is a progressive arrhythmia. Eventually, in 14% to 24% of patients with paroxysmal AF, persistent AF will develop, even in the absence of progressive underlying heart disease. Furthermore, conversion of AF to NSR, electrically or pharmacologically, becomes more difficult when the arrhythmia has been present for a longer period. In fact, the arrhythmia itself results in a cascade of electrical and structural changes in the atria that are themselves conducive to the perpetuation of the arrhythmia ("AF begets AF"), a process known as remodeling.[20] Recurrent AF can potentially lead to irreversible atrial remodeling and eventually permanent structural changes that account for the progression of paroxysmal to persistent and finally to permanent AF, characterized by the failure of electrical cardioversion or pharmacological therapy, or both, to restore and maintain NSR. Even after cessation of AF, these abnormalities persist for periods that vary in proportion to the duration of the arrhythmia.[17,21]

Changes in atrial EP features that are induced by AF can occur through alterations in ion channel activities that cause partial depolarization and abbreviation of atrial refractoriness. These changes promote the initiation and perpetuation of AF (electrical remodeling) and the modification of cellular Ca^{2+} handling, which causes contractile dysfunction (contractile remodeling), as well as atrial dilation with associated structural changes (structural remodeling). Electrical remodeling can potentially begin within a few hours after the onset of AF, whereas the structural changes are slower, likely starting after several weeks.[17]

Electrical remodeling results from the high rate of electrical activation. The EP changes typical of atrial myocytes during AF are shortening of the atrial refractory period and action potential duration, reduction in the amplitude of the action potential plateau, and loss of response of action potential duration to changes in rate (abnormal restitution). Whereas the normal atrial action potential duration shortens in response to pacing at shorter CLs, AF results in loss of this rate dependence of atrial action potential duration, and the atrial refractory period fails to lengthen appropriately at slow rates (e.g., with return to NSR). These changes can explain the increased duration of AF because, according to the multiple wavelet theory, a short wavelength results in smaller wavelets, which increase the maximum number of wavelets, given a certain atrial mass.[2,20] Tachycardia-induced changes in refractoriness are spatially heterogeneous, and there is increased variability both within and among various atrial regions that may promote atrial vulnerability and AF maintenance and provide a substrate for reentry.

The mechanism for electrical remodeling and shortening of the atrial refractory period is not entirely clear. Several potential explanations exist, including ion channel remodeling, angiotensin II, and atrial ischemia. Shortening of the atrial action potential can be caused by a net decrease of inward ionic currents (Na^+ or Ca^{2+}), a net increase of outward currents (K^+), or a combination of both. The decrease of I_{CaL} seems to be responsible for shortening of the atrial action potential, whereas the decrease of I_{to} is considered to result in loss of physiological rate adaptation of the action potential. The reduction in I_{CaL} can be explained by a decreased expression of the L-type Ca^{2+} channel α_{1C} subunit, likely as a compensatory mechanism to minimize the potential for cytosolic Ca^{2+} overload secondary to increased Ca^{2+} influx during the rapidly repetitive action potentials during AF. Verapamil, an L-type Ca^{2+} channel blocker, was shown to prevent electrical remodeling and hasten complete recovery without affecting inducibility of AF, whereas intracellular Ca^{2+} overload, induced by hypercalcemia or digoxin, enhances electrical remodeling. Electrical remodeling can be attenuated by the sarcoplasmic reticulum's release of the Ca^{2+} antagonist ryanodine, a finding suggesting the importance of increased intracellular Ca^{2+} to the maladaptation of the atrial myocardium during AF. Angiotensin II may also be involved in electrical and atrial myocardial remodeling, and angiotensin II inhibitors may prevent atrial electrical remodeling. Angiotensin-converting enzyme inhibitors reduce the incidence of AF in patients with left ventricular (LV) dysfunction after myocardial infarction and in patients with chronic ischemic cardiomyopathy. Atrial ischemia is another possible contributor to electrical remodeling and shortening of the atrial refractory period via activation of the Na^+-H^+ exchanger.[10,11]

Furthermore, persistent AF can result in other changes within the atria, including gap junctional remodeling, cellular remodeling, and sinus node remodeling. Gap junctional remodeling is manifest as an increase in the expression and distribution of connexin 43 and heterogeneity in the distribution of connexin 40, both of which are intercellular gap junction proteins.[20] Cellular remodeling is caused by the apoptotic death of myocytes with myolysis, which may not be entirely reversible. AF results in marked changes in atrial cellular substructures, including loss of myofibrils, accumulation of glycogen, changes in mitochondrial shape and size, fragmentation of sarcoplasmic reticulum, and dispersion of nuclear chromatin.[20]

Sustained AF has also been associated with structural changes, such as myocyte hypertrophy, myocyte death, impaired atrial contractility, and atrial stretch and dilation, which act to reduce conduction velocity.[20] Atrial dilation increases electrical instability by shortening the effective refractory period and slowing atrial conduction.[10] These structural changes, many of which probably are irreversible, appear to occur more slowly, over periods of weeks to months.

Contractile remodeling is likely caused by downregulation of I_{CaL} (resulting in reduced release of Ca^{2+} during systole), as well as myolysis (loss of sarcomeres). Contractile remodeling can potentially cause thrombus formation and atrial dilation. Contractile remodeling starts early after onset of AF, and its recovery generally takes longer than reversal of electrical remodeling, likely because of the time it takes for the atria to replace lost sarcomeres.

In addition to remodeling of the atria, the sinus node can undergo remodeling, resulting in sinus node dysfunction and bradyarrhythmias caused by reduced sinus node automaticity or prolonged sinoatrial conduction. The phenomenon of sinus node remodeling may contribute to the episodes of bradycardia seen in the tachycardia-bradycardia syndrome and may reduce sinus rhythm stability and increase the stability of AF.[20] As mentioned earlier, elements of the sinus bradycardia appear to be functionally reversible if the tachycardia is prevented.

Studies suggest that the PVs are more susceptible to electrical alterations resulting from AF than the atria. Although the PVs display significantly longer refractory periods at baseline than the atria, they exhibit more prominent shortening of refractoriness after a brief episode of pacing-induced AF. Moreover, the short-term presence of AF does influence PV EP features by slowing the conduction velocity without affecting the conduction times of the atria. Structural changes in the atria after remodeling, such as stretch, can also result in increased PV activity. Atrial stretch can lead to increased intraatrial pressure, causing a rise in the rate and spatiotemporal organization of electrical waves originating in the PVs. These changes imply that electrical and structural remodeling increases the likelihood of ectopic PV automaticity and AF maintenance. Therefore, rather than AF begets AF, one can vary that theme: "PV-induced paroxysmal AF begets PV-induced chronic AF."[22]

Atrial tachycardia (AT)–induced remodeling can potentially underlie various clinically important phenomena, such as the tendency of patients with other forms of supraventricular arrhythmias to develop AF, the tendency of AF to recur early after electrical cardioversion, the resistance of longer duration AF to antiarrhythmic medications, and the tendency of paroxysmal AF to become persistent.[2]

If NSR is restored within a reasonable period of time, EP changes and atrial electrical remodeling appear to normalize gradually, atrial size decreases, and atrial mechanical function is restored. These observations lend support to the idea that the negative downhill spiral in which AF begets AF can be arrested with NSR that perpetuates NSR, and restoration of NSR may forestall progressive remodeling and the increase in duration and frequency of arrhythmic episodes by reverse remodeling.

Role of Autonomic Nervous System in Atrial Fibrillation

Cardiac function is modulated by both the extrinsic and the intrinsic cardiac autonomic nervous systems. The extrinsic (central) system is composed of the vagosympathetic system from the brain and spinal cord to the heart. The intrinsic system is composed of a large network of autonomic cardiac ganglia buried throughout the epicardial fat within the pericardial space. Groups of several cardiac ganglia comprise plexuses that coalesce in specific locations, and different groups of ganglia have different sites of innervation throughout the heart. Atrial ganglia contain afferent neurons from the atrial myocardium and from the central autonomic nervous system, and efferent cholinergic and adrenergic neurons, with heavy innervation of the PV myocardium and the atrial myocardium surrounding the ganglionic plexuses. Additionally, an extensive array of interconnecting neurons creates a communication network among the different ganglionic plexuses, as well as between the ganglionic plexuses and the atrium and PV myocardium. The intrinsic system receives input from the extrinsic system but acts independently to modulate numerous cardiac functions, including automaticity, contractility, and conduction.[23,24]

Several studies have suggested that both divisions of the autonomic nervous system are involved in the initiation, maintenance, and termination of AF, with a predominant role of the parasympathetic system. Electrical stimulation of autonomic nerves on the heart itself can facilitate the induction of AF. Increased vagal tone is frequently involved in the onset of AF in patients with structurally normal hearts. Parasympathetic stimulation shortens the atrial refractory period, increases the dispersion of refractoriness, and decreases the wavelength of reentrant circuits that facilitate initiation and perpetuation of AF. Long-term vagal denervation of the atria renders AF less easily inducible in animal experiments, presumably because of increased EP homogeneity. On the other hand, vagal stimulation results in maintenance of AF, and catheter ablation of the parasympathetic autonomic nerves entering the RA from the SVC prevents vagally induced AF in animal models. Sympathetic stimuli also shorten the atrial refractory period and increase the vulnerability to AF.[23,25]

Spatial heterogeneity of refractoriness can also be produced by the heterogeneity of autonomic innervation. It has been well established that vagal innervation of the atria is heterogeneous and vagal stimulation can precipitate AF as a result of heterogeneity of atrial refractoriness. Heterogeneity of sympathetic neural inputs also plays a role in AF. In animal models, sympathetic atrial denervation facilitates sustained AF, and AF induced by rapid RA pacing is associated with nerve sprouting and a heterogeneous increase in sympathetic innervation. Enhanced sympathetic activity can promote automaticity, delayed afterdepolarization–related AT, and focal AF. Sympathetic stimulation also shortens atrial refractoriness and may facilitate the induction of AF in patients with structural heart disease, in whom possible heterogeneous sympathetic denervation leads to increased refractoriness heterogeneity.

Experimental evidence suggests that the electrical properties of the PVs are also modulated by changes in autonomic tone.[6] Anatomical studies revealed that the LA and PVs are innervated by adrenergic and cholinergic nerve fibers. A collection of ganglia is localized on the posterior wall of the LA between the superior PVs. Subsequent studies found that ganglionated plexuses clustered at the PV entrances (within fat pads) could be stimulated without atrial excitation. For patients with PV foci, a primary increase in adrenergic tone followed by a marked vagal predominance was reported just prior to the onset of paroxysmal AF. A similar pattern of autonomic tone was reported in an unselected group of patients with paroxysmal AF and various cardiac conditions.[25] Activation of the ganglionic plexuses at the PV-LA junction can potentially result in conversion of PV ectopy to AF. Furthermore, ablation of the ganglionated plexuses located at the atrial entrances or antra of the PVs can potentially abolish or reduce AF inducibility.

Role of the Pulmonary Veins in Atrial Fibrillation

There is little controversy now that the PVs play a major role in triggering and maintaining AF, as established by animal and human models, especially in the setting of paroxysmal AF. First, fibrillatory

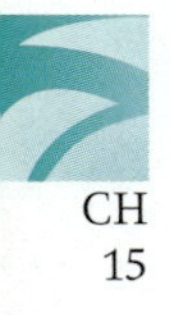

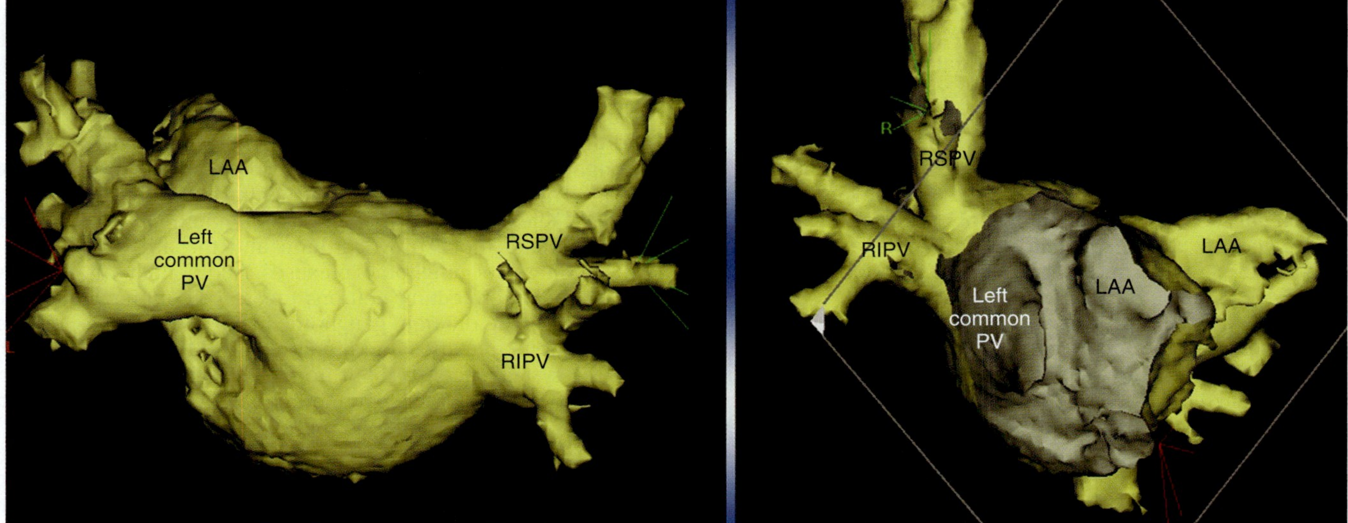

FIGURE 15-3 Cardiac CT angiogram (posteroanterior and cardioscopic views) showing a common ostium for the left pulmonary veins (PVs). LAA = LA appendage; RIPV = right inferior pulmonary vein; RSPV = right superior pulmonary vein.

conduction is likely initiated by rapid discharges from one or several focal sources within the atria; in most patients with AF (94%), the focus is in one of the PVs (Fig. 15-1). Extra-PV sites can also trigger AF, but this occurs in a few cases, likely no more than 6% to 10% of patients. AF is also perpetuated by microreentrant circuits, or rotors, that exhibit high-frequency periodic activity from which spiral wavefronts of activation radiate into surrounding atrial tissue. Conduction becomes slower and less organized with increasing distance from the rotors, likely because of atrial structural remodeling, resulting in fibrillatory conduction. Interestingly, the dominant rotors in AF are localized primarily in the junction between the LA and PVs. One study also demonstrated that the PV-LA region has heterogeneous EP properties capable of sustaining reentry (microreentry or macroreentry). Finally, vagal inputs may be important in triggering and maintaining AF, and many of these inputs are clustered close to the PV-LA junction. Thus, the PVs play a critical role in triggering and maintaining AF.

The role of PVs in the initiation and perpetuation of persistent AF seems less prominent than in the setting of paroxysmal AF, likely secondary to the electrical and structural remodeling associated with persistent AF. Non-PV triggers occur more commonly, and the reentry sites required for AF perpetuation are more often found outside the PV-LA junction in persistent AF than in paroxysmal AF.

PULMONARY VEIN ANATOMY

PVs can have variable anatomy. Most hearts examined are found to have four PVs with discrete ostia, but the remainder (approximately 25%) has a common ostium, either on the left or on the right (Fig. 15-3).[4] The PV ostia are ellipsoid with a longer superoinferior dimension, and funnel-shaped ostia are frequently noted in patients with AF. The right superior PV is located close to the SVC or RA, and the right inferior PV projects horizontally. The left superior PV is close to the vicinity of the LA appendage, and the left inferior PV courses near the descending aorta. PVs are larger in patients with AF than in normal subjects, in men than in women, and in persistent versus paroxysmal AF. Significant variability of PV morphologies exists, however, including supernumerary right PVs (in 8% to 29% of patients; Fig. 15-4), multiple ramification and early branching (especially of the right inferior PV), and common ostium of left-sided or, less frequently, right-sided PVs.

The PVs are covered by myocardial sleeves formed by one or more layers of myocardial fibers oriented in a circular, longitudinal, oblique, or spiral direction. These sleeves, continuing from the LA into the PV, vary from 2 to 25 mm in length, with a mean extent of 13 mm. The length of the myocardial sleeves usually has a distinctive distribution; superior PVs have longer and better developed myocardial sleeves than inferior PVs, which may explain why arrhythmogenic foci are found more often in the superior PVs than in the inferior PVs.[4,5] It should be noted that all PVs in all individuals have such myocardial sleeves, regardless of the presence or absence of AF.

The walls of the PVs are composed of a thin endothelium, a media of smooth muscle, and a thick outer fibrous adventitia. The transition from atrial to venous walls is gradual because the myocardial sleeves from the LA overlap with the smooth muscle of the venous wall. The myocardial sleeves are thickest at the venoatrial junction (mean, 1.1 mm) and then gradually taper distally. Furthermore, the thickness of the sleeves is not uniform, with the inferior walls of the superior veins and the superior walls of the inferior veins having the thicker sleeves. Throughout the PV, and even at the venoatrial junction, there are gaps in the myocardial sleeves mainly composed of fibrous tissue. The arrangement of the myocyte bundles within the sleeves is rather complex. There appears to be a mesh-like arrangement of muscle fascicles made up of circularly oriented bundles (spiraling around the long axis of the vein) that interconnect with bundles that run in a longitudinal orientation (along the long axis of the vein). Such an arrangement, together with the patchy areas of fibrosis seen, may be relevant to the role of the PVs in the initiation of AF.[4]

ELECTROPHYSIOLOGY OF PULMONARY VEIN MUSCULATURE

As noted, the PVs play a crucial role in the initiation and maintenance of AF. However, it is not clear what makes this region so susceptible to the arrhythmia.[4,6] There are, at present, limited data available on the ionic mechanisms that may underlie the arrhythmogenicity of PVs. Detailed mapping studies have suggested that reentry within the PVs is most likely responsible for their arrhythmogenicity, although focal or triggered activity cannot be excluded.

The EP features of the PV, with its distinct area of slow conduction, decremental conduction, nonuniform anisotropy, and heterogeneous repolarization, are potential substrates for reentry. The heterogeneous fiber orientation in the transition from the LA to the PV sleeve results in unique conduction properties in this area.[4,6] It is possible that the complex arrangement of muscle fibers within the myocardial sleeves and the uneven distribution of interspersed connective and adipose tissue account for the greater degree of decremental conduction observed in the myocardial sleeves than in the LA and for the heterogeneity in conduction properties and

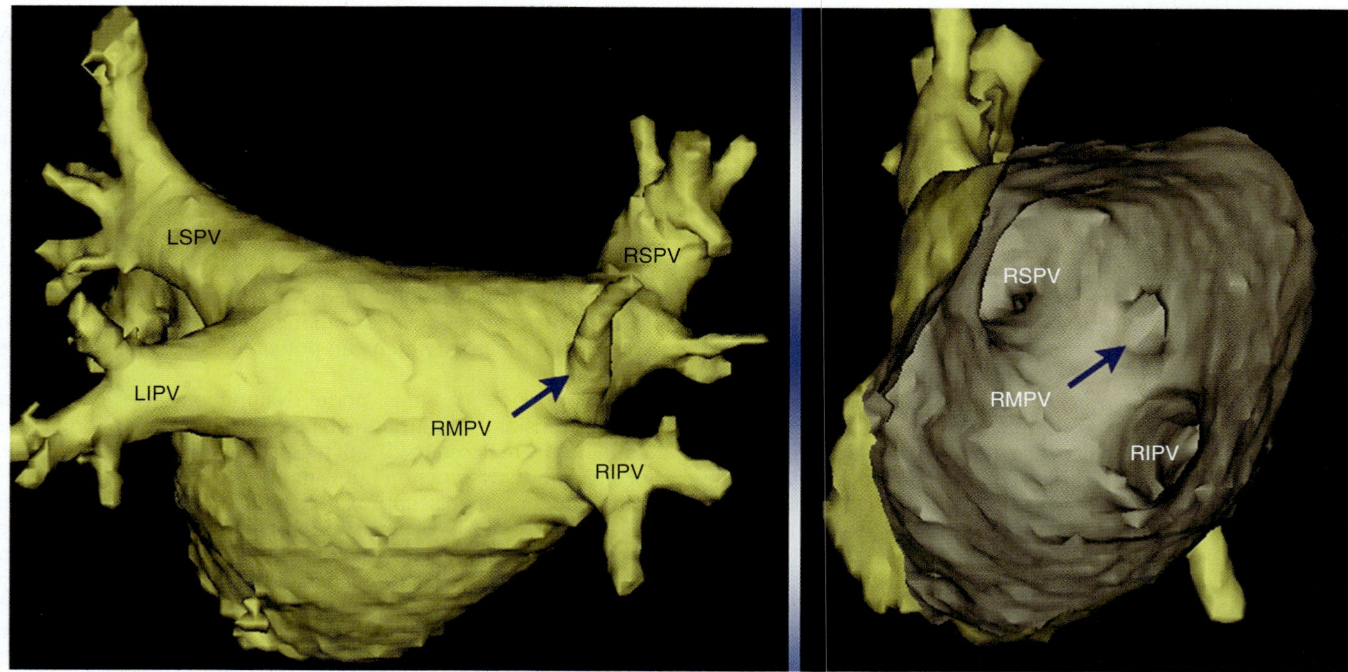

FIGURE 15-4 Cardiac CT angiogram (posteroanterior and cardioscopic views) showing the right middle pulmonary vein (RMPV). LIPV = left inferior pulmonary vein; LSPV = left superior pulmonary vein; RIPV = right inferior pulmonary vein; RSPV = right superior pulmonary vein.

refractory periods among the fascicles in the myocardial sleeves. Therefore, the fractionation of PV potentials commonly observed during premature stimulation (which usually indicates local slowing of conduction) is consistent with anisotropic properties that can be attributable to the complex arrangement of muscle fascicles within the myocardial sleeves.[5]

Several studies suggested that abnormal automaticity or triggered activity, either alone or in combination with the reentrant mechanisms described previously, can play a role in the initiation of AF. These studies suggested that the propensity of PVs to exhibit focal or triggered activity is enhanced by pathological conditions.[4] Further work also implicated the posterior LA in the genesis of AF. Studies suggested that the PVs, together with the posterior LA, have an important role in the persistent form of AF. However, the nature of the relationship between this arrhythmogenic region and the pathological conditions that provide a substrate for AF has not been elucidated. Whether the critical region is the posterior LA, the PVs, or both, has been the source of ongoing debate.[6]

PULMONARY VEIN TACHYCARDIA VERSUS PULMONARY VEIN FIBRILLATION

In patients with paroxysmal AF originating from the PVs, a wide spectrum of atrial arrhythmias can coexist. Extensive monitoring frequently documents coexisting paroxysms of AT and AF. Furthermore, patients with paroxysmal AF usually have multiple PV foci in multiple veins, and many of these foci originate distally in those veins.

In patients whose only clinical arrhythmia is PV AT, the clinical course is more comparable to that in patients with AT from other anatomical locations than to patients with PV AF. Those patients demonstrate a largely focal process, without evidence of a more progressive and diffuse process as observed in the population with paroxysmal AF, and they have no tendency to develop further atrial arrhythmias during long-term follow-up. Notably, when patients with PV AT present with recurrence, in almost all cases this is from the original focus. In contrast, patients with paroxysmal AF have recurrences from foci in other PVs and from within the body of the LA. Importantly, in most patients with PV AT, the focus is located at the ostium of the vein (or within 1 cm of the designated ostium), rather than from further distally (2 to 4 cm). These observations suggest that patients with focal PV AT may represent a different population from those with PV AF. PV AT patients have a discrete and focally curable process, in contrast to the more diffuse process involving multiple PVs and the LA seen in AF.

The spontaneous onset of focal AT from the PVs and its lack of inducibility with programmed stimulation suggest that this arrhythmia is more likely to be caused by abnormal automaticity or triggered activity rather than reentry. However, attempts to classify the arrhythmia mechanism of focal AT definitively in the EP laboratory are limited because of the significant overlap in the arrhythmia characteristics (initiation, response to drugs).

Clinical Considerations

Epidemiology

AF is the most common sustained arrhythmia encountered in clinical practice. It accounts for approximately one-third of hospitalizations for cardiac rhythm disturbance. AF affects 1% to 2% of the general population, and it has been estimated that 2.3 million people in the United States and 4.5 million in the European Union have paroxysmal or persistent AF. However, the true prevalence of AF is probably higher given the common occurrence of asymptomatic (silent) AF.[26]

The prevalence of AF increases with age. AF is uncommon in childhood except after cardiac surgery. It occurs in less than 1% of individuals younger than 60 years, but in approximately 6% of those older than 65 years, and in more than 10% of those older than 80 years. The median age of patients with AF is approximately 75 years, and approximately 75% of patients with AF are 65 years of age or older.

The lifetime risk of the development of AF at age 40 years has been estimated to be approximately 25%. The age-adjusted prevalence is higher in men. Blacks have less than half the age-adjusted risk of developing AF than whites.[27] Given the increasing prevalence of AF with age, coupled with our aging population, the number of affected U.S. residents is expected to increase to nearly 16 million by 2050.

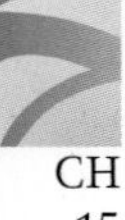

AF is a progressive disease. Approximately half of individuals who experience an initial episode of AF will eventually develop recurrent AF, typically within the first 2 years of follow-up. AF progresses from paroxysmal to persistent despite antiarrhythmic therapy in approximately 10% at 1 year, in 25% to 30% at 5 years, and in more than 50% beyond 10 years. Furthermore, progression from paroxysmal and persistent AF to permanent AF occurs in up to 34% of patients at 4 years after initial diagnosis. Maintenance of sinus rhythm is progressively more difficult as the duration of persistent AF increases. Only 40% to 60% of patients with persistent AF of less than 1 year's duration remain in sinus rhythm 1 year after initiation of antiarrhythmic drug therapy, despite multiple cardioversions, whereas patients with persistent AF of more than 3 year's duration have only a 15% likelihood of long-term sinus rhythm. Increased age, diabetes, and heart failure are among potential predictors of progression to permanent AF. Lone AF is less likely to progress.[28]

AF is associated with an increased long-term risk of stroke, heart failure, hospitalization, and all-cause mortality, especially in women, even after controlling for $CHADS_2$ score and other covariables. The mortality rate of patients with AF is approximately double that of patients in NSR and is linked to the severity of underlying heart disease.[27,29]

Clinical Risk Factors Predisposing to Atrial Fibrillation

As noted, AF can be related to a transient reversible cause, such as thyrotoxicosis, acute myocardial infarction, acute pericarditis, recent cardiac surgery, acute pulmonary disease, alcohol intake, or electrocution. In these cases, AF is generally eliminated by treatment of the underlying precipitating condition.

AF is thought to be secondary to underlying structural heart disease in more than 70% of patients and is the final arrhythmic expression of a diverse family of diseases. AF derives from a complex continuum of predisposing factors that appear to involve disease processes that contribute to the triggering of AF (e.g., sympathetic and parasympathetic nervous systems [neurogenic AF], predisposing arrhythmias, ectopic foci in PVs), increase atrial distention (e.g., valvular heart disease, hypertension, and heart failure), decrease the ratio of atrial myocyte to fibrotic tissue, possibly including an increased rate of apoptotic cell death (e.g., hypertension and ischemic heart disease), disrupt transmyocyte communications (e.g., pericarditis and edema), increase inflammatory mediators (e.g., pericarditis and myocarditis), or alter energy and redox states that modulate the function of ion channels and gap junctions.

The most frequent causes of acute AF are myocardial infarction (5% to 10% of patients with infarct) and cardiothoracic surgery (up to 50% of patients). The most common clinical settings for permanent AF are hypertension and ischemic heart disease, with the subset of patients having congestive heart failure most likely to experience the arrhythmia. In the developing world, hypertension and rheumatic valvular (usually mitral) and congenital heart diseases are the most commonly related conditions.[30]

Heart failure is present in 34% of patients with AF, and AF develops in up to 42% of patients with heart failure. AF and heart failure have a grim prognosis, with a 1-year mortality of 9.5% and worsening of heart failure in almost 25%.[31] In patients with heart failure who are undergoing defibrillator implantation, a history of AF at time of procedure identifies additional risk of heart failure and death, and the new detection of AF afterward is associated with even higher rates of death.[32]

There is accumulating evidence demonstrating an independent association between sleep apnea and AF, likely related to the effects of sleep apnea and nocturnal hypoxemia on LA electrical remodeling, fibrosis, and chamber enlargement. AF occurs in 5% of persons with severe sleep apnea and only 1% of those without sleep apnea. The prevalence of at least moderate sleep apnea was reported in up to 32% of patients with lone AF. Furthermore, cross-sectional studies demonstrated that patients with AF had a significantly higher risk of obstructive sleep apnea than matched controls (49% versus 33%), and multivariate analysis demonstrated a strong independent association between sleep apnea and AF (odds ratio, 2.2). Additionally, several prospective studies showed that obstructive sleep apnea predicts the occurrence of future AF. Untreated obstructive sleep apnea was associated with a remarkably high rate of AF recurrence at 1 year compared with patients with unknown sleep apnea status (83% versus 53%). The presence of sleep apnea can also predict a higher rate of early recurrence of PV conduction and AF following catheter ablation of AF.[33] Several investigations identified obesity (found in approximately 25% of patients with AF) as a risk factor for the development of AF, and there exists a linear association between the body mass index and AF risk. Obesity is associated with increased LA size and impaired LV diastolic function, which can potentially explain its predisposition to AF.[34]

The presence of sinus node dysfunction also predicts an increased risk for AF. Atrial high-rate episodes lasting longer than 5 minutes were noted in 29% of the patients receiving pacemakers for sinus node dysfunction but with no prior history of AF.

In younger patients, approximately 30% to 45% of paroxysmal cases and 20% to 25% of persistent cases of AF occur in the absence of any chronic or acute risk factors for the arrhythmia, a condition referred to as lone AF. Adrenergic and vagotonic forms of paroxysmal AF are uncommon. Nonetheless, patients with lone AF often have attacks against the background of parasympathetic predominance, whereas paroxysms in patients with structural heart disease more usually occur in a sympathetic setting.

Clinical Presentation

AF can be symptomatic or asymptomatic, even in the same patient. Asymptomatic, or silent, AF occurs frequently. In patients with paroxysmal AF; up to 90% of episodes can be unrecognized by the patient, including some lasting more than 48 hours. On the other hand, continuous monitoring with a pacemaker with dedicated functions for AF detection and electrogram storage showed that as many as 40% of patients experienced AF-like symptoms in the absence of AF, whereas 38% of patients with a history of AF had episodes of AF lasting more than 48 hours noted at the time of interrogation even though these patients were asymptomatic. In more than 10% to 25% of patients, however, AF is discovered in the absence of symptoms or after a complication attributable to AF.

Symptoms associated with AF vary, depending on the ventricular rate, the underlying functional status, the duration of AF, the presence and degree of structural heart disease, and the individual patient's perception. The hemodynamic consequences of AF are related to loss of coordinated atrial contraction, irregularity of ventricular response, and fast heart rate, as well as long-term consequences such as atrial and ventricular cardiomyopathy. Loss of effective atrial contraction can potentially reduce cardiac output by 15% to 20%. These consequences are magnified in the presence of impaired diastolic ventricular filling, hypertension, mitral stenosis, LV hypertrophy, and restrictive cardiomyopathy. Irregularity of the cardiac cycle, especially when accompanied by short coupling intervals, and rapid heart rates in AF can lead to reduction in diastolic filling, stroke volume, and cardiac output.[27]

Most patients with AF complain of palpitations, chest discomfort, dyspnea, generalized fatigue, or dizziness. Although palpitation, or awareness of the irregularity of the heartbeat, is prominent in more than half of patients with AF, its correlation with documented arrhythmia is unimpressive.[35] Furthermore, AF with a chronically rapid heart rate (more than 120 to 130 beats/min) can lead to tachycardia-mediated cardiomyopathy and heart failure. Syncope is an uncommon complication of AF that can occur on conversion in patients with sinus node dysfunction or because of rapid ventricular rates in patients with hypertrophic cardiomyopathy, in patients with valvular aortic stenosis, or in patients with ventricular preexcitation over an accessory pathway. The first presentation of asymptomatic AF can be catastrophic—an embolic complication or acute decompensation of heart failure.[27,35]

In some patients, paroxysmal AF can be classified as either *vagal* or *adrenergic*, depending on the types of triggers and the temporal distribution of the arrhythmic episodes. Vagal AF typically occurs in young male patients without structural heart disease and characteristically develops during sleep or postprandial. In contrast, patients with adrenergic AF are usually older, often with evidence of underlying heart disease, and the episodes of AF usually occur during the day and are associated with physical or emotional stress. In patients with paroxysmal AF, the prevalence of vagal AF probably ranges between 6% and 25%, whereas that of adrenergic AF ranges between 7% and 16%. Approximately 12% of patients with paroxysmal AF exhibit features of mixed vagal and adrenergic patterns.[25]

Many patients with persistent or permanent AF have one or more comorbid conditions that can considerably contribute to specific complaints and to overall quality of life. Therefore, it is important to establish a correlation between any symptoms and AF, as well as ventricular response rates. The effect of regulation of ventricular rate during persistent AF or conversion to NSR on a patient's symptoms and quality of life can help assess the relative contribution of AF to the patient's complaints. The Canadian Cardiovascular Society Severity in Atrial Fibrillation (CCS-SAF) scale is a simple, five-point semiquantitative scale (Table 15-1) that has been proposed for use at the bedside to assess the functional consequences of symptoms during AF and can provide objective assessment of the patient's subjective state (analogous to the New York Heart Association [NYHA] congestive heart failure functional class and the CCS angina severity class).[35]

Risk of Thromboembolism

AF is a major risk factor for thromboembolism, causing approximately 15% of the ischemic strokes in the United States and up to 25% of those in patients older than 80 years. In the Framingham Heart Study, patients with rheumatic heart disease and AF had a 17-fold increased risk of stroke compared with age-matched controls, and the attributable risk was 5 times greater than in those with nonrheumatic AF. For nonvalvular AF, the risk of stroke is estimated to be 2 to 7 times that of subjects without arrhythmia, thus resulting in an average incidence of stroke of 5% per year. This rate may increase to 7% per year when silent cerebral ischemic events and transient ischemic attacks are taken into account.[27] Patients with paroxysmal and persistent AF appear to have a stroke risk similar to that in patients with permanent AF.

Although patients with AF in the setting of rheumatic valvular disease are accepted to be at high risk of stroke, stroke risk in nonvalvular AF is not homogeneous across the various subgroups of patients. The risk ranges from less than 1.5% per year in patients with lone AF who are less than 59 years old to more than 10% per year in older patients, especially when AF is associated with specific conditions or comorbidities. Prior history of stroke, transient ischemic attack, or thromboembolism, age, gender, hypertension, diabetes, coronary artery disease, peripheral artery disease, cardiomyopathy, and heart failure are important risk factors. Also, smoking was identified on multivariate analysis in one study as a significant predictor of thromboembolism.[36-38] The presence of moderate to severe LV systolic dysfunction on transthoracic echocardiography is the only independent echocardiographic risk factor for stroke on multivariable analysis. On transesophageal echocardiography (TEE), the presence of an LA thrombus (relative risk, 2.5), complex aortic plaques (relative risk, 2.1), spontaneous echo contrast (relative risk, 3.7), and low LA appendage velocities (up to 20 cm/sec; relative risk, 1.7) are independent predictors of stroke and thromboembolism.[36] Limited data suggest that large LA appendage dimensions on magnetic resonance imaging (MRI) may predict a higher risk of thromboembolism.[39]

Several prominent risk stratification schemes have been developed to help distinguish those patients with AF who are at high risk of ischemic stroke and other systemic thromboembolism from those with a risk sufficiently low that anticoagulation may not be beneficial when considering the associated bleeding risks. Two schemes were developed from multivariable analyses of pooled data from randomized trial participants: the Atrial Fibrillation Investigators (AFI) and the Stroke Prevention in Atrial Fibrillation (SPAF) risk schemes. The $CHADS_2$ index, named for a combination of clinical risk factors (Congestive heart failure, Hypertension, Age 75 years or more, Diabetes mellitus, and prior Stroke or transient ischemic attack), was subsequently developed using data from the AFI and SPAF studies and was validated in a retrospective cohort of hospitalized patients with AF. The $CHADS_2$ score assigns two points to a history of prior cerebral ischemia and one point for the presence of congestive heart failure, hypertension, age 75 years or more, or diabetes mellitus. The $CHADS_2$ score has been associated with higher rates of thromboembolic stroke in a linear fashion for patients, both those taking anticoagulants and those not receiving anticoagulation. The stroke rate per 100 patient-years without antithrombotic therapy increases by a factor of approximately 1.5 for each one-point increase in the $CHADS_2$ score: from 1.9% for a score of 0 to 18.2% for a score of 6.[40]

TABLE 15-1 Canadian Cardiovascular Society Severity of Atrial Fibrillation Scale

Step 1: *Symptoms*	
Identify the presence of the following symptoms: • Palpitation • Dyspnea • Dizziness, presyncope, or syncope • Chest pain • Weakness or fatigue	
Step 2: *Association*	
Is AF, when present, associated with the foregoing symptoms? For example: Ascertain whether any of the foregoing symptoms are present during AF and are likely caused by AF (as opposed to some other cause).	
Step 3: *Functionality*	
Determine whether the symptoms associated with AF (or the treatment of AF) affect the patient's functionality (subjective QOL).	
CCS-SAF Class Definitions	
Class 0	Asymptomatic with respect to AF
Class 1	Symptoms attributable to AF have *minimal* effect on patient's general QOL • Minimal and/or infrequent symptoms, or • Single episode of AF without syncope or heart failure
Class 2	Symptoms attributable to AF have *minor* effect on patient's general QOL • Mild awareness of symptoms in patients with persistent or permanent AF, or • Rare episodes (e.g., less than a few per year) in patients with paroxysmal or intermittent AF
Class 3	Symptoms attributable to AF have a moderate effect on patient's general QOL • Moderate awareness of symptoms on most days in patient with persistent or permanent AF, or • More common episodes (e.g., more than every few months) or more severe symptoms, or both, in patients with paroxysmal or intermittent AF
Class 4	Symptoms attributable to AF have a severe effect on patient's general QOL • Very unpleasant symptoms in patients with persistent or paroxysmal AF and/or • Frequent and highly symptomatic episodes in patients with paroxysmal or intermittent AF, and/or • Syncope thought to result from AF, and/or • Congestive heart failure secondary to AF

AF = atrial fibrillation; CCS = Canadian Cardiovascular Society; QOL = quality of life; SAF = severity of atrial fibrillation.

From Dorian P, Guerra PG, Kerr CR, et al: Validation of a new simple scale to measure symptoms in atrial fibrillation: the Canadian Cardiovascular Society Severity in Atrial Fibrillation (CCS-SAF) scale, *Circ Arrhythm Electrophysiol* 2:268-275, 2009.

The $CHADS_2$ score was compared with four other risk stratification schemes to predict thromboembolism in persons with nonvalvular AF. No risk scheme was superior, and all of them had relatively poor ability to predict thromboembolism. Nonetheless, the $CHADS_2$ scheme remains the most widely used because of its simplicity and ease, and it is useful for assessment of when a patient has sufficiently high risk ($CHADS_2$ score of 2 or higher) to warrant anticoagulation. However, the $CHADS_2$ scheme does not incorporate other stroke risk factors and can lead to inadequate discrimination of risk. In fact, many patients (more than 60%) are classified as having intermediate risk, for whom the ideal thromboprophylaxis strategy is uncertain.[40]

A newer scheme (the CHA_2DS_2-VASc score or Birmingham 2009 schema) incorporates additional risk factors, including vascular disease, female gender, and age 65 to 74 years (Table 15-2). This scheme showed a modest improvement of thromboembolic risk stratification over the $CHADS_2$ score and classified a much smaller proportion of patients (15.1%) into the intermediate risk category than the original $CHADS_2$ score (61.9%), hence allowing less uncertainty regarding treatment decisions. Also, those in the low-risk category in the CHA_2DS_2-VASc system were truly at low risk, with a 0% rate of thromboembolic events at 1 year, in contrast to the subjects classified as low risk using the $CHADS_2$ schema (i.e., a score of 0) who still had an annual event rate of 1.4%.[38]

The CHA_2DS_2-VASc score was validated in a cohort of more than 1000 patients with nonvalvular AF followed during 1 year without anticoagulation, as well as in a large anticoagulated clinical trial cohort (Table 15-3).[37,38] The risk of thromboembolism for patients with a CHA_2DS_2-VASc score of 1 who were not receiving anticoagulation was 0.6% in the first year, but in those with a score of 0, no thromboembolic events were observed. Nonetheless, it is important to recognize that all the available clinical prediction tools have only modest predictive ability.[36]

In patients with AF who are undergoing implantation of a dual-chamber pacemaker, risk stratification for thromboembolic events can be improved by combining the $CHADS_2$ score with data on the presence and duration of AF episodes detected by the pacemaker. Patients with a $CHADS_2$ score of 2 or less who have no or only very short (less than 5 minutes' duration) episodes of AF, those with a $CHADS_2$ score of 1 or less who have AF episodes lasting between 5 minutes and 24 hours, and those with a $CHADS_2$ score of 0 regardless of the duration of AF episodes all appear to exhibit a low risk of stroke (0.8% per year).[41]

Importantly, the assessment of stroke risk is independent of the type of AF (i.e., paroxysmal, persistent or permanent). Although current guidelines consider patients with paroxysmal AF as having a stroke risk similar to those with persistent or permanent AF, in the presence of risk factors, the threshold burden of paroxysmal AF required to justify chronic anticoagulant therapy has not been clearly defined. In patients with AF who have implanted pacemakers or defibrillators, the risk for thromboembolism appears to be quantitatively linked to AF burden as quantified by the implanted devices. An AF burden for more than 5.5 hours on any day in the most recent 30 days seems to confer a doubling of the risk of thromboembolism compared with an AF burden of less than 5.5 hours, even after adjusting for baseline stroke risk factors and antithrombotic therapy. Further research is necessary to identify precisely the amount of AF burden associated with a significantly increased risk of stroke.[36,42]

It is still unclear how to assess the risk of thromboembolism and guide antithrombotic therapy in patients with implanted pacemakers or defibrillators (but no prior clinical history of AF) in whom atrial high-rate episodes consistent with AT or AF have been detected by the implanted devices. Limited data suggest that any strategy of anticoagulation therapy should take into consideration not only the duration of the atrial arrhythmias but also the individual's risk factor profile according to the previously mentioned risk stratification schemes.[26] Importantly, episodes detected by the device and designated as indicative of AF must be validated because some detection algorithms are overly sensitive and diagnose AF episodes when apparent rapid atrial recordings are, in fact, caused by atrial noncapture during NSR, erroneous counting of far-field R waves, or other phenomena.

Initial Evaluation

The initial evaluation of a patient with suspected or documented AF includes characterizing the pattern of the arrhythmia (e.g., paroxysmal or persistent), determining underlying causes (e.g., heart failure, pulmonary problems, hypertension, or hyperthyroidism), defining associated cardiac and extracardiac conditions, and identifying potential complications of AF. Additionally, a thorough history should be obtained to estimate of the risk of stroke (using the $CHADS_2$ or CHA_2DS_2-VASc schemes) and quantify AF-related

TABLE 15-2 2009 Birmingham (CHA_2DS_2-VASc) Scoring System for Predicting Stroke and Thromboembolism in Atrial Fibrillation

RISK FACTOR	SCORE
Congestive heart failure or left ventricular dysfunction	1
*H*ypertension	1
*A*ge ≥75 yr	2
*D*iabetes mellitus	1
*S*troke, transient ischemic attack, or thromboembolism	2
*V*ascular disease (prior myocardial infarction, peripheral artery disease, or aortic plaque)	1
*A*ge 65-74 yr	1
*S*ex *c*ategory (i.e., female gender)	1

CHA_2DS_2-VASc = updated version of the $CHADS_2$ (*c*ongestive heart failure, *h*ypertension, *a*ge, *d*iabetes, and *s*troke [doubled]) system, with additional risk factors.

From Lip GY, Nieuwlaat R, Pisters R, et al: Refining clinical risk stratification for predicting stroke and thromboembolism in atrial fibrillation using a novel risk factor-based approach, *Chest* 137:263-272, 2010.

TABLE 15-3 Stroke or Other Thromboembolism Events Based on the CHA_2DS_2-VASc Scoring System

	Cohort of Patients on Anticoagulation		*Cohort of Patients off Anticoagulation*	
CHA_2DS_2-VASc SCORE	PATIENTS (*N* = 7239)	ADJUSTED STROKE RATE* (% PER YR)	PATIENTS (*N* = 1084)	ADJUSTED STROKE RATE† (% PER YR)
0	1	0	103	0
1	422	1.3	162	0.7
2	1230	2.2	184	1.9
3	1730	3.2	203	4.7
4	1718	4.0	208	2.3
5	1159	6.7	95	3.9
6	679	9.8	57	4.5
7	294	9.6	25	10.1
8	82	6.7	9	14.2
9	14	15.2	1	100

*Theoretical thromboembolism rates without anticoagulation therapy: assuming that warfarin provides a 64% reduction in thromboembolic risk. Data from Lip GY, Frison L, Halperin JL, Lane DA: Identifying patients at risk of stroke despite anticoagulation, *Stroke* 41: 2731-2738, 2010.

†Theoretical thromboembolism rates without antiplatelet therapy: assuming that aspirin provides a 22% reduction in thromboembolic risk. Data from Lip GY, Nieuwlaat R, Pisters R, et al: Refining clinical risk stratification for predicting stroke and thromboembolism in atrial fibrillation using a novel risk factor-based approach, *Chest* 137:263-272, 2010.

CHA_2DS_2-VASc = updated version of the $CHADS_2$ (*c*ongestive heart failure, *h*ypertension, *a*ge, *d*iabetes, and *s*troke [doubled]) system, with additional risk factors.

symptoms (e.g., CCS-SAF score). A careful history results in a well-planned focused work-up that serves as an effective guide to therapy.

The physical examination can suggest AF on the basis of irregular pulse, irregular jugular venous pulsations, and variation in the intensity of the first heart sound. Examination can also disclose associated valvular heart disease, myocardial abnormalities, or heart failure.

Exercise testing is often used to assess the adequacy of rate control with exercise in permanent AF, to reproduce exercise-induced AF, and to evaluate for associated ischemic heart disease. Although ischemic heart disease is not a common cause of AF, identifying underlying coronary artery disease is particularly important if the use of a class IC antiarrhythmic drug is being considered. Ambulatory cardiac monitoring can also be required for documentation of AF, its relation to symptoms, and evaluation of the adequacy of heart rate control.[27]

Assessment for hyperthyroidism is indicated for all patients with a first episode of AF, when the ventricular response to AF is difficult to control, or when AF recurs unexpectedly after cardioversion. Serum should be obtained for measurement of thyroid-stimulating hormone (TSH) and free thyroxine (T4), even if there are no symptoms suggestive of hyperthyroidism, because the risk of AF is increased up to threefold in patients with subclinical hyperthyroidism.

Rarely, EP testing can be required, especially in patients with wide QRS complex tachycardia or a possible predisposing arrhythmia, such as AFL or paroxysmal SVT. Hints to the presence of paroxysmal SVT include a history of episodes of regular rapid palpitations dating from teenage or early adult years (unusual for AF to occur de novo in this age group) and termination of episodes of palpitations with vagal maneuvers or adenosine (which should not occur with AF).

Principles of Management

Management of AF should be aimed at identifying and treating underlying causes of the arrhythmia, as well as reducing symptoms, improving quality of life, and preventing cardiovascular morbidity and mortality associated with AF. There are two main issues that must be addressed in the treatment of AF: (1) prevention of systemic embolization, and (2) control of symptoms related to AF, typically involving rate or rhythm control. The choice of therapy is influenced by patient preference, associated structural heart disease, severity of symptoms, and whether the AF is recurrent paroxysmal, recurrent persistent, or permanent. In addition, patient education is critical, given the potential morbidity associated with AF and its treatment. For control of symptoms, a safety-driven approach is of paramount importance because most treatments (drug, surgery, ablation) have the capacity to produce significant morbidity and even mortality.[27]

PREVENTION OF SYSTEMIC EMBOLIZATION

As noted, AF significantly increases the risk of stroke, and the stroke risk appears to be equivalent in paroxysmal and persistent AF and equivalent with a rate control or rhythm control management strategy.

ANTIPLATELET THERAPY. Aspirin is associated with only modest (22%) reduction in the incidence of stroke, corresponding to an absolute stroke risk reduction of 1.5% per year as compared with placebo. Thus, except in the lowest risk patients, aspirin alone is not a viable treatment option for stroke prevention. The combination of aspirin plus clopidogrel is superior to aspirin therapy alone (28% relative risk reduction), but it is associated with a significantly increased risk of major bleeding (2.0% versus 1.3% per year) to levels generally similar to those associated with warfarin therapy.

VITAMIN K ANTAGONISTS. Oral anticoagulation therapy with vitamin K antagonists (warfarin) reduces stroke risk by approximately 64%, corresponding to an absolute annual risk reduction in all strokes of 2.7% as compared with placebo. Warfarin is superior to aspirin, with relative risk reduction of 39% for stroke and 29% for cardiovascular events. However, warfarin increases the risk of major bleeding by approximately 70% compared with aspirin. Although the risk of intracranial hemorrhage is doubled with adjusted-dose warfarin compared with aspirin, the absolute risk increase appears to be small (0.2% per year). Furthermore, randomized clinical trials have shown that warfarin is superior to the combination of aspirin plus clopidogrel for prevention of vascular events in patients with AF at high risk of stroke (relative risk reduction of 40%), with similar risks for major bleeding events. Combinations of warfarin (international normalized ratio [INR], 2.0 to 3.0) with antiplatelet therapy offer no incremental benefit in stroke risk reduction while they increase the risk of bleeding.[36,43,44]

The reduction in ischemic stroke with warfarin in patients with paroxysmal AF is probably similar to that in patients with persistent or permanent AF. The benefit of warfarin is greatest for patients at higher risk of stroke, and there appears to be little benefit for those with no risk factors. The true efficacy of warfarin is likely to be even higher than suggested by trial results because many of the strokes in the warfarin-treated groups occurred in patients who were noncompliant at the time of the stroke.[27] It has been found that if a patient's INR is not maintained in the therapeutic range at least 65% of the time, the advantage of taking warfarin over aspirin is nullified.

Warfarin therapy, however, has several problems that limit the enthusiasm of patients and clinicians: a narrow therapeutic window that requires periodic INR monitoring and frequent dose adjustments, multiple drug and dietary interactions, genetic variability in response (accounting for 39% to 56% of the variability in the warfarin dose), long half-life (36 to 42 hours), and slow onset of action. In several trials, more than one-third of the patients refused warfarin therapy, largely because of the life-style changes required, the inconvenience of INR monitoring, and concern about bleeding risk. These issues have contributed to the underutilization of anticoagulation therapy in patients who can stand to derive benefit from it. In fact, it is estimated that less than 50% of eligible patients are being treated with warfarin. Additionally, more than one-third of patients taking warfarin are not maintained in the therapeutic range, thus exposing them to increased risk of either stroke or bleeding.

Furthermore, it is estimated that up to 44% of patients with AF have one or more absolute or relative contraindications for long-term oral anticoagulation therapy, most commonly related to increased risk of bleeding. The estimated annual incidence of bleeding associated with oral anticoagulation is 0.6% for fatal bleeding, 3.0% for major bleeding, and 9.6% for major or minor bleeding. The risk of bleeding appears to be especially high during the first year of treatment. Notably, the risk of major bleeding in older patients (at least 80 years of age) receiving warfarin therapy, although higher than younger patients, is acceptably low (2.5% per year), and these patients can still benefit from warfarin prophylaxis when a good quality of anticoagulation is obtained.[42] The risk of falling and intracranial bleeding should be considered but not overstated, because a patient may need to fall almost 300 times per year for the risk of intracranial hemorrhage to outweigh the benefit of warfarin therapy in stroke prevention.

DIRECT THROMBIN INHIBITORS. Dabigatran, an oral direct thrombin inhibitor, was compared with warfarin therapy in a large (18,113 patients) randomized controlled trial in patients with nonvalvular AF and a mean $CHADS_2$ score of 2. Dabigatran was superior to warfarin for stroke prevention, with similar risk of bleeding at a higher dabigatran dose (150 mg twice daily). A lower dose (110 mg twice daily) of dabigatran was associated with stroke rates similar to those seen with warfarin, with lower bleeding risk.

Disadvantages of dabigatran include lack of long-term safety data, twice-daily dosing, tolerability issues secondary to dyspepsia, lack of an antidote, and when compared with warfarin, a trend toward increased incidence of myocardial infarction and higher cost. Bleeding with dabigatran remains a hazard and increases over time, out to 2.5 years of follow-up, albeit at a lower rate than with warfarin.

Dabigatran was approved by the U.S. Food and Drug Administration (FDA) for stroke prevention in nonvalvular AF and is likely to improve compliance by obviating the need for dietary restrictions and frequent blood monitoring required for warfarin therapy.[45]

FACTOR Xa INHIBITORS. Several oral factor Xa inhibitors are being considered. Rivaroxaban was shown to be noninferior to warfarin in stroke prevention in patients with AF and two or more stroke risk factors, and it seems to be associated with a lower risk of intracranial and fatal bleeding.[46] In patients for whom vitamin K–antagonist therapy was considered unsuitable, apixaban was found more than 50% superior to aspirin for the prevention of stroke or systemic embolism, with a similar risk of bleeding.[47] Also, when compared with warfarin for stroke prevention in patients with AF with one or more additional stroke risk factors, apixaban was found superior to warfarin for stroke and systemic embolism in patients with AF with one or more additional stroke risk factors, thus reducing the risk, with less risk of major bleeding and lower mortality.[48]

NONPHARMACOLOGICAL INTERVENTIONS. Given that the LA appendage is the most common site of thrombi in patients with nonvalvular AF, several approaches have targeted exclusion of the LA appendage from the systemic circulation to help prevent systemic thromboembolism. These approaches can potentially become important clinical options in many patients, given the fact that up to 44% of patients with AF have one or more absolute or relative contraindications for chronic oral anticoagulation therapy, most commonly related to increased risk of bleeding.[49,50]

Open surgical LA appendage amputation, suture ligation, or stapling is commonly performed in patients with AF who are undergoing valvular or coronary artery bypass surgery or as an adjunct to the maze procedure. LA excision appears more efficacious than ligation or stapling, largely because achieving complete LA appendage closure with suture ligation or stapling is quite challenging and operator dependent.[50]

Additionally, various minimally invasive thoracoscopic LA appendage exclusion techniques (LA appendage excision, stapling, and clipping) have emerged as isolated surgical procedures or in conjunction with minimally invasive maze procedures for ablation of AF. However, data are still limited regarding its efficacy and safety.[51]

Percutaneous catheter-based closure of the LA appendage using various closure devices (e.g., the Watchman device [Atritech, Plymouth, Minn.], PLAATO implant [ev3 Endovascular, Inc., North Plymouth, Minn.], or Amplatzer cardiac plug [AGA Medical Corporation, Golden Valley, Minn.]) is an emerging approach. The feasibility, safety, and efficacy of these interventions have been demonstrated in experimental and clinical studies; however, further evaluation is required to demonstrate long-term efficacy.[49,50]

RECOMMENDATIONS FOR LONG-TERM STROKE PREVENTION. The choice of therapy (oral anticoagulation versus aspirin) varies with the estimated thromboembolic risk. Patients with valvular AF (those with mitral stenosis or valvular prosthesis) should be managed with oral anticoagulation. For nonvalvular AF, the $CHADS_2$ (Table 15-4) and CHA_2DS_2-VASc (see Tables 15-2 and 15-3) scoring systems are currently the best validated and most clinically useful for risk stratification. Patients with a $CHADS_2$ score of 2 or higher are at high risk and should be managed with oral anticoagulation therapy, unless contraindicated. Most patients with AF, however, have a $CHADS_2$ score of less than 2, and a more comprehensive risk factor–based approach, such as the CHA_2DS_2-VASc scheme, can be used for better risk assessment. Patients with a CHA_2DS_2-VASc score higher than 1 should be considered for oral anticoagulation, whereas patients with a score of 0 have very low risk and can be managed with aspirin therapy (75 to 325 mg daily). Patients with a score of 1 probably represent an intermediate-risk category and can be managed with either aspirin or oral anticoagulation. When possible, patients at intermediate risk should be considered for oral anticoagulation rather than for aspirin because undertreatment is more harmful than overtreatment. Importantly, those recommendations apply to all patients with AF irrespective of the type of AF.[27,38]

TABLE 15-4 Stroke Risk in Patients with Nonvalvular Atrial Fibrillation According to $CHADS_2$ Index*

$CHADS_2$ RISK CRITERIA		POINT(S)
Prior stroke or transient ischemic attack		2
Age >75 yr		1
Hypertension		1
Diabetes mellitus		1
Heart failure		1
PATIENTS (*N*= 1,733)	**ADJUSTED STROKE RATE† (5%/YR) (95% CI)**	**$CHADS_2$ SCORE**
120	1.9 (1.2-3.0)	0
463	2.8 (2.0-3.8)	1
523	4.0 (3.1-5.1)	2
337	5.9 (4.6-7.3)	3
220	8.5 (6.3-11.1)	4
65	12.5 (8.2-17.5)	5
5	18.2 (10.5-27.4)	6

*Not treated with anticoagulation.
†The adjusted stroke rate was derived from multivariate analysis assuming no aspirin usage.
$CHADS_2$ = congestive heart failure, *h*ypertension, *a*ge, *d*iabetes, and stroke (doubled); CI = confidence interval.
From Gage BF, Waterman AD, Shannon W, et al: Validation of clinical classification schemes for predicting stroke: results from the National Registry of Atrial Fibrillation, *JAMA* 285: 2864-2870, 2010.

An INR between 2.0 and 3.0 is recommended for most patients with AF who receive warfarin therapy. The risk of stroke doubles when the INR falls to 1.7, and values up to 3.5 do not convey an increased risk of bleeding complications.[27] A higher goal (INR between 2.5 and 3.5) is reasonable for patients at particularly high risk for embolization (e.g., prior thromboembolism, rheumatic heart disease, prosthetic heart valves). Similarly, in patients who sustain ischemic stroke or systemic embolism during treatment with therapeutic doses of warfarin (INR, 2.0 to 3.0), raising the intensity of anticoagulation to a higher INR range of 3.0 to 3.5 should be considered. This approach is probably preferable to adding an antiplatelet agent because an appreciable risk in major bleeding is seen with warfarin only when the INR is greater than 3.5 and is likely to be less than that associated with combination therapy.

Oral anticoagulation is associated with increased risk of bleeding; therefore, an assessment of bleeding risk should be part of the patient assessment before starting anticoagulation. At therapeutic INR levels, the rates of intracerebral hemorrhage are typically between 0.1% and 0.6%, with no increment in bleeding risk with INR values between 2.0 and 3.0 compared with lower INR levels. However, an appreciable increase in bleeding risk is observed with higher INR values (more than 3.5 to 4.0). The risk of bleeding should be weighed against the potential benefit of stroke prevention in individual patients considered for anticoagulation therapy. Various bleeding risk scores have been validated for bleeding risk in anticoagulated patients. Among those is the HAS-BLED score, which was found to correlate well with the risk of major bleeding, hospitalization, or death (Table 15-5). Patients are categorized as low, intermediate, and high bleeding risk according to HAS-BLED scores 0 to 1, 2, and 3 or higher, respectively. A score higher than 2 suggests a risk of major bleeding of 1.9% per year, whereas a score of 5 is associated with a risk of major bleeding of up to 12.5% per

TABLE 15-5 Clinical Characteristics Comprising the HAS-BLED Bleeding Risk Score

LETTER	CLINICAL CHARACTERISTIC*	POINTS AWARDED
H	Hypertension	1
A	Abnormal renal and liver function (1 point each)	1 or 2
S	Stroke	1
B	Bleeding	1
L	Labile INR	1
E	Older patients (e.g., age >65 years)	1
D	Drugs or alcohol use (1 point each)	1 or 2
		Maximum 9 points

*Hypertension is defined as systolic blood pressure higher than160 mmHg. Abnormal kidney function is defined as the presence of long-term dialysis or renal transplantation or serum creatinine concentration of at least 200 µmol/liter. Abnormal liver function is defined as chronic hepatic disease (e.g., cirrhosis) or biochemical evidence of significant hepatic derangement (e.g., bilirubin more than twice the upper limit of normal, in association with aspartate aminotransferase, alanine aminotransferase, and alkaline phosphatase more than three times the upper limit of normal). Bleeding refers to previous bleeding history or predisposition to bleeding, or both (e.g., bleeding diathesis, anemia). Labile INRs refers to unstable or high INRs or poor time in therapeutic range (e.g., less than 60%). Drugs or alcohol use refers to concomitant use of drugs (e.g., antiplatelet agents, nonsteroidal antiinflammatory drugs, or alcohol abuse).

INR = international normalized ratio.

From Pisters R, Lane DA, Nieuwlaat R, et al: A novel user-friendly score (HAS-BLED) to assess 1-year risk of major bleeding in patients with atrial fibrillation: the Euro Heart Survey, *Chest* 138:1093-1100, 2010.

year.[52] One report also proposed a simple 5-variable risk score for quantifying the risk of warfarin-associated hemorrhage, including anemia (3 points), severe renal disease (3 points), age 75 years or more (2 points), prior bleeding (1 point), and hypertension (1 point). Major bleeding annual rates were 0.8% for the low-risk group (0 to 3 points), 2.6% for the intermediate-risk group (4 points), and 5.8% for the high-risk group (5 to 10 points).[53]

In high-risk patients who cannot be treated with oral anticoagulation because of poor tolerance or noncompliance issues or because of strong patient preference, dual antiplatelet therapy (aspirin plus clopidogrel) can be used. However, dual antiplatelet therapy is not an alternative to oral anticoagulation in patients at high bleeding risk because the risk of major bleeding associated with dual antiplatelet therapy is broadly similar to that with oral anticoagulation. In the latter group, aspirin monotherapy is associated with lesser bleeding risk, although at the expense of less protection from systemic thromboembolism.[36,43,44] Percutaneous LA appendage exclusion procedures may become an important therapeutic alternative to long-term antithrombotic therapy in these patients.[36]

The new antithrombotic agents have many potential advantages over the vitamin K antagonists, including their rapid onset of action, predictable therapeutic effect, less complex pharmacodynamics, and limited dietary and drug interactions. These advantages will likely promote greater use of anticoagulants, enhance patients' compliance, allow for routine therapy without monitoring, and possibly eliminate the need for anticoagulation with parenteral agents such as heparin ("bridge therapy"). However, warfarin will remain the mainstay of treatment for patients with valvular AF and those with mechanical heart valves because studies in this population have not been started. Warfarin may also hold favor with patients who are considered noncompliant with therapy and as an option for those patients who "fail" or develop an event while taking one of the new agents.

ANTICOAGULATION IN PATIENTS WITH CORONARY ARTERY DISEASE. The combined use of antiplatelet and anticoagulant drugs can be required in patients with AF and coronary artery disease. In these patients, it is a common practice to add low-dose aspirin therapy in conjunction with warfarin. Although this strategy appears to be appropriate in patients with acute coronary syndromes, it is important to recognize that in patients with AF with stable coronary, carotid artery disease, or peripheral artery disease, adding aspirin to warfarin does not reduce the risk of stroke, systemic embolism, or myocardial infarction, but it substantially increases the risk of major bleeding (3.9% per year versus 2.3% per year).[54]

After percutaneous coronary interventions, dual antiplatelet therapy with aspirin plus clopidogrel is superior to aspirin alone, warfarin alone, or warfarin plus aspirin, for reduction of the risk for myocardial infarction and cardiovascular death. On the other hand, the omission of warfarin therapy in eligible patients with AF following percutaneous coronary interventions can result in increased rates of mortality and ischemic stroke, a finding suggesting the importance of maintaining anticoagulation in this population. Importantly, triple therapy (aspirin plus clopidogrel plus warfarin) has been associated with major bleeding rates as high as 7% per year.

In the absence of randomized trials, antithrombotic therapy should be individualized, taking into account the risks of bleeding, thromboembolism, and stent thrombosis. It appears reasonable to resume anticoagulation as soon as feasible after percutaneous coronary interventions and to use triple therapy (aspirin [75 to 100 mg] plus clopidogrel [75 mg] plus warfarin) in patients with AF with moderate or high stroke risk in the initial period following an acute coronary syndrome (3 to 6 months) and following placement of coronary stents (4 weeks for a bare-metal stent, 6 to 12 months for a drug-eluting stent), especially in patients with low risk of serious bleeding. Afterward, warfarin is continued in addition to a single antiplatelet agent (either aspirin or clopidogrel). During triple therapy, it is advisable to target a lower INR (approximately 2.0), limit the duration of triple therapy to the period required for stent endothelialization, consider prophylactic proton pump inhibition, and follow patients closely to help minimize the high risk of bleeding. Additionally, it is advisable to avoid drug-eluting stents (which are associated with delayed endothelialization and an apparently higher incidence of late stent thrombosis) in patients requiring anticoagulation to reduce the need for prolonged triple therapy.[36,54]

ANTICOAGULATION IN THE PERICARDIOVERSION PERIOD. Patients without a contraindication to oral anticoagulation who have been in AF for more than 48 hours should receive 3 to 4 weeks of warfarin prior to and after cardioversion. This approach is also recommended for patients with AF who have valvular disease, evidence of LV dysfunction, recent thromboembolism, or AF of unknown duration.[27]

The rationale for anticoagulation prior to cardioversion is based on observational studies showing that more than 85% of LA thrombi resolve after 4 weeks of warfarin therapy. Thromboembolic events have been reported in 1% to 7% of patients who did not receive anticoagulation before cardioversion. The recommended target INR is 2.0 to 3.0. It has been suggested that it may be prudent to aim for an INR greater than 2.5 before cardioversion to provide the greatest protection against embolic events. Probably more important is to document that the INR has consistently been higher than 2.0 in the weeks before cardioversion.[27]

An alternative approach that eliminates the need for prolonged anticoagulation prior to cardioversion, particularly in low-risk patients who would benefit from earlier cardioversion, is the use of TEE-guided cardioversion. Cardioversion is performed if TEE excludes the presence of intracardiac clots. Anticoagulation after cardioversion, however, is still necessary.

After cardioversion, it is recommended to continue warfarin therapy for at least 4 weeks, with a target INR of 2.5 (range, 2.0 to 3.0). This recommendation deals only with protection from embolic events related to the cardioversion period. Subsequently, the long-term recommendations for patients who have been cardioverted to NSR but are at high risk for thromboembolism are similar to those for patients with chronic AF, even though the patients are in NSR.[27]

A different approach with respect to anticoagulation can be used in low-risk patients (no mitral valve disease, severe LV dysfunction, or history of recent thromboembolism) in whom there is reasonable certainty that AF has been present for less than 48 hours. Such patients have a low risk of clinical thromboembolism if converted early (0.8% in one study), even without screening TEE. The American College of Cardiology/American Heart Association guidelines do not recommend long-term anticoagulation prior to cardioversion in such patients, but they do recommend heparin use at presentation and during the pericardioversion period. The optimal therapy after cardioversion in this group is uncertain. A common practice is to administer aspirin for a first episode of AF that converts spontaneously and warfarin for at least 4 weeks to all other patients. Aspirin should not be considered for patients with AF of less than 48 hours' duration if there is associated rheumatic mitral valve disease, severe LV dysfunction, or recent thromboembolism. Such patients should be treated the same as patients with AF of longer duration: 3 to 4 weeks of oral anticoagulation with warfarin or shorter term anticoagulation with screening TEE prior to elective electrical or pharmacological cardioversion, followed by prolonged warfarin therapy after cardioversion.[27]

RATE CONTROL

Rate control during AF is important to prevent hemodynamic instability or symptoms such as palpitations, heart failure, lightheadedness, and poor exercise capacity and, over the long-term, to prevent tachycardia-mediated cardiomyopathy and improve quality of life. Beta blockers (e.g., atenolol or metoprolol), diltiazem, and verapamil are recommended for rate control during rest and exercise. Digoxin is not effective during exercise but can be used in patients with heart failure or hypotension or as a second-line agent.

Adequacy of rate control should be assessed at rest and with exertion. However, parameters for optimal rate control in AF remain controversial. It appears reasonable to target a resting heart rate of 60 to 80 beats/min and 90 to 115 beats/min during moderate exercise. Additionally, ambulatory monitoring can help assess adequacy of rate control; goals of therapy include a 24-hour average heart rate lower than 100 beats/min and no heart rate higher than 100% of the maximum age-adjusted predicted exercise heart rate. Also, a maximum heart rate of 110 beats/min during a 6-minute walk test is a commonly used target.[27,47]

Nevertheless, one study found that a more lenient rate control (resting heart rate less than 110 beats/min) is not inferior to strict rate control (heart rate less than 80 beats/min at rest and less than 110 beats/min during moderate exercise). Such an approach can be more convenient in clinical practice and may be considered especially in asymptomatic patients with permanent AF and no significant structural heart disease, but periodic monitoring of LV function is necessary to evaluate for the potential risk of tachycardia-mediated cardiomyopathy.[47,55] Of note, lenient rate control does not seem to increase the risk of adverse atrial or ventricular remodeling.

In some patients with tachycardia-bradycardia syndrome, pacemaker implantation can be required to protect from severe bradycardia while allowing the use of AV nodal (AVN) blockers for adequate control of fast ventricular rates during AF (see Fig. 8-4).

AVN ablation and permanent pacemaker implantation are highly effective means of improving symptoms in patients with AF who experience symptoms related to a rapid ventricular rate during AF that cannot be adequately controlled with antiarrhythmic or AVN blockers. AV junction ablation is especially useful when excessive ventricular rates induce a tachycardia-mediated decline in LV systolic function, despite appropriate medical therapy. Additionally, in patients with AF and advanced heart failure requiring cardiac resynchronization therapy, AVN ablation can potentially improve long-term survival, NYHA class, and LV systolic function, even in patients with mean ventricular rates lower than 100 beats/min during AF. In these patients, AVN ablation ensures a high percentage of resynchronized QRS complexes and attenuates cardiac output impairment resulting from R-R interval variability.[56]

RHYTHM CONTROL

Restoration and maintenance of sinus rhythm in patients with AF can have several potential benefits, including relief of symptoms, improved functional status and quality of life, prevention of systemic thromboembolism, and avoidance of cardiomyopathy. Reduction in atrial remodeling and retardation of progression of AF, and improvement in LV function also have been described. The impact of rhythm control on mortality, however, remains to be determined.[21]

Unfortunately, complete restoration of sinus rhythm (100% freedom from AF recurrence) often is unachievable with current drug therapies and remains an impractical treatment goal. It has been estimated that the average 1-year recurrence rate associated with amiodarone approximates 35%, and the recurrence rate for other currently available antiarrhythmic drug therapies is even higher (approximately 50%). However, it is likely that individuals with AF can derive benefit from even partial restoration of sinus rhythm, including improvements in symptoms and attenuation of electrical and structural atrial remodeling associated with AF and hence retardation of progression of AF.[21]

REVERSION TO NORMAL SINUS RHYTHM. When rhythm control is chosen, both electrical and pharmacological cardioversion methods are appropriate options. The timing of attempted cardioversion is influenced by the duration of AF. As noted, in patients with AF of a duration longer than 48 hours or unknown duration, cardioversion should be delayed until the patient has been anticoagulated at appropriate levels for 3 to 4 weeks or TEE has excluded atrial thrombi.[27]

Electrical cardioversion is indicated for patients with rapid ventricular rates not responding promptly to medical therapy and ongoing myocardial ischemia, hypotension, acute heart failure, or ventricular preexcitation. In stable patients in whom spontaneous reversion caused by correction of an underlying condition is not likely, electrical or pharmacological cardioversion can be performed. Electrical cardioversion is usually preferred because of greater efficacy and a low risk of proarrhythmia; however, it requires conscious sedation or anesthesia. Importantly, electrical cardioversion is contraindicated in patients with ongoing toxic reactions from digitalis or patients with hypokalemia.[57]

The overall success rate of electrical cardioversion (at any level of energy) for AF is 75% to 93% and is related inversely to the duration of AF and LA size. Occasionally, electrical cardioversion can fail to terminate AF, or AF recurs shortly after transient restoration of sinus rhythm. When AF fails to terminate, using higher energy levels, applying external pressure on the cardioversion patches, and performing cardioversion during exhalation can improve effectiveness. When AF recurs early after a successful cardioversion, pretreatment with amiodarone, dofetilide, flecainide, ibutilide, propafenone, or sotalol can facilitate successful electrical cardioversion.[57,58] It is important to distinguish failure to terminate AF with a certain shock energy (the solution for which is higher energy shock) from successful termination of AF with nearly immediate recurrence (for which repeated shocks at any energy are unlikely to have greater benefit). Sinus pauses or transient sinus arrest after successful cardioversion are common; rarely, several-second pauses result from sinus node dysfunction and the effect of sedation. Almost all external defibrillators have the capability of back-up bradycardia pacing through the defibrillation patches, which can be used transiently if needed. The need for more prolonged pacing after cardioversion is rare.

Certain antiarrhythmic drugs have been found to be more effective than placebo for chemical cardioversion of AF, by converting 30% to 60% of patients. Evidence of efficacy from randomized trials has been best established for dofetilide, ibutilide, flecainide, propafenone, amiodarone, and quinidine. The benefit from specific antiarrhythmic drugs varies with the duration of AF: dofetilide, flecainide, ibutilide, propafenone or, to a lesser degree, amiodarone if less than 7 days' duration; and dofetilide or, to a lesser degree, amiodarone or ibutilide if AF is more prolonged. Flecainide and propafenone should be avoided in patients with abnormal LV function and ischemia.[57]

Rate control with an AVN blocker (beta blockers, diltiazem, verapamil, digoxin) should be attained before instituting a class IA or

IC drug because of possible conversion to AFL and a very rapid ventricular rate.[27] Importantly, continuous cardiac monitoring is required (to detect sinus node dysfunction, AV block, ventricular arrhythmias, and conversion into AFL) for an interval that is dependent on the agent used (usually approximately half the drug elimination half-life). Once the safety of pharmacological conversion with propafenone or flecainide has been established, repeat patient-administered cardioversion using oral propafenone (450 to 600 mg) or flecainide (200 to 300 mg) may be appropriate on an outpatient basis ("pill-in-the-pocket" approach).[36,57]

MAINTENANCE OF NORMAL SINUS RHYTHM. Only 20% to 30% of patients who are successfully cardioverted maintain NSR for more than 1 year without chronic antiarrhythmic therapy. This is more likely to occur in patients with AF for less than 1 year, no enlargement of the LA (less than 4.0 cm), and a reversible cause of AF, such as hyperthyroidism, pericarditis, pulmonary embolism, or cardiac surgery. It has been thought that the drugs most likely to maintain NSR suppress triggering ectopic beats and arrhythmias and affect atrial EP properties to diminish the likelihood of AF. There is therefore a strong rationale for prophylactic antiarrhythmic drug therapy in patients who have a moderate to high risk of recurrence, provided that the therapy is effective and that toxic and proarrhythmic effects are low. Prophylactic drug treatment is seldom indicated in patients with a first-detected episode of AF and can also be avoided in patients with infrequent and well-tolerated paroxysmal AF.[27]

Evidence of efficacy from randomized trials is best for amiodarone, propafenone, disopyramide, sotalol, flecainide, dofetilide, dronedarone, and quinidine. Amiodarone is the most effective agent but is associated with substantial noncardiac toxic effects. The relative efficacy of the other antiarrhythmic drugs for the management of AF remains unknown. Drug selection is largely driven by the safety profile. The presence and extent of concomitant cardiovascular disease have to be carefully considered. A safer, although possibly less efficacious, drug is usually recommended before resorting to more effective but less safe therapies (Fig. 15-5).[36]

In patients with AF with and minimal or no heart disease (lone AF), flecainide, propafenone, sotalol, and dronedarone are preferred. In patients with adrenergically mediated AF, beta blockers represent first-line treatment, followed by sotalol. The anticholinergic activity of long-acting disopyramide makes it a relatively attractive choice for patients with vagally mediated AF. In contrast, propafenone is not recommended in vagally mediated AF because its (weak) intrinsic beta-blocking activity may aggravate this type of paroxysmal AF. In patients with lone AF, amiodarone should be chosen later in the sequence of drug therapy because of its potential toxicity.[36]

In patients with substantial LV hypertrophy (LV wall thickness greater than 1.4 cm), sotalol is thought to be associated with an increased incidence of proarrhythmia. It is also reasonable to avoid flecainide and propafenone because of concern of increased proarrhythmic risk. Dronedarone, although not specifically tested in this population, is likely to be safe. Amiodarone is usually considered when symptomatic AF recurrences continue to affect the quality of life of these patients.[27,36]

Flecainide and propafenone are contraindicated in patients with coronary artery disease. Sotalol, dofetilide, or dronedarone are recommended as first-line therapy. Amiodarone is considered the drug of last resort in this population because of its potential toxicity.[36]

Dronedarone, dofetilide, and amiodarone are the only agents available for patients with AF with concomitant heart failure; other antiarrhythmic agents can be associated with substantial toxicity and proarrhythmia. Dronedarone is contraindicated in patients with NYHA Class III to IV or recently (within the previous month) decompensated heart failure, especially when the LV ejection fraction is 35% or lower. In such patients, dofetilide and amiodarone are preferred. Importantly, concerning results emerged from a study (the Permanent Atrial fibriLLAtion Outcome Study Using

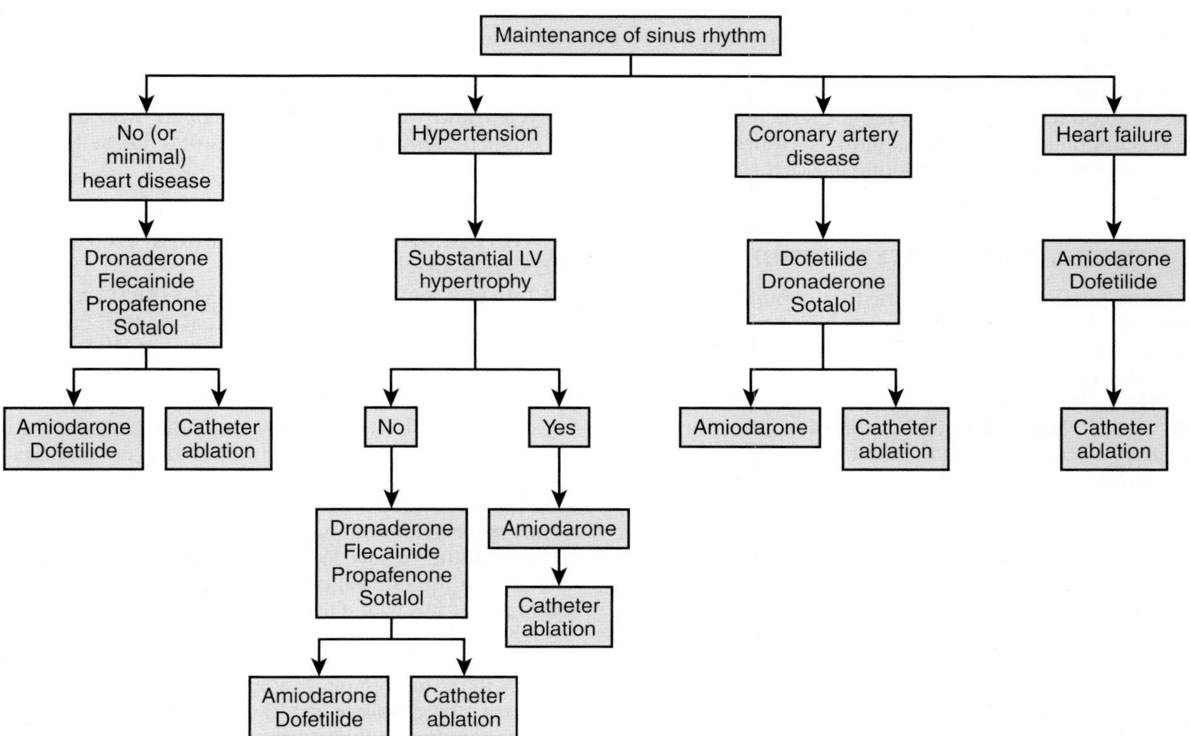

FIGURE 15-5 Therapy to maintain sinus rhythm in patients with recurrent paroxysmal or persistent atrial fibrillation. Drugs are listed alphabetically and not in order of suggested use. The seriousness of heart disease progresses from left to right, and selection of therapy in patients with multiple conditions depends on the most serious condition present. LV = left ventricle. *(With permission from Wann LS, Curtis AB, January CT, et al: 2011 ACCF/AHA/HRS Focused update on the management of patients with atrial fibrillation [updating the 2006 guideline], Heart Rhythm 8:157-176, 2011.)*

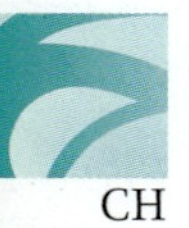

Dronedarone on Top of Standard Therapy [PALLAS]) conducted to assess the potential clinical benefit of dronedarone in patients more than 65 years of age with permanent AF in the reduction of major cardiovascular events (stroke, systemic arterial embolism, myocardial infarction, or cardiovascular death), or unplanned cardiovascular hospitalization or death from any cause. The study was stopped early because of a twofold increase in death, as well as twofold increases in stroke and hospitalization for heart failure in patients receiving dronedarone compared with patients taking a placebo. These data currently are being reviewed by the FDA to determine whether those results apply to patients who use dronedarone for the approved indications in nonpermanent (paroxysmal or persistent) AF.

Although amiodarone is associated with organ toxicity, it appears to have a lower risk of proarrhythmia than other agents. Class IC agents can be associated with substantial toxicity in patients with heart failure because of their proarrhythmic and negative inotropic effects.[36]

Quinidine is associated with increased mortality, likely the result of ventricular proarrhythmia secondary to QT interval prolongation. Hence, this drug has largely been abandoned for AF therapy.

When treatment with a single drug fails, combinations of antiarrhythmic drugs can be tried. Useful combinations include a beta blocker, sotalol, or amiodarone, in addition to a class IC agent.[27] When AF recurrences are infrequent and tolerated, patients experiencing breakthrough arrhythmias may not require a change in antiarrhythmic drug therapy.

UPSTREAM THERAPY. Given the limited effectiveness and marked risks of serious complications associated with currently available antiarrhythmic drug therapy, the role of therapies targeting the atrial substrate underlying AF ("upstream therapy") is of particular clinical interest. The goal of this approach is attenuation and reversal of atrial structural remodeling. Given the role of fibrosis and inflammation in the pathogenesis of AF, drugs that suppress fibrosis, as well as antiinflammatory and antioxidative drugs, are being investigated both alone and in combination with traditional antiarrhythmic drugs. Among these drugs are several angiotensin-converting enzyme inhibitors, angiotensin II type 1 receptor blockers, antialdosterone agents, statins (3-hydroxy-3-methylglutaryl-coenzyme A reductase inhibitors), and omega-3 poly-unsaturated fatty acids. These agents seem to reduce atrial fibrosis and were found potentially to reduce structural remodeling and AF susceptibility in various AF models. Nonetheless, current evidence does not support the routine use of these agents for the sole purpose of preventing or treating AF.[13,16,59,60]

RHYTHM CONTROL VERSUS RATE CONTROL

In the past, many physicians preferred rhythm control to rate control. Reversion of AF and maintenance of NSR restores normal hemodynamics and had been thought to reduce the frequency of embolism. However, two major clinical trials—AFFIRM (Atrial Fibrillation Follow-Up Investigation of Rhythm Management) and RACE (RAte Control versus Electrical Cardioversion for Persistent Atrial Fibrillation)— compared rhythm and rate control and found that embolic events occurred with equal frequency, regardless of whether a rate control or rhythm control strategy was pursued, and this occurred most often after warfarin had been stopped or when the INR was subtherapeutic. Both studies also showed an almost significant trend toward a lower incidence of the primary endpoint with rate control. There was no difference in the functional status or quality of life. Thus, both rhythm control and rate control are acceptable approaches, and both require long-term anticoagulation for stroke prevention. The trials provided supportive evidence for the rate control option in most patients. The AF-Congestive Heart Failure (AF-CHF) study demonstrated similar results among patients with AF with concomitant heart failure.[61]

In a worldwide, prospective, observational survey of management of AF in unselected, community-based patients, clinical outcomes were not influenced by the choice of rhythm control versus rate control. Major cardiovascular outcomes were driven mainly by hospitalizations for arrhythmia or proarrhythmia and other cardiovascular causes and were more dependent on comorbidity than the choice of cardiac rhythm management. Nevertheless, patients receiving rhythm control progressed less rapidly to permanent AF.

However, it would be incorrect to extrapolate that NSR offers no benefit over AF and that effective treatments to maintain NSR need not be pursued. First, these trials were not comparisons of NSR and AF. They compared a rate control strategy to a rhythm control strategy that attempted to maintain NSR but fell short. The failure of AFFIRM and RACE in showing any difference between rate and rhythm control is not so much a positive statement for rate control but rather a testimony to the ineffectiveness of the rhythm control methods used. Failure of rhythm control to demonstrate superiority over rate control is caused by failure to achieve maintenance of NSR over the long term. Several trials demonstrated that the success of antiarrhythmic therapy in maintaining NSR is borderline, at best, with increasing failure rates over time. When the data from these trials were analyzed according to the patient's actual rhythm (as opposed to his or her treatment strategy), the benefit of NSR over AF became apparent: the presence of NSR was found to be one of the most powerful independent predictors of survival, along with the use of warfarin, even after adjustment for all other relevant clinical variables. Patients in NSR are almost half as likely to die compared with those with AF. This benefit, however, is offset by the use of antiarrhythmic drug therapy, which increases the risk of death.[21,61,62]

Achieving and maintaining sinus rhythm remain viable and important treatment goals. However, because currently available antiarrhythmic agents commonly fail to suppress AF completely and have safety profiles that are less than ideal, it is reasonable to reserve it to the populations of patients likely to derive the greatest benefit from rhythm control. The selection of appropriate rhythm control or rate control strategies should be individualized and take into consideration the nature, intensity, and frequency of symptoms, patient preferences, comorbid conditions, and the risk of recurrent AF. According to analyses of available data, these groups may include young patients and those with newly diagnosed AF, significant symptoms, poorly controlled ventricular response, or tachycardia-mediated cardiomyopathy. On the other hand, asymptomatic or mildly symptomatic patients, especially those older than 65 years, and women with persistent AF who have hypertension or other underlying heart diseases may be better suited for rate control therapy.[21,61,62]

NONPHARMACOLOGICAL APPROACHES FOR RHYTHM CONTROL

CATHETER ABLATION OF ATRIAL FIBRILLATION. Currently, the mainstay of nonpharmacological rhythm control is catheter ablation of AF, which can help maintain NSR without the risk associated with long-term antiarrhythmic therapy and has been shown to significantly improve symptoms, exercise capacity, quality of life, and LV function, even in the presence of concurrent heart disease and when ventricular rate control has been adequate before ablation. Because no mortality benefit of catheter ablation of AF has so far been demonstrated, the procedure is currently reserved for patients with symptomatic AF.

Several studies have found catheter ablation superior to medical therapy for the control of AF. In a meta-analysis of 6 randomized, controlled trials with a total of 693 patients with AF that compared catheter ablation (PV isolation) and medical therapy, the efficacy of PV isolation for the maintenance of NSR was more than twofold greater than that of antiarrhythmic drug therapy (77% versus 29% at 12 months of follow-up). The benefit of PV isolation was even greater in patients with paroxysmal AF. Moreover, catheter ablation was associated with a two-thirds reduction in hospitalization for cardiovascular causes, with a relatively small (2.6%) risk of major procedural complications.[25] Nonetheless, in the absence of large, well-designed, multicenter randomized trials of catheter ablation as a first-line therapy for AF in symptomatic or asymptomatic patients, a history of symptoms, despite therapeutic doses of antiarrhythmic medication (type IA, IC, or III), is widely accepted as the minimum qualifying criterion for catheter ablation. With improved efficacy of ablation techniques, however, the threshold for ablation will continue to fall.

Catheter ablation was also found to be associated with better quality of life, higher rates of freedom from both AF and antiarrhythmic medications, and lower rates of AF progression when compared with AVN ablation and biventricular pacing in symptomatic patients with AF and cardiomyopathy (LV ejection fraction 40% or less).[63]

SURGICAL ABLATION OF ATRIAL FIBRILLATION. The classic Cox-maze procedure involves creating a series of incisions in both the left and right atria that were originally designed to direct the propagation of the sinus impulse through both atria while interrupting the multiple macroreentrant circuits thought to be responsible for AF. This procedure is the most effective means of curing this arrhythmia, eliminating AF in 75% to 95% up to 15 years after surgery. Improvements and simplifications culminated in the Cox-maze III procedure, which became the gold standard for the surgical treatment of AF. Nonetheless, because of its complexity, technical difficulty, and risk of mortality and other complications, the maze procedure did not gain widespread acceptance.[64]

To simplify the procedure, the standard cut-and-sew surgical technique has been replaced with linear epicardial ablation using unipolar or bipolar RF ablation, cryoablation, laser, high-frequency ultrasound, and microwave energy. Most surgical epicardial ablation procedures have been performed in conjunction with mitral valve surgery; the combination of mitral valve repair and cure of AF can enable selected patients to avoid life-long anticoagulation.[64,65]

Current surgical instrumentation now enables minimally invasive approaches to be performed epicardially on the beating heart through mini-thoracotomies with video assistance. However, despite elimination of the need for median sternotomy and cardiopulmonary bypass, these procedures are still relatively invasive. To minimize the invasiveness of the procedure further, a totally thoracoscopic approach has been developed. Bipolar RF is the predominant energy source used, and bilateral PV isolation is the most common lesion set, with some approaches adding ganglionic plexus ablation, as well as exclusion of the LA appendage. Although multiple series described high success rates for paroxysmal AF (89% at 12 months of follow-up), success has been limited in patients with persistent and longstanding persistent AF (25% to 87%).[64,65] Limited follow-up has left uncertainty about overall results.

More extensive ablation lines, in addition to PV antral isolation and ganglionic plexus ablation, as well as documentation of complete PV isolation by demonstration of EP entrance or exit block, conduction block across ablation lines, and the detection and confirmation of ablation of the parasympathetic component of the ganglionic plexuses, are being evaluated to improve outcome. Some series reported a single procedure success rate of 86% at 1 year without the use of antiarrhythmic drugs.[66,67]

Currently, stand-alone surgical epicardial AF ablation may be considered for symptomatic patients with AF who were refractory to one or more attempts at catheter ablation or who are not candidates for catheter ablation (e.g., patients not candidates for long-term anticoagulation and those with an LA thrombus). There have been no randomized studies comparing surgical and catheter ablation of AF. Hence, the decision to recommend surgical AF ablation before considering catheter ablation for patients with symptomatic AF refractory to drug therapy and no other indication for cardiac surgery remains controversial, and it should be based on each institution's experience with both techniques, the relative outcomes and risks of each in the individual patient, and patient preference.[64,65] Given the degree of patient discomfort, longer hospitalizations and recovery times, and the risk of bleeding following LA appendage excision, most patients prefer catheter to surgical ablation.[68]

DEVICE THERAPY. Atrial defibrillators and pacemakers have demonstrated poor efficacy in treating AF. Burst atrial pacing can effectively convert AT or AFL but fails to terminate or minimize AF. Atrial defibrillators can terminate AF with high acute success rates, but the need for repeated shocks and the resulting patient discomfort often render this option intolerable. Similarly, dual-site atrial pacing has failed to demonstrate any consistent reduction in AF burden or improvement in AF symptoms.

Electrocardiographic Features

Atrial Activity

AF is characterized by rapid and irregular atrial fibrillatory waves (f waves) and a lack of clearly defined P waves, with an undulating baseline that may alternate between recognizable atrial activity and a nearly flat line (Fig. 15-6). Atrial fibrillatory activity is generally best seen in lead V_1 and in the inferior leads. Less often, the f waves are most prominent in leads I and aVL.

The rate of the fibrillatory waves is generally between 350 and 600 beats/min. With up to 600 pulses generated every minute, syncytial contraction of the atria is replaced by irregular atrial twitches. Therefore, the fibrillating atria look like a bag of worms in that the contractions are very rapid and irregular. The f waves vary in amplitude, morphology, and intervals, thus reflecting the multiple potential types of atrial activation that may be present at the same time at different locations throughout the atria. The f waves can be fine (amplitude less than 0.5 mm on ECG) or coarse (amplitude more than 0.5 mm). On occasion, the f waves can be inapparent on the standard and precordial leads, which is most likely to occur

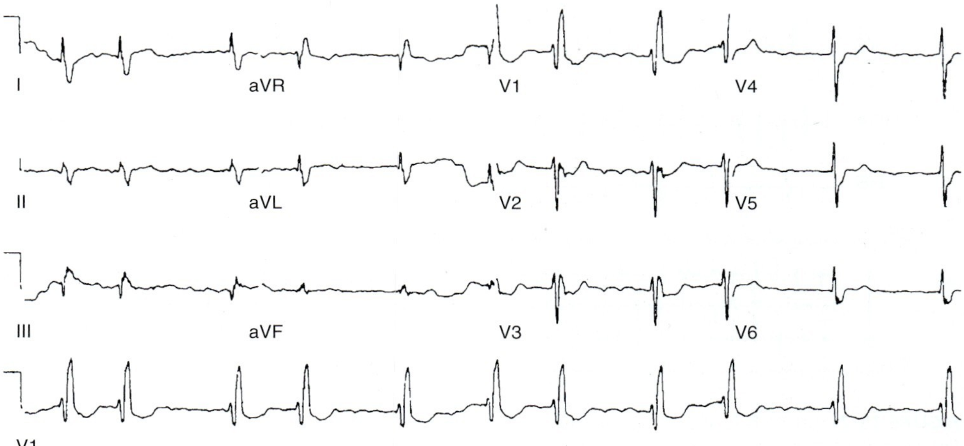

FIGURE 15-6 Surface ECG of atrial fibrillation with chronic right bundle branch block.

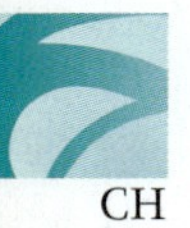

in permanent AF. It was initially thought that the amplitude of the f waves correlated with increasing atrial size; however, echocardiographic studies have failed to show a correlation among the amplitude of the f waves, the size of the atria, and the type of heart disease. The amplitude, however, may correlate with the duration of AF.

AF should be distinguished from other rhythms in which the R-R intervals are irregularly irregular. These include multifocal AT (see Fig. 11-1), wandering atrial pacemaker, multifocal PACs, and AT or AFL with varying AV block (see Fig. 12-4). In general, distinct (although often abnormal and possibly variable) P (or flutter) waves are present during these arrhythmias, in contrast to AF. Patients with rheumatic mitral stenosis often demonstrate large-amplitude fibrillatory waves in the anterior precordial leads (V_1 and V_2), which can be confused with AFL. However, careful examination of the fibrillatory waves reveals them to have a varying CL and morphology. The distinction between AF and AFL can also be confusing in patients who demonstrate a transition between these arrhythmias. Thus, AF may organize to AFL or AFL may degenerate to AF (Fig. 15-7). Occasionally, extracardiac artifacts (e.g., 60 cycle/min muscle tremors, as in parkinsonism) can mimic f waves.

Intracardiac recordings demonstrate variability in the atrial electrogram morphology, amplitude, and CL from beat to beat. The different patterns of conduction during AF may be reflected in the morphology of atrial electrograms recorded with mapping during induced AF. Single potentials usually indicate rapid uniform conduction, short intervals between double potentials may indicate collision, long intervals between double potentials are usually indicative of conduction block, and fragmented potentials and complex fractionated atrial electrograms (CFAEs) are markers for pivoting points or slow conduction.

Atrioventricular Conduction during Atrial Fibrillation

The ventricular response in AF is typically irregularly irregular, and the ventricular rate depends on multiple factors, including the EP properties of the AVN, the rate and organization of atrial inputs to the AVN, the level of autonomic tone, the effects of medications that act on the AV conduction ystem, and the presence of preexcitation over an AV BT.

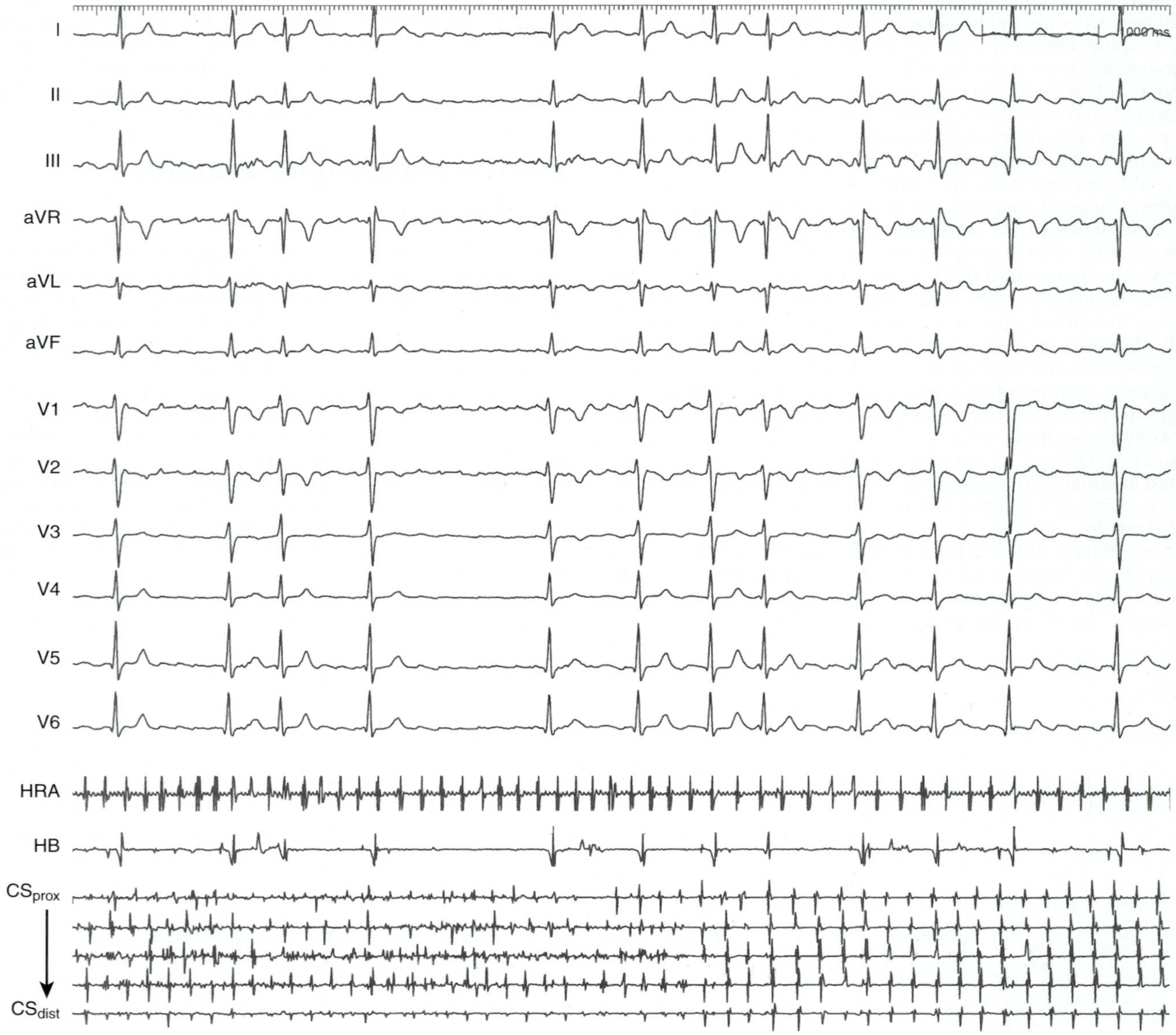

FIGURE 15-7 Surface ECG and intracardiac recordings demonstrating spontaneous conversion of atrial fibrillation (at left) into typical atrial flutter (right). CS_{dist} = distal coronary sinus; CS_{prox} = proximal coronary sinus; HB = His bundle = HRA = high right atrium.

The ventricular rate in untreated patients usually ranges from 90 up to 170 beats/min. Ventricular rates that are clearly outside this range suggest some concurrent problem. Ventricular rates slower than 60 beats/min are seen with AVN disease and can be associated with the sick sinus syndrome, drugs that affect conduction, and high vagal tone, as can occur in a well-conditioned athlete. The ventricular rate in AF can become rapid (more than 200 beats/min) during exercise, with catecholamine excess (Fig. 15-8), parasympathetic withdrawal, thyrotoxicosis, or preexcitation (Fig. 15-9). The ventricular rate can be very rapid (more than 300 beats/min) in patients with the Wolff-Parkinson-White syndrome, with conduction over AV BTs having short anterograde refractory periods.

The compact AVN is located anteriorly in the triangle of Koch. There are two distinct atrial inputs to the AVN, anteriorly via the interatrial septum and posteriorly via the crista terminalis. Experiments in a rabbit AVN preparation demonstrated that propagation of impulses during AF through the AVN to the His bundle (HB) is critically dependent on the relative timing of activation of septal inputs to the AVN at the crista terminalis and interatrial septum. Other investigators showed that the ventricular response also depends on atrial input frequency.

Concealed conduction likely plays the predominant role in determining ventricular response during AF. The constant bombardment of atrial impulses into the AVN creates substantial and varying degrees of concealed conduction, with atrial impulses that enter the AVN but do not conduct to the ventricle, thus leaving a wake of refractoriness encountered by subsequent impulses. This also accounts for the irregular ventricular response during AF. Although the AVN would be expected to conduct whenever it recovers excitability after the last conducted atrial impulse, which would then be at regular intervals, the ventricular response is irregularly irregular because of the varying depth of penetration of the numerous fibrillatory impulses approaching the AVN, leaving it refractory in the face of subsequent atrial impulses.

Alterations of autonomic tone can have profound effects on AVN conduction. Enhanced parasympathetic and sympathetic tone have negative and positive dromotropic effects, respectively, on AVN conduction and refractoriness. An additional factor is the use of AVN blocking agents such as digoxin, Ca^{2+} channel blockers, or beta blockers. There also may be a circadian rhythm for both AVN refractoriness and concealed conduction that accounts for the circadian variation in ventricular rate.

PREEXCITATION DURING ATRIAL FIBRILLATION. The presence of a grossly irregular, very rapid ventricular response (more than 250 beats/min) with QRS longer than 120-millisecond duration during AF rarely results from conduction over the AVN and strongly implies conduction over an AV BT, with rare exceptions (see Fig. 15-9). At very fast heart rates, there is usually a tendency toward regularization of the R-R intervals; therefore, distinguishing the preexcited AF from ventricular tachycardia (VT) or preexcited SVT can be difficult. However, careful measurement always discloses definite irregularities. Moreover, very rapid and irregular VTs are usually unstable and quickly degenerate into VF. Thus, when a rapid, irregular wide QRS complex tachycardia is noted in a patient who has a reasonably stable hemodynamic state, preexcited AF is the most likely diagnosis.

The ability to conduct rapidly over an AV BT is determined primarily by the intrinsic conduction and refractoriness properties of the AV BT. However, as with AVN conduction, factors such as spatial and temporal characteristics of atrial wavefronts during AF, autonomic tone, and concealed conduction influence activation over the AV BT. Very rapid AV conduction during AF can occur in the presence of AV BTs with very short refractoriness, especially when normal conduction through the AVN and His-Purkinje system (HPS) is blocked (as occurs with AVN blocking drugs) and ventricular activation occurs only via the rapidly conducting BT, which would then eliminate retrograde concealment into the BT. This would result in extremely rapid ventricular rates, possibly more than 300 beats/min, which may occasionally degenerate into VF.

REGULAR VENTRICULAR RATE DURING ATRIAL FIBRILLATION. Regular ventricular rate during AF indicates associated abnormalities. A regular, slow ventricular rhythm during AF suggests a junctional, subjunctional, or ventricular rhythm, either as an escape mechanism with complete AV block or as an accelerated pacemaker activity with AV dissociation (see Fig. 9-27). Rarely, the R-R interval can be regularly irregular and show group beating with the combination of complete heart block and a lower nodal pacemaker with a Wenckebach type of exit block. Patients with severe underlying heart disease may develop the combination of AF and VT, leading to a rapid, regular, wide QRS complex tachycardia.

EFFECT OF DIGITALIS TOXICITY ON THE VENTRICULAR RESPONSE. With increasing degrees of digitalis toxicity, high-grade but not complete AV block during AF initially leads to single junctional, subjunctional, or ventricular escape beats.

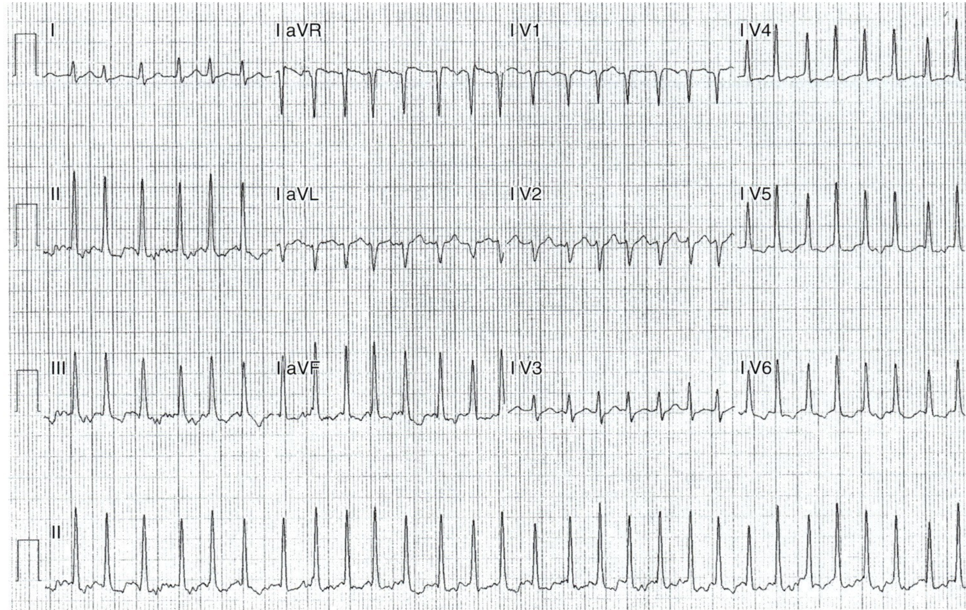

FIGURE 15-8 Surface ECG of atrial fibrillation with rapid ventricular response (207 beats/min) in a patient with septic shock on dopamine infusion.

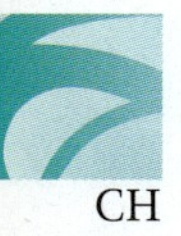

Higher degrees of AV block result in so few atrial impulses being conducted that the lower pacemaker takes over, thus leading to an escape junctional, subjunctional, or ventricular rhythm with a regular R-R interval for two or more cycles. On occasion, the junctional rate can increase, possibly because of digitalis-induced triggered activity, and it is called nonparoxysmal junctional tachycardia. Increasing digitalis toxicity can result in a Wenckebach exit block and give the appearance of an irregular ventricular rhythm with restoration of AF conduction, but the rhythm shows repetitive group beating as a result of the exit block. Complete AV block is marked by a regular escape rhythm with no conducted beats, a finding that may lead to the erroneous assumption that the patient has converted to NSR. Infrequently, impulses from the lower pacemaker travel alternately down the right and left bundle branches or alternate fascicles of the left bundle branch, resulting in a bidirectional tachycardia. This arrhythmia, which is also frequently a reflection of marked digitalis toxicity, may appear to be ventricular bigeminy. In true bigeminy, however, the ventricular beat in the bigeminal pattern is premature. In comparison, the R-R interval is regular with a bidirectional tachycardia, because all the beats arise from a single pacemaker.

QRS Morphology

The QRS complexes during AF are narrow and normal unless AV conduction is abnormal because of functional (rate-related) aberration, preexisting bundle branch block (BBB; see Fig. 15-6), or preexcitation over an AV BT (see Fig. 15-9).

Aberrant conduction commonly occurs during AF. Aberrancy is caused by the physiological changes of the conduction system refractory periods that are associated with sudden changes in heart rate. The refractoriness of the HPS tissue is directly related to the preceding R-R interval. Thus, there can be aberrant conduction as the result of a long R-R interval followed by a short cycle. In this scenario, the refractory period of the bundles increases during the long R-R interval (long cycle). The QRS complex that ends the long pause will be conducted normally but is followed by a prolonged refractory period of the bundle branches. If the next QRS complex occurs after a short coupling interval, it can be conducted aberrantly because one of the bundle branches is still refractory as a result of a lengthening of the refractory period (the Ashman phenomenon). The gross irregularity of ventricular response during AF yields an abundance of different R-R intervals; therefore, the long-short cycle sequence occurs commonly, and the Ashman phenomenon is seen frequently during AF. Right BBB (RBBB) aberrancy is more common than left BBB (LBBB) aberrancy, because the right bundle branch has a longer refractory period at slower heart rates. The left anterior fascicle is also frequently involved, often in combination with RBBB. In contrast, functional aberration is uncommon in the HB, the left posterior fascicle, or the main left bundle. Moreover, CLs preceding the pause may also affect the chance for aberrancy after the pause.

The aberrancy caused by the Ashman phenomenon can be present for one beat and have a morphology that resembles a premature ventricular complex (PVC), or it can involve several sequential complexes, suggesting VT. The persistence of aberrancy may reflect a time-dependent adjustment of refractoriness of the

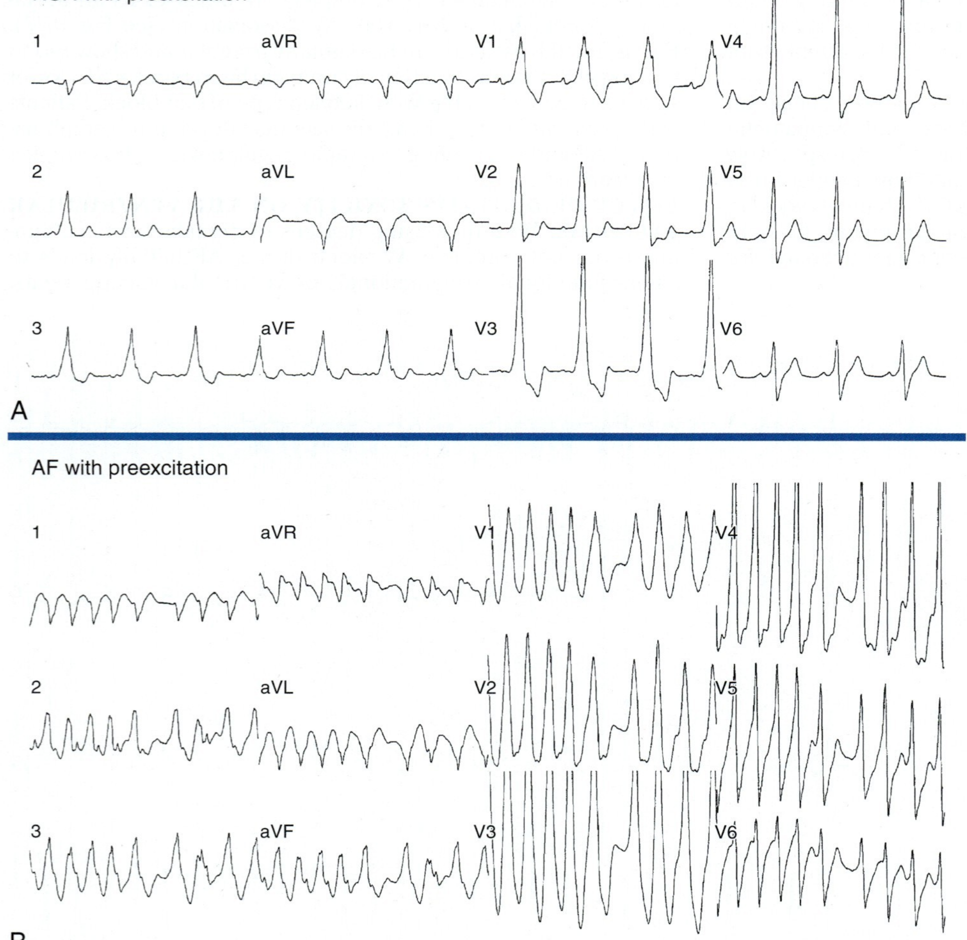

FIGURE 15-9 Preexcited atrial fibrillation (AF). **A,** ECG showing normal sinus rhythm (NSR) with a Wolff-Parkinson-White pattern and preexcitation using a left lateral bypass tract (BT). **B,** ECG showing preexcited AF (i.e., AF with conduction over the BT).

bundle branch to an abrupt change in CL, or it may be the result of concealed transseptal activation.

Although functional BBB is common in AF, PVCs are even more frequent, and it is important to differentiate between aberrant ventricular conduction and VT when repetitive wide QRS complexes occur during AF. The presence or absence of a long-short cycle sequence may not be helpful in differentiating aberration from ectopy for two reasons. Although a long cycle (pause) sets the stage for the Ashman phenomenon, it also tends to precipitate ventricular ectopy. Moreover, concealed conduction occurs frequently during AF, and therefore it is never possible to determine exactly when a bundle branch is activated from the surface ECG.

The proper diagnosis of aberrant conduction is a continuing challenge, but it can usually be accomplished by careful analysis of the rhythm strip and application of certain criteria. An aberrantly conducted beat caused by BBB generally has the pattern of a classic bundle branch or fascicular block. A PVC is usually followed by a longer R-R cycle, indicating the occurrence of a compensatory pause, the result of retrograde conduction into the AVN and anterograde block of the impulse originating in the atrium. The presence of long R-R cycles after the wide QRS complex that have identical CLs also suggests a ventricular origin (see Fig. 10-3). Furthermore, the absence of a long-short cycle sequence associated with the wide or aberrant QRS complex suggests that it is of ventricular origin. Aberrancy is not present if, with inspection of a long ECG rhythm strip, there are R-R interval combinations that are longer and shorter than those associated with the wide QRS complex. Also, a ventricular origin is likely if there is a fixed coupling interval between the normal and wide QRS complexes (Fig. 15-10).

Catheter Ablation of Atrial Fibrillation

Evolution

Since 1990, catheter ablation for the treatment of AF has evolved from an investigational procedure to one that is now performed on thousands of patients annually in many medical centers worldwide. The growing acceptance of this procedure has been brought about by a steadily increasing number of reports showing the safety and efficacy of catheter ablation of AF targeting the PVs and posterior LA.

CATHETER ABLATION OF ATRIAL FIBRILLATION: SUBSTRATE MODIFICATION

Cox and colleagues developed a series of techniques for the surgical disruption of AF. The final iteration, the maze III procedure, was based on a model of AF in which maintenance of the arrhythmia requires persistence of a critical number of circulating wavelets of reentry, each of which requires a critical mass of atrial tissue to sustain it. The concept behind the maze III, in which a series of complete, transmural incisions are made in the left and right atria, was that by dividing the atria into small enough electrically isolated compartments, reentrant activity was no longer possible and maintenance of AF could be prevented, regardless of the mode of initiation. However, application of the maze III operation has been limited by the morbidity and risk associated with sternotomy-thoracotomy and cardiopulmonary bypass, as well as by limited adoption by cardiothoracic surgeons. With the success of the Cox-maze procedure, multiple variations of the procedure have been performed, most of which have involved the use of a smaller lesion set. The LA lesion set was found to be fairly adequate to prevent AF, whereas RA lesions were required to prevent the development of AFL. Isolation of the PVs and posterior LA was a feature common to all successful iterations of the maze procedure. Therefore, this and other similar compartmentalization procedures have evolved over time and now predominantly involve the LA. In general, all these approaches have lower success rates than the maze III procedure.[64,65]

The success of surgical linear lesions led to the development of the catheter-based approach to perform linear ablation. Initial attempts at delivering long lines of RF ablation aimed at mimicking the lines of the surgical maze. Schwartz and associates reported recreation of the maze III lesion set in a small series of patients by using specially designed sheaths and standard RF catheters.[69] Although the efficacy was modest, complication rates were high, and procedure and fluoroscopy times were exceedingly long, this

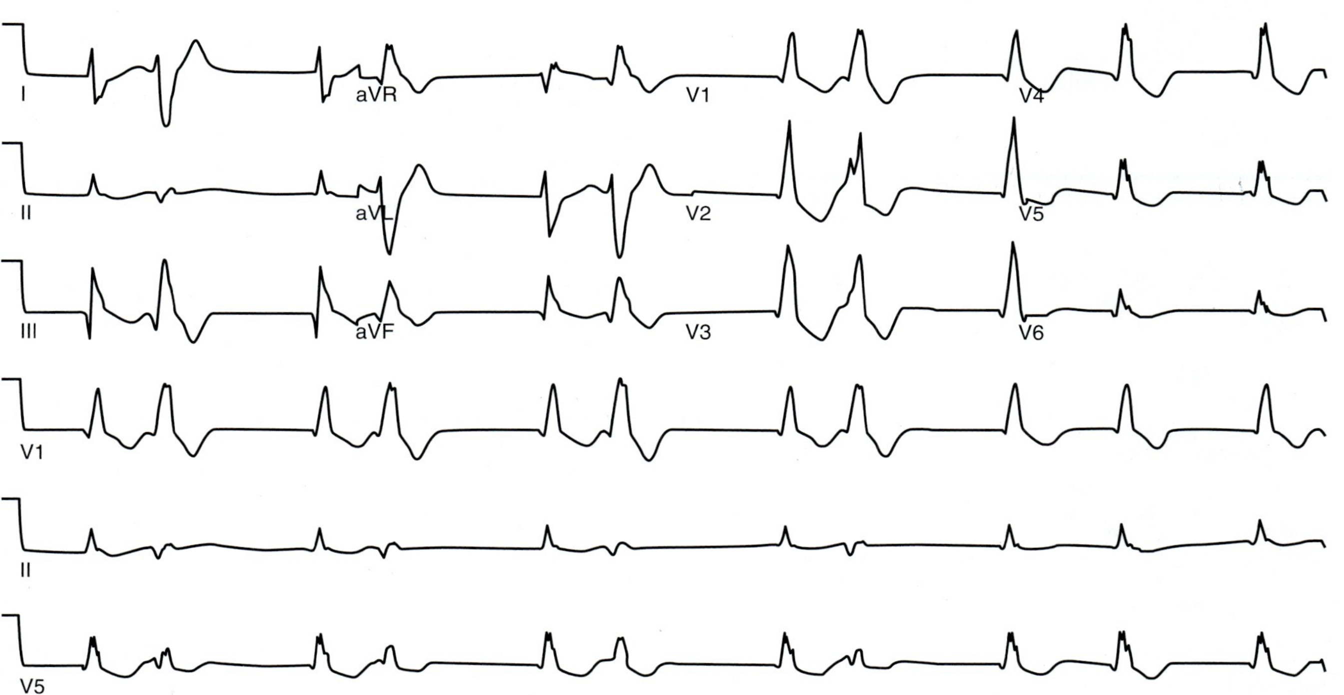

FIGURE 15-10 Surface ECG of atrial fibrillation with right bundle branch block. Ventricular bigeminy is present. Note the fixed coupling interval of the premature ventricular complexes (PVCs). Also, QRS morphology during PVCs is different from that during conducted AF complexes and is inconsistent with aberration.

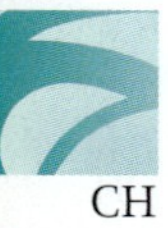

report demonstrated a proof of concept that led others to try to improve the catheter-based approach. Further refinement of the linear catheter ablation technique involved creating a series of ablation lesions using RF catheters to create specific lesion sets in the RA (two lines) and LA (three or four lines). The RA lesion sets consisted of an intercaval line along the interatrial septum and a cavotricuspid isthmus line to prevent AFL. LA lesions were designed to connect the four PVs to each other and to the mitral annulus. As increasing evidence emerged regarding the importance of the LA in the maintenance of AF, ablation targets became limited to the LA.

In the late 1990s, Pappone and coworkers developed the wide-area circumferential ablation approach using three-dimensional (3-D) electroanatomical mapping.[70] RF ablation was performed circumferentially around ipsilateral PVs, with the endpoint of ablation being the absence or marked reduction (80%) in the amplitude of electrical signals within the encircling lesions (Fig. 15-11). Despite lack of evidence showing that PVs treated in this way are electrically isolated from the LA, this group began reporting results for paroxysmal AF which were just as good as or better than those working with the ostial segmental PV isolation approach (see later). Furthermore, patients with persistent or permanent AF treated with the Pappone approach achieved freedom from AF almost as good as in patients with paroxysmal AF and far better than reports of patients treated with segmental PV isolation. Further improvements have required a strategy closer to the surgical maze—that is, lines to connect the ipsilateral pairs of the PVs and a line to link the left PV encircling lesion to the mitral annulus, which can be described as the *catheter maze*. Such lines further improved the outcomes of paroxysmal AF and have produced good results for ablation of longstanding persistent AF as well. It became clear that producing lines with proven transmural conduction block leads to a lower rate of recurrence of AF. However, achieving this is technically challenging and requires long, arduous procedures. Also, gaps in these lines could promote macroreentrant AT.[71]

More recently, fractionated electrograms and autonomic responses have been used to guide substrate modification for AF ablation (see Fig. 15-11).[72-74] The ablation of all fractionated electrograms in the RA and LA was based on the hypothesis that these are consistent sites where fibrillating wavefronts turn or split. By ablating these areas, the propagating random wavefronts are progressively restricted until the atria can no longer support AF. Other studies have also provided strong presumptive evidence that hyperactivity of the intrinsic autonomic nervous system constitutes a dysautonomia that can lead to a greater propensity for AF, both paroxysmal and sustained forms. Targeting autonomic nerves at a few specific sites on the heart that are directly related to arrhythmia formation may help limit the extent of damage to healthy myocardium while curtailing the ability to induce or maintain AF.[75,76]

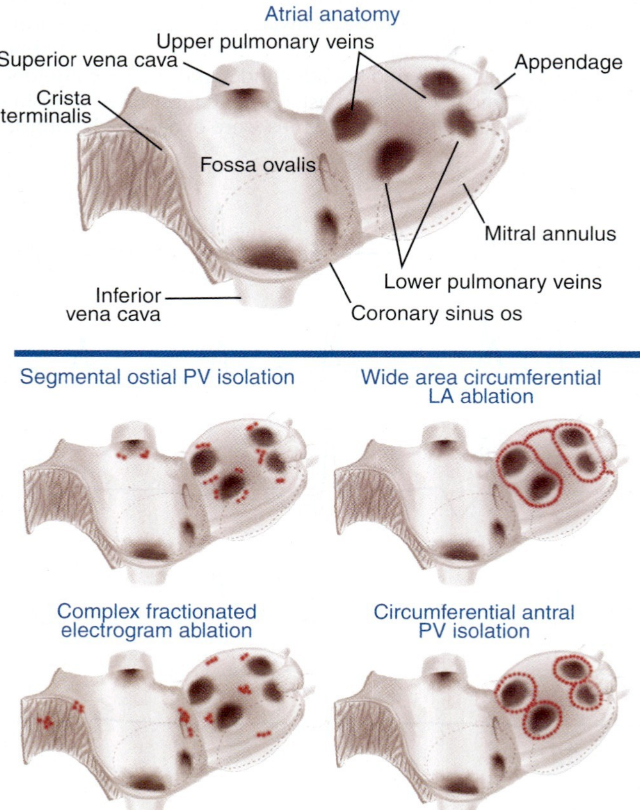

FIGURE 15-11 Catheter ablation of atrial fibrillation (AF). Atrial anatomy is shown at top; both atria are opened and viewed from the front. Various procedures for catheter ablation of AF are shown (red dots are ablation lesions). See text for further discussion. LA = left atrium; PV = pulmonary vein.

CATHETER ABLATION OF ATRIAL FIBRILLATION: ELIMINATION OF TRIGGERS

FOCAL ABLATION OF TRIGGERS. The landmark publication of Haissaguerre and colleagues in 1998 demonstrated that paroxysmal episodes of AF are consistently initiated by spontaneous triggers or atrial extrasystoles.[4] Remarkably, 94% of those triggers originated within the PVs, most within 2 to 4 cm of the ostium. The EP basis of these focal sources appeared to be the sleeves of LA muscle investing the PVs. One or more veins developed abnormal, paroxysmal, rapid automaticity, triggering AF as a result. AF was initiated with a burst of rapid firing from the foci and was abolished with RF ablation at the site of origin. The initial technique was to identify and ablate the culprit focus within the PV, but this approach was limited by the complication of PV stenosis and the recognition that multiple veins are involved in most patients, which leads to frequent recurrences after a "successful" procedure. Moreover, it is frequently difficult to elicit PV arrhythmia in the EP laboratory to allow adequate mapping and ablation.[4]

PULMONARY VEIN ISOLATION. Recognition of major limitations of focal ablation has led to the development of the PV electrical isolation technique. Recognizing that PV musculature conducts to LA musculature by discrete connections has allowed investigators to target those connections using multipolar catheters shaped into rings or baskets. Ablation is performed with a separate roving catheter at the site of earliest activation sequentially until PV electrical activity disappears or becomes dissociated from the LA activity (see Fig. 15-11). Using this strategy, between 20% and 60% of the PV circumference is targeted by ablation. PV isolation has the additional advantage of simultaneously treating all triggering foci within the vein, thereby obviating the need to elicit and map those foci individually. For the same reason, investigators were soon led to attempt to isolate as many PVs as possible at the initial ablation session. Comparative case series ultimately demonstrated that empirical isolation of the four PVs led to superior outcomes over isolating fewer veins.[36,37]

It was subsequently found that by ablating at or just outside the PV ostia, the incidence of PV stenosis could be reduced significantly. Using this approach, ablation is performed circumferentially around the antrum of each of the four PVs (see Fig. 15-11). In patients in whom the inferior and superior veins were closely spaced or shared a common ostium, a single large circumferential RF lesion set was performed.[77,78]

With further research, it was also observed that non-PV foci were an important source of AF in some patients, although percentages varied among different groups. Among the sources identified are the vein of Marshall, the CS, and the SVC, all of which are, like the PVs, thoracic veins. Targeting those triggers by electrical isolation of the involved thoracic veins has been attempted in selected patients.[79]

Periprocedural Management

ANTIARRHYTHMIC AGENTS

Antiarrhythmic medications are frequently stopped more than 5 days (more than five half-lives) before the ablation procedure because they can suppress spontaneous firing and fractionation of the electrograms that can be used to guide ablation. However, a longer period (approximately 6 months) is required for amiodarone, which may not be practical. Hence, amiodarone may be continued or discontinued before or after ablation.

One report suggested that, in patients with persistent AF, it may be reasonable to attempt electrical cardioversion and maintenance of sinus rhythm using antiarrhythmic medications as a prelude to ablation. Restoration of sinus rhythm, even for a relatively short time, can potentially result in reverse electrical atrial remodeling and hence improve the outcome of the ablation procedure.[80]

Continuing antiarrhythmic drug therapy after ablation can potentially reduce the incidence of early recurrences of symptomatic atrial arrhythmias and the need for cardioversion or hospitalization for arrhythmia management. However, this strategy does not seem to improve long-term freedom from AF. Therefore, it seems unnecessary to continue antiarrhythmic drug therapy following ablation with a view to the prevention of long-term arrhythmia recurrences. Nonetheless, the early short-term prophylactic use of antiarrhythmic drugs may be reasonable to help reduce morbidity.[81] Alternatively, antiarrhythmic treatment can be initiated in select patients, such as those with incomplete or unsuccessful ablation procedures and patients with early recurrences of AF or AFL after ablation.

In patients discharged with antiarrhythmic drug therapy, such therapy is usually discontinued after 1 to 3 months if no recurrence of AF is observed. In patients discharged without antiarrhythmic drug therapy who develop recurrent AF, antiarrhythmic drug therapy is initiated unless the patient is satisfied with the extent of symptomatic improvement or elects to undergo a repeat ablation procedure.

ANTICOAGULATION

Patients with a high risk of thromboembolism are anticoagulated with warfarin (INR, 2 to 3) for more than 4 to 6 weeks before the ablation procedure. Warfarin is usually stopped 2 to 5 days before the procedure, and replaced with enoxaparin or intravenous heparin once the INR is lower than 2.0. Enoxaparin is stopped 12 to 24 hours and heparin is stopped 4 to 6 hours before ablation (because transseptal catheterization is frequently required).

An alternative strategy is the continuation of warfarin at a therapeutic INR at the time of ablation without the use of heparin or enoxaparin for bridging. This approach appears to be a safe and efficacious periprocedural anticoagulation strategy and a potentially better alternative to strategies that use bridging with heparin or enoxaparin. The reasons are that it eliminates a period of inadequate anticoagulation immediately following the ablation procedure (a critical period for thromboembolic risk as a result of the inflammation and irritation associated with ablation), and it potentially reduces the risk of acute bleeding complications by obviating the need for heparin or enoxaparin therapy after ablation. Furthermore, a therapeutic INR at the time of the ablation procedure is associated with lower heparin requirements to achieve the target activated clotting time (ACT) and more consistent maintenance of a goal ACT value during the ablation procedure.[82,83]

Notably, continuation of warfarin through the ablation procedure was not associated with an increase in the incidence of cardiac tamponade. However, patients who developed pericardial effusion are likely to have a larger amount of blood removed from their pericardium for stabilization and require more blood transfusion units, but without an increase in the need to undergo emergency surgical exploration as compared with patients with normal INR levels. Nevertheless, this approach has been predominantly used by experienced operators, and the transseptal puncture is typically performed under the guidance of intracardiac echocardiography (ICE). Using this approach, warfarin is started (or continued) several weeks before ablation, and the INR is maintained at therapeutic levels. On the day of ablation, an INR of 2.0 to 4.0 is considered acceptable. TEE is performed in patients with a subtherapeutic INR in the 3 weeks prior to ablation. The procedure is cancelled in patients with an INR greater than 4.0.[82-85]

Once vascular access is achieved, intravenous heparin (bolus of 100 units/kg, then infusion of 10 units/kg/hr) is administered to all patients during the ablation procedure, even those fully anticoagulated with therapeutic INR at the time of the procedure. During the initial experience with AF ablation, anticoagulation with heparin was delayed until after the LA access had been achieved because of fear of complications with the transseptal puncture. Later, it became evident that such a strategy can allow thrombus formation on sheaths, catheters, and high-profile wires in the RA before transseptal puncture, and these thrombi could potentially travel to the LA. More recently, experienced operators have favored complete heparinization after vascular access, and clearly before transseptal puncture. The ACT should be checked at 10- to 15-minute intervals during the procedure and the heparin dose is adjusted to achieve an ACT of 300 to 400 seconds; then the ACT is checked at 30-minute intervals. To reduce the risk of bleeding complications, it is preferable to avoid antiplatelet therapy (especially glycoprotein IIb/IIIa receptor blockers and clopidogrel) if possible.[3]

At the conclusion of the ablation procedure, sheath removal requires interruption of anticoagulation to achieve adequate hemostasis. Heparin infusion can be discontinued and the sheaths removed when the ACT is less than 200 seconds. Alternatively, protamine can be administered to reverse heparin effects (1 mg of protamine for every 100 units of heparin received in the previous 2 hours). Warfarin is restarted after the procedure and is continued for a minimum of 2 to 3 months in all patients, regardless of stroke risk factors. Intravenous heparin (therapeutic loading doses) or subcutaneous enoxaparin (0.5 mg/kg twice daily) is administered 4 to 6 hours after sheath removal and continued until the INR reaches therapeutic levels. In patients undergoing the ablation procedure while fully anticoagulated with warfarin, no heparin or enoxaparin is required following ablation as long as INR levels are maintained in the therapeutic range.[84] In patients who have not taken warfarin before the procedure, it may be initiated the day of the procedure or even the day before, because the INR will not increase immediately. Bridging its effect with enoxaparin is routine in these cases. Alternatively, some centers use dabigatran at therapeutic doses starting at the time of sheath removal to minimize the duration of suboptimal anticoagulation. There are as yet no data on the safety and efficacy of the latter strategy.

When cardiac perforation or major bleeding occurs, protamine is administered intravenously to reverse the effects of heparin. For patients with therapeutic INR levels, fresh frozen plasma, vitamin K, and higher doses of protamine can be required for reversal of anticoagulation. Activated factor VII also can be used to reverse the effects of warfarin. Type and crossmatch for packed red blood cells and fresh frozen plasma should be universally performed and readily available to be infused, along with cardiothoracic surgical back-up if emergency interventions are needed.[84,85]

Decisions regarding the use of warfarin more than 2 to 3 months following ablation should be based on the patient's risk factors for stroke and not on the presence or absence of AF. Discontinuation of warfarin therapy after ablation is generally not recommended in patients who have a $CHADS_2$ score of 2 or higher.[3] Although one study showed that discontinuation of warfarin therapy 3 months after successful catheter ablation can be safe over medium-term follow-up in some subsets of patients, this was never confirmed by a large prospective randomized trial and therefore remains unproven.[3] Even when discontinuation of warfarin therapy is being considered, recurrences of AF should be excluded with confidence. Reliance only on symptoms as an indicator for AF recurrence or ambulatory monitoring can be misleading and can

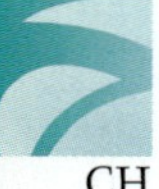

underestimate the incidence of recurrence. With transtelephonic ECGs, the rate of recurrent AF is much higher (28% versus 14% with serial ECG and Holter monitoring in one report). Moreover, a high rate of asymptomatic AF episodes, with some lasting more than 48 hours, has also been noted in patients with paroxysmal AF, even in patients who were significantly symptomatic before the ablation procedure. Therefore, without reliable documentation of the absence of AF recurrences, patients should be anticoagulated according to the guidelines for other patients with AF. The $CHADS_2$ or CHA_2DS_2-VASc score is recommended for risk stratification to determine which patients require long-term warfarin and which patients can be treated with aspirin. One exception is that patients who would be treated with aspirin receive warfarin anticoagulation for 2 to 3 months after the ablation procedure. In high-risk patients with previous stroke or other indications for anticoagulation, warfarin should be continued indefinitely. Some investigators have also suggested continuation of anticoagulation therapy if significant PV stenosis (more than 50%) is detected.

TRANSESOPHAGEAL ECHOCARDIOGRAPHY

TEE is performed in most patients undergoing AF ablation to screen for LA thrombus. Although it is optional in patients with paroxysmal AF and no structural heart disease, preablation TEE is often performed in patients who are in AF at the time of the procedure, regardless of the anticoagulation status prior to ablation. The presence of intracardiac thrombus should prompt cancellation of the procedure and mandate 4 to 8 more weeks of anticoagulation, followed by another TEE. The technique of 64-slice computed tomographic (CT) scanning has been used to identify LA thrombus, but TEE remains the gold standard.

Some reports suggested that a TEE may not be necessary in patients receiving warfarin therapy if therapeutic INR is present on the day of the procedure and has been verified every week in the 4 weeks preceding the ablation.[84] However, other studies reported a substantial prevalence of LA appendage clots (up to 3.6%) among patients with full anticoagulation and in those with paroxysmal AF and suggested that TEE should be performed in all patients prior to ablation. Therefore, until more data are available, the risk of a thromboembolic event must be weighed against relatively low risk of moderate sedation and TEE, by taking into consideration the type of AF (paroxysmal versus persistent), anticoagulation status, $CHADS_2$ score, LA diameter, and LV function. At this time, it may be reasonable to perform TEE in all patients, with the possible exception of those with paroxysmal AF *and* a $CHADS_2$ score of 0.[86,87]

CARDIAC MONITORING

Patients are generally hospitalized the night after the procedure, with cardiac monitoring, and discharged home the following day. After discharge, patients who report symptoms compatible with an arrhythmia should undergo ambulatory cardiac monitoring. Because early recurrences of atrial arrhythmias are common during the first 1 to 3 months following ablation and many of them resolve spontaneously, arrhythmia monitoring to assess the efficacy of the ablation procedure is typically delayed for at least 3 months following ablation. Periodic Holter monitoring to screen for asymptomatic occurrences of atrial arrhythmias can be considered. Event monitoring, even in asymptomatic patients, can also help screen for recurrent episodes of AF. The patient is encouraged to activate the event monitor whenever he or she develops symptoms and randomly a few times a day. Patients are also encouraged to take their pulse periodically and monitor for irregularity. Twelve-lead ECGs should be obtained at all follow-up visits.[3]

PULMONARY VEIN IMAGING

MRI or contrast-enhanced, multislice CT scanning of the LA with 3-D reconstruction is performed to define the anatomy of the PVs before the procedure (see Figs. 15-3 and 15-4). After ablation, CT or MRI is important to evaluate for evidence of PV stenosis in patients in whom there is a clinical suspicion. Although many investigators recommend routine follow-up imaging for detection of asymptomatic PV stenosis 3 to 4 months after ablation of AF, it is unknown whether early diagnosis and treatment of asymptomatic PV stenosis provide any long-term advantage to the patient.[88] Nevertheless, follow-up PV imaging should be considered during the initial experience of a new AF ablation procedure for quality assurance.

Technical Aspects Common to Different Methods of Ablation

SEDATION DURING ABLATION

In most patients, conscious sedation or general anesthesia is used; the choice is determined by the institutional preference and also by assessment of the patient's suitability for conscious sedation. General anesthesia is typically used for patients at risk of airway obstruction, those with history of sleep apnea, and those at increased risk of pulmonary edema. General anesthesia may also be used electively in healthy patients to improve patient tolerance of the procedure.[3]

LEFT ATRIAL ACCESS

Mapping and ablation in the LA are performed through a transseptal approach. A search for a patent foramen ovale is initially performed. If one is absent, a transseptal puncture is performed (see detailed discussion in Chap. 4). Generally, one or two transseptal punctures are performed under fluoroscopic (with or without ICE) guidance, and one or two long vascular sheaths (SR0, SL1, or Mullins sheath, St. Jude Medical, Minnetonka, Minn.) are introduced into the LA. The long sheaths are flushed with heparinized saline at a low infusion rate during the entire procedure, whether or not they are withdrawn into the RA during the LA mapping and ablation portion of the procedure.

IDENTIFICATION OF THE PULMONARY VEINS

Initial approaches of focal ablation targeting arrhythmic foci within the PVs were associated with high incidences of PV stenosis. To avoid this serious complication, the ablation procedure has evolved over time to an increasingly proximal ablation, first at the venous ostium or venoatrial junction and most recently proximal to the PV to encompass the antral region. However, the more proximal ablation approaches require correct identification of the ostia and PV-LA junction, and given the marked variation in PV anatomy, assessment of the number of PVs and anatomy of the ostia is essential when planning an ablation strategy. Various imaging techniques have been developed in an attempt to identify the PV ostium more accurately, but exact localization of this structure remains difficult, and the exact definition of the PV ostium varies, depending on the imaging modality used. Ultimately, however, the choice of imaging modality is dictated by local availability.

FLUOROSCOPY. Entry into the PV is clearly identified as the catheter leaves the cardiac shadow on fluoroscopy and electrical activity disappears; however, the ostium is located more proximally. The inferior portion of the PV ostia can be localized by advancing the catheter into the PV with downward deflection of the tip and then dragging back while fluoroscopically monitoring the drop off the ostial edge of the catheter.

IMPEDANCE MAPPING. Impedance monitoring can be used to identify the LA-PV junction. With catheter entry into the PV, the impedance usually rises to more than 140 to 150 Ω. At the PV ostium, the impedance typically is more than 4 Ω higher than the mean LA impedance.

PULMONARY VEIN ANGIOGRAPHY. PV angiography can be used at the time of catheter ablation to detail PV anatomy. Selective PV angiography is performed using a 5- to 10-mL hand injection of contrast medium through a long sheath (for angiography of right superior, left superior, and left inferior PVs) or NIH catheter (for angiography of right inferior PV; Fig. 15-12). Alternatively, PV angiography is performed by injecting contrast in the left and right pulmonary arteries or the pulmonary trunk; PVs are then assessed during the venous phase of pulmonary arteriography. A third technique used for PV angiography involves contrast injection in the body of the LA or at the roof of the right or left superior PV ostium immediately after administration of an adenosine intravenous bolus to induce AV block; the contrast medium will fill the LA body, PV antrum, and proximal part of the PV during the phase of ventricular asystole. An important limitation of PV angiography is that it images only the tubular portion and does not adequately define the full posterior extension of the PV. Studies of PV anatomy from pathological specimens and 3-D CT scans have shown that the PV is funnel-shaped, with a tube that fans out into a proximal cup that blends into the posterior atrial wall, referred to as the antrum. Furthermore, the PV antrum connects to the LA wall at an oblique angle. The posterior aspect of each PV is more proximal, whereas the anterior segments of the PVs are more distal.

INTRACARDIAC ECHOCARDIOGRAPHY. Phased-array ICE can be used to visualize the antrum and ostium of the PVs (see detailed discussion in Chap. 6). ICE has the advantage of providing real-time imaging of the PVs. In contrast to angiography, ICE can define the proximal edge of the PV antrum (see Fig. 6-22).

ELECTROANATOMICAL MAPPING. The CARTO (Biosense Webster, Inc., Diamond Bar, Calif.) and EnSite NavX (St. Jude Medical, St. Paul, Minn.) electroanatomical mapping systems have been used to construct a 3-D shell of the LA and identify the PVs. However, definition of the true PV ostium using these systems alone can be difficult because of variants in 3-D vein morphology.

COMBINING ELECTROANATOMICAL MAPPING SYSTEMS WITH CARDIAC CT OR MRI. Cardiac CT and MRI provide critical information regarding the number, location, and size of the PVs, which is needed in planning the ablation and selecting appropriately sized mapping and ablation devices. In addition, preacquired CT and MRI scans have the advantage of allowing full integration with 3-D mapping systems and real-time catheter navigation on a 3-D CT or MRI image, which can facilitate identification of PV ostia and ablation targets (see detailed discussion in Chap. 6).

CATHETERIZATION OF THE PULMONARY VEINS

In the anteroposterior fluoroscopic view, the PV ostia are situated on both sides of the spine. Clockwise rotation of the catheter inside the LA directs its tip posteriorly and toward the PVs. It is frequently necessary to apply clockwise torque to both the catheter and its long sheath. For catheterization of the left PVs, the catheter should be directed anteroposteriorly in the right anterior oblique (RAO) view and to the left in the left anterior oblique (LAO) view. Care must be taken to avoid advancing the catheter into the LA appendage, in which case the catheter is directed to the right (anteriorly) in the RAO view and not anteroposteriorly. Advancing a catheter into the LA appendage results in an increase in electrogram amplitude (rather than decreasing amplitude, when advancing into a PV). For catheterization of the right PVs, the catheter is rotated further clockwise and is directed to the right in the RAO view and anteroposteriorly in the LAO view. An alternative method for reaching the ostia of the right PVs is to loop the catheter around the lateral, inferior, and then septal LA walls, laying the catheter down along the wall, and dragging the catheter by withdrawing it along the posterior right ostia. Forming a tight loop with maximal deflection of the catheter and using rotational movements can provide greater stability during ablation, particularly at the anterior aspect of the PVs. Counterclockwise rotation of the catheter inside the LA would lead the catheter into the LV. Care must be taken not to allow the circular (Lasso) catheter to cross the mitral annulus because it can then become trapped with the mitral valve apparatus. Usually, reversal of the catheter movement (clockwise torque) that resulted in this situation helps correct it.

Focal Ablation of Pulmonary Vein Triggers

Rationale

There are two different types of arrhythmias that can play a role in generating AF, and both may be addressed by focal ablation. One type is a PAC (or runs of PACs) that triggers self-sustained AF (focal triggers). Ablation of a focal trigger does not terminate AF but prevents its reinitiation (see Fig. 15-1).[4,70] A second type is a focal tachycardia that either induces fibrillation in the atria or mimics AF by creating a pattern of rapid and irregular depolarization wavefronts in the atria. Such a tachycardia acts as a focal driver and is necessary for the continuation and maintenance of AF. Ablation of a focal driver results in the termination of AF and prevention of its reinitiation. Focal tachycardias that initiate or mimic AF can be recognized in the EP laboratory because they are frequently associated with exit block between the site of origin of the tachycardia and the rest of the atria (Fig. 15-13).[4]

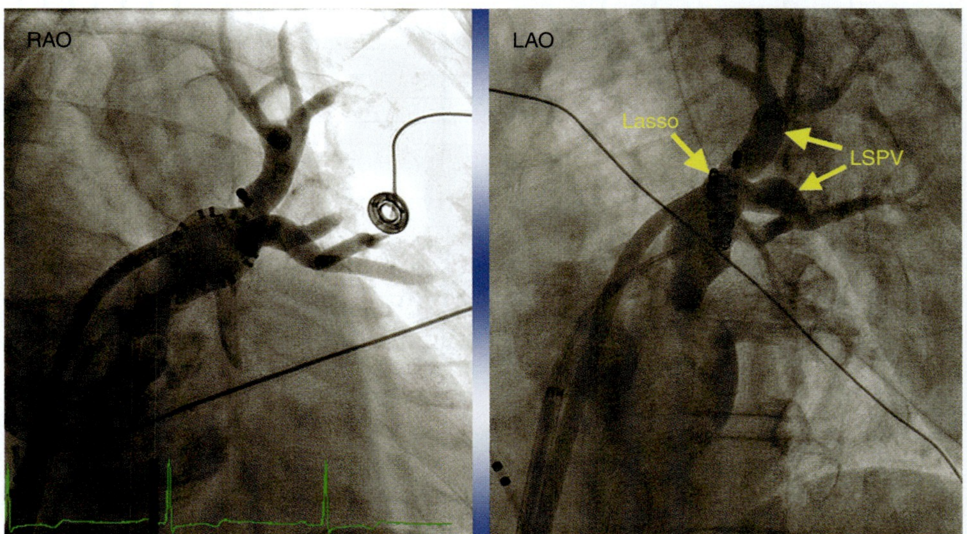

FIGURE 15-12 Pulmonary vein (PV) angiography. Fluoroscopic (right anterior oblique [RAO] and left anterior oblique [LAO]) views of the left superior PV (LSPV). The ring catheter is positioned at the PV ostium.

Several observations have provided evidence that the electrical activity that arises in the PVs plays a role in the maintenance of AF. By analyzing surface ECG and 24-hour Holter recordings, studies have shown that most paroxysmal AF episodes are initiated by a single PAC.[70] Although focal sources of AF may be found in the RA, LA, CS, SVC, or vein of Marshall, 94% of foci are located within a PV. It is possible that intermittent bursts of PV tachycardia serve to perpetuate AF in the same fashion as aconitine-induced rapid firing or bursts of rapid atrial pacing (see Fig. 15-13).[4]

There may be a subset of patients with focally induced AF in whom ablation of a single dominant focus can result in cure, without the need for empirical isolation of all PVs. A more limited ablation approach requires shorter procedure and fluoroscopy times and may be safer. These are important considerations in a relatively young patient population.

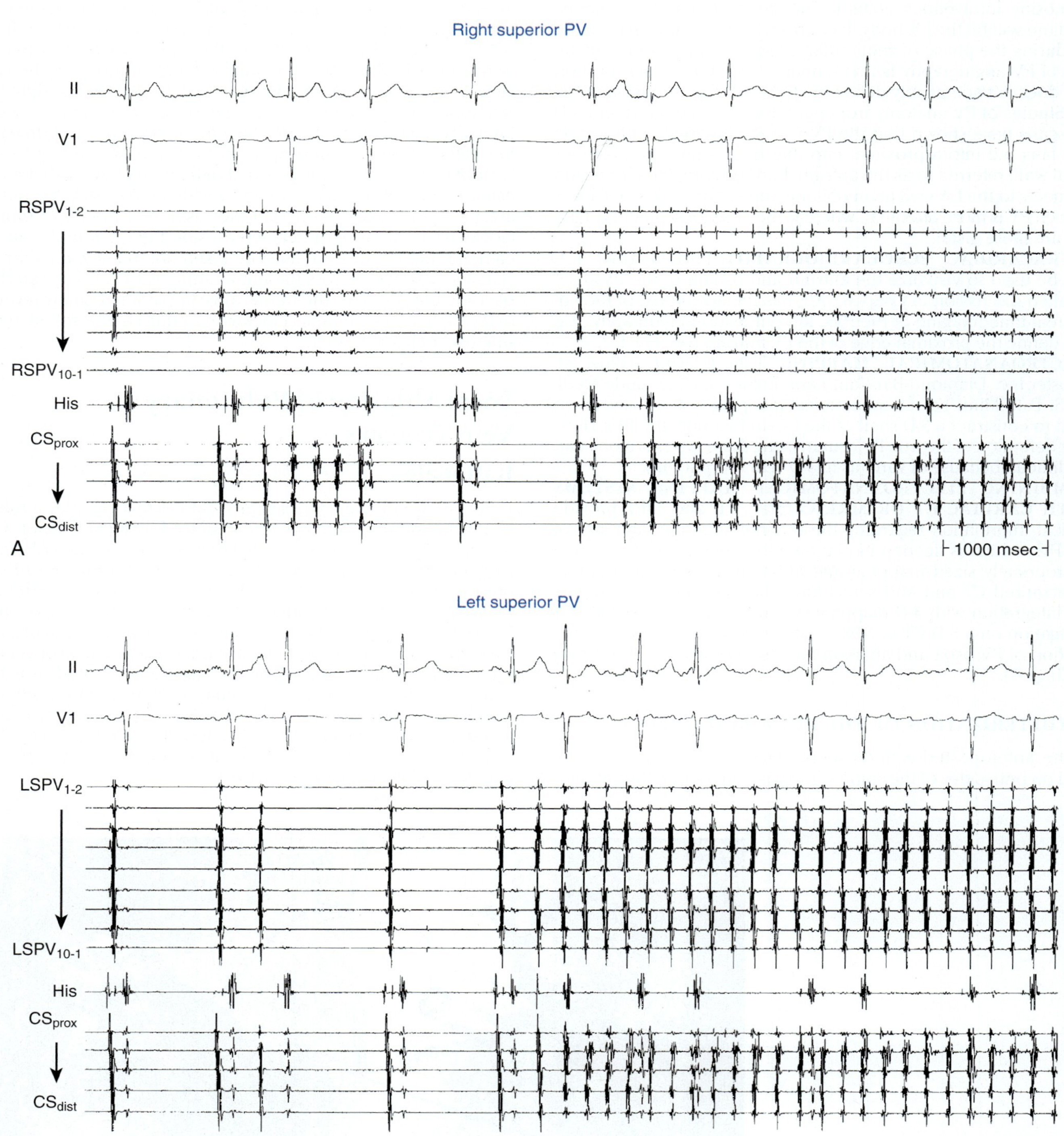

FIGURE 15-13 Atrial fibrillation (AF) initiation from the right superior pulmonary vein (RSPV). **A,** A burst of nonsustained PV tachycardia followed by a second sustained episode. Note that the local cycle length (CL) in the ring catheter recordings from the RSPV is significantly shorter than atrial CL recorded in the coronary sinus (CS) during AF, indicating that this PV is most probably the source and driver of AF. **B,** Recording from the left superior PV (LSPV) in the same patient during spontaneous initiation of AF showing LSPV activity with a CL similar to the atrial CL, a finding suggesting that this PV is activated passively. CS_{dist} = distal coronary sinus; CS_{prox} = proximal coronary sinus.

Identification of Arrhythmogenic Pulmonary Veins

DEFINITION OF AN ARRHYTHMOGENIC PULMONARY VEIN

An arrhythmogenic PV is defined by single or multiple ectopic discharges originating from the vein, with or without conduction to the LA. During ectopy from an arrhythmogenic PV, there is a reversal in activation sequence, from the distal PV trunk (source) to the ostium and LA (exit), with the PV potential preceding the LA potential (Figs. 15-14 and 15-15). Conversely, if the explored PV is not the origin of ectopy, it is passively activated, as in NSR, with a proximal-to-distal sequence and a PV potential after or fusing with the LA potential.[89]

Ectopic discharges with a short coupling interval may not be conducted to the LA, thus producing isolated PV potentials confined within the PV. These can be recognized as a PV potential coincident with or just after the ventricular electrogram and can be distinguished from a potential of ventricular origin by their spontaneous disappearance (intermittent PV potential) or suppression during atrial pacing.

During an episode of AF, rapid rhythms arising in the PVs (variably referred to as rapid focal activity, repetitive rapid activity, intermittent PV tachycardia, or paroxysmal CL shortening) are common and can play an important role in the maintenance of AF or may be markers of an arrhythmogenic PV that triggers AF during NSR. The CL of local activity within the arrhythmogenic PV is shorter than that of the atrium. In contrast, the local CL in passively activated PVs is similar to or longer than that of the atrium (see Fig. 15-13).

PROVOCATION OF PULMONARY VEIN ECTOPY

If PV ectopy does not spontaneously develop during EP monitoring or is not sufficiently sustained, one or a combination of several provocative maneuvers can be tried to induce the arrhythmia, including physiological procedures (e.g., Valsalva maneuvers, carotid sinus massage, or deep breathing), pharmacological agents (isoproterenol, 1 to 8 μg/min; and adenosine, rapid intravenous injection, 12 mg and then 18 mg, up to 20 to 60 mg), and slow-rate atrial pacing (bursts of 3 to 10 stimuli at 100 to 200 beats/min for postpause ectopy). Additionally, in patients who present with AF at the time of ablation, electrical cardioversion of AF can reproducibly induce PACs from the same location as spontaneous PACs, and those PACs that follow cardioversion may reinitiate AF. In fact, there is a high degree of correlation between spontaneous and postcardioversion PACs or PACs inducing AF. If AF is not present at baseline, rapid burst atrial pacing to induce AF, followed by electrical cardioversion, may also be attempted to identify early postcardioversion PV triggers.[89]

Mapping of Pulmonary Vein Ectopy

ECG LOCALIZATION OF PULMONARY VEIN ECTOPY

ATs arising from the PVs are characterized by entirely positive P waves in lead V_1 in 100% of cases, isoelectric or negative in aVL in 86%, and negative in lead aVR in 96%; lead aVL can be biphasic or positive in right-sided PV ATs (Fig. 15-16).[90]

Left PV ATs have several characteristics (as compared with right PV ATs), including positive notching in the P waves in two or more surface leads, isoelectric or negative P wave in lead I, P wave

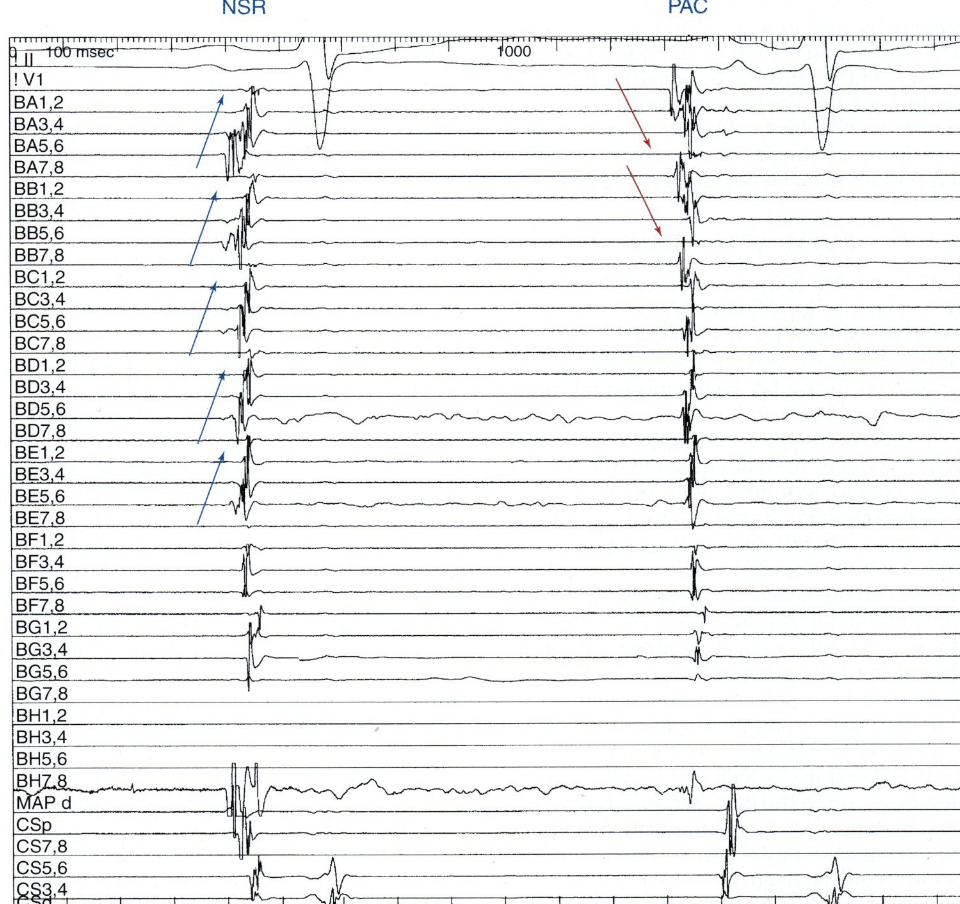

FIGURE 15-14 Mapping of pulmonary vein (PV) ectopy using a basket catheter. The basket catheter is positioned in the left superior PV. Bipolar recordings are obtained from the eight electrodes (1-2, 3-4, 5-6, 7-8) on each of the eight splines (BA through BH) of the basket catheter. **Left,** During normal sinus rhythm (NSR), PV activation propagates from proximal (ostial) to distal, as reflected by earlier activation timing on the proximal basket electrodes than the distal ones (blue arrows). **Right,** In contrast, during a premature atrial complex (PAC) originating from this PV, activation occurs earliest deep in the vein and progressively later toward the ostium and the left atrial (LA) exit, resulting in distal to proximal venous activation on the basket catheter recordings (red arrows). Note that the PV potentials precede the onset of the P wave on the surface ECG during PV ectopy, but they occur late after P wave onset during NSR.

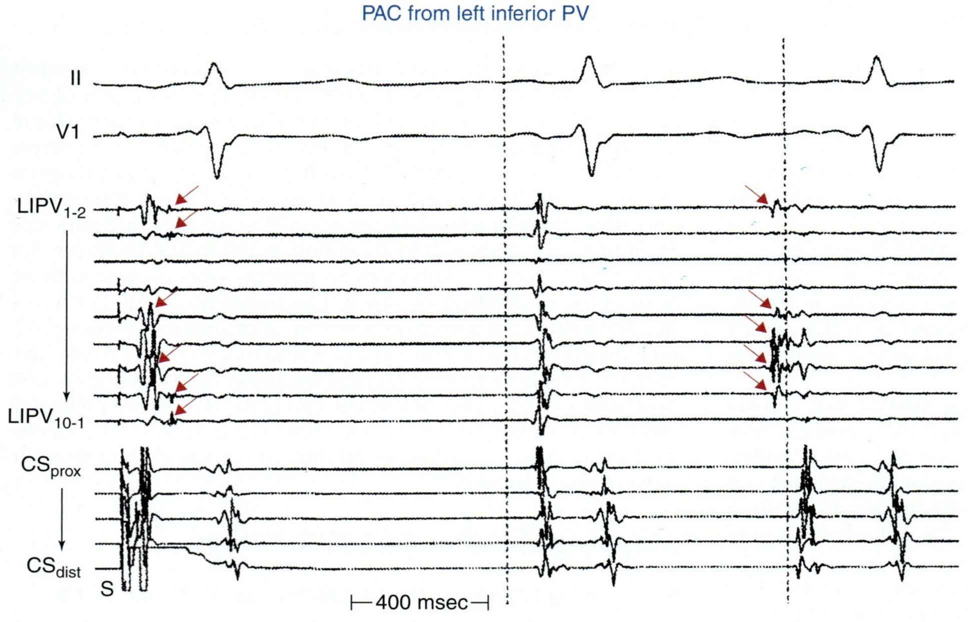

FIGURE 15-15 Mapping pulmonary vein (PV) ectopy using a ring catheter. The ring catheter is positioned at the ostium of the left inferior PV (LIPV). **Left,** During pacing from the distal coronary sinus (CS) (at left), PV potentials (red arrows) follow the left atrium (LA) potentials. During normal sinus rhythm (NSR; middle complex), LA and PV potentials overlap, and they occur in the second half of the P wave. **Right,** During a premature atrial complex (PAC) originating from the LIPV, reversal of the electrogram sequence in the ring catheter recording is observed, with the PV potentials (red arrows) preceding the LA potentials and occurring well before the onset of the P wave on the surface ECG (dashed line). CS_{dist} = distal coronary sinus; CS_{prox} = proximal coronary sinus.

amplitude in the lead III/II ratio greater than 0.8, and broad P waves in lead V1 (see Fig. 15-16).

ATs arising from superior PVs have larger amplitude P waves in inferior leads than those in ATs arising from inferior PVs (see Fig. 15-16). However, P wave morphology generally is of greater accuracy in distinguishing right-sided from left-sided veins, in contrast to superior from inferior.

During right superior PV ATs, the P waves are narrow, positive in inferior leads, of equal amplitude in leads II and III, biphasic or slightly positive in lead V_1, and isoelectric in lead I (see Fig. 15-16). The right superior PV is a common site of origin for LA ATs. It is only a few centimeters from the sinus node. Activation rapidly crosses the septum via the Bachmann bundle to activate the RA in a fashion similar to NSR, thus explaining the similarities in P wave morphology. However, whereas the P wave is biphasic in lead V_1 during NSR, it is positive in that lead during right superior PV AT (see Fig. 15-16).[90]

ENDOCARDIAL ACTIVATION MAPPING

Initially, the PV of interest is identified based on earliest activation of triggers in the CS and RA catheters. If no sharp bipolar activity is recorded in the RA at least 10 milliseconds before the onset of the ectopic P wave, the ectopic beats are considered to have originated in the LA. Following initial identification, the ablation catheter is placed and maneuvered to the appropriate PV.

Activation mapping within the PV is performed during ectopy. It is important to have adequate frequency of PACs from each focus, to be able to acquire enough points and identify the earliest activation sequence. Electroanatomical mapping or multielectrode mapping catheters, such as the ring catheter (a decapolar catheter with a distal ring configuration) or basket catheter positioned in the PV, can be of value in mapping the source of ectopy (Fig. 15-17). The ectopic focus is localized inside the selected PV according to the earliest atrial activity relative to the reference electrogram or the onset of the ectopic P wave. PV depolarization during ectopy is marked by a spike (an electrogram of sharp onset and short duration) preceding the onset of the ectopic P wave by 106 ± 24 milliseconds (range, 40 to 160 milliseconds; see Figs. 15-14 and 15-15). The spike is typically localized, and its amplitude rapidly decreases when the catheter tip is turned or moved a few millimeters. Bystander or far-field activity from contiguous branches can be distinguished by temporal delay or lower amplitude. The spike occurs earliest deep in the vein and progressively later toward the ostium and LA exit, thus resulting in distal-to-proximal venous activation during multipolar recordings (see Fig. 15-14). A second electrogram component with a slow deflection (depolarization rate [dV/dt] of less than 0.5 mV/msec), reflecting later LA activation, is temporally distinct from the spike inside the vein and then approaches and becomes continuous with the spike at the ostium.

Mechanically induced beats can be prevented by avoiding manipulation of the catheters during the recordings. These beats are excluded by comparing the ECG pattern and intracardiac activation sequence with the confirmed spontaneous ectopic beats.

If still insufficient spontaneous or induced ectopy is present, focal mapping and ablation of AF can become difficult. In these cases, the use of a multielectrode basket catheter mapping (see Fig. 15-14) or noncontact mapping (EnSite) system can map a single beat and help identify the origin of spontaneously occurring PACs and PACs induced following the cardioversion of spontaneous or induced AF.

Following successful ablation of the initially targeted PV triggers, a second PV is usually targeted if there are either significant spontaneous isolated PACs (at least five per minute), at least two separate PACs inducing AF, or PACs originating from the same PV inducing AF following cardioversion on at least two occasions.

Target of Ablation

The site showing the earliest atrial activity relative to the reference electrogram or onset of the ectopic P wave is targeted by ablation. If more than one PV is arrhythmogenic, the PV producing the most repetitive ectopy and/or AF-triggering ectopy is targeted first. If ablation of the ectopic focus fails, electrical isolation of the arrhythmogenic PV should be considered (see later). In addition, ablation may be performed at sites with catheter-induced repetitive ectopy, manifesting as a burst of rapid PACs starting on touching the wall, sustained irritability while at the site, and acute termination of rapid activity on release of the catheter.[89]

Ablation Technique

RF energy is delivered using a 4-mm-tip catheter with a target temperature of 45°C to 50°C and a maximal power output of 25 to 30 W to reduce the risk of PV stenosis. At successful ablation sites, a rapid burst of PACs originating from that site often develops during RF energy delivery, or an abrupt disappearance of triggering PACs is observed.[89] Cryoablation has also been used to target these sites although the precision of mapping is less (6-mm catheter tip).

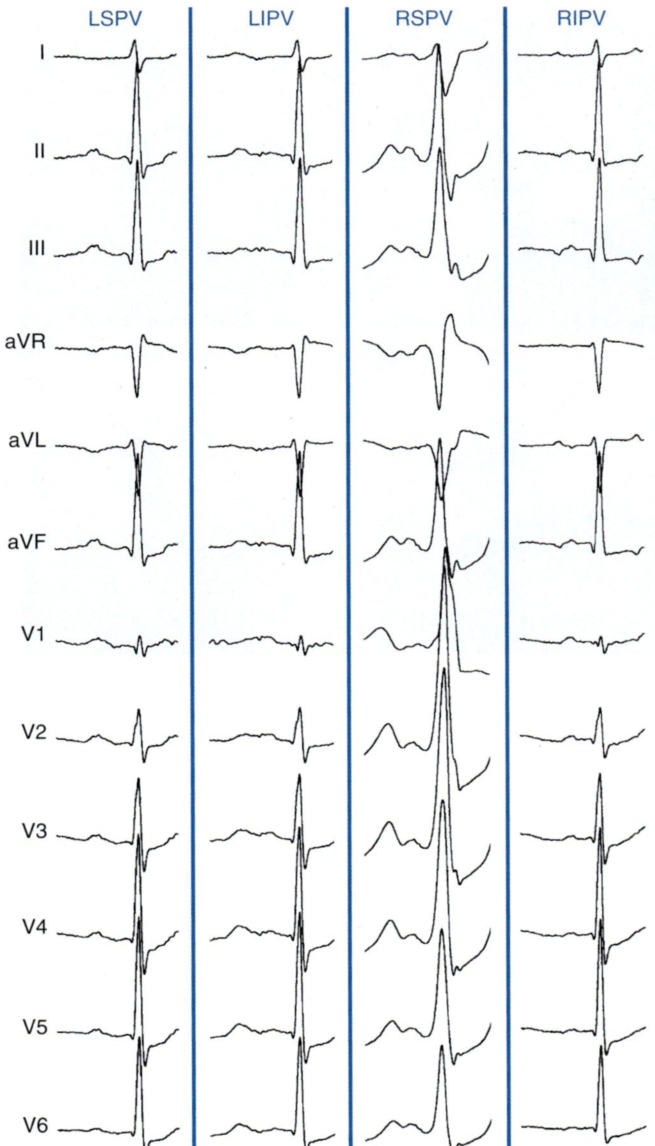

FIGURE 15-16 Surface ECG of spontaneous premature atrial complexes originating from the pulmonary veins. LIPV = left inferior pulmonary vein; LSPV = left superior pulmonary vein; RIPV = right inferior pulmonary vein; RSPV = right superior pulmonary vein.

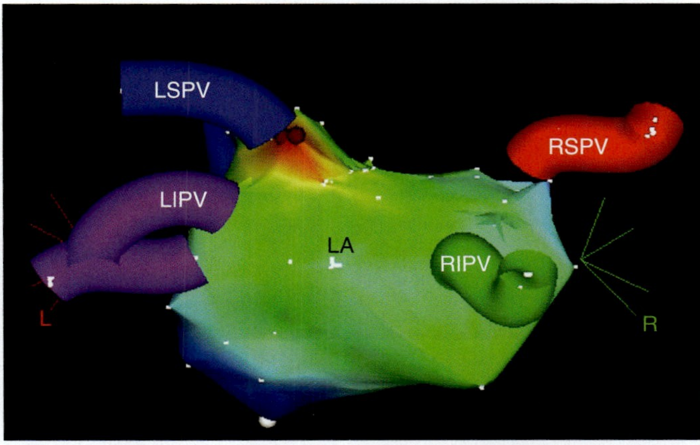

FIGURE 15-17 CARTO (Biosense Webster, Inc., Diamond Bar, Calif.) activation map of the left atrium (LA) (posteroanterior view) during premature atrial complexes (PACs) originating from the left superior pulmonary vein (LSPV). Focal ablation (red dots) at the PV ostium eliminated those PACs. LIPV = left inferior pulmonary vein; RIPV = right inferior pulmonary vein; RSPV = right superior pulmonary vein.

Endpoints of Ablation

The endpoint is elimination of ectopy, spontaneous or induced by provocative maneuvers (using both the same provocative maneuvers and defibrillation protocols as before the ablation). Elimination or dissociation of PV potentials from atrial activity is also a satisfactory endpoint.

Outcome

Early experience with the focal ablation of PV arrhythmias has indicated that the recurrence rate is high and the success rate is only modest, even in experienced laboratories. The suboptimal results can be attributed to the limitations of the technique. Many patients have multiple foci in the same PV or in multiple PVs. Multiple arrhythmogenic PVs are usually associated with older age, longer AF duration, and larger atrial dimensions. In addition, there may be a paucity of spontaneous or inducible arrhythmias during the procedure. The spontaneous occurrence of ectopic beats and paroxysms of AF is unpredictable, and provocative procedures are not consistently effective. Mapping can also be made difficult by frequent recurrences of persistent AF requiring multiple cardioversions. Furthermore, after a successful procedure, new foci may emerge. Remapping usually shows new foci in the ablated vein or in other veins, rather than recurrence of the original focus.

It is also important to recognize that RF ablation inside the PVs carries a significant risk of PV stenosis, which limits the amount of RF energy that can be safely delivered within a PV. Some degree of PV stenosis was detected by increased PV flow velocity on TEE in 42% of cases in one report. An increased risk of PV stenosis has been associated with the use of RF power more than 45 W.

Focal ablation has been successful only in highly selected patients with frequently recurring paroxysmal AF. Reported rates of a positive outcome using a focal ablation approach to eliminate AF triggers have varied from 38% to 80%. AF recurrences appear to be related to recovery of initially targeted foci or emergence of new nontargeted ones in the same or in a different PV. Because of these safety and efficacy limitations, this method is generally not used currently.

Segmental Ostial Pulmonary Vein Isolation

Rationale

ELECTRICAL ISOLATION OF PULMONARY VEINS

On the basis of the knowledge of the AF initiation mechanism by focal discharges in the PVs, electrical disconnection at the PV ostium seemed to be a better ablative technique than focal ablation to inactivate focal triggers of AF. Ablation guided by mapping focal ectopy has a high recurrence rate and low long-term success and is limited by unpredictability, inconsistent inducibility, and the risk of inducing AF requiring cardioversion multiple times during the procedure. Moreover, the appearance of multiple sources of AF triggers and the high recurrence rate argue for more extensive ablation strategy. PV isolation has been introduced to address these issues.

PV potentials identify muscular sleeves that extend from the LA into the PVs. These muscular bands are responsible for transmitting triggering impulses from the vein to the LA. The myocardial fibers that envelop the PVs may not be present along the entire circumference of the PV ostia. Therefore, to eliminate conduction

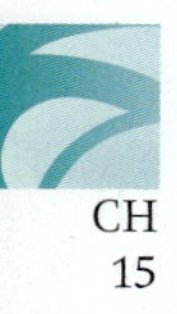

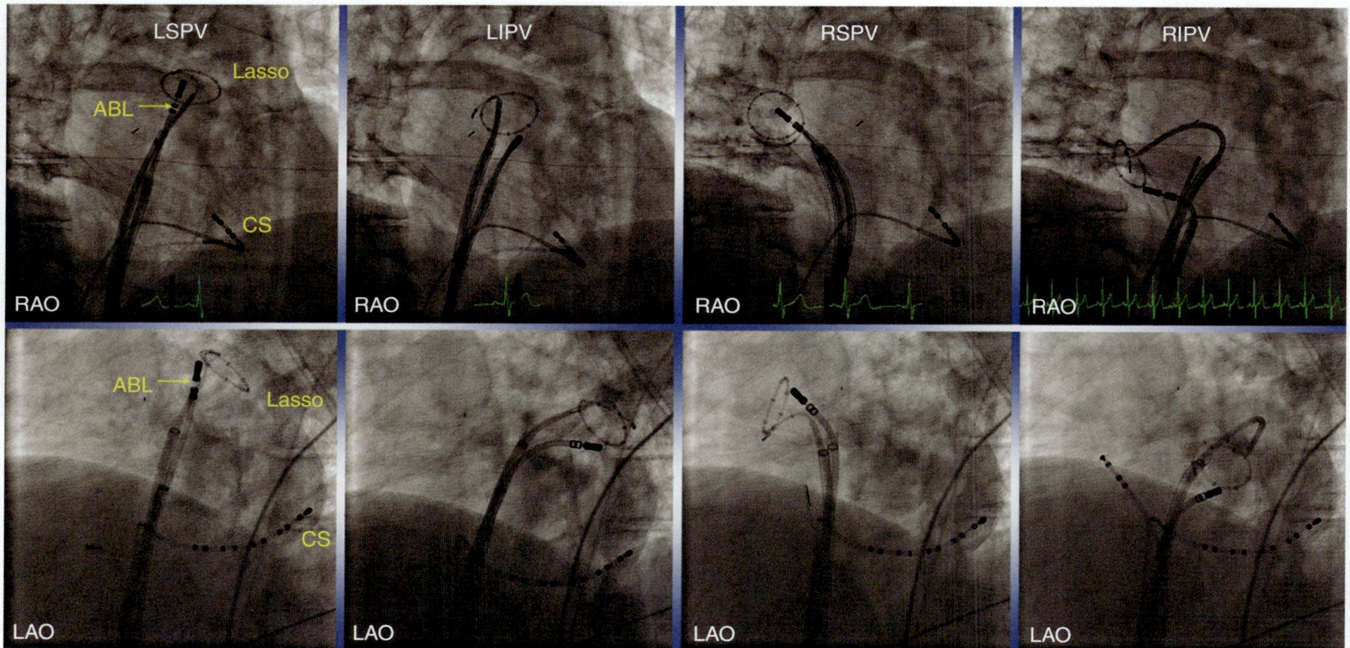

FIGURE 15-18 Fluoroscopy views (right anterior oblique [RAO] and left anterior oblique [LAO]) of the ring catheter positioned at the ostium of the four pulmonary veins (PVs). **Panels from left to right,** Left superior PV (LSPV), left inferior PV (LIPV), right superior PV (RSPV), and right inferior PV (RIPV). Note that during ablation, the ablation catheter (ABL) is always positioned at the atrial side of the ring catheter. CS, coronary sinus.

in and out of a PV, ablation along the entire circumference of the ostium may not be necessary. Instead, RF energy can be targeted to the segments of the ostium at which muscle fibers are present, which typically involves RF application to 30% to 80% of the circumference of the PVs. These sites are identified by the presence of high-frequency depolarizations, which likely represent PV muscle potentials.[89]

The major advantages of this technique are that it eliminates the need for detailed mapping of all PV foci and that there is a clear-cut endpoint of ablation, even when spontaneous arrhythmias are absent, and PV stenosis is far less likely to occur (although it is still possible).

WHICH PULMONARY VEINS TO ISOLATE

ONLY ARRHYTHMOGENIC PULMONARY VEINS. Focal ablation deep in a PV carries a risk of PV stenosis. Restricting RF delivery to the ostium of the arrhythmogenic PV, as in segmental ostial PV isolation, may help reduce this risk. Furthermore, a more limited ablation approach (as compared with isolation of all PVs) requires shorter procedure and fluoroscopy times and can potentially be safer.[89]

ALL FOUR PULMONARY VEINS. PV isolation of only the arrhythmogenic PV was shown to have a limited success rate. Furthermore, identification of the arrhythmogenic PV can be difficult and time consuming, because focal activity can be difficult to observe or induce during the ablation procedure. Additionally, the prevalence of multiple arrhythmogenic PVs is high (greater than 70%).[89] Therefore, isolation of only the culprit PV identified during the procedure may allow the emergence of focal ectopy from other PVs, which can potentially cause AF recurrence after the procedure. Moreover, electrical disconnection may not be achieved by ostial ablation to only the targeted PV in patients with electrical connections between the PVs (i.e., across the carina between left PVs).

Evidence has suggested that almost all PVs are capable of generating the premature depolarizations that trigger AF, and the upper PVs are responsible for most AF triggers (the left superior PV is the vein with the longest muscular sleeve). Only a few (0% to 30%) foci have been identified in the inferior PVs (the right inferior PV is the least important source of triggers). The relatively infrequent importance of the right inferior PV in patients with AF is consistent with prior anatomical studies demonstrating that the muscle sleeves around the right inferior PV are less prominent than the muscle sleeves that surround the other PVs. Although cannulation of the right inferior PV with a distal ring catheter electrode can be challenging in some patients, in most patients this vein can be successfully isolated with little prolongation in the total PV isolation procedural time. Therefore, unless no PV potentials are present at its ostium (a rare finding), all four PVs should be targeted, whenever feasible.

Circumferential Mapping of Pulmonary Vein Potentials

LASSO CATHETER MAPPING

A deflectable decapolar catheter with a distal ring configuration (Lasso catheter) is advanced sequentially into each PV and is used for ostial mapping (Fig. 15-18). The ring catheter enables circumferential mapping of the PV ostia perpendicular to the axis of the vein. Lasso catheters are of different sizes. The selection of a 15-, 20-, or 25-mm-diameter Lasso catheter is guided by the estimated size of the PVs angiographically and/or with CT (see Fig. 15-12). Because of the highly variable sizes of PV ostia, fixed-diameter catheters may not always achieve catheter stability and optimal electrogram recordings. In some cases, suboptimal positioning, poor wall contact, and poor stability of an inappropriately sized circumferential catheter underestimate the number of PV potentials and can result in failure to isolate the PV completely because of undetected residual PV-atrial electrical connections. Some of those issues can be addressed by using an expandable 15- to 25-mm-diameter ring catheter. The expandable ring catheter is introduced into each PV and withdrawn to the most proximal stable position, with optimal wall contact ensured by progressive loop expansion. These catheters may enable more proximal and stable placement and optimal wall contact at the PV ostia. This is important because the ablation target is not within the ostia, but in the atrial tissue proximal to the LA-PV junction.

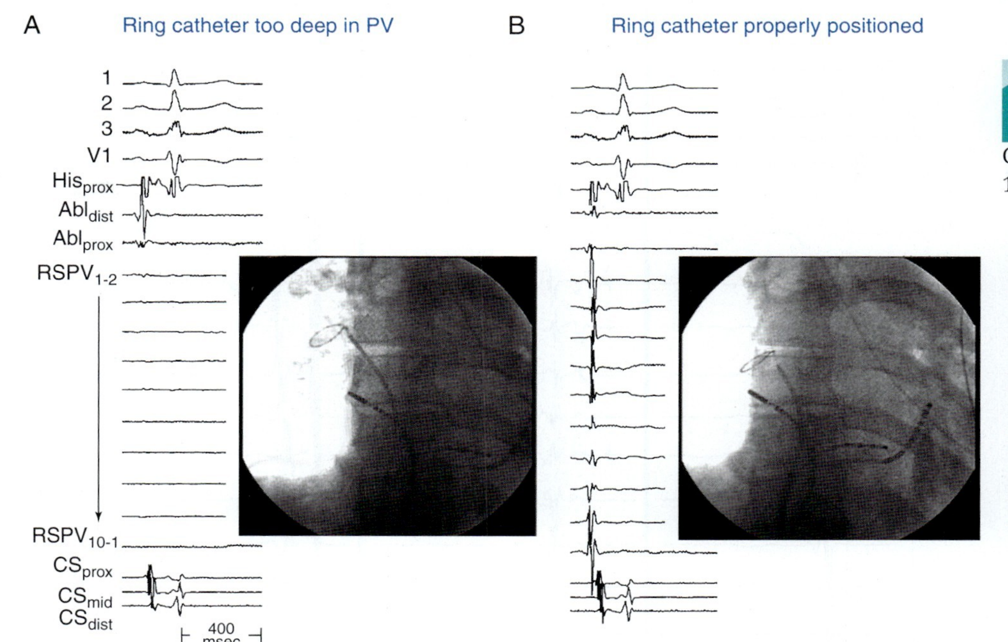

FIGURE 15-19 Recordings from a ring catheter in the right superior pulmonary vein (RSPV). **A,** The ring catheter is situated too deep in the vein; recordings suggest no pulmonary vein (PV) potentials. **B,** The ring catheter pulled back 1.5 cm, showing abundant PV potentials. Abl_{dist} = distal ablation site; Abl_{prox} = proximal ablation site; CS_{dist} = distal coronary sinus; CS_{mid} = middle coronary sinus; CS_{prox} = proximal coronary sinus; His_{prox} = proximal His bundle.

The ring catheter is positioned in the left superior PV, left inferior PV, and right superior PV. If accessible, the right inferior PV is usually mapped last because of the technical difficulty and the risk of dislodgment of the mapping catheters from the LA to the RA. The ring catheter is positioned within a PV and gradually withdrawn to within 5 mm of the ostium. It is important to position the ring catheter at the ostium of the PV; when it is positioned too deeply in the PV, PV potentials can be missed (Fig. 15-19). Subsequently, circumferential mapping of the PV is performed by obtaining 10 bipolar electrograms (1-2, 2-3, up to 10-1 electrode pairs) with the circular arranged electrodes of the ring catheter. The band-pass settings for the bipolar recordings are 30 to 500 Hz. Pacing from each pair of electrodes from the ring catheter has been used by some to ensure appropriate ring catheter sizing (80% of electrode pairs resulting in capture) and to demonstrate conduction from the veins to the atrium before ablation.

Ring catheters with 20 poles are also available and can offer higher resolution circumferential mapping and improve the differentiation of PV from LA potentials. The conventional wide bipolar electrograms record the PV potentials, as well as the larger LA potentials, which can obscure or mimic the PV potentials. In contrast, the high-resolution electrograms minimize the extent of far-field electrogram detection and display very small or completely absent LA potentials. In the context of PV isolation during sustained AF, improved discrimination between atrial and PV potentials can facilitate the recognition of complete PV disconnection and possibly limit the number of unnecessary RF applications. On the other hand, when a ring catheter and closely spaced electrodes make poor contact with the PV wall or are placed deep within the PV, near-field potentials may not be seen, which leads to underdetection of PV potentials.

The use of a navigational system (CARTO-3 or EnSite NavX) in ostial segmental PV isolation provides accurate nonfluoroscopic visualization of multiple catheter tips and curves (including the ring catheter) and allows a real-time assessment of wall contact and catheter stability, as well as assessment of the spatial relationship between ablation and ring catheters. Furthermore, the NavX technology enables taking a shadow of the stable position of the ring catheter and, hence, accurate repositioning of the catheter in the case of displacement to its original location. Also, the system enables labeling the electrodes on the ring catheters, thus allowing precise navigation of the ablation catheter to the labeled pole of the ring catheter without the assistance of fluoroscopy.

MAPPING DURING NORMAL SINUS RHYTHM

It is preferable to perform PV mapping during NSR or atrial pacing whenever possible because AF reduces PV potential amplitude and makes PVs more difficult to identify. Therefore, if the patient is in AF, electrical cardioversion is usually performed to restore NSR. Ibutilide (1 mg) or amiodarone (300 mg) may also be administered intravenously to prevent immediate recurrences of AF after cardioversion.

PV mapping during NSR typically shows double or multiple potentials that are usually recorded in a progressively later temporal sequence, synchronous with the first (right PVs) or second (left PVs) half of the sinus P wave (Fig. 15-20). The first low-frequency potential reflects activation of the adjacent LA. The latest high-frequency electrograms indicate PV potentials.

IDENTIFICATION OF PULMONARY VEIN POTENTIALS USING PACING MANEUVERS. PV potentials often are fused with the far-field LA electrograms but can be identified by their high-frequency appearance. Not uncommonly, an isoelectric interval separates the far-field LA electrogram and the near-field PV potential. The basis for this separation is unclear; however, evidence has suggested that there is an area of slow conduction at the proximal PV. The interval between the far-field electrogram and the PV potential may differ based on the site of pacing. The reasons for this phenomenon may be related to fiber orientation (anisotropy), which can make it easier to enter the vein from certain wavefront directions or because the far-field electrogram is not actually coming from the LA but is arising from a neighboring structure. Therefore, pacing from different atrial sites (most commonly high RA or distal CS) can help separate PV potentials from far-field atrial signals (Fig. 15-21; see Fig. 15-20). Furthermore, incremental rate atrial pacing and premature atrial stimulation from the same atrial site can sometimes result in conduction delay between the LA and PV at the PV ostium, which often exhibits decremental conduction properties (Fig. 15-22). Thus, if a complex electrogram is seen on a PV mapping catheter and, with faster or premature pacing, one of the potentials is seen to occur later after the far-field atrial electrogram, the delayed signal likely is a PV potential.

Right-sided PVs are typically mapped during NSR or RA pacing. For left PVs, the ostial PV potentials are sometimes not obvious during NSR because of the superimposed LA potential; therefore, pacing from the distal CS (at a CL of 500 to 600 milliseconds) allows

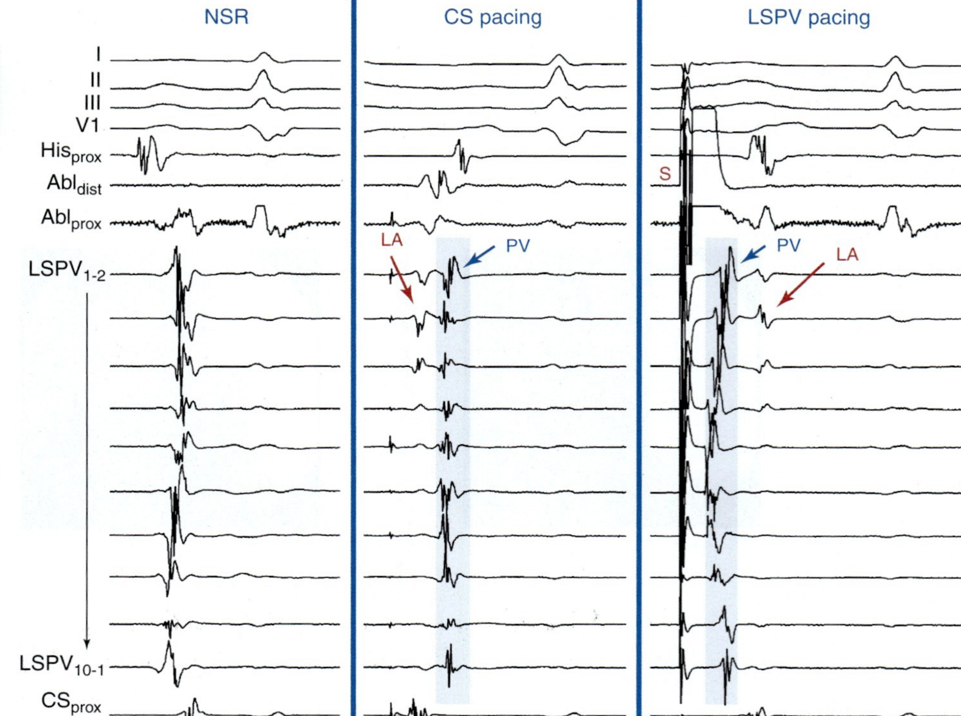

FIGURE 15-20 Differential atrial pacing to identify pulmonary vein (PV) potentials. **Left panel,** During normal sinus rhythm (NSR), the atrial and left superior PV (LSPV) potentials are superimposed and distinction of PV potentials from left atrial (LA) electrograms is difficult, if not impossible. **Middle panel,** During coronary sinus (CS) pacing, PV potentials (shaded area) are delayed relative to LA potentials and are thus readily discerned. **Right panel,** Pacing from within the LSPV also shows a clear delineation of PV versus LA potentials; in this case, PV potentials precede LA potentials. Abl_{dist} = distal ablation site; Abl_{prox} = proximal ablation site; CS_{dist} = distal coronary sinus; CS_{mid} = middle coronary sinus; CS_{prox} = proximal coronary sinus; His_{prox} = proximal His bundle.

their separation and easy recognition of PV potentials (see Fig. 15-20). However, even during CS pacing, the atrial and PV potentials still can overlap in approximately 50% to 60% of left PVs (see Fig. 15-22). The separation can be less evident in the posterior PV antrum, which is closer to the CS. Pacing from the LA appendage can help in this situation.

Because of the anatomical proximity of the PVs to several other structures that are electrically active, complex signals may be recorded by a catheter placed in the PV. For example, a catheter placed in the left superior PV may record electrical activity in the LA, LA appendage, ipsilateral PV, and ligament of Marshall. Similarly, a mapping catheter placed in the right superior PV may record electrical activity in the right middle PV, right inferior PV (particularly a superior branch), RA, LA, and SVC (Fig. 15-23). When a typical PV potential is recorded in a left PV, the far-field electrogram usually is coming from the LA. When mapping catheters are placed in the right-sided PV, often the main far-field electrogram is the RA electrogram, and the second far-field electrogram, if seen, is the LA electrogram.[91] In general, only the PV potential itself is near-field; all other structures picked up by the antenna of the mapping catheter are blunted and far-field. However, this criterion alone is insufficient for identifying the true PV potential. For example, if a catheter is deep within the left superior PV, where no PV musculature is present, the LA appendage electrograms will appear relatively near-field. Similarly, when RF ablation has already been performed, edema near the PV os and inadvertent ablation within the PV (more frequent than generally realized) will cause PV potentials to be less sharp and less near-field in character.[91] Various pacing maneuvers can differentiate from among these possibilities and can help exclude or prove a relationship of various components of the electrogram recorded from a PV to anatomical structures surrounding that particular PV. An important feature of far-field potentials is that they should be seen only on electrodes that "face" the structure in question; for instance, with a catheter in the left superior PV, signals that are recorded on electrodes adjacent to the LA appendage may represent far-field recordings from that structure, whereas signals visible only on electrodes at the posterior aspect of the left superior PV cannot be far-field LA appendage potentials (Fig. 15-24).

One pacing maneuver commonly used when complex electrograms are recorded on a mapping catheter placed in a PV is pacing at specific sites likely to be responsible for the components of the electrogram. The premise of such a maneuver is that pacing from a particular site causes the electrogram originating from that site to occur earlier, close to the pacing stimulus. For example, because of the proximity of the LA appendage to the left PVs (especially the left superior PV), far-field LA appendage potentials can be recorded in these PVs, and PV potentials can be confused with LA appendage potentials. These potentials are distinguished from PV potentials by differential pacing from the distal CS and LA appendage. If a pacing catheter is placed in the LA appendage and LA appendage capture is documented, the LA appendage component of the complex electrogram will occur early and will be drawn toward the pacing artifact (Fig. 15-25). Thus, the electrogram that moves the closest to the pacing stimulus can be diagnosed as originating from the LA appendage. Similar reasoning can be applied when pacing in an ipsilateral PV—if a component of the electrogram recorded in the left superior PV is, in fact, a left inferior PV potential—or when pacing in the SVC and vein of Marshall.[91]

LA electrograms, particularly when fragmented secondary to partial ablation, can also be mistaken for a PV potential, and pacing from a site in the LA close to, but not within, the PV (perivenous pacing) can help define the LA electrogram component of a complex PV recording. When pacing from a perivenous location, the LA signal will occur very close to, and often will merge with, the saturation artifact related to the pacing spike. However, because pacing is being performed proximal to the site of ostial delay, the PV potential remains unchanged or may occur with slightly more delay. The shift of the LA signal, which now is being captured by perivenous pacing, toward the pacing spike indicates the origin of that component of a complex signal. Differentiation of RA, LA, and PV potentials recorded within right-sided PVs can also be achieved using similar maneuvers (Fig. 15-26).[91]

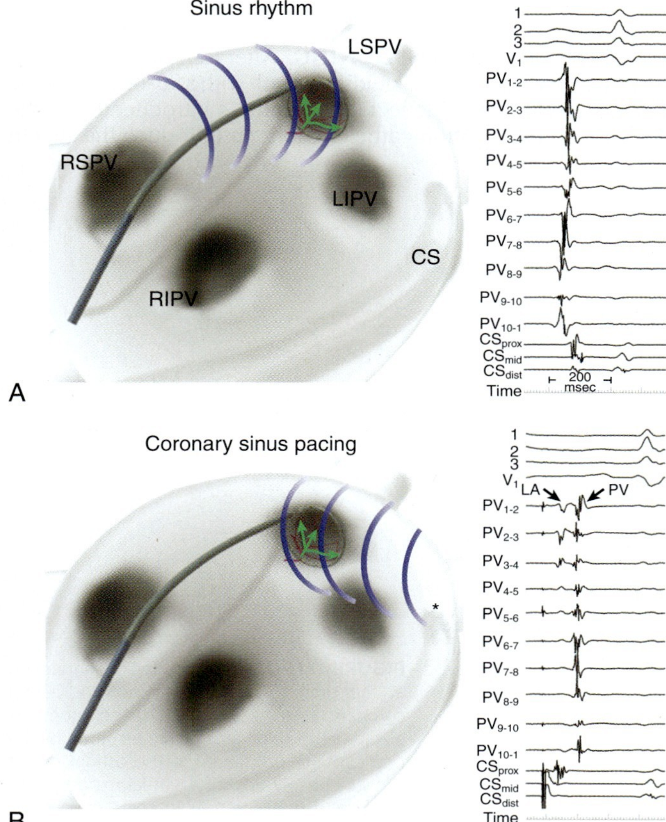

FIGURE 15-21 Depiction of differential activation of left atrial (LA) and pulmonary vein (PV) potentials. The LA is opened from the front, showing orifices of PVs; a ring catheter is in the left superior PV (LSPV). Red strands indicate a muscular PV fascicle extending into the LSPV; green arrows indicate propagation into the PV over the fascicle. **A,** During sinus rhythm, the wavefront propagates as indicated by blue curved lines and activates LA tissue around the PV and the PV fascicle at almost the same time, yielding a summated electrogram at right. **B,** During pacing from the coronary sinus (CS, at asterisk), the wavefront approaches from a different direction and activates LA muscle well before the PV fascicle is entered, accounting for the delay in PV potential inscription at right. CS_{dist} = distal coronary sinus; CS_{mid} = middle coronary sinus; CS_{prox} = proximal coronary sinus; LIPV, left inferior pulmonary vein; RIPV, right inferior pulmonary vein; RSPV, right superior pulmonary vein.

Multisite simultaneous pacing is an extension of the basic concept that pacing from a particular site will cause earlier occurrence of the electrogram arising from that site. For example, pacing from the CS alone is compared with simultaneous pacing from both the CS and LA appendage, with specific attention paid to the transition in the recorded electrogram between single-site (e.g., CS only) and dual-site (e.g., CS and LA appendage) pacing, which can help immediate distinction of the various components of a complex signal recorded within the PV.[91]

ABLATION TARGET SITES. Target sites for ablation are selected by identifying the earliest bipolar PV potentials or the unipolar electrograms with the most rapid (sharpest) intrinsic deflection on high-speed recordings (150 to 200 mm/sec) that have equivalent or earlier activation relative to the earliest PV potential recorded on the adjacent ring catheter recording sites (Fig. 15-27).

Electrogram polarity reversal can also be used as an additional indicator of breakthroughs from the LA to the PVs and identify potential ablation targets. *Polarity reversal* is defined as a sudden change in the main deflection of the PV potential. The reversal occurs as the wavefront of activation propagates radially in the PV from its connection with the LA, thus reaching contiguous bipolar recording electrodes in opposing directions (Fig. 15-28; see also Fig. 15-27).

MAPPING DURING ATRIAL FIBRILLATION

Although segmental ostial PV isolation is accomplished most efficiently during NSR, maintenance of NSR during an ablation procedure may not be readily achievable, particularly in patients with chronic AF. During an ongoing episode of AF, PV potentials can be obscured during the chaotic electrical activity of AF. Nevertheless, segmental ostial PV isolation was found to be as feasible and successful during AF as during NSR. An advantage of mapping during AF is that it obviates the need for the administration of antiarrhythmic drugs and for multiple electrical cardioversions in patients with immediately recurrent AF after cardioversion. Two approaches have been described for PV isolation during AF: the first uses intermittent bursts of PV tachycardia to guide PV isolation, and the second uses organized PV potentials during AF to guide PV isolation.

INTERMITTENT PULMONARY VEIN TACHYCARDIA. Prior studies demonstrated that rapid rhythms arising in the PVs (intermittent PV tachycardia) are common during AF (recorded during AF in 90% to 97% of PVs) and can play an important role in the maintenance of AF, or they can be a marker of an arrhythmogenic PV that triggers AF. Those intermittent bursts of PV tachycardia indicate the presence of an underlying arrhythmogenic muscle fascicle near the ostial recording sites and therefore can be used to guide segmental ostial ablation to isolate the PVs during AF.

During AF, the PVs are sequentially mapped with the ring catheter to assess the presence of intermittent PV tachycardia, defined as a PV rhythm that intermittently has a CL shorter than the AF CL recorded in the adjacent LA. When intermittent PV tachycardia is recorded by several electrodes, the ostial site corresponding to the most rapid intrinsic deflection of the unipolar electrogram should be targeted by RF applications. If PV tachycardia is not observed, ostial sites that display a high-frequency bipolar PV potential or rapid unipolar intrinsic deflection during AF, or both, can alternatively be targeted for ablation.

If AF terminates during ablation, PV potentials are then assessed during NSR and atrial pacing. If there is evidence of residual conduction over a PV fascicle, RF energy is delivered at these ostial sites during NSR or atrial pacing. On the other hand, if AF is still present after isolation of a PV, electrical cardioversion is performed. If AF recurs, other PVs are isolated during AF and, if NSR is maintained, the remaining PVs are isolated during NSR or atrial pacing.

ORGANIZATION OF PULMONARY VEIN POTENTIALS. PV potentials are classified at baseline as organized (have a consistent activation sequence for more than 10 seconds) or disorganized (activation sequence on the ring catheter varies from beat to beat). Approximately 37% of PVs have organized PV potentials (more for inferior than superior PVs—53% versus 26%; Fig. 15-29). When the PV activation pattern is organized (from the beginning or after some anatomically guided RF applications), the area showing the earliest activation or demonstrating polarity reversal on the ring catheter is targeted.

For disorganized PV potentials, ablation is performed circumferentially around the ring catheter on the ostial side of the PV. The top and bottom segments of the PV are targeted first because of the high prevalence of LA-PV breakthroughs at these sites. In most cases, initial RF applications result in organization of PV activity. This activity is probably secondary to progressive reduction of LA-PV breakthroughs that diminishes the mass of fibrillatory conduction within the PV and channels the electrical activity through the last remaining fascicles connecting the LA to the PV, thereby activating the PV in an organized fashion. This consequently enables EP-guided PV isolation.

Organized PV activity can represent fewer LA-PV connections and therefore may require fewer RF applications than PVs with disorganized activity. This may explain the greater frequency of organized activity in the inferior PVs, presumably because of the presence of less extensive muscular sleeves in these veins as demonstrated by pathological studies.

BASKET CATHETER MAPPING

The basket catheter (Constellation, Boston Scientific, Natick, Mass.) is composed of 64 electrodes mounted on 8 flexible, self-expanding splines (see Fig. 4-4). Each spline is identified by a letter (from A to H) and each electrode by a number (distal 1 to proximal 8). The 32 bipolar electrograms provide 3-D mapping of PV activation.

BASKET CATHETER POSITIONING. After transseptal access is gained, an 8.5 Fr soft-tipped guiding sheath with a 90- or 120-degree curve or, preferably, a deflectable sheath, is introduced into the PVs. A steerable ablation catheter can help introduce the sheath

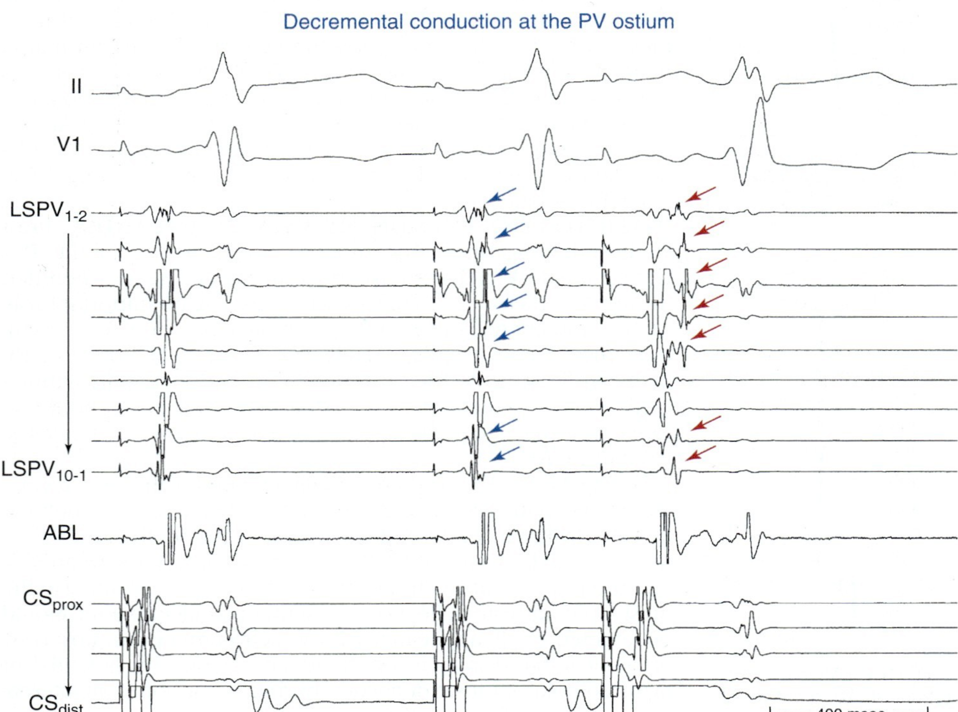

FIGURE 15-22 Decremental conduction at the pulmonary vein (PV) ostium. During coronary sinus (CS) drive pacing, complex electrograms (blue arrows) are recorded by the ring catheter positioned at the ostium of the left superior PV (LSPV). An atrial extrastimulus from the distal CS results in conduction delay between the left atrium (LA) and the PV at the PV ostium. Therefore, PV potentials (red arrows) become delayed and separated from atrial electrograms. ABL = ablation site; CS_{dist} = distal coronary sinus; CS_{prox} = proximal coronary sinus.

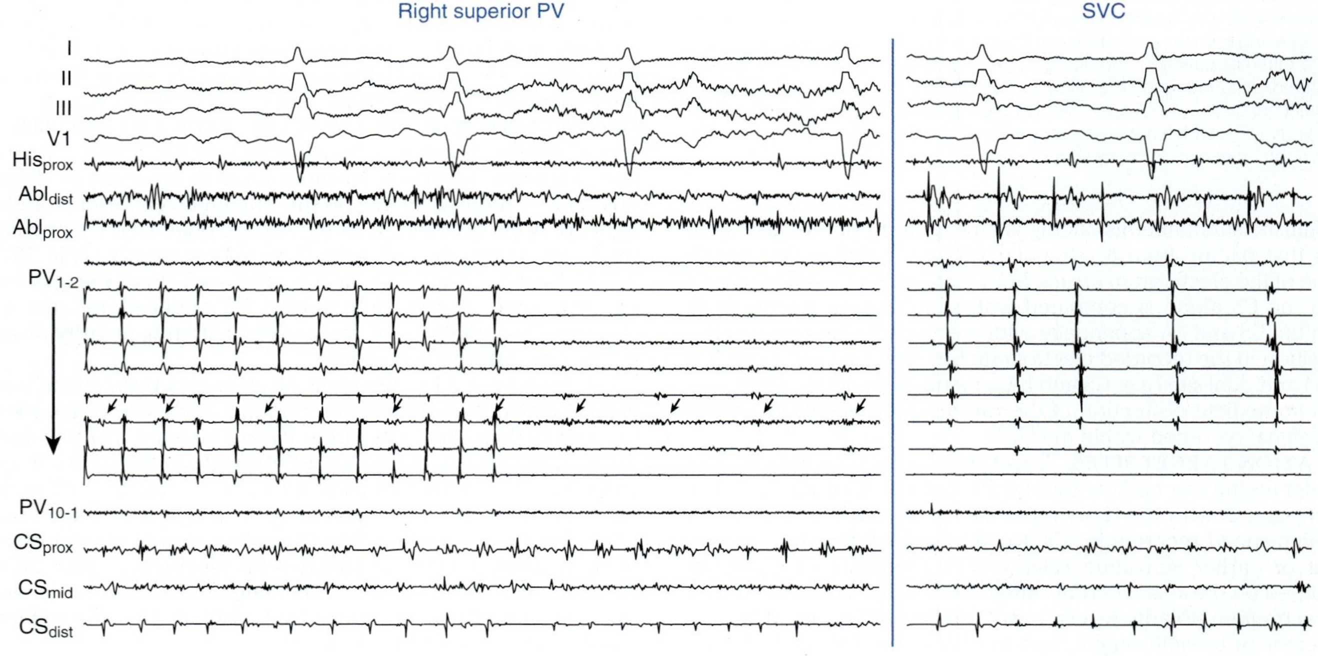

FIGURE 15-23 Superior vena cava (SVC) activity recorded in the right superior pulmonary vein (PV). **Left panel,** Recordings from a ring catheter positioned at the ostium of the right superior PV showing high-amplitude PV potentials that disappear midway through the recording because of isolation of the vein with radiofrequency ablation. Another set of lower amplitude signals (arrows) remains and was present prior to PV isolation. **Right panel,** These potentials represent far-field SVC recordings, shown as sharp near-field recordings after the ring catheter is positioned in the SVC. Abl_{dist} = distal ablation site; Abl_{prox} = proximal ablation site; CS_{dist} = distal coronary sinus; CS_{mid} = middle coronary sinus; CS_{prox} = proximal coronary sinus; His_{prox} = proximal His bundle.

into the PVs (especially the inferior PVs). The ablation catheter is introduced through the sheath, and once it is engaged in the PV, the sheath is advanced over the ablation catheter. Once the sheath is in place in the PV, the steerable catheter is removed and is replaced by the basket catheter. The basket catheter is introduced into the sheath so that the tip of the basket catheter reaches the tip of the sheath; the sheath is then pulled back to allow expansion of the basket catheter (Fig. 15-30). Alternatively, the basket catheter is inserted directly into the PVs directly with the sheath positioned in the LA. However, although this technique was found to be safe because of the very flexible splines of the basket catheter, extreme caution is required to avoid venous perforation by the stiff catheter tip.

A basket catheter with a diameter of 31 mm is chosen when the diameter of the main PV trunk is 26 mm or smaller, and a basket catheter with a diameter of 38 mm is used when the PV diameter is greater than 26 mm or when there is a common ostium. The PV diameter is determined by preacquired MRI, CT scanning, or PV angiography. The position of the basket catheter in relation to the PV ostium can be determined by PV angiography (Fig. 15-31). If necessary, the basket catheter is retracted to obtain optimal contact to the main trunk and ostium of the PV.

BASKET CATHETER MAPPING. The basket catheter is deployed within the target PV with its most proximal electrodes positioned at the PV ostium, as determined by selective PV angiography. PV activation can be followed during NSR or CS pacing propagating through the four levels of bipolar electrograms from proximal ostial (7/8) to distal (1/2) inside the PV. During ectopic beats or initiation of AF, the activation can be followed from the source of ectopy to its exit to the LA (see Fig. 15-14).[91]

A computerized 3-D mapping system (QMS2, CathData Inc., Toronto, Canada) has been introduced to construct a 3-D color isochronal or isopotential map from a total of 56 bipolar electrograms recorded by the basket catheter. This 3-D mapping system has been found useful for identifying a preferential electrical connection and determining its elimination accurately because it enables not only a visualization of the activation sequence of the PV potentials but also an adequate evaluation of the activation sequence between the splines. An animation of a 3-D potential map, which can reflect a series of electrical activations, is used to reveal the style of breakthrough, distribution of the PV musculature, and activation pattern within the PV. A color setup with a gradation that corresponds to the relative size of the potential amplitude can be arranged variously on the QMS map. For example, in the detection of an AF focus, the color setup needs to be arranged to emphasize the small PV potentials triggering the AF. In contrast, for PV isolation, it is essential to minimize the low-amplitude LA potentials and emphasize the

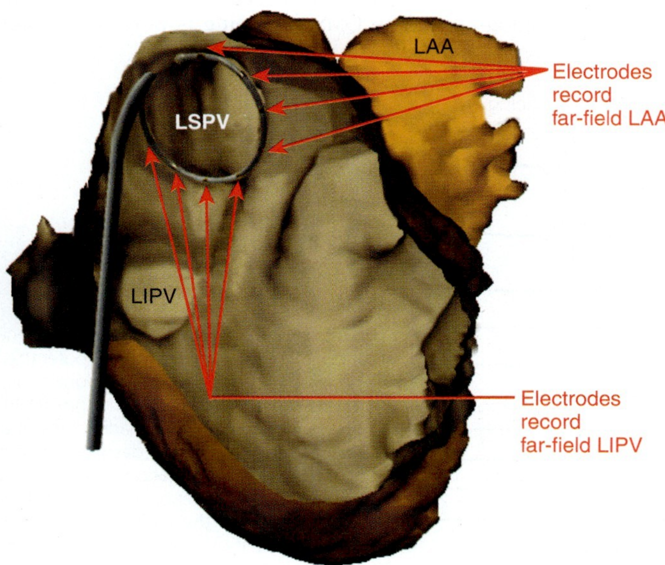

FIGURE 15-24 Left pulmonary veins versus left atrial appendage (LAA). Cutaway view of the left atrium showing the inside of the lateral aspect. A ring catheter is depicted in the left superior pulmonary vein (LSPV). Far-field recordings can be made from adjacent structures on certain electrodes of the ring catheter as indicated, such as LAA or left inferior pulmonary vein (LIPV).

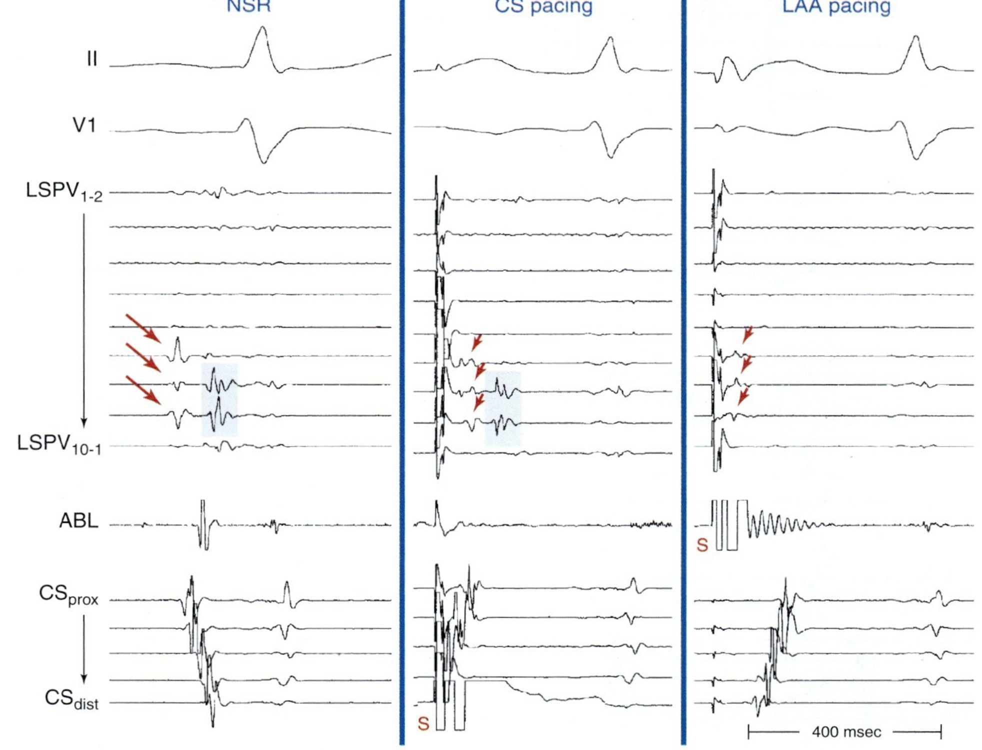

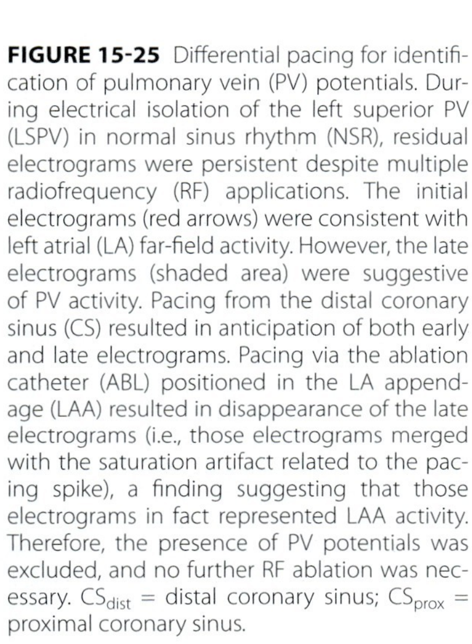

FIGURE 15-25 Differential pacing for identification of pulmonary vein (PV) potentials. During electrical isolation of the left superior PV (LSPV) in normal sinus rhythm (NSR), residual electrograms were persistent despite multiple radiofrequency (RF) applications. The initial electrograms (red arrows) were consistent with left atrial (LA) far-field activity. However, the late electrograms (shaded area) were suggestive of PV activity. Pacing from the distal coronary sinus (CS) resulted in anticipation of both early and late electrograms. Pacing via the ablation catheter (ABL) positioned in the LA appendage (LAA) resulted in disappearance of the late electrograms (i.e., those electrograms merged with the saturation artifact related to the pacing spike), a finding suggesting that those electrograms in fact represented LAA activity. Therefore, the presence of PV potentials was excluded, and no further RF ablation was necessary. CS_{dist} = distal coronary sinus; CS_{prox} = proximal coronary sinus.

high-amplitude PV potentials to construct a clear 3-D map of the PV potentials. When the small potentials need to be emphasized, the color threshold is decreased to 30% of the largest amplitude of all the related potentials. The short stay of the activation wavefront near the outer frame of the 3-D PV potential map before the longitudinal propagation, which reflects a conduction delay, indicates the LA-PV junction where continuous fractionated potentials connecting the LA potentials and PV potentials are observed. The serial activation patterns moving around the outer frame of the 3-D PV isopotential map before the longitudinal propagation are defined to indicate the LA-PV junction. The onset of a centrifugal activation on the LA-PV junction is identified as an electrical connection.

BASKET CATHETER–GUIDED PULMONARY VEIN ISOLATION. With a multipolar basket catheter, ostial PV isolation can be performed by RF application to the breakthrough site identified by the 3-D PV potential map. The Astronomer system (Boston Scientific) is used for navigation of the ablation catheter inside the basket catheter.[92] Ablation is performed at the junction between the PV and the LA, as ostial as catheter stability allows, at the site of earliest PV potential recording or shortest atrial-PV potential delay. The location of the ostium is determined by electrogram morphology and by noting the shape of the basket catheter because it conforms to the PV, and ostial anatomy can be confirmed by angiography. The QMS recording is performed after

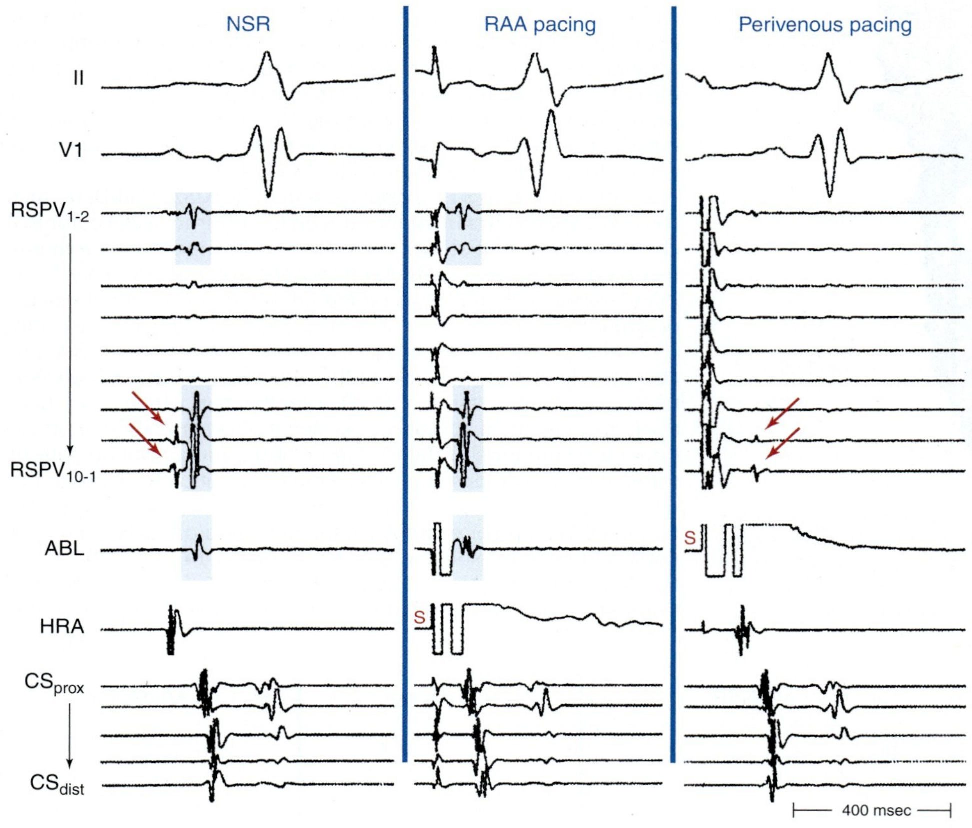

FIGURE 15-26 Differential pacing for identification of pulmonary vein (PV) potentials. During electrical isolation of the right superior PV (RSPV) in normal sinus rhythm (NSR), residual electrograms (blue shaded area and red arrows) were persistent despite multiple radiofrequency (RF) applications. Pacing from the right atrial (RA) appendage (RAA) resulted in disappearance of the earlier electrograms (red arrows; i.e., those electrograms merged with the saturation artifact related to the pacing spike), a finding suggesting that those electrograms in fact represented RA activity. During pacing just outside the ostium of the RSPV (using the ablation catheter), the second set of electrograms (shaded area) disappeared, whereas the RA electrograms (red arrows) persisted in the ring catheter recordings, indicating that the second set of electrograms in fact represented left atrial (LA) activity. Therefore, the presence of PV potentials was excluded, and no further radiofrequency ablation was necessary. ABL = ablation site; CS_{dist} = distal coronary sinus; CS_{prox} = proximal coronary sinus; HRA = high right atrium.

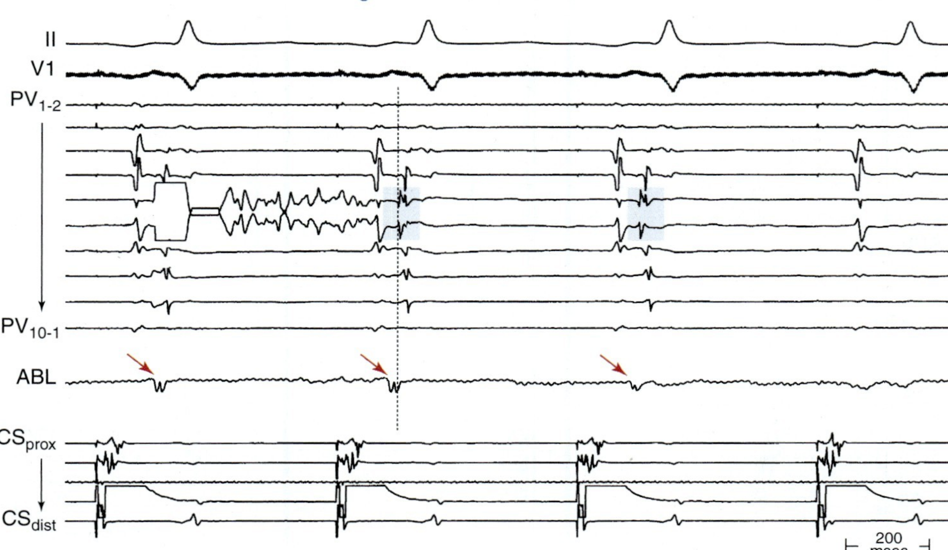

FIGURE 15-27 Segmental ostial pulmonary vein (PV) isolation. During circumferential ostial PV mapping using a ring catheter, electrical connections between the left atrium (LA) and the PV (target sites for ablation) are identified by recording the earliest bipolar PV potentials with electrogram polarity reversal on adjacent poles (shaded electrograms). Note that the distal bipoles of the ablation catheter record even an earlier sharp PV potential (arrows). The presence of ablation artifact on the recording from a specific ring catheter pole confirms the pole the catheter is on and that the catheter is in the same plane as the ring catheter. Catheter ablation at that site results in complete elimination of PV potentials and LA-PV block (last complex). ABL = ablation site; CS_{dist} = distal coronary sinus; CS_{prox} = proximal coronary sinus.

every RF application and, if the elimination of a target breakthrough is confirmed, another breakthrough is identified and ablated.

ADVANTAGES OF THE BASKET CATHETER. The basket catheter is currently the mapping tool with the highest resolution available for endovascular mapping of the LA-PV junction in humans. In addition, the basket catheter provides information about the anatomy of the PV, such as exact ostium localization, because the basket catheter takes the shape of the PV (see Fig. 15-31) and allows 3-D reconstruction of the PV activation from the ostium to deep inside the PV.

The Astronomer navigation system permits precise and reproducible guidance of the ablation catheter tip to areas identified as LA to PV conduction pathways and thereby allows efficient PV isolation. The distal poles of the basket catheter can be used to monitor changes in the activation sequence in real time and to demonstrate the effects of ablation at the ostium as lesions are created. They also provide an immediate indication of successful PV isolation by the disappearance of the distal PV potentials. The system also helps identify areas near the PV ostium with fragmented potentials and with discharging ostial foci, which can be localized in a single beat.

The risk of PV stenosis seems to be low (1.2%) with the use of basket catheter–guided PV isolation. This technology can potentially minimize the risk of PV stenosis, first by reducing the number of RF applications and second by avoiding ablation inside the PV, because the basket catheter allows localization of the PV ostium during the entire procedure. Thus, the use of complementary navigation systems or ICE appears to be nonessential when using the basket catheter for PV isolation.

DISADVANTAGES OF THE BASKET CATHETER. Carbonizations can form after ablation on the splines of the basket catheter, which can potentially cause embolism. Carbonizations, which appear as dark material attached to the basket catheter electrodes or splines, are thought to be caused by the concentration of RF energy on the thin splines that results in very high local temperatures that induce denaturization of serum proteins. However, carbonization can be greatly diminished with the use of an irrigated-tip catheter as opposed to conventional ablation catheters.

Another disadvantage is that the basket catheter is nondeflectable and has limited maneuverability, and it requires a special sheath with a limited number of preshaped curves. Sometimes, it can be challenging to introduce a basket catheter into the inferior PVs. The use of a deflectable transseptal sheath can facilitate catheterization of the PVs.

Additionally, the splines may contact one another when the basket catheter is positioned within a relatively small PV, thereby inducing electrical artifact (see Fig. 15-31). Similarly, the splines may not always be equally spaced relative to the circumference of the PV. As a result, areas in which several splines are clustered may be densely mapped, whereas other regions are less densely recorded.

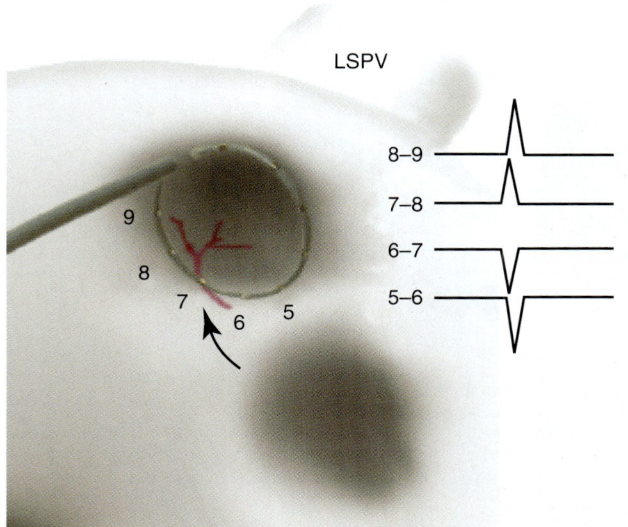

FIGURE 15-28 Bipolar electrogram polarity reversal. The ring electrode catheter (electrodes numbered) is situated in the ostium of the left superior pulmonary vein (LSPV); a strand of atrial muscle crosses from the left atrium (LA) to the PV (red) and branches within the vein. The arrow indicates propagation of the wavefront of activation from the LA to the PV. The strand crosses at electrode 7; recordings from surrounding bipoles indicate the direction of propagation away from (negative deflection) or toward (positive deflection) the bipole. The point at which the polarity reverses from positive to negative is where the strand crosses into the PV.

Target of Ablation

The objective of the mapping and ablation procedure is to identify PV potentials along the circumference of the PV ostium and ablate to eliminate these potentials completely. Isolation of all PVs is performed without attempting to identify the PVs demonstrating arrhythmogenicity. RF ablation is targeted to the ostial portion of the breakthrough segments (electrical connections) connecting the LA to the PV, which are identified as the earliest PV potentials recorded from the ring catheter. The PV potential reflects

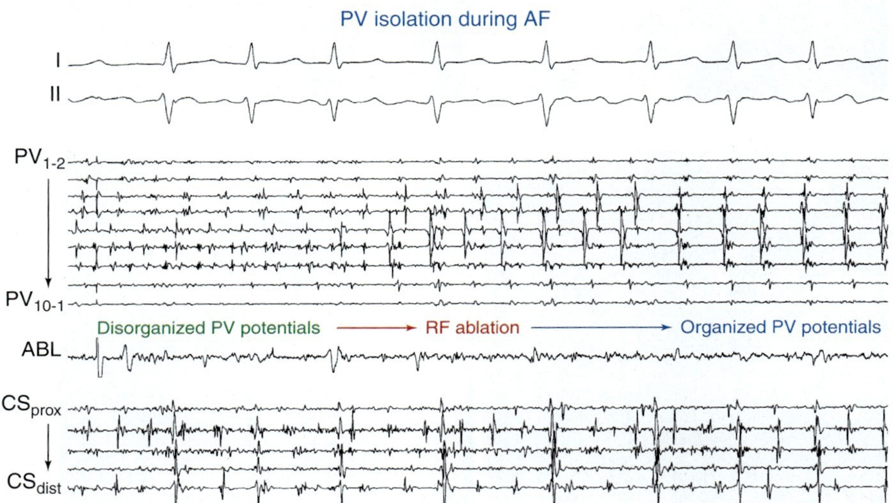

FIGURE 15-29 Pulmonary vein (PV) isolation during atrial fibrillation (AF). Initially (at left), PV potentials are disorganized. During radiofrequency (RF) application at the PV ostium, the PV potentials become organized. See text for discussion. ABL = ablation site; CS_{dist} = distal coronary sinus; CS_{prox} = proximal coronary sinus.

the activation of muscular LA bands extending into the PV with longitudinal, oblique, or complex courses and ending in a cul-de-sac or even looping back in the LA. The source, its course within the PV, and its exit into the LA may all be considered appropriate individual targets for ablation. The PV potential is recorded over a broader area proximally, but with great variability. Therefore, a few seconds of energy application may be sufficient at some proximal sites to eliminate downstream PV muscle activity, whereas wide or repeated RF applications may have been required in others.

Once the presence of the PV potentials along the PV circumference is defined on the ring catheter, target sites for ablation are selected by identifying the earliest bipolar PV potentials or the unipolar electrograms with the most rapid (sharpest) intrinsic deflection on high-speed recordings (150 to 200 mm/sec) that had equivalent or earlier activation relative to the earliest PV potential recorded on the adjacent ring catheter recording sites (see Fig. 15-27). The ablation catheter then is maneuvered to a position adjacent to the target electrode pair of the ring catheter and withdrawn to the edge of the ostium (the ostial side of the ring catheter). RF ablation is performed within 5 to 15 mm of the PV ostium; the exact location usually depends on catheter stability. This is safer (regarding the risk of PV stenosis) than more distal applications, especially in smaller veins.

Several PV potential electrogram characteristics predict a successful ablation site: (1) timing of the (unipolar and bipolar) PV potential electrogram recorded by the ablation catheter equal to or earlier than the earliest PV potential recorded by the ring catheter (see Fig. 15-27); (2) larger (unipolar and bipolar) electrogram amplitude; (3) steeper intrinsic deflection of the unipolar electrogram; and (4) identical morphologies of the unipolar electrograms recorded by the ablation catheter and by the contiguous electrode of the ring catheter.

Ablation Technique

A temperature-controlled, 4- or 8-mm-tip deflectable catheter or a 3.5-mm irrigated-tip ablation catheter can be used. For 8-mm-tip catheters, RF ablation is performed with the maximum temperature set at 45°C to 55°C, the power set at 70 W or lower, and for a duration of 20 to 60 seconds. Power limit is usually reduced to 25 W

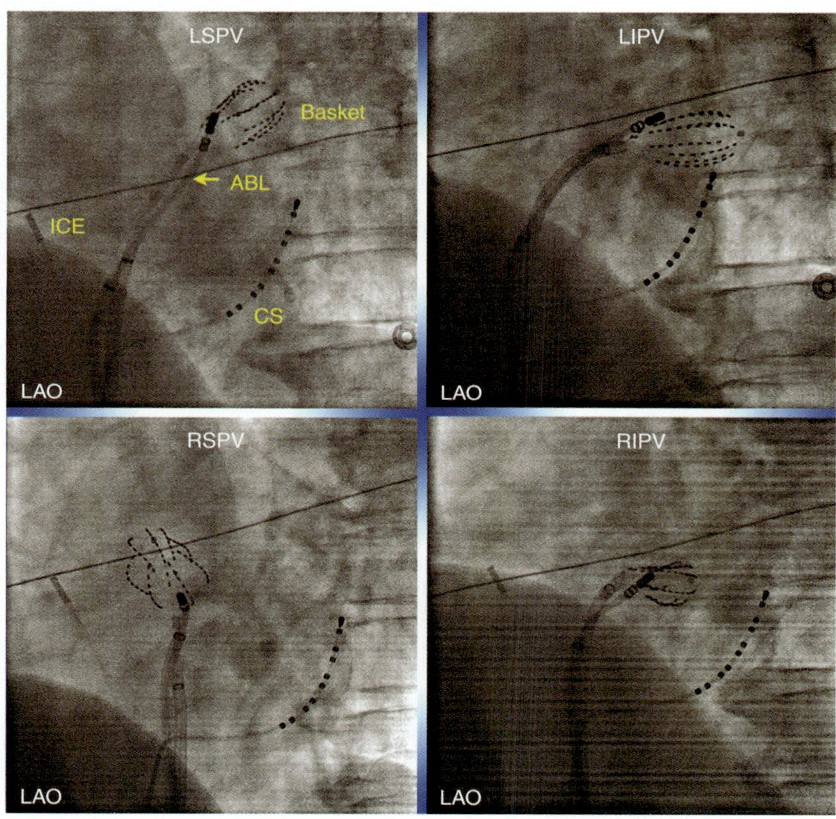

FIGURE 15-30 Left anterior oblique (LAO) fluoroscopic views of basket catheter positioned in the four pulmonary veins (PVs). A long deflectable sheath is used to help position the basket catheter in the different PVs. CS = coronary sinus; ICE = intracardiac echocardiography; LIPV = left inferior pulmonary vein; LSPV = left superior pulmonary vein; RIPV = right inferior pulmonary vein; RSPV = right superior pulmonary vein.

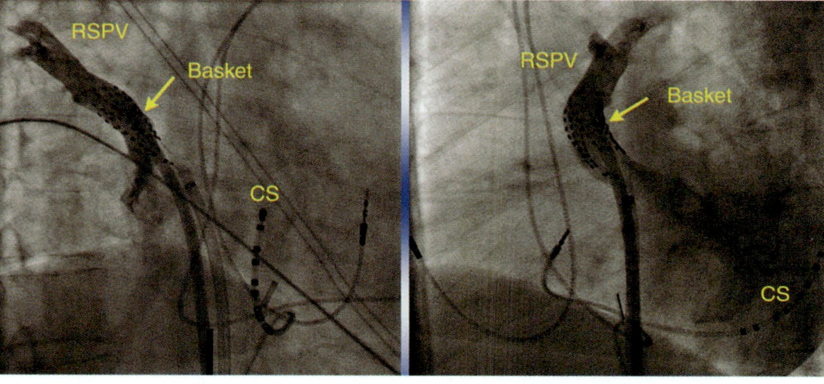

FIGURE 15-31 Fluoroscopic right anterior oblique (RAO) and left anterior oblique (LAO) views of angiography of the right superior pulmonary vein (RSPV) with a basket catheter positioned in the vein. Note that the basket catheter takes the shape of the PV and provides anatomical information about the location of the ostium and size of the PV. CS = coronary sinus.

for the case of a left inferior PV and to 20 W if the PV diameter is less than 15 mm. For irrigated-tip catheters, power is set at 50 W or lower and temperature at 40°C or lower. Ablation lesions are delivered for a maximum of 60 seconds to achieve an impedance drop of 5 to 10 Ω at the ablation site. RF application may be repeated or prolonged when a change occurs in activation or morphology of the PV potentials, or both, as determined by circumferential mapping recorded downstream. Additional ostial applications targeting fragmented electrograms are performed after PV isolation to eliminate any ostial PV potentials, thus reducing the risk of recurrence caused by ostial foci. The presence of high-amplitude electrical artifact on the recording from a specific ring catheter pole confirms the pole with which the ablation catheter is in contact and that the catheter is in the same plane as the ring catheter (see Fig. 15-27).

A successful ablation site is defined as a site at which an application of RF energy results in elimination of a PV potential at more than one ring catheter recording sites or delay (shift) of a PV potential by at least 10 milliseconds at more than two ring catheter recording sites (Fig. 15-32). Once a shift or elimination of PV potentials at some ring catheter poles is achieved, the ablation catheter is adjusted to target the new ring catheter pole recording the now earliest PV potential. This maneuver is repeated until the whole PV is electrically isolated. Complete electrical isolation of the PV is defined as complete entrance block into the PV during AF and elimination or dissociation of all ostial PV potentials during NSR and atrial pacing (see Fig. 15-32), as well as exit block from the vein (see later).

The extent of the circumference ablated is variable among PVs. When ablation is performed proximally to the PV ostium or during AF, more circumferential ablation is often required to achieve PV isolation. Occasionally, electrical connections exist between ipsilateral PVs, and elimination of these connections is important only when isolation of one PV is the goal of the ablation procedure. The electrical connections between PVs are defined as the identification of the earliest activation at the ostium of an untargeted PV during pacing inside the targeted PV; thus, ablation is performed at this untargeted PV ostium to achieve electrical disconnection.

When a multielectrode basket catheter is used for PV mapping, it is recommended to use an irrigated-tip catheter at a maximum temperature of 45°C, maximum power of 30 W, and flow rate during ablation of 17 mL/min.

CRYOABLATION

Although RF energy has become the gold standard for catheter ablation in most cardiac arrhythmias, PV isolation by heating has potential limitations. RF energy produces tissue disruption, which increases the risk of perforation and thromboembolism. Moreover, RF energy induces inhomogeneous, dense fibrosis and shrinking of the tissue, leading to PV stenosis. Cryothermal energy is an alternative energy source that may overcome these limitations. Cryothermal energy creates minimal endothelial and endocardial disruption and preserves the underlying tissue architecture. Therefore, the lesions are minimally thrombogenic and arrhythmogenic, and cryoablation of the PV should have a low risk of PV stenosis.

Initial experiences of EP-guided segmental ostial PV isolation by using cryothermal energy application with a 10.5 Fr (CryoCor, San Diego, Calif.) or 7 Fr (Freezor, CryoCath Technologies, Montreal, Canada) focal ablation catheter showed that PV isolation is feasible with a comparable number of applications and clinical outcome with regard to RF ablation. Importantly, the early cryoablation experience has not evidenced, so far, development of PV stenosis following ablation. On the other hand, cryothermal injury is sensitive to surrounding thermal conditions. The high flow of the PVs can present a considerable heat load to cryothermal technologies, which can limit the size and depth of the lesion produced by cryothermal energy at the PV ostium and thus limit the ability of achieving complete and permanent PV isolation. Additionally, the longer application times (2.5 to 5.0 minutes) required when cryothermal energy is used may relevantly reflect on the procedure duration, thus limiting the clinical use of this theoretically optimal energy source.

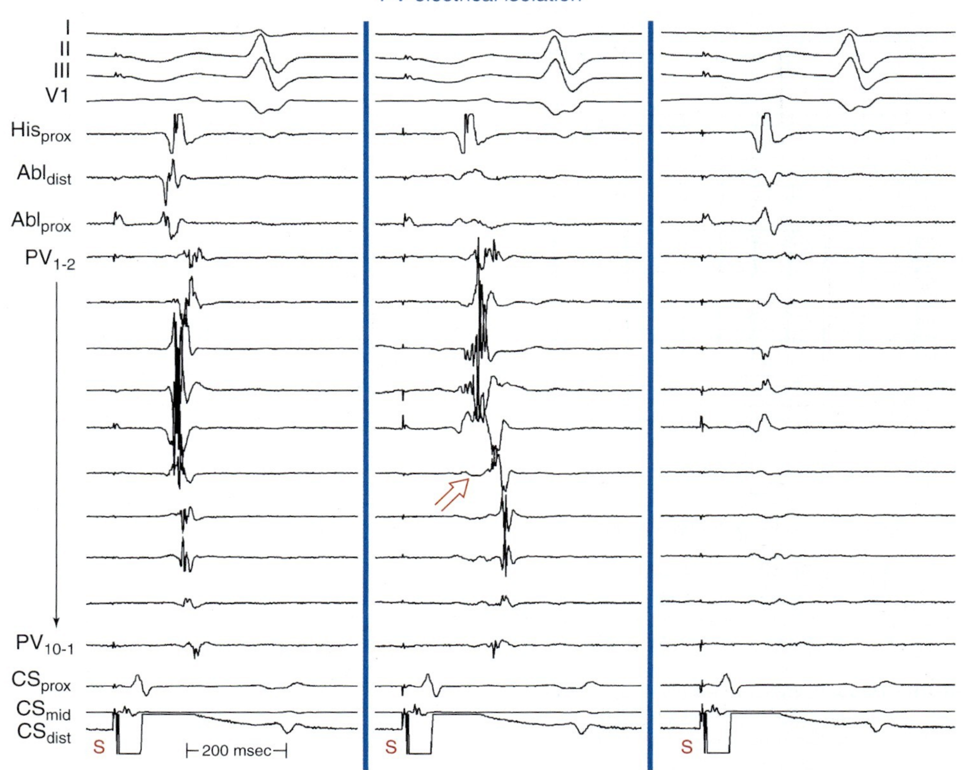

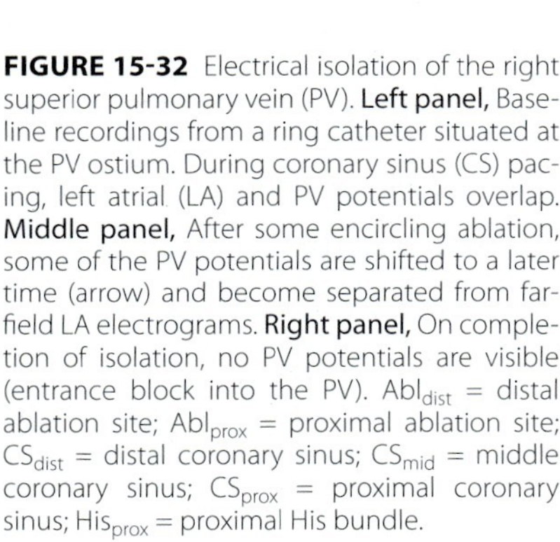

FIGURE 15-32 Electrical isolation of the right superior pulmonary vein (PV). **Left panel,** Baseline recordings from a ring catheter situated at the PV ostium. During coronary sinus (CS) pacing, left atrial (LA) and PV potentials overlap. **Middle panel,** After some encircling ablation, some of the PV potentials are shifted to a later time (arrow) and become separated from far-field LA electrograms. **Right panel,** On completion of isolation, no PV potentials are visible (entrance block into the PV). Abl_{dist} = distal ablation site; Abl_{prox} = proximal ablation site; CS_{dist} = distal coronary sinus; CS_{mid} = middle coronary sinus; CS_{prox} = proximal coronary sinus; His_{prox} = proximal His bundle.

Endpoints of Ablation

ELECTRICAL DISCONNECTION OF THE PULMONARY VEIN

Complete PV electrical disconnection is verified by (1) complete entrance block into the PV during AF and the elimination or dissociation of all ostial PV potentials recorded by the ring catheter during NSR and atrial pacing (i.e., LA-PV conduction block) (Fig. 15-33; see also Fig. 15-32) and (2) complete exit block from the PV to the PV ostium and LA during intra-PV pacing (i.e., PV-LA conduction block; Fig. 15-34).[93] Evidence suggests that demonstration of only entrance block is an insufficient endpoint. In one report, less than 60% of PVs demonstrated exit block after achieving entrance block (Fig. 15-35). The fact that tachycardias can be induced in isolated PV segments highlights the importance of achieving PV exit block. PV pacing is performed from multiple sites in as circumferential a manner as possible by using the bipoles of the ring catheter or mapping-ablation catheter and with the minimal output that constantly captures the PV potential. This maneuver also can unmask electrical connections between ipsilateral PVs, which manifest as intact LA conduction during intra-PV pacing after elimination of all potentials in that PV, thus indicating unidirectional block. This is relevant when only one (and not all) PV is targeted for isolation.

Early PV reconduction can be observed in up to 93% of patients and 50% of PVs, with 33% of the PVs demonstrating a first recurrence at 30 minutes and 17% showing a first recurrence at 60 minutes. Notably, recovery of PV conduction is more frequently observed in the left superior PV as compared with the other PVs. Therefore, reconfirmation of PV isolation after a 30- or even 60-minute waiting period after initial PV isolation or pharmacological provocation with adenosine (20 to 30 mg rapid intravenous bolus) or isoproterenol (20 μg/min intravenous infusion) has been suggested to improve outcome. Incorporation of shorter waiting time (20 to 30 minutes) in conjunction of adenosine administration may also be reasonable. Of note, each of those methods seems to have unique features in uncovering PV reconnection, and the results of the different methods may not be in agreement. In other words, PV reconnection may be unmasked only after a waiting period but not by administration of adenosine, and vice versa. Even the sites of PV reconnection uncovered by one method can be different from those uncovered by the other methods.[93-95]

INABILITY TO ISOLATE A PULMONARY VEIN

More than 90% of PVs can be electrically isolated from the LA by conventional applications of RF energy along segments of the ostia, guided by PV potentials. The inability to abolish the arrhythmogenic PV potential or its recovery (even in a very discrete area and with a prolonged conduction time) is associated with a higher AF recurrence rate.

The inability to disconnect the PV has been demonstrated in 3% to 24% of targeted PVs in previous studies and may be attributable to anatomical variations in the geometry of the ostia that could limit optimal recording of PV potentials with the ring catheter. Using an expandable ring catheter or using ICE to guide positioning of the ring catheter aids in stabilizing the mapping catheter. Additionally, some fascicles can be too thick to be ablated with conventional RF energy, and the use of high-power output or an irrigated-tip ablation catheter, which creates deeper lesions than a conventional ablation catheter, can be required to isolate those PVs. Also, the inability to isolate a PV can be caused by the presence of electrical connections between PVs. Approximately 14% of the patients have electrical connections between ipsilateral PVs. In these patients, ostial ablation of an untargeted PV is required for successful disconnection of the targeted PV. Recognition of

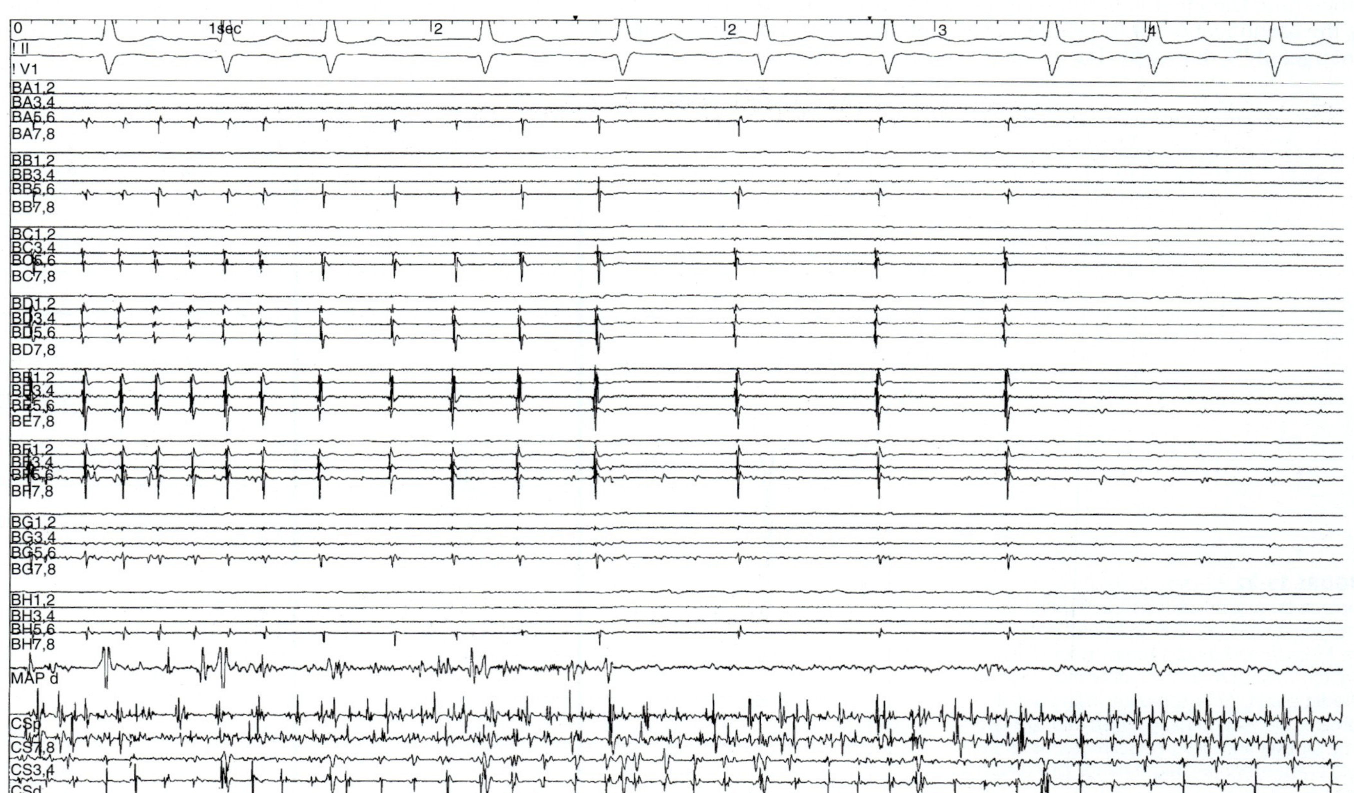

FIGURE 15-33 Pulmonary vein (PV) isolation during atrial fibrillation (AF) using a basket catheter. Bipolar recordings from the eight electrodes (1-2, 3-4, 5-6, 7-8) on each of the eight splines (BA through BH) of the basket catheter positioned in the left superior PV initially show sharp PV potentials. Radiofrequency ablation during AF results in gradual slowing and then disappearance of all PV potentials and persistence of residual low-amplitude, far-field, left atrial (LA) electrograms, consistent with LA-PV entrance block. AF continues in the coronary sinus (CS) recordings.

electrical connections between PVs during ostial ablation of PVs prevents unnecessary or excessive RF applications that probably produce postablation PV stenosis. Occasionally, the proximity of a targeted PV to an important extracardiac structure (esophagus, phrenic nerve) limits the ability to isolate the vein fully.

Outcome

Segmental ostial PV isolation represents an important advance in catheter treatment of AF and was found more efficacious than focal ablation for the control of paroxysmal AF. As compared with focal ablation, PV isolation eliminates the need for detailed mapping of spontaneous ectopy, and there is a clear-cut endpoint of ablation, even when spontaneous arrhythmias are absent. Importantly, the risk of PV stenosis is less than that with focal PV ablation.

On the other hand, the benefit of empiric isolation of all PVs over the identification and selective isolation of arrhythmogenic veins is less clear. Previous comparative case series demonstrated that empirical all-PV isolation led to superior outcomes over isolating fewer veins, which is expected given that most (up to 71%) patients

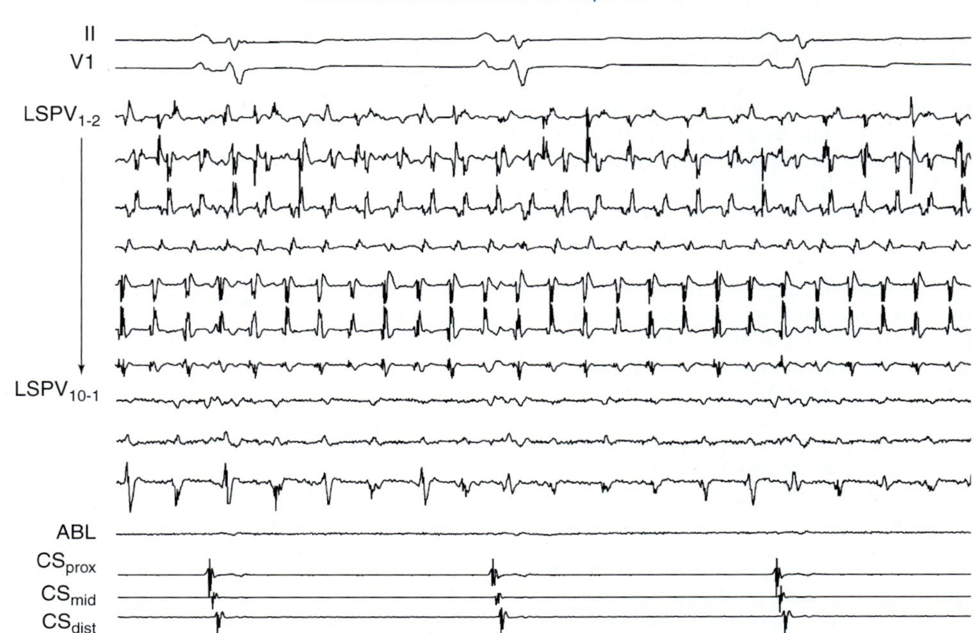

FIGURE 15-34 Electrical isolation of the left superior pulmonary vein (LSPV). Complete electrical isolation of the LSPV resulted in termination of atrial fibrillation (AF) and conversion to normal sinus rhythm (NSR) on the surface ECG and coronary sinus (CS) recordings, whereas AF continued in the LSPV (PV–left atrial exit block). ABL = ablation site; CS_{dist} = distal coronary sinus; CS_{mid} = middle coronary sinus; CS_{prox} = proximal coronary sinus.

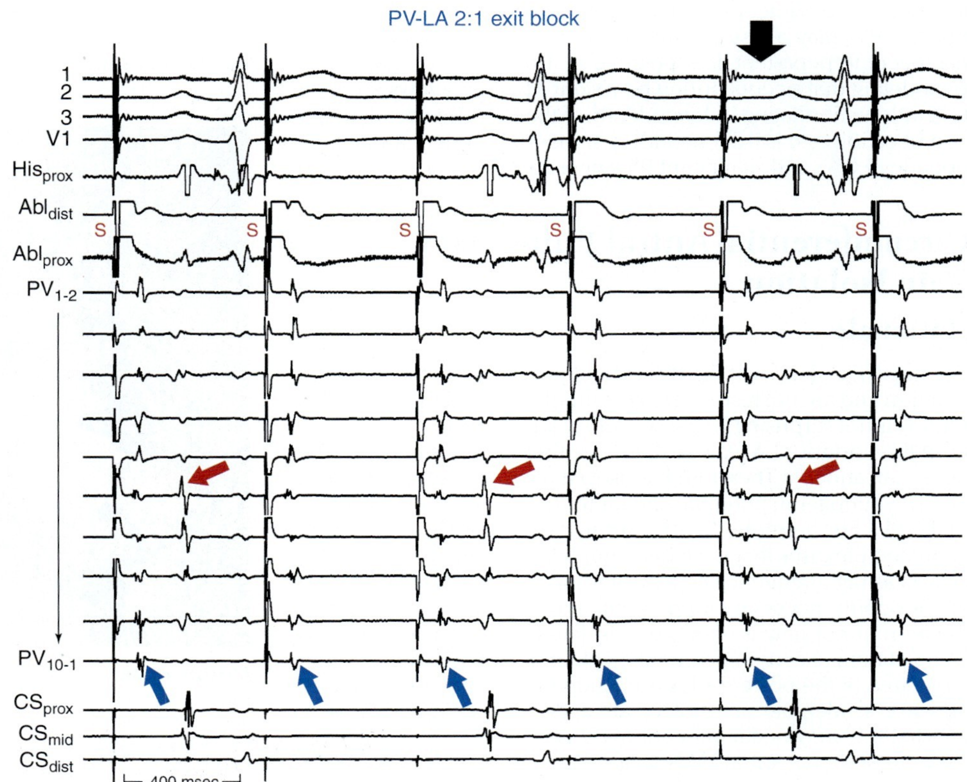

FIGURE 15-35 Pulmonary vein (PV)–left atrium (LA) 2:1 exit block. The ring catheter is positioned at the ostium of the left superior PV. During pacing using the ablation catheter positioned more distally in the vein, consistent capture of PV potentials is shown (blue arrows) but only every other PV potential conducts to LA (red arrows). Note very long delay between the stimulus and the P wave of the conducted complex (black arrow). Abl_{dist} = distal ablation site; Abl_{prox} = proximal ablation site; CS_{dist} = distal coronary sinus; CS_{mid} = middle coronary sinus; CS_{prox} = proximal coronary sinus; His_{prox} = proximal His bundle.

prove to have three or more arrhythmogenic PVs.[89] Nevertheless, in a study in patients with predominantly paroxysmal AF, isolation of arrhythmogenic veins identified using a comprehensive stimulation protocol was found as effective as empiric isolation of all PVs in achieving long-term arrhythmia control after a single ablation procedure. Of interest, limiting ablation to the arrhythmogenic PV did not yield any significant benefit over isolation of all PVs in terms of serious adverse events or procedure and fluoroscopy times.[89,93]

Reconnection of previously isolated PVs (caused by recovery of conduction through inadequately ablated fascicles in the muscle sleeves surrounding the PVs) is probably the most common reason for recurrent AF after PV isolation, at least among patients with paroxysmal AF. Other causes include ectopy from PVs not targeted or that could not be isolated at the initial procedure and the presence of non-PV triggers. In one study on the recurrence of AF following PV electrical isolation, most triggers were found to originate from previously targeted PVs (54%), whereas one-third of recurrent triggers (32%) originated from PVs that were not ablated during the initial session. Notably, 61% of previously isolated PVs in that series had evidence of recovered PV potentials. Therefore, successful PV isolation does not confer permanent disconnection of the PV musculature from the LA, and in most isolated PVs residual conduction remains or recurs with time.

Predictors of early recurrence of AF include older age (65 years or more), the presence of associated cardiovascular disease, the presence of multiple AF foci, the presence of AF foci from LA free wall, LA enlargement, and longstanding persistent AF. Predictors of late recurrence of AF include the presence of early recurrence of AF and the presence of multiple AF foci.

In most reports, a successful outcome was defined as the absence of any symptomatic atrial arrhythmias beyond the first 2 to 3 months after ablation without the use of antiarrhythmic drugs. Medium-term success has reportedly been achieved in up to 70% of patients with paroxysmal AF but in only 30% of patients with persistent AF. This finding suggests that intervention with PV isolation in patients with drug-refractory paroxysmal AF should not be postponed until the AF becomes persistent. Once AF has become persistent, it is likely that PV isolation will have to be supplemented by some other type of ablation procedure directed at the atrial myocardium. The less satisfactory outcome of PV isolation in persistent AF suggests that the PVs play a less critical role in generating AF once the AF has become persistent. It is possible that the EP and anatomical remodeling that occurs during persistent AF often allows the atria to continue fibrillating independently of the PVs. The overall major complication rate is 6.3%, including stroke (0.7%), pericardial tamponade (1.2%), and significant PV stenosis (4.3%).

Circumferential Antral Pulmonary Vein Isolation

Rationale

The muscular sleeves of the PVs extend proximally to the antral-LA junction and are not restricted to the tubular portion of the PV. This finding is not surprising, because embryologically the PVs originate from the posterior LA wall, so that a continuum exists between the atrial wall and PVs. Therefore, it is likely that the PV antrum also has an arrhythmogenic potential similar to that of the tubular portion of the PVs. Furthermore, the PV antrum can potentially harbor ganglionated plexuses that have been implicated in the genesis of AF, as well as high-frequency activity or rotors that are thought to have anchor points necessary for perpetuation of AF. Hence, ablation at the antrum not only is effective to isolate PVs electrically, but also it can eliminate certain potential mechanisms of AF. Additionally, a large area of the posterior LA is included inside the ablation lines and a considerable amount of atrial debulking (approximately 25% to 30%) may occur after antral PV isolation.

Circumferential antral PV isolation has several additional advantages over segmental ostial PV isolation. This technique does not rely on localizing the sites of electrical breakthroughs into the PV, and thus it is easier to perform during AF. Furthermore, this approach reduces the risk of PV stenosis because ablation is performed in the LA, away from the PV ostia (Fig. 15-36). In addition, in some patients with PV anatomical variations, this approach can be more favorable. One such variation is the presence of a common ostium of the left PVs, occurring in up to 32% of patients undergoing PV isolation. Such common ostia typically are too large to allow a stable position of the ring catheter (see Fig. 15-3). Another anatomical variation is the presence of a right middle PV, present in up to 21% of patients, which typically is separated from the right superior PV and right inferior PV by a narrow rim of atrial tissue (see Fig. 15-3). This would predispose to sliding of the ablation catheter into the PV during ablation. Another anatomical finding that renders extraostial PV isolation more favorable is a PV ostial diameter of less than 10 mm. RF application at a small ostium carries a higher risk of PV stenosis.

Circumferential antral PV isolation has been shown to be more effective in preventing AF recurrence than segmental ostial PV isolation, and this procedure has become a preferred ablation strategy in patients with paroxysmal and persistent AF. The preferred ablation target is the outmost atrial side of the PV ostium.

Identification of Pulmonary Vein Antra

The objective of the mapping and ablation procedure is to identify PV potentials along the perimeter of the PV antrum and ablate to eliminate these potentials completely. Reliable definition of the anatomy of PV antra is crucial to provide an effective set of lesions. A navigation system is used to provide 3-D anatomical images that allow safe maneuvering of the ablation catheter to complete the lesions at the antrum and eliminate conduction to PVs. However, the use of these systems does not replace the use of circumferential mapping and an EP endpoint to the procedure. More importantly, none of these systems can exclude the risk of RF delivery within the PVs and therefore the risk of PV stenosis.

RING CATHETER MAPPING

The ring catheter is used for circumferential ostial mapping of PV potentials, as described for segmental ostial PV isolation. However, the breakthrough segments (electrical connections) connecting

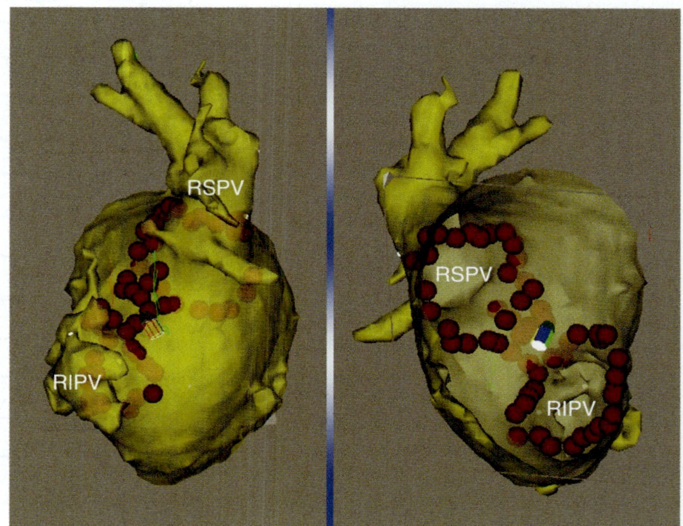

FIGURE 15-36 Circumferential antral pulmonary vein (PV) isolation. Registered three-dimensional surface reconstructions of the left atrium (LA; right lateral and cardioscopic views) during circumferential antral PV isolation of the right PVs are illustrated. Contiguous radiofrequency lesions are deployed in the LA proximal to the ostia of the PVs, creating a circumferential line around each PV ostium. RIPV, right inferior pulmonary vein; RSPV, right superior pulmonary vein.

the LA to the PV, identified as the earliest PV potentials recorded from the ring catheter, are not specifically mapped or targeted. Instead, the entire perimeter of the PV ostium is the target for the ablation procedure. Using the ring catheter enables circumferential mapping of the PV ostia perpendicular to the axis of the vein and serves as a landmark for the PV ostium around which RF lesions are delivered. In addition, the ring catheter is vital for confirming complete electrical isolation of the PV, an important endpoint of this ablation strategy.

BASKET CATHETER MAPPING

The technique of positioning the basket catheter into the PVs is described earlier in this chapter (see Fig. 15-30). For antral PV isolation, the basket catheter is introduced toward the distal PV under fluoroscopy guidance and then is pulled back as proximally as possible without dislodgment until its most proximal electrodes are positioned at the PV antrum, which is identified by selective angiography. The basket catheter can help identify the true junction between the PVs and LA anatomically and electrically. Because the basket catheter conforms to the shape of the PV, it provides information about the anatomy of the PV.[92]

Furthermore, longitudinal mapping with a basket catheter can help identify the transition zone between the PV and LA potentials. Far-field LA potentials are normally recorded almost simultaneously all over the PV, whereas the activation sequence of the PV potentials is from proximal to distal when the activation propagates from the LA to the distal PV. Consequently, the interval between the LA potentials and PV potentials is shorter at the proximal PV than at the distal PV. At the transition zone, total fusion of the PV and LA potentials occurs (Fig. 15-37). Therefore, the potential recorded at the transition zone may reflect the activation of the PV antrum. A transverse activation pattern, indicated by simultaneous activation recorded by some neighboring electrode pairs along the spline, sometimes occurs around the LA-PV junction before the longitudinal activation pattern within the PVs. This pattern may reflect the activation of the circle of myocardium at the PV antrum.[92]

On the basis of these findings, PV antrum potentials are defined as single sharp potentials formed by the total fusion of the PV and LA potentials around the PV ostium or single sharp potentials with a transverse activation pattern around the PV ostium (see Fig. 15-37). Targeting those potentials by RF ablation would target the transition zone between the PV ostium and LA. When potentials conforming to the definition of PV antrum potentials are observed from some electrode pairs on the same spline, the antrum potential recorded from the most proximal electrode pair is targeted. RF applications are also delivered to the gap between the targeted electrode pairs on the neighboring splines to produce a continuous RF lesion at the PV antrum.[92]

ELECTROANATOMICAL MAPPING

Different navigation tools, such as the EnSite NavX and CARTO systems, have been used to facilitate circumferential PV isolation. These systems can provide a high-resolution reconstruction of the LA and defining PV ostia and antra and allow real-time visualization of the ablation catheter within the reconstructed 3-D geometry. Additionally, ablation lesions can be tagged, thus facilitating creation of lines of block with considerable accuracy by serial RF lesion placement and allowing verification of the continuity of ablation line.

CARTO. The CARTO-3 system, the third-generation platform from Biosense Webster, allows visualization of up to five catheters (with and without the magnetic sensors) simultaneously with clear distinction of all electrodes. Unlike point-by-point electroanatomical mapping required in the older CARTO versions, volume data can be collected with Fast Anatomical Mapping (FAM), which permits rapid creation of anatomical maps by movement of a sensor-based catheter throughout the cardiac chamber (Fig. 15-38, see Video 15). Proprietary catheters besides the ablation catheter (e.g., the Lasso catheter) can further enhance the collection of points and increase the mapping speed.

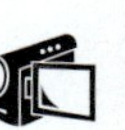

ENSITE NAVX. Similar to the CARTO system, the EnSite NavX system can provide a high-resolution reconstruction of the PV antrum and its anatomical variations. NavX-guided procedures are performed using the same catheter setup as conventional approaches, and the system does not need any special catheter. The system also works with most manufacturers' ablation catheters and RF or cryogenerators. The NavX system allows real-time visualization of the position of up to 64 electrodes on up to 8 standard EP catheters. Any electrode can be used to gather data, create static isochronal and voltage maps, and perform ablation procedures. A shadow can be displayed on the catheters of interest (e.g., the reference CS catheter and the ring catheter) to record the catheter's spatial position to realize displacement during the procedure. In case of displacement, the catheter can be returned easily to its original location under the guidance of NavX.

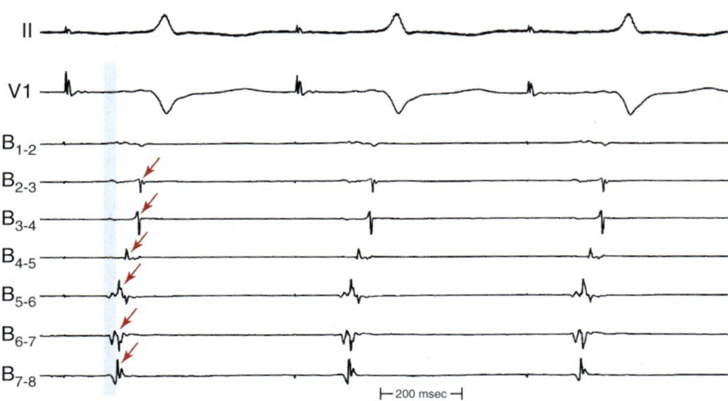

FIGURE 15-37 Identification of the pulmonary vein (PV) antrum using the basket catheter. The basket catheter is positioned in the left superior PV. Shown are seven bipolar recordings obtained from the eight electrodes (1-2, 2-3, to 7-8) on one of the eight splines (B1-2 through B7-8) of the basket catheter. During coronary sinus pacing, far-field left atrial (LA) potentials are normally recorded almost simultaneously all over the PV (shaded area). In contrast, PV activation propagates from proximal (ostial) to distal, and the interval between the LA potentials and the PV potentials is shorter at the proximal PV than at the distal PV. At the transition zone (PV antrum), a total fusion of the PV and LA potentials occurs (B7-8).

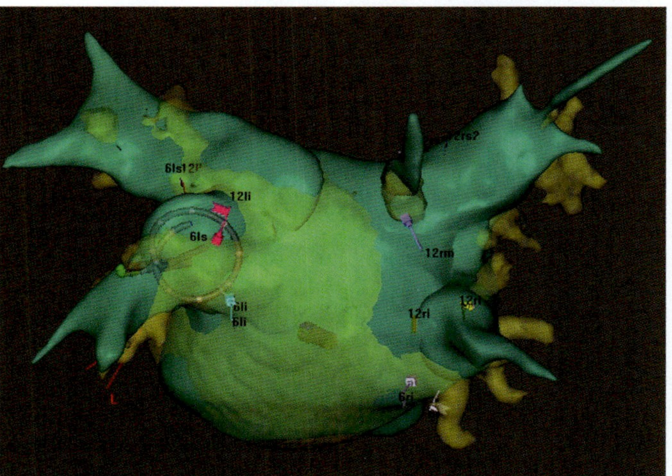

FIGURE 15-38 Three-dimensional reconstruction of the left atrium (LA, posterior view) using the CARTO-3 (Biosense Webster, Inc., Diamond Bar, Calif.) electroanatomical system (fast anatomical mapping [FAM]) and integration with preacquired computed tomography. The ring catheter is visualized in the left inferior pulmonary vein.

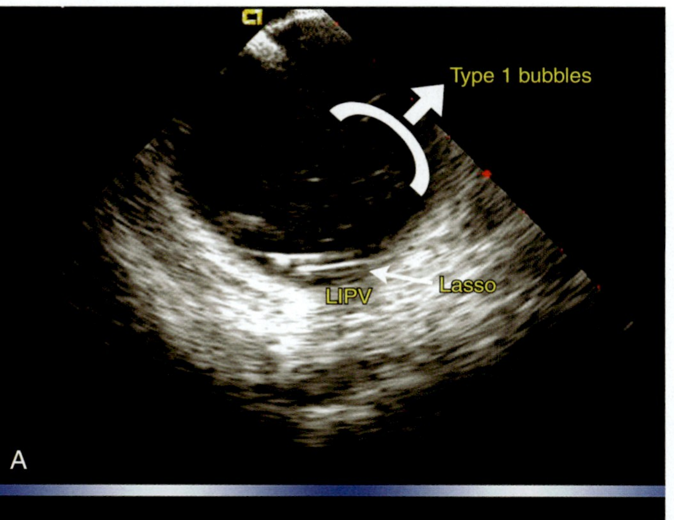

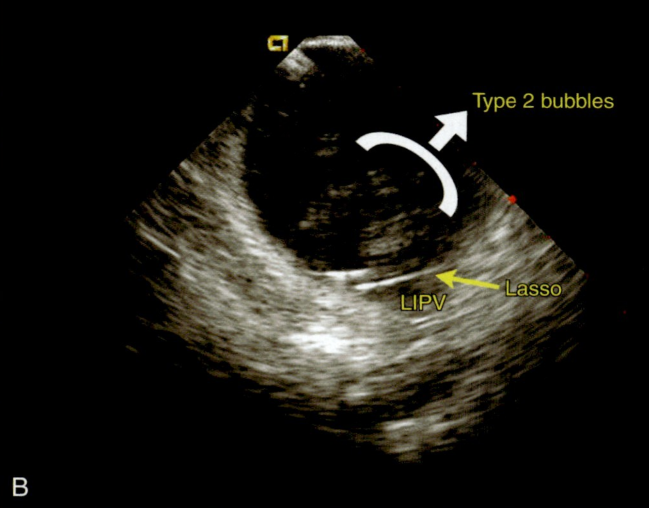

FIGURE 15-39 Intracardiac echocardiography (ICE)-guided radiofrequency (RF) energy delivery (microbubble monitoring). These are phased-array ICE views of the left atrium (LA) across the interatrial septum with the ring (Lasso) catheter positioned at the ostium of the left inferior pulmonary vein (LIPV). **A,** Localized microbubbles (type 1 bubbles) are observed during radiofrequency (RF) delivery. **B,** Showers of dense microbubbles extending to the LA cavity (type 2 bubbles) are observed during RF delivery. See text for discussion.

Using either the CARTO or NavX system, the 3-D shell representing the LA and PVs is constructed using the ablation or ring catheter, or both. Initially, fixed anatomical points are acquired at the four PV ostia, the LA appendage is demarcated, and three locations are recorded along the mitral isthmus to tag the valve orifice (Fig. 15-39; see Fig. 15-36). To acquire the PVs, entry into the vein is clearly identified as the catheter leaves the cardiac shadow on fluoroscopy, the impedance usually rises to more than 140 to 150 Ω, and electrical activity disappears. Because of the orientation of some veins and the limitations of catheter shape, it can be difficult to enter deeply into some veins, but the impedance still rises when the catheter is in the mouth of the vein. To differentiate between PVs and LA more clearly, voltage criteria (fractionation of local bipolar electrogram) and impedance (rise more than 4 Ω higher than the mean LA impedance) can be used to define the PV ostium. Mapping of each PV is performed by placing the mapping catheter 2 to 4 cm inside the PV and slowly pulling it back to the LA under fluoroscopy guidance. Care should be taken to reconstruct each PV ostium and the transition toward the LA (antrum), posterior free wall, mitral isthmus, and left interatrial septum. Subsequently, the system is allowed to create the geometry automatically while the ablation (or ring) catheter is moved throughout the LA. Sequential positioning of a catheter at multiple sites along the endocardial surface of the LA establishes that chamber's geometry.

COMPUTED TOMOGRAPHY AND MAGNETIC RESONANCE IMAGING

CT and MRI provide critical information regarding the number, location, and size of PVs, as needed for planning the ablation and selecting appropriately sized ablation devices. Resulting images also identify branching patterns of potentially arrhythmogenic PVs, disclose the presence of fused superior and inferior veins into antral structures, and clarify the potentially confounding origins of far-field electrograms that masquerade as PV potentials.

Furthermore, the segmented CT/MRI volumes can be downloaded on the CARTO and NavX platforms. The 3-D electroanatomical maps can be simultaneously displayed side-by-side with CT/MRI segmented cardiac scans to confirm cardiac structures and guide ablation. These systems also enable registration of the preacquired 3-D CT/MRI images of LA reconstructions on the real-time 3-D electroanatomical maps reconstructed from multiple endocardial locations. This allows real-time visualization of the location and orientation of the catheter tip within the registered CT/MRI anatomical framework and can potentially improve the quality of lesion sets, reduce complications, and shorten procedure and fluoroscopy times (see Video 13 and Figs. 15-39 and 3-45).

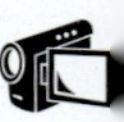

A novel application (EP Navigator prototype, Philips Healthcare, Best, The Netherlands) has been developed to superimpose a preacquired segmented 3-D CT image of the LA over a real-time fluoroscopy system (CT overlay), to help in guiding ablation of AF.

The process of image integration—preprocedural CT and MRI image acquisition, image segmentation and extraction, and image registration—is discussed in Chapter 6.

INTRACARDIAC ECHOCARDIOGRAPHY

Phased-array ICE has been used in AF ablation procedures for several purposes: to assist with transseptal puncture, to identify the number and position of PVs, to identify the true border of the PV antrum, to determine the branching patterns of the right PVs needed for total PV isolation, to guide the positioning of the ring and ablation catheters at the antrum of the PV, to verify ablation catheter tip to tissue contact, to assess the degree of PV occlusion during balloon-based ablative interventions, and to detect procedural complications (e.g., pericardial effusion, LA thrombus, and PV stenosis).

For ICE imaging, a 10 or 8 Fr 64-element phased-array ultrasound catheter is positioned in the middle of the RA via an 11 or 9 Fr left femoral venous access. The ICE catheter remains in the RA for the entire procedure to guide transseptal puncture, define PV anatomy, and monitor for microbubble formation during RF ablation. A 7.5- or 8.5-MHz imaging frequency optimizes visualization of LA structures and PVs beyond the interatrial septum. PV imaging is uniformly possible by first visualizing the membranous fossa from a middle to low RA catheter tip position. From this view, clockwise catheter rotation allows visualization of the LA appendage, followed by long-axis views of the left superior and inferior PVs (see Figs. 4-13 and 6-22). Further clockwise rotation of the catheter brings the orifice of the right superior and inferior PVs into view. The LA ostia of these veins are typically viewed en face, to yield an owl's eye appearance at the vein's orifice.

As the operator images each vein, the ring and ablation catheters can be positioned at the antral-LA interface for ablation. Because the PV antrum is a large-diameter structure, its circumference cannot be mapped using a stationary ring catheter fixed in one position. Instead, the ring catheter must be sequentially positioned along each segment of the antral circumference to look for PV potentials. ICE can identify the true border of the PV antrum and guide positioning of the ring and ablation catheters. Therefore, the ring catheter is a roving catheter in this procedure. An operator's assistant often must hold the ring catheter in position around the antrum because the ring catheter is not wedged into the tubular ostium for stability. When mapping the anterior segments of the left PVs or septal segments of the right PVs, the ring catheter must be advanced slightly because of the oblique nature of the antral-LA interface.

Additionally, ICE can help with the registration process of the CT/MRI image with the electroanatomical mapping system. Furthermore, the CARTOSound Image Integration Module (Biosense Webster, Inc.) allows for 3-D reconstruction of the LA using real-time ICE and incorporates the electroanatomical map to the map derived from ICE (see Chap. 6 and Video 14).

Target of Ablation

The ablation procedure is based on electrical isolation of all PVs. The objective is to identify PV potentials along the circumference of the PV antrum and ablate to eliminate these potentials completely. However, unlike segmental ostial PV isolation, the ostial portion of the breakthrough segments (electrical connections) connecting the LA to the PV, identified as the earliest PV potentials recorded from the ring catheter, is not the sole target of ablation. Complete encirclement of each PV antrum with ablation lesions is the goal of the ablation procedure, which would consequently result in PV isolation (see Fig. 15-36). All PVs are targeted.

Ablation lines consist of contiguous focal lesions deployed in the LA at a distance 5 mm or more proximal to the ostia of the PVs, to create a circumferential line of conduction block around each PV (see Fig. 15-36). PV isolation is performed 1 cm from the ostium of the right PVs, as well as for the posterior and superior aspects of the left PVs, to enhance efficacy and prevent PV stenosis. However, ablation at the anterior portions of the left PVs usually requires energy be delivered less than 5 mm from the ostium of the PV to achieve catheter stability. Ablation is started randomly in the right or left PVs and is performed individually.

When two or three ipsilateral PV ostia are coalescent, en bloc encirclement of those ostia is performed (i.e., one encirclement for the right-sided or left-sided PVs), and no line between the ipsilateral PVs is deployed (Fig. 15-40). The use of two ring catheters within the ipsilateral PVs may be considered in such an approach. With this double-Lasso technique, electrical isolation of ipsilateral PVs occurs simultaneously in most (more than 80%) cases. The simultaneous use of two ring catheters provides insights into the electrical interactions of the ipsilateral PVs and helps identify conduction gaps in the complete circumferential ablation lines in case of redoing the ablation procedure for recurrent AF. However, this approach involves obtaining a third transseptal access, which rendered its use uncommon. Importantly, single encirclement of ipsilateral PVs predisposes to breakthrough conduction of both ipsilateral PVs in case of a single gap in the en bloc circle. Furthermore, one report found that AF triggers originate frequently from the carina region of the PVs; hence, ablation in this area between ipsilateral PVs, in addition to being frequently necessary for complete electrical isolation of PVs, can be effective for targeting the source of the PV triggers.[96]

Ablation Technique

Several ablation technologies have been used for circumferential PV isolation. Most commonly, RF ablation is performed with an irrigated-tip ablation catheter. Alternatively, an 8-mm-tip standard ablation catheter can be used. Technological evolution is now aimed at developing new catheter designs for circumferential ablation of the PVs as an alternative for the conventional point-by-point RF ablation. A novel ablation system using duty-cycled and alternating unipolar and bipolar RF energy is currently undergoing clinical evaluation. Furthermore, balloon-based ablation devices using different energy sources (e.g., cryothermal energy, laser energy, RF energy ["hot balloon" and mesh technologies], and high-intensity focused ultrasound [HIFU]) have been evaluated. The cryoballoon has proven feasibility, safety, and efficacy in the treatment of AF. The laser balloon is currently undergoing evaluation, and preliminary clinical results are promising. Because of severe complications in the form of atrioesophageal fistula, the HIFU balloon is no longer in clinical use (see Chap. 7). The clinical evaluation of the RF hot balloon catheter is still in its initial stages. Another novel ablation catheter system delivers RF energy through a flexible mesh electrode (C.R. Bard, Inc., Billerica, Mass.) that is deployed in the PV ostium. This system is undergoing investigation for PV isolation.[97-99]

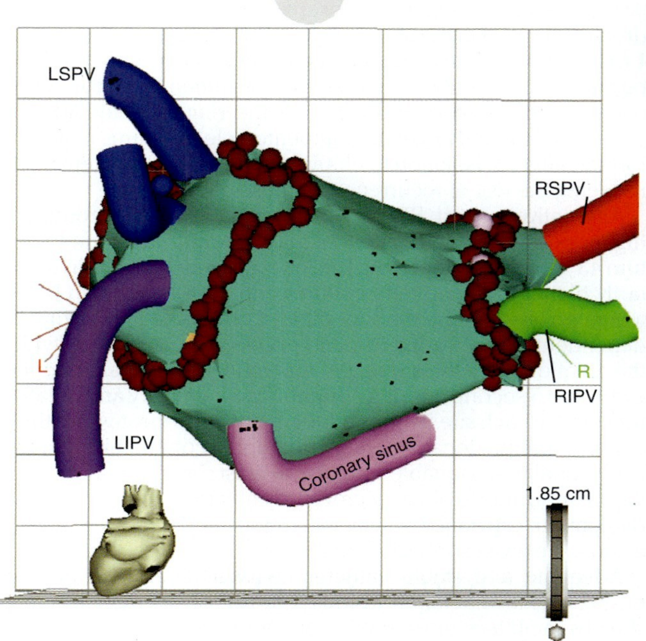

FIGURE 15-40 Circumferential antral pulmonary vein (PV) isolation. This posterior view of the electroanatomical map of the left atrium (LA) at the conclusion of the PV isolation procedure shows closely spaced red dots denoting locations at which radiofrequency ablation was performed. En bloc encirclement of the PV ostia (one encirclement for the right-sided and a second encirclement of left-sided PVs) was performed without ablation lines between the ipsilateral PVs. LIPV = left inferior pulmonary vein; LSPV = left superior pulmonary vein; RIPV = right inferior pulmonary vein; RSPV = right superior pulmonary vein.

CONVENTIONAL RADIOFREQUENCY ABLATION

Ablation is started at the posterior wall of each PV, usually fluoroscopically facing the border of the spine in the anteroposterior projection, and continued around the venous perimeter. The posterior wall of the right PV is reached by counterclockwise torque of the catheter and the left PV by clockwise torque. For ablation at the anterior portions of the left PVs, energy must usually be delivered within a few millimeters of the vein (because of a relatively narrow border between the left PVs and the LA appendage, and the difficulty to balance the catheter tip on the narrow rim of tissue separating these structures) to achieve effective disconnection. RF ablation sites are tagged on the reconstructed 3-D map. This tagging helps ensure coalescence of the ablation lesions to ensure continuity of the ablation line (see Fig. 15-36).

RF energy is delivered using an irrigated-tip catheter, with power output limited to 25 to 30 W (or even less) on the posterior LA wall where the atrial wall is thin and esophageal proximity presents potential danger, and 30 to 50 W on the left PV-LA appendage ridge and anterior LA wall, and a target temperature of less than 41°C and irrigation rates of 5 to 20 mL/min (0.9% heparinized saline). Alternatively, ablation may be performed using an 8-mm-tip conventional ablation catheter, with a maximum power of up to 70 W and a target temperature of 50°C to 55°C.

RF energy is delivered for 30 to 60 seconds at each point, until the maximal local electrogram amplitude is decreased by 50% to 90% or double potentials are observed or to achieve an impedance drop of 5 to 10 Ω at the ablation site. RF application is prolonged for 1 to 2 minutes when a change occurs in the activation or morphology, or both, of the PV potentials, as determined by circumferential mapping recorded downstream on the ring catheter. Additional ostial applications targeting fragmented electrograms may be performed after PV isolation to eliminate any ostial PV potentials, thus reducing the risk of recurrence because of ostial foci.

Alternatively, short RF applications (for 2 to 5 seconds) at a higher power (50 W, irrigation rate 30 mL/min, maximum temperature 43°C) can be employed. The latter approach results in momentarily higher LA tissue temperatures and allows the tip to be set at a high power to injure the superficial tissue while minimizing time-dependent deep heating through excessive heat transfer. Typically, the ablation catheter is dragged continuously in small increments every 2 to 5 seconds during continuous RF delivery, and ablation is repeated at each site, if required, for many times throughout the procedure until the local atrial electrogram is completely eliminated. It is probably reasonable to allow at least 2-minute time intervals before returning to ablate a previously ablated site to allow for heat dissipation, especially when ablating at the LA posterior wall, to avoid excessive esophageal heating.[100]

Adequate and stable catheter tip-tissue contact is critical to ensure effective ablation lesions. The use of steerable transseptal sheaths facilitates more stable catheter positioning and access to all desired ablation targets for PV isolation. Additionally, ICE can provide detailed anatomical information and real-time information of the location of the tip electrode of the ablation catheter and can help confirm catheter stability. Real-time measurements of the contact force of the ablation tip have been introduced using different technologies, especially in conjunction with robotic navigation systems.

INTRACARDIAC ECHOCARDIOGRAPHY–GUIDED ABLATION

INTRACARDIAC ECHOCARDIOGRAPHY–GUIDED CATHETER POSITIONING. The ring and ablation catheters are positioned at the antral-LA interface for ablation. The ring catheter is then sequentially positioned along each segment of the antral circumference (guided by ICE) to look for PV potentials. As the ring catheter is moved from one segment of the LA-antral interface to the next, ablation is performed at the poles demonstrating PV potentials. The ablation catheter is moved to the target pole on the ring catheter, while care is taken to keep the catheter in the same plane as the ring catheter. Ablation is performed only along the specific antral segment that the ring catheter is mapping. Because the PV antrum is a large structure, multiple movements of the ring catheter around the PV antrum are needed. After all segments of a PV are ablated, the ring catheter is used to again map the vein's interface with the LA to confirm the absence of PV potentials at the antral-LA interface. During NSR or CS pacing, the ring catheter is advanced deep into the PV tube to confirm an absence of electrogram recordings, which represents entrance block into the PV.

Using ICE to define the PV antrum and guide RF ablation, the anatomical region within the ablation circles typically encompasses the entire posterior wall, LA roof, and anteroseptal extension of the right PVs.

INTRACARDIAC ECHOCARDIOGRAPHY–GUIDED RADIOFREQUENCY ENERGY DELIVERY (MICROBUBBLE MONITORING). ICE can help visualize evolving lesions during RF energy delivery and image microbubble formation during tissue heating. The latter is important because microbubble formation during ablation can indicate excessive tissue heating, which could lead to thrombus or char formation, tissue disruption, or PV stenosis.

Observation by ICE of microbubbles during ablation was previously proposed as a method of titrating RF power delivery. Two types of bubble patterns are seen with ICE: scattered microbubbles (type 1) and a brisk shower of dense microbubbles (type 2) (see Fig. 15-39). It has been hypothesized that type 1 microbubbles indicate early tissue overheating (i.e., subcritical heating of the myocardium with imminent risk of steam pop formation), whereas type 2 microbubbles indicate excessive heating. Microbubbles seen on ICE directly correlate with cerebral microembolic events detected by transcranial Doppler, tissue disruption, and char formation. Restricting power output to avoid microbubble formation on ICE increases the efficacy of antral PV isolation while minimizing severe PV stenosis and cerebroembolic complications. Absolute temperature and impedance readings do not correlate with microbubbles and cannot reliably predict tissue disruption and cerebroembolic events.

By using these principles, RF energy is initially set at 30 W and 55°C using a nonopen irrigated ablation catheter. Subsequently, RF power is titrated up to a maximum of 70 W by 5-W increments every few seconds while monitoring for microbubble formation on ICE. When type 1 (scattered) microbubbles are seen, energy is titrated down by 5-W decrements every 5 seconds until microbubble generation has subsided. Energy delivery is terminated immediately when type 2 (dense showers) microbubbles are seen. The operator should aggressively avoid any microbubble formation. Ablation is continued in one spot until no more PV potentials are seen. Each lesion typically lasts 30 to 50 seconds.

Microbubble formation, however, is not a straightforward surrogate for tissue heating. Experimental animal studies revealed that, particularly with the use of an irrigated ablation electrode, the abrupt occurrence of steam popping can occur without prior development of any bubbles on ICE. Thus, caution is warranted in interpretation of the absence of bubble formation on ICE as an indicator of inadequate intramyocardial heating. The absence of microbubble formation does not indicate that tissue heating is inadequate or that the power level should be increased, nor does the presence of scattered microbubbles indicate safe tissue heating. This marker is fairly specific for tissue heating as judged by tissue temperatures, but it is not routinely sensitive. Specifically, scattered microbubbles are noted to occur over the entire spectrum of tissue temperatures, whereas dense showers of microbubbles occur only at tissue temperatures higher than 60°C. Scattered microbubbles may represent an electrolytic phenomenon, whereas dense showers of microbubbles suggest steam formation, with associated tissue disruption and impedance rises. Furthermore, it must be recognized that bubbles are typically present during open-irrigated ablation and can also be seen during high-output pacing and infusion of saline through the transseptal sheath side port.

DUTY-CYCLED BIPOLAR AND UNIPOLAR RADIOFREQUENCY CATHETER ABLATION

A novel ablation system (GENius, Medtronic Inc., Minneapolis, Minn.) has been developed for AF ablation, in which duty-cycled and alternating unipolar and bipolar (between adjacent electrodes) nonirrigated RF energy is used to create contiguous ablation lesions in the PV antrum using a circular multielectrode PV ablation catheter (PVAC, Ablation Frontiers, Inc., Carlsbad, Calif.) (Figs. 7-4 and 7-5).

The PVAC is a circular decapolar 9 Fr bidirectional over-the wire catheter with a 25-mm diameter array at the distal tip, 3-mm-long platinum electrodes, and interelectrode spacing of 3 mm. The multielectrode catheter allows selective mapping, pacing, and ablation through any or all electrodes as required. Each electrode is supplied with a thermocouple, and a software algorithm modulates power to reach the user-defined target temperature (usually 60°C), but it limits power to a maximum of 8 W per electrode when using the PVAC in a 4:1 power setting or 10 W in all other settings.[101]

The PVAC is advanced over a guidewire into the LA via a steerable transseptal sheath. Initially, the PVAC itself is maneuvered within each PV to map PV potentials. Once the region of interest is localized and good contact of the PVAC with antral tissue is achieved (as indicated by local electrogram interpretation and enhanced fluoroscopy), RF energy is delivered in a combination of one or more of the five bipolar channels. When ablating large common PV ostia, some electrode pairs that have no or suboptimal contact to the atrial tissue are deactivated to avoid ineffective energy delivery. Bipolar and unipolar RF delivery is typically set in a 4:1 configuration (i.e., 80% bipolar and 20% unipolar), to create a 3- to 4-mm wide and deep lesion. After several RF applications over all electrode pairs, the PVAC is rotated around the PV ostium to look for the earliest PV potential to isolate the vein completely.

ADVANTAGES. The PVAC represents a reasonable alternative for point-by-point circumferential PV isolation. Preliminary studies found the PVAC system very successful in achieving complete PV isolation in most patients and veins, and it was associated with shorter procedure and fluoroscopy times. The short-term and intermediate-term efficacy is comparable to that of a conventional antral ablation technique. This system is still undergoing investigation. One advantage of the PVAC system is the simultaneous application of RF energy across the electrode array, thus creating contiguous lesions.[101,102]

LIMITATIONS. This system has several limitations. The PVAC diameter is unadjustable; large vein ostia can be difficult to isolate. Additionally, it is not feasible to monitor PV potentials during RF energy delivery. The PVAC is primarily designed for PV isolation, and mapping of extra-PV triggers usually requires a second ablation catheter. Other catheter designs, which use the same multichannel duty-cycled RF generator, also have been developed for ablation of fractionated electrograms in the LA (MAAC, Ablation Frontiers), septal ablation (MASC, Ablation Frontiers), as well as linear ablation (TVAC, Ablation Frontiers) (see Fig. 7-4).[101,102] Ablation with the PVAC has been associated with a high incidence of subclinical cerebral microemboli detected by MRI in a small number of patients, compared with other technologies (37% of cases, versus 7% for standard irrigated RF and 4% for cryoablation). The significance of this finding remains to be determined.

CRYOBALLOON ABLATION

Clinical studies indicate an acceptable efficacy rate of PV isolation using the cryoballoon, with 1-year freedom from AF demonstrated in 73% in patients with paroxysmal AF and in 45% for those with persistent AF. Further studies, including direct comparison with conventional RF ablation, are ongoing and will provide important insight into long-term efficacy and safety.[103,104]

The cryothermal balloon ablation system (CryoCath Technologies) consists of a nondeflectable, over-the-wire, 10 Fr two-lumen catheter with double inner-outer cooling balloons (outer balloon maximum diameter, 23 mm; total length, 20 mm; see Fig. 7-11). The refrigerant nitrous oxide (N_2O) is delivered under pressure from the console into the inner balloon chamber via a lumen within 2 mm of the catheter tip, where it undergoes a liquid to gas phase change, resulting in inner balloon cooling to temperatures of −80°C or lower. During cryotherapy, temperature is monitored via a thermocouple located at the inner balloon.[103]

The deflated cryoballoon is advanced via a steerable transseptal sheath over either an extrarigid 0.032-mm guidewire or a small six-pole microcircular mapping catheter placed inside of each PV. Initially, PV angiography is performed to delineate PV anatomy and guide balloon positioning. The cryoballoon is inflated outside of the PV (to avoid any mechanical damage) and then is advanced into the PV to occlude the vein. Achieving complete mechanical occlusion of the PV is important to prevent the heating effect of residual PV flow during freezing. In fact, the degree of PV occlusion at the tip of the inflated balloon has been correlated with electrical isolation. Complete PV occlusion is confirmed by the lack of contrast medium runoff into the LA during contrast injection into the distal lumen of the cryoballoon or the disappearance of flow on color Doppler obtained by ICE or TEE. If PV occlusion is not achieved, the device can be turned clockwise and counterclockwise or even slightly withdrawn until PV flow disappears. Also, the guidewire can be positioned in a different PV branch to change the orientation of the balloon at the PV ostium. Among the other maneuvers used to facilitate PV occlusion by the cryoballoon is the "hockey stick technique," which allows for an optimized tissue contact at the inferior circumference of the inferior PVs. This technique involves advancing the sheath via a guidewire placed in the PV with a maximal bend to the superoposterior LA and pushing the balloon into the inferior part of the PV ostium. The "pull-down technique" is used if angiography indicates perfect contact of the balloon only at the superior circumference of the PV but not at the lower PV circumference. The pull-down involves waiting for the balloon to adhere to the superior aspect of the targeted vein (generally after 60 seconds), followed by catheter and shaft deflection to pull the frozen balloon downward to achieve contact with the inferior portion of the vein and thereby eliminate the inferior gap.[103,104]

After confirmation of PV occlusion by contrast injection, the 5-minute freezing cycle is initiated. During ablation of the right superior PV, maintenance of phrenic nerve activity is ensured by continuous monitoring of spontaneous breathing or by continuous pacing of the right phrenic nerve from a catheter positioned in the SVC. In case of loss of capture or weakening of right hemidiaphragmatic movements, freezing should be immediately stopped.

After two freezing cycles, the balloon is deflated, and a conventional circular mapping catheter is inserted into the PV to assess for isolation. Although a small six-pole microcircular mapping catheter can be introduced through the lumen of the cryoballoon and can help with real-time PV mapping during freezing, this catheter often lacks the mechanical support needed for adequate mapping and confirmation of complete PV isolation.[104]

If PV isolation is not achieved, the cryoballoon is repositioned, and additional freezes are applied. If remnant ostial potentials are still recorded, electrical isolation is segmentally completed by focal cryoablation using an 8-mm cryoablation catheter (Freezor Max, CryoCath Technologies).

ADVANTAGES. Cryoablation can offer several potential advantages, including elimination of coagulum formation, which should reduce stroke risk, and absence of coagulative necrosis of the ablated tissue, which can potentially reduce the risk of tamponade, PV stenosis, and pericarditis. Although the highly variable anatomy of the PVs provides a significant challenge for any balloon-based technology (it requires the shaft of the catheter to be directed coaxially to the PV), the cryothermal balloon overcomes this problem because the entire balloon can freeze and adhere to the adjacent tissue. As such, the perimeter of the balloon in closest apposition to the vein becomes the source of ablation, irrespective of the orientation in the vein. Also, compared with other balloon-based ablation technologies (HIFU and endoscopic laser), the cryoballoon is less direction dependent, because the refrigerant jet inside the balloon is directed to produce the lowest ablation temperatures in a large circular zone on the anterior third of the balloon. As such, cryoballoon ablation may be expected to isolate the muscular PV sleeves, as well as the PV antrum.

LIMITATIONS. Cryoablation of the right inferior PV remains challenging. The most important complication of cryoballoon ablation is phrenic nerve palsy, which occurs in up to 11.2% of patients, even with close monitoring of phrenic movement. Phrenic nerve palsy is transient, with complete resolution observed within 1 year in most cases. It has become evident that cryoballoon ablation can be associated with PV stenosis (the rate of symptomatic PV stenosis or PV stenosis requiring intervention was 0.17%). A distal position of the cryoballoon with respect to the PV ostium, especially when using the smaller 23-mm balloon, can potentially increase the risk of these complications. It is possible that using the big (28-mm) cryoballoon for all veins can help direct cryothermal lesions proximal to the PV ostium at the antral level and thereby reduce the risk of phrenic nerve injury and PV stenosis.[104]

LASER ABLATION

The laser ablation catheter technology (CardioFocus, Inc., Marlborough, Mass.) is still in clinical trials. The initial clinical experience

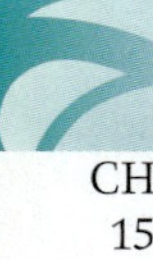

Pulmonary vein isolation using balloon-delivered laser

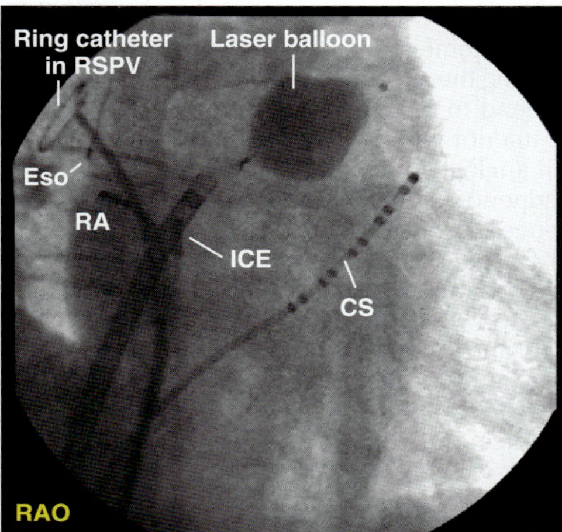

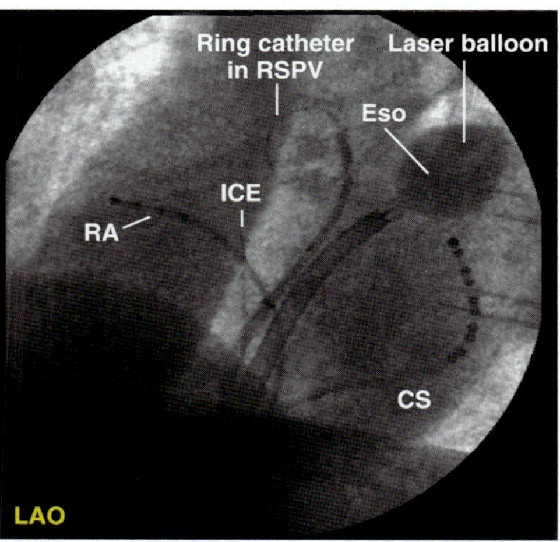

FIGURE 15-41 Pulmonary vein (PV) isolation using the laser balloon technology. The laser balloon is inflated in the left superior PV. The ring catheter is positioned in the right superior PV (RSPV) during balloon inflation. CS = coronary sinus catheter; Eso = esophageal temperature probe; ICE = phased-array intracardiac echocardiography catheter; RA = right atrial catheter.

with this technology suggests the ability to create discrete point-by-point ablation and a configurable ablation line design and achieve reliable and lasting circumferential PV electrical isolation in patients with highly variable PV shapes and sizes.[98,99]

The endoscopic ablation system consists of a nonsteerable, compliant balloon catheter with an adjustable diameter that allows treatment of PVs of 9 to 32 mm in diameter. The laser balloon is inserted at the PV antrum through a steerable 12 Fr transseptal sheath. Selective PV angiography or ICE, or both, can be used to verify appropriate position of the balloon. The balloon is filled with a mixture of contrast and deuterium dioxide (D_2O) and is irrigated internally at 20 mL/min to minimize absorption of laser energy.

The efficacy of the laser balloon ablation depends on good contact around the balloon circumference. Hence, the laser ablation catheter system incorporates a 2 Fr fiberoptic endoscope positioned at the proximal end of the balloon that, once the balloon is deployed, enables direct visualization of the face of the balloon at the targeted PV antrum and monitoring for the intrusion of blood into the space between the balloon and the tissue.

The arc generator consists of an optical fiber located within the central shaft that projects a 30-degree arc of light onto regions of balloon-tissue contact guided by an endoscopic view of the PV antrum (areas of balloon-tissue contact are visualized as blanched white, whereas contact with blood is visualized as red). This arc serves as an aiming beam for laser delivery. It can be steered along the balloon face with endoscopic visualization, independently of the balloon itself, thus facilitating individual lesion application in an anatomically flexible lesion design that adapts to the highly variable PV anatomy. Once the proper location is identified, a diode laser is used to deliver laser energy at 980 nm. The laser fiber can be advanced or withdrawn to shift the site of lasing along the longitudinal axis of the catheter. Lesions are deployed in a point-by-point fashion. Each individual ablation lesion covers 30 degrees of a circle, and lesions are overlapped by 30% to 50% to minimize gaps between adjacent lesions. Rotating and advancing and retracting the aiming beam, and consequently the laser beam, facilitate individual lesion application and individual line design. The balloon inflation pressure and diameter can be adjusted to optimize sealing of the PV antrum and maximize tissue exposure to the laser arc. Laser energy is delivered at power output of 5.5 to 18 W for 20 to 30 seconds, depending on the thickness of tissue or the proximity of the esophagus, or both. Because the catheter shaft obscures one-fifth of the circumference, catheter rotation is required to complete ablation at a particular PV.[98]

Importantly, the laser balloon does not have the capability of simultaneous mapping and ablation. Mapping of PV potential is performed using a ring catheter before and after ablation. Initially, the ring catheter should not be left in the same PV while the laser balloon is deployed and during circumferential ablation because its shaft can impede balloon-tissue contact (Fig. 15-41). After completion of the ablation circle, the balloon is deflated, and the ring catheter is inserted into the PV to assess for electrical isolation. However, if PV isolation is incomplete after a single ablation, the ring catheter may be placed distally to the inflated laser balloon to visualize PV electric activity online during laser energy application. However, the shaft of the ring catheter is positioned opposite to the presumed electrical gap to avoid incomplete PV sealing at the targeted ablation site.

Preliminary studies of PV isolation using the laser ablation catheter technology in patients with paroxysmal AF found the short-term and 1-year success rates similar to those of other ablation techniques and other ablation energies (Fig. 15-42). Procedure times also were comparable with those of established balloon-based ablation systems. No PV stenosis has been observed. The incidence of phrenic nerve palsies after laser ablation seems to be moderate compared with other balloon-based ablation systems, but it needs further investigation. Larger studies evaluating the long-term efficacy and safety of this system are required.[98,99]

ADVANTAGES. An advantage of the laser balloon system is the ability to visualize the substrate for ablation directly, thus superseding the need for additional imaging. Additionally, in comparison with the cryoballoon and HIFU balloon, the size of the laser balloon is adjustable to the individual PV anatomy in a broad range, which allows for treatment of virtually any PV with a single device. The laser arc of 30 degrees allows for very discrete lesions, and the laser energy is titratable, to enable flexible lesion deployment and freedom to create the preferred ablation line design. Moreover, unlike the cryoballoon and HIFU balloon systems in which energy titration is not possible, the ability to titrate laser energy can potentially decrease injury to adjacent structures.[98]

LIMITATIONS. One of the limitations of the laser balloon system is an observed trend toward higher esophageal temperatures, resulting in more severe mucosal damage, as known from other energy sources, although no atrioesophageal fistula has been reported. Therefore, esophageal temperature monitoring is essential with the use of this system. However, the optimal esophageal cutoff temperature is still not known. Additionally, defining the appropriate laser energy setting will require further investigation. Because the laser balloon system is not designed as an over-the-wire system, it is sometimes challenging to direct and stabilize the balloon catheter within the LA or the respective PV.[99]

Endpoints of Ablation

Common intraprocedural endpoints of circumferential antral PV isolation include electrical isolation of all PVs, noninducibility of

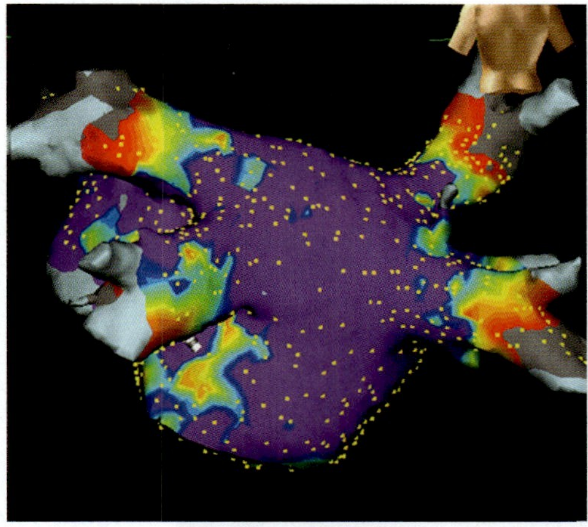

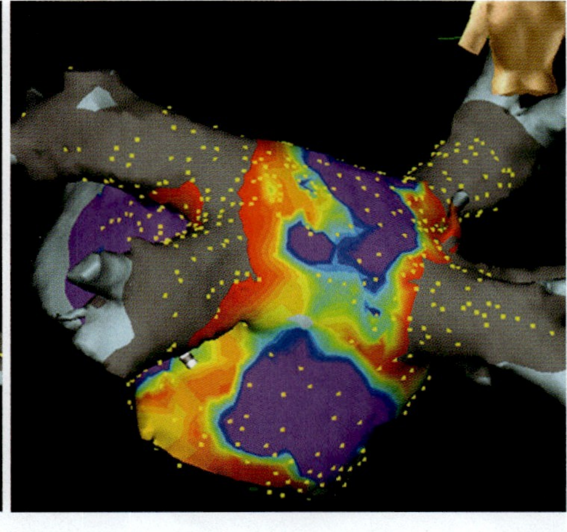

FIGURE 15-42 Three-dimensional electroanatomical voltage map of the left atrium before **(left)** and after **(right)** circumferential pulmonary vein isolation using the laser balloon. Sites with voltage lower than 0.5 mV are red on the map, and those with voltage higher than 1.5 mV are purple, with interpolation of color for intermediate amplitudes. The gray area denotes no detectable signal (scar). Note the voltage abatement at the level of the antrum of each of the pulmonary veins, indicating the level of ablation achieved using the laser balloon catheter system. *(Courtesy of CardioFocus, Inc., Marlborough, Mass.)*

AF, and elimination of residual potentials inside the circumferential ablation lines. Importantly, these endpoints, even when successfully achieved during the procedure, often do not persist over time, both in patients with and in those without AF recurrences. Nevertheless, there is a consensus on the importance of the complete bidirectional electrical isolation of all PVs as a procedural endpoint. On the other hand, less agreement exists on the value of the other endpoints.[105]

ELECTRICAL DISCONNECTION OF ALL PULMONARY VEINS

The endpoint of ablation is complete bidirectional electrical isolation of all four PVs, as described earlier for segmental ostial PV isolation.

NONINDUCIBILITY OF ATRIAL FIBRILLATION

Induction of sustained AF is thought to indicate the presence of a potential atrial substrate capable of maintaining AF; however, its value as a predictor for clinical outcome remains controversial. Elimination of PV potentials correlates with clinical success better than the acute suppression of AF inducibility. However, a successful outcome is sometimes observed without complete PV potential elimination, and some supposedly unsuccessfully treated patients experience remarkable improvement with a previously ineffective drug.

Different pacing protocols and definitions of inducibility of AF have been employed in different studies. Aggressive pacing protocols can decrease the specificity, yet more conservative pacing protocols can potentially decrease the predictive value. In fact, aggressive atrial pacing (at CLs shorter than 180 milliseconds) can induce AF in up to 26% of patients without a history of AF. Further investigation is needed to optimize the specificity of using AF induction as an endpoint for AF ablation.[106]

Commonly, induction of AF is attempted by burst pacing at a CL of 250 milliseconds with sequential decrement down to 200 milliseconds (as long as 1:1 capture is maintained) for 5 to 10 seconds at least three times from the CS and then repeated from the RA. If AF is not inducible, isoproterenol (10 to 20 µg/min intravenous infusion) is then administered, and atrial pacing is repeated. Also, AF induction by a 30-joule external biphasic shock delivered during the vulnerable period of atrial refractoriness (i.e., synchronized to the R wave) may predict recurrent AF after PV isolation. This predictor of AF recurrence can provide additive information over inducibility with burst atrial pacing alone.[107]

Many (up to 57%) patients with paroxysmal AF have no inducible AF after PV isolation. This subset can represent a group that can potentially benefit from PV isolation alone and do not require additional substrate modification. Induction of AF should prompt reconfirmation of PV isolation in all veins. If AF remains inducible despite complete PV isolation, additional substrate-based atrial ablation may be considered (see later discussion).

ELIMINATION OF RESIDUAL POTENTIALS INSIDE THE CIRCUMFERENTIAL ABLATION LINES

The value of complete voltage abatement (i.e., reduction of the atrial electrogram amplitude by >80% or a decrease to less than 0.1 mV as determined by local electrogram analysis and voltage mapping) inside the circumferential ablation lines in preventing the recurrence of AF remains controversial and requires further investigation. Some studies suggested that the elimination of residual potentials inside the LA-PV junctions or carina after PV isolation offer an incremental benefit on the recurrence of AF. In contrast, other studies showed no additional benefit of this approach.[93,108]

Outcome

Circumferential antral PV isolation offers a better outcome compared with ostial segmental PV isolation for paroxysmal AF (approximately 71% versus 64%). The incremental clinical benefit of adjuvant linear LA ablation or CFAE ablation, or both, in patients with paroxysmal AF has been controversial and is likely to be small or negligible. For patients with persistent AF, the success rates of circumferential antral PV isolation (approximately 50% to 70%) are less than for paroxysmal AF but are still better than those achieved by ostial segmental PV isolation, and adjuvant substrate modification seems to offer additional benefit in AF control, although this remains controversial.[78,109,110]

Circumferential Left Atrial Ablation

Rationale

Attempts to replicate the results of the maze procedure in the EP laboratory have consisted of the creation of linear lesions in the LA or RA, or both. In the past, multiple catheters with coil electrodes positioned against the atrial wall were used to create the linear lesions without having to reposition the catheter repeatedly. Currently, linear ablation lesions are created with individual contiguous applications of RF energy on a point-by-point basis. RF ablation is performed circumferentially around the ipsilateral PVs, with the endpoint of ablation being the absence or marked reduction (80%) in the amplitude of electrical signals within the encircling lesions.

Whereas the efficacy of PV isolation depends on complete and lasting PV disconnection from the LA, the efficacy of circumferential LA ablation does not. This finding highlights the fact that circumferential LA ablation (also referred to as wide-area LA ablation or circumferential PV ablation) eliminates AF by mechanisms other than complete PV isolation. Several mechanisms of action can be involved. First, there is substrate modification by LA compartmentalization.

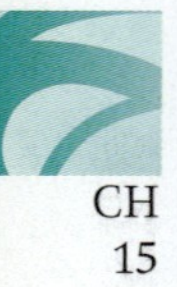

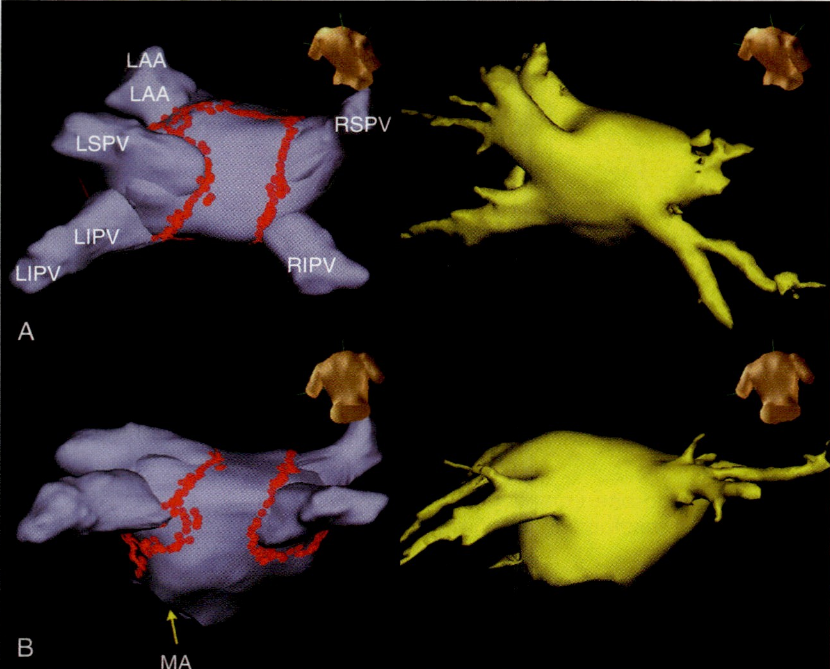

FIGURE 15-43 Wide-area circumferential left atrial (LA) ablation. Shown are cephalic **(A)** and caudal **(B)** posteroanterior views of three-dimensional (3-D) reconstruction of the LA and pulmonary veins (PVs) using EnSite NavX (St. Jude Medical, Austin, Tex.; **left**) and synchronized 3-D reconstruction of the LA and PVs using cardiac CT angiography **(right).** Red dots indicate the sites of ablation, with circumferential LA ablation in addition to the LA roof and mitral isthmus lines. LAA = left atrial appendage; LIPV = left inferior pulmonary vein; LSPV = left superior pulmonary vein; MA, mitral annulus; RIPV = right inferior pulmonary vein; RSPV = right superior pulmonary vein.

Approximately 25% to 30% of the LA myocardium is excluded by the encircling lesions, thereby limiting the area available for circulating wavelets needed to perpetuate AF. The ablation lines can also eliminate anchor points for rotors or mother waves that drive AF and make reentry pathways unsuitable. Autonomic denervation by ablation of vagal inputs to the posterior LA wall is another potential mechanism. Furthermore, the Marshall ligament or Bachmann bundle, which can be involved in the initiation and maintenance of AF, may be excluded by the circumferential ablation lines. The ligament of Marshall, which inserts in close proximity to the left superior PV and can be a source of triggers for AF, can potentially be eliminated by the ablation line that encircles the left-sided PVs. Additionally, promotion of atrial electroanatomical remodeling involving the LA posterior wall may result, to the point that the substrate for AF is no longer present. Modification of PV arrhythmogenic activity can also be operative. By encircling the PVs, LA ablation can potentially eliminate the triggers and driving mechanisms of paroxysmal AF that arise in the PVs. Although complete conduction block across the encircling lesions may not be achieved, decremental conduction can occur, particularly at shorter CLs, and it may impede the conduction of PV tachycardias to the LA.[111,112]

There are several differences between circumferential LA ablation and PV isolation strategies. From a mechanistic standpoint, segmental ostial ablation electrically isolates the PVs, thereby eliminating the arrhythmogenic activity in the PVs that triggers or perpetuates episodes of paroxysmal AF. However, sources of AF that do not originate in the PVs and the substrate that supports the maintenance of AF are not addressed by PV isolation. From a technical aspect, segmental ostial and circumferential antral PV isolation techniques require the insertion of two catheters into the LA, whereas linear LA ablation requires only a single catheter in the LA. Also, although PV isolation requires the identification of PV potentials, which can be difficult to distinguish from atrial electrograms, circumferential LA ablation is primarily an anatomical approach to ablation. Furthermore, the risk of PV stenosis, which is a major concern during ostial PV isolation, is minimized during circumferential LA ablation because most ablation sites are more than 1 cm away from PV ostia.[111,112]

Electroanatomical Mapping

The ablation catheter is advanced into the LA through a transseptal puncture. A ring or basket catheter is unnecessary; therefore, only one transseptal puncture is required. A nonfluoroscopic 3-D electroanatomical CARTO or NavX navigation system is used for generating and validating the continuity of the circular ablation lines (Fig. 15-43). Integration of CT and MRI scans into the electroanatomical mapping system improves visualization of complex LA geometries and can potentially improve the safety and success of catheter ablation for AF (see Fig. 15-39). CT/MRI integration offers the added benefit of displaying the atrial configuration, thus allowing completion of a ring of ablation lesions that follows the patient's own anatomy rather than empirical encirclement.[111]

The ostium of each PV is identified based on the results of selective biplane PV angiography (if performed) and fluoroscopic visualization of the catheter tip entering the cardiac silhouette, with a simultaneous decrease in impedance and appearance of the atrial potential (see previous discussion).

If validation of the circumferential lesions around PVs and the completeness of conduction block across the ablation lines are to be used as endpoints for the ablation procedure, propagation maps have to be created before and after RF ablation. Additionally, the collected data can be displayed as voltage maps, which can be useful to define scar areas and electrically diseased tissues. In patients in NSR at the beginning of the procedure, maps are acquired during pacing from the CS or RA at a CL of 600 milliseconds. In patients in AF at the end of the mapping procedure, electrical cardioversion to restore NSR is performed to allow stimulation maneuvers.

Target of Ablation

The ablation lines are typically created with encircling lesions around the left- and right-sided PVs, 1 to 2 cm from the PV ostia. The circumferential ablation lines may surround each of the PVs, or, instead of encircling each PV, one big circle is placed around the PVs of each side (Fig. 15-44; see also Fig. 15-43). An ablation line is also created across the LA roof to connect the two circumferential ablation lines and often another ablation line across the mitral isthmus between the inferior portion of the left-sided encircling lesion and the lateral mitral annulus (see later discussion). In some patients, additional ablation lines are created in the septum and anterior wall that extend from the roof line to the mitral isthmus. At present, the number and location of LA linear lesions should be tailored to the individual patient. The ideal configuration would combine technical ease and safety with long-term control of AF.[111,112]

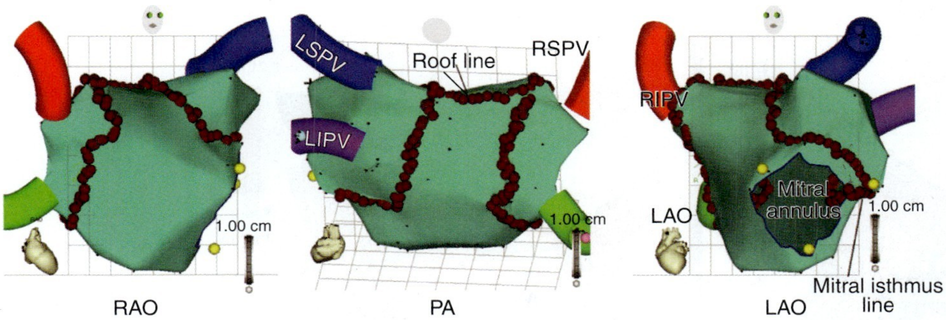

FIGURE 15-44 Wide-area circumferential left atrial (LA) ablation. Shown are multiple (right anterior oblique [RAO], posteroanterior [PA], and left anterior oblique [LAO]) views of anatomical "shell" rendering of the LA anatomy and pulmonary veins (PVs) using CARTO (Biosense Webster, Inc., Diamond Bar, Calif.). Red dots indicate sites of ablation. LA roof and mitral isthmus lines, connecting anatomical barriers, are as shown. LIPV = left inferior pulmonary vein; LSPV = left superior pulmonary vein; RIPV = right inferior pulmonary vein; RSPV = right superior pulmonary vein.

Ablation Technique

Once an electroanatomical map of the main PVs and LA has been adequately reconstructed, RF ablation is performed 1 to 2 cm from the PV ostia to encircle the left- and right-sided PVs. However, because there is a narrow rim of atrial tissue between the anterior aspect of the left superior PV and the LA appendage in approximately 50% of patients, ablation within 1 cm of the ostium of this vein sometimes is required.

Circumferential ablation lines are usually created starting at the lateral mitral isthmus and withdrawing the ablation catheter tip posteriorly and then anteriorly to the left-sided PVs, passing between the left superior PV and the LA appendage before completing the circumferential line on the posterior wall of the LA. The ridge between the left superior PV and the LA appendage can be identified by fragmented electrograms caused by collision of activity from the LA appendage and left superior PV-LA. The LA appendage is identifiable by a significantly higher impedance (more than 4 Ω higher than the LA mean), a high-voltage local bipolar electrogram, with characteristically organized activity in fibrillating patients. The right PVs are ablated in a similar fashion. Ablation sites are tagged on the model of the LA created with the electroanatomical mapping system, and that system is used for generating and validating the continuity of circular lines.

An irrigated 3.5- to 4-mm-tip catheter is typically used with power settings of 20 to 30 W on the posterior wall, 35 to 40 W elsewhere, with a temperature limit of less than 42°C. Alternatively, a solid 8-mm-tip ablation catheter may be used, with RF energy set to a target temperature of 55°C to 65°C and a power limit of 70 to 100 W. The power and temperature limits are reduced in the posterior LA wall to 50 W and 55°C to minimize the risk of injury to the surrounding structures. A series of RF applications is delivered until the maximum local bipolar electrogram amplitude decreases by 80% to 90% or to less than 0.05 to 0.1 mV, or to a maximum RF duration of 40 milliseconds, whichever comes first. Alternatively, RF energy is applied continuously on the planned circumferential ablation lines as the catheter is gradually dragged along the line, with repositioning of the catheter tip every 10 to 20 seconds. Continuous catheter movement, often in a to-and-fro fashion over a point, helps keep the catheter tip temperature down as a result of passive cooling.

Power, impedance, and electrical activity are monitored continuously during navigation and ablation. Impedance can increase suddenly if a thrombus forms on the catheter tip. A much more useful indicator is a 40% to 50% reduction in the power delivered to reach target temperature. If thrombus formation is suspected, catheter withdrawal from the LA without advancing the transseptal sheath can be necessary to avoid stripping any thrombus present on the catheter tip as the catheter is withdrawn into the sheath, which can result in systemic embolization.

RF application should be immediately terminated when the catheter position deviates significantly from the planned line or falls into a PV, when impedance rises suddenly, or when the patient develops cough, burning pain, or severe bradycardia.

After completion of the circular lesions around the left- and the right-sided PVs, the area within the ablation lines is explored with the ablation catheter. RF energy is applied at sites that have a local electrogram amplitude greater than 0.1 mV. In addition, when AF is still present, sites inside the encircling ablation lines where the CL is shorter than the atrial CL in the CS also are ablated.

Endpoints of Ablation

To date, circumferential LA ablation for AF has stood apart from most other types of ablation procedures in that a clear-cut EP endpoint has not been defined. The only endpoint of ablation used in most studies has been voltage abatement. Although one study suggested that complete block across the ablation lines is a useful EP endpoint, this was not confirmed in two other studies.

VOLTAGE MAPPING. The primary endpoint for circumferential ablation is the reduction in voltage within the isolated regions by more than 80% to 90% or the recording of low (less than 0.05 to 0.1 mV) peak-to-peak bipolar potentials inside the lesion, as determined by local electrogram analysis and voltage mapping (Fig. 15-45).

Postablation voltage mapping is performed using the preablation map for the acquisition of new points (on the existing LA geometry) to permit accurate comparison of preablation and postablation bipolar voltage maps. After completion of the circular lesions around the left- and right-sided PVs, the area within the ablation lines is explored with the ablation catheter, and RF energy is applied at sites that have a local electrogram amplitude greater than 0.1 mV. As an anatomy-based ablation strategy, this may be the only required endpoint.

ACTIVATION MAPPING. Another endpoint used for lesion validation requires the acquisition of two activation-propagation maps during CS and RA pacing for left- and right-sided PVs, respectively. The rationale behind this setting is to pace from a site close to the lesions and shorten conduction time to the ablation site, thereby allowing detection of delayed activation inside the circular line.

Several criteria are used to define line continuity: (1) low peak-to-peak bipolar potentials (less than 0.1 mV) inside the lesion, as determined by local electrogram analysis and voltage mapping; (2) local activation time delay of more than 30 milliseconds between contiguous points lying in the same axial plane on the external and internal sides of the line, as assessed by activation mapping; and (3) gaps in the ablation lines, defined as breakthroughs in an ablated area and identified by sites with single potentials and by early local activation. Changes in activation spread are also evaluated with propagation mapping. Incomplete block is revealed by impulse propagation across the line; in this case, further RF applications are given to complete the line of block.

Importantly, the only predictive criterion for a successful ablation seems to be the amount of postablation low-voltage encircled area.

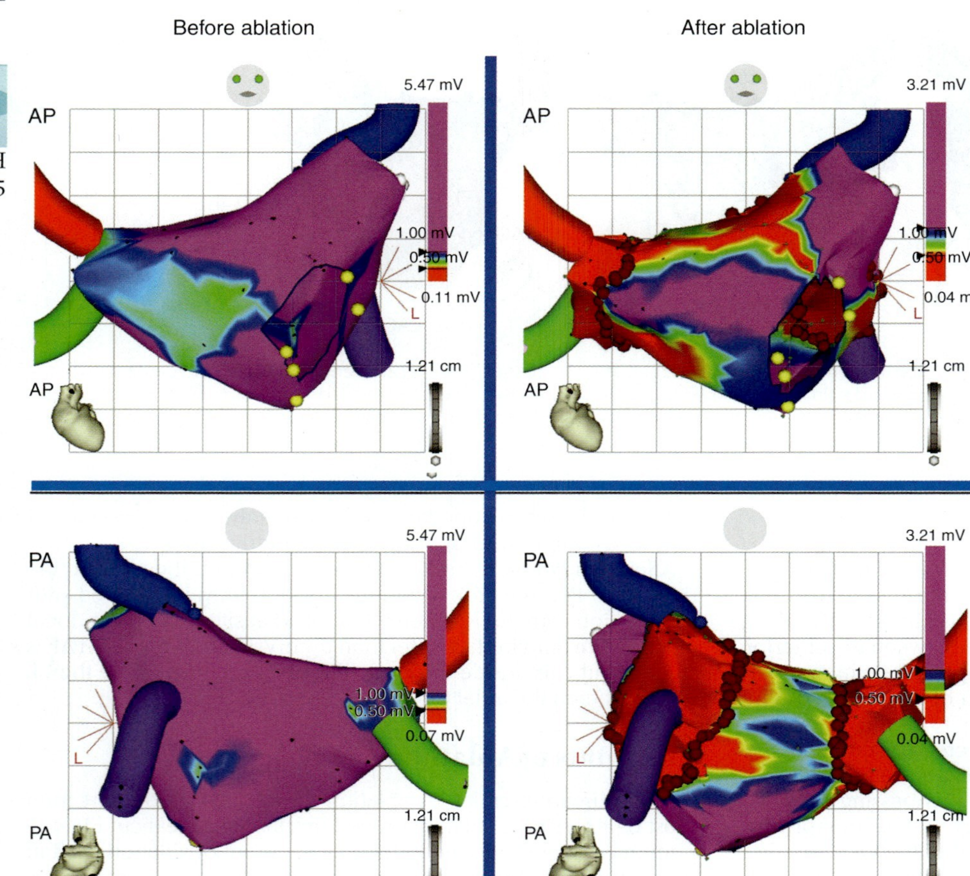

FIGURE 15-45 CARTO (Biosense Webster, Inc., Diamond Bar, Calif.) voltage map after wide-area circumferential left atrial (LA) ablation. Anteroposterior (AP) and posteroanterior (PA) views of electroanatomical voltage maps before **(left)** and after **(right)** wide-area circumferential LA ablation depict peak-to-peak bipolar electrogram amplitude. Red represents lowest voltage, and purple represents the highest voltage. In postablation maps, areas within and around the ablation lines, involving to some extent the LA posterior wall, show low-amplitude (less than 0.5 mV) electrograms.

Therefore, validation of the circumferential lesions around PVs by pacing maneuvers, the completeness of conduction block across the ablation lines, and the search for gaps in the ablation lines are not routinely performed.

PULMONARY VEIN ISOLATION. Controversial data have been published regarding the influence of PV disconnection during circumferential LA ablation. Several reports showed that complete electrical isolation of the PVs is not necessary for a successful outcome. Hence, complete PV isolation is not required as an endpoint for circumferential LA ablation.[112] In fact, this ablation strategy typically is associated with incomplete PV isolation. Nonetheless, although PV potentials were still present in one or more PVs in 80% of patients, there usually is a conduction delay between the LA and PVs, and the prevalence of PV tachycardias is markedly reduced after circumferential LA ablation.

Of interest, conduction gaps in the ablation lines and LA-PV connection sites can be characterized by multicomponent electrograms without isoelectric lines during sinus rhythm and by multicomponent electrograms or continuous activity during AF. In one report, targeting those sites with ablation was shown to increase the PV disconnection rate during circumferential LA ablation to more than 85% of PVs, which can potentially improve clinical outcome.[111]

TERMINATION OF PERSISTENT ATRIAL FIBRILLATION. Termination of AF during the procedure occurs in approximately one-third of patients. If AF does not terminate during RF, transthoracic cardioversion is performed at the conclusion of ablation. If AF recurs immediately after the cardioversion, the completeness of the lines is reassessed, and additional ablation lines should be considered. Additional ablation consists of ablation lines created along the LA septum, roof, posterior mitral isthmus, or anterior wall, on the basis of the presence of fractionated or rapid atrial activity (see later discussion).

ORGANIZED ATRIAL ARRHYTHMIAS. When LA ablation is performed during an ongoing episode of AF, the AF converts to NSR or to a more organized type of atrial tachyarrhythmia in approximately 20% to 30% of patients. LA ablation can create macroreentrant circuits in the LA, thus mediating conversion of AF into AT. The most common type of macroreentry is mitral isthmus–dependent AT. Additionally, macroreentrant circuits (single or multiple-loop reentry as well as small-loop reentry) can be created by gaps in the ablation lines that encircle the PVs, mostly located on the ridge between the LA appendage and the left superior PV. Entrainment and activation mapping should be performed during organized ATs, and detailed online mapping to search for gaps in the ablation lines should be performed. RF applications at the gaps in the circumferential ablation lines or linear ablation across the lateral mitral isthmus or LA roof can be required for elimination of those ATs.[113]

NONINDUCIBILITY OF ATRIAL FIBRILLATION. Whether noninducibility of AF can be used as a clinical endpoint of ablation in patients with AF who have undergone circumferential LA ablation is still controversial. Some reports found that inducibility of AF after ablation was an independent predictor of recurrent AF. One study suggested performing additional ablation when AF is still inducible after the initial procedure. Circumferential LA ablation renders AF noninducible by rapid atrial pacing in approximately 40% of patients with paroxysmal AF. With additional LA ablation lines, the percentage of patients in whom AF was rendered noninducible increases to approximately 90%, and such an endpoint is associated with a better clinical efficacy than when AF was still inducible. Conversely, other reports showed a rather low predictive accuracy of the postablation stimulation test that prohibited its use as a reliable procedural endpoint for individual patients; these reports suggested that continuation of ablation caused by a positive stimulation test or AF persistence may lead to overtreatment in a substantial proportion of patients.[106]

Outcome

In multiple reports, long-term success was achieved in approximately 74% of patients with paroxysmal AF and in 49% of patients with persistent or permanent AF.

One study suggested that circumferential LA ablation to encircle the PVs is preferable to segmental ostial PV isolation as the first approach in patients with symptomatic paroxysmal AF. In contrast, another prospective randomized study comparing the two strategies showed the opposite results. Not unexpectedly, the opposite results in the two studies were obtained because of the large variability in the success rate observed in patients undergoing circumferential LA ablation (88% versus 47%), whereas the success rates in patients undergoing segmental ostial PV isolation were similar (67% versus 71%).

Although some studies reported that PV electrical isolation was not related to the success of the procedure, more recent studies found that rigorously achieving complete PV electrical isolation improved the success of circumferential LA ablation as compared with the purely anatomical endpoint of abatement of electrical activity by the ablation catheter recording within the encircled regions.[112,114] Currently, the Heart Rhythm Society's consensus statement on AF ablation strongly urges demonstration of PV isolation with whatever ablation strategy used.

Linear Atrial Ablation

Linear ablation lesions in the LA in conjunction with circumferential LA ablation were proposed to improve the clinical outcome of AF ablation by modifying the atrial substrate. Additionally, linear atrial ablation can potentially reduce the risk of postablation macroreentrant ATs. Ablation strategies may involve the LA roof line, the LA mitral isthmus line, and the RA cavotricuspid isthmus line in conjunction with circumferential LA ablation or PV isolation.[93]

Left Atrial Roof Line

RATIONALE

Although the exact mechanism by which the LA roof supports the fibrillatory process is unclear, evidence has implicated this region in the substrate for AF. In addition, the LA roof represents a region demonstrating highly fragmented electrograms, perhaps indicating the presence of substrate capable of sustaining localized reentry or focal activity that may maintain fibrillation, and it also has the potential for supporting macroreentry around the PVs using the LA roof.

Ablation at the LA roof was found to have a direct effect on the fibrillation process, by prolonging the fibrillatory CL and terminating the arrhythmia in some patients and rendering AF noninducible in patients with inducible or sustained arrhythmia after PV isolation. This finding implicated the LA roof in the substrate maintaining AF after PV isolation.[115]

Linear ablation was previously performed posteriorly or anteriorly across the LA. However, a posterior ablation line between the two superior PVs carries a higher risk of atrioesophageal fistula. Transection of the anterior LA results in significantly delayed activation of the lateral LA during NSR, which has potentially deleterious hemodynamic consequences. Therefore, these lines are currently substituted with the LA roof line (see Fig. 15-44).[115]

ABLATION TECHNIQUE

LA roof ablation is performed after circumferential LA ablation or circumferential antral PV isolation. Commencing at the encircling lesion at the left superior PV, the sheath and catheter assembly are rotated clockwise posteriorly and are dragged toward the right superior PV. To achieve stability along the cranial LA roof, the catheter may be directed toward the left superior PV and the sheath rotated to face the right PVs, or vice versa. Two alternative methods can also be used to reach the LA roof for ablation. First, the catheter can be looped around the lateral, inferior, septal, and then cranial walls, then laying the catheter down along the cranial wall of the LA to allow dragging of the catheter by withdrawal from the left to the right superior PV ostia. Second, the catheter can be maximally deflected to form a tight loop near the left superior PV, with the tip facing the right PVs. Releasing the curve positions the catheter tip adjacent to the right superior PV ostia and allows dragging back to the left PV.[115]

The stability of the catheter is monitored during RF applications with the use of the proximal electrograms, intermittent fluoroscopy, or a navigation system to recognize inadvertent displacement of the catheter. Electroanatomical mapping is used for real-time monitoring and to tag the ablation sequence. RF energy is delivered for 60 to 120 seconds at each point while the local atrial electrograms are monitored. Local potential elimination or formation of double potentials during pacing or AF signifies the effectiveness of ablation locally.

ENDPOINTS OF ABLATION

The EP endpoint of ablation is the demonstration of a complete line of block joining the two superior PVs. Following the restoration of NSR, complete linear block is defined by point-by-point mapping of an online corridor of double potentials along the entire length of the LA roof during pacing from the anterior LA (from the LA appendage or the distal CS) or during NSR and by demonstration of an activation detour circumventing the right and left PVs to activate the posterior wall caudocranially (instead of the craniocaudal activation typically observed during NSR and LA appendage pacing), with no conduction through the LA roof. When residual conduction is demonstrated, detailed mapping is performed to identify and ablate gaps in the linear lesion.[116]

OUTCOME

Ablation of the LA roof in conjunction with circumferential antral PV isolation was shown in one study to affect results significantly. The clinical outcome was improved compared with PV isolation alone in patients with paroxysmal AF. Additional roof line ablation with complete conduction block was associated with 87% of patients being arrhythmia-free without antiarrhythmic medications compared with 69% undergoing PV isolation alone. The clinical benefit was similar to other described lines (e.g., mitral isthmus line); however, the roof line could be achieved with shorter RF application and procedural durations. With a mean of 12 ± 6 minutes of RF energy, complete block at the LA roof could be achieved in 96% of cases.

Although the addition of a complete line of block at the LA roof can potentially improve efficacy for the suppression of atrial arrhythmia compared with PV isolation alone, this requires additional ablation and can be associated with a proarrhythmic risk. Whether such linear ablation should be empirically performed in all patients with AF or applied selectively on the basis of clinical or procedural variables, notably persistent inducibility after PV isolation, remains to be determined prospectively.

Left Atrial Posterior Wall Isolation (Box Isolation)

RATIONALE

The role of the LA posterior wall in initiation and perpetuation of AF has been suggested by both human and animal studies. Focal discharges from the posterior LA are important in the initiation of AF as non-PV foci. Furthermore, the LA posterior wall can harbor rotors that can participate in maintaining AF. Several

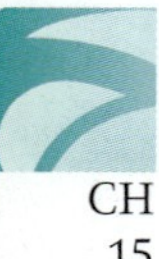

studies suggested that deployment of linear lesions along the LA to exclude the LA posterior wall in addition to PV ablation was shown to improve the success rate. Electrical isolation of the LA posterior wall after PV isolation was shown to result in further prolongation of the AF CL with termination of longstanding AF achieved in approximately 20%. After isolation of this region, the LA posterior wall demonstrates automatic activity, independent of the PVs, in up to 30% of patients.[117,118]

ABLATION TECHNIQUE

Following circumferential PV ablation, isolation of the LA posterior wall is achieved by an ablation line joining the two superior PVs (roof line) and a second ablation line joining the two inferior PVs (inferior line). The lateral boundaries of the box isolation are formed by the contiguous lesions previously created by circumferential PV ablation (Fig. 15-46).[117,118]

Ablation of the LA roof is performed as described earlier. Following the roof line, a contiguous line of ablation lesions joins the inferior PVs to isolate the LA posterior wall. Commencing at the lesion at the left inferior PV, the sheath and catheter are rotated clockwise posteriorly and dragged toward the right inferior PV. RF power output is limited to 20 to 30 W to minimize the risk of atrioesophageal fistula.[117,118]

During ablation, the slowing of LA posterior wall activity with progressive completion of the posterior LA rectangle and termination of AF can be observed in some patients. Complete linear block can be verified by the demonstration of no conduction through the LA roof and inferior lines by point-by-point sequential mapping either conventionally or by electroanatomical mapping. Persistent conduction across to the posterior wall should prompt meticulous online mapping to identify and ablate gaps in the linear lesions.[118]

ENDPOINTS OF ABLATION

The endpoints of box isolation are the demonstration of the absence or dissociation of electrical activity within the ablated zone (i.e., entrance block), as well as failure to capture the LA outside the isolated region (i.e., exit block) during pacing from the posterior LA and all PVs (after the restoration of NSR).[117-119]

OUTCOME

Initial studies showed that exclusion of the LA posterior wall is feasible and results in incremental improvement to the effect of PV isolation. In patients with longstanding AF, box isolation resulted in further prolongation of the fibrillatory CL (independent of PV isolation) with termination of AF in approximately 20%. At 2 years following ablation, 63% of these patients with longstanding persistent AF have remained in NSR.[117] However, one prospective randomized study showed that isolation of the LA posterior wall did not offer additional benefit over a single LA roof line with respect to the risk of arrhythmia recurrence after circumferential PV ablation. This finding suggests that the benefits demonstrated in previous reports may represent a general debulking of the atria rather than a specific role of electrical isolation of the posterior wall.[119]

Left Atrial Mitral Isthmus Line

Emerging evidence has implicated regions of conduction slowing and block associated with atrial remodeling in the substrate predisposing to AF. In the LA, studies demonstrated preferential propagation that is closely correlated with muscle fiber orientation along the posterior LA and circumferentially around the mitral annulus. Such preferential propagation occurring in response to functional or anatomical conduction block (perhaps exacerbated by AF or conditions predisposing to AF) is capable of facilitating reentry using the mitral isthmus, as recognized with common forms of LA macroreentry, and thus can have a role in the milieu that maintains AF.

Because of the contiguity with the left PVs and LA appendage, ablation of the mitral isthmus results in a long (functional) line of conduction block that transects the lateral LA from the mitral isthmus to the roof. Its EP consequences can be considered analogous to those produced by cavotricuspid isthmus ablation, in which a short line is amplified by the crista terminalis to result in a long line of functional conduction block. It is thus likely that ablation of the mitral isthmus, as an adjunct to other ablation strategies for AF, helps modify a large region of the LA substrate for AF by eliminating anatomical or functional reentry involving the mitral isthmus or PVs. Additionally, it can eliminate arrhythmogenic triggers arising from the ligament of Marshall.

LA macroreentrant ATs can develop following catheter ablation of AF in up to 50% of cases. The most common type of macroreentry is mitral isthmus–dependent AT, and it seems more likely that this type of AT is a direct result of LA ablation. The potential of this complication underscores the importance of an ablation line across the mitral isthmus. Ablation of the mitral isthmus is discussed in detail in Chapter 13.

In one report, the outcome of 100 consecutive patients with paroxysmal AF undergoing circumferential PV isolation alone was compared with that of an equal number of consecutive patients undergoing circumferential PV isolation and mitral isthmus ablation. Mitral isthmus block was achieved in 92% of patients after 20 ± 10 minutes of endocardial RF application (additional 5 ± 4 minutes of epicardial RF application from within the CS was required in 68%). One year after the last procedure, 87% of patients with mitral isthmus ablation and 69% without ablation ($p = 0.002$) were arrhythmia-free in the absence of antiarrhythmic drugs. Another study showed a significant improvement of

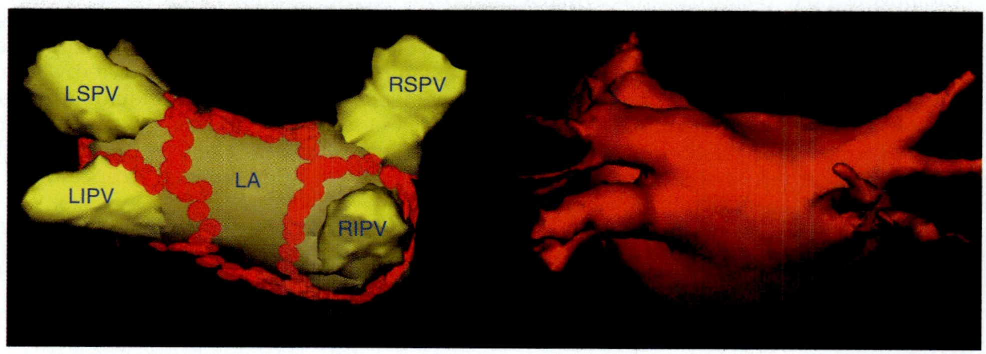

FIGURE 15-46 Three-dimensional reconstruction of the left atrium (LA, posterior view) using ESI EnSite NavX (St. Jude Medical, Austin, Tex.) electroanatomical system **(left)** and computed tomography **(right).** Small red circles are tagged sites at which radiofrequency energy was applied to isolate the pulmonary veins (PVs). Electrical isolation of the LA posterior wall (box isolation) is performed by an ablation line joining the two superior PVs (roofline) and a second ablation line joining the two inferior PVs (inferior line). LIPV = left inferior pulmonary vein; LSPV = left superior pulmonary vein; RIPV = right inferior pulmonary vein; RSPV = right superior pulmonary vein.

long-term sinus rhythm maintenance with the combination of bidirectional block along the left mitral isthmus and circumferential PV isolation in patients with both paroxysmal (76% versus 62%) and persistent (74% versus 36%) AF.

Importantly, continuous linear lesions are difficult to achieve, even under direct visualization during intraoperative ablation. It has been shown that creating transmural permanent lines of block across the mitral isthmus line in particular is technically challenging and sometimes requires ablation deep within the CS. Gaps within the ablation lines, whether secondary to areas of recovery or areas missed initially, can produce areas of slow conduction and a substrate for macroreentry. Therefore, when linear LA ablation is applied, complete bidirectional conduction block across the ablation lines should be verified to reduce the risk of development of macroreentrant ATs related to gaps in the ablation lines.

Right Atrial Cavotricuspid Isthmus Line

AF and AFL frequently coexist in the same patient. Clinical AFL occurs in more than one-third of patients with AF. AF often precedes the onset of AFL and can also develop after the successful catheter ablation of AFL. AFL, usually induced either by atrial pacing or by AF, can be observed in up to two-thirds of patients undergoing PV isolation for AF. Approximately 80% of these episodes are typical AFL.

Although typical AFL and AF frequently coexist, their precise interrelationship is unclear. It may be that the same premature depolarizations that trigger AF also trigger AFL, or the EP and structural remodeling that accompany AF may also promote the occurrence of AFL, or vice versa. Evidence suggests that AF plays an important role in the genesis of typical AFL. Commonly, spontaneous or induced typical AFL does not start immediately after a premature beat or burst rapid atrial pacing; rather, its onset is generally preceded by a transitional rhythm (AF) of variable duration.[120] AF can promote the formation of an intercaval functional line of block in the RA, which can be critical for the initiation of AFL. Also, class IC and IA antiarrhythmic drugs and amiodarone used to suppress AF commonly promote AFL.

On the other hand, it is also possible that at least some episodes of AFL can degenerate into AF. AFL with a short CL can result in fibrillatory conduction. Additionally, AFL can induce atrial electrical remodeling that predisposes to development of AF.

Catheter ablation techniques targeting the cavotricuspid isthmus for typical AFL or the initiating triggers within the PVs for AF were independently shown to offer a potential cure for the two arrhythmias. However, more recent studies suggested that successful ablation of typical AFL does not improve the natural history of AF. The occurrence rates of AF following ablation of typical AFL alone have been shown to range from 38% to 50% when preprocedural AFL is the dominant arrhythmia over AF to 86% when AF is the dominant arrhythmia. In most patients, AF develops within the first year after AFL ablation.[121] These observations suggest that AFL may be initiated by bursts of AF and that in the absence of AFL substrate the AF continues to progress, or, alternatively, the atrial electrical remodeling caused by AFL can provide the substrate for subsequent AF development. Hence, some investigators have proposed additional PV isolation at the time of cavotricuspid isthmus ablation in patients with AFL but no documented AF before ablation to help improve long-term freedom of AF recurrences. Although small studies suggested some value of this approach, this strategy cannot be recommended for general adoption before confirmation by larger studies because of the increased risk and procedure duration when PV isolation is added.[121,122]

In patients with AF and no known history of AFL, ablation of the cavotricuspid isthmus at the time of AF ablation was proposed in some studies to reduce the risk of subsequent typical AFL, as well as AF, after ablation. However, as was shown in one study, although cavotricuspid isthmus ablation can potentially reduce early recurrences of AFL, those early recurrences do not represent a long-term problem in most patients and require only short-term therapy. Additionally, the potential benefit of adjunctive cavotricuspid isthmus ablation on risk of recurrence of AF after PV isolation has not been confirmed by large studies. Therefore, routinely performing typical AFL ablation in all patients undergoing AF ablation may not provide added clinical benefit but can potentially add time, cost, and risk.[123]

In patients with paroxysmal AF who had periods of typical AFL, the effect of PV isolation alone on the risk of recurrence of AFL remains controversial. It has been reported that ablation of AF in these patients, although not interrupting the reentrant circuit in typical AFL, can potentially control both arrhythmias, a finding suggesting that AF initiated by PV triggers can be the precursor rather than the consequence of AFL. This is consistent with the observation that AFL commonly starts after a transitional rhythm of variable duration, usually AF. However, these findings were not confirmed by other studies that showed no benefit of PV isolation on the risk of recurrence of typical AFL. Therefore, in patients undergoing AF ablation, it is likely beneficial to ablate the cavotricuspid isthmus whenever typical AFL is observed clinically. Additionally, the occurrence of typical AFL in the course of a catheter ablation procedure aimed at elimination of AF was shown to be predictive of symptomatic AFL during follow-up after PV isolation, even in patients who had no prior clinical history of AFL, a risk that was lowered by combining AF and AFL ablation in those patients. Thus, supplementary cavotricuspid isthmus ablation in conjunction with AF ablation seems reasonable in these patients.[123]

Ablation of Complex Fractionated Atrial Electrograms

Rationale

Evaluation of the complexity and frequency of intracardiac electrograms can help in understanding the pathophysiology of AF. Atrial electrograms during sustained AF have three distinct patterns: single potentials, double potentials, and complex fractionated potentials. Continuous propagation of multiple wavelets in the atria and wavelets as offspring of atrial reentry circuits has been suggested as the mechanism by which AF can be perpetuated without continuous focal discharge. Fractionated and continuous electrical activity has been assumed to indicate the presence of wave collision, slow conduction, or pivot points where the wavelets turn around at the end of the arcs of functional blocks. Thus, areas of CFAEs during AF can potentially represent continuous reentry of the fibrillation waves into the same area or overlap of different wavelets entering the same area at different times, although the mapping resolution to discern whether such rotors even exist in human AF is still limited.[124,125]

Such complex electrical activity has a relatively short CL and heterogeneous temporal and spatial distribution. A relatively short CL may indicate the presence of a driver, analogous to the frequency gradient from the drivers or rotors to the rest of the atria observed in experimental models of AF, in which the central core of these rotors can have high-frequency electrical activity, whereas the periphery of the rotors can display complex electrograms because of wave break and fibrillatory conduction. Importantly, regions of CFAEs have been shown to remain spatially and temporally stable in individual patients, particularly when these regions were measured over several seconds, a surprising finding considering the earlier observation that the underlying mechanism for AF is random reentry and that the reentrant wavelets are expected to meander.[124,125]

Data have suggested that areas of CFAEs are critical sites for AF perpetuation and can serve as target sites for AF ablation. It has been proposed that once CFAEs are eliminated by ablation, AF can no longer be sustained because the random reentry paths are altered or eliminated so that the fibrillation wavelets can no longer reenter the ablated areas.[126] Whereas PV isolation targets the triggering foci, ablation of CFAEs targets the substrate for AF. However,

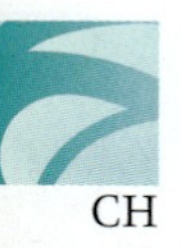

some connections between both approaches probably exist. Data indicate that PVs are the key areas where CFAEs are located; these areas need to be ablated to achieve conversion of AF to NSR. It is thus very likely that many patients may respond to ablation in the PV regions because of both trigger elimination and substrate modification.[124,126]

Mapping of Complex Fractionated Atrial Electrograms

Mapping of CFAEs is performed during AF. In patients in NSR at the time of study, AF is induced by isoproterenol infusion or rapid atrial pacing. In patients with persistent AF or with induced AF sustained for more than 5 minutes, biatrial electroanatomical (CARTO or NavX) mapping is performed.[126] The CS or RA appendage recording is used for electrical reference during mapping. Atrial CLs are monitored and recorded from the reference and mapping catheters. Electroanatomical mapping systems enable the operator to associate areas of CFAEs with the anatomy of both atria. Sites with CFAEs can be tagged and associated with the atrial geometry created by the electroanatomical mapping system and thereby serve as target sites for ablation. During AF, the local activation time of the arrhythmia is of no value in guiding activation sequence mapping.

The definition of CFAEs has not been consistent. Initially, CFAEs were defined as: (1) atrial electrograms that are fractionated and composed of at least two deflections and/or have a perturbation of the baseline with continuous deflection of a prolonged activation complex over a 10-second recording period; or (2) atrial electrograms with a very short CL (up to 120 milliseconds) averaged over a 10-second recording period (Fig. 15-47). More recently, CFAEs have been defined as having any of the following: (1) a magnitude of less than 0.5 mV; (2) a duration longer than 50 milliseconds with multiple deflections from the isoelectric line (more than three deflections); or (3) continuous electrical activity without an isoelectric line, verified visually. Some investigators, using unipolar mapping, defined fragmented potentials as electrograms exhibiting two or more negative deflections within 50 milliseconds. The limit of 50 milliseconds was based on the assumption that the atrial refractory period during AF and the interval between two successive fibrillation waves were 50 milliseconds or more.[124,125,127]

An important limitation of this approach is that the visual appearance of CFAEs is variable, and they are often of very low amplitude (less than 0.25 to 0.5 mV); therefore, their identification by visual inspection can be challenging and is highly subjective and investigator dependent (Fig. 15-48). To improve the accuracy of CFAE mapping, custom software was developed with algorithms that enable automated detection and tagging of areas of CFAEs with the anatomical shell of both atria. This software offers valuable advantages in the detection, quantification, and regionalization of CFAEs.

Currently, the automatic algorithms are variable and are dependent on the recording technology (NavX and CARTO). With CARTO, the CFAE complex is identified using an algorithm that quantifies the CFAE phenomenon in two parameters. First is the "interval confidence level," which characterizes the repetitiveness of the electrogram peaks within the recorded intracardiac signal. The assumption is that the more repetitions are recorded in a given time duration (2.5 milliseconds), the more confident is the categorization of a site as harboring CFAEs. The second parameter is either the "shortest complex interval," which is the shortest interval found in milliseconds out of all the intervals identified between consecutive CFAE complexes, or the "average complex interval," which is the average of all the intervals identified between consecutive CFAE complexes for each 2.5-second electrogram. CFAE areas are displayed on the whole-chamber map in a color-coded manner according to the degree of fractionated signals and their CLs for easier identification (Fig. 15-49). The algorithm allows the operator to exclude both noise and high-voltage signal from the analysis (default values, 0.05 mV and 0.15 mV).[128]

With the NavX system, CFAEs are characterized using the "CFAE-mean" contact mapping tool. The CFAE-mean is defined as the average time duration between consecutive deflections (–dV/dt) in a local AF intracardiac bipolar electrogram recorded over a specified length of time (at least 5 seconds). The mean interdeflection time interval (i.e., the mean CL) is then projected onto the LA anatomical shell as a color-coded display. The shorter the mean CL is, the more rapid and fractionated the local electrogram will be. Regions with mean CLs shorter than 120 milliseconds are considered to correspond to CFAE. To optimize algorithm accuracy, bipolar recordings are filtered at 30 to 500 Hz, and electrogram width

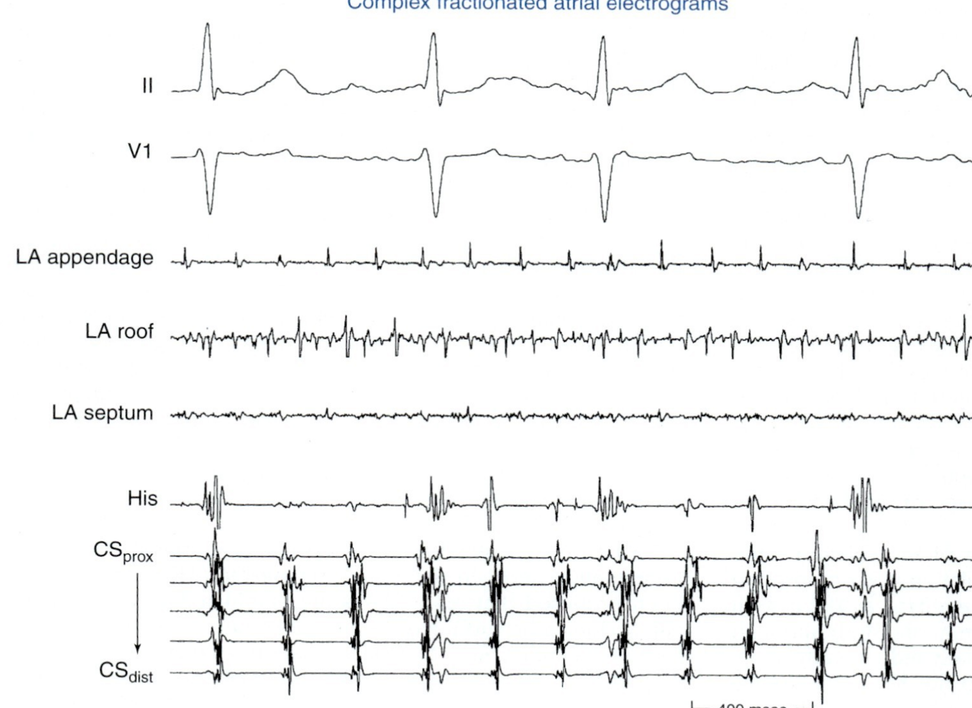

FIGURE 15-47 Examples of complex fractionated atrial electrograms. Fractionated atrial electrograms with a very short cycle length, compared with the rest of the atria, were recorded in the left atrial (LA) roof. In the LA septum, fractionated electrograms with continuous prolonged activation complex were observed. See text for discussion. CS_{dist} = distal coronary sinus; CS_{prox} = proximal coronary sinus.

and "refractory" period are typically set at 10 to 20 milliseconds and 30 to 50 milliseconds, respectively, to avoid multiple detections on a single deflection or counting of ventricular far-field signals. Additionally, the baseline signal noise level is determined, and the peak-to-peak electrogram amplitude detection limit is set just higher than the noise level (typically, 0.03 to 0.05 mV) to minimize noise detection while allowing detection of CFAEs, which are typically of very low amplitude (less than 0.5 mV). This algorithm is probably most analogous to the "average complex interval" map from the CARTO software. Advantages of the NavX system include an adjustable duration of recording from 1 to 8 seconds and the ability to record electrograms from multiple poles of several catheters simultaneously, which can potentially occupy a significant proportion of local AF CL.[124,129]

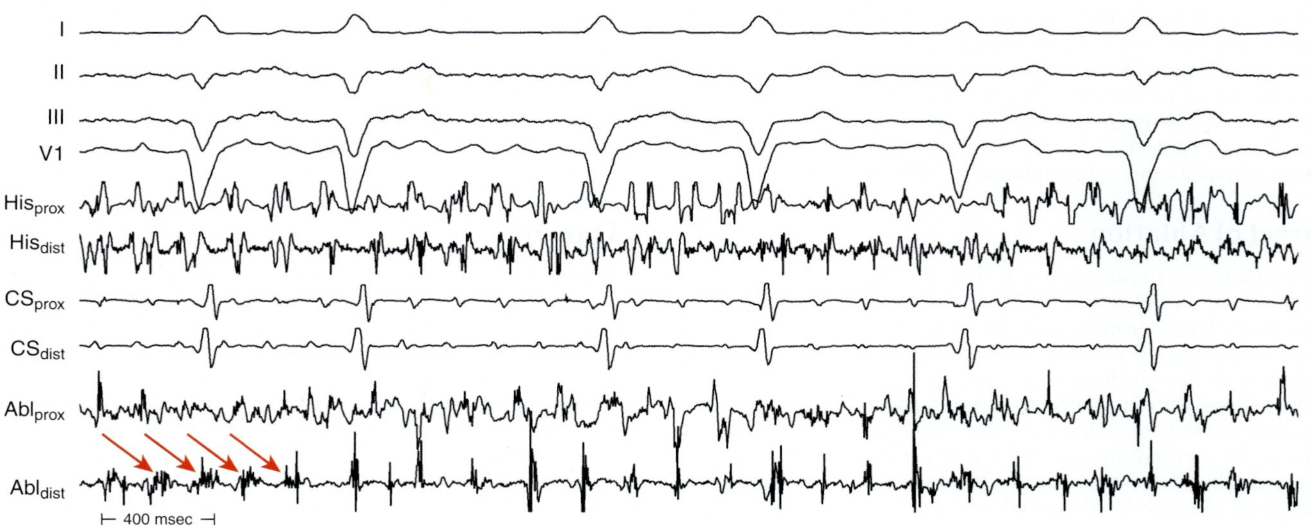

FIGURE 15-48 Recordings from near ligament of Marshall (Abl) showing complex fragmented atrial electrograms (high-frequency, somewhat repetitive spikes [arrows]); these are not consistently present over the duration of the recording, whereas similar activity is intermittently seen in the His recordings (right atrial). Abl_{dist} = distal ablation site; Abl_{prox} = proximal ablation site; CS_{dist} = distal coronary sinus; CS_{prox} = proximal coronary sinus; His_{dist} = distal His bundle; His_{prox} = proximal His bundle.

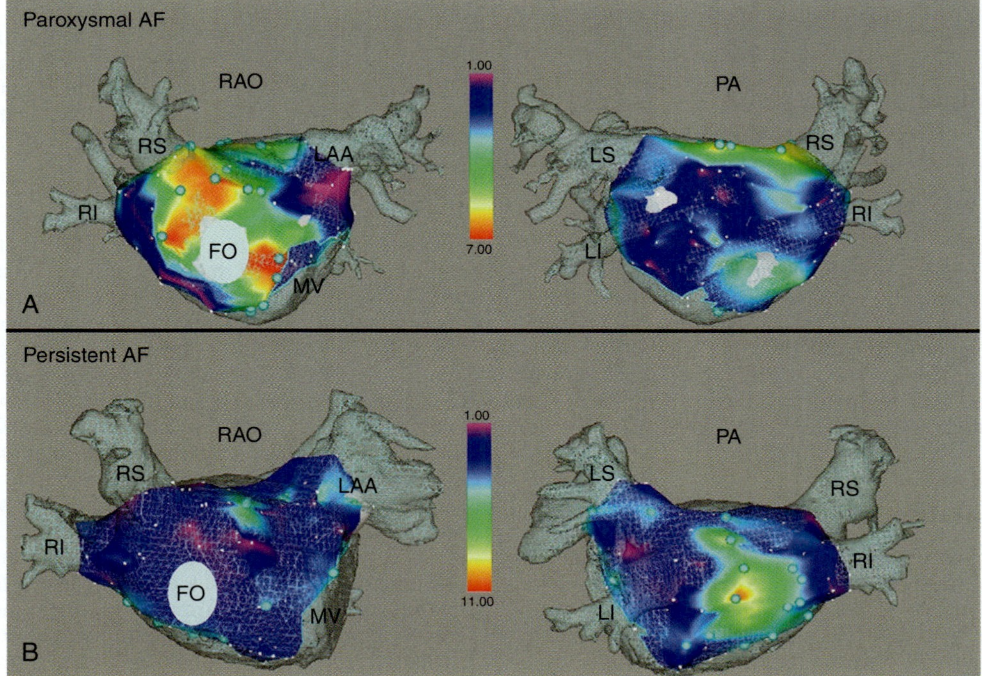

FIGURE 15-49 CARTO (Biosense Webster, Inc., Diamond Bar, Calif.) maps of complex fractionated atrial electrograms (CFAEs). CFAE maps with registered left atrial (LA) CT surface reconstruction (shown as wire frame), shown in right anterior oblique (RAO) view (left-sided images) and posteroanterior (PA) view (right-sided images), in patients with paroxysmal atrial fibrillation (AF) **(A)** and persistent AF **(B)**. The CFAE maps are color-coded, with red representing the highest interval confidence level (ICL) and purple representing the lowest ICL. Highly repetitive CFAE sites (ICL ≥ 5) are tagged with light blue dots on the CFAE maps. As shown in this example, the highly repetitive CFAE sites are more likely located at the pulmonary vein (PV) ostia, interatrial septum, and mitral annulus area in patients with paroxysmal AF, whereas patients with persistent AF have highly repetitive CFAE sites predominantly identified on the LA posterior wall. FO = fossa ovalis; LAA = left atrial appendage; LI = left inferior pulmonary vein; LS = left superior pulmonary vein; MV = mitral valve; RI = right inferior pulmonary vein; RS = right superior pulmonary vein. *(From Scherr D, Dalal D, Cheema A, et al: Automated detection and characterization of complex fractionated atrial electrograms in human left atrium during atrial fibrillation, Heart Rhythm 4:1013, 2007.)*

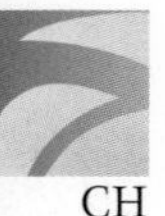

Importantly, assessment of fractionated electrograms during AF requires a recording duration of at least 5 seconds at each site to obtain a consistent fractionation and accurate analysis. A small mapping catheter tip (4 mm), good atrial contact, and stable mapping catheter positions for several seconds while mapping at each location are important to obtain high-quality recordings.[124]

CFAEs usually can be identified in most (80%) areas of the LA, but they appear to be predominantly located in the interatrial septum, LA roof, posterior wall, mitral annulus, and PV ostia. Less commonly, CFAEs are located in the RA, involving the septal region, crista terminalis, and cavotricuspid isthmus, as well as the CS os. Notably, patients with paroxysmal AF appear to have more CFAE sites identified around the PV ostia, whereas CFAEs detected in patients with persistent AF appear to be more evenly distributed over all areas of the LA. However, these findings have not been consistent across studies using different CFAE detection methods.[124]

Target of Ablation

Atrial ablation is performed at all sites displaying continuous electrical activity, complex and fractionated electrograms, regions with a gradient of activation (significant electrogram offset between the distal and proximal recording bipoles on the map electrode), or regions with shorter CL activity compared with the LA appendage. CFAE regions with the shortest CL and highest degrees of fractionation are the regions of most interest; sites displaying a greater percentage of continuous activity or a temporal activation gradient are more likely to be associated with slowing or termination of AF after local ablation.[127] The atrial septum, followed by the regions of the PVs, is the most common site for CFAEs. The most common localizations for termination and regularization of AF during CFAE ablation are the regions of the PV ostia, the interatrial septum, and the LA anterior wall close to the roof of the LA appendage.

After ablation of CFAEs in the LA, those in the CS and RA are targeted. RA ablation aimed at termination of AF can potentially offer a clinical benefit in patients with longstanding persistent AF, but it does not seem to improve outcome in patients with persistent AF of shorter durations.[130]

Ablation Technique

The ablation typically begins at sites at which CFAEs have the shortest interval and preferably also have a high interval confidence level. RF energy is applied using an 8-mm-tip or, preferably, an irrigated-tip catheter. Lower power output is applied in the CS and along the posterior LA.

A mean of 64 ± 36 RF applications was required in one study. In a second study, the mean duration of RF energy application was 36 ± 13 minutes. When the areas with CFAEs are completely eliminated, but the arrhythmia organizes into AFL or AT, the atrial tachyarrhythmias are mapped and ablated (occasionally in conjunction with ibutilide, 1 mg infused over 10 minutes). If the arrhythmias are not successfully terminated by ablation or ibutilide, external cardioversion is performed.

Endpoints of Ablation

The ablation endpoints when targeting CFAEs are uncertain. In most studies, the primary endpoints were complete elimination of the areas with CFAEs or organization slowing of local electrograms, conversion of AF to NSR (either directly or first to an AT) for patients with persistent AF, or noninducibility of AF (with isoproterenol and atrial pacing) for patients with paroxysmal AF.[126] When areas with CFAEs are completely eliminated, but arrhythmias continue as organized AFL or AT, those arrhythmias are mapped and ablated.

However, arrhythmia termination (conversion to AT or NSR) in patients with persistent AF can potentially be a challenging endpoint to achieve and generally requires very long procedure times. Reports demonstrated the limited ability of CFAE ablation to terminate persistent AF. Furthermore, although AF termination during ablation can potentially predict the mode of recurrence (AT versus AF), its correlation with long-term success is still controversial. AF recurrence rates of more than 50% were observed even in patients in whom AF was terminated during CFAE ablation. Thus, ablation of all areas displaying the electrogram of interest in the LA and CS can be a reasonable alternative endpoint when ablation fails to terminate AF.[130-134]

Preliminary reports suggested the clinical utility of monitoring dominant frequency in real time to guide catheter ablation of AF. A critical decrease (11% or higher, measured in lead V_1 and the CS) of dominant frequency following CFAE ablation can potentially indicate adequate elimination of drivers of AF and is associated with clinical efficacy that is as high as when AF is terminated by ablation. However, these findings require validation in prospective studies.[135]

Outcome

Although initial single-center studies using CFAE ablation as a stand-alone strategy for ablation of AF showed high success rates (up to 92% freedom from AF at 1 year follow-up after one or two ablation procedures), these results were not reproducible, and several more recent trials achieved only modest short-term efficacy. These findings suggest that CFAE ablation alone is not a sufficient strategy for successful treatment of AF.[72-74,125,128]

On the other hand, CFAE ablation can potentially be of value as an adjunct strategy in combination with PV isolation, particularly in patients with persistent AF whose response to other ablation strategies is suboptimal, as well as in patients with recurrent AF who are undergoing a second ablation procedure. Nonetheless, different studies produced conflicting results, partly because of variability of mapping techniques, the inconsistencies in CFAE electrogram interpretations, differences in the type and size of the mapping-ablation electrode, and differences in the accompanying lesion set. Whether ablating sites with CFAEs in paroxysmal AF has any additional effect on long-term outcome is even less clear. A meta-analysis (7 controlled trials with a total of 622 patients) found that, as compared with PV antral isolation alone, additional CFAE ablation after the PV isolation procedure slightly increased the rate of sinus rhythm maintenance in patients with persistent or longstanding persistent AF but did not show benefit in patients with paroxysmal AF.[136,137]

The benefits of AF substrate ablation have to be balanced against the potential risks in individual patients, especially given that CFAE ablation involves additional ablation lesions that can encompass extensive amounts of the atrial surface area, which can potentially compromise long-term atrial contractile function, produce arrhythmogenic atrial scarring, prolong procedure and radiation times, and increase risks of acute procedural complications. When adjunctive CFAE ablation is planned, it may be reasonable to target CFAEs after, rather than before, PV electrical isolation because that latter strategy can itself reduce the burden of CFAEs and minimize the consequent need for extensive LA ablation.[124,138]

In its current iteration, the CFAE ablation approach is limited by uncertainties regarding the mechanistic significance, efficacy, and endpoint of the ablation strategy. The lack of standardization in CFAE definition and differences in mapping technologies and electrogram measurements, especially given the lack of comparative information for the current technologies, adds to the challenge. Furthermore, although multiple studies have found that ablation at sites of CFAEs could prolong the CL or terminate AF, their true significance in the pathophysiology of AF remains to be determined, and the sensitivity and specificity of CFAEs in identifying sites critical to perpetuation of AF are uncertain. The mechanistic relevance of all sites of CFAEs in specific clinical contexts and in individual patients can potentially differ. Some CFAE sites can simply result from passive atrial activation and reflect shortening in the AF CL, random collision of fibrillatory waves, wave disruption adjacent to rapidly firing foci or rotors, or nonuniform anisotropic conduction.

In fact, significant spatiotemporal variability of CFAEs exists across studies for uncertain reasons. Whether all CFAE sites need to be targeted for catheter ablation is still not known, and reliable criteria to distinguish active from passive electrogram patterns and define optimal ablation targets are lacking.[124,127]

In addition to the time-domain (fractionation) mapping method, which involves scanning the atrium for CFAEs, the electrical substrate during AF can be described using the frequency mapping method. Frequency-domain (spectral) analysis of the atrial electrograms uses the fast Fourier transform algorithm to break down the AF signals into their different frequency components, distill the local activation frequency from highly complex electrograms, and determine the dominant frequency of the signal. Experimental evidence suggests that sites with high dominant frequencies can potentially be more specific than CFAEs at identifying the rotor regions driving the fibrillation process. Additionally, monophasic action potentials can identify local activation and repolarization in AF and help exclude CFAEs resulting from far-field signals that may be less attractive ablation sites. However, the clinical role of targeting the sites with high dominant frequency or monophasic action potentials by ablation is still under investigation.[124,139]

Pulmonary Vein Denervation

Rationale

Experimental and clinical data suggest that the autonomic nervous system plays a critical role in the initiation and maintenance of AF.[126] High-frequency stimulation of epicardial autonomic plexuses can induce triggered activity from the PVs and potentially shorten the atrial refractory periods to provide a substrate for the conversion of PV firing into sustained AF. Clinical studies found that ablation of the ganglionated plexuses located at the antra of the PVs (by specifically targeting the ganglionated plexuses or inadvertently during standard PV ablation procedures) can potentially reduce the risk of recurrence of AF.[25,93,140]

Localization of Ganglionated Plexuses

Autonomic inputs to the heart converge at several locations; these convergence points are typically embedded in the epicardial fat pads and form ganglionated plexuses that contain autonomic ganglia and nerves. In the LA, there are four major ganglionated plexuses located around the antral regions of the PVs and in the crux. The superior left ganglionated plexus is located on the roof of the LA, medial to the left superior PV, and often extends to the medial aspect of LA appendage. The anterior right ganglionated plexus is located just anterior to the right superior PV and often extends inferiorly, to the region anterior to the right inferior PV. The inferior left ganglionated plexus is located at the inferior aspect of the posterior wall of the LA, 1 to 3 cm below the left inferior PV. The inferior right ganglionated plexus is also located at the inferior aspect of the posterior wall of the LA below the right inferior PV and may extend toward the area adjacent to the crux of the heart, where another atrial ganglionated plexus (the crux ganglionated plexus) is located.[24,76]

High-frequency electrical nerve stimulation allows for precise determination of the location, threshold, and predominance of the parasympathetic or sympathetic response of the ganglionated plexuses. The distal electrode of the mapping-ablation catheter is used to deliver high-frequency stimulation (1200 beats/min [20 Hz], at 12 to 24 V and pulse width 1 to 10 milliseconds) using a Grass stimulator (S88X dual output square pulse stimulator, Grass Instruments Division, Astro Med Inc., Warwick, R.I.). Tolerance of the conscious patient to the stimulation still must be determined, because most reports have described use of this approach in deeply sedated patients.[75,76,141]

High-frequency stimulation of a ganglionated plexus can elicit both parasympathetic and sympathetic responses. A parasympathetic response is typically elicited immediately (within to 4 seconds) following stimulation, but a sympathetic response requires longer stimulation durations (8 to 10 seconds). A predominant efferent parasympathetic response is defined as induction of sinus bradycardia (slower than 40 beats/min), AV block (second- or third-degree AV block during sinus rhythm or a 50% or higher increase in mean R-R interval during AF), and/or hypotension (20 mm Hg or greater reduction of systolic blood pressure), following a 5-second application of high-frequency stimulation, with return to baseline values on cessation of stimulation. The sites of positive parasympathetic responses to high-frequency stimulation are marked on the electroanatomical map. If no response occurs, the catheter is positioned at adjacent sites. It is important to limit high-frequency stimulation to only 2 to 5 seconds, to avoid eliciting a sympathetic response that can otherwise mask or attenuate the parasympathetic response (e.g., by facilitating AV conduction and increasing blood pressure).[75,76]

Before applying high-frequency stimulation to inferior ganglionated plexuses, it is important to ensure that the catheter tip is not close to the ventricle to avoid induction of VF. When high-frequency stimulation is applied during NSR, AF generally occurs and usually terminates within seconds or minutes. Repeated stimulation usually results in sustained AF, at least in patients with a clinical history of AF.[76]

Alternatively, ganglia identification and ablation can be accomplished by a purely anatomical technique without the need for specific ganglionated plexus identification with high-frequency stimulation. The suboptimal sensitivity of high-frequency stimulation in identifying *all* LA ganglionated plexuses can result in partial and nonhomogeneous atrial denervation. Additionally, high-frequency stimulation commonly requires general anesthesia and carries the risk of induction of AF. The anatomical approach is based on studies in humans demonstrating that the largest accumulation of PV-related cardiac neural structures is localized to the inferior and posterior surface of the roots of both left and right inferior PVs, as well as on the anterior surface of the root of the right superior PV.[75,140]

Target of Ablation

During ablation of AF, the LA ganglionated plexuses are specifically targeted by ablation, as identified by high-frequency stimulation or on an anatomical basis, as described previously.

Ablation Technique

High-frequency stimulation is performed in the LA adjacent to the antral region of the PVs and the region of the LA crux. Once identified, the location of a ganglionated plexus is tagged on the electroanatomical map. Generally, the four major LA ganglionated plexuses can be identified and localized using high-frequency stimulation in the majority of patients; though, it is not uncommon that one or more ganglionated plexuses cannot be identified, especially in patients with persistent AF. RF is delivered after all ganglionated plexus sites have been identified.[76]

RF ablation is usually performed using an irrigated-tip catheter (25 to 35 W for 40 to 60 seconds). RF power and duration are reduced at sites close to the esophagus (15 to 20 W for 20 to 30 seconds). After each RF application, high-frequency stimulation is repeated immediately at the same site. If a positive parasympathetic response is still elicited, RF applications are repeated until a positive parasympathetic response is no longer elicited. Notably, RF energy delivery does not usually elicit a parasympathetic response, even at sites with positive response to high-frequency stimulation. Thus, the absence of an autonomic response should not prompt termination of RF application.[75,76,140] Because there is experimental evidence that ablation of the inferior right ganglionated plexus can potentially attenuate the parasympathetic response of other ganglionated plexuses to high-frequency stimulation and hence render subsequent localization of other ganglionated plexuses challenging,

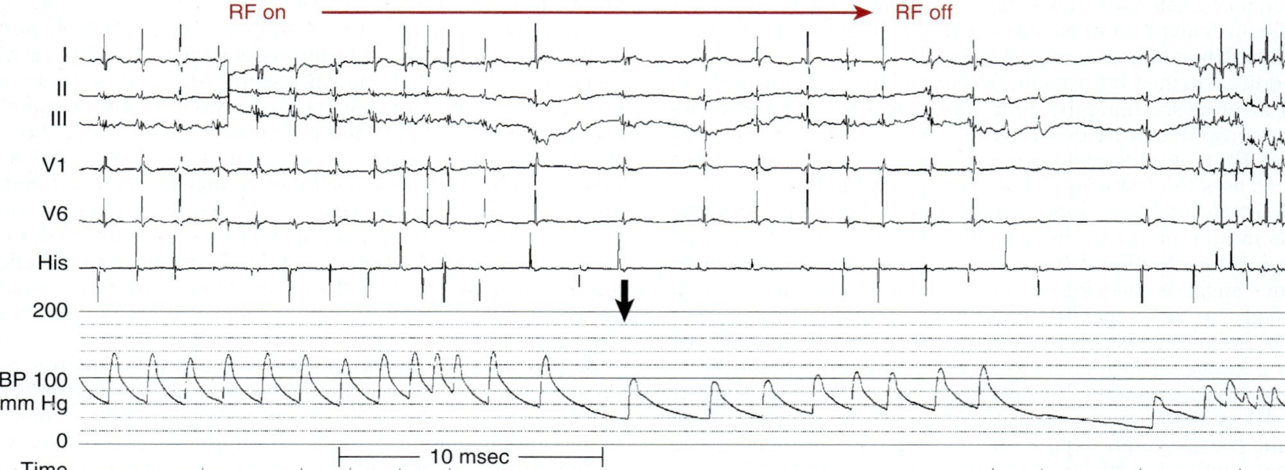

FIGURE 15-50 Vagal reflex during pulmonary vein (PV) isolation. Sinus rhythm is present at the beginning of the tracing; when radiofrequency (RF) energy is applied ("RF on"), blood pressure (BP) and heart rate decrease markedly (sinus bradycardia and nonconducted P wave). After energy is stopped ("RF off"), a short episode of atrial fibrillation ensues.

it is preferred to stimulate and ablate the inferior right ganglionated plexus last.

When using an anatomical approach for localization of the ganglionated plexuses, the presumed ganglionated plexus clusters near the PV antra are targeted by RF ablation. Because the exact anatomical borders of ganglionated plexus clusters are unknown and their location can vary slightly in different patients, a relatively extensive regional ablation is performed by delivering RF energy at multiple sites in and around the presumed anatomical location of each ganglionated plexus. Using this approach, vagal reflexes can be observed in at least one-third of patients, typically within a few seconds of the onset of RF application (Fig. 15-50). When a vagal reflex is observed during RF application, RF energy should be delivered until these reflexes are abolished, or for up to 30 seconds. It is important to recognize that the specificity and sensitivity of eliciting such vagal responses during RF application are not known. Similar responses can be triggered by pericardial pain during RF energy delivery. Additionally, as noted previously, vagal responses are not usually observed during RF ablation directly over the location of the ganglionated plexuses identified by high-frequency stimulation or even while applying RF energy to the plexuses during epicardial surgical ablation.[75,76,140]

Endpoints of Ablation

The endpoint of ablation is the abolition of all vagal reflexes evoked by high-frequency stimulation over the ganglionated plexus sites marked on the electroanatomical map. For anatomically guided atrial autonomic denervation, the endpoint of the ablation procedure is elimination of electrical activity (peak-to-peak bipolar electrogram less than 0.1 mV) in the specified areas and abolition of any vagal effects during RF energy delivery.[75]

Outcome

At present, no reports have suggested that targeting of ganglionated plexuses as a stand-alone procedure will consistently terminate AF or prevent its reinitiation. On the other hand, several studies incorporating ganglionated plexus mapping and ablation with PV-based ablation procedures for the treatment of AF have produced promising but variable results. Although modification of LA autonomic ganglia by epicardial or endocardial ablation has been proposed as an adjunctive procedure in association with PV-directed ablation procedures for the treatment of AF, only limited data have been available on the long-term benefit of vagal denervation, and the effectiveness of LA ganglionated plexus ablation requires more evaluation. Because the ganglionated plexuses are predominantly located near the PV antra, regions that are typically targeted by the different AF ablation strategies, whether the clinical benefits of ablation in these regions are related to selective ganglionated plexus modification and parasympathetic denervation, as opposed to interference with other AF-related mechanisms, is not known. On the other hand, some type of atrial denervation is likely to be inadvertently achieved after PV-based ablation procedures, which can potentially underlie, at least in part, the efficacy of these procedures.[76] Approximately 10% of patients undergoing PV isolation have subacute (weeks to months) acceleration of the sinus rate (to 80 to 95 beats/min) following ablation, a finding suggesting at least some effect on ganglionated plexuses.

Given the limitations of high-frequency stimulation in identifying all neural cardiac elements, some investigators have proposed that expanded regional LA ablation at the anatomical sites of the LA ganglionated plexuses can promote a more homogeneous and complete autonomic atrial denervation and can potentially offer higher clinical efficacy as compared with ablation guided by high-frequency stimulation.[75]

Ablation of Non–Pulmonary Vein Triggers

Rationale

Although the PVs are the major site of ectopic foci initiating AF, evidence has demonstrated the important role of non-PV ectopic beats initiating AF. Investigators have debated the frequency of the non-PV sources, with an incidence ranging from 3.2% to 47%; the incidence was found to be higher in chronic AF. The non-PV ectopic beats can arise from the SVC (most common, especially in female patients), LA posterior free wall (especially in patients with LA enlargement), crista terminalis, CS, ligament of Marshall, interatrial septum, or, rarely, a persistent left SVC. Additionally, SVTs such as AVN reentrant tachycardia (AVNRT) and AV reentrant tachycardia (AVRT) can be identified in up to 4% in unselected patients referred for AF ablation and can serve as a triggering mechanism for AF (see Fig. 15-2).[79]

Additionally, the presence of non-PV ectopic beats can play an important role in the recurrence of AF after PV isolation. Several investigators have reported focal AT originating from the LA after isolating all four PVs or circumferential LA ablation in up to 3% to 10% of patients. The locations of focal ATs were around the PV ostium, LA appendage, or LA free wall. Those findings support the concept that non-PV triggers actually exist before the AF ablation, and that they become the drivers of the AF or AT after part of the LA tissue is ablated or the LA-PV conduction is interrupted. Previous studies have also shown that wide-area circumferential LA ablation may be more effective than simple PV isolation, in part because some LA posterior free wall foci may be eliminated and/or isolated during circumferential ablation.

At the present time, most PV ablation procedures are performed anatomically by isolating all PV ostia. However, it is currently unclear whether an attempt should be made before and after PV isolation to observe the spontaneous or provoked ectopic beats initiating AF to evaluate for non-PV sources of this ectopy during initial and repeat ablation procedures.

Mapping of Non–Pulmonary Vein Triggers

PROVOCATION OF ECTOPY

The initial step is to locate the spontaneous onset of ectopic beats initiating AF in the baseline state or after infusion of isoproterenol (up to 4 to 8 μg/min for 5 minutes). If spontaneous AF does not develop, intermittent atrial pacing (8 to 12 beats) with a CL of 200 to 300 milliseconds from the high RA or CS is used to facilitate spontaneous initiation of AF after a pause in the atrial pacing. If spontaneous AF does not occur, burst pacing from the high RA or CS is used to induce sustained AF. After an episode of pacing-induced AF is sustained for 5 to 10 minutes, external cardioversion is attempted to convert the AF to NSR and observe the spontaneous reinitiation of AF. A bolus of high-dose adenosine (24 to 84 mg) may also be used to provoke the spontaneous onset of AF.

The onset pattern of spontaneous AF is analyzed, and the earliest ectopic site is considered to be the initiating focus of AF. The method used to provoke spontaneous AF is repeated at least twice to ensure reproducibility.

LOCALIZATION OF ECTOPY

Mapping of endocardial atrial activation sequences from the high RA, HB, and CS catheters can predict the location of AF initiation foci. The difference in the time interval between the high RA and HB atrial activation obtained during sinus beats and PACs is a good method to identify whether the ectopic focus is from the RA or LA. When the difference in the time interval is less than 0 millisecond, the accuracy for discriminating RA from LA ectopy approximates 100%.

If the initiating focus of the AF is considered to be from the RA, a duodecapolar catheter is placed along the crista terminalis, so that it would reach to the top of the SVC. The polarity of the P wave of the ectopic beat in the inferior leads is a useful method to differentiate the location of the ectopic beats. Ectopy from the SVC and upper crista exhibits upright P waves in the inferior leads, whereas ectopy from the coronary sinus ostium (CS os) exhibits a negative P wave polarity in the inferior leads and ectopy from the midcrista exhibits biphasic P waves. During RA ectopy, the P wave can be biphasic or positive in lead V_1, whereas it is predominantly positive in the case of right superior PV ectopy.

If the RA ectopy cannot be confirmed by the activation time, P wave morphology on the surface ECG, or intracardiac signals, transseptal access is obtained and two multipolar catheters are placed in the right superior PV and at the LA posterior wall simultaneously. Unusual ectopy from the RA septal region also requires biatrial mapping to confirm the location, especially in cases with a shorter activation time (less than 15 milliseconds) preceding P wave onset or a monophasic, narrow, and positive P wave in lead V_1 during ectopy. Multielectrode basket catheter, balloon catheter (EnSite noncontact mapping), and 3-D electroanatomical mapping systems can be of value in localization of the origin of AF triggers, especially in patients with infrequent PACs.

Mapping and Ablation of the Ligament of Marshall

The ligament of Marshall is an epicardial vestigial fold that marks the location of the embryological left SVC; it contains the nerve, vein (vein of Marshall), and muscle tracts, and it encompasses portions of the embryonic sinus venosus and left cardinal vein, running between the left superior and left inferior PVs along the left side of the parietal pericardium. The ligament of Marshall leads to the earliest tributaries of the CS and the transition from a ligamentous structure to a vein occurs in the region between the left superior PV and base of the LA appendage. The proximal portions of the muscle tracts connect directly to the CS myocardial sleeves. The connecting point is the landmark that separates the great cardiac vein from the CS (the origin of the ligament of Marshall often corresponds to the location of the tip of a CS catheter advanced to the wedge position as far distally as possible in the CS). The distal portions of the muscle tracts extend upward into the PV region.

Studies demonstrated electrical activity within the ligament of Marshall, and the two terminal ends of this atrial tract can have insertions into the LA musculature and CS. Also, more recently, the ligament of Marshall was shown to have electrically active myocardial tissue capable of generating focal automatic activity and can potentially contribute to the development of AF. It seems that isoproterenol infusion is usually required to provoke ectopy or bursts of AF originating from the ligament of Marshall.

Several attributes of the ligament of Marshall have been proposed to explain its mechanistic role in AF. Multiple connections among the Marshall bundle, LA, and CS can potentially create paths for reentrant excitation, leading to more complex and rapid activations. In fact, electrograms recorded from the ligament of Marshall during AF often exhibit short CLs, high dominant frequency, and CFAEs. Furthermore, rich innervation of the ligament of Marshall, predominantly by sympathetic fibers at its PV junction and parasympathetic ganglia at its CS junction, has been observed.

The ligament of Marshall should be considered as a source of paroxysmal AF, especially in young patients with a history compatible with adrenergic AF. Additionally, whenever an ectopic beat is mapped to the region around the posterolateral mitral annulus or a left-sided PV ostium, an origin from the ligament of Marshall should be considered. The P wave morphology associated with vein of Marshall ectopic activity is characterized by an isoelectric P wave in leads I and aVL, positive in leads III, aVF, and V_2 to V_5, and it is similar to that seen with ectopic beats arising from the left PVs. The P waves can be biphasic or negative in lead II.[79]

MAPPING OF THE LIGAMENT OF MARSHALL

The ligament of Marshall can be mapped epicardially or endocardially. The endocardial approach involves cannulation of the CS (preferably via an internal jugular venous access) with a 7 Fr luminal decapolar CS catheter. A venogram of the CS is obtained in the RAO 30-degree view to visualize the vein of Marshall and its ostium inside the CS. A 7 Fr luminal CS catheter is then directly engaged into the ostium of the vein of Marshall, and a 1.4 Fr mapping catheter is inserted into the inner lumen of the CS catheter and advanced toward the vein of Marshall.[79]

However, cannulation of the vein of Marshall is not always successful because of various anatomical and technical reasons. In patients whose vein of Marshall either is not visible on a CS venogram or is visible but cannot be cannulated, the percutaneous (subxiphoid) epicardial approach may result in successful mapping and ablation (Fig. 15-51). This latter approach has the advantage of free catheter movement and is not limited by the size of the

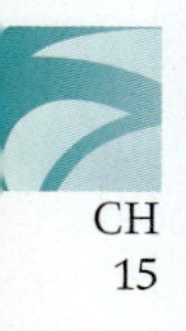

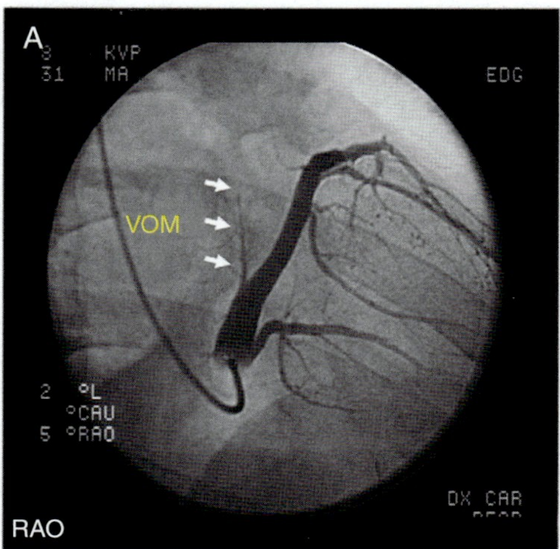

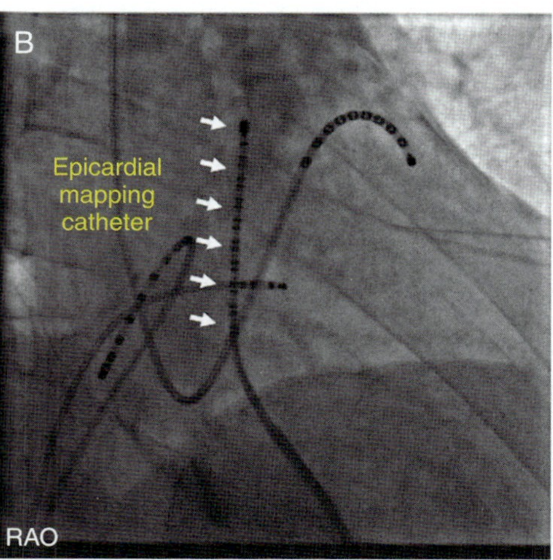

FIGURE 15-51 Two different approaches to mapping of the ligament of Marshall, right anterior oblique (RAO) views. **A,** Vein of Marshall (VOM) visualized by balloon occlusion coronary sinus (CS) angiogram. A 1.5 Fr mapping catheter can be inserted via the CS into this VOM for endocardial mapping. **B,** Epicardial mapping catheter inserted via a subxiphoid pericardial puncture. *(From Hwang C, Fishbein MC, Chen P: How and when to ablate the ligament of Marshall, Heart Rhythm 3:1505, 2006.)*

vein of Marshall. However, the endocardial approach is the best method for differentiating ligament of Marshall ectopy from other sources.

Certain observations and pacing maneuvers can indicate vein of Marshall activation, including (1) unexpected PV activation sequence during NSR, (2) unexpected PV activation sequence during low-output CS pacing, and (3) unexpectedly early exit from PV ectopy.[79]

During NSR, PV activation spreads from proximal (PV ostium) to distal. If earlier activation is seen in the middle or distal PV electrodes than near the ostium, a bypass of the ostium with direct activation of the middle or distal PV is likely. One explanation is epicardial activation via the myocardial tissue within the vein of Marshall.

With high-output pacing in the mid-CS, there is capture of both the myocardium of the CS itself and the adjacent LA. With lower-output pacing, in most cases there will be capture of the myocardium of the CS only, with the LA activated from the CS through a CS-to-LA connection. In some patients, the CS-to-LA connection is small and discrete and, if the connection is not close to the site of pacing within the CS, there can be considerable delay between the CS myocardial electrograms and adjacent LA tissue electrograms (Fig. 15-52). This observation can be used to determine whether PV activation is occurring via the vein of Marshall. During low-output CS pacing, the LA is not directly activated. Because PV activation depends on LA activation, in most cases, when the LA electrogram is delayed, PV potentials also are delayed. When the time from stimulus to PV potential remains fixed regardless of whether direct capture of the LA occurs, PV activation is dependent only on CS muscular activation and a vein of Marshall connection very likely is present (see Fig. 15-52).

Because the ligament of Marshall can have multiple insertion sites in the LA posterior free wall or near the PV ostium, it can be difficult to differentiate ligament of Marshall ectopy from PV or LA posterior free wall ectopy. Ectopy or rapid tachycardias arising from the PV typically demonstrate an early near-field potential on catheters placed within the PV and a late far-field electrogram consistent with LA activation. Often, the exit delay (interval between the early near-field potential and late far-field potential) exceeds the entrance delay seen in sinus rhythm with activation from the LA to the PV. Despite this exit delay, however, the earliest atrial activation should be in the perivenous area. If earlier activation is noted in the CS rather than the perivenous LA, direct conduction from the PV to the CS through the musculature of an atrial epicardial vein, usually the vein of Marshall, is likely (Fig. 15-53).

Furthermore, the possibility of ligament of Marshall ectopy should be considered when the so-called triple potentials (a discrete sharp potential preceding the LA and PV potentials) are recorded around the PV ostium. Furthermore, in patients with ectopic beats from the ligament of Marshall, double potentials are

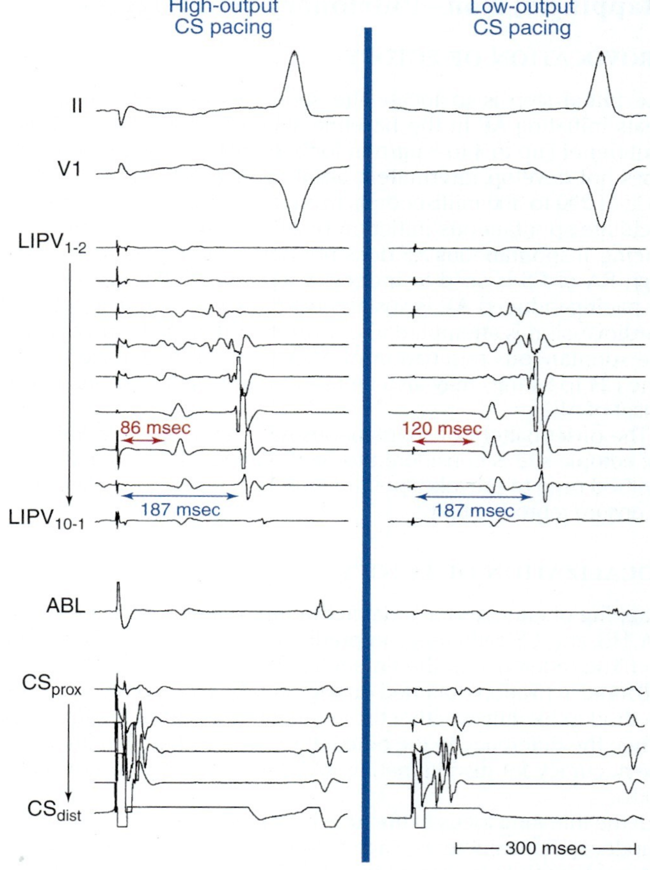

FIGURE 15-52 Identification of vein of Marshall activation using differential-output coronary sinus (CS) pacing. **Left panel,** During high-output CS pacing, both the left atrium (LA) and CS musculature are captured directly. **Right panel,** During low-output CS pacing, only the CS musculature is captured directly; the LA is activated from the CS through a CS to LA connection. In this case, the CS-LA connection is not close to the site of pacing within the CS; therefore, considerable delay is observed between the CS myocardial electrograms and the adjacent LA tissue electrograms. Despite the delay in LA activation (as reflected by the interval between the pacing artifact and the LA electrograms) during low-output versus high-output CS pacing, the timing of left inferior pulmonary vein (LIPV) activation remains constant (as reflected by the fixed interval between the pacing artifact and the PV potentials in both cases), thus indicating that PV activation is occurring via the vein of Marshall and is independent of LA activation. ABL = ablation site; CS_{dist} = distal coronary sinus; CS_{prox} = proximal coronary sinus.

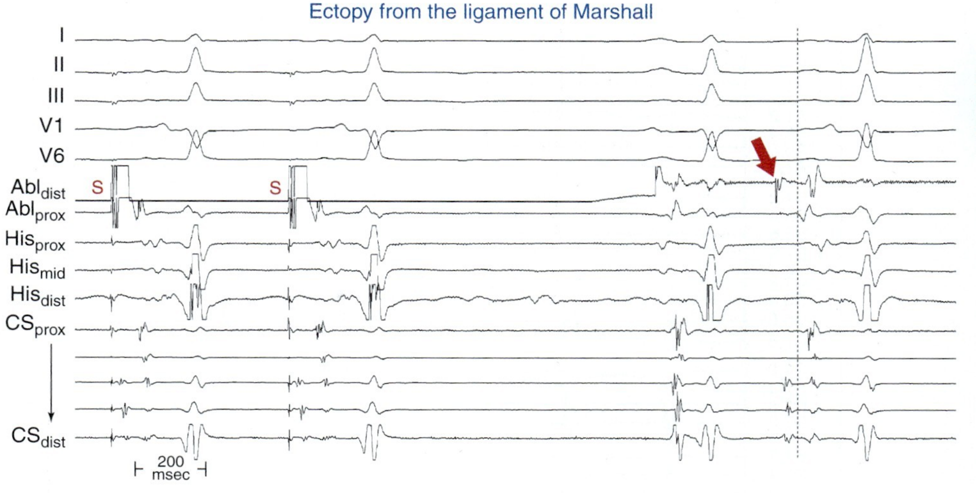

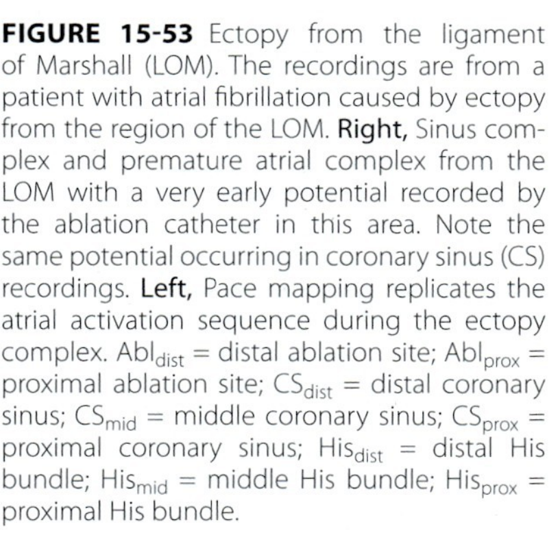

FIGURE 15-53 Ectopy from the ligament of Marshall (LOM). The recordings are from a patient with atrial fibrillation caused by ectopy from the region of the LOM. **Right,** Sinus complex and premature atrial complex from the LOM with a very early potential recorded by the ablation catheter in this area. Note the same potential occurring in coronary sinus (CS) recordings. **Left,** Pace mapping replicates the atrial activation sequence during the ectopy complex. Abl_{dist} = distal ablation site; Abl_{prox} = proximal ablation site; CS_{dist} = distal coronary sinus; CS_{mid} = middle coronary sinus; CS_{prox} = proximal coronary sinus; His_{dist} = distal His bundle; His_{mid} = middle His bundle; His_{prox} = proximal His bundle.

present at the orifice of or inside the left PVs, and distal CS pacing can help differentiate the ligament of Marshall potential from the PV musculature potential. If the second deflection of double potentials is attributable to the activation of the ligament of Marshall, the interval between the CS os and the second deflection will be shorter during distal CS pacing compared with NSR. In contrast, if the second deflection is attributable to activation of the PV musculature, the interval between the CS os and the second deflection will be longer during distal CS pacing compared with NSR.

Finally, the persistence of ectopic triggers of AF consistent with origins from the left-sided PVs despite complete electrical isolation of those veins should alert the operator to the ligament of Marshall as the source of ectopy.[79]

ABLATION OF THE LIGAMENT OF MARSHALL

Cannulation of the vein of Marshall and direct recording of the ligament of Marshall potentials from the vein of Marshall can be used as the anatomical targets for endocardial ablation and to confirm successful elimination of the ligament of Marshall potentials. Even when cannulation of the vein of Marshall is not feasible, obtaining a CS venogram to visualize the vein of Marshall can be used as an indirect method to trace the possible route of the ligament of Marshall to help guide ablation (see Fig. 15-51).[79]

The site having the shortest distance from the LA endocardium to the ligament of Marshall is located at the inferior region of the left antrum, just under the left inferior PV ostium. RF energy application from the endocardium to this region eliminates ligament of Marshall potentials in more than 90% of the cases, as confirmed by the mapping catheter inside the vein of Marshall. The elimination of ligament of Marshall electrograms along the entire length of the ligament and the presence of exit block between the ligament of Marshall and the LA during pacing from multiple sites within the vein of Marshall help confirm successful ablation.[79]

To simplify the procedure, a large-diameter (20 to 25 mm) ring catheter can be placed at the antrum of the left inferior PV to guide and then confirm simultaneous isolation of the antrum and ligament of Marshall. Complete isolation or disconnection of the entire left PV and antrum can be confirmed by pacing from the inside of the left PV. If PV potentials are dissociated from the LA potentials, these findings will confirm elimination of all connections to the LA, including the left PVs and ligament of Marshall.

Infrequently, endocardial ablation alone cannot eliminate all connecting fibers, as evidenced by the ability to still record ligament of Marshall potentials. In these situations, most of the remaining connections are located in the ridge between the anterior border of the left PVs and the posterior wall of the appendage. In some patients, the ridge can be as thick as 10 mm. Even using an irrigated-tip catheter and a high-power setting, complete isolation still may not be possible. In these difficult cases, a combined endocardial and epicardial approach can be used to ablate ligament of Marshall ectopy initiating AF and is associated with a higher success rate. Cannulation of the vein of Marshall can be used to guide epicardial ablation sites.

Electrical Isolation of the Superior Vena Cava

RATIONALE

The proximal SVC contains cardiac muscle fibers connected to the RA, and atrial excitation can propagate into the SVC. SVC cardiomyocytes can acquire pacemaker activity, and enhanced automaticity and afterdepolarization play a role in the arrhythmogenic activity of SVC (Fig. 15-54). The SVC myocardial extension harbors most (up to 55%) non-PV triggers of AF (especially in female patients), and elimination of SVC triggers is associated with improved long-term maintenance of sinus rhythm after AF ablation. Of interest, a long SVC sleeve greater than 30 mm long and a large SVC potential greater than 1.0 mV were proposed in one report to indicate an SVC source of AF triggers.

Electrical isolation of SVC from the RA can be a better strategy than focal ablation of ectopy inside SVC. It obviates the need for detailed mapping of the exact origin of the ectopy focus, as well as the need for RF ablation inside the SVC, which may carry the risk of SVC stenosis. Nevertheless, injury to the sinus node and phrenic nerve remains a concern. The value of empirical isolation of the SVC as an adjunctive strategy for AF ablation needs further evaluation.[142]

MAPPING OF SUPERIOR VENA CAVA ECTOPY

To localize the accurate site of SVC ectopy, 3-D electroanatomical, ring catheter, or basket catheter mapping can be useful (Fig. 15-55). During NSR or atrial pacing, the intracardiac recordings from inside the lower level of the SVC (near the SVC-RA junction) frequently exhibit a blunted far-field atrial electrogram followed by a sharp and discrete SVC potential. At a more cranial level of the SVC, the SVC potential precedes the atrial electrogram during the SVC ectopic beat (Fig. 15-56). Furthermore, the intracardiac recordings in the higher SVC frequently exhibit double potentials. The first potential represents the SVC potential, and the second potential represents the far-field right superior PV potential. Simultaneous recordings from the right superior PV also exhibit a double potential during SVC ectopy. The recording from the right superior PV shows that the first potential is a far-field potential from the SVC, and the second potential is true activation of the right superior PV.

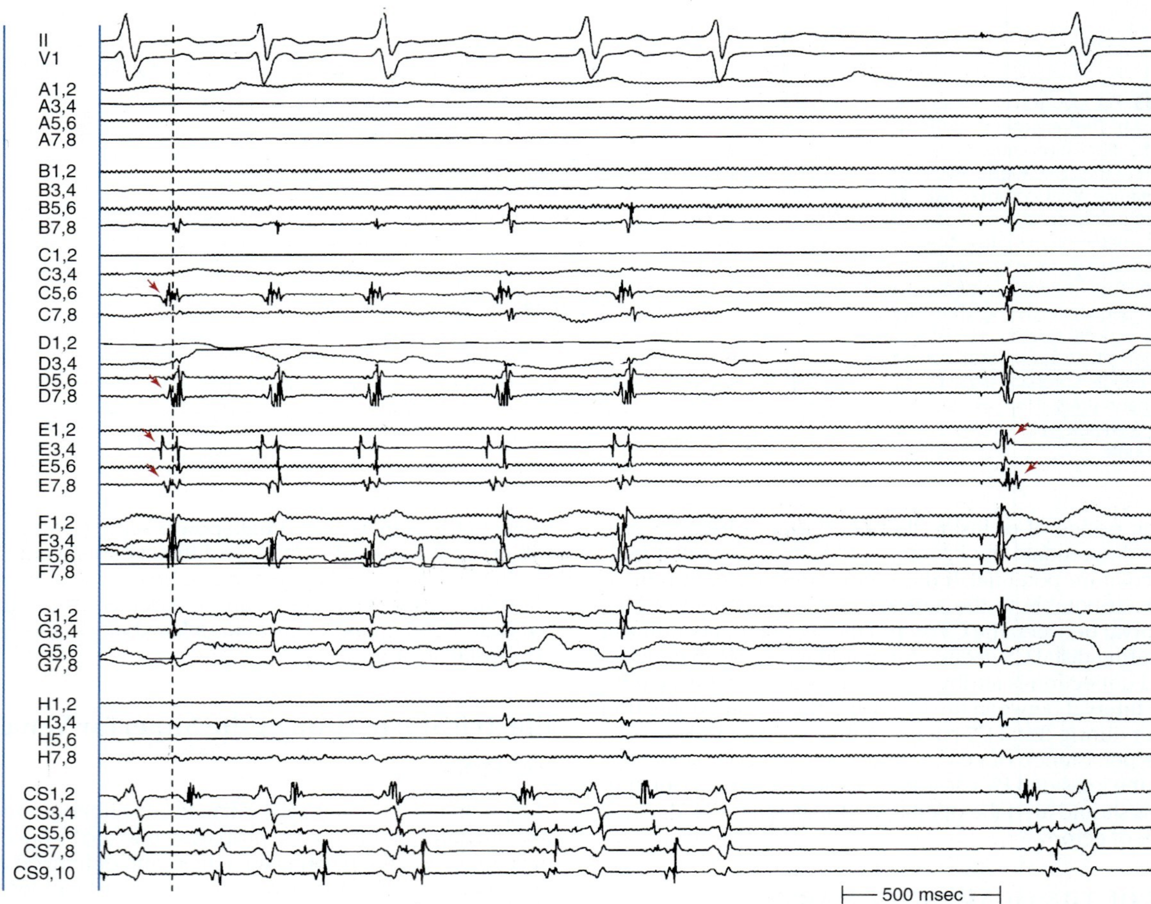

FIGURE 15-54 Focal atrial tachycardia (AT) originating from the superior vena cava (SVC). The basket catheter is positioned in the SVC–right atrial (RA) junction. Bipolar recordings are obtained from the eight electrodes (1-2, 3-4, 5-6, 7-8) on each of the eight splines (A through H) of the basket catheter. During AT (at left), SVC potentials (arrowheads) precede RA potentials and also precede P wave onset on the surface ECG (dashed line). During RA pacing (at right), SVC potentials overlap with or follow RA potentials.

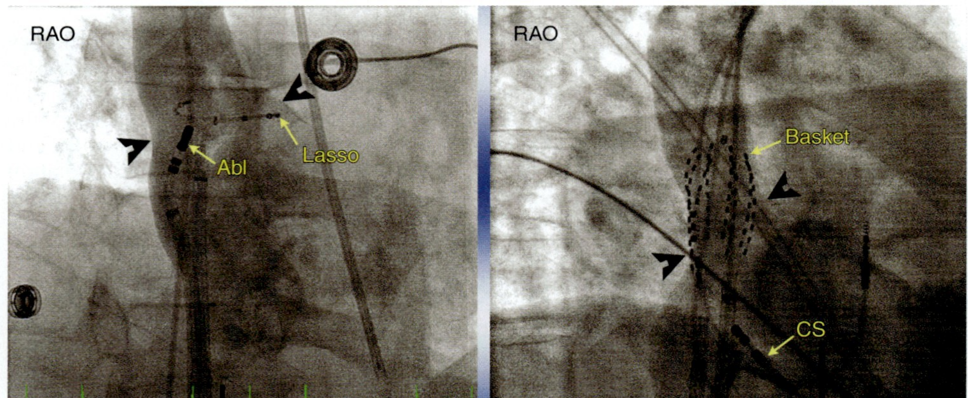

FIGURE 15-55 Superior vena cava (SVC) angiogram. Fluoroscopic right anterior oblique (RAO) views of SVC angiography with the ring (Lasso) catheter (at left) and basket catheter (at right) positioned at the SVC–right atrial (RA) junction (black arrowheads). Note that the size of the ring catheter is usually smaller than the circumference of the SVC, and repositioning of the ring catheter is typically required for circumferential mapping and electrical isolation of the SVC. Abl = ablation site; CS = coronary sinus.

ABLATION TECHNIQUE

The SVC is isolated using the same technique and endpoint as used for segmental ostial PV isolation. The SVC-RA junction (defined as the point below which the cylindrical SVC flares into the RA) can be confirmed by SVC venography (see Fig. 15-55), ICE (Fig. 15-57), or by the electrical signals. SVC venography can be performed by placing a pigtail catheter at the top of the SVC and using a contrast injector (a total of 40 mL of contrast medium over 2 seconds) and biplane fluoroscopic views (RAO, 30 degrees; LAO 60 degrees). The overlapping of the anterior wall of the SVC and RA appendage is near the level of the SVC-RA junction. The ring catheter is placed just above the RA-SVC junction at the level of the lower border of the pulmonary artery, as seen by ICE (see Fig. 15-57). The size of the ring catheter is usually smaller than the circumference of the SVC, and repositioning of the ring catheter is typically required for circumferential mapping and electrical isolation of the SVC (see Fig. 15-55).

Compared with PV isolation, it is easier to interrupt the conduction between the RA and the SVC. Most patients exhibit only two

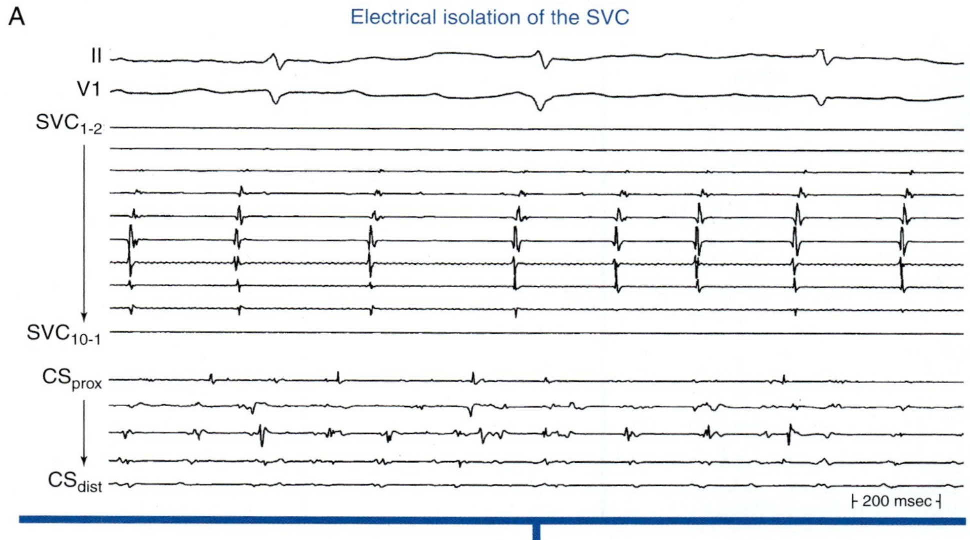

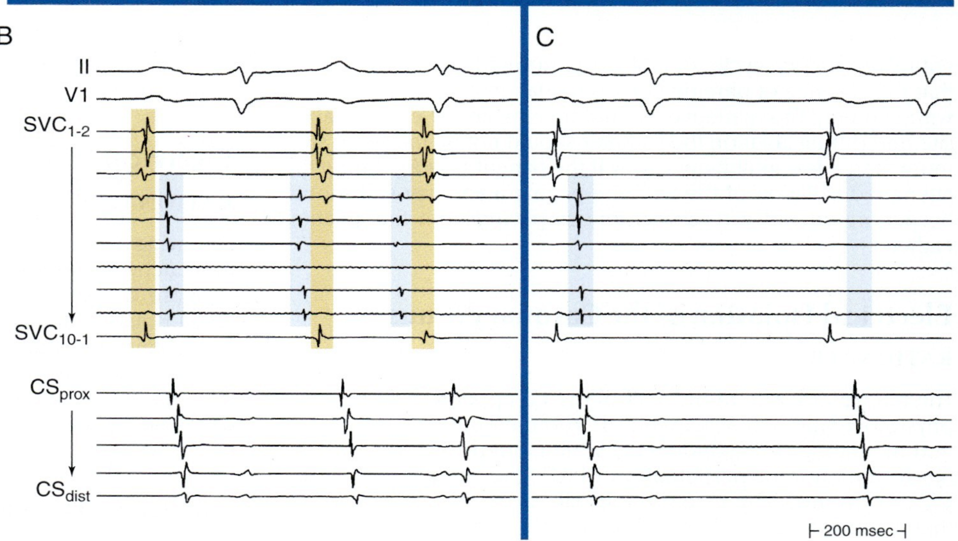

FIGURE 15-56 Electrical isolation of the superior vena cava (SVC). This recording was obtained from a ring catheter positioned at the SVC–right atrium (RA) junction during electrical isolation of the SVC. **A,** During atrial fibrillation, SVC potentials are observed at a cycle length (CL) longer than the atrial CL observed in the coronary sinus (CS) recordings. **B,** The first complex is normal sinus, during which SVC potentials (blue shading) are observed following RA potentials (orange shading). The second and third complexes are premature atrial complexes originating from the SVC, during which SVC potentials precede RA potentials. **C,** Radiofrequency energy application at a single site results in the disappearance of SVC potentials (at right) and complete SVC entrance block. CS_{dist} = distal coronary sinus; CS_{prox} = proximal coronary sinus.

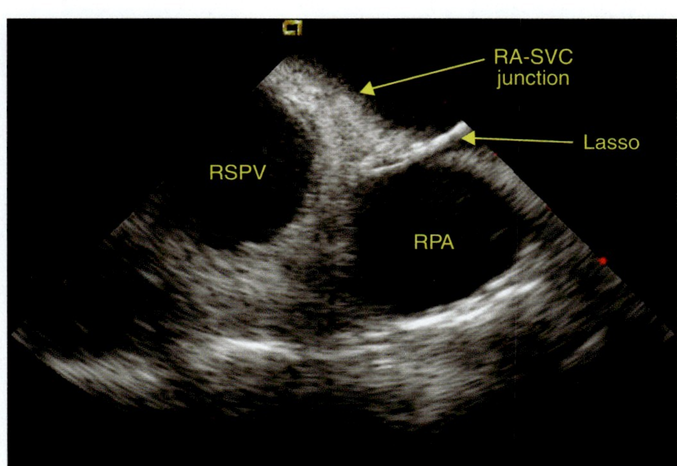

FIGURE 15-57 Electrical isolation of the superior vena cava (SVC). The intracardiac echocardiography catheter positioned in the high right atrium (RA) is used to guide positioning of the ring catheter at the RA-SVC junction (at the level of the lower border of the right pulmonary artery [RPA]). RSPV = right superior pulmonary vein.

breakthrough sites. A ring or basket catheter can be used for mapping SVC potentials (see Fig. 15-56). The SVC-RA junction exhibits an eccentric, not a round, shape; thus, the basket or ring catheter may not contact the wall well. Therefore, one needs to manipulate the catheter to contact the whole SVC-RA circumference to confirm the presence or disappearance of SVC potentials. The circumference of the SVC-RA junction is mapped to determine the region of earliest activation during NSR characterized by an initial negative rapid deflection or fusion, or both, of the major atrial electrogram and the SVC muscular potential. Those regions are then targeted by RF ablation.

RF energy should be applied at the level approximately 5 mm below the entire circumference of the SVC-RA junction. Although application of RF energy inside the SVC makes it easier to interrupt the SVC-RA myocardial sleeve, it carries a higher risk of SVC narrowing or stenosis. RF energy is set at a power setting of 45 to 55 W, targeting a temperature of 50°C to 55°C and applied for a duration of 20 to 40 seconds. Acceleration of the sinus rate during RF delivery is a sign that heat injury to the sinus node is occurring and should prompt discontinuation of RF application.

The phrenic nerve often courses posterolaterally at the level of the SVC-RA junction. Pacing prior to ablation along the circumference of this vein at an output between 5 and 10 mA is mandatory before energy delivery. The patient should not receive a paralytic agent if general anesthesia is to be used, and both mechanical palpation for diaphragmatic stimulation and fluoroscopy of an

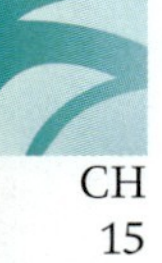

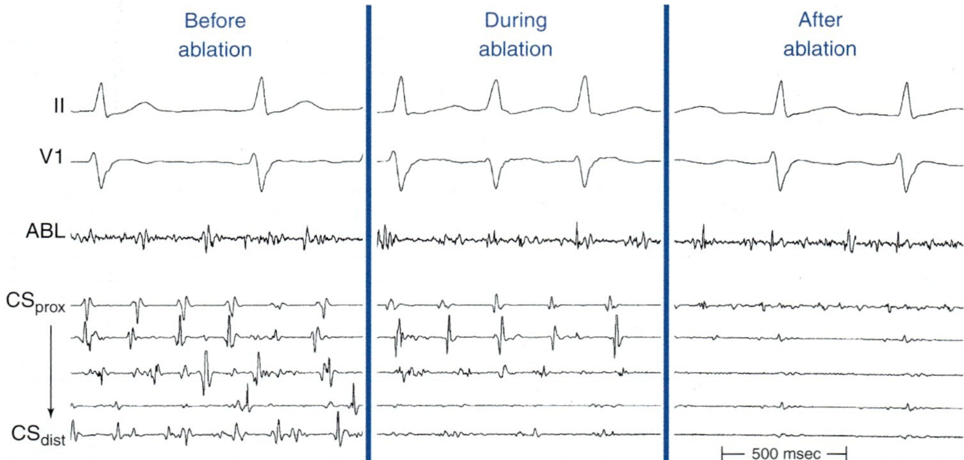

FIGURE 15-58 Electrical isolation of the coronary sinus (CS). Intracardiac recordings illustrating CS electrograms during atrial fibrillation before, during, and after successful electrical isolation of the CS. Following complete electrical isolation, the local sharp potentials within the CS are eliminated. ABL = ablation site; CS_{dist} = distal coronary sinus; CS_{prox} = proximal coronary sinus.

entire respiratory cycle should be performed during pacing so that the absence of phrenic nerve stimulation can be determined with certainty. The maneuver should be repeated at each ablation site, and during ablation the catheter should not be moved to sites more than a few millimeters away. If the patient is in AF during the attempted isolation of the SVC, the pacing maneuver still should be performed, but with asynchronous pacing from the ablation catheter.

Electrical Isolation of the Coronary Sinus

RATIONALE

The muscular tissue in the wall of the CS appears to be electrophysiologically active, capable of spontaneous depolarization and mediating slow conduction, which can potentially contribute to initiation or perpetuation of AF. The venous wall of the CS is surrounded by a continuous sleeve of atrial myocardium that extends for 25 to 51 mm from the CS os. This muscle is continuous with the RA myocardium proximally, but it is usually separated from the LA by adipose tissue. This separation can be bridged by muscular strands producing electrical continuity between the CS musculature and the LA. These connections are targeted by RF ablation for electrical isolation of the CS from the LA.[143]

ABLATION TECHNIQUE

Isolation of the CS is commenced along the endocardial aspect and completed from within the CS, as required. The ablation catheter is dragged along the endocardium of the inferior LA after looping the catheter to position it parallel to the CS catheter. After achieving a 360-degree loop in the LA, the catheter is gradually withdrawn initially along the septal area anterior to the right PVs and ablation commenced at the inferior LA along the posterior mitral annulus from a site adjacent to the CS os progressing to the lateral LA (at the 4-o'clock position in the LAO projection). The endpoint is elimination of local endocardial electrograms bordering the mitral isthmus in an attempt to eliminate or prolong the CL of sharp potentials present within the CS (Fig. 15-58). Ablation within the CS is started distally (at the 4-o'clock position in the LAO projection) and pursued along the CS up to the ostium by targeting local sharp potentials at individual sites or as a continuous drag. During AF, ablation within the CS is performed at all sites showing persistent or intermittent rapid activity, either continuous electrograms or discrete electrograms displaying CLs shorter than the CL measured in the LA appendage. Finally, additional RF applications are continued around the CS orifice from the RA. CS disconnection is confirmed by the dissociation or abolition of sharp potentials in its first 3 cm.

Electrical Isolation of the Left Atrial Appendage

RATIONALE

Following extensive LA ablation, some patients have focal or reentrant tachycardias arising in the region of the LA appendage (base or more deeply in the appendage). Some operators have advocated isolation of the appendage as a means of eliminating these arrhythmias without entering the deeper part of the appendage, which typically turns back medially toward the midline (limiting catheter reach) and where muscle is very thin. The appendage is occasionally inadvertently isolated during roof or mitral isthmus line ablation.

ABLATION TECHNIQUE

The ring catheter may be carefully situated in the mouth of the appendage, with ablation targeting earliest sites of propagation into or out of the appendage (similar to selective ostial isolation of PVs). Alternatively, anatomically based ablation around the ostium or the appendage can be performed, guided by a mapping system, because much of the line will have already been made with prior ablation.

Outcome

The success rate of AF elimination varies, depending on the site of ectopy. A higher success rate is noted when the triggering foci are located in the RA, including the SVC and crista terminalis. The LA posterior free wall has a higher recurrence rate because of anatomical limitations and multiple ectopic foci. The success rate of curing ligament of Marshall ectopy initiating AF is low when ablation is limited only to the endocardial area. A combined endocardial and epicardial approach to ablate ligament of Marshall ectopy has a higher success rate (60% to 70%). Isolation of the LA appendage, resulting in an akinetic or competitively contracting structure (if it retains an automatic rhythm), has not been associated with adverse hemodynamic outcomes although data are limited.

Non-PV foci triggering AF appear to be the mechanism of recurrences of AF after PV isolation procedures in only a small proportion (approximately 10%) of patients undergoing repeat ablation. Given the fact that inducing those triggers is usually challenging and time consuming, it is unclear whether to incorporate a routine search for these triggers into an initial ablation procedure.

Outcome of Catheter Ablation of Atrial Fibrillation

Success Rates

There are several hypothetical benefits of ablation of AF and restoration of sinus rhythm: improvement in quality of life, reduction of stroke risk, reduction in heart failure risk, and improved survival. Several randomized trials demonstrated the benefit of ablation in the reduction of the burden of AF and improvement in quality of life. However, no studies demonstrated that these findings translate into reduction in overall mortality. Therefore, the primary justification for an AF ablation procedure at this time is the presence of symptomatic AF.

Interestingly, the quality of life improvement after AF ablation is not entirely dependent on efficacy of the procedure. In fact, up to 65% of patients with documented recurrences of AF after ablation exhibit improvement of symptoms during the AF episodes and report significant improvement of the physical component of the quality of life.[144,145] Reduction of symptomatic episodes after ablation may arise from a placebo effect or autonomic denervation.

With time, operator experience, and greater consistency in the technique, AF ablation has proved itself to be a very effective treatment for symptomatic AF. Reportedly, current techniques of RF catheter ablation can achieve a 60% to 90% improvement in selected patients with medically refractory AF, with similar success rates being reported by several different groups. Although success rates are not perfect, they are two- to threefold better than anything achievable by antiarrhythmic medications. Furthermore, successful control of AF by ablation seems to be durable, given the long follow-up (almost 3 years) reported by some groups and the observation that most recurrences tend to occur early in the follow-up period, and they only infrequently occur late after ablation.

Variations in success rates for similar procedural techniques for catheter ablation of AF reported by different centers can potentially arise from several factors, including variation in study design, different patient population characteristics (age, cardiac disease, LA size), different types of AF (paroxysmal versus persistent versus longstanding), differences in follow-up duration and strategy, and differences in definition of success (complete freedom from all atrial arrhythmias versus AF versus symptomatic arrhythmias, with or without antiarrhythmic agents). Also, the efficacy of AF ablation can be largely influenced by the operator's experience and the volume of ablations.[131]

Consideration also needs to be given to the adoption of a subclassification of AF based on clinical criteria if the magnitude of the therapeutic impact of catheter ablation on patients' quality of life is to be meaningfully assessed. For a patient whose condition is transformed from a predominant pattern of highly symptomatic persistent AF, with occasional spontaneous terminations before ablation, to a pattern of asymptomatic or symptomatic short-lived episodes of transient AF (lasting a few minutes) after ablation, the procedure could be deemed clinically successful. In contrast, a binary outcome analysis limited to whether a patient has any recurrence of AF at any time or is free of AF recurrence would classify the ablation as a failed procedure, and any clinical benefit to the patient would not be recognized.

ABLATION OF PAROXYSMAL ATRIAL FIBRILLATION. In the setting of paroxysmal AF, RF ablation of AF (generally PV isolation with little to no adjuvant ablation) was found superior to antiarrhythmic drug therapy in several studies, with a success rate of approximately 77% over 12 months. In many of these studies, a single repeat ablation procedure was required in 10% to 25% of patients. Circumferential antral PV isolation appears more effective than segmental ostial PV isolation. The role of adjunctive substrate-based ablation techniques (linear ablation, CFAE ablation, and vagal denervation) is controversial, but these approaches appear to have little value, if any, over antral PV isolation alone in patients with paroxysmal AF.[78,109,110]

ABLATION OF NONPAROXYSMAL ATRIAL FIBRILLATION. In patients with persistent AF, segmental ostial PV isolation is inadequate for arrhythmia control, with single-procedure, drug-free success rates of approximately 22%, and multiple-procedure success rates lower than 55%. In contrast, circumferential antral PV isolation offers better success rates (32% to 44% after a single procedure and 59% to 77% after multiple procedures). Several studies found an incremental benefit of adding LA linear ablation (LA roof line and mitral isthmus ablation) to antral PV isolation, especially in patients with longstanding AF. The data are not convincing regarding the additive benefit of posterior wall isolation. Importantly, linear LA ablation can be proarrhythmic, increasing the risk of LA macroreentrant ATs, especially if the presence of bidirectional block across the ablation lines has not been verified. The role of CFAE ablation is more controversial. Although some studies achieved higher success rates with PV isolation when combined to CFAE ablation, other studies showed no incremental benefit. CFAE ablation as a stand-alone strategy appears inadequate for successful treatment of AF (pooled success rate of only 26%). Purely anatomical techniques of PV ablation (with or without adjunctive CFAE ablation) have been found to be inferior to techniques that rigorously confirm complete PV electrical isolation (single procedure success rate of 27% versus 57% at 2 years of follow-up). Importantly, regardless of the ablation strategy, multiple procedures appear to be required in nearly half of patients with persistent AF. Prospective, randomized trials comparing ablative strategies are much needed.[74,78,146,147]

A stepwise ablation strategy has been proposed for patients with persistent AF, whereby antral PV isolation is followed by CFAE ablation and linear ablation until AF termination. This approach results in a single-procedure success rate of 25% to 62%. More than half of all patients undergo at least one repeat ablation procedure, and when all are complete the success rate is approximately 70% to 88%.[78,131,148]

Recurrence of Atrial Fibrillation

Recurrences of AF are common and can be observed in more than 50% of patients within the first 3 months following catheter ablation, regardless of the ablation technique. The incidence of recurrent AF seems to be higher in patients with persistent AF (47%) as compared with paroxysmal AF (33%), in patients older than 65 years (48%) versus patients younger than 65 years (28%), and in patients with structural heart disease (47% to 74%) versus patients without structural heart disease (29% to 50%).[3] Less consistent predictors of AF recurrence include the presence of comorbidities such as hypertension, sleep apnea, and diabetes. Gender and obesity do not appear to predict AF recurrence.[105,149,150]

The incidence of AF recurrences increases with increasing follow-up duration and intensity. Considering the intermittent nature of the arrhythmia and the inconsistency of symptoms, the exclusive reliance on patient reporting of symptomatic recurrences results in an underestimation of recurrence of the arrhythmia. To obtain reliable information about the success of AF ablation, repeated ambulatory monitoring with automatic detection of arrhythmias is necessary.[151]

Most recurrences occur within the first 12 months, and most patients who remain free of AF at 1 year after ablation are likely to remain in NSR at long-term follow-up. Among patients who develop recurrent AF, approximately 76% do so within the first 6 months after ablation, 86% by 12 months, and 92% by 24 months. Although there continues to be an ongoing risk of recurrent AF, new recurrences of AF are infrequent beyond 12 to 24 months following ablation.[152]

EARLY RECURRENCES. Early (within 3 months after ablation) AF recurrences peak within the first few weeks and then gradually decrease to lower levels in the period of 3 months after ablation. The mechanism of early postablation AF is unclear but seems to be different from that of the patient's preablation arrhythmia. Several mechanisms have been implicated, including local inflammation in response to RF thermal injury or pericarditis, systemic inflammation, heightened adrenergic tone, changes in medicines, fluid and electrolyte imbalances, and a delayed therapeutic effect of RF ablation likely attributable to lesion growth or maturation. Additionally, failure to identify and modify AF triggers (e.g., failure to isolate the PVs) can manifest with early AF recurrences.[153,154]

LATE RECURRENCES. Beyond the early postablation period, recurrent AF following ostial segmental or circumferential antral PV isolation is predominantly caused by PV ectopy originating from previously isolated PVs rather than non-PV foci. Recurrence of PV-LA conduction is almost universal (more than 80%), and reisolation of the PVs is recommended in these patients. However, additional linear LA ablation, substrate modification, or targeting non-PV foci should also be considered. Additionally, a significant subset of recurrences can be iatrogenic, resulting from macroreentry secondary to gaps in ablation lines or tissue recovery, or both.[155]

VERY LATE RECURRENCES. The incidence of very late AF recurrences after long-lasting (more than 12 months) arrhythmia-free intervals following catheter ablation is approximately 4% to 10%. These recurrences appear still to be triggered by foci from reconnected PVs in most cases; however, non-PV triggers can play a more dominant role in AF initiation in this setting. The insidious and progressive arrhythmogenic substrate formation during a period of apparent AF elimination is also a likely cause. Most studies have reported that patients in whom an initial attempt at ablation fails and who undergo a repeat ablation procedure demonstrate recurrent conduction in previously isolated PVs, rather than new arrhythmogenic foci from nontargeted PVs or outside the PVs. In patients with AF caused by reconduction from the PVs, reisolation of the PV is frequently sufficient. Other patients may require targeting non-PV triggers or ablation strategies directed at the AF substrate, including additional linear ablation lesions or ablation of CFAEs.[105,155]

Late recurrences of AF after initial arrhythmia-free intervals argue against AF ablation as a curative procedure and also suggest that a decision regarding discontinuation of anticoagulation after AF ablation should be based on the stroke risk stratification rather than the apparent efficacy of the AF ablation procedure.[147]

MANAGEMENT OF RECURRENT ATRIAL FIBRILLATION. As noted previously, administration of antiarrhythmic drug therapy to patients who undergo catheter ablation for AF can decrease early recurrence of atrial arrhythmias. However, the long-term risk of AF recurrence does not seem to be affected by early, prophylactic, short-term use of antiarrhythmic drugs.[81] Nonetheless, because early recurrences of AF are common and do not necessarily predict long-term recurrences, some operators choose to treat all patients with suppressive antiarrhythmic drugs during the first 1 to 3 months following ablation, a strategy that can potentially help decrease morbidity related to symptomatic arrhythmia episodes and the need for cardioversion or hospitalization. Typically, a class IC agent, sotalol, dofetilide, or amiodarone, is used. In patients discharged with antiarrhythmic drug therapy, such therapy is discontinued if no recurrence of AF is observed after 1 to 3 months.

In patients discharged without antiarrhythmic drug therapy who develop paroxysmal episodes of AF, antiarrhythmic drug therapy is initiated unless the patient is satisfied with the extent of symptomatic improvement. Catheter ablation of AF can be partially effective and allow a patient with AF that was previously refractory to antiarrhythmic drug therapy to become responsive to drugs. Therefore, if AF recurs following discontinuation of antiarrhythmic medications, it is common practice to reinitiate the antiarrhythmic drug. For persistent AF, the early restoration of sinus rhythm can improve the likelihood of long-term maintenance of sinus rhythm, regardless of when the arrhythmia first recurs after the ablation procedure.[154]

Although early recurrence of AF carries an independent risk for ablation failure, its occurrence should not prompt immediate reablation attempts because many patients experiencing recurrences within the first months after ablation will not have any further arrhythmias during long-term follow-up. Repeat ablation procedures should be deferred for at least 3 months following the initial procedure, except in patients with poorly tolerated atrial arrhythmias refractory to medical therapy.[3] Many patients with satisfactory control of AF with drugs prefer to continue antiarrhythmic drug therapy rather than undergo a repeat ablation procedure, in which case drug therapy is an acceptable long-term management strategy. However, in other patients it is desirable to eliminate all arrhythmias and possibly eliminate antiarrhythmic drug therapy; hence, repeat ablation may be considered in the setting of AF recurrence following the initial procedure. In general, recurrences of AF or AT after an initial AF ablation procedure lead to a reablation procedure in 20% to 40% of patients.

Atrial Tachycardia and Flutter Following Ablation of Atrial Fibrillation

LA tachycardia or flutter is a known complication of surgical and catheter-based therapies of AF. Originally reported in association with LA scar following mitral valve or maze surgical procedures, several reports demonstrated focal and macroreentrant ATs occurring after linear LA ablation and circumferential and segmental PV isolation, with an incidence ranging between 2% and 50%. The incidence seems to be lower following segmental ostial PV isolation than circumferential PV isolation and much higher following circumferential or linear LA ablation (more than 30%). Targeting CFAEs without linear lesions or PV isolation is associated with a moderate risk (8.3%) of postablation ATs. Following stepwise approaches of catheter ablation incorporating extensive lesions in the LA and RA to terminate persistent AF, ATs can be observed in more than 50% of patients.[156,157] Although typical AFL should be considered in the differential diagnosis of regular tachycardias (even in the presence of atypical ECG patterns) observed following AF ablation, most of these arrhythmias arise from the LA and can be focal or macroreentrant.[158]

LA tachycardias tend to occur at variable time intervals after AF ablation procedures. AT (macroreentrant or focal) can develop in the course of the ablation procedure or up to 1 year after the procedure, but the most common timing appears to be 1 to 2 months after ablation.[159,160] This time course suggests that healing of ablation lines likely contributes to the substrate for atrial reentry. The occurrence of ATs early after ablation is common and potentially, but not necessarily, predicts later recurrences of both AT and AF.[159,160] These tachycardias can be problematic because they frequently are incessant and are associated with rapid ventricular rates, and they are more likely to require electrical cardioversion when compared with the episodes of AF prior to ablation.

The three predominant catheter-based techniques for AF ablation appear to be associated with different rates and types of postprocedure ATs. Segmental ostial PV isolation is associated with a lower incidence of atrial tachyarrhythmias (less than 5%). When they do occur, these arrhythmias tend to be focal ATs, often originating from ostial segments of reconnected PVs. Reisolation of the PV and ablation of non-PV foci are usually sufficient to treat this proarrhythmia. Macroreentrant ATs (LA flutters) have been reported after segmental PV isolation, but this situation appears to be significantly less common. Most reentrant circuits use the ablated zone as a central obstacle, resulting in perimitral or peri-PV reentry, with the latter more prevalent in patients with larger atria.

Circumferential antral PV isolation has also been complicated by LA tachyarrhythmias, both focal and macroreentrant, and PV-LA conduction recovery is frequently a critical element in these arrhythmias. The area of recovery within an ablated region of the antrum can potentially create a region of slow conduction and the substrate for reentry (Fig. 15-59). When this area is a critical limb of the macroreentry circuit, reisolation of the PVs by ablation within the antrum terminates the tachycardia. In some cases, it is also possible that the recovered PV conduction allows PV triggers to induce a tachycardia that does not involve the PV antra. These patients also benefit from PV reisolation and elimination of PV triggers.

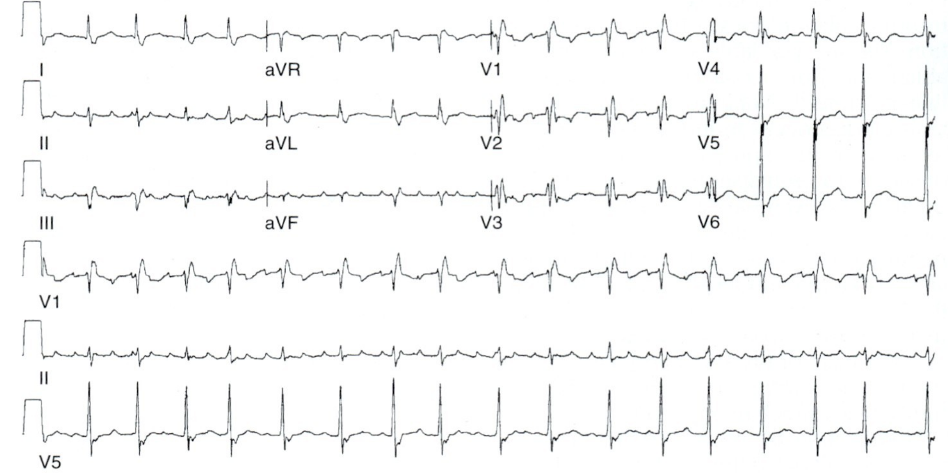

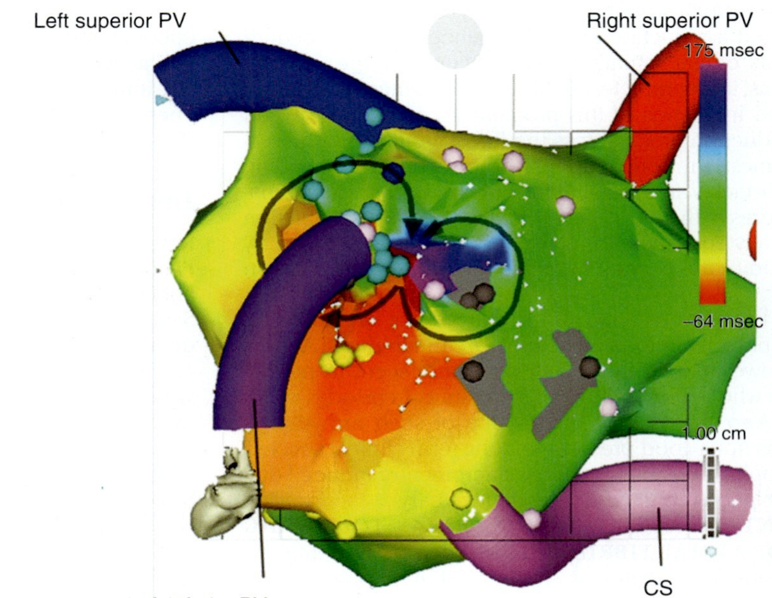

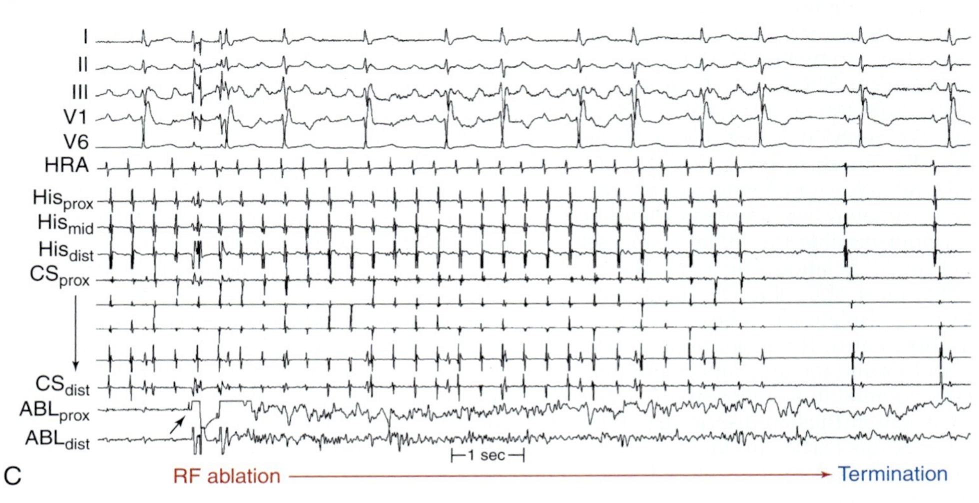

FIGURE 15-59 Macroreentrant atrial tachycardia (AT) after atrial fibrillation ablation. **A,** ECG of incessant AT occurring months following circumferential antral pulmonary vein (PV) isolation. **B,** Electroanatomical activation map (posterolateral view) of the same AT. Figure-of-8 reentry is seen involving the orifice of the left inferior PV and scar tissue (gray patches) resulting from the prior ablation. **C,** Intracardiac recordings during the AT. A single radiofrequency application at the site of the diastolic potential terminates the AT within a few seconds after onset of power delivery. Abl_{dist} = distal ablation site; Abl_{mid} = middle ablation site; Abl_{prox} = proximal ablation site; CS_{dist} = distal coronary sinus; CS_{prox} = proximal coronary sinus; His_{dist} = distal His bundle; His_{mid} = middle His bundle; His_{prox} = proximal His bundle.

Wide-area circumferential LA ablation is frequently complicated by LA macroreentrant ATs. Most of those ATs are related to gaps in prior ablation lines, a finding that implies that most postablation ATs are avoidable, either by limiting the amount of linear ablation and/or by confirming complete conduction block across linear lesions.[161] Not infrequently, multiple (three to four) different tachycardias occur in individual patients. The long linear lesions required in this approach to prevent AF also create new fixed obstacles to propagation, adjacent areas of block, and slow conduction, and eventual discontinuities represent ideal substrates for large reentrant circuits. Perimitral macroreentrant AT traversing the mitral isthmus is the most common, accounting for approximately 40% of macroreentrant ATs, and macroreentrant circuits traversing the LA roof account for approximately 20%. Less common sites of macroreentry involve the LA septum, the cavotricuspid isthmus, and the base of the LA appendage.[157] Focal ATs also have been reported following circumferential LA ablation, but macroreentrant ATs are much more common.

Modification of the original circumferential LA ablation technique has involved the addition of linear ablation connecting the superior PVs (roof line) and connecting the left inferior ablation line to the mitral annulus (mitral isthmus line). Whereas some studies demonstrated a reduction in the incidence of postprocedure LA tachycardias, others actually raised concern that the addition of linear lesions, if incomplete, could lead to an increased rather than decreased incidence of this problem. As noted, even when complete conduction block across the linear lesions is achieved, the ablation lines can potentially promote reentry by providing conduction obstacles and protected isthmuses with adjacent anatomical structures in the LA.[110] Therefore, these additional ablation lines can actually contribute to, rather than prevent, macroreentry, and further studies are needed to define their role in the ablation strategy.[162]

Importantly, LA macroreentry can be induced in a large percentage (38%) of patients immediately after circumferential LA ablation for AF; however, such inducibility does not seem to predict those patients who subsequently develop clinical episodes of LA tachycardias. Also, the lack of inducibility of such arrhythmias after ablation is not a good predictor of long-term clinical success. Therefore, mapping and ablation of LA macroreentry induced during catheter ablation for AF do not seem necessary.

MANAGEMENT OF ATRIAL TACHYCARDIAS FOLLOWING ABLATION OF ATRIAL FIBRILLATION. There is currently no well-defined standard treatment strategy for ATs following AF ablation procedures, and treatment should be tailored to the potential arrhythmia mechanism. It is important to recognize that many of these arrhythmias are self-limited and resolve spontaneously in up to two-thirds of patients within the first 3 to 6 months of follow-up. Therefore, efforts should be focused at suppressing these arrhythmias with antiarrhythmic medications or controlling the ventricular response with AVN blocking drugs. Despite the often more severe symptoms associated with these arrhythmias, ablation for LA macroreentrant ATs should be postponed for approximately 3 to 4 months after diagnosis.[3]

Understanding the initial lesion set is critical before embarking on AT ablation. For focal ATs following PV isolation procedures, most of the foci are located in a PV or in the antrum of a PV, and reisolation of all reconnected PVs appears to be sufficient in most cases. The septal aspect of ablation lines encircling the right PVs and the area anterior to the left superior PV are particularly vulnerable to recovery of conduction after circumferential PV isolation, thus predisposing patients to the development of LA tachycardia. Particular attention should be paid at these sites to ensure continuous transmural lesions. If the PVs are excluded as the site of origin of a focal AT, mapping then should focus on the other most likely sites of origin, including the posterior LA, mitral annulus, CS, SVC, and crista terminalis.[157] Nonetheless, PV isolation is still appropriate if there is evidence of PV conduction, even if the focal AT is not arising in the PV, to minimize the possibility of recurrent AF.[163]

Mapping and ablation of LA macroreentry following circumferential LA ablation or circumferential antral PV isolation are frequently challenging. Detailed mapping with a high density of points is necessary to elucidate the mechanism of the arrhythmias (see Chap. 13). Current treatment of macroreentrant ATs primarily involves electrical isolation of all reconnected PVs and, if needed, empirical linear lesions within the AT circuit, often including a line between the mitral annulus and left inferior PV and a line between the superior PVs. However, when the macroreentrant circuit can be mapped, ablation lesions should be tailored to interrupt the path of the reentrant circuit (see Fig. 15-59). The mitral isthmus, LA roof, and septum account for 75% of the ablation target sites for macroreentrant ATs from the LA. Successful catheter ablation has been reported in approximately 85% of macroreentrant ATs arising in the LA in highly experienced laboratories; however, ablation of macroreentrant ATs occurring in the septal wall is challenging and less successful.[161,163]

Multiple macroreentrant circuits and multiple-loop reentrant circuits are not infrequently encountered after catheter ablation of AF, especially following extensive ablation strategies. Transition from one tachycardia to another tachycardia incorporating a different loop of the same circuit or using a different circuit can be encountered during mapping or after successful ablation of the initial tachycardia.[157,161] Additionally, localized reentrant circuits are not uncommon, especially following ablation of longstanding AF. These small circuits usually arise from the vicinity of the isolated PVs or linear lesions.[164]

Impact on Cardiac Structure and Function

Restoration of sinus rhythm is expected to improve atrial mechanical function as compared with AF; however, the impact of catheter ablation of AF on LA transport function is still under investigation. Several studies demonstrated an increase in the LA voltage and a decrease in the LA volume following AF ablation. Reversal of atrial electrical remodeling following restoration of NSR can happen within 1 week, and reverse structural remodeling has been demonstrated by imaging studies during long-term follow-up after successful AF ablation.[165]

On the other hand, extensive ablation of atrial tissue replaces myocardium with scar and prolongs intraatrial conduction, which can potentially result in asynchronized contraction of the LA, possibly attenuating atrial contractile performances. The decline in LA systolic function appears to be strongly correlated with the volume of RF ablation scar.[166] Furthermore, extensive septal ablation can potentially damage the Bachmann bundle and delay LA activation, attenuating LA contribution to LV filling, especially when the latest activity in the LA occurs after the QRS, because of closure of the mitral valve before completion of LA contraction.[167] It is likely that the smaller the surface area occupied by scar tissue, the greater the probable benefit for atrial contractile function. One report described pulmonary hypertension with LA diastolic dysfunction with preserved atrial systolic function (so-called stiff LA syndrome) occurring in 1.4% of patients following AF ablation. Patients with extensive atrial scarring, small LA (45 mm or less), diabetes mellitus, obstructive sleep apnea, and high LA pressure seem to be more prone to develop this syndrome. Symptomatic patients manifest with dyspnea and congestive heart failure and experience symptomatic improvement after diuretic therapy. Further refinement of techniques to identify sites crucial for maintenance of AF or subsequent AT on an individual basis is therefore necessary to minimize the extent of LA injury and to maximize the mechanical benefit of catheter ablation therapy for AF.

In patients with heart failure and an LV ejection fraction of less than 45%, AF ablation was shown to produce significant improvement in LV function, LV dimensions, exercise capacity, symptoms, and quality of life. However, larger studies are needed to determine exactly which component of this improvement in LV function results from improvement in rate control as compared with restoration of sinus rhythm per se. Of note, restoration of NSR by AF ablation was found to improve LV function even in patients with preserved LV ejection fraction.[168]

Complications of Catheter Ablation of Atrial Fibrillation

Catheter ablation of AF is one of the most complex interventional EP procedures, and the risk associated with such a procedure is higher than for the ablation of most other arrhythmias. Complications include local vascular complications, cardiac perforation, valvular injury, systemic embolism, esophageal injury, PV stenosis, and proarrhythmia resulting from reentrant tachycardias arising from incomplete ablative lesions.

Numerous studies have reported complication rates following catheter ablation for AF ranging from 3.9% to 6%. A voluntary worldwide survey of AF ablation in 8745 patients (181 centers) collected in 2002 to 2003 reported an overall complication rate of 6%, including both early and late complications, and an updated survey from 2003 to 2006 (32,569 patients undergoing 45,115 procedures in 262 centers) reported a complication rate of 4.5% and an overall mortality rate of approximately 1 per 1000. The most frequent causes of mortality were tamponade (25%), stroke (16%), and atrioesophageal fistula (16%).[169-171] A more recent Italian multicenter registry reported a lower complication rate of 3.9%.[172] In an analysis of Medicare claims data for fiscal years 2001 to 2006, the annual probability of an in-hospital complication increased significantly from 6.7% to 10.1% during this time interval, driven mainly by the occurrence of vascular access complications and cardiac perforation/tamponade. Baseline demographic and clinical variables and hospital procedural volume had relatively little impact on the overall risk of complications. However, an association between hospital procedural volume and in-hospital death was observed.[173]

PULMONARY VEIN STENOSIS

PV stenosis after AF ablation has been reported with a wide range of incidence (0% to 42%), depending on the ablation technique, the operator's experience, and the method for detection of PV stenosis (see Fig. 32-7). Focal ablation and then ostial PV ablation carry the highest risk for PV stenosis. Circumferential LA ablation, with ablation limited to atrial tissue outside the PV orifice, seems to have the lowest rates of PV stenosis, whereas the use of an individual encircling lesion set that requires RF ablation between the ipsilateral PVs carries a higher risk. Stenosis seems to be more common in the left-sided PVs. Delivery of energy inside the PV during ablation, although undesirable, is more likely in the left PVs because the ablation catheter moves easily into them when patients breathe.[88]

The prevalence of this complication has decreased because of various factors, including abandonment of in-vein ablation at the site of the AF focus, limiting of ablation to the extraostial portion of the PV or PV antrum, use of advanced imaging techniques to guide catheter placement and RF application, reduction in target ablation temperature and energy output, and increased operator experience. Nonetheless, PV stenosis remains an important complication, affecting approximately 1.0 % to 1.4% of procedures (see Chap. 32 and Videos 24, 25, and 26).[174,175]

Although PV angiography, electroanatomical mapping, and impedance monitoring have been used in an attempt to avoid delivery of RF energy to the PV ostia or within the PVs, these techniques are still imperfect. Electroanatomical mapping, for example, relies on the patient's position remaining unchanged throughout the procedure. With patient movement, the 3-D electroanatomical reconstruction of the LA and PVs may not accurately reflect true, contemporaneous anatomy. Similarly, PV angiography is typically performed immediately prior to the start of PV ablation. Not only does this provide a crude two-dimensional representation of true PV anatomy, but patient movement later in the procedure can also result in misalignment of the true PV anatomy with that reflected by the PV angiograms. Although impedance monitoring provides online feedback to the location of the ablation catheter relative to the PV, one study found no significant difference in impedance between PV ostial and LA sites. Therefore, it is possible for movement of the ablation catheter into the PV ostia to be missed.[88]

Cryothermal ablation has unique characteristics that may prove to be desirable when lesions are required within the PV. Specifically, there is less endothelial disruption, maintenance of extracellular collagen matrix without collagen denaturation, and no collagen contracture related to thermal effects. These characteristics may translate into a reduction in PV stenosis as compared with RF ablation. Nonetheless, cryoballoon ablation for PV isolation still can be associated with PV stenosis (the rate of symptomatic PV stenosis or PV stenosis requiring intervention was 0.17%). A distal position of the cryoballoon with respect to the PV ostium, especially when using the smaller 23-mm balloon, can potentially increase the risk of these complications.[104]

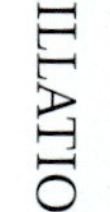

ATRIOESOPHAGEAL FISTULA

The formation of an atrioesophageal fistula is the most feared complication of catheter ablation of AF (see Fig. 32-9 and Video 27). Although rare (with an incidence estimated at 0.03% to 0.2%), this complication is highly fatal, accounting for 15.6% of cases with fatal outcome, the second leading cause of mortality following AF ablation, following cardiac tamponade (see Chap. 32).[170-172]

On the other hand, esophageal mucosal changes consistent with thermal injury are much more common, reported in up to 47% of the patients following AF ablation, and esophageal ulcerations confirmed by esophagogastroscopy or capsule endoscopy can be observed in 14% to 18%.[176,177]

The risk of esophageal injury likely is enhanced by increasing magnitude and duration of local tissue heating (i.e., the total ablation energy delivered to cardiac tissue near the esophagus), which is related to catheter tip size, contact pressure, catheter orientation, and energy power output and duration. Additionally, ablation strategies incorporating extensive ablation in the LA posterior wall, the type of AF (persistent more than paroxysmal AF, possibly because of the additional linear ablation lesions), the use of nasogastric tubes, and general anesthesia have been associated with an increased rate of esophageal ulcerations.[178,179]

Cryoballoon ablation commonly causes significant decreases in esophageal temperature in most patients, especially during cryoablation of the inferior PVs, resulting in esophageal ulcerations. Although no instances of atrioesophageal fistula formation after cryoballoon PV isolation have yet been reported, the total number of cryoballoon ablation cases performed is relatively small to detect this rare complication reliably. Furthermore, esophageal ulcerations have been observed following cryoballoon ablation at a rate similar to those seen with RF ablation (17% of patients). Factors associated with ulcerations were the mean nadir and the cumulative decrease of luminal esophageal temperature, as well as the number of lesions with an observed esophageal temperature lower than 30°C. Although there is no definitive proof that esophageal ulcer formation is predictive of fistulas, it is reasonable to assume that esophageal ulcerations can represent the first step on the way to atrioesophageal fistula. Therefore, cryoballoon ablation should not be considered completely safe with regard to atrioesophageal fistula formation.[180]

PV electrical isolation with HIFU ablation can cause excessive esophageal heating. Studies showed that power modulation did not prevent esophageal temperature to exceed levels higher than 40°C at the end of the ablation. In fact, elevated esophageal temperature prompting cessation of energy delivery occurred in 9% of PVs. Despite use of the safety algorithm, the occurrence of esophageal thermal damage and lethal atrioesophageal fistula could not be prevented, which occurred in 1 of 28 patients. PV isolation with HIFU has proven to be successful but is not yet safe for clinical use.[181]

Various strategies can be used to avoid the development of an atrioesophageal fistula. However, because of the rarity of this complication, it remains unproven whether the use of these approaches lowers or eliminates the risk of esophageal perforation or fistula formation, and the optimal technique has not yet been determined. Therefore, it appears prudent to apply a combination of these preventive techniques during AF ablation.[182]

AVOIDING ABLATION IN THE VICINITY OF THE ESOPHAGUS. The most effective measure to prevent atrioesophageal fistula formation is to avoid ablation in the LA posterior wall at sites close to the esophagus. However, effective treatment of AF and PV isolation typically require ablation at those sites, and complete avoidance of the LA posterior wall usually is not feasible. Nonetheless, inclusion of a linear lesion connecting the PV encirclements in the posterior LA wall is no longer advised. If such a connection is thought to be clinically necessary, it should be performed superiorly in the dome of the LA instead of the posterior wall.

ASSESSMENT OF THE ESOPHAGUS POSITION. Newer imaging techniques have been used to visualize the anatomical relationship between the esophagus and the LA during AF catheter ablation. Esophageal imaging is not part of the usual CT or MRI of the LA and PVs. Visualization of the esophagus can be achieved during the CT angiography by the use of barium sulfate or Gastrografin and swallowing instructions, which help the contrast substance to lodge in the middle and distal esophagus, rather than in the stomach (Fig. 15-60). Visualization of the esophagus during CT or MRI can also be achieved by combining the barium sulfate paste with gadolinium diglutamate. The barium cream helps the gadolinium lodge in the esophagus. However, these approaches have several limitations. The esophagus is a mobile structure, and CT and MRI scans of the esophagus are static and not real-time images, acquired on a previous session; therefore, these images may be an unreliable guide to the position of the esophagus during the ablation procedure. This may be particularly true for procedures performed while the patient is under conscious sedation, when esophageal peristalsis is likely to occur. Furthermore, the image of the esophagus is obtained with a barium sulfate paste, and the real dimensions of the esophagus depend on the volume of contrast media injected. During ablation, the esophagus is empty, and the real dimension and probably the exact location can be misinterpreted.[178,182] The use of 3-D mapping systems that allow the integration of preacquired 3-D CT scans or MRI of the LA, PVs, and esophagus provides a visualization tool that permits a rapid understanding of complex cardiac anatomical relationships. The location of the esophagus can also be tagged by the electroanatomical system (CARTO or NavX). A nasogastric tube is inserted into the esophagus, and the mapping catheter is coated with lubricant and passed down the nasogastric tube under fluoroscopy guidance. Alternatively, a special catheter (EsophaStar, Biosense Webster) is currently available for esophageal mapping combined with the CARTO system. Acquisition of the catheter tip location is made during pull-back of the catheter out of the nasogastric tube; these data points are saved as a separate map in the electroanatomical mapping system. After LA chamber reconstruction is made, the esophageal map is displayed in 3-D space in relation to the LA reconstruction (see Fig. 15-60). The EsophaStar catheter can be left in the esophagus and used as a fluoroscopic guide to esophageal location during the ablation procedure (see Fig. 15-60). It is important to recognize, however, that the catheter used for tagging can be positioned eccentrically in the esophageal lumen, thus providing misleading information.[182]

Phased-array ICE has been evaluated as a diagnostic tool for rapid real-time localization of the esophageal location in relation to the posterior LA wall (Fig. 15-61). The location of the esophagus determined by ICE during the ablation procedure was found to correlate well with the location determined by MRI before the procedure.[178] This technique has the advantage of providing real-time information on the location of the esophagus, especially when movement occurs.

Another strategy to limit the risk of esophageal injury is real-time imaging of the anatomical course of the esophagus during the ablation procedure by placement of a radiopaque esophageal monitoring probe or use of a viscous radiopaque contrast paste. Orally administered barium provides a simple, inexpensive, and safe way to keep track of the esophagus accurately during an ablation procedure (Fig. 15-62). In most patients, barium paste coats the wall of the esophagus, and residual barium often allows visualization of the esophagus for 1 to 2 hours after the initial barium swallow. However, to avoid the risk of aspiration, patients should receive little or no sedation before swallowing the barium. The ablation procedure can also be performed with the patient under general anesthesia with orotracheal intubation and esophagography during the procedure. General anesthesia guarantees enough esophageal immobilization because the swallow reflex is abolished. Placement of an orogastric tube to allow esophageal localization is carried out before anticoagulation to avoid any risk of trauma and bleeding. At the end of the procedure, the contrast is totally removed. This technique allows visualization of the esophagus position in real

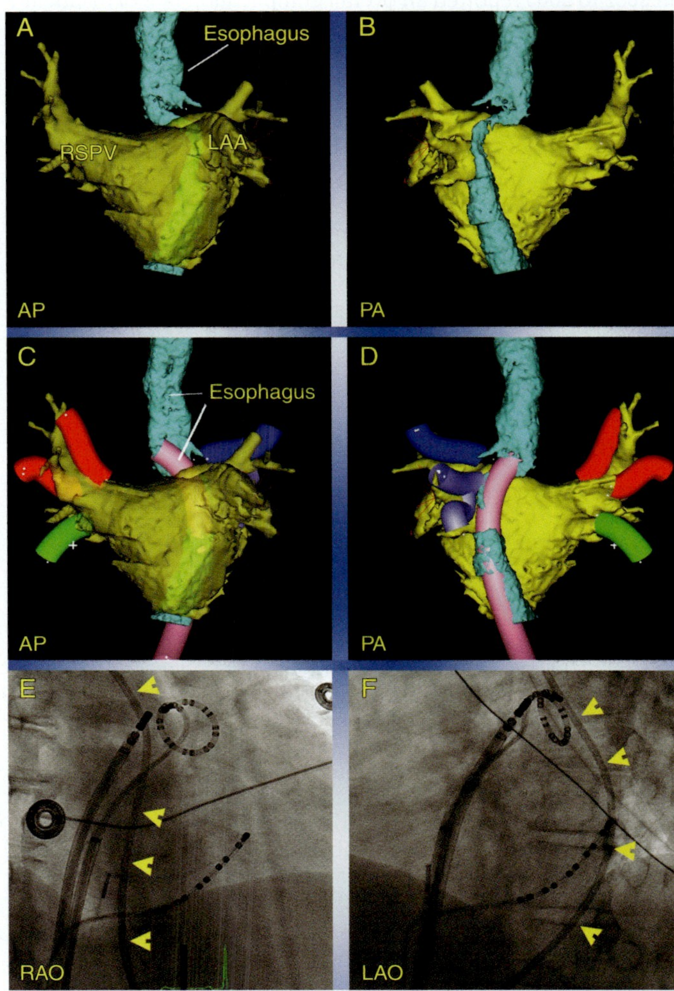

FIGURE 15-60 Esophageal imaging. **A** and **B**, Anteroposterior (AP) and posteroanterior (PA) views of a CT image of the left atrium and esophagus. The esophagus is visualized during CT scanning by the use of Gastrografin (contrast medium). Note that the real dimensions of the midsegment are not very clear because of peristaltic movements and inadequate filling of the esophagus. **C** and **D**, AP and PA views of integrated CT image and electroanatomical mapping system (CARTO, Biosense Webster, Inc., Diamond Bar, Calif.). The esophagus is tagged by passing the esophageal mapping catheter (EsophaStar) through the esophagus. Note that the position of the esophagus during the ablation procedure (as marked by the CARTO system) correlates well with the position on the preacquired CT image. Note the close proximity of the esophagus to the ostia of the left pulmonary veins (PVs). **E** and **F**, Fluoroscopic (right anterior oblique [RAO] and left anterior oblique [LAO]) views in the same patient with the esophageal mapping catheter (arrowheads) left in the esophagus during the ablation procedure to provide a real-time guide to the location of the esophagus. LAA = left atrial appendage; RSPV = right superior pulmonary vein.

time. The operator visualizes any subsequent esophageal movement immediately. Nonetheless, the use of nasogastric tubes can potentially increase the risk by pressing the anterior esophageal wall against the LA posterior wall.

MECHANICAL DISPLACEMENT OF THE ESOPHAGUS. When ablation cannot be performed in certain LA regions because of proximity of the ablation site to the esophagus, mechanical displacement of the esophagus to the contralateral side from the ablation catheter by an endoscope has been suggested to facilitate safe energy delivery. However, the risk of esophageal perforation by the endoscope should be recognized, and the safety of this strategy needs to be determined before implementation into clinical practice. Furthermore, apparent displacement of the esophagus with an endoscope can potentially represent mere distortion rather than anatomical displacement, in which setting the esophagus can be rendered more vulnerable to injury. Additionally, the presence of the endoscope probe can increase the diameter of the esophagus and increase its contact with the posterior LA wall.[183]

ESOPHAGEAL TEMPERATURE MONITORING. Thermal monitoring of the esophagus during ablation can be of value.[100] Measurement of esophageal temperature involves the placement of a monotherm temperature probe, which is advanced under fluoroscopy guidance to the lower third of the esophagus directly posterior to the LA. This technique requires general anesthesia to allow tolerability of the esophageal probe. Adjustment of the position of the temperature probe during ablation to keep the probe in close vicinity to the ablation catheter tip is crucial to obtain reliable information on the real current esophageal temperature. The probe is used to identify the general location of the esophagus in relation to the posterior LA and PVs based on a 3°C to 4°C rise in temperature from baseline and assuming a linear degree of heating from the external esophagus relative to the lumen. However, discrepancies between the temperatures of the external and internal esophagus and thermal latency in heat transfer from the atrium to the esophagus can limit the utility of esophageal temperature monitoring. Also, because the esophagus is broad, a lateral position of the temperature probe may not align with the ablation electrode. The possibility of heating of the esophageal wall without recording a change in central luminal esophageal temperature can be harmful by providing a false sense of safety.[178,182] It is important to note that esophageal temperature can continue to increase for several seconds after discontinuation of RF delivery; thus, energy application must be stopped as soon as there is any increase in esophageal temperature.

Although studies demonstrated the absence of esophageal lesions in patients with a maximal esophageal luminal temperature lower than 41.8°C, the safety zone of temperature rise from baseline has not been validated.[184]

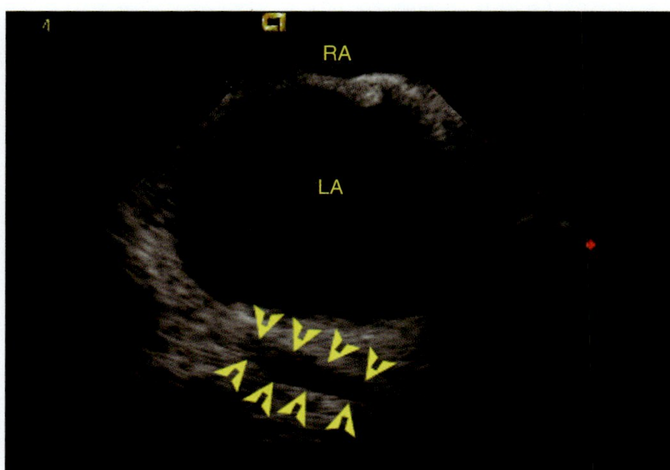

FIGURE 15-61 Intracardiac echocardiography (ICE) imaging of the esophagus. This phased-array ICE image with the transducer placed in the right atrium (RA) showing the esophagus (between arrowheads). Note that the left atrial (LA) posterior wall is contiguous with the esophagus.

LIMITING ABLATION ENERGY. Modification of RF application parameters at sites close to the esophagus is the most widely utilized strategy to avoid atrioesophageal fistula formation. Limitation of power and duration of RF applications, particularly in the posterior LA, even if a significant reduction in bipolar electrogram amplitude is not recorded, can be the most important safety considerations for the avoidance of fistula formation. Although no data exist on which to make specific recommendations, there is widespread agreement that prolonged RF applications in the posterior LA are to be avoided and that low power settings should be used. When standard RF energy is to be applied close to the esophagus, the RF power is typically reduced to 20 to 30 W and 55°C for no more than 20 seconds. Also, direct perpendicular orientation of the ablating electrode and forward pressure against the posterior LA wall should be avoided, particularly if an 8-mm or irrigated electrode is used. It is preferable to maintain frequent movements of the ablation catheter when RF energy is applied at the posterior LA wall in the vicinity of the esophagus. Open irrigation RF ablation may be associated with less risk of esophageal injury compared with standard RF ablation using an 8-mm-tip catheter. When using open-irrigated RF ablation, lower energy outputs (15 W compared with 25 W) were found to be associated with a decreased rate of esophageal ulcerations.[179]

The value of limiting the duration of RF application without energy output reduction for prevention of ulcerations remains to be evaluated.[179] Although many investigators recommend the use of lower power settings for longer periods of time (25 W for 20 to 30 seconds), some investigators suggest that short RF applications

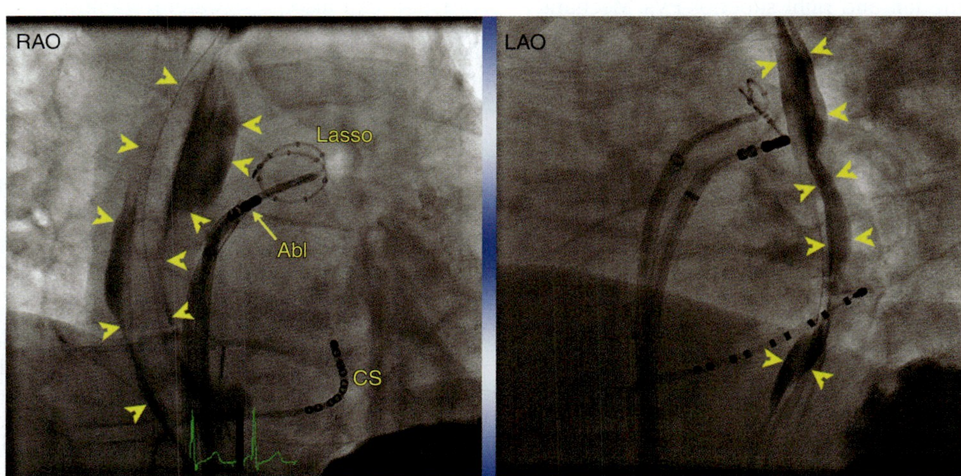

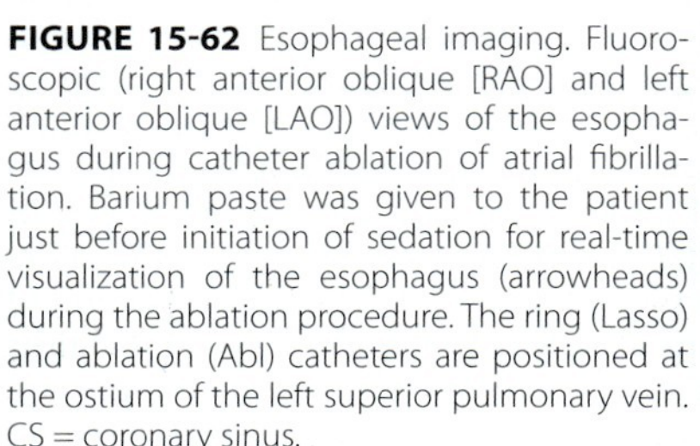

FIGURE 15-62 Esophageal imaging. Fluoroscopic (right anterior oblique [RAO] and left anterior oblique [LAO]) views of the esophagus during catheter ablation of atrial fibrillation. Barium paste was given to the patient just before initiation of sedation for real-time visualization of the esophagus (arrowheads) during the ablation procedure. The ring (Lasso) and ablation (Abl) catheters are positioned at the ostium of the left superior pulmonary vein. CS = coronary sinus.

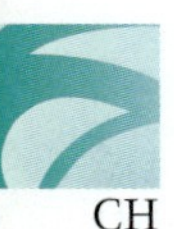

(for 2 to 5 seconds) at a higher power (50 W, irrigation rate 30 mL/min, maximum temperature 43°C) result in momentarily higher LA tissue temperatures and allow the tip to be set at a high power to injure the superficial tissue while minimizing time-dependent deep heating through excessive heat transfer. The latter approach can compromise lesion efficacy because the time-dependent variable of "total heat transferred" is decreased. Typically, the ablation catheter is dragged continuously in small increments every 2 to 5 seconds during continuous RF delivery, and ablation is repeated at each site, if required, for many times throughout the procedure until the local atrial electrogram is completely eliminated. It is probably reasonable to allow at least 2-minute time intervals before returning to ablate a previously ablated site to allow for heat dissipation and complete cooling of potential esophageal heating.[100]

Importantly, using light conscious sedation during the procedure can allow the use of pain as an indicator for potential esophageal injury; RF application should be interrupted promptly and the catheter moved to a different site on the development of significant or sharp pain during energy delivery.

PROPHYLACTIC PROTON PUMP INHIBITORS. The value of routine prophylactic administration of proton pump inhibitors after AF ablation to reduce the risk of fistula formation is unknown. However, this therapy is commonly offered to patients in whom esophageal lesions are detected by endoscopy or capsule endoscopy following the procedure. Because fistula tracts develop over the first 2 to 4 weeks after the procedure, when the patient is already home and recovering in other regards, it is important that patients be aware of and report symptoms of dysphagia, fever, stroke-like symptoms, new chest discomfort, or gastrointestinal bleeding. Early diagnosis of atrioesophageal fistula is critical to give the best chance for survival and recovery.

CARDIAC TAMPONADE

The risk of pericardial tamponade during AF ablation (averaging 0.8% to 2.9% and up to 6% in some reports) is higher than that associated with other EP procedures, likely secondary to the common need for two or more transseptal punctures, extensive intracardiac catheter manipulation and ablation, and prolonged high-dose heparinization during the procedure. Cardiac tamponade is the most common cause of death following AF ablation.[175,185]

Several factors can affect the risk of developing cardiac tamponade. High RF power output may increase the risk of cardiac perforation. An audible pop associated with an abrupt rise in impedance is heard in many patients who develop tamponade. Popping occurs because of tissue boiling causing endocardial tissue rupture, and it is increased by irrigated-tip ablation, high tissue-catheter interface flow, poor or unstable tissue contact, and high catheter tip temperature. Notably, the atrial dome is susceptible to perforation injury during transitioning the catheter tip between the left and right superior PVs. Mechanical perforation can also occur from inadvertent movement of the catheter inside the LA appendage while it is being positioned during left superior PV or mitral isthmus ablation. In one report, pericardial effusion developed in 20% of patients undergoing antral PV isolation using an irrigated-tip ablation catheter at high power (50 W), but no cases were reported when lower power (35 W) or a standard 8-mm-tip catheter was used.[175,185]

Although the use of ICE can potentially limit the risk of cardiac perforation by guiding transseptal puncture and visualizing microbubbles in the LA during RF ablation, perforations remain relatively common. New anatomical approaches, such as linear LA ablation or ablation of sites of highly fractionated electrograms that maintain the catheter in the muscular atrium, may affect perforation rates. The thickness of the atrium averages 4 mm, but decreases from 3.7 to 2.5 mm at the venoatrial junction. The PV further decreases in thickness by 1 to 2 mm outside the PV orifice. However, one report showed a higher risk of tamponade during linear LA ablation strategies as compared with PV isolation.[175,185]

Although most perforations occur in the LA, few (13.3% in one report) require surgical closure. Percutaneous pericardiocentesis effectively restores hemodynamic function in the majority of cases. The LA dome seems to be especially susceptible to perforation that may not be responsive to conservative therapy. The atrial dome may be more susceptible to persistent bleeding because the pericardium is not closely adherent to the atrium, and a tight seal of these structures is difficult to achieve by applying negative pressure through the percutaneous pigtail catheter.[175]

As noted previously, continuation of warfarin through the ablation procedure does not appear to increase the risk of cardiac tamponade. Although patients with therapeutic INR levels who develop cardiac perforation are likely to have a larger amount of blood removed from their pericardium for stabilization and require more blood transfusion units, the need to undergo emergency surgical exploration is not increased as compared with patients with normal INR levels.[82,83]

The occurrence of cardiac perforation is associated with short-term recurrent AF in most patients, in part because the ablation procedure is interrupted by the complication prior to achieving electrical endpoints. Other patients probably have a higher rate of arrhythmia recurrence because of pericardial inflammation, but in most patients this appears to be transient. Most patients with completed ablations have favorable long-term rates of AF elimination, although still lower than expected with uncomplicated cases.

THROMBOEMBOLISM

Systemic thromboembolism is a serious complication of AF ablation, with a reported incidence of 0.5 to 2.8%. In a worldwide report, the rate of stroke was approximately 0.25% and that of transient ischemic attacks was 0.66%. Prior history of stroke or transient ischemic attack is the most potent individual risk factor for cerebrovascular accidents complicating AF ablation; patients with a history of cerebrovascular accidents had a ninefold increased risk of periprocedural stroke. Additionally, the incidence of periprocedural stroke increases in a stepwise fashion with an increasing $CHADS_2$ score.[186]

Thromboembolic events typically occur within 24 hours of the ablation procedure, with the high-risk period extending for the first 2 weeks following ablation. Cerebral thromboembolism is most common, but emboli can also involve the coronary, abdominal, or peripheral vascular circulations. Although silent cerebral thromboembolism has been reported, its incidence is unknown.

Potential sources of emboli include thrombus formation on the LA catheters and sheaths, char formation at the tip of the ablation catheter or at the site of ablation, endocardial disruption from the ablation lesions, embolization of air, dislodgment of a preexisting LA thrombus by catheter manipulation, development of thrombi in the LA appendage after conversion of AF to sinus rhythm, or thrombus formation over the disrupted endothelium.[186]

Careful attention to anticoagulation before, during, and after the ablation procedure is critical to minimize the risk of stroke. TEE should be considered in most patients undergoing AF ablation to screen for LA thrombus. Aggressive intraprocedural anticoagulation, including early heparin administration (preferably before the transseptal puncture), is followed by continuous infusion to maintain the ACT above 300 seconds.[186] Anticoagulation with warfarin should be started before and continued for at least 2 to 3 months after ablation. Furthermore, continuation of warfarin at a therapeutic INR at the time of AF ablation can potentially be a better alternative to strategies that use bridging with heparin or enoxaparin because this approach eliminates a period of inadequate anticoagulation immediately following the ablation procedure. This period is critical for thromboembolic risk as a result of the inflammation and irritation inherently associated with ablation.[82,83] Additionally, meticulous attention to sheath management is paramount to prevent thrombus formation and air embolization, with visualized aspiration and flushing whenever catheters are inserted into the sheaths and continuous flushing of transseptal sheaths with heparinized saline.[71] Open irrigated-tip RF ablation catheters or cryoablation can potentially decrease the formation of char and thrombus at the tip of the ablation catheter. Also, the use of ICE can enable detection of intracardiac thrombi and accelerated bubble formation consistent with endocardial tissue disruption with RF application.[186]

AIR EMBOLISM

The most common cause of air embolism is introduction of air into the transseptal sheath. Although air can be introduced through the infusion line, air embolism can also occur with suction when catheters are removed. Careful sheath management, including constant infusion of heparinized saline and air filters, should be observed. Whenever catheters are removed, they need to be withdrawn slowly to minimize suction effects and the fluid column within the sheath should be aspirated simultaneously. The sheath should then be aspirated and irrigated to ascertain that neither air nor blood has collected in the sheath.[3,175]

Arterial air emboli can distribute to almost any organ, but they have devastating clinical sequelae when they enter the end arteries (see Chap. 32). This situation can lead to the hypoxic manifestations of myocardial injury and cerebrovascular accidents. A common presentation of air embolism during AF ablation is acute inferior ischemia or heart block. This reflects preferential downstream migration of air emboli into the right coronary artery. Air embolism to the cerebral vasculature can be associated with altered mental status, seizures, and focal neurological signs. The central nervous system dysfunction is attributable to both mechanical obstruction of the arterioles and thrombotic-inflammatory responses of air-injured endothelium.[3]

CATHETER ENTRAPMENT IN THE MITRAL VALVE APPARATUS

There are several reports of the ring catheter becoming entrapped in the mitral valve apparatus during AF ablation, resulting in valve injury that required thoracic surgery and valve replacement. The risk of this complication can be minimized by preventing anterior displacement of the ring catheter during the ablation. Catheter position can be monitored by using a combination of orthogonal fluoroscopy (ensuring that the ring catheter remains behind the CS on the RAO view) and ICE, as well as by paying close attention to the characteristics of the electrograms recorded on the catheter.[71,187]

Catheters entangled in the valve apparatus may be difficult to free by clockwise and counterclockwise rotation of the shaft, especially after significant tugging has occurred. To prevent this, prior to pulling on the catheter, one may consider advancing the catheter toward the LV apex. Advancing the sheath over the catheter may facilitate the effort further and is also recommended so that the catheter can be withdrawn into the sheath and the whole assembly withdrawn to the LA.[71,187]

Forcible traction of the catheter may damage the valve and ultimately lead to mitral valve replacement. Therefore, when gentle manipulation and moderate traction are unsuccessful, removing the catheter by thoracic surgery may be preferable.[187]

RADIATION EXPOSURE

Catheter ablation of AF is associated with markedly prolonged fluoroscopy duration (60 to 100 minutes of fluoroscopy exposure delivered to patients in both the RAO and LAO projections), which exceeds that of patients undergoing catheter ablation of AFL or AVNRT by approximately fourfold.[3,71] The use of CT scanning before and after AF ablation procedures further increases patient exposure to radiation.

During AF ablation, the patient tissue receiving the greatest radiation dose is the skin area of the back at the entrance point of the x-ray beam, which can cause skin injuries (see Chap. 32).[188,189]

The estimated lifetime risk of a fatal malignant disease after PV ablation using a modern low-frame pulsed fluoroscopy system is relatively low (0.15% for female patients and 0.21% for male patients in one report), and it is higher than, although within the range of, previously reported risk to result from the ablation of standard types of supraventricular arrhythmias (0.03% to 0.26%). It has been estimated that for every 60 minutes of fluoroscopy, the mean total lifetime excess risk of a fatal malignant disease is 0.03% to 0.065%.

One study found that patient body mass index is a more important determinant of the effective radiation dose than total fluoroscopy time, and obese patients receive more than twice the effective radiation dose of normal-weight patients during AF ablation procedures. Therefore, obesity needs to be considered in the risk-to-benefit ratio of AF ablation and should prompt further measures to reduce radiation exposure.

The use of 3-D mapping systems can significantly reduce fluoroscopy time. The use of remote navigation systems also is likely to reduce fluoroscopy exposure to the patient and certainly to the operator.[188,189]

PHRENIC NERVE INJURY

Fortunately, phrenic nerve injury has been an infrequent complication of AF catheter ablation. Injury to the right phrenic nerve can occur during ablation in and around the right superior PV and electrical isolation of the SVC. The reported incidence of phrenic nerve injury secondary to AF ablation varies from 0% to 0.48%. Although it is much less common, left phrenic nerve injury can also occur during RF delivery at the proximal aspect of the roof of the LA appendage.[24,190]

The use of a non-RF source of energy is unlikely to prevent this complication because phrenic nerve injury has been reported with ultrasound, laser, and cryotherapy. Furthermore, phrenic nerve injury occurs independently of the strategy of AF ablation used (PV isolation versus wide-area circumferential LA ablation). Fortunately, phrenic nerve injury has been an infrequent complication of AF catheter ablation. Complete or partial recovery of diaphragmatic function was observed in most patients (more than 80%).[24,190] Diaphragmatic paralysis may develop 1 to 2 days following the procedure despite normal function at the end of the ablation protocol; this may reflect inflammation rather than direct injury to the phrenic nerve.

Studies indicated that transient phrenic nerve injury occurs early and uniformly before permanent injury. Therefore, in areas at high risk of phrenic nerve injury (inferoanterior part of right PV ostium, posteroseptal part of the SVC, and proximal LA appendage roof) that require ablation, high-output pacing should be performed before energy delivery. When diaphragmatic stimulation is observed, energy application at this site should be avoided. Early suspicion of phrenic nerve injury should be considered in the case of hiccup, cough, or decrease in diaphragmatic excursion during energy delivery. Early recognition of phrenic nerve injury during RF delivery allows the immediate interruption of the application prior to the onset of permanent injury, which is associated with the rapid recovery of phrenic nerve function.[24,190]

Diaphragmatic electromyography during continuous pacing of the right phrenic nerve with a catheter in the SVC has been used for monitoring phrenic nerve integrity during ablation. A progressive decline in compound motor action potential amplitude heralded phrenic nerve palsy, with a 30% decrease yielding the best predictive value, preceding hemidiaphragmatic paralysis. The clinical application of this approach to prevent phrenic nerve palsy induced by cryoballoon ablation of the right superior PV is still in its preliminary stages, and further evaluation is required to validate and optimize this approach.

OTHER COMPLICATIONS

Vagal denervation, resulting in gastroparesis, has been rarely reported. This is usually transient, resolving over the course of 1 to 3

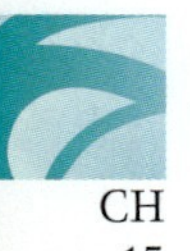

weeks following the procedure. Sinus node dysfunction and heart block are rare but can occur sporadically. The stiff LA syndrome, characterized by LA diastolic dysfunction and pulmonary hypertension, is also uncommon and seems associated with more extensive ablation.

Recommendations and Controversies

Determination of Candidates for Catheter Ablation

The ideal candidate for catheter ablation of AF has symptomatic episodes of paroxysmal or persistent AF, has not responded to one or more class I or III antiarrhythmic drugs, does not have severe comorbid conditions or severe structural heart disease, has an LA diameter smaller than 50 to 55 mm, and, for those with longstanding AF, has had AF for less than 5 years. Catheter ablation of AF is likely to be of little or no benefit in patients with end-stage cardiomyopathy or massive enlargement of the LA (more than 60 mm), or in patients who have severe mitral regurgitation or stenosis and are deemed inappropriate candidates for valvular intervention.

The introduction into clinical practice of the various techniques described earlier has contributed to the expansion of inclusion criteria for catheter ablation of AF. Expanded indications at many centers now include patients with permanent AF and those with cardiomyopathy. It is controversial whether patient preference to discontinue anticoagulation should be considered an indication for AF catheter ablation; however, it is important to recognize that there are still no randomized controlled data demonstrating that a patient's stroke risk is reduced by ablation. It is currently recommended to continue long-term anticoagulation with warfarin in all patients with a $CHADS_2$ score of 2 or higher, even those with a successful catheter ablation procedure.[3] Nonetheless, it is probably reasonable to consider ablation in patients in whom anticoagulation is indicated secondary to AF but who cannot tolerate, or whose occupations or activities preclude, long-term anticoagulation.

Several reports attempted to identify preprocedural markers of the extent of pathological atrial tissue remodeling and predictors of success (e.g., quantification of atrial fibrosis and scar burden on MRI and severity of LA enlargement) that may help improve selection criteria. Although the LA size and duration of longstanding AF, among other markers, can potentially predict lower procedure success rates, most of these markers do not adequately distinguish subjects in whom ablation should categorically be avoided. The question of how to identify patients in whom structural remodeling and scarring have become irreversible and it is too late to intervene remains unanswered, although preliminary data from cardiac MRI, assessing the degree of LA scarring, hold promise. Nonetheless, it is now well recognized that intervention relatively early in the course of persistent AF helps achieve a better outcome.[191]

Complications of catheter ablation can have catastrophic outcomes in certain patients, including those with severe obstructive carotid artery disease, cardiomyopathy, aortic stenosis, nonrevascularized left main or three-vessel coronary artery disease, severe pulmonary arterial hypertension, or hypertrophic cardiomyopathy with severe LV outflow obstruction. Another relative contraindication is a history of major lung resection because of the severe impact of potential PV stenosis. Furthermore, because the risk of thromboembolic events during the procedure and in the early postoperative period, patients who cannot be anticoagulated during and for at least 2 months after the ablation procedure should not be considered for catheter ablation of AF. Also, catheter ablation should not be performed in patients with an LA appendage thrombus or a recently implanted LA appendage closure device.

It is also important to realize that surgical intervention can be lifesaving should a severe mechanical complication, such as rupture or massive cardiac perforation or catheter entrapment, occur. Therefore, catheter ablation of AF should not be performed, particularly in higher risk patients, if surgical back-up is not readily available. In addition, catheter ablation of AF should not be performed in patients who are scheduled to undergo cardiac surgery for another indication when surgical ablation of AF also can be performed.

At the current time, criteria for selection of patients for AF ablation should include weighing risks and potential benefits associated with the procedure, as well as consideration of other factors such as severity of symptoms, quality of life, presence and severity of structural heart disease and other comorbidities, and availability of other reasonable treatment options. Additionally, the projected ablation success rate with the operator's own experience and the tools available to him or her should be taken into consideration.

Whether catheter ablation will provide a more effective approach than antiarrhythmic therapy as a primary strategy for control of AF, and reduce attendant morbidity and mortality, is the subject of a 3000-patient multicenter trial, CABANA (Catheter ABlation versus ANtiarrhythmic Drug Therapy for Atrial Fibrillation). A similar study, CASTLE-AF (Catheter Ablation versus Standard Conventional Treatment in Patients with LEft Ventricular Dysfunction and AF), is under way in Europe.

Importantly, recurrence of AF after the initial ablation procedure should not prompt automatic reablation. Because improvement in quality of life and reduction of symptoms are the main goals of ablation, the mere recurrence of AF after the initial ablation procedure should not be the only basis for recommending reablation. Reassessment of the degree of improvement the patient experienced following the initial procedure, the severity of symptoms during AF recurrences, the burden of AF, and the potential response to antiarrhythmic drugs should all be taken into consideration before recommending a redo ablation. For example, some patients experience a substantial palliative effect of ablation whereby AF recurrences cause minor or no symptoms, whereas others achieve satisfactory control with antiarrhythmic drugs that previously failed in the treatment of AF. Those patients may benefit from noninvasive management without the need for further ablation procedures.

Determination of the Necessity of Pulmonary Vein Electrical Isolation

Several investigators addressed this issue and came to differing conclusions. There is evidence that short-term efficacy can occasionally be observed in the presence of conduction recurrence across all previously disconnected PVs. In these cases, it is possible that the extent of conduction delay developed in response to the changes induced by chronic lesions prevents, at least for some time during follow-up, the occurrence of arrhythmia relapses. Conversely, patients with recurrence of AF invariably show restored conduction across one or more previously disconnected PVs, and reisolation of the reconnected PVs was found to be an effective treatment strategy. More recent reports strongly suggest that achievement of complete PV isolation improves outcome with the circumferential LA ablation approach.[112,114]

In conclusion, although the importance of achieving isolation of the PVs remains unclear, it is acknowledged that electrical isolation of the PVs should be at least as effective as not achieving isolation. Furthermore, it is clear that if wide-area circumferential ablation is performed, complete PV isolation is also the most desirable endpoint. As long as PV stenosis is avoided, there are no deleterious effects of complete PV isolation as an additional endpoint in wide-area circumferential LA ablation techniques.

Currently, PV electrical isolation is considered central to any AF ablation strategy, and most centers performing AF ablation are empirically isolating all four PVs, without mapping or specific targeting of the trigger of the focus causing the arrhythmia. Furthermore, most groups are ablating outside the tubular portion of the PV (i.e., antral ablation as opposed to ostial ablation) to avoid the risk of PV stenosis and improve the efficacy of the procedure. The antrum blends into the posterior wall of the LA, and, on the posterior wall, there is little space between adjacent antra. Therefore, to encompass as much of the PV structure as possible, ablation needs to be performed around the entire antrum, along the posterior LA wall. Although different groups may refer to ablation in this region by different names, such as wide-area LA ablation, circumferential antral PV ablation, or extraostial isolation, the lesion sets produced by the procedures are all similar. There is less consensus, however, on the distance from the PV ostia at which the optimal circumferential lesions should be placed. The greater the distance is, the greater the number of applications and density of lesions will be required to achieve isolation, but the lower the likelihood of PV stenosis. Furthermore, the greater the distance is from the ostia, the larger will be the area encircled and the greater the potential impact of the lesion set on atrial rotors and sites within the posterior LA, which can potentially contribute to the maintenance of AF. However, it is clear that wide-area circumferential LA ablation minimizes the risk of PV stenosis, but at the cost of a higher incidence of macroreentrant ATs and more extensive LA ablation with possible deleterious hemodynamic effects.

Determination of the Necessity of Adjunctive Substrate Modification

While elimination of PV triggers appears to be an adequate initial ablation strategy for patients with paroxysmal AF, atrial substrate modification takes on a more important role in the setting of persistent AF. However, current techniques of substrate modification (linear ablation, CFAE ablation, vagal denervation) are technically challenging and lack robust procedural endpoints to determine when enough ablation has been performed to modify the atrial substrate sufficiently. Additionally, these approaches involve more extensive ablation that can potentially increase the risk of complications, impair LA mechanical properties, and predispose to the development of LA macroreentry. Therefore, to balance efficacy and safety, it may not be advisable to use such an approach for all patients. A rational approach that targets a particular patient profile, rather than a unified strategy used for all patients, may be advisable.

For paroxysmal AF, circumferential antral electrical isolation of all PVs is the procedure of choice. If a focal trigger is identified outside the PVs, it should be targeted if possible. The clinical value of adjunctive substrate-based techniques has not been definitively proven, and these approaches are likely unnecessary, especially during the initial ablation procedure.[78,93,152]

Circumferential antral isolation of all PVs also is recommended as the cornerstone of most ablation procedures in patients with persistent AF. In addition to elimination of the most common AF triggers, this technique incorporates substrate modification by considerable debulking of the atrium as well as elimination of CFAEs, rotors, and ganglionated plexuses commonly located within the circumferential ablation lesions around the PV antra. Nevertheless, adjunctive substrate-based ablation techniques can potentially play an important role in improving ablation efficacy. Supplementary linear LA ablation (roof and mitral isthmus lines) or CFAE ablation can be considered especially in patients with longstanding persistent AF or during redo ablation after failure of an initial PV-based ablation procedure. If additional linear ablation lesions are applied, complete bidirectional block across the ablation lines should be verified by mapping and pacing maneuvers to reduce the risk of proarrhythmias. Also, when CFAE ablation is being considered, it is reasonable to target CFAEs after, rather than before, PV electrical isolation, because that latter strategy can itself reduce the burden of CFAEs and minimize the consequent need for extensive LA ablation. The role of ablation of ganglionated plexuses in patients with AF remains to be determined in well-designed future studies, and it has not yet been adopted as a routine strategy in the treatment of patients with persistent AF.[93,112,138]

In patients with longstanding AF, several stepwise or tailored approaches have implemented increasing ablation lesions until persistent AF is terminated by ablation or until AF is rendered noninducible by rapid atrial pacing or infusion of isoproterenol or adenosine. A common approach involves starting with circumferential antral PV isolation, which is then followed by linear ablation across the LA roof, CS isolation, ablation of CFAEs, mitral isthmus ablation, and RA-SVC ablation in a stepwise fashion whereby each step is started if AF still persists after completion of earlier steps. It should be recognized, however, that despite the best efforts with various combinations of several ablation strategies, converting chronic AF to sinus rhythm solely by ablation may not occur in most patients. Hence, an endpoint of acute termination of chronic AF may not be practical. Moreover, whether acute termination of chronic AF by RF ablation is a predictor of long-term clinical efficacy remains to be evaluated.[78,131,148]

Importantly, substrate-based ablation techniques are typically used in conjunction with PV isolation. Their use as a stand-alone procedure for either paroxysmal or persistent AF without any attempt to isolate the PVs electrically has been associated with high rates of recurrence, and this approach has been abandoned by many centers.

Atrioventricular Junction Ablation

Rationale

AF may not be amenable to ablation procedures and may require multiple pharmacological agents for management. In some of these patients, medical therapy is poorly tolerated or unsuccessful. In these cases, AVN ablation combined with permanent pacemaker implantation (the "ablate and pace" approach) is a possible treatment strategy, with rate control as the goal. The pacemaker may be single-chamber (VVI) for permanent AF, dual-chamber (DDD) for paroxysmal or recurrent persistent AF, or biventricular for patients with LV dysfunction. This procedure is successful in almost 100% of cases, and late recovery of AV conduction is rare. However, this procedure still mandates anticoagulation and possibly requires antiarrhythmic therapy to control the AF.

The timing of AVN ablation in relation to pacing is debatable, mainly in the setting of paroxysmal AF. In most EP laboratories, permanent pacemaker implantation is performed prior to the ablation procedure. Long-term pacemaker function does not seem to be affected by RF ablation; however, the pacemaker may develop a transient unpredictable response during RF application in up to 50% of patients, including inhibition, switching to back-up mode, oversensing, undersensing, loss of capture, exit block, and electromechanical interference. These responses may argue for the use of an external pacemaker during the ablation procedure. In patients with paroxysmal AF, a dual-chamber pacemaker may be implanted first, and the need for AV junction ablation is reassessed after 1 to 3 months of intensification of medical therapy (i.e., AVN blocking drugs).

Target of Ablation

The target site of this approach is located closer to the compact AVN than the HB in the anterosuperior region of the triangle of Koch. This approach selectively ablates the AVN, and not the HB. This ensures ablation of the proximal part of the AV junction to preserve underlying automatism and to avoid complete pacemaker dependency. Occasionally, when ablation of the AVN is unsuccessful, RF ablation of the HB may be performed using a right- or left-sided approach.

Ablation Technique

A 4- or 8-mm-tip ablation catheter is initially positioned at the AV junction to obtain the maximal amplitude of the bipolar His potential recorded from the distal pair of the electrodes. The catheter is then withdrawn while maintaining clockwise torque on the catheter to maintain septal contact until the His potential becomes small or barely visible, or disappears while recording a relatively

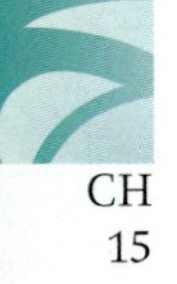

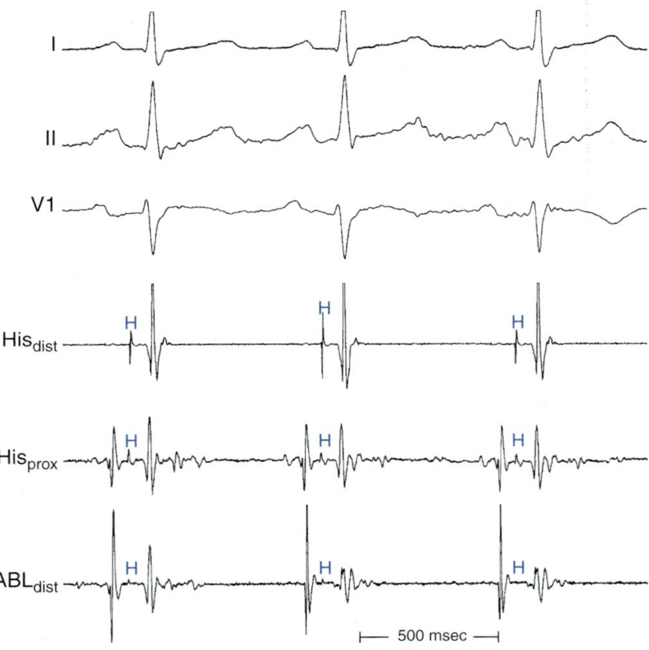

FIGURE 15-63 Optimal ablation site for atrioventricular junction ablation during normal sinus rhythm. The distal ablation electrodes (Abl_{dist}) record a small His potential and a large atrial electrogram (atrial-ventricular [A/V] ratio greater than 1). More prominent His potentials, such as recorded by the proximal or distal His bundle catheter bipoles, suggest inappropriate site for ablation. His_{dist} = distal His bundle; His_{prox} = proximal His bundle.

large atrial electrogram (A/V ratio greater than 1) or, in patients with AF, until the His potential disappears under the fibrillatory waves (Fig. 15-63).

An alternative approach is to position a quadripolar catheter at the HB position. The tip of the ablation catheter is then withdrawn to approximately 2 cm below and to the left of the tip of the HB catheter in the RAO view (Fig. 15-64). Occasionally, in 5% to 15% of patients, when the right-sided approach is undesirable or unsuccessful, a left-sided approach to ablate the HB may be used. The ablation catheter is advanced retrogradely through the aorta into the LV, withdrawn so that the catheter tip lies against the membranous septum just below the aortic valve, and records a large HB electrogram and small atrial electrogram (Fig. 15-65). Often, no atrial electrogram is seen. A large atrial electrogram suggests that the catheter tip is close to the LA above the aortic valve; ablation should not be attempted at this site. The left-sided approach typically requires fewer RF applications than the right-sided approach.

One report described the feasibility of AV junction ablation performed from the axillary vein concurrent with the implantation of a dual-chamber pacemaker.[192] This approach involves placing two separate introducer sheaths into the axillary or subclavian vein. The first sheath is used for implantation of the pacemaker ventricular lead, which is then connected to the pulse generator or a temporary pacemaker. Subsequently, a standard ablation catheter is introduced through the second venous sheath and used for ablation of the AV junction. The ablation catheter is advanced into the right ventricle (RV) and is positioned near the HB region by deflection of the tip superiorly to form a J shape; the catheter is then withdrawn so that it lies across the superior margin of the tricuspid annulus (Fig. 15-66). Alternatively, the catheter can be looped in the RA (figure-of-6) and the body of the loop advanced in the RV so

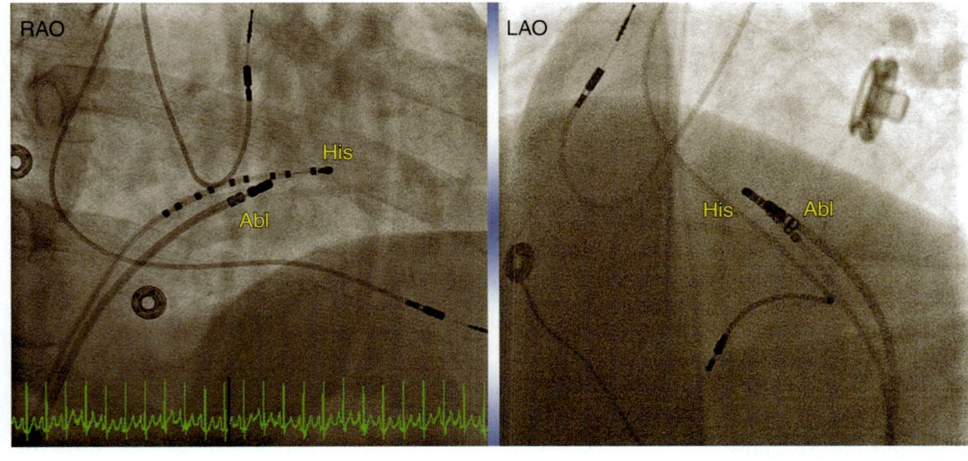

FIGURE 15-64 Fluoroscopic (right anterior oblique [RAO] and left anterior oblique [LAO]) views of the ablation catheter position (Abl) in relation to the His bundle (HB) catheter at the optimal site of atrioventricular junction ablation. The distal ablation electrode is positioned just proximal and inferior to the proximal HB electrodes.

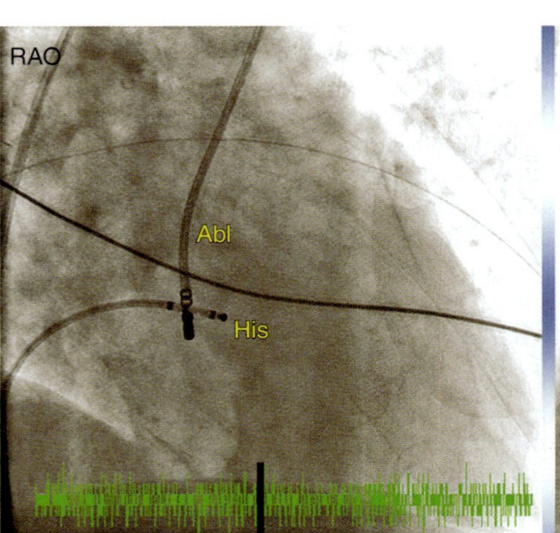

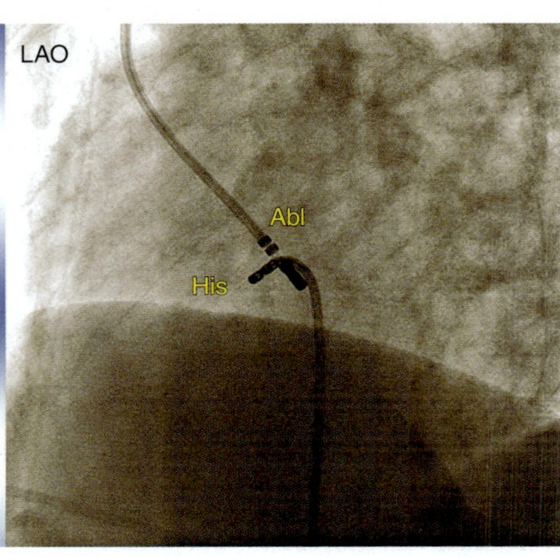

FIGURE 15-65 Fluoroscopic (right anterior oblique [RAO] and left anterior oblique [LAO]) views of the ablation catheter introduced via a transaortic approach in relation to the His bundle (HB) catheter at the optimal site for atrioventricular junction ablation (Abl). The distal ablation electrode is positioned just inferior to the aortic cusp in the left ventricular outflow tract, opposite the HB catheter in the right ventricle.

that the tip of the catheter is pointing toward the RA and lying on the septal aspect of the RA. Gentle withdrawal of the catheter can increase the size of the loop and allow the catheter tip to rest on the HB location (see Fig. 15-66). After successful ablation, the ablation catheter is withdrawn, and the atrial pacing lead is advanced through that same sheath.[192]

RF energy is delivered with a power output of 50 W, targeting a temperature of 60°C to 70°C, and for a duration of 30 to 120 seconds. AV block may appear immediately or after several RF applications. Typically, at good ablation sites, an accelerated junctional rhythm is induced during RF application (Fig. 15-67).

Endpoints of Ablation

The endpoint of ablation is achieving complete AV block. It is preferable to achieve AVN block with a junctional escape rhythm to avoid pacemaker dependency; however, sometimes this is difficult to achieve, and HB ablation with fascicular or no escape rhythm is the end result (see Fig. 15-67).

Outcome

Complete AV block can be achieved in almost 100% of patients, with a 3% risk of recurrence of AV conduction. Achieving complete AVN block specifically, however, is less successful (80% to 90%). Ablation of the AV junction may be difficult to achieve in patients with atrial enlargement or hypertrophy, as seen with longstanding heart failure or hypertension.

Most patients who undergo RF ablation of the AV junction are pacemaker dependent after the procedure, as defined by lack of an escape rhythm that is faster than 40 beats/min. Following AV junction ablation, an escape rhythm develops in 70% to 100% of cases, and the absence of escape rhythm immediately after ablation seems to be the only predictor for long-term pacemaker dependency. Although the appearance of an escape rhythm does not obviate the need for pacing, it may provide reassurance in case of pacemaker failure.

Malignant ventricular arrhythmias and sudden cardiac death have been observed in the early phase following AV junction ablation. Polymorphic VTs are related to electrical instability caused by an initial prolongation and then slow adaptation of repolarization caused by changes in the heart rate and activation sequence. Most polymorphic VTs, VF, and torsades de pointes that have been reported seem to be consistent with a pause or bradycardia-dependent mechanism. Anomalous dynamics of the paced QT intervals have been observed until the second day after AV junction ablation in patients with rapid refractory AF, resulting in prolongation of the QT interval when the heart rate is less than 75 beats/min. This finding may explain the ventricular arrhythmias occurring after AV junction ablation and may also explain the beneficial effects of temporary relatively rapid pacing. On the other hand, bradycardia may not be the sole factor. Sympathetic tone augmentation following AV junction ablation has been described in patients paced at 60 beats/min, thus causing prolongation of action potential duration and RV refractoriness, whereas sympathetic tone was reduced in patients paced at 90 beats/min. Such an increase in sympathetic activity and prolongation in action potential duration may favor early afterdepolarization and triggered activity, which may mediate torsades de pointes and polymorphic VT. To reduce the risk of these arrhythmias, routine pacing at 80 beats/min has been recommended following AV junction ablation. Patients with high-risk factors for arrhythmias, such as congestive heart failure or impaired LV function, may require pacing at higher rates (e.g., at 90 beats/min for 1 to 3 months) as well as in-hospital monitoring for at least 48 hours. Adjustment of the pacing rate, although rarely to less than 70 beats/min, is usually undertaken after 1 week in most patients, preferably after an ECG evaluation for repolarization abnormalities at the lower rate.

Another adverse effect of the ablate and pace approach is ventricular dyssynchrony induced by RV pacing, which may result in impairment of LV systolic function. Positioning the ventricular

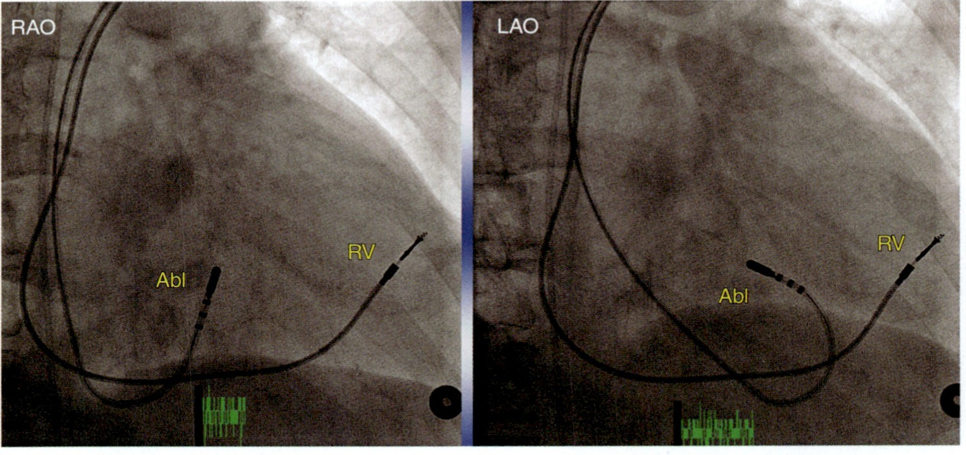

FIGURE 15-66 Fluoroscopic (right anterior oblique) views of the ablation (Abl) catheter introduced via the left axillary vein. Implantation of the pacemaker ventricular lead is initially performed. The ablation catheter is positioned near the His bundle region by deflection of the tip superiorly to form a J shape and then withdrawing the catheter so that it lies across the superior margin of the tricuspid annulus **(left)**, or by looping the catheter in the right atrium (RA; figure-of-6) and then advancing the body of the loop into the right ventricle so that the tip of the catheter is pointing toward the RA and lying on the septal aspect of the RA **(right)**. LAO = left anterior oblique; RAO = right anterior oblique; RV = right ventricle.

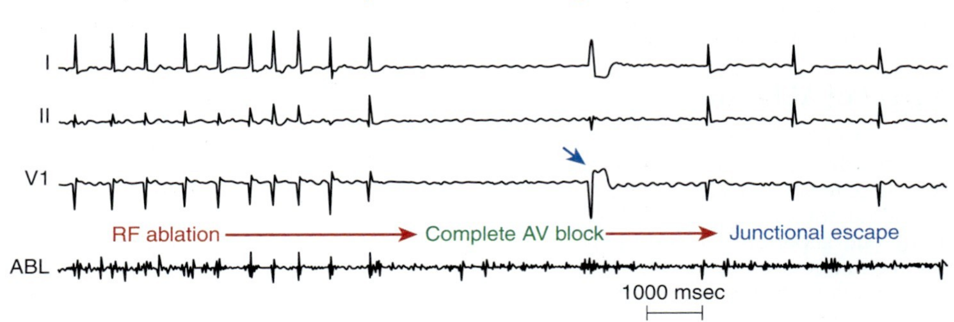

FIGURE 15-67 Atrioventricular (AV) junction ablation (ABL) during atrial fibrillation (AF). A ventricular pacemaker was implanted prior to ablation and programmed to VVI pacing mode at 30 beats/min. Radiofrequency (RF) application results in complete AV block with an escape ventricular paced complex (blue arrow) followed by the emergence of a junctional escape rhythm at 35 beats/min.

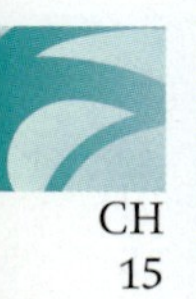

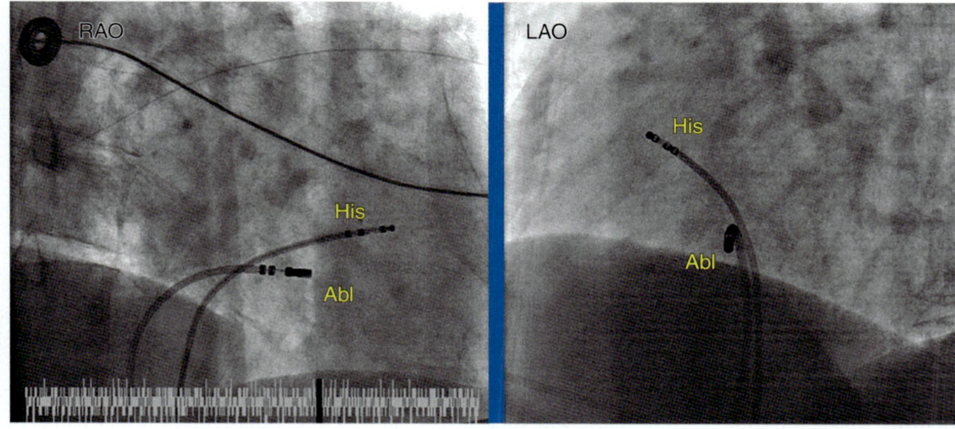

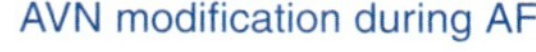

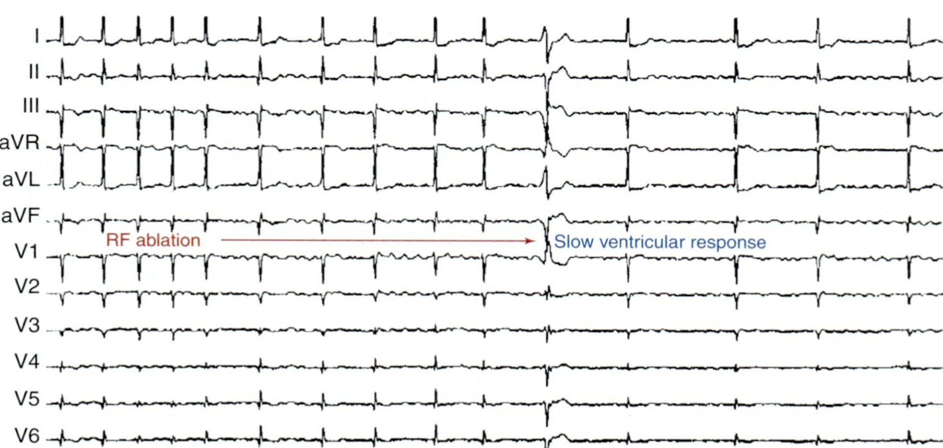

FIGURE 15-68 Atrioventricular node (AVN) modification during atrial fibrillation (AF). **Upper panel,** Fluoroscopic (right anterior oblique [RAO] and left anterior oblique [LAO]) views of the ablation catheter position (Abl) in relation to the His bundle (HB) catheter at the optimal site of AVN modification. The distal ablation electrode is positioned in the posteroatrial or midatrial septum near the tricuspid annulus, close to the coronary sinus ostium. **Lower panel,** AF with rapid ventricular response is initially observed (at left). Radiofrequency (RF) application results in slowing of the ventricular rate (at right) but not complete AV block, as indicated by irregularity of the rhythm.

pacing electrode over the RV septum, HB pacing, and biventricular pacing are being evaluated to reduce the impact of this potential problem.

Atrioventricular Nodal Modification

Rationale

AVN modification is performed to injure the AVN to reduce the ventricular rate during AF without producing complete heart block. As compared with ablation of the AV junction, AVN modification has the advantage in that it results in adequate control of the ventricular rate in most patients while obviating the need for a permanent pacemaker. Therefore, it may be appropriate to attempt first to modify AV conduction in patients with AF and rapid ventricular rates who are appropriate candidates for ablation of the AV junction. Because the risk of inadvertent complete AV block is approximately 20%, the use of the procedure should be limited at present to patients with AF who are symptomatic enough for ablation of the AV junction and implantation of a permanent pacemaker to be justified.

Target of Ablation

The right posteroseptal area along the tricuspid annulus extending from the CS os to the recording site of the HB can be divided into three regions: posterior, medial, and anterior. The conventional technique for ablation of the AV junction uses sites located anteriorly and superiorly on the tricuspid annulus. In contrast, with the technique used to modify AV conduction, the target sites are located inferiorly and posteriorly near the tricuspid annulus close to the CS os (i.e., in the posterior or midatrial septum) (Fig. 15-68). In the presence of dual AVN physiology, the slow AVN pathway is targeted, as described for ablation of AVNRT.

Ablation Technique

Two quadripolar-electrode catheters are inserted into a femoral vein and positioned at the HB and in the RV. An ablation catheter with a 4-mm tip is used. In patients with no demonstrable dual AVN physiology, RF energy is delivered during AF under continuous infusion of isoproterenol (4 µg/min) to permit immediate assessment of the effect of each RF application. The ventricular rate during AF, obtained after administration of isoproterenol, is presumed to simulate the maximal rate of clinical AF. If NSR is present, AF is induced by rapid atrial pacing before the delivery of RF energy. The ablation catheter is initially positioned against the posterior RA septum, at the level of or lower than the CS os, to record a stable electrogram for at least 10 seconds, with a maximal A/V electrogram amplitude ratio of 0.5 or lower.

RF energy is delivered for 20 seconds at 30 W. If there is no change in the ventricular rate or no accelerating junctional rhythm within 20 seconds, higher energy (an increment of 5 W every 20 seconds, up to 40 W) is delivered to the same site. Whenever there is an abrupt lengthening of the R-R interval or appearance of an accelerated junctional rhythm, the application of energy is immediately discontinued (see Fig. 15-68). If the ventricular rate is still higher than the endpoint ventricular rate (i.e., more than 130 beats/min), higher energy is delivered to the effective site, or the ablation site is changed and the catheter is repositioned in progressively upward (more superior and anterior) positions along the tricuspid annulus until the endpoint is achieved. RF energy should not be delivered at the upper third of the atrial septum, where a HB potential is visible.

If the endpoint ventricular rate could not be achieved after RF application to the posterior and midatrial septum, a decision should be made about whether to attempt complete ablation of AVN. In the presence of dual AVN physiology, RF energy is delivered during NSR to eliminate a slow AVN pathway. The ablation technique is similar to that described for ablation of AVNRT.

Endpoints of Ablation

The endpoint of the procedure is an average ventricular rate of 120 to 130 beats/min or 70% to 75% of the maximum ventricular rate during infusion of isoproterenol (4 µg/min).

Outcome

SHORT-TERM RESULTS

The immediate success of AVN modification to control the ventricular rate without inducing pathological AV block is approximately 75% to 92%.

LONG-TERM RESULTS

In one report, 92% of patients with paroxysmal AF and uncontrolled ventricular rates refractory to antiarrhythmic drugs achieved adequate slowing of the ventricular rate and were free of symptoms without any antiarrhythmic drug or the need for a permanent pacemaker. The mean resting, ambulatory, and minimal ventricular rates during AF usually remained stable during an interval from 2 days to 3 months after the modification procedure. However, the mean maximal ventricular rate tended to increase (by up to 25%) during this period, which may reflect partial recovery of AV conduction from the immediate effects of RF energy. Nevertheless, the mean maximal ventricular rate during exercise or isoproterenol infusion at 3 months of follow-up remained approximately 25% lower than at baseline, a degree of attenuation adequate to result in the persistent resolution of symptoms.

ATRIOVENTRICULAR BLOCK

Inadvertent complete AV block occurs in approximately 20% to 25% of patients. Of those patients who develop transient AV block during RF application, approximately two-thirds develop persistent AV block within the first 36 to 72 hours after the procedure. It may be that transient thermal injury to the AV conduction system results in an inflammatory reaction responsible for the delayed occurrence of permanent injury. Regardless of the mechanism, if transient AV block occurs during an attempt to modify AV conduction, continuous ECG monitoring on an inpatient basis is appropriate for 3 to 4 days to watch for a recurrence of AV block.

LIMITATIONS

The AVN modification approach is applicable only to patients who do not have symptoms caused by irregular heart rhythm. An irregular rhythm may be hemodynamically less efficient than a regular paced rhythm. Additionally, at least 25% of patients in whom AVN modification is attempted develop inadvertent complete AV block that necessitates implantation of a permanent pacemaker.

REFERENCES

1. Lubitz SA, Benjamin EJ, Ruskin JN, et al: Challenges in the classification of atrial fibrillation, *Nat Rev Cardiol* 7:451–460, 2010.
2. Nattel S, Ehrlich JR: Atrial fibrillation. In Zipes DP, Jalife J, editors: *Cardiac electrophysiology: from cell to bedside*, ed 4, Philadelphia, 2004, Saunders, pp 512–522.
3. Calkins H, Brugada J, Packer DL, et al: HRS/EHRA/ECAS expert consensus statement on catheter and surgical ablation of atrial fibrillation: recommendations for personnel, policy, procedures and follow-up. A report of the Heart Rhythm Society (HRS) Task Force on catheter and surgical ablation of atrial fibrillation, *Heart Rhythm* 4:816–861, 2007.
4. Olgin JE: Electrophysiology of the pulmonary veins: mechanisms of initiation of atrial fibrillation. In Zipes DP, Jalife J, editors: *Cardiac electrophysiology: from cell to bedside*, ed 4, Philadelphia, 2004, Saunders, pp 355–362.
5. Chen PS, Chou CC, Tan AY, et al: The mechanisms of atrial fibrillation, *J Cardiovasc Electrophysiol* 17(Suppl 3):S2–S7, 2006.
6. Chen YJ, Chen SA: Electrophysiology of pulmonary veins, *J Cardiovasc Electrophysiol* 17:220–224, 2006.
7. Moe GK, Rheinboldt WC, Abildskov JA: A computer model of atrial fibrillation, *Am Heart J* 67:200–220, 1964.
8. Krummen DE, Narayan SM: Mechanisms for the initiation of human atrial fibrillation, *Heart Rhythm* 6(Suppl):S12–S16, 2009.
9. Aldhoon B, Melenovsky V, Peichl P, Kautzner J: New insights into mechanisms of atrial fibrillation, *Physiol Res* 59:1–12, 2010.
10. Casaclang-Verzosa G, Gersh BJ, Tsang TS: Structural and functional remodeling of the left atrium: clinical and therapeutic implications for atrial fibrillation, *J Am Coll Cardiol* 51:1–11, 2008.
11. Workman AJ, Kane KA, Rankin AC: Cellular bases for human atrial fibrillation, *Heart Rhythm* 5(Suppl):S1–S6, 2008.
12. Stiles MK, John B, Wong CX, et al: Paroxysmal lone atrial fibrillation is associated with an abnormal atrial substrate: characterizing the "second factor," *J Am Coll Cardiol* 53:1182–1191, 2009.
13. Burstein B, Nattel S: Atrial fibrosis: mechanisms and clinical relevance in atrial fibrillation, *J Am Coll Cardiol* 51:802–809, 2008.
14. Ravelli F, Mase M, Del GM, et al: Acute atrial dilatation slows conduction and increases AF vulnerability in the human atrium, *J Cardiovasc Electrophysiol* 22:394–401, 2011.
15. Kuijpers NH, ten Eikelder HM, Bovendeerd PH, et al: Mechanoelectric feedback leads to conduction slowing and block in acutely dilated atria: a modeling study of cardiac electromechanics, *Am J Physiol Heart Circ Physiol* 292:H2832–H2853, 2007.
16. Patel P, Dokainish H, Tsai P, Lakkis N: Update on the association of inflammation and atrial fibrillation, *J Cardiovasc Electrophysiol* 21:1064–1070, 2010.
17. Issac TT, Dokainish H, Lakkis NM: Role of inflammation in initiation and perpetuation of atrial fibrillation: a systematic review of the published data, *J Am Coll Cardiol* 50:2021–2028, 2007.
18. Li J, Solus J, Chen Q, et al: Role of inflammation and oxidative stress in atrial fibrillation, *Heart Rhythm* 7:438–444, 2010.
19. Liuba I, Ahlmroth H, Jonasson L, et al: Source of inflammatory markers in patients with atrial fibrillation, *Europace* 10:848–853, 2008.
20. Schoonderwoerd BA, Van Gelder IC, Van Veldhuisen DJ, et al: Electrical and structural remodeling: role in the genesis and maintenance of atrial fibrillation, *Prog Cardiovasc Dis* 48:153–168, 2005.
21. Cohen M, Naccarelli GV: Pathophysiology and disease progression of atrial fibrillation: importance of achieving and maintaining sinus rhythm, *J Cardiovasc Electrophysiol* 19:885–890, 2008.
22. Rostock T, Steven D, Lutomsky B, et al: Atrial fibrillation begets atrial fibrillation in the pulmonary veins on the impact of atrial fibrillation on the electrophysiological properties of the pulmonary veins in humans, *J Am Coll Cardiol* 51:2153–2160, 2008.
23. Nakagawa H, Scherlag BJ, Patterson E, et al: Pathophysiologic basis of autonomic ganglionated plexus ablation in patients with atrial fibrillation, *Heart Rhythm* 6(Suppl):S26–S34, 2009.
24. Lachman N, Syed FF, Habib A, et al: Correlative anatomy for the electrophysiologist, part II: cardiac ganglia, phrenic nerve, coronary venous system, *J Cardiovasc Electrophysiol* 22:104–110, 2011.
25. Rosso R, Sparks PB, Morton JB, et al: Vagal paroxysmal atrial fibrillation: prevalence and ablation outcome in patients without structural heart disease, *J Cardiovasc Electrophysiol* 21:489–493, 2010.
26. Lim HS, Lip GY: Asymptomatic atrial fibrillation on device interrogation, *J Cardiovasc Electrophysiol* 19:891–893, 2008.
27. Fuster V, Ryden LE, Cannom DS, et al: ACC/AHA/ESC 2006 guidelines for the management of patients with atrial fibrillation—executive summary: a report of the American College of Cardiology/American Heart Association Task Force on Practice Guidelines and the European Society of Cardiology Committee for Practice Guidelines (writing committee to revise the 2001 guidelines for the management of patients with atrial fibrillation), *J Am Coll Cardiol* 48:854–906, 2006.
28. Pappone C, Radinovic A, Manguso F, et al: Atrial fibrillation progression and management: a 5-year prospective follow-up study, *Heart Rhythm* 5:1501–1507, 2008.
29. Crandall MA, Horne BD, Day JD, et al: Atrial fibrillation significantly increases total mortality and stroke risk beyond that conveyed by the $CHADS_2$ risk factors, *Pacing Clin Electrophysiol* 32:981–986, 2009.
30. Haywood LJ, Ford CE, Crow RS, et al: Atrial fibrillation at baseline and during follow-up in ALLHAT (Antihypertensive and Lipid-Lowering Treatment to Prevent Heart Attack Trial), *J Am Coll Cardiol* 54:2023–2031, 2009.
31. Nieuwlaat R, Eurlings LW, Cleland JG, et al: Atrial fibrillation and heart failure in cardiology practice: reciprocal impact and combined management from the perspective of atrial fibrillation. Results of the Euro Heart Survey on atrial fibrillation, *J Am Coll Cardiol* 53:1690–1698, 2009.
32. Bunch TJ, Day JD, Olshansky B, et al: Newly detected atrial fibrillation in patients with an implantable cardioverter-defibrillator is a strong risk marker of increased mortality, *Heart Rhythm* 6:2–8, 2009.
33. Gami AS, Somers VK: Implications of obstructive sleep apnea for atrial fibrillation and sudden cardiac death, *J Cardiovasc Electrophysiol* 19:997–1003, 2008.
34. Tedrow UB, Conen D, Ridker PM, et al: The long- and short-term impact of elevated body mass index on the risk of new atrial fibrillation the WHS (Women's Health Study), *J Am Coll Cardiol* 55:2319–2327, 2010.
35. Dorian P, Guerra PG, Kerr CR, et al: Validation of a new simple scale to measure symptoms in atrial fibrillation: the Canadian Cardiovascular Society Severity in Atrial Fibrillation scale, *Circ Arrhythm Electrophysiol* 2:218–224, 2009.
36. Camm AJ, Kirchhof P, Lip GY, et al: Guidelines for the management of atrial fibrillation: the Task Force for the Management of Atrial Fibrillation of the European Society of Cardiology (ESC), *Eur Heart J* 31:2369–2429, 2010.

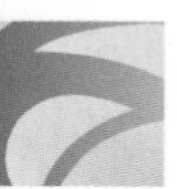

37. Lip GY, Frison L, Halperin JL, Lane DA: Identifying patients at high risk for stroke despite anticoagulation: a comparison of contemporary stroke risk stratification schemes in an anticoagulated atrial fibrillation cohort, *Stroke* 41:2731–2738, 2010.
38. Lip GY, Nieuwlaat R, Pisters R, et al: Refining clinical risk stratification for predicting stroke and thromboembolism in atrial fibrillation using a novel risk factor-based approach: the Euro Heart Survey on atrial fibrillation, *Chest* 137:263–272, 2010.
39. Beinart R, Heist EK, Newell JB, et al: Left atrial appendage dimensions predict the risk of stroke/TIA in patients with atrial fibrillation, *J Cardiovasc Electrophysiol* 22:10–15, 2011.
40. Fang MC, Go AS, Chang Y, et al: Comparison of risk stratification schemes to predict thromboembolism in people with nonvalvular atrial fibrillation, *J Am Coll Cardiol* 51:810–815, 2008.
41. Botto GL, Padeletti L, Santini M, et al: Presence and duration of atrial fibrillation detected by continuous monitoring: crucial implications for the risk of thromboembolic events, *J Cardiovasc Electrophysiol* 20:241–248, 2009.
42. Glotzer TV, Daoud EG, Wyse DG, et al: The relationship between daily atrial tachyarrhythmia burden from implantable device diagnostics and stroke risk: the TRENDS study, *Circ Arrhythm Electrophysiol* 2:474–480, 2009.
43. Hohnloser SH, Pajitnev D, Pogue J, et al: Incidence of stroke in paroxysmal versus sustained atrial fibrillation in patients taking oral anticoagulation or combined antiplatelet therapy: an ACTIVE W substudy, *J Am Coll Cardiol* 50:2156–2161, 2007.
44. Connolly S, Pogue J, Hart R, et al: Clopidogrel plus aspirin versus oral anticoagulation for atrial fibrillation in the Atrial fibrillation Clopidogrel Trial with Irbesartan for prevention of Vascular Events (ACTIVE W): a randomised controlled trial, *Lancet* 367:1903–1912, 2006.
45. Connolly SJ, Ezekowitz MD, Yusuf S, et al: Dabigatran versus warfarin in patients with atrial fibrillation, *N Engl J Med* 361:1139–1151, 2009.
46. Patel MR, Mahaffey KW, Garg J, et al: Rivaroxaban versus warfarin in nonvalvular atrial fibrillation, *N Engl J Med* 365:883–891, 2011.
47. Wann LS, Curtis AB, January CT, et al: 2011 ACCF/AHA/HRS focused update on the management of patients with atrial fibrillation (updating the 2006 guideline): a report of the American College of Cardiology Foundation/American Heart Association Task Force on Practice Guidelines, *Heart Rhythm* 8:157–176, 2011.
48. Granger CB, Alexander JH, McMurray JJ, et al: Apixaban versus warfarin in patients with atrial fibrillation, *N Engl J Med* 365:981–992, 2011.
49. Holmes DR, Reddy VY, Turi ZG, et al: Percutaneous closure of the left atrial appendage versus warfarin therapy for prevention of stroke in patients with atrial fibrillation: a randomised non-inferiority trial, *Lancet* 374:534–542, 2009.
50. Singh IM, Holmes DR Jr: Left atrial appendage closure, *Curr Cardiol Rep* 12:413–421, 2010.
51. Friedman PA, Asirvatham SJ, Dalegrave C, et al: Percutaneous epicardial left atrial appendage closure: preliminary results of an electrogram guided approach, *J Cardiovasc Electrophysiol* 20:908–915, 2009.
52. Pisters R, Lane DA, Nieuwlaat R, et al: A novel user-friendly score (HAS-BLED) to assess 1-year risk of major bleeding in patients with atrial fibrillation: the Euro Heart Survey, *Chest* 138:1093–1100, 2010.
53. Fang MC, Go AS, Chang Y, et al: A new risk scheme to predict warfarin-associated hemorrhage: the ATRIA (Anticoagulation and Risk Factors in Atrial Fibrillation) study, *J Am Coll Cardiol* 58:395–401, 2011.
54. Rothberg MB, Celestin C, Fiore LD, et al: Warfarin plus aspirin after myocardial infarction or the acute coronary syndrome: meta-analysis with estimates of risk and benefit, *Ann Intern Med* 143:241–250, 2005.
55. Van Gelder IC, Groenveld HF, Crijns HJ, et al: Lenient versus strict rate control in patients with atrial fibrillation, *N Engl J Med* 362:1363–1373, 2010.
56. Dong K, Shen WK, Powell BD, et al: Atrioventricular nodal ablation predicts survival benefit in patients with atrial fibrillation receiving cardiac resynchronization therapy, *Heart Rhythm* 7:1240–1245, 2010.
57. Reiffel JA: Cardioversion for atrial fibrillation: treatment options and advances, *Pacing Clin Electrophysiol* 32:1073–1084, 2009.
58. Singh SN, Tang XC, Reda D, Singh BN: Systematic electrocardioversion for atrial fibrillation and role of antiarrhythmic drugs: a substudy of the SAFE-T trial, *Heart Rhythm* 6:152–155, 2009.
59. Schneider MP, Hua TA, Bohm M, et al: Prevention of atrial fibrillation by renin-angiotensin system inhibition: a meta-analysis, *J Am Coll Cardiol* 55:2299–2307, 2010.
60. Mason PK, DiMarco JP: New pharmacological agents for arrhythmias, *Circ Arrhythm Electrophysiol* 2:588–597, 2009.
61. Roy D, Talajic M, Nattel S, et al: Rhythm control versus rate control for atrial fibrillation and heart failure, *N Engl J Med* 358:2667–2677, 2008.
62. Guglin M, Chen R, Curtis AB: Sinus rhythm is associated with fewer heart failure symptoms: insights from the AFFIRM trial, *Heart Rhythm* 7:596–601, 2010.
63. Khan MN, Jais P, Cummings J, et al: Pulmonary-vein isolation for atrial fibrillation in patients with heart failure, *N Engl J Med* 359:1778–1785, 2008.
64. Shen J, Bailey MS, Damiano RJ Jr: The surgical treatment of atrial fibrillation, *Heart Rhythm* 6(Suppl):S45–S50, 2009.
65. Mack MJ: Current results of minimally invasive surgical ablation for isolated atrial fibrillation, *Heart Rhythm* 6(Suppl):S46–S49, 2009.
66. Lockwood D, Nakagawa H, Peyton MD, et al: Linear left atrial lesions in minimally invasive surgical ablation of persistent atrial fibrillation: techniques for assessing conduction block across surgical lesions, *Heart Rhythm* 6(Suppl):S50–S63, 2009.
67. Krul SP, Driessen AH, van Boven WJ, et al: Thoracoscopic video-assisted pulmonary vein antrum isolation, ganglionated plexus ablation, and periprocedural confirmation of ablation lesions: first results of a hybrid surgical-electrophysiological approach for atrial fibrillation, *Circ Arrhythm Electrophysiol* 4:262–270, 2011.
68. Han FT, Kasirajan V, Wood MA, Ellenbogen KA: Minimally invasive surgical atrial fibrillation ablation: patient selection and results, *Heart Rhythm* 6(Suppl):S71–S76, 2009.
69. Khargi K, Hutten BA, Lemke B, Deneke T: Surgical treatment of atrial fibrillation: a systematic review, *Eur J Cardiothorac Surg* 27:258–265, 2005.
70. Pappone C, Rosanio S, Oreto G, et al: Circumferential radiofrequency ablation of pulmonary vein ostia: a new anatomic approach for curing atrial fibrillation, *Circulation* 102:2619–2628, 2000.
71. Dixit S, Marchlinski FE: How to recognize, manage, and prevent complications during atrial fibrillation ablation, *Heart Rhythm* 4:108–115, 2007.
72. Estner HL, Hessling G, Ndrepepa G, et al: Acute effects and long-term outcome of pulmonary vein isolation in combination with electrogram-guided substrate ablation for persistent atrial fibrillation, *Am J Cardiol* 101:332–337, 2008.
73. Verma A, Mantovan R, Macle L, et al: Substrate and Trigger Ablation for Reduction of Atrial Fibrillation (STAR AF): a randomized, multicentre, international trial, *Eur Heart J* 31:1344–1356, 2010.
74. Khaykin Y, Skanes A, Champagne J, et al: A randomized controlled trial of the efficacy and safety of electroanatomic circumferential pulmonary vein ablation supplemented by ablation of complex fractionated atrial electrograms versus potential-guided pulmonary vein antrum isolation guided by intracardiac ultrasound, *Circ Arrhythm Electrophysiol* 2:481–487, 2009.
75. Pokushalov E, Romanov A, Shugayev P, et al: Selective ganglionated plexi ablation for paroxysmal atrial fibrillation, *Heart Rhythm* 6:1257–1264, 2009.
76. Po SS, Nakagawa H, Jackman WM: Localization of left atrial ganglionated plexi in patients with atrial fibrillation, *J Cardiovasc Electrophysiol* 20:1186–1189, 2009.
77. Callahan TD, Natale A: Procedural end points in pulmonary vein antrum isolation: are we there yet? *Circulation* 117:131–133, 2008.
78. Verma A: The techniques for catheter ablation of paroxysmal and persistent atrial fibrillation: a systematic review, *Curr Opin Cardiol* 26:17–24, 2011.
79. Hwang C, Chen PS: Ligament of Marshall: why it is important for atrial fibrillation ablation, *Heart Rhythm* 6(Suppl):S35–S40, 2009.
80. Khan A, Mittal S, Kamath GS, et al: Pulmonary vein isolation alone in patients with persistent atrial fibrillation: an ablation strategy facilitated by antiarrhythmic drug induced reverse remodeling, *J Cardiovasc Electrophysiol* 22:142–148, 2011.
81. Leong-Sit P, Roux JF, Zado E, et al: Antiarrhythmics after ablation of atrial fibrillation (5A Study): six-month follow-up study, *Circ Arrhythm Electrophysiol* 4:11–14, 2011.
82. Gautam S, John RM, Stevenson WG, et al: Effect of therapeutic INR on activated clotting times, heparin dosage, and bleeding risk during ablation of atrial fibrillation, *J Cardiovasc Electrophysiol* 22:248–254, 2011.
83. Hussein AA, Martin DO, Saliba W, et al: Radiofrequency ablation of atrial fibrillation under therapeutic international normalized ratio: a safe and efficacious periprocedural anticoagulation strategy, *Heart Rhythm* 6:1425–1429, 2009.
84. Gopinath D, Lewis WR, Biase LD, Natale A: Pulmonary vein antrum isolation for atrial fibrillation on therapeutic Coumadin: special considerations, *J Cardiovasc Electrophysiol* 22:236–239, 2011.
85. Latchamsetty R, Gautam S, Bhakta D, et al: Management and outcomes of cardiac tamponade during atrial fibrillation ablation in the presence of therapeutic anticoagulation with warfarin, *Heart Rhythm* 8:805–808, 2011.
86. Wallace TW, Atwater BD, Daubert JP, et al: Prevalence and clinical characteristics associated with left atrial appendage thrombus in fully anticoagulated patients undergoing catheter-directed atrial fibrillation ablation, *J Cardiovasc Electrophysiol* 21:849–852, 2010.
87. Puwanant S, Varr BC, Shrestha K, et al: Role of the $CHADS_2$ score in the evaluation of thromboembolic risk in patients with atrial fibrillation undergoing transesophageal echocardiography before pulmonary vein isolation, *J Am Coll Cardiol* 54:2032–2039, 2009.
88. Baranowski B, Saliba W: Our approach to management of patients with pulmonary vein stenosis following AF ablation, *J Cardiovasc Electrophysiol* 22:364–367, 2011.
89. Dixit S, Gerstenfeld EP, Ratcliffe SJ, et al: Single procedure efficacy of isolating all versus arrhythmogenic pulmonary veins on long-term control of atrial fibrillation: a prospective randomized study, *Heart Rhythm* 5:174–181, 2008.
90. Kistler PM, Sanders P, Fynn SP, et al: Electrophysiologic and electroanatomic changes in the human atrium associated with age, *J Am Coll Cardiol* 44:109–116, 2004.
91. Asirvatham SJ: Pulmonary vein-related maneuvers: part I, *Heart Rhythm* 4:538–544, 2007.
92. Yamada T, Murakami Y, Okada T, et al: Electrophysiological pulmonary vein antrum isolation with a multielectrode basket catheter is feasible and effective for curing paroxysmal atrial fibrillation: efficacy of minimally extensive pulmonary vein isolation, *Heart Rhythm* 3:377–384, 2006.
93. Katritsis D, Merchant FM, Mela T, et al: Catheter ablation of atrial fibrillation: the search for substrate-driven end points, *J Am Coll Cardiol* 55:2293–2298, 2010.
94. Jiang CY, Jiang RH, Matsuo S, et al: Early detection of pulmonary vein reconnection after isolation in patients with paroxysmal atrial fibrillation: a comparison of ATP-induction and reassessment at 30 minutes postisolation, *J Cardiovasc Electrophysiol* 20:1382–1387, 2009.
95. Ninomiya Y, Iriki Y, Ishida S, et al: Usefulness of the adenosine triphosphate with a sufficient observation period for detecting reconduction after pulmonary vein isolation, *Pacing Clin Electrophysiol* 32:1307–1312, 2009.
96. Valles E, Fan R, Roux JF, et al: Localization of atrial fibrillation triggers in patients undergoing pulmonary vein isolation: importance of the carina region, *J Am Coll Cardiol* 52:1413–1420, 2008.
97. Sohara H, Takeda H, Ueno H, et al: Feasibility of the radiofrequency hot balloon catheter for isolation of the posterior left atrium and pulmonary veins for the treatment of atrial fibrillation, *Circ Arrhythm Electrophysiol* 2:225–232, 2009.
98. Schmidt B, Metzner A, Chun KR, et al: Feasibility of circumferential pulmonary vein isolation using a novel endoscopic ablation system, *Circ Arrhythm Electrophysiol* 3:481–488, 2010.
99. Metzner A, Schmidt B, Fuernkranz A, et al: One-year clinical outcome after pulmonary vein isolation using the novel endoscopic ablation system in patients with paroxysmal atrial fibrillation, *Heart Rhythm* 8:988–993, 2011.
100. Bunch TJ, Day JD: Novel ablative approach for atrial fibrillation to decrease risk of esophageal injury, *Heart Rhythm* 5:624–627, 2008.
101. Bittner A, Monnig G, Zellerhoff S, et al: Randomized study comparing duty-cycled bipolar and unipolar radiofrequency with point-by-point ablation in pulmonary vein isolation, *Heart Rhythm* 8:1383–1390, 2011.
102. Duytschaever M, Anne W, Papiashvili G, et al: Mapping and isolation of the pulmonary veins using the PVAC catheter, *Pacing Clin Electrophysiol* 33:168–178, 2010.
103. Andrade JG, Khairy P, Guerra PG, et al: Efficacy and safety of cryoballoon ablation for atrial fibrillation: a systematic review of published studies, *Heart Rhythm* 8:1444–1451, 2011.

104. Kuck KH, Furnkranz A: Cryoballoon ablation of atrial fibrillation, *J Cardiovasc Electrophysiol* 21:1427–1431, 2010.
105. Pratola C, Baldo E, Notarstefano P, et al: Radiofrequency ablation of atrial fibrillation: is the persistence of all intraprocedural targets necessary for long-term maintenance of sinus rhythm? *Circulation* 117:136–143, 2008.
106. Huang W, Liu T, Shehata M, et al: Inducibility of atrial fibrillation in the absence of atrial fibrillation: what does it mean to be normal? *Heart Rhythm* 8:489–492, 2011.
107. Wylie JV Jr, Essebag V, Reynolds MR, Josephson ME: Inducibility of atrial fibrillation with a synchronized external low energy shock post-pulmonary vein isolation predicts recurrent atrial fibrillation, *J Cardiovasc Electrophysiol* 20:29–36, 2009.
108. Kim YH, Lim HE, Pak HN, et al: Role of residual potentials inside circumferential pulmonary veins ablation lines in the recurrence of paroxysmal atrial fibrillation, *J Cardiovasc Electrophysiol* 21:959–965, 2010.
109. Terasawa T, Balk EM, Chung M, et al: Systematic review: comparative effectiveness of radiofrequency catheter ablation for atrial fibrillation, *Ann Intern Med* 151:191–202, 2009.
110. Sawhney N, Anousheh R, Chen W, Feld GK: Circumferential pulmonary vein ablation with additional linear ablation results in an increased incidence of left atrial flutter compared with segmental pulmonary vein isolation as an initial approach to ablation of paroxysmal atrial fibrillation, *Circ Arrhythm Electrophysiol* 3:243–248, 2010.
111. Arenal A, Atea L, Datino T, et al: Identification of conduction gaps in the ablation line during left atrium circumferential ablation: facilitation of pulmonary vein disconnection after endpoint modification according to electrogram characteristics, *Heart Rhythm* 5:994–1002, 2008.
112. Stabile G, Bertaglia E, Turco P, et al: Role of pulmonary veins isolation in persistent atrial fibrillation ablation: the pulmonary vein isolation in persistent atrial fibrillation (PIPA) study, *Pacing Clin Electrophysiol* 32(Suppl 1):S116–S119, 2009.
113. Zheng L, Yao Y, Zhang S, et al: Organized left atrial tachyarrhythmia during stepwise linear ablation for atrial fibrillation, *J Cardiovasc Electrophysiol* 20:499–506, 2009.
114. Tamborero D, Mont L, Berruezo A, et al: Circumferential pulmonary vein ablation: does use of a circular mapping catheter improve results? A prospective randomized study, *Heart Rhythm* 7:612–618, 2010.
115. Weerasooriya R, Jais P, Wright M, et al: Catheter ablation of atrial tachycardia following atrial fibrillation ablation, *J Cardiovasc Electrophysiol* 20:833–838, 2009.
116. Sang C, Jiang C, Dong J, et al: A new method to evaluate linear block at the left atrial roof: is it reliable without pacing? *J Cardiovasc Electrophysiol* 21:741–746, 2010.
117. Sanders P, Hocini M, Jais P, et al: Complete isolation of the pulmonary veins and posterior left atrium in chronic atrial fibrillation: long-term clinical outcome, *Eur Heart J* 28:1862–1871, 2007.
118. Kumagai K, Muraoka S, Mitsutake C, et al: A new approach for complete isolation of the posterior left atrium including pulmonary veins for atrial fibrillation, *J Cardiovasc Electrophysiol* 18:1047–1052, 2007.
119. Tamborero D, Mont L, Berruezo A, et al: Left atrial posterior wall isolation does not improve the outcome of circumferential pulmonary vein ablation for atrial fibrillation: a prospective randomized study, *Circ Arrhythm Electrophysiol* 2:35–40, 2009.
120. Waldo AL, Feld GK: Inter-relationships of atrial fibrillation and atrial flutter mechanisms and clinical implications, *J Am Coll Cardiol* 51:779–786, 2008.
121. Luria DM, Hodge DO, Monahan KH, et al: Effect of radiofrequency ablation of atrial flutter on the natural history of subsequent atrial arrhythmias, *J Cardiovasc Electrophysiol* 19:1145–1150, 2008.
122. Navarrete A, Conte F, Moran M, et al: Ablation of atrial fibrillation at the time of cavotricuspid isthmus ablation in patients with atrial flutter without documented atrial fibrillation derives a better long-term benefit, *J Cardiovasc Electrophysiol* 22:34–38, 2011.
123. Shah DC, Sunthorn H, Burri H, Gentil-Baron P: Evaluation of an individualized strategy of cavotricuspid isthmus ablation as an adjunct to atrial fibrillation ablation, *J Cardiovasc Electrophysiol* 18:926–930, 2007.
124. Singh JP, Ptaszek LM, Verma A: Elusive atrial substrate: complex fractionated atrial electrograms and beyond, *Heart Rhythm* 7:1886–1890, 2010.
125. Nademanee K, Schwab MC, Kosar EM, et al: Clinical outcomes of catheter substrate ablation for high-risk patients with atrial fibrillation, *J Am Coll Cardiol* 51:843–849, 2008.
126. Oral H, Chugh A, Good E, et al: A tailored approach to catheter ablation of paroxysmal atrial fibrillation, *Circulation* 113:1824–1831, 2006.
127. Takahashi Y, O'Neill MD, Hocini M, et al: Characterization of electrograms associated with termination of chronic atrial fibrillation by catheter ablation, *J Am Coll Cardiol* 51:1003–1010, 2008.
128. Wu J, Estner H, Luik A, et al: Automatic 3D mapping of complex fractionated atrial electrograms (CFAE) in patients with paroxysmal and persistent atrial fibrillation, *J Cardiovasc Electrophysiol* 19:897–903, 2008.
129. Verma A, Novak P, Macle L, et al: A prospective, multicenter evaluation of ablating complex fractionated electrograms (CFEs) during atrial fibrillation (AF) identified by an automated mapping algorithm: acute effects on AF and efficacy as an adjuvant strategy, *Heart Rhythm* 5:198–205, 2008.
130. Takahashi Y, Takahashi A, Kuwahara T, et al: Clinical characteristics of patients with persistent atrial fibrillation successfully treated by left atrial ablation, *Circ Arrhythm Electrophysiol* 3:465–471, 2010.
131. Elayi CS, Verma A, Di BL, et al: Ablation for longstanding permanent atrial fibrillation: results from a randomized study comparing three different strategies, *Heart Rhythm* 5:1658–1664, 2008.
132. Rostock T, Steven D, Hoffmann B, et al: Chronic atrial fibrillation is a biatrial arrhythmia: data from catheter ablation of chronic atrial fibrillation aiming arrhythmia termination using a sequential ablation approach, *Circ Arrhythm Electrophysiol* 1:344–353, 2008.
133. O'Neill MD, Wright M, Knecht S, et al: Long-term follow-up of persistent atrial fibrillation ablation using termination as a procedural endpoint, *Eur Heart J* 30:1105–1112, 2009.
134. Elayi CS, Di BL, Barrett C, et al: Atrial fibrillation termination as a procedural endpoint during ablation in long-standing persistent atrial fibrillation, *Heart Rhythm* 7:1216–1223, 2010.
135. Yoshida K, Chugh A, Good E, et al: A critical decrease in dominant frequency and clinical outcome after catheter ablation of persistent atrial fibrillation, *Heart Rhythm* 7:295–302, 2010.
136. Li WJ, Bai YY, Zhang HY, et al: Additional ablation of complex fractionated atrial electrograms after pulmonary vein isolation in patients with atrial fibrillation: a meta-analysis, *Circ Arrhythm Electrophysiol* 4:143–148, 2011.
137. Di BL, Elayi CS, Fahmy TS, et al: Atrial fibrillation ablation strategies for paroxysmal patients: randomized comparison between different techniques, *Circ Arrhythm Electrophysiol* 2:113–119, 2009.
138. Roux JF, Gojraty S, Bala R, et al: Effect of pulmonary vein isolation on the distribution of complex fractionated electrograms in humans, *Heart Rhythm* 6:156–160, 2009.
139. Narayan SM, Wright M, Derval N, et al: Classifying fractionated electrograms in human atrial fibrillation using monophasic action potentials and activation mapping: evidence for localized drivers, rate acceleration, and nonlocal signal etiologies, *Heart Rhythm* 8:244–253, 2011.
140. Vaitkevicius R, Saburkina I, Rysevaite K, et al: Nerve supply of the human pulmonary veins: an anatomical study, *Heart Rhythm* 6:221–228, 2009.
141. Lu Z, Scherlag BJ, Lin J, et al: Autonomic mechanism for initiation of rapid firing from atria and pulmonary veins: evidence by ablation of ganglionated plexi, *Cardiovasc Res* 84:245–252, 2009.
142. Arruda M, Mlcochova H, Prasad SK, et al: Electrical isolation of the superior vena cava: an adjunctive strategy to pulmonary vein antrum isolation improving the outcome of AF ablation, *J Cardiovasc Electrophysiol* 18:1261–1266, 2007.
143. Habib A, Lachman N, Christensen KN, Asirvatham SJ: The anatomy of the coronary sinus venous system for the cardiac electrophysiologist, *Europace* 11(Suppl 5):V15–V21, 2009.
144. Pontoppidan J, Nielsen JC, Poulsen SH, Hansen PS: Symptomatic and asymptomatic atrial fibrillation after pulmonary vein ablation and the impact on quality of life, *Pacing Clin Electrophysiol* 32:717–726, 2009.
145. Wokhlu A, Monahan KH, Hodge DO, et al: Long-term quality of life after ablation of atrial fibrillation: the impact of recurrence, symptom relief, and placebo effect, *J Am Coll Cardiol* 55:2308–2316, 2010.
146. Tilz RR, Chun KR, Schmidt B, et al: Catheter ablation of long-standing persistent atrial fibrillation: a lesson from circumferential pulmonary vein isolation, *J Cardiovasc Electrophysiol* 21:1085–1093, 2010.
147. Gaita F, Caponi D, Scaglione M, et al: Long-term clinical results of 2 different ablation strategies in patients with paroxysmal and persistent atrial fibrillation, *Circ Arrhythm Electrophysiol* 1:269–275, 2008.
148. Rostock T, Salukhe TV, Steven D, et al: Long-term single and multiple procedure outcome and predictors of success after catheter ablation for persistent atrial fibrillation, *Heart Rhythm* 8:1391–1397, 2011.
149. Matsuo S, Lellouche N, Wright M, et al: Clinical predictors of termination and clinical outcome of catheter ablation for persistent atrial fibrillation, *J Am Coll Cardiol* 54:788–795, 2009.
150. Balk EM, Garlitski AC, Sheikh-Ali AA, et al: Predictors of atrial fibrillation recurrence after radiofrequency catheter ablation: a systematic review, *J Cardiovasc Electrophysiol* 21:1208–1216, 2010.
151. Pokushalov E, Romanov A, Corbucci G, et al: Ablation of paroxysmal and persistent atrial fibrillation: 1-year follow-up through continuous subcutaneous monitoring, *J Cardiovasc Electrophysiol* 22:369–375, 2011.
152. Medi C, Sparks PB, Morton JB, et al: Pulmonary vein antral isolation for paroxysmal atrial fibrillation: results from long-term follow-up, *J Cardiovasc Electrophysiol* 22:137–141, 2011.
153. Joshi S, Choi AD, Kamath GS, et al: Prevalence, predictors, and prognosis of atrial fibrillation early after pulmonary vein isolation: findings from 3 months of continuous automatic ECG loop recordings, *J Cardiovasc Electrophysiol* 20:1089–1094, 2009.
154. Baman TS, Gupta SK, Billakanty SR, et al: Time to cardioversion of recurrent atrial arrhythmias after catheter ablation of atrial fibrillation and long-term clinical outcome, *J Cardiovasc Electrophysiol* 20:1321–1325, 2009.
155. Hussein AA, Saliba WI, Martin DO, et al: Natural history and long-term outcomes of ablated atrial fibrillation, *Circ Arrhythm Electrophysiol* 4:271–278, 2011.
156. Matsuo S, Lim KT, Haissaguerre M: Ablation of chronic atrial fibrillation, *Heart Rhythm* 4:1461–1463, 2007.
157. Morady F, Oral H, Chugh A: Diagnosis and ablation of atypical atrial tachycardia and flutter complicating atrial fibrillation ablation, *Heart Rhythm* 6(Suppl):S29–S32, 2009.
158. Kron J, Kasirajan V, Wood MA, et al: Management of recurrent atrial arrhythmias after minimally invasive surgical pulmonary vein isolation and ganglionic plexi ablation for atrial fibrillation, *Heart Rhythm* 7:445–451, 2010.
159. Themistoclakis S, Schweikert RA, Saliba WI, et al: Clinical predictors and relationship between early and late atrial tachyarrhythmias after pulmonary vein antrum isolation, *Heart Rhythm* 5:679–685, 2008.
160. Choi JI, Pak HN, Park JS, et al: Clinical significance of early recurrences of atrial tachycardia after atrial fibrillation ablation, *J Cardiovasc Electrophysiol* 21:1331–1337, 2010.
161. Chae S, Oral H, Good E, et al: Atrial tachycardia after circumferential pulmonary vein ablation of atrial fibrillation: mechanistic insights, results of catheter ablation, and risk factors for recurrence, *J Am Coll Cardiol* 50:1781–1787, 2007.
162. Schmidt M, Daccarett M, Segerson N, et al: Atrial flutter ablation in inducible patients during pulmonary vein atrium isolation: a randomized comparison, *Pacing Clin Electrophysiol* 31:1592–1597, 2008.
163. Knecht S, Veenhuyzen G, O'Neill MD, et al: Atrial tachycardias encountered in the context of catheter ablation for atrial fibrillation part II: mapping and ablation, *Pacing Clin Electrophysiol* 32:528–538, 2009.
164. Takahashi Y, Takahashi A, Miyazaki S, et al: Electrophysiological characteristics of localized reentrant atrial tachycardia occurring after catheter ablation of long-lasting persistent atrial fibrillation, *J Cardiovasc Electrophysiol* 20:623–629, 2009.
165. Lo LW, Tsao HM, Lin YJ, et al: Different patterns of atrial remodeling after catheter ablation of chronic atrial fibrillation, *J Cardiovasc Electrophysiol* 22:385–393, 2011.
166. Wylie JV Jr, Peters DC, Essebag V, et al: Left atrial function and scar after catheter ablation of atrial fibrillation, *Heart Rhythm* 5:656–662, 2008.
167. Jiang CX, Sang CH, Dong JZ, et al: Significant left atrial appendage activation delay complicating aggressive septal ablation during catheter ablation of persistent atrial fibrillation, *Pacing Clin Electrophysiol* 33:652–660, 2010.

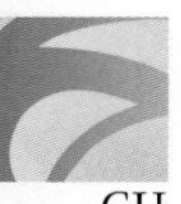

168. Tops LF, Den Uijl DW, Delgado V, et al: Long-term improvement in left ventricular strain after successful catheter ablation for atrial fibrillation in patients with preserved left ventricular systolic function, *Circ Arrhythm Electrophysiol* 2:249–257, 2009.
169. Cappato R, Calkins H, Chen SA, et al: Worldwide survey on the methods, efficacy, and safety of catheter ablation for human atrial fibrillation, *Circulation* 111:1100–1105, 2005.
170. Cappato R, Calkins H, Chen SA, et al: Updated worldwide survey on the methods, efficacy, and safety of catheter ablation for human atrial fibrillation, *Circ Arrhythm Electrophysiol* 3:32–38, 2010.
171. Cappato R, Calkins H, Chen SA, et al: Prevalence and causes of fatal outcome in catheter ablation of atrial fibrillation, *J Am Coll Cardiol* 53:1798–1803, 2009.
172. Dagres N, Hindricks G, Kottkamp H, et al: Complications of atrial fibrillation ablation in a high-volume center in 1,000 procedures: still cause for concern? *J Cardiovasc Electrophysiol* 20:1014–1019, 2009.
173. Ellis ER, Culler SD, Simon AW, Reynolds MR: Trends in utilization and complications of catheter ablation for atrial fibrillation in Medicare beneficiaries, *Heart Rhythm* 6:1267–1273, 2009.
174. Barrett CD, Di Biase L, Natale A: How to identify and treat patients with pulmonary vein stenosis post atrial fibrillation ablation, *Curr Opin Cardiol* 24:42–49, 2009.
175. Doppalapudi H, Yamada T, Kay N: Complications during catheter ablation of atrial fibrillation: identification and prevention, *Heart Rhythm* 6(Suppl):S18–S25, 2009.
176. Halm U, Gaspar T, Zachaus M, et al: Thermal esophageal lesions after radiofrequency catheter ablation of left atrial arrhythmias, *Am J Gastroenterol* 105:551–556, 2010.
177. Schmidt M, Nolker G, Marschang H, et al: Incidence of oesophageal wall injury post-pulmonary vein antrum isolation for treatment of patients with atrial fibrillation, *Europace* 10:205–209, 2008.
178. Bahnson TD: Strategies to minimize the risk of esophageal injury during catheter ablation for atrial fibrillation, *Pacing Clin Electrophysiol* 32:248–260, 2009.
179. Martinek M, Bencsik G, Aichinger J, et al: Esophageal damage during radiofrequency ablation of atrial fibrillation: impact of energy settings, lesion sets, and esophageal visualization, *J Cardiovasc Electrophysiol* 20:726–733, 2009.
180. Ahmed H, Neuzil P, d'Avila A, et al: The esophageal effects of cryoenergy during cryoablation for atrial fibrillation, *Heart Rhythm* 6:962–969, 2009.
181. Neven K, Schmidt B, Metzner A, et al: Fatal end of a safety algorithm for pulmonary vein isolation with use of high-intensity focused ultrasound, *Circ Arrhythm Electrophysiol* 3:260–265, 2010.
182. Dagres N, Anastasiou-Nana M: Prevention of atrial-esophageal fistula after catheter ablation of atrial fibrillation, *Curr Opin Cardiol* 26:1–5, 2011.
183. Chugh A, Rubenstein J, Good E, et al: Mechanical displacement of the esophagus in patients undergoing left atrial ablation of atrial fibrillation, *Heart Rhythm* 6:319–322, 2009.
184. Tilz RR, Chun KR, Metzner A, et al: Unexpected high incidence of esophageal injury following pulmonary vein isolation using robotic navigation, *J Cardiovasc Electrophysiol* 21:853–858, 2010.
185. McElderry HT, Yamada T: How to diagnose and treat cardiac tamponade in the electrophysiology laboratory, *Heart Rhythm* 6:1531–1535, 2009.
186. Scherr D, Sharma K, Dalal D, et al: Incidence and predictors of periprocedural cerebrovascular accident in patients undergoing catheter ablation of atrial fibrillation, *J Cardiovasc Electrophysiol* 20:1357–1363, 2009.
187. Kesek M, Englund A, Jensen SM, Jensen-Urstad M: Entrapment of circular mapping catheter in the mitral valve, *Heart Rhythm* 4:17–19, 2007.
188. Lickfett L, Mahesh M, Vasamreddy C, et al: Radiation exposure during catheter ablation of atrial fibrillation, *Circulation* 110:3003–3010, 2004.
189. Frazier TH, Richardson JB, Fabre VC, Callen JP: Fluoroscopy-induced chronic radiation skin injury: a disease perhaps often overlooked, *Arch Dermatol* 143:637–640, 2007.
190. Vatasescu R, Shalganov T, Kardos A, et al: Right diaphragmatic paralysis following endocardial cryothermal ablation of inappropriate sinus tachycardia, *Europace* 8:904–906, 2006.
191. Akoum N, Daccarett M, McGann C, et al: Atrial fibrosis helps select the appropriate patient and strategy in catheter ablation of atrial fibrillation: a DE-MRI guided approach, *J Cardiovasc Electrophysiol* 22:16–22, 2011.
192. Issa ZF: An approach to ablate and pace: AV junction ablation and pacemaker implantation performed concurrently from the same venous access site, *Pacing Clin Electrophysiol* 30:1116–1120, 2007.

CHAPTER 16 Inappropriate Sinus Tachycardia

Pathophysiology

Sinus tachycardia is a physiological response to sympathetic activation and/or parasympathetic withdrawal, such as during exercise, anxiety, pain, hypovolemia, orthostatic hypotension, fever, infections, hyperthyroidism, hypoglycemia, anemia, myocardial infarction, heart failure, pericarditis, diabetes-related autonomic dysfunction, drug abuse, catecholamine infusions, anticholinergic drugs, tobacco, caffeine, alcohol, and beta-blocking agent withdrawal. Inappropriate sinus tachycardia (IST) is a nonparoxysmal tachyarrhythmia characterized by a persistent increase in resting sinus rate unrelated to, or out of proportion with, the level of physical, emotional, pathological, or pharmacological stress or an exaggerated heart rate response to minimal exertion or a change in body posture.[1] IST is neither a response to a pathological process (e.g., heart failure, hyperthyroidism, or drug effects) nor a result of physical deconditioning.

The underlying mechanism of IST remains poorly understood. Several potential mechanisms have been suggested, including enhanced automaticity of the sinus node, altered sinus nodal intrinsic regulation, disorder of autonomic responsiveness of the sinus node, and sympathovagal imbalance, with excessive sympathetic drive or reduced vagal influence on the sinus node, or both. A primary abnormality of sinus node function has been suggested, as evidenced by a higher intrinsic heart rate (after muscarinic and beta-receptor blockade) than that found in normal controls or a blunted response to adenosine with less sinus cycle length prolongation than in control subjects (with and without autonomic blockade).[2,3] In addition, beta-adrenergic receptor hypersensitivity, alpha-adrenergic receptor hyposensitivity, M_2 muscarinic receptor abnormalities, brain stem dysregulation, depressed efferent cardiovagal reflex, and impaired baroreflex control are likely explanations. Chronic beta-receptor stimulation by autoantibodies and autonomic neuritis or autonomic neuropathy can play a role in some cases. The extent to which each of these mechanisms contributes to tachycardia and associated symptoms is unknown, but the underlying mechanisms are likely multifactorial and complex.[4-7]

In some patients, there can be an overlap between IST and disorders such as chronic fatigue syndrome and neurocardiogenic syncope, and other patients can have a psychological component of hypersensitivity to somatic input.[8] Other groups with similar or overlapping laboratory findings and clinical course include patients with hyperadrenergic syndrome, idiopathic hypovolemia,[9] orthostatic hypotension, and mitral valve prolapse syndrome.[2,3]

Clinical Considerations

Epidemiology

Almost all patients afflicted with IST are young women (mean age, 38 ± 12 years), and many of them are hypertensive. IST affects people working in health care in disproportionate numbers. The explanation for these findings is lacking.[3,10] The prevalence of IST in a middle-aged population (up to 1.16% in one report) appears to be higher than previously assumed. Despite the chronic nature of the disorder and long-lasting symptoms, the natural course and prognosis of IST are benign.[10]

Clinical Presentation

The most prominent symptoms are palpitations, fatigue, and exercise intolerance. IST can also be associated with a host of other symptoms, including chest pain, dyspnea, lightheadedness, dizziness, presyncope, and syncope. The clinical presentation of the arrhythmia is highly variable, ranging from totally asymptomatic patients identified during routine medical examination to those with paroxysmal short episodes of palpitations to individuals with chronic, incessant, and incapacitating symptoms.[2,10] The risk of tachycardia-induced cardiomyopathy in untreated patients is unknown but is likely to be low.[1,10,11]

Initial Evaluation

IST is an ill-defined clinical syndrome with diverse clinical manifestations. There is no gold standard to make a definitive diagnosis of IST, and the diagnosis remains a clinical one after exclusion of other causes of symptomatic tachycardia. Clinical examination and routine investigations allow elimination of secondary causes for the tachycardia but are generally not helpful in establishing the diagnosis of IST.[1-3]

The syndrome of IST is characterized by the following: (1) a relative or absolute increase in sinus rate out of proportion to the physiological demand (there can be an increased resting sinus rate of more than 100 beats/min or an exaggerated heart rate response to minimal exertion or change in body posture); (2) P wave axis and morphology during tachycardia that are similar or identical to those noted during normal sinus rhythm; (3) lack of secondary causes of sinus tachycardia; and (4) markedly distressing symptoms of palpitations, fatigue, dyspnea, and anxiety during tachycardia, with an absence of symptoms during normal sinus rates.[1-4,12]

Ambulatory Holter recordings characteristically demonstrate a mean heart rate of more than 90 to 95 beats/min (Fig. 16-1). However, some patients have either a physiological or normal heart rate at rest (less than 85 beats/min) with an inappropriate tachycardia response to a minimal physiological challenge or a moderately elevated resting heart rate (more than 85 beats/min) with an accentuated (inappropriate) heart rate response to minimal exertion.[2,3,13] However, this quantitative definition of inappropriate is arbitrary, and validation of the reproducibility of the heart rate and activity correlation can be challenging.[12,14]

Exercise ECG testing typically shows an early and excessive increase of heart rate in response to minimal exercise (heart rate greater than 130 beats/min within 90 seconds of exercise; Bruce protocol). This heart rate response is differentiated from physical deconditioning by chronicity and the presence of associated symptoms.[2]

Isoproterenol provocation helps demonstrate sinus node hypersensitivity to beta-adrenergic stimulation. Isoproterenol is

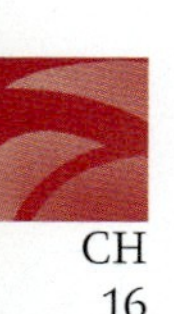

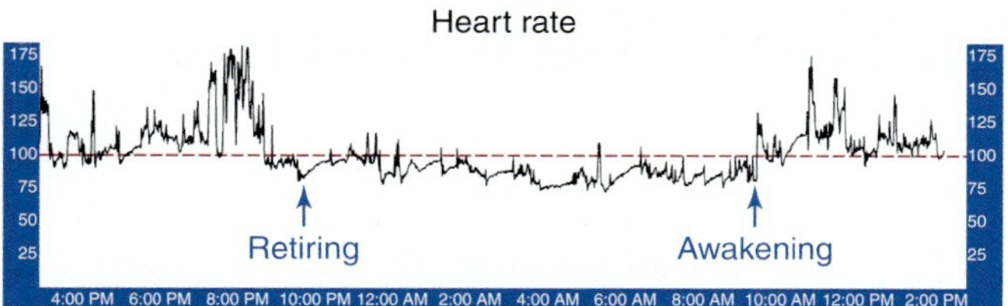

FIGURE 16-1 A 24-hour trend of the long-term ECG showing inappropriate sinus tachycardia throughout usual activity and on awakening.

administered as escalating intravenous boluses at 1-minute intervals, starting at 0.25 μg, with doubling of the dose every minute, until a target heart rate increase of 35 beats/min higher than baseline or a maximum heart rate of 150 beats/min is reached. In patients with IST, the target heart rate is reached with an isoproterenol dose of 0.29 ± 0.1 μg (versus 1.27 ± 0.4 μg in normal controls).[2]

Invasive electrophysiological (EP) testing may be considered when other arrhythmias are suspected or when a decision to proceed with catheter ablation is undertaken. It is important to recognize that sinus node modification to target IST is a clinical decision, and it must be made prior to the invasive EP study itself. The diagnosis of IST and the treatment approach have to be established before the patient is brought to the EP laboratory.[2,3]

IST shares several characteristics with postural orthostatic tachycardia syndrome (POTS), and it is sometimes challenging to differentiate between the two conditions. POTS is characterized by the presence of symptoms of orthostatic intolerance (i.e., the provocation of symptoms on standing that are relieved by recumbence) associated with a heart rate increase of 30 beats/min (or a rate that exceeds 120 beats/min) that occurs within the first 10 minutes of standing or upright tilt and is not associated with other chronic debilitating conditions such as prolonged bed rest or the use of medications known to diminish vascular or autonomic tone. Patients with POTS tend to display a more pronounced degree of postural change in heart rate than do those with IST. Additionally, in the supine position, the heart rate in patients with POTS rarely exceeds 100 beats/min, whereas in IST the resting heart rate is often higher than 100 beats/min. Patients with IST do not display the same degree of postural change in norepinephrine levels as do patients with hyperadrenergic POTS. The distinction between IST and POTS is important because catheter ablation of the sinus node rarely improves, and can even worsen, symptoms in patients with POTS.[15]

Principles of Management

The treatment of IST is predominantly symptom driven. Medical management remains the mainstay of therapy. Beta-blockers can be useful and should be prescribed as first-line therapy for most patients. Nondihydropyridine calcium channel blockers (verapamil and diltiazem) can also be effective.[1] However, pharmacological therapy for IST has been limited by the poor long-term tolerance to the drugs and the disappointing long-term outcome.

Ivabradine is a novel selective inhibitor of cardiac pacemaker I_f ion current, which is highly expressed in the sinus node and contributes to sinus node automaticity. Ivabradine selectivity induces heart rate reduction in humans and animals without any modification in cardiac contractility and atrioventricular and intraventricular conduction times. Blockade of the I_f current induced by ivabradine is dose and heart rate dependent, resulting in greater effects during fast heart rates and limiting the risk of symptomatic bradycardia. This agent is commonly used to relieve pain in patients affected by chronic stable angina. Preliminary data suggest that orally administered ivabradine lowers the mean daily and maximal heart rates in patients with IST, improves symptoms, enhances exercise-stress tolerance, and markedly improves quality of life, even in patients refractory to beta-blocking therapy. This pharmacological treatment could be considered a second-line therapy in patients refractory to and intolerant of beta-blockers and nondihydropyridine calcium channel blockers. However, more large-cohort studies are needed to confirm these preliminary results.[11,16,17]

Despite advances in ablation technologies, the long-term success of catheter ablation for IST remains disappointing. Nevertheless, sinus node modification by catheter ablation remains a potentially important therapeutic option in the most refractory cases of IST.[1,2]

Electrophysiological Testing

The goals of EP testing in patients with IST are to exclude other tachycardias that can mimic sinus tachycardia, such as atrial tachycardia (AT) originating near the superior aspect of the crista terminalis or right superior pulmonary vein, and to ensure that the tachycardia occurring spontaneously or, more likely with isoproterenol infusion, acts in a manner consistent with an exaggeration of normal sinus node physiology.[2,3]

For activation sequence mapping, a multipolar (20-pole) crista catheter is placed along the crista terminalis in addition to the catheters used for a routine EP evaluation (coronary sinus, His bundle, and right ventricular apex). The crista catheter is positioned on the crista terminalis from the superomedial aspect originating at the junction of the superior vena cava (SVC) and right atrial (RA) appendage, with continuation along the crista toward the junction of the inferior vena cava and RA inferolaterally. Catheter contact with the crista terminalis can be enhanced by using a long sheath (Fig. 16-2). Intracardiac echocardiography (ICE) may also be used to identify the crista terminalis and guide mapping catheter positioning as well as radiofrequency (RF) ablation (see later).[2,3]

Induction of Tachycardia

Programmed electrical stimulation is performed before and after isoproterenol infusion. Isoproterenol infusion is started at 0.5 to 1.0 μg/min and titrated every 3 to 5 minutes to a maximum of 6 μg/min. Atropine (1 mg) can also be administered to assess maximum sinus cycle length. It is important to document failure to induce AT and other supraventricular tachycardias during programmed stimulation. IST cannot be initiated with atrial rapid pacing or extrastimulation, but it can be induced by adrenergic stimulation. Initiation of IST is associated with a gradual increase of the sinus rate, with a gradual shift of the earliest atrial activation site up the crista terminalis.

EP phenomena such as dual atrioventricular nodal physiology or atrioventricular nodal echo beats should be cautiously evaluated in patients in whom the only documented symptomatic tachycardia appears to have a sinus mechanism. The relevance of these phenomena should be carefully assessed.

Tachycardia Features

The atrial activation sequence during IST is characterized by a craniocaudal activation sequence along the crista, with the site of earliest atrial activation shifting up the crista at faster rates and down the crista at slower rates. The earliest atrial activation site always occurs along the crista terminalis (as confirmed by the multipolar catheter placed on the crista) despite a changing tachycardia rate or autonomic modulation (isoproterenol and atropine).

In contrast focal AT, IST is characterized by a gradual increase and decrease in heart rate with changes in autonomic tone or at the initiation and termination of the tachycardia. Additionally, adrenergic stimulation reproducibly causes an increase in IST rate and a cranial shift in atrial activation along the crista terminalis, whereas vagal stimulation causes slowing of the IST rate with caudal shift.

Exclusion of Other Arrhythmia Mechanisms

Both sinus node reentrant tachycardia and focal AT have to be excluded. Sinus node reentry is easily and reproducibly initiated with atrial extrastimulation, and AT can be initiated with atrial extrastimulation, burst pacing, or adrenergic stimulation, whereas IST cannot

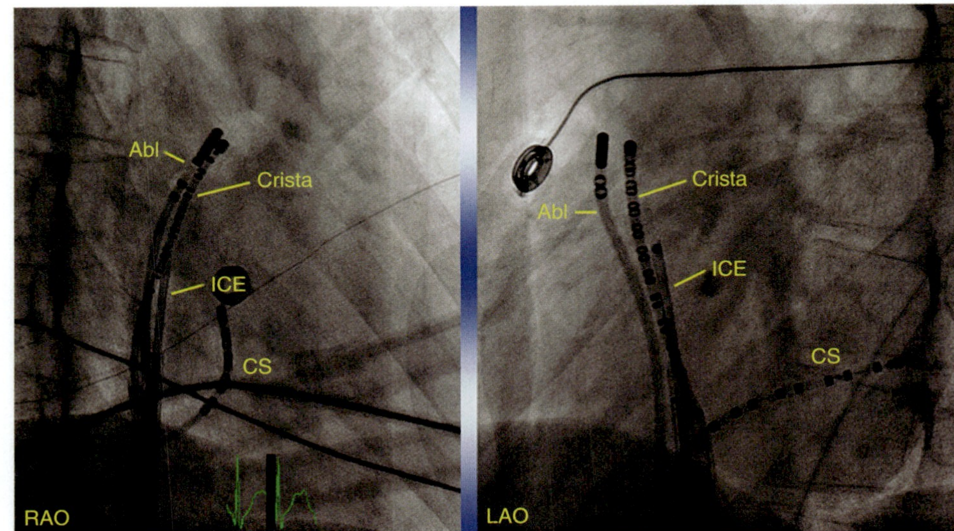

FIGURE 16-2 Right anterior oblique (RAO) and left anterior oblique (LAO) fluoroscopic view during sinus node modification. Multipolar (crista) catheter is placed along the crista terminalis with intracardiac echocardiography (ICE) guidance. Abl = ablation; CS = coronary sinus.

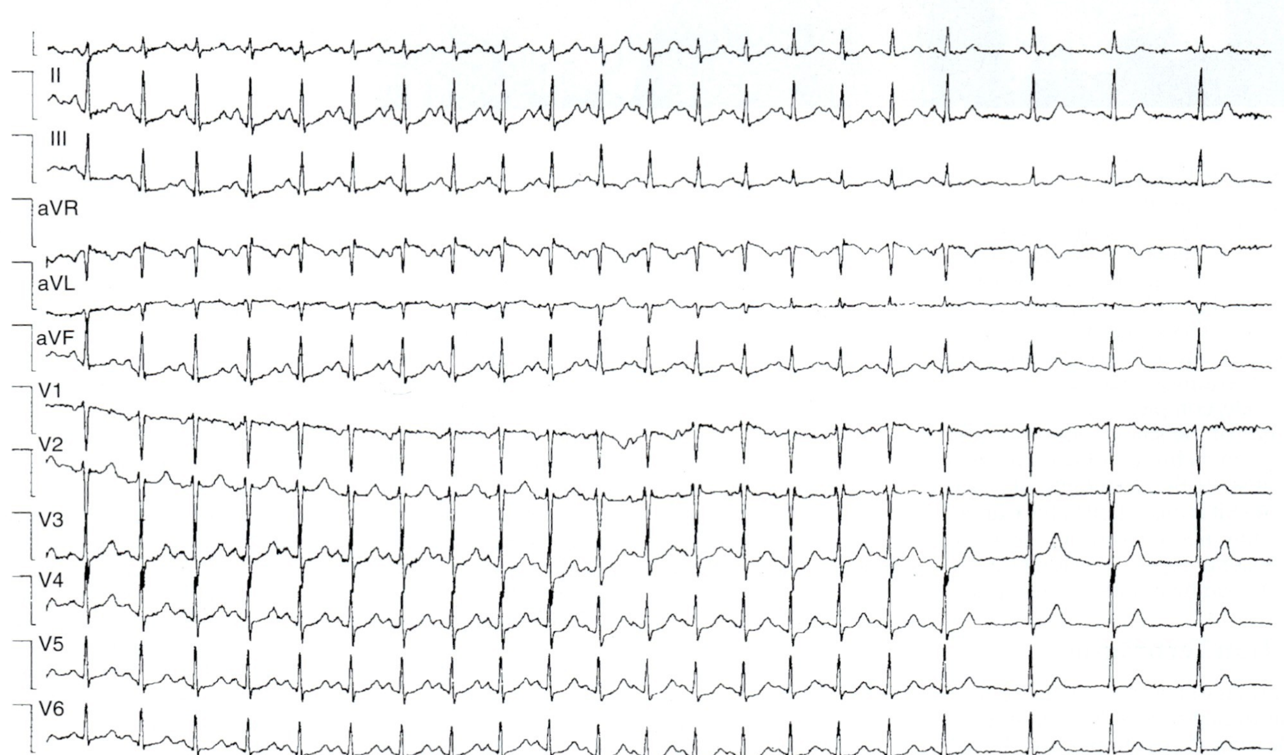

FIGURE 16-3 A 12-lead ECG showing perinodal focal atrial tachycardia (or sinus node reentrant tachycardia) with abrupt termination and restoration of normal sinus rhythm. Note the similarities between the tachycardia and sinus P wave morphology.

be initiated with programmed electrical stimulation. Furthermore, AT and the sinus node reentrant tachycardia rate can shift suddenly at initiation, although AT can then warm up over a few beats, as opposed to the gradual increase of the IST rate over seconds to minutes.

The atrial activation sequence shifts suddenly at the onset of AT or sinus node reentrant tachycardia, as opposed to a gradual cranial shift of the earliest atrial activation up the crista terminalis with adrenergic stimulation as the sinus rate increases during IST. Although the rate of focal AT can continue to increase with continued adrenergic stimulation, this is not associated with a further shift in the atrial activation sequence.

Sinus node reentry is easily and reproducibly terminated with programmed stimulation, whereas IST cannot be terminated with programmed stimulation. Termination of focal AT and sinus node reentry is sudden, as opposed to gradual slowing (cooldown) of the IST rate (Fig. 16-3). Vagal maneuvers result in abrupt termination of sinus node reentry and in either no effect or abrupt termination of AT, as opposed to gradual slowing and inferior shift down the crista terminalis of the site of origin of IST. Abrupt termination of the tachycardia with a single RF application suggests AT, because IST originates from a widespread area involving the superior crista terminalis.

Ablation

Target of Ablation

Understanding the anatomy and physiology of the sinus node (see Chap. 8) is critical for identifying the target of ablation for sinus node

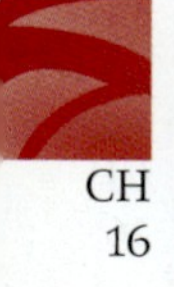

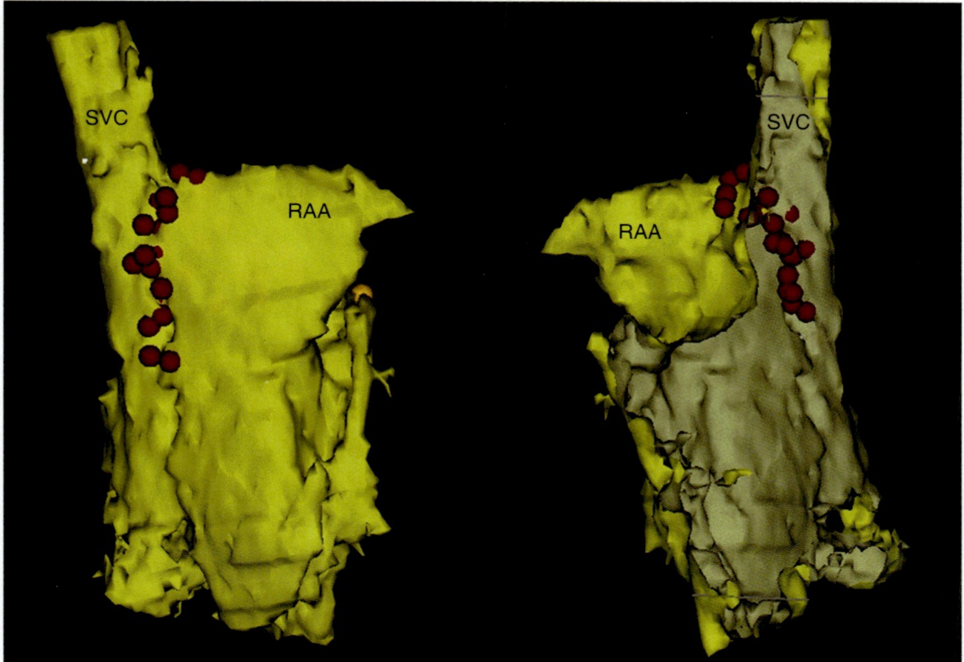

FIGURE 16-4 Integrated computed tomography (CT) and electroanatomical (CARTO) map of the right atrium acquired during sinus node modification. Right anterior oblique and cardioscopic views of the CT scan are shown. Note the area targeted by radiofrequency ablation (red dots) starting cranially at the medial portion of the crista as it courses in front of the superior vena cava (SVC). RAA = right atrial appendage.

modification. The sinus node region is a distributed complex characterized by rate-dependent site differentiation (i.e., there is anatomical distribution of impulse generation with changes in sinus rate), which allows for targeted ablation to eliminate the fastest sinus rates while maintaining some degree of sinus node function.[18]

Sinus node modification targets the site of most rapid discharge, generally at the superior aspect of the crista terminalis. One must recognize, however, that sinus node modification is not a focal ablation, but requires complete abolition of the cranial portion of the sinus node complex (Fig. 16-4). Ideally, this procedure eliminates the areas of the sinus node responsible for rapid rates while preserving some chronotropic competence.

Because of the possibility of unsatisfactory results of ablation (see later), it is important to have an understanding with the patient and family about likely outcomes and implications (needing a pacemaker or repeat ablation procedure, persistence of symptoms despite good heart rate control) prior to an ablation procedure.

Ablation Technique

The crista terminalis is not visible on fluoroscopy and has a varied course among patients. Therefore, some operators prefer using ICE to help identify the crista, position the tip of the ablation catheter with firm contact on the crista, and assess the RF lesion (see Fig. 11-23).[19,20]

A three-dimensional mapping system (CARTO, NavX) can also help delineate relevant anatomical structures (SVC, boundaries of atrium), define the extent of the earliest site of activation during IST, delineate the course of the phrenic nerve (sites at which pacing stimulates the diaphragm), and catalog sites of ablation.[21,22]

A multipolar catheter is placed along the crista terminalis (with or without ICE guidance; see Fig. 16-2). A standard ablation catheter with a 4- or 8-mm-tip or an irrigated-tip catheter is used for RF application. RF power is adjusted to achieve a tip temperature of 50° to 60°C or an impedance drop of 5 to 10 Ω, or both. RF lesions are applied as guided by the earliest atrial activation time, usually along superior regions of the crista terminalis using the guidance of the crista catheter. The local endocardial activation time recorded by the ablation catheter at successful sites typically precedes the onset of the surface P wave during the tachycardia by 25 to 45 milliseconds (Fig. 16-5).

RF ablation is performed under maximal adrenergic stimulation with isoproterenol (with or without parasympathetic blockade with atropine) to reveal the superior portions of the crista terminalis as the earliest sites of atrial activation. The medial portion of the crista as it courses in front of the SVC is usually the site of earliest activation for the fastest sinus rates; this portion of the crista should be targeted by RF ablation first. Progressively inferior portions of the crista are then ablated until target heart rate reduction is achieved. This technique often requires ablating an estimated area of 12 ± 4 × 19 ± 5 mm.[21]

RF energy delivery at any one site should probably be limited to 30 seconds because these are usually closely spaced applications, which carry the risk of char formation with longer applications. Pacing from the ablation catheter tip at high output (5 to 10 mA) before each RF application to verify the absence of diaphragmatic stimulation is necessary to avoid phrenic nerve injury. Rarely, pericardial access with epicardial ablation has been necessary. Then, avoidance of the phrenic nerve can be even more problematic and require instilling saline into the pericardial space or placing a balloon catheter through a second pericardial access to separate the phrenic nerve physically from the ablation zone.[2,3,20,22]

Acceleration of the sinus rate followed by a marked subsequent rate reduction or the appearance of a junctional rhythm during ablation is an indicator of successful ablation sites, and thereafter delivery of RF energy should be continued for at least 60 to 90 seconds. Most patients demonstrate a stepwise reduction in sinus rate during the course of ablation, associated with migration of the site of earliest atrial activation in a craniocaudal direction along the crista terminalis (see Fig. 16-5). However, it is not uncommon to observe an abrupt reduction in the sinus rate in response to RF ablation at a focal site of earliest atrial activation (Fig. 16-6).[22] Echocardiographic lesion characteristics using ICE can also provide a guide for directing additional RF lesions. The effective RF lesion has an increased or changed echodensity completely extending to the epicardium with the development of a trivial linear low-echodensity or echo-free interstitial space, which suggests a transmural RF lesion.[23]

Endpoints of Ablation

Acute procedural success is defined as the following: (1) abrupt reduction of the sinus rate by 30 beats/min or more during RF delivery or a 30% decline in maximum heart rate during infused isoproterenol and atropine; (2) persistence of a reduced sinus rate; (3) maintenance of a superiorly directed P wave (negative P wave in lead

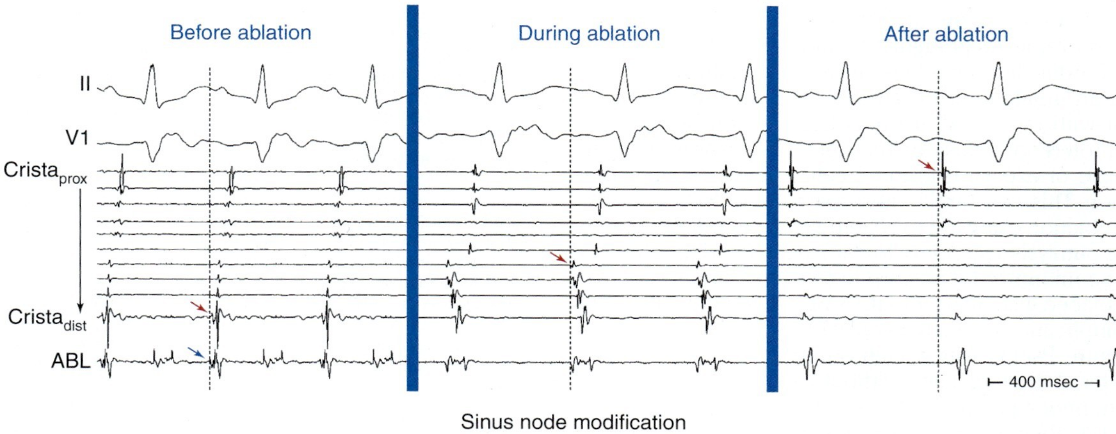

FIGURE 16-5 Intracardiac recordings during sinus node modification. **Left panel,** Before ablation (ABL) and under adrenergic stimulation, sinus tachycardia is observed, with the earliest local activation (red arrows) recorded by the most distal (cranial) electrodes of the crista catheter, just anterior to the superior vena cava–right atrial junction. Note that local activation recorded by the ablation catheter (blue arrow) precedes the onset of the P wave (indicated by the vertical dashed line) by 20 to 30 milliseconds. **Middle panel,** Following ablation of the most cranial part of the sinus node, the sinus rate becomes slower, and the activation sequence shifts toward more proximal (caudal) electrodes 7 to 8 on the crista catheter. **Right panel,** Following successful sinus node modification, the sinus rate (under constant adrenergic stimulation) is reduced by more than 30%, and the atrial activation sequence shifts to the most proximal (caudal) crista catheter electrodes. Note the P wave is now inverted in lead II. dist = distal; prox = proximal.

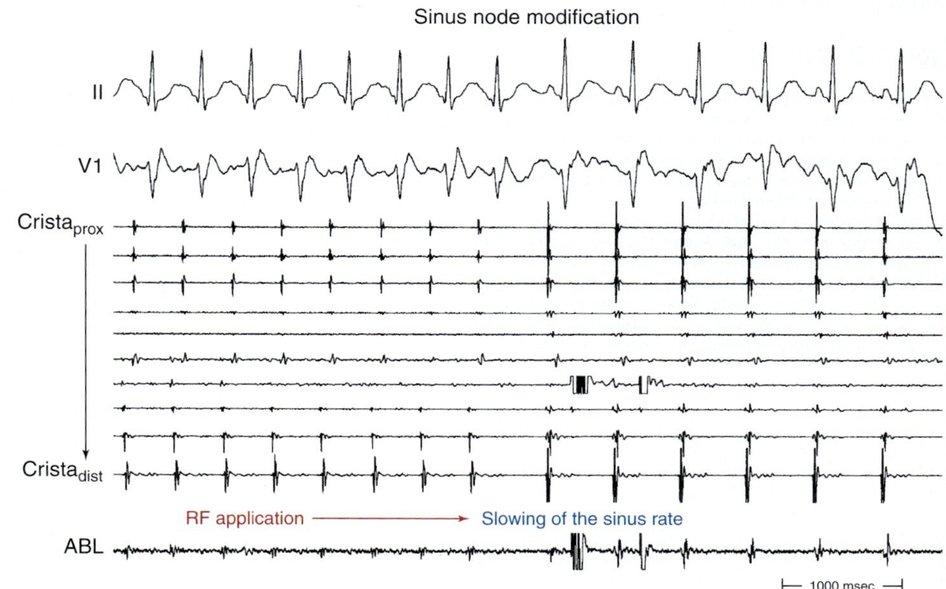

FIGURE 16-6 Intracardiac recordings during sinus node modification. An abrupt reduction in the sinus rate is observed in response to radiofrequency (RF) ablation (ABL) at a focal site of earliest atrial activation. dist = distal; prox = proximal.

III); and (4) inferior shift of the site of earliest atrial activation down the crista terminalis, even with maximal adrenergic stimulation.[2,3,22]

RF ablation of IST often is difficult and requires multiple RF applications; a mean of 12 RF applications (range, 6 to 92) was required in one study (see Fig. 16-4).[19] The resilience of the sinus node to endocardial catheter ablation can be explained, in part, by the architectural features of the node—the dense matrix of connective tissue in which the specialized sinus node cells are packed; the cooling effect of the nodal artery; the subepicardial nodal location; and the thick terminal crest, particularly in relation to the nodal portion caudal to the sinus node artery. Additionally, the length of the sinus node, the absence of an insulating sheath, the presence of nodal radiations, and caudal fragments offer a potential for multiple breakthroughs of the nodal wavefront.[18]

Outcome

Prior to undertaking ablation of the sinus node for IST, the physician and patient should have realistic expectations and understanding of the goals of ablation and potential outcomes. Relatively few patients will achieve the desired combination of relief of symptoms and normal resting heart rate and chronotropic response without the need for implantation of a permanent pacemaker. In some patients, symptoms persist despite an acceptable technical result.[2,3]

RF ablation is at best only a modestly effective technique for managing patients with IST. The long-term success rate is variable, ranging between 23% and 83%.[8] Complete ablation of the sinus node resulting in junctional rhythm has better long-term success (72%) but requires pacemaker insertion. Most recurrences occur 1 to 6 months after the procedure and are typically related to tachycardia recurrence after an initially successful procedure. A repeat procedure may be necessary in patients with intolerable symptoms. Symptomatic recurrence or persistence of symptoms in the absence of documented IST and despite persisting evidence of a successful EP outcome has been observed in some cases. Persistent symptoms despite heart rate reduction may be suggestive of a more global dysautonomia that also happens to affect the sinus node.[2,3,20-22]

Complications of sinus node modification include cardiac tamponade, SVC syndrome, diaphragmatic paralysis, and sinus node dysfunction.[24] Cardiac tamponade is rare and is usually caused by penetration of an unattended right ventricular catheter in a thin female patient with rapid and vigorous heart action because of high-dose isoproterenol infusion. Transient SVC syndrome can develop because of extensive lesion creation and edema at the SVC-RA junction. This can rarely cause permanent SVC stenosis. More targeted ablation using ICE may help avoid this complication. Diaphragmatic paralysis secondary to damage to the right phrenic nerve should be minimized if ablative lesions are confined to the crista itself or placed just anterior to it. Using ICE to guide ablation makes this complication unlikely because the phrenic nerve is a posterior structure. Pacing with a high output of 10 mA from the ablation catheter at the target site without capture of the phrenic nerve and continuous pacing in the SVC to capture the phrenic nerve during RA ablation are reassuring, but their efficacy has never been assessed. Additionally, suspicion of phrenic nerve injury should be considered in the case of hiccup, cough, or decrease in diaphragmatic excursion during energy delivery. Early recognition of phrenic nerve injury during RF delivery allows the immediate interruption of the application prior to the onset of permanent injury and is associated with rapid recovery of phrenic nerve function. Persistent junctional rhythm requiring pacemaker insertion is rare. Such junctional rhythm usually disappears with the return of sinus rhythm within several days.[2,3,22]

REFERENCES

1. Blomstrom-Lundqvist C, Scheinman MM, Aliot EM, et al: ACC/AHA/ESC guidelines for the management of patients with supraventricular arrhythmias—executive summary: a report of the American College of Cardiology/American Heart Association Task Force on Practice Guidelines and the European Society of Cardiology Committee for Practice Guidelines (Writing Committee to Develop Guidelines for the Management of Patients With Supraventricular Arrhythmias), *Circulation* 108:1871–1909, 2003.
2. Line D, Callans D: Sinus rhythm abnormalities. In Zipes DP, Jalife J, editors: *Cardiac electrophysiology: from cell to bedside*, ed 4, Philadelphia, 2004, Saunders, pp 479–484.
3. Desh M, Karch M, Kalman J, et al: Ablation of inappropriate sinus tachycardia. In Huang S, Wilber D, editors: *Radiofrequency catheter ablation of cardiac arrhythmias: basic concepts and clinical applications*, ed 2, Armonk, NY, 2000, Futura, pp 165–174.
4. Leon H, Guzman JC, Kuusela T, et al: Impaired baroreflex gain in patients with inappropriate sinus tachycardia, *J Cardiovasc Electrophysiol* 16:64–68, 2005.
5. Nattel S: Inappropriate sinus tachycardia and beta-receptor autoantibodies: a mechanistic breakthrough? *Heart Rhythm* 3:1187–1188, 2006.
6. Chiale PA, Garro HA, Schmidberg J, et al: Inappropriate sinus tachycardia may be related to an immunologic disorder involving cardiac beta adrenergic receptors, *Heart Rhythm* 3:1182–1186, 2006.
7. Zhou J, Scherlag BJ, Niu G, et al: Anatomy and physiology of the right interganglionic nerve: implications for the pathophysiology of inappropriate sinus tachycardia, *J Cardiovasc Electrophysiol* 19:971–976, 2008.
8. Shen WK, Low PA, Jahangir A, et al: Is sinus node modification appropriate for inappropriate sinus tachycardia with features of postural orthostatic tachycardia syndrome? *Pacing Clin Electrophysiol* 24:217–230, 2001.
9. Goldstein DS, Holmes C, Frank SM, et al: Cardiac sympathetic dysautonomia in chronic orthostatic intolerance syndromes, *Circulation* 106:2358–2365, 2002.
10. Still AM, Raatikainen P, Ylitalo A, et al: Prevalence, characteristics and natural course of inappropriate sinus tachycardia, *Europace* 7:104–112, 2005.
11. Winum PF, Cayla G, Rubini M, et al: A case of cardiomyopathy induced by inappropriate sinus tachycardia and cured by ivabradine, *Pacing Clin Electrophysiol* 32:942–944, 2009.
12. Shen WK: Modification and ablation for inappropriate sinus tachycardia: current status, *Card Electrophysiol Rev* 6:349–355, 2002.
13. Brady PA, Low PA, Shen WK: Inappropriate sinus tachycardia, postural orthostatic tachycardia syndrome, and overlapping syndromes, *Pacing Clin Electrophysiol* 28:1112–1121, 2005.
14. Vatasescu R, Shalganov T, Kardos A, et al: Right diaphragmatic paralysis following endocardial cryothermal ablation of inappropriate sinus tachycardia, *Europace* 8:904–906, 2006.
15. Grubb BP: Postural tachycardia syndrome, *Circulation* 117:2814–2817, 2008.
16. Schulze V, Steiner S, Hennersdorf M, Strauer BE: Ivabradine as an alternative therapeutic trial in the therapy of inappropriate sinus tachycardia: a case report, *Cardiology* 110:206–208, 2008.
17. Calo L, Rebecchi M, Sette A, et al: Efficacy of ivabradine administration in patients affected by inappropriate sinus tachycardia, *Heart Rhythm* 7:1318–1323, 2010.
18. Sanchez-Quintana D, Cabrera JA, Farre J, et al: Sinus node revisited in the era of electroanatomical mapping and catheter ablation, *Heart* 91:189–194, 2005.
19. Ren JF, Marchlinski FE, Callans DJ, Zado ES: Echocardiographic lesion characteristics associated with successful ablation of inappropriate sinus tachycardia, *J Cardiovasc Electrophysiol* 12:814–818, 2001.
20. Mantovan R, Thiene G, Calzolari V, Basso C: Sinus node ablation for inappropriate sinus tachycardia, *J Cardiovasc Electrophysiol* 16:804–806, 2005.
21. Marrouche NF, Beheiry S, Tomassoni G, et al: Three-dimensional nonfluoroscopic mapping and ablation of inappropriate sinus tachycardia: procedural strategies and long-term outcome, *J Am Coll Cardiol* 39:1046–1054, 2002.
22. Man KC, Knight B, Tse HF, et al: Radiofrequency catheter ablation of inappropriate sinus tachycardia guided by activation mapping, *J Am Coll Cardiol* 35:451–457, 2000.
23. Ren JF, Callans D: Intracardiac echocardiography imaging in radiofrequency catheter ablation for inappropriate sinus tachycardia and atrial tachycardias. In Ren JF, Marchlinski FE, Callans D, editors: *Practical intracardiac echocardiography in electrophysiology*, Malden, Mass, 2006, Blackwell Futura, pp 74–87.
24. Leonelli FM, Pisano E, Requarth JA, et al: Frequency of superior vena cava syndrome following radiofrequency modification of the sinus node and its management, *Am J Cardiol* 85:771–774, A9, 2000.

CHAPTER 17 Atrioventricular Nodal Reentrant Tachycardia

Pathophysiology

Anatomy and Physiology of the Atrioventricular Node

The atrioventricular (AV) junction is a complex structure, located within an area called the triangle of Koch (Fig. 17-1).[1] The triangle of Koch is bounded by the coronary sinus ostium (CS os) posteriorly, the tricuspid annulus (the attachment of the septal leaflet of the tricuspid valve) inferiorly, and the tendon of Todaro anteriorly and superiorly. The triangle of Koch is septal in location and constitutes the right atrial (RA) endocardial surface of the muscular AV septum. The compact AV node (AVN) lies just beneath the RA endocardium, at the apex of the triangle of Koch, anterior to the CS os, and directly above the insertion of the septal leaflet of the tricuspid valve, where the tendon of Todaro merges with the central fibrous body. Slightly more anteriorly and superiorly is where the His bundle (HB) lies. The mean distances from the HB electrogram recording site to the upper and lower lips of the CS os are 10 mm (range, 0 to 23 mm), and 20 to 25 mm (range, 9 to 46 mm), respectively. However, the contour of the Koch triangle may be small or even horizontal in some patients.[2-4]

Functionally, based on activation times during anterograde or retrograde propagation, or both, and on the action potential characteristics from microelectrode recordings in the rabbit AV junction, the cells of the AVN region are frequently described as AN (atrionodal), N (nodal), and NH (nodal-His). The transition from one cell area to the other is gradual, with intermediate cells exhibiting intermediate action potentials with great changes related to the autonomic tone.[2-6]

The AN region corresponds to the cells in the transitional zone, which are activated shortly after the atrial cells. The transitional cell zone represents the inferior, more open portion of the AVN into which atrial bands gradually merge (i.e., the approaches from the working atrial myocardium to the AVN). Transitional cells are histologically distinct from both the cells of the compact AVN and the working atrial myocytes. Transitional cells are not insulated from the surrounding myocardium but tend to be separated from one another by thin fibrous strands. The connections between atrial and transitional cells are so gradual that no clear anatomical demarcations can be detected.[7] Transitional cells do not represent conducting tracts, but rather a bridge funneling of atrial depolarization into the compact AVN through discrete AVN inputs (approaches). In humans and animals, two such inputs are commonly recognized in the right septal region: the anterior (superior) approaches, which travel from the anterior limbus of the fossa ovalis and merge with the AVN closer to the apex of the triangle of Koch, and the posterior (inferior) approaches, located in the inferoseptal RA and which serve as a bridge with the atrial myocardium at the CS os. Although both inputs have traditionally been assumed to be RA structures, growing evidence supports the AV conduction apparatus as a transseptal structure that reaches both atria. A third, middle group of transitional cells has also been identified to account for the nodal connections with the septum and left atrium (LA).[2,5,8-12]

The N region corresponds to the compact AVN, the region where transitional cells merge with midnodal cells. The N cells represent the most typical of the nodal cells because they are characterized by a less negative resting membrane potential and low action potential amplitude (mediated by the L-type calcium [Ca^{+2}] current), slow rates of depolarization and repolarization, few intercellular connections such as gap junctions, and reduced excitability compared with surrounding cells. The N cells in the compact AVN appear to be responsible for the major part of AV conduction delay. Sodium channel density is lower in the midnodal zone of the AVN than in the AN and NH cell zones, and the inward L-type Ca^{2+} current is the basis of the upstroke of the N cell action potential. Therefore, conduction is slower through the compact AVN than through the AN and NH cell zones.[1,6] Fast pathway conduction through the AVN apparently bypasses many of the N cells by transitional cells, whereas slow pathway conduction traverses the entire compact AVN. Importantly, the recovery of excitability after conduction of an impulse is faster for the slow pathway than for the fast pathway for reasons that are unclear.[5,6,13]

The NH region corresponds to the lower nodal cells, typically distal to the site of Wenckebach block, connecting to the insulated penetrating portion of the HB. The action potentials of the NH cells are closer in appearance to the fast-rising and long action potentials of the HB.

When traced inferiorly, toward the base of the triangle of Koch, the compact AVN area separates into two extensions, usually with the artery supplying the AVN running between them. The prongs bifurcate toward the CS os and tricuspid annulus (right posterior extension) and toward the mitral annulus (left posterior extension). The right posterior nodal extension has been implicated as the anatomical substrate for the so-called slow pathway in the AVN reentrant tachycardia (AVNRT) circuit. The tachycardia circuit may seldom involve the left posterior nodal extension (see later). The fast pathway is less well defined from an anatomical and structural standpoint. The probable anatomical substrate of this pathway consists of the transitional cell layers located around the compact AVN at the interface between the compact node and transitional cells.[3,4,12,14] The HB connects with the distal part of the compact AVN and passes through the fibrous core of the central fibrous body in a leftward direction (away from the RA endocardium and

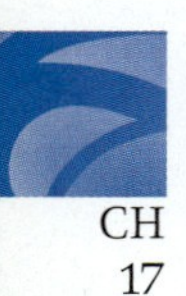

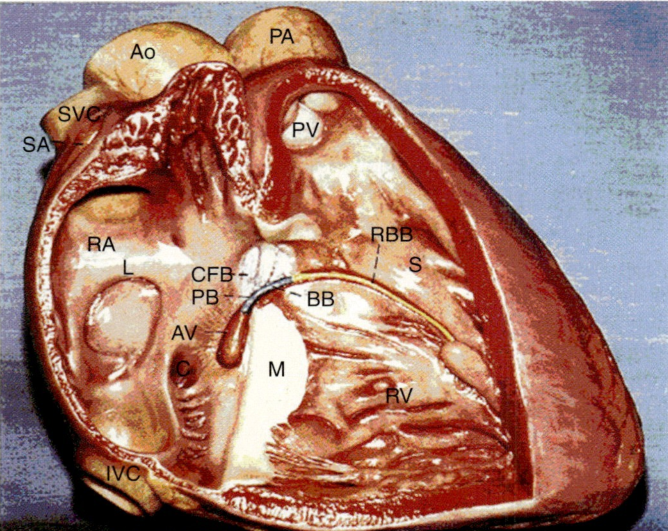

FIGURE 17-1 Right lateral view of the right atrium (RA). Ao = aorta; AV = atrioventricular node; BB = bundle of His, branching portion; C = coronary sinus; CFB = central fibrous body; IVC = inferior vena cava; L = limbus of the fossa ovalis; M = medial (septal) leaflet of the tricuspid valve; PA = pulmonary artery; PB = bundle of His, penetrating portion; PV = pulmonic valve; RBB = right bundle branch; RV = right ventricle; S = septal band of the crista supraventricularis; SA = sinoatrial node; SVC = superior vena cava. *(From Saffitz J, Zimmerman F, Lindsay B: In Braunwald E, McManus BM, editors: Atlas of cardiovascular pathology for the clinician, Philadelphia, 2000, Wiley-Blackwell, p 21.)*

toward the ventricular septum). The HB then continues through the annulus fibrosis, where it is called the nonbranching portion as it penetrates the membranous septum, along the crest of the left side of the interventricular septum, for 1 to 2 cm and then divides into the right bundle branch (RB) and left bundle branch (LB). The HB is insulated from the atrial myocardium by the membranous septum and from the ventricular myocardium by connective tissue of the central fibrous body.[1] Viewed from the left ventricle (LV), the HB is marked by the area of fibrous continuity between the aortic and mitral valves adjacent to the membranous septum. Viewed from the aorta, the HB passes beneath the part of the membranous septum that adjoins the interleaflet fibrous triangle between the right and noncoronary sinuses.[12]

Tachycardia Circuit

The concept of AVN reentry is related, but not identical, to the so-called dual pathway electrophysiology. It is well established that dual AVN physiology is the underlying substrate for AVNRT; however, it is important to recognize that dual AVN physiology characterizes the normal AVN electrophysiology, and the presence of dual (or multiple) AVN pathways is not necessarily indicative of the existence of functional reentry, although it is required to maintain the reentry circuit. Nevertheless, the presence of dual AVN physiology provides the natural substrate for the occurrence of AVN reentry. In the absence of an animal model, however, the exact pathophysiological substrate for AVNRT remains uncertain.[4]

The AVNRT circuit does not involve the ventricles, but whether the circuit is confined to the compact AVN (subatrial) or involves a component of perinodal atrial myocardium is controversial. There is good evidence that the distal junction of the slow and fast pathways is located in the AVN, with the existence of a region of AVN tissue extending between the distal junction of the two pathways and the HB (called the lower common pathway), at least in a subset of patients (Table 17-1). However, the nature of the proximal link between these pathways is unclear, and the existence of an upper common pathway is still a matter of controversy (Tables 17-2 and 17-3). Based on rare cases of dissociation of atrial activation from the tachycardia (e.g., persistence of AVNRT during different patterns of VA block) and on similarities between fast-slow AV conduction and longitudinal-transverse conduction in nonuniform anisotropy, early studies proposed that AVNRT results from reentry within the compact AVN because of functional longitudinal

TABLE 17-1 Evidence against the Necessity of Ventricle in Reentrant Circuit*

VA Wenckebach CL during ventricular pacing longer than the tachycardia CL
HA interval during ventricular pacing at the tachycardia CL longer than that during AVNRT
AV block occurring without interruption of AVNRT
AES during AVNRT resulting in changes in the relative activation of HB and atrium (i.e., varying HA intervals)
VES during AVNRT prematurely depolarizing the HB without affecting the tachycardia

*Supporting the presence of a lower common pathway.
AES = atrial extrastimulation; AV = atrioventricular; AVNRT = atrioventricular nodal reentrant tachycardia; CL = cycle length; HA = His bundle–atrial; HB = His bundle; VA = ventriculoatrial; VES = ventricular extrastimulation.
From Josephson ME: Supraventricular tachycardias. In Josephson ME, editor: *Clinical cardiac electrophysiology,* ed 3, Philadelphia, 2002, Lippincott Williams & Wilkins, pp 168-271.

TABLE 17-2 Evidence for the Necessity of Atrium in Reentrant Circuit*

The finding that AES delivered to the inferior atrial septum close to the CS os during AVNRT just before the expected time of retrograde fast pathway conduction can activate the slow pathway and advance the SVT
The finding that cure of AVNRT can be produced by placing ablative lesions in the perinodal atrial myocardium, as much as 10 mm or more from the compact AVN
Differences in the site of earliest atrial activation between retrograde conduction over the fast and slow pathways
Microelectrode and extracellular recordings and optical mapping of AVN reentrant echo beats in animals

*That is, against the presence of an upper common pathway.
AES = atrial extrastimulation; AVN = atrioventricular node; AVNRT = atrioventricular nodal reentrant tachycardia; CS os = coronary sinus ostium; SVT = supraventricular tachycardia.
From Josephson ME: Supraventricular tachycardias. In Josephson ME, editor: *Clinical cardiac electrophysiology,* ed 3, Philadelphia, 2002, Lippincott Williams & Wilkins, pp 168-271.

TABLE 17-3 Evidence against the Necessity of Atrium in Reentrant Circuit*

Initiation of AVNRT in the absence of an atrial echo
AV Wenckebach CL during atrial pacing longer than the tachycardia CL
AH interval during atrial pacing at the tachycardia CL longer than that during AVNRT
Retrograde VA block occurring without interruption of AVNRT
AVNRT occurrence in the presence of AF
Depolarization of the atria surrounding the AVN without affecting the tachycardia
Resetting of the tachycardia by ventricular stimulation in the absence of atrial activation
Heterogeneous atrial activation during AVNRT that is incompatible with atrial participation
Changing VA relationship with minimal or no change in the tachycardia CL (suggesting that atrial activation is determined by the functional output to the atrium from the tachycardia and not causally related to it)

*Supporting the presence of an upper common pathway.
AF = atrial fibrillation; AH = atrial–His bundle; AV = atrioventricular; AVN = atrioventricular node; AVNRT = atrioventricular nodal reentrant tachycardia; CL = cycle length; VA = ventriculoatrial.
From Josephson ME: Supraventricular tachycardias. In Josephson ME, editor: *Clinical cardiac electrophysiology,* ed 3, Philadelphia, 2002, Lippincott Williams & Wilkins, pp 168-271.

TABLE 17-4 Functional Differences between Fast and Slow Atrioventricular Node Pathways
The fast pathway forms the normal physiological conduction axis, and the AH interval during conduction over the fast pathway is usually no longer than 220 msec. Longer AH intervals can be caused by conduction over the slow pathway.
Anterograde ERP of the fast pathway is usually longer than that of the slow pathway. However, many exceptions exist.
Adrenergic stimulation tends to shorten the anterograde and retrograde ERP of the fast pathway to a greater extent than that of the slow pathway. Conversely, beta blockers tend to prolong ERP of the fast pathway more than that of the slow pathway.
The earliest atrial activation site during retrograde conduction over the fast pathway is in the anterior apex of the triangle of Koch at the same site recording the proximal His potential (although some studies showed the earliest site of atrial activation occurring in the anterior interatrial septum above the tendon of Todaro, outside the triangle of Koch), whereas that over the slow pathway is in the base of the triangle of Koch.

AH = atrial–His bundle; ERP = effective refractory period.

dissociation within the AVN into fast and slow pathways and suggested the presence of an upper common pathway, at least in a subset of patients.[13,15]

Current evidence, derived from multielectrode recordings and optical mapping studies, supports the role of perinodal tissue and suggests that the fast and slow pathways involved in the reentrant circuit of AVNRT represent conduction over different atrionodal connections, thus making at least a small amount of atrial tissue a necessary part of the reentrant circuit (Video 19). As noted, the compact AVN is surrounded by transitional cells whose structure and function are intermediate between those of atrial and compact nodal cells. If one considers the compact AVN and the surrounding transitional cells as a functional AVN unit, which implies that the AVN tissue occupies the bulk of the triangle of Koch, then the AVN reentrant circuit may be considered as confined to the AVN. Therefore, much of the disagreement on the presence or absence of an upper common pathway and the role of the atrium in the genesis of the reentrant circuit may, in part, be related to the definition of the extent of the AVN.[16]

Nevertheless, the understanding of the AVN as having superior (anterior) and inferior (posterior) inputs that form the fast and slow pathways, respectively, is a simple conceptual framework that seems to enable the clinician to confront most cases. Reentry occurring along these pathways is the basic mechanism for the various subtypes of AVNRT. The proximal atrial insertions of the fast and slow pathways are anatomically distinct during retrograde conduction, and several important functional differences exist between the two pathways (Table 17-4).[13,14]

Multiple slow pathways (as demonstrated by multiple discontinuities in the AVN function curves; see later) are present in up to 14% of patients with AVNRT, although not all these pathways are involved in the initiation and maintenance of AVNRT. Whether these pathways represent discrete anatomically distinct circuits or are functionally present because of nonuniform anisotropy is unclear. Frequently, multiple slow pathways are in close proximity within the triangle of Koch, and elimination of multiple slow pathways with radiofrequency (RF) ablation at one site is observed in approximately 42% of cases. Slow pathways with longer conduction times have a more inferior location in the triangle of Koch when compared with locations producing a shorter atrial-HB (AH) interval.

Types of Atrioventricular Nodal Reentry

SLOW-FAST (TYPICAL, COMMON) ATRIOVENTRICULAR NODAL REENTRANT TACHYCARDIA

Typical AVNRT accounts for 90% of AVNRTs. The reentrant circuit uses the slow AVN pathway anterogradely and the fast pathway retrogradely. The earliest atrial activation during typical AVNRT is usually in the apex of the triangle of Koch; however, retrograde atrial activation over the fast pathway is heterogeneous and may be found at the CS os or on the left side of the septum in up to 9% of patients (Fig. 17-2).[8,13,17,18]

During typical AVNRT, atrial and ventricular activations occur almost simultaneously. The AH interval is relatively long (more than 200 milliseconds) and the HA interval is relatively short (less than 70 milliseconds), resulting in a short RP tachycardia.

The presence of a lower common pathway in typical AVNRT remains controversial. Although some studies suggested the existence of a lower common pathway in most patients with typical AVNRT, others demonstrated that most patients with AVNRT without evidence of a substantial lower common pathway had typical AVNRT (i.e., the lower turnaround is within the proximal HB), and the presence of a lower common pathway was strongly associated with the atypical variants of AVNRT. Nevertheless, it is recognized that the lower common pathway in typical AVNRT, if present, is very short (as assessed by the degree of HB prematurity required for a ventricular extrastimulus [VES] to reset the tachycardia, and by comparing the HB-atrial (HA) interval during AVNRT with that during ventricular pacing at the tachycardia cycle length [CL]).[8]

FAST-SLOW (ATYPICAL, UNCOMMON) ATRIOVENTRICULAR NODAL REENTRANT TACHYCARDIA

In this variant of AVNRT, the reentrant circuit uses the fast AVN pathway anterogradely and the slow pathway retrogradely. Although fast-slow AVNRT is thought of as using the same circuit as typical AVNRT but in the reverse direction, two previous studies reported different anatomical sites for the anterograde and retrograde slow pathways, and the fast-slow form of AVNRT may not be exactly the reverse form of the slow-fast form of AVNRT in some patients.

The earliest retrograde atrial activation during fast-slow AVNRT is usually in the inferoposterior part of the triangle of Koch. The AH interval is shorter than the HA interval (30 to 185 milliseconds versus 135 to 435 milliseconds), resulting in long RP tachycardia. The lower common pathway is relatively long.[8,19]

SLOW-SLOW (POSTERIOR-TYPE) ATRIOVENTRICULAR NODAL REENTRANT TACHYCARDIA

In slow-slow AVNRT, the reentrant circuit uses a slow or an intermediate pathway anterogradely and a second slow pathway retrogradely. The earliest retrograde atrial activation occurs along the roof of the proximal CS or, less commonly, at the inferoposterior part of the triangle of Koch.

The AH interval is long (more than 200 milliseconds). The HA interval is often short, but it has a much wider range than that in typical AVNRT (–30 to 260 milliseconds, usually more than 70 milliseconds). The ventriculoatrial (VA) interval (as measured from the onset of ventricular activity to the onset of atrial activity by whichever electrode recorded the earliest interval) may be prolonged, ranging from 76 to 168 milliseconds. The AH/HA ratio, however, remains greater than 1. Therefore, this type is sometimes called slow-intermediate AVNRT. The lower common pathway is significantly longer than that in typical AVNRT, a finding that explains the short HA interval seen in many patients with slow-slow AVNRT. These patients often exhibit multiple AH interval jumps during atrial extrastimulus (AES) testing, consistent with multiple slow pathways.[8]

LEFT VARIANT OF ATRIOVENTRICULAR NODAL REENTRANT TACHYCARDIA

It has been known for some time that the slow pathway may be composed of both rightward and leftward posterior nodal extensions. The rightward extensions travel anatomically in the triangle of Koch between the tricuspid annulus and the CS os. The leftward extensions travel within the myocardial coat of the proximal CS

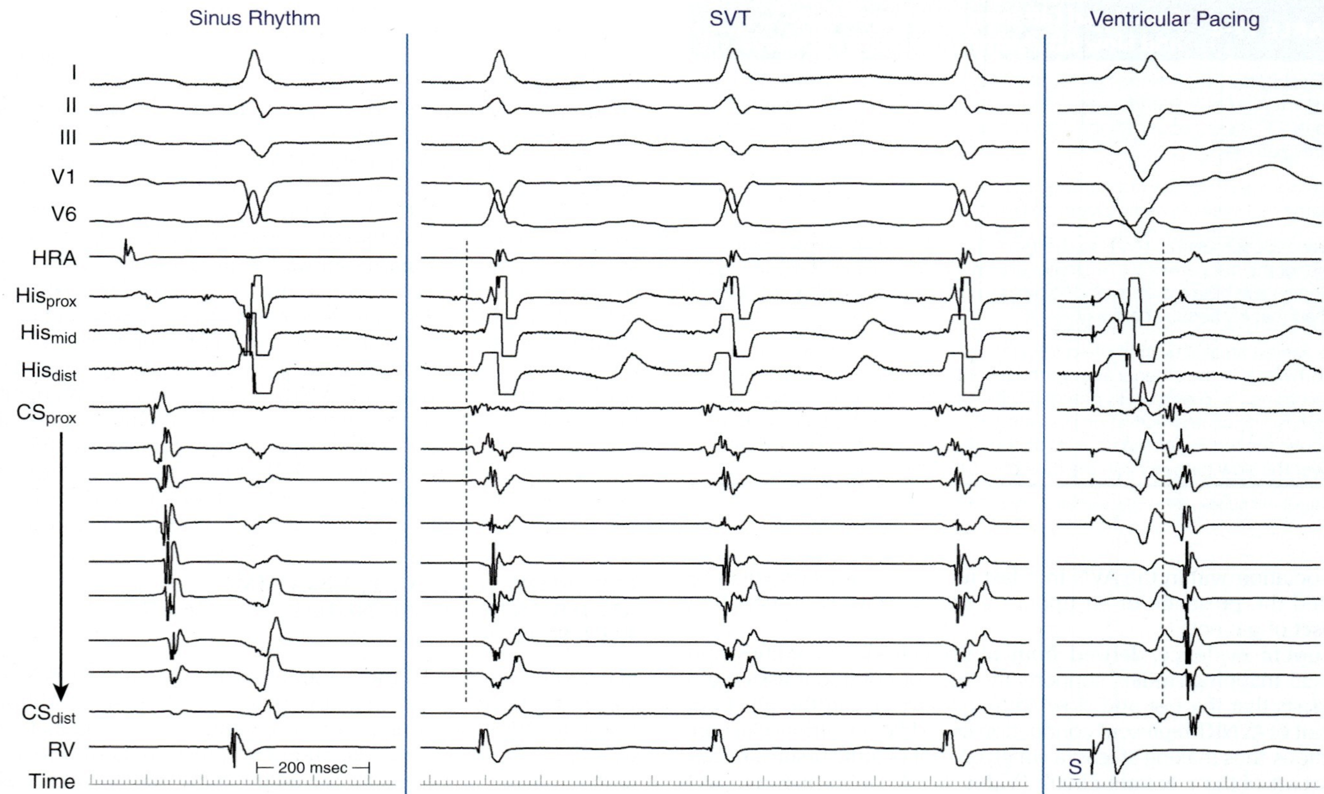

FIGURE 17-2 Atrioventricular nodal reentrant tachycardia (AVNRT) with early atrial activation in the coronary sinus (CS) ostium region. Sinus rhythm is shown on the **left**, slow-fast AVNRT is shown in the **center**, and ventricular pacing during sinus rhythm appears on the **right**. The dashed line denotes earliest atrial activation (proximal CS, near ostium), significantly before the His bundle atrial activation (most visible during ventricular pacing). CS_{dist} = distal coronary sinus; CS_{prox} = proximal coronary sinus; His_{dist} = distal His bundle; His_{mid} = middle His bundle; His_{prox} = proximal His bundle; HRA = high right atrium; RV = right ventricle.

leftward (transseptally) toward the left inferoseptal region and mitral annulus. These leftward extensions can then connect with the rightward extensions in the triangle of Koch anterior to the CS os. The leftward inferior extension can provide an LA input to the AVN, as suggested by functional studies showing preferential access to the AVN from the left inferior septum. Clinically, the leftward inferior nodal extension can behave as the slow pathway and lead to AVNRT. In the typical (slow-fast) form of AVNRT, this would render ablation in the usual inferoseptal RA ineffective and lead to the necessity of ablating inside the CS or on the posterior mitral annulus.[8] In atypical forms of AVNRT, if the leftward inferior extension serves as the slow pathway conducting retrogradely, then the earliest atrial activation would be recorded in the LA, thus leading to eccentric CS activation.[9]

Eccentric retrograde atrial activation sequences that are suggestive of leftward atrionodal extensions of the slow AVN pathway have been described in AVNRT, but the exact incidence is unknown. Various reports have shown a higher incidence of the eccentric CS activation pattern among patients with atypical (14% to 80%) than those with typical (0% to 8%) forms of AVNRT.[8,18,20,21] However, even in the presence of eccentric retrograde atrial activation during AVNRT, the significance of such leftward extensions to the AVNRT circuit has been debated. Whether the retrograde left-sided atrionodal connection constitutes the critical component of the reentrant circuit or is only an innocent bystander in atypical AVNRT with the eccentric CS activation pattern is controversial. It may be possible for both the leftward and rightward extensions, either together or separately, to participate in nodal reentry. Right-sided ablation is probably sufficient for most of these patients. However, in some patients, the slow pathway participating in the reentrant circuit cannot be ablated from the posteroseptal RA or the CS os, but it can be eliminated by ablation along the roof of the CS, as much as 5 to 6 cm from the CS os, or mitral annulus. In one report, direct left-sided ablation to the earliest retrograde activation site inside the CS (without ablation at the conventional site of the slow pathway) rendered the tachycardias noninducible in all 18 patients, a finding suggesting that the left-sided slow pathway constituted critical parts of the reentrant circuit.[8,22]

SUPERIOR VARIANT OF ATRIOVENTRICULAR NODAL REENTRANT TACHYCARDIA

The superior variant of AVNRT uses a slowly conducting retrograde pathway with a superoseptal atrial exit as a retrograde limb and is associated with evidence of a lower common pathway. The anterograde limb of the circuit is likely the fast pathway. The superior variant of atypical AVNRT has been observed in 3% of all forms of AVNRT, and it is characterized by a shorter AH and longer HA interval during the tachycardia, a longer HA interval during ventricular pacing, and earliest retrograde atrial activation in the superoseptal RA. Whereas classical slow pathway ablation in the inferoseptal RA or proximal CS is highly successful in eliminating most types of AVNRT, it is inefficient in eliminating the superior variant of AVNRT. Instead, the tachycardia was eliminated in most patients in one report by ablation in the midseptal RA (where no His potential is recorded). Those observations suggest that the entire components of the tachycardia circuit in the superior type of atypical AVNRT may be localized to the superior part of the Koch triangle as compared with those in the inferior type. The mechanism by which ablation in the midseptal RA, not in the superoseptal RA where the earliest retrograde atrial activation was recorded, modified the retrograde slow pathway conduction properties and eliminated the tachycardia inducibility of the superior type is unclear.[23]

Clinical Considerations

Epidemiology

AVNRT is the most common form of paroxysmal supraventricular tachycardia (SVT). The absolute number of patients with AVNRT and its proportion of paroxysmal SVT increase with age. The reason may be related to the normal evolution of AVN physiology over the first two decades of life, as well as to age-related changes in atrial and nodal physiology observed in later decades.[24] AVNRT is unusual in children less than 5 years of age, and it typically initially manifests in early life (e.g., in the teens). Conversely, atrioventricular reentrant tachycardia (AVRT) manifests earlier, with an average of more than 10 years separating the time of clinical presentation of AVRT and that of AVNRT. There is also a striking 2:1 predominance of AVNRT in women, in whom symptoms start at a significantly younger age.[24,25] In fact, female sex and older age (i.e., teens versus newborns or young children) favor the diagnosis of AVNRT over AVRT.[26] Gender differences in the anterograde and retrograde AVN electrophysiological (EP) properties have been observed and may contribute to the pathogenesis of AVNRT.[25]

Clinical Presentation

Patients with AVNRT typically present with the clinical syndrome of paroxysmal SVT. This is characterized as regular rapid tachycardia of abrupt onset and termination. Patients commonly describe palpitations and dizziness. Rapid ventricular rates can be associated with complaints of dyspnea, weakness, angina, or even frank syncope and can at times be disabling. Episodes can last from seconds to several hours. Patients often learn to use certain maneuvers such as carotid sinus massage or the Valsalva maneuver to terminate the arrhythmia, although many require pharmacological treatment. There is no significant association of AVNRT with other types of structural heart disease.

About half of patients with typical AVNRT report experiencing a pounding sensation in the neck during tachycardia, which is caused by simultaneous contraction of the atria and ventricles against closed mitral and tricuspid valves. The physical examination correlate of this phenomenon is continuous pulsing cannon A waves in the jugular venous waveform (described as the "frog" sign). This clinical feature has been reported to distinguish paroxysmal SVT resulting from AVNRT from that caused by orthodromic AVRT. Although atrial contraction during AVRT occurs against closed AV valves, the longer VA interval results in separate ventricular and then atrial contraction and a relatively lower RA and venous pressure; therefore, the presence of palpitations in the neck is experienced less commonly (about 17%) in patients with AVRT.[26]

Initial Evaluation

History, physical examination, and 12-lead ECG constitute an appropriate initial evaluation. In patients with brief, self-terminating episodes, an event recorder is the most effective way to obtain ECG documentation. An echocardiographic examination should be considered in patients with documented sustained SVT to exclude the possibility of structural heart disease.[27] Further diagnostic studies (e.g., cardiac stress testing) are indicated only if there are signs or symptoms that suggest structural heart disease.[8]

The diagnosis of AVNRT as the mechanism of SVT can be strongly suspected based on the surface ECG but is often difficult to confirm, especially when only single-lead rhythm strips are available during the SVT. EP testing, however, is not indicated unless a decision to proceed with catheter ablation is undertaken.

Principles of Management

ACUTE MANAGEMENT

Because maintenance of AVNRT is dependent on AVN conduction, maneuvers or drugs that slow AVN conduction can be used to terminate the tachycardia. Initially, maneuvers that increase vagal tone (e.g., Valsalva maneuvers, gagging, carotid sinus massage) are used.[27] When vagal maneuvers are unsuccessful, termination can be achieved with antiarrhythmic drugs whose primary effects increase refractoriness and/or decrease conduction (negative dromotropic effect) over the AVN. Adenosine is the drug of choice and is successful in almost 100% of cases.[27] Verapamil, diltiazem, and beta blockers also can terminate AVNRT and prevent induction. Digoxin, which has a slower onset of action than the other AVN blockers, is not favored for the acute termination of AVNRT, except if there are relative contraindications to the other agents. Class IA and IC sodium channel blockers can also be used in treating an acute event of AVNRT, a strategy that is rarely used when other regimens have failed. If AVNRT cannot be terminated with intravenous drugs, electrical cardioversion can always be used. Energies in the range of 10 to 50 J are usually adequate.[8]

CHRONIC MANAGEMENT

Because AVNRT is generally a benign arrhythmia that does not influence survival, the primary indication for its treatment relates to its impact on a patient's quality of life. Factors that contribute to the therapeutic decision include the frequency and duration of tachycardia, tolerance of symptoms, the effectiveness and tolerance of antiarrhythmic drugs, the need for lifelong drug therapy, and the presence of concomitant structural heart disease. Patients who develop a highly symptomatic episode of paroxysmal SVT, particularly if it requires an emergency room visit for termination, can elect to initiate therapy after a single episode. In contrast, a patient who presents with minimally symptomatic episodes of paroxysmal SVT that terminate spontaneously or in response to Valsalva maneuvers may elect to be followed clinically without specific therapy.[8,27]

Once it is decided to initiate treatment for AVNRT, the question arises whether to initiate pharmacological therapy or to use catheter ablation. Because of its high efficacy (greater than 95%) and low incidence of complications, catheter ablation has become the preferred therapy over long-term pharmacological therapy and can be offered as an initial therapeutic option. It is reasonable to discuss catheter ablation with all patients suspected of having AVNRT. However, patients considering RF ablation must be willing to accept the risk, albeit low, of AV block and pacemaker implantation. For patients in whom ablation is not desirable or available, long-term pharmacological therapy may be effective.[27]

Most pharmacological agents that depress AVN conduction (including beta blockers and calcium channel blockers) can reduce the frequency of recurrences of AVNRT. If those agents are ineffective, class IA, IC, or III antiarrhythmic agents may be considered. In general, drug efficacy is in the range of 30% to 50%.[8]

Outpatients can use a single dose of verapamil, propranolol, or flecainide to terminate an episode of AVNRT effectively. This so-called pill in the pocket approach (i.e., administration of a drug only during an episode of tachycardia for the purpose of termination of the arrhythmia when vagal maneuvers alone are not effective) is appropriate to consider for patients with infrequent episodes of AVNRT that are prolonged but well tolerated, and it obviates exposure of patients to long-term and unnecessary therapy between rare arrhythmic events. This approach necessitates the use of a drug that has a short onset of action (i.e., immediate-release preparations).[27] Candidate patients should be free of significant LV dysfunction, sinus bradycardia, and preexcitation. Single-dose oral therapy with diltiazem (120 mg) plus propranolol (80 mg) has been shown to be superior to both placebo and flecainide in terminating AVNRT.[8,27]

Electrocardiographic Features

P Wave Morphology

In typical (slow-fast) AVNRT, the P wave is usually not visible because of the simultaneous atrial and ventricular activation. The P wave can distort the initial portion of the QRS (mimicking a q wave

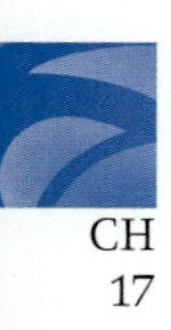

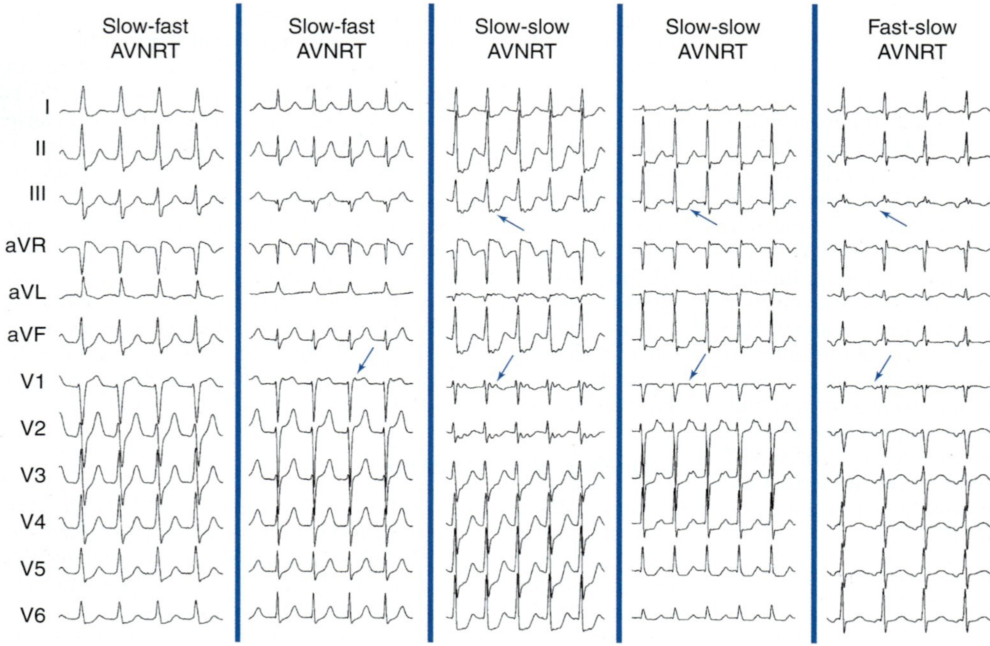

FIGURE 17-3 Surface ECG of the different types of atrioventricular nodal reentrant tachycardia (AVNRT). Arrows mark the P waves. In slow-fast (typical) AVNRT, the P wave may lie within the QRS (invisible, **first panel**) or distort the terminal portion of the QRS (mimicking an r wave in V_1, **second panel**). In slow-slow AVNRT, the P wave lies outside the QRS in the ST-T wave, and the RP interval is longer than that in slow-fast AVNRT. In fast-slow AVNRT, the P wave lies before the QRS with a long RP interval. In all varieties of AVNRT, the P wave is relatively narrow, negative in the inferior leads, and positive in V_1.

in the inferior leads), lie just within the QRS (inapparent), or distort the terminal portion of the QRS (mimicking an s wave in the inferior leads or an r wave in lead V_1) (Fig. 17-3).[8] When apparent, the P wave is significantly narrower than the sinus P wave and is negative in the inferior leads, findings consistent with concentric retrograde atrial activation over the fast AVN pathway.[8] In atypical (fast-slow) AVNRT, the P wave is relatively narrow, negative in the inferior leads, and positive in lead V_1 (see Fig. 17-3).[8]

QRS Morphology

QRS morphology during AVNRT is usually the same as in normal sinus rhythm (NSR). The development of prolonged functional aberration during AVNRT is uncommon, and it usually occurs following induction of AVNRT by ventricular stimulation more frequently than by atrial stimulation, or following resumption of 1:1 conduction to the ventricles after a period of block below the tachycardia circuit.[8] At times, alternans of QRS amplitude can occur when the tachycardia rates are rapid. Occasionally, AVNRT can coexist with ventricular preexcitation over an AV bypass tract (BT), whereby the BT is an innocent bystander.[8]

P-QRS Relationship

In typical (slow-fast) AVNRT, the RP interval is very short (–40 to 75 milliseconds). Variation of the P-QRS relationship with or without block can occur during AVNRT, especially in atypical or multiple-form tachycardias.[8] This phenomenon usually occurs when the conduction system and the reentry circuit are unstable during initiation or termination of the tachycardia, likely secondary to decremental conduction in the lower common pathway. The ECG manifestation of P-QRS variations with or without AV block during tachycardia, especially at the initiation of tachycardias or in cases of nonsustained tachycardias, should not be misdiagnosed as atrial tachycardias (ATs); these variations may represent atypical or, rarely, typical forms of AVNRT. Moreover, the variations can be of such magnitude that long RP tachycardia can masquerade for brief periods of time as short RP tachycardia.

Usually, the A/V ratio during AVNRT is equal to 1; however, 2:1 AV block can be present because of block below the reentry circuit (usually below the HB and, infrequently, in the lower common pathway). In such cases, narrow, inverted P wave morphology in the inferior leads inscribed exactly between QRS complexes strongly suggests AVNRT (Fig. 17-4). The incidence of reproducible sustained 2:1 AV block during induced episodes of AVNRT is approximately 10%. Rarely, VA block can occur because of block in an upper common pathway.[8]

In atypical (fast-slow) AVNRT, the RP interval is longer than the PR interval. In slow-slow AVNRT, the RP interval is usually shorter than, and sometimes equal to, the PR interval. Occasionally, the P wave is inscribed in the middle of the cardiac cycle, thus mimicking atrial flutter or AT with 2:1 AV conduction (Fig. 17-5).[19] Slow-slow AVNRT can be associated with RP intervals and P wave morphology similar to that during orthodromic AV reentrant tachycardia (AVRT) using a posteroseptal AV BT. However, although both SVTs have the earliest atrial activation in the posteroseptal region, conduction time from that site to the HB region is significantly longer in AVNRT than in orthodromic AVRT. The results are a significantly longer RP interval in lead V_1 and a significantly larger difference in the RP interval between lead V_1 and inferior leads during AVNRT. Therefore, ΔRP interval (V_1 – III) of more than 20 milliseconds suggests slow-slow AVNRT (sensitivity, 71%; specificity, 87%).

Electrophysiological Testing

EP testing is used to study the inducibility and mechanism of the SVT and to guide catheter ablation. Typically, three quadripolar catheters are positioned in the high RA, the right ventricular (RV) apex, and the HB region, and a decapolar catheter is positioned in the CS (see Fig. 4-7).

Baseline Observations during Normal Sinus Rhythm

ATRIAL EXTRASTIMULATION AND ATRIAL PACING DURING NORMAL SINUS RHYTHM

ANTEROGRADE DUAL ATRIOVENTRICULAR NODAL PHYSIOLOGY. Demonstration of anterograde dual AVN pathway conduction curves requires a longer effective refractory period (ERP) of the fast pathway than the slow pathway ERP and atrial functional refractory period (FRP), as well as a sufficient difference in conduction times between the two pathways. Dual AVN physiology can be diagnosed by demonstrating the following: (1) a "jump" in the AH interval in response to progressively more premature AES; (2) two ventricular responses to a single atrial impulse;

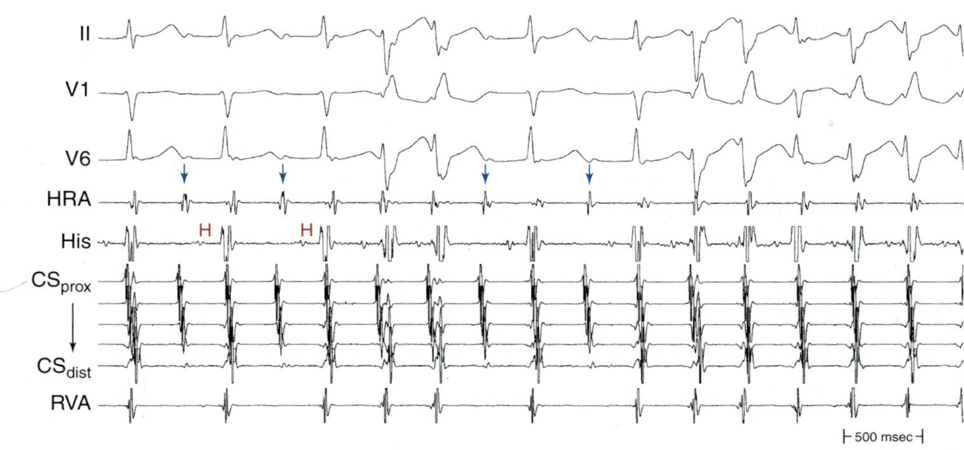

FIGURE 17-4 Typical atrioventricular nodal reentrant tachycardia (AVNRT) with intermittent 2:1 AV block. His potential (H) is observed following conducted atrial impulses, but not after blocked atrial impulses, thus indicating AV block in the lower common pathway or in the portion of the His bundle proximal to the recording site. Note that intermittent AV block results in long-short cycle sequences associated with a right bundle branch block (RBBB) pattern during complexes conducted following a short cycle. RBBB is also observed intermittently during supraventricular tachycardia with 1:1 AV conduction. Note the lack of effect of RBBB on the tachycardia cycle length (A-A interval) or ventricular-atrial (VA) interval. CS_{dist} = distal coronary sinus; CS_{prox} = proximal coronary sinus; HRA = high right atrium; RVA = right ventricular apex.

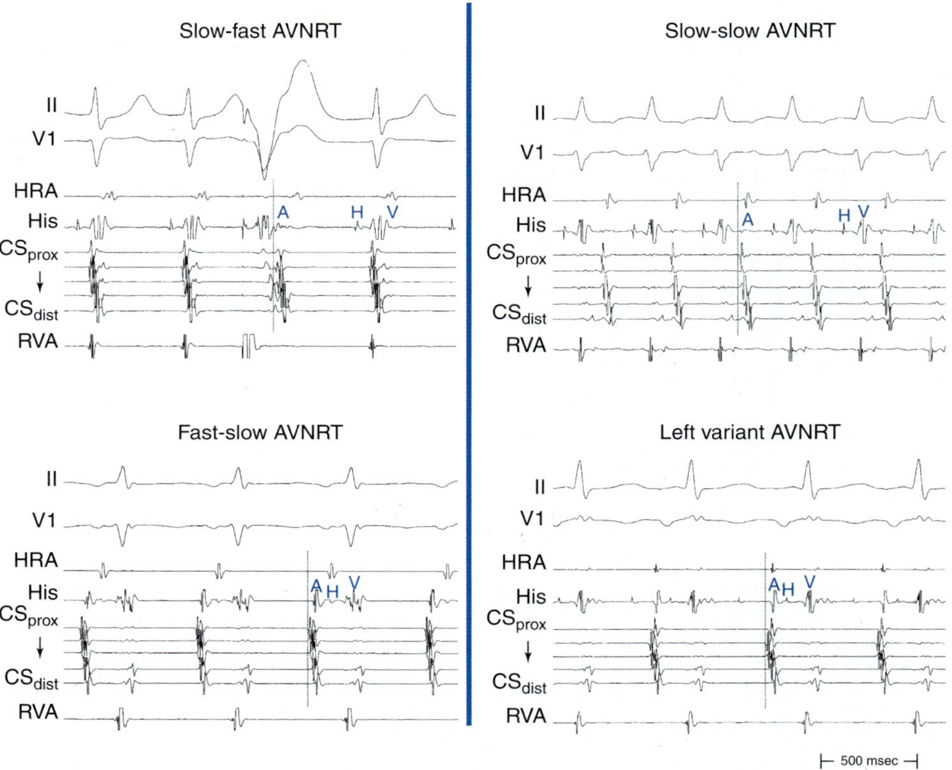

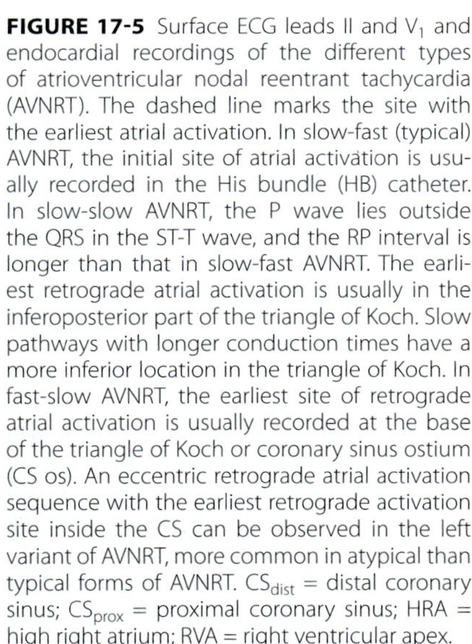

FIGURE 17-5 Surface ECG leads II and V_1 and endocardial recordings of the different types of atrioventricular nodal reentrant tachycardia (AVNRT). The dashed line marks the site with the earliest atrial activation. In slow-fast (typical) AVNRT, the initial site of atrial activation is usually recorded in the His bundle (HB) catheter. In slow-slow AVNRT, the P wave lies outside the QRS in the ST-T wave, and the RP interval is longer than that in slow-fast AVNRT. The earliest retrograde atrial activation is usually in the inferoposterior part of the triangle of Koch. Slow pathways with longer conduction times have a more inferior location in the triangle of Koch. In fast-slow AVNRT, the earliest site of retrograde atrial activation is usually recorded at the base of the triangle of Koch or coronary sinus ostium (CS os). An eccentric retrograde atrial activation sequence with the earliest retrograde activation site inside the CS can be observed in the left variant of AVNRT, more common in atypical than typical forms of AVNRT. CS_{dist} = distal coronary sinus; CS_{prox} = proximal coronary sinus; HRA = high right atrium; RVA = right ventricular apex.

(3) a PR interval exceeding the R-R interval during rapid atrial pacing; and/or (4) different PR or AH intervals during NSR or fixed-rate atrial pacing.[28]

ATRIAL-HIS INTERVAL JUMP. In contrast to the normal pattern of AVN conduction, in which the AH interval gradually lengthens in response to progressively shorter AES coupling intervals, patients with dual AVN physiology usually demonstrate a sudden increase (jump) in the AH interval at a critical AES (A_1-A_2) coupling interval (Fig. 17-6). Conduction with a short PR or AH interval reflects fast pathway conduction, whereas conduction with a long PR or AH interval reflects slow pathway conduction. The AH interval jump signals block of anterograde conduction of the progressively premature AES over the fast pathway (once the AES coupling interval becomes shorter than the fast pathway ERP) and anterograde conduction over the slow pathway (which has an ERP shorter than the AES coupling interval), with a longer conduction time (i.e., longer A_2-H_2 interval). A jump in the A_2-H_2 (or H_1-H_2) interval of 50 milliseconds or more in response to a 10-millisecond shortening of either the A_1-A_2 interval (i.e., AES coupling interval) or the A_1-A_1 interval (i.e., pacing CL) is defined as a discontinuous AVN function curve and is considered evidence of dual anterograde AVN pathways (see Fig. 4-23).[8]

1:2 RESPONSE. Rapid atrial pacing or AES can result in two ventricular complexes to a single paced atrial impulse. The first ventricular complex is caused by conduction of the atrial

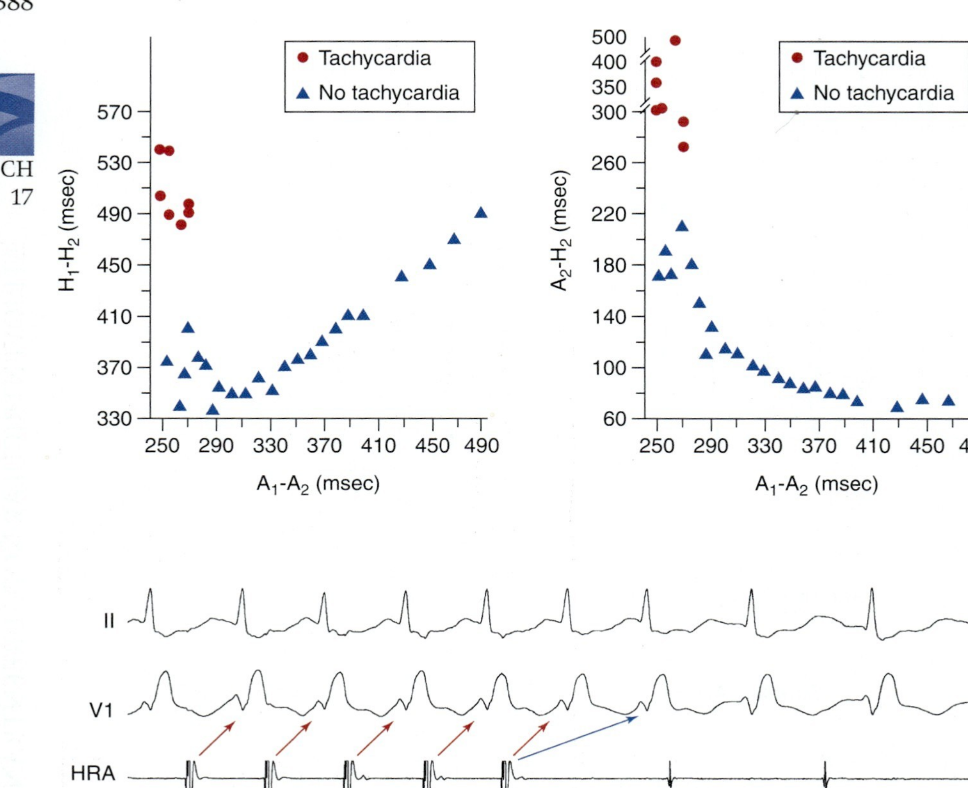

FIGURE 17-6 Dual atrioventricular node (AVN) physiology. H_1-H_2 intervals **(left)** and A_2-H_2 intervals **(right)** are at various A_1-A_2 intervals, with a discontinuous AVN curve. At a critical A_1-A_2 interval, the H_1-H_2 and A_1-H_2 intervals increase markedly. At the break in the curves, atrioventricular nodal reentrant tachycardia is initiated. *(From Olgin JE, Zipes DP: Specific arrhythmias: diagnosis and treatment. In Libby P, Bonow RO, Mann DL, Zipes DP, editors: Braunwald's heart disease: a textbook of cardiovascular medicine, ed 7, Philadelphia, 2008, Saunders, p 880.)*

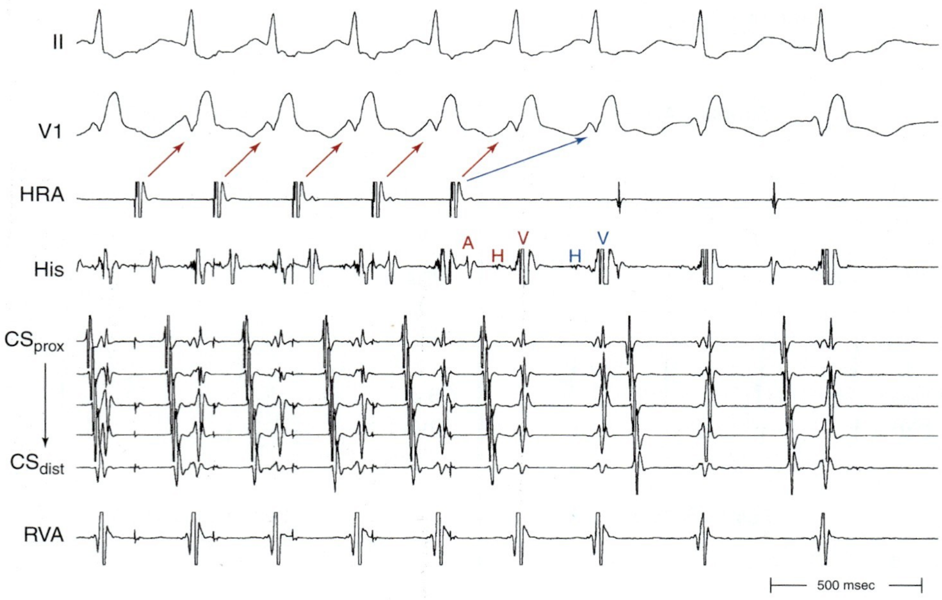

FIGURE 17-7 Rapid atrial pacing during normal sinus rhythm (NSR). Each paced atrial impulse conducts anterogradely over the fast atrioventricular node (AVN) pathway (red arrows). The last paced impulse, however, conducts anterogradely over both the fast (red arrow) and slow (blue arrow) pathways, resulting in two His bundle and ventricular responses. CS_{dist} = distal coronary sinus; CS_{prox} = proximal coronary sinus; HRA = high right atrium; RVA = right ventricular apex.

impulse over the fast AVN pathway, and the second complex is caused by conduction over the slow AVN pathway (Fig. 17-7). This response requires unidirectional retrograde block in the slow AVN pathway. Typically, in the presence of dual AVN pathways, conduction propagates simultaneously over both fast and slow AVN pathways. However, the wavefront conducting down the fast pathway reaches the distal junction of the two pathways before the impulse conducting down the slow pathway, and, subsequently, it conducts retrogradely up the slow pathway to collide with the impulse conducting anterogradely down that pathway. Thus, the anterograde impulse conducting down the slow pathway does not have the opportunity to reach the HB and ventricle. Rarely, the slow pathway conducts anterogradely only or has a very long retrograde ERP. In this setting, the wavefront traveling anterogradely down the fast pathway blocks (but does not conceal) in the slow pathway retrogradely and fails to retard the impulse traveling anterogradely down that pathway. Consequently, the wavefront traveling down the slow pathway can reach the HB and ventricle to produce a second His potential and QRS in response to a single atrial impulse. Because retrograde block in the slow pathway is a prerequisite to a 1:2 response, when such a phenomenon is present, it indicates that the slow pathway cannot support reentrant tachycardia using the slow pathway as the retrograde limb (i.e., atypical AVNRT cannot be operative). The 1:2 response should be differentiated from pseudo–simultaneous fast and slow pathway conduction, which is a much more common phenomenon during rapid atrial pacing. In the latter case, all paced atrial impulses block anterogradely in the fast pathway and conduct exclusively down the slow pathway with prolonged AH intervals (with PR intervals longer than atrial pacing CL), so that the last paced atrial impulse falls before the His potential caused by conduction of the preceding paced atrial impulse. Thus, the last paced atrial impulse is followed by two His potentials and two ventricular complexes. The last response may then be followed by induction of AVN echo beats or AVNRT, mimicking simultaneous fast and slow pathway conduction (Fig. 17-8).[8,29]

PR INTERVAL LONGER THAN PACING CYCLE LENGTH DURING ATRIAL PACING. The PR interval gradually prolongs as the atrial pacing rate increases. When a critical pacing rate is reached, the PR interval typically exceeds the R-R interval, with all AVN conduction over the slow AVN pathway (see Fig. 17-8). This manifests as *crossing over* of the pacing stimulus artifacts and QRSs; that is, the paced atrial complex is conducting not to the QRS immediately following it, but rather to the next QRS, because of a very long PR interval. There should be consistent 1:1 AV conduction that remains stable over the span of several cycles for this observation to be interpreted (i.e., without Wenckebach

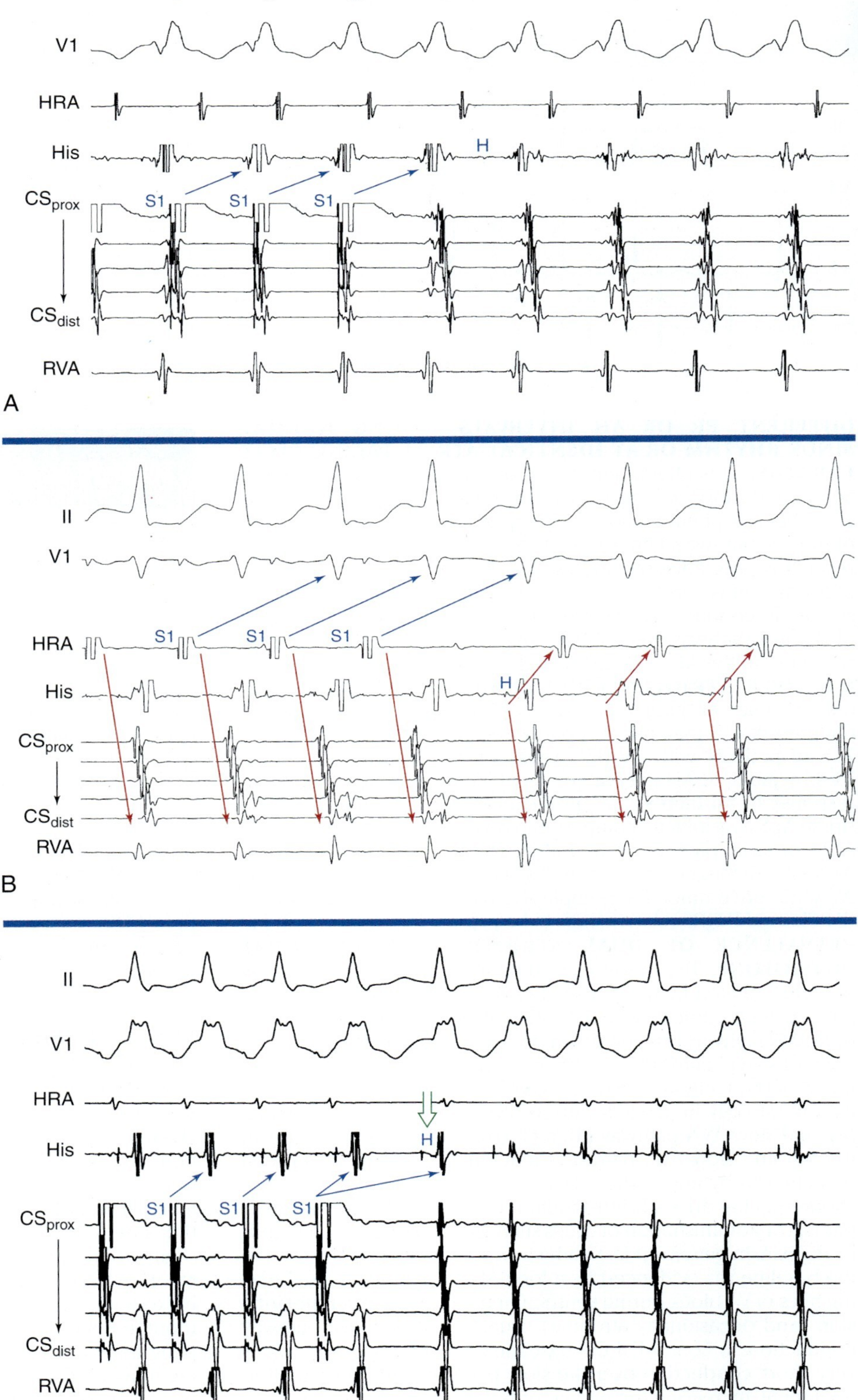

FIGURE 17-8 Induction of typical atrioventricular nodal reentrant tachycardia (AVNRT) with atrial pacing. **A,** Each of the atrial paced impulses (S1) conducts anterogradely over the slow AVN pathway. The last paced impulse, following anterograde conduction down the slow pathway, also conducts retrogradely up the fast AVN pathway to initiate typical AVNRT with right bundle branch block (RBBB). **B,** Each of the atrial paced impulses conducts anterogradely over the slow AVN pathway with a long PR interval (blue arrows); this is longer than the pacing cycle length (CL), resulting in crossing over, which can mimic a 1:2 AV response caused by anterograde conduction over both the fast and slow AVN pathways. Following anterograde conduction down the slow pathway, the last paced impulse also conducts retrogradely over the fast pathway, initiating typical AVNRT. Red arrows illustrate atrial activation sequence during atrial pacing versus AVNRT. **C,** Atrial pacing from the coronary sinus ostium (CS os) induces typical AVNRT. Each of the atrial paced impulses (S1) conducts over the fast AVN pathway except for the last paced impulse, which conducts over both the fast and slow AVN pathways (blue arrows), resulting in a 1:2 response (i.e., 2 ventricular responses); this is followed by induction of typical AVNRT with RBBB. The possibility of conduction of the paced atrial beats over the slow AVN pathway with a long atrial–His bundle (AH) interval (longer than the paced CL) is unlikely because the His potential preceding the first tachycardia complex (indicated by the green arrow) occurs later (i.e., at a longer AH interval) than what would be expected if that His potential was actually a result of conduction of the last atrial stimulus (as compared with the previous AH intervals). CS_{dist} = distal coronary sinus; CS_{prox} = proximal coronary sinus; HRA = high right atrium; RVA = right ventricular apex.

block). Such slow AVN conduction is seen only when conduction propagates over a slow AVN pathway, and it is not seen in the absence of dual AVN physiology. This phenomenon is diagnostic of the presence of dual AVN physiology, even in the absence of an AH interval jump and therefore is very helpful in patients with smooth AVN function curves. In fact, 96% of patients with AVNRT and smooth AVN function curves have a PR interval/RR interval ratio greater than 1 (i.e., PR interval longer than pacing CL) during atrial pacing at the maximal rate with consistent 1:1 AV conduction (versus 11% in controls).

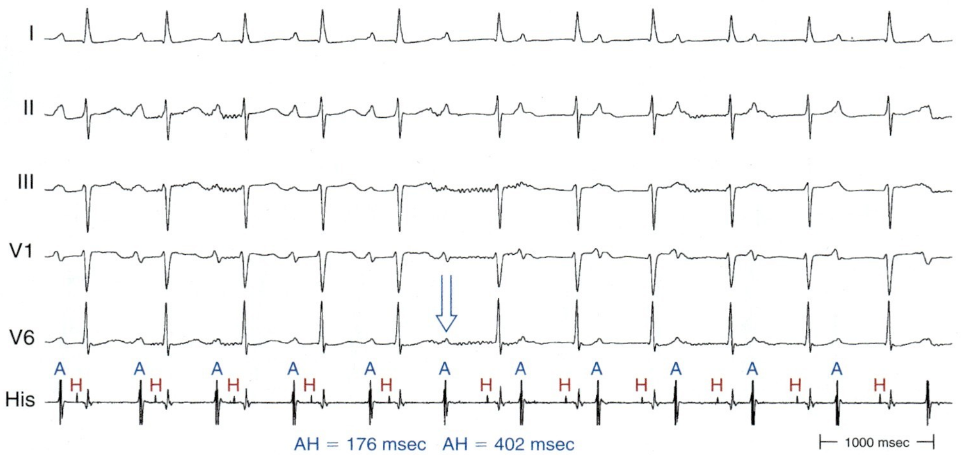

FIGURE 17-9 Dual atrioventricular node (AVN) physiology manifesting as two different PR intervals during normal sinus rhythm. Note that the shift in AV conduction from the fast to the slow AVN pathway (arrow) occurs without any changes in the sinus cycle length (CL) (680 milliseconds). This phenomenon indicates that the fast pathway anterograde effective refractory period is long relative to the sinus CL.

DIFFERENT PR OR AH INTERVALS DURING NORMAL SINUS RHYTHM OR AT IDENTICAL ATRIAL PACING CYCLE LENGTHS. This phenomenon can occur when the fast pathway anterograde ERP is long relative to the sinus or paced CL (Fig. 17-9). Such a phenomenon also requires a long retrograde ERP of the fast pathway. Otherwise, AVN echo beats or AVNRT would result, because once the impulse blocks anterogradely in the fast pathway and is conducted down the slow pathway, it would subsequently conduct retrogradely up the fast pathway if the ERP of the fast pathway were shorter than the conduction time (i.e., shorter than the AH interval) over the slow pathway.[8]

MULTIPLE ATRIOVENTRICULAR NODAL PATHWAYS. Multiple AH interval "jumps" in response to AES, a finding suggesting the presence of multiple AVN pathways, can be observed in up to 14% of patients with AVNRT. These phenomena are characterized by multiple AH interval jumps of 50 milliseconds or more in response to an increasingly premature AES. In these patients, a single AES may initiate multiple jumps in only 68%, whereas double AESs or atrial pacing is required in 32%. Such patients can have AVNRT with longer tachycardia CLs and longer ERP and FRP of the AVN. It is uncommon for multiple AVNRTs with different tachycardia CLs and P-QRS relationships to be present in the same patient.

PREVALENCE OF DUAL ATRIOVENTRICULAR NODAL PHYSIOLOGY. The presence of dual AVN pathways can usually be demonstrated by using a single AES or atrial pacing in 85% of patients with clinical AVNRT. In 95% of patients, the presence of dual AVN pathways can be shown by using multiple AESs, multiple-drive CLs (typically 600 and 400 milliseconds), and multiple pacing sites (typically high RA and CS). Failure to demonstrate dual AVN physiology in patients with AVNRT can be caused by similar fast and slow AVN pathway ERPs. Dissociation of refractoriness of the fast and slow AVN pathways may then be required. This can be achieved by any of the following: introduction of an AES at a shorter pacing drive CL; introduction of multiple AESs; burst atrial pacing; or administration of drugs such as beta blockers, verapamil, or digoxin. In general, if fast pathway conduction is suppressed in the baseline (as evidenced by a long AH interval at all atrial pacing rates or VA block during ventricular pacing), isoproterenol infusion (and occasionally atropine) usually facilitates fast pathway conduction. In contrast, if the baseline ERP of the fast pathway is very short, conduction over the slow pathway can be difficult to document. Increasing the degree of sedation or infusion of esmolol can prolong the fast pathway ERP and allow recognition of slow pathway conduction.

Another potential reason for the inability to demonstrate dual AVN physiology is block in the fast AVN pathway at the pacing drive CL (i.e., pacing drive CL is shorter than fast pathway ERP). Additionally, atrial FRP can limit the prematurity of the AES. Consequently, AVN activation cannot be adequately advanced to produce block in the fast pathway because a more premature AES would result in more intraatrial conduction delay and less premature stimulation of the AVN. This obstacle can be overcome by the introduction of an AES following a shorter pacing drive CL, introduction of multiple AESs, burst atrial pacing, or stimulation from multiple atrial sites. A typical programmed electrical stimulation protocol used for EP testing in patients with AVNRT is outlined in Table 17-5.[28]

TABLE 17-5 Programmed Stimulation Protocol for Electrophysiology Testing of Atrioventricular Nodal Reentrant Tachycardia

Atrial burst pacing from the RA and CS (down to AV Wenckebach CL)
Single and double AESs at multiple CLs (600-400 msec) from the high RA and CS (down to atrial ERP)
Ventricular burst pacing from the RV apex (down to VA Wenckebach CL)
Single and double VESs at multiple CLs (600-400 msec) from the RV apex (down to ventricular ERP)
Administration of isoproterenol infusion as needed to facilitate tachycardia induction (0.5-4 µg/min)

AES = atrial extrastimulus; AV = atrioventricular; CL = cycle length; CS = coronary sinus; ERP = effective refractory period; RA = right atrium; RV = right ventricle; VA = ventriculoatrial; VES = ventricular extrastimulus.

VENTRICULAR EXTRASTIMULATION AND VENTRICULAR PACING DURING NORMAL SINUS RHYTHM

RETROGRADE DUAL ATRIOVENTRICULAR NODAL PHYSIOLOGY. Demonstration of retrograde dual AVN pathway conduction curves requires a longer retrograde ERP of the fast pathway than slow pathway ERP and ventricular and His-Purkinje system (HPS) FRP, as well as a sufficient difference in conduction times between the two pathways. In a pattern analogous to that of anterograde dual AVN physiology, ventricular stimulation can result in discontinuous retrograde AVN function curves, manifesting as a jump in the H_2-A_2 (or A_1-A_2) interval of 50 milliseconds or more in response to a 10-millisecond decrement of the VES coupling interval (V_1-V_2) or ventricular pacing CL (V_1-V_1). This finding must be distinguished from sudden VA prolongation caused by VH interval (but not HA interval) prolongation related to retrograde functional block in the RB and transseptal activation of HB through the LB (see Fig. 4-27). A 1:2 response (i.e., two atrial responses to a single ventricular stimulus) can also be observed.[28]

Failure to demonstrate retrograde dual AVN physiology in patients with atypical AVNRT can be caused by similar fast and slow AVN pathway ERPs. Dissociation of refractoriness of the fast and slow AVN pathways may be required and usually can be achieved by any of the following: introduction of VESs at a shorter pacing drive CL; introduction of multiple VESs; burst ventricular pacing; or administration of drugs such as beta blockers, verapamil, or digoxin. In addition, retrograde block in the fast AVN pathway at the pacing drive CL (i.e., the pacing CL is shorter than the fast pathway ERP) and ventricular or HPS FRP interval limiting the prematurity of the VES can also account for such failure.[28]

Induction of Tachycardia

INITIATION BY ATRIAL EXTRASTIMULATION OR ATRIAL PACING

TYPICAL (SLOW-FAST) ATRIOVENTRICULAR NODAL REENTRANT TACHYCARDIA. Clinical AVNRT almost always can be initiated with an AES that blocks anterogradely in the fast pathway, conducts down the slow pathway, and then conducts retrogradely up the fast pathway. Only when anterograde conduction down the slow pathway is slow enough (critical AH interval) to allow for recovery of the fast pathway to conduct retrogradely does reentry occur (see Fig. 17-6). This critical AH interval is not a fixed interval. It can change with changes in pacing drive CL, changes in autonomic tone, or after drug administration, thus reflecting changes in the fast pathway retrograde ERP.[28]

There is a zone of AES coupling intervals (A_1-A_2) associated with AVNRT induction called the tachycardia zone. This zone usually begins at coupling intervals associated with marked prolongation of the AH intervals. This AVN conduction delay (AH interval prolongation), and not the AES coupling interval, is of prime importance for the genesis of AVNRT.

Atrial pacing can initiate AVNRT at pacing CLs associated with sufficient AVN conduction delay (see Fig. 17-8), especially during the atypical Wenckebach periodicity, when anterograde block occurs in the fast pathway and conduction shifts to the slow pathway.

Rarely, AES or atrial pacing can produce a 1:2 response with anterograde conduction over both the fast and slow pathways, as explained earlier (see Fig. 17-8).[29] Such a response predicts easy induction of slow-fast AVNRT by ventricular stimulation because poor slow pathway retrograde conduction would increase the opportunity for the ventricular stimulus to block in the slow pathway and conduct up the fast pathway to return down the slow pathway and initiate AVNRT.

The site of atrial stimulation can affect the ease of inducibility of AVNRT, probably because of different atrial inputs to the AVN or different atrial FRPs. Therefore, it is important to perform atrial stimulation from both the high RA and CS.

Atrial echoes and AVNRT usually occur at the same time that dual pathways are revealed (see Fig. 4-23). In 20% of patients, the dual AVN pathway AH interval jump occurs without concurrent occurrence of echo beats or AVNRT because of failure of retrograde conduction up the fast pathway. This failure can be caused by the absence of a distal connection between the two AVN pathways, a long retrograde ERP of the fast AVN pathway, or concealment of the AES anterogradely into the fast AVN pathway (i.e., the AES propagates some distance into the fast pathway before being blocked). The last event results in anterograde postdepolarization refractoriness, which would consequently make the fast pathway refractory to the wavefront invading it in the retrograde direction. The latter phenomenon can be diagnosed by demonstrating that the AH interval following the AES that fails to produce an echo beat is longer than the shortest ventricular pacing CL with 1:1 retrograde conduction. Such a pacing CL is a marker of the fast pathway retrograde ERP. This finding implies that an AES blocking in the fast pathway and conducting over the slow pathway, with an AH interval exceeding fast pathway ERP and still not conducting retrogradely over the fast pathway, is caused by anterograde concealment (and not just block) into the fast pathway.[28]

Markers of poor retrograde conduction over the fast AVN pathway predict low inducibility of AVNRT. These markers include the absence of VA conduction, poor VA conduction (manifest as retrograde AVN Wenckebach CL longer than 500 milliseconds), and retrograde dual pathways (indicative of long retrograde ERP of the fast pathway, which must exceed the refractoriness of the slow pathway for retrograde dual pathways to be demonstrable). In fact, retrograde fast AVN pathway characteristics (i.e., ERP) are the major determinant of whether reentry (AVN echoes or AVNRT, or both) occurs, whereas conduction delay anterogradely over the slow pathway (i.e., "critical AH interval") determines when reentry is to occur.

Although isolated AVN echoes can occur as long as VA conduction is present, the ability to initiate sustained AVNRT also requires the capability of the slow pathway to sustain repetitive anterograde conduction. In other words, sustenance of AVNRT requires that the tachycardia CL be longer than the ERP of all components of the circuit. Typically, for AVN reentry to occur, the fast pathway should be able to support 1:1 VA conduction at a ventricular pacing CL shorter than 400 milliseconds (i.e., retrograde Wenckebach CL shorter than 400 milliseconds), and the slow pathway should be able to support 1:1 AV conduction at an atrial pacing CL shorter than 350 milliseconds (i.e., anterograde Wenckebach CL shorter than 350 milliseconds). The shorter the AH interval during anterograde conduction over the fast pathway, the better the retrograde conduction over the same pathway (i.e., the shorter the HA interval), and the better the inducibility of AVNRT. Nevertheless, it is important to recognize that during EP testing, these criteria are dependent on the cardiac autonomic tone at that moment, and they can change dramatically by changing the level of patient sedation or the use of isoproterenol or by prolonged periods of rapid pacing (particularly ventricular) that cause hypotension and a reflex increase in adrenergic tone, which then affect inducibility of AVNRT.[28]

ATYPICAL (FAST-SLOW) ATRIOVENTRICULAR NODAL REENTRANT TACHYCARDIA. Anterograde dual AVN physiology is usually not demonstrable in patients with atypical AVNRT. Additionally, as noted, the presence of a 1:2 response to AES predicts noninducibility of atypical AVNRT because it indicates failure of the slow pathway to support retrograde conduction, a prerequisite for the atypical AVNRT circuit.[19]

When atypical AVNRT is initiated with atrial stimulation, it is usually with modest prolongation of the AH interval over the fast pathway and anterograde block in the slow pathway, followed by retrograde slow conduction over the slow pathway (Fig. 17-10). Therefore, a critical AH interval delay is not obvious.[19]

INITIATION BY VENTRICULAR EXTRASTIMULATION OR VENTRICULAR PACING

TYPICAL (SLOW-FAST) ATRIOVENTRICULAR NODAL REENTRANT TACHYCARDIA. Ventricular stimulation induces typical AVNRT by different mechanisms. The most common mechanism involves retrograde block of the ventricular stimulus in the slow pathway and retrograde conduction up the fast pathway, followed by anterograde conduction down the slow pathway. This occurs when the retrograde ERP of the slow pathway exceeds that of the fast pathway. This means that induction occurs without the demonstration of retrograde dual AVN physiology, and no critical VA or HA interval is required for induction. Occasionally, an interpolated premature ventricular complex (PVC) can block in the slow pathway retrogradely and penetrate into the fast pathway and cause concealment, so that the fast pathway will be refractory when the next sinus beat occurs. The sinus beat would then block in the fast pathway and conduct down the slow pathway and initiate typical AVNRT. This mechanism is uncommon. Retrograde VA conduction over the fast AVN pathway is usually good, and VA block rarely occurs in patients with typical AVNRT initiated by ventricular stimulation.[28]

Ventricular stimulation is less effective than atrial stimulation in inducing typical AVNRT (success rate is approximately 10% with VES and 40% with ventricular pacing), whereas atypical AVNRT can be induced almost as frequently by ventricular stimulation as

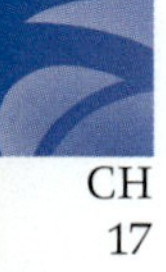

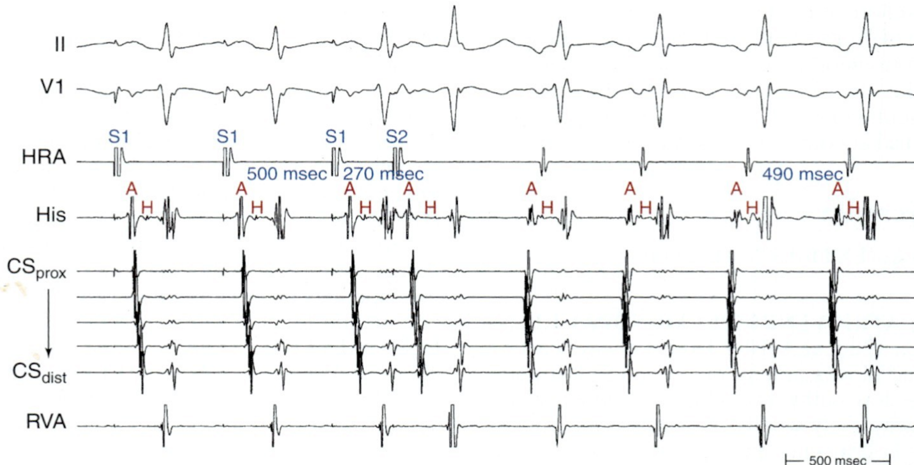

FIGURE 17-10 Induction of atypical atrioventricular nodal reentrant tachycardia (AVNRT) with atrial extrastimulation (AES). AES delivered from the high right atrium (HRA) at a coupling interval of 270 milliseconds after a drive cycle length (CL) of 500 milliseconds initiated atypical AVNRT with a CL of 490 milliseconds. Note that the AES conducted with only a modest prolongation of the atrial–His bundle (AH) interval. Additionally, comparing the AH interval between atrial drive pacing and that during the SVT (because the tachycardia CL approximates the pacing CL) reveals that ΔAH ($AH_{pacing} - AH_{SVT}$) is more than 40 milliseconds, thus favoring AVNRT over atrial tachycardia and orthodromic atrioventricular reentrant tachycardia. CS_{dist} = distal coronary sinus; CS_{prox} = proximal coronary sinus; RVA = right ventricular apex.

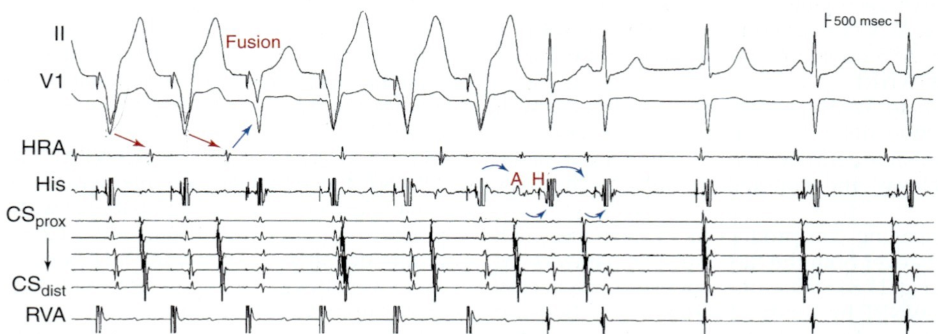

FIGURE 17-11 Ventricular pacing inducing atrioventricular nodal (AVN) echo beats. Note that ventriculoatrial conduction during ventricular pacing is occurring up the slow AVN pathway (red arrows). This results in AVN echo beats caused by anterograde conduction over the fast pathway, which results in occasional QRS fusion (i.e., fusion between the echo beat and the paced impulse) during the pacing drive. Cessation of ventricular pacing is followed by double AVN echo beats (blue arrows). CS_{dist} = distal coronary sinus; CS_{prox} = proximal coronary sinus; HRA = high right atrium; RVA = right ventricular apex.

by atrial stimulation. It is difficult for VES to induce typical AVNRT because the prematurity with which the VES arrives at the AVN can be limited by conduction delay in the HPS or in the lower common pathway. The ERP of the HPS may exceed that of the slow AVN pathway. This limitation can usually be overcome by the introduction of multiple VESs, use of a shorter drive CL, or ventricular pacing, which results in adaptation and shortening of the HPS ERP. Additionally, the anterograde ERP of the slow pathway may exceed the ventricular pacing CL so that the slow pathway is incapable of anterograde conduction of the ventricular impulse conducting retrogradely over the fast pathway. Similar retrograde ERPs of the slow and fast pathways also can limit the successful initiation of AVNRT by ventricular stimulation. As noted, manipulation of the autonomic tone with vagal maneuvers or drugs can facilitate dissociation of those ERPs. Another explanation for the lower success rate of AVNRT induction by ventricular stimulation is that the ventricular stimulus can penetrate (and not just block) in the slow pathway retrogradely, thus causing concealment that renders that pathway refractory and incapable of anterograde conduction of the ventricular impulse traveling retrogradely over the fast pathway.[28]

Burst ventricular pacing can overcome many of the problems imposed by HPS refractoriness in the induction of typical AVNRT (Fig. 17-11). During ventricular pacing, the AVN is the primary site of conduction delay. However, block in the lower common pathway and repetitive concealment (not just block) in the slow AVN pathway can still limit the success of ventricular pacing in inducing typical AVNRT.

Of note, a VES that initiates an SVT with an HA interval longer than the HA (or VA) interval during the SVT, even though the H-H interval following that particular VES is longer than the H-H interval during the SVT, indicates that the SVT is AVNRT and not orthodromic AVRT. The reason is that both the HA interval during orthodromic AVRT and that following the VES represent sequential conduction duration from the HB up the lower common pathway and fast pathway to the atrium (Fig. 17-12). In contrast, during AVNRT, the HB and the atrium are activated in parallel, resulting in a shortened HA interval.[28]

ATYPICAL (FAST-SLOW) ATRIOVENTRICULAR NODAL REENTRANT TACHYCARDIA. Ventricular stimulation can induce atypical AVNRT by different mechanisms. The ventricular impulse can block in the fast pathway and conduct retrogradely over the slow pathway, with a long HA interval, thus allowing for recovery of the fast pathway and subsequent anterograde conduction down this pathway, initiating atypical AVNRT (see Fig. 17-12). This requires the retrograde ERP of the fast pathway to exceed that of the slow pathway. In this case, dual retrograde AVN pathways would be demonstrated with ventricular stimulation. Both VES and ventricular pacing are equally effective in inducing atypical AVNRT by this mechanism. Occasionally, a VES can conduct over both AVN pathways, to produce a 1:2 response, which is

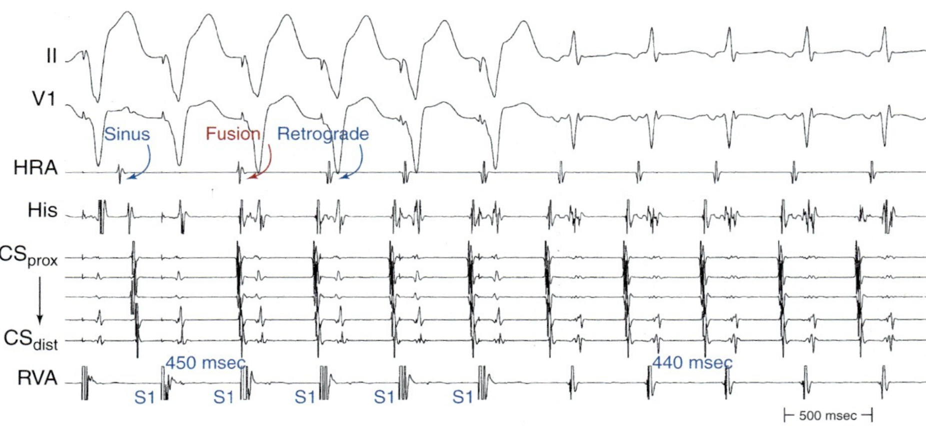

FIGURE 17-12 Induction of atypical atrioventricular nodal reentrant tachycardia (AVNRT) with ventricular pacing. Right ventricular apical (RVA) pacing (cycle length [CL] = 450 milliseconds) induces atypical AVNRT (CL = 440 milliseconds). Retrograde atrial activation sequence during ventricular pacing is similar to that during the supraventricular tachycardia (SVT), and the ventriculoatrial (VA) interval during ventricular pacing is longer than during the SVT; both criteria favor AVNRT over orthodromic atrioventricular reentrant tachycardia. Note that the first atrial complex on the left of the tracing is actually a sinus P wave, and the second is a fusion between retrograde VA conduction and a sinus impulse; a pure retrograde atrial activation sequence is observed only after the third ventricular stimulus. CS_{dist} = distal coronary sinus; CS_{prox} = proximal coronary sinus; HRA = high right atrium.

subsequently followed by the induction of atypical AVNRT. Ventricular pacing can initiate atypical AVNRT at pacing CLs associated with sufficient retrograde AVN conduction delay, especially during Wenckebach cycles, when retrograde block occurs in the fast pathway and conduction shifts to the slow pathway.[19]

Inducibility of atypical AVNRT is mostly determined by the retrograde slow pathway conduction.The reason is that the anterograde fast pathway conduction is usually sufficiently fast and its ERP is sufficiently short to allow anterograde conduction of the impulse arriving from the slow pathway.[28]

Tachycardia Features

TYPICAL (SLOW-FAST) ATRIOVENTRICULAR NODAL REENTRANT TACHYCARDIA

ATRIAL ACTIVATION SEQUENCE. The initial site of atrial activation is usually recorded in the HB catheter at the apex of the triangle of Koch. In general, the shorter the HA interval is, the more likely the earliest atrial activation is to be recorded in the HB electrograms. As the HA interval prolongs, the earliest atrial activation moves closer to the base of the triangle of Koch or in the CS. However, significant heterogeneity in atrial activation exists, with multiple breakthrough points (unlike AT or orthodromic AVRT). In addition, in approximately 60% of patients, retrograde atrial activation during typical AVNRT can be slightly discordant quantitatively and qualitatively from that during ventricular pacing. Subsequently, the wave of atrial activation propagates radially cephalad and laterally to activate both atria (i.e., concentric atrial activation). This results in a relatively narrow P wave. In fact, the narrowest P wave during any arrhythmia is seen when the atrial activation begins at the apex of the triangle of Koch. The site of earliest atrial activation is not always obvious during AVNRT because of superimposition of atrial and ventricular electrograms. Delivering a VES that advances ventricular activation but does not reset atrial activation usually helps unmask the atrial activation sequence.[8]

ATRIAL-VENTRICULAR RELATIONSHIP. The onset of atrial activation appears before or coincides with the onset of the QRS in approximately 70% of cases. The RP interval is very short (−40 to 75 milliseconds); however, variation of the A/V relationship (with changes in AH, HA, and AH/HA interval ratio) can occasionally occur during initiation or termination of the tachycardia, likely because of decremental conduction in the lower common pathway. Usually, the A/V ratio equals 1. However, AV block can be present because of block below the reentry circuit (usually below the HB and infrequently in the lower common pathway), which can occur especially at the onset of the SVT, during acceleration of the SVT, and following a PVC or VES. Moreover, Wenckebach-type block can occur in the lower common pathway and can result in a changing relationship between the His potential and the atrial electrogram (i.e., retrograde atrial electrogram moves closer to or actually precedes the His potential, until block occurs with no His potential apparent). Reproducible, sustained 2:1 AV block during induced episodes of AVNRT can be observed in approximately 10% of cases (see Fig. 17-4). The His potential is absent in blocked beats in approximately 40% of patients who have 2:1 AV block. In the remaining patients, the His potential can range from being rudimentary to large in amplitude. However, irrespective of whether a His potential is present in blocked beats, the AV block persists after the administration of atropine, a finding suggesting that the site of block is not in the AVN. In addition, a VES introduced during the 2:1 AV block consistently results in 1:1 conduction, indicating that the AV block is functional and that the level of block is infranodal. Therefore, what was previously thought to be 2:1 AVN block in the lower common pathway of the AVNRT circuit (because of the absence of visible His potentials) is more likely to be intra-Hisian block. Rarely, VA block can occur during AVNRT because of block in the upper common pathway (see Fig. 17-11).[8,15]

OSCILLATION IN THE TACHYCARDIA CYCLE LENGTH. When CL variability is observed during typical AVNRT, it is generally caused by changes in anterograde conduction over the slow AVN pathway. Because retrograde conduction through the fast AVN pathway generally is much less variable, the changes in the ventricular CL that result from variability in anterograde AVN conduction precede the subsequent changes in the atrial CL (Fig. 17-13), and changes in the atrial CL do not predict changes in the subsequent ventricular CL, as is the case in orthodromic AVRT.[30]

EFFECT OF BUNDLE BRANCH BLOCK. The development of prolonged functional aberration during AVNRT is uncommon, and it usually occurs at initiation of the tachycardia or after resumption of 1:1 AV conduction after a period of block in the HB or lower common pathway (see Fig. 17-4). When BBB does occur during AVNRT, it does not influence the tachycardia CL (A-A or H-H intervals) because the ventricles are not required for the tachycardia circuit.

TERMINATION AND RESPONSE TO PHYSIOLOGICAL AND PHARMACOLOGICAL MANEUVERS. The tachycardia CL is correlated best to the conduction time down the slow pathway.Spontaneous or pharmacologically mediated changes in the tachycardia CL are also more closely associated with changes in slow pathway conduction. Spontaneous termination of typical AVNRT occurs because of block in the fast or the slow pathway. However, the better the retrograde fast pathway conduction is, the less likely it is to

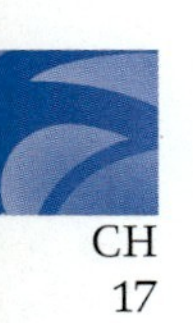

CH 17

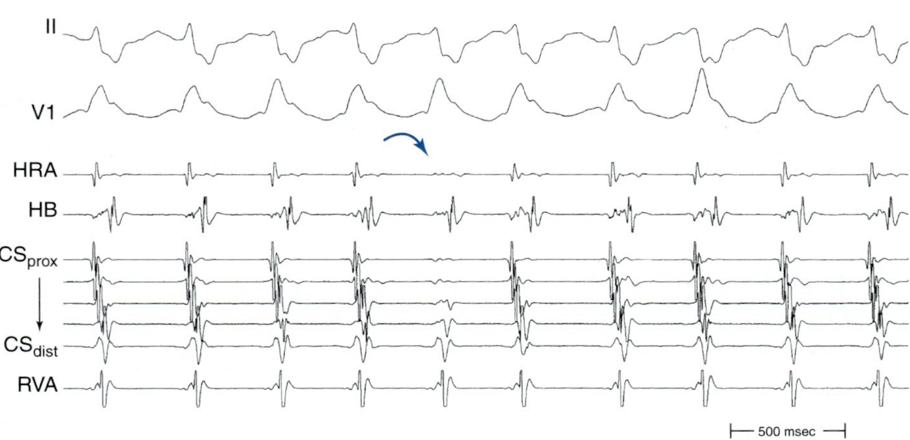

FIGURE 17-13 Typical atrioventricular nodal reentrant tachycardia (AVNRT) with right bundle branch block. Intermittent ventriculoatrial (VA) block is observed (arrow) secondary to block in an upper common pathway. Oscillation of the tachycardia cycle length (CL) is observed before the block. Note the changes in the H-H and V-V intervals preceding similar changes in the A-A interval. Both atrial tachycardia and orthodromic atrioventricular reentrant tachycardia are excluded by the fact that the atrium is not necessary for continuation of the tachycardia. CS_{dist} = distal coronary sinus; CS_{prox} = proximal coronary sinus; HRA = high right atrium; RVA = right ventricular apex.

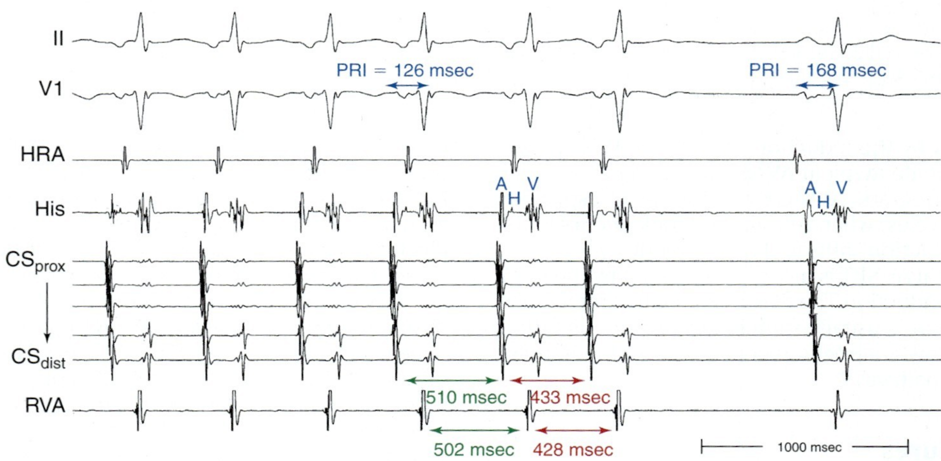

FIGURE 17-14 Atypical (fast-slow) atrioventricular nodal reentrant tachycardia (AVNRT) terminating spontaneously. Oscillation of the tachycardia cycle length (CL) is observed just before termination. Note that changes in the atrial CL predict changes in the subsequent ventricular CL because CL variability during atypical AVNRT is usually caused by changes in retrograde conduction over the slow AVN pathway, whereas anterograde conduction occurs over the more stable fast AVN pathway and is less subject to variability. Additionally, the PR interval (PRI) and atrial–His bundle (AH) interval are shorter during AVNRT than those during normal sinus rhythm (NSR) because both the atrium and the ventricle are activated in parallel with simultaneous conduction up an upper common pathway and down the anterograde fast pathway in atypical AVNRT but in sequence during NSR. CS_{dist} = distal coronary sinus; CS_{prox} = proximal coronary sinus; HRA = high right atrium; RVA = right ventricular apex.

be the site of block. Carotid sinus massage and vagal maneuvers can terminate typical AVNRT with gradual anterograde slowing and then block in the slow pathway, whereas block in the fast pathway is uncommon. AVN blockers (digoxin, calcium channel blockers, and beta blockers) prolong the refractoriness of the fast and slow pathways to similar or different degrees. Such effects mediate termination of AVNRT. However, they can occasionally help dissociate the ERP of the fast and slow pathways and unmask dual AVN physiology, and they can also facilitate inducibility of the AVNRT. Adenosine blocks the slow pathway and terminates AVNRT, but it does not affect the fast pathway. Class IA and IC agents and amiodarone affect both the fast and the slow pathways.[28]

ATYPICAL (FAST-SLOW) ATRIOVENTRICULAR NODAL REENTRANT TACHYCARDIA

The earliest site of retrograde atrial activation during atypical AVNRT is usually recorded at the base of the triangle of Koch or CS os, and CS breakthrough is observed in most patients. The CS breakthrough is likely part of or very close to the reentry circuit, as demonstrated by entrainment mapping.[21]

The RP interval during atypical AVNRT is longer than the PR interval. Additionally, the PR and AH intervals are shorter during AVNRT than during NSR because the atrium and ventricle are activated in parallel with simultaneous conduction up the upper common pathway and down the anterograde fast pathway in atypical AVNRT, but in sequence during NSR (Fig. 17-14).

Usually, the A/V ratio equals 1, as is the case for typical AVNRT. BBB can occur but does not influence the tachycardia CL. In contrast to typical AVNRT, CL variability during atypical AVNRT is usually caused by changes in retrograde conduction over the slow AVN pathway. Anterograde conduction occurs over the more stable fast AVN pathway and is less subject to variability (see Fig. 17-14). Therefore, during atypical AVNRT, changes in the atrial CL predict changes in the subsequent ventricular CL (as is the case in AT).[30] Carotid sinus massage, vagal maneuvers, adenosine, and AVN blockers (e.g., digoxin, calcium channel blockers, and beta blockers) generally terminate atypical AVNRT by gradual slowing and then block in the retrograde slow pathway (see Fig. 17-14). Termination of atypical AVNRT with adenosine can also result from block in the fast AVN pathway; however, the value of this observation in distinguishing between atypical AVNRT and orthodromic AVRT using a slow retrograde BT is questionable.

Diagnostic Maneuvers during Tachycardia

ATRIAL EXTRASTIMULATION AND ATRIAL PACING DURING SUPRAVENTRICULAR TACHYCARDIA

A late-coupled AES usually fails to reach the AVN with adequate prematurity and thus fails to affect the tachycardia, and a full

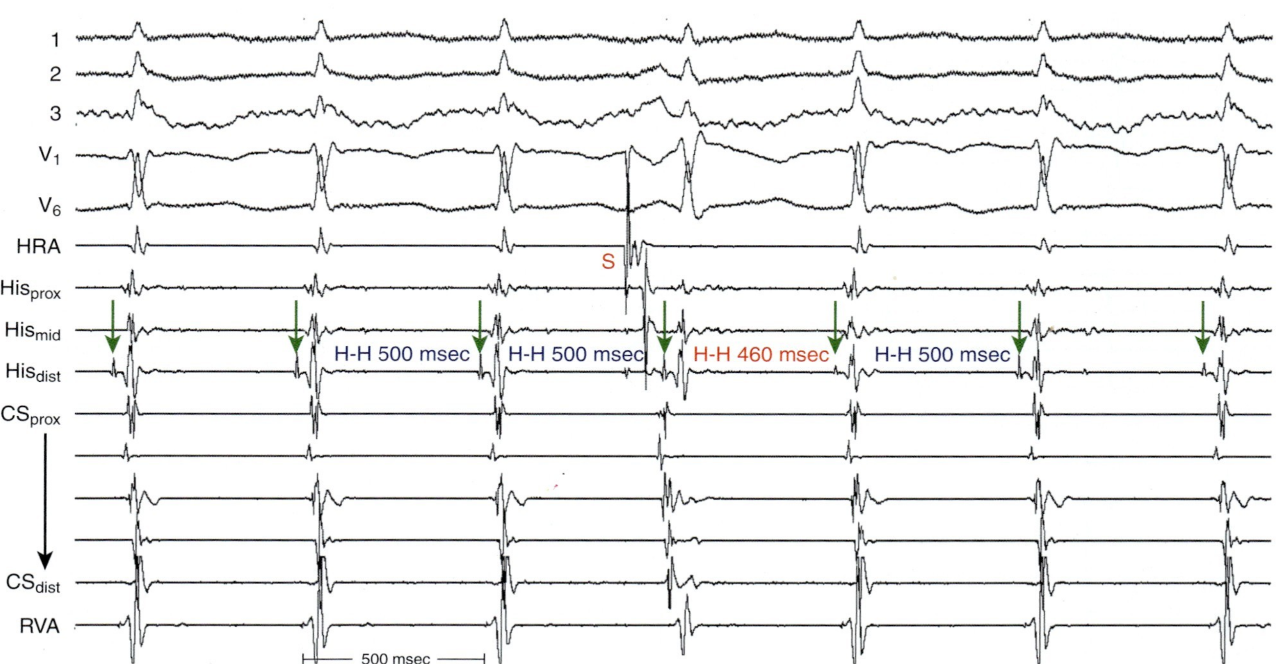

FIGURE 17-15 Atrial extrastimulus during atrioventricular nodal reentrant tachycardia has no effect on the timing of the immediately following His potential (H-H interval = 500 milliseconds) but advances the timing of the following His potential (H-H interval = 460 milliseconds). Arrows mark His potentials. CS_{dist} = distal coronary sinus; CS_{prox} = proximal coronary sinus; His_{dist} = distal His bundle; His_{mid} = middle His bundle; His_{prox} = proximal His bundle; HRA = high right atrium; RVA = right ventricular apex.

compensatory pause results. However, the AES can anterogradely conceal in the upper common pathway, thereby retarding conduction of the impulse traveling retrogradely up the fast pathway and resulting in a delay in the timing of the next atrial activation. This is usually manifested by an AES that delays the subsequent atrial activation but without affecting the timing of HB and ventricular activation.[28]

In typical AVNRT, an early-coupled AES frequently penetrates the AVN and resets the reentry circuit, with a resulting compensatory pause that is less than, equal to, or greater than a full compensatory pause, depending on the degree of anterograde conduction delay that the AES encounters down the slow pathway (because of the decremental conduction properties of the AVN). The AES orthodromically propagates through the anterograde slow pathway, with a resulting alteration of the subsequent H-H' interval, whereas it antidromically collides with the preceding tachycardia wavefront traveling retrogradely up the fast pathway (Fig. 17-15). Progressively premature AESs encounter progressive anterograde conduction delay in the slow pathway, and an increasing resetting response pattern occurs. Theoretically, the degree of conduction delay in the slow pathway can exactly compensate for the prematurity of the AES, thus producing a pause that is equal to a full compensatory pause. To verify whether that pause was fully compensatory because the AES failed to penetrate the AVN or because the degree of anterograde conduction delay in the AVN was exactly sufficient to compensate for the prematurity of the AES, the return cycles are evaluated after delivery of additional AESs with different coupling intervals. Similarly, a delay in the slow pathway causes delay in the subsequent His potential timing, and such a delay can be equal to, greater, or smaller than what is needed to compensate for the prematurity of the AES. Therefore, the His potential following an AES can occur early, late, or on time relative to the expected tachycardia His potential. An early-coupled AES can also impinge on the relative refractory period of the lower common pathway and can cause slowed conduction and delay in the timing of the next His potential (i.e., longer A_2-H_2 than the baseline tachycardia A_1-H_1). This can occur even without affecting the timing of the next atrial activation, if conduction delay occurs only in the lower common pathway but not in the slow pathway.[28] In atypical AVNRT, an early-coupled AES can reset the SVT in a fashion to that seen in typical AVNRT. However, the delay in conduction that the AES will engender is mainly in the retrograde limb of the circuit (i.e., the slow pathway). An AES that accelerates the next His potential and resets tachycardia is indicative of focal junctional tachycardia (Fig. 17-16).

Resetting with fusion (a hallmark of macroreentrant tachycardias) cannot be demonstrated in AVNRT. For atrial fusion (i.e., fusion of atrial activation from both the tachycardia wavefront and the AES) to occur, the AES should be able to enter the reentrant circuit, while at the same time the tachycardia wavefront should be able to exit the circuit. This requires spatial separation between the entry and exit sites to the reentrant circuit, a condition that seems to be lacking in the setting of AVNRT. Once the tachycardia wavefront exits the reentry circuit to activate the atrium, any AES delivered beyond that time and resulting in atrial fusion is not capable of reaching the reentry circuit because the entry-exit site is already refractory in response to activation by the exiting wavefront, and the AES has no alternative way of reaching the circuit. Similarly, once an AES is capable of reaching the reentry circuit, the shared entry-exit site is made refractory and incapable of allowing a simultaneous exit of the tachycardia wavefront.

During typical AVNRT, a very early-coupled AES can block anterogradely in the slow pathway, and it usually collides with a retrograde wavefront in the fast pathway to terminate the SVT. However, if the tachycardia CL is sufficiently long, with a wide fully excitable gap, and the AES is appropriately timed, the AES can block anterogradely in the slow pathway and still conduct down the fast pathway to capture the HB and ventricle and terminate the SVT before the SVT wavefront traveling down the slow pathway reaches the lower turnaround point. Therefore, the last HB and ventricular electrograms before termination are advanced and premature, in contrast to termination secondary to an AES blocking anterogradely in the slow and fast pathways, whereby the last HB and ventricular electrograms of the SVT occur on time. This phenomenon occurs more commonly in atypical AVNRT.[28] In atypical AVNRT, a very early-coupled AES can conduct down the fast pathway during retrograde slow pathway activation and block retrogradely in

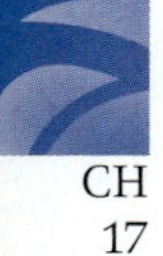

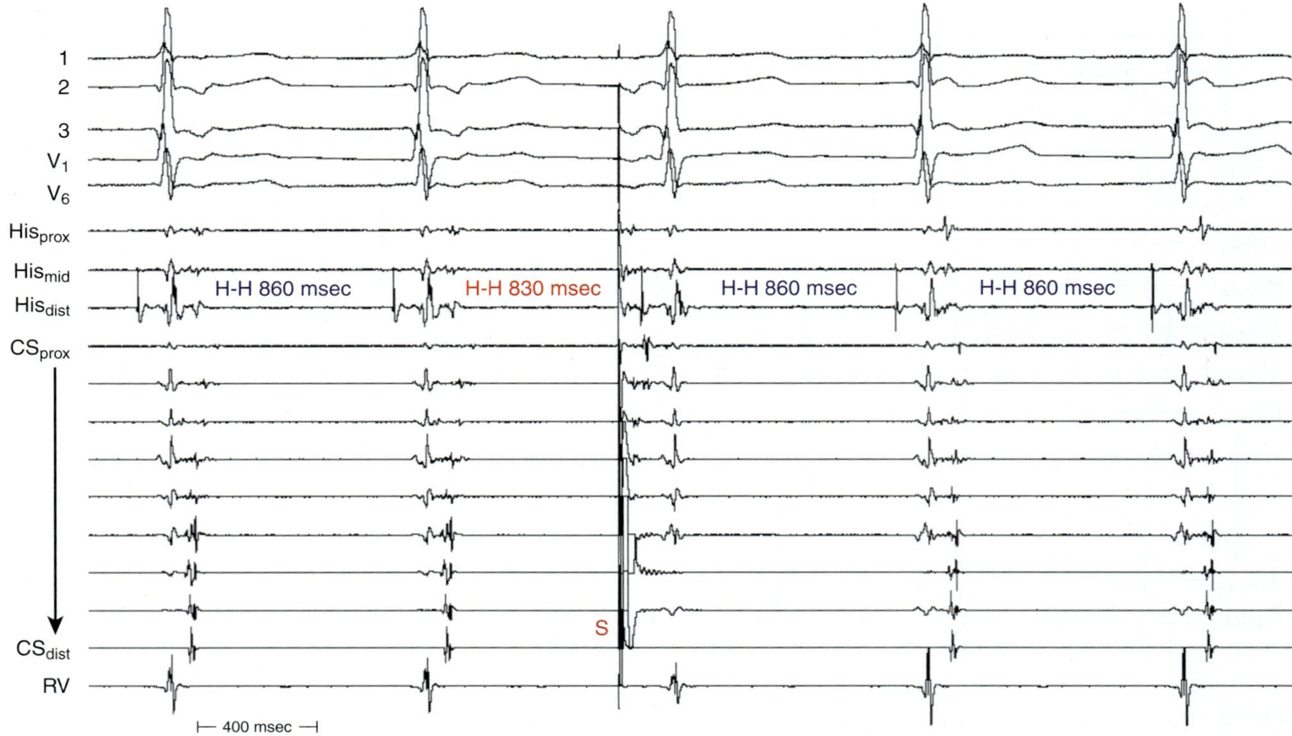

FIGURE 17-16 Atrial extrastimulus during focal junctional rhythm advances the timing of the immediately following His potential (H-H interval = 830 milliseconds) and resets the timing of the following His potential (H-H interval = 860 milliseconds). CS_{dist} = distal coronary sinus; CS_{prox} = proximal coronary sinus; His_{dist} = distal His bundle; His_{mid} = middle His bundle; His_{prox} = proximal His bundle; RV = right ventricle.

the slow pathway. In this case, the AES results in a premature HB and ventricular activation, and the AVNRT is terminated before the expected atrial activation.

TERMINATION. The ability of an AES to terminate AVNRT depends on the following: (1) the tachycardia CL (AVNRT with a CL shorter than 350 milliseconds is rarely terminated by a single AES, unless atrial stimulation is performed close to the AVN); (2) the distance of the site of atrial stimulation from the AVN (which would influence the ability of the AES to arrive to the AVN with adequate prematurity); (3) the refractoriness of the intervening atrial tissue (which can be overcome by delivery of multiple AESs); (4) atrial conduction velocity resulting from the AES; and (5) the size of the excitable gap in the reentrant circuit.[28]

ENTRAINMENT. Atrial pacing at a CL approximately 10 to 30 milliseconds shorter than the tachycardia CL is usually able to entrain AVNRT. In contrast to orthodromic AVRT, entrainment with atrial fusion cannot be demonstrated during AVNRT, a finding suggesting that the reentrant circuit in AVNRT does not have widely separate atrial entry and exit sites. Therefore, during entrainment of AVNRT by atrial pacing, the atrial activation sequence and P wave morphology are always those of pure paced morphology. The inability to demonstrate entrainment with manifest atrial fusion suggests a purely intranodal location of the AVNRT circuit. On the other hand, one study showed orthodromic capture of the atrial electrogram at the HB recording site (i.e., the bipolar HB electrogram morphology is identical to that during the tachycardia and is unaffected by pacing, and the first post-pacing interval [PPI] is identical to the pacing CL) during entrainment from the CS os region, a finding consistent with intracardiac atrial fusion. This suggests the absence of an upper common pathway between a reentrant circuit and atrial tissue surrounding the AVN and supports the concept that the reentrant circuit in AVNRT incorporates the atrial tissue surrounding the AVN. The AH interval during entrainment is usually longer than that during AVNRT because the atrial and the His electrograms are activated in parallel during AVNRT and in sequence during atrial pacing entraining the AVNRT (in response to the presence of intervening atrial tissue and, potentially, an upper common pathway separating the site of atrial stimulation from the reentry circuit).[28]

VENTRICULOATRIAL LINKING The initial atrial complex following cessation of atrial pacing entraining typical AVNRT is *linked* to, and cannot be dissociated from, the last captured ventricular complex. As a consequence, the post-pacing VA intervals are fixed and similar to those during tachycardia (with less than 10 milliseconds variation) after different attempts at SVT entrainment, regardless of the site, duration, or CL of the entraining atrial pacing drive. VA linking occurs in the setting of typical AVNRT because the timing of atrial activation is dependent on ventricular activation and is the result of retrograde VA conduction over the AVN fast pathway, which is relatively fixed and constant. VA linking can also be observed in orthodromic AVRT. In contrast, in the setting of AT, the first atrial return cycle following cessation of pacing is dependent on the distance between the AT origin and pacing site, the atrial conduction properties, and the mode of the resetting response of the AT, and it is not related to the preceding ventricular activation. Hence, the post-pacing VA intervals following different attempts at entrainment can vary especially when pacing at different rates or durations or from different atrial sites.[31,32]

VENTRICULAR EXTRASTIMULATION AND VENTRICULAR PACING DURING SUPRAVENTRICULAR TACHYCARDIA

RESETTING. For a VES to reset the AVNRT circuit, it needs to advance (prematurely activate) the HB timing by a degree that is dependent on the following: (1) the tachycardia CL, (2) the local ventricular ERP, (3) the time needed for the VES to reach the HB, and (4) the length of the lower common pathway. The longer the lower common pathway is, the more the timing of HB activation must be advanced so that the VES will be able to activate the AVNRT circuit prematurely. Therefore, in slow-fast and slow-slow

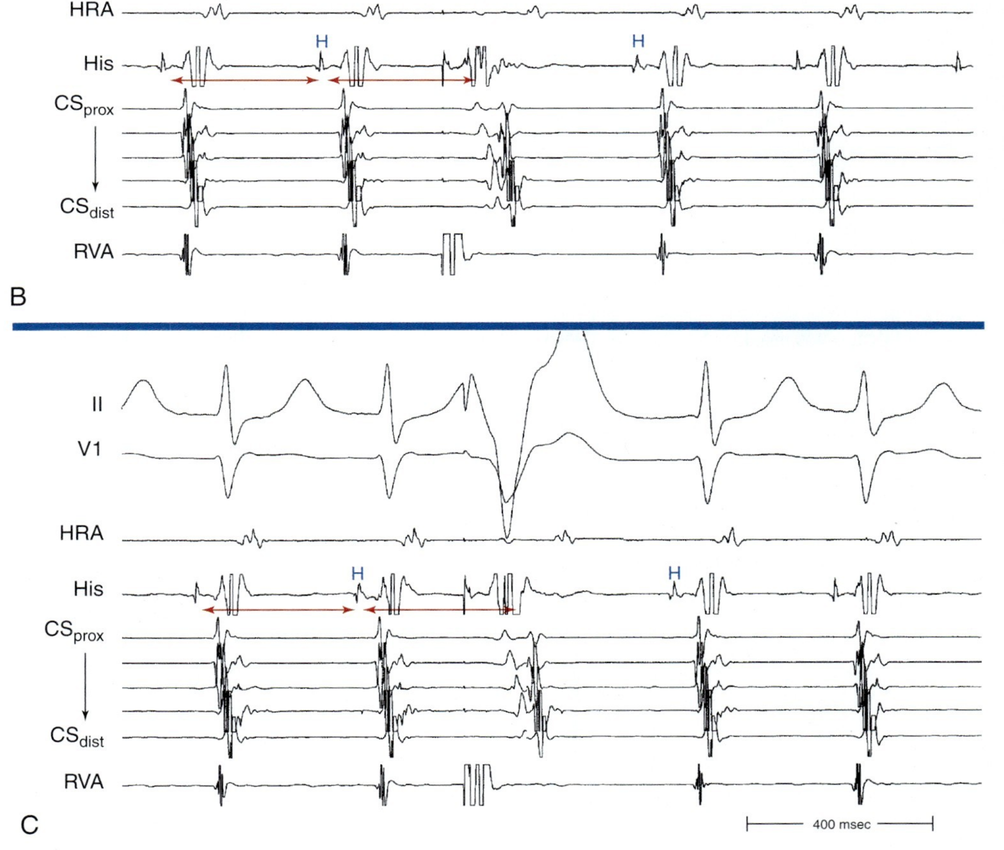

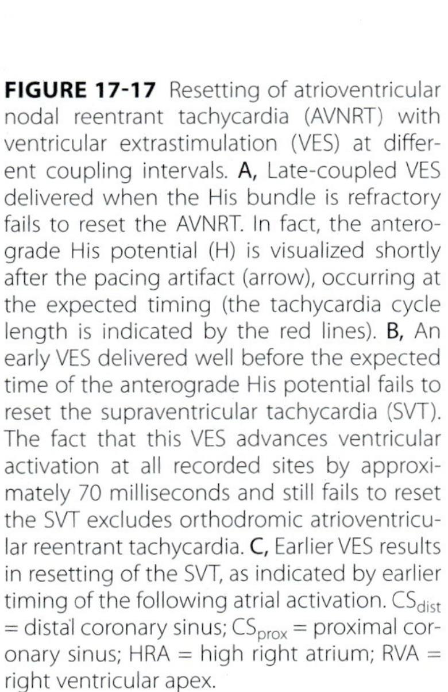

FIGURE 17-17 Resetting of atrioventricular nodal reentrant tachycardia (AVNRT) with ventricular extrastimulation (VES) at different coupling intervals. **A,** Late-coupled VES delivered when the His bundle is refractory fails to reset the AVNRT. In fact, the anterograde His potential (H) is visualized shortly after the pacing artifact (arrow), occurring at the expected timing (the tachycardia cycle length is indicated by the red lines). **B,** An early VES delivered well before the expected time of the anterograde His potential fails to reset the supraventricular tachycardia (SVT). The fact that this VES advances ventricular activation at all recorded sites by approximately 70 milliseconds and still fails to reset the SVT excludes orthodromic atrioventricular reentrant tachycardia. **C,** Earlier VES results in resetting of the SVT, as indicated by earlier timing of the following atrial activation. CS_{dist} = distal coronary sinus; CS_{prox} = proximal coronary sinus; HRA = high right atrium; RVA = right ventricular apex.

AVNRT, which typically has a long lower common pathway, the HB activation must be advanced by more than 30 to 60 milliseconds. In contrast, in slow-fast AVNRT, the lower common pathway is shorter, and the tachycardia is typically reset by the VES as soon as the HB activation is advanced.[28]

A late-coupled VES may block in the HPS or lower common pathway and may not affect the SVT (Fig. 17-17A). A late-coupled VES that resets the SVT without first retrogradely activating the HB (i.e., VES delivered at, after, or within 50 milliseconds of the expected inscription of the anterograde His potential) excludes AVNRT.

An early-coupled VES can reset AVNRT, especially when the tachycardia CL is relatively long (more than 350 milliseconds). The resetting VES antidromically collides with the preceding tachycardia wavefront traveling anterogradely and is conducted through the retrograde pathway to reset the tachycardia (see Fig. 17-17). Resetting of AVNRT with fusion of the QRS cannot be demonstrated because of the shared entry-exit site from the ventricle to the circuit, as discussed earlier.

A VES can reset the AVNRT circuit without resulting in subsequent atrial activation (i.e., advances the subsequent His potential and QRS and blocks in the upper common pathway). This latter phenomenon excludes AT and orthodromic AVRT as the mechanism of SVT, because it proves that the atrium is not part of the SVT circuit.

TERMINATION. Termination of AVNRT with VES is difficult (more so than termination with AES) and is rare when the tachycardia CL is shorter than 350 milliseconds. Such termination favors the diagnosis of orthodromic AVRT. In typical AVNRT, when termination occurs, it is usually caused by block of the VES in the anterograde or retrograde limb of the AVNRT circuit. The slower the SVT is, the more likely the block will be to occur in the anterograde slow pathway. Ventricular pacing can terminate AVNRT more easily than VES because rapid ventricular pacing can modulate and overcome the refractoriness of the intervening HPS. VES always terminates atypical AVNRT by blocking retrogradely in the slow pathway.[28]

ENTRAINMENT. Ventricular pacing at a CL approximately 10 to 30 milliseconds shorter than the tachycardia CL is usually able to entrain AVNRT. Visualization of the His potential before atrial activation during entrainment helps differentiate AVNRT from orthodromic AVRT. If the His potential cannot be visualized during ventricular pacing, two other parameters can be helpful to distinguish AVNRT from orthodromic AVRT: the VA interval during ventricular pacing and the PPI. The VA interval during ventricular pacing is significantly longer than that during AVNRT (ΔVA [$VA_{pacing} - VA_{SVT}$] is usually more than 85 milliseconds) because both the ventricle and the atrium are activated in parallel during AVNRT but in sequence during ventricular pacing entraining the AVNRT (Figs. 17-18 and 17-19).

The PPI after entrainment of AVNRT from the RV apex is significantly longer than the tachycardia CL (the [PPI − SVT CL] difference is usually more than 115 milliseconds) because the reentrant circuit in AVNRT (confined above the HB and does not involve the ventricle) is far from the pacing site. In AVNRT, the PPI reflects the conduction time from the pacing site through the RV muscle and HPS, once around the reentry circuit and back to the pacing site. Therefore, the difference between the PPI and tachycardia CL reflects twice the sum of the conduction time through the RV muscle, the HPS, and the lower common pathway. In orthodromic AVRT using a septal BT, the PPI reflects the conduction time through the RV to the septum, once around the reentry circuit and back. In other words, the difference between the PPI and tachycardia CL reflects

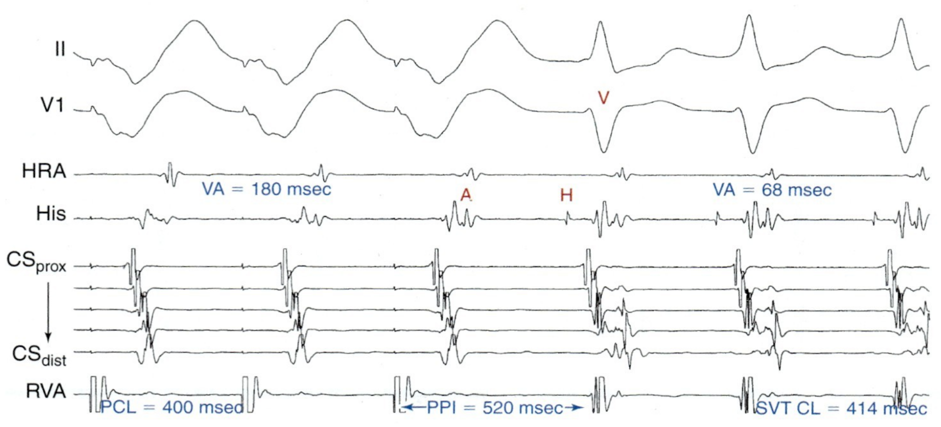

FIGURE 17-18 Entrainment of typical atrioventricular nodal reentrant tachycardia (AVNRT) with right ventricular (RV) apical pacing. The post-pacing interval (PPI) minus supraventricular tachycardia (SVT) cycle length (CL) (PPI − SVT CL) is more than 115 milliseconds, and the ΔVA interval (ventriculoatrial [$VA]_{pacing} - VA_{SVT}$) is more than 85 milliseconds. The atrial activation sequence during ventricular pacing is identical to that during AVNRT. No QRS fusion is observed. Cessation of ventricular pacing is followed by an AV response. CS_{dist} = distal coronary sinus; CS_{prox} = proximal coronary sinus; HRA = high right atrium; PCL = pacing CL; RVA = right ventricular apex.

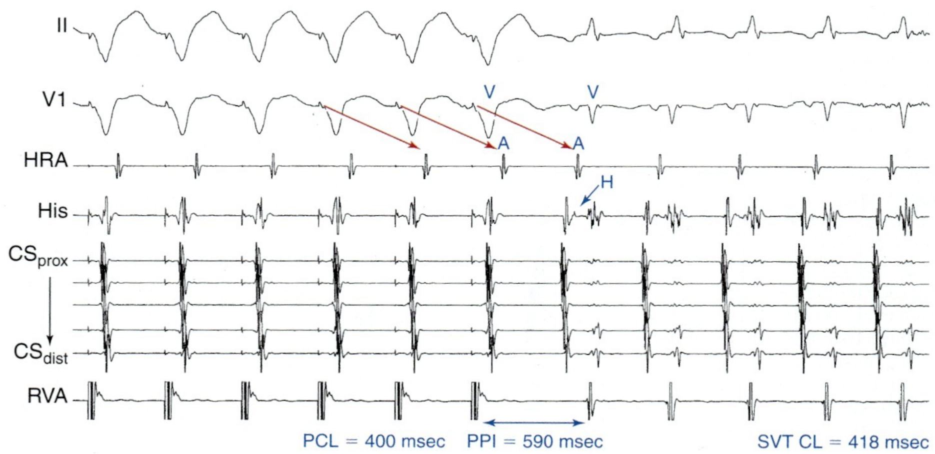

FIGURE 17-19 Entrainment of atypical atrioventricular nodal reentrant tachycardia (AVNRT) with right ventricular (RV) apical pacing. The post-pacing interval (PPI) minus supraventricular tachycardia (SVT) cycle length (CL) (PPI − SVT CL = 172 milliseconds) is long, and the ΔVA ($VA_{pacing} - VA_{SVT}$) interval is also long (188 milliseconds); both criteria favor AVNRT over orthodromic atrioventricular reentrant tachycardia. Note that the atrial activation sequence during RV pacing is similar to that during the SVT, again favoring AVNRT over other types of SVT. Additionally, a pseudo–A-A-V response is observed following cessation of ventricular pacing because retrograde conduction occurs through the slow pathway during ventricular pacing with a long VA interval (red arrows), longer than the pacing CL (PCL); hence, the last ventricular paced impulse is followed first by the P wave conducted slowly from the previous paced QRS and then by the P wave resulting from the last paced QRS, thus mimicking an A-A-V response. This is confirmed by the observation that the last atrial activation resulting from conduction of the last paced ventricular complex follows the preceding P wave with an A-A interval equal to the ventricular PCL. CS_{dist} = distal coronary sinus; CS_{prox} = proximal coronary sinus; HRA = high right atrium; RVA = right ventricular apex.

twice the conduction time from the pacing catheter through the ventricular myocardium to the reentry circuit. Because the ventricle is an essential component of the AVRT circuit, the RV apex is closer to the tachycardia circuit. Therefore, the PPI more closely approximates the SVT CL in orthodromic AVRT using a septal BT ([PPI – SVT CL] difference is usually less than 115 milliseconds) compared with AVNRT. This maneuver was studied specifically for differentiation between atypical AVNRT and orthodromic AVRT using a septal BT, but the principle also applies to typical AVNRT (see Figs. 17-18 and 17-19). For borderline values, ventricular pacing at the RV base can help exaggerate the difference between the PPI and tachycardia CL in the case of AVNRT, but without significant changes in the case of orthodromic AVRT. The reason is that the site of pacing at the RV base is farther from the AVNRT circuit than the RV apex (the paced wavefront has to travel first to near the RV apex before engaging the HPS and conducting retrogradely to the AVN), but it is still close to an AVRT circuit using a septal BT (and in fact is closer to the ventricular insertion of the BT).[33]

However, there are several potential pitfalls to those criteria. The tachycardia CL and VA interval are often perturbed for a few cycles after entrainment. For this reason, care should be taken not to measure unstable intervals immediately after ventricular pacing. In addition, spontaneous oscillations in the tachycardia CL and VA intervals can be seen. The discriminant points chosen may not apply when the spontaneous variability is more than 30 milliseconds. In addition, it is possible to mistake isorhythmic VA dissociation for entrainment if the pacing train is not sufficiently long or the pacing CL is too close to the tachycardia CL. Finally, those criteria may not apply to BTs with significant decremental properties, although small decremental intervals are unlikely to provide a false result.

Additionally, overdrive ventricular pacing during entrainment can induce decremental anterograde AVN conduction. Subtracting the increment in AVN conduction time in the first PPI (post-pacing AH interval – prepacing AH interval) from the [PPI – SVT CL] difference ("corrected" [PPI – SVT CL]) has been found to improve the accuracy of this criterion. The difference between the AV intervals (post-pacing AV interval – prepacing AV interval) can be taken for the latter adjustment when a clear His deflection is lacking. A corrected [PPI – SVT CL] of less than 110 milliseconds was found to be highly accurate in identifying orthodromic AVRT from AVNRT.[34-36]

Again, no QRS fusion is manifest during ventricular entrainment of AVNRT, and QRS morphology is that of pure paced morphology. Fusion during resetting or entrainment of AVNRT with ventricular stimulation would require the paced ventricular wavefronts to enter the circuit propagating through the HB at the time that impulses are exiting through this structure. The HB is also the site of exit of the tachycardia circuit to the ventricular tissue. Therefore, collision of the antidromic wavefront and the orthodromic wavefront from the preceding beat occurs in AVN tissue and not in the ventricle. Under such circumstances, constant fusion during entrainment is almost impossible (unless a second connection exists between the atria and ventricles; i.e., an innocent bystander BT). Manifest ventricular fusion during entrainment of SVT indicates that the reentrant circuit includes ventricular tissue (diagnostic of AVRT), thus excluding both AVNRT and AT.

DIFFERENTIAL RIGHT VENTRICULAR ENTRAINMENT. Differential-site RV entrainment (from RV apex versus RV base) can help distinguish AVNRT from orthodromic AVRT. Because the reentrant circuit in AVNRT is confined above the HB and does not involve the ventricle, the base of the RV is electrically more distant (although anatomically closer) than the RV apex to the tachycardia circuit, given that the His-Purkinje network directly inserts in the RV apex. Consequently, the PPI after entrainment of AVNRT from the RV base is longer than that following entrainment from the RV apex. The difference in PPI from RV base versus RV apex is largely composed of the extra time required to reach the circuit from the base versus the apex (approximately 30 milliseconds). Conversely, in orthodromic AVRT, in which the ventricles are an obligatory part of the circuit, the basal pacing site relative to the RV apex is variably related to the circuit, closer than the RV apex with septal BTs and equidistant with free wall BTs, but the paced wavefront from either RV apex or RV base tends to have, on average, approximately equal access and EP proximity to the reentrant circuit involved in orthodromic AVRT. Therefore, the time taken to reach the circuit (and hence the PPI) tends to be similar, irrespective of the location of the BT.

As noted, decremental conduction can occur during entrainment of either AVNRT or orthodromic AVRT, and most commonly it occurs during conduction through the AVN, especially the AVN slow pathway. The degree of decrement is dependent on both the pacing rate and the functional refractory properties of the AVN. Therefore, the PPI will prolong if decrement occurs, but the degree of decrement is not expected to be materially different from basal rather than apical pacing as long as the pacing rates are the same or similar. To avoid potential error introduced by decremental conduction within the AVN, correction of the PPI is preferred, and it is obtained by subtracting any increase in the AV interval of the return cycle beat (as compared with the AV interval during SVT). In one study, a differential corrected [PPI – SVT CL] of more than 30 milliseconds after transient entrainment was observed in all cases of AVNRT (i.e., corrected PPI following pacing from the RV base was consistently at least 30 milliseconds longer than that following pacing from the RV apex), and corrected [PPI – SVT CL] of less than 30 milliseconds was observed in all cases of orthodromic AVRT. Additionally, differential VA interval (ventricular stimulus-to-atrial interval during entrainment from RV base versus RV septum) of more than 20 milliseconds was consistent with AVNRT, whereas a differential VA interval of less than 20 milliseconds was consistent with orthodromic AVRT.[37]

LENGTH OF PACING DRIVE REQUIRED FOR ENTRAINMENT. Careful analysis of the beginning of RV pacing during the SVT can aid in the tachycardia diagnosis. Assessing the timing and type of response of SVT to RV pacing also can help differentiate orthodromic AVRT from AVNRT with high positive and negative predictive values. In the setting of orthodromic AVRT, ventricular tissue is the only intervening tissue between the pacing wavefront and the ventricular insertion site of the BT. Therefore, once ventricular capture is achieved during RV pacing, the paced wavefront propagates to the ventricular insertion site of the BT quickly and resets the tachycardia. Consequently, RV pacing results in a faster response of resetting the tachycardia. In the setting of AVNRT, on the other hand, the pacing wavefront has to penetrate the HPS and AVN tissue prior to resetting the tachycardia. This results in delayed resetting of the tachycardia compared with orthodromic AVRT. After initiation of synchronized RV pacing during SVT at a CL 10 to 40 milliseconds shorter than the tachycardia CL, once constant-appearing paced RV complexes (either pure capture or fixed fusion) are observed (as evidenced by fixed pacing morphology of the surface ECG), the number of RV paced beats required to accelerate the SVT to the pacing CL is determined. The first atrial capture beat accelerated to the pacing CL is identified by demonstrating a fixed ventricular stimulus–to–atrial capture interval. One report demonstrated that using a cutoff of one beat to accelerate the SVT to the pacing CL could identify all orthodromic AVRT cases and essentially exclude all cases of AVNRT with high accuracy. On the contrary, if two beats are required to accelerate SVT to the pacing CL, this can distinguish AVNRT from orthodromic AVRT with very high confidence as well. The major advantage of this method is its independence of tachycardia continuation after cessation of pacing. However, it is likely that these criteria may not be applicable at faster pacing CLs because resetting of the tachycardia may occur earlier in AVNRT in response to a greater degree of penetration into the tachycardia circuit. In addition, these findings may not apply in cases in which AVNRT occurs in the setting of a bystander BT because SVT may be reset using the bystander BT.[38]

ATRIAL RESETTING DURING THE TRANSITION ZONE. On initiation of RV pacing trains during the SVT at a rate slightly faster than the SVT CL, there is a transition zone during which the

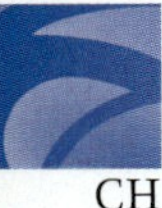

pacing train fuses with anterograde ventricular activation (i.e., the zone in which the paced QRS complexes show progressive fusion with the SVT complexes) until stable QRS morphology is observed (either completely paced or constantly fused). In patients with AVNRT or AT, acceleration of the timing of atrial activation cannot occur through the AVN during the transition zone. The reason is that the HB is expected to be refractory, as indicated by at least some ventricular activation still occurring by anterograde conduction over the HPS, similar to the concept of entrainment with manifest fusion discussed previously. If perturbation of atrial timing occurs during the transition zone, it indicates the presence of a retrogradely conducting BT, which can be an integral part of the SVT circuit (i.e., orthodromic AVRT) or a bystander. In one report, these criteria showed excellent diagnostic accuracy and could be applied regardless of whether entrainment was achieved or whether the SVT terminated during pacing. Perturbation of atrial timing for 15 milliseconds or longer or a fixed S-A interval measured from last beat of the transition zone was seen in all the patients with orthodromic AVRT and in none of the patients with AVNRT or AT.[39]

ATRIAL AND VENTRICULAR ELECTROGRAM SEQUENCE FOLLOWING CESSATION OF VENTRICULAR PACING. Following ventricular entrainment of typical AVNRT, an "A-V" electrogram sequence is observed after the last paced QRS (see Fig. 17-18). In contrast, following overdrive ventricular pacing (1:1 VA conduction) during AT, retrograde conduction occurs through the AVN. In this setting, the last retrograde P wave resulting from ventricular pacing is unable to conduct back to the ventricle because the AVN is still refractory to anterograde conduction, and the result is an A-A-V response (as discussed in detail in Chap. 11). Importantly, this maneuver is not useful when 1:1 VA conduction during ventricular pacing is absent (see Fig. 11-14). Additionally, a pseudo–A-A-V response can occur during atypical AVNRT because retrograde conduction during ventricular pacing occurs through the slow pathway. This can result in a VA interval that is longer than the pacing CL; hence, the last ventricular paced impulse is followed first by the P wave conducted slowly from the previous paced QRS and then by the P wave resulting from the last paced QRS, thus mimicking an A-A-V response (see Fig. 17-19). Careful identification of the last atrial electrogram that resulted from VA conduction during ventricular pacing avoids this potential pitfall. The last atrial activation resulting from conduction of the last paced ventricular complex follows the preceding P wave with an A-A interval equal to the ventricular pacing CL. A pseudo–A-A-V response can also occur during typical AVNRT with long HV intervals or short HA intervals, or both, in which atrial activation precedes ventricular activation. In the latter setting, using HB activation instead of ventricular activation (i.e., characterizing the response as A-A-H or A-H instead of A-A-V or A-V, respectively) can be more accurate and can help eliminate the pseudo–A-A-V response.[40]

Diagnostic Maneuvers during Normal Sinus Rhythm after Tachycardia Termination

ATRIAL PACING AT THE TACHYCARDIA CYCLE LENGTH

Atrial pacing at the tachycardia CL can result in an AH interval during atrial pacing that is longer than the AH interval during AVNRT. The AH interval during AVNRT can appear artificially shortened because both the atrium and the HB are activated in parallel with simultaneous conduction up an upper common pathway (if present) and down the anterograde AVN pathway (the slow pathway in typical AVNRT and the fast pathway in atypical AVNRT). In contrast, during AT and orthodromic AVRT, the atrium and HB are activated in sequence, and, consequently, the AH interval during SVT approximates that during atrial pacing.

Under comparable autonomic tone status, 1:1 AV conduction over the AVN may or may not be maintained during atrial pacing at the tachycardia CL. AV block can occur during atrial pacing but not during AVNRT because of anterograde block in an upper common pathway. Retrograde conduction properties of the upper common pathway may allow 1:1 conduction from the AVNRT circuit up to the atrium, but the anterograde conduction properties may not allow 1:1 anterograde conduction from the atrium down to the ventricle during atrial pacing at a similar CL. In contrast, 1:1 AV conduction, under comparable autonomic tone status, is typically maintained during atrial pacing at the tachycardia CL in the case of AT and orthodromic AVRT.[28] Typically, atrial pacing at the tachycardia CL yields an AH shorter than that during AVNRT as a result of preferential conduction over the fast pathway. To compare slow pathway conduction intervals between AVNRT and atrial pacing more directly, one may have to initiate pacing at a CL less than the tachycardia CL to block in the fast pathway, engage the slow pathway, and then increase the pacing CL to the tachycardia CL.

VENTRICULAR PACING AT THE TACHYCARDIA CYCLE LENGTH

Ventricular pacing at the tachycardia CL results in HA and VA intervals that are longer during pacing than those during AVNRT when assessed with standard 5-mm spacing quadripolar catheters in the His position. With more closely spaced His recording electrodes, the HA interval during pacing (HA_{pacing}) may be less than that during tachycardia (HA_{SVT}), a finding implying that part of the proximal HB is part of the AVNRT circuit. Whether or not the HA interval during pacing is longer than that during tachycardia thus depends in large part on how proximal an HB recording is made. The ΔHA interval ($HA_{pacing} - HA_{SVT}$) is typically more than −10 milliseconds, because the HA interval during AVNRT is shortened by parallel activation of both the HB and the atrium during the tachycardia, whereas the HB and atrium are activated sequentially during ventricular pacing (Fig. 17-20). The ΔHA interval is even more pronounced in atypical AVNRT, which has a lower common pathway that is longer than that in typical AVNRT. In focal junctional tachycardia, the ΔHA interval is typically close to 0 (see Fig. 17-20).[28]

When pacing the atrium or ventricle at the tachycardia CL, it is important that the autonomic tone be similar to its state during the tachycardia because alterations of autonomic tone can independently influence AV or VA conduction. Under comparable autonomic tone, 1:1 VA conduction over the AVN may or may not be maintained during ventricular pacing at the tachycardia CL because of possible retrograde block in the lower common pathway. Anterograde conduction properties of the lower common pathway may allow 1:1 conduction from the AVNRT circuit down to the ventricle, but its retrograde conduction properties may not allow 1:1 retrograde conduction from the ventricle up to the atrium during ventricular pacing at a CL similar to the tachycardia CL. When VA block is present, orthodromic AVRT is excluded, and AT or AVNRT with lower common pathway physiology is more likely.

The atrial activation sequence during ventricular pacing is similar to that during AVNRT. A different atrial activation sequence suggests the presence of a retrogradely conducting BT, which may or may not be related to the SVT.

PARA-HISIAN PACING

Para-Hisian pacing helps exclude the presence of a septal AV BT, which can mediate an orthodromic AVRT with a retrograde atrial activation sequence similar to that during AVNRT. In the absence of a BT, para-Hisian pacing results in a shorter S-A interval when the HB-RB is captured (S-H = 0 and S-A = HA) than the S-A interval when only the ventricle is captured (S-A = S-H+HA) with no change in the atrial activation sequence or HA interval. This response to para-Hisian pacing is termed *pattern 1* or *AVN/AVN pattern*.[28]

A change in the retrograde atrial activation sequence with loss of HB-RB capture indicates the presence of a retrogradely conducting BT. Similarly, an S-A (VA) interval that is constant

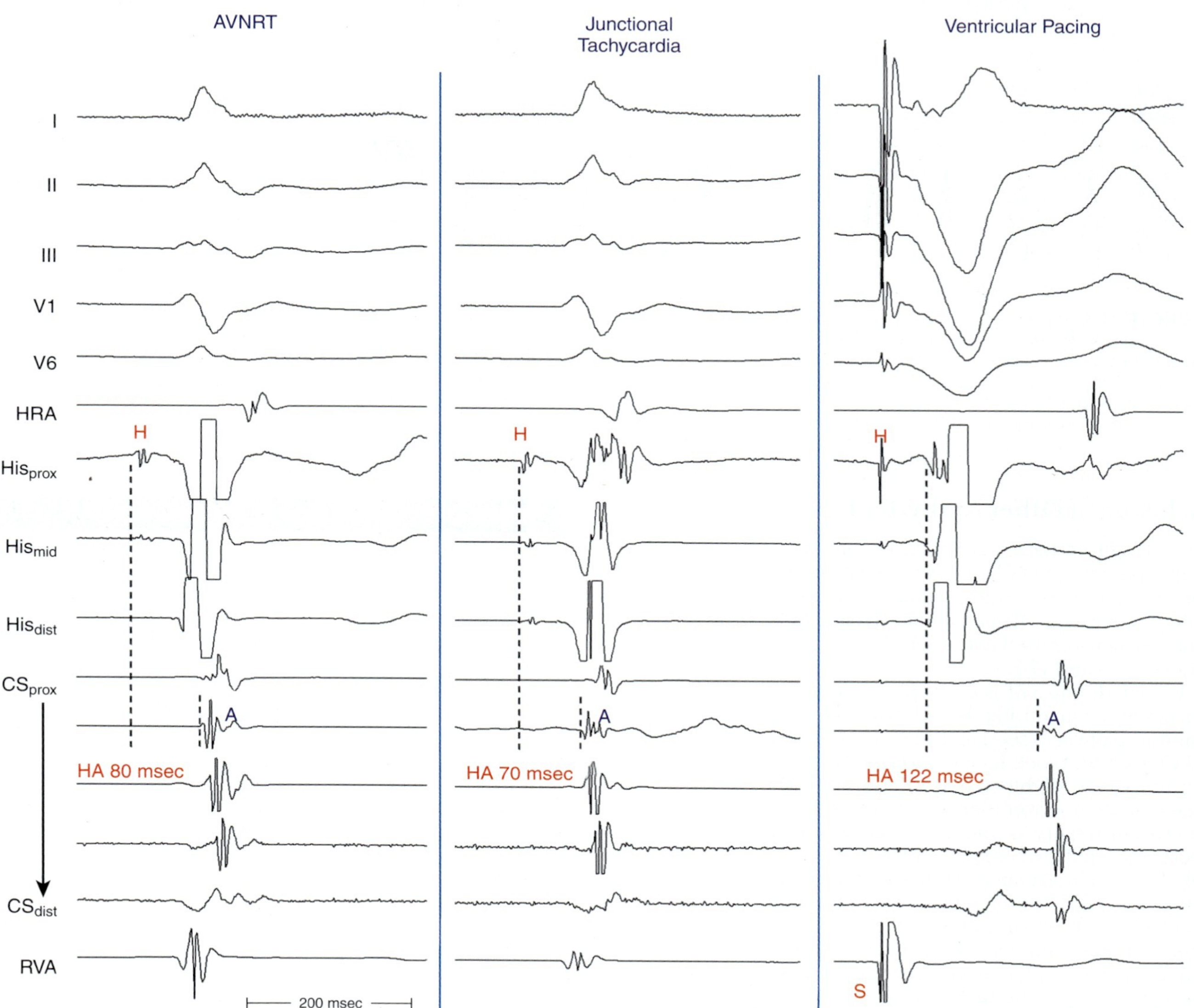

FIGURE 17-20 HA intervals during atrioventricular nodal reentrant tachycardia (AVNRT) **(left)**, junctional tachycardia during radiofrequency application **(center)**, and ventricular pacing at tachycardia cycle length in the same patient **(right)**, measured from His potential onset to onset of atrial activation (near-proximal coronary sinus) as indicated by dashed lines. CS_{dist} = distal coronary sinus; CS_{prox} = proximal coronary sinus; His_{dist} = distal His bundle; His_{mid} = middle His bundle; His_{prox} = proximal His bundle; HRA = high right atrium; RVA = right ventricular apex.

regardless of whether the HB RB is being captured indicates the presence of a BT, whereas prolongation of the S-A (VA) interval on loss of HB capture, compared with that during HB capture, excludes the presence of a retrogradely conducting BT, except for slowly conducting and far free-wall BTs. Please refer to Chapter 18 for a more detailed discussion of para-Hisian pacing.[28]

DIFFERENTIAL RIGHT VENTRICULAR PACING

The response to differential RV pacing can be evaluated by comparing two variables between RV basal and RV apical pacing: the VA interval and atrial activation sequence. In the absence of a septal AV BT, pacing at the RV apex results in rapid access of the paced wavefront to the RB, HB, and AVN, and in a shorter VA interval compared with pacing at the RV base. In the presence of a retrogradely conducting septal AV BT, pacing at the RV base allows the wavefront to access the BT rapidly and activate the atrium with a shorter VA interval than during RV apical pacing, which is farther from the BT ventricular insertion site.[28]

Occurrence of RB block (RBBB) (but not LB block [LBBB]) can alter the significance of the VA interval criterion, especially when VA conduction propagates over the HPS-AVN. In the presence of retrograde RBBB, VA conduction occurs over the LB-HB. Therefore, the VA interval depends on the distance between the pacing site and the LB rather than the RB, and access of the paced wavefront to the LB can be faster for RV basal or septal pacing compared with pacing from the RV apex (Fig. 17-21).

The atrial activation sequence is similar during RV apical and RV basal pacing in the absence of a retrogradely conducting AV BT because the atrium is activated over the AVN in both cases. In contrast, in the presence of a septal AV BT, the atrial activation sequence may or may not be similar during pacing from the RV apex versus RV base. Atrial activation may propagate only over the AV BT in both situations, or it may propagate over the AV BT during RV basal pacing and over the AVN (or a fusion of conduction over both the AVN and AV BT) during RV apical pacing. Please refer to Chapter 18 for a more detailed discussion on differential RV pacing.

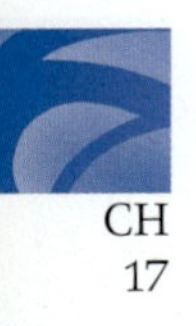

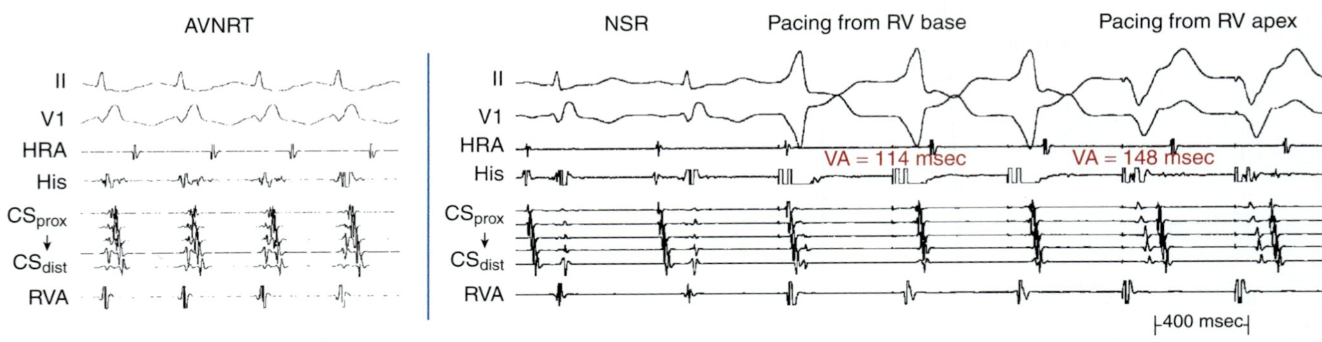

FIGURE 17-21 Comparison between right ventricular (RV) basal versus apical pacing during normal sinus rhythm (NSR, **right panel**) in a patient with typical atrioventricular nodal reentrant tachycardia (AVNRT) and right bundle branch block (RBBB, **left panel**) but no bypass tracts (BTs). RBBB is also observed during NSR **(beginning of right panel).** In the absence of a retrogradely conducting BT, pacing from the RV apex is expected to result in a shorter ventriculoatrial (VA) interval than pacing from the RV base. However, in this case, the presence of RBBB produces misleading results because retrograde VA conduction occurs over the left bundle branch (LB)–His bundle, and the VA interval depends on the distance between the pacing site to the LB, as opposed to the right bundle branch. CS_{dist} = distal coronary sinus; CS_{prox} = proximal coronary sinus; HRA = high right atrium; RVA = right ventricular apex.

Exclusion of Other Arrhythmia Mechanisms

ATs arising from the anteroseptal region and orthodromic AVRT using superoparaseptal BTs can mimic typical AVNRT. Additionally, ATs arising from the posteroseptal region and orthodromic AVRT using posteroseptal BTs can mimic atypical AVNRT. The various EP testing maneuvers used to exclude these tachycardias are outlined in Tables 17-6 and 17-7.

VA block during SVT is a rare phenomenon. As noted, VA block can rarely occur during AVNRT because of block in an upper common pathway (see Fig. 17-13). Other potential mechanisms of SVT with VA block include automatic junctional tachycardia with retrograde VA block and orthodromic AVRT using a nodofascicular or nodoventricular BT for retrograde conduction.[41] Intra-Hisian reentry is another potential mechanism, but it is a theoretical entity whose clinical occurrence has not convincingly been demonstrated. All these tachycardias are associated with a concentric atrial activation sequence, mimicking AVNRT. Nonetheless, several criteria can distinguish AVNRT from the other SVT mechanisms. Automatic junctional tachycardia typically cannot be induced or terminated by programmed stimulation; initiation of the tachycardia is usually spontaneous with absence of a critical AH delay and often requires catecholamines. Additionally, automatic junctional tachycardia is characterized by a gradual increase in tachycardia rate (warm-up) following initiation, marked CL variation, and slow decrease in tachycardia rate (cool-down), rather than an abrupt termination. The presence of nodofascicular (nodoventricular) tachycardia should be suspected when intermittent anterograde preexcitation is recorded, when AES fails to capture the tachycardia circuit, and when the SVT can be initiated with a single AES producing two ventricular complexes (mimicking the 1:2 response observed in patients with dual AVN physiology) or by a VES without a retrograde His deflection. Orthodromic AVRT can be diagnosed by demonstrating changes in the tachycardia CL with the development of BBB, and resetting or termination of the SVT by a late-coupled VES delivered when the HB is refractory.[15,42]

TABLE 17-6 Exclusion of Atrial Tachycardia

Oscillations in SVT CL	• Changes in atrial CL that are predicted by the change in the preceding ventricular CL argue against AT. • Spontaneous changes in tachycardia CL accompanied by constant VA interval (VA linking) exclude AT.
VES delivered during SVT	• VES that terminates the SVT without atrial activation excludes AT. • VES that delays the next atrial activation excludes AT.
Overdrive ventricular pacing during SVT	• The presence of A-V electrogram sequence following cessation of pacing is consistent with AVNRT and generally excludes AT.
Overdrive atrial pacing during SVT	• An ΔAH interval ($AH_{pacing} - AH_{SVT}$) >40 msec excludes AT. • If the VA interval following the last entrained QRS is reproducibly constant (with <10 msec variation), despite pacing at different CLs or for different durations (VA linking) and similar to that during SVT CL, AT is unlikely. • If the VA interval following the last entrained QRS is reproducibly constant (with <14-msec variation), despite pacing at different atrial sites (VA linking), AT is unlikely.
Atrial pacing during NSR at tachycardia CL	• An ΔAH interval ($AH_{pacing} - AH_{SVT}$) >40 msec excludes AT. • AV block during atrial pacing argues against AT.
SVT termination	• Reproducible termination of the SVT (spontaneous or with adenosine) with a P wave not followed by a QRS excludes AT.

AH = atrial–His bundle; AT = atrial tachycardia; AV = atrioventricular; A-V = atrium-ventricle; AVNRT = atrioventricular nodal reentrant tachycardia; CL = cycle length; NSR = normal sinus rhythm; SVT = supraventricular tachycardia; VA = ventriculoatrial; VES = ventricular extrastimulus.

Ablation

Target of Ablation

Ablation of the slow pathway is indicated in patients with documented AVNRT during EP testing, but it also can be performed in patients with documented SVT that is morphologically consistent with AVNRT on preprocedure ECG or rhythm strip but in whom only dual AVN physiology (but not tachycardia) is demonstrated during an EP study. Slow pathway ablation may also be considered at the discretion of the physician when sustained (more than 30 seconds) AVNRT is induced incidentally during an ablation procedure directed at a different clinical tachycardia.

Historically, the initial approach of RF ablation of AVNRT was modification of AVN conduction by lesions created near the anterosuperior aspect of the triangle of Koch (fast pathway ablation or the "anterior approach"). However, because the fast pathway constitutes the physiological conduction axis and is located in close proximity to the compact AVN and HB, this procedure was associated with an unacceptable risk of AV block or unphysiologically long PR intervals and was consequently abandoned. Since the early 1990s, selective ablation of the slow AVN pathway by lesions created near the posteroinferior base

TABLE 17-7	Exclusion of Orthodromic Atrioventricular Reentrant Tachycardia
VA interval	• A VA interval <70 msec or a V–high RA interval <95 msec during SVT excludes orthodromic AVRT.
AV block	• Spontaneous or induced AV block with continuation of the SVT excludes orthodromic AVRT.
VES delivered during the SVT	• Failure to reset (advance or delay) atrial activation with early-coupled VES on multiple occasions and at different VES coupling intervals, despite advancement of the local ventricular activation at all sites (including the site of the suspected BT) by >30 msec, excludes orthodromic AVRT and the presence of AV BT.
Entrainment of SVT by ventricular pacing	• A ΔVA ($VA_{pacing} - VA_{SVT}$) >85 msec argues against orthodromic AVRT. • A PPI – SVT CL >115 msec argues against orthodromic AVRT. • A corrected PPI – SVT CL >110 msec argues against AVRT. • Manifest ventricular fusion during entrainment indicates AVRT and excludes AVNRT. • Acceleration of the SVT to the pacing CL occurring only after two or more captured paced RV complexes is consistent with AVNRT and excludes orthodromic AVRT. • A differential corrected PPI – SVT CL of >30 msec after transient entrainment from the RV apex versus the RV base is consistent with AVNRT and excludes orthodromic AVRT. • A differential VA interval (ventricular stimulus-to-atrial interval during entrainment from RV base versus RV septum) of >20 msec is consistent with AVNRT and excludes orthodromic AVRT.
Entrainment of SVT by atrial pacing	• An ΔAH ($AH_{pacing} - AH_{SVT}$) >40 msec excludes orthodromic AVRT.
Ventricular pacing during NSR at the tachycardia CL	• A ΔHA ($HA_{pacing} - HA_{SVT}$) > −10 msec excludes orthodromic AVRT.
Atrial pacing during NSR at the tachycardia CL	• An ΔAH ($AH_{pacing} - AH_{SVT}$) >40 msec excludes orthodromic AVRT. • AV block during atrial pacing argues against orthodromic AVRT.
Differential RV pacing during NSR	• Pacing at the RV base producing a longer VA interval and identical atrial activation sequence compared with that during pacing at the RV apex excludes the presence of a septal AV BT mediating an orthodromic AVRT.
Para-Hisian pacing	• Loss of HB RB capture resulting in an increase in the S-A interval in all electrograms (equal to the increase in the S-H interval), with no change in the atrial activation sequence or HA interval, excludes the presence of a septal AV BT mediating an orthodromic AVRT.

AH = atrial–His bundle interval; AV = atrioventricular; AVRT = atrioventricular reentrant tachycardia; BT = bypass tract; CL = cycle length; HA = His bundle–atrial; HB = His bundle; NSR = normal sinus rhythm; PPI = post-pacing interval; RA = right atrium; RB = right bundle branch; RV = right ventricle; S-A = stimulus-to-atrial; S-H = stimulus-to-His bundle; SVT = supraventricular tachycardia; VA = ventriculoatrial; VES = ventricular extrastimulation.

of the triangle of Koch between the CS os and tricuspid annulus (the "posterior approach") has proved to be a more successful and safer procedure. Additionally, in patients with multiple slow pathways, ablation of the fast pathway can be associated with persistently inducible AVNRT with anterograde conduction over a second slowly conducting pathway. In contrast, successful ablation of the slow pathway can eliminate all variants of AVNRT.[43,44]

The target for the posterior approach is the site of the slow pathway. This target can be defined by one of two approaches: a purely anatomical approach and an electroanatomical approach. Despite the lack of precise knowledge of the pathophysiological substrate for AVNRT, ablation procedures have fortunately been successful.

ANATOMICAL APPROACH

The target of ablation is the isthmus of tissue between the tricuspid annulus and the CS os (Fig. 17-22).[28] The sequence of ablation sites chosen for RF delivery is related to the probability of successful slow pathway ablation at each site and the risk of impairing AV conduction. The most common site for effective and safe ablation is along the tricuspid annulus immediately anterior to the CS os; this site has a success rate of 95%. Occasionally, successful ablation can require the catheter positioned along the tricuspid annulus inferior to the CS os. If ablation is not successful at these locations, the catheter is then moved more cephalad along the tricuspid annulus superior to the CS os. Finally, if those sites are unsuccessful, RF delivery at more superior sites (more than halfway between the CS os and HB) can be considered only if the risk of complete AV block can be justified by the severity of clinical symptoms.[28]

If slow pathway ablation cannot be achieved in the inferoseptal RA, it may be worthwhile to deliver RF energy at sites within the proximal CS, close to the os, with the ablation catheter pointing toward the LV with counterclockwise torque. Rarely, successful slow pathway ablation may require an application of energy on the left side of the posterior septum, along the mitral annulus.[28,43]

Catheter-induced AVN block occasionally occurs during mapping (approximately 2%). This may indicate the presence of a relatively small compact AVN that may be more susceptible to heart block during ablation. Catheter-induced AV block typically resolves after seconds to minutes. Careful catheter positioning to avoid sites at which catheter-induced block occurs generally results in successful ablation without AV block.

ELECTROANATOMICAL APPROACH (SLOW PATHWAY POTENTIALS)

The electroanatomical approach is guided by the identification of slow pathway potentials in conjunction with anatomical landmarks. These potentials have been used by some to define the site of the slow pathway within the triangle of Koch, and they can be used effectively as a guide to target ablation.[28]

It has been suggested that activation of the slow pathway is associated with inscription of discrete electrical potentials, often referred to as slow pathway potentials. The origin of these potentials is uncertain. Whether they represent nodal tissue activation, anisotropic conduction through muscle bundles in various sites in the triangle of Koch, or a combination of both is unclear. The electrogram morphology of the slow potentials has been variously described as sharp and rapid (representing the atrial connection to the slow pathway; see Fig. 17-22), or slow and broad with low amplitude (representing slow potentials; see Fig. 17-22). The timing of slow potentials during NSR was reported to follow closely (within 10 to 40 milliseconds) local atrial activation near the CS os or to span the AH interval (it can occur as late as the His potential). However, such potentials are specific neither to the triangle of Koch nor to patients with AVNRT and can be recorded near the tricuspid annulus at sites distant from the slow pathway. Despite these observations, the probability of recording putative slow potentials at the site of effective slow ablation is more than 90%.[28] For ablation of slow-slow and fast-slow AVNRT, the slow pathway used for retrograde conduction during the tachycardia should be targeted by ablation, and this target can be different from the slow AVN pathway used for

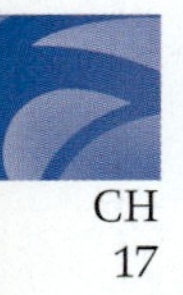

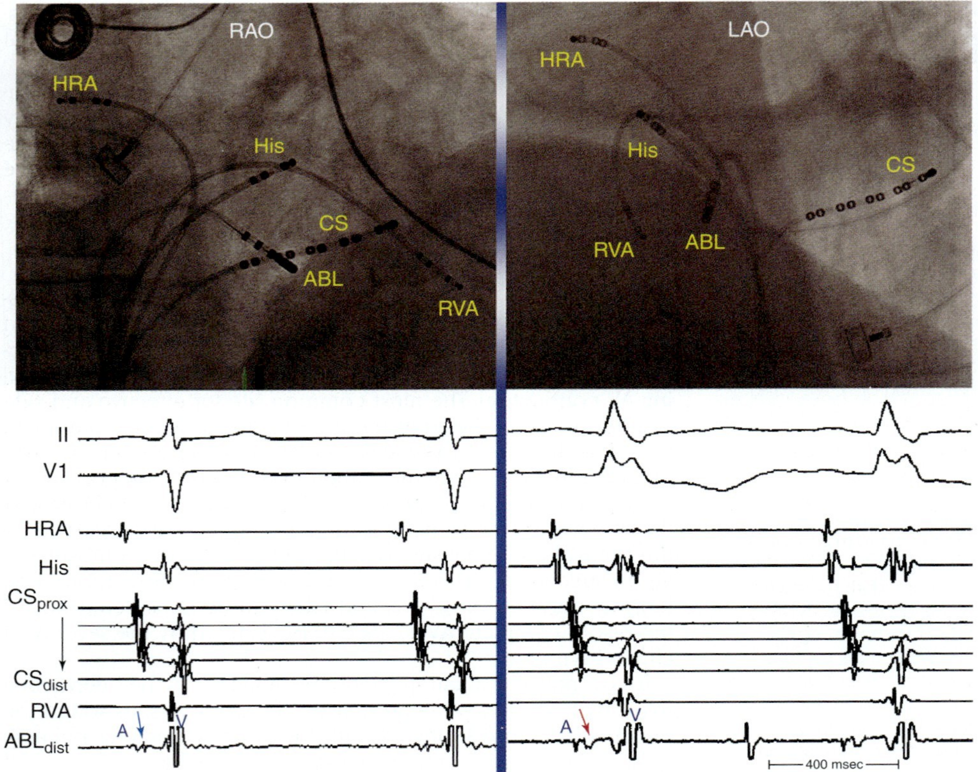

FIGURE 17-22 Ablation of the slow atrioventricular node (AVN) pathway. **Upper panel,** Right anterior oblique (RAO) and left anterior oblique (LAO) fluoroscopic views of a typical catheter setup during atrioventricular nodal reentrant tachycardia (AVNRT) ablation. The ablation catheter (ABL) is positioned at the slow pathway location in the lower portion of the triangle of Koch, away from the His bundle (His) and anterior to the coronary sinus (CS) (those landmarks are defined by the His bundle and CS catheters, respectively). **Lower panel,** Intracardiac recordings during ablation of the slow pathway. Note the sharp (blue arrow, **left lower panel**) and broad (red arrow, **right lower panel**) potentials recorded between the atrial and ventricular electrograms at the ablation sites. Those potentials were suggested to reflect activation of the slow pathway (slow pathway potentials). ABL_{dist} = distal ablation site; CS_{dist} = distal coronary sinus; CS_{prox} = proximal coronary sinus; HRA = high right atrium; RVA = right ventricular apex.

anterograde conduction. Therefore, ablation can be guided by the site of earliest retrograde atrial activation during AVNRT or ventricular pacing, which is usually localized to the isthmus of tissue between the tricuspid annulus and the CS os in fast-slow AVNRT and along the anterior aspect of the CS in slow-slow AVNRT (Fig. 17-23).[44,45]

Ablation Technique

For slow pathway ablation, a quadripolar, 4-mm-tip, deflectable ablation catheter is advanced through a femoral vein. Rarely, a superior vena caval approach (through the internal jugular or subclavian vein) is required because of inferior vena caval obstruction or barriers, and one report demonstrated the feasibility of this approach.[46] The target site can be mapped using the anatomical or electroanatomical approach. Large-tip and irrigated-tip catheters have no role in catheter ablation of the slow pathway because the larger lesions they create can increase the risk of AV block.

ANATOMICAL APPROACH

As noted, the target of slow pathway ablation is the isthmus of tissue between the tricuspid annulus and the CS os.[28] Using the right anterior oblique fluoroscopy view, which best displays the triangle of Koch in profile, the ablation catheter is advanced into the RV, moved inferiorly so that it lies anterior to the CS os, and then withdrawn until the distal pair of electrodes records small atrial and large ventricular electrograms (with an A/V electrogram amplitude ratio during NSR of 0.1 to 0.5). Gentle clockwise torque is maintained to keep the catheter in contact with the low atrial septum. This positions the catheter along the tricuspid annulus immediately anterior to the CS os (see Fig. 17-22). Positioning is best performed during NSR, rather than AVNRT, because the atrial and ventricular electrograms at the tricuspid annulus are more easily discerned. The catheter often slips into the CS when one applies even a small amount of torque because the CS is large in many of these patients. If the catheter does not easily reach far enough into the ventricle, yielding an A/V ratio of only 1:1, or if catheter stability is inadequate or falls into the CS repeatedly, a long sheath with a slight septal angulation can be helpful. Moreover, some ablation catheters have asymmetrical bidirectional deflection curves, an option that can prove to be of value for catheter reach and stability in some cases.[43]

ELECTROANATOMICAL APPROACH

The target site is identified by slow pathway potentials (see Fig. 17-22).[28] Initially, the triangle of Koch is mapped from the apex (where the HB is recorded) and then moved toward the CS os. This approach also helps evaluate the extension of the zone recording a His potential. Slow pathway potentials are usually recorded at the midanteroseptal position, where they are located in the middle of the isoelectric line connecting the atrial and ventricular electrograms. Moving the mapping catheter inferiorly, the slow pathway potential moves toward the atrial electrogram, and when the optimal site for slow pathway ablation is reached, it merges with the atrial electrogram. Because electrograms with these characteristics can be recorded near the tricuspid annulus at sites distant from the slow pathway, the region explored with the ablation catheter should be limited to the posterior septum, near the CS os.[28] In the left anterior oblique fluoroscopy view, using the HB and CS os positions (as defined by the HB and CS catheters) as landmarks, the most common area where the slow potentials are recorded is in the posterior third of the line connecting those two landmarks.[45]

Validation of slow pathway potentials can be useful and can be achieved by demonstrating that they represent slow and decremental conduction properties. Typically, brief runs of incremental atrial pacing or AES produce a decline in the amplitude and slope, an increase in the duration, and a separation of the slow potential from the preceding atrial electrogram until disappearance of any consistent activity. This is especially helpful in the presence of a sharp slow pathway potential, to distinguish it from a proximal HB recording (Fig. 17-24). Catheter-induced junctional ectopy, when present, indicates that the catheter tip is at a good ablation site. In patients with slow-slow and slow-fast AVNRT, mapping during

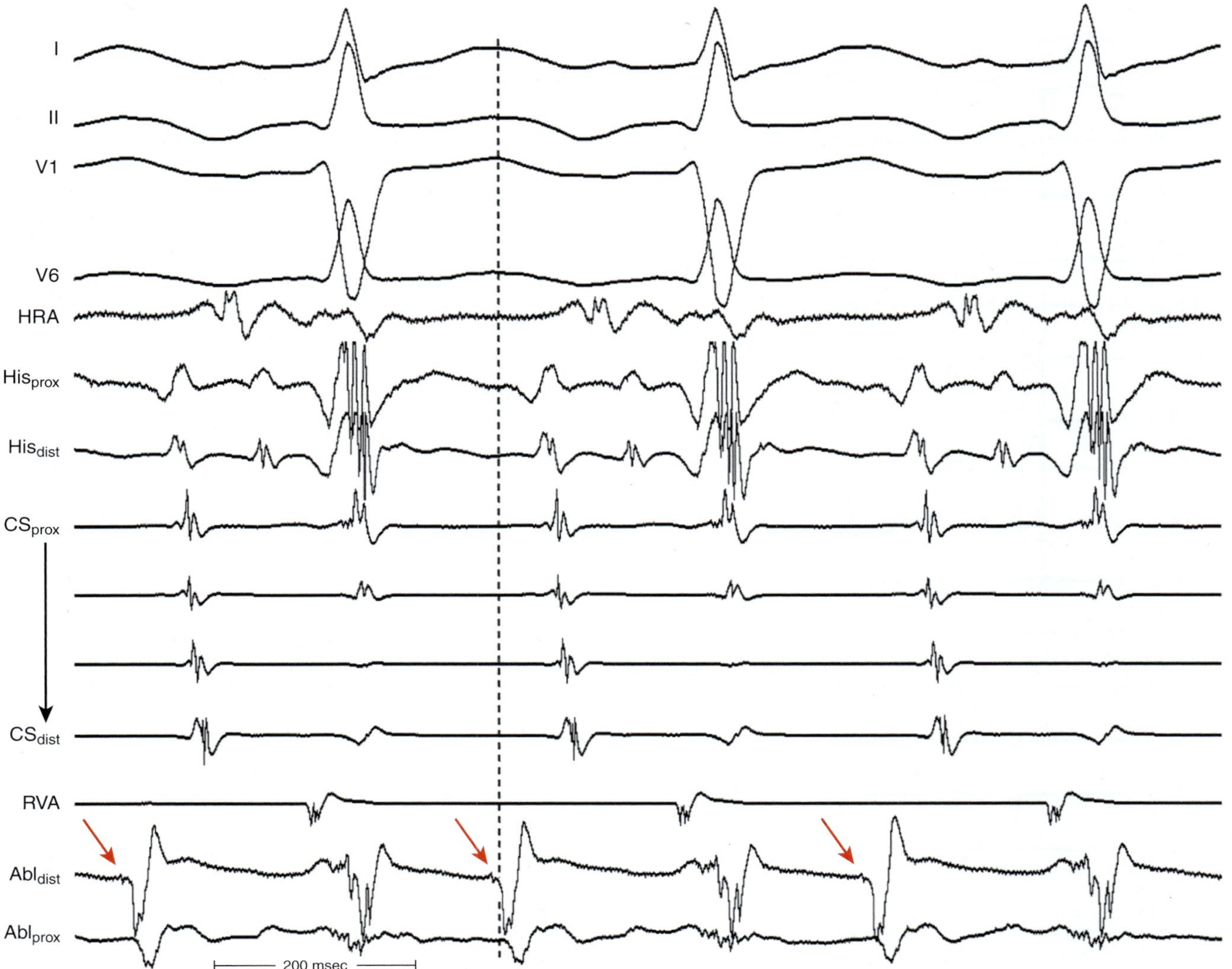

FIGURE 17-23 Ablation site in atypical (fast-slow) atrioventricular nodal reentrant tachycardia; a small spike (arrow) precedes the earliest atrial electrogram. ABL$_{dist}$ = distal ablation site; ABL$_{prox}$ = proximal ablation site; CS$_{dist}$ = distal coronary sinus; CS$_{prox}$ = proximal coronary sinus; His$_{dist}$ = distal His bundle; His$_{prox}$ = proximal His bundle; HRA = high right atrium; RVA = right ventricular apex.

AVNRT often shows a discrete potential 20 to 40 milliseconds prior to the earliest atrial electrogram; this may indicate the slow pathway and signify a good target site.[45]

RADIOFREQUENCY ENERGY DELIVERY

Catheter stability should be optimized before starting RF energy application, to avoid inadvertent AV block. This may require cessation of isoproterenol infusion if hyperdynamic contractility is present. Additionally, good positioning of the other EP catheters defining the anatomical landmarks demarcating the triangle of Koch and the location of HB is mandatory.

Ablation should be performed during NSR, when it is easier to maintain a stable catheter position. When ablation is carried out during AVNRT, sudden termination of the tachycardia during RF delivery can result in any combination of dislodgment of the ablation catheter, inadvertent AV block, or an incomplete RF lesion.[28]

Typical RF settings consist of a maximum power of 50 W and a maximum temperature of 55° to 60°C, continued for 30 to 60 seconds, or until the junctional rhythm extinguishes (see later).[28] Impedance and ECG should be carefully monitored throughout RF application. However, in the case of slow pathway ablation, the decrement in impedance associated with successful energy applications is usually small (approximately 2.5 Ω); such a small change precludes the clinical usefulness of impedance monitoring.

JUNCTIONAL RHYTHM

An accelerated junctional rhythm typically develops within a few seconds of RF delivery at the effective ablation site (Fig. 17-25). The mechanism of this rhythm is unclear but is likely to be secondary to enhanced automaticity in AVN tissue because of thermal injury. Accelerated junctional rhythm during RF ablation is usually associated with subtle changes in retrograde atrial activation sequence (compared with that during AVNRT). Occurrence of this rhythm is strongly correlated with and sensitive to successful ablation sites; it occurs more frequently (94% versus 64%) and for a longer duration (7.1 versus 5.0 seconds) during successful compared with unsuccessful RF applications. Such a rhythm is, however, not specific for slow pathway ablation and is routinely observed during intentional fast pathway and AVN ablation. More rapid junctional tachycardia, on the other hand, is probably caused by thermal injury of the HB and heralds impending AV block (Fig. 17-26).[44,47,48]

When an accelerated junctional rhythm occurs, careful monitoring of VA conduction during this rhythm is essential, and

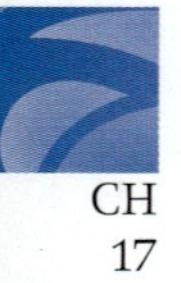

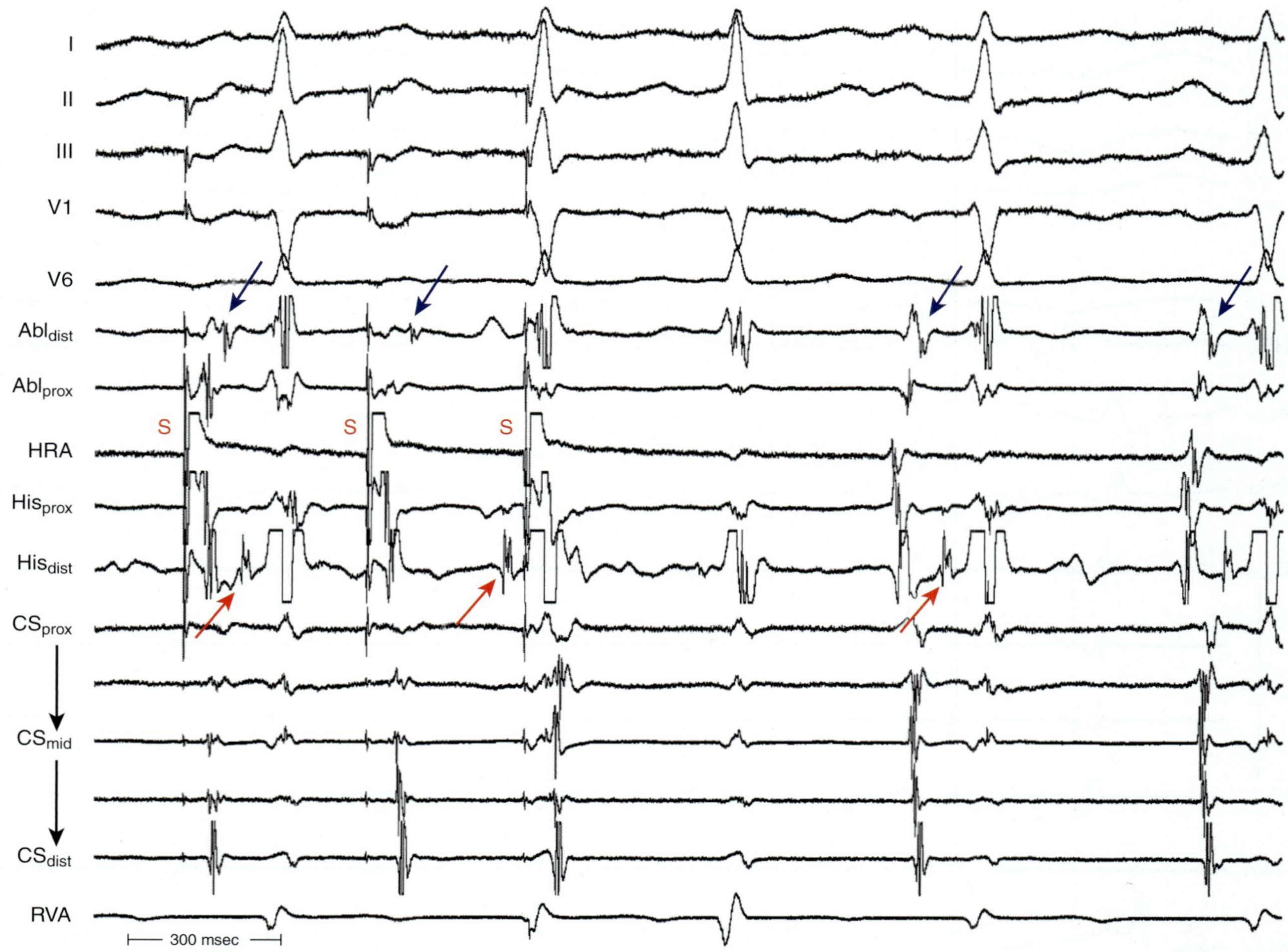

FIGURE 17-24 A putative slow pathway potential (blue arrows) is validated as being distinct from the His bundle potential (red arrows) by a burst of atrial stimulation. ABL_{dist} = distal ablation site; ABL_{prox} = proximal ablation site; CS_{dist} = distal coronary sinus; CS_{prox} = proximal coronary sinus; His_{dist} = distal His bundle; His_{prox} = proximal His bundle; HRA = high right atrium; RVA = right ventricular apex; S = stimulus.

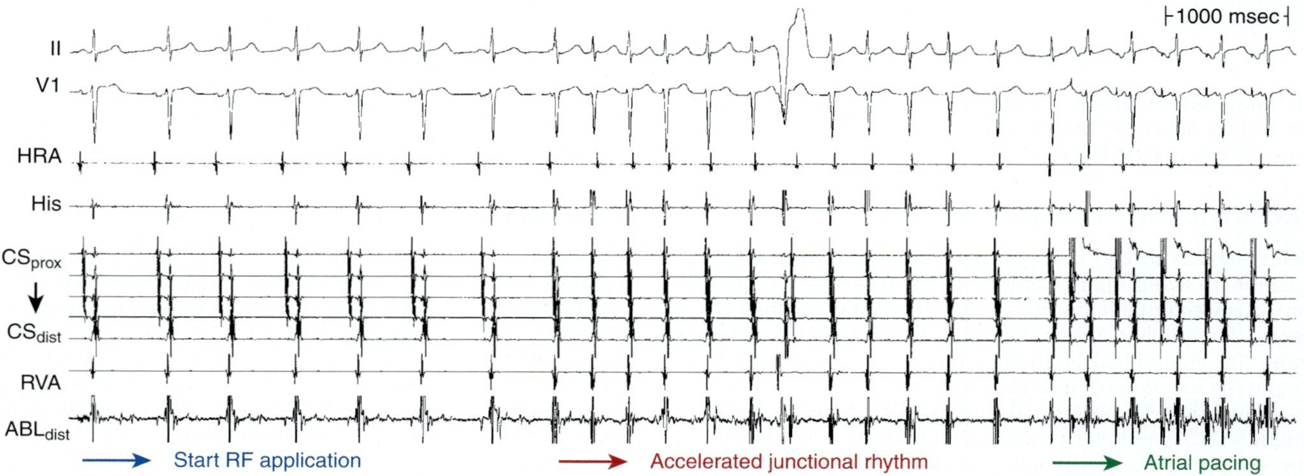

FIGURE 17-25 Catheter ablation of the slow atrioventricular nodal pathway. Radiofrequency (RF) energy delivery during normal sinus rhythm results in accelerated junctional rhythm with intact ventriculoatrial conduction. Overdrive atrial pacing at a rate faster than the junctional rhythm rate was started and confirmed intact atrioventricular conduction. This observation can indicate a good ablation site, with no injury to the fast pathway. ABL_{dist} = distal ablation site; CS_{dist} = distal coronary sinus; CS_{prox} = proximal coronary sinus; HRA = high right atrium; RVA = right ventricular apex.

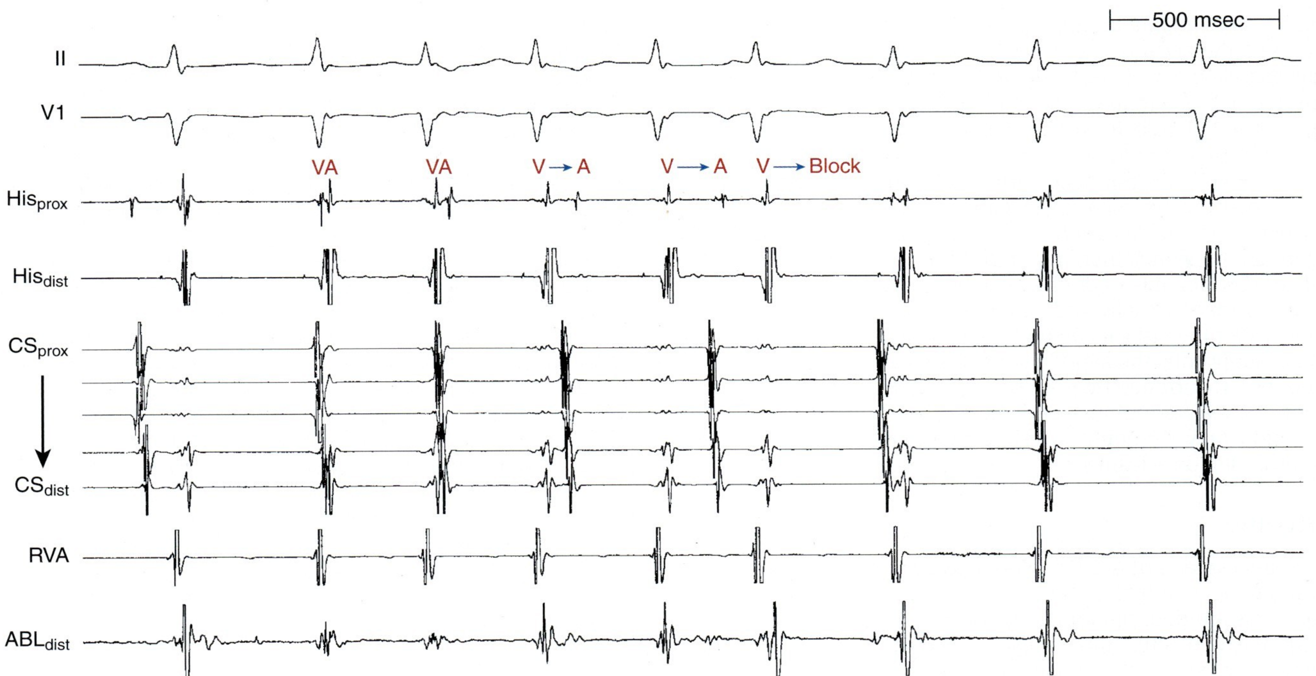

FIGURE 17-26 Junctional tachycardia observed during slow pathway ablation. Wenckebach ventriculoatrial (VA) block is observed during the junctional rhythm, a sign that heralds injury to the His bundle and should prompt immediate termination of radiofrequency application. ABL_{dist} = distal ablation site; CS_{dist} = distal coronary sinus; CS_{prox} = proximal coronary sinus; His_{dist} = distal His bundle; His_{prox} = proximal His bundle; RVA = right ventricular apex.

overdrive atrial pacing may be performed to ensure maintenance of 1:1 anterograde AV conduction (see Fig. 17-25). Occasionally, atrial pacing at a rate sufficiently fast to override the junctional rhythm results in AV Wenckebach block at baseline, even before the onset of RF energy delivery. In this case, isoproterenol can be used to shorten the AV block CL and maintain 1:1 AV conduction during pacing.[48]

The absence of junctional rhythm during RF application corresponds to an unsuccessful ablation site. When an accelerated junctional rhythm does not develop within 10 to 20 seconds of RF delivery, RF application should be stopped, and the catheter tip should be repositioned to a slightly different site or until better contact is verified, and a new RF application is attempted. Nevertheless, a junctional rhythm may not occur in several situations, including atypical forms of AVNRT (fast-slow and slow-slow) and some cases of typical (slow-fast) AVNRT undergoing repeat ablation.

After an RF application that results in an accelerated junctional rhythm, programmed electrical stimulation (atrial and ventricular stimulation) is performed to determine the presence or absence of slow pathway conduction, AVN echoes, or inducible AVNRT. If the result is unsatisfactory, the catheter is moved to a slightly different site (usually a few millimeters anteriorly), and RF is reapplied.[44,48]

Several observations should prompt immediate discontinuation of RF application, including sudden impedance rise (more than 10 Ω), prolongation of the PR interval (during NSR or atrial pacing), development of AV block, fast junctional tachycardia (CL shorter than 350 milliseconds), and retrograde conduction block during junctional ectopy (see Fig. 17-26). Although the last observation may herald anterograde AV bock in the case of typical AVNRT and necessitates immediate discontinuation of RF delivery, retrograde block over the fast pathway is a common occurrence in patients with atypical AVNRT, even before ablation. In this setting, the occurrence of junctional rhythm with no VA conduction may not be such an ominous sign; in fact, such an occurrence may indicate successful ablation of the slow pathway and thus should prompt ongoing RF delivery.[28] As noted earlier, atrial pacing at a rate sufficient to overdrive junctional rhythm allows monitoring of anterograde fast pathway conduction and helps ensure safe RF application.

Endpoints of Ablation

The optimal endpoint for slow pathway ablation is the complete elimination of slow pathway conduction and dual AVN physiology without impairing the fast pathway. This is evidenced by loss of conduction over the slow pathway (i.e., disappearance of discontinuous AV conduction curves), alteration of Wenckebach CL (shorter or longer), an increase in the ERP of the AVN, and preservation of intact anterograde and retrograde AVN (fast pathway) conduction.[49] In many cases, the ERP of the fast pathway can actually shorten, likely secondary to the withdrawal of electrotonic inhibition imposed on the fast pathway by the slow pathway. For atypical AVNRT, elimination of retrograde fast pathway conduction (i.e., complete VA block) is an important additional endpoint.[43,44]

However, elimination of all evidence of slow pathway conduction is not a necessary requirement for a successful slow pathway ablation procedure.[28] It suffices to eliminate inducibility of AVNRT and 1:1 anterograde conduction over the slow pathway, with and without isoproterenol infusion. Complete elimination of all anterograde slow conduction is not essential for clinical success and is actually associated with a slightly higher risk of AV block. In patients with a successful slow pathway ablation procedure, 40% to 50% will still have dual AVN physiology, and 75% of those patients will have single AVN echoes, but AVNRT is not inducible (these patients are said to have undergone slow pathway modification). In most patients who no longer have inducible AVNRT after ablation in the slow pathway region, residual discontinuous AVN function curves and single AVN echoes do not predict an increased risk of AVNRT recurrence.

Therefore, noninducibility of AVNRT (with and without isoproterenol infusion), with residual evidence of dual AVN pathways (AH interval jump) and single AVN echoes with an echo zone shorter than 30 milliseconds, is an acceptable endpoint. However, double AVN echoes or single echoes produced over a wide range of coupling intervals usually predict inducibility of AVNRT with the addition of isoproterenol or atropine, as well as late clinical recurrence of SVT. Therefore, additional RF applications are recommended.[43] When AVNRT or dual AVN physiology, or both, is rarely inducible at baseline, it may not be possible to confirm the efficacy of RF ablation. In this case, other parameters can be indicative of a successful

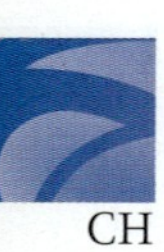

ablation, including the disappearance of a PR/RR ratio greater than 1 during rapid atrial pacing with 1:1 AV conduction, prolongation of the Wenckebach CL, and a decrease in fast pathway ERP.[8,28,43] If isoproterenol was required for initiation of SVT prior to ablation, isoproterenol should be discontinued during ablation and readministered afterward to assess the efficacy of ablation adequately. If isoproterenol was not necessary for SVT initiation prior to ablation, it need not be used for postablation testing. However, if the presence of single AVN echoes is accepted as an endpoint, isoproterenol infusion is then required during postablation testing to verify noninducibility of double echoes or AVNRT.[43,44]

Reassessment of tachycardia inducibility is typically repeated 30 minutes after the last successful RF application. However, there are no data supporting the hypothesis that such a waiting period leads to reduced recurrence rates following acutely successful ablation. In fact, one report demonstrated that a procedure-prolonging waiting period may be omitted without compromising the patient's long-term outcome results.[50]

Outcome

Acute success rates of AVNRT ablation using the posterior approach are approximately 97% to 99%, and they are similar whether the ablation is guided anatomically or electroanatomically.[49] The recurrence rate after apparently successful ablation is approximately 2% to 5%. In 40% of patients with AVNRT recurrences, slow pathway conduction recovers after initial evidence of its abolition. Most AVNRT recurrences take place within the first days to months after ablation.[44,49]

The most important complication of AVNRT ablation is AV block. AV block occurs in approximately 0.2% to 0.8% of patients who undergo slow pathway ablation using the posterior approach, it generally occurs during RF delivery or within the first 24 hours after ablation, and it is almost always preceded by junctional ectopy with VA block. The level of block is usually in the AVN. Predictors of AV block include proximity of the anatomical ablation site to the compact AVN, the occurrence of fast junctional tachycardia (CL shorter than 350 milliseconds) during RF application, the occurrence of junctional rhythm with VA block, the number of RF applications (related to the amount of tissue damage), and significant worsening of anterograde AV conduction during the ablation procedure.[49,51]

Palpitations occur in 20% to 30% of patients following ablation of AVNRT. These are generally transient and usually are not caused by recurrent AVNRT. Most are caused by premature atrial or ventricular complexes, which subside spontaneously and require no treatment other than reassurance. Inappropriate sinus tachycardia can develop in some patients after AVNRT ablation, a finding suggesting disruption of the parasympathetic or sympathetic inputs into the sinus node and AVN.

Subclinical activation of the coagulation system (e.g., elevated plasma levels of the D-dimer) is common during RF ablation. Nevertheless, clinically detectable embolic events are uncommon (0.7%). Aspirin is usually recommended for 6 to 8 weeks following ablation, to minimize the risk of thrombus formation in the RA or vena cavae. Other complications include cardiac tamponade (in 0.2% of patients), hematoma (in 0.2%), and femoral artery pseudoaneurysm (in 0.1%).[44]

There are several advantages of selective slow pathway ablation over fast pathway ablation, including a significantly lower risk of AV block and avoidance of a long postablation PR interval, which can cause symptoms similar to those of the pacemaker syndrome. Furthermore, in patients with multiple slow pathways, as demonstrated by AVN function curves, ablation of the fast pathway can be associated with persistently inducible AVNRT, with anterograde conduction over a second slowly conducting pathway.[44]

Selective slow pathway ablation can be technically challenging in several clinical situations. For example, in patients with evidence of impaired fast pathway conduction (usually older patients with tachycardia CL longer than 400 milliseconds), ablation of the slow pathway can result in mandatory conduction through the impaired fast pathway, and Wenckebach block during rest can develop. Whether the fast pathway should be targeted by ablation instead of the slow pathway in these patients is controversial. Similarly, some patients with AVNRT have a markedly prolonged PR interval during NSR, a finding suggesting the possibility of absent anterograde fast pathway conduction and a high risk of complete AV block if the slow pathway is ablated. However, in such patients, the fast pathway can be affected by an electrotonic interaction with the slow pathway, and elimination of this effect by slow pathway ablation often shortens the ERP of the fast pathway. In fact, in many of these patients, the AH interval remains stable or even shortens after slow pathway ablation. Another challenging situation may be experienced in patients with prior unsuccessful attempts at fast pathway ablation, with persistent AVNRT. Slow pathway ablation may then result in high-degree AV block because of impairment of the fast pathway related to the prior ablation attempt. In such patients, it may be wise to confine further ablation efforts to the pathway originally targeted for ablation.[43,44]

It is also important to know that in some cases of typical AVNRT, the fast pathway can have a more posterior location, and the earliest atrial activation site during the tachycardia is near the CS os. In such cases, ablation should be performed with caution because RF application at the usual slow pathway anatomical site can result in PR interval prolongation or heart block. Cryoablation can be of advantage in these situations.

Fast Pathway Modification (Anterior Approach)

TARGET OF FAST PATHWAY ABLATION

The target site of this approach is located closer to the compact AVN and HB in the anterosuperior region of the triangle of Koch. The anterior approach selectively ablates or modifies fast pathway retrograde conduction; however, it can also cause damage to fast or slow pathway anterograde conduction.[43,44] Fast pathway ablation is hardly ever the treatment of choice, with the rare exception of patients with clear AVNRT who have a long PR in sinus rhythm (i.e., slow pathway conduction) and no evidence of anterograde fast pathway conduction.

FAST PATHWAY ABLATION TECHNIQUE

The ablation catheter is initially positioned at the AV junction to obtain the maximal amplitude of the bipolar His potential recorded from the distal pair of electrodes. The catheter is then withdrawn while a firm clockwise torque is maintained until the His potential becomes small or barely visible or disappears while recording a relatively large atrial electrogram (with an A/V electrogram amplitude ratio greater than 1; see Fig. 15-63). At the optimal ablation site, retrograde atrial activation timing occurs earlier or simultaneously with the atrial electrogram in the catheter at the HB position. At this point, the ablation catheter is held steadily, and RF energy is applied (starting at low power outputs of 5 to 10 W) until one of the following events occurs: impedance rise, transient high-grade AV block, prolongation of the PR interval by more than 30% to 50%, or appearance of very rapid junctional rhythm associated with retrograde conduction block. Overdrive atrial pacing may be performed to monitor AV conduction in case a junctional escape rhythm occurs during RF application.[43,44]

ENDPOINTS OF FAST PATHWAY ABLATION

The endpoint of ablation is noninducibility of AVNRT or development of AV block. Frequently, fast pathway ablation is associated with retrograde VA block over both the slow and fast pathways. Occasionally, dual AVN physiology can still be present.

OUTCOME OF FAST PATHWAY ABLATION

Short-term success rates are greater than 95%. However, the anterior approach has a small safety margin and is associated with a higher risk of inadvertent complete AV block (approximately 10%, but ranging from 2% to 20%). Careful monitoring of AV conduction during RF application and prompt discontinuation of energy delivery on evidence of AV block are the keys to minimize the incidence of AV block.

Cryoablation of the Slow Pathway

TARGET OF CRYOABLATION

The target of ablation is the region of the slow pathway, and it is identified anatomically or electroanatomically, as described for standard RF ablation. The target site should be identified during NSR whether cryoablation is to be performed during NSR or AVNRT, because the A/V ratio and electrogram morphology usually are obscured during AVNRT.

CRYOABLATION TECHNIQUE

Cryomapping

Cryomapping (ice mapping) is designed to verify that ablation at the chosen site will have the desired effect (i.e., block in the slow pathway) and to reassure the absence of complications (i.e., AV block). Cryomapping is performed at a temperature of –30°C. At this temperature, the cryolesion is reversible (for up to 60 seconds), and the catheter is stuck to the atrial endocardium within an ice ball that includes the tip of the catheter (cryoadherence). Formation of an ice ball at the catheter tip and adherence to the underlying myocardium are signaled by the appearance of electrical noise recorded from the ablation catheter's distal bipole. In the cryomapping mode, the temperature is not allowed to drop to less than –30°, and the duration of energy application is limited to 60 seconds. Once an ice ball is formed, various pacing protocols are performed to test the modification or disappearance of slow pathway conduction.[52]

Cryomapping is usually performed during NSR in patients with discontinuous anterograde dual AVN conduction curve. For patients without a clear discontinuity in the AVN conduction curve, cryomapping may be performed during AVNRT, which is feasible without the risk of catheter dislodgment on termination of the tachycardia (because of cryoadherence).[52]

During cryoablation of the slow pathway, no junctional rhythm is observed. Thus, other parameters must be used to validate the potential effectiveness of the ablation site. In fact, the absence of junctional rhythm can be advantageous because it allows the maintenance of NSR during ablation and enables monitoring of the PR interval throughout the procedure. Additionally, the maintenance of NSR during cryoablation allows various pacing maneuvers to be performed during ongoing cryoenergy application, to evaluate the effect of the ablation on slow pathway conduction. Disappearance of the dual AVN physiology, noninducibility of AVNRT, and modification of the fast pathway ERP predict a successful ablation site. When cryoablation is performed during AVNRT, progressive AH interval lengthening followed by termination of AVNRT indicates slow pathway block.[52]

Slow pathway block usually occurs quickly (within 10 to 20 seconds) at the optimal target site. If cryomapping does not yield the desired result within 20 to 30 seconds or causes unintended AV conduction delay or block, the cryomapping procedure is interrupted. After a few seconds, to allow the catheter to thaw and become dislodged from the tissue, the catheter is moved to a different site, and cryomapping is repeated.[52]

Cryoablation

When sites of successful cryomapping are identified by demonstrating satisfactory slow pathway block or modification with no modification of the basal anterograde AV conduction, the cryoablation mode is activated, during which a target temperature lower than –75°C is sought (a temperature of approximately –75° to –80°C is generally achieved). The application is then continued for 4 minutes, to create an irreversible lesion. If the catheter tip is in close contact with the endocardium, a prompt drop in catheter tip temperature should be seen as soon as the cryoablation mode is activated. A slow decline in temperature or a very high flow rate of refrigerant during ablation suggests poor catheter tip tissue contact; in such cases, cryoablation should be interrupted and the catheter repositioned.[52]

The successful site for cryomapping and cryoablation of the slow pathway frequently is found in the midseptal region of the Koch triangle, more superiorly than the usual site of successful RF ablation. Rarely, AV block does not appear during cryomapping at a particular site but occurs during cryoablation at the same site. Fortunately, this resolves quickly if the cryoablation is interrupted promptly.

ENDPOINTS OF CRYOABLATION

The goal of cryoablation is the complete elimination of slow pathway function. This usually requires delivery of several cryoapplications at closely adjacent sites. If a discontinuity in the anterograde AVN conduction curve and single AVN echoes persist despite multiple cryoapplications, this is still a reasonable endpoint, provided that multiple echoes or SVT are not inducible, even during isoproterenol infusion. If acute procedural success cannot be achieved with a standard 4-mm-tip catheter, a 6-mm-tip catheter can be used, which can help yield larger and deeper cryolesions.[52]

OUTCOME OF CRYOABLATION

Previously published reports with cryoablation of AVNRT in pediatric patients demonstrated procedural success rates of 83% to 97% and recurrence rates ranging from 0% to 20%. Although the use of bonus cryoapplications to consolidate the acutely successful cryoablation and the choice of larger-tip cryocatheters (8-mm and 6-mm versus 4-mm tips) to create larger lesions have been associated with fewer recurrences on long-term follow-up without compromising safety, the overall procedural success rate has remained consistently lower than that of RF ablation.[51,53-56]

The safety of cryoablation is indisputable. Not a single case of persistent AV block has been reported, even when using large-tip cryocatheters, despite the fact that transient AV block occurs in up to 11% of patients during cryomapping at –30°C or during cryoablation at –75°C.

ADVANTAGES OF CRYOABLATION

One of the distinct advantages of cryothermal technology is the ability to demonstrate loss of function of tissue with cooling reversibly (ice mapping or cryomapping), thereby demonstrating the functionality of prospective ablation sites without inducing permanent injury. Furthermore, once the catheter tip temperature is reduced to less than 0°C, progressive ice formation at the catheter tip causes adherence to the adjacent tissue (cryoadherence), which maintains stable catheter contact at the site of ablation and minimizes the risk of catheter dislodgment during changing cardiac rhythm.[52] A disadvantage of cryoablation is that the cryocatheter is not yet as steerable as the conventional RF catheter, and this can potentially limit proper positioning of the catheter tip.[52] The procedure is also slightly longer than standard RF ablation.

Cryoablation can be of particular advantage in patients with AVNRT with posterior displacement of the fast pathway or AVN, and those with a small space in the triangle of Koch between the HB and the CS os, when ablation must be performed in the midseptum. However, given the high success rate and low risk of RF slow pathway ablation, it may be difficult to demonstrate a clinical advantage of cryoablation over RF ablation of unselected AVNRT cases. Therefore, the use of cryoablation may be recommended in specific circumstances in which the use of RF can be more likely to cause AVN damage. These circumstances include patients with unusual cardiac anatomy that makes safe RF delivery difficult, those with evidence of impaired AV conduction at baseline, those who need ablation in the close vicinity of the compact AVN following unsuccessful RF ablation at more posterior sites, pediatric patients, and patients in whom even the small risk of AV block associated with RF ablation is considered unacceptable.[51-53]

REFERENCES

1. Tawara SL: Das Reitzleitungssystem des Saugetierherzens. In Fischer G, editor: *Handbuch der vergleichenden und experimentellen entwicklungslehre der wirbeltiere,* Jena, Germany, 1906, Semper Bonis Artibus, pp 136–137.
2. Anderson R, Ho S: The anatomy of the atrioventricular node. Heart Rhythm Society, 2008, http://www.hrsonline.org/Education/SelfStudy/Articles/AndersonHo_Anatomy_AVNode.pdf.
3. Kurian T, Ambrosi C, Hucker W, et al: Anatomy and electrophysiology of the human AV node, *Pacing Clin Electrophysiol* 33:754–762, 2010.
4. Lee PC, Chen SA, Hwang B: Atrioventricular node anatomy and physiology: implications for ablation of atrioventricular nodal reentrant tachycardia, *Curr Opin Cardiol* 24:105–112, 2009.
5. Mazgalev T: AV nodal physiology. Heart Rhythm Society, 2008, http://www.hrsonline.org/Education/Self Study/Articles/mazgalev.cfm.
6. Shryock J, Belardinelli L: *Pharmacology of the AV node. Heart Rhythm Society*, 2008, http://www.hrsonline.org/Education/SelfStudy/Articles/shrbel.cfm.
7. Luc PJ: Common form of atrioventricular nodal reentrant tachycardia: do we really know the circuit we try to ablate? *Heart Rhythm* 4:711–712, 2007.
8. Lockwood D, Nakagawa H, Jackman W: Electrophysiological characteristics of atrioventricular nodal reentrant tachycardia: implications for the reentrant circuit. In Zipes DP, Jalife J, editors: *Cardiac electrophysiology: from cell to bedside*, ed 5, Philadelphia, 2009, Saunders, pp 615–646.
9. Valderrabano M: Atypical atrioventricular nodal reentry with eccentric atrial activation: is the right target on the left? *Heart Rhythm* 4:433–434, 2007.
10. Racker DK, Kadish AH: Proximal atrioventricular bundle, atrioventricular node, and distal atrioventricular bundle are distinct anatomic structures with unique histological characteristics and innervation, *Circulation* 101:1049–1059, 2000.
11. Mazgalev TN: The specialized rings and the endless saga of the AV node puzzle, *Heart Rhythm* 6:681–683, 2009.
12. Basso C, Ho SY, Thiene G: Anatomical and histopathological characteristics of the conductive tissues of the heart. In Gussak I, Antzelevitch C, editors: *Electrical diseases of the heart: genetics, mechanisms, treatment, prevention*, London, 2008, Springer, pp 37–51.
13. Katritsis DG, Becker A: The atrioventricular nodal reentrant tachycardia circuit: a proposal, *Heart Rhythm* 4:1354–1360, 2007.
14. Mazgalev TN, Ho SY, Anderson RH: Anatomic-electrophysiological correlations concerning the pathways for atrioventricular conduction, *Circulation* 103:2660–2667, 2001.
15. Morihisa K, Yamabe H, Uemura T, et al: Analysis of atrioventricular nodal reentrant tachycardia with variable ventriculoatrial block: characteristics of the upper common pathway, *Pacing Clin Electrophysiol* 32:484–493, 2009.
16. Otomo K, Okamura H, Noda T, et al: Unique electrophysiologic characteristics of atrioventricular nodal reentrant tachycardia with different ventriculoatrial block patterns: effects of slow pathway ablation and insights into the location of the reentrant circuit, *Heart Rhythm* 3:544–554, 2006.
17. Katritsis DG, Ellenbogen KA, Becker AE: Atrial activation during atrioventricular nodal reentrant tachycardia: studies on retrograde fast pathway conduction, *Heart Rhythm* 3: 993–1000, 2006.
18. Otomo K, Okamura H, Noda T, et al: "Left-variant" atypical atrioventricular nodal reentrant tachycardia: electrophysiological characteristics and effect of slow pathway ablation within coronary sinus, *J Cardiovasc Electrophysiol* 17:1177–1183, 2006.
19. Lee PC, Hwang B, Tai CT, et al: The electrophysiological characteristics in patients with ventricular stimulation inducible fast-slow form atrioventricular nodal reentrant tachycardia, *Pacing Clin Electrophysiol* 29:1105–1111, 2006.
20. Verma A: Guilty culprit or innocent bystander? *J Cardiovasc Electrophysiol* 17:1184–1186, 2006.
21. Nam GB, Rhee KS, Kim J, et al: Left atrionodal connections in typical and atypical atrioventricular nodal reentrant tachycardias: activation sequence in the coronary sinus and results of radiofrequency catheter ablation, *J Cardiovasc Electrophysiol* 17:171–177, 2006.
22. Otomo K, Nagata Y, Uno K, et al: Atypical atrioventricular nodal reentrant tachycardia with eccentric coronary sinus activation: electrophysiological characteristics and essential effects of left-sided ablation inside the coronary sinus, *Heart Rhythm* 4:421–432, 2007.
23. Otomo K, Nagata Y, Taniguchi H, et al: Superior type of atypical AV nodal reentrant tachycardia: incidence, characteristics, and effect of slow pathway ablation, *Pacing Clin Electrophysiol* 31:998–1009, 2008.
24. Porter MJ, Morton JB, Denman R, et al: Influence of age and gender on the mechanism of supraventricular tachycardia, *Heart Rhythm* 1:393–396, 2004.
25. Suenari K, Hu YF, Tsao HM, et al: Gender differences in the clinical characteristics and atrioventricular nodal conduction properties in patients with atrioventricular nodal reentrant tachycardia, *J Cardiovasc Electrophysiol* 21:1114–1119, 2010.
26. Gonzalez-Torrecilla E, Almendral J, Arenal A, et al: Combined evaluation of bedside clinical variables and the electrocardiogram for the differential diagnosis of paroxysmal atrioventricular reciprocating tachycardias in patients without pre-excitation, *J Am Coll Cardiol* 53:2353–2358, 2009.
27. Blomstrom-Lundqvist C, Scheinman MM, Aliot EM, et al: ACC/AHA/ESC guidelines for the management of patients with supraventricular arrhythmias: executive summary: a report of the American College of Cardiology/American Heart Association Task Force on Practice Guidelines and the European Society of Cardiology Committee for Practice Guidelines (writing committee to develop guidelines for the management of patients with supraventricular arrhythmias), *Circulation* 108:1871–1909, 2003.
28. Josephson ME: Supraventricular tachycardias. In Josephson ME, editor: *Clinical cardiac electrophysiology*, ed 4, Philadelphia, 2008, Lippincott Williams & Wilkins, pp 175–284.
29. Kertesz NJ, Fogel RI, Prystowsky EN: Mechanism of induction of atrioventricular node reentry by simultaneous anterograde conduction over the fast and slow pathways, *J Cardiovasc Electrophysiol* 16:251–255, 2005.
30. Crawford TC, Mukerji S, Good E, et al: Utility of atrial and ventricular cycle length variability in determining the mechanism of paroxysmal supraventricular tachycardia, *J Cardiovasc Electrophysiol* 18:698–703, 2007.
31. Maruyama M, Kobayashi Y, Miyauchi Y, et al: The VA relationship after differential atrial overdrive pacing: a novel tool for the diagnosis of atrial tachycardia in the electrophysiologic laboratory, *J Cardiovasc Electrophysiol* 18:1127–1133, 2007.
32. Knight BP, Ebinger M, Oral H, et al: Diagnostic value of tachycardia features and pacing maneuvers during paroxysmal supraventricular tachycardia, *J Am Coll Cardiol* 36:574–582, 2000.
33. Platonov M, Schroeder K, Veenhuyzen GD: Differential entrainment: beware from where you pace, *Heart Rhythm* 4:1097–1099, 2007.
34. Gonzalez-Torrecilla E, Arenal A, Atienza F, et al: First postpacing interval after tachycardia entrainment with correction for atrioventricular node delay: a simple maneuver for differential diagnosis of atrioventricular nodal reentrant tachycardias versus orthodromic reciprocating tachycardias, *Heart Rhythm* 3:674–679, 2006.
35. Veenhuyzen GD, Stuglin C, Zimola KG, Mitchell LB: A tale of two post pacing intervals, *J Cardiovasc Electrophysiol* 17:687–689, 2006.
36. Kannankeril PJ, Bonney WJ, Dzurik MV, Fish FA: Entrainment to distinguish orthodromic reciprocating tachycardia from atrioventricular nodal reentry tachycardia in children, *Pacing Clin Electrophysiol* 33:469–474, 2010.
37. Segal OR, Gula LJ, Skanes AC, et al: Differential ventricular entrainment: a maneuver to differentiate AV node reentrant tachycardia from orthodromic reciprocating tachycardia, *Heart Rhythm* 6:493–500, 2009.
38. Dandamudi G, Mokabberi R, Assal C, et al: A novel approach to differentiating orthodromic reciprocating tachycardia from atrioventricular nodal reentrant tachycardia, *Heart Rhythm* 7:1326–1329, 2010.
39. Al Mahameed ST, Buxton AE, Michaud GF: New criteria during right ventricular pacing to determine the mechanism of supraventricular tachycardia, *Circ Arrhythm Electrophysiol* 3:578–584, 2010.
40. Vijayaraman P, Lee BP, Kalahasty G, et al: Reanalysis of the "pseudo A-A-V" response to ventricular entrainment of supraventricular tachycardia: importance of His-bundle timing, *J Cardiovasc Electrophysiol* 17:25–28, 2006.
41. Lau EW: Infraatrial supraventricular tachycardias: mechanisms, diagnosis, and management, *Pacing Clin Electrophysiol* 31:490–498, 2008.
42. Issa ZF: Mechanism of paroxysmal supraventricular tachycardia with ventriculoatrial conduction block, *Europace* 11:1235–1237, 2009.
43. McElderry H, Kay GN: Ablation of atrioventricular nodal reentrant tachycardia and variants guided by intracardiac recordings. In Huang S, Wood MA, editor: *Catheter ablation of cardiac arrhythmias*, Philadelphia, 2006, Saunders, pp 347–367.
44. Snowdon RL, Kalman JM: Catheter ablation of supraventricular arrhythmias. In Zipes DP Jalife J, editor: *Cardiac electrophysiology: from cell to bedside*, ed 5, Philadelphia, 2009, Saunders, pp 1083–1092.
45. Gonzalez MD, Rivera J: Ablation of atrioventricular nodal reentry by the anatomical approach. In Huang S, Wood MA, editor: *Catheter ablation of cardiac arrhythmias*, Philadelphia, 2006, Saunders, pp 325–346.
46. Salem YS, Burke MC, Kim SS, et al: Slow pathway ablation for atrioventricular nodal reentry using a right internal jugular vein approach: a case series, *Pacing Clin Electrophysiol* 29: 59–62, 2006.
47. Lee SH, Tai CT, Lee PC, et al: Electrophysiological characteristics of junctional rhythm during ablation of the slow pathway in different types of atrioventricular nodal reentrant tachycardia, *Pacing Clin Electrophysiol* 28:111–118, 2005.
48. McGavigan AD, Rae AP, Cobbe SM, Rankin AC: Junctional rhythm: a suitable surrogate endpoint in catheter ablation of atrioventricular nodal reentry tachycardia? *Pacing Clin Electrophysiol* 28:1052–1054, 2005.
49. Estner HL, Ndrepepa G, Dong J, et al: Acute and long-term results of slow pathway ablation in patients with atrioventricular nodal reentrant tachycardia: an analysis of the predictive factors for arrhythmia recurrence, *Pacing Clin Electrophysiol* 28:102–110, 2005.
50. Steven D, Rostock T, Hoffmann BA, et al: Favorable outcome using an abbreviated procedure for catheter ablation of AVNRT: results from a prospective randomized trial, *J Cardiovasc Electrophysiol* 20:522–525, 2009.
51. Opel A, Murray S, Kamath N, et al: Cryoablation versus radiofrequency ablation for treatment of atrioventricular nodal reentrant tachycardia: cryoablation with 6-mm-tip catheters is still less effective than radiofrequency ablation, *Heart Rhythm* 7:340–343, 2010.
52. Friedman PL: How to ablate atrioventricular nodal reentry using cryoenergy, *Heart Rhythm* 2:893–896, 2005.
53. Chanani NK, Chiesa NA, Dubin AM, et al: Cryoablation for atrioventricular nodal reentrant tachycardia in young patients: predictors of recurrence, *Pacing Clin Electrophysiol* 31: 1152–1159, 2008.
54. Silver ES, Silva JN, Ceresnak SR, et al: Cryoablation with an 8-mm tip catheter for pediatric atrioventricular nodal reentrant tachycardia is safe and efficacious with a low incidence of recurrence, *Pacing Clin Electrophysiol* 33:681–686, 2010.
55. Rivard L, Dubuc M, Guerra PG, et al: Cryoablation outcomes for AV nodal reentrant tachycardia comparing 4-mm versus 6-mm electrode-tip catheters, *Heart Rhythm* 5:230–234, 2008.
56. Drago F, Russo MS, Silvetti MS, et al: Cryoablation of typical atrioventricular nodal reentrant tachycardia in children: six years' experience and follow-up in a single center, *Pacing Clin Electrophysiol* 33:475–481, 2010.

CHAPTER 18 Atrioventricular Reentrant Tachycardia

Types of Bypass Tracts

Bypass tracts (BTs) are remnants of the atrioventricular (AV) connections caused by incomplete embryological development of the AV annuli and failure of the fibrous separation between the atria and ventricles. There are several types of BTs. Atrioventricular BTs are strands of working myocardial cells connecting atrial and ventricular myocardium across the electrically insulating fibrofatty tissues of the AV junction bypassing the atrioventricular node–His-Purkinje system (AVN-HPS). In the older literature, these BTs were called Kent bundles, although incorrectly (Kent described AVN-like tissue in the right atrial [RA] free wall that did not connect to the ventricle). Thus, the use of the term *bundle of Kent* should be discouraged.[1] Atrionodal BTs connect the atrium to the distal or compact AVN. They have been called James fibers and are of uncertain physiological significance. Atrio-Hisian BTs connect the atrium to the His bundle (HB); these BTs are rare.[2,3] Atypical BTs include various types of Hisian-fascicular BTs, which connect the atrium (atriofascicular pathways), AVN (nodofascicular pathways), or HB (fasciculoventricular) to distal Purkinje fibers or ventricular myocardium, in addition to slowly conducting short atrioventricular BTs and long atrioventricular BTs. These atypical BTs are sometimes collectively referred to as Mahaim fibers, a term to be discouraged because it is more illuminating to name the precise BT according to its connections.

Types of Preexcitation Syndromes

Several patterns of preexcitation can occur, depending on the anatomy of the BT and the direction in which impulses are conducted. Conduction from the atria to the ventricles normally occurs via the AVN-HPS. Patients with preexcitation have an additional or alternative pathway, the BT, which directly connects the atria and ventricles and bypasses the AVN. The term *syndrome* is used when the anatomical variant is responsible for tachycardia.

In the Wolff-Parkinson-White (WPW) syndrome, AV conduction occurs, partially or entirely, through an AV BT, which results in earlier activation (preexcitation) of the ventricles than if the impulse had traveled through the AVN.[1] In the setting of Lown-Ganong-Levine (LGL) syndrome, preexcitation purportedly occurs via atrio-Hisian BTs or, alternatively, no BT is present and enhanced AVN conduction accounts for the electrocardiographic (ECG) findings. The net effect is a short PR interval without delta wave or QRS prolongation. It is important to stress, however, that LGL is not a recognized syndrome with an anatomical basis, but only an ECG description, and the use of the term should be discouraged.[2,3] The so-called Mahaim variant of preexcitation does not typically result in a delta wave, because these pathways, which usually terminate in the conducting system or in the ventricular myocardium close to the conducting system, conduct slowly, and the AVN-HPS has adequate time to activate most of the ventricular muscle mass. Concealed AV BTs refer to AV BTs that do not manifest anterograde conduction and therefore do not result in ventricular preexcitation. Because they do not result in alteration of the QRS complex in the ECG, they cannot be detected by inspection of the surface ECG; they are called *concealed*. However, the concealed BT can conduct in a retrograde fashion, thereby creating a reentrant circuit with impulses traveling from the atrium to the AVN, HPS, ventricle, and then back to the atrium via the BT.

Pathophysiology

Wolff-Parkinson-White Syndrome

WPW pattern refers to the constellation of ECG abnormalities related to the presence of an AV BT (short PR interval, delta wave) in asymptomatic patients.[1] *WPW syndrome* refers to a WPW ECG pattern associated with tachyarrhythmias.

Because the AV BT typically conducts faster than the AVN, the onset of ventricular activation is earlier than if depolarization occurred only via the AVN, resulting in a shortened PR (P-delta) interval. Additionally, because the BT exhibits practically nondecremental conduction, the early activation (and P-delta interval) remains almost constant at all heart rates. Preexcited intraventricular conduction in WPW propagates from the insertion point of the AV BT in the ventricular myocardium via direct muscle-to-muscle conduction. This process is inherently slower than ventricular depolarization resulting from rapid HPS conduction. Thus, although the initial excitation of the ventricles (via the BT) occurs earlier, it is followed by slower activation of the ventricular myocardium than occurs normally. The net effect is that the QRS complex consists of fusion between the early ventricular activation caused by preexcitation with the later ventricular activation resulting from impulse propagation through the AVN and HPS to the ventricles. The initial part of ventricular activation resulting in the upstroke of the QRS complex is slurred because of slow muscle-to-muscle conduction; this is termed a *delta wave*. The more rapid the conduction along the BT in relation to the AVN, the greater the amount of myocardium depolarized via the BT, resulting in a more prominent or wider delta wave and increasing prolongation of the QRS complex duration.

Atrioventricular Bypass Tracts

The AV junctions are the areas of the heart where the atrial musculature connects to the annuli of the mitral and tricuspid valves. The AVN-HPS, which lies in the septal component of the AV junction, is the only normal electrical connection between the atria and the ventricles. The fibrous skeleton and AV valvular annuli act as an insulator to prevent electrical impulses from getting into the ventricles by any other route. The main function of the AVN is modulation of atrial impulse transmission to the ventricles, thereby coordinating atrial and ventricular contractions; it receives, slows down, and conveys atrial impulses to the ventricles.

AV BTs are aberrant muscle bundles that connect the atria to the ventricles outside of the normal AV conduction system. AV BTs are found most often in the parietal AV junctional areas, including the paraseptal areas. They breach the insulation provided by the fibrofatty tissues of the AV groove (sulcus tissue) and the hinge lines (fibrous annulus) of the valves. They are rarely found in the area of fibrous continuity between the aortic and mitral valves because in this area, there is usually a wide gap between the atrial myocardium and ventricular myocardium to accommodate the aortic outflow tract.[4,5] The remainder of the AV groove may be divided into quadrants consisting of the left free wall, right free wall, and posteroseptal and anteroseptal spaces. The distribution of BTs within these regions is not homogeneous—46% to 60% of BTs are found within the left free wall space; 25% are within the posteroseptal space; 13% to 21% of BTs are within the right free wall space; and 2% are within the right superoparaseptal (formerly called anteroseptal) space (Fig. 18-1).

BTs are usually very thin muscular strands (rarely thicker than 1 to 2 mm) but can occasionally exist as broad bands of tissue. The AV BT can run in an oblique course rather than perpendicular to the transverse plane of the AV groove. As a result, the fibers can have an atrial insertion point that is transversely from less than one to several centimeters removed from the point of ventricular attachment.[6] Some posteroseptal pathways insert into coronary sinus (CS) musculature rather than atrial myocardium and can be associated with the coronary venous system or diverticula from a CS branch vein.

Multiple AV BTs occur in 5% to 10% of patients. BTs are defined as multiple when they are separated by more than 1 to 3 cm. The most common combination of widely spaced multiple BTs is posteroseptal and right free wall BTs. The incidence of multiple BTs is particularly high in patients with antidromic atrioventricular reentrant tachycardia (AVRT) (50% to 75%), patients in whom AF resulted in ventricular fibrillation (VF), and patients with Ebstein anomaly.

Although the majority (approximately 60%) of AV BTs conduct both anterogradely and retrogradely (i.e., bidirectionally), some AV BTs are capable of propagating impulses in only one direction. BTs that conduct only in the anterograde direction are uncommon (<5%), often cross the right AV groove, and frequently possess decremental conduction properties.[3] On the other hand, BTs that conduct only in the retrograde direction occur more frequently, accounting for 17% to 37% of all BTs. When the BT is capable of anterograde conduction, ventricular preexcitation is usually evident during normal sinus rhythm (NSR), and the BT is referred to as *manifest.* BTs capable of retrograde-only conduction are referred to as *concealed.*

Because working myocardial cells make up the vast majority of AV BTs, conduction over those BTs is mediated by the rapid inward sodium current, similar to normal His-Purkinje tissue and atrial and ventricular myocardium. Therefore, AV BTs have rather constant anterograde and retrograde conduction at all rates until the refractory period is reached, at which time conduction is completely blocked (nondecremental conduction). Thus, conduction over AV BTs usually behaves in an all-or-none fashion. In contrast, the AVN, which depends on the slow inward calcium current for generation and propagation of its action potential, exhibits what has been called *decremental conduction*, in which the conduction time of the impulse propagating through the AVN prolongs as the atrial cycle length (CL) shortens. Thus, AV conduction is more rapid through the AV BT than through the AVN, a difference that is increased at a fast heart rate. This difference has potentially great clinical importance. A primary function of the AVN is to limit the number of impulses conducted from the atria to the ventricles, which is particularly important during fast atrial rates (e.g., AF or atrial flutter [AFL]) when only a fraction of impulses are conducted to the ventricles, whereas the remainder are blocked in the AVN. However, in the presence of nondecrementally conducting AV BTs with short refractory periods, these arrhythmias can lead to very fast ventricular rates that can degenerate into VF.

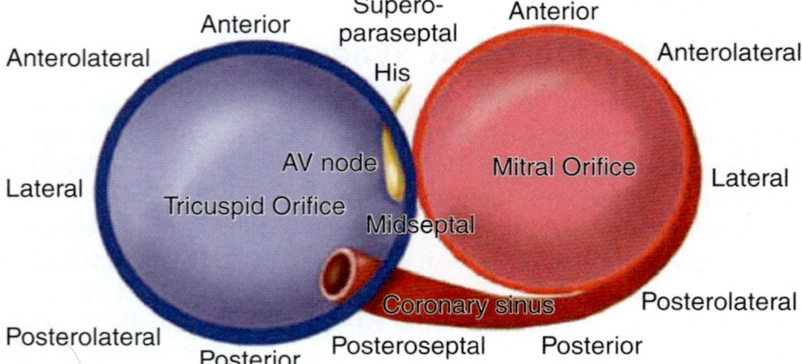

FIGURE 18-1 Locations of atrioventricular bypass tracts (AV BTs) by anatomical region. Tricuspid and mitral valve annuli are depicted in a left anterior oblique view. Locations of the coronary sinus, AV node, and His bundle are shown. AV BTs may connect atrial to ventricular myocardium in any of the regions shown. *(From Miller JM, Zipes DP: Therapy for cardiac arrhythmias. In Libby P, Bonow R, Mann DL, Zipes DP, editors: Braunwald's heart disease: a textbook of cardiovascular medicine, ed 8, Philadelphia, 2007, WB Saunders, pp 779-830.)*

Atrioventricular Reentry

AVRT is a macroreentrant tachycardia with an anatomically defined circuit that consists of two distinct pathways, the normal AV conduction system and an AV BT, linked by common proximal (atrial) and distal (ventricular) tissues. If sufficient differences in conduction time and refractoriness exist between the normal conduction system and the BT, a properly timed premature impulse of atrial or ventricular origin can initiate reentry. AVRTs are the most common (80%) tachycardias associated with the WPW syndrome. AVRT is divided into orthodromic and antidromic according to the direction of conduction in the AVN-HPS (Fig. 18-2). Orthodromic indicates normal direction (anterograde) of conduction over AVN-HPS during the AVRT.

ORTHODROMIC ATRIOVENTRICULAR REENTRANT TACHYCARDIA

In orthodromic AVRT, the AVN-HPS serves as the anterograde limb of the reentrant circuit (i.e., the pathway that conducts the impulse from the atria to the ventricles), whereas an AV BT serves as the retrograde limb (see Fig. 18-2). Approximately 50% of BTs participating in orthodromic AVRT are manifest (able to conduct bidirectionally) and 50% are concealed (able to conduct retrogradely only). Therefore, a WPW pattern may or may not be present on the surface ECG during NSR. When preexcitation is present, the delta wave seen during NSR is lost during orthodromic AVRT, because anterograde conduction during the tachycardia is not via the BT (i.e., the ventricle is not preexcited) but over the normal AV conduction system. Orthodromic AVRT accounts for approximately 95% of AVRTs and 35% of all paroxysmal supraventricular tachycardias (SVTs).

ANTIDROMIC ATRIOVENTRICULAR REENTRANT TACHYCARDIA

In antidromic AVRT, an AV BT serves as the anterograde limb of the reentrant circuit (see Fig. 18-2). Consequently, the QRS complex during antidromic AVRT is fully preexcited (i.e., the ventricles are activated totally by the BT with no contribution from the normal conduction system). The BT involved in the antidromic AVRT circuit must be capable of anterograde conduction and, therefore, preexcitation is typically observed during NSR. During classic antidromic AVRT, retrograde VA conduction occurs over the AVN-HPS. Other less frequent, nonclassic forms of antidromic AVRT can use a second BT as the retrograde limb of the reentrant circuit or a combination of one BT plus the AVN-HPS in either direction (Fig. 18-3). Antidromic AVRT occurs in 5% to 10% of patients with WPW syndrome. Susceptibility to antidromic AVRT appears to be facilitated by a distance of at least 4 cm between the BT and the normal AV conduction system. Consequently, most antidromic AVRTs use a lateral (right or left) BT as the anterograde route for conduction. Because posteroseptal BTs are in close proximity to the AVN, those BTs are less commonly part of antidromic AVRT if the other limb is the AVN and not a second free wall BT.[3] Up to 50% to 75% of patients with spontaneous antidromic AVRT have multiple BTs (manifest or concealed), which may or may not be used as the retrograde limb during the tachycardia. Antidromic SVT is thus a subset of preexcited tachycardias.

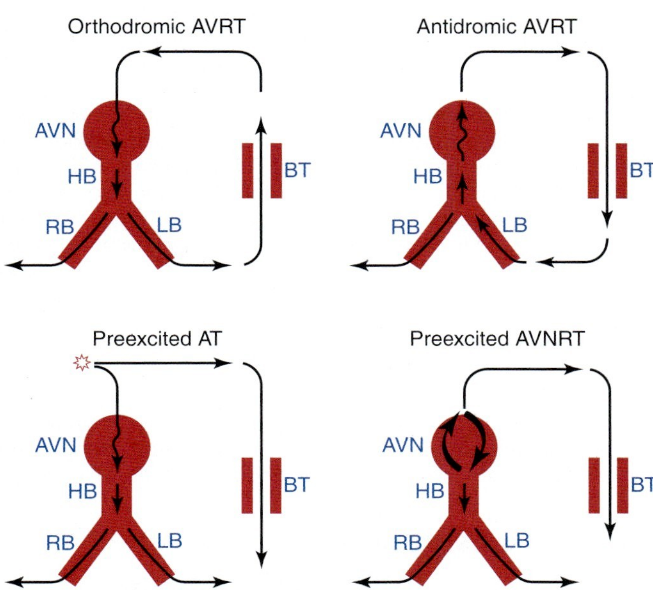

FIGURE 18-2 Schematic representation of the reentrant circuit during orthodromic atrioventricular reentrant tachycardia (AVRT), antidromic AVRT, preexcited atrial tachycardia (AT), and preexcited atrioventricular nodal reentrant tachycardia (AVNRT) using a left-sided bypass tract (BT). HB = His bundle; LB = left bundle branch; RB = right bundle branch.

PERMANENT JUNCTIONAL RECIPROCATING TACHYCARDIA

Permanent junctional reciprocating tachycardia (PJRT) is an orthodromic AVRT mediated by a concealed, retrogradely conducting AV BT that has slow and decremental conduction properties. Conduction properties of this retrograde BT are slower than the anterograde conduction properties of the AVN and those of typical fast BTs found in patients with AVRT. The BT in PJRT is most often located in the posteroseptal region, although other portions of the AV groove can also harbor this unusual pathway. Because these BTs are almost always concealed and have slow conduction, all elements necessary for reentry are present at all times, and thus PJRT can be present much of the time (i.e., incessant), with only short interludes of sinus rhythm.

Other Arrhythmias Associated with Wolff-Parkinson-White Syndrome

Atrial tachycardia (AT), AFL, AF, and atrioventricular nodal reentrant tachycardia (AVNRT) can all coexist with a BT. In these preexcited tachycardias, the BT serves as a bystander route for ventricular or atrial activation, and is not required for the initiation or maintenance of the arrhythmia.

ATRIOVENTRICULAR NODAL REENTRANT TACHYCARDIA AND ATRIAL TACHYCARDIA

Physiology consistent with dual AVN physiology has been reported in 8% to 40% of patients with WPW syndrome, although spontaneous sustained AVNRT is less frequent. Both AVNRT and AT can use the bystander BT to transmit impulses to the ventricle (see Fig. 18-2). When AVNRT occurs in the WPW syndrome, the arrhythmia can be difficult to distinguish from AVRT without electrophysiological (EP) testing.

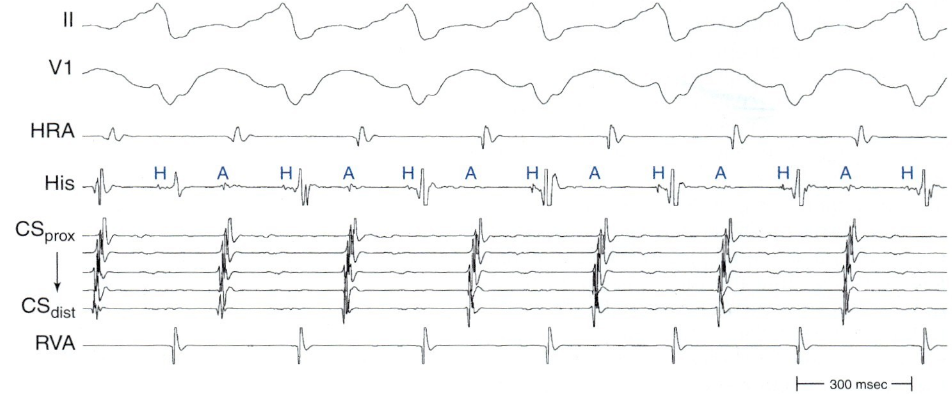

FIGURE 18-3 The presence of multiple bypass tracts (BTs) is indicated by an eccentric atrial activation sequence during antidromic atrioventricular reentrant tachycardia using a right lateral BT anterogradely and a left lateral BT retrogradely. A = atrial electrogram; H = His bundle potential.

ATRIAL FIBRILLATION

Paroxysmal AF occurs in 50% of patients with WPW, and is the presenting arrhythmia in 20%. Chronic AF, however, is rare in these patients.[3] Spontaneous AF is most common in patients with anterograde conduction through the BT. Patients with antidromic AVRT, multiple BTs, and BTs that have a short anterograde effective refractory period (ERP) are more liable to develop AF.[3] In individuals with WPW, AF is often preceded by AVRT that degenerates into AF.

The frequency with which intermittent AF occurs in patients with the WPW syndrome is striking because of the low prevalence of coexisting structural heart disease, which is a major predisposing factor for AF in subjects without a BT. This observation suggests that the AV BT itself can be related to the genesis of AF.

The mechanisms by which AVRT precipitates AF are not well understood. The rapid atrial rate can cause disruption in atrial activation and reactivation, creating an electrophysiological substrate conducive to AF. The observation that most patients with BT and AF who undergo BT ablation are cured of both AVRT and AF is compatible with this hypothesis. Another possibility is that the complex geometry of networks of BTs predisposes to AF by fractionation of the activation wavefronts. Localized reentry has been recorded in some patients, using direct recordings of the activation of the BTs. Hemodynamic changes, atrial stretch caused by atrial contraction against closed AV valves during ventricular systole, can also play a role. Ablation of the BT can cure AF in more than 90% of patients; however, vulnerability to AF persists in up to 56%, and the response to atrial extrastimulation (AES) is also unaltered by ablation.

ATRIAL FLUTTER

AFL is the most common (60%) regular preexcited tachycardia in patients with WPW syndrome. AFL is caused by a reentrant circuit within the RA and therefore exists independently of the BT, and AFL does not have the same causal association to AV BTs as AF. In some patients with WPW syndrome who develop AFL, AVRT is the initiating event. This relationship can be mediated by contraction-excitation feedback into the atria during the AVRT.

AFL, like AF, can conduct anterogradely via a BT causing a preexcited tachycardia. Depending on the various refractory periods of the normal and pathological AV conduction pathways, AFL potentially can conduct 1:1 to the ventricles during a preexcited tachycardia, making the arrhythmia difficult to distinguish from ventricular tachycardia (VT; see Fig. 12-6).

VENTRICULAR FIBRILLATION AND SUDDEN CARDIAC DEATH

The mechanism of sudden cardiac death (SCD) in most patients with WPW is likely the occurrence of AF with a very rapid ventricular rate that leads to VF. Although the frequency with which AF having rapid AV conduction via a BT degenerates into VF is unknown, the incidence of SCD in patients with WPW syndrome is rather low, ranging from 0% to 0.39% annually in several large case series. The trigger for AF in this population of patients (who usually are otherwise healthy individuals and are expected to have a low rate of AF) is generally an episode of SVT. In fact, most patients who have been resuscitated from VF secondary to preexcitation have previous history of AVRT, AF, or both (although in some patients, SCD may be the presenting symptom), and induction of SVT during EP testing is also predictive of clinical symptoms in some asymptomatic individuals.[7-11]

Several factors can help identify the patient with WPW who is at increased risk for VF, including symptomatic SVT, septal location of the BT, presence of multiple BTs, and male gender.[8] Nonetheless, it is clear that the most important factor for the occurrence of VF in these patients is the ability of the BT to conduct rapidly to the ventricles. This is best measured by determining the shortest and average preexcited intervals during AF or alternatively by measuring the anterograde ERP of the BT. If the BT has a very short anterograde effective refractory period (ERP <250 milliseconds), a rapid ventricular response can occur with degeneration of the rhythm to VF. A short preexcited R-R interval during AF (≤220 milliseconds) appears to be a sensitive clinical marker for identifying patients at risk for SCD in children, although its positive predictive value in adults is only 19% to 38%.[9,10,12]

Drug therapy can be an additional determinant of the risk of VF in patients with preexcitation. As an example, intravenous verapamil can increase the ventricular response to AF and has resulted in VF in some patients. Several mechanisms are probably involved; hypotension produced by verapamil-induced vasodilation is followed by a sympathetic discharge that enhances BT conduction. Furthermore, verapamil slows AVN conduction directly and increases AVN refractoriness, resulting in less concealed penetration of the BT by normally conducted beats. Additionally, the increased rate, irregular rate, hypotension, and sympathetic discharge probably result in fractionation of the ventricular wavefront and VF. For these reasons, intravenous verapamil is contraindicated for the acute treatment of AF in patients with WPW. Other intravenous drugs that block the AVN also should be avoided, including beta blockers, adenosine, diltiazem, and digoxin. Both oral and intravenous digoxin has been associated with the degeneration of AF into VF in patients with preexcitation syndromes. Some of these patients had a history of previously benign AF. How digitalis might promote the development of VF is uncertain. One possible mechanism is that shortening of the atrial and BT ERP, plus increasing AVN block, results in decreased concealed retrograde penetration of the BT by normally conducted beats, thereby preventing its inactivation.

Intravenous adenosine, given appropriately to treat orthodromic AVRT, can also precipitate AF episodes. This is unusual and should not be viewed as a contraindication to adenosine use, but one should be prepared for emergency cardioversion before administering adenosine to SVT patients. Lidocaine, for reasons that are unclear, has also been associated with degeneration of AF into VF. It is occasionally used in patients with WPW who have a wide QRS complex tachycardia that might be misinterpreted as VT.

VENTRICULAR TACHYCARDIA

Coexisting VT is uncommon because patients with WPW syndrome infrequently have structural heart disease. Naturally, older patients are subject to coronary artery and other diseases that can cause VT.

Clinical Considerations

Epidemiology of Wolff-Parkinson-White Syndrome

WOLFF-PARKINSON-WHITE PATTERN

The prevalence of WPW pattern on the surface ECG is 0.15% to 0.25% in the general population. The prevalence is increased to 0.55% among first-degree relatives of affected patients, suggesting a familial component. The yearly incidence of newly diagnosed cases of preexcitation in the general population was substantially lower, 0.004% in a diverse population of residents from Olmsted County, Minnesota, 50% of whom were asymptomatic.[12] The incidence in men is twice that in women and highest in the first year of life, with a secondary peak in young adulthood.

The WPW pattern on the ECG can be intermittent and can even permanently disappear (in up to 40% of cases) over time. Intermittent and/or persistent loss of preexcitation may indicate that the BT has a relatively longer baseline ERP, which makes it more susceptible to age-related degenerative changes and variations in autonomic tone. Consistent with this hypothesis is the observation that, compared with patients with a persistent WPW pattern, those in whom anterograde conduction via the BT disappeared were older (50 versus 39 years) and had a longer ERP of the BT at initial EP study (414 versus 295 milliseconds). The lifetime risk of mortality related to this in asymptomatic individuals can never be accurately known but has been estimated at 0.1% annual risk, with the majority of patients identified between the ages of approximately 10 and 40 years.

In a recent report, about 90% of 293 adults who were asymptomatic at the time of diagnosis of WPW ECG pattern had no arrhythmic events, remaining totally asymptomatic over a median follow-up of 67 months, and 30% of them had disappearance of preexcitation. Only a minority of young adult patients (10%) developed a first arrhythmic event, which was potentially life-threatening in approximately 5%, but no one died. Compared with patients who experienced potentially life-threatening events, those who did not showed a characteristic EP profile (older age, lower tachyarrhythmia inducibility, longer anterograde refractory ERP of BTs, and low likelihood of baseline retrograde BT conduction or multiple BTs).[10]

In a similar report in 184 children (8 to 12 years of age) with WPW ECG pattern who were totally asymptomatic at the time of diagnosis (which was made incidentally in the majority of cases either at a routine medical examination or on a screening ECG before admission to sports), during a median follow-up of 57 months, no child lost preexcitation, more than 70% had no arrhythmic events, and about 30% developed a first arrhythmic event, which was potentially life-threatening in 10%. Compared with children who experienced potentially life-threatening tachyarrhythmias, those who did not showed a characteristic electrophysiological profile (lower tachyarrhythmia inducibility, longer anterograde refractory period of BTs, and low likelihood of baseline retrograde AP conduction or multiple BTs).[9]

WOLFF-PARKINSON-WHITE SYNDROME

The prevalence of the WPW syndrome is substantially lower than that of the WPW ECG pattern. In a review of 22,500 healthy aviation personnel, the WPW pattern on surface ECG was seen in 0.25%; only 1.8% of these patients had documented arrhythmias. In another report of 228 subjects with WPW ECG pattern followed for 22 years, the overall incidence of arrhythmia was 1% per patient-year. The occurrence of arrhythmias is related to the age at the time preexcitation was discovered. In the Olmsted County population, one-third of asymptomatic individuals younger than 40 years at the time of diagnosis of WPW eventually had symptoms, compared with none of those who were older than 40 years at diagnosis. In a recent report, of 293 asymptomatic adults with the WPW ECG pattern who underwent EP testing without ablative intervention, almost 90% remained asymptomatic over a median follow-up of 67 months, whereas 31 patients had an arrhythmic event, and 17 had a "potentially" life-threatening event (AF with mean rate of 250 beats/min or faster).[10] In another report, of 188 asymptomatic children (between 8 and 12 years of age) with the WPW ECG pattern who underwent EP testing without ablative intervention, 72% remained asymptomatic over a median follow-up of 57 months, whereas 31 patients had an arrhythmic event.[9] Symptomatic arrhythmias developed more commonly in initially asymptomatic patients with a WPW ECG pattern who had inducible SVTs in the EP laboratory compared with those with no inducible tachycardias. In one report, less than 4% of patients developed clinical SVT over a 37.7-month follow-up period, compared with 67% of those with inducible SVT on EP testing.

A recent report demonstrated that women more commonly had right-sided BTs compared with men and that Asians had right free wall BTs substantially more frequently than other races. These relationships may suggest a potential inherited component of development of the AV annuli.[13]

ASSOCIATED CARDIAC ABNORMALITIES

Most patients with AV BTs do not have coexisting structural cardiac abnormalities, except for those that are age-related. Associated congenital heart disease, when present, is more likely to be right-sided than left-sided in location. Ebstein anomaly is the congenital lesion most strongly associated with the WPW syndrome. As many as 10% of such patients have one or more BTs; most of these are located in the right free wall and right posteroseptal space. An association between mitral valve prolapse and left-sided BTs has also been reported. However, this association may simply reflect the random coexistence of two relatively common conditions.

FAMILIAL WOLFF-PARKINSON-WHITE SYNDROME

Among patients with the WPW syndrome, 3.4% have first-degree relatives with a preexcitation syndrome. A familial form of WPW has infrequently been reported and is usually inherited as an autosomal dominant trait. The genetic cause of a rare form of familial WPW syndrome has been described.[14,15] The clinical phenotype is characterized by the presence of preexcitation on the ECG; frequent SVTs, including AF; progressive conduction system disease; and cardiac hypertrophy. Patients typically present in late adolescence or the third decade with syncope or palpitations. Premature SCD occurred in 10% of patients. Paradoxically, by the fourth decade of life, progression to advanced sinus node dysfunction or AV block (with the loss of preexcitation) requiring pacemaker implantation was common. Approximately 80% of the patients older than 50 years had chronic AF. Causative mutations in the *PRKAG2* gene were identified in these families. The *PRKAG2* gene encodes the gamma-2 regulatory subunit of the adenosine monophosphate (AMP)–activated protein kinase, which is a key regulator of metabolic pathways, including glucose metabolism. The penetrance of the disease for WPW syndrome was complete, but the expression was variable. The described phenotype of this syndrome is similar to the autosomal recessive glycogen storage disease, Pompe disease. Given the function of the AMP-activated protein kinase and this similarity, the PRKAG2 syndrome is likely a cardiac-specific glycogenosis syndrome. This syndrome thus belongs to the group of genetic metabolic cardiomyopathies, rather than to the congenital primary arrhythmia syndromes.

CONCEALED BYPASS TRACTS

The true prevalence of concealed BTs is unknown because, unlike the situation with the WPW ECG pattern, these BTs are concealed on the surface ECG and are only expressed during AVRT; only symptomatic patients undergo EP testing. As noted, orthodromic AVRT accounts for approximately 95% of AVRTs and 35% of all paroxysmal SVTs, and 50% of the BTs that participate in orthodromic AVRT are concealed. SVTs using a concealed BT have no gender predilection and tend to occur more frequently in younger patients than in those with AVNRT; however, significant overlap exists. PJRT most often occurs in early childhood, although clinically asymptomatic patients presenting later in life are not uncommon.

Clinical Presentation

Most patients with preexcitation are asymptomatic and are discovered incidentally on an ECG obtained for unrelated reasons. When symptomatic arrhythmias occur in the WPW patient, the disorder is called the WPW syndrome. The two most common types of arrhythmias in the WPW syndrome are AVRT and AF. Patients with AVRT experience symptoms characteristic of paroxysmal SVT with sudden onset and termination, including rapid and regular palpitations, chest pain, dyspnea, presyncope, and rarely, syncope. Symptoms are usually mild and short-lived and terminate spontaneously or with vagal maneuvers. However, occasionally patients present with disabling symptoms, especially in the presence of structural heart disease. Of note, clinical symptoms are not usually helpful in differentiating AVRT from other forms of paroxysmal SVTs.

An AVRT that in general is well tolerated by the patient when additional heart disease is absent can deteriorate into AF. AF can be a life-threatening arrhythmia in the WPW syndrome if the BT has a short anterograde ERP, resulting in very fast ventricular rates, with possible deterioration into VF and SCD.

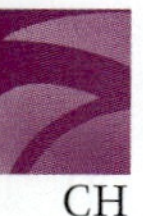

The incidence of SCD in patients with the WPW syndrome has been estimated to range from 0.15% to 0.39% over a 3- to 10-year follow-up. It is unusual for cardiac arrest to be the first symptomatic manifestation of WPW syndrome. Conversely, in about 50% of cardiac arrest cases in WPW patients, it is the first manifestation of WPW.

PJRT commonly presents as a frequently recurring or incessant tachycardia that is refractory to drug therapy and can lead to cardiomyopathy and congestive heart failure symptoms.

Initial Evaluation

History, physical examination, and 12-lead ECG constitute an appropriate initial evaluation. In patients with brief, self-terminating episodes of palpitations, an event recorder is the most effective way to obtain ECG documentation. Echocardiographic examination is often useful to exclude structural heart disease.

Several other noninvasive tests have been proposed as useful for evaluating symptomatic patients and risk-stratifying patients for SCD risk. However, the sensitivity and specificity of noninvasive testing have been shown to be limited. Invasive EP testing may be considered in patients with arrhythmias and those with a WPW ECG pattern when noninvasive testing does not lead to the conclusion that the anterograde ERP of the BT is relatively long.

EP testing can help risk-stratify asymptomatic patients with WPW pattern for developing symptoms and SCD secondary to preexcitation. As noted, inducibility of AVRT, a shorter BT ERP (<250 milliseconds), a shorter preexcited R-R interval during induced AF (<220 milliseconds), the presence of multiple pathways, and septal and right-sided pathway locations appear to identify a higher risk group.[9-11] However, a strategy to perform an EP study for all asymptomatic patients with the WPW ECG pattern for the purpose of risk stratification is still controversial and not widely accepted.[16]

METHODS FOR EVALUATION OF BYPASS TRACT REFRACTORY PERIOD

DEMONSTRATION OF INTERMITTENT PREEXCITATION. Observation of intermittent loss of the preexcitation pattern in a Holter monitor or serial ECGs is generally correlated with a long BT ERP and essentially ensures that the BT has a low "margin of safety" for conduction and hence is likely to block during AF, resulting in a slower ventricular response. Intermittent preexcitation, however, has to be distinguished from inapparent preexcitation (see later) and from a bigeminal ventricular rhythm with a long coupling interval.

ASSESSING ABILITY OF ANTIARRHYTHMIC AGENTS TO PRODUCE ANTEROGRADE BLOCK IN BYPASS TRACTS. When, during NSR, the intravenous injection of ajmaline (1 mg/kg over 3 minutes) or procainamide (10 mg/kg over 5 minutes) results in complete block of the BT, a long anterograde ERP (>270 milliseconds) of the BT is likely. The shorter the BT ERP, the less likely it would be blocked by these drugs. Furthermore, the amount of ajmaline required to block conduction over the BT correlates with the duration of the anterograde ERP of the BT. However, the incidence of BT block in response to these drugs is low and, although the occurrence of block predicts a long ERP of the BT, failure to produce block does not necessarily suggest a short ERP. Moreover, pharmacological testing is carried out at rest and therefore does not indicate what effect the drug will have on the BT ERP during sympathetic stimulation, such as exercise, emotion, anxiety, and recreational drug use.[8,17,18]

RESPONSE OF PREEXCITATION TO EXERCISE. Demonstration of a sudden loss of preexcitation (indicated by abrupt loss of the delta wave associated with prolongation of the PR interval and normalization of the QRS) during exercise is consistent with block in the BT and is indicative of a long BT ERP (>300 milliseconds). This is a good predictor that the patient is not at risk for VF, even during sympathetic stimulation. However, the frequency of block in the BT during exercise is low (approximately 10%), and thus sensitivity of this test is poor.

EVALUATION OF VENTRICULAR RESPONSE DURING ATRIAL FIBRILLATION. During spontaneous or induced AF, the propensity for rapid AV conduction can be judged by the interval between consecutively preexcited QRS complexes. A mean preexcited R-R interval of more than 250 milliseconds and a shortest preexcited R-R of more than 220 milliseconds predict low risk for SCD, with a negative predictive value of more than 95%; however, the positive predictive value is low (20%).

RESPONSE OF PREEXCITATION TO TRANSESOPHAGEAL ATRIAL STIMULATION. There is good correlation between the value of the anterograde ERP of the BT obtained during single-test programmed atrial stimulation and atrial pacing at increasing rates and the ventricular rate during AF. Programmed electrical stimulation of the atrium can be performed by the transesophageal route and the value of the anterograde ERP of the BT can be determined.

ELECTROPHYSIOLOGICAL TESTING. Programmed atrial stimulation is used to evaluate the BT ERP. Because BT refractoriness shortens with decreasing pacing CL, the ERP should be determined at multiple pacing CLs (preferably ≤400 milliseconds). Additionally, atrial stimulation should be performed close to the BT atrial insertion site to obviate the effect of intraatrial conduction delay. Incremental rate atrial pacing is performed to determine the maximal rate at which 1:1 conduction over the BT occurs. Induction of AF should be performed to determine the average and the shortest R-R interval during preexcited AF. Atrial and ventricular stimulation is also performed to evaluate inducibility of AVRT as well as the number and location of BTs.

Principles of Management

MANAGEMENT OF ASYMPTOMATIC PATIENTS WITH PREEXCITATION

The role of EP testing and catheter ablation in asymptomatic patients with preexcitation is still controversial. Guidelines of the American College of Cardiology and European Society of Cardiology on the management of asymptomatic WPW patients suggest restricting catheter ablation of BTs to those in high-risk occupations (e.g., school bus drivers, police, and pilots) and professional athletes.[19] Catheter ablation in asymptomatic preexcitation was classified as a class IIA indication with a B level of evidence. This means essentially that it is "reasonable" to offer ablation in selected patients but is not mandated in all patients. According to the North American Society of Pacing and Electrophysiology (NASPE; now the Heart Rhythm Society [HRS]) Expert Consensus Conference, asymptomatic WPW pattern on the ECG without recognized tachycardia is a class IIB indication for catheter ablation in children older than 5 years and a class III indication in younger children.[20]

This approach has several justifications; one-third of asymptomatic individuals younger than 40 years when preexcitation was identified eventually developed symptoms, whereas no patients in whom preexcitation was first uncovered after the age of 40 years developed symptoms. Additionally, most patients with asymptomatic preexcitation have a good prognosis; cardiac arrest is rarely the first manifestation of the disorder. The positive predictive value of invasive EP testing is considered to be too low to justify routine use in asymptomatic patients.

Some studies, however, have questioned the approach discussed above.[8,17,18] Those studies have shown that in the asymptomatic WPW population, a negative EP study with no AVRT or AF inducibility identifies subjects at very low risk for the development of spontaneous arrhythmias. Inducibility of sustained preexcited AF with a fast ventricular response, particularly in the presence of multiple BTs, may help select asymptomatic WPW subjects at definite risk for dying suddenly, and catheter ablation of the BT(s) appears to be required to prevent SCD. Because extensive studies have reported extremely rare complications from EP testing and radiofrequency (RF) ablation in experienced centers, it has been suggested that all asymptomatic patients with WPW pattern should undergo EP testing for risk stratification, and those with inducible AVRT or AF or who have a short BT ERP should be considered for catheter ablation of the BT, whereas patients who are noninducible and have a long BT ERP may be followed without treatment.[8-10,21] This argument is further supported by the fact that assessment of the future VF risk in an asymptomatic patient with WPW is not easy. Noninvasive markers of lower risk such as intermittent loss of preexcitation, sudden loss of BT conduction on exercise stress testing, and loss of BT conduction after treatment with antiarrhythmic drugs are limited by inadequate sensitivity or specificity and the low incidence of future adverse events. With this approach, prophylactic ablation of BTs in high-risk subjects may be justified but is not an acceptable option for low-risk individuals. The physician involved needs to use special care and discretion in making the decision to proceed to ablation and must especially consider his or her own success and complication rates for ablation of the specific location of the BT identified.

In summary, the potential value of EP testing in identifying high-risk patients who may benefit from catheter ablation must be balanced against the approximately 2% risk of a major complication associated with catheter ablation.[22] If RF catheter ablation were a totally risk-free procedure, one would logically advise such a procedure to the asymptomatic WPW patient with a short anterograde ERP. However, complications such as AV block, stroke, tamponade, and even death have been reported. It is not difficult to envision a small potential mortality benefit, if present, erased or eclipsed by a small complication rate if thousands of patients with BTs in various locations undergo ablation.[16] Although complications of a diagnostic EP study are minor and non–life-threatening and are less common than those of catheter ablation, if routine EP testing of all asymptomatic WPW patients were considered, many patients would proceed immediately to RF ablation and, in others, there would be a strong temptation to ablate when catheters are in place (regardless of predicted SCD risk), especially given the fact that the criteria for ablation usually will not be black or white. This greatly increases the risk to the patient. Furthermore, invasive EP assessment has drawbacks, because no single factor has both a high sensitivity and specificity for identifying at-risk individuals. For example, a shortest preexcited R-R interval of less than 250 milliseconds during sustained induced AF is a very sensitive but not specific marker of the risk of VF in WPW patients, because approximately one-third of patients will have a shortest R-R interval of less than 250 milliseconds during induced AF. In fact, the addition of isoproterenol to the baseline study may shorten the ERP of the accessory pathway to levels of potential concern in the majority of individuals with WPW. In view of those considerations, prudence dictates that noninvasive testing with a Holter monitor and (if the Holter monitor does not show intermittent preexcitation) exercise testing should be considered before the EP study to identify the low-risk patient because of a long anterograde ERP of the BT.[21,22]

For the low-risk patient, it may be appropriate to pursue a strategy of follow-up with ECGs and reevaluation at selected intervals with a high degree of suspicion for new arrhythmia symptoms. This strategy is supported by recent prospective studies of asymptomatic patients with WPW pattern; although "potentially" life-threatening arrhythmias were observed during follow-up, no patients had actually died. This observation implies that patient education about the potential risks associated with preexcitation and about the symptoms of arrhythmias that should prompt them to seek attention can prove very important at reducing the risk of mortality without necessarily exposing the patient to the risks of catheter ablation.[10,16] It is also advisable to give the patient a copy of his or her ECG and a short note about the fact that the WPW pattern is present to prevent the misdiagnosis of myocardial infarction (MI) and to explain the basis of cardiac arrhythmias in case they develop later. Patients should also be encouraged to seek medical expertise whenever arrhythmia-related symptoms occur.

In patients not showing block in their BT during noninvasive studies, esophageal pacing may be performed to determine the anterograde ERP of the BT and the ability to induce sustained arrhythmias. This procedure is neither pleasant for patients nor often definitive, but if arrhythmias can be induced, the benefits and risk of an invasive investigation and catheter ablation should be based on individual considerations such as age, gender, occupation, and athletic involvement. This should be discussed with the patient or, in the case of a child, with the parents. Because knowledge about the success and complication rate at the EP center plays a major role in decision making, that information should be made available so that the appropriate place for invasive diagnosis and treatment can be selected. If an EP study is performed for risk stratification, the combination of inducible AVRT and a shortest preexcited R-R interval during AF of less than 250 milliseconds provides the most compelling indications for ablation. The key is a clear understanding by the patient of the relative merits of each strategy. The well-informed patient needs to choose between a very small risk of potentially life-threatening arrhythmia over a long period of time and a one-time small procedural risk associated with EP testing and catheter ablation. Certain patients such as athletes and those in higher risk occupations will generally choose ablation. Others, especially patients older than 30 years, may prefer the small risk of a conservative strategy.[10,16,21,22]

MANAGEMENT OF SYMPTOMATIC PATIENTS

ACUTE MANAGEMENT. Patients with AVRT are treated in a similar fashion as those with paroxysmal SVT. In patients with orthodromic and antidromic AVRT, drug treatment can be directed at the BT (ibutilide, procainamide, flecainide) or at the AVN (beta blockers, diltiazem, verapamil) because both are critical components of the tachycardia circuit. Adenosine should be used with caution because it can induce AF with a rapid ventricular rate in patients with preexcited tachycardias.[19]

AVN blocking drugs are ineffective in patients with antidromic AVRT who have anterograde conduction over one BT and retrograde conduction over a separate BT because the AVN is not involved in the circuit.[19] Additionally, caution is advised against AVN blocking agents for the treatment of preexcited tachycardias occurring in patients with AT, AFL, or AF with a bystander BT. Antiarrhythmic drugs such as ibutilide, procainamide, or flecainide, which prevent rapid conduction through the bystander pathway, are preferable, even if they may not convert the atrial arrhythmia. When drug therapy fails or hemodynamic instability is present, electrical cardioversion should be considered.

CHRONIC MANAGEMENT. The NASPE policy statement on catheter ablation states that catheter ablation is considered first-line therapy (class I) and the treatment of choice for patients with the WPW syndrome—that is, patients with manifest preexcitation along with symptoms.[20] It is curative in more than 95% of patients and has a low complication rate. It also obviates the unwanted side effects of antiarrhythmic agents. For patients with preexcitation who are not candidates for ablation, antiarrhythmic drugs to block BT conduction should be used, such as sodium or potassium channel blockers.[23] However, there have been no controlled trials of pharmacological therapy in patients with AVRT, but small nonrandomized trials have reported the safety and efficacy of drug therapy. Despite the absence of data from clinical trials, chronic oral beta blocker therapy can be used for the treatment of patients with WPW syndrome, particularly if their BT has been demonstrated during EP testing to be incapable of rapid anterograde conduction. Verapamil, diltiazem, and digoxin, on the other hand, generally should not be used as the sole long-term therapy for patients with BT that might be capable of rapid conduction during AF.

Catheter ablation is also considered first-line therapy (class I) for patients with paroxysmal SVT involving a concealed BT. However, because concealed BTs are not associated with an increased risk of SCD in these patients, catheter ablation can be presented as one of a number of potential therapeutic approaches, including pharmacological therapy and clinical follow-up alone.[19] When pharmacological therapy is selected for patients with concealed BTs, it is reasonable to consider a trial of beta blocker therapy, calcium channel blockers, or a class IC antiarrhythmic agent.

Electrocardiographic Features

Electrocardiography of Preexcitation

Anterogradely conducting AV BTs produce the classic WPW ECG pattern characterized by a fusion between conduction via the BT and the normal AVN-HPS: (1) short PR (P-delta) interval (<120 milliseconds); (2) slurred upstroke of the QRS (delta wave); and (3) wide QRS (>120 milliseconds) (Fig. 18-4).

The degree of preexcitation depends on several factors, including conduction time over the AVN-HPS, conduction time from the sinus node to the atrial insertion site of the BT (which depends on the distance, conduction, and refractoriness of the intervening atrial tissue), and conduction time through the BT (which depends on the length, thickness, and conduction properties of the BT).

Pharmacological and/or physiological maneuvers (e.g., carotid sinus massage, Valsalva maneuvers, adenosine, beta blockers) that alter AVN conduction can be used to alter the degree of preexcitation, thereby confirming the diagnosis of the presence of an AV BT.

The ECG pattern displayed by some patients with the WPW syndrome can simulate the pattern found in other cardiac conditions

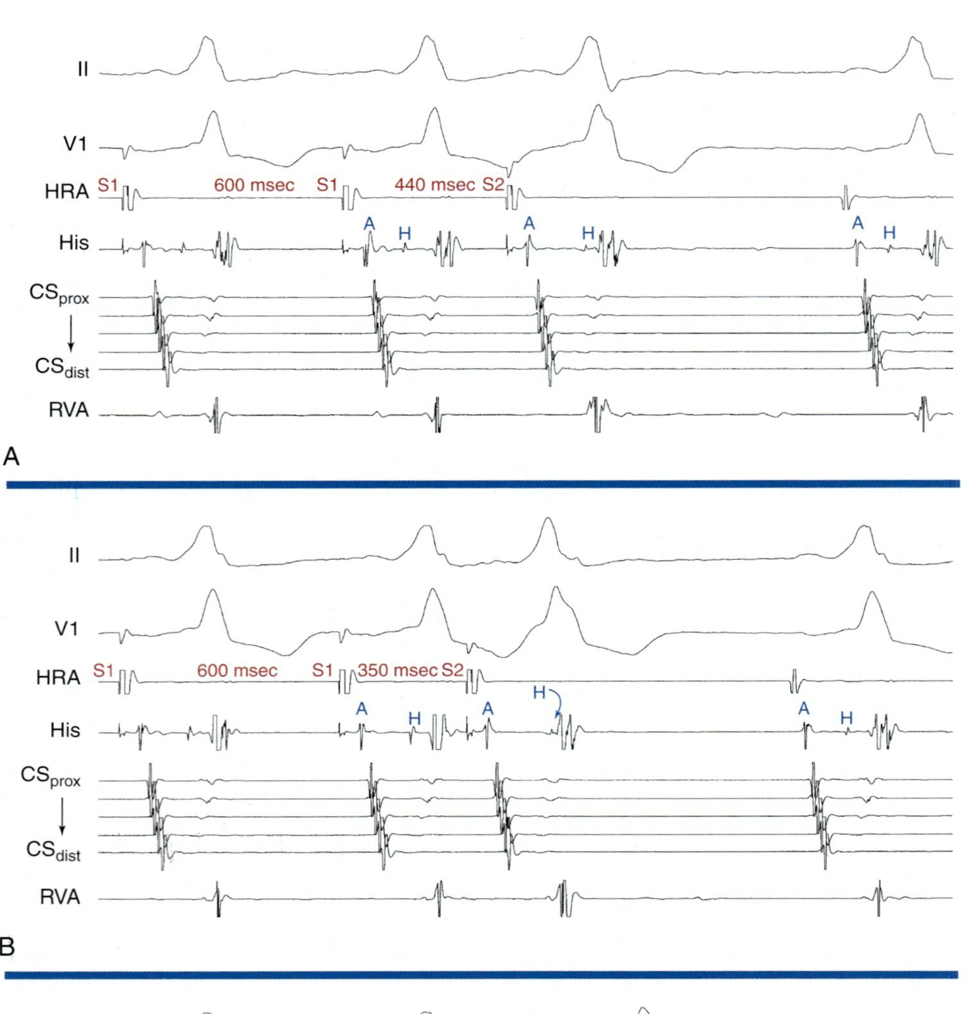

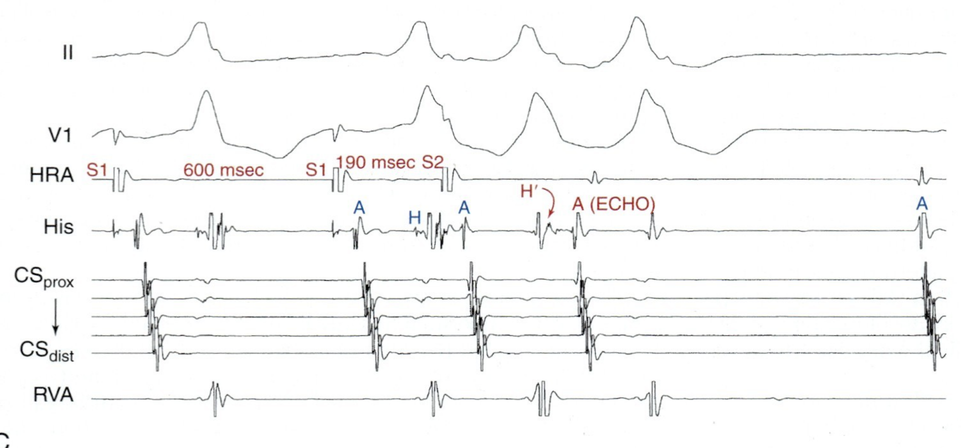

FIGURE 18-4 Effect of atrial extrastimulation (AES) on preexcitation. **A,** Preexcitation is manifest during normal sinus rhythm (NSR) and atrial pacing associated with a short His bundle–ventricular (HV) interval (−11 milliseconds). AES produces decremental conduction over the atrioventricular node (AVN) (with prolonged atrial–His bundle [AH] interval) but not over the bypass tract (constant P-delta interval), increasing the degree of preexcitation with the His potential inscribed within the QRS (HV interval of −64 milliseconds). **B,** An earlier coupled AES produces more pronounced preexcitation and an HV interval of −93 milliseconds. **C,** A more premature AES produces full preexcitation with the HB activated retrogradely (H′), followed by ventriculoatrial conduction over the AVN and an echo beat (atrioventricular reentry).

and can alter the pattern seen in the presence of other cardiac disease. A negative delta wave (presenting as a Q wave) can mimic an MI pattern. Conversely, a positive delta wave can mask the presence of a previous MI. Intermittent WPW can also be mistaken for frequent premature ventricular complexes (PVCs; Fig. 18-5). If the WPW pattern persists for several beats, the rhythm can be misdiagnosed as an accelerated idioventricular rhythm. The WPW pattern is occasionally seen on alternate beats and may suggest ventricular bigeminy. An alternating WPW and normal pattern can occasionally suggest electrical alternans. On the other hand, late-coupled PVCs (Fig. 18-6) and ventricular pacing (Fig. 18-7) with inapparent pacing artifacts can occasionally mimic ventricular preexcitation.

INAPPARENT VERSUS INTERMITTENT PREEXCITATION

INAPPARENT PREEXCITATION. With inapparent preexcitation, preexcitation is absent on the surface ECG despite the presence of an anterogradely conducting AV BT, because conduction over the AVN-HPS reaches the ventricle faster than that over the BT. In this setting, the PR interval is shorter than what the P-delta interval would be if preexcitation were present. Therefore, when preexcitation becomes inapparent, the PR interval becomes shorter, reflecting the now better AVN-HPS conduction.[3]

Inapparent preexcitation is usually caused by (1) enhanced AVN conduction, so that it is faster than conduction over the BT; (2) prolonged intraatrial conduction from the site of atrial stimulation to the atrial insertion site of BT (most often left lateral), favoring anterograde conduction over the AVN-HPS; and/or (3) prolonged conduction over the BT, so that it is slower than AVN-HPS conduction.

INTERMITTENT PREEXCITATION. Intermittent preexcitation is defined as the presence and absence of preexcitation on the same tracing (Fig. 18-8). True intermittent preexcitation is characterized by an abrupt loss of the delta wave (independently of how fast or slow is AVN conduction), with prolongation (normalization) of the PR interval (reflecting the loss of the faster BT conduction, and the subsequent conduction over the slower AVN-HPS), and normalization of the QRS in the absence of any significant change in heart rate.

Intermittent preexcitation is usually caused by (1) phase 3 (i.e., tachycardia-dependent) or phase 4 (i.e., bradycardia-dependent) block in the BT (see Chap. 10); (2) anterograde or retrograde concealed conduction produced by PVCs, premature atrial complexes (PACs), or atrial arrhythmias; (3) BTs with long ERP and the gap phenomenon in response to PACs; and/or (4) BTs with long ERP and supernormal conduction.

Intermittent preexcitation is generally a reliable sign that the AV BT has a relatively long anterograde ERP and is not capable of excessively rapid impulse conduction, such as during AF. Maneuvers that slow AVN conduction (e.g., carotid sinus massage, AVN blockers) would unmask inapparent preexcitation but would not affect intermittent preexcitation.

Preexcitation alternans is a form of intermittent preexcitation in which a QRS complex manifesting a delta wave alternates with a normal QRS complex (see Fig. 18-5). *Concertina preexcitation* is another form of intermittent preexcitation in which the PR intervals and QRS complex durations show a cyclic pattern; that is, preexcitation becomes progressively more prominent over a number of QRS complex cycles followed by a gradual diminution in the degree of preexcitation over several QRS cycles, despite a fairly constant heart rate.

Differentiation between intermittent preexcitation and inapparent preexcitation on an ECG showing QRS complexes with and without preexcitation can be achieved by comparing the P-delta interval during preexcitation and the PR interval when preexcitation is absent. Loss of preexcitation associated with a PR interval longer than the P-delta interval is consistent with intermittent preexcitation (see Fig. 18-8), whereas loss of preexcitation associated with a PR interval shorter than the P-delta interval is consistent with inapparent preexcitation.

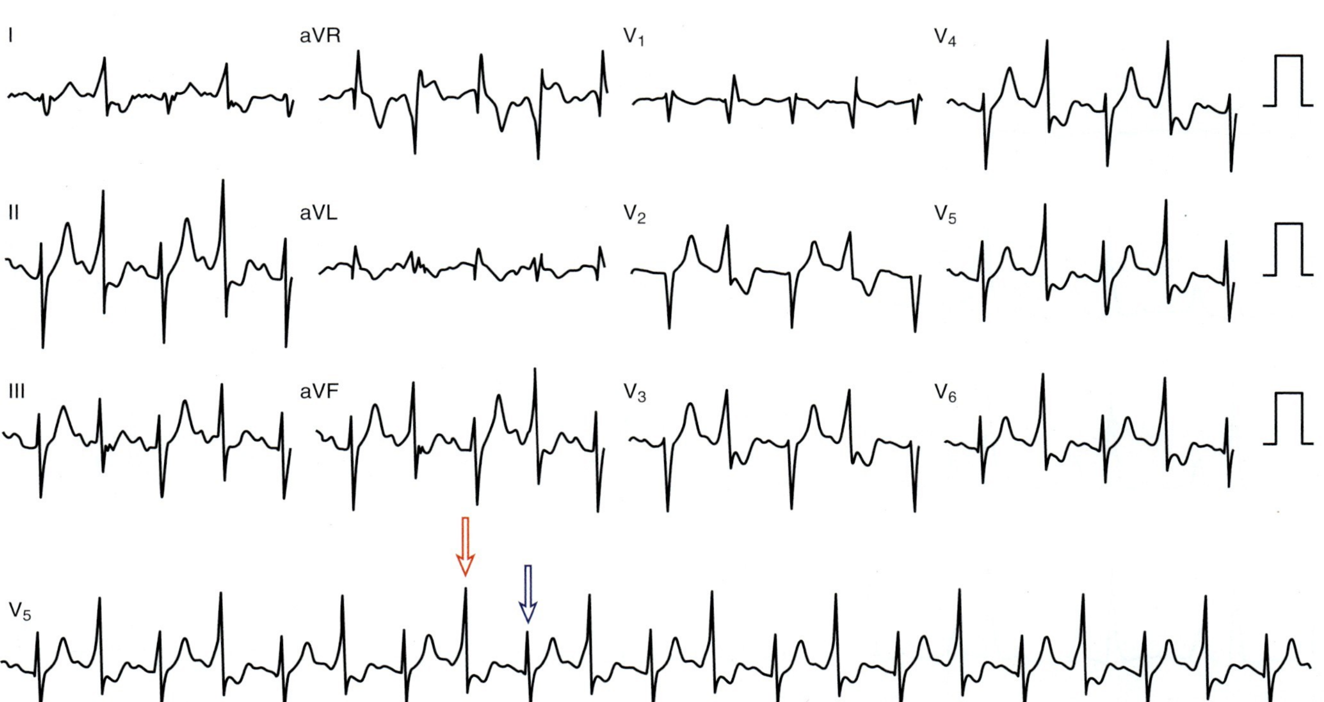

FIGURE 18-5 Preexcitation alternans. Surface ECG during sinus tachycardia demonstrating intermittent preexcitation in which a QRS complex manifesting a delta wave (red arrow) alternates with a normal QRS complex (blue arrow) (i.e., preexcitation alternans). Note the intermittent abrupt loss of delta wave associated with prolongation of the PR interval and the presence of a stable sinus rate, indicating that loss of preexcitation is secondary to anterograde block in the bypass tract (i.e., intermittent preexcitation) rather than enhanced atrioventricular nodal conduction.

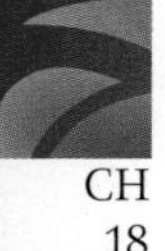

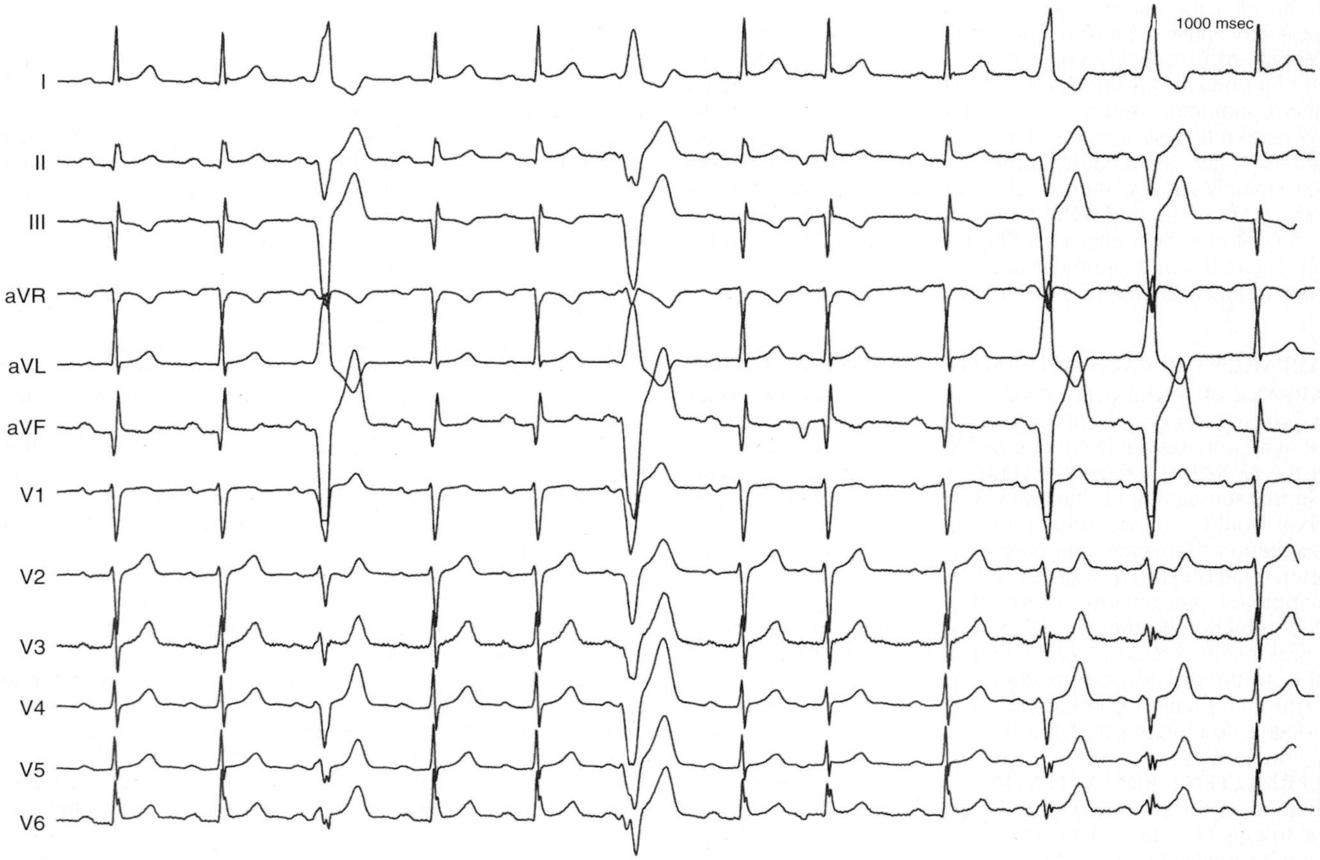

FIGURE 18-6 Surface ECG of normal sinus rhythm with late-coupled premature ventricular complexes, which are inscribed shortly after the sinus P waves, resulting in a short PR interval and wide QRS complexes mimicking intermittent ventricular preexcitation. Note that the degree of widening of the QRS and the variability of the QRS morphology and the varying relationship to the preceding P waves all argue against ventricular preexcitation.

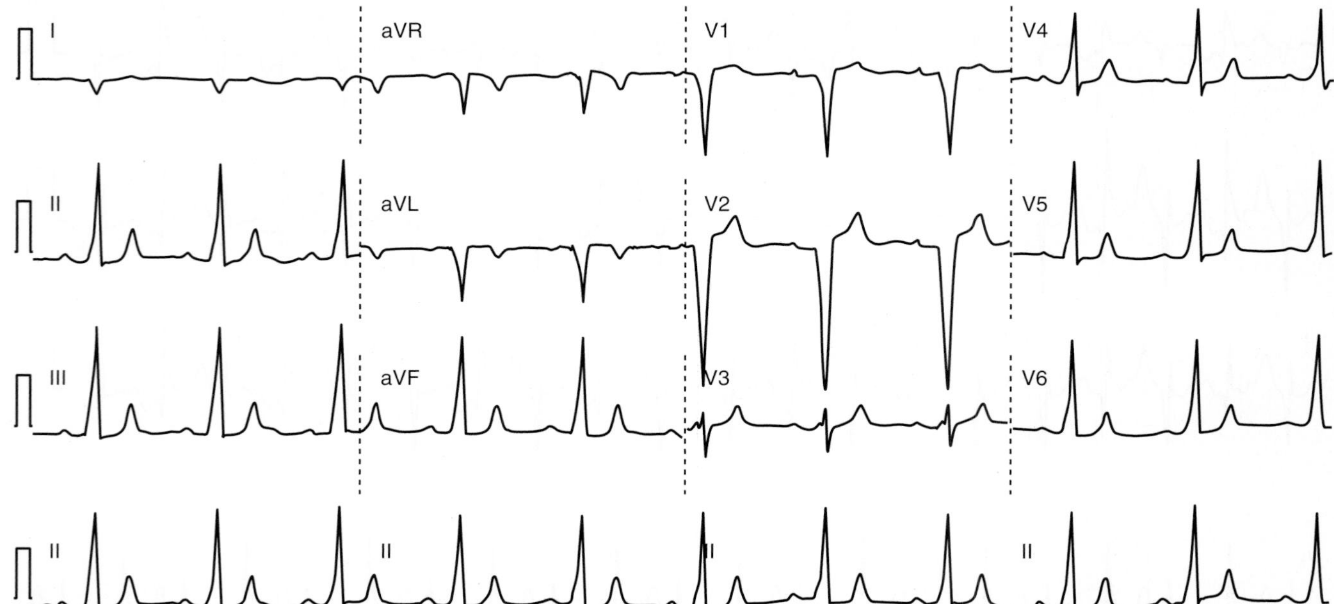

FIGURE 18-7 Surface ECG of normal sinus rhythm with atrial-tracking ventricular pacing. The QRS complexes are the result of fusion from ventricular pacing and conduction over the normal atrioventricular conduction axis, resulting in a pseudo-delta wave, mimicking a Wolff-Parkinson-White ECG pattern. The pacing artifacts are very small, but careful inspection reveals those artifacts most clearly in lead III.

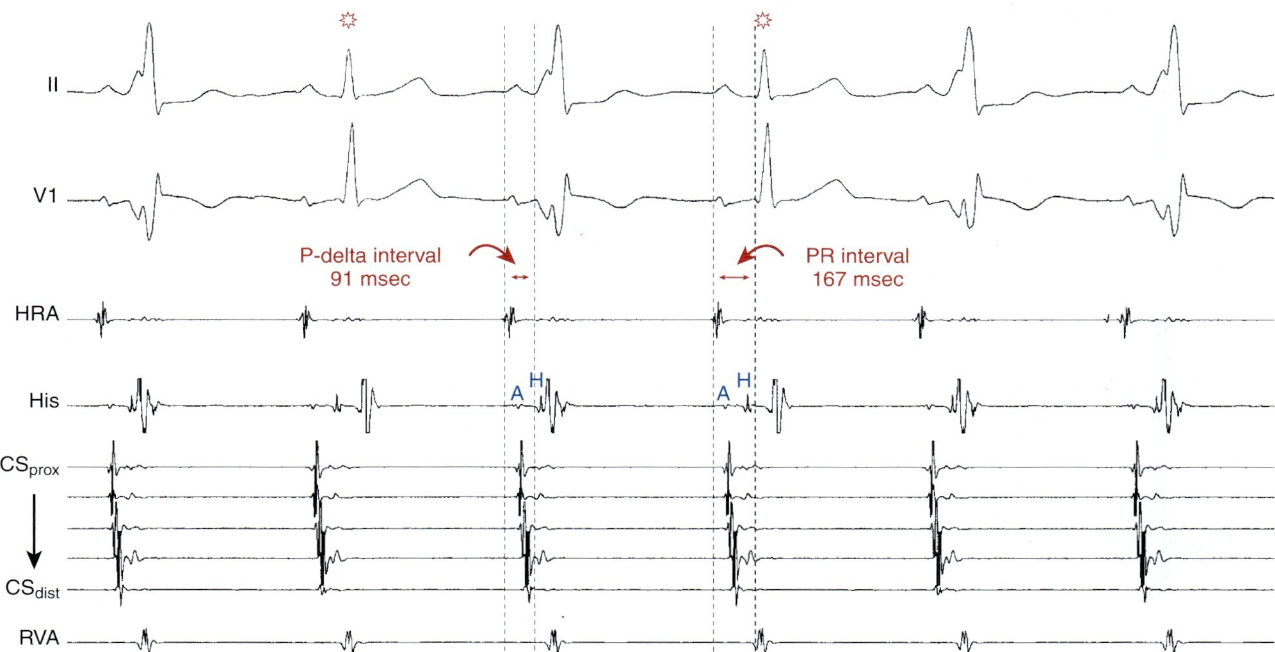

FIGURE 18-8 Intermittent preexcitation. Surface ECG leads II and V_1 and intracardiac recordings in a patient with Wolff-Parkinson-White syndrome and a right anterior bypass tract (BT). Note the intermittent abrupt loss of delta wave (stars) associated with prolongation of the PR interval and normalization of the His bundle–ventricular (HV) interval, despite the presence of a constant atrial–His bundle (AH) interval (atrioventricular node [AVN] conduction) and a stable sinus rate, indicating that loss of preexcitation is secondary to anterograde block in the BT (i.e., intermittent preexcitation) rather than enhanced AVN conduction.

Supraventricular Tachycardias Associated with Wolff-Parkinson-White Syndrome

ORTHODROMIC ATRIOVENTRICULAR REENTRANT TACHYCARDIA

The ECG during orthodromic AVRT shows P waves inscribed within the ST-T wave segment with an RP interval that is usually less than half of the tachycardia R-R interval (i.e., RP interval < PR interval) (Fig. 18-9). The RP interval remains constant, regardless of the tachycardia CL, because it reflects the nondecremental conduction over the BT. QRS morphology during orthodromic AVRT is generally normal and not preexcited, even when preexcitation is present during NSR (Fig. 18-10). Functional bundle branch block (BBB) can be observed frequently during orthodromic AVRT (see Fig. 18-9). The presence of BBB during SVT in a young person (<40 years) should raise the suspicion of orthodromic AVRT incorporating a BT ipsilateral to the blocked bundle, because the longer conduction time through the involved ventricle engendered by the BBB facilitates orthodromic reentry by enabling all portions of the circuit enough time to recover excitability from the prior cycle. This is particularly true with left bundle branch block (LBBB), which is very uncommon in younger patients.

Orthodromic AVRT tends to be a rapid tachycardia, with rates ranging from 150 to more than 250 beats/min. A beat-to-beat oscillation in QRS amplitude (QRS alternans) is present in up to 38% of cases and is most commonly seen when the rate is very rapid. The mechanism for QRS alternans is not clear but can partly result from oscillations in the relative refractory period of the distal portions of the HPS.

Ischemic-appearing ST segment depression also can occur during orthodromic AVRT, even in young individuals who are unlikely to have coronary artery disease. An association has been observed between repolarization changes (ST segment depression or T wave inversion) and the underlying mechanism of the tachycardia, because such changes are more common in orthodromic AVRT than AVNRT (57% versus 25%). Several factors can contribute to ST segment depression in these arrhythmias, including changes in autonomic tone, intraventricular conduction disturbances, a longer ventricular-atrial (VA) interval, and a retrograde P wave of longer duration that overlaps into the ST segment. The location of the ST segment changes can vary with the location of the BT; ST segment depression in leads V_3 to V_6 is almost invariably seen with a left lateral BT, whereas ST segment depression and a negative T wave in the inferior leads is associated with a posteroseptal or posterior BT. A negative or notched T wave in leads V_2 or V_3 with a positive retrograde P wave in at least two inferior leads suggests an anteroseptal BT. However, ST segment depression occurring during orthodromic AVRT in an older patient mandates consideration of possible coexisting ischemic heart disease.

ANTIDROMIC ATRIOVENTRICULAR REENTRANT TACHYCARDIA

Antidromic AVRT is characterized by a wide (fully preexcited) QRS complex, usually regular R-R intervals, and ventricular rates of up to 250 beats/min. The width of the preexcited QRS complex and the amplitude of the ST-T wave segment usually obscure the retrograde P wave on the surface ECG. When the P waves can be identified, they are inscribed within the ST-T wave segment with an RP interval that may be more than half of the tachycardia R-R interval because retrograde conduction occurs slowly via the AVN-HPS. The PR (P-delta) interval remains constant, regardless of the tachycardia CL, because it reflects nondecremental conduction over the BT.

PERMANENT JUNCTIONAL RECIPROCATING TACHYCARDIA

PJRT tends to be incessant, stopping and starting spontaneously every few beats without initiating PACs or PVCs. The heart rate is usually between 120 and 200 beats/min and the QRS duration is generally normal. Slow retrograde conduction over the BT causes the RP interval during PJRT to be long, usually more than half of the tachycardia R-R interval (Fig. 18-11). The P waves resulting from retrograde conduction are easily seen on the ECG and are inverted in leads II, III, aVF, and V_3 to V_6.

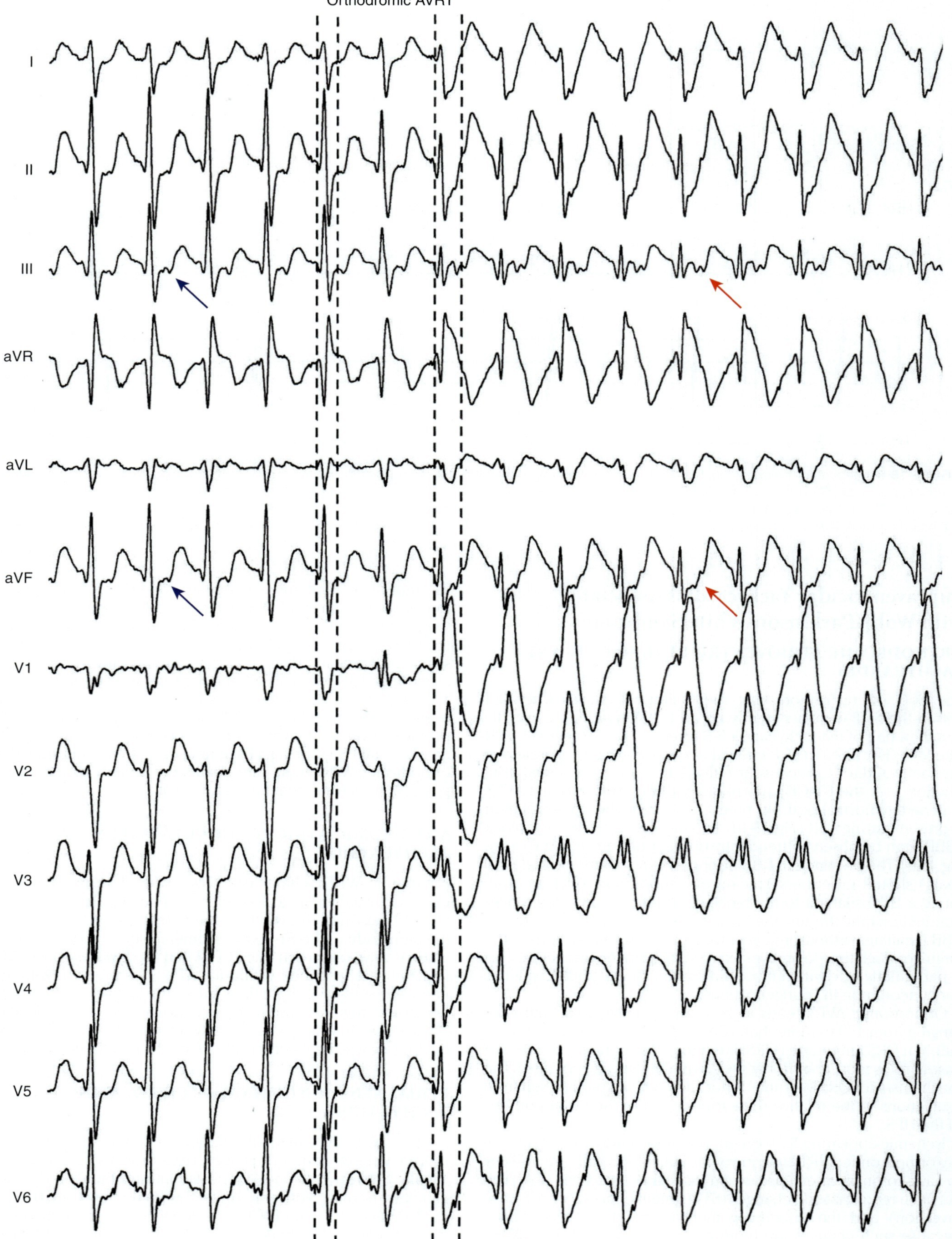

FIGURE 18-9 Surface ECG of orthodromic atrioventricular reentrant tachycardia (AVRT) using a concealed superoparaseptal bypass tract (BT). Note the P waves (arrows) inscribed within the ST-T wave segment (short RP interval). Ischemic-appearing ST segment depression is also observed. Functional right bundle branch block occurs in the right side of the tracing, with prolongation of the RP (ventriculoatrial [VA]) interval, suggesting that retrograde VA conduction during the supraventricular tachycardia is mediated by a right-sided BT. The dashed lines denote the QRS onset and P wave onset.

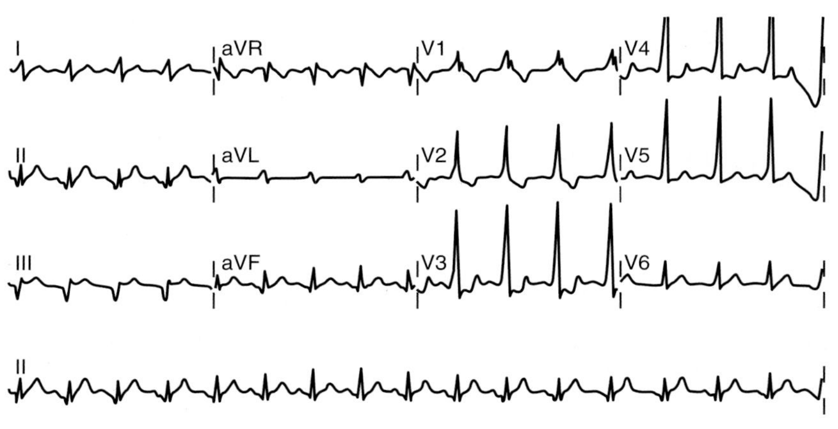

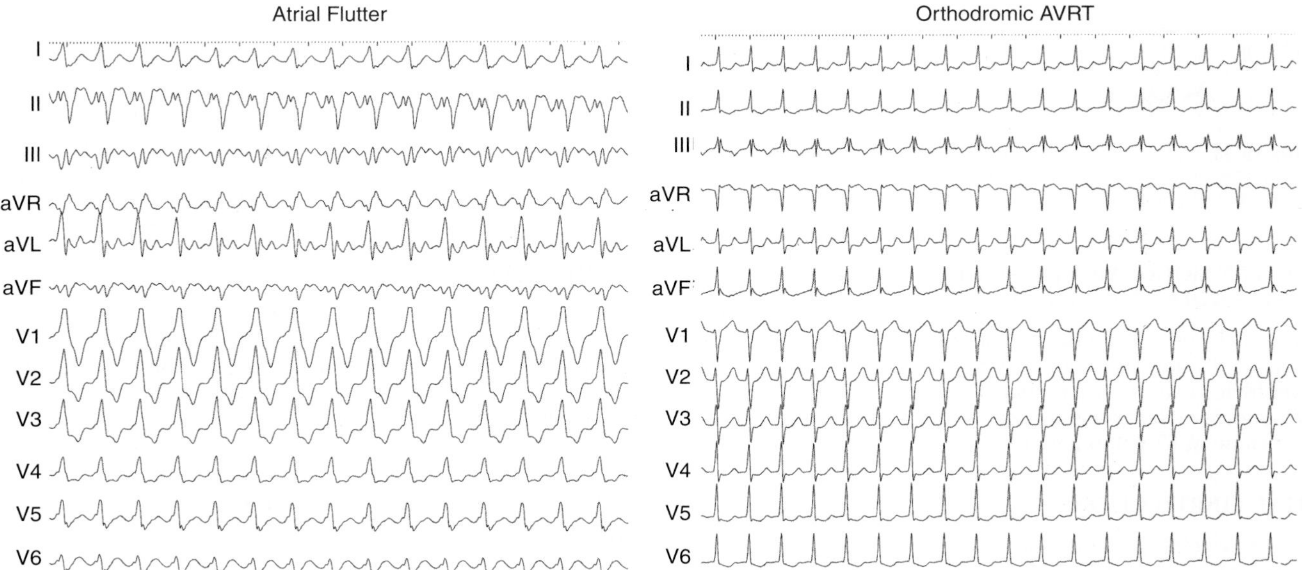

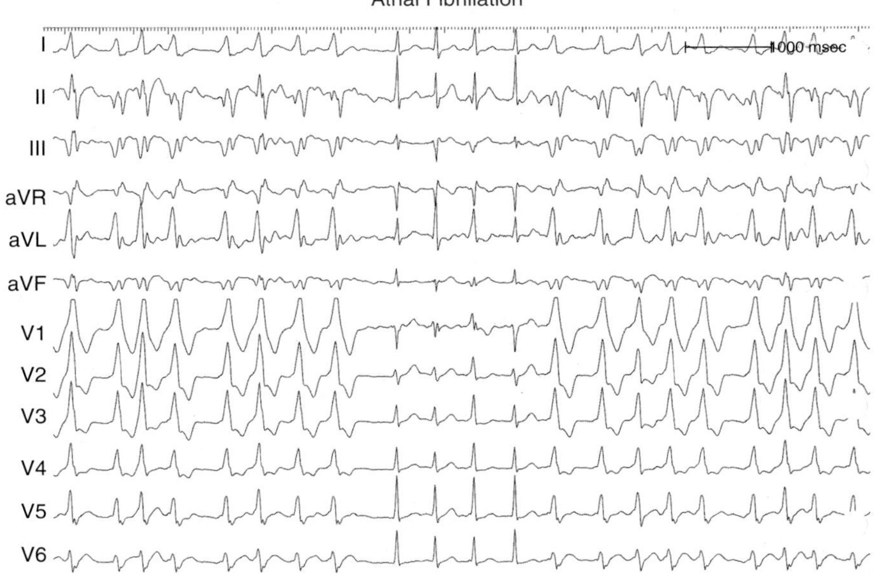

FIGURE 18-10 Surface ECG of multiple supraventricular arrhythmias in a patient with a bidirectional left posteroseptal bypass tract (BT). Ventricular preexcitation is evident during normal sinus rhythm (NSR). Atrial flutter with 2:1 atrioventricular (AV) conduction over the BT results in a wide complex tachycardia. The narrow complex tachycardia represents orthodromic atrioventricular reentrant tachycardia (AVRT) using the BT as the retrograde limb of the reentrant circuit. Atrial fibrillation results in an irregularly irregular rhythm with "clumping" of the preexcited (wide) and normal QRS complexes.

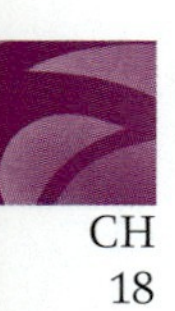

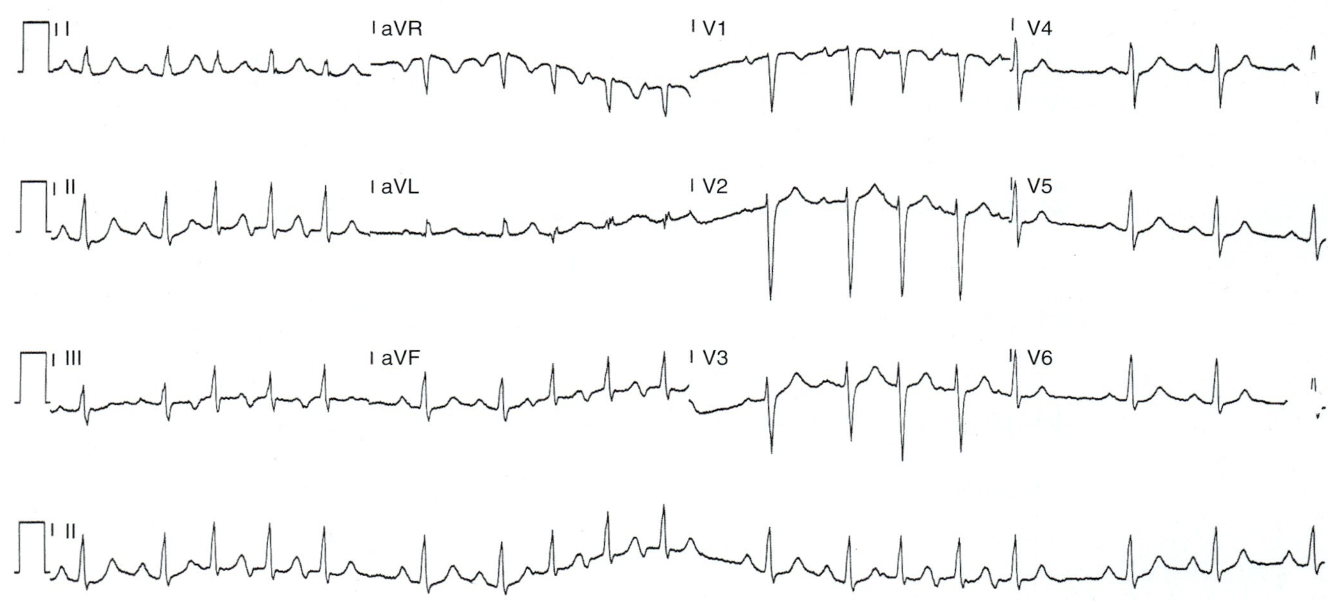

FIGURE 18-11 Surface ECG of permanent junctional reciprocating tachycardia (PJRT). Note the incessant nature of the arrhythmia, stopping and starting spontaneously every few beats without initiating atrial or ventricular ectopic beats. Slow retrograde conduction over the bypass tract causes the RP interval during PJRT to be long (long RP tachycardia). The P waves resulting from retrograde conduction are easily seen on the ECG and are inverted in the inferior leads.

ATRIOVENTRICULAR NODAL REENTRANT TACHYCARDIA AND ATRIAL TACHYCARDIA

Both AVNRT and AT can be associated with partially or fully preexcited QRS complex secondary to anterograde conduction to the ventricles over the bystander BT. When AVNRT occurs in the WPW syndrome, the arrhythmia can be difficult to distinguish from orthodromic AVRT without EP testing.

ATRIAL FIBRILLATION

There are several characteristic findings on the ECG in patients with AF conducting over a BT, so-called preexcited AF (see Fig. 18-10). The rhythm is irregularly irregular, and can be associated with very rapid ventricular response caused by the nondecremental anterograde AV conduction over the BT. However, a sustained rapid ventricular rate of more than 180 to 200 beats/min will often create pseudo-regularized R-R intervals when the ECG is recorded at 25 mm/sec. Although the QRS complexes are conducted aberrantly, resembling those during preexcited NSR, their duration can be variable and they can become normalized. This is not related to the R-R interval (i.e., it is not a rate-related phenomenon), but rather is related to the variable relationship between conduction over the BT and AVN-HPS. Preexcited and normal QRS complexes often appear "clumped" (see Fig. 18-10). This can result from concealed retrograde conduction into the BT or the AVN.

The QRS complex during preexcitation is a fusion between the impulse that preexcites the ventricles caused by rapid conduction through a BT and the impulse that takes the usual route through the AVN. The number of impulses that can be transmitted through the BT and the amount of preexcitation depend on the refractoriness of both the BT and AVN. The shorter the anterograde ERP of the BT, the more rapid is anterograde impulse conduction and, because of more preexcitation, the wider the QRS complexes. Patients who have a BT with a very short ERP and rapid ventricular rates represent the group at greatest risk for development of VF.

Anterograde block in the BT abolishes retrograde conduction into the AVN, which in turn allows the AVN to recover its excitability and conduct anterogradely. These conducted impulses through the AVN can result in retrograde concealment into the BT, causing anterograde block of the BT, thereby slowing the ventricular rate.

ATRIAL FLUTTER

AFL, like AF, can conduct anterogradely via a BT resulting in a preexcited tachycardia (see Fig. 18-10). Depending on the various refractory periods of the normal and pathological AV conduction pathways, AFL potentially can conduct 1:1 to the ventricles during a preexcited tachycardia, making the arrhythmia difficult to distinguish from VT (see Fig. 12-6).

Electrocardiographic Localization of the Bypass Tract

LOCALIZATION USING THE DELTA WAVE

Careful analysis of the preexcitation pattern during sinus rhythm can potentially allow an accurate approximation of the location of the BT. This provides the electrophysiologist with important information that can guide patient counseling with regard to risks and benefits of ablation, in particular, providing some guidance about the proximity of the BT to the normal conduction system and the subsequent risk of AV block associated with an ablation attempt, as well as the need for left heart catheterization and atrial septal puncture and their potential complications. Additionally, it can also allow planning the subsequent catheter ablation, such as the use of cryoablation for septal BTs or the need for special equipment for atrial septal puncture for left-sided BTs.[24]

The delta wave vector is helpful in approximating BT location, especially when maximal preexcitation is present. However, during NSR, only partial ventricular preexcitation is usually present, which limits the accuracy of ECG localization of the BT. Additionally, the degree of preexcitation may vary in an individual, depending on heart rate, autonomic tone, and AVN function, as well as BT location and EP characteristics. Therefore, it is important first to assess the degree of preexcitation visible throughout the entire ECG and then use only the delta wave polarity for localization (the first 40 milliseconds of the QRS in most cases, unless fully preexcited) rather than the overall QRS polarity, which may vary from each other.[25-29]

Several algorithms have been developed to precisely locate a BT to a specific anatomic location, using the delta wave polarity (Table 18-1; Figs. 18-12 and 18-13).[25,26] Although these algorithms

TABLE 18-1 Delta Wave Characteristics during Preexcitation According to Bypass Tract Location*

Left Lateral/Left Anterolateral BTs
A. R/S ≥1 in V_2 and positive delta in III, or R/S <1 in V_2 and positive delta in III and V_1
B. RS transition ≤V_1 and >2 positive delta in the inferior leads or S > R in aVL
C. QS or QR morphology in aVL and no negative QRS in III and V_1
Left Posterior/Left Posterolateral BTs
A. R/S ≥1 in V_1 and V_2, no positive delta in III and positive delta in V_1
B. R/S transition ≤V_1, no ≥2 positive delta in the inferior leads, no S > R in aVL, in lead I R <(S 0.8 mV), and the sum of the inferior delta is not negative
C. Positive QRS in aVL and an equiphasic QRS or positive in V_1 and no negative QRS in III
Left Posteroseptal BTs
A. R/S ≥1 in V_2, no positive delta in III, and positive delta and R/S <1 in V_1
B. R/S transition ≤V_1, no ≥2 positive delta in the inferior leads, no S > R in aVL, in lead I R <(S 0.8 mV), and the sum of the inferior delta is negative
C. Negative QRS in III, V_1, and aVF, tallest precordial R wave in V_2-V_4 and R wave width in V_1 >0.06 msec
Midseptal BTs
A. R/S <1 in V_2, no positive delta in III, and negative delta in V_1
B. R/S transition between V_2 and V_3 or between V_3 and V_4 but the delta amplitude in lead II ≥1.0 mV (septal location), and the sum of delta polarities in inferior leads is −1, 0, or +1 mV
C. Negative QRS in leads III, V_1, and aVF, tallest precordial R in leads V_2-V_4 and R wave width in V_1 <0.06 msec
Right Posteroseptal BTs
A. R/S ≥1 in V_2 and no positive delta in III and V_1
B. The sum of delta polarities in inferior leads is less than or equal to −2 mV
C. Negative QRS in leads III, V_1, and aVF and tallest precordial R in V_5 or V_6
Right Posterior/Right Posterolateral BTs
A. R/S <1 in V_2, no positive delta in III and no negative delta in V_1, and negative delta polarity in aV_F
B. R/S transition between V_3 and V_4 with delta amplitude in lead II <1.0 mV or≥V_4 and the delta axis is <0 degrees and the R in lead III is ≤0 mV
C. Positive QRS in III, negative in V_1, and RS morphology in aVL
Right Lateral/Right Anterolateral BTs
A. R/S<1 in V_2, no positive delta in III and no negative delta in V_1 and negative or biphasic delta in aVF
B. R/S transition between leads V_3 and V_4 with delta amplitude in lead II <1.0 mV or>V_4 and the delta axis is <0 degrees and the R amplitude in lead III is <0 mV
C. Positive QRS in leads aVL and III and negative in V_1
Right Anterior/Right Superoparaseptal BTs
A. R/S <1 in V_2, positive delta in III and no positive delta in V_1
B. The sum of delta polarities in inferior leads is ≥2
C. Positive QRS in aVF and negative in leads III and V_1

*A, algorithm of Chiang and colleagues[27]; B, algorithm of Fitzpatrick and colleagues[25]; C, algorithm of Xie and colleagues.[28]

BT = bypass tract; R/S = R-S wave ratio.

From Katsouras CS, Greakas GF, Goudevenos JA, et al: Localization of accessory pathways by the electrogram, *Pacing Clin Electrophysiol* 27:189, 2004.

facilitate prediction of the location of a BT, they are inherently limited by biological variability in anatomy (e.g., rotation of the heart within the thorax), variable degree of preexcitation and QRS fusion, the presence of more than one manifest BT, intrinsic ECG abnormalities (such as prior myocardial infarction and ventricular hypertrophy), as well as technical variability in ECG acquisition and electrode positioning. These factors can subject all algorithms to exceptions and inaccuracies.[24]

No single published algorithm offers extremely high sensitivity and specificity for all BT locations, particularly when differentiating septal BTs. Therefore, it may be more realistic to initially identify a general area in which the BT is located, and then to apply more subtle criteria from one or more of the algorithms to attempt a more precise localization.

The mere presence and the degree of preexcitation can sometimes help in predicting the location of the BT. In fact, an apparently normal ECG does not fully rule out anterograde conducting left lateral BTs or rate-dependent or decremental BTs. Posteroseptal and right-sided BTs tend to be associated with a prominent degree of preexcitation because of the proximity to the sinus node, whereas left lateral BTs are often associated with subtle preexcitation. Nevertheless, when preexcitation is prominent, the accuracy of surface ECG localization of manifest BTs tends to be higher for the diagnosis of left free wall BTs than for BTs in other locations. The presence of multiple manifest BTs may result in fusion of preexcitation patterns or predominance of right-sided conduction.[24]

LOCALIZATION USING POLARITY OF THE RETROGRADE P WAVE DURING ORTHODROMIC ATRIOVENTRICULAR REENTRANT TACHYCARDIA

The polarity of the retrograde P waves during orthodromic AVRT is dependent on the location of the atrial insertion of the BT, and is helpful to localize the BT. However, the P wave is usually inscribed within the ST segment and its morphology may not be easily determined.[3,30,31]

In general, P wave morphology in leads I and V_1 and in the inferior leads is most helpful. Negative P wave vector in lead I is highly suggestive of left free wall BTs, whereas a positive P wave is suggestive of right free wall BTs. On the other hand, a negative P wave in lead V_1 is highly suggestive of right-sided BTs. P wave polarity in the inferior leads, positive or negative, suggests superior or inferior location of the BT, respectively.[3,30,31]

Posteroseptal BTs have positive P waves in leads V_1, aVR, and aVL and negative P waves in the inferior leads. Left posterior BTs also have negative P waves in the inferior leads, but the P waves are more negative in lead II than in lead III and are more positive in lead aVR than in lead aVL, which is often isoelectric. Left lateral BTs have negative P waves in leads I and aVL, with a tendency for more positive P waves in lead III than in leads II and aVF as the location of the BT moves more superiorly.[3,30,31]

Electrophysiological Testing

EP testing is used to study the features, location, and number of BTs and the tachycardias, if any, associated with them (Table 18-2). Typically, three quadripolar catheters are positioned in the high RA, right ventricle (RV) apex or septum, and HB region, and a decapolar catheter is positioned in the CS (see Fig. 4-7). If a right-sided BT is suspected, a duo-decapolar (Halo; Biosense Webster, Diamond Bar, Calif.) catheter along the tricuspid annulus can be helpful.

Baseline Observations during Normal Sinus Rhythm

Preexcitation is associated with a short His bundle–ventricular (HV) or H-delta interval during NSR. The HV interval can even be negative or the His potential can be buried in the local ventricular electrogram (see Fig. 18-4). The QRS is a fusion between conduction over the BT and that over the AVN-HPS. The site of earliest ventricular activation is near the ventricular insertion site of the BT (i.e., near the tricuspid annulus or mitral annulus at the base of the heart). Slowing of conduction in the AVN by carotid sinus massage, AVN blockers, or rapid atrial pacing unmasks and increases the degree of preexcitation, because these maneuvers do not affect the conduction over the BT. Dual AVN pathways are present in 8% to 40% of patients.

ATRIAL PACING AND ATRIAL EXTRASTIMULATION DURING NORMAL SINUS RHYTHM

In the presence of a manifest AV BT, atrial stimulation from any atrial site can help unmask preexcitation if it is not manifest during

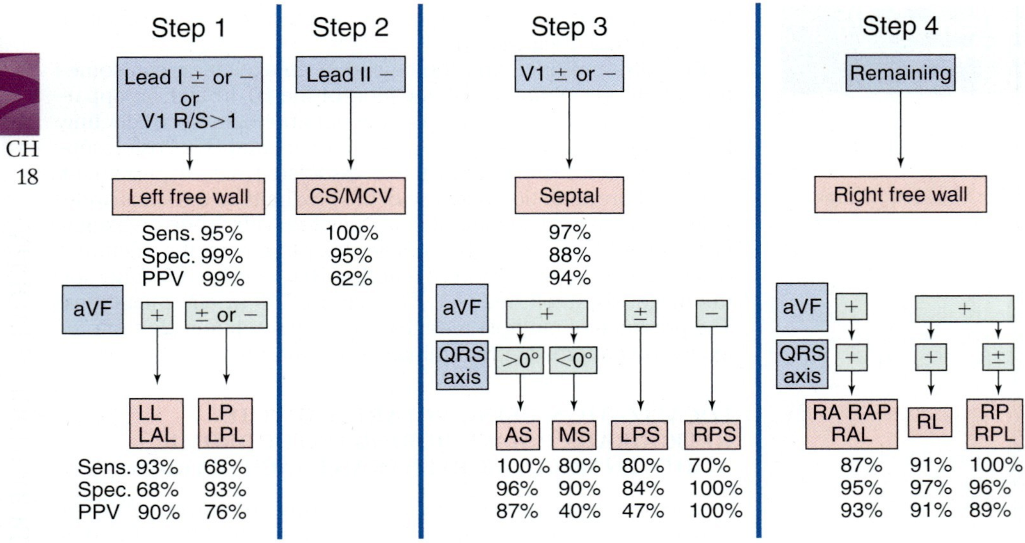

FIGURE 18-12 Algorithm for localization of bypass tract (BT) using delta wave morphology on the surface ECG. + = positive delta wave; ± = isoelectric delta wave; – = negative delta wave; AS = right anteroseptal; CS/MCV = coronary sinus/middle cardiac vein; LAL = left anterolateral; LL = left lateral; LP = left posterior; LPL = left posterolateral; LPS = left posteroseptal; MS = midseptal; PPV = positive predictive value; RA = right anterior; RAL = right anterolateral; RAP = right anterior paraseptal; RL = right lateral; RP = right posterior; RPL = right posterolateral; RPS = right posteroseptal; R/S = R-S wave ratio; Sens. = sensitivity; Spec. = specificity. *(From Arruda M, Wang X, McClelland J: ECG algorithm for predicting sites of successful radiofrequency ablation of accessory pathways [abstract], Pacing Clin Electrophysiol 16:865, 1993.)*

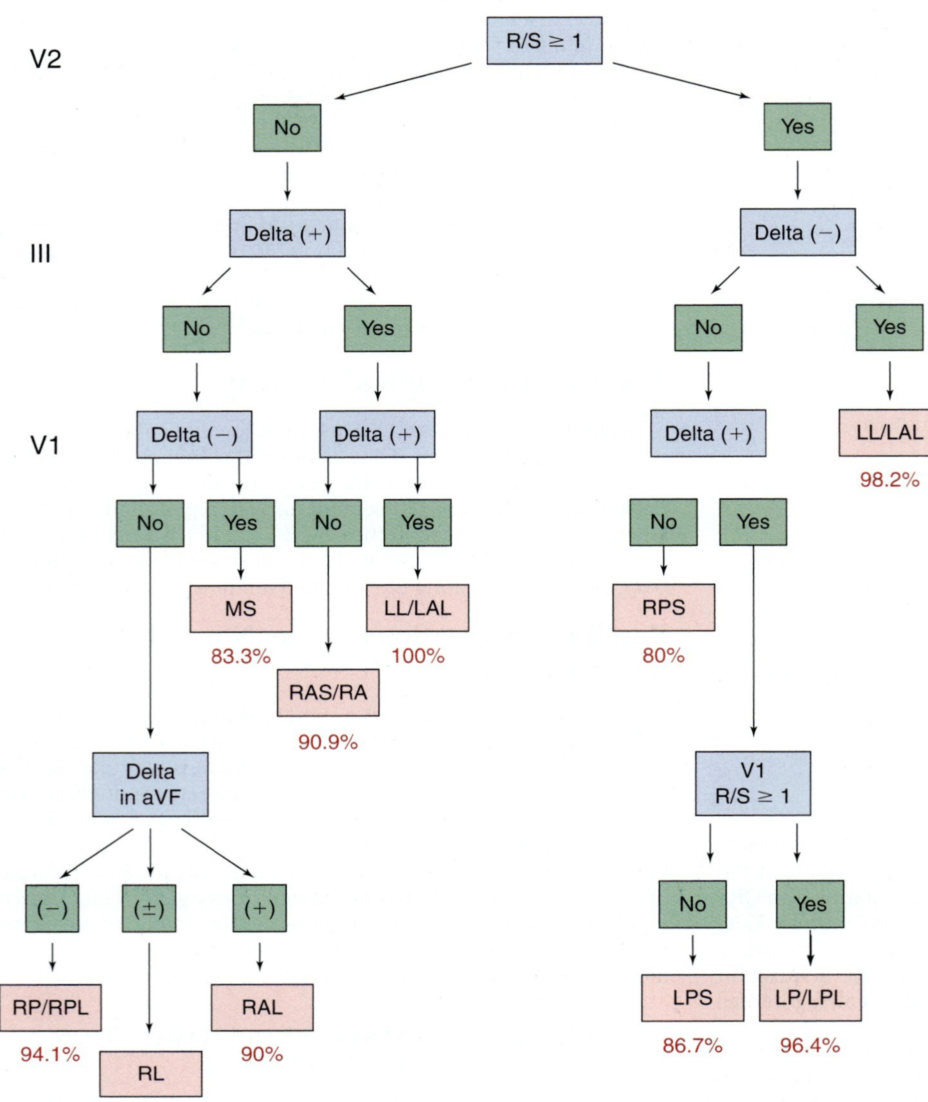

FIGURE 18-13 Stepwise algorithm for localization of the bypass tract (BT) by delta wave polarity. Numbers indicate the accuracy of the algorithm for each BT location. LAL = left anterolateral; LL = left lateral; LP = left posterior; LPL = left posterolateral; LPS = left posteroseptal; MS = midseptal; RA = right anterior; RAL = right anterolateral; RAS = right anteroseptal; RL = right lateral; RP = right posterior; RPL = right posterolateral; RPS = right posteroseptal; R/S = R-S wave ratio. *(From Chiang CE, Chen SA, Teo WS, et al: An accurate stepwise electrocardiographic algorithm for localization of accessory pathways in patients with Wolff-Parkinson-White syndrome from a comprehensive analysis of delta waves and R/S ratio during sinus rhythm, Am J Cardiol 6:40, 1995.)*

TABLE 18-2 Goals of Electrophysiological Evaluation in Patients with Wolff-Parkinson-White Syndrome

- Confirming the presence of an atrioventricular bypass tract (BT)
- Evaluation for the presence of multiple BTs
- Localization of the BT(s)
- Evaluation of the refractoriness of the BT and its implications for life-threatening arrhythmias
- Induction and evaluation of tachycardias
- Demonstration of the BT role in the tachycardia
- Evaluation of other tachycardias not dependent on the presence of the BT
- Termination of the tachycardias

NSR because of fast AVN conduction. Incremental rate atrial pacing and progressively premature AES produce decremental conduction over the AVN (but not over the BT), increasing the degree of preexcitation and shortening the HV interval, until the His potential is inscribed within the QRS. The His potential is still activated anterogradely over the AVN until anterograde block in the AVN occurs; the QRS then becomes fully preexcited, and the His potential becomes retrogradely activated (see Fig. 18-4).

Atrial stimulation close to or at the AV BT insertion site results in maximal preexcitation and the shortest P-delta interval because of the lack of intervening atrial tissue whose refractoriness may otherwise limit the ability of atrial stimulation to activate the AV BT as early (Fig. 18-14). The failure of atrial stimulation to increase the amount of preexcitation can be caused by markedly enhanced AVN conduction, the presence of another AV BT, a pacing-induced block in the AV BT because of a long ERP of the BT (longer than that of the AVN), total preexcitation already present at the basal state caused by prolonged or absent AVN-HPS conduction, and/or decremental conduction in the BT. Atrial pacing can reveal the presence of multiple BTs (Fig. 18-15). Rare cases of catecholamine-dependent BTs have been reported that require isoproterenol infusion to manifest preexcitation that is absent at baseline.

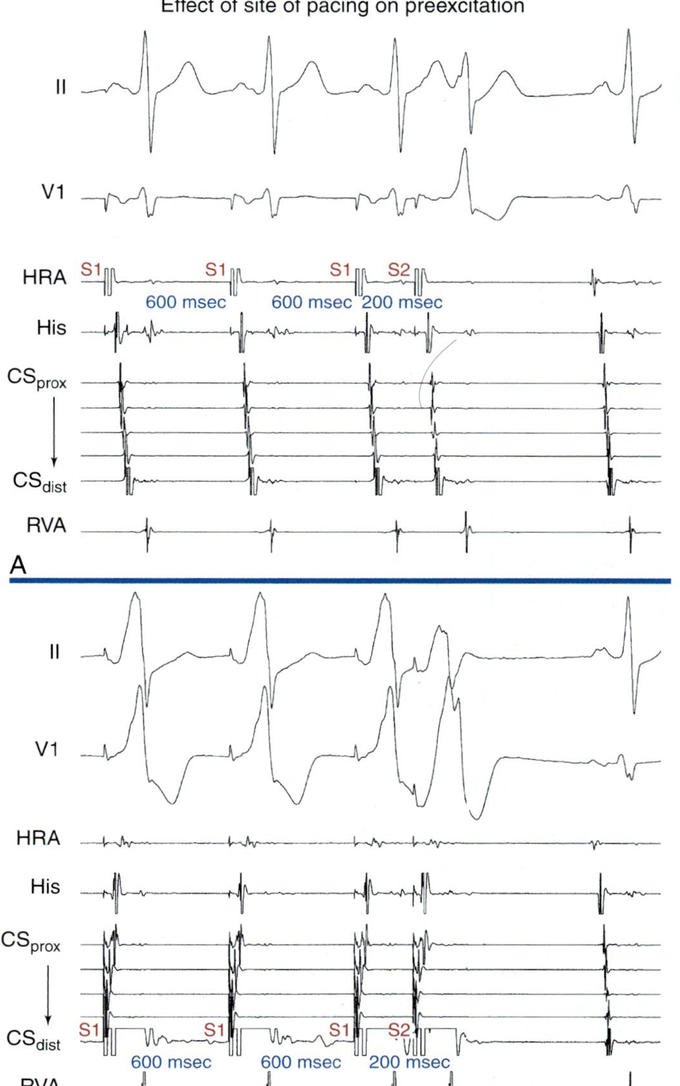

FIGURE 18-14 Effect of site of pacing on preexcitation. **A,** In the presence of a manifest left lateral bypass tract (BT), pacing from the high right atrium at a cycle length (CL) of 600 milliseconds produces minimal preexcitation. The degree of preexcitation increases with premature stimulation because of delay in atrioventricular nodal conduction. **B,** In the same patient, pacing at the same CLs from the distal coronary sinus (CS), close to or at the BT insertion site, results in a larger degree of preexcitation and shorter P-delta interval because of the lack of intervening atrial tissue whose refractoriness might otherwise limit the ability of atrial stimulation to activate the BT as early.

VENTRICULAR PACING AND VENTRICULAR EXTRASTIMULATION DURING NORMAL SINUS RHYTHM

In the presence of a retrogradely conducting AV BT (whether manifest or concealed), ventricular extrastimulation (VES) during NSR can result in VA conduction over the BT, AVN, both, or neither (Fig. 18-16). Conduction over the BT alone is the most common pattern at short pacing CLs or short VES coupling intervals. In this setting, the VA conduction time is fairly constant over a wide range of pacing CLs and VES coupling intervals, in the absence of intraventricular conduction abnormalities or additional BTs. On the other hand, retrograde conduction over the BT and HPS-AVN is especially common when RV pacing is performed in the presence of a left-sided BT at long pacing CLs or long VES coupling intervals. This occurs because it is easier to engage the right bundle branch (RB) and conduct retrogradely through the AVN than it is to reach a distant left-sided BT. In this setting, the atrial activation pattern depends on the refractoriness and conduction times over both pathways and usually exhibits a variable degree of fusion. In addition, VA conduction can proceed over the HPS-AVN alone, resulting in a normal pattern of VA conduction, or can be absent because of block in both the HPS-AVN and BT, which is especially common with short pacing CLs and very early VES.

Ventricular stimulation during NSR also helps prove the presence of a retrogradely conducting AV BT. Ventricular stimulation resulting in retrograde VA conduction not consistent with normal conduction over the AVN (i.e., eccentric atrial activation sequence; see Fig. 18-16) and a VES delivered when the HB is refractory that results in atrial activation are indicators of the presence of a retrogradely conducting AV BT. However, if a VES delivered when the HB is refractory does not result in atrial activation, this does not necessarily exclude the presence of a retrogradely conducting AV BT, because such a VES can be associated with retrograde block in the BT itself (see Fig. 18-16). Additionally, the lack of such a response does not exclude the presence of unidirectional (anterograde-only) AV BTs. A VES that conducts to the HB and results in an atrial activation that either precedes HB activation (Fig. 18-17) or is associated with an apparent His bundle–atrial (HA) interval shorter than that during drive complexes indicates the presence of a BT. Ventricular pacing can also reveal the presence of multiple BTs (Fig. 18-18).

During the delivery of progressively premature single VESs, an abrupt increase in the VA conduction interval is often observed. This may be due to a variety of reasons including a change in activation from a BT block to the AVN or a change from fast to slow pathway conduction; or it may be the result of an abrupt change when the refractory period of the RB has been reached. Retrograde right bundle branch block (RBBB) occurs frequently during VES testing,

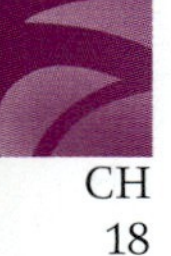

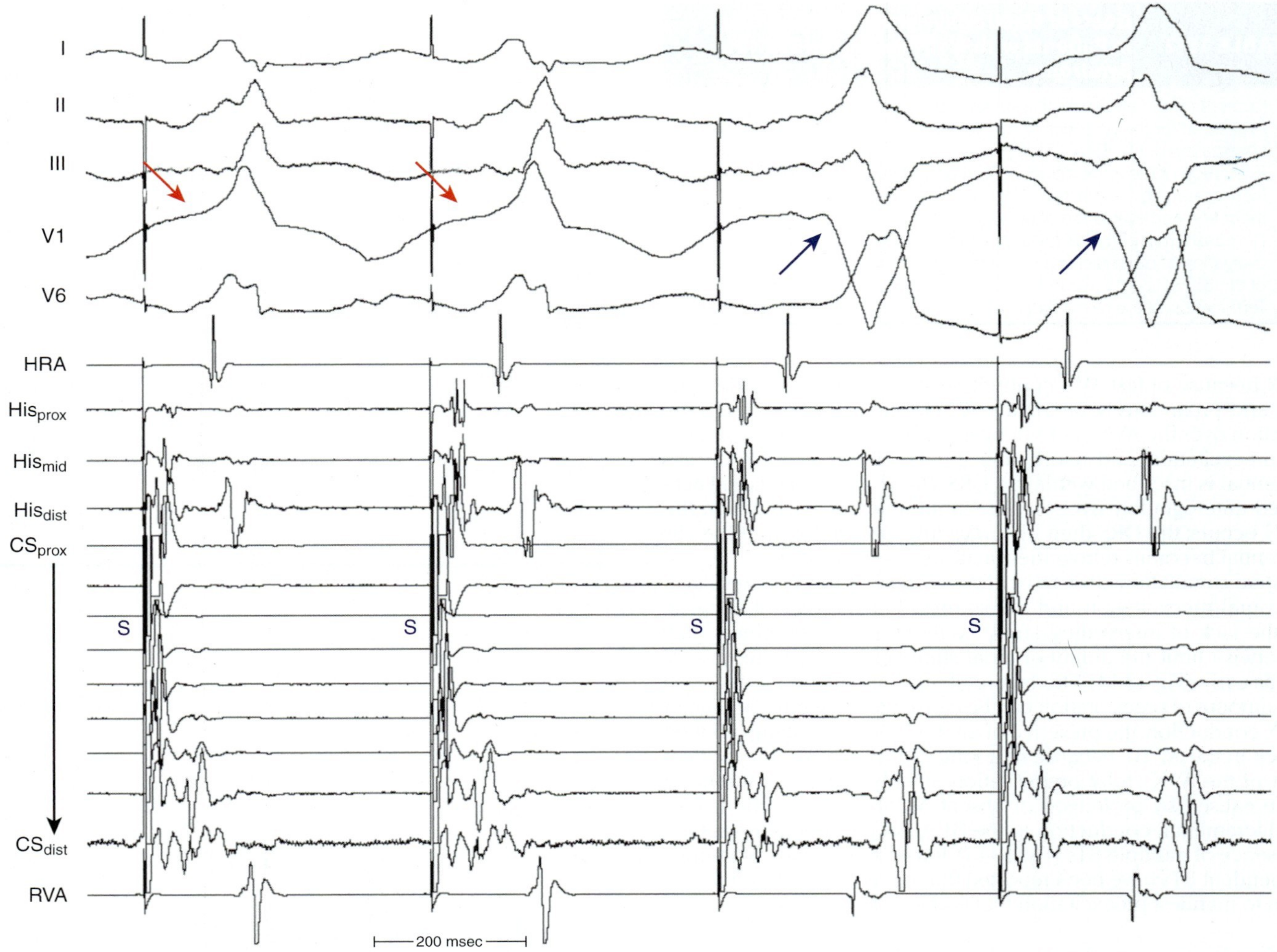

FIGURE 18-15 Surface ECG and intracardiac recordings during coronary sinus (CS) pacing (S) in a patient with both right and left lateral BTs. The first two complexes show a left lateral preexcitation pattern (red arrows), whereas this pathway fails to conduct on the last two complexes, which show a right lateral preexcitation pattern (blue arrows).

and can be diagnosed by observing the retrograde His potential during the drive train and its abrupt delay following the VES. Often, however, it is difficult to visualize the retrograde His potential during the pacing train; nevertheless, the sudden appearance of an easily distinguished retrograde His potential, separate from the ventricular electrogram following the VES, may be sufficient to recognize retrograde RBBB. Prolongation of the V-H interval is observed on development of retrograde RBBB, because conduction must traverse the interventricular septum (which requires approximately 60 to 70 milliseconds in normal hearts), enter retrograde via the left bundle branch (LB), and ascend to reach the HB. Although an increase in the V-H interval necessarily occurs with retrograde RBBB, whether a similar increase occurs in the VA interval depends on the nature of VA conduction. Measurement of the effect of retrograde V-H and VA intervals on the development of retrograde RBBB during VES can help the distinction between retrograde AVN and BT conduction. In the absence of a BT, the AVN can be activated in a retrograde fashion only after retrograde activation of the HB; as a consequence, VA activation will necessarily be delayed with retrograde RBBB, and the increase in the VA interval will be at least as much as the increase in the V-H interval. On the other hand, when retrograde conduction is via a BT, there will be no expected increase in the VA interval when retrograde RBBB is induced. Thus, the increase in the VA interval is minimal and always less than the increase in the V-H interval.[32]

During retrograde conduction over the BT, the VA interval may increase slightly in response to incremental rate ventricular pacing or progressively premature VES. At short ventricular pacing CLs or VES coupling intervals, intramyocardial conduction delay can occur, resulting in prolongation in the VA interval; however, the local VA interval at the BT location remains unchanged. Furthermore, short ventricular pacing CLs or VES coupling intervals can encroach on the BT refractoriness, causing some decremental conduction, with a consequent increase in total and local VA intervals. The VA interval can also change with changing the site of ventricular stimulation, because the VA interval represents the sum of conduction time over the BT and conduction time through the ventricular tissue intervening between the site of stimulation and ventricular insertion site of the BT. BTs with retrograde decremental conduction properties can also exhibit prolongation of conduction time and VA interval with ventricular pacing or VES.

The absence of VA conduction (at long pacing CLs) or the presence of decremental VA conduction at baseline makes the presence of a retrogradely conducting BT unlikely, except for the rare catecholamine-dependent BTs that require isoproterenol infusion for demonstration.

Induction of Tachycardia

INITIATION BY ATRIAL EXTRASTIMULATION OR ATRIAL PACING

ORTHODROMIC ATRIOVENTRICULAR REENTRANT TACHYCARDIA: MANIFEST ATRIOVENTRICULAR BYPASS TRACT. In the presence of a manifest AV BT, initiation of orthodromic AVRT with an AES requires the following: (1) anterograde block in the AV BT; (2) anterograde conduction over the AVN-HPS; and (3) slow

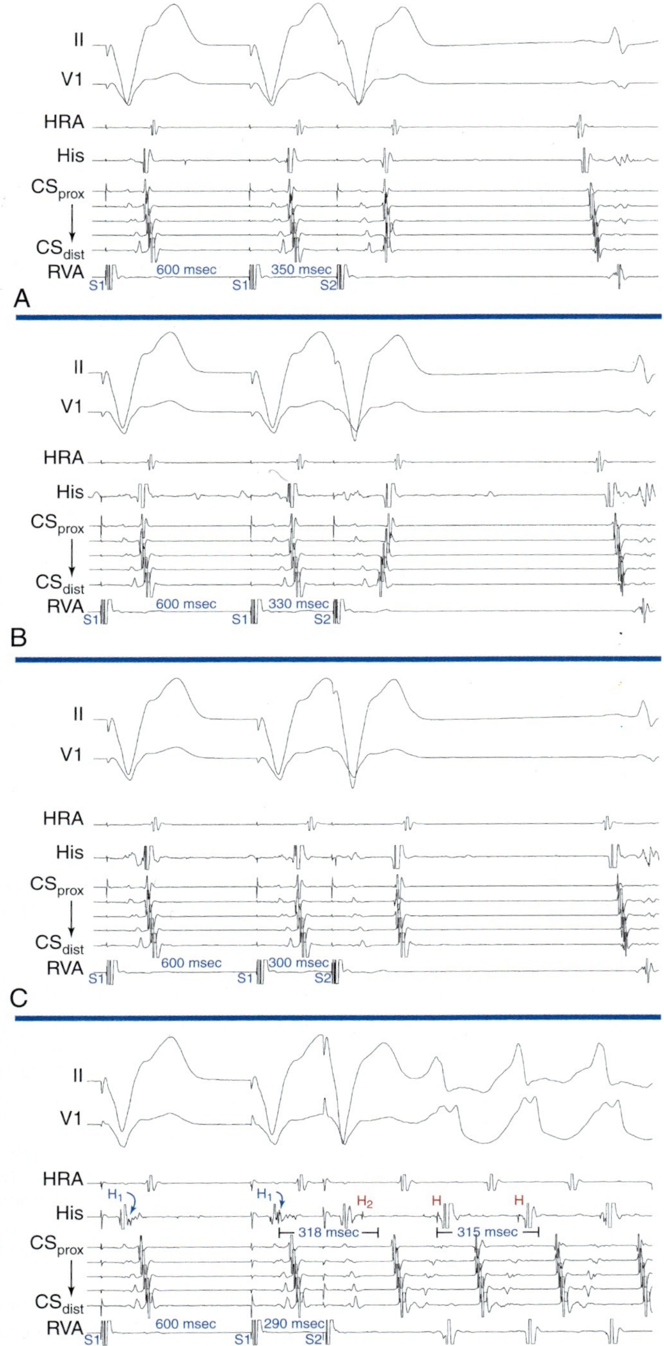

FIGURE 18-16 Retrograde conduction during ventricular extrastimulation (VES) in a patient with a bidirectional left lateral bypass tract (BT). **A,** The ventricular pacing drive is conducted retrogradely over the atrioventricular node (AVN) with a concentric atrial activation sequence. The VES is conducted over both the AVN and BT (atrial fusion). **B,** An earlier VES encounters delay in the His-Purkinje system (HPS)–AVN and conducts solely over the BT with an eccentric atrial activation sequence. **C,** An early-coupled VES blocks retrogradely in the BT and conducts solely over the AVN. **D,** The VES conducts only over the HPS-AVN with more pronounced ventriculoatrial (VA) delay, which allows recovery of the BT and anterograde conduction, initiating antidromic atrioventricular reentrant tachycardia (AVRT). The VA delay is provided by conduction delay, not only within the AVN but also within the HPS. Note that the VES encounters retrograde block in the right bundle branch (RB), and His bundle (HB) activation is mediated by retrograde conduction over the left bundle branch (LB). Consequently, the His potential is visible after the ventricular electrogram. Note that despite the fact that the H_1-H_2 interval following VES approximates the H-H interval during supraventricular tachycardia (SVT), the His bundle–atrial (HA) interval following the initiating VES is shorter than that during the SVT, which favors antidromic AVRT over preexcited atrioventricular nodal reentrant tachycardia (AVNRT) as the mechanism of the SVT.

conduction over the AVN-HPS, with adequate delay to allow for the recovery of the atrium and AV BT and subsequent retrograde conduction over the BT (see Fig. 3-10).[3] The reason this occurs is that, whereas the BT conducts more rapidly than the AVN, it has a longer ERP, so the early atrial impulse blocks anterogradely in the BT but conducts over the AVN. The site of AV delay is less important; it is most commonly in the AVN, but it can occur also in the HB, bundle branches, or ventricular myocardium. Because the coupling intervals of the AES required to achieve anterograde block in the BT are usually short, sufficient AVN delay is usually present so that orthodromic AVRT is initiated once anterograde BT block occurs. The presence of dual AVN physiology can facilitate the initiation of orthodromic AVRT by providing adequate AV delay by mediating anterograde conduction over the slow AVN pathway. BBB ipsilateral to the AV BT provides an additional AV delay that can facilitate tachycardia initiation.

Induction of orthodromic AVRT is easier with atrial stimulation at a site in close proximity to the AV BT insertion site; the closer the stimulation site to the BT, the easier it is to encroach on the refractory period of the BT and achieve block, because it is not limited by the refractoriness of intervening atrial tissue. Furthermore, the earlier the atrial insertion of the BT is activated, the more likely it will recover before arrival of the retrograde atrial activation wavefront to the BT atrial insertion site, thereby facilitating reentry. Thus, one may actually require less anterograde AV delay if recovery of excitability is shifted earlier in time. In addition, different sites of atrial stimulation can produce different AVN conduction velocities and refractoriness (even at the same AES coupling intervals).

If SVT induction fails, the use of multiple AESs, rapid atrial pacing, and pacing closer to the BT would achieve block in the BT and produce adequate AV delay.

AES can also result in a 1:2 response caused by conduction over both the AV BT and the AVN-HPS (i.e., a single AES resulting in two ventricular complexes; the first is fully preexcited and the second is normal). For this response to occur, significant delay in AVN-HPS conduction should be present to allow for recovery of the ventricle after its activation via the BT. AES can also produce sinus nodal or AVN echo beats that in turn may block in the BT and achieve adequate AV delay to initiate orthodromic AVRT.

ORTHODROMIC ATRIOVENTRICULAR REENTRANT TACHYCARDIA: CONCEALED ATRIOVENTRICULAR BYPASS TRACT. Orthodromic AVRT in patients with concealed BTs is identical to that in patients with WPW. The only difference is that in patients with concealed BTs anterograde block in the BT is already present. Consequently, the only condition needed to induce orthodromic AVRT is adequate AV delay (in the AVN or HPS) to allow for recovery of the atrium and atrial insertion site of the AV BT. Therefore, orthodromic AVRT initiation requires less premature coupling intervals of the AESs in patients with concealed BTs than in patients with WPW.

ORTHODROMIC ATRIOVENTRICULAR REENTRANT TACHYCARDIA: SLOWLY CONDUCTING CONCEALED ATRIOVENTRICULAR BYPASS TRACT (PERMANENT JUNCTIONAL RECIPROCATING TACHYCARDIA). PJRT is usually incessant and is initiated by spontaneous shortening of the sinus CL, without a triggering PAC or PVC. The tachycardia can be transiently terminated by PACs or PVCs but usually resumes after a few sinus beats (Fig. 18-19). This phenomenon has three potential mechanisms: a rate-related decrease in the retrograde ERP of the BT, a rate-related decrease in atrial refractoriness that allows the impulse to reactivate the atrium retrogradely over the BT, or a concealed Wenckebach block with block at the atrial-BT junction terminating the Wenckebach cycle, relieving any anterograde concealed conduction that may have prevented retrograde conduction up the BT. The latter is the most likely mechanism, because such slow BTs actually demonstrate decremental conduction at rapid rates and, in most cases, the atrial ERP at the atrial-BT junction is shorter than the RP (VA) interval. Thus, some sort of anterograde concealment during NSR in the BT must be operative, preventing tachycardia from always occurring.[3] Late-coupled AESs can also readily initiate PJRT.

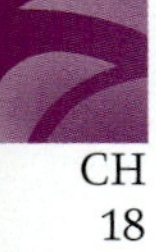

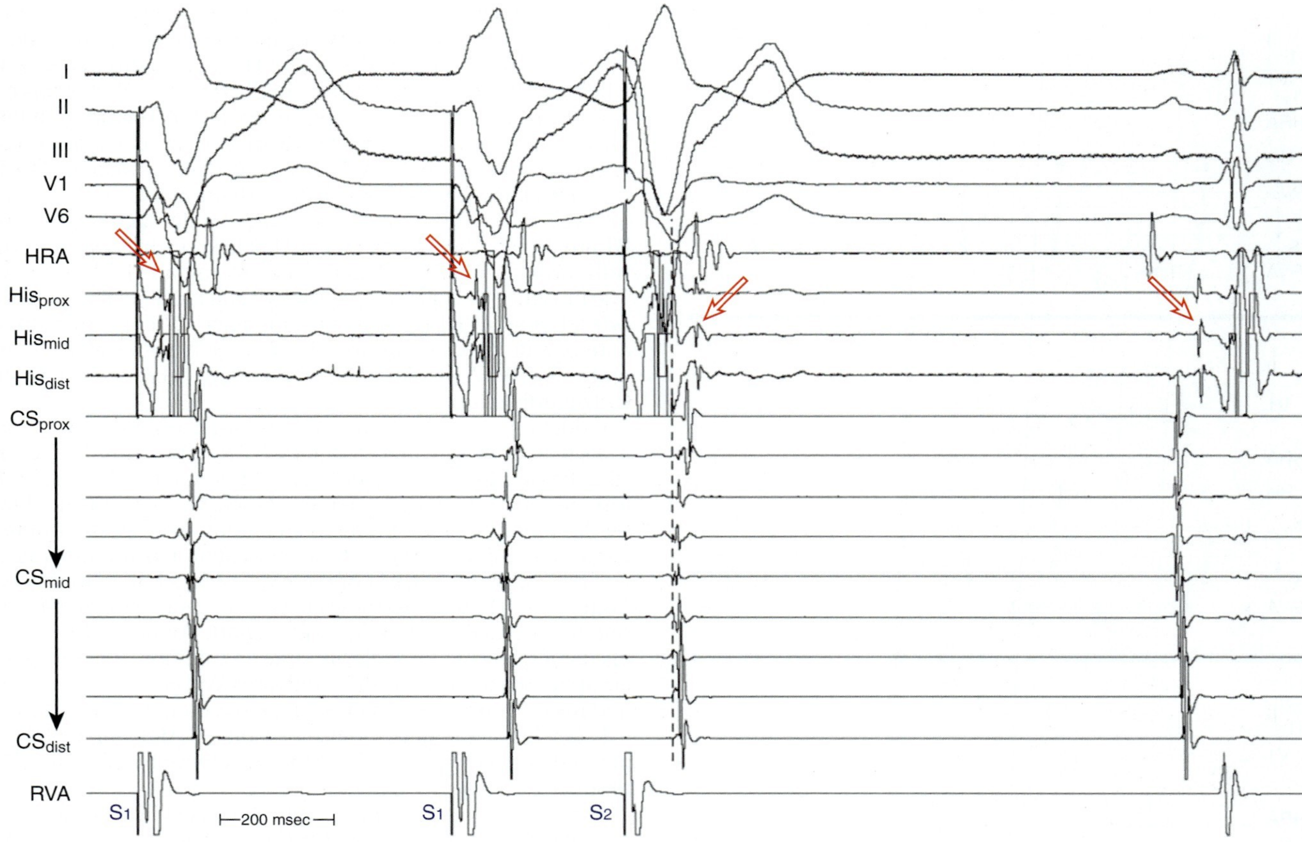

FIGURE 18-17 Ventricular pacing with a single ventricular extrastimulus (S_2) showing the presence of a bypass tract (BT). A retrograde His potential is present on both drive complexes (S_1) as well as following the extrastimulus (arrows); although atrial activation also follows each stimulus, it occurs (dashed line) before the inscription of the His potential on the extrastimulus complex. Thus, a BT is present because atrial activation is not dependent on His bundle–atrioventricular (HB-AVN) activation.

ANTIDROMIC ATRIOVENTRICULAR REENTRANT TACHYCARDIA. The initiation of classic antidromic AVRT by an AES requires the following: (1) intact anterograde conduction over the BT; (2) anterograde block in the AVN or HPS; and (3) intact retrograde conduction over the HPS-AVN once the AVN resumes excitability following partial anterograde penetration (see Fig. 18-4). The latter is usually the limiting factor for the initiation of antidromic AVRT. A delay of more than 150 milliseconds between atrial insertion of the BT and HB is probably required for the initiation of antidromic AVRT.[3]

Several mechanisms of antidromic AVRT initiation can be operative.[3] The AES may block in the AVN with anterograde conduction down the BT and subsequent retrograde conduction over the HPS-AVN. In this setting, ventricular–His bundle (V-H) delay is required to allow recovery of the AVN. Because antidromic AVRTs have relatively short VA intervals, this mechanism of initiation is probably uncommon, except with left-sided BTs, which would potentially provide sufficient V-H delay to allow retrograde conduction. Tachycardia initiation can be facilitated by a short retrograde AVN ERP, a common finding in patients with these SVTs. Alternatively, the AES may block in the AVN, with anterograde conduction down the BT and subsequent retrograde conduction over a different BT. Subsequent complexes can conduct retrogradely over the AVN-HPS or the second BT. Changing tachycardia CL (and VA interval) may relate to whether retrograde conduction proceeds over the AVN-HPS or the second BT. A third potential mechanism for the initiation of antidromic AVRT involves AES conduction over the BT and simultaneously over the slow pathway of a dual AVN pathway situation, with anterograde block in the fast AVN pathway. Conduction beyond the HB to the ventricle is not possible because of ventricular refractoriness, yet an AVN echo to the atrium may occur, which in turn may conduct anterogradely over the BT, when the ventricle would have recovered excitability, and subsequently back up the now-recovered AVN, initiating antidromic AVRT. AVN reentry may not persist or may be preempted by retrograde conduction up the fast AVN pathway because of the premature ventricular activation over the BT. In this scenario, the location of the His potential will depend on whether or not it was anterograde or retrograde.

In general, if atrial stimulation induces antidromic AVRT, multiple BTs are often operative. Whether or not they are operative throughout the SVT depends on the relative retrograde activation times over the additional BTs and HPS-AVN and the varying degree of anterograde and/or retrograde concealment into the additional BTs, HPS-AVN, or both during the SVT.

The site of atrial stimulation plays an important role in inducibility of AVRT, and can also determine the type of AVRT initiated in patients with bidirectional BTs. The closer the stimulation site to the BT, the more likely anterograde block in the BT will occur and orthodromic AVRT will result. Conversely, antidromic AVRT is more likely to occur with atrial stimulation close to the AVN.

INITIATION BY VENTRICULAR EXTRASTIMULATION OR VENTRICULAR PACING

ORTHODROMIC ATRIOVENTRICULAR REENTRANT TACHYCARDIA: MANIFEST OR CONCEALED ATRIOVENTRICULAR BYPASS TRACT. Ventricular stimulation is usually able to induce orthodromic AVRT (inducibility rate of 60% with VES and 80% with ventricular pacing), and is similar in patients with manifest or concealed BTs (Fig. 18-20). Initiation of orthodromic AVRT by ventricular stimulation requires the following: (1) retrograde block of the ventricular impulse in the HPS-AVN; (2) retrograde conduction only over the AV BT; and (3) adequate VA conduction delay to allow for recovery of the AVN-HPS from any concealment

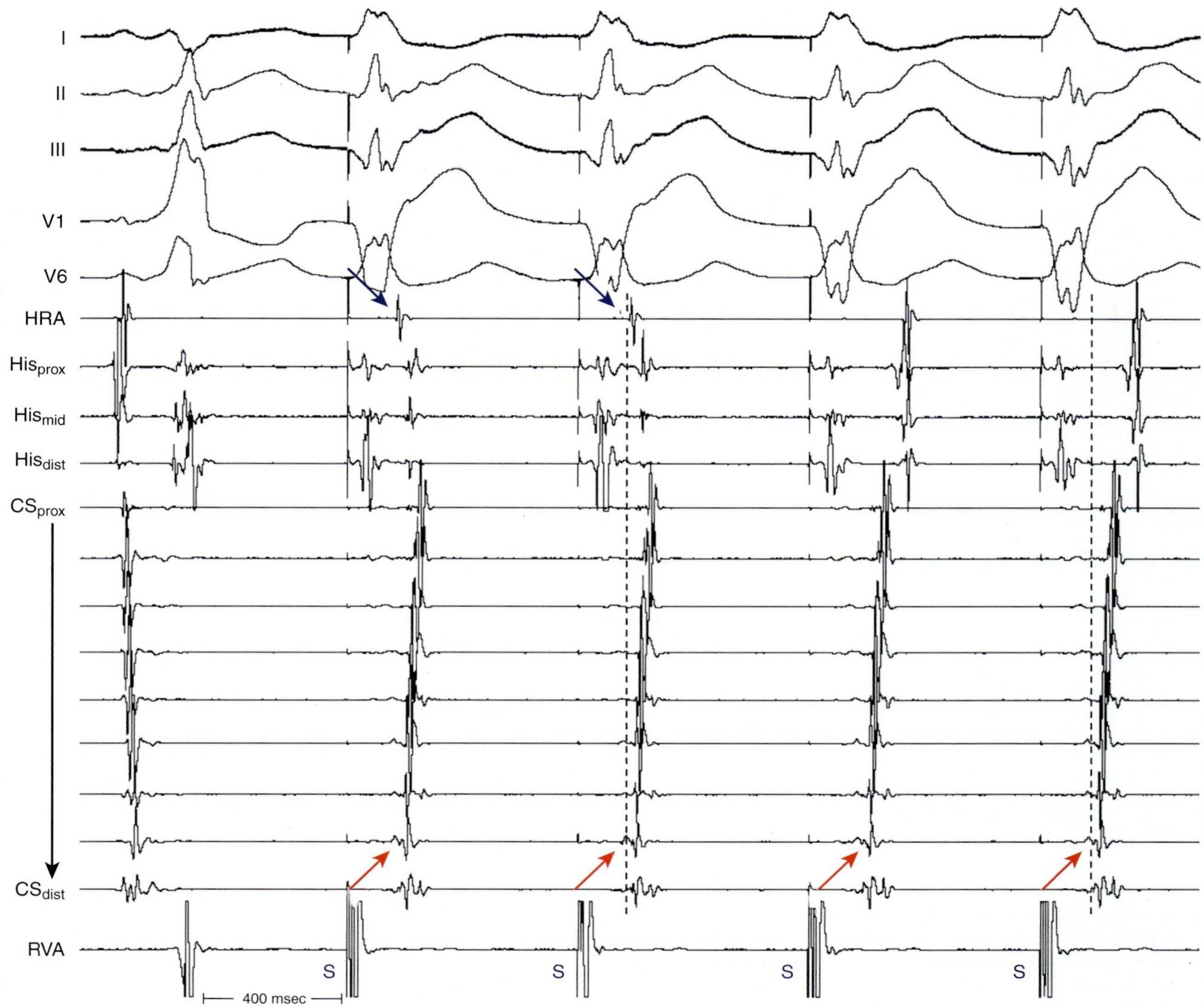

FIGURE 18-18 Surface ECG and intracardiac recordings in a patient with both right and left free wall bypass tracts (BTs). The first complex shows sinus rhythm with preexcitation, showing a left free wall pattern. Four complexes of right ventricular pacing follow, the first two of which show fusion of retrograde activation over both a left lateral BT (red arrows), which is present in each complex, as well as a right lateral BT (blue arrows) that is present in the first two paced complexes but fails to conduct on the last two complexes. Dashed lines aid in comparison of activation sequences.

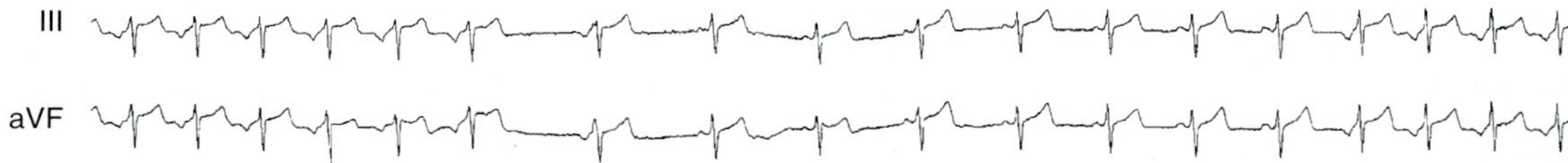

FIGURE 18-19 Two surface ECG leads are shown during permanent junctional reciprocating tachycardia. Carotid sinus pressure is applied at left, resulting in termination of supraventricular tachycardia (SVT) caused by block in the bypass tract (the SVT terminates with a QRS). Several escape and sinus complexes follow, and then the SVT resumes. This phenomenon gives rise to the use of the term *permanent* or *incessant*.

produced by ventricular stimulation, so it can support anterograde conduction of the reentrant impulse. Because the BT retrograde ERP is usually very short, the prime determinant of orthodromic AVRT initiation is the extent of retrograde conduction and/or concealment in the HPS-AVN.[3]

Multiple modes of initiation of orthodromic AVRT can be present, depending on the pacing CL or VES coupling interval, conduction velocities, and refractoriness of the HPS-AVN and BT, as well as the site of ventricular stimulation.[3] Ventricular pacing at a CL or a VES with a coupling interval shorter than the ERP of the AVN but longer than that of the HPS and AV BT would block retrogradely in the AVN and conduct over the AV BT to initiate orthodromic AVRT. Block in the AVN, which is more likely to occur with rapid ventricular pacing or VES delivered after a short pacing drive CL, can cause concealment and subsequent delay in anterograde conduction of the first SVT impulse over the AVN, resulting in longer AH and PR intervals of the first SVT beat compared with subsequent beats (see Fig. 18-20). On the other hand, a VES with a coupling interval or ventricular

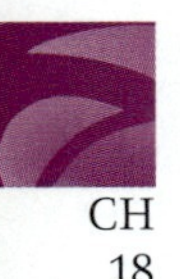

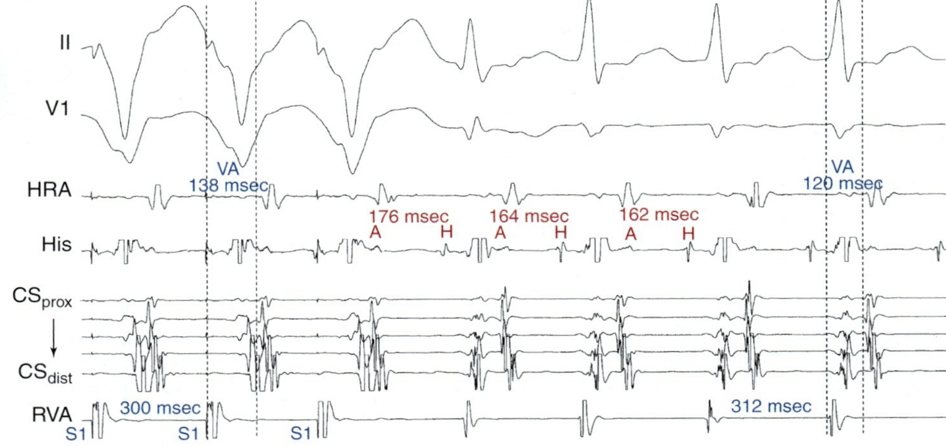

FIGURE 18-20 Induction of an orthodromic atrioventricular reentrant tachycardia (AVRT) using a concealed posteroseptal bypass tract with ventricular pacing. Note that although the ventricular pacing cycle length (CL) approximates the supraventricular tachycardia (SVT) CL, the ventriculoatrial (VA) interval (dashed lines) during ventricular pacing is only slightly longer than that during SVT, which favors orthodromic AVRT over atrioventricular nodal reentrant tachycardia (AVNRT) as the mechanism of the SVT. Additionally, the atrial–His bundle interval of the first SVT complex is longer than that of subsequent beats, indicating retrograde concealment in the AVN produced by the last ventricular stimulus.

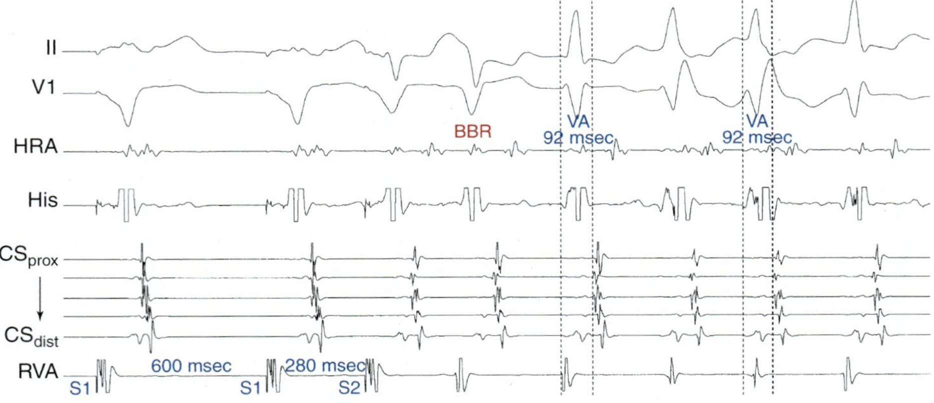

FIGURE 18-21 Induction of an orthodromic atrioventricular reentrant tachycardia (AVRT) using a concealed left posteroseptal bypass tract (BT) with ventricular extrastimulation (VES). The VES conducts retrogradely over the BT, but also results in a bundle branch reentrant (BBR) beat, which in turn conducts to the atrium over the BT and initiates orthodromic AVRT. Note that right bundle branch block (RBBB) develops shortly after initiation of the SVT; however, the ventriculoatrial (VA) interval (dashed lines) remains constant, regardless of the presence or absence of RBBB, because the BT is in the contralateral ventricle.

pacing at a CL shorter than the ERP of the HPS, but longer than that of the AV BT, would block retrogradely in the HPS and conduct over the AV BT to initiate orthodromic AVRT. When block occurs in the HPS, which is more likely to occur with a VES delivered during NSR or after a long pacing drive CL, the first SVT beat will approach a fully recovered AVN and conduct with short AH and PR intervals equal to subsequent SVT beats. In this case, adequate prolongation of the HV interval may be required to allow for the recovery of ventricular refractoriness for the ventricle to be activated and support reentry, because AVN delay may have not been sufficient. When HV interval prolongation is required to initiate orthodromic AVRT, it is almost invariably associated with LBBB. A short-coupled VES, especially following a pacing drive with a long CL, that blocks retrogradely in both the AV BT and RB and conducts transseptally and then retrogradely over the LB, can result in a bundle branch reentrant (BBR) beat that conducts to the ventricle down the RB, and then retrogradely to the atrium over the AV BT, mediating the initiation of orthodromic AVRT. The long HV interval often associated with BBR beats, plus the LBBB pattern, facilitate the induction of orthodromic AVRT using a left-sided BT (Fig. 18-21).

ORTHODROMIC ATRIOVENTRICULAR REENTRANT TACHYCARDIA: SLOWLY CONDUCTING CONCEALED ATRIOVENTRICULAR BYPASS TRACT (PERMANENT JUNCTIONAL RECIPROCATING TACHYCARDIA). Ventricular stimulation is less effective in initiating PJRT because of the already impaired conduction in the BT, such that an early VES produces block in the BT. A late-coupled VES (when the HB is refractory) can initiate SVT in some cases.

ANTIDROMIC ATRIOVENTRICULAR REENTRANT TACHYCARDIA. Initiation of classic antidromic AVRT by ventricular pacing and VES requires the following: (1) retrograde block in the BT; (2) retrograde conduction over the AVN or HPS; and (3) adequate VA delay to allow for recovery of the atrium and BT so it can support subsequent anterograde conduction (see Fig. 18-16).[3]

When induction of the SVT is achieved by ventricular pacing at a CL similar to the tachycardia CL or by a VES that activates the HB at a coupling interval (i.e., H_1-H_2 interval) similar to the H-H interval during the SVT, the HA interval following the initiating ventricular stimulus is always equal to or shorter than that during the antidromic AVRT. This is because the His potential and atrium are activated in sequence during antidromic AVRT and in parallel during ventricular stimulation. Therefore, an HA interval of the initiating ventricular stimulus longer than the HA interval during SVT favors AVNRT and excludes antidromic AVRT (see Fig. 18-16). Moreover, because the AVN usually exhibits greater decremental conduction with repetitive engagement of impulses than to a single impulse at a similar coupling interval, the more prolonged the HA interval with the initiating ventricular stimulus, the more likely that the SVT is AVNRT.

Tachycardia Features

ORTHODROMIC ATRIOVENTRICULAR REENTRANT TACHYCARDIA: MANIFEST OR CONCEALED ATRIOVENTRICULAR BYPASS TRACT

ATRIAL ACTIVATION SEQUENCE. The initial site of atrial activation during orthodromic AVRT depends on the location of the AV BT, but is always near the AV groove and without multiple breakthrough points. The atrial activation sequence during orthodromic AVRT should be identical to that during ventricular pacing at comparable CLs when VA conduction occurs exclusively over the AV BT. However, retrograde conduction during ventricular pacing may proceed over the AVN or over both the BT and AVN, resulting in fusion of atrial activation, depending on the site of

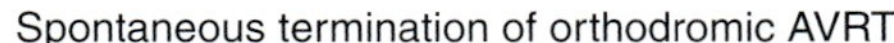

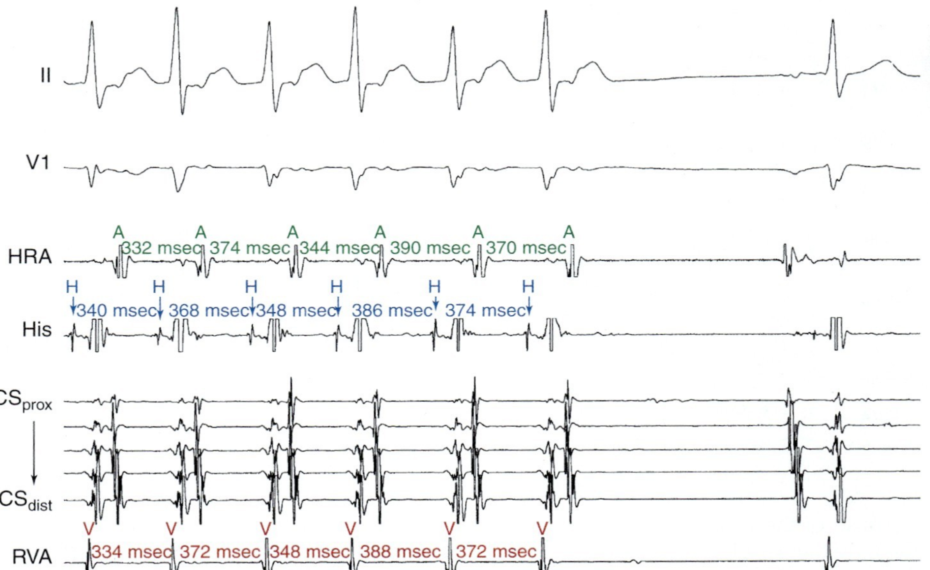

FIGURE 18-22 Spontaneous termination of orthodromic atrioventricular reentrant tachycardia (AVRT) using a concealed superoparaseptal bypass tract. Note that the supraventricular tachycardia (SVT) terminates with an atrial complex not followed by a QRS, consistent with anterograde block in the atrioventricular node (AVN). Also, note the oscillation in the SVT cycle length (CL) preceding termination. Changes in H-H and V-V intervals precede the subsequent changes in A-A intervals, and the ventriculoatrial (VA) interval remains constant despite oscillation of the CL. This indicates that the variability in the tachycardia CL is secondary to changes in the anterograde conduction over the AVN, whereas VA conduction over the retrograde limb of the reentrant circuit (the bypass tract) remains constant.

ventricular stimulation relative to the BT and HPS, and on retrograde conduction and refractoriness of the HPS-AVN.

ATRIAL–VENTRICULAR RELATIONSHIP. Conduction time over the classic (fast) BTs is approximately 30 to 120 milliseconds. Therefore, the RP interval during orthodromic AVRT is short, but longer than that during typical AVNRT, because in the setting of orthodromic AVRT the wavefront has to activate the ventricle before it reaches the AV BT ventricular insertion site at the AV groove and subsequently conduct to the atrium. Consequently, a very short VA interval (<70 milliseconds) or V–high RA interval (<95 milliseconds) largely excludes orthodromic AVRT, and is consistent with typical AVNRT.[33] The RP and VA intervals remain constant during orthodromic AVRT regardless of oscillations in tachycardia CL from whatever cause or changes in the PR interval (AH interval); as a consequence, the tachycardia CL is most closely associated with the PR interval (i.e., anterograde slow conduction) and the RP/PR ratio may vary (Fig. 18-22).

A 1:1 A-V relationship is a prerequisite for maintenance of AVRT, because parts of both the atrium and the ventricle are essential components of the reentrant circuit. If an SVT persists despite the presence of AV block, orthodromic AVRT is excluded.

When dual AVN pathways are present, the slow AVN pathway functions in most cases as the anterograde limb during orthodromic AVRT. An AH interval of more than 180 milliseconds during orthodromic AVRT suggests a slow AVN pathway mediating the anterograde limb of the reentrant circuit, whereas an AH interval of less than 160 milliseconds suggests a fast AVN pathway mediating anterograde conduction. Obviously, orthodromic AVRT using the slow pathway will have a longer tachycardia CL.

Slow-slow AVNRT is associated with an RP interval and P wave morphology similar to that during orthodromic AVRT using a posteroseptal AV BT. However, although both SVTs have the earliest atrial activation in the posteroseptal region, conduction time from that site to the HB region is significantly longer in AVNRT than in orthodromic AVRT, resulting in a significantly longer RP interval in lead V_1 and a larger difference in the RP interval between lead V_1 and the inferior leads. Therefore, a ΔRP interval (V_1 – III) longer than 20 milliseconds suggests slow-slow AVNRT with a sensitivity of 71%, specificity of 87%, and positive predictive value of 75%.

EFFECTS OF BUNDLE BRANCH BLOCK. The presence of BBB during SVT is much more common in orthodromic AVRT than AVNRT or AT (90% of SVTs with sustained LBBB are orthodromic AVRTs). Two reasons have been proposed to explain why prolonged aberration occurs less commonly during AVNRT than

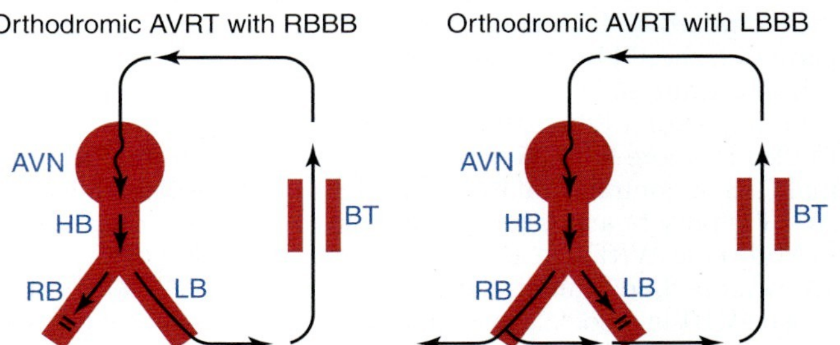

FIGURE 18-23 Schematic illustration of the effect of bundle branch block (BBB) on the reentrant circuit during orthodromic atrioventricular reentrant tachycardia (AVRT) using a left-sided bypass tract (BT). Block in the left bundle branch (LB) (ipsilateral to the BT) results in prolongation of the reentrant pathway and, therefore, prolongation of the ventriculoatrial interval. In contrast, block in the right bundle branch (RB) (contralateral to the BT) has no effect on the reentrant circuit. AVN = atrioventricular node; HB = His bundle; LBBB = left bundle branch block; RBBB = right bundle branch block.

orthodromic AVRT. First, the induction of AVNRT requires significant AVN delay, which makes the H_1-H_2 interval longer and makes aberration unlikely, whereas in orthodromic AVRT, AVN conduction need not be slow, resulting in a shorter AH interval and an impulse encroaching on HPS refractoriness, in turn resulting in BBB. Second, LBBB facilitates the induction of orthodromic AVRT when a left-sided AV BT is present.[34]

BBB is more common when AVRT is initiated by an AES that is delivered during NSR or after long-drive CLs, whereby HPS refractoriness is longest and AVN conduction and refractoriness are shortest. When AVRT is induced by atrial stimulation, RBBB is more common than LBBB (2:1). In contrast, when AVRT is induced by ventricular stimulation, LBBB is much more common than RBBB (because of concealment in the LB). Additionally, the incidence of BBB is more common in AVRTs induced by ventricular stimulation than those induced by atrial stimulation (75% versus 50%).

BBB ipsilateral to the AV BT results in prolongation of the surface VA interval because more time is needed for the impulse to travel from the AVN down the HB and contralateral bundle branch, and transseptally to the ipsilateral ventricle to reach the AV BT and then activate the atrium (Fig. 18-23). However, the local VA interval (measured at the site of BT insertion) remains constant. On the other hand, the tachycardia CL usually increases in concordance with the increase in the surface VA interval as a result of ipsilateral BBB,

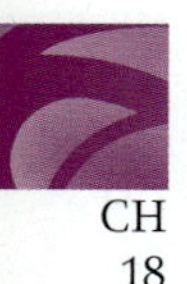

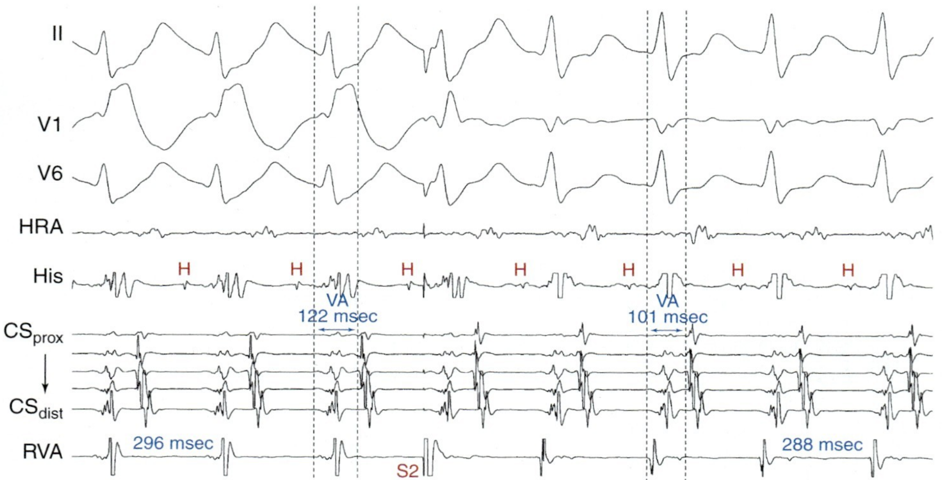

FIGURE 18-24 Effect of right bundle branch block (RBBB) on orthodromic atrioventricular reentrant tachycardia (AVRT). RBBB is initially present during an orthodromic AVRT using a concealed superoparaseptal bypass tract (BT). Introduction of a ventricular extrastimulus (S_2) from the right ventricular apex during the tachycardia is followed by resolution of RBBB (peeling of refractoriness). Note that the loss of RBBB is associated with shortening of the ventriculoatrial (VA) interval (by 21 milliseconds) and a milder degree of shortening of the tachycardia cycle length (by 8 milliseconds), indicating the presence and participation of a septal BT in the reentrant circuit.

because of the now larger tachycardia circuit; however, because the time the wavefront spends outside the AVN is now longer, AVN conduction may improve, resulting in shortening of the AH interval (PR interval), which can be sufficient to overcome the prolongation of the VA interval. This can consequently result in shortening of the tachycardia CL. Thus, the surface VA interval and not the tachycardia CL should be used to assess the effects of BBB on the SVT (Fig. 18-24; and see Fig. 18-23).

Prolongation of the surface VA interval during SVT in response to BBB by more than 35 milliseconds compared to that with normal QRS or contralateral BBB indicates that an ipsilateral free wall AV BT is present and is participating in the SVT (i.e., diagnostic of orthodromic AVRT). On the other hand, prolongation of the surface VA by more than 25 milliseconds suggests a septal AV BT (posteroseptal AV BT in association with LBBB, and superoparaseptal AV BT in association with RBBB; see Fig. 18-24). In contrast, BBB contralateral to the AV BT does not influence the VA interval or tachycardia CL (because the contralateral ventricle is not part of the reentrant circuit; see Figs. 18-21 and 18-23). Prolongation of the VA interval by more than 45 milliseconds in response to RV pacing entraining the orthodromic AVRT is also diagnostic of a left-sided BT, whereby RV pacing results in effects analogous to those created by LBBB and, as a consequence, VA interval prolongation.

OSCILLATIONS IN THE TACHYCARDIA CYCLE LENGTH. Oscillation of the tachycardia CL during orthodromic AVRT can occur and generally is caused by changes in the anterograde conduction over the AVN (see Fig. 18-22). Because retrograde conduction through the BT is much less variable, the changes in ventricular CL that result from variability in the anterograde AVN conduction precede the subsequent changes in atrial CL, and changes in atrial CL do not predict changes in subsequent ventricular CL (similar to observations during typical AVNRT). Contrariwise, changes in atrial CL predict the changes in subsequent ventricular CL during atypical AVNRT and AT.[35]

Additionally, orthodromic AVRT in the presence of dual AVN physiology can be associated with anterograde conduction alternating over the slow and fast AVN pathways, resulting in a regular irregularity of the tachycardia CL (alternating long and short cycles). Alternatively, the presence of dual AVN pathways can lead to two separate stable tachycardia CLs. In either setting, the RP interval during the SVT remains constant.

QRS ALTERNANS. Alternans of the QRS complex amplitude during relatively slow SVTs is almost always indicative of orthodromic AVRT (Fig. 18-25). On the other hand, although QRS alternans during fast SVTs is most commonly seen in orthodromic AVRT, it can also be seen with other types of SVTs.

TERMINATION AND RESPONSE TO PHYSIOLOGICAL AND PHARMACOLOGICAL MANEUVERS. Spontaneous termination of orthodromic AVRT is usually caused by gradual slowing and then block in the AVN (see Fig. 18-22), sometimes causing initial oscillation in the tachycardia CL, with alternate complexes demonstrating a Wenckebach periodicity before block. However, termination with block in the AV BT without any perturbations of the tachycardia CL can occur during very rapid AVRT or following a sudden shortening of the tachycardia CL.

Carotid sinus massage can terminate orthodromic AVRT by gradual slowing and then block in the AVN. Adenosine, digoxin, calcium channel blockers, and beta blockers terminate orthodromic AVRT by block in the AVN; therefore, the SVT terminates with a P wave not followed by a QRS. Verapamil rarely produces block in the AV BT and, when it does, block is usually preceded by oscillation in the tachycardia CL produced by changes in AVN conduction, leading to long-short sequences. Class IA and IC antiarrhythmic agents can produce block in the AV BT with variable effect on the AVN-HPS. Amiodarone can terminate AVRT by block in the AVN, HPS, or AV BT. Sotalol affects the AVN with little or no effect on the AV BT.

ORTHODROMIC ATRIOVENTRICULAR REENTRANT TACHYCARDIA: SLOWLY CONDUCTING CONCEALED ATRIOVENTRICULAR BYPASS TRACT (PERMANENT JUNCTIONAL RECIPROCATING TACHYCARDIA)

ATRIAL ACTIVATION SEQUENCE. The initial site of atrial activation is most often in the posteroseptal part of the triangle of Koch near the CS os, similar to that in atypical AVNRT (Fig. 18-26).

ATRIAL–VENTRICULAR RELATIONSHIP. Because the retrograde limb of the reentry circuit is the slow BT (which conducts more slowly than the AVN), the RP interval is longer than the PR interval, similar to atypical AVNRT (see Figs. 18-11 and 18-26). In contrast to the classic fast BTs, the RP interval during PJRT is not fixed, because the BT serving as the retrograde limb of the reentrant circuit has decremental properties. Similar to all types of AVRTs, a 1:1 A-V relationship is a prerequisite to sustenance of the tachycardia.

OSCILLATIONS IN THE TACHYCARDIA CYCLE LENGTH. The tachycardia rate typically fluctuates (100 to 220 beats/min) in response to autonomic tone and physical activity, and the rate changes result from modulation of the PR and RP intervals. The tachycardia CL is often just longer than the shortest CL at which the BT can conduct retrogradely.

EFFECTS OF BUNDLE BRANCH BLOCK. BBB affects PJRT in a manner analogous to that described for orthodromic AVRT.

TERMINATION AND RESPONSE TO PHYSIOLOGICAL AND PHARMACOLOGICAL MANEUVERS. Carotid sinus massage and AVN blockers (adenosine, digoxin, calcium channel blockers, and beta blockers) usually terminate PJRT by block in the AVN (two-thirds) or in the BT (one-third) (see Fig. 18-19). Although the mode of tachycardia termination by adenosine has

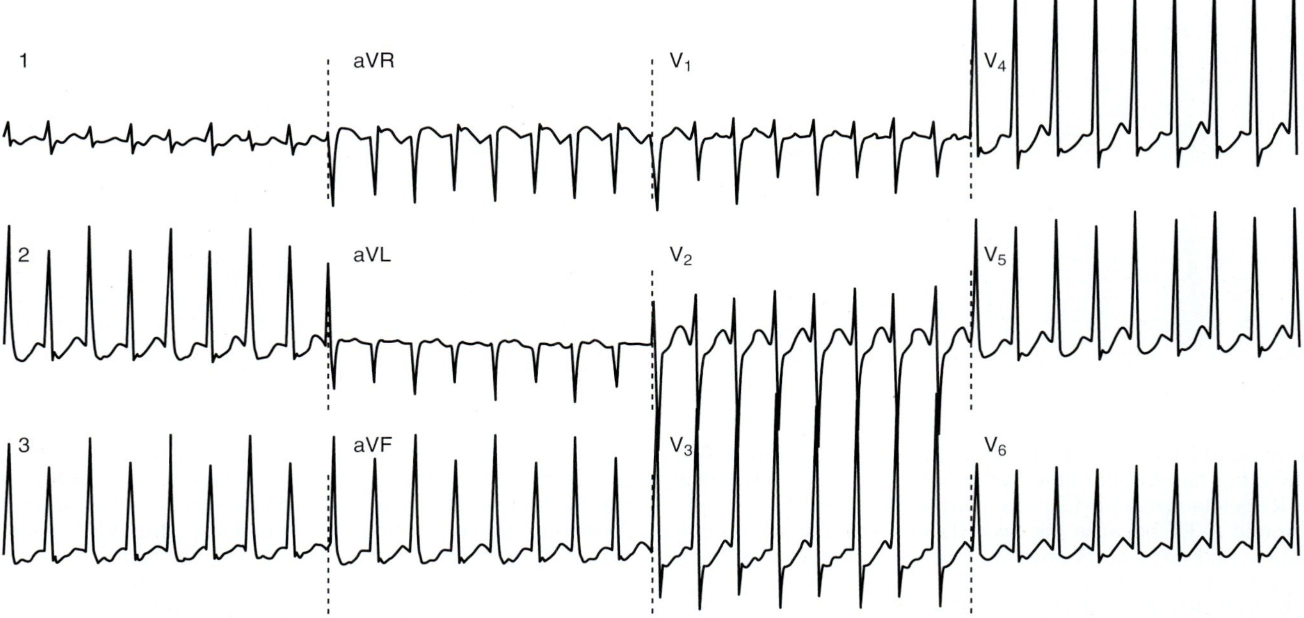

FIGURE 18-25 Surface 12-lead ECG of orthodromic atrioventricular reentrant tachycardia showing QRS alternans in multiple ECG leads.

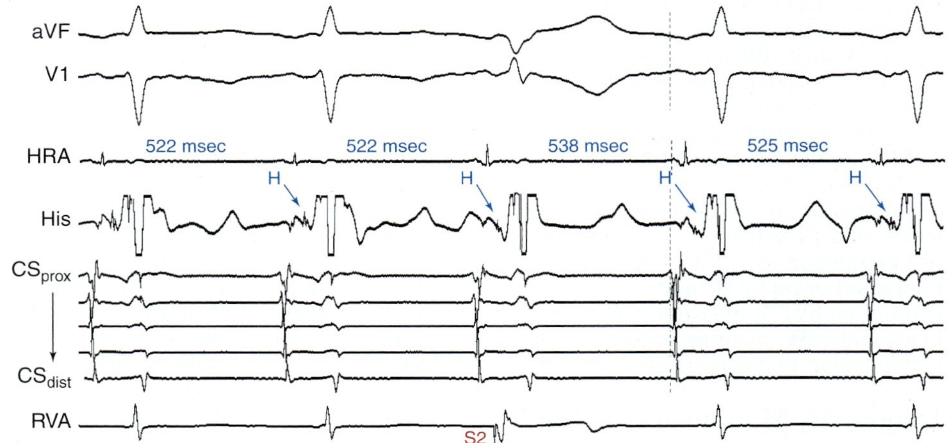

FIGURE 18-26 Ventricular extrastimulation (VES) during permanent junctional reciprocating tachycardia. The supraventricular tachycardia has a stable baseline cycle length (522 milliseconds). A single VES (S_2) introduced during His bundle refractoriness retards the timing of the next atrial complex (538 milliseconds) (postexcitation). The anticipated timing of the high RA electrogram is indicated by the dashed line.

been suggested to distinguish between PJRT and atypical AVNRT, one report has shown that termination of atypical AVNRT with adenosine can also result from block in the fast AVN pathway and therefore its value in distinguishing between atypical AVNRT and PJRT is questionable.

ANTIDROMIC ATRIOVENTRICULAR REENTRANT TACHYCARDIA

ATRIAL ACTIVATION SEQUENCE. The initial site of atrial activation in classic antidromic AVRT is consistent with retrograde conduction over the AVN. If the antidromic AVRT is using a second BT for retrograde conduction, then the atrial activation sequence will depend on the location of that BT (see Fig. 18-3). Additionally, ventricular activation precedes HB activation during classic antidromic AVRT. Therefore, during preexcited SVT, a positive HV interval or a V-H interval not more than 10 milliseconds, especially when the HA interval is not more than 50 milliseconds, favors preexcited AVNRT over antidromic AVRT.

ATRIAL-VENTRICULAR RELATIONSHIP. Conduction time over classic (fast) BTs is approximately 30 to 120 milliseconds. Therefore, the PR is short and fixed, regardless of oscillations in the tachycardia CL from whatever cause. Similar to all types of AVRT, the A/V ratio is always equal to 1. If the SVT persists in the presence of AV block, antidromic AVRT is excluded.

OSCILLATIONS IN THE TACHYCARDIA CYCLE LENGTH. Antidromic AVRT can be irregular. Tachycardia CL changes are usually caused by changes in retrograde conduction over different fascicles of the HPS with different VA intervals (regardless of the type and degree of changes in the V-H or HA intervals), retrograde conduction over dual AVN pathways (with different HA intervals), different routes of anterograde conduction (with different AV intervals), and/or retrograde conduction over different BTs (with different VA intervals). When the change in the tachycardia CL can be ascribed to a change in the V-H interval and/or the subsequent HA interval, it suggests that retrograde conduction occurs over the HPS and AVN and not over a second BT.

The tachycardia CL tends to be shorter during classic antidromic AVRT than orthodromic AVRT when these arrhythmias occur in the same patient. This may be explained by the fact that antidromic AVRT uses the fast AVN pathway (of a dual AVN physiology) retrogradely, whereas orthodromic AVRT uses the slow pathway anterogradely or, in the absence of dual AVN physiology, this may be merely supportive evidence that retrograde conduction during

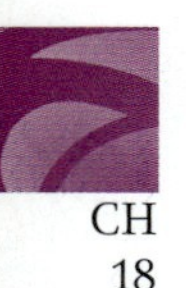

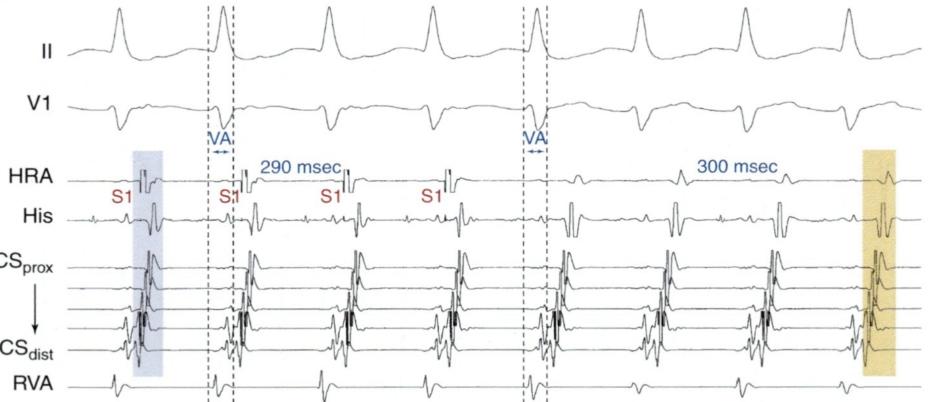

FIGURE 18-27 Atrial entrainment of orthodromic atrioventricular reentrant tachycardia (AVRT) using a left lateral bypass tract (BT). Atrial fusion (between the paced and tachycardia wavefronts; compare shaded areas) is observed during entrainment, which is consistent with AVRT and excludes both focal atrial tachycardia and atrioventricular nodal reentrant tachycardia. Note that the ventriculoatrial (VA) interval (dashed lines) of the return cycle after cessation of atrial pacing is similar to that of the supraventricular tachycardia (V-A linking), because retrograde VA conduction of the last entrained QRS is mediated by the BT.

antidromic AVRT uses another fast BT instead of the slower AVN. On the other hand, antidromic AVRTs using two or more BTs may have longer tachycardia CLs than orthodromic AVRT or classic antidromic AVRT because the two BTs are typically in opposite chambers and are incorporated in a larger reentrant circuit than one involving a midline AVN.[3]

EFFECTS OF BUNDLE BRANCH BLOCK. Retrograde BBB affects antidromic AVRT in a manner analogous to that described for orthodromic AVRT.

TERMINATION AND RESPONSE TO PHYSIOLOGICAL AND PHARMACOLOGICAL MANEUVERS. Various physiological and pharmacological maneuvers affect the AV BT and AVN during antidromic AVRT in a fashion similar to that described for orthodromic AVRT. Carotid sinus massage and adenosine terminate classic antidromic AVRT after ventricular activation, secondary to retrograde block up the AVN. In contrast, preexcited typical AVNRT terminates after atrial activation, secondary to anterograde block down the slow AVN pathway.

Termination or prolongation of the VA (and V-H) interval and tachycardia CL with transient RBBB, caused by mechanical trauma or introduction of VES, is diagnostic of antidromic AVRT using a right-sided or septal BT and excludes preexcited AVNRT. Continuation of an SVT at the same tachycardia CL, despite anterograde block in the BT (by drugs, mechanical trauma caused by catheter manipulation, or ablation), excludes antidromic AVRT.

Diagnostic Maneuvers during Tachycardia

ATRIAL EXTRASTIMULATION AND ATRIAL PACING DURING SUPRAVENTRICULAR TACHYCARDIA

ORTHODROMIC ATRIOVENTRICULAR REENTRANT TACHYCARDIA. Atrial pacing at a CL slightly shorter than the tachycardia CL generally can entrain orthodromic AVRT (Fig. 18-27). If the P waves on the surface ECG can be seen, which usually is not the case, they may appear to be fusion beats resulting from intraatrial collision of the impulse propagating from the paced site with the one emerging from the BT. In general, when pacing is initiated orthodromically to the zone of slow conduction (the AVN in this case), conduction time within the area of slow conduction is long enough to allow a wide atrial antidromic wavefront to generate surface ECG fusion (see Fig. 18-27).

The initial atrial complex following cessation of atrial pacing entraining orthodromic AVRT is *linked* to, and cannot be dissociated from, the last captured ventricular complex. As a consequence, the VA intervals of the return cycle after cessation of atrial pacing are fixed and similar to those during tachycardia (with <10 milliseconds of variation) after different attempts at SVT entrainment (see Fig. 18-27). The post-pacing VA intervals typically remain constant regardless of the site, duration, or CL of the entraining atrial pacing drive because retrograde VA conduction of the last entrained QRS is mediated by the BT, which is fixed and constant. VA linking can also be observed in typical AVNRT but not AT.[33,36]

It is difficult for AES not to affect the SVT because of the large size and large excitable gap of the reentrant circuit. However, this can be influenced by the distance between the site of atrial stimulation and the atrial region incorporated in the AVRT circuit (i.e., atrial myocardium between the BT and the AVN). Because only parts of the atrium ipsilateral to the BT are requisite components of the orthodromic AVRT circuit, AES delivered in the contralateral atrium may not affect the circuit, whereas AESs delivered at sites in close proximity to the BT or the AVN have the highest success at resetting the reentrant circuit.

AES over a wide range of coupling intervals can reset orthodromic AVRT via conduction down the AVN-HPS. In this setting, atrial activation is a fusion of the AES and the SVT impulse traveling retrogradely up the AV BT. The next QRS can be early or late, depending on the degree of slowing of conduction of the AES anterogradely down the AVN (i.e., the degree of prolongation of the A_2-H_2 interval).

An early-coupled AES can terminate the SVT, usually by block in the AVN-HPS. In this setting, the SVT terminates with an AES not followed by a QRS (i.e., AV block). Alternatively, the AES can render the atrium refractory to the SVT impulse traveling retrogradely up the AV BT, in which case the SVT terminates with an AES followed by a QRS (i.e., VA block). The AES can also anterogradely penetrate the AV BT and collide with the retrogradely traveling SVT wavefront (VA block). Lastly, the AES can conduct down the AVN-HPS and advance the next QRS, which then blocks in the still-refractory AV BT or atrium (VA block).

ANTIDROMIC ATRIOVENTRICULAR REENTRANT TACHYCARDIA. AES is of value in distinguishing antidromic AVRT from preexcited AVNRT. A late-coupled AES, delivered close to the BT atrial insertion site during SVT when the AV junctional atrium is refractory (i.e., when the atrial electrogram is already manifest in the HB recording at the time of AES delivery) that advances (accelerates) the timing of both the next ventricular activation as well as the subsequent atrial activation, proves that the SVT is an antidromic AVRT using an AV BT anterogradely, and excludes preexcited AVNRT (Fig. 18-28A). Because the AV junctional atrium is refractory at the time of the AES, the AES cannot penetrate the AVN, and resetting of the SVT by such an AES is therefore incompatible with AVNRT.

Also, an AES delivered during the SVT that advances ventricular activation and does not influence the VA interval excludes preexcited AVNRT and is diagnostic of antidromic AVRT (see Fig. 18-28A). The VA interval should change in the setting of preexcited AVNRT because the AES penetrates the AVN, producing slower conduction down the AVN before resumption of the tachycardia, which, in the presence of a fixed AV interval (caused by conduction down the BT) in response to the AES, would lead to a longer VA interval. In addition, the advanced QRS could invade and capture the HB retrogradely and conduct up the fast AVN pathway and reset the AVN circuit. Then the V-H interval of the advanced QRS plus the HA interval in response to this QRS

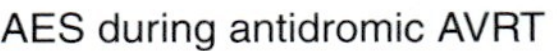

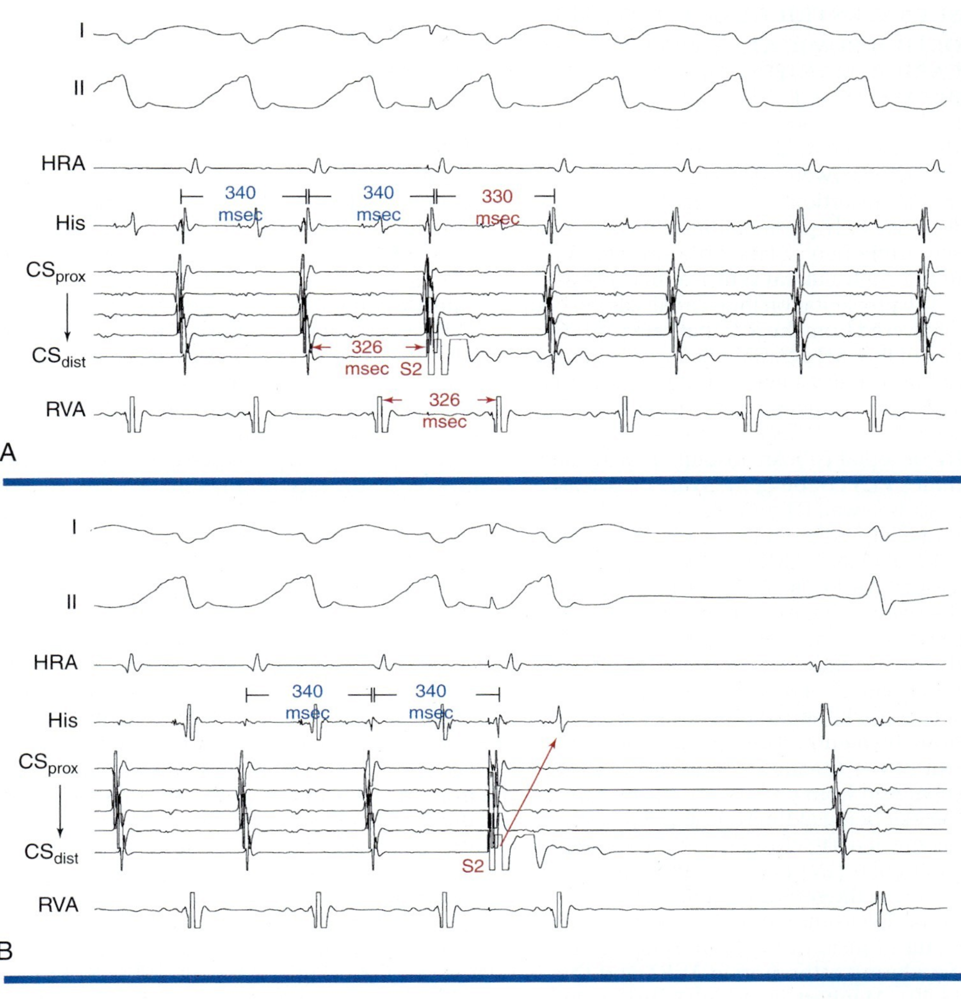

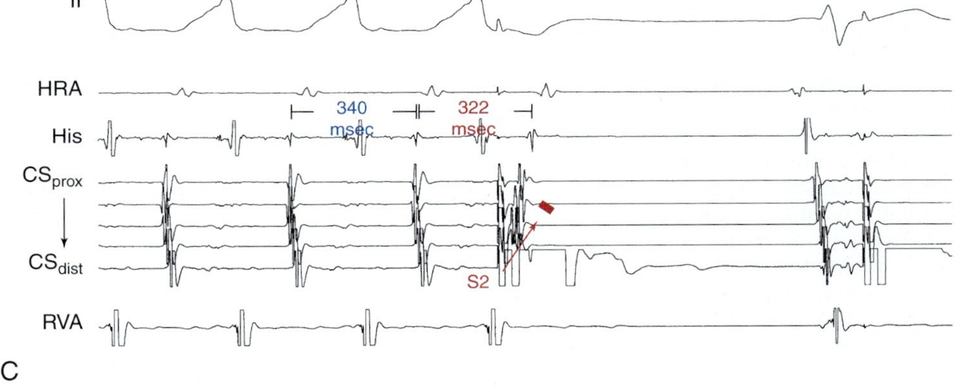

FIGURE 18-28 Atrial extrastimulation (AES) during antidromic atrioventricular reentrant tachycardia (AVRT) using a left lateral bypass tract (BT). **A,** A late-coupled AES delivered when the atrioventricular (AV) junction is refractory (as indicated by lack of advancement of the timing of the local atrial electrogram recording by the His bundle catheter) resets both the next ventricular activation and the subsequent atrial activation. This proves that the supraventricular tachycardia (SVT) is an antidromic AVRT using an AV BT anterogradely, and excludes preexcited atrioventricular nodal reentrant tachycardia (AVNRT). Additionally, the reset ventricular activation occurs at a coupling interval identical to the AES coupling interval (i.e., exact coupling phenomenon), and the ventriculoatrial (VA) interval following the AES remains similar to that during SVT, which is consistent with antidromic AVNRT. **B,** Late-coupled AES delivered when the AV junction is refractory advances the subsequent QRS and terminates the SVT by retrograde block in the His-Purkinje system–atrioventricular node. **C,** An earlier AES terminates the SVT without conduction to the ventricle (i.e., anterograde block in the BT). The AES advances the timing of AV junctional atrial activation.

should add up to the same VA interval on an undisturbed AVNRT, which is clearly unlikely.

Exact atrial and ventricular capture by an AES delivered when the AV junction is depolarized excludes AVNRT (see Fig. 18-28A). An AES that captures the ventricle at the same coupling interval as that of the AES indicates that the atrial stimulation site is inside the reentrant circuit, because if there were intervening atrial tissue between the stimulation site and the tachycardia circuit (as is the case during AVNRT), the AV interval would increase, and consequently, the V-V interval would exceed the AES coupling interval.[3]

The presence of a fixed and short V-H interval during entrainment of the SVT with atrial pacing suggests antidromic AVRT, and makes AVNRT unlikely (but does not exclude AVNRT). Moreover, failure of entrainment by atrial pacing to influence the VA interval during SVT excludes preexcited AVNRT.

An early-coupled AES can terminate the SVT by retrograde block in the AVN-HPS (the SVT terminates with an AES followed by a QRS; i.e., VA block; Fig. 18-28B) or by anterograde block in the BT (the SVT terminates with an AES not followed by a QRS; i.e., AV block; Fig. 18-28C).

VENTRICULAR EXTRASTIMULATION AND VENTRICULAR PACING DURING SUPRAVENTRICULAR TACHYCARDIA

ORTHODROMIC ATRIOVENTRICULAR REENTRANT TACHYCARDIA: MANIFEST OR CONCEALED ATRIOVENTRICULAR BYPASS TRACT. VES and ventricular pacing can easily reset, entrain, and may terminate orthodromic AVRT (Fig. 18-29).[33] However, the ability of the VES to affect the SVT depends on the distance between the site of ventricular stimulation to the ventricular insertion site of the BT and on the VES coupling interval. Because only parts of the ventricle ipsilateral to the BT are requisite components of the orthodromic AVRT circuit, a VES delivered in the contralateral ventricle may not affect the circuit.

The preexcitation index analyzes the coupling interval of the VES (delivered from the RV) that resets orthodromic AVRT as a percentage of the tachycardia CL. A relative preexcitation index (the ratio of the coupling interval to the tachycardia CL) more than 90% of a VES that advances atrial activation during orthodromic AVRT suggests that the BT is close to the site of ventricular stimulation (i.e., RV or septal BT). An absolute preexcitation index (tachycardia CL minus VES coupling interval) of at least 75 milliseconds suggests a left free wall BT, an index of less than 45 milliseconds suggests a septal BT, and an index of 45 to 75 milliseconds is indeterminate.

RESETTING AND/OR ENTRAINMENT WITH MANIFEST VENTRICULAR FUSION. The relative proximity (conduction time) of the pacing site, the site of entrance to a reentrant circuit, and the site of exit from the circuit to the paced chamber is critical for the occurrence of fusion during resetting and/or entrainment. A requirement for the presence of fusion, independent of the pacing site, is spatial separation between the sites of entrance to and exit from the reentrant circuit. In orthodromic AVRT, the entrance and exit of the reentrant circuit (to and from ventricular tissue) are separated from each other, the entrance being from the HPS and the exit being at the ventricular insertion site of the BT. Therefore, pacing at a site closer to the BT ventricular insertion site (e.g., left ventricular [LV] pacing in the setting of left free wall BTs, and RV pacing in the setting of right-sided or septal BTs) than the entrance of the reentrant circuit to ventricular tissue (i.e., the HPS) would result in fusion of QRS morphology between baseline morphology during orthodromic AVRT and that of fully paced QRS (Fig. 18-30). Manifest ventricular fusion during entrainment is proof that the ventricle is a part of the SVT circuit because fusion is due to collision of the antidromic stimulated wavefront with the orthodromic wavefront from the preceding beat occurring within ventricular myocardium. On the other hand, such phenomena cannot occur during AVNRT because of the lack of spatial separation of the entrance and exit to the AVNRT circuit and because the ventricles are not an obligatory part of the AVNRT circuit.

ENTRAINMENT BY RIGHT VENTRICULAR APICAL PACING. This technique can help differentiate orthodromic AVRT with a right lateral or septal BT from AVNRT. The VA interval during ventricular pacing is compared with that during SVT. The ventricle and atrium are activated in sequence during orthodromic AVRT and during ventricular pacing, whereas during AVNRT the ventricle and atrium are activated in parallel. Therefore, the VA interval during orthodromic AVRT approximates that during ventricular pacing. On the other hand, the VA interval during AVNRT is much shorter than that during ventricular pacing (see Fig. 18-30). Therefore, a ΔVA interval (VA interval during ventricular pacing minus VA interval during SVT) of more than 85 milliseconds is consistent with AVNRT, whereas a ΔVA interval of less than 85 milliseconds is consistent with orthodromic AVRT. In addition, evaluation of the post-pacing interval (PPI) versus the tachycardia CL is of value. In AVNRT (typical or atypical), the PPI reflects conduction time from the RV pacing site through the RV muscle and HPS, once around the reentry circuit and back. Therefore, the [PPI – tachycardia CL] difference represents twice the sum of the conduction time through the RV muscle and HPS. In orthodromic AVRT using a septal BT, the PPI reflects the conduction time through the RV to the septum, once around the reentry circuit and back. Hence, the PPI more closely approximates the tachycardia CL in orthodromic AVRT using a septal BT compared with AVNRT (see Fig. 18-30). Therefore, a [PPI – tachycardia CL] difference of more than 115 milliseconds is consistent with AVNRT, whereas a [PPI – tachycardia CL] difference of less than 115 milliseconds is consistent with orthodromic AVRT. For borderline values, ventricular pacing at the RV base can help exaggerate the difference between the PPI and tachycardia CL in the setting of AVNRT, but without significant changes in the setting of orthodromic AVRT, because the site of pacing at the RV base is farther from the AVNRT circuit than the RV apex, but is still close to an AVRT circuit using a septal BT (and in fact is closer to the ventricular insertion of the BT).[37]

However, there are several potential pitfalls to the criteria discussed above. The tachycardia CL and VA interval are often perturbed for a few cycles after entrainment. For this reason, care should be taken not to measure unstable intervals immediately after ventricular pacing. In addition, spontaneous oscillations in the tachycardia CL and VA intervals can be seen. The discriminant points chosen may not apply when the spontaneous variability is greater than 30 milliseconds. Also, it is possible to mistake isorhythmic VA dissociation for entrainment if the pacing train is not long enough or the pacing CL is too close to the tachycardia CL. Furthermore, this test is less reliable and should be used with caution in patients with left lateral BTs. Additionally, these criteria may not apply to BTs with significant decremental properties, although small decremental intervals are unlikely to provide a false result.

A relatively common phenomenon encountered during entrainment of orthodromic AVRT by ventricular pacing is the prolongation of the AH interval because of either decremental conduction properties of the AVN or (in the presence of dual AVN physiology) a jump of anterograde conduction from the fast pathway to the slow pathway. The prolonged AH interval on the last entrained beat will contribute to prolongation of the PPI that is not reflective of the distance of the pacing site from the circuit. Thus, the [PPI – SVT CL] differences obtained after entrainment of orthodromic AVRT employing a septal BT can actually overlap with those observed after entrainment of AVNRT. Subtracting the increment in AVN conduction time in the first PPI (post-pacing AH interval minus pre-pacing AH interval) from the [PPI – SVT CL] difference ("corrected" [PPI – SVT CL]) has been found to improve the accuracy of this criterion. The difference between AV intervals (post-pacing AV interval minus pre-pacing AV interval) can be taken for the latter adjustment when a His deflection is not clearly visible (assuming the HV interval remains constant). In a study of patients with both typical and atypical forms of AVNRT, as well as orthodromic using septal and free wall BTs, a corrected [PPI – SVT CL] difference of less than 110 milliseconds was found more accurate in identifying orthodromic AVRT from AVNRT than the uncorrected [PPI – SVT CL] difference. The use of change in the VA interval is of course not influenced by prolongation of the AV interval during pacing and does not require correction.[38-40]

DIFFERENTIAL RIGHT VENTRICULAR ENTRAINMENT. As discussed in Chapter 17, differential-site RV entrainment (from RV apex versus RV base) can help distinguish AVNRT from orthodromic AVRT. In orthodromic AVRT, in which the ventricles are an obligatory part of the circuit, the basal pacing site relative to the RV apex is variably related to the circuit, being closer than the RV apex with septal BTs and equidistant with free wall BTs, but the paced wavefront from either RV apex or RV base tends to have, on average, approximately equal access and proximity (electrophysiologically) to the reentrant circuit involved in orthodromic AVRT and, therefore, the time taken to reach the circuit (and hence the PPI) tends to be similar, irrespective of the location of the BT. Conversely, the base of the RV is electrically more distant than the RV apex (where the His-Purkinje network directly inserts) from the AVNRT circuit. Hence, following ventricular entrainment of AVNRT, the difference in PPI from RV base versus RV apex will largely be composed of the extra time required to reach the circuit from the base versus the apex (approximately 30 milliseconds).

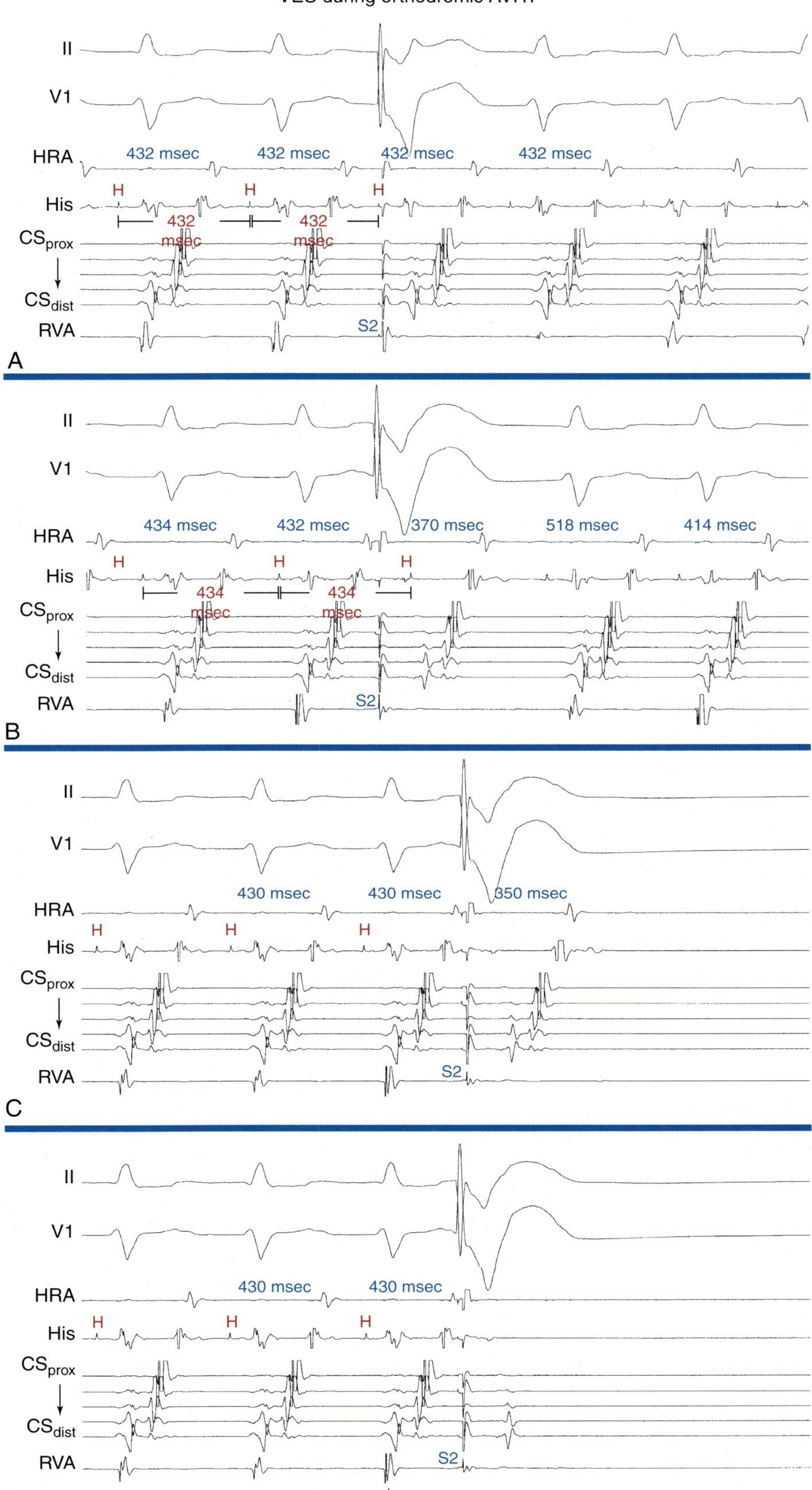

FIGURE 18-29 Ventricular extrastimulation (VES) during orthodromic atrioventricular reentrant tachycardia (AVRT) using a left lateral bypass tract (BT). **A,** A late-coupled VES delivered when the His bundle (HB) is refractory, as indicated by lack of advancement of the timing of the His potential, fails to reset the supraventricular tachycardia (SVT). **B,** An earlier VES fails to advance the timing of the HB but advances the subsequent atrial activation, indicating orthodromic AVRT and excluding atrioventricular nodal reentrant tachycardia (AVNRT). Note that the reset atrial impulse is followed by a prolonged atrial–His bundle (AH) interval caused by decremental anterograde conduction in the atrioventricular node (AVN). However, the local ventriculoatrial (VA) interval (retrograde BT conduction) remains constant. **C,** An earlier VES delivered before the HB is refractory resets the subsequent atrial activation and terminates the SVT by anterograde atrioventricular (AV) block in the AVN. **D,** A more premature VES terminates the SVT by retrograde VA block in the BT, excluding atrial tachycardia (AT), but can still occur in AVNRT because the VES is delivered before anterograde activation of the HB and could potentially penetrate the AVN.

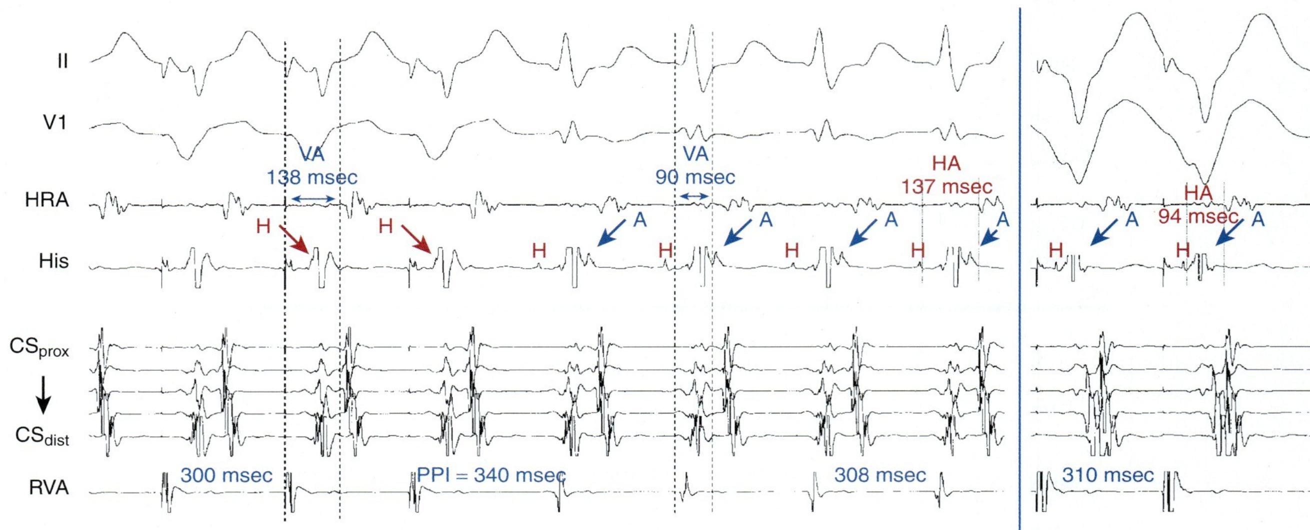

FIGURE 18-30 Ventricular entrainment of an orthodromic atrioventricular reentrant tachycardia (AVRT) using a concealed superoparaseptal bypass tract. Note that the ΔVA interval (ventriculoatrial interval during ventricular pacing minus VA interval during supraventricular tachycardia [SVT]) is less than 85 milliseconds and the post-pacing interval minus SVT cycle length [PPI – SVT CL] is less than 115 milliseconds, both of which favor orthodromic AVRT over atrioventricular nodal reentrant tachycardia (AVNRT). Additionally, ventricular fusion (between the paced and tachycardia wavefronts) is observed during entrainment (**right,** pure paced QRS morphology), which is consistent with AVRT and excludes AVNRT. Comparing the His bundle–atrial (HA) interval during the SVT **(left)** with that during ventricular pacing during normal sinus rhythm at the tachycardia CL **(right)** demonstrates that the ΔHA interval (HA interval during ventricular pacing minus HA interval during SVT) is −43 milliseconds, which favors orthodromic AVRT over AVNRT; the HA interval is measured from the end of the His potential to the atrial electrogram in the high RA.

Correction of the PPI (to avoid potential error introduced by decremental conduction within the AVN during ventricular pacing) increases the accuracy of this method. The "corrected PPI" is obtained by subtracting any increase in the AV interval of the return cycle beat (as compared with the AV interval during SVT). A differential corrected [PPI – SVT CL] difference of more than 30 milliseconds after transient entrainment was found to be consistent with AVNRT (i.e., corrected [PPI – SVT CL] difference following pacing from the RV base was consistently at least 30 milliseconds longer than that following pacing from the RV apex), and a corrected [PPI – SVT CL] difference of less than 30 milliseconds was observed in all cases of orthodromic AVRT. Additionally, a differential VA interval (ventricular stimulus-to-atrial interval during entrainment from RV base versus RV septum) of more than 20 milliseconds was consistent with AVNRT, whereas a differential VA interval of less than 20 milliseconds was consistent with orthodromic AVRT.[41]

LENGTH OF PACING DRIVE REQUIRED FOR ENTRAINMENT. As discussed in Chapter 17, assessing timing and type of response of SVT to RV pacing also can help differentiate orthodromic AVRT from AVNRT with high positive and negative predictive values. In the setting of orthodromic AVRT, once ventricular capture is achieved during RV pacing, the paced wavefront propagates to the ventricular insertion site of the BT quickly and resets the tachycardia. In the setting of AVNRT, on the other hand, where the pacing wavefront has to penetrate the HPS followed by AVN tissue prior to resetting the tachycardia, resetting of the tachycardia is delayed as compared with orthodromic AVRT. When resetting of the SVT occurs after a single paced beat orthodromic AVRT is suggested and AVNRT is generally excluded. On the contrary, if resetting occurs only after at least two beats AVNRT is suggested.[42]

ATRIAL RESETTING DURING THE TRANSITION ZONE. Similar to the concept discussed earlier for entrainment with manifest QRS fusion, perturbation (at least 15 milliseconds) of atrial timing during "transition zone" on initiation of RV pacing (the zone during which the pacing train fuses with anterograde ventricular activation) indicates the presence of a retrogradely conducting BT, and cannot occur in AT or AVNRT unless a bystander retrogradely conducting BT is present (see Chap. 17).[43]

TERMINATION. Termination of orthodromic AVRT by VES can occur secondary to block of the VES retrogradely in the AV BT, conduction of the VES retrogradely over the AVN-HPS with or without conduction up the BT, or retrograde conduction of the VES up the BT and preexcitation of the atrium and subsequent anterograde block in the AVN-HPS (the most common mechanism) (see Fig. 18-29). Termination of SVT with a single VES strongly suggests orthodromic AVRT as the mechanism of SVT in three settings: when the VES is late-coupled (>80% of tachycardia CL), when the tachycardia CL is less than 300 milliseconds, and when the VES is delivered during HB refractoriness and is associated with no atrial activation.

MANEUVERS TO PROVE PRESENCE OF AN ATRIOVENTRICULAR BYPASS TRACT. When VES or ventricular pacing results in eccentric atrial activation sequence, the presence of a BT is strongly suggested. A VES delivered when the HB is refractory (i.e., when the His potential is already manifest or within 35 to 55 milliseconds before the time of the expected His potential) that advances (accelerates) the next atrial activation is diagnostic of the presence of a retrogradely conducting BT. Such a VES has to conduct and advance atrial activation via an AV BT because the HPS-AVN is already refractory and cannot mediate retrograde conduction of the VES to the atrium (see Fig. 18-29). Although such an observation excludes AVNRT, it does not exclude AT or prove orthodromic AVRT, and the preexcited atrial activation can reset or even terminate an AT, whereby the AV BT is an innocent bystander. However, if this VES advances atrial activation with an activation sequence identical to that during the SVT, this suggests that the SVT is orthodromic AVRT and the AV BT is participating in the SVT, although it does not exclude the rare case of an AT originating at a site close to the atrial insertion site of a bystander AV BT. Furthermore, a VES delivered when the HB is refractory may not affect the next atrial activation if the ventricular stimulation site is far from the BT. Conduction from the ventricular stimulation site to the BT, local ventricular refractoriness, and the tachycardia

CL all determine the ability of a VES to reach the reentrant circuit before ventricular activation over the normal AVN-HPS.[33]

MANEUVERS TO PROVE PRESENCE AND PARTICIPATION OF ATRIOVENTRICULAR BYPASS TRACT IN THE SUPRAVENTRICULAR TACHYCARDIA. One maneuver is a VES delivered when the HB is refractory that delays the next atrial activation. Although such a VES can advance atrial activation during AT through fast retrograde conduction over a bystander BT, it should not be able to delay an AT beat by conduction over the AV BT. Such delay indicates that the VES was conducted with some delay over the AV BT and that the next atrial activation was dependent on this slower conduction; thus, the AV BT is participating in the SVT, proving orthodromic AVRT as the mechanism of the tachycardia. Similarly, a VES delivered when the HB is refractory that terminates the SVT without atrial activation is diagnostic of AVRT. Furthermore, entrainment of the SVT by ventricular pacing that results in prolongation in the surface VA interval indicates that the SVT is orthodromic AVRT mediated by an AV BT in the ventricle contralateral to the site of ventricular pacing; this is analogous to the influence of ipsilateral BBB on the VA interval during orthodromic AVRT (see Fig. 18-30). Exact and paradoxical capture phenomena are also diagnostic of AVRT. VES that captures the atrium at the same coupling interval as that of the VES (exact capture phenomenon) indicates that the ventricular stimulation site is inside the reentrant circuit, because if there were intervening tissue involved, the VA interval would increase and, subsequently, the A-A interval would exceed the VES coupling interval. Similarly, a VES that captures the atrium at a shorter coupling interval than that of the VES (paradoxical capture phenomenon) indicates that the ventricular stimulation site is not only inside the reentrant circuit but also closer to the ventricular insertion site of the AV BT than the initial site of ventricular activation over the AVN-HPS during the SVT, so that the VA interval following the VES is shorter than that during the SVT. This is easier to demonstrate with RV apical pacing during orthodromic AVRT mediated by a right-sided BT.[3]

ORTHODROMIC ATRIOVENTRICULAR REENTRANT TACHYCARDIA: SLOWLY CONDUCTING CONCEALED ATRIOVENTRICULAR BYPASS TRACT (PERMANENT JUNCTIONAL RECIPROCATING TACHYCARDIA). A VES delivered during PJRT can produce decremental conduction in the BT and prolongation of the VA interval, resulting in possible delay of the next atrial activation (i.e., postexcitation or delay of excitation; see Fig. 18-26). Such a response excludes AT, and when this occurs in response to a VES delivered when the HB is refractory, it is diagnostic of orthodromic AVRT, and excludes both AT and AVNRT. Additionally, a late-coupled VES introduced when the HB is refractory frequently blocks retrogradely in the BT and reproducibly terminates the tachycardia without reaching the atrium, again excluding both AT and AVNRT.

The ability to preexcite the atrium with a VES introduced when the HB is refractory is difficult to demonstrate in PJRT because of the long conduction time over the BT, the decremental conduction properties of the BT, and the fact that the tachycardia CL is just longer than the shortest length at which the BT is capable of retrograde conduction. This can be facilitated by introduction of the PVC at a site closer to the BT ventricular insertion.

ANTIDROMIC ATRIOVENTRICULAR REENTRANT TACHYCARDIA. Failure of entrainment by ventricular pacing to influence the surface VA interval during SVT excludes AVNRT. In addition, when a VES introduced during the SVT results in retrograde RBBB (i.e., blocks retrogradely in the RB), such RBBB will not change the timing of the next atrial activation in the setting of AVNRT. However, in antidromic AVRT using a right-sided BT, such RBBB will increase the size of the reentrant circuit, because the impulse cannot reach the HB through the RB and has to travel transseptally and then retrogradely over the LB. This results in prolongation in the VA interval and delay in the timing of the next atrial activation. The increment in the VA interval is caused by prolongation of the V-H interval and, if RBBB persists, the SVT will have a long V-H interval.

Antidromic AVRT usually can be terminated by ventricular pacing. Termination occurs by retrograde invasion and concealment in the BT, resulting in anterograde block over the BT following conduction to the atrium through the AVN.

Diagnostic Maneuvers during Normal Sinus Rhythm after Tachycardia Termination

ATRIAL PACING AT THE TACHYCARDIA CYCLE LENGTH

Under comparable autonomic tone, 1:1 AV conduction over the AVN should be maintained during atrial pacing at a CL similar to the tachycardia CL. If AV block develops during atrial pacing, AT and orthodromic AVRT are less likely, and AVNRT is the likely mechanism of the SVT. Additionally, the PR and AH intervals during atrial pacing at a CL similar to the tachycardia CL should be comparable to those during orthodromic AVRT. These findings are also observed in the setting of AT. In contrast, the AH and PR intervals during atrial pacing would be longer than those during tachycardia in the setting of AVNRT, assuming the slow pathway has been engaged.

VENTRICULAR PACING AT THE TACHYCARDIA CYCLE LENGTH

Under comparable autonomic tone status, 1:1 VA conduction over the AVN should be maintained during ventricular pacing at a CL similar to the tachycardia CL. If VA block develops during ventricular pacing, orthodromic AVRT is unlikely, and AT and AVNRT are favored.

It is important to recognize that the atrial activation sequence during ventricular pacing can be mediated by retrograde conduction over the BT, over the AVN, or a fusion of both, and consequently it can be similar to or different from that during orthodromic AVRT.

Ventricular pacing during NSR at a CL similar to the tachycardia results in HA and VA intervals that are shorter than those during orthodromic AVRT, because the HB and atrium are activated sequentially during orthodromic AVRT but in parallel during ventricular pacing (see Fig. 18-30). To help distinguish between orthodromic AVRT and AVNRT, the HA interval is measured from the *end* of the His potential (where the impulse leaves the HB to enter the AVN) to the atrial electrogram in the high RA recording and the ΔHA interval (HA interval during ventricular pacing minus HA interval during SVT) is calculated. In the setting of orthodromic AVRT the ΔHA interval is typically less than −10 milliseconds. In contrast, in the setting of AVNRT the ΔHA interval is more than −10 milliseconds. This criterion has 100% specificity and sensitivity and positive predictive accuracy for differentiation between AVNRT and orthodromic AVRT. The main limitation of the ΔHA interval criterion is the ability to record the retrograde His potential during ventricular pacing. Retrograde His potential generally appears before the local ventricular electrogram in the HB tracing, and can be verified by the introduction of a VES that causes the His potential to occur after the local ventricular electrogram. Moreover, pacing from different sites (e.g., midseptum) may allow earlier penetration into the HPS and facilitate observation of a retrograde His potential. When the retrograde His potential is not visualized, using the ΔVA interval instead of the ΔHA interval is not as accurate in discriminating orthodromic AVRT from AVNRT. Another limitation is that VA conduction during ventricular pacing may not occur over the BT but propagates preferentially over the HPS-AVN, leading to earlier atrial activation over this pathway than over the BT. If this were the case, the HA interval during ventricular pacing would be shorter than that observed if the atrium were activated via the BT. This would yield a more negative ΔHA interval.

PARA-HISIAN PACING DURING NORMAL SINUS RHYTHM

TECHNIQUE. Ideally, two quadripolar catheters (one for pacing and one for recording) or a single octapolar catheter (for both

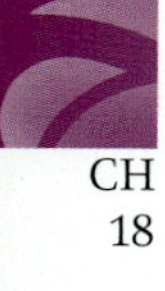

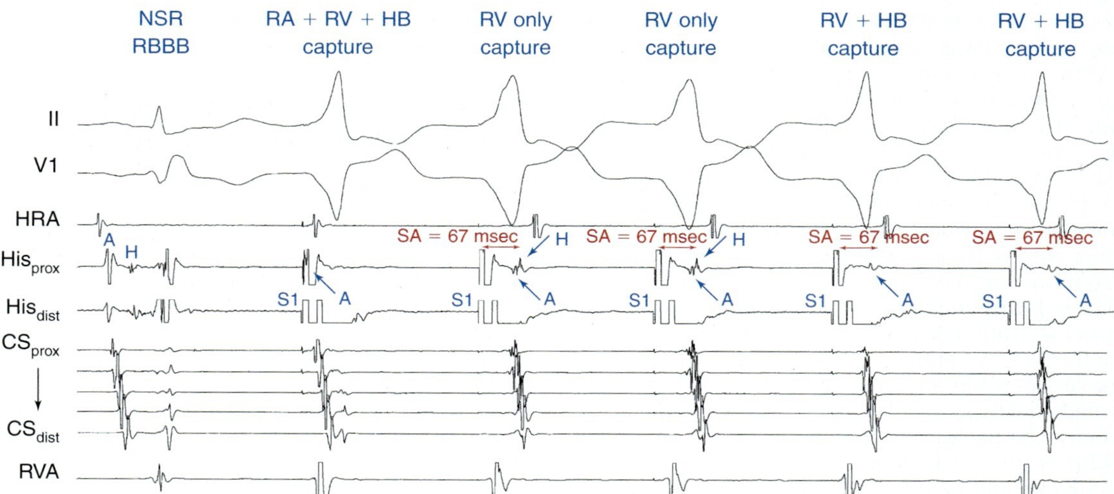

FIGURE 18-31 Para-Hisian pacing in a patient with concealed midseptal bypass tract and right bundle branch block (RBBB). The first complex is a sinus beat with RBBB. The second complex shows capture of the atrium, ventricle, and His bundle–right bundle branch (HB-RB). Atrial capture is indicated by immediate inscription of atrial electrogram following the pacing artifact. It is important to identify this occurrence to avoid erroneous interpretation of the results of para-Hisian pacing. The third and fourth complexes show right ventricle (RV)–only capture, and the last two complexes show RV and HB-RB capture but without atrial capture. Note that the atrial activation sequence and stimulus-atrial (SA) intervals remain unchanged, regardless of whether HB-RB capture occurs, because retrograde ventriculoatrial (VA) conduction occurs over the bypass tract in either case. During RV-only capture, the HB activation occurs after atrial activation, indicating that VA conduction is independent of the atrioventricular node (AVN). Note that para-Hisian pacing could be performed successfully even in the presence of RBBB if capture of the HB-RB is achieved proximal to the site of block. NSR = normal sinus rhythm.

pacing and recording) is placed at the distal His bundle–right bundle branch (HB-RB) region. Alternatively, a single quadripolar HB catheter (which is typically used during a diagnostic EP study) is used, taking into account that such an approach would limit the ability to record the retrograde His potential and HA interval.[44]

Overdrive ventricular pacing is performed (from the pair of electrodes on the HB catheter that records activation of the distal HB-RB) at a long pacing CL (>500 milliseconds) and high output. During pacing, direct HB-RB capture is indicated by narrowing of the paced QRS width. The pacing output and pulse width are then decreased until the paced QRS widens, which is associated with a delay in the timing of the retrograde HB potential, indicating loss of HB-RB capture. The pacing output is increased and decreased to gain and lose HB-RB capture, respectively, while local ventricular capture is maintained. Occasionally, the HB can be captured uniquely (without myocardial capture), resulting in a QRS identical to the patient's normally conducted QRS.[44]

CONCEPT OF PARA-HISIAN PACING. The para-Hisian pacing site is unique because it is anatomically close but electrically distant from the HB. Para-Hisian pacing at high output simultaneously captures the HB or proximal RB, as well as the adjacent ventricular myocardium. At lower output, direct HB-RB capture is lost and retrograde activation of the HB is delayed because the HB and RB are insulated from the adjacent myocardium and the peripheral inputs to the Purkinje system are located far from the para-Hisian pacing site. By maintaining local ventricular capture while intermittently losing HB-RB capture, retrograde VA conduction can be classified as dependent on the timing of local ventricular activation (BT), HB activation (AVN), or both (fusion).

Para-Hisian pacing can result in capture of the ventricle (indicated by a wide paced QRS), the atrium (indicated by atrial activation in the HB region immediately following the pacing artifact), the HB (indicated by narrow paced QRS), or any combination of these (Fig. 18-31).[44] Careful attention must be given to minimize the atrial signal seen on the recording from the pacing electrode pair to ensure that local atrial capture does not occur during pacing.

RESPONSE TO PARA-HISIAN PACING. When the ventricle and HB are captured simultaneously, the wavefront activates the ventricles over the HPS and results in a relatively narrow QRS. The wavefront can also travel retrogradely over the AVN to activate the atrium with an S-A interval (i.e., the interval from the pacing stimulus to the atrial electrogram) that represents conduction time over the proximal part of the HB and AVN (i.e., S-A interval = HA interval) because the onset of ventricular activation occurs simultaneously to that of HB activation (i.e., S-H interval = 0).

When the ventricle is captured but not the atrium or HB, the wavefront activates the ventricles by muscle-to-muscle conduction, resulting in a wide QRS with LBBB morphology caused by pacing in the RV. Once the wavefront reaches the RV apex, it conducts retrogradely up the RB and then over the HB and AVN to activate the atrium. In this setting, the S-A interval represents the conduction time from the RV base to the HB (S-H interval) plus the conduction time over the HB and AVN (HA interval). Thus, normally (in the absence of a retrogradely conducing BT), para-Hisian pacing results in a shorter S-A interval when the HB (or HB plus RV) is captured than the S-A interval when only the ventricle is captured (because of the delayed conduction of the impulse to the HB [i.e., S-H interval] when only the RV is captured).

In the presence of a septal AV BT, the S-A interval usually remains fixed regardless of whether or not the HB is being captured, because in both situations the paced impulse travels retrogradely over the AV BT, with constant conduction time to the atrium as long as local ventricular myocardium is being captured. Atrial activation in this setting can be secondary to activation over the BT, especially when only the ventricle is captured, or a result of fusion of conduction over both the AV BT and AVN, especially when both the ventricle and the HB are captured. Nevertheless, because VA conduction time over the BT is faster than that over the AVN, the timing of the earliest atrial activation remains constant (i.e., the S-A and local VA intervals), regardless of whether or not HB-RB capture occurs and regardless of whether or not atrial activation occurs exclusively over the AV BT or as a fusion of conduction over both the AV BT and AVN.

Seven patterns of response to para-Hisian pacing can be observed (Table 18-3 and Fig. 18-32; and see Fig. 18-31). In patients with retrogradely conducing AV BTs, in whom retrograde conduction occurs over both the AVN and BT during para-Hisian pacing, the amount of atria activated by each of the two pathways (atrial

TABLE 18-3 Response Patterns to Para-Hisian Pacing

Pattern 1 (AVN/AVN Pattern)

- Retrograde conduction occurs exclusively over the AVN regardless of whether the HB-RB is captured.
- Loss of HB-RB capture results in an increase in the S-A interval in all electrograms equal to the increase in the S-H interval, with no change in the atrial activation sequence. The HA interval remains essentially the same.
- This response indicates that retrograde conduction is dependent on HB activation and not on local ventricular activation.
- This pattern is observed in all patients with AVNRT and is not observed in any patient with a septal or right free wall BT. However, this pattern can be observed in some patients with a left free wall BT or PJRT, in which case retrograde AVN conduction masks the presence of retrograde BT conduction.

Pattern 2 (BT-BT Pattern)

- Retrograde conduction occurs exclusively over a single BT.
- The S-A interval is identical during HB-RB capture and noncapture, indicating that retrograde conduction is dependent on local ventricular activation and not on HB activation.
- This pattern does not exclude the presence of retrograde conduction over the AVN with longer conduction time or a second BT with longer conduction time or located far from the pacing site.

Pattern 3 (BT-BT_L Pattern)

- Retrograde conduction occurs exclusively over a BT.
- Loss of HB-RB capture is associated with a delay in the timing of ventricular activation close to the BT. This results in an increase in the S-A interval in all electrograms, with no change in the atrial activation sequence. The local VA interval, recorded close to the BT, remains approximately the same. The increase in S-A interval is less than the increase in the S-H interval. Therefore, the HA interval is shortened with loss of HB-RB capture, indicating that retrograde conduction cannot be occurring over the AVN. Two mechanisms have been identified accounting for the delay in timing of ventricular activation close to the BT.
- Activation of the HPS results in earlier ventricular activation near some BTs located far from the para-Hisian pacing site, such as left lateral or anterolateral BTs.
- Decreasing the pacing output to lose HB-RB capture occasionally results in a small delay in ventricular activation close to the pacing site.
- Pattern 3 is referred to as the BT-BT_L pattern, where BT_L refers to a lengthening of the S-A interval with loss of HB-RB capture.

Pattern 4 (AVN-BT Pattern)

- Loss of HB-RB capture is associated with atrial activation exclusively over the BT.
- Loss of HB-RB capture results in an increase in S-A and local VA intervals in all electrograms, with the least increase occurring in the electrogram closest to the BT.
- The HA interval shortens, indicating that the atrium near the AVN is activated by the BT before retrograde conduction over the AVN is complete.

Pattern 5 (AVN-Fusion Pattern)

- Loss of HB-RB capture results in activation of part of the atria by the AVN and part by the BT.
- Loss of HB-RB capture is associated with an increase in S-A and local VA intervals in all electrograms.
- The HA interval remains constant, indicating that part of the atria was still activated by the AVN.

Pattern 6 (Fusion-BT Pattern)

- Loss of HB-RB capture results in atrial activation exclusively over the BT.
- Loss of HB-RB capture is associated with no change in the S-A or local VA intervals recorded near the BT.
- In the HB electrogram, the S-A interval increases, but not as much as the S-H interval, leading to a decrease in the HA interval. This indicates that the atrial myocardium in that region is no longer activated by the AVN.

Pattern 7 (Fusion-Fusion Pattern)

- The atria continue to be activated by both the AVN and the BT during loss of HB-RB capture, with more of the atria activated by the BT than during HB-RB capture.
- Like pattern 6, loss of HB-RB capture is associated with minimal change in the S-A or local VA intervals recorded close to the BT; however, the HA interval remains essentially the same, indicating that part of the atria is still activated by the AVN.

AVN = atrioventricular node; AVNRT = atrioventricular nodal reentrant tachycardia; BT = bypass tract; HA = His bundle–atrial; HB-RB = His bundle–right bundle branch; HPS = His-Purkinje system; PJRT = permanent junctional reciprocating tachycardia; S-A = stimulus-atrial; S-H = stimulus–His bundle; VA = ventriculoatrial.

fusion) is dependent on four variables: (1) the magnitude of delay in retrograde activation of the HB (i.e., S-H interval); (2) retrograde conduction time over the AVN (HA interval); (3) intraventricular conduction time from the para-Hisian pacing site to the ventricular end of the BT (S-V_{BT}); and (4) retrograde conduction time over the BT (V-A_{BT}). The first two variables (S-H plus HA) form the S-A interval resulting from retrograde VA conduction over the AVN, and the latter two variables (S-V_{BT} plus V-A_{BT}) form the S-A interval resulting from retrograde VA conduction over the BT. The amount of the atria activated by the AVN is greater during HB-RB capture, secondary to a minimal S-H interval (i.e., S-A interval = HA interval). Loss of HB-RB capture results in prolongation of the S-H interval and, therefore, an increase in the amount of atria activated by the BT, resulting in a change in the retrograde atrial activation sequence. Consequently, a change in the retrograde atrial activation sequence with loss of HB-RB capture always indicates the presence of retrograde conduction over both the BT and AVN. There are four such patterns (patterns 4 through 7). In patterns 4 and 5, HB-RB capture is associated with activation of the atria exclusively by retrograde conduction over the AVN. In patterns 6 and 7, HB-RB capture results in atrial activation over both the AVN and the BT.[44]

INTERPRETATION OF RESULTS OF PARA-HISIAN PACING. The response to para-Hisian pacing can be determined by comparing the following four variables between HB-RB capture and noncapture while maintaining local ventricular capture and no atrial capture: (1) atrial activation sequence, (2) S-A interval, (3) local VA interval, and (4) HA interval (see Figs. 18-31 and 18-32).

The S-A interval is defined as the interval between the pacing stimulus and atrial electrogram. It should be recorded at multiple sites, including close to the site of earliest atrial activation during SVT.

The local VA interval is defined as the local ventricular to atrial electrogram interval in the electrode position with the earliest retrograde atrial activation time. For the local VA to be relied on, it actually has to be measured at the site of earliest atrial activation (this requires positioning a catheter at the site of earliest atrial activation recorded during SVT). The high RA catheter, for example, may not be satisfactory for evaluation of the local VA interval in the presence of a septal BT.

The HA interval is recorded in the HB electrogram; however, this measurement can be obtained only if two catheters are placed

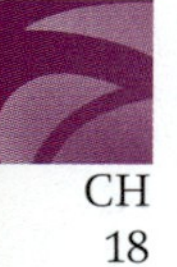

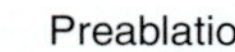

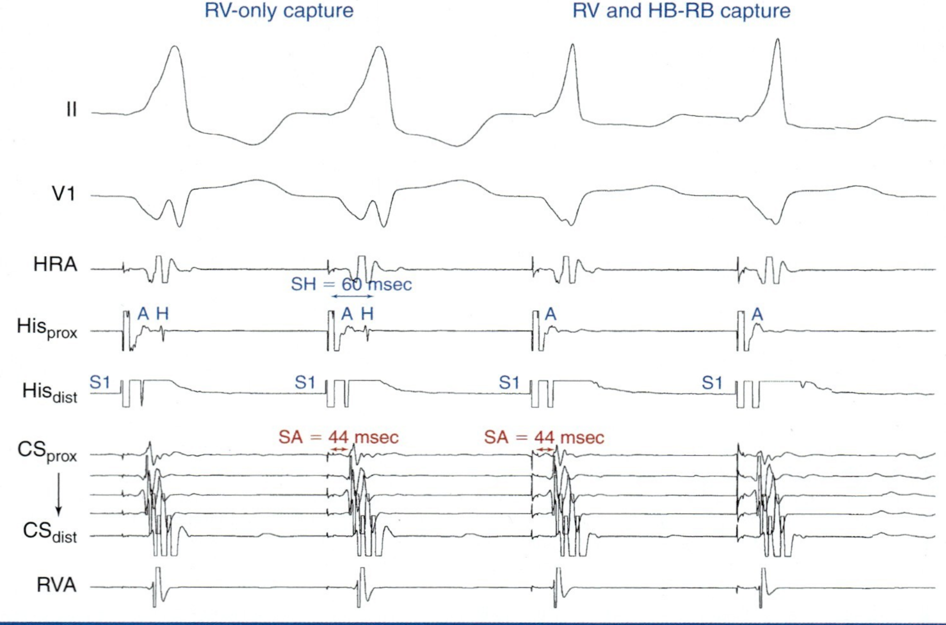

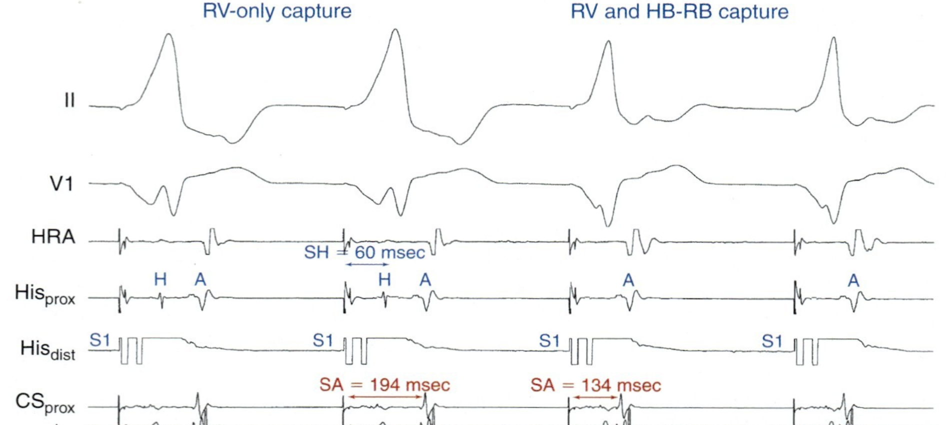

FIGURE 18-32 Para-Hisian pacing in a patient with a concealed superoparaseptal bypass tract (BT). In each panel, the first two complexes show right ventricle (RV)-only capture, and the last two complexes show RV and His bundle–right bundle branch (HB-RB) capture. The loss of HB-RB capture is identified by delay in the HB activation (S-H interval = 60 milliseconds) and widening of the QRS. The His potential is not visible during HB-RB capture. **A,** Para-Hisian pacing is performed before ablation of the BT, and the S-A interval remains unchanged regardless of whether HB-RB capture occurs, because retrograde ventriculoatrial (VA) conduction occurs over the BT in either case. In fact, during RV-only capture, the S-A interval is shorter than the S-H interval, indicating that VA conduction is independent of the atrioventricular node (AVN). **B,** Para-Hisian pacing is performed after successful ablation of the BT; the S-A interval is longer than before ablation, and it prolongs further on loss of HB-RB capture, concomitant with delay in HB activation (i.e., prolongation in the S-H interval) and a constant HA interval, indicating that VA conduction is mediated only by the AVN. Note that the activation sequence before ablation (VA conduction occurring over the BT) is slightly different from after ablation (VA conduction occurring over the AVN). However, in each case, the atrial activation sequence occurs over the same pathway and remains constant, regardless of whether HB-RB occurs.

in the HB position (one for pacing and one for recording) or if an octapolar catheter is used for pacing and sensing around the HB. The use of a single quadripolar HB catheter, which is typically used during a diagnostic EP study, negates the ability to record the retrograde His potential and HA interval during pacing. However, the combination of the S-A and local VA intervals is sufficient to identify the presence of retrograde BT.

If the S-A (and local VA) interval at any site remains fixed, regardless of whether or not HB-RB capture occurs, while the HA interval shortens, retrograde conduction is occurring only over an AV BT. In this setting, the HA interval shortens on loss of HB-RB capture because the HB and atrium are activated in parallel and HB activation is delayed because of prolongation of the S-H interval, while atrial activation timing remains unchanged because it results from retrograde conduction over the AV BT and is independent of timing of HB activation. On the other hand, if the S-A (and local VA) interval increases in all electrograms (including the electrode recording the earliest atrial activation) coincident with loss of HB-RB capture, while the HA interval remains essentially the same, retrograde conduction is occurring only over the AVN.

An identical retrograde atrial activation sequence during HB-RB capture and noncapture indicates that retrograde conduction is occurring over the same system (either the BT or AVN) and does not help prove or exclude the presence of a BT (especially a septal BT; see Fig. 18-32). A change in retrograde atrial activation sequence with loss of HB-RB capture, however, indicates the presence of retrograde conduction over both a BT and the AVN. Morphological change in the atrial electrogram recorded at the AV junction without overlapping the ventricular electrogram also seems to have diagnostic significance, indicating the presence of both BT and AVN conduction.

LIMITATIONS OF PARA-HISIAN PACING. The location of the BT, as well as retrograde conduction time over the BT, must be taken into account when interpreting the results of para-Hisian pacing. For superoparaseptal BTs, the S-V_{BT} interval is short. For BTs located progressively farther from the para-Hisian pacing site, the $S\text{-}V_{BT}$ increases progressively. This is not a significant factor for midseptal, posteroseptal, or most right free wall BTs. However, for left free wall BTs, which are located far from the pacing site, the $S\text{-}V_{BT}$ interval can be sufficiently long to have the entire atria activated by the AVN, even during loss of HB-RB capture. In this setting, para-Hisian pacing can produce an AVN retrograde conduction pattern, regardless of whether or not the HB-RB is captured (pattern 1: AVN-AVN), failing to identify the presence of retrograde BT conduction (because of the long $S\text{-}V_{BT}$). However, a left lateral BT should not be a diagnostic challenge because of the obvious eccentric retrograde atrial activation sequence during orthodromic AVRT, and para-Hisian pacing is performed mainly to investigate the presence of a septal BT. Additionally, for BTs located far from the para-Hisian pacing site, it is important to record atrial activation close to the suspected site of the BT. Otherwise, without recording electrograms near the BT, the change in atrial activation sequence may not be identified, incorrectly suggesting that retrograde conduction is occurring over just the AVN. This is most likely to occur in patients with short retrograde AVN conduction (short HA interval) and a BT located far from the pacing site.

Para-Hisian pacing may fail to identify retrograde conduction over a slowly conducting BT (e.g., PJRT) because of the long $V\text{-}A_{BT}$ interval. Performing para-Hisian entrainment or resetting during SVT can help in these situations (see later). Additionally, although para-Hisian pacing during NSR can help prove the presence of an AV BT, it does not show whether that BT is operative during the SVT.

In patients with very proximal retrograde RBBB, RB capture may fail to produce early retrograde activation of the HB, limiting the use of para-Hisian pacing in these patients. This observation suggests that HB-RB capture actually represents capture of the proximal RB and not HB capture. This is supported by the observation that, during HB-RB capture, the HB potential is often recorded 10 to 20 milliseconds after the pacing stimulus. Importantly, para-Hisian pacing has been performed successfully in many patients with more distal RBBB (see Fig. 18-31).

Assurance of lack of atrial capture by the pacing stimulus is important to interpret the results of para-Hisian pacing. Atrial capture is indicated by a very short S-A interval in the electrodes just proximal to the pacing electrodes. It is sometimes helpful to withdraw the para-Hisian pacing catheter until atrial capture alone is seen; if the S-A interval in the presence of ventricular capture is not longer than this, atrial capture was also present and the test should be repeated at a more distal pacing site.

PARA-HISIAN PACING DURING SUPRAVENTRICULAR TACHYCARDIA (PARA-HISIAN ENTRAINMENT OR RESETTING)

TECHNIQUE. Entrainment of the tachycardia is performed by pacing at the para-Hisian region using the HB catheter, as described previously, at a pacing CL 10 to 30 milliseconds shorter than the tachycardia CL. Entrainment is confirmed when the atrial CL accelerates to the pacing CL, without a change in the atrial activation sequence, and the tachycardia continues after pacing is discontinued.[45]

Para-Hisian entrainment is performed by alternately pacing at high-energy output for HB-RB capture or lower energy output for HB-RB noncapture. Entrainment with HB-RB capture is recorded separately from that without HB-RB capture. The S-A and local VA intervals during HB-RB capture and noncapture are then examined.[45]

One must be cautious about performing the para-Hisian entrainment maneuver by simply decreasing the pacing energy output during the same run to achieve HB-RB noncapture. That is, even though the SVT may have been entrained during HB-RB capture, on loss of HB-RB capture, the initial paced complexes typically do not entrain the SVT. This initial failure of entrainment occurs because of the sudden increase in the distance from the pacing site to the actual reentrant circuit. During HB-RB capture of AVNRT, the pacing site is near the circuit (the HB-RB); however, the pacing site (the basal RV myocardium) is well outside the circuit during HB-RB noncapture. This limitation would not apply if HB-RB noncapture is performed *prior* to HB-RB capture. That is, if the pacing output is increased while the SVT is being entrained during HB-RB noncapture, the circuit almost certainly will be entrained on HB-RB capture (unless the SVT terminates).

If para-Hisian entrainment cannot be performed because of repetitive termination of the tachycardia during entrainment attempts, isoproterenol infusion may be used to help sustain the rhythm. Alternatively, single or double VESs can be given to reset the tachycardia (para-Hisian resetting). These VESs are delivered at progressively shorter coupling intervals until the first VES that reliably advances or resets the tachycardia. This is performed alternately with high- or low-energy outputs to achieve HB-RB capture and noncapture, respectively. As with para-Hisian entrainment, the retrograde atrial activation sequence and timing are compared during para-Hisian resetting to characterize the response.

INTERPRETATION OF RESULTS OF PARA-HISIAN ENTRAINMENT OR RESETTING. In AVNRT (typical or atypical), the AVN-AVN pattern is observed in response to para-Hisian entrainment/resetting. Both the S-A and the local VA intervals increase during HB-RB noncapture compared with HB-RB capture.[45]

In orthodromic AVRT, the BT-BT pattern or $BT\text{-}BT_L$ pattern is observed. In the setting of a BT-BT pattern, the S-A and local VA intervals are usually not significantly different between HB-RB capture and noncapture. Conversely, in the case of a $BT\text{-}BT_L$ pattern, the S-A interval increases on HB-RB noncapture, but without significant change in the local VA interval.[45]

A ΔS-A interval of less than 40 milliseconds was found to be a reasonable guide to separating the AVN-AVN from the BT-BT response; patients with AVNRT uniformly have a ΔS-A interval of greater than 40 milliseconds, and only rare patients with AVRT (with a left lateral BT) have a ΔS-A interval less than 40 milliseconds. However, the Δ local VA interval is a more accurate parameter.

An AVN-AVN or fusion pattern during para-Hisian entrainment or resetting has not been observed in patients with AVNRT, a potential advantage over para-Hisian pacing during NSR in identifying the presence of a BT. Because retrograde VA conduction can only proceed over a single route during entrainment of the SVT (assuming that a complex scenario such as multiple BTs is not present), the various forms of retrograde fusion that might be seen during para-Hisian pacing during NSR cannot occur during para-Hisian entrainment or resetting.[45]

DIFFERENTIAL RIGHT VENTRICULAR PACING

The response to differential-site RV pacing can be evaluated by comparing the VA interval and atrial activation sequence during pacing at the RV base versus the RV apex (Fig. 18-33). The RV apex, although anatomically more distant from the atrium than the RV base, is nonetheless electrically closer because of the proximity of the distal RB to the pacing site. Consequently, in the absence of a retrogradely conducting septal AV BT, pacing at the RV apex allows entry into the rapidly conducting HPS and results in a shorter stimulus-to-atrial (S-A) interval during pacing from the apex than from the base. Pacing from the RV base requires the paced wavefront to travel a longer distance by muscle-to-muscle conduction to reach the RV apex and then propagate retrogradely through the RB and HB. In other words, the V-H interval is shorter with pacing at the RV apex versus the RV base. In the presence of a septal AV BT, pacing at the RV base allows the wavefront to access the AV BT rapidly and activate the atrium with a shorter S-A interval than during pacing at the RV apex, which is distant from the ventricular insertion site of AV BT (i.e., because the V-BT interval is shorter with pacing at the RV base versus the RV apex).

In the absence of a retrogradely conducting AV BT, atrial activation sequence will be similar during pacing both at the RV apex and at the RV base because the atrium is activated over the AVN in both settings. On the other hand, if a septal AV BT is present,

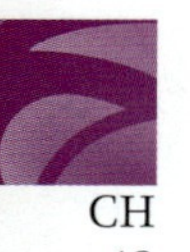

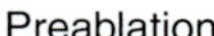

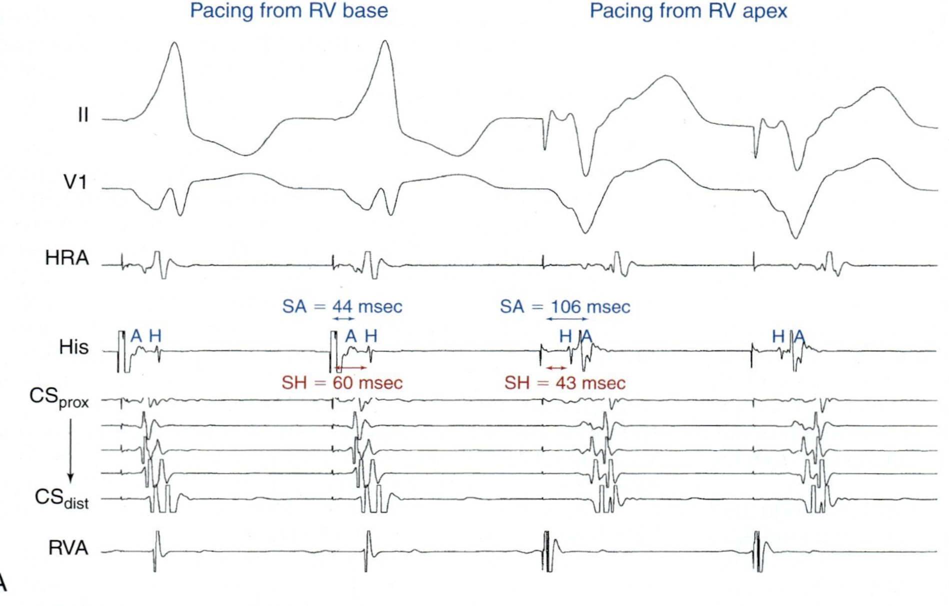

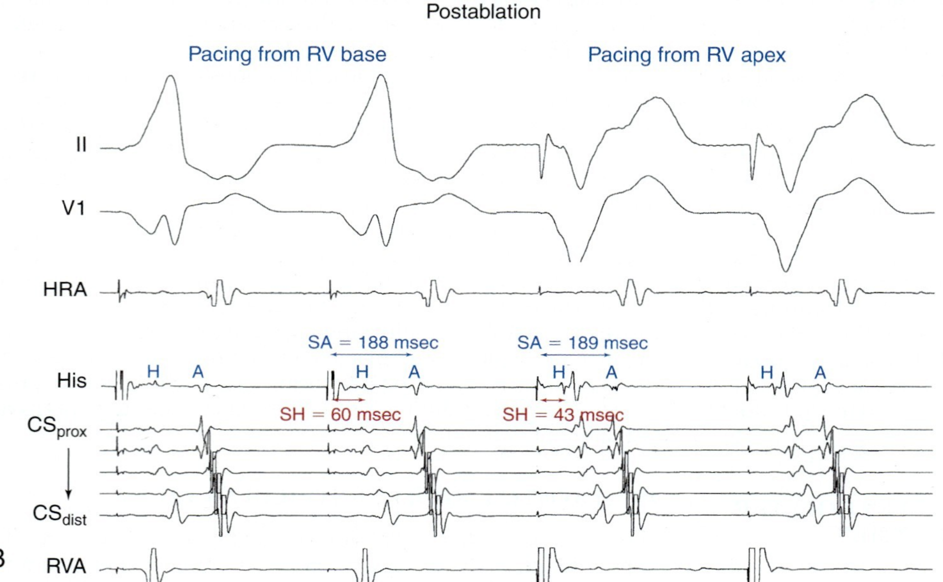

FIGURE 18-33 Differential-site right ventricular (RV) pacing in a patient with concealed superoparaseptal bypass tract (BT). In each panel, the first two complexes show RV basal-septal pacing, and the last two complexes show RV apical pacing. **A,** RV pacing is performed before ablation of the BT. The S-A (ventriculoatrial [VA]) interval is shorter during pacing at the RV base than during pacing at the RV apex, suggesting VA conduction occurring over a BT. Note that atrial activation occurs even before His bundle (HB) activation during pacing from the RV base, suggesting that VA conduction is independent of the AVN. **B,** RV pacing is performed after successful ablation of the BT. During pacing from the RV apex, the S-A interval is longer than before ablation, and it prolongs further by pacing at the RV base, consistent with the occurrence of VA conduction exclusively over the AVN. Note that in both panels the S-H (V-H) interval during RV apical pacing is shorter than that during RV basilar pacing because of the faster access of the paced wavefront to the right bundle branch–His bundle (RB-HB) during pacing at the RV apex. However, when VA conduction occurs over a BT (upper panel), the S-A interval remains constant; in contrast, in the absence of a BT (lower panel), the S-A interval shortens, coinciding with shortening of the S-H interval during pacing at the RV apex compared with pacing at the RV base.

atrial activation results from VA conduction over the AV BT during pacing at the RV base, and over either the AVN, the AV BT, or a fusion of both during pacing at the RV apex. Therefore, a variable retrograde atrial activation sequence in response to differential RV pacing (RV base versus RV apex) is indicative of the presence of an AV BT, but a constant atrial activation sequence is not helpful in excluding the presence of an AV BT.

This maneuver, however, does not exclude the presence of a distant right or left free wall AV BT, because the site of pacing is far from the AV BT; as a consequence, pacing from the RV apex or RV base may result in preferential VA conduction exclusively over the AVN and a constant atrial activation sequence. Similarly, this maneuver does not exclude the presence of a slowly conducting BT. The VA interval criterion identifies the actual route of VA conduction and therefore the fastest path of this conduction; hence, a slowly conducting BT would be missed in the presence of fast VA conduction over the HPS-AVN.

Conflicting results can also occur if conduction occurs simultaneously over a BT and HPS-AVN or, alternatively, over these two routes, depending on the pacing site. To help in these situations, calculation of the VA interval should be performed at several pacing CLs (the VA index should be independent of the pacing rate and, consequently, different values of the index at different rates would suggest more than one conducting path), after verapamil infusion (which would block the AVN and allow preferential VA conduction over the BT, if one is present), or during entrainment of the SVT (which would then ensure that VA conduction is occurring over the same path as that during the SVT).

The occurrence of RBBB (but not LBBB) also can alter the significance of the VA interval criterion, especially when VA conduction propagates over the HPS-AVN. In the presence of retrograde RBBB, VA conduction occurs over the LB-HB; therefore, the VA interval depends on the distance between the pacing site and the LB rather than the RB, and access of the paced wavefront to the LB can be faster for RV basilar or septal pacing compared with pacing from the RV apex (see Fig. 17-21).

DUAL-CHAMBER SEQUENTIAL EXTRASTIMULATION

Although the various ventricular pacing maneuvers described previously can expose an eccentric or nondecremental atrial activation pattern that suggests retrograde conduction over a BT rather than the AVN, in certain circumstances, these maneuvers may not be adequate to confirm the presence or absence of BT conduction, especially when the BT has an ERP, retrograde atrial activation pattern, and conduction time similar to the AVN. In particular, identification, mapping, and verification of success of ablation of BT function can be challenging in the setting of septal BTs with a retrograde activation pattern similar to retrograde AVN conduction, slowly conducting BTs, as well as BTs with decremental properties.[46]

Dual-chamber sequential extrastimulation is a useful maneuver for identifying concealed slowly conducting BTs not revealed with standard pacing maneuvers. This maneuver relies on concealed AVN conduction during a critically timed AES to cause transient retrograde AVN blockade at the time a VES is delivered, thereby allowing the BT to become manifest with the VES (analogous to delivering a VES during SVT while the HB is refractory).[46]

The dual-chamber sequential extrastimulation maneuver consists of an eight-beat drive train of simultaneous atrial and RV pacing at 600 milliseconds, followed by an AES (A_2) delivered at a coupling interval equal to the AVN ERP, followed by a VES (V_2) delivered at a coupling interval equal to the drive train CL (600 milliseconds). Repeat drives are then performed with decrements of 10 milliseconds for V_2 until VA block is observed.[46]

The critically timed A_2 prolongs the AVN refractory period via concealed anterograde conduction, causing V_2 to block in the AVN when it would have conducted had A_2 not been delivered. If a BT is present, V_2 conducts back to the atrium while the AVN remains refractory, resulting in a retrograde atrial activation pattern consistent with exclusive BT conduction. Although there can also be some degree of concealed anterograde conduction into the BT during A_2 stimulation, the more pronounced decremental properties of AVN tissue should prolong AVN refractoriness to a greater degree than that of the BT, allowing exclusive retrograde conduction over the BT to remain intact during V_2 stimulation.[46]

This maneuver has several potential limitations. First, atrial ERP may exceed anterograde AVN ERP. Additionally, local atrial ERP at the site of BT insertion can render the atrium refractory to the wavefront traveling retrogradely over the BT. Therefore, atrial pacing during this maneuver ideally should be performed at a site in close proximity to the atrial insertion of the BT if possible. Furthermore, the AES may cause anterograde concealed conduction in the BT, potentially resulting in BT conduction block during delivery of V_2. The success of this pacing maneuver relies on the differential effects of concealed conduction into the AVN and BT, with greater extension of refractoriness in the former than the latter.[46]

EXCLUSION OF OTHER ARRHYTHMIA MECHANISMS

AVNRT and AT arising near the AV groove can mimic orthodromic AVRT and, in the presence of a manifest BT, those tachycardias can be associated with ventricular preexcitation mimicking antidromic AVRT, whereby the BT is functioning as an innocent bystander. Therefore, EP testing is required, not just to identify the presence of a BT, but also to define its role in any clinical or inducible arrhythmia. Tables 18-4 and 18-5 summarize the EP findings indicative of the presence of a BT and its potential participation in an inducible SVT. Exclusion of other SVT mechanisms is necessary, because the mere presence of a BT is not adequate to make a diagnosis and a treatment strategy (Tables 18-6, 18-7, and 18-8).

Furthermore, the presence of multiple BTs is not infrequent, and careful EP testing is required to evaluate this possibility. Several clinical and EP findings are indicative of the presence of multiple BTs (Table 18-9 and Fig. 18-34; and see Fig. 18-3). However, despite these various methods, many BTs are not identified until after catheter ablation of the first BT. Failure to detect the presence of multiple BTs during EP testing has been reported in as many as 5% to 15% of patients. This may be explained by the fact that changes in the preexcitation pattern can be subtle in shifting from one BT to another. Furthermore, one BT can preferentially conduct during atrial pacing or participate in preexcited tachycardias while another BT can be responsible for the retrograde limb during orthodromic AVRT or ventricular pacing. Additionally, there may be fusion of BT conduction, anterograde or retrograde. Repetitive concealed conduction into the BT during AVRT also may preclude identification of that BT before ablation of the first BT.

TABLE 18-4 Electrophysiological Findings Indicating Presence of Retrograde Atrioventricular Bypass Tract Function

- Eccentric atrial activation sequence during ventricular pacing
- RV apical pacing producing longer VA interval and/or different atrial activation sequence compared with that during RV basilar pacing
- Para-Hisian pacing producing similar VA interval with and without HB capture or producing different atrial activation sequence depending on whether the HB is captured
- VES delivered when the HB is refractory advances the next atrial activation during SVT

HB = His bundle; RV = right ventricle; SVT = supraventricular tachycardia; VA = ventriculoatrial; VES = ventricular extrastimulus.

TABLE 18-5 Electrophysiological Findings Indicating Presence and Participation of Atrioventricular Bypass Tract in Supraventricular Tachycardia

- VES delivered during SVT when the HB is refractory terminates the SVT without atrial activation.
- VES delivered during SVT when the HB is refractory delays the next atrial activation.
- VES during SVT captures the atrium at the same coupling interval as that of the VES (exact capture phenomenon).
- VES delivered during SVT captures the atrium at a shorter coupling interval than that of the VES (paradoxical capture phenomenon).
- VA interval (with or without concomitant prolongation in tachycardia CL) prolonged during the SVT secondary to the development of BBB.
- Entrainment of the SVT by ventricular pacing results in prolongation of the VA interval ($VA_{pacing} > VA_{SVT}$).

BBB = bundle branch block; CL = cycle length; HB = His bundle; SVT = supraventricular tachycardia; VA = ventriculoatrial; VES = ventricular extrastimulus.

Localization of the Bypass Tract

Pacing from Multiple Atrial Sites

The closer the pacing site to the BT atrial insertion, the more rapidly the impulse will reach the BT relative to the AVN and thus the greater is the degree of preexcitation and the shorter is the P-delta interval. This method is especially helpful when the BT cannot conduct retrogradely, prohibiting localization with atrial mapping during SVT or ventricular pacing.

Preexcitation Index

As noted, the preexcitation index analyzes the coupling interval of the VES (delivered from the RV) that resets orthodromic AVRT as a percentage of the tachycardia CL. A relative preexcitation index (the ratio of coupling interval to the tachycardia CL) of more than 90% of a VES that advances atrial activation during orthodromic AVRT suggests that the BT is close to the site of ventricular stimulation (i.e., RV or septal BT). An absolute preexcitation index (tachycardia CL minus VES coupling interval) of at least 75 milliseconds suggests a left free wall BT, an index of less than 45 milliseconds suggests a septal BT, and an index of 45 to 75 milliseconds is indeterminate.

TABLE 18-6 Exclusion of Atrial Tachycardia

Effects of BBB

- Prolongation of surface VA interval during SVT (with or without tachycardia CL prolongation) on development of BBB excludes AT.

Oscillations in SVT CL

- Spontaneous changes in tachycardia CL accompanied by constant VA interval (VA linking) exclude AT.
- Changes in atrial CL that are predicted by the change in the preceding ventricular CL argue against AT.

VES Delivered during SVT

- VES that terminates the SVT without atrial activation excludes AT.
- VES that delays next atrial activation excludes AT.
- VES during SVT that captures the atrium at the same coupling interval as that of the VES (exact capture phenomenon) excludes AT.
- VES delivered during SVT that captures the atrium at a shorter coupling interval than that of the VES (paradoxical capture phenomenon) excludes AT.
- Ventricular fusion during resetting indicates AVRT and excludes AT.

Overdrive Ventricular Pacing during SVT

- If atrial activation sequence during ventricular entrainment is similar to that during the SVT, AT is less likely.
- Presence of A-V electrogram sequence at cessation of ventricular pacing generally excludes AT.
- Ventricular fusion during entrainment indicates AVRT and excludes AT.

Overdrive Atrial Pacing during SVT

- If the VA interval following the last entrained QRS is reproducibly constant (with <10-msec variation), despite pacing at different CLs or for different durations (VA linking) and similar to that during SVT CL, AT is unlikely.
- If the VA interval following the last entrained QRS is reproducibly constant (with <14-msec variation), despite pacing at different atrial sites (VA linking), AT is unlikely.

Atrial Pacing during NSR at Tachycardia CL

- If the VA interval following the last entrained QRS is reproducibly constant (with <10-msec variation), despite pacing at different CLs or for different durations (VA linking) and similar to that during SVT CL, AT is unlikely.
- If the VA interval following the last entrained QRS is reproducibly constant (with <14-msec variation), despite pacing at different atrial sites (VA linking), AT is unlikely.

Ventricular Pacing during NSR at Tachycardia CL

- If retrograde atrial activation sequence during ventricular pacing is similar to that during SVT, AT is less likely.

AT = atrial tachycardia; AVRT = atrioventricular reentrant tachycardia; BBB = bundle branch block; CL = cycle length; NSR = normal sinus rhythm; SVT = supraventricular tachycardia; VA = ventriculoatrial; VES = ventricular extrastimulus.

TABLE 18-7 Exclusion of Atrioventricular Nodal Reentrant Tachycardia

Atrial Activation Sequence

- Eccentric atrial activation sequence during the SVT excludes AVNRT (with the exception of left variant AVNRT).

Effects of BBB

- Prolongation of VA interval or tachycardia CL on development of BBB excludes AVNRT.

Oscillations in SVT CL

- Spontaneous changes in tachycardia CL accompanied by constant VA interval (VA linking) make AVNRT unlikely.

VES Delivered during SVT

- VES delivered during SVT when the HB is refractory that resets or terminates the SVT excludes AVNRT.
- VES during SVT that conducts to the atrium at the same coupling interval as that of the VES (exact capture phenomenon) excludes AVNRT.
- VES delivered during SVT that conducts to the atrium at a shorter coupling interval than that of the VES (paradoxical capture phenomenon) excludes AVNRT.

Entrainment of SVT by Atrial Pacing

- $AH_{pacing} - AH_{SVT} < 20$ msec excludes AVNRT.

Entrainment of SVT by Ventricular Pacing

- $VA_{pacing} - VA_{SVT} < 85$ msec argues against AVNRT.
- PPI – SVT CL < 115 msec argues against AVNRT.
- Corrected PPI – SVT CL < 110 msec argues against AVNRT.
- Manifest ventricular fusion during entrainment indicates AVRT and excludes AVNRT.
- Acceleration of the SVT to the pacing CL occurring after a single captured paced RV complex is consistent with orthodromic AVRT and essentially excludes AVNRT.
- A differential corrected PPI – SVT CL of <30 msec after transient entrainment from the RV apex versus the RV base is consistent with orthodromic AVRT and excludes AVNRT.
- A differential VA interval (ventricular stimulus-to-atrial interval during entrainment from RV base versus RV septum) of <20 msec is consistent with orthodromic AVRT and excludes AVNRT.

Atrial Pacing during NSR at Tachycardia CL

- $AH_{pacing} - AH_{SVT} < 20$ msec excludes AVNRT.

Ventricular Pacing during NSR at Tachycardia CL

- If $HA_{pacing} - HA_{SVT}$ is less than −10 msec, the SVT excludes AVNRT.

Differential RV Pacing

- If the atrial activation sequence changes during pacing at the RV apex versus pacing at the RV base, AVNRT is less likely.
- If the S-A interval is shorter with pacing from the base than from the apex, AVNRT is less likely.

Para-Hisian Pacing

- Para-Hisian pacing producing similar VA interval, regardless of whether HB capture occurs, and/or different atrial activation sequence, depending on whether HB capture occurs, makes AVNRT unlikely.

AH = atrial–His bundle; AVNRT = atrioventricular nodal reentrant tachycardia; AVRT = atrioventricular reentrant tachycardia; BBB = bundle branch block; CL = cycle length; HA = His bundle–atrial interval; HB = His bundle; NSR = normal sinus rhythm; PPI = post-pacing interval; RV = right ventricle; SVT = supraventricular tachycardia; VA = ventriculoatrial; VES = ventricular extrastimulus.

Effects of Bundle Branch Block during Orthodromic Atrioventricular Reentrant Tachycardia

Prolongation of the tachycardia CL and, more importantly, the surface VA interval by more than 35 milliseconds following the development of BBB is diagnostic of AVRT using a free wall BT ipsilateral to the BBB (LBBB with left-sided BT, and RBBB with right-sided BT).[33,34] Superoparaseptal and posteroseptal BTs are associated with a lesser degree of prolongation of the VA interval (approximately 5 to 25 milliseconds) on the development of BBB (RBBB with superoparaseptal BT, and LBBB with posteroseptal BT). In an analogous fashion, entrainment of the SVT by ventricular pacing that results in prolongation of the VA interval ($VA_{pacing} > VA_{SVT}$) suggests that the SVT is orthodromic AVRT mediated by an AV BT in the ventricle contralateral to the site of ventricular pacing.

Earliest Ventricular Activation Site during Anterograde Bypass Tract Conduction

During ventricular preexcitation (preexcited sinus or atrial paced rhythm, or antidromic AVRT), the surface ECG lead with the earliest onset of the delta wave, preferably with a relatively sharp delineation of its onset, should be selected and used as the timing reference during mapping (Fig. 18-35). The site of earliest ventricular activation (preceding the onset of the delta wave) along the tricuspid and

TABLE 18-8 Differentiation Between Antidromic AVRT and Preexcited AVNRT

SVT Features

- HA_{SVT} < 70 msec excludes antidromic AVRT.
- Positive HV or V-H interval ≤10 msec (especially when HA interval is ≤50 msec) suggests AVNRT.

Termination of SVT

- Continuation of the SVT at the same tachycardia CL, despite anterograde block in the BT (by drugs, mechanical trauma, or ablation), is diagnostic of AVNRT and excludes antidromic AVRT.
- Block of the BT by drugs and subsequent induction of narrow-complex SVT with the same tachycardia CL, HA interval, and retrograde atrial activation sequence as that of the preexcited SVT induced before the BT block is diagnostic of preexcited AVNRT and excludes antidromic AVRT.
- Termination of SVT in response to carotid sinus massage or adenosine:
  - AVNRT terminates after atrial activation (secondary to anterograde block down the slow pathway).
  - Classic antidromic AVRT terminates after ventricular activation (secondary to retrograde block up the AVN).

Effects of BBB

- Prolongation of VA interval or tachycardia CL on development of BBB excludes AVNRT.

SVT Induction with Ventricular Stimulation

- Induction of the SVT by ventricular pacing at a pacing CL similar to the tachycardia CL or by a VES that advances the timing of the His potential by a coupling interval (i.e., H_1-H_2 interval) similar to the H-H during the SVT, the HA interval following such a VES is compared with that during the SVT:
  - $HA_{VES\ or\ ventricular\ pacing}$ > HA_{SVT} is diagnostic of AVNRT and excludes antidromic AVRT.
  - $HA_{VES\ or\ ventricular\ pacing}$ ≤ HA_{SVT} is diagnostic of antidromic AVRT and excludes AVNRT.

AES Delivered during SVT

- Late-coupled AES is delivered close to the BT atrial insertion site during SVT when the AV junctional atrium is refractory. If it advances the timing of both the next ventricular activation and the subsequent atrial activation, it proves that the SVT is antidromic AVRT using an AV BT anterogradely, and excludes preexcited AVNRT.
- AES during the SVT that advances ventricular activation and does not affect VA interval excludes AVNRT and is diagnostic of antidromic AVRT.
- Exact atrial and ventricular capture by AES delivered when the AV junction is depolarized excludes AVNRT.

Entrainment of SVT by Atrial Pacing

- Failure of entrainment by atrial pacing to influence the VA interval during SVT excludes AVNRT.
- The presence of a fixed short V-H interval during entrainment of the SVT with atrial pacing suggests antidromic AVRT, and makes AVNRT unlikely (but does not exclude AVNRT).

Entrainment of SVT by Ventricular Pacing

- Failure of entrainment by ventricular pacing to influence the VA interval during SVT excludes AVNRT.

Ventricular Pacing during NSR at the Tachycardia CL

- Pacing at the RV apex at tachycardia CL is performed, and the HA interval during RV pacing is compared with the HA interval during SVT. (It is important to verify that VA conduction occurred only over the AVN and not over the BT for this analysis to be valid.)
- HA_{pacing} > HA_{SVT} is diagnostic of AVNRT and excludes antidromic AVRT.
- HA_{pacing} ≤ HA_{SVT} is diagnostic of antidromic AVRT and excludes AVNRT.
- VA block during RV apical pacing excludes antidromic AVRT.

AES = atrial extrastimulus; AV = atrioventricular; AVNRT = atrioventricular nodal reentrant tachycardia; AVRT = atrioventricular reentrant tachycardia; BBB = bundle branch block; BT = bypass tract; CL = cycle length; HA = His bundle–atrial; HV = His bundle–ventricular; NSR = normal sinus rhythm; RV = right ventricle; SVT = supraventricular tachycardia; VA = ventriculoatrial; VES = ventricular extrastimulus; V-H = ventricular–His bundle.

TABLE 18-9 Electrophysiological Findings Indicating Presence of Multiple Atrioventricular Bypass Tracts

During Preexcited Rhythms (NSR, PACs, Spontaneous or Induced AF, RA, and LA Pacing)

- Changing anterograde delta wave (i.e., variations in preexcited QRS morphology). Atrial pacing from different sites (high RA and CS) may accentuate preexcitation over one BT and not the other, help unmask the changes in the delta wave
- Atypical pattern of preexcitation (i.e., does not conform to an expected QRS morphology for a given location)
- Changing anterograde delta wave following antiarrhythmic agents (e.g., amiodarone or class I agents) that may block one BT and not the other or following ablation of one BT

During Ventricular Pacing at Different CLs and from Multiple Pacing Sites

- Evidence of multiple routes of retrograde atrial activation:
  - Changing P wave morphology or atrial activation sequence
  - Multiple atrial breakthrough sites
  - Changing VA interval
  - Evidence of mismatch of site of anterograde preexcitation and site of retrograde atrial activation observed during ventricular pacing

During Orthodromic AVRT

- Evidence of multiple routes of retrograde atrial activation:
  - Changing P wave morphology or atrial activation sequence
  - Multiple atrial breakthrough sites
  - Changing VA interval
  - Failure to delay atrial activation at all sites with the development of BBB ipsilateral to the BT
- Evidence of multiple routes of anterograde ventricular activation:
  - Intermittent anterograde fusion (preexcited) complexes
  - Evidence of mismatch of site of anterograde preexcitation and site of retrograde atrial activation observed during orthodromic AVRT

During Antidromic AVRT

- Eccentric atrial activation sequence
- Varying degrees of anterograde fusion
- Changing V-H interval without any change in the tachycardia CL or atrial activation sequence (suggesting that the HPS is not part of the reentrant circuit)
- Tachycardia CL during antidromic AVRT slower than orthodromic AVRT in the same patient (in absence of dual AVN pathways)
- Anterograde ventricular activation over posteroseptal BT
- The mere presence of antidromic AVRT

AF = atrial fibrillation; AVN = atrioventricular node; AVRT = atrioventricular reentrant tachycardia; BBB = bundle branch block; BT = bypass tract; CL = cycle length; CS = coronary sinus; HPS = His-Purkinje system; LA = left atrium; NSR = normal sinus rhythm; PAC = premature atrial complex; RA = right atrium; VA = ventriculoatrial.

mitral annuli identifies the BT ventricular insertion site. Both bipolar and unipolar recordings on the ablation catheter should be used for mapping (Fig. 18-36). Bipolar electrograms display electrogram components and timing and may demonstrate a BT potential. The unfiltered (0.05 to ≥300 Hz) unipolar signal morphology should show a monophasic QS complex with a rapid negative deflection if the site was at the origin of impulse formation in the ventricle (i.e., BT insertion site). Concordance of the timing of the onset of the bipolar electrogram with that of the filtered or unfiltered unipolar electrogram (with the rapid downslope of the S wave of the unipolar QS complex coinciding with the initial peak of the bipolar signal) helps ensure that the tip electrode, which is the ablation electrode, is responsible for the early component of the bipolar electrogram. If only bipolar recordings are used, one does not know which of the two poles is responsible for the earliest component of the bipolar electrogram.[6]

Earliest Atrial Activation Site during Retrograde Bypass Tract Conduction

During orthodromic AVRT or during ventricular pacing with retrograde conduction over the BT, the site of earliest atrial activation

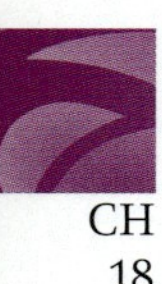

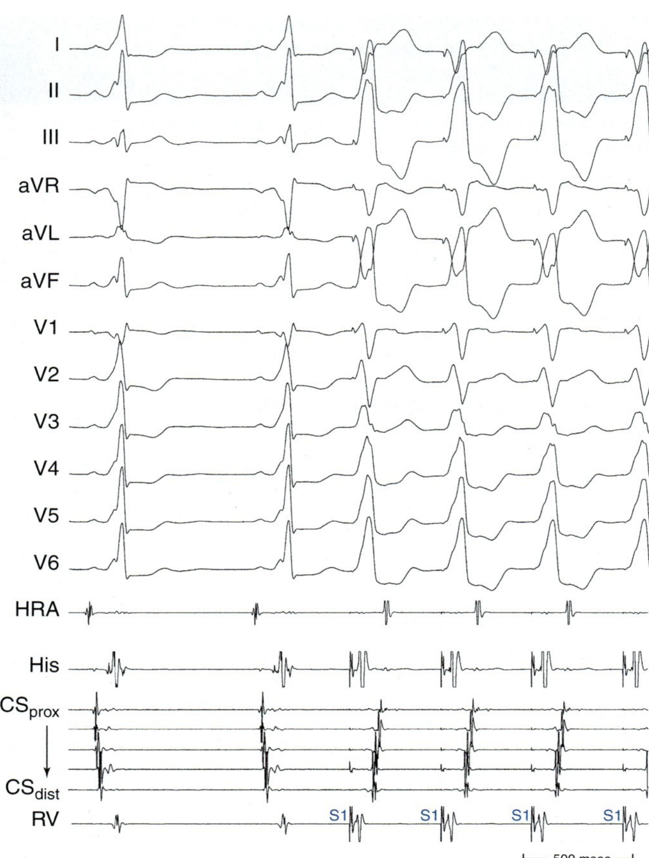

FIGURE 18-34 The presence of multiple bypass tracts (BTs) is indicated by the mismatch of sites of anterograde preexcitation during normal sinus rhythm (the delta wave morphology is consistent with anterograde conduction over a right anterior BT) and site of retrograde atrial activation observed during ventricular pacing (the atrial activation sequence is consistent with VA conduction over a left lateral BT).

along the tricuspid and mitral annuli identifies the BT atrial insertion site. When mapping is performed during ventricular pacing, fusion of atrial activation, caused by simultaneous retrograde conduction over both the AVN and the BT, has to be considered, because it can affect the accuracy of mapping. This can be an issue in the setting of septal BTs whereby retrograde atrial activation sequence over the BT may not be very different from that over the AVN. Dissociation of retrograde conduction over the BT from that over the AVN is required in these situations, and can usually be achieved with ventricular stimulation from sites closer to the BT and with the use of AVN blockers (e.g., adenosine) to ensure preferential retrograde conduction over the BT.[3] As with ventricular mapping, both bipolar and unipolar recordings on the distal ablation electrode should be used for atrial mapping (Fig. 18-37). Determining what components of a complex ablation electrode recording is atrial versus ventricular can be facilitated by either rapid burst ventricular pacing that does not conduct 1:1 retrogradely (Fig. 18-38) or introduction of a VES that does not conduct retrogradely during fixed rate ventricular pacing (Fig. 18-39). In either case, the principle is to compare the electrogram that is known to have no atrial component with the electrogram in question (with some atrial component), any difference being due to the contribution of the atrial electrogram.

Mapping Atrial Electrogram Polarity Reversal during Retrograde Bypass Tract Conduction

The morphology and amplitude of the bipolar electrograms are influenced by the orientation of the bipolar recording axis to the direction of propagation of the activation wavefront. Although the direction of wavefront propagation cannot be reliably inferred from the morphology of the bipolar signal, a change in morphology can be a useful finding, and the unfiltered bipolar electrogram with the electrodes oriented parallel to the axis of the annulus can be used to localize the atrial insertion site of the BT.

During retrograde BT conduction (orthodromic AVRT or ventricular pacing), BT atrial insertion is identified as the site where the polarity of the atrial potential reverses. Because the site of BT atrial insertion is usually discrete, atrial activation propagates in two opposite directions along the annulus from the insertion site. Consequently, an RS configuration electrogram will be present on one side of the BT, where the wavefront is propagating from the distal electrode toward the proximal electrode, and a QR morphology electrogram on the other side, where the wavefront is propagating from the proximal electrode toward the distal electrode (see Fig. 5-5).

This technique is typically used for localization of left free wall BTs via the transseptal approach, which allows an electrode orientation parallel with atrial activation along the mitral annulus. As the ablation catheter is moved along the mitral annulus during retrograde BT conduction, the amplitude and polarity of the atrial electrogram are examined. With the tip electrode negative, and the catheter lying on the mitral annulus from anterior to posterior, an upright atrial electrogram indicates a catheter position anterior to the insertion site, whereas a negative electrogram indicates positions posterior to the insertion site. When the bipole approaches and then passes directly over the atrial insertion site, the atrial electrogram becomes diminished in amplitude, isoelectric, and fractionated. As the catheter moves from one side of the insertion site to the other side, reversal of the atrial electrogram polarity is observed. This maneuver has a sensitivity of 97%, specificity of 46%, and positive predictive value of 75%.[23] For BTs at other locations, mapping can be facilitated by using a multipolar catheter positioned in the CS or around the tricuspid annulus (e.g., Halo catheter); the site of the BT atrial insertion is enclosed between the two adjacent bipoles, demonstrating atrial electrogram polarity reversal.

Direct Recording of Bypass Tract Potential

The BT potential manifests as a sharp narrow spike on both unipolar and bipolar recordings 10 to 30 milliseconds before the onset of the delta wave during anterograde preexcitation or between the ventricular and atrial electrograms at the earliest site of retrograde atrial activation during orthodromic AVRT or ventricular pacing. The BT potential amplitude averages 0.5 to 1 mV at successful ablation sites (see Figs. 18-36 and 18-37). Similar electrical signals, however, can be a component of the atrial or ventricular electrogram, and proof that an electrical signal actually is a BT potential is difficult, because it needs to be dissociated from the local atrial and ventricular electrograms.

DISSOCIATION OF BYPASS TRACT POTENTIAL FROM LOCAL ATRIAL POTENTIAL

During orthodromic AVRT or ventricular pacing, introduction of a VES may cause retrograde block near the BT-atrial interface. This would result in loss of the atrial potential while maintaining the BT potential, providing evidence that this potential is not a component of the atrial electrogram. Additionally, during ventricular pacing, introduction of a late-coupled AES can advance the timing of the local atrial potential without affecting the retrograde BT potential, providing evidence that the BT potential is not related to atrial activation. Alternatively, during atrial pacing, introduction of a late-coupled VES may advance ventricular and BT activation without affecting atrial activation, providing additional evidence that the BT potential is not related to atrial activation (Fig. 18-40).

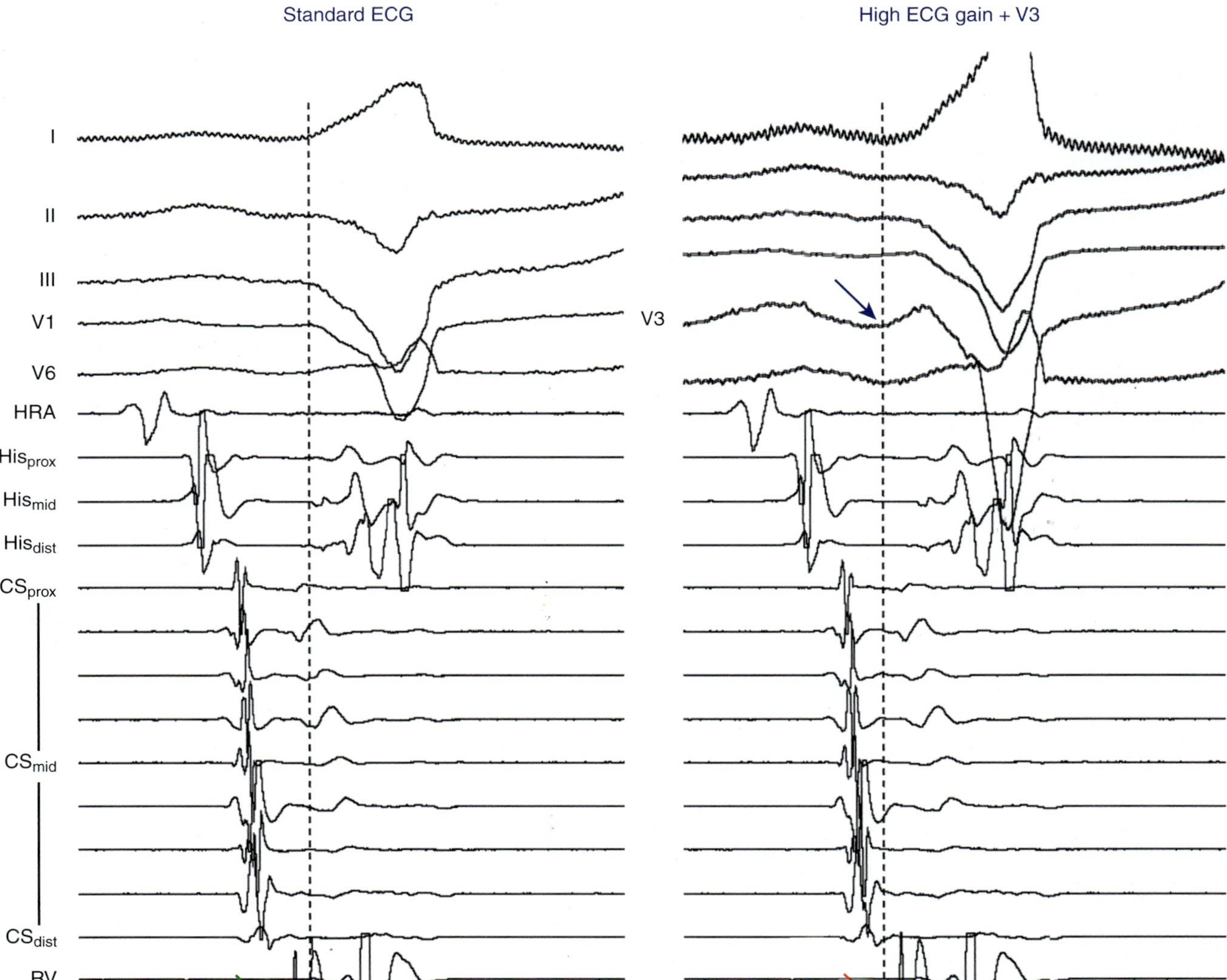

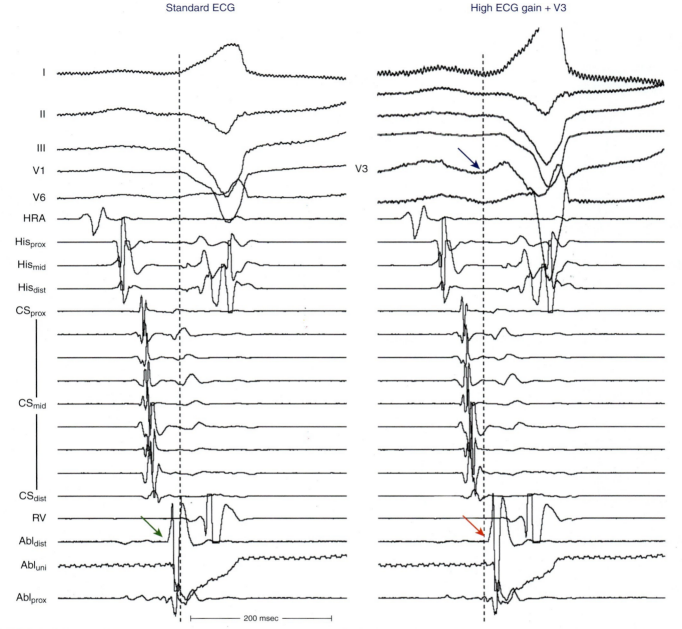

FIGURE 18-35 Surface ECG and intracardiac recordings of possible ablation site. On the **left,** with standard ECG recordings, the features of the ablation site electrograms (Abl) suggest this would be a good ablation site (green arrow) because they occur well before the onset of the delta wave (dashed line). However, on the **right,** the very same complex is shown, but with increased gain on surface ECG leads as well as an addition of lead of V_3 (showing sharp delineation of delta wave onset, blue arrow). Now, the dashed line that denotes the true onset of surface preexcitation reveals that the putative ablation site is not attractive (red arrow).

DISSOCIATION OF BYPASS TRACT POTENTIAL FROM LOCAL VENTRICULAR POTENTIAL

During AVRT or ventricular pacing, introduction of a late-coupled VES may block retrogradely in the BT near the ventricular-BT interface. This would result in loss of the BT potential while maintaining the ventricular potential, providing evidence that the BT potential is not related to ventricular activation. Additionally, during preexcited atrial pacing, introduction of a late-coupled VES (occurring at the time of the anterograde BT potential) that advances the local ventricular electrogram but does not alter the BT potential dissociates this potential from local ventricular activation. Moreover, during ventricular pacing, introduction of a critically timed AES may anterogradely activate the BT, advancing the timing of the BT potential without affecting the timing or morphology of the ventricular potential, providing evidence that the BT potential does not result from atrial activation (Fig. 18-41).

However, these criteria for validation of BT potentials are often difficult to achieve. Therefore, validation of BT potentials by programmed electrical stimulation is often not practical in clinical settings; instead, such a potential is called *possible* or *probable* BT potential.

Targeting an isolated BT potential has been associated with the highest frequency of ablation success. The usefulness of this criterion, however, has been limited by difficulty in locating or validating a BT potential. The difficulty in identifying the BT potential is often related to the oblique course of the BT. A ventricular or atrial wavefront propagating concurrently with the BT can overlap and mask the BT potential. Pacing from the site producing the shorter

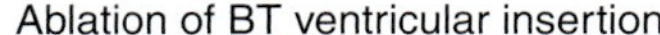

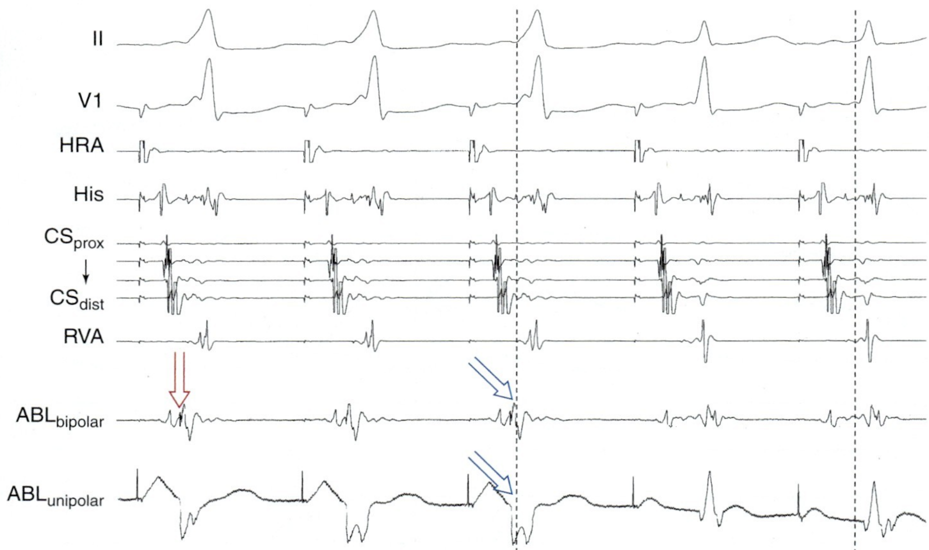

FIGURE 18-36 Catheter ablation of a left anterolateral bypass tract (BT) during anterograde conduction. Ablation is performed during preexcited atrial pacing. Preexcitation is observed during the first three complexes. The dashed line indicates the onset of the delta wave. Note the sharp negative deflection (QS morphology) in the unipolar recording. Also, note the concordance of the timing of the unipolar and bipolar electrograms (blue arrows), which precedes the onset of the delta wave by 10 to 15 milliseconds. A sharp potential (possible BT potential, red arrow) is recorded between the atrial and ventricular electrograms. RF application at this site successfully eliminated preexcitation (last two complexes).

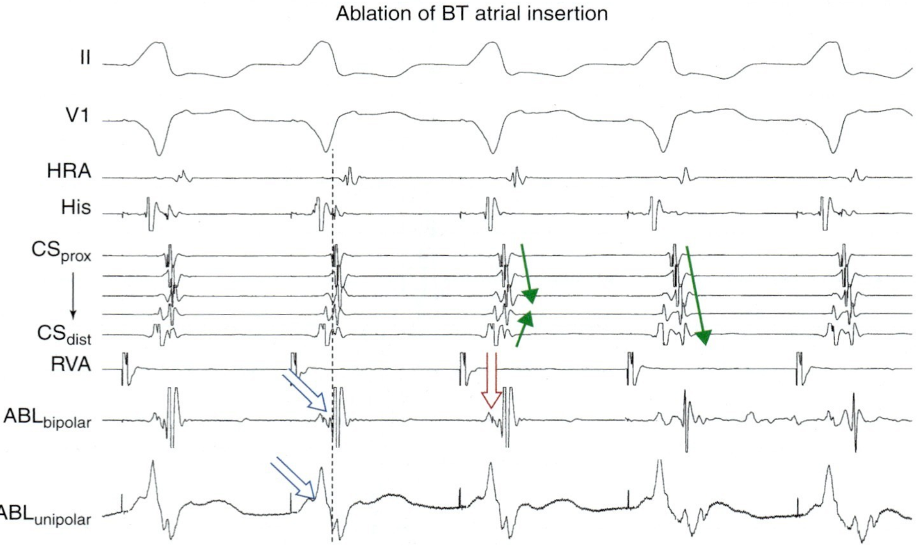

FIGURE 18-37 Catheter ablation of a left lateral bypass tract (BT) during retrograde conduction. Ablation is performed during ventricular pacing with atrial fusion (ventriculoatrial conduction occurring over both the BT and atrioventricular node [AVN]). The dashed line indicates the onset of the earliest atrial activation. Note the sharp negative deflection (QS morphology) in the unipolar recording. The timing of the unipolar electrogram coincides with the bipolar electrogram (blue arrows) and precedes the delta wave by 5 to 10 milliseconds. The atrial and ventricular electrograms merge together, and the true morphology of the ventricular electrogram is unmasked after successful ablation (last two complexes). A sharp potential (possible BT potential, red arrow) is recorded between the two electrograms. After successful elimination of the BT function, atrial activation occurs exclusively over the AVN (last two complexes, green arrows).

local VA or local AV intervals helps identify the BT potential in most of these cases.

Local Atrioventricular (or Ventriculoatrial) Interval

Although the site of the shortest local VA interval during retrograde BT conduction and the site of the shortest local AV interval during anterograde BT conduction are often considered the optimal target for BT ablation, the reliability of this criterion has been debated and can be misleading in the setting of oblique BTs.[3,6] Short local VA intervals can occur at sites along the valve annulus distant from the BT because atrial and ventricular activation wavefronts can propagate circumferentially along the annulus, and the timing of local atrial and ventricular activation can be close to one another at multiple sites along the annulus (Fig. 18-42). Furthermore, with oblique BTs, the shortest local VA interval can be shifted away from the BT in the direction of the ventricular wavefront if the velocity of the ventricular wavefront along the annulus is less than the velocity of the atrial wavefront. Similarly, the site of the shortest local AV interval can be shifted away from the BT in the direction of the atrial wavefront if the atrial wavefront is slower than the ventricular wavefront.

With an oblique course, the local VA and AV intervals at the site of earliest ventricular activation varies by reversing the direction of the paced ventricular and atrial wavefronts, respectively.[6] During ventricular pacing, a ventricular wavefront propagating from the direction of the ventricular end (concurrently with BT activation) produces a short local VA interval, because activation along the BT propagates to the site of earliest atrial activation concomitant with the ventricular wavefront. Contrariwise, a ventricular wavefront propagating in the opposite (countercurrent) direction produces a longer local VA interval because the ventricular wavefront must pass the site of earliest atrial activation before reaching the ventricular end of the BT (Fig. 18-43). This has important implications for localizing oblique AV BTs. With a concurrent wavefront, the ventricular potential may overlap and mask the BT potential and overlap the atrial potential, masking the site of earliest atrial activation. If the velocity of the ventricular wavefront along the annulus were slower than the BT and atrial wavefronts, the shortest local VA interval would be shifted away from the BT. A countercurrent wavefront should expose the atrial activation sequence and BT potential.

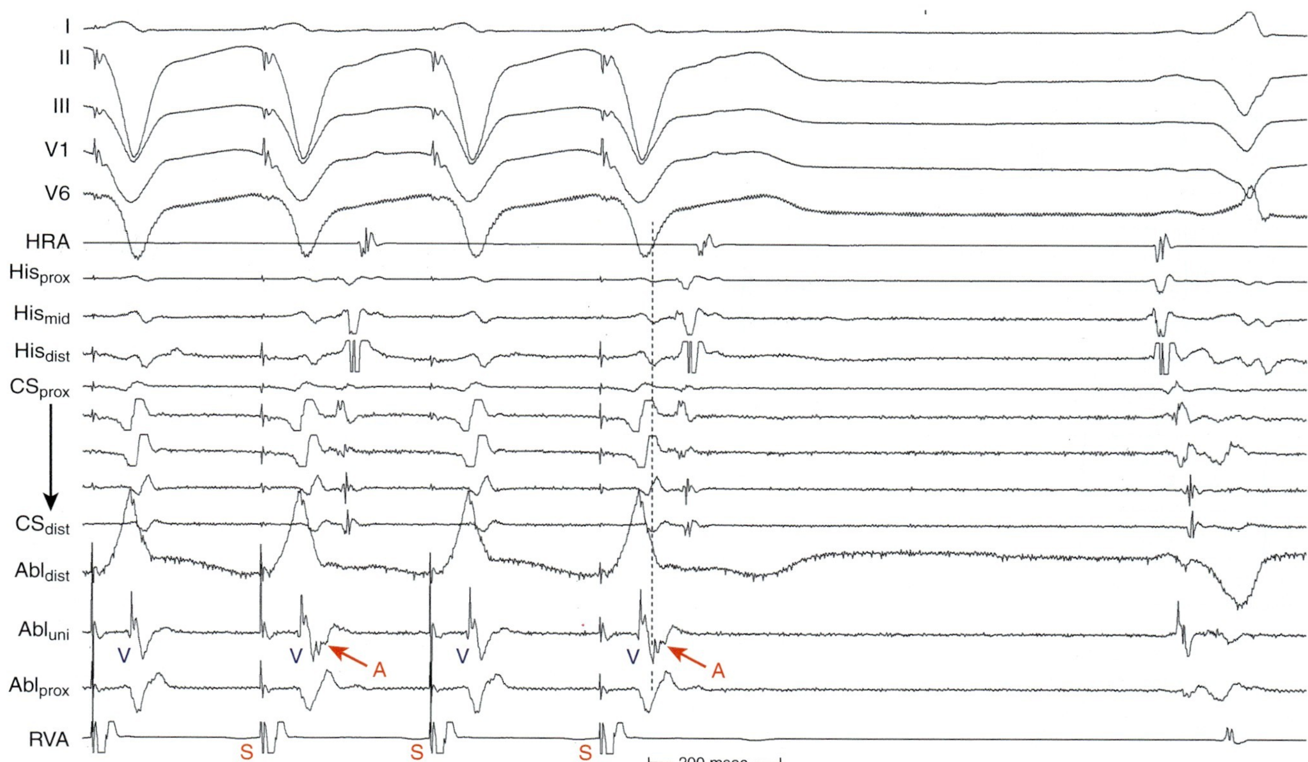

FIGURE 18-38 Using ventricular pacing to evaluate ablation site electrogram components. Burst ventricular pacing is shown at a rate that produces 2:1 retrograde conduction over the bypass tract (BT). This facilitates determination of what portion of the ablation site recording is atrial versus ventricular, because whatever is present in recordings on cycles during which retrograde conduction is present, but absent when retrograde conduction fails, is the atrial (or BT plus atrial) recording (red arrows).

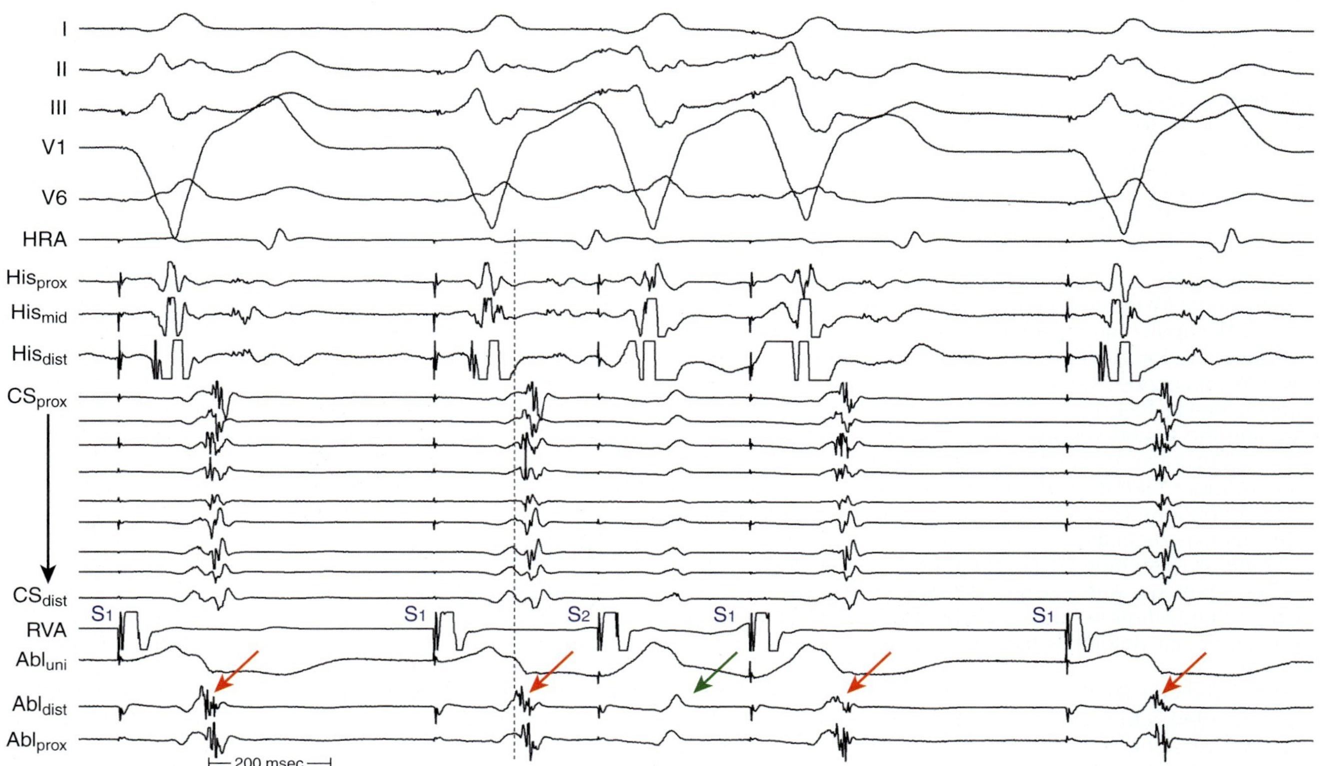

FIGURE 18-39 Using ventricular extrastimuli to evaluate ablation site electrogram components. Determining what part of a complex ablation site recording is atrial or bypass tract (BT) is aided by introducing an extrastimulus (S_2) during a fixed-rate drive, which fails to conduct retrogradely while drive complexes do conduct. The portion of the electrogram that is absent on this complex (green arrow), but present on others (red arrows), is the atrial (±BT) component.

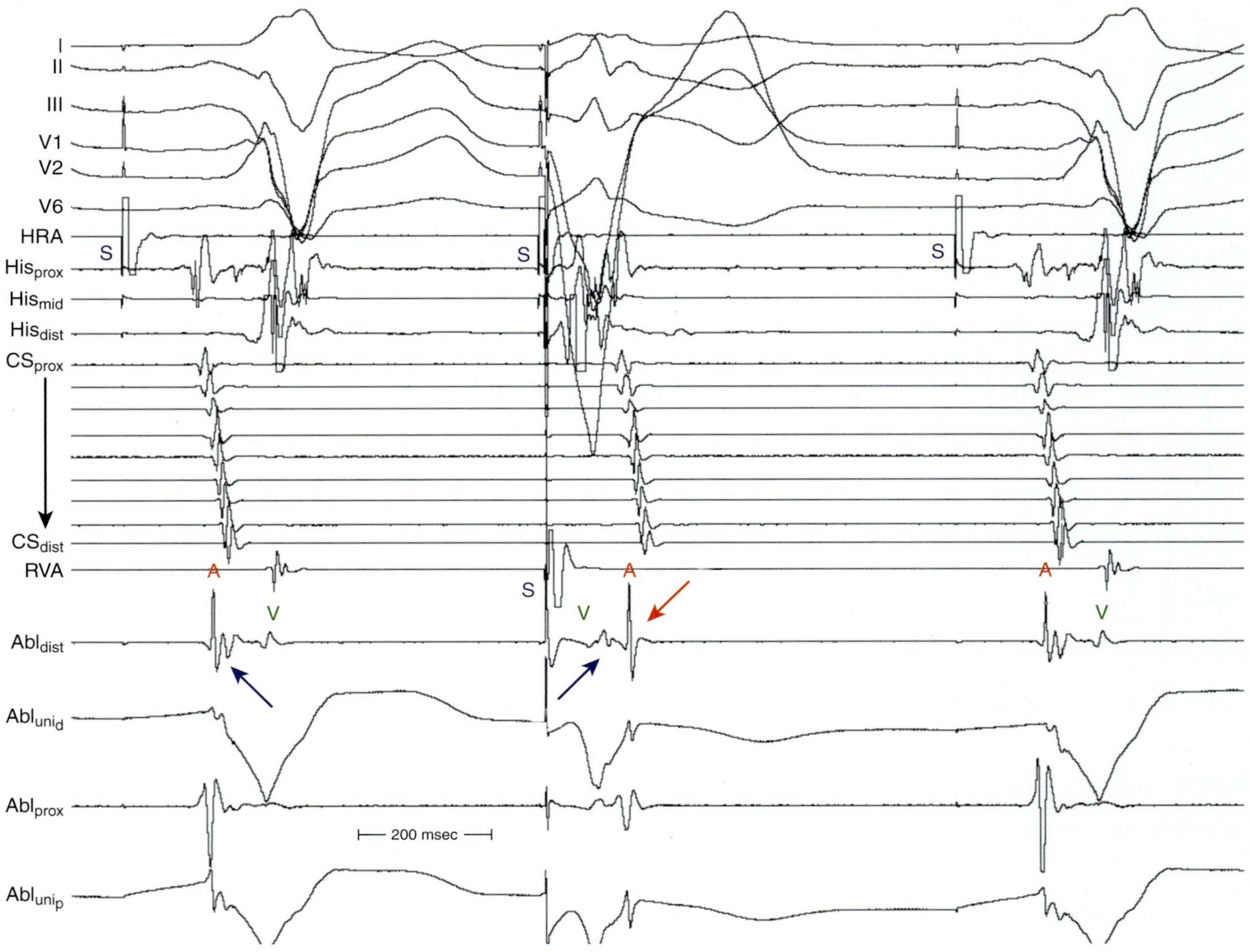

FIGURE 18-40 Dissociation of bypass tract (BT) potential from local atrial potential. Surface ECG and intracardiac recordings evaluate possible BT potential. Fixed-rate atrial pacing is present on all three complexes shown. On the first complex, a blue arrow points to a possible BT potential following the sharp atrial potential (A). This same sharp atrial potential is seen at the same rate as atrial pacing on all three complexes. On the middle complex, a single ventricular extrastimulus is delivered almost simultaneously with the atrial drive stimulus (S). Here, the blue arrow shows that the putative BT potential does not follow the sharp atrial recording (red arrow indicates its absence), and thus is not part of the atrial electrogram.

Similarly, during atrial pacing, a concurrent atrial wavefront would shorten the local AV interval at the site of earliest ventricular activation (local AV) and could mask the BT potential and site of earliest ventricular activation. A countercurrent wavefront should lengthen the local AV and expose the BT potential and ventricular activation sequence (see Fig. 18-43).

Reversing the paced ventricular or atrial wavefronts increases the local VA or local AV interval, respectively, by at least 15 milliseconds in more than 85% of patients, which suggests that most BTs have an oblique course. The increase in the local VA or local AV intervals may facilitate identification of the BT potential.[6] An anterograde or retrograde BT potential can be recorded in more than 85% of patients with oblique BTs, which is much more frequent than that with nonoblique BTs, because fusion of the atrial, BT, and ventricular potentials may be expected with nonoblique BT.

During retrograde BT conduction, the earliest atrial activation may be recorded 3 to 5 mm (or possibly more) from the actual BT insertion. Ablation is likely to be successful if the electrode is located 3 to 5 mm from the atrial insertion in the direction of the ventricular insertion and unsuccessful if located in the opposite direction. During anterograde BT conduction, ablation at a site recording earliest ventricular activation is likely to be successful, even if the electrode is located 3 to 5 mm from the ventricular end but in the direction of the atrial insertion and unsuccessful if located in the opposite direction. This explains the 40% ablation success for the criterion of local ventricular activation preceding the onset of the delta wave by less than 0 millisecond during anterograde BT conduction, even though ventricular activation usually can be recorded as much as 30 milliseconds before the delta wave in right-sided BTs and 15 to 20 milliseconds in left-sided BTs.

Ablation

Target of Ablation

The BT is the target of ablation. The best site of ablation of a BT is where it crosses the annulus. Localization of the BT can be achieved with different mapping methods, as described earlier. Ablation should be performed at the same side of the annulus to the one being mapped (i.e., ablation on the atrial side during mapping of the atrial insertion site during retrograde BT conduction, and ablation on the ventricular side during mapping of the earliest ventricular activation during anterograde BT conduction). This is especially important in the presence of oblique BTs, whereby

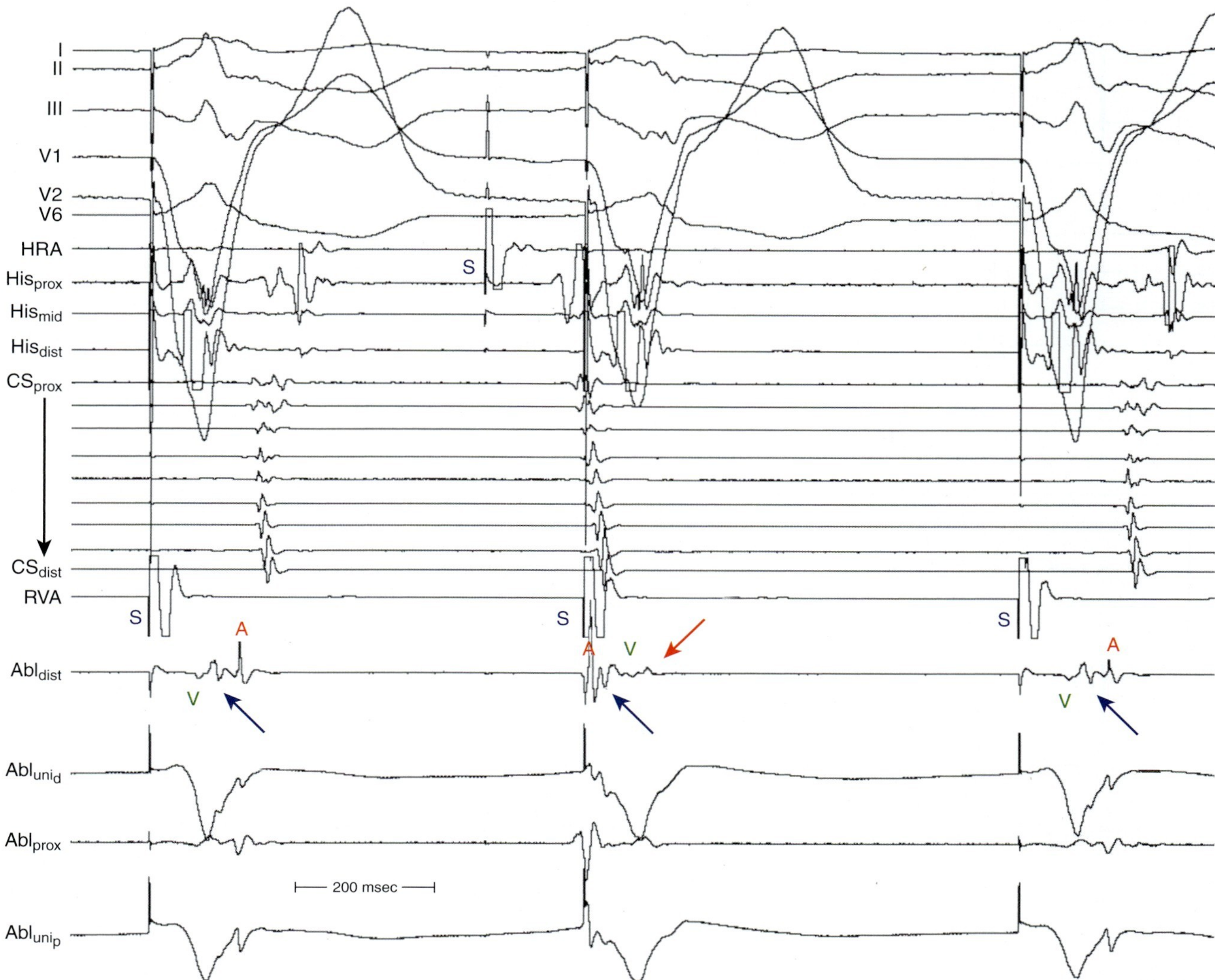

FIGURE 18-41 Dissociation of bypass tract (BT) potential from local ventricular potential. Surface ECG and intracardiac recordings evaluate possible BT potential in the same patient as in Figure 18-40. Fixed-rate ventricular pacing is shown in all three complexes, with a single atrial extrastimulus (AES) introduced during the middle complex. The blue arrow in the first complex points to a putative BT potential between ventricular (V) and atrial (A) electrograms. In the middle complex, the AES is timed such that the BT potential follows the atrial electrogram (blue arrow), and not the ventricular recording (red arrow). Thus, it is not part of the ventricular electrogram.

the earliest ventricular activation site during anterograde BT conduction from the atrial aspect of the annulus can be distant from the atrial insertion site of the BT, and ablation would not then be successful.

Although BT conduction can be eliminated by ablation anywhere between the atrial and ventricular ends, RF applications targeted to the atrial end (site of earliest atrial activation during retrograde BT conduction) or ventricular end (site of earliest ventricular activation during anterograde BT conduction) can occasionally fail. This observation suggests that the recording range of the 4-mm electrode (unipolar or bipolar configuration) commonly used for RF ablation is greater than the RF lesion radius.

Criteria of successful ablation sites during anterograde or retrograde activation mapping of BTs are presented in Table 18-10 (and see Figs. 18-36 and 18-37).

Ablation Technique: General Considerations

Some investigators have advocated a simplified approach to ablation using one or two catheters. Although often successful, 10% of patients with preexcitation have multiple arrhythmias, and 10% to 20% of such patients have multiple BTs that can result in a very complex procedure. Because it is difficult to know beforehand in any given patient whether the procedure will be straightforward or complex, the single-catheter approach to ablation of arrhythmias should be discouraged.

For most free wall BTs, complete bidirectional block can be achieved with a conventional 4-mm-tip ablation catheter, using a power setting of 50 W and targeting a temperature of 60°C. If BT conduction block is transient, permanent BT block can usually be obtained with better and more consistent contact at the same site. It is rare that an 8-mm- or irrigated-tip ablation catheter is necessary, except when ablating in small branches of the CS, at which time irrigated-tip catheters can be helpful, because power delivery with a standard 4-mm electrode is limited because of less passive cooling in small vessels.

RADIOFREQUENCY ENERGY DELIVERY

A temperature of 55°C to 60°C should be sought. Transient loss of BT function is seen at roughly 50°C, and permanent loss of function occurs at 60°C. Therefore, sites with favorable electrogram

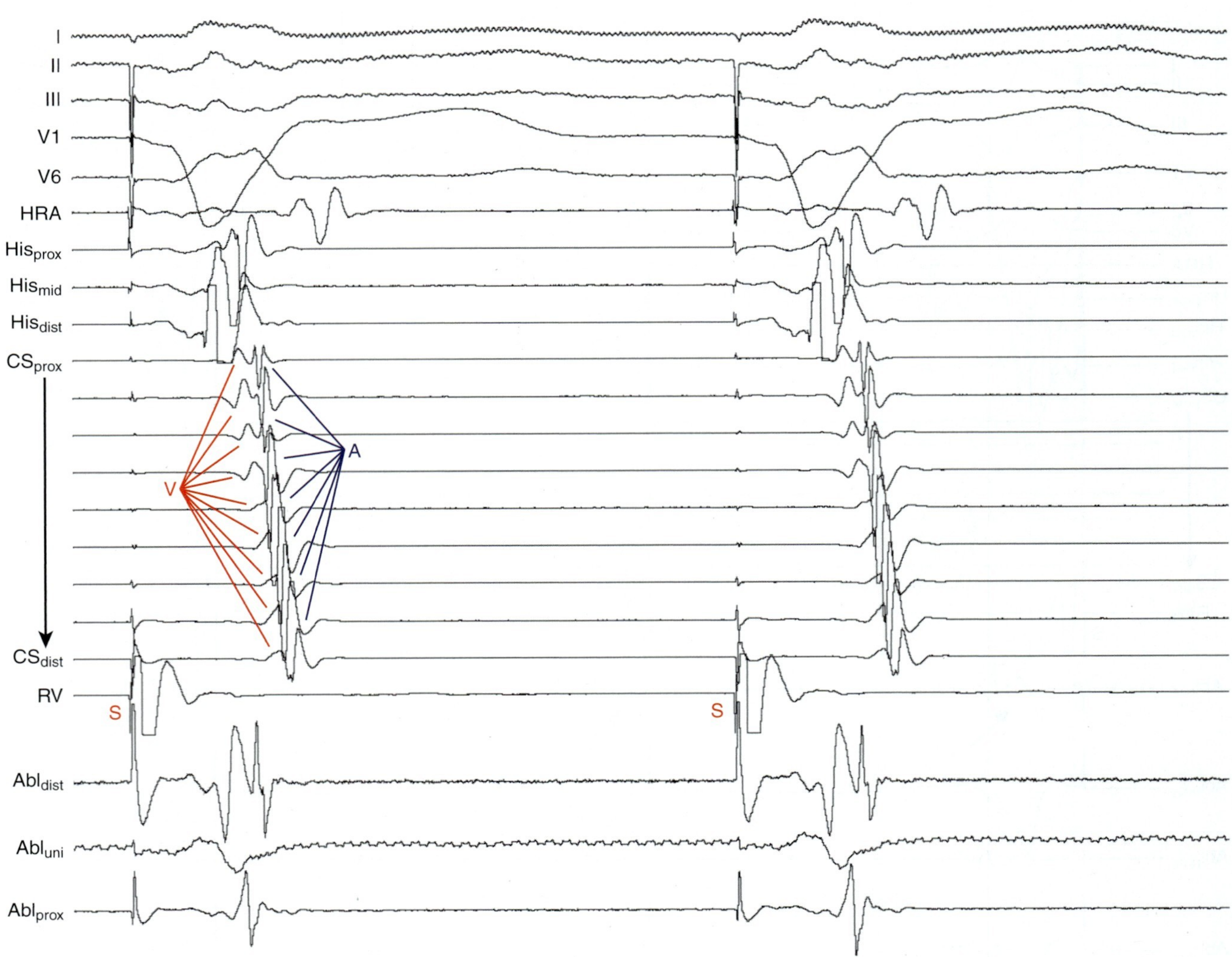

FIGURE 18-42 Two ventricular paced complexes with retrograde conduction are shown. Ventricular (V) and atrial (A) recordings are as designated by lines. Of the recordings indicated, the earliest atrial electrogram is at CS_{prox} (proximal coronary sinus), whereas the shortest local VA interval is far more distal in the coronary sinus recordings; in fact, in CS_{dist} (distal coronary sinus), the VA interval is negative.

characteristics should not be abandoned until a temperature higher than 50°C to 55°C is reached. Conversely, repeated energy applications at the same location after achieving a temperature of 55°C or higher are unlikely to succeed.[47]

Loss of BT conduction is expected within 1 to 6 seconds of RF application (once the target temperature and power delivery have been reached) for most successful lesions. If no effect is seen after 15 seconds of RF delivery, energy delivery should be discontinued because it is unlikely to be beneficial, and mapping criteria and catheter contact should be reexamined. If BT conduction is eliminated during the application, RF delivery should be continued for up to 60 seconds. BT conduction may be eliminated in one direction only (most typically loss of anterograde but persistence of retrograde conduction). Thus, testing for conduction in each direction is mandatory after what appears to be a successful RF application.

If preexcitation is present, ablation should be performed during NSR or, preferably, atrial pacing. For concealed BTs, RF energy is delivered during ventricular pacing, which usually allows for detection of an altered retrograde atrial activation sequence. RF energy delivery during AVRT should be avoided because of potential catheter dislodgment from its critical position on abrupt tachycardia termination. This event can be associated with transient loss of conduction over the BT for a variable period of time without resulting in permanent damage to the BT caused by premature interruption of the RF application. Occasionally, BT conduction may resume hours to days after the procedure; therefore, one may not find a suitable target to complete the RF lesion if not addressed adequately during the initial attempt. Ablation during continuous pacing prevents this problem. For incessant AVRT, energy may be delivered during ventricular pacing entraining the tachycardia. Also, the use of an electroanatomical mapping system can obviate this problem by tagging the initial site of ablation, allowing precise return to that site.[47]

If BT function is not eliminated at a site with apparent favorable electrographic features, catheter contact with the tissue may be inadequate. Adequacy of catheter contact can be verified by evaluating the electrode temperature, catheter stability on fluoroscopy, electrogram stability, and ST elevation on the unipolar electrogram (Fig. 18-44). If the electrode temperature is consistently more than 50°C with more than 25 W of energy delivered to the tissue during the RF application, good catheter contact is likely; however, if electrode temperature reaches more than 50°C but with very low power (<10 W), coagulum may have formed at the catheter tip. Also, catheter "shimmering" on fluoroscopy suggests poor contact. Similarly, changing electrographic amplitudes before or during ablation suggest inadequate catheter contact. Furthermore, ablation-related injury usually yields ST elevation on the unipolar electrogram; if absent, inadequate tissue heating is likely.[47]

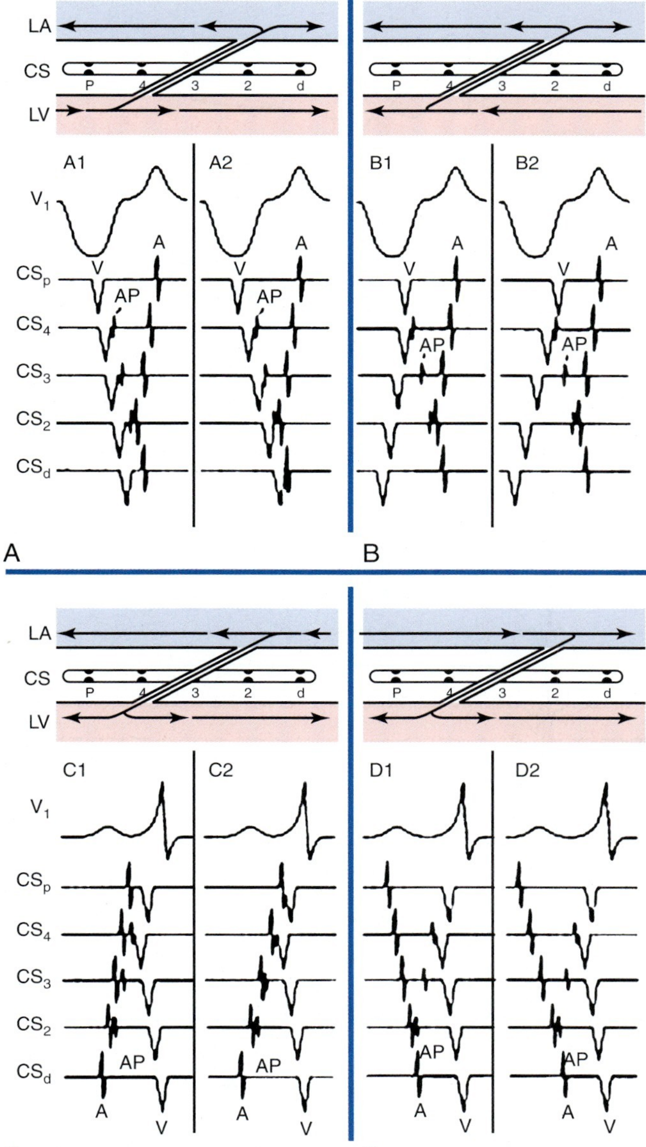

FIGURE 18-43 Schematic representation of anterograde and retrograde activation of a left free wall bypass tract. The oblique course illustrates change in electrogram timing with the reversal of the paced ventricular wavefront (**A** and **B**) and reversal of the paced atrial wavefront (**C** and **D**). AP = accessory pathway potential; p = proximal; d = distal. *(From Otomo K, Gonzalez MD, Beckman KJ, et al: Reversing the direction of paced ventricular and atrial wavefronts reveals an oblique course in accessory AV pathways and improves localization for catheter ablation, Circulation 104:550, 2001.)*

TABLE 18-10 Electrophysiological Criteria of Successful Bypass Tract Ablation Sites

Criteria of Successful Ablation Sites during Anterograde Activation Mapping

- Stable catheter position, as confirmed fluoroscopically and by observing a stable electrogram (<10% change in amplitude in atrial and ventricular electrograms over 5-10 beats).
- Atrial electrogram amplitude >0.4 mV, or A/V ratio >0. Both atrial and ventricular electrogram components should be recorded from the ablation (tip) electrode. When ablating from the atrial aspect of the annulus, the atrial electrogram is usually equal to or larger than the ventricular electrogram. Sometimes, the two can merge and it may be difficult to determine whether both components are present. Rapid atrial or ventricular pacing resulting in block in the BT can help eliminate ventricular or atrial electrogram (respectively) so that the exact morphology of the other component can be visualized.
- Local AV interval on the ablation catheter is usually short (25-50 msec, except for previously damaged, slowly conducting, oblique, or epicardial BTs).
- The local ventricular electrogram on the ablation catheter should precede the onset of the delta wave on the ECG by a mean of 0-10 msec for left-sided BTs and 10-30 msec for right-sided BTs (the local ventricular electrogram is measured from the peak of the bipolar electrogram or the maximal dV/dT in the unipolar electrogram).
- QS (or, less preferably, rS) morphology of the unipolar electrogram. Right-sided BTs usually have unipolar recordings that show more pronounced (rapid and deeper) QS configuration than left-sided BTs.
- Continuous electrical activity (defined as isoelectric interval of <5 msec between ventricular and atrial electrograms).
- Presence of BT potential.

Criteria of Successful Ablation Sites during Retrograde Activation Mapping

- Stable catheter position, as confirmed fluoroscopically and by observing a stable electrogram (<10% change in amplitude in atrial and ventricular electrograms over 5-10 beats).
- Local VA interval during retrograde activation of the BT is short (25-50 msec, except for previously damaged, slowly conducting, oblique, or epicardial BTs), usually resulting in inscription of the atrial electrogram on the ascending portion of the terminal ventricular electrogram. The "pseudo-disappearance" of the atrial electrogram within the terminal portion of the ventricular electrogram (forming a W sign) during orthodromic AVRT is a manifestation of an extremely short local VA interval, which correlates with successful ablation sites.
- Surface QRS to local atrial electrogram interval ≤70 msec (during orthodromic AVRT).
- The local VA interval remains constant regardless of which direction the ventricular wavefront engaging the BT is traveling (i.e., despite pacing from different ventricular sites). If one uses the ventricular approach to ablate a concealed BT, the ventricular insertion site can be identified as one that maintains a constant local VA interval, despite differences in direction of activation to the ventricular site.
- Continuous electrical activity (defined as isoelectric interval <5 msec between ventricular and atrial electrograms).
- Presence of BT potential.

A/V = atrium to ventricle; AVRT = atrioventricular reentrant tachycardia; BT = bypass tract; VA = ventriculoatrial.

Ablation of Left Free Wall Bypass Tracts

ANATOMICAL CONSIDERATIONS

Although the atrial insertion of the BT is typically discrete in size (1 to 3 mm) and close to the mitral annulus, the ventricular insertion site tends to ramify over the region of tissue and can be displaced a small distance away from the mitral annulus, toward the ventricular apex.[48] Additionally, most left free wall BTs cross the mitral annulus obliquely, with the atrial insertion typically 4 to 30 mm proximal (posterior) to the more distal (anterior) ventricular insertion site (as mapped from within the CS).[6]

Conduction at the insertion sites of the BT is markedly anisotropic because of almost horizontal orientation of the atrial and ventricular fibers as they insert into the mitral annulus. In addition, the atrial fibers run parallel to the annulus, giving rise to rapid conduction away from the insertion site, parallel to the annulus, and slow conduction to the free wall of the atrium, perpendicular to the annulus.

Although the CS is useful as a guide for mapping the mitral annulus in the left anterior oblique (LAO) fluoroscopy view, it has a variable relationship to the mitral annulus. The CS lies 2 cm superior to the annulus as it empties into the RA. Anterolaterally, the CS frequently overrides the LV. Thus, depending on the distance from the ostium, the CS can lie above the mitral annulus and be associated with the left atrium (LA), or can cross over the LV side of the mitral annulus. Therefore, electrograms recorded from the CS can only provide a reference for atrial and/or ventricular insertion sites of the BT and can only be used to guide the ablation catheter to areas in which more detailed mapping needs to be performed.[48]

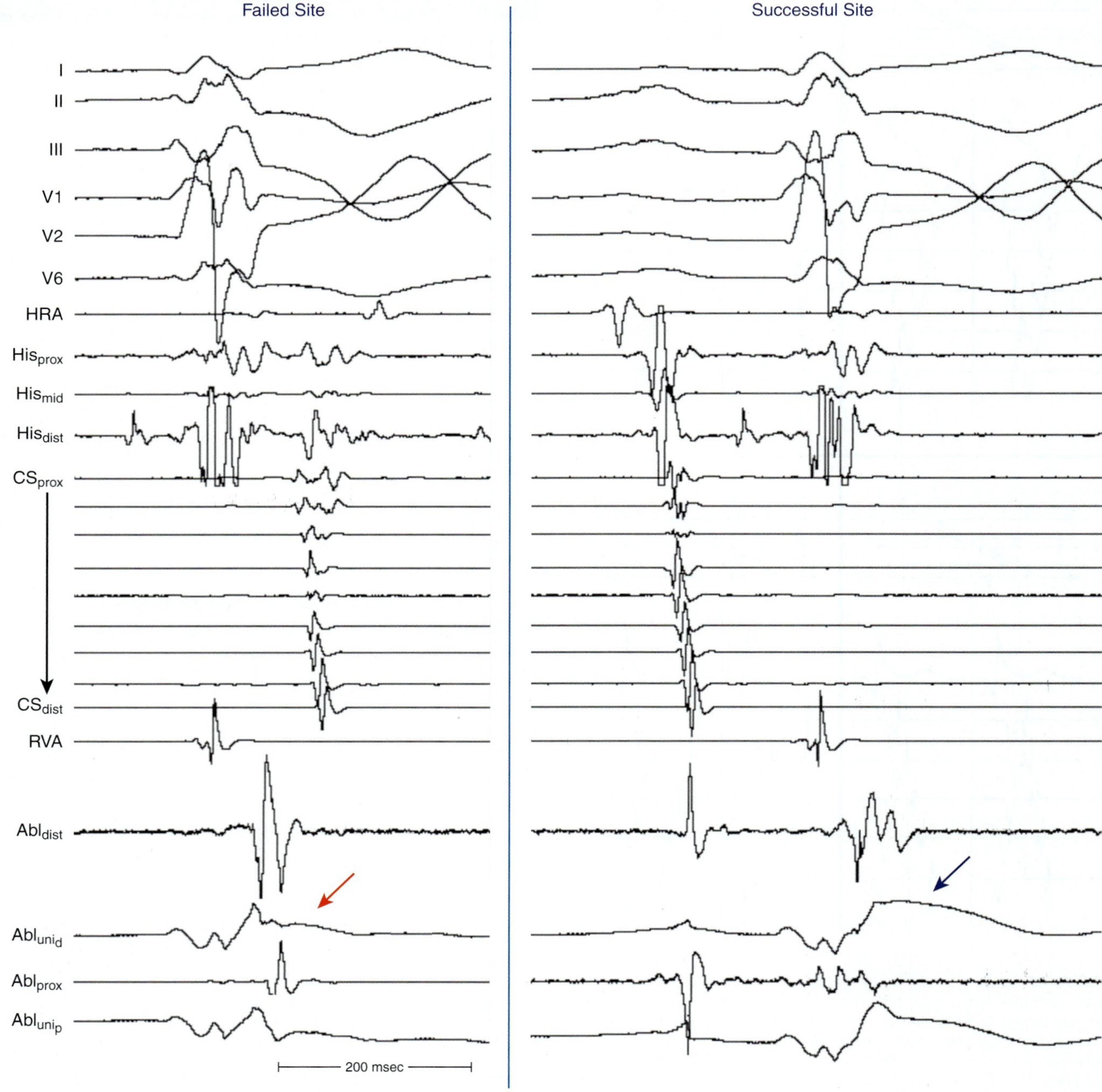

FIGURE 18-44 Effect of ablation on unipolar ST segment. On the **left** ("Failed Site"), recordings during orthodromic atrioventricular reentrant tachycardia are shown following an unsuccessful ablation attempt. The distal ablation unipolar (Abl_{unid}) recording shows minimal, if any, ST segment shift in the ventricular recording (red arrow). On the **right** ("Successful Site"), a single complex of sinus rhythm is shown with significant ST elevation (blue arrow), indicating injury has occurred at that site.

TECHNICAL CONSIDERATIONS

TRANSAORTIC (RETROGRADE) APPROACH. The right femoral artery is the most commonly used access for the transaortic approach. A long vascular sheath may provide added catheter stability, although with a possibly increased risk of thromboembolism. Anticoagulation is started before the LV is accessed (with heparin, 5000 U IV bolus, followed by 1000 U/hr infusion), to maintain the activated clotting time (ACT) between 250 and 300 seconds. The ablation catheter is advanced to the descending aorta and, in this position, a tight **J** curve is formed with the catheter tip before passage to the aortic root to minimize catheter manipulation in the arch. In the right anterior oblique (RAO) fluoroscopy view, the curved catheter is advanced through the aortic valve with the J curve opening to the right, so the catheter passes into the LV oriented anterolaterally. The straight catheter tip must never be used to cross the aortic valve, because of the risk of leaflet perforation. Once in the LV, and while maintaining a tight curve, the catheter is rotated counterclockwise and withdrawn in the LA as the tip turns posteriorly. By opening the **J** curve slightly, the tip can easily map the mitral annulus; clockwise torque moves the tip anteriorly (distally along the CS), and counterclockwise torque returns the tip posteriorly (proximally along the CS). Alternatively, after crossing the aortic valve, the catheter can be straightened and steered directly under the mitral annulus to the BT location or withdrawn in the LV outflow tract, rotated posteriorly with a slight curve, and then advanced under the posterior mitral annulus for left paraseptal or posterior BTs. When the ablation catheter is approximated along the mitral annulus, the catheter tip is simultaneously withdrawn and straightened slightly to slip under the annulus for fine manipulation. For left lateral and anterior BTs, extended-reach catheters may be required.[48]

Catheter positions beneath the annulus between the ventricular myocardium and mitral leaflet are most stable for ablation of the BT ventricular insertion, but manipulation can be constrained by the chordae. Catheter positions above or along the annulus provide more freedom to map along the mitral annulus but are sometimes too unstable for successful energy delivery. Initial mapping is performed with the ablation electrode on the annulus. From this general area, the catheter is then positioned beneath the mitral annulus for more precise mapping. Catheter tip positions beneath the mitral annulus are suggested by proximity to the CS catheter, motion concomitant with the CS catheter, and an A/V electrogram ratio of less than 1.

Because the transaortic approach targets the ventricular insertion site of the BT, it is best suited for mapping anterograde BT activation (i.e., preexcitation). Mapping retrograde activation from the subannular position is more difficult than for anterograde mapping because of obscuration of the low-amplitude atrial electrogram following the large ventricular electrogram.

Although BT locations are commonly defined by mapping along the CS catheter, this only approximates localization of the subannular ablation site because of the oblique course of left free wall BTs, displacement of the CS above the mitral annulus, variable basilar-apical ventricular insertion of the BT, and BT location beyond the distal CS electrode.

TRANSSEPTAL APPROACH. Transseptal and transaortic approaches are equally effective for ablation of left free wall BTs.[49] However, the transseptal approach is primarily used for mapping of the BT atrial insertion site during retrograde BT conduction (orthodromic AVRT or ventricular pacing). On the other hand, ventricular mapping of manifest BTs (during preexcitation) using the transseptal approach is limited.[47]

The transseptal approach has several advantages over the transaortic approach.[49] The transseptal approach provides better access to far lateral and anterolateral BT locations, easier catheter maneuverability in the LA, and less risk of coronary injury. Additionally, no arterial access is required with the transseptal approach, and vascular recovery is therefore shorter. However, the transseptal approach provides less catheter stability and is associated with a higher risk of cardiac perforation and air embolism. Furthermore, the transseptal approach entails higher cost if intracardiac echocardiography is used.[49]

Before introducing the standard transseptal sheath, its curvature can be modified according to BT location. The curve is left intact for left posterior BTs. The sheath is progressively withdrawn toward the RA for lateral BT locations, and it is almost entirely withdrawn toward the RA for anterior BTs. Alternatively, preformed or deflectable sheaths may be used. Ablation catheters with bidirectional asymmetric deflections also can be of value.

Once the ablation catheter is positioned on the mitral annulus in a 30-degree RAO view, mapping is performed in the LAO view. In the absence of preformed septal sheaths, gentle clockwise torque is needed to maintain the catheter on the posterior mitral annulus. No torque is needed for lateral positions. As the catheter is moved anteriorly, counterclockwise torque is necessary to keep the catheter tip on the annulus. In the anterior positions, the catheter tip can dislodge into the LA appendage or LV, and attention to intracardiac electrograms is necessary when mapping anterior regions, because the CS catheter rarely provides an accurate fluoroscopic reference in this setting. The goal is to maintain the catheter tip on the atrial aspect of the mitral annulus, so that the mitral annulus can be easily mapped by advancing and withdrawing the catheter, causing it to slide along the mitral annulus freely in parallel to the CS catheter. Advancing the catheter moves the tip posteriorly; withdrawing it moves the tip anteriorly. The ventricular aspect of the mitral annulus can be mapped by passing the catheter tip across the mitral valve and deflecting the tip toward the annulus.

The transseptal approach facilitates mapping of the atrial aspect of the mitral annulus. Catheter position on the atrial aspect of the annulus can be verified by recording a bipolar A/V electrogram amplitude ratio of greater than 1, and a unipolar electrogram PR segment displacement from baseline without ST segment displacement. The stability of the catheter can be assessed by PR segment elevation (confirming good atrial tissue contact), consistent local electrographic amplitudes, and concordant motion of the CS and ablation catheters.

Because of the mobility of the ablation catheter and the electrode orientation parallel with atrial activation along the mitral annulus, a unique vectorial mapping technique is possible with the transseptal approach. As noted, using the unfiltered bipolar electrogram with the electrodes oriented parallel to the axis of the mitral annulus, the BT atrial insertion can be identified as the site at which the polarity of the atrial potential reverses.

Ablation of Right Free Wall Bypass Tracts

ANATOMICAL CONSIDERATIONS

Unique features of the tricuspid annulus and important anatomic differences as compared with the mitral annulus have often rendered ablation of right-sided BTs more challenging than that of left free wall BTs. Additionally, transient interruption of BT conduction during RF delivery, with subsequent resumption of conduction within seconds or minutes, and recurrence rates over the first few weeks after initially successful BT ablation, are more common with right-sided BTs compared with left-sided BTs.

A significantly larger endocardial area is present along the tricuspid ring because of the larger circumference compared with the mitral ring (12 versus 10 cm). Additionally, BTs may occur anywhere around the tricuspid annulus whereas the mitral ring has an area of fibrous continuity with the left and posterior leaflets of the aortic valve (the aortomitral continuity) where BTs are rarely found. Despite these facts, right-sided BTs are much less common than left-sided BTs (12% versus 59%).

In contrast to the mitral valve, which attaches to its fibrous annulus at a right angle, the tricuspid valve attaches to its annulus at an acute angle oriented toward the RV, making it more difficult to wedge an ablation catheter underneath the tricuspid valve. Additionally, unlike left parietal AV BTs, which tend to pass close to the hinge line of the mitral valve, the AV groove between the RA and RV is much deeper than on the left side. The deep groove can allow the RA wall to fold over onto the RV wall, and the BT muscle bundles can cross at any depth.[4] Hence, the right-sided BTs can be somewhat removed from the tricuspid annulus. In fact, atrial insertion of the BT can be as far as 1 cm away from the annulus in the folded-over atrial sac. The folded-over atrium and the bizarre angle required for mapping of the inferior and posterolateral aspect of the RA by a catheter passed through the RA from the inferior vena cava (IVC) can make it difficult to achieve a stable catheter position at the tricuspid annulus because of a tendency of the catheter to fall into the folded-over sac. Thus, sometimes the superior vena cava (SVC) approach is required to allow full exploration of the folded-over atrial sac and the inferior-inferolateral positions around the tricuspid annulus. The standard IVC approach, however, is usually adequate to map the superior aspects of the tricuspid annulus. If the IVC approach is used, a guiding sheath can be especially helpful for better catheter stability and tissue contact. The use of a multipolar (Halo) catheter positioned around the tricuspid annulus can provide good regional localization to guide the ablation catheter.

Furthermore, closely adjacent but anatomically discrete sites of catheter ablation can be necessary to eliminate anterograde and retrograde BT conduction in up to 10% of patients—the incidence is highest (18.6%) with right free wall BTs. The explanation for this phenomenon is not clear but probably relates to the complexity of fiber orientation, possibly branching over 1 to 2 cm along the annulus. This factor emphasizes the importance of identifying and targeting both the atrial and the ventricular BT insertion sites.[50] Right-sided

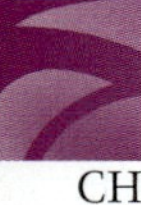

AV BTs are associated with higher incidences of anatomic variations and congenital abnormalities along the tricuspid annulus. Ebstein anomaly is an abnormality of the tricuspid valve in which the septal leaflet and often the posterior leaflet are displaced a variable distance into the RV and the anterior leaflet is usually malformed, excessively large, and abnormally attached or adherent to the RV free wall. Thus, a portion of the RV is "atrialized" in that it is located on the atrial side of the tricuspid valve, and the remaining functional RV is small. The atrialized portion of the RV is morphologically and electrically ventricular but functionally atrial. Right-sided BTs have been reported in 10% to 30% of patients with Ebstein anomaly, and they often are multiple. The BTs bridge the true anatomical tricuspid annulus, regardless of where the valve is located, and ablation can be challenging as electrical signals recorded from the atrialized portion of the RV can be complex and fractionated, and identification of the true AV groove, along which BTs are targeted, can be difficult. Coronary angiography or insertion of a thin multielectrode catheter in the right coronary artery may be necessary to help identify the true AV groove. Ablation is usually accomplished at the true tricuspid annulus, above the displaced valve leaflet, although some patients may undergo successful ablation from the ventricular side of the tricuspid annulus (but still above the valve leaflet).[50]

TECHNICAL CONSIDERATIONS

Characteristics of successful ablation sites for right-sided BTs include the following: the local AV interval is shorter than that for BTs elsewhere, the local ventricular electrogram precedes the onset of the delta wave by an interval longer than that for BTs elsewhere (18 ± 10 milliseconds for right-sided BTs versus 0 ± 5 milliseconds for left-sided BTs), and the unipolar recording shows more pronounced (rapid and deeper) QS configuration.

Most commonly, ablation of the BT is approached from the atrial aspect. The optimal site of ablation is the earliest atrial activation site during retrograde BT conduction (during orthodromic AVRT or ventricular pacing), preferably with a BT potential present. The earliest site of atrial activation is identified using a roving catheter or a multipolar (Halo) catheter along the tricuspid annulus. If mapping is performed during ventricular pacing, conduction over both the BT and AVN can occur, resulting in atrial fusion, which can interfere with localization of the BT. Ventricular pacing performed close to the BT ventricular insertion site can accentuate atrial activation over the BT.[50]

Occasionally, the BT may be better approached from the ventricular side. Ventricular activation mapping is performed during preexcited NSR, atrial pacing, preexcited SVT, or antidromic AVRT.[50] The site of the earliest ventricular activation during preexcitation, preferably with a BT potential present, would be the optimal site. The earliest onset of ventricular activation recorded on the ablation catheter (using unipolar or bipolar electrograms) should precede the onset of the delta wave by at least 10 to 25 milliseconds. For concealed BTs, the ventricular insertion site cannot be determined by ventricular activation mapping because of the lack of preexcitation. In this setting, recording of a BT potential can be especially useful to help guide ablation.

The tricuspid annulus is usually mapped in the LAO fluoroscopy view. The right posterior, posterolateral, and lateral regions are usually best mapped from the IVC approach. The right anterior and anterolateral regions can also often be ablated using the IVC approach, but the SVC approach can offer more stable and better catheter-tissue contact in these areas. The catheter can be prolapsed across the tricuspid valve to help stabilize the tip on the tricuspid annulus. In the LAO view, the HB is located at about 1 o'clock and the CS at 5 o'clock; right free wall BTs span from approximately 6 to 12 o'clock. Right anterior BTs are at the most superior aspect of the tricuspid annulus, right superoparaseptal BTs are located near the HB catheter, and right posterior free wall BTs are located at the most posterior aspect of the tricuspid annulus, whereas right posteroseptal BTs are located near the CS.[50] Although the location of the mitral annulus is reasonably indicated by the CS catheter, the location of the tricuspid annulus is not as easily discerned because there is no analogous venous structure to mark with a catheter. Furthermore, because the mitral and tricuspid annuli are not always in the same plane, the CS catheter is only a rough guide to the location of the tricuspid annulus in the RAO view.

Attempts at providing an endocardial reference catheter along the tricuspid annulus have been made using a 20-pole Halo catheter. This approach has had limited success, as the catheter often does not position directly on the AV groove. Introducing the Halo catheter through a preformed sheath can provide better catheter stability along the tricuspid annulus. Occasionally, a fine angioplasty wire may be passed into the right coronary artery to delineate the location of the tricuspid annulus. The latter approach, however, has not been widely adopted, possibly in part because of concerns of prolonged instrumentation of the right coronary artery during the procedure. Another approach is to create a three-dimensional electroanatomical map (EnSite-NavX; St. Jude Medical, St. Paul, Minn.) of the right coronary artery. After right coronary artery angiography, a 2.3 French (Fr) octapolar microcatheter (Cardima Inc., Fresno, Calif.) is inserted in the right coronary artery. The EnSite NavX system is used because it is nonproprietary with respect to catheter recognition. Mapping and acquisition of the bipolar electrograms recorded by the microcatheter are performed during anterograde or retrograde BT conduction. This map allows for early removal of the catheter from the coronary artery while continuously displaying electroanatomic information to assist with mapping of the BT.[51]

To target the ventricular aspect of the tricuspid annulus, the catheter is introduced across the tricuspid valve and looped back on itself in the RV underneath the valve until a small atrial electrogram and a larger ventricular electrogram are recorded, confirming adequate proximity to the tricuspid annulus. A long sheath may be used to stabilize the body of the catheter and direct the catheter to several different locations along the tricuspid annulus.

RF energy may be delivered during NSR, atrial pacing, or ventricular pacing. Delivery during AVRT can result in sudden termination of the SVT, which can cause dislodgment of the ablation catheter, resulting in an inadequate RF application. Therefore, if retrograde mapping during orthodromic AVRT is used to determine the optimal atrial ablation site, especially for concealed BTs, it is preferable to entrain the orthodromic AVRT with ventricular pacing at a slightly shorter CL so that block in the BT and termination of the SVT during RF energy delivery will be followed by ventricular pacing at a rate similar to that of the SVT, minimizing catheter movement. If BT function does not disappear despite good catheter stability, adequate catheter-tissue contact, and good temperature rise (>50°C), the catheter is probably located at the wrong site. Although transient interruption of BT conduction during RF delivery, with subsequent reappearance of conduction within seconds or minutes after energy delivery is completed, is more common with right than left free wall BTs, the use of multisite "insurance lesions" is discouraged, and the use of one or two ablation sites should be the goal, which requires careful mapping to achieve.

Three-dimensional electroanatomical mapping can help ablation of right-sided BTs, and is especially useful in the presence of multiple BTs or complicated anatomy. An electroanatomical color-coded activation map along the tricuspid annulus can be constructed, either along the atrial side, during orthodromic AVRT or ventricular pacing, or along the ventricular side, during anterograde preexcitation. Sites of interest can be tagged for further reference, so that the ablation catheter can be returned to any of them with precision. Information with regard to catheter stability and movement can also be provided.

Ablation of Posteroseptal (Inferoparaseptal) Bypass Tracts

ANATOMICAL CONSIDERATIONS

The posteroseptal region corresponds to a complex anatomic region where the four cardiac chambers reach their maximal proximity posteriorly (i.e., the crux), and incorporates the converging segments of the AV rings as well as the CS with its proximal branches. The posteroseptal region spans the area between the central fibrous body (superiorly), the interventricular septum (anteriorly), the right posterior paraseptal (right lateral border), and the left posterior paraseptal (left lateral border) regions. Posteroseptal BTs may be located in a relatively wide area either at an epicardial site around the proximal CS or the middle cardiac vein or at an endocardial site along the tricuspid ring in the immediate vicinity of the CS os or along the posteromedial ventricular aspect of the mitral annulus. Because the posteroseptal region is actually posterior to the septum and not a septal structure, posteroseptal BTs are more appropriately referred to as right- or left-sided inferoparaseptal or posterior paraseptal BTs.[52,53]

Because the interatrial sulcus is displaced to the far left of the interventricular sulcus, and because the AV valves are not isoplanar (the attachment of the septal leaflet of the tricuspid valve into the most anterior part of the central fibrous body is displaced a few millimeters apically relative to the attachment of the septal leaflet of the mitral valve), the true septal part of the AV junction (the RA-LV sulcus) actually separates the inferomedial RA from the posterior superior process of the LV. The undersurface of the CS is about 1 cm above the mitral annulus, and the CS os abuts the superior margin of the RA-LV sulcus.[48] The right margin of the posteroseptal space includes the area surrounding the CS os and the inferior portion of the triangle of Koch; the left margin (the junction of the posterior septum and left free wall) lies as far as 2 to 3 cm from the CS os. The epicardial dimension of the posteroseptal space at the level of the valve annuli extends a mean of 3.4 ± 0.5 cm. BTs can be located anywhere within this relatively large space or in the adjacent right or left free walls. BTs located close to the edges of the septum can be ablated from the adjacent atrial or ventricular cavity, but BTs located deep within the posteroseptal space or near the epicardial aspect require ablation from within the CS or cardiac veins. BTs located in the proximal 1.5 cm of the CS are almost always in the posterior septum. Those located between 1.5 and 3 cm from the CS os can be in the left free wall or posterior septum, and those located more than 3 cm from the CS os are almost invariably in the left free wall.[48] Most posteroseptal BTs are believed to be RA-to-LV BTs, with the ventricular insertion attaching onto the posterior superior process of the LV, but some posteroseptal BTs are considered to be left paraseptal (connecting the LA to the LV) or right paraseptal (connecting the RA to the RV).[53-55]

Although epicardial BTs can be found at any location, they are most common in the posteroseptal and left posterior paraseptal regions.[49] Approximately 20% of all posteroseptal BTs and 40% of those in patients referred after a failed ablation procedure are epicardial. One hypothesis for this predilection is that those BTs connect the myocardial coat of the CS, which is connected anatomically and electrically to both the RA and LA, and to the LV (see later discussion).

TECHNICAL CONSIDERATIONS

Ablation of posteroseptal BTs usually is more difficult than other BT locations because of the complexity of the anatomical structures involved.[48] Mapping and ablation may be required at either the mitral or the tricuspid annulus, or inside the CS or its proximal branches. Therefore, the ability to discriminate—without instrumentation of the left heart—BTs amenable to ablation from the right side (on the tricuspid ring or inside the coronary venous system) from those requiring ablation on the mitral ring can potentially have great impact on procedure outcome and safety by reducing procedural and fluoroscopy times, reducing the number of unsuccessful RF applications, as well as avoiding unnecessary left atrial access and its potential complications.[54,55]

Generally, a right-sided endocardial approach is initially adopted for mapping and ablation of BTs in the posteroseptal region. The posteroseptal tricuspid annulus, including the CS os and its most proximal part, and inferomedial RA are carefully mapped. If the ablation site fails or no appropriate ablation site can be obtained, the left posteroseptal area is mapped (with a transaortic or transseptal approach, as described for left-sided BTs). A primary left-sided approach can also be considered if multiple ECG and EP features suggest a left-sided location of the BT. If endocardial mapping fails, an epicardial approach via the CS is then considered (see later).

Prediction of the site of successful ablation of posteroseptal BTs into either the right or the left heart has been attempted by the analysis of the preexcitation pattern on the surface ECG. In addition to the obvious limitation of the surface ECG in the case of concealed BTs (47.5% in a recent report), reports on the accuracy of surface ECG features to differentiate BTs associated with the three compartments of the inferior paraseptal space have been conflicting.

Previous reports found that, in patients with preexcitation, a negative delta wave polarity in lead V_1 and positive polarity in lead V_2 favors right-sided localization of a posteroseptal BT, whereas left posteroseptal BTs were associated with biphasic or positive delta wave polarity in leads V_1 and V_2. Recent reports, however, have questioned the predictive value for such a criterion. The vast majority of posteroseptal BTs can be successfully ablated at the tricuspid annulus or within the proximal CS although the delta wave polarity on the ECG suggests a left ventricular origin. This phenomenon can be explained by the fact that many posteroseptal BTs are "RA-to-LV" fibers and an RA approach would suffice even though the delta wave polarity in lead V_1 is suggestive of left posteroseptal BTs.[54,55]

On the other hand, the R/S ratio in lead V_1 was found to be an accurate ECG parameter to predict the site of successful posteroseptal BT ablation. This finding might be related to the observation that the ventricular insertion of "RA-to-LV" posteroseptal BTs attaches onto the posterosuperior process of the LV, resulting in earlier activation of the posterobasal LV with positive delta wave and predominantly negative QRS morphology (R/S ratio <1) in lead V_1. In contrast, the ventricular insertion of "LA-to-LV" BTs attaches to the posteromedial aspect of the mitral annulus, resulting in a positive delta wave and a predominantly positive QRS morphology (R/S ratio >1) in lead V_1.[55]

Invasive EP findings also have been used to predict the successful ablation site of manifest or concealed posteroseptal BTs. The prolongation of the VA interval in response to the development of LBBB during orthodromic AVRT has been regarded as suggestive of a left-sided BT. However, many posteroseptal BTs associated with this phenomenon can be ablated from the right side, sometimes even when the prolongation is more than 30 milliseconds.[54]

Additionally, measurement of the ΔVA interval during orthodromic AVRT (the difference in VA intervals measured at the HB catheter and the site of earliest atrial activation in the CS) was found to be useful for predicting the successful approach. A ΔVA interval greater than or equal to 25 milliseconds suggests a left endocardial BT, whereas a ΔVA interval less than 25 milliseconds favors a right endocardial BT. This suggests that atrial activation is relatively early in the HB region during retrograde conduction through both right endocardial and CS-associated BTs, compared with left endocardial ones.[54]

Furthermore, a previous report found that a VA interval less than 50 milliseconds recorded at the left posteroseptal region during RV pacing identified 71% of patients with left posteroseptal BTs, with 100% specificity. In patients with a VA interval greater than or equal to 50 milliseconds, a difference in the VA intervals of less than 20 milliseconds recorded at the HB region and left posteroseptal region during RV pacing predicted right posteroseptal BT with a sensitivity of 97%, a specificity of 85%, and a positive predictive value of 91%.[52]

PJRT is usually caused by a slowly conducting BT, commonly located in the posteroseptal region. Although the mere presence of a long-RP AVRT has been suggested to favor a right endocardial BT, in 50% of cases, such BTs can be located in the left posterior or free wall (>4 cm inside the CS). In the remaining 50%, it is located between the base of the pyramidal space formed by the points of pericardial deflection that contact the posterior RA and LA. None have been reported in the anteroseptal region.[54]

An earliest atrial activation during orthodromic AVRT in the middle CS favors a left endocardial ablation site. However, recent studies found that a large proportion (more than one-third) of patients with an earliest site distal at or distal to the mid-CS required ablation inside the CS after a failed left endocardial approach, and 35% of all BTs ablated from the right side produced such an eccentric retrograde atrial activation.[54] Therefore, the ability of the site of earliest atrial activation during AVRT to predict the successful approach seems very limited, mainly because CS-associated BTs can produce a very much eccentric retrograde atrial activation sequence.

"Atrial" electrograms recorded from inside the proximal CS originate not only from LA myocardium, but also from activation of the CS myocardial coat. This results in "fragmented" or double potentials, with a low-amplitude, blunt "far field" LA component and a larger, sharp "near field" signal from the CS musculature. The sequence of LA and CS myocardial coat activation at the earliest "atrial" electrograms in the CS recorded during retrograde BT conduction by a catheter placed inside the CS can guide mapping of these BTs into right- or left-sided compartments of the inferoparaseptal space. An activation wavefront traveling from the posteroseptal RA toward the left (e.g., by pacing posterior to the CS os) will first activate the muscle coat covering the proximal CS, producing a large, sharp signal recorded by the electrodes inside the CS. Discrete connections of the CS musculature with the LA will activate the LA myocardium, producing a lower amplitude, blunt, "far field" signal on the CS electrodes. Thus two-component "fragmented" or double potentials will be recorded in the proximal CS, with the sharp component preceding the blunt signal (sharp/blunt sequence). The same sequence (sharp/blunt) of potentials is expected to happen when a retrogradely conducting right-sided "endocardial" BT first activates RA myocardium as well as when a BT inserts directly into the CS musculature (as is the case with epicardial CS-associated BTs). Contrariwise, when pacing is performed from the lateral LA, the sequence is the opposite (blunt/sharp), with CS musculature activation following activation of LA myocardium. This sequence should be produced if a BT connects to LA myocardium (i.e., left-sided "endocardial" AV BTs), the first signal recorded in the CS being a "far field" potential followed by later activation of the CS musculature resulting in a blunt/sharp sequence of potentials. Different conduction velocities of LA myocardium and CS musculature can cause the sequence of potentials to change farther away from the insertion site of the BT, explaining the importance of analyzing the electrograms recorded at the earliest site. The recording of double potentials inside the CS has been found to be especially common during retrograde conduction through posteroseptal BTs.[54]

Ablation of Superoparaseptal and Midseptal Bypass Tracts

ANATOMICAL CONSIDERATIONS

The midseptum is the only true muscular septal area between the offset attachments of the mitral and tricuspid valves, and it corresponds roughly to the location of the triangle of Koch. The triangle of Koch is bounded by the CS os posteriorly, the tricuspid annulus (the attachment of the septal leaflet of the tricuspid valve) inferiorly, and the tendon of Todaro anteriorly and superiorly. The compact AVN is located anteriorly at its apex, where the tendon of Todaro merges with the central fibrous body. Slightly more anteriorly and superiorly is where the HB penetrates the AV junction through the central fibrous body and posterior aspect of the membranous AV septum (see Fig. 17-1). The triangle of Koch constitutes the RA endocardial surface of the muscular AV septum. BTs with an atrial insertion in the floor of the triangle of Koch, posteroinferior to the compact AVN and HB and above the anterior portion of the CS os, have been labeled as midseptal; these BTs are the only truly septal BTs; hence, they can be referred to simply as septal BTs.[56]

The previously named anteroseptal and posteroseptal areas are not septal but are parts of the parietal AV junction that are anterior and posterior to the true septum. Anterosuperior to the AV septum and compact AVN and HB, the tricuspid annulus diverges laterally away from membranous part of the septum to course along the supraventricular crest of the RV (crista supraventricularis). This muscular structure interposes between the attachments of the leaflets of the tricuspid and pulmonic valves in the roof of the RV. BTs in this area (at the apex of the triangle of Koch) are labeled anteroseptal, but they must be considered "superoparaseptal" right free wall BTs, because anatomically they do not belong to the septum. There is no atrial septum in the region anterior to the HB recording site; the aortic root separates the right and left atrial walls here.[53]

TECHNICAL CONSIDERATIONS

BTs are classified as superoparaseptal if the BT potential and His potential are simultaneously recorded from the diagnostic catheter placed at the HB region. The precise location of the BT is verified by mapping this space in a 30-degree LAO fluoroscopy view using the ablation catheter, advanced via the right internal jugular vein or IVC. The use of a long vascular sheath may help stabilize the catheter tip during mapping and ablation in the superoparaseptal region. The optimal site of ablation is one from which the atrial and ventricular electrograms are recorded in conjunction with a BT potential, but with no or only a tiny His potential (<0.1 mV).[57] Preferably, the ventricular insertion site of the BT is targeted with ablation to minimize the risk of damage to the AVN. Rarely, ablation is required in the presence of a marked (>0.1 mV) His potential recorded through the ablation catheter (true para-Hisian BTs).

BTs are classified as midseptal if ablation is achieved through the mapping-ablation catheter located in an area bounded superiorly by the electrode recording the His potential, and posteroinferiorly by the CS os, as marked by the vortex of curvature in the CS catheter. The optimal site of ablation for a right midseptal BT is one from which atrial and ventricular electrograms are recorded simultaneously with a BT potential in between. Ablation is first attempted from the right side. If it is ineffective or early recurrence occurs after termination of RF application, then the left-sided approach is attempted. The combination of a negative delta wave in lead V_1 and R-S transition in leads V_3-V_4 suggests right-sided midseptal BT, whereas a biphasic delta wave in lead V_1 and earlier QRS transition (in leads V_1-V_2) suggest a left-sided location of the midseptal BT.[58] Midseptal BTs can be differentiated from superoparaseptal and para-Hisian BTs by a negative delta wave in lead III and a biphasic delta wave in lead aVF.[26,57]

Ablation in the region of the triangle of Koch is associated with a 5% incidence of AV block and, to decrease this risk, such BTs should be ablated with the catheter placed on the tricuspid annulus or on the ventricular side of the tricuspid annulus, preferably with the use of lower RF power. Titrated RF energy output can be used for true para-Hisian BTs, starting with 5 W, and increasing by 5 W every 10 seconds of energy application, up to a maximum of 40 W. For other superoparaseptal BTs, ablation can be started at 30 W, targeting a temperature of 50°C to 60°C. During RF ablation within the triangle of Koch, the occurrence of junctional tachycardia is not uncommon and is associated with loss of preexcitation; this should not be misinterpreted as successful ablation leading to continuing RF energy delivery. Instead, overdrive atrial pacing should be performed to monitor AV conduction or RF application should be stopped and other sites sought (Fig. 18-45).[57] RF application should be stopped after 10 to 15 seconds if no block in the BT is achieved to minimize potential damage to the AVN-HB.

For manifest BTs, RF application is performed during NSR or atrial pacing. In the setting of concealed para-Hisian BTs, it is challenging to assess the success of RF application and monitor AV conduction simultaneously, an important parameter when performing RF ablation near the HB. When RF delivery is performed during ventricular

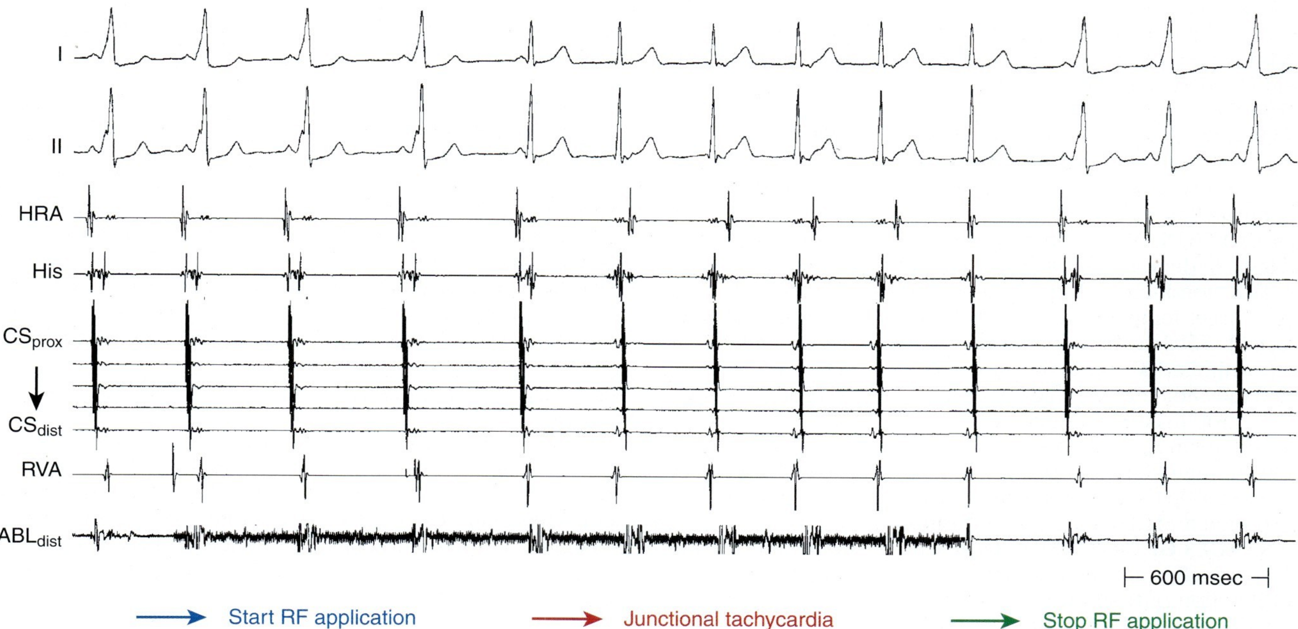

FIGURE 18-45 Junctional tachycardia during radiofrequency (RF) ablation of a superoparaseptal bypass tract. The first few complexes demonstrate normal sinus rhythm with preexcitation. A few seconds after starting RF energy delivery, junctional tachycardia develops, with loss of preexcitation. This prompted immediate termination of RF application, after which preexcitation resumed.

pacing, monitoring the success of RF application is not possible because the retrograde atrial activation sequence during ventricular pacing can be similar with BT and AVN conduction. Although atrial pacing during RF delivery helps monitor AV conduction and override junctional rhythms that may occur during RF delivery, it is not helpful for assessing the efficacy of RF application because the BT is retrograde only. RF delivery during orthodromic AVRT is an option; however, this will certainly have the potential for catheter dislodgment on SVT termination, as stated earlier, and such dislodgment can endanger the AVN-HB. Moreover, application of RF energy during orthodromic AVRT will not allow monitoring of AV conduction. In this setting, monitoring of the mode of termination of orthodromic AVRT during RF delivery is essential. Termination of orthodromic AVRT with an atrial electrogram signifies potential damage to the anterograde limb of the SVT circuit (i.e., the AVN), and therefore RF delivery should be immediately stopped. On the other hand, termination of orthodromic AVRT with a ventricular electrogram suggests successful block in the retrograde limb of the SVT circuit (i.e., the BT), and therefore RF delivery should be continued, with careful monitoring of AV conduction during NSR following termination of the SVT. Another valuable option is RF delivery during atrial-entrained orthodromic AVRT with manifest atrial fusion. This technique enables continuous monitoring of effects of RF application on BT function and also obviates a sudden change in ventricular rate on termination of the SVT. In addition, this technique allows monitoring of AV conduction during RF application once the orthodromic AVRT is terminated, and therefore reduces the risk of damage to the AVN-HB. During successful RF application, termination of orthodromic AVRT will be indicated by transformation from the tachycardia P wave morphology and atrial activation sequence into a fully paced atrial activation sequence at the same rate.

To reduce the risk of AV block, RF delivery should be immediately discontinued when the following occur: (1) the impedance rises suddenly (>10 Ω); (2) the PR interval (during NSR or atrial pacing) prolongs; (3) AV block develops; (4) retrograde conduction block is observed during junctional ectopy; or (5) fast junctional tachycardia (tachycardia CL <350 milliseconds) occurs, which may herald imminent heart block.

CRYOABLATION OF SUPEROPARASEPTAL AND MIDSEPTAL BYPASS TRACTS

Cryothermal ablation of BTs in the superoparaseptal and midseptal areas, both at high risk of complete permanent AV block when standard RF energy is performed, is extremely safe and successful. Cryoablation can also be successfully and safely used to ablate selected cases of epicardial left-sided BTs within the CS, well beyond the middle cardiac vein, once attempts using the transseptal and transaortic approaches have failed. The experience with cryoablation in unselected BTs, however, is more limited and less satisfactory; this is likely related to multiple factors, including the learning curve and the smaller size of the lesion produced by cryoablation. In addition, all the peculiarities of cryothermal energy, which are optimal for septal ablation, are less important or even useless for ablation of BTs located elsewhere.[59,60]

CRYOMAPPING. Cryomapping, or ice mapping, is designed to verify that ablation at the chosen site will have the desired effect (i.e., block in the BT) and to ensure the absence of complications (i.e., AV block). Cryomapping is performed at −30°C in the selected site. At this temperature, the lesion is reversible (for up to 60 seconds) and the catheter is "stuck" to the endocardium in an ice ball that includes the tip of the catheter (cryoadherence). This permits programmed electrical stimulation to test the disappearance of BT conduction during ongoing ablation and also allows ablation to be performed during AVRT without the risk of catheter dislodgment on tachycardia termination.

In the cryomapping mode, the temperature is not allowed to drop below −30°C, and the time of application is limited to 60 seconds. Formation of an ice ball at the catheter tip and adherence to the underlying myocardium are signaled by the appearance of electrical noise recorded from the ablation catheter's distal bipole. Once an ice ball is formed, programmed electrical stimulation is repeated to verify that the BT has been blocked. If cryomapping does not yield the desired result within 30 seconds or results in unintended AV conduction delay or block, cryomapping is interrupted and, after a few seconds, allowing the catheter to thaw and become dislodged from the tissue, the catheter can be moved to a different site and cryomapping repeated. Alternatively, if the test application is unsuccessful, after rewarming, further 30-second applications are tested, decreasing the temperature by 10°C for every step of the application, up to the last application at −70°C. This is because the amount of cryothermal energy required for permanent ablation is individualized, ranging from an application of −40°C for 40 seconds to one of −75°C for 480 seconds; limiting test applications to only −30°C can limit the applicability of cryoablation for these patients. Additionally, the use of cryothermal energy at temperatures lower than −30°C should be considered safer than RF energy at these critical sites.

CRYOABLATION. When sites of successful cryomapping are identified by demonstrating BT block with no modification of basal AVN conduction, the cryoablation mode is activated, in which a target temperature below about 75°C is sought (a temperature of −75°C to −80°C is generally achieved). The application is then continued for up to 480 seconds, creating an irreversible lesion. If the catheter tip is in close contact with the endocardium, a prompt drop in catheter tip temperature should be seen as soon as the cryoablation mode is activated. A slow decline in temperature or very high flow rates of refrigerant during ablation suggests poor catheter tip tissue contact and, in such a case, cryoablation is interrupted and the catheter is repositioned.

ADVANTAGES OF CRYOABLATION. One of the distinct advantages of cryothermal technology is the ability to demonstrate loss of function of tissue reversibly with cooling (cryomapping), thereby demonstrating the functionality of prospective ablation sites without inducing permanent injury. Furthermore, once the catheter tip temperature is reduced below 0°C, progressive ice formation at the catheter tip causes adherence to the adjacent tissue (cryoadherence). A disadvantage of cryoablation is that the cryocatheter is not yet as steerable as the conventional RF catheter, which can potentially limit proper positioning of the catheter tip. In addition, the larger electrodes decrease the specificity of mapping.

OUTCOME OF CRYOABLATION. In recent series, the acute success rate of cryoablation of BTs in the superoparaseptal and midseptal regions exceeded 90%; however, resumption of BT conduction with palpitation recurrences can occur in up to 20% of patients, and overall success rates have been lower than those of AVNRT cryoablation. Nevertheless, whereas RF ablation of some superoparaseptal and midseptal BTs may otherwise be abandoned because of a prohibitive risk of AV block, cryoablation is a viable, and often successful, option to eliminate those BTs. Although transient modifications of the normal AVN conduction pathways can be observed during cooling, no permanent modifications have been observed. RBBB has occurred on occasion, but inadvertent AV block has yet to be reported. In fact, immediate discontinuation of cryothermal energy application at any temperature on observation of modification of conduction over normal pathways results in return to baseline conditions soon after discontinuation.[60]

Ablation of Epicardial Bypass Tracts

ANATOMICAL CONSIDERATIONS

As noted, epicardial BTs can be found at any location, but they are most common in the posteroseptal and left posterior regions.[49] Epicardial BTs also account for 4% of left lateral ablation cases and 10% of those in patients referred after a failed ablation attempt.

Embryologically, the CS develops from the sinus venosus, together with the smooth part of the RA. As a remnant of sinus venosus musculature, a cuff of striated muscle covers the proximal CS, continuous with RA myocardium at the CS os. The CS muscle coat has electrical connections with both the right and the left atria and may extend for several millimeters over the necks of the middle cardiac vein and posterior coronary vein in 3% and 2% of hearts, respectively. Additionally, myocardial cords extending around the AV groove branch of the distal left circumflex coronary artery can be found in 6% of hearts. These myocardial sleeves or cords do not usually extend into the ventricular myocardium. In variations, where a continuation into the epicardial surface of the ventricle is formed, however, an AV BT (referred to as an "epicardial" BT) is formed in the posteroseptal and left posterior region.[61,62] In some cases, the muscle creating this connection is found in the neck of a CS diverticulum. The prevalence of CS-associated epicardial BTs is approximately 22% to 36% among patients with posteroseptal or left posterior BTs, and is up to 47% among patients with a previous failed ablation attempt. This highlights the difficulty of localizing these BTs.[54,63] Other types of unusual BTs that cannot be ablated with a standard endocardial approach at the annulus have been described. These include BTs that connect an atrial appendage to its respective ventricle, which can be successfully ablated using a transcutaneous pericardial approach or endocardial ablation over a large area. Another example is BTs closely associated with the ligament of Marshall, which can be ablated by targeting this ligament.

TECHNICAL CONSIDERATIONS

ECG predictors of epicardial posteroseptal BTs include the following: (1) steep negative delta wave in lead II; (2) steep positive delta wave in aV_R; and (3) deep S wave in V_6. A negative delta wave in lead II has highest sensitivity and a positive delta in aV_R has highest specificity for prediction of the presence of epicardial (i.e., requiring ablation within the CS and its branches) versus endocardial posteroseptal BTs.[55]

An epicardial location of the BT is suggested if the earliest site of endocardial ventricular activation does not precede the onset of the delta wave, and if a very large BT potential can be easily recorded on the CS electrodes.

Additionally, as noted previously, the CS activation sequence can be of value in distinguishing between CS-associated epicardial BTs from left-sided "endocardial" AV BTs. During retrograde conduction either over a CS-associated BT (which inserts directly into the CS musculature) or over a right-sided "endocardial" BT, the CS muscular coat is activated prior to the LA myocardium, and the high-frequency component precedes the low-frequency component. Thus, a sharp/blunt sequence in the CS electrogram indicates that the BT can be ablated using a right-sided approach. In contrast, with left-sided "endocardial" BTs, the impulse activates the LA before the CS and the low-frequency, far-field signal from the LA will precede the sharp, CS component.[54]

During anterograde conduction over a CS-ventricular BT, ventricular activation within a branch of the CS precedes endocardial activation, and CS muscle extension potentials usually are recorded in the venous branch, producing a pattern similar to a BT potential.[49] The closer proximity of these BTs to the CS than the mitral annulus results in large BT potentials recorded within the CS and susceptibility to ablation from within the CS. Such large BT potentials usually exceed the local atrial and/or ventricular electrogram amplitude. Furthermore, the earliest endocardial anterograde ventricular activation (as indicated by a rapid downstroke on the unfiltered unipolar electrogram) may be recorded more than 15 milliseconds after the onset of the far-field ventricular potential and at a site 1 to 3 cm apical to the mitral and tricuspid annuli. Elimination of these requires ablation of the ventricular end at the insertion of the middle cardiac vein or posterior coronary vein into the CS, because ablation at the site of earliest retrograde atrial activation often produces only a shift in the site of earliest atrial activation (mimicking multiple BTs) because of the multiple connections of the CS myocardial coat to both atria.[54,63] BTs in the inferior pyramidal space can be approached through the CS and also the middle cardiac vein, but proximity to important structures must be borne in mind. This is an important issue, particularly given the close proximity of the right coronary artery with the middle cardiac vein in the vast majority of individuals.

The CS provides a useful route for mapping and ablation of left-sided AV BTs around the mitral valve and those traversing the inferior pyramidal space, the inferior BTs. Epicardial BTs resulting from connections between the muscular coat of the CS and ventricle are generally ablatable only within a branch of the CS, most commonly the middle cardiac vein, on the floor of the CS at the orifice of a venous branch, or within a CS diverticulum. Nevertheless, BTs located very close to the hinge of the mitral valve may be difficult to ablate because the CS is some distance away. Rarely, a transcutaneous pericardial approach is required to ablate epicardial BTs that are posteroseptal or right-sided.[61,62]

The middle (or "posterior interventricular") cardiac vein is a well-established site for posterior epicardial BTs, and is useful for approaching AV BTs located in the inferior pyramidal space. This vein courses with the posterior descending coronary artery in the posterior interventricular groove and enters the CS close to the RA orifice or, rarely, enters directly into the RA apical to the septal attachment of the tricuspid valve. At its junction with the CS, the venous entrance is very occasionally dilated, forming a venous diverticulum. The proximity and crossover relationship of the middle cardiac vein with the right coronary artery and its branch to the AVN should be appreciated to avoid inadvertent damage to these structures.[61,62]

CS venography is typically required to help delineate its anatomy and guide ablation. Also, coronary angiography should be performed before delivering RF energy near or within a branch of the CS to determine whether there are any branches of the right or left coronary artery in proximity to the ablation site. If there is a branch of the right coronary artery within 2 mm of the ablation site, there may be a high risk of coronary artery injury if RF energy is delivered. In this situation, cryoablation can be performed with little or no risk of coronary artery injury.

A 4-mm-tip, 7 Fr (for CS), or 6 Fr (for CS branches), ablation catheter is generally used. However, a conventional ablation catheter may completely occlude a branch of the CS, preventing cooling of the ablation electrode and resulting in high impedance when RF energy is delivered. This markedly reduces the amount of power that can be delivered and may result in adherence of the ablation electrode to the wall of the vein. An external saline-cooled ablation catheter allows more consistent delivery of RF energy, with less heating at the electrode-tissue interface.

RF energy of 20 to 30 W and a temperature of 55°C to 60°C for 30 to 60 seconds is delivered at sites within the CS, with the ablation catheter tip directed toward the ventricle within the CS (by maintaining a gentle counterclockwise torque on the ablation catheter). RF energy is stopped if impedance rises significantly (>130 to 140 Ω).

Epicardial posteroseptal BTs are most successfully ablated from the terminal segment of the middle cardiac vein or posterior coronary vein at the site recording the largest, sharpest unipolar BT potential. If ablation is unsuccessful, the catheter can be withdrawn slightly to a more proximal part of the vein. This is relevant in that RF application in a small vein may occlude it at that point, precluding advancement of the catheter to more distal portions of the vein if the RF application was unsuccessful and further mapping is needed. However, the distal right (or left) coronary artery is frequently located within 2 mm of the ideal ablation site, increasing the risk of acute arterial injury.

Causes of Failed Bypass Tract Ablation

Technical difficulties are the most common cause of failed BT ablation. These difficulties are typically related to catheter manipulation and stability (Fig. 18-46) or inability to access the target site, and are occasionally caused by inability to deliver sufficient energy to the optimal target site. They are more common with right-sided BTs because of the smooth atrial aspect of the tricuspid annulus. Such difficulties can be overcome by using preformed guiding sheaths to help stabilize the catheter, using different catheter curvatures and shaft stiffness, changing the approach for ablation (e.g., from transseptal to transaortic, or from IVC to SVC), or changing the ablation modality. Cryoablation can help achieve better catheter stability and target sites that might otherwise be avoided because of the risk of damage to neighboring structures. Large (8-mm) ablation electrodes and cooled RF ablation can also help generate large RF lesions. However, other causes of ablation failure should be considered first before shifting to those approaches, which are only rarely required for BT ablation because the target tissue (BT) is generally a thin strand, ablation of which should not require a large amount of damage.

Mapping errors are the second most common cause of ablation failure. Mapping pitfalls are largely related to inaccurate localization of a BT that has an oblique course. This is more likely to occur when retrograde atrial activation mapping is performed with the ablation catheter positioned at the ventricular side of the annulus; because of the oblique course of the BT, the site of earliest atrial activation recorded from the ventricular aspect of the annulus does not correspond to the ventricular insertion site. Similar situations can occur when the ablation catheter is positioned on the atrial aspect of the annulus and RF applications are delivered where the earliest ventricular activation is recorded. In these situations, mapping for the earliest atrial activation site with the catheter on the atrial side of the annulus, or mapping for the earliest ventricular activation site with the catheter on the ventricular side of the annulus, should be undertaken. Occasionally, ablation at an atrial site proximal to the BT's actual atrial insertion site can cause a substantial shift in atrial activation sequence simulating the presence of a second BT.

Failure to recognize that a posteroseptal BT is left-sided rather than right-sided, and epicardial location of a left-sided or a posteroseptal BT, are other potential causes of failed ablation of those BTs. Detailed mapping in the CS should be considered in such situations. Furthermore, some BTs insert in the ventricle at a distance from the annulus, in which case a search for a presumed BT potential within the ventricle adjacent to the region of the earliest ventricular activation recorded at the annulus can be helpful. Unusual BTs (e.g., atriofascicular BTs) and anatomical abnormality (e.g., congenital heart disease) also account for some failures in BT ablation.

Catheter-induced trauma to the BT also can lead to ablation failure. Catheter-induced BT trauma is often persistent, leading to discontinuation of the mapping and ablation procedure in many cases, and the long-term risk for recovery of BT function is high. Superoparaseptal and atriofascicular BTs exhibit the highest susceptibility to mechanical trauma, followed by left free wall BTs. The outcome can still be improved in these situations by close observation of the ECG recordings to recognize catheter-induced trauma of a BT promptly and, whenever conduction block in the BT does not resolve within 1 minute, by immediate application of RF energy, provided that the catheter has not moved from the site of presumed trauma.

Endpoints of Ablation

Confirmation of complete loss of BT function, and not just noninducibility of tachycardias, is essential. Confirmation of loss of anterograde BT function using AES and atrial pacing is achieved by demonstrating lack of preexcitation and marked prolongation of the local AV interval at the ablation site. Atrial stimulation should be performed at sites and rates that were associated with preexcitation before ablation. It is possible to have loss of anterograde conduction with persistence of retrograde conduction (less commonly the opposite). Care must be taken to ensure bidirectional conduction block.

Confirmation of complete loss of retrograde BT function using VES and ventricular pacing is achieved by demonstrating concentric and decremental retrograde atrial activation, consistent with VA conduction over the AVN, VA dissociation, and/or marked prolongation of the local VA interval at the ablation site. Ventricular stimulation should be performed at sites and rates that were associated with retrograde VA conduction over the BT before ablation. Para-Hisian pacing and RV apical versus RV basilar pacing can also help confirm the absence of septal and paraseptal BTs.

Outcome

RF ablation is a highly effective and curative treatment for AVRT (>95%). Initially successful RF ablation is persistent and late recurrence of BT conduction after ablation is rare (4%).[49] Short runs of

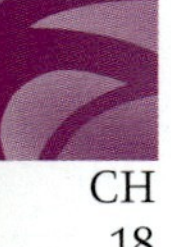

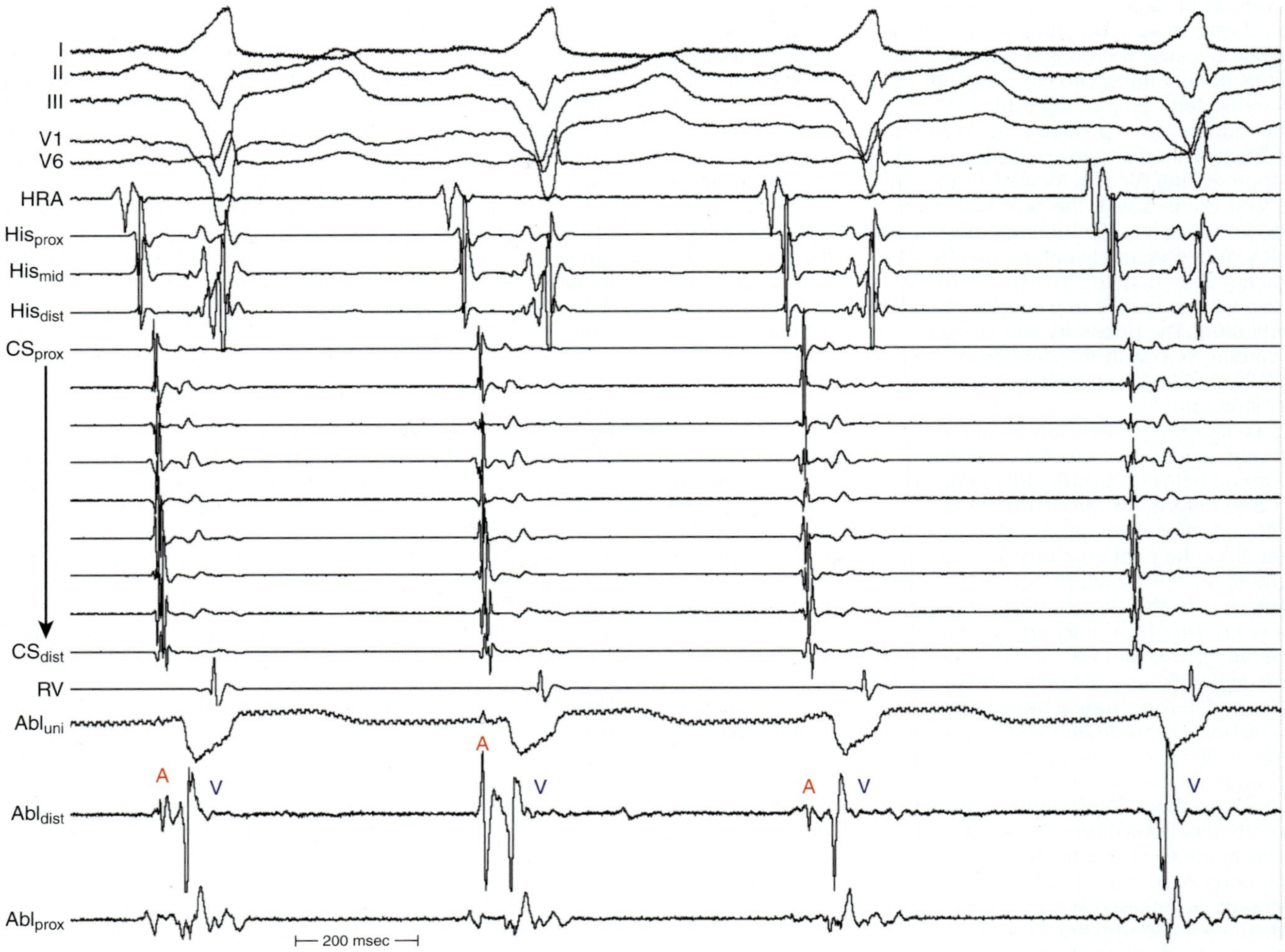

FIGURE 18-46 Poor choice of ablation sites because of unstable recordings. In the distal ablation bipolar (Abl$_{dist}$) recording, the atrial and ventricular electrograms have constantly changing amplitudes, signifying unstable electrode contact with tissue. Ablation should not be performed until the recordings are stable.

palpitations are frequent, usually caused by isolated or short runs of PACs or PVCs and not by recurrence of BT conduction, and can be easily managed with symptomatic treatment without further investigation. Recurrence of BT-mediated tachycardia is usually observed during the first month after ablation, whereas later symptoms (palpitations appearing more than 3 months after the ablation) are highly suggestive of SVTs not related to the ablated BT and justify a thorough evaluation (e.g., event monitoring, long-term ECG monitoring, new EP study).

In a survey of 6065 patients, the long-term success rate was 98% and a repeat procedure was necessary in 2.2% of cases. Serious complication (e.g., cardiac tamponade, AV block, coronary artery injury, retroperitoneal hemorrhage, stroke) occurred in 0.6% of patients, with one fatality (0.02%).[49] Therefore, the one-time risk of catheter ablation appears to be considerably lower than the cumulative annual risk associated with the WPW syndrome. It is clear that the treatment of choice for patients with the WPW syndrome who may be at risk for life-threatening arrhythmias is catheter ablation. In addition, the highly favorable risk-benefit ratio justifies the use of catheter ablation as first-line therapy for any patient with BT-dependent tachycardia requiring treatment.

Success rates and risk of complications vary with different BT locations. Ablation of right free wall BT is associated with a success rate of 93% to 98%, a recurrence rate of 21%, and a complication rate less than that with other BT locations. Ablation of posteroseptal BTs is also associated with a high success rate (98%) and a recurrence rate of 12%. With ablation of superoparaseptal BTs, the reported success rate is up to 97%, with a risk of RBBB in 5% to 10% of cases. Similarly, ablation of midseptal BTs is associated with a success rate of 98%, with an incidence of first-degree AV block in 2% and second-degree AV block in 2%. Although with superoparaseptal BT ablation RF energy is frequently applied at locations with visible His potential, the risk of high-grade AV block is higher for ablation of midseptal BTs because the compact AVN is located in the midseptum. In contrast to the well-insulated HB, the compact AVN is fragile and more vulnerable to damage during ablation.[53]

The immediate success rate of transaortic ablation of left free wall BTs is 86% to 100% (highest with anterograde BT activation), and the recurrence rate is 2% to 5%, less frequent than for BTs at other locations. Complications of this approach include vascular complications (50% of all complications: groin hematoma, aortic dissection, and thrombosis), cardiac tamponade, stroke, coronary dissection (from direct catheter trauma), injury to the left circumflex coronary artery (from subannular RF application), valvular damage, and systemic embolism (from aortic atherosclerosis, catheter tip coagulum, or ablation site thrombosis). The transseptal approach, on the other hand, is associated with a success rate of 85% to 100%, a recurrence rate of 3% to 6.6%, and a complication rate of 0% to 6%. Such complications include coronary spasm, cardiac tamponade, systemic embolization (0.08%), and death (0.08%).

The ablation of epicardial BTs (within the CS) is associated with a success rate of 62% to 100% and a complication rate of 0% to 6%. Complications associated with this approach include CS spasm, cardiac tamponade, pericarditis, and right coronary artery spasm or occlusion. The overall incidence of coronary artery injury is low (0.1%) and it can present immediately or several weeks after ablation.[64]

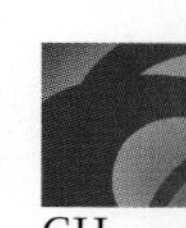

REFERENCES

1. Wolff L, Parkinson J, White PD: Bundle branch block with a short P-R interval in healthy young people prone to paroxysmal tachycardia, *Am Heart J* 5:685, 1930.
2. Lown B, Ganong WF, Levine SA: The syndrome of short P-R interval, normal QRS complex and paroxysmal rapid heart action, *Circulation* 5:693–706, 1952.
3. Josephson ME: Preexcitation syndromes. In Josephson ME, editor: *Clinical cardiac electrophysiology*, ed 3, Philadelphia, 2008, Lippincott Williams & Wilkins, pp 322–424.
4. Ho SY: Accessory atrioventricular pathways: getting to the origins, *Circulation* 117: 1502–1504, 2008.
5. Liew R, Ward D: Two cases of accessory pathways located at the aortomitral continuity: clues from the 12-lead ECG where the algorithms have failed, *Heart Rhythm* 5:1206–1209, 2008.
6. Otomo K, Gonzalez MD, Beckman KJ, et al: Reversing the direction of paced ventricular and atrial wavefronts reveals an oblique course in accessory AV pathways and improves localization for catheter ablation, *Circulation* 104:550–556, 2001.
7. Fitzsimmons PJ, McWhirter PD, Peterson DW, Kruyer WB: The natural history of Wolff-Parkinson-White syndrome in 228 military aviators: a long-term follow-up of 22 years, *Am Heart J* 142:530–536, 2001.
8. Pappone C, Santinelli V, Rosanio S, et al: Usefulness of invasive electrophysiologic testing to stratify the risk of arrhythmic events in asymptomatic patients with Wolff-Parkinson-White pattern: results from a large prospective long-term follow-up study, *J Am Coll Cardiol* 41:239–244, 2003.
9. Santinelli V, Radinovic A, Manguso F, et al: The natural history of asymptomatic ventricular pre-excitation a long-term prospective follow-up study of 184 asymptomatic children, *J Am Coll Cardiol* 53:275–280, 2009.
10. Santinelli V, Radinovic A, Manguso F, et al: Asymptomatic ventricular preexcitation: a long-term prospective follow-up study of 293 adult patients, *Circ Arrhythm Electrophysiol* 2: 102–107, 2009.
11. Harahsheh A, Du W, Singh H, Karpawich PP: Risk factors for atrioventricular tachycardia degenerating to atrial flutter/fibrillation in the young with Wolff-Parkinson-White, *Pacing Clin Electrophysiol* 31:1307–1312, 2008.
12. Munger TM, Packer DL, Hammill SC, et al: A population study of the natural history of Wolff-Parkinson-White syndrome in Olmsted County, Minnesota, 1953-1989, *Circulation* 87: 866–873, 1993.
13. Hsu JC, Tanel RE, Lee BK, et al: Differences in accessory pathway location by sex and race, *Heart Rhythm* 7:52–56, 2010.
14. Gollob MH, Green MS, Tang AS, et al: Identification of a gene responsible for familial Wolff-Parkinson-White syndrome, *N Engl J Med* 344:1823–1831, 2001.
15. Gollob MH, Seger JJ, Gollob TN, et al: Novel PRKAG2 mutation responsible for the genetic syndrome of ventricular preexcitation and conduction system disease with childhood onset and absence of cardiac hypertrophy, *Circulation* 104:3030–3033, 2001.
16. Klein GJ, Gula LJ, Krahn AD, et al: WPW pattern in the asymptomatic individual: has anything changed? *Circ Arrhythm Electrophysiol* 2:97–99, 2009.
17. Pappone C, Santinelli V, Manguso F, et al: A randomized study of prophylactic catheter ablation in asymptomatic patients with the Wolff-Parkinson-White syndrome, *N Engl J Med* 349:1803–1811, 2003.
18. Pappone C, Manguso F, Santinelli R, et al: Radiofrequency ablation in children with asymptomatic Wolff-Parkinson-White syndrome, *N Engl J Med* 351:1197–1205, 2004.
19. Blomstrom-Lundqvist C, Scheinman MM, Aliot EM, et al: ACC/AHA/ESC guidelines for the management of patients with supraventricular arrhythmias—executive summary: a report of the American College of Cardiology/American Heart Association Task Force on Practice Guidelines and the European Society of Cardiology Committee for Practice Guidelines (Writing Committee to Develop Guidelines for the Management of Patients With Supraventricular Arrhythmias), *Circulation* 108:1871–1909, 2003.
20. Scheinman M, Calkins H, Gillette P, et al: NASPE policy statement on catheter ablation: personnel, policy, procedures, and therapeutic recommendations, *Pacing Clin Electrophysiol* 26:789–799, 2003.
21. Pappone C, Santinelli V: Should catheter ablation be performed in asymptomatic patients with Wolff-Parkinson-White syndrome? Catheter ablation should be performed in asymptomatic patients with Wolff-Parkinson-White syndrome, *Circulation* 112:2207–2215, 2005.
22. Wellens HJ: Should catheter ablation be performed in asymptomatic patients with Wolff-Parkinson-White syndrome? When to perform catheter ablation in asymptomatic patients with a Wolff-Parkinson-White electrocardiogram, *Circulation* 112:2201–2207, 2005.
23. Knight B, Morady F: Atrioventricular reentry and variants. In Zipes DP, Jalife J, editors: *Cardiac electrophysiology: from cell to bedside*, ed 4, Philadelphia, 2004, WB Saunders, pp 528–536.
24. Fox DJ, Klein GJ, Skanes AC, et al: How to identify the location of an accessory pathway by the 12-lead ECG, *Heart Rhythm* 5:1763–1766, 2008.
25. Fitzpatrick AP, Gonzales RP, Lesh MD, et al: New algorithm for the localization of accessory atrioventricular connections using a baseline electrocardiogram, *J Am Coll Cardiol* 23:107–116, 1994.
26. Arruda M, Wang X, McClennand J: ECG algorithm for predicting sites of successful radiofrequency ablation of accessory pathways [abstract], *Pacing Clin Electrophysiol* 16:865, 1993.
27. Chiang CE, Chen SA, Teo WS, et al: An accurate stepwise electrocardiographic algorithm for localization of accessory pathways in patients with Wolff-Parkinson-White syndrome from a comprehensive analysis of delta waves and R/S ratio during sinus rhythm, *Am J Cardiol* 76:40–46, 1995.
28. Xie B, Heald SC, Bashir Y, et al: Localization of accessory pathways from the 12-lead electrocardiogram using a new algorithm, *Am J Cardiol* 74:161–165, 1994.
29. Katsouras CS, Greakas GF, Goudevenos JA, et al: Localization of accessory pathways by the electrocardiogram: which is the degree of accordance of three algorithms in use? *Pacing Clin Electrophysiol* 27:189–193, 2004.
30. Tai CT, Chen SA, Chiang CE, et al: A new electrocardiographic algorithm using retrograde P waves for differentiating atrioventricular node reentrant tachycardia from atrioventricular reciprocating tachycardia mediated by concealed accessory pathway, *J Am Coll Cardiol* 29:394–402, 1997.
31. Fitzgerald DM, Hawthorne HR, Crossley GH, et al: P wave morphology during atrial pacing along the atrioventricular ring. ECG localization of the site of origin of retrograde atrial activation, *J Electrocardiol* 29:1–10, 1996.
32. Kapa S, Henz BD, Dib C, et al: Utilization of retrograde right bundle branch block to differentiate atrioventricular nodal from accessory pathway conduction, *J Cardiovasc Electrophysiol* 20:751–758, 2009.
33. Knight BP, Ebinger M, Oral H, et al: Diagnostic value of tachycardia features and pacing maneuvers during paroxysmal supraventricular tachycardia, *J Am Coll Cardiol* 36:574–582, 2000.
34. Yang Y, Cheng J, Glatter K, et al: Quantitative effects of functional bundle branch block in patients with atrioventricular reentrant tachycardia, *Am J Cardiol* 85:826–831, 2000.
35. Crawford TC, Mukerji S, Good E, et al: Utility of atrial and ventricular cycle length variability in determining the mechanism of paroxysmal supraventricular tachycardia, *J Cardiovasc Electrophysiol* 18:698–703, 2007.
36. Maruyama M, Kobayashi Y, Miyauchi Y, et al: The VA relationship after differential atrial overdrive pacing: a novel tool for the diagnosis of atrial tachycardia in the electrophysiologic laboratory, *J Cardiovasc Electrophysiol* 18:1127–1133, 2007.
37. Platonov M, Schroeder K, Veenhuyzen GD: Differential entrainment: beware from where you pace, *Heart Rhythm* 4:1097–1099, 2007.
38. Gonzalez-Torrecilla E, Arenal A, Atienza F, et al: First postpacing interval after tachycardia entrainment with correction for atrioventricular node delay: a simple maneuver for differential diagnosis of atrioventricular nodal reentrant tachycardias versus orthodromic reciprocating tachycardias, *Heart Rhythm* 3:674–679, 2006.
39. Veenhuyzen GD, Stuglin C, Zimola KG, Mitchell LB: A tale of two post pacing intervals, *J Cardiovasc Electrophysiol* 17:687–689, 2006.
40. Kannankeril PJ, Bonney WJ, Dzurik MV, Fish FA: Entrainment to distinguish orthodromic reciprocating tachycardia from atrioventricular nodal reentry tachycardia in children, *Pacing Clin Electrophysiol* 33:469–474, 2010.
41. Segal OR, Gula LJ, Skanes AC, et al: Differential ventricular entrainment: a maneuver to differentiate AV node reentrant tachycardia from orthodromic reciprocating tachycardia, *Heart Rhythm* 6:493–500, 2009.
42. Dandamudi G, Mokabberi R, Assal C, et al: A novel approach to differentiating orthodromic reciprocating tachycardia from atrioventricular nodal reentrant tachycardia, *Heart Rhythm* 7:1326–1329, 2010.
43. AlMahameed ST, Buxton AE, Michaud GF: New criteria during right ventricular pacing to determine the mechanism of supraventricular tachycardia, *Circ Arrhythm Electrophysiol* 3:578–584, 2010.
44. Nakagawa H, Jackman WM: Para-Hisian pacing: useful clinical technique to differentiate retrograde conduction between accessory atrioventricular pathways and atrioventricular nodal pathways, *Heart Rhythm* 2:667–672, 2005.
45. Reddy VY, Jongnarangsin K, Albert CM, et al: Para-Hisian entrainment: a novel pacing maneuver to differentiate orthodromic atrioventricular reentrant tachycardia from atrioventricular nodal reentrant tachycardia, *J Cardiovasc Electrophysiol* 14:1321–1328, 2003.
46. Sauer WH, Lowery CM, Cooper JM, Lewkowiez L: Sequential dual chamber extrastimulation: a novel pacing maneuver to identify the presence of a slowly conducting concealed accessory pathway, *Heart Rhythm* 5:248–252, 2008.
47. Wood MA, Swartz JF: Ablation of left-free wall accessory pathways. In Huang D, Wilber DJ, editors: *Radiofrequency catheter ablation of cardiac arrhythmias: basic concepts and clinical applications*, ed 2, Armonk, NY, 2000, Futura, pp 509–540.
48. Chen SA, Chiang CE, Tai CT, Chang MS: Ablation of posteroseptal accessory pathways. In Huang D, Wilber DJ, editors: *Radiofrequency catheter ablation of cardiac arrhythmias: basic concepts and clinical applications*, ed 2, Armonk, NY, 2000, Futura, pp 495–508.
49. Morady F: Catheter ablation of supraventricular arrhythmias: state of the art, *J Cardiovasc Electrophysiol* 15:124–139, 2004.
50. Miles W: Ablation of right free wall accessory pathways. In Huang D, Wilber DJ, editors: *Radiofrequency catheter ablation of cardiac arrhythmias: basic concepts and clinical applications*, ed 2, Armonk, NY, 2000, Futura, pp 465–494.
51. Fishberger SB, Hernandez A, Zahn EM: Electroanatomic mapping of the right coronary artery: a novel approach to ablation of right free-wall accessory pathways, *J Cardiovasc Electrophysiol* 20:526–529, 2009.
52. Takenaka S, Yeh SJ, Wen MS, et al: Algorithm for differentiation of left and right posterior paraseptal accessory pathway, *J Electrocardiol* 37:75–81, 2004.
53. Macedo PG, Patel SM, Bisco SE, Asirvatham SJ: Septal accessory pathway: anatomy, causes for difficulty, and an approach to ablation, *Indian Pacing Electrophysiol J* 10:292–309, 2010.
54. Pap R, Traykov VB, Makai A, et al: Ablation of posteroseptal and left posterior accessory pathways guided by left atrium-coronary sinus musculature activation sequence, *J Cardiovasc Electrophysiol* 19:653–658, 2008.
55. Haghjoo M, Mahmoodi E, Fazelifar AF, et al: Electrocardiographic and electrophysiologic predictors of successful ablation site in patients with manifest posteroseptal accessory pathway, *Pacing Clin Electrophysiol* 31:103–111, 2008.
56. Basso C, Ho SY, Thiene G: Anatomical and histopathological characteristics of the conductive tissues of the heart. In Gussak I, Antzelevitch C, editors: *Electrical diseases of the heart: genetics, mechanisms, treatment, prevention*, London, 2008, Springer, pp 37–51.
57. Schluter M, Cappato R, Ouyang F, Kuck KH: Ablation of anteroseptal and midseptal accessory pathways. In Huang D, Wilber DJ, editors: *Radiofrequency catheter ablation of cardiac arrhythmias: basic concepts and clinical applications*, ed 2, Armonk, NY, 2000, Futura, pp 541–558.
58. Chang SL, Lee SH, Tai CT, et al: Electrocardiographic and electrophysiologic characteristics of midseptal accessory pathways, *J Cardiovasc Electrophysiol* 16:237–243, 2005.
59. Tai CT, Chen SA, Chiang CE, et al: Electrocardiographic and electrophysiologic characteristics of anteroseptal, midseptal, and para-Hisian accessory pathways: implication for radiofrequency catheter ablation, *Chest* 109:730–740, 1996.
60. Lemola K, Dubuc M, Khairy P: Transcatheter cryoablation. II. Clinical utility, *Pacing Clin Electrophysiol* 31:235–244, 2008.
61. Habib A, Lachman N, Christensen KN, Asirvatham SJ: The anatomy of the coronary sinus venous system for the cardiac electrophysiologist, *Europace* 11(Suppl 5):V15–V21, 2009.
62. Ho SY, Sanchez-Quintana D, Becker AE: A review of the coronary venous system: a road less travelled, *Heart Rhythm* 1:107–112, 2004.
63. Sun Y, Arruda M, Otomo K, et al: Coronary sinus-ventricular accessory connections producing posteroseptal and left posterior accessory pathways: incidence and electrophysiological identification, *Circulation* 106:1362–1367, 2002.
64. Roberts-Thomson KC, Steven D, Seiler J, et al: Coronary artery injury due to catheter ablation in adults: presentations and outcomes, *Circulation* 120:1465–1473, 2009.

CHAPTER 19 Variants of Preexcitation

Variants of Preexcitation (Atypical Bypass Tracts)

A working definition of an atypical bypass tract (BT) is a conduction pathway that bypasses all or part of the normal conduction system but is not a rapidly conducting pathway connecting atrium and ventricle near the mitral or tricuspid annulus. Thus, pathways that connect the atrium to the His bundle (HB), the atrioventricular node (AVN) to the His-Purkinje system (HPS) or the ventricle, or the HPS to the ventricle fit into this designation (Fig. 19-1).

"Mahaim Fibers"

In 1937, during pathological examination of the heart, Mahaim and Benatt identified islands of conducting tissue extending from the HB into the ventricular myocardium. These fibers were called Mahaim fibers or fasciculoventricular fibers.[1-3] This description was subsequently expanded to include connections between the AVN and the ventricular myocardium (nodoventricular fibers). Later, it was recognized that BTs could arise from the AVN and insert into the right bundle branch (RB; nodofascicular fibers).[2,3] This classification for Mahaim fibers persisted until evidence suggested that the anatomical substrate of tachycardias with characteristics previously attributed to nodoventricular and nodofascicular fibers is actually atrioventricular (AV) and atriofascicular BTs with decremental conduction properties (i.e., conduction slows at faster heart rates) (see Fig. 19-1). Although these BTs are sometimes collectively referred to as "Mahaim fibers," the use of this term is discouraged because it is more illuminating to name the precise BT according to its connections. In this chapter, these BTs are referred to as *atypical* BTs to differentiate them from the more common *(typical)* rapidly conducting AV BTs that result in the Wolff-Parkinson-White (WPW) syndrome.[4]

"Mahaim Tachycardia"

The term *Mahaim tachycardia* is used to describe the typical constellation of electrophysiological (EP) features that characterize the unusual form of reentrant tachycardia using an atypical BT, without implication about the underlying anatomical cause. It should be noted that, because the term was originally applied to an anatomical finding and subsequently (incorrectly) applied to physiology that matched what would be expected from this anatomy, it has given rise to more confusion than understanding. Hence, the use of the term *Mahaim tachycardia* should generally be discouraged; instead, one should simply describe the physiological characteristics of the tachyarrhythmia.[5]

Types of Atypical Bypass Tracts

LONG DECREMENTALLY CONDUCTING ATRIOVENTRICULAR AND ATRIOFASCICULAR BYPASS TRACTS

These BTs comprise the majority (80%) of atypical BTs; their atrial insertion site is in the right atrial (RA) free wall.[6,7] These BTs tend (84%) to cross the tricuspid annulus in the lateral, anterolateral, or anterior region. They extend along the right ventricular (RV) free wall to the region where the moderator band usually inserts at the apical third of the RV free wall, inserting into the distal part of the RB (atriofascicular BT) or into the ventricular myocardium close to the RB (long decrementally conducting AV BT). These BTs are functionally similar to the normal AV junction, with an AVN-like structure leading to a His bundle (HB)–like structure. In essence, those BTs function as an auxiliary conduction system parallel to the normal conduction system (AVN–HPS). Similar to the normal AVN, these BTs demonstrate decremental conduction (related to the slow rate of recovery of excitability) and Wenckebach-type block in response to rapid atrial pacing and are sensitive to adenosine. The conduction delay in these BTs has been localized to the intraatrial portion of the BT (the AVN-like portion), whereas the interval from the inscription of the BT potential at the tricuspid annulus and the onset of ventricular activation (BT-V interval) remains constant.[4-6,8,9]

SHORT DECREMENTALLY CONDUCTING ATRIOVENTRICULAR BYPASS TRACTS

These BTs are analogous to decrementally conducting concealed BTs responsible for the permanent form of junctional reciprocating tachycardia (PJRT; see Chap. 18) in that they bridge the AV rings and insert proximally into ventricular myocardium in close proximity to the AV annulus.[7,10] These BTs primarily arise from the RA free wall, but can also arise from the posterior or septal region. Left-sided BTs with decremental conduction characteristics have rarely been described. Although these BTs demonstrate decremental conduction and Wenckebach-type block in response to rapid atrial pacing, they do not consistently appear to be responsive to adenosine, which suggests that their structure is not composed of AVN-like tissue.[10]

NODOVENTRICULAR AND NODOFASCICULAR BYPASS TRACTS

Nodoventricular BTs arise in the normal AVN and insert into ventricular myocardium near the AV junction.[7] Nodofascicular BTs arise in the normal AVN and insert into the RB. These BTs are sensitive to adenosine, probably because of their AVN connection.[5]

FASCICULOVENTRICULAR BYPASS TRACTS

Fasciculoventricular BTs are the rarest form of preexcitation (1.2% to 5.1% of atypical BTs). These BTs have different features from the other atypical BTs, and are discussed separately (see later).[5]

Arrhythmias Associated with Atypical Bypass Tracts

Atypical BTs in patients with clinical arrhythmias have the following characteristics: (1) unidirectional (anterograde-only) conduction (with rare exceptions); (2) long conduction times; and (3) decremental conduction (i.e., cycle length [CL]-dependent slowing of conduction).

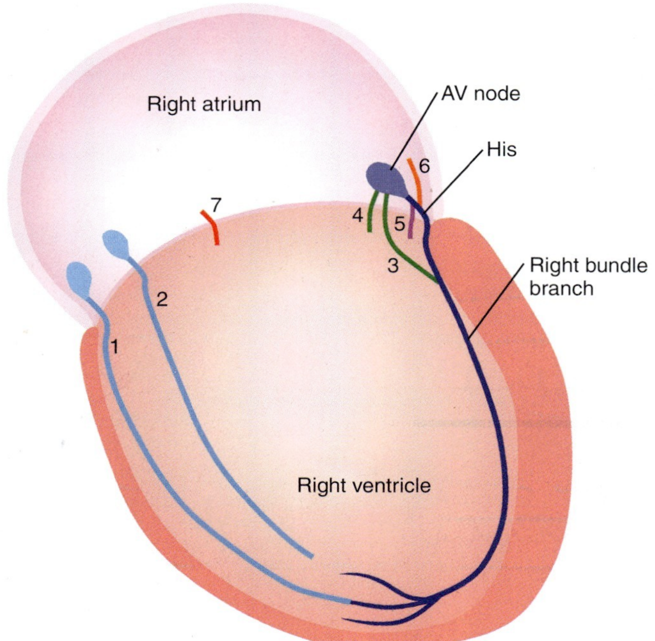

FIGURE 19-1 Variants of preexcitation. Right atrium and ventricle are depicted. *1,* Atriofascicular bypass tract (BT); *2,* long atrioventricular BT; *3,* nodofascicular BT; *4,* nodoventricular BT; *5,* fasciculoventricular BT; *6,* atrio-Hisian BT; *7,* typical short atrioventricular BT.

Atypical BTs comprise 3% to 5% of all BTs. The incidence is slightly higher (6%) in patients presenting with supraventricular tachycardia (SVT) with a left bundle branch block (LBBB) morphology.[7] Multiple BTs occur in 10% of patients with atypical BTs. In some cases, a typical, rapidly conducting AV BT can mask the presence of an atypical BT, which only becomes apparent after ablation of the typical BT. Dual AVN pathways or multiple BTs occur in 40% of patients with atypical BTs. Atypical BTs can also be associated with Ebstein anomaly.

SUPRAVENTRICULAR TACHYCARDIAS REQUIRING AN ATRIOVENTRICULAR BYPASS TRACT FOR INITIATION AND MAINTENANCE

Antidromic atrioventricular reentrant tachycardia (AVRT) can use the atypical BT anterogradely and the HPS-AVN retrogradely. Antidromic AVRT can also use the atypical BT anterogradely and a second AV BT retrogradely. In the latter case, the AVN can participate as an innocent bystander mediating anterograde or retrograde fusion. Because these atypical BTs almost always conduct anterogradely only, they cannot mediate orthodromic AVRT, but can mediate antidromic AVRT or can be an innocent bystander during other SVTs (e.g., atrioventricular nodal reentrant tachycardia [AVNRT]). However, they can coexist with typical rapidly conducting AV BTs. AVRTs using a nodoventricular or nodofascicular BT as the anterograde limb generally use a second AV BT as the retrograde limb of the reentrant circuit.[5] Right free wall atriofascicular BTs capable of both anterograde and retrograde conduction that participate in both antidromic and orthodromic AVRT have rarely been reported.[11]

SUPRAVENTRICULAR TACHYCARDIAS NOT REQUIRING AN ATRIOVENTRICULAR BYPASS TRACT FOR INITIATION AND MAINTENANCE

AVNRT, atrial tachycardia (AT), atrial flutter (AFL), or atrial fibrillation (AF) can coexist with atypical BTs, in which case the atypical BTs function as bystanders, wholly or partly responsible for ventricular activation during the tachycardia.

Electrocardiographic Features

NORMAL SINUS RHYTHM

During normal sinus rhythm (NSR), the ECG shows normal QRS or minimal preexcitation in most patients with atypical BTs. Subtle preexcitation can be suspected by the absence of the normal septal forces (small q waves) in leads I, aVL, V_5, and V_6 and the presence of an rS complex in lead III in the setting of a narrow QRS.[12] The degree of preexcitation depends on the relative conduction time over the AVN and BT. Maneuvers that prolong conduction over the AVN (e.g., atrial pacing, vagal maneuvers, or drugs) to a greater degree than BT conduction will increase the degree of preexcitation. Because atypical BTs exhibit decremental conduction, increasing the atrial pacing rate results in prolongation of the P-delta interval. In contrast, in the setting of typical rapidly conducting AV BTs, the P-delta interval remains relatively constant regardless of the degree of preexcitation; whereas prolonging the AVN conduction time results in more preexcitation. The P-delta interval remains constant or exhibits mild prolongation because conduction over the typical BT displays less decrement than does the AVN.[5,7,12-14]

PREEXCITED QRS MORPHOLOGY

For atriofascicular and nodofascicular BTs, the QRS is relatively narrow (133 ± 10 milliseconds), and its morphology is classic for typical LBBB with a QRS axis between 0 and −75 degrees and a late precordial R/S transition zone (at V_4 or V_5, and sometimes V_6). However, for long decrementally conducting AV BTs, the QRS is relatively wider (166 ± 26 milliseconds) and the LBBB pattern is less typical (with broad initial R in V_1). The QRS is even wider and the LBBB pattern is less typical with nodoventricular and decrementally conducting short AV BTs than that with atriofascicular or long decrementally conducting AV BTs.[5,12,14]

SUPRAVENTRICULAR TACHYCARDIAS

Arrhythmias associated with atypical BTs are associated with an LBBB pattern and, most often, in the setting of long decrementally conducting AV and atriofascicular BTs, left axis deviation on the surface ECG (Fig. 19-2). There are several ECG features that suggest (although are not diagnostic of) atypical BTs as the cause of an SVT with LBBB pattern. These include (1) QRS axis between 0 and −75 degrees, (2) QRS duration of 150 milliseconds or less, (3) R wave in lead I, (4) rS complex in lead V_1, and (5) precordial R wave transition in lead V_4 or later.[5,12,14]

Electrophysiological Testing

BASELINE OBSERVATIONS DURING NORMAL SINUS RHYTHM

In the baseline state, minimal or no preexcitation can be present; thus, the His bundle–ventricular (HV) interval is normal or slightly short.

Atrial Pacing and Atrial Extrastimulation during Normal Sinus Rhythm

Progressively shorter atrial pacing CLs or atrial extrastimulus (AES) coupling intervals produce decremental conduction in both the atypical BT and, to a greater degree, the AVN (Fig. 19-3).[12] Consequently, the atrial–His bundle (AH) interval increases, the QRS morphology gradually shifts to a more preexcited LBBB morphology, and the AV (A-delta) interval increases. However, the AV (A-delta) interval increases to a lesser degree than the AH interval. This is in contrast to the setting of typical rapidly conducting AV BTs, in which the AV (A-delta) interval remains constant despite prolongation of the AH interval and exaggeration of the degree of preexcitation, because the A-delta interval represents conduction time over the BT. Typical AV BTs maintain constant conduction time during

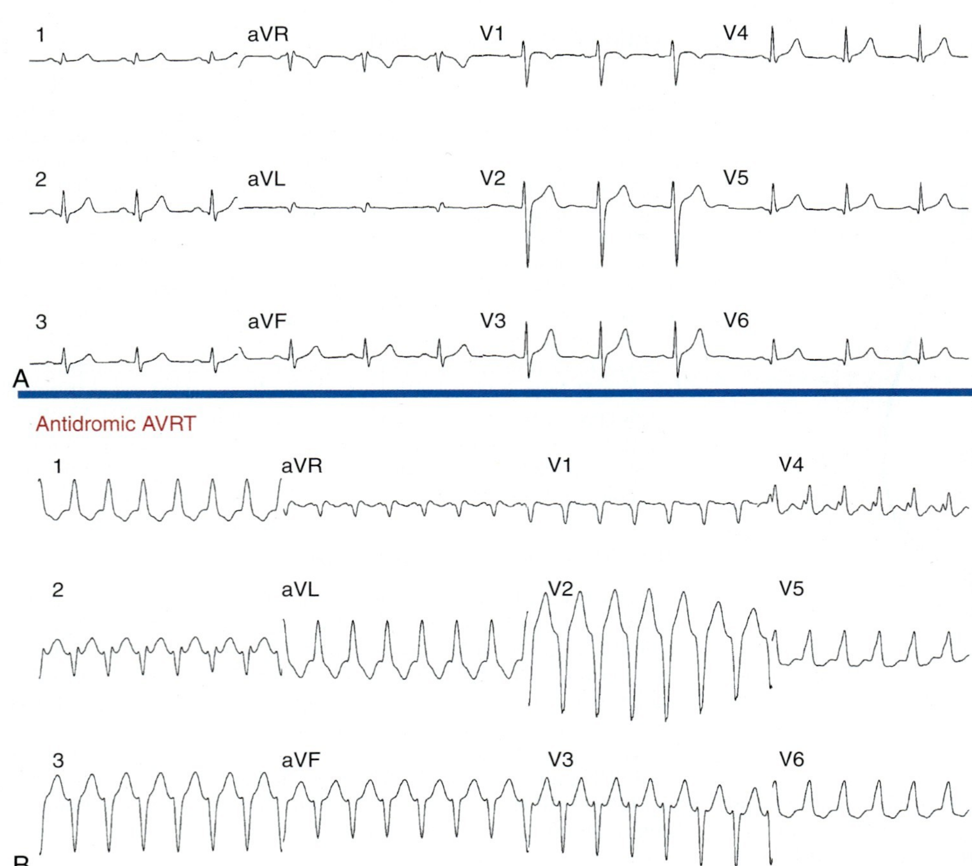

FIGURE 19-2 Atriofascicular bypass tracts (BTs). **A,** Normal sinus rhythm (NSR) with no evidence of preexcitation. **B,** Antidromic atrioventricular reentrant tachycardia (AVRT) using an atriofascicular BT. QRS morphology during tachycardia resembles left bundle branch block aberration because of anterograde activation over the atriofascicular BT. Retrograde P waves can be seen after the end of the QRS.

different pacing rates and AES coupling intervals—that is, nondecremental conduction.[5]

With progressively shorter atrial pacing CLs or AES coupling intervals, the HV interval decreases as the His potential becomes progressively inscribed into the QRS (usually within the first 5 to 25 milliseconds after the onset of the QRS). The His potential eventually becomes activated retrogradely as the wavefront travels anterogradely down the BT and then retrogradely up the RB to the HB (see Fig. 19-3). When the His potential is lost within the QRS, it is unclear whether anterograde AV conduction continues to propagate over the HB or block has occurred.[7]

At the point of maximal preexcitation, the AV (A-delta) interval continues to prolong with more rapid pacing because of the decremental conduction properties of the BT, and the His potential–QRS relationship remains unaltered because the HB is activated retrogradely until block in the BT occurs. The fixed ventricular–His bundle (VH) interval, despite shorter pacing CLs or AES coupling intervals, suggests that the BT inserts into or near the distal RB at the anterior free wall of the RV with retrograde conduction to the HB. Whenever the VH interval is less than 20 milliseconds, insertion into the RB (i.e., atriofascicular or nodofascicular BT) is likely. On the other hand, with long decrementally conducting AV BTs, which insert into the ventricular myocardium close to the RB, the VH interval approximates the HV interval minus the duration of the His potential (because the His potential is activated retrogradely).[5,7]

For short decrementally conducting BTs, the HB is activated anterogradely, and retrograde conduction to the HB is only seen following AV block or during antidromic AVRT. Decremental conduction (progressive prolongation of the AV interval) and Wenckebach-type block develop in the BT. The conduction delay in these BTs is localized to the intraatrial portion of the BT; the interval from the inscription of the BT potential at the tricuspid annulus to the onset of ventricular activation (BT-V interval) remains constant.[5]

Dual AVN physiology is common in patients with atypical BTs. Sometimes, during AES, a jump from the fast to the slow AVN pathway prolongs the AH interval to a degree sufficient to unmask preexcitation over the BT, at which time the His potential becomes inscribed within the QRS.

The site of the earliest ventricular activation during preexcitation is at the RV apex for long, decrementally conducting AV BTs and atriofascicular BTs, but adjacent to the annulus near the base of the RV for short, decrementally conducting AV BTs.

The site of atrial stimulation does not influence the degree of preexcitation in the setting of nodofascicular and nodoventricular BTs. Contrariwise, preexcitation becomes more prominent when atrial stimulation is performed closer to the atrial insertion site of AV or atriofascicular BTs.

Ventricular Pacing and Ventricular Extrastimulation during Normal Sinus Rhythm

Because these BTs rarely have retrograde conduction, ventricular stimulation cannot help in mapping of the BT location. VA conduction during ventricular pacing should propagate over the HPS-AVN with concentric atrial activation sequence and decremental properties in response to progressively shorter ventricular pacing CLs or ventricular extrastimulation (VES) coupling intervals. If rapid and fixed VA conduction is present, a separate retrogradely and rapidly conducting AV BT should be excluded. Retrograde dual AVN pathways may be present.

Effects of Adenosine

Adenosine produces conduction delay in most atypical BTs except for short decrementally conducting AV BTs. The conduction delay has been localized to the intraatrial portion of the BT; the interval from the inscription of the BT potential at the tricuspid annulus and the onset of ventricular activation remains constant.[7,13] When

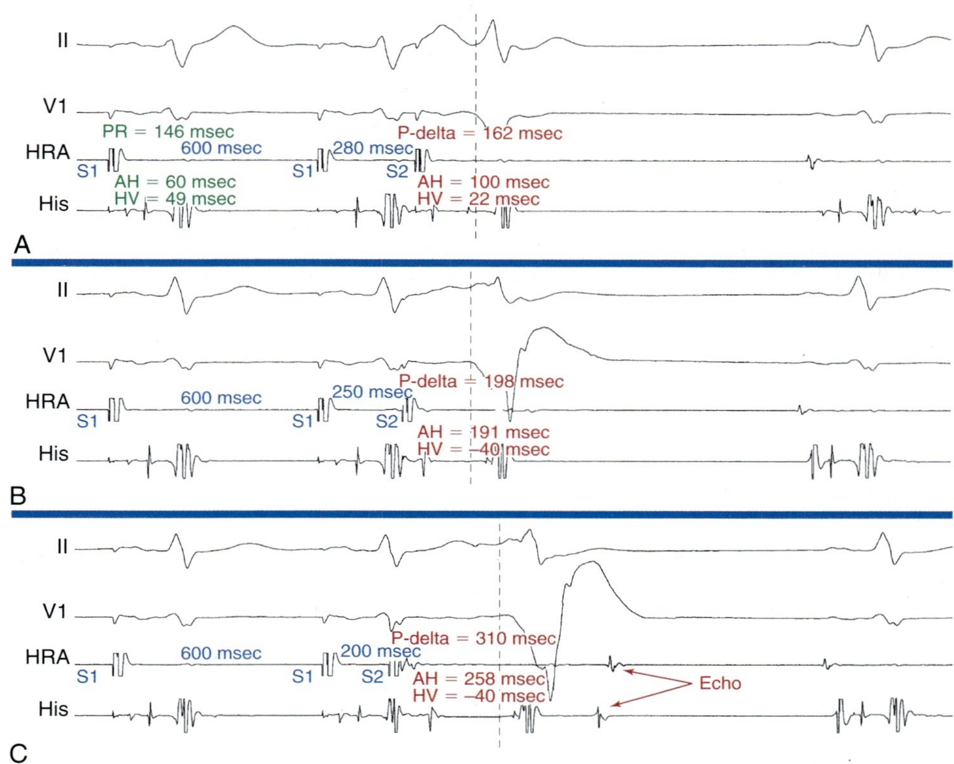

FIGURE 19-3 Effect of atrial extrastimulation (AES) on preexcitation via a long atrioventricular (AV) bypass tract (BT). No preexcitation is observed during normal sinus rhythm and during the pacing drive at a cycle length of 600 milliseconds (normal PR and His bundle–ventricular [HV] intervals). **A,** AES produces decremental conduction in the atrioventricular node (AVN) with prolongation of the atrial–His bundle (AH) interval (from 60 to 100 milliseconds), associated with manifest preexcitation and shortening of the HV interval (from 49 to 22 milliseconds). **B** and **C,** Progressively shorter AES coupling intervals produce decremental conduction in the BT and, to a greater degree, in the AVN. Consequently, the AH interval prolongs, the QRS morphology gradually shifts to a more preexcited left bundle branch block morphology, and the AV (P-delta) interval prolongs. However, the P-delta interval prolongs to a lesser degree than the AH interval. The HV interval decreases (becomes negative) but remains fixed (**B** and **C**) although the P-delta interval continues to prolong with more premature AES because of decremental conduction over the BT. The fixed ventricular–His bundle (VH) interval, despite shorter AES coupling intervals, suggests that the BT inserts into or near the distal right bundle branch (RB) at the anterior free wall of the right ventricle, with retrograde conduction to the His bundle (HB). However, because the VH interval is modestly long (40 milliseconds), a long decrementally conducting AV BT inserting into the ventricle close to the RB is more likely than an atriofascicular BT. **C,** AV reentrant echo complex (red arrows) secondary to anterograde conduction over the BT and retrograde conduction over the AVN.

adenosine administration slows AVN conduction, an increase in the degree of preexcitation is noted in all types of BTs (as long as adenosine does not block the BT).

INDUCTION OF TACHYCARDIA

Initiation by Atrial Extrastimulation or Atrial Pacing

Initiation of antidromic AVRT by an AES requires the following: (1) intact anterograde conduction over the BT; (2) anterograde block in the AVN or HPS; and (3) intact retrograde conduction over the HPS-AVN once the AVN resumes excitability following partial anterograde penetration. Whereas the latter is usually the limiting factor for the initiation of antidromic AVRT using typical rapidly conducting AV BTs, it is readily available in the setting of atypical BTs. This is because of the slow decremental conduction anterogradely over the atypical BT, providing adequate delay for full recovery of the HPS-AVN.

As noted, progressively shorter atrial pacing CLs (especially from the RA) result in progressive AV (A-delta) interval prolongation and a greater degree of preexcitation until maximal. Often, once maximal preexcitation has been achieved, cessation of pacing is followed by preexcited SVT. Progressively shorter AES coupling intervals similarly result in progressive AV (A-delta) interval prolongation and a greater degree of preexcitation until maximal. When anterograde AVN conduction fails but conduction persists over the BT, the HPS-AVN can be activated retrogradely to initiate antidromic AVRT.[7]

The sudden appearance of preexcitation associated with a "jump" from the fast to the slow AVN pathway with a His potential inscribed before ventricular activation or with a VH interval of less than 10 milliseconds strongly favors AVNRT. Although a slowly conducting atriofascicular BT that becomes manifest with a jump to the slow AVN pathway cannot be excluded, a consistent pattern of dual pathway dependence and an HV relationship too short to be retrograde from the distal RB would be unlikely.[7] Induction of AVNRT with AES is almost always associated with a dual pathway response, which may not be seen if the impulse conducts anterogradely over the BT and captures the HB before it is activated by the impulse traversing the slow AVN pathway anterogradely. In other cases, a jump can be seen so that the anterograde His potential follows the QRS with a typical AVN echo to initiate SVT, analogous to 1:2 conduction initiating antidromic AVRT.

Initiation by Ventricular Extrastimulation or Ventricular Pacing

Initiation of antidromic AVRT by ventricular pacing or VES requires the following: (1) retrograde block in the BT, which is almost always available, because the atypical BTs are usually unidirectional (anterograde only); (2) retrograde conduction over the HPS-AVN; and (3) adequate VA delay to allow for recovery of the atrium and BT so it can support subsequent anterograde conduction.

Ventricular pacing can initiate SVT in 85% of cases. Initiation is almost always associated with retrograde conduction up a relatively fast AVN pathway, followed by anterograde conduction down a slow pathway, which is associated with preexcitation. The anterograde slow pathway can be a BT (i.e., antidromic AVRT) or a slow AVN pathway (i.e., AVNRT with an innocent bystander BT). During induction of the SVT by ventricular pacing at a CL similar to the tachycardia CL or by a VES that advances the His potential by a coupling interval similar to the H-H interval during the SVT, the His bundle–atrial (HA) interval following the ventricular stimulus is compared with that during the SVT—an HA interval that is longer with ventricular pacing or VES initiating the SVT than that during the SVT suggests AVNRT. This occurs despite the fact that the H-H interval of the VES (i.e., the interval between the His potential activated anterogradely by the last sinus beat to the His potential activated retrogradely by the VES initiating the SVT) exceeds the H-H interval during the SVT. Because the AVN usually exhibits greater decremental conduction with repetitive engagement of impulses than in response to a single impulse at a similar coupling interval, the more prolonged the HA with the initiating ventricular stimulus, the more likely the SVT is AVNRT. If the SVT uses the BT for anterograde conduction, the HA interval during ventricular pacing or the VES initiating the SVT, at a comparable coupling interval as the tachycardia CL, should have the same HA interval as during the SVT.

TACHYCARDIA FEATURES

Antidromic Atrioventricular Reentrant Tachycardia Using an Atypical Bypass Tract Anterogradely

SITE OF EARLIEST VENTRICULAR ACTIVATION. In the setting of atriofascicular, nodofascicular, and long decrementally conducting AV BTs, the earliest ventricular activation occurs at or near the RV apex. In contrast, for nodoventricular and short decrementally conducting AV BTs, the earliest ventricular activation occurs adjacent to the tricuspid annulus.

VENTRICULAR–HIS BUNDLE INTERVAL. For atriofascicular and nodofascicular BTs, the VH interval is short (16 ± 5 milliseconds), much shorter than the nonpreexcited HV interval and also shorter than the VH interval during ventricular pacing, because the BT inserts into the RB, hence, the HB and ventricle are activated in parallel, not in sequence. Conduction time to the distal RB is short (V-RB = 3 ± 5 milliseconds).[13] For long decrementally conducting AV BTs, the VH interval is short (37 ± 9 milliseconds) but longer than that of atriofascicular BTs because the ventricle and HB are activated in sequence, not in parallel. However, the VH interval is still shorter than the nonpreexcited HV interval. In this setting, the VH interval approximates the HV interval minus the duration of the His potential, because the BT inserts close to the RB and the His potential is activated retrogradely. In the presence of long decrementally conducting AV BTs, conduction time to the distal RB (V-RB = 25 ± 6 milliseconds) is longer than that for atriofascicular BTs. During antidromic AVRT using a nodoventricular or a short decrementally conducting AV BT, intermediate VH intervals are observed, whereby the His potential is inscribed within the QRS. The VH interval during the AVRT is longer than the nonpreexcited HV interval and than the VH interval during RV apical pacing, exceeding it by the time it takes the impulse to travel from the ventricular insertion site of the BT at the RV base to the distal RB (i.e., because of the long V-RB interval).[7,13] When antidromic AVRT occurs in the presence of retrograde right bundle branch block (RBBB), the VH interval is long (the His potential is inscribed after the QRS and the VH interval is longer than the nonpreexcited HV interval). Retrograde block over the RB results in anterograde conduction over the distal RB (in the setting of atriofascicular BTs) or RV and transseptal impulse propagation with subsequent retrograde conduction over the left bundle branch (LB) into the HB and AVN. This results in an antidromic AVRT with a macroreentrant circuit incorporating the LB retrogradely and either an atriofascicular, a long decrementally conducting, or a short decrementally conducting AV BT anterogradely.[7,13]

ATRIAL-VENTRICULAR RELATIONSHIP. For atriofascicular BTs, long decrementally conducting AV BTs, and short decrementally conducting AV BTs, a 1:1 A-V relationship is a prerequisite for the maintenance of antidromic AVRT, because parts of both the RA and the RV are incorporated in the reentrant circuit. However, in the setting of nodofascicular and nodoventricular BTs, the atrium is neither part of nor required for the reentrant circuit, and AV block or dissociation can (although rarely) be present without disrupting the SVT.[7,13]

RESPONSE TO DRUGS. These SVTs are very responsive to and terminate easily with adenosine, calcium channel blockers, and beta blockers.

CHANGES IN TACHYCARDIA CYCLE LENGTH. Changes in the rate of antidromic AVRT using an atriofascicular or a long AV BT as the anterograde limb of the circuit can occur secondary to changes in the VA conduction time, due to either retrograde RBBB or shift of retrograde conduction over a fast AVN pathway to conduction over a slow AVN pathway. The prolongation of the tachycardia CL will be in the VH interval in the former setting, but in the HA interval in the latter setting. Additionally, VA conduction over the HB-AVN axis changing into VA conduction over a second BT can alter the tachycardia CL. When this occurs, the change in the tachycardia CL will depend on the location of the ventricular end of the second BT and the conduction properties of that BT. Therefore, there may be a shortening or a prolongation of the CL. The behavior of the V-RB and VH interval in that situation will depend on where the block is located in the bundle branch–HB-AVN axis.[15]

Preexcited Atrioventricular Nodal Reentrant Tachycardia Using an Atypical Bypass Tract as an Innocent Bystander

The site of earliest ventricular activation depends on the type of the atypical BT mediating preexcitation (see previous discussion). A positive HV interval or VH interval of 10 milliseconds or less (especially when the HA interval is 50 milliseconds or less) is characteristic of AVNRT, because the HB is usually activated anterogradely. However, the HB can become activated retrogradely when conduction over the anterograde slow AVN pathway is very slow; then the VH interval will depend on the type of the atypical BT mediating preexcitation (see earlier).[7,13]

DIAGNOSTIC MANEUVERS DURING TACHYCARDIA

Atrial Extrastimulation and Atrial Pacing during Tachycardia

To prove the presence of a BT and its participation in the SVT, a late-coupled AES is delivered from the lateral RA (close to the BT) when the AV junctional portion of the atrium is refractory, so that the AES does not penetrate the AVN, as indicated by the lack of advancement of local atrial activation in the HB or coronary sinus ostium (CS os) recording. Therefore, such an AES cannot conduct to the ventricle over the AVN; this maneuver is analogous to the introduction of VES when the HB is refractory during orthodromic AVRT. If this AES advances (or delays) the timing of the next ventricular activation, it indicates that an anterogradely conducting AV or atriofascicular BT is present, and excludes nodoventricular and nodofascicular BTs. If the AES advances (or delays) the timing of the next ventricular activation and the advanced (or delayed) QRS morphology is identical to that during the SVT, this proves that the AV or atriofascicular BT also mediates preexcitation during the SVT, either as an integral part of the SVT circuit or as an innocent bystander. On the other hand, if the AES advances the timing of both the next ventricular activation and subsequent atrial activation, it proves that the SVT is an antidromic AVRT using an AV or atriofascicular BT anterogradely, and excludes preexcited AVNRT (Fig. 19-4). Advancement of both ventricular and atrial activation by such an AES requires anterograde conduction over the BT followed by retrograde conduction over the AVN. This can occur during antidromic AVRT but not in AVNRT, because in the setting of AVNRT the HB would be refractory because of anterograde activation by the time the advanced ventricular impulse invades the HPS retrogradely, with subsequent failure of the advanced ventricular activation to penetrate the HPS-AVN and affect the timing of subsequent atrial activation.[7,13]

During entrainment of the SVT by atrial pacing at a CL slightly shorter than the tachycardia CL, the presence of a fixed short VH interval suggests antidromic AVRT, but does not exclude AVNRT. Atrial pacing can usually terminate the SVT, whereby anterograde block is always produced in the AVN, with or without block in the BT. A short-coupled AES can block in the BT, terminating the SVT

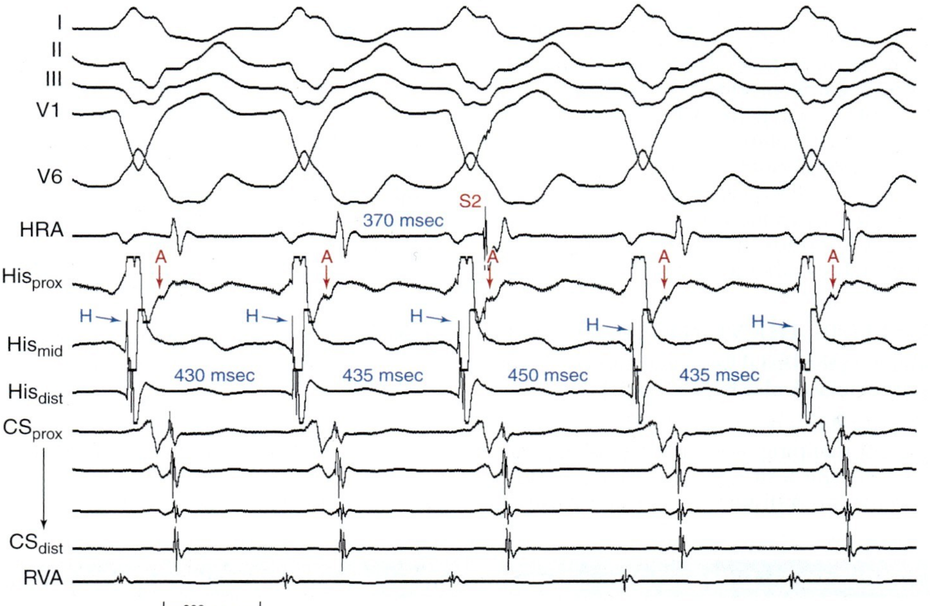

FIGURE 19-4 Atrial extrastimulation (AES) during antidromic atrioventricular reentrant tachycardia (AVRT) using an atriofascicular bypass tract. A late-coupled AES (S_2) delivered from the right atrium (RA) when the AV junctional atrium is refractory (as evidenced by the failure of the AES to affect the timing of atrial activation recorded by the proximal His bundle and proximal coronary sinus electrodes) results in a delay in the timing of the next QRS ("postexcitation"), as well as a delay in the timing of the following atrial activation. This confirms the diagnosis of antidromic AVRT and excludes preexcited atrioventricular nodal reentrant tachycardia and ventricular tachycardia as potential mechanisms of this wide QRS complex tachycardia.

(in the setting of antidromic AVRT) or changing the SVT to a narrow QRS complex SVT at the same CL and same HA interval (in the setting of preexcited AVNRT).

Ventricular Extrastimulation and Ventricular Pacing during Tachycardia

Introduction of a VES during the SVT that results in RBBB can be of diagnostic value. During AVNRT, such RBBB will not change the time of the next atrial activation, because the ventricle and HPS are not parts of the AVNRT circuit. Conversely, during antidromic AVRT, retrograde block in the RB increases the size of the reentrant circuit, because the impulse cannot reach the HB through the RB, and it has to travel transseptally and then retrogradely over the LB. This results in prolongation in the VA interval and delay in the timing of the next atrial activation. The increment in the VA interval occurs because of prolongation of the VH interval, and, if RBBB persists, the SVT will have a long VH interval.

Ventricular pacing can usually terminate the SVT. Termination occurs by retrograde invasion and concealment in the BT, resulting in anterograde block over the BT following conduction to the atrium through the AVN.

DIFFERENTIAL DIAGNOSIS

The goals of programmed electrical stimulation during SVT are evaluation of the relationship among the His potential, the QRS, and the VH interval during atrial pacing and during SVT and differentiation between the different types of atypical BTs (Table 19-1). In addition, exclusion of a separate BT is necessary, especially if a rapid and fixed VA interval exists during incremental rate ventricular pacing. Furthermore, it is important to differentiate between antidromic AVRT using the BT anterogradely and preexcited AVNRT, in which the BT is an innocent bystander (Table 19-2).

Localization of the Bypass Tract

Mapping principles for typical AV BTs—searching for sites with the earliest atrial activation during retrograde BT conduction and earliest ventricular activation during anterograde BT conduction—are largely inapplicable in the case of atypical BTs because of their unusual course and conduction properties. Therefore, different approaches are used.

Mapping of the ventricular insertion site of atriofascicular and long decrementally conducting AV BTs is difficult because of the long intracardiac course and distal insertion of these BTs, which shows extensive arborization over a wide area of ventricular muscle, with a diameter of up to 0.5 to 2 cm. A propensity to temporary loss of conduction of the atypical BT because of catheter trauma further complicates ventricular mapping.[5]

Mapping of the atrial insertion site can be performed by (1) P-delta interval mapping by stimulation at different atrial sites, (2) recording of the BT potential at the tricuspid annulus, and (3) AES from the RA during antidromic AVRT.[8]

Careful mapping of the tricuspid annulus and the anterior free wall of the RV typically demonstrates discrete potentials with complexes comparable to those recorded at the AV junction. The BT potential is analogous to the His potential. Atrial pacing, AES, and adenosine produce delay proximal to BT potential with a constant BT potential to QRS (BT-V) interval. Faster atrial pacing produces Wenckebach block proximal to the BT potential.[13]

MAPPING THE ATRIAL INSERTION SITE

Mapping the Shortest Atrial Stimulus to Delta (S-V) Interval

The mapping catheter is advanced from site to site along the atrial aspect of the tricuspid annulus while pacing from its distal tip. The resulting interval between the stimulus and the onset of the delta wave (S-V interval) should decrease progressively as the BT atrial insertion site is approached, and increase as it is passed. Thus, the atrial pacing site associated with the shortest S-V interval is the site closest to the BT atrial insertion site. It is essential that pacing at different sites be performed at a constant CL to avoid rate-dependent conduction slowing in the BT as a reason for changing the S-V interval. This method is rarely used because of several limitations: (1) a constant distance of the mapping-pacing catheter from the tricuspid annulus must be maintained to reduce the influence of the time spent traversing intervening atrial tissue; (2) catheter manipulation during pacing can result in initiation of tachycardia, which must then be terminated to continue mapping; (3) optimal sites can be overlooked if they cannot be consistently paced because of unstable catheter contact; and (4) this method cannot be applied in the setting of incessant tachycardia or when AF is present.[13]

Atrial Extrastimulation Mapping during Supraventricular Tachycardias

The BT atrial insertion site is close to the site from which the longest coupled AES delivered during preexcited tachycardia advances the timing of the next ventricular activation. Alternatively, the BT atrial insertion site is close to the site from which the greatest amount of advancement of the next ventricular activation occurs when using a fixed AES coupling interval. This method is rarely used because of several limitations: (1) it is time-consuming, and cannot be used if the SVT is difficult to initiate or nonsustained; (2) it is not particularly useful in cases of true nodofascicular BTs; (3) a constant distance of the mapping-pacing catheter from the tricuspid annulus must be maintained to reduce the influence of the time spent traversing intervening atrial tissue; and (4) optimal sites can be overlooked if they cannot be consistently paced because of unstable catheter contact.[13]

MAPPING THE VENTRICULAR INSERTION SITE

Mapping the Distal Fascicular Insertion Site (for Atriofascicular Bypass Tracts)

The distal insertion site of atriofascicular BTs can be localized by careful mapping along the lateral RV wall toward the apex, seeking the earliest site of ventricular activation during anterograde BT conduction. A distal RB recording is usually present at this site. This method can be used to map any rhythm during which consistent preexcitation is present (atrial pacing, AF, and preexcited SVT). However, seeking the distal insertion is less precise because a distal RB recording may be localized, but not the portion into which the atriofascicular fiber inserts. It is most useful if the course of the atriofascicular BT can be traced from the tricuspid annulus to its insertion into the RB. Additionally, ablation at the distal site offers no advantage unless catheter stability is better at that location as opposed to the tricuspid annulus. If the RB is ablated rather than the BT, RBBB will result. Not only will this fail to eliminate the BT function, but it can also facilitate induction and maintenance of the SVT by increasing the reentrant circuit size.[8,13]

Mapping the Distal Ventricular Insertion Site (for Slowly Conducting Atrioventricular Bypass Tracts)

Mapping is performed in the same fashion as for typical rapidly conducting AV BTs—seeking the ventricular site with the earliest unipolar or bipolar ventricular electrogram recording. However, there is evidence that a variable degree of arborization of the distal insertion site occurs in some patients. This feature makes the

TABLE 19-1 Differentiation among Different Types of Atypical Bypass Tracts

Preexcited QRS Morphology

- **Atriofascicular BTs:** The QRS is relatively narrow (133 ± 10 msec), and is classic for typical LBBB morphology.
- **Long decrementally conducting AV BTs:** The QRS is wider (166 ± 26 msec) and the LBBB pattern is less typical (with broad initial R in V_1) than that with atriofascicular BTs.
- **Nodofascicular BTs:** Same as for atriofascicular BTs.
- **Nodoventricular BTs:** The QRS is significantly wider and the LBBB pattern is less typical than that with atriofascicular or long decrementally conducting AV BTs.
- **Short decrementally conducting AV BTs:** The QRS is significantly wider and the LBBB pattern is less typical than that with atriofascicular or long decrementally conducting AV BTs.

Site of Earliest Ventricular Activation

- **Atriofascicular BTs:** The earliest ventricular activation occurs at or near the RV apex.
- **Long decrementally conducting AV BTs:** The earliest ventricular activation occurs at or near the RV apex.
- **Nodofascicular BTs:** The earliest ventricular activation occurs at or near the RV apex.
- **Nodoventricular BTs:** The earliest ventricular activation occurs adjacent to the tricuspid annulus.
- **Short decrementally conducting AV BTs:** The earliest ventricular activation occurs adjacent to the tricuspid annulus.

Influence of Site of Atrial Stimulation

- **Atriofascicular BTs:** Preexcitation increases when atrial stimulation is performed closer to the atrial insertion site.
- **Long decrementally conducting AV BTs:** Preexcitation increases when atrial stimulation is performed closer to the atrial insertion site.
- **Nodofascicular BTs:** The degree of preexcitation is not influenced by the site of atrial stimulation.
- **Nodoventricular BTs:** The degree of preexcitation is not influenced by the site of atrial stimulation.
- **Short decrementally conducting AV BTs:** Preexcitation increases when atrial stimulation is performed closer to the atrial insertion site.

AES Delivered from Lateral RA During Antidromic AVRT when AV Junctional Atrium Is Refractory

- **Atriofascicular BTs:** The AES can advance or delay the next ventricular activation.
- **Long decrementally conducting AV BTs:** The AES can advance or delay the next ventricular activation.
- **Nodofascicular BTs:** The AES cannot advance the next ventricular activation.
- **Nodoventricular BTs:** The AES cannot advance the next ventricular activation.
- **Short decrementally conducting AV BTs:** The AES can advance or delay the next ventricular activation.

VH Interval during Maximal Preexcitation or Antidromic AVRT

- **Atriofascicular BTs:** The VH interval is short (VH interval = 16 ± 5 msec and V-RB interval = 3 ± 5 msec; VH interval < HV interval and < VH interval during RV pacing).
- **Long decrementally conducting AV BTs:** The VH interval is short but longer than that with atriofascicular BTs (VH interval = 37 ± 9 msec and V-RB interval = 25 ± 6 msec).
- **Nodofascicular BTs:** The VH interval is short, as for atriofascicular BTs.
- **Nodoventricular BTs:** The VH interval is intermediate (His potential is inscribed in the QRS, VH interval ≥ HV interval; VH interval > HV interval and > VH interval during RV pacing).
- **Short decrementally conducting AV BTs:** The VH interval is intermediate, as for nodoventricular BTs.
- **Antidromic AVRT in presence of retrograde RBBB:** The VH interval is long (His potential is inscribed after the QRS, VH interval > HV interval).

Presence of VA Block or AV Dissociation

- VA block or AV dissociation during the SVT excludes atriofascicular, short decrementally conducting AV BTs, and long decrementally conducting AV BTs, but does not exclude nodofascicular and nodoventricular BTs.

Effects of Adenosine

- Adenosine produces conduction delay in most atypical BTs (except for short decrementally conducting BTs).
- When adenosine administration slows AVN conduction but not the BT, an increase in the degree of preexcitation is noted in all types of BTs except for fasciculoventricular BTs, whereby the degrees of preexcitation and HV interval remain fixed.

AES = atrial extrastimulation; AV = atrioventricular; AVRT = atrioventricular reentrant tachycardia; HV = His bundle–ventricular; LBBB = left bundle branch block; RA = right atrium; RBBB = right bundle branch block; RV = right ventricle; SVT = supraventricular tachycardia; VA = ventriculoatrial; VH = ventricular–His bundle; V-RB = ventricular–right bundle branch.

TABLE 19-2 Differentiation between Antidromic AVRT and Preexcited AVNRT Using an Atypical BT

SVT Induction

- Induction of the SVT by ventricular pacing at a CL similar to the tachycardia CL, or by a VES that advances the His potential by a coupling interval similar to the H-H interval during the SVT—the HA interval following such a ventricular stimulus is compared with that during the SVT:
  - $HA_{VES} > HA_{SVT}$ is diagnostic of AVNRT and excludes antidromic AVRT.
  - $HA_{VES} \leq HA_{SVT}$ is diagnostic of antidromic AVRT and excludes AVNRT.

Features of the SVT

- Positive HV interval or VH interval ≤10 msec (especially when HA interval is ≤50 msec) suggests AVNRT.
- Continuation of the SVT at the same tachycardia CL, despite anterograde block in the BT (by extrastimuli, drugs, mechanical trauma caused by catheter manipulation, or ablation), is diagnostic of AVNRT and excludes antidromic AVRT.
- Termination of the SVT or prolongation of the VA (and VH) interval and tachycardia CL with transient RBBB (caused by mechanical trauma or introduction of VES) is diagnostic of antidromic AVRT and excludes AVNRT.

AES Delivered from Lateral RA when AV Junction Is Refractory

- If the AES advances the timing of both the following ventricular activation and the subsequent atrial activation, it proves that the SVT is an antidromic AVRT using an AV or atriofascicular BT anterogradely, and excludes preexcited AVNRT.

Entrainment of the SVT with Atrial Pacing

- The presence of a fixed short VH interval during entrainment of the SVT with atrial pacing suggests antidromic AVRT and makes AVNRT unlikely (but does not exclude AVNRT).

RV Apical Pacing during NSR

- RV apical pacing at the tachycardia CL is performed, and the HA interval during RV apical pacing versus the HA interval during SVT are compared:
  - $HA_{SVT} < HA_{pacing}$ is diagnostic of AVNRT and excludes antidromic AVRT.
  - $HA_{SVT} \geq HA_{pacing}$ is diagnostic of antidromic AVRT and excludes AVNRT.

AES = atrial extrastimulation; AV = atrioventricular; AVNRT = atrioventricular nodal reentrant tachycardia; AVRT = atrioventricular reentrant tachycardia; BT = bypass tract; CL = cycle length; HA = His bundle–atrial; NSR = normal sinus rhythm; RA = right atrium; RBBB = right bundle branch block; RV = right ventricle; SVT = supraventricular tachycardia; VA = ventriculoatrial; VES = ventricular extrastimulation; VH = ventricular–His bundle.

ventricular insertion site a less attractive ablation target because of the potential of requiring ablation of a relatively large amount of ventricular myocardium to be effective.[13]

MAPPING THE BYPASS TRACT POTENTIAL

Direct recording of the BT potential at the tricuspid annulus is the most precise and preferred method of localizing the atypical BT. The BT potential is usually a low-amplitude, high-frequency recording made at the tricuspid annulus, which resembles a His potential (Fig. 19-5). Only the annular and subannular portions of the BT have been successfully recorded; attempts to record potentials from the atrial portion (corresponding to nodal-like tissue) have been unsuccessful. Distinct atrial, BT, and ventricular potentials can be found at the BT atrial insertion site. Recording a BT potential can be successful during NSR, atrial pacing, or preexcited SVT. However, recording of a BT potential along the tricuspid annulus may not be successful in up to 48% of cases. Furthermore, because of the low amplitude of the BT potential, it is difficult or impossible to record it during AF. Additionally, this technique presents the risk of producing mechanical block in the BT. Nevertheless, this method is less time-consuming and more precise than the previous ones.[8,13]

MAPPING SITES OF MECHANICALLY INDUCED LOSS OF PREEXCITATION

Atypical BTs are particularly sensitive to mechanical trauma, and catheter manipulation along the tricuspid annulus during mapping of the BT may result in loss of BT function, even as a result of gentle pressure from the catheter tip. When mapping is performed during preexcited atrial pacing or SVT, damage to the BT is indicated by a sudden, transient loss of preexcitation. This phenomenon can be used to localize the BT precisely (bump mapping). Conduction block typically occurs while a BT potential is still recorded; thus, conduction is interrupted within the ventricular course of the BT. Block usually lasts from a few beats to a few minutes but can last for hours, after which preexcitation resumes. This method can be used during any consistently preexcited rhythm (atrial pacing, AF, and antidromic AVRT). However, if it occurs during antidromic AVRT, termination of the tachycardia may result in catheter displacement and loss of the exact location of the BT. Additionally, interruption of BT conduction can occur as the catheter is passing the area, and

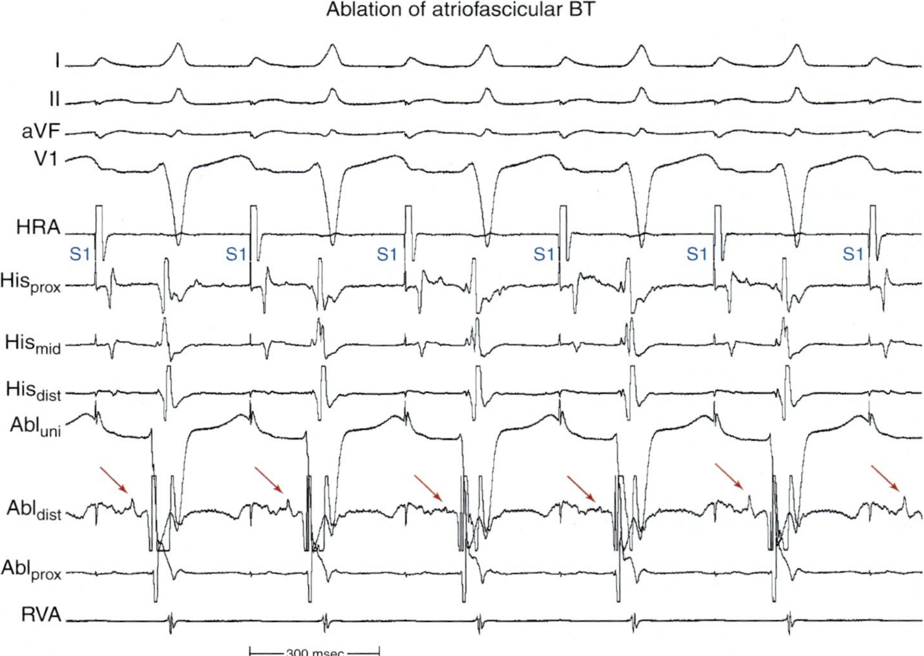

FIGURE 19-5 Ablation of an atriofascicular bypass tract (BT). A discrete potential (arrows) is shown in the ablation recording during atrial pacing, with a small His potential occurring just after the onset of the preexcited QRS. Ablation at this site eliminated this BT in 2 seconds.

where the catheter comes to rest may not be the same site as where loss of BT function occurred; in this situation, the target cannot be relocated until BT conduction resumes. Delivery of radiofrequency (RF) energy at a site at which catheter pressure caused loss of preexcitation may successfully eliminate conduction in the BT; however, it is best to wait to deliver energy until preexcitation resumes, because of the possibility that the catheter position may have changed. Electroanatomical mapping (e.g., CARTO, NavX) can help tag sites of interest, facilitating precise relocation of the ablation catheter to these sites if it has been determined that they are a good ablation target. Atriofascicular BTs are more susceptible to mechanically induced block, probably suggesting that these BTs are composed of thinner strands or are located closer to the endocardium.[13]

Ablation

TARGET OF ABLATION

Direct recording of the BT potential at the tricuspid annulus is the most precise and preferred method of localizing the BT and serves as the target of ablation (see Fig. 19-5).[7,13] Ablation at the ventricular insertion site of the BT offers no advantage over targeting the atrial insertion site because there is evidence that a variable degree of arborization of the distal insertion site occurs in some patients, with the potential of requiring ablation of a relatively large amount of ventricular myocardium to be effective.[5,8]

However, when a BT potential along the tricuspid annulus cannot be recorded, ablation of the distal insertion sites of atriofascicular BTs becomes an alternative and has been found to be highly effective, but is commonly (57%) associated with the development of RBBB. Ablation of the RB can carry a proarrhythmic effect and facilitate induction of the SVT or cause incessant tachycardia; however, this is not a concern as long as the BT itself is also successfully ablated.[8,13]

Using these methods, the locations of successful ablation of atypical BTs are found to be mostly along the lateral tricuspid annulus, with a minority along the septal aspect of the tricuspid annulus or within the ventricle. Atriofascicular and long decrementally conducting AV BTs tend (84%) to cross the tricuspid annulus in a lateral, anterolateral, or anterior region, whereas short decrementally conducting AV BTs are roughly equally distributed between these and a posterior or septal region.

ABLATION TECHNIQUE

Once an appropriate target site for ablation has been identified, RF energy may be applied during NSR, atrial pacing, or antidromic AVRT. Atrial pacing is preferred to ensure that adequate preexcitation is evident (unlike NSR) to be able to assess the efficacy of ablation, and that the rhythm remains the same after elimination of preexcitation (unlike antidromic AVRT) to prevent catheter dislodgment.[5,8]

The use of long curved sheaths can help achieve good catheter positioning and stability along the tricuspid annulus. Typical RF settings consist of a maximal power of 50 W and a maximal temperature of 55°C to 60°C, continued for 30 to 60 seconds after elimination of the BT function (i.e., after disappearance of preexcitation). During RF energy delivery, an accelerated preexcited rhythm is often observed. This so-called *Mahaim automatic tachycardia* is analogous to the accelerated junctional rhythm observed during AVN modification, and is presumably secondary to heating-related automaticity of nodal-like tissue of the BT. Accelerated automatic beats during RF ablation have been considered a marker of a successful result, and RF energy delivery should be continued for a sufficient duration after termination of this rhythm.[13] Heat-induced automaticity during RF ablation is observed less commonly in short decrementally conducting AV BTs as compared with atriofascicular BTs (50% versus 91%).[16,17]

ENDPOINTS OF ABLATION

Complete loss of BT function, not just noninducibility of tachycardias, is an essential endpoint. BT block is confirmed by demonstrating loss of preexcitation with atrial pacing and AES and noninducibility of AVRT. Atrial stimulation should be performed at sites and rates that were associated with preexcitation before ablation.[13]

OUTCOME

The acute success rate is approximately 90% to 100%, and the short-term recurrence rate is less than 5%.[13]

Fasciculoventricular Bypass Tracts

General Considerations

Fasciculoventricular BTs are the rarest form of preexcitation (1.2% to 5.1% of atypical BTs). They connect the HB to ventricular myocardium in the anteroseptal location. These fibers do not give rise to any reentrant tachycardia, and appear to be only an ECG and EP curiosity. Even during AF and AFL, a rapid ventricular response is not expected in the presence of a normal AVN proximal to the BT. However, it is important to distinguish fasciculoventricular BTs from superoparaseptal BTs to avoid unnecessary invasive EP procedures and potential harm to the AVN-HB if such a BT is mistakenly targeted by ablation, because this form of preexcitation does not require treatment.[7]

Electrocardiographic Features

In patients with fasciculoventricular BTs, preexcitation is always present during NSR. The ECG preexcitation pattern can mimic that of manifest WPW pattern, especially that of superoparaseptal AV BTs, with a normal frontal plane axis between 0 and 75 degrees and precordial RS transitional zone in leads V_2-V_3. With fasciculoventricular BTs, the PR interval is normal despite the presence of preexcitation (Fig. 19-6). This is in contrast to superoparaseptal AV BTs, which result in the WPW pattern with significant shortening of the PR interval because of the relative proximity of the BT location to the sinus node.

Several ECG findings in lead V_1 favor fasciculoventricular BTs as the cause of preexcitation, including: (1) PR interval greater than 110 milliseconds; (2) R wave width less than 35 milliseconds; (3) S wave amplitude less than 20 mm; (4) flat or negative delta wave; and (5) notching in the descending limb of the S wave (see Fig. 19-6).[18]

Electrophysiological Testing

With fasciculoventricular BTs, preexcitation is present during NSR with a normal AH interval and short HV interval. The earliest ventricular activation occurs at the HB region (Table 19-3).

Progressively shorter atrial pacing CLs or AES coupling intervals produce progressive prolongation of the PR and AH intervals but with a fixed degree of preexcitation, a constant and short HV interval, and a fixed relationship between the His potential and RB potential (Fig. 19-7). AVN Wenckebach block can develop, which is then associated with a fixed degree of preexcitation and a constant, short HV interval. The loss of AV conduction is associated with loss of preexcitation. AES can result in block in the fasciculoventricular BT, producing a sudden loss of preexcitation and prolongation of the HV interval to normal values (see Fig. 19-7).

HB pacing normalizes the HV interval and eliminates preexcitation in all types of BTs except for fasciculoventricular BTs, in which a fixed degree of preexcitation and a constant short HV interval remain unchanged during HB pacing (see Fig. 19-6).

When adenosine administration slows AVN conduction, an increase in the degree of preexcitation is noted in all types of BTs, as long as adenosine does not block the BT, except for fasciculoventricular BTs, in which the degree of preexcitation and HV interval remain fixed. Moreover, adenosine administration can be associated with complete AV block and junctional escape beats and, in the setting of fasciculoventricular BTs, these beats are associated with the same degree of preexcitation and the same HV interval as during NSR, even when these ectopic beats are associated with retrograde VA block and no atrial depolarization.

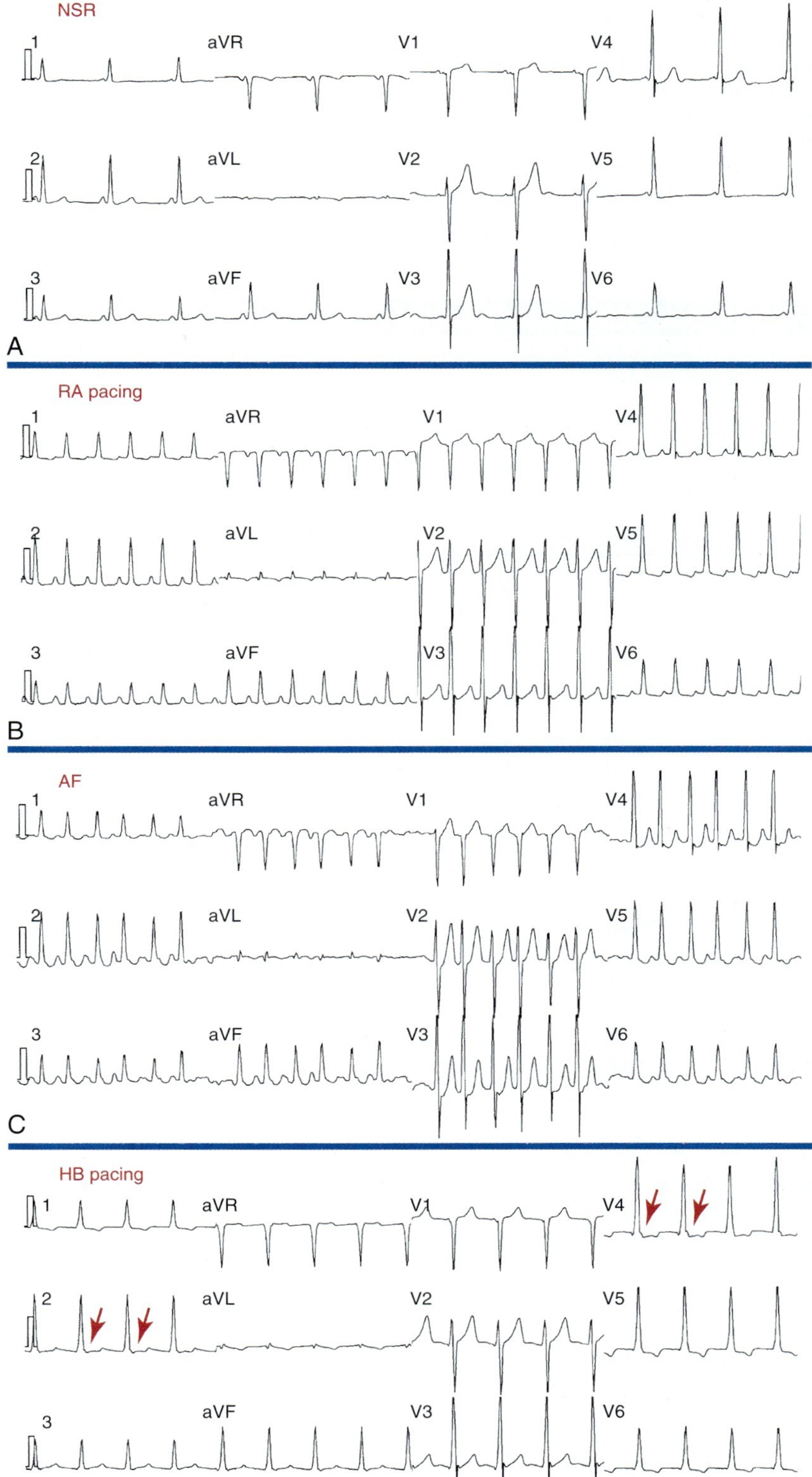

FIGURE 19-6 ECG of fasciculoventricular bypass tracts. **A,** Surface ECG of normal sinus rhythm (NSR) with preexcitation over a fasciculoventricular pathway. Note the short PR and slight slurring of the QRS upstroke in several leads. **B,** Pacing from the right atrium (RA) at the shortest cycle length associated with 1:1 atrioventricular (AV) conduction results in no change in the mild degree of preexcitation compared with NSR despite atrioventricular nodal conduction delay (longer PR interval). **C,** Atrial fibrillation (AF) is present, with no change in the mild degree of preexcitation compared with NSR regardless of the R-R interval. **D,** Surface ECG during His bundle (HB) pacing in the same patient. The same degree of preexcitation persists as in NSR. Retrograde P waves are visible (arrows), deforming the end of QRS complexes.

Atrio-Hisian Bypass Tracts

General Considerations

Patients with palpitations who had a short PR interval but normal QRS complex in the resting ECG were first described in 1938 and then further evaluated by Lown and colleagues in 1952.[19] The latter report consisted of a retrospective examination of 13,500 ECGs and identified short PR intervals in a mixed group of 200 subjects, most of whom had a normal QRS complex (Fig. 19-8). The authors described a "syndrome" characterized by short PR interval, narrow QRS complex, and recurrent paroxysmal SVTs. They initially ascribed this syndrome to the presence of an AV nodal BT.[7,19] A variety of explanations were later offered to account for the short PR interval.

Although the incidence of palpitations was significantly higher in these patients with short PR intervals when compared with a control group with a normal PR interval (17% versus 0.5%), most contemporary electrophysiologists do not consider the "Lown-Ganong-Levine syndrome" to be a recognized syndrome consisting of a single entity but an electrocardiographic description. It probably represents one end of the normal spectrum of AVN conduction properties. Therefore, the use of the term is inappropriate and should be discouraged and the mechanism responsible for the short PR interval should be used instead. The persistence of the term probably relates to the appealing parallel with the initials of the WPW syndrome.

The short PR interval can have different mechanisms: (1) enhanced AVN conduction (perhaps using specialized intranodal fibers), which is believed responsible for most cases of short PR interval and is secondary to an anatomically small AVN, enhanced sympathetic tone, or a variant of normal; (2) atrio-Hisian BT (rare), in which case AF or AFL with a rapid ventricular response is the presenting arrhythmia; (3) ectopic atrial rhythm with differential input into the AVN; and (4) isorhythmic AV dissociation, whereby the short PR interval is not caused by a conducted P wave.[7]

TABLE 19-3 Features of Fasciculoventricular Bypass Tracts

- Preexcitation is present in NSR with a normal PR interval with a transitional zone in V_2-V_3.
- The earliest ventricular activation occurs at the HB region.
- The degree of preexcitation is not influenced by the site of atrial stimulation.
- Incremental rate atrial pacing results in progressive prolongation in the P-delta interval, but the degree of preexcitation is not influenced by the pacing rate.
- HB pacing does not change the degree of preexcitation or the HV interval.

HB = His bundle; HV = His bundle–ventricular; NSR = normal sinus rhythm.

Supraventricular Tachycardias in Patients with Short PR Intervals

PATIENTS WITH ENHANCED ATRIOVENTRICULAR NODE CONDUCTION

The mechanism(s) of SVTs in patients with enhanced AVN conduction does not appear to differ significantly from those in patients with normal PR intervals (AVNRT being the most common, followed by orthodromic AVRT). The tachycardia CL of AVNRT occurring in patients with short PR intervals is not different from that in patients with normal PR intervals. This is expected, because the tachycardia CL of AVNRT is determined by conduction over the slow AVN pathway, which is similar in these patients and those with a normal

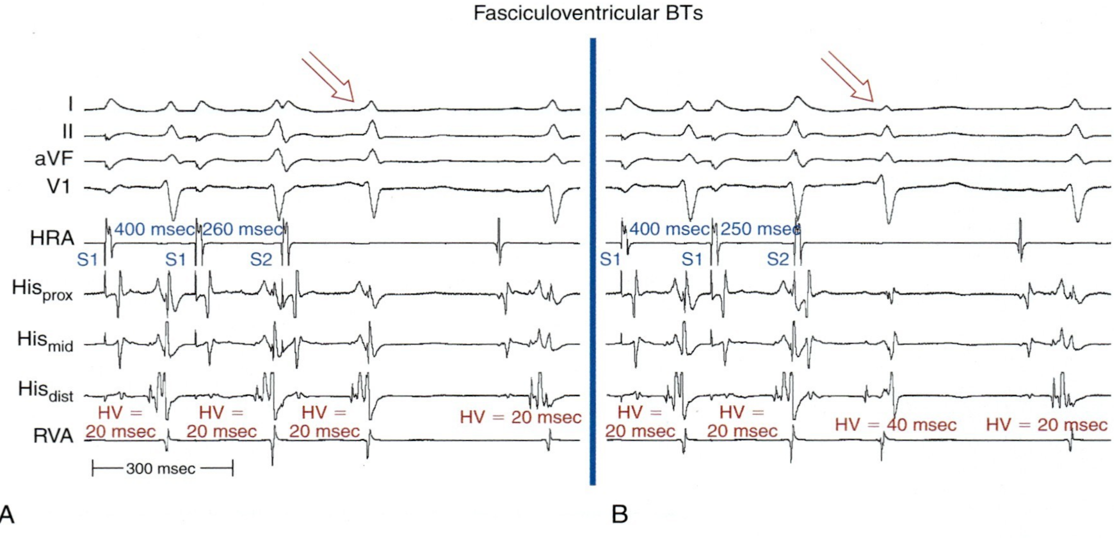

FIGURE 19-7 Effect of atrial stimulation of fasciculoventricular bypass tracts (BTs). **A,** Minimal preexcitation is present during normal sinus rhythm (NSR), with the same during atrial pacing and following an atrial extrastimulus (AES) that lengthens the atrial–His bundle (AH) interval, but the His bundle–ventricular (HV) interval remains fixed at only 20 milliseconds. These features are consistent with a fasciculoventricular pathway. **B,** A more premature AES results in block in the fasciculoventricular pathway, resulting in a narrow QRS complex and normal HV interval (40 milliseconds). Note the difference in QRS complex morphology following the AESs (arrows).

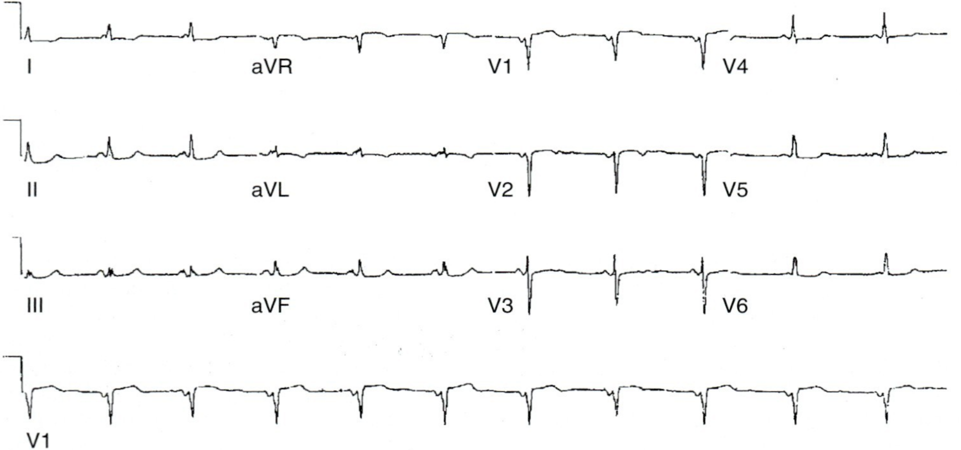

FIGURE 19-8 Surface ECG of an asymptomatic patient with short PR interval and no preexcitation.

PR interval. In contrast, the tachycardia CL of orthodromic AVRT tends to be much shorter in these patients compared with patients with normal PR intervals, which is expected because the circuit of orthodromic AVRT uses the fast AVN pathway for anterograde conduction. In fact, in any SVT with a tachycardia CL shorter than 250 milliseconds enhanced AVN conduction and orthodromic AVRT should be suspected. In such patients, bundle branch block (BBB) is common during SVT, resulting in wide complex tachycardia.[7]

PATIENTS WITH ATRIO-HISIAN BYPASS TRACTS

These patients primarily present with AF and AFL with a rapid ventricular response, and do not develop reentrant SVTs using the AV junction as one limb.[7] Rapid ventricular response during AF depends on refractoriness of the tissue responsible for AV conduction (i.e., AVN or BT) and not on the site of insertion for that tissue.

Electrophysiological Testing

BASELINE OBSERVATIONS DURING NORMAL SINUS RHYTHM

Enhanced AVN conduction is characterized by a short AH interval (<60 milliseconds) and normal HV interval.[7] In rare cases in which the AVN is completely bypassed by an atrio-Hisian BT, the HV interval is short. The HV interval in these cases is artifactually short because the proximal HB and the ventricle are activated in parallel since the atrio-Hisian BT inserts into the distal HB (i.e., the proximal HB is activated retrogradely).

ATRIAL PACING AND ATRIAL EXTRASTIMULATION

Patients with Enhanced Atrioventricular Node Conduction

The AH interval prolongs with progressively shorter atrial pacing CLs and AES coupling intervals.[7] The prolongation in the AH interval is smooth, continuous, and blunted, with a maximal increase in the AH interval of 100 milliseconds or less during pacing at a CL of 300 milliseconds compared with the value measured during NSR. The maximal AH interval (at any pacing rate) is rarely longer than 200 milliseconds and 1:1 conduction typically is maintained to pacing rates greater than 200 beats/min.

The AH interval response can be characteristic of dual AVN physiology, with an initial blunted small prolongation in the AH interval followed by a significant jump at a critical pacing CL or AES coupling interval, while maintaining 1:1 conduction at a pacing rate greater than 200 beats/min. In such patients, the maximal AH interval can be greater than 200 milliseconds, and the maximal prolongation in the AH interval can be greater than 100 milliseconds.[7] Atrial pacing from the CS is associated with shorter AH intervals, shorter Wenckebach CLs, and shorter AVN effective refractory periods, suggesting a preferential input into the AVN.

Patients with Atrio-Hisian Bypass Tracts

The AH interval remains short with no or minimal prolongation in response to progressively shorter atrial pacing CLs and AES coupling intervals. Block in the BT, which can usually be achieved by antiarrhythmic agents or occasionally by the induction of AF, is associated with a simultaneous increase in the PR and AH intervals and normalization of the HV interval.[7]

VENTRICULAR PACING AND VENTRICULAR EXTRASTIMULATION

Patients with Enhanced Atrioventricular Node Conduction

Retrograde AVN conduction is extremely rapid in these patients. In general, the HA interval is shorter than the AH interval at comparable pacing CLs. The HA interval typically remains relatively short with little prolongation in response to progressively shorter ventricular pacing CLs and VES coupling intervals.[7] A concealed AV BT mediating retrograde VA conduction should be excluded, which can be achieved by a variety of pacing maneuvers (see Chap. 18).

Patients with Atrio-Hisian Bypass Tracts

VA conduction is unpredictable in these patients. In many cases, VA conduction is absent and, even when present, it is not as good as AV conduction.[7]

RESPONSE TO PHARMACOLOGICAL AND PHYSIOLOGICAL MANEUVERS

Patients with Enhanced Atrioventricular Node Conduction

The AH interval prolongs in response to beta blockers, verapamil, digoxin, carotid sinus massage, and vagal maneuvers. Complete autonomic blockade results in increases in the AH interval and AVN functional refractory period, but a minimal change in the AVN effective refractory period (suggesting sympathetic tone predominance in these patients, in contrast to individuals with normal AVN conduction in whom vagal tone predominates).[7]

Patients with Atrio-Hisian Bypass Tracts

AV conduction over the atrio-Hisian BT is not affected by autonomic modulation. Conduction block in the BT requires class IA or IC agents or amiodarone. Conduction block is associated with an immediate, sudden, and marked prolongation of the AH and HV intervals to normal values.

REFERENCES

1. Mahaim I, Benatt A: Nouvelles recherches sur les connections superieures de la branche du faisceau de His-Tawara avec cloison interventriculaire, *Cardiologia* 1:61, 1937.
2. Mahaim I, Winston MR: Recherches d'anatomie comparee et de pathologie experimentale sur les connexions hautes des His-Tawara, *Cardiologia* 33:651–653, 1941.
3. Mahaim I: Kent's fibers and the A-V paraspecific conduction through the upper connections of the bundle of His-Tawara, *Am Heart J* 33:651–653, 1947.
4. Benditt DG, Lu F: Atriofascicular pathways: fuzzy nomenclature or merely wishful thinking? *J Cardiovasc Electrophysiol* 17:261–265, 2006.
5. Miller J, Olgin JE: Catheter ablation of free-wall accessory pathways and "Mahaim" fibers. In Zipes DP, Haissaguerre M, editors: *Catheter ablation of arrhythmias*, Armonk, NY, 2002, Futura, pp 277–303.
6. Sternick EB, Lokhandwala Y, Timmermans C, et al: The atrioventricular interval during pre-excited tachycardia: a simple way to distinguish between decrementally or rapidly conducting accessory pathways, *Heart Rhythm* 6:1351–1358, 2009.
7. Josephson ME: Preexcitation syndromes. In Josephson ME, editor: *Clinical cardiac electrophysiology*, ed 4, Philadelphia, 2008, Lippincott Williams & Wilkins, pp 339–445.
8. Kothari S, Gupta AK, Lokhandwala YY, et al: Atriofascicular pathways: where to ablate? *Pacing Clin Electrophysiol* 29:1226–1233, 2006.
9. Davidson NC, Morton JB, Sanders P, Kalman J: Latent Mahaim fiber as a cause of antidromic reciprocating tachycardia: recognition and successful radiofrequency ablation, *J Cardiovasc Electrophysiol* 13:74–78, 2002.
10. Sternick EB, Fagundes ML, Cruz FE, et al: Short atrioventricular Mahaim fibers: observations on their clinical, electrocardiographic, and electrophysiologic profile, *J Cardiovasc Electrophysiol* 16:127–134, 2005.
11. Kalbfleisch S, Bowman K, Augostini R: A single Mahaim fiber causing both antidromic and orthodromic reciprocating tachycardia, *J Cardiovasc Electrophysiol* 19:740–742, 2008.
12. Sternick EB, Timmermans C, Sosa E, et al: The electrocardiogram during sinus rhythm and tachycardia in patients with Mahaim fibers: the importance of an "rS" pattern in lead III, *J Am Coll Cardiol* 44:1626–1635, 2004.
13. Miller JM, Rothman SA, Hsia HH, Buxton AE: Ablation of Mahaim fibers. In Huang SKS, Wilber DJ, editors: *Radiofrequency catheter ablation of cardiac arrhythmias: basic concepts and clinical applications*, Armonk, NY, 2000, Futura, pp 559–578.
14. Bogun F, Krishnan S, Siddiqui M, et al: Electrogram characteristics in postinfarction ventricular tachycardia: effect of infarct age, *J Am Coll Cardiol* 46:667–674, 2005.
15. Sternick EB, Rodriguez LM, Timmermans C, et al: Effects of right bundle branch block on the antidromic circus movement tachycardia in patients with presumed atriofascicular pathways, *J Cardiovasc Electrophysiol* 17:256–260, 2006.
16. Sternick EB, Gerken LM, Vrandecic M: Appraisal of "Mahaim" automatic tachycardia, *J Cardiovasc Electrophysiol* 13:244–249, 2002.
17. Sternick EB, Sosa EA, Timmermans C, et al: Automaticity in Mahaim fibers, *J Cardiovasc Electrophysiol* 15:738–744, 2004.
18. Oh S, Choi YS, Choi EK, et al: Electrocardiographic characteristics of fasciculoventricular pathways, *Pacing Clin Electrophysiol* 28:25–28, 2005.
19. Lown B, Ganong WF, Levine SA: The syndrome of short P-R interval, normal QRS complex and paroxysmal rapid heart action, *Circulation* 5:693–706, 1952.

CHAPTER 20 Approach to Paroxysmal Supraventricular Tachycardias

Clinical Considerations

A "supraventricular" origin of a tachycardia implies the obligatory involvement of one or more cardiac structures above the bifurcation of the His bundle (HB), including the atrial myocardium, the atrioventricular node (AVN), the proximal HB, the coronary sinus (CS), the pulmonary veins (PVs), the venae cavae, or abnormal atrioventricular (AV) connections other than the HB (i.e., bypass tracts, BTs).[1]

Epidemiology

Narrow QRS complex supraventricular tachycardia (SVT) is a tachyarrhythmia with a rate greater than 100 beats/min and a QRS duration of less than 120 milliseconds. Narrow QRS complex SVTs include sinus tachycardia, inappropriate sinus tachycardia, sinoatrial nodal reentrant tachycardia, atrial tachycardia (AT), multifocal AT, atrial fibrillation (AF), atrial flutter (AFL), junctional ectopic tachycardia, nonparoxysmal junctional tachycardia, atrioventricular nodal reentrant tachycardia (AVNRT), and atrioventricular reentrant tachycardia (AVRT).

Narrow QRS complex tachycardias can be divided into those that require only atrial tissue for their initiation and maintenance (sinus tachycardia, AT, AF, and AFL), and those that require the AV junction (junctional tachycardia, AVNRT, and AVRT).

Paroxysmal SVT is the term generally applied to intermittent SVT other than AF, AFL, and multifocal AT. The major causes are AVNRT (approximately 50% to 60% of cases), AVRT (approximately 30% of cases), and AT (approximately 10% of cases).

Paroxysmal SVT with sudden onset and termination is relatively common; the estimated prevalence in the normal population is 2.25/1000, with an incidence of 35/100,000 person-years. Paroxysmal SVT in the absence of structural heart disease can present at any age but most commonly first presents between ages 12 and 30 years. Women have a twofold greater risk of developing this arrhythmia than men.

The mechanism of paroxysmal SVT is significantly influenced by both age and gender. In a large cohort of patients with symptomatic paroxysmal SVT referred for ablation, as patients grew older there was a significant and progressive decline in the number of patients presenting with AVRT, which was the predominant mechanism in the first decade, and a striking increase in AVNRT and AT (Fig. 20-1). These trends were similar in both genders, although AVNRT replaced AVRT as the predominant mechanism much earlier in women.[2] The early predominance of AVRT is consistent with the congenital nature of the substrate and with the fact that symptom onset occurs earlier in patients with AVRT than AVNRT, most commonly in the first two decades of life. However, a minority of patients have relatively late onset of symptoms associated with AVRT and thus continue to account for a small proportion of ablations in older patients. Men account for a higher proportion of AVRT at all ages.

AVNRT is the predominant mechanism overall in patients undergoing ablation and after the age of 20 years accounts for the largest number of ablations in each age group. AVNRT is unusual in children under 5 years of age, and typically initially manifests in early life, often in the teens. AVRT presents earlier, with an average of more than 10 years separating the time of clinical presentation of AVRT versus AVNRT. There is a striking 2:1 predominance of women in the AVNRT group, which remains without clear physiological or anatomical explanation. Female sex and older age, that is, teens versus early childhood years, favor the diagnosis of AVNRT over AVRT.[3]

ATs comprise a progressively greater proportion of those with paroxysmal SVT with increasing age, accounting for 23% of patients older than 70 years. Although there is a greater absolute number of women with AT, the proportion of AT in both genders is similar. Age-related changes in the atrial electrophysiological (EP) substrate (including cellular coupling and autonomic influences) can contribute to the increased incidence of AT in older individuals.

Clinical Presentation

The clinical syndrome of paroxysmal SVT is characterized as a regular rapid tachycardia of abrupt onset and termination. Episodes can last from seconds to several hours. Patients commonly describe palpitations and dizziness. Dizziness can occur initially because of hypotension, but it then disappears when the sympathetic response to the SVT stabilizes the blood pressure. Rapid ventricular rates can be associated with complaints of dyspnea, weakness, angina, or even frank syncope, and can at times be disabling. Neck pounding can occur during tachycardia because of simultaneous contraction of the atria and ventricles against closed mitral and tricuspid valves. The latter is more common in patients with typical AVNRT, occurring in approximately 50% of patients.

Patients often learn to use certain maneuvers such as carotid sinus massage or the Valsalva maneuver to terminate the arrhythmia, although many require pharmacological treatment to achieve this. In patients without structural heart disease, the physical examination is usually remarkable only for a rapid, regular heart rate. At times, because of the simultaneous contraction of atria and ventricles, cannon A waves can be seen in the jugular venous waveform (described as the "frog" sign). This clinical feature has been reported to distinguish paroxysmal SVT resulting from AVNRT from that caused by orthodromic AVRT. Although the atrial contraction during AVRT will occur against closed AV valves, the longer VA interval results in separate ventricular and then atrial contraction and a relatively lower right atrial (RA) and venous pressure; therefore, the presence of palpations in the neck is experienced less commonly (up to 17%) in patients with AVRT.[3] In patients with an

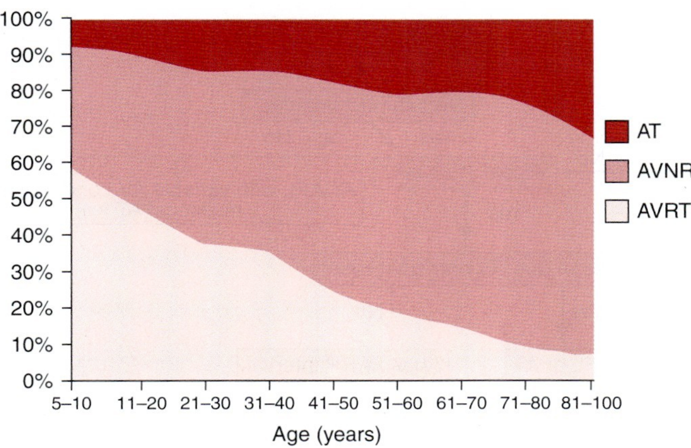

FIGURE 20-1 Proportion of paroxysmal supraventricular tachycardia mechanisms by age. AT = atrial tachycardia; AVNRT = atrioventricular nodal reentrant tachycardia; AVRT = atrioventricular reentrant tachycardia. *(From Porter MJ, Morton JB, Denman R, et al: Influence of age and gender on the mechanism of supraventricular tachycardia, Heart Rhythm 1:393, 2004.)*

AT exhibiting AV block, usually of the Wenckebach type, the ventricular rate is irregular.

Initial Evaluation

History, physical examination, and an electrocardiogram (ECG) constitute an appropriate initial evaluation of paroxysmal SVT. However, clinical symptoms are not usually helpful in distinguishing different forms of paroxysmal SVT. A 12-lead ECG during tachycardia can be helpful for defining the mechanism of paroxysmal SVT. Ambulatory 24-hour Holter recording can be used for documentation of the arrhythmia in patients with frequent (i.e., several episodes per week) but self-terminating tachycardias. A cardiac event monitor is often more useful than a 24-hour recording in patients with less frequent arrhythmias. Implantable loop recorders can be helpful in selected cases with rare episodes associated with severe symptoms of hemodynamic instability (e.g., syncope).

An echocardiographic examination should be considered in patients with documented sustained SVT to exclude the possibility of structural heart disease. Exercise testing is rarely useful for diagnosis unless the arrhythmia is clearly triggered by exertion. Further diagnostic studies are indicated only if there are signs or symptoms that suggest structural heart disease.

Transesophageal atrial recordings and stimulation can be used in selected cases for diagnosis or to provoke paroxysmal tachyarrhythmias if the clinical history is insufficient or if other measures have failed to document an arrhythmia. Esophageal stimulation is not indicated if invasive EP investigation is planned. Invasive EP testing with subsequent catheter ablation may be used for diagnosis and therapy in cases with a clear history of paroxysmal regular palpitations. It may also be considered in patients with preexcitation or disabling symptoms without ECG documentation of an arrhythmia.

Principles of Management

ACUTE MANAGEMENT

Most episodes of paroxysmal SVT require intact 1:1 AVN conduction for continuation and are therefore classified as AVN-dependent. AVN conduction and refractoriness can be modified by vagal maneuvers and by many pharmacological agents and thus are the weak links targeted by most acute therapies. Termination of a sustained episode of SVT is usually accomplished by producing transient block in the AVN.

Vagal maneuvers such as carotid sinus massage, Valsalva maneuvers, or the dive reflex are usually used as the first step and generally terminate the SVT. Valsalva is the most effective technique in adults, but carotid sinus massage can also be effective. Facial immersion in water is the most reliable method in infants. Vagal maneuvers are less effective once a sympathetic response to paroxysmal SVT has become established, so patients should be advised to try them soon after onset of symptoms. Vagal maneuvers present the advantage of being relatively simple and noninvasive, but their efficacy seems to be lower compared with pharmacological interventions, with the incidence of paroxysmal SVT termination ranging from 6% to 22% following carotid sinus massage.

When vagal maneuvers are unsuccessful, termination can be achieved with antiarrhythmic drugs whose primary effects increase AVN refractoriness, decrease AVN conduction (negative dromotropic effect), or both. These drugs can have direct (e.g., verapamil and diltiazem block the slow inward calcium current of the AVN) or indirect effects (e.g., digoxin increases vagal tone to the AVN). In most patients, the drug of choice is either adenosine or verapamil.

The advantages of adenosine include its rapid onset of action (usually within 10 to 25 seconds via a peripheral vein), short half-life (<10 seconds), and high degree of efficacy. The effective dose of adenosine is usually 6 to 12 mg, given as a rapid bolus. Doses up to 12 mg terminate over 90% of paroxysmal SVT episodes. Sequential dosing can be given at 60-second intervals because of adenosine's rapid metabolism. In AVNRT, termination is usually caused by block in the anterograde slow pathway. In AVRT, termination occurs secondary to block in the AVN. Termination can also occur indirectly, that is, because of adenosine-induced premature atrial complexes (PACs) or premature ventricular complexes (PVCs). Adenosine shortens the atrial refractory period, and atrial ectopy can induce AF. This can be dangerous if the patient has a BT capable of rapid anterograde conduction, and sometimes subsequently requires immediate electrical cardioversion. Because adenosine is cleared so rapidly, reinitiation of paroxysmal SVT after initial termination can occur. Either repeated administration of the same dose of adenosine or substitution of a calcium channel blocker will be effective.

The AVN action potential is calcium channel–dependent, and the non–dihydropyridine calcium channel blockers verapamil and diltiazem are effective for terminating AVN-dependent paroxysmal SVT. The recommended dosage of verapamil is 5 mg intravenously over 2 minutes, followed in 5 to 10 minutes by a second 5- to 7.5-mg dose. The recommended dose of diltiazem is 20 mg intravenously followed, if necessary, by a second dose of 25 to 35 mg. Paroxysmal SVT termination should occur within 5 minutes of the end of the infusion, and over 90% of patients with AVN-dependent paroxysmal SVT respond. As with adenosine, transient arrhythmias, including atrial and ventricular ectopy, AF, and bradycardia, can be seen after paroxysmal SVT termination with calcium channel blockers. Hypotension can occur with calcium channel blockers, particularly if the paroxysmal SVT does not terminate. Adenosine and verapamil have been reported to have a similar high efficacy in terminating paroxysmal SVT, with a rate of success ranging from 59% to 100% for adenosine and from 73% to 98.8% for verapamil, according to the dose and mode of administration. However, data also suggest that the efficacy of adenosine and verapamil is affected by the arrhythmia rate. Increasing SVT rates are significantly associated with higher percentages of sinus rhythm restoration following treatment with adenosine. In contrast, the efficacy of verapamil in restoring sinus rhythm was inversely related to the rate of paroxysmal SVT.[4]

Intravenous beta blockers including propranolol (1 to 3 mg), metoprolol (5 mg), and esmolol (500 µg/kg over 1 minute and a 50-µg/kg/min infusion) are also useful for acute termination. Digoxin (0.5 to 1.0 mg) is considered the least effective of the four categories of drugs available, but is a useful alternative when there is a contraindication to the other agents.

AVN-dependent paroxysmal SVT can present with a wide QRS complex in patients with fixed or functional aberration, or if a BT is used for anterograde conduction. Most wide complex tachycardias, however, are caused by mechanisms that can worsen after intravenous administration of adenosine and calcium channel blockers. Unless there is strong evidence that a wide QRS tachycardia is AVN-dependent, adenosine, verapamil, and diltiazem should not be used.

Limited data are available on the acute pharmacological therapy of ATs. Automatic or triggered tachycardias and sinus node reentry should respond to adenosine, verapamil, diltiazem, or beta-adrenergic blockers. Other ATs can respond to class I or III antiarrhythmic drugs given orally or parenterally.

CHRONIC MANAGEMENT

Because most paroxysmal SVTs are generally benign arrhythmias that do not influence survival, the main reason for treatment is to alleviate symptoms. The threshold for initiation of therapy and the decision to treat SVT with oral antiarrhythmic drugs or catheter ablation depends on the frequency and duration of the arrhythmia, severity of symptoms, and patient preference. The threshold for treatment will also reflect whether the patient is a competitive athlete, a woman considering pregnancy, or someone with a high-risk occupation. Catheter ablation is an especially attractive option for patients who desire to avoid or are unresponsive or intolerant to drug therapy.

For patients requiring therapy who are reluctant to undergo catheter ablation, antiarrhythmic drug therapy remains a viable alternative. For AVN-dependent paroxysmal SVT, calcium channel blockers and beta blockers will improve symptoms in 60% to 80% of patients. A comparison of verapamil, propranolol, and digoxin has shown equivalent efficacy in a small group of patients. However, in general, calcium channel blockers and beta blockers are preferred to digoxin. In patients who do not respond, class IC and III drugs can be considered. Flecainide and propafenone affect the AVN and BTs and reduce SVT frequency. Sotalol, dofetilide, and amiodarone are second-line agents. Because sympathetic stimulation can antagonize the effects of many antiarrhythmic agents, concomitant therapy with a beta blocker can improve efficacy.

Patients with well-tolerated episodes of paroxysmal SVT that always terminate spontaneously or with vagal maneuvers do not require chronic prophylactic therapy. Selected patients may be treated only for acute episodes. Outpatients may use a single oral dose of verapamil, propranolol, or propafenone to terminate an episode of AVRT or AVNRT effectively. This so-called "pill in the pocket" or "cocktail therapy" is a reasonable treatment option for patients who have tachycardia episodes that are sustained but infrequent enough that daily preventive therapy is not desired. Oral antiarrhythmic drug tablets are not reliably absorbed during rapid paroxysmal SVT, but some patients can respond to self-administration of crushed medications.

Pharmacological management of ATs has not been well evaluated in controlled clinical trials. Depending on the mechanism responsible for the arrhythmia, beta blockers, calcium channel blockers, and class I or III antiarrhythmic drugs may reduce or eliminate symptoms.

Electrocardiographic Features

Assessment of Regularity of the Supraventricular Tachycardia

Most SVTs are associated with a regular ventricular rate. If the rhythm is irregular, the ECG should be scrutinized for discrete atrial activity and for any evidence of a pattern to the irregularity (e.g., grouped beating typical of Wenckebach periodicity). If the rhythm is irregularly irregular (i.e., no pattern can be detected), the mechanism of the arrhythmia is either multifocal AT or AF (Fig. 20-2). Multifocal AT is an irregularly irregular atrial rhythm characterized by more than three different P wave morphologies, with the P waves separated by isoelectric intervals and associated with varying P-P, R-R, and PR intervals (see Fig. 11-1). On the other hand,

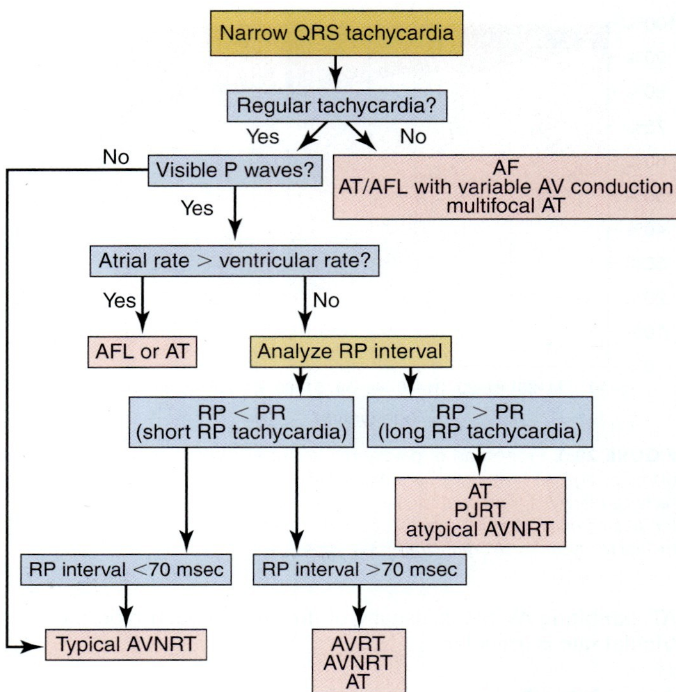

FIGURE 20-2 Differential diagnosis of narrow QRS tachycardia. AF = atrial fibrillation; AFL = atrial flutter; AT = atrial tachycardia; AV = atrioventricular; AVNRT = atrioventricular nodal reentrant tachycardia; AVRT = atrioventricular reentrant tachycardia; PJRT = permanent junctional reciprocating tachycardia. *(From Blomström-Lundqvist C, Scheinman MM, Aliot EM, et al: American College of Cardiology; American Heart Association Task Force on Practice Guidelines; European Society of Cardiology Committee for Practice Guidelines [Writing Committee to Develop Guidelines for the Management of Patients with Supraventricular Arrhythmias]: ACC/AHA/ESC guidelines for the management of patients with supraventricular arrhythmias—executive summary: a report of the American College of Cardiology/American Heart Association Task Force on Practice Guidelines and the European Society of Cardiology Committee for Practice Guidelines [Writing Committee to Develop Guidelines for the Management of Patients with Supraventricular Arrhythmias], Circulation;108:1871, 2003.)*

AF is characterized by rapid and irregular atrial fibrillatory activity and, in the presence of normal AVN conduction, by an irregularly irregular ventricular response. P waves cannot be detected in AF, although coarse fibrillatory waves and prominent U waves can sometimes give the appearance of P waves. At times, the fibrillatory activity is so fine as to be undetectable.

Atrial Activity

IDENTIFICATION

If the patient's rhythm is regular or has a clearly discernible pattern, the ECG should next be assessed for P waves (atrial activity).[5] The P waves may be easily discernible; however, frequently, comparison with a normal baseline ECG is needed and can reveal a slight alteration in the QRS, ST segment, or T waves, suggesting the presence of the P wave. If the P waves cannot be clearly identified, carotid sinus massage or the administration of intravenous adenosine may help clarify the diagnosis. These maneuvers may also terminate the SVT.

Carotid Sinus Massage

Carotid sinus massage can result in one of four possible effects: (1) temporary decrease in the atrial rate in patients with sinus tachycardia or automatic AT; (2) slowing of AVN conduction and AVN block, which can unmask atrial electrical activity—that is, reveal P waves or flutter waves in patients with AT or AFL by decreasing the number of QRS complexes that obscure the electrical baseline; (3) with some SVTs that require AVN conduction, especially AVNRT and AVRT, the transient slowing of AVN conduction can terminate the arrhythmia by interrupting the reentry circuit; less commonly, carotid sinus massage can cause some ATs to slow and terminate; or (4) in some cases, no effect is observed.

Adenosine Administration

Adenosine results in slowing of the sinus rate and AVN conduction. In the setting of SVT, the effects of adenosine are similar to those seen with carotid sinus massage described earlier. For intravenous adenosine administration, the patient should be supine and should have ECG and blood pressure monitoring. The drug is administered by rapid intravenous injection over 1 to 2 seconds at a peripheral site, followed by a normal saline flush. The usual initial dose is 6 mg, with a maximal single dose of 12 mg. If a central intravenous access site is used, the initial dose should not exceed 3 mg and may be as little as 1 mg. Adenosine can precipitate AF and AFL because it shortens atrial refractoriness. In patients with Wolff-Parkinson-White (WPW) syndrome and AF, adenosine can result in a rapid ventricular response that can degenerate into VF. However, this problem has not been observed frequently, and the use of adenosine for diagnosis and termination of regular SVTs, including AVRT, is appropriate as long as close patient observation and preparedness to treat potential complications, such as with immediate electrical cardioversion/defibrillation, are maintained.

Termination of the Arrhythmia

Carotid sinus massage or adenosine can terminate the SVT, especially if the rhythm is AVNRT or AVRT. A continuous ECG tracing should be recorded during these maneuvers, because the response can aid in the diagnosis.[5] Termination of the tachycardia with a P wave after the last QRS complex is most common in AVRT and typical AVNRT and is rarely seen with AT (see Fig. 18-22), whereas termination of the tachycardia with a QRS complex is more common with AT, atypical AVNRT, and permanent junctional reciprocating tachycardia (PJRT; see Fig. 18-19). If the tachycardia continues despite development of AV block, the rhythm is almost certainly AT or AFL; AVRT is excluded and AVNRT is very unlikely.

CHARACTERIZATION

Atrial Rate

An atrial rate greater than 250 beats/min is usually caused by AFL. However, overlap exists, and AT and AVRT can occasionally be faster than 250 beats/min. AVRT tends to be faster than AVNRT and AT; again, significant overlap exists and this criterion does not usually help in distinguishing among different SVTs.

P Wave Morphology

A P wave morphology identical to sinus P wave suggests sinus tachycardia, inappropriate sinus tachycardia, sinoatrial nodal reentrant tachycardia, or AT arising close to the region of the sinus node. An abnormal P wave morphology can be observed during AVNRT (P wave is concentric; see Fig. 17-3), AVRT (P wave can be eccentric or concentric; see Fig. 18-9), AT (P wave can be eccentric or concentric), and AFL (lack of distinct isoelectric baselines between atrial deflections is suggestive of AFL, but can also be seen occasionally in AT; see Fig. 12-2).[5]

The P waves may not be discernible on ECG, which suggests typical AVNRT or, less commonly, AVRT (especially in the presence of bundle branch block [BBB] contralateral to the BT).

CHARACTERIZATION OF THE P/QRS RELATIONSHIP

RP/PR Intervals

SVTs are classified as short or long RP interval SVTs (see Fig. 20-2). During short RP SVTs, the ECG will show P waves inscribed within the ST-T wave with an RP interval that is less than half the tachycardia R-R interval. Such SVTs include typical AVNRT (most common), orthodromic AVRT, AT with prolonged AV conduction, and slow-slow AVNRT. A very short RP interval (<70 milliseconds) excludes AVRT.[5,6]

In typical AVNRT, the P wave is usually not visible because of the simultaneous atrial and ventricular activation. The P wave may distort the initial portion of the QRS (mimicking a q wave in inferior leads) or lie just within the QRS (inapparent) or distort the terminal portion of the QRS (mimicking an s wave in inferior leads or r′ in V_1; see Fig. 17-3).

Long RP SVTs include AT, atypical (fast-slow) AVNRT, and AVRT using a slowly conducting AV BT (e.g., PJRT). If the PR interval during the SVT is shorter than that during normal sinus rhythm (NSR), AT and AVRT are very unlikely, and atypical AVNRT, which is associated with an apparent shortening of the PR interval, is the likely diagnosis. ATs originating close to the AV junction are also a possibility.

Atrial-Ventricular Relationship

SVTs with an A/V ratio of 1 (i.e., equal number of atrial and ventricular events) include AVNRT, AVRT, and AT. On the other hand, an A/V ratio during the SVT of greater than 1 indicates the presence of AV block and that the ventricles are not required for the SVT circuit, thereby excluding AVRT and suggesting either AT (most common; see Fig. 11-2) or AVNRT (rare; see Fig. 17-4). AV dissociation (i.e., complete AV block) can be observed during AT (most common) or AVNRT (rare).

QRS Morphology

The QRS morphology during SVT is usually the same as in NSR. However, functional aberration can occur at rapid rates. Functional aberration occurs frequently in AF, AFL, and AVRT, is less common in AT, and is very uncommon in AVNRT.

Electrophysiological Testing

Discussion in this section will focus on differential diagnosis of narrow QRS complex paroxysmal SVTs, including AT, orthodromic AVRT, and AVNRT. The goals of EP testing in these patients include the following: (1) evaluation of baseline cardiac electrophysiology; (2) induction of SVT; (3) evaluation of the mode of initiation of the SVT; (4) definition of atrial activation sequence during the SVT; (5) definition of the relationship of the P wave to the QRS at the onset and during the SVT; (6) evaluation of the effect of BBB on the tachycardia cycle length (CL) and ventriculoatrial (VA) interval; (7) evaluation of the SVT circuit and requirement for the atria, His bundle (HB), and/or ventricles in the initiation and maintenance of the SVT; (8) evaluation of the SVT response to programmed electrical stimulation and overdrive pacing from the atrium and ventricle; and (9) evaluation of the effects of drugs and physiological maneuvers on the SVT.

Baseline Observations during Normal Sinus Rhythm

The presence of preexcitation during NSR suggests AVRT as the likely diagnosis; however, it does not exclude other causes of SVT during which the AV BT is an innocent bystander. Furthermore, the absence of preexcitation during NSR does not exclude the presence of an AV BT or the diagnosis of AVRT mediated by either a concealed or a slowly conducting BT. The presence of intraatrial conduction delay suggests AT, but does not exclude other types of SVTs.

Programmed Electrical Stimulation during Normal Sinus Rhythm

The programmed stimulation protocol should include (1) ventricular burst pacing from the right ventricular (RV) apex (down to pacing CL at which VA block develops); (2) single and double ventricular extrastimuli (VESs, down to the ventricular effective refractory period, ERP) at multiple CLs (600 to 400 milliseconds) from the RV apex; (3) atrial burst pacing from the high right atrium (RA) and coronary sinus (CS; down to the pacing CL at which 2:1 atrial capture occurs); (4) single and double atrial extrastimuli (AESs, down to the atrial ERP) at multiple CLs (600 to 400 milliseconds) from the high RA and CS; and (5) administration of isoproterenol infusion (0.5 to 4 μg/min) as needed to facilitate tachycardia induction.

ATRIAL EXTRASTIMULATION AND ATRIAL PACING DURING NORMAL SINUS RHYTHM

Dual Atrioventricular Nodal Physiology

Although the demonstration of dual AVN physiology during programmed atrial stimulation favors AVNRT as the mechanism of SVT, it is not an uncommon finding in patients with other types of SVTs. Furthermore, failure to demonstrate dual AVN physiology does not exclude the possibility of AVNRT, and might be related to similar fast and slow AVN pathway ERPs. Dissociation of refractoriness of the fast and slow AVN pathways can then be necessary (see Chap. 17).

Ventricular Preexcitation

Atrial stimulation can help unmask preexcitation if it is not manifest during NSR because of fast AVN conduction, slow BT conduction, or both. AES and atrial pacing from any atrial site result in slowing of AVN conduction and, consequently, unmask or increase the degree of preexcitation over the AV BT (see Fig. 18-4). Moreover, atrial stimulation close to the AV BT insertion site results in maximal preexcitation and the shortest P-delta interval because of the ability to advance the activation of the AV BT down to its ERP from pacing at this site caused by the lack of intervening atrial tissue, whose conduction time and refractoriness can otherwise limit the ability of the AES to stimulate the BT prematurely (see Fig. 18-14).

Failure of atrial stimulation to increase the amount of preexcitation can occur because of markedly enhanced AVN conduction, the presence of another AV BT, or pacing-induced block in the AV BT due to the long ERP of the BT (longer than that of the AVN). It can also occur because total preexcitation is already present in the basal state as a result of prolonged AVN/His-Purkinje system (HPS) conduction.

Extra Atrial Beats

AES and atrial pacing can trigger extra atrial beats or echo beats. Those beats can be caused by different mechanisms.

INTRAATRIAL REENTRANT BEATS. These beats usually occur at short coupling intervals, and can originate anywhere in the atrium. Therefore, the atrial activation sequence depends on the site of origin of the beat. The more premature the AES, the more likely it will induce nonspecific intraatrial reentrant beats and short runs of irregular AT or AF.

CATHETER-INDUCED ATRIAL BEATS. These beats usually have the earliest activation site recorded at that particular catheter tip and have the same atrial activation sequence as the atrial impulse produced by pacing from that catheter. Portions of the catheter proximal to the tip usually do not elicit mechanically induced ectopic impulses.

ATRIOVENTRICULAR NODAL ECHO BEATS. These beats occur in the presence of anterograde dual AVN physiology (see Fig. 4-23). Such beats require anterograde block of the atrial stimulus in the fast AVN pathway, anterograde conduction down the slow pathway, and then retrograde conduction up the fast pathway. AVN echo beats have several features: they appear reproducibly after a critical AH interval; the atrial activation sequence is consistent with retrograde conduction over the fast pathway, with the earliest atrial activation site in the HB; and the VA interval is very short, but it can be longer if the atrial stimulus causes anterograde concealment (and not just block) in the fast pathway.

ATRIOVENTRICULAR ECHO BEATS. AV echo beats occur secondary to anterograde conduction of the atrial stimulus over the AVN-HPS and retrograde conduction over an AV BT (concealed or bidirectional BT). If preexcitation is manifest during atrial stimulation, the last atrial impulse inducing the echo beat will demonstrate loss of preexcitation because of anterograde block in the AV BT, and atrial activation sequence and P wave morphology of the echo beat will depend on the location of the BT (see Fig. 3-10). These beats have a relatively short VA interval, but always longer than 70 milliseconds. Moreover, the VA interval of the AV echo beat remains constant, regardless of the varying coupling interval of the AES triggering the echo beat (VA linking). Alternatively, AV echo beats can occur secondary to anterograde conduction of the atrial stimulus over a manifest AV BT and retrograde conduction over an AVN, in which setting the last paced beat is associated with anterograde block in the AVN and fully preexcited QRS complex.

VENTRICULAR EXTRASTIMULATION AND VENTRICULAR PACING DURING NORMAL SINUS RHYTHM

Retrograde Dual Atrioventricular Nodal Physiology

Demonstration of retrograde dual AVN physiology during programmed ventricular stimulation suggests AVNRT (occurring most commonly during atypical AVNRT), but it can also be observed with other SVTs.[7] Importantly, failure to demonstrate retrograde dual AVN physiology in patients with AVNRT can be the result of similar fast and slow AVN pathway ERPs, in which setting dissociation of refractoriness of the fast and slow AVN pathways is required (see Chap. 17).

VA block at a ventricular pacing CL greater than 600 milliseconds or decremental VA conduction during ventricular pacing makes the presence of a retrogradely conducting BT unlikely, except for decrementally conducting BTs and the rare catecholamine-dependent BTs. In addition, development of VA block during ventricular pacing in response to adenosine suggests the absence of BT.

Retrograde Atrial Activation Sequence

VA conduction over the AVN produces a classic concentric atrial activation sequence starting in the anteroseptal or posteroseptal region of the RA because of retrograde conduction over either the fast or the slow AVN pathways, respectively. In the presence of a retrogradely conducting AV BT, atrial activation can result from conduction over the AV BT, over the AVN, or a fusion of both (see Fig. 18-16). An eccentric atrial activation sequence in response to ventricular stimulation suggests the presence of an AV BT mediating VA conduction (see Fig. 18-16). The presence of a concentric retrograde atrial activation sequence, however, does not exclude the presence of a retrogradely conducting BT that could be septal in location or located far from the pacing site, allowing for preferential VA conduction over the AVN.

Extra Ventricular Beats

Ventricular stimulation can trigger extra ventricular beats or echo beats. These beats can be caused by different mechanisms.

BUNDLE BRANCH REENTRANT BEATS. During RV stimulation at close coupling intervals, progressive retrograde conduction delay and block occur in the right bundle branch (RB), so that retrograde HB activation occurs via the left bundle branch (LB). At this point, the His potential usually follows the local ventricular electrogram. Further decrease in the coupling interval produces an increase in retrograde HPS conduction delay. When a critical degree of HPS delay (S_2-H_2) is attained, the impulse can return down the initially blocked RB and result in a QRS of similar morphology to the paced QRS at the RV apex—specifically, it will look like a typical left bundle branch block (LBBB) pattern with left axis deviation because ventricular activation originates from conduction over the RB. The His bundle–ventricular (HV) interval of the bundle branch reentrant (BBR) beat is usually longer than or equal to the HV interval during NSR. Retrograde atrial activation, if present, follows the His potential (see Fig. 4-27).

ATRIOVENTRICULAR NODE ECHO BEATS. These beats are caused by reentry in the AVN in patients with retrograde dual AVN physiology (see Fig. 17-11). The last paced beat conducts retrogradely up the slow AVN pathway and then anterogradely down the fast pathway to produce the echo beat. AVN echoes appear reproducibly after a critical H_2-A_2 interval (or V_2-A_2 interval, when the His potential cannot be seen), and manifest as extra beats with a normal anterograde QRS morphology and atrial activity preceding the His potential before the echo beat. This phenomenon can occur at long or short coupling intervals and depends only on the degree of retrograde AVN conduction delay. In most cases, this delay is achieved before the appearance of a retrograde His potential beyond the local ventricular electrogram (i.e., before retrograde block in the RB).

ATRIOVENTRICULAR ECHO BEATS. These beats occur secondary to retrograde block in the HPS-AVN and VA conduction over an AV BT, followed by anterograde conduction over the AVN, or secondary to retrograde block in the AV BT and VA conduction over the AVN-HPS, followed by anterograde conduction over the AV-BT. In the latter setting, the echo beat is fully preexcited (see Fig. 18-16).

INTRAVENTRICULAR REENTRANT BEATS. This response occurs most commonly in the setting of a cardiac pathological condition, especially coronary artery disease, and usually occurs at short coupling intervals. It can have any QRS morphology, but more often right bundle branch block (RBBB) than LBBB in patients with prior myocardial infarction (MI). These responses are usually nonsustained (1 to 30 complexes) and typically polymorphic. In patients without prior clinical arrhythmias, such responses are of no clinical significance.

CATHETER-INDUCED VENTRICULAR BEATS. Such beats usually have the earliest ventricular activation site recorded at that particular catheter tip and have the same QRS morphology as the QRS produced by pacing from that catheter.

Right Bundle Branch Block during Ventricular Extrastimulation

During the delivery of progressively premature single VESs, an abrupt increase in the VA conduction interval is often seen. This may be due to a variety of reasons including a change in activation from a BT block to the AVN or a change from fast to slow pathway conduction, or it may be the result of an abrupt change when the refractory period of the RB has been reached.

Retrograde RBBB occurs frequently during VES testing, and can be diagnosed by observing the retrograde His potential during the drive train and its abrupt displacement with the VES. Often, however, it is difficult to visualize the retrograde His potential during the pacing train; even then, the sudden appearance of an easily distinguished retrograde His potential, separate from the ventricular electrogram, may be sufficient to recognize retrograde RBBB.

The VH interval prolongation occurs because, following RBBB, conduction must traverse the interventricular septum (which requires approximately 60 to 70 milliseconds in normal hearts), enter retrogradely via the LB, and ascend to reach the HB. Although an increase in the VH interval necessarily occurs with retrograde RBBB, whether a similar increase occurs in the VA interval depends on the nature of VA conduction. Measurement of the retrograde VH and VA intervals on development of retrograde RBBB during VES can help the distinction between retrograde AVN and BT conduction.

In the absence of a BT, the AVN can be activated in a retrograde fashion only after retrograde activation of the HB; as a consequence, VA activation will necessarily be delayed with retrograde RBBB, and the increase in the VA interval will be at least as much as the increase in the VH interval. In contrast, when retrograde conduction is via a BT, there will be no expected increase in the VA interval when retrograde RBBB is induced. Thus, the increase in the VA interval is minimal and always less than the increase in the VH interval.[8]

Induction of Tachycardia

INITIATION BY ATRIAL EXTRASTIMULATION OR ATRIAL PACING

Inducibility

All types of paroxysmal SVTs can be inducible with atrial stimulation (except automatic AT). SVT initiation that is reproducibly dependent on a critical AH interval is classic for typical AVNRT (see Fig. 17-8). Atypical AVNRT is usually initiated with modest prolongation of the AH interval along the fast pathway with anterograde block in the slow pathway, followed by retrograde slow conduction over the slow pathway. Therefore, a critical AH interval delay is not obvious (see Fig. 17-10). AT initiation also can be associated with AV delay, but that is not a prerequisite for initiation. Orthodromic AVRT usually requires some AV delay for initiation; however, the delay can occur anywhere along the AVN-HPS axis. In patients with baseline manifest preexcitation, initiation of orthodromic AVRT is usually associated with anterograde block in the AV BT and loss of preexcitation following the initiating atrial stimulus, which would then allow that BT to conduct retrogradely during the SVT.[9] Initiation may require catecholamines (isoproterenol) with any type of SVT, and this observation does not help for differential diagnosis.

Warm-Up

Progressive shortening of the tachycardia CL for several beats (warm-up) before its ultimate rate is achieved is characteristic of automatic AT, but may occur in other SVTs as well.

Ventriculoatrial Interval

If the VA interval of the first tachycardia beat is reproducibly identical to that during the rest of the SVT, AT is very unlikely, and such "VA linking" is suggestive of typical AVNRT and orthodromic AVRT.

INITIATION BY VENTRICULAR EXTRASTIMULI OR VENTRICULAR PACING

Inducibility

Ventricular stimulation commonly induces AVRT, typical and atypical AVNRT, and less frequently AT.

His Bundle–Atrial Interval

During induction of the SVT by ventricular pacing at a CL similar to the tachycardia CL or by a VES that advances the His potential by a coupling interval (i.e., H_1-H_2) similar to the H-H interval during the SVT (i.e., similar to the tachycardia CL), the His bundle–atrial (HA) or VA interval following the initiating ventricular stimulus then is compared with that during the SVT. During AVNRT, the HA interval of the ventricular stimulus initiating the SVT is longer than that during the SVT, because both the HB and atrium are activated in sequence during ventricular stimulation and in parallel during AVNRT. This is even exaggerated by the fact that the AVN usually exhibits greater decremental conduction with repetitive engagement of impulses than to a single impulse at a similar coupling interval. Therefore, the more prolonged the HA interval with the initiating ventricular stimulus, the more likely the SVT is AVNRT. On the other hand, if the SVT uses an AV BT for retrograde conduction, the HA interval during the initiating ventricular stimulus (at a coupling interval comparable to the tachycardia CL) should approximate that during the SVT, because the atrium and ventricle are activated in sequence in both scenarios (see Fig. 18-16).[9]

Tachycardia Features

ATRIAL ACTIVATION SEQUENCE

During typical AVNRT, the initial site of atrial activation is usually recorded in the HB catheter at the apex of the triangle of Koch.[10] In contrast, the initial site of atrial activation during atypical AVNRT is usually recorded at the base of the triangle of Koch or coronary sinus ostium (CS os) (see Fig. 17-5).[10] On the other hand, in orthodromic AVRT, the initial site of atrial activation depends on the location of the AV BT, but is always near the AV groove, without multiple breakthrough points. It is comparable to that during ventricular pacing when VA conduction occurs exclusively over the AV BT. The atrial activation sequence during AT depends on the origin of the AT, and can simulate that of other types of SVTs. In summary, eccentric atrial activation during SVT excludes typical and atypical

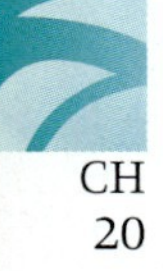

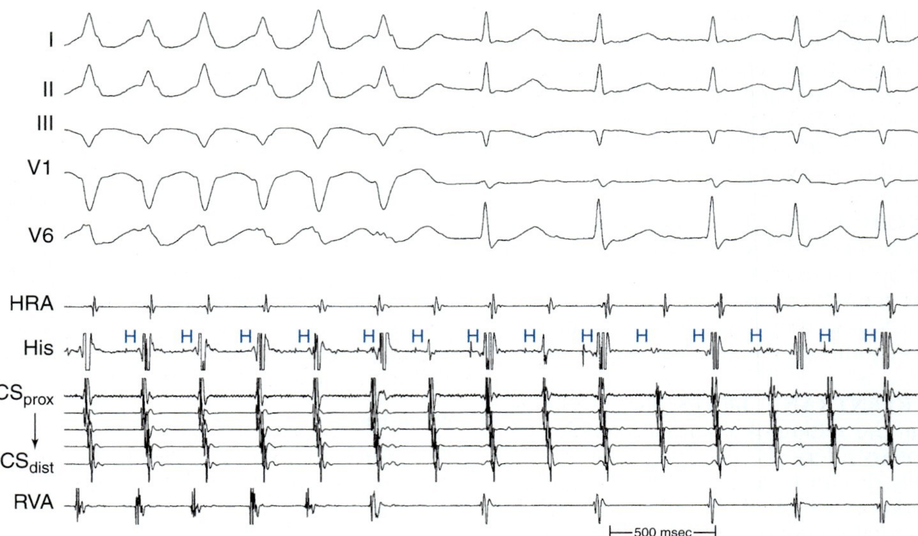

FIGURE 20-3 Supraventricular tachycardia (SVT) with concentric atrial activation sequence and intermittent atrioventricular (AV) block. At **left,** a wide complex tachycardia with left bundle branch block (LBBB) pattern and 1:1 AV ratio is shown. Simultaneous atrial and ventricular activation is observed, excluding atrioventricular reentrant tachycardia (AVRT) as the mechanism of the tachycardia, and favoring typical atrioventricular nodal reentrant tachycardia (AVNRT) or atrial tachycardia (AT) with a long PR interval. At **right,** 2:1 AV block is observed without disruption of the tachycardia. Normalization of QRS morphology is observed during the period of 2:1 AV block, suggesting that wide QRS morphology during 1:1 AV conduction was a result of functional LBBB. The development of AV block with continuation of the tachycardia confirms that the ventricle is not part of the tachycardia circuit and, thus, excludes AVRT. The presence of His potentials, even during the blocked beats, suggests that the block is infra-Hisian. The observation of AV block favors AT, but does not exclude AVNRT. The ventriculoatrial (VA) interval remains constant following both the narrow and wide QRS complexes, which suggests AVNRT. Other pacing maneuvers confirmed that this SVT was in fact typical AVNRT.

AVNRT, except for the left variant of AVNRT, during which the earliest atrial activation occurs in the proximal or mid-CS. Moreover, an eccentric atrial activation sequence that originates away from the AV rings is diagnostic of AT and excludes both AVNRT and AVRT.[9]

ATRIAL-VENTRICULAR RELATIONSHIP

PR/RP

During AT, the PR interval is appropriate for the AT rate and is usually longer than that during NSR. The faster the AT rate, the longer the PR interval. Thus, the PR interval can be shorter, longer, or equal to the RP interval. The PR interval can also be equal to the R-R and the P wave can then fall within the preceding QRS, mimicking typical AVNRT. During typical AVNRT, the RP interval is very short (–40 to 75 milliseconds); in contrast, during atypical AVNRT, the RP interval is longer than the PR interval. On the other hand, during orthodromic AVRT, the RP interval is short but longer than that in typical AVNRT (>70 milliseconds), because the wavefront has to activate the ventricle before it reaches the AV BT and subsequently conduct retrogradely to the atrium. Thus, the ventricle and atrium are activated in sequence, in contrast to AVNRT, during which the ventricle and atrium are activated in parallel, resulting in abbreviation of the VA interval.[6]

Atrioventricular Block

The presence of AV block during SVT excludes AVRT, is uncommon during AVNRT, and strongly favors AT (Fig. 20-3). AV block occurs commonly during AT, with either Wenckebach periodicity or fixed-ratio block. AV block may also occur during AVNRT because of block below the reentry circuit, usually below the HB and infrequently in the lower common pathway, which can occur especially at the onset of the SVT, during acceleration of the SVT, and following a PVC or a VES (see Fig. 17-4).

Ventriculoatrial Block

VA block during SVT is a rare phenomenon, and may occasionally be observed in infraatrial SVTs, including junctional ectopic tachycardia, orthodromic AVRT using a nodofascicular or nodoventricular BT for retrograde conduction, as well as infra-atrial AVNRT. VA block can rarely occur during AVNRT because of block in an upper common pathway (see Fig. 17-13). Intra-Hisian reentry is another potential mechanism, but it is a theoretical entity whose clinical occurrence has not been convincingly demonstrated.[1,11-13]

Variation of the P/QRS Relationship

Spontaneous changes in the PR and RP intervals with fixed A-A interval favor AT and exclude orthodromic AVRT (Fig. 20-4, see Fig. 11-13). On the other hand, spontaneous changes in tachycardia CL accompanied by constant VA interval suggest orthodromic AVRT (see Fig. 18-22). During orthodromic AVRT, the RP interval remains fixed, regardless of oscillations in tachycardia CL from whatever cause or changes in the PR (AH) interval. Thus, the RP/PR ratio may change, and the tachycardia CL is most closely associated with the PR interval (i.e., anterograde slow conduction). Variation of the P/QRS relationship (with changes in the AH interval, HA interval, and AH/HA ratio), with or without block, can occur during AVNRT, especially in atypical or slow-slow AVNRT. This phenomenon usually occurs when the conduction system, the reentry circuit, or both are unstable during initiation or termination of the tachycardia or in cases of nonsustained tachycardias. The ECG manifestation of P/QRS variations, with or without AV block during tachycardia, should not be misdiagnosed as AT; they can be atypical or, rarely, typical forms of AVNRT. Moreover, the variations could be of such magnitude that a long RP tachycardia can masquerade for brief periods of time as short RP tachycardia.

OSCILLATION IN TACHYCARDIA CYCLE LENGTH

Analysis of tachycardia CL variability can provide useful diagnostic information that is available even when episodes of SVT are nonsustained. SVT CL variability of at least 15 milliseconds in magnitude was found to occur in up to 73% of paroxysmal SVTs and was equally prevalent in AT, AVNRT, and orthodromic AVRT. Changes in atrial CL preceding similar changes in subsequent ventricular CL strongly favor AT or atypical AVNRT (see Fig. 17-14). In contrast, when the change in atrial CL is predicted by the change in preceding ventricular CL, typical AVNRT or orthodromic AVRT is the most likely mechanism (see Fig. 18-22).

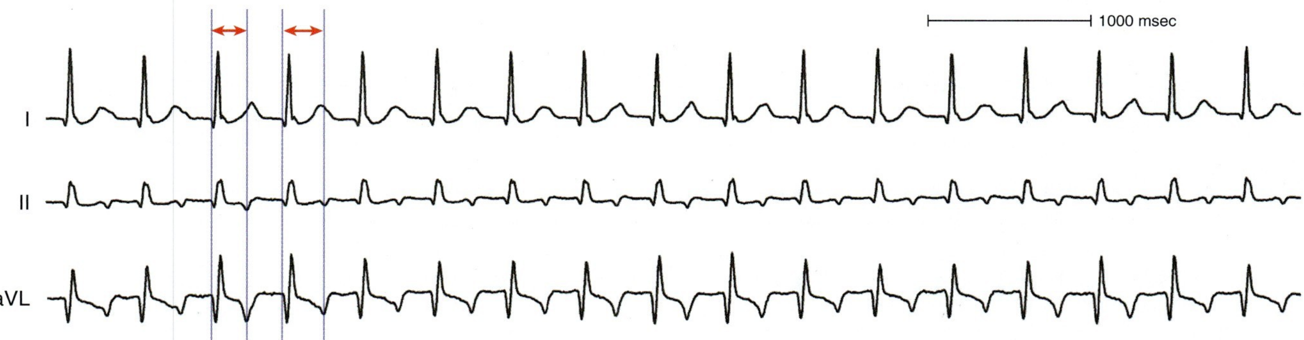

FIGURE 20-4 Narrow complex supraventricular tachycardia (SVT) with variable RP intervals. Three surface ECG leads are shown. The P waves are inscribed within the T waves, and are more discernible with negative polarity in lead aV_L. Note that the RP interval varies during the SVT (arrows) with constant A-A intervals, consistent with atrial tachycardia as the mechanism of the SVT and excludes orthodromic atrioventricular reentrant tachycardia.

The AVN participates either actively or passively in all types of SVTs and the AV interval can vary depending on the preceding atrial CL and autonomic tone. A change in anterograde or retrograde AVN conduction can result in tachycardia CL variability in AVNRT or orthodromic AVRT. In contrast, CL variability in AT is a result of changes in the CL of the atrial reentrant or focal tachycardia, or changes in AVN conduction. Therefore, when there is CL variability in both the atrium and ventricle, changes in atrial CL during AT would be expected to precede and predict the changes in ventricular CL. However, ventricular CL variability can be caused by changes in AV conduction instead of changes in the CL of an AT, in which case ventricular CL variability may not be predicted by a prior change in atrial CL during AT. Nevertheless, because there is no VA conduction during AT, ventricular CL variability by itself would not be expected to result in atrial CL variability during AT.

In contrast to AT, typical AVNRT and orthodromic AVRT generally have CL variability because of changes in anterograde AVN conduction. Because retrograde conduction through a fast AVN pathway or a BT generally is much less variable than anterograde conduction through the AVN, the changes in ventricular CL that result from variability in anterograde AVN conduction would be expected to precede the subsequent changes in atrial CL. This explains why the change in atrial CL does not predict the change in subsequent ventricular CL in typical AVNRT and orthodromic AVRT. On the other hand, in atypical AVNRT, anterograde conduction occurs over the more stable fast AVN pathway and retrograde conduction is more subject to variability. This explains the finding that changes in atrial CL predict the changes in subsequent ventricular CL in atypical AVNRT, as was the case in AT.

EFFECTS OF BUNDLE BRANCH BLOCK

The development of BBB during SVT that neither influences the tachycardia CL (A-A or H-H interval) nor the VA interval is consistent with AT, AVNRT (see Fig. 17-4), and orthodromic AVRT using a BT in the ventricle contralateral to the BBB (see Fig. 18-21), but excludes orthodromic AVRT using a BT ipsilateral to the BBB.

BBB ipsilateral to the AV BT mediating orthodromic AVRT results in prolongation of the surface VA interval because of the extra time required for the impulse to travel from the AVN down the HB and contralateral bundle branch, and transseptally to the ipsilateral ventricle to reach the AV BT and then activate the atrium (see Fig. 18-23). However, the local VA interval (measured at the site of BT insertion) remains constant. Additionally, the tachycardia CL usually increases in concordance with the increase in the surface VA interval as a result of ipsilateral BBB, because of the now-larger tachycardia circuit; however, because the time the wavefront spends outside the AVN is now longer, AVN conduction may improve, resulting in shortening in the AH interval (PR interval), which can be of a magnitude sufficient to overcome the prolongation of the VA interval. This can consequently result in shortening in the tachycardia CL. Thus, the surface VA interval and not the tachycardia CL should be used to assess the effects of BBB on the SVT (see Fig. 18-9).

Prolongation of the VA interval during SVT in response to BBB by more than 35 milliseconds indicates that an ipsilateral free wall AV BT is present and is participating in the SVT (i.e., diagnostic of orthodromic AVRT). On the other hand, prolongation of the surface VA by more than 25 milliseconds suggests a septal AV BT (posteroseptal AV BT in association with LBBB, and superoparaseptal AV BT in association with RBBB; see Fig. 18-24). In contrast, BBB contralateral to the AV BT does not influence the VA interval or tachycardia CL because the contralateral ventricle is not part of the reentrant circuit (see Figs. 18-21 and 18-23).

Since the occurrence of BBB during SVT is much more common in orthodromic AVRT than AVNRT or AT (90% of SVTs with sustained LBBB are orthodromic AVRTs), the mere presence of LBBB aberrancy during SVT is suggestive of orthodromic AVRT, but can still occur in other types of SVTs.[6,9]

QRS ALTERNANS

QRS alternans during relatively slow SVTs is almost always consistent with orthodromic AVRT. However, QRS alternans during fast SVTs is most commonly seen in orthodromic AVRT but can also be seen with other types of SVTs as well.

TERMINATION AND RESPONSE TO PHYSIOLOGICAL AND PHARMACOLOGICAL MANEUVERS

Spontaneous Termination

Spontaneous termination of orthodromic AVRT usually occurs because of anterograde gradual slowing and then block in the AVN, sometimes causing initial oscillation in the tachycardia CL, with alternate complexes demonstrating a Wenckebach periodicity before block. However, termination with retrograde block in the AV BT can occur without any perturbations of the tachycardia CL during very rapid orthodromic AVRT or with sudden shortening of the tachycardia CL. Spontaneous termination of AVNRT occurs because of block in the fast or slow pathway. However, the better the retrograde fast pathway conduction, the less likely that it is the site of block. Spontaneous termination of AT is usually accompanied by progressive prolongation of the A-A interval, with or without changes in AV conduction. During AT with 1:1 AV conduction, the last beat of AT is conducted to the ventricle. Spontaneous termination of SVT with a P wave not followed by a QRS practically excludes AT, except coincidentally or in the case of a nonconducted PAC terminating the AT (neither of which will be reproducible).[9]

Termination with Adenosine

The mere termination of SVT in response to adenosine is usually not helpful in differentiating SVTs. However, the pattern of SVT termination can be helpful in two situations: First, reproducible

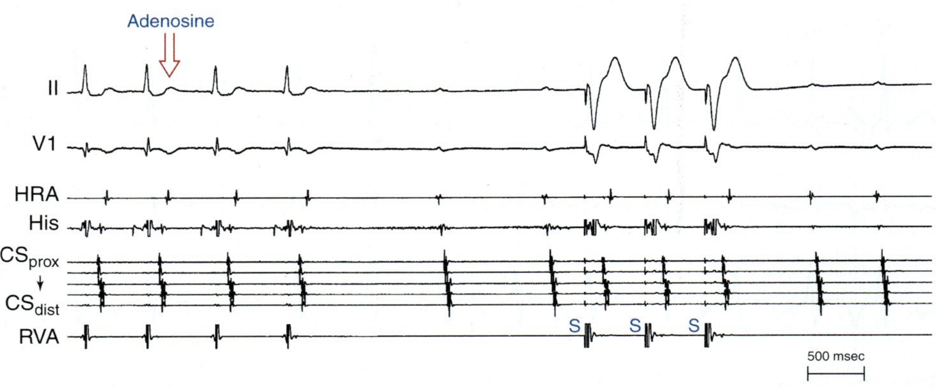

FIGURE 20-5 Termination of supraventricular tachycardia (SVT) with adenosine. Administration of adenosine during an SVT with concentric atrial activation sequence and short RP interval results in termination of the SVT with an atrial complex not followed by a QRS, which is inconsistent with atrial tachycardia. Following termination of the SVT, complete atrioventricular (AV) block during sinus rhythm is observed; however, ventricular pacing is associated with intact ventriculoatrial (VA) conduction and retrograde atrial activation sequence identical to that during the SVT, which suggests that VA conduction is not mediated by the atrioventricular node (AVN) but by an AV bypass tract (BT). The SVT is in fact an orthodromic atrioventricular reentrant tachycardia using a concealed septal BT, and termination with adenosine was the result of block in the AVN. Retrograde conduction over the BT was not affected by adenosine.

termination of the SVT with a QRS not followed by a P wave excludes orthodromic AVRT using a rapidly conducting AV BT as the retrograde limb (adenosine blocks the AVN and not the BT), is unusual in typical AVNRT (adenosine blocks the slow pathway but does not affect the fast pathway), and is consistent with AT, PJRT, or atypical AVNRT. Second, reproducible termination of the SVT with a P wave not followed by a QRS excludes AT, because it occurs in AT only if adenosine terminates the AT at the same moment it causes AV block, which is an unlikely coincidence (Fig. 20-5). Most ATs (50% to 80%) can be terminated by adenosine, typically (80%) prior to the onset of AV block. Response to adenosine does not help differentiate between atypical AVNRT and PJRT.

Termination with Vagal Maneuvers

Carotid sinus massage and vagal maneuvers reproducibly slow or terminate up to 25% of ATs. Orthodromic AVRT usually terminates with gradual slowing and then block in the AVN. Typical AVNRT usually terminates with gradual anterograde slowing and then block in the slow pathway; block in the fast pathway is uncommon. Additionally, carotid sinus massage and vagal maneuvers terminate atypical AVNRT by gradual slowing and then block in the retrograde slow pathway.[9]

Diagnostic Maneuvers during Tachycardia

ATRIAL EXTRASTIMULATION DURING SUPRAVENTRICULAR TACHYCARDIA

Resetting

An AES can reset AT, AVNRT, and orthodromic AVRT, and demonstration of resetting by itself is not helpful in distinguishing among the different types of SVTs. However, resetting with manifest atrial fusion can be demonstrated only in orthodromic AVRT and macroreentrant AT, but not with AVNRT or focal AT. For atrial fusion (i.e., fusion of atrial activation from both the tachycardia wavefront and the AES) to occur, the AES should be able to enter the reentrant circuit while at the same time the tachycardia wavefront should be able to exit the circuit. This requires spatial separation between the entry and exit sites to the reentrant circuit, a condition that seems to be lacking in the setting of AVNRT and focal AT.

Additionally, the resetting curve can help differentiate the different subtypes of SVT. Reentrant AT, AVNRT, and orthodromic AVRT are characterized by an increasing or mixed response curve, whereas triggered activity AT exhibits a decreasing resetting response curve and automatic AT exhibits an increasing resetting response curve. It is difficult for an AES not to affect orthodromic AVRT because of the large size of the reentrant circuit, and an AES over a wide range of coupling intervals can reset the SVT via conduction down the AVN-HPS. However, for AVNRT, more premature AESs are needed to demonstrate resetting.[9]

Termination

Termination of SVT with an AES is not usually helpful for the differential diagnosis. An AES can reproducibly terminate reentrant AT, AVNRT, and orthodromic AVRT, but not automatic AT. Termination of triggered activity AT is less reproducible.[9]

ATRIAL PACING DURING SUPRAVENTRICULAR TACHYCARDIA

Entrainment

Overdrive atrial pacing can entrain reentrant AT, AVNRT, and orthodromic AVRT but not triggered activity or automatic ATs. Entrainment with manifest fusion, on the other hand, can be seen only in AVRT and macroreentrant AT, but not with AVNRT or focal AT (see Fig. 18-27). However, it is important to understand that overdrive pacing of focal AT and AVNRT can result in a certain degree of fusion, especially when the pacing CL is only slightly shorter than the tachycardia CL. Such fusion, however, is unstable during the same pacing drive at a constant CL, because the pacing stimuli fall on a progressively earlier portion of the tachycardia cycle, producing progressively less fusion and more fully paced morphology. Such phenomena should be distinguished from entrainment, and sometimes this requires pacing for long intervals to demonstrate variable degrees of fusion.

During entrainment at a pacing CL close to the tachycardia CL, the AH interval during entrainment is longer than that during AVNRT because the atrium and HB are activated in parallel during AVNRT and in sequence during atrial pacing entraining the AVNRT (because of the presence of an upper common pathway). In contrast, in the setting of AT and orthodromic AVRT, the AH interval is comparable during SVT and entrainment with atrial pacing.[9]

Acceleration

Overdrive pacing during triggered activity AT generally produces acceleration of the tachycardia CL.

Overdrive Suppression

Automatic AT cannot be entrained by atrial pacing; however, rapid atrial pacing results in overdrive suppression of the AT rate, with the return CL following the pacing train prolonging with increasing the duration and/or rate of overdrive pacing, in contrast to constant return cycles following entrainment of reentrant circuits, regardless of the length of the pacing drive. The AT resumes following cessation of atrial pacing but at a slower rate, gradually speeding up (warming up) back to pre-pacing tachycardia CL.[9]

Termination

Termination of SVT with atrial pacing is not usually helpful for differential diagnosis. Atrial pacing can reproducibly terminate reentrant AT, AVNRT, and orthodromic AVRT, but not automatic AT. Termination of triggered activity AT is less reproducible.

Ventriculoatrial Linking

On cessation of overdrive atrial pacing, if the VA interval following the last entrained QRS is reproducibly constant (<10 milliseconds in variation), despite pacing at different CLs or for different durations ("VA linking") and is similar to that during SVT, AT is unlikely. If no VA linking is demonstrable, AT is more likely than other types of SVTs (see Fig. 18-27).[6] VA linking occurs in the setting of typical AVNRT and orthodromic AVRT because the timing of atrial activation is dependent on the preceding ventricular activation and is the result of retrograde VA conduction over the AVN fast pathway (during typical AVNRT) or the AV BT (during orthodromic AVRT), which is relatively fixed and constant. Contrariwise, following cessation of overdrive pacing (with 1:1 AV conduction) during focal AT, the VA interval can vary significantly from the VA interval during AT, because the timing of the tachycardia atrial return cycle is not related to the preceding QRS.[2,6]

Differential-Site Atrial Pacing

As discussed in Chapter 11, differential site atrial pacing can help distinguish AT from other mechanisms of SVT. When the ΔVA interval (i.e., the maximal difference in the post-pacing VA intervals following cessation of pacing from the high RA and proximal CS) is more than 14 milliseconds, AT is suggested. On the other hand, in orthodromic AVRT and AVNRT, the initial atrial complex following cessation of atrial pacing entraining the SVT is *linked* to, and cannot be dissociated from, the last captured ventricular complex; hence, the ΔVA interval is typically less than 14 milliseconds.[14]

VENTRICULAR EXTRASTIMULATION DURING SUPRAVENTRICULAR TACHYCARDIA

Resetting

During orthodromic AVRT, a VES can usually reset the SVT. However, the ability of the VES to affect the SVT depends on the distance between the site of ventricular stimulation to the ventricular insertion site of the BT and on the VES coupling interval. Because only parts of the ventricle ipsilateral to the BT are requisite components of the orthodromic AVRT circuit, a VES delivered in the contralateral ventricle may not affect the circuit (see Fig. 18-29). On the other hand, the inability of early single or double VESs to reset the SVT despite advancement of all ventricular electrograms (including the local electrogram in the electrode recording the earliest atrial activation during the SVT, which would be close to the potential BT ventricular insertion site) by more than 30 milliseconds excludes orthodromic AVRT. Several other findings can help confirm the presence of BT function and whether it is participating in the SVT or is only a bystander (see Tables 18-4 and 18-5).

For AVNRT, the ability of a VES to affect the SVT depends on its ability to activate the HB prematurely and penetrate the AVN, which in turn depends on the tachycardia CL, local ventricular ERP, and the time needed for the VES to reach the HB. Even when HB activation is advanced by the VES, the ability of the paced impulse to invade the AVN will depend on the length of the lower common pathway; the longer the lower common pathway, the more the timing of HB activation must be advanced. In fast-slow or slow-slow AVNRT, which typically has a long lower common pathway, the HB activation must be advanced by more than 30 to 60 milliseconds. In contrast, in slow-fast AVNRT, the lower common pathway is shorter and the tachycardia is typically reset by the VES as soon as the HB activation is advanced. Therefore, a late VES, delivered when the HB is refractory, would not be able to penetrate the AVN and reset AVNRT. During AT, a VES can advance the next atrial activation when given the chance to conduct retrogradely and prematurely to the atrium. However, it would never be able to delay the next AT beat.

Although resetting the SVT by a VES is not diagnostic by itself of a specific type of SVT, it can be helpful in certain situations. First, the ability of a late VES delivered while the HB is refractory (i.e., when the anterograde His potential is already manifest or within 35 to 55 milliseconds before the time of the expected His potential) to affect (reset or terminate) the SVT excludes AVNRT, because such a VES would not have been able to penetrate the AVNRT circuit (Fig. 20-6; and see Fig. 18-29). It also excludes AT, except for cases of AT associated with the presence of innocent bystander BT, in which case the presence of such a BT is usually easy to exclude with ventricular pacing during NSR. Second, the ability of a VES to delay the next atrial activation excludes AT (see Fig. 18-26). Third, the ability of a VES to reset the SVT without atrial activation (i.e., the VES advances the subsequent His potential and QRS and blocks in the upper common pathway) excludes AT and orthodromic AVRT, because it proves that the atrium is not part of the SVT circuit. Fourth, failure of early single or double VESs to reset the SVT, despite advancement of ventricular electrograms in the electrode recording the earliest atrial activation by more than 30 milliseconds, excludes orthodromic AVRT. Fifth, resetting with manifest QRS fusion can be observed during orthodromic AVRT, especially during pacing at a site closer to the BT ventricular insertion site than the entrance of the reentrant circuit to ventricular tissue (i.e., the HPS). Such a phenomenon, on the other hand, cannot occur during AVNRT or focal AT because of the lack of spatial separation of the entrance and exit to the tachycardia circuit. Sixth, retrograde atrial activation sequence following a VES that resets the tachycardia is usually similar to that during SVT in the setting of AVNRT and orthodromic AVRT, because it should conduct over the tachycardia retrograde limb (except in the presence of a bystander retrogradely conducting AV BT). In contrast, a retrograde atrial activation sequence during the VES is usually different from that during AT, except for ATs originating close to the AV junction.

Termination

Termination of AVNRT with a single VES is difficult and occurs rarely when the tachycardia CL is less than 350 milliseconds; such termination favors the diagnosis of orthodromic AVRT, which can usually be readily terminated by single or double VESs. Termination of the SVT with a VES delivered when the HB is refractory excludes AVNRT (see Fig. 20-6). It also excludes AT, except for cases of AT associated with the presence of an innocent bystander BT mediating VA conduction. Reproducible termination of the SVT with a VES not followed by atrial activation excludes AT (see Fig. 18-29) and, if this occurs with a VES delivered while the HB is refractory, it excludes both AT and AVNRT (see Fig. 20-6).

VENTRICULAR PACING DURING SUPRAVENTRICULAR TACHYCARDIA

Ventricular pacing is performed at a CL 10 to 30 milliseconds shorter than the tachycardia CL; the pacing CL is then progressively reduced by 10 to 20 milliseconds in a stepwise fashion with discontinuation of ventricular pacing after each pacing CL to verify continuation versus termination of the SVT. The presence of ventricular capture during ventricular pacing should be verified. Additionally, the presence of 1:1 VA conduction and acceleration of the atrial rate to the pacing CL should be carefully examined (Fig. 20-7). It is also important to verify the continuation of the SVT following cessation of ventricular pacing and whether SVT termination, with or without reinduction of the SVT, has occurred during ventricular pacing.

Ventriculoatrial Dissociation

When overdrive ventricular pacing during SVT fails to accelerate the atrial CL to the pacing CL (i.e., the ventricles are dissociated

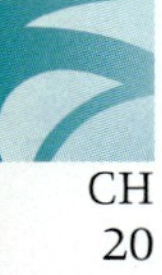

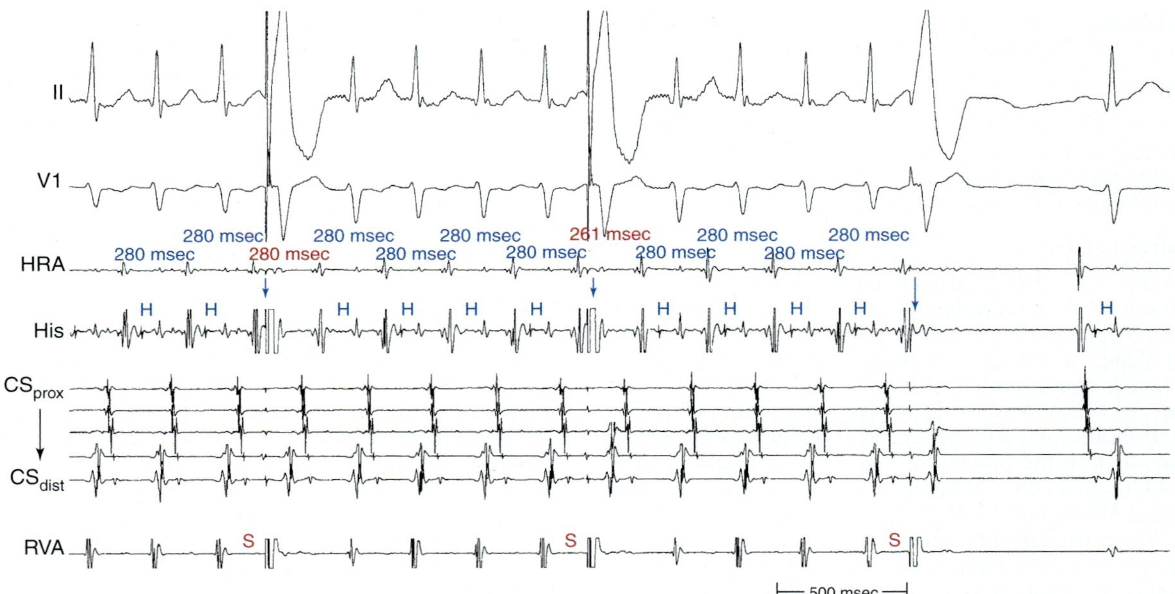

FIGURE 20-6 Ventricular extrastimulation (VES) during supraventricular tachycardia (SVT). VESs were delivered at progressively shorter coupling intervals during a narrow complex SVT with concentric atrial activation sequence. Timing of the anticipated anterograde His bundle (HB) activation is indicated by the blue arrows. The first VES is delivered during HB refractoriness and fails to reset the tachycardia, a phenomenon that does not help in the differential diagnosis. The second VES is delivered slightly earlier but still during HB refractoriness, and it does accelerate the following atrial activation. Atrial activation sequence during the reset atrial complex is identical to that during SVT. This observation excludes atrioventricular nodal reentrant tachycardia (AVNRT), and favors orthodromic atrioventricular reentrant tachycardia (AVRT), but does not exclude the rare example of atrial tachycardia (AT) with a bystander bypass tract (BT) with atrial insertion close to the AT focus. The third VES is delivered during HB refractoriness (within 40 milliseconds before the anticipated anterograde HB activation) and it terminates the tachycardia without conducting to the atrium. This observation, when reproducible, excludes both AVNRT and AT, and proves that the tachycardia is an orthodromic AVRT.

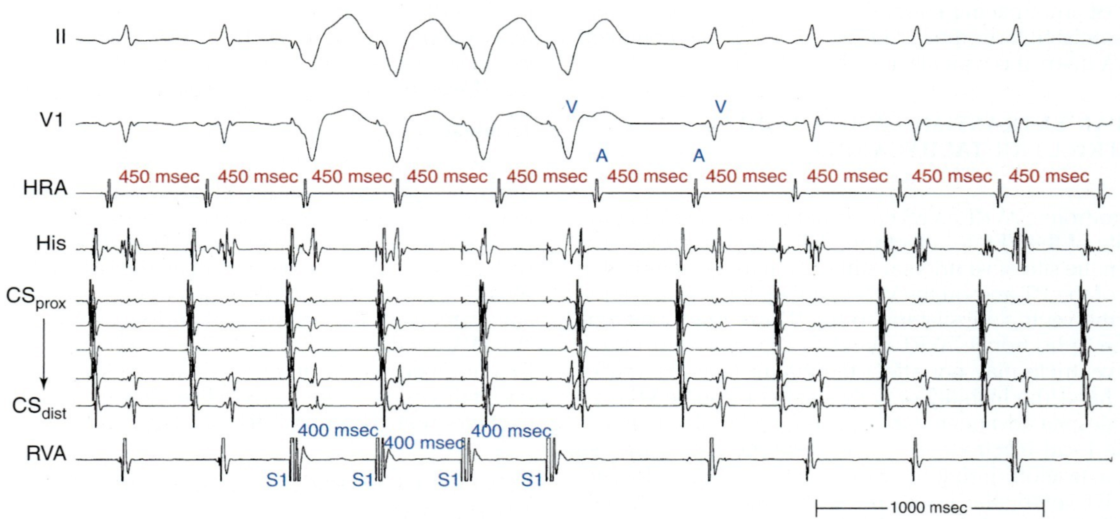

FIGURE 20-7 Overdrive ventricular pacing during supraventricular tachycardia (SVT). The SVT has a long RP interval and concentric atrial activation sequence, which favors atypical atrioventricular nodal reentrant tachycardia (AVNRT), atrial tachycardia (AT) originating close to the AV junction, or orthodromic AVRT using a slowly conducting septal bypass tract. Overdrive ventricular pacing during the tachycardia fails to entrain the tachycardia or capture the atrium (no ventriculoatrial [VA] conduction), because the tachycardia atrial cycle length (CL; 450 milliseconds) remains stable and unaltered by the faster ventricular pacing CL (400 milliseconds). Therefore, analysis of the post-pacing interval or VA interval during pacing versus SVT is invalid. Analysis of the response sequence following cessation of pacing (A-V versus A-A-A-V response) is also invalid in view of the lack of 1:1 VA conduction during ventricular pacing (resulting in a pseudo–A-A-V response). Nonetheless, the fact that ventricular pacing has dissociated the atrium from the ventricle excludes AVRT. However, other pacing maneuvers are required for differentiation between atypical AVNRT and AT.

from the tachycardia), AVRT is excluded, AT is the most likely diagnosis, but AVNRT is still possible.

Atrial Activation Sequence

As noted, the retrograde atrial activation sequence during ventricular pacing during the SVT is usually similar to that during the SVT in the setting of AVNRT and orthodromic AVRT, because it should conduct over the tachycardia retrograde limb. On the other hand, the retrograde atrial activation sequence during ventricular pacing is usually different from that during AT, except for ATs originating close to the AV junction. A pitfall of this criterion is the presence of a bystander AV BT, which can provide another retrograde route capable of mediating retrograde conduction during ventricular pacing without being part

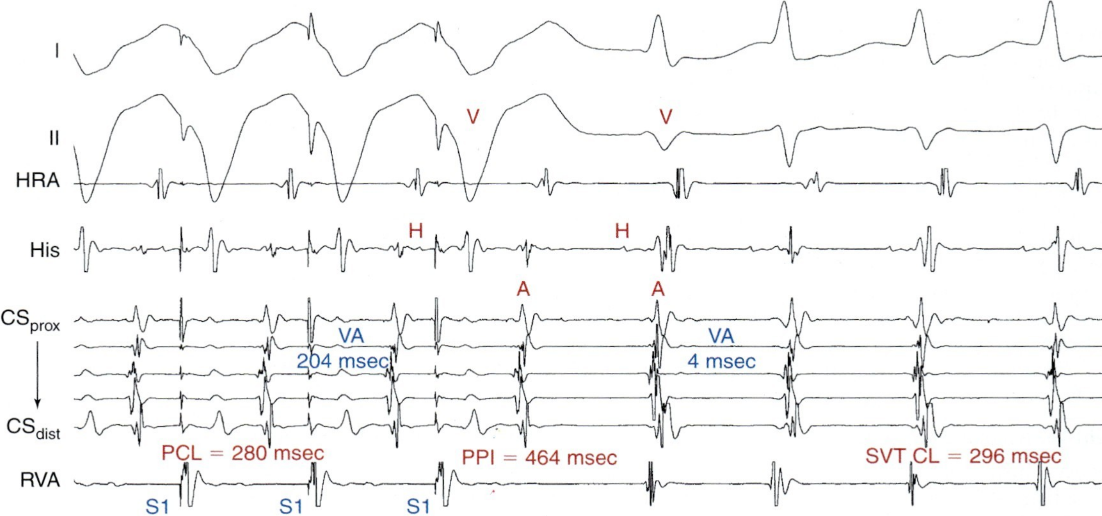

FIGURE 20-8 Entrainment of narrow QRS supraventricular tachycardia (SVT) with right ventricular (RV) apical pacing. Several features in this tracing can help in the differential diagnosis of the SVT. First, atrial and ventricular activation occur simultaneously during the SVT, which excludes atrioventricular reentrant tachycardia (AVRT). Second, atrial activation during the SVT is eccentric, with earliest activation in the mid–coronary sinus (CS), which favors atrial tachycardia (AT) over AVNRT. Third, the atrial activation sequence during ventricular pacing is identical to that during SVT, which favors AVNRT and AVRT over AT. Fourth, following cessation over ventricular pacing, the post-pacing interval (PPI) minus SVT cycle length (CL), [PPI – SVT CL], is more than 115 milliseconds, and the ΔVA interval ($VA_{pacing} - VA_{SVT}$) is more than 85 milliseconds, which favors AVNRT over AVRT. Fifth, although characterization of the activation sequence following cessation of ventricular pacing (A-A-V versus A-V response) is unclear (because of the simultaneous occurrence of atrial and ventricular activation in the first tachycardia complex, replacing ventricular activation with HB activation [i.e., characterizing the response as A-A-H or A-H instead of A-A-V or A-V, respectively]) reveals an A-H response, which favors AVRT and AVNRT over AT. In summary, AVRT can be reliably excluded by the simultaneous atrial and ventricular activation. AT is excluded by the A-H response following cessation of ventricular pacing and by the identical atrial activation sequence during the SVT and ventricular pacing. The left variant of typical AVRT (with an eccentric atrial activation sequence) is the mechanism of the SVT.

of the SVT circuit. In this setting, ventricular pacing can result in a retrograde atrial activation sequence different from that of AVNRT or orthodromic AVRT. The presence of such an AV BT, however, is generally easy to verify with ventricular stimulation during NSR.

Entrainment

Ventricular pacing is almost always able to entrain AVNRT and orthodromic AVRT and, if 1:1 VA conduction is maintained, reentrant AT. Entrainment of the SVT by RV pacing can help differentiate orthodromic AVRT from AVNRT by evaluating the VA interval during SVT versus that during pacing, and also by evaluating the post-pacing interval (PPI). The ventricle and atrium are activated in sequence during orthodromic AVRT and during ventricular pacing, but in parallel during AVNRT. Therefore, the VA interval during orthodromic AVRT approximates that during ventricular pacing (see Fig. 18-30). In contrast, the VA interval during AVNRT would be much shorter than that during ventricular pacing (see Fig. 17-18). In general, a difference in the VA interval (ΔVA [$VA_{pacing} - VA_{SVT}$]) greater than 85 milliseconds is consistent with AVNRT, whereas a ΔVA of less than 85 milliseconds is consistent with orthodromic AVRT (Fig. 20-8).

Additionally, the PPI after entrainment of AVNRT from the RV apex is significantly longer than the tachycardia CL (the [PPI – SVT CL] difference is usually >115 milliseconds), because the reentrant circuit in AVNRT is above the ventricle and far from the pacing site (see Fig. 17-18). In AVNRT, the PPI reflects the conduction time from the pacing site through the RV muscle and HPS, once around the reentry circuit and back to the pacing site. Therefore, the difference between the PPI and the SVT CL [PPI – SVT CL] reflects twice the sum of the conduction time through the RV muscle, the HPS, and any lower common pathway (see Fig. 20-8). In orthodromic AVRT using a septal BT, the PPI reflects the conduction time through the RV to the septum, once around the reentry circuit and back. In other words, the [PPI – SVT CL] reflects twice the conduction time from the pacing catheter through the ventricular myocardium to the reentry circuit. Therefore, the PPI more closely approximates the SVT CL in orthodromic AVRT using a septal BT, compared with AVNRT (see Fig. 18-30). This maneuver was studied specifically for differentiation between atypical AVNRT and orthodromic AVRT, but the principle also applies to typical AVNRT. In general, a [PPI – SVT CL] difference greater than 115 milliseconds is consistent with AVNRT, whereas a [PPI – SVT CL] difference greater than 115 milliseconds is consistent with orthodromic AVRT. For borderline values, ventricular pacing at the RV base can help exaggerate the difference between the PPI and tachycardia CL in the setting of AVNRT, but without significant changes in the setting of orthodromic AVRT, because the site of pacing at the RV base is farther from the AVNRT circuit than the RV apex (because the paced wavefront has to travel first to the RV apex before engaging the HPS and conducting retrogradely to the AVN), but is still close to an AVRT circuit using a septal BT (and, in fact, it is closer to the ventricular insertion of the BT).[15,16]

However, there are several potential pitfalls to the criteria discussed above. The tachycardia CL and VA interval are often perturbed for a few cycles after entrainment. For this reason, care should be taken not to measure unstable intervals immediately after ventricular pacing. In addition, spontaneous oscillations in the tachycardia CL and VA intervals can be seen. The discriminant points chosen may not apply when the spontaneous variability is more than 30 milliseconds. Also, it is possible to mistake isorhythmic VA dissociation for entrainment if the pacing train is not long enough or the pacing CL is too close to the tachycardia CL. Finally, those criteria may not apply to BTs with significant decremental properties, although small decremental intervals are unlikely to provide a false result.

Another limitation is that the [PPI – SVT CL] difference does not account for potential decremental anterograde AVN conduction that may be induced by overdrive pacing, which can significantly affect diagnostic interpretations of the PPI. The prolonged AH interval on the last entrained beat will contribute to prolongation of the PPI that is not reflective of the distance of the pacing site from the circuit. Thus, [PPI – SVT CL] differences obtained after entrainment of orthodromic AVRT employing a septal BT can actually overlap with those observed after entrainment of AVNRT. Correction of the [PPI – SVT CL] difference for the degree of decrement in the AVN (by subtracting the difference in AH [or AV] interval during tachycardia and on the return cycle from the [PPI – SVT CL]) has been shown to improve the accuracy of this criterion for distinction between AVNRT and orthodromic AVRT. In a study of patients with both typical and atypical forms of AVNRT, as well as orthodromic using septal and free wall BTs, a corrected [PPI – SVT CL] difference of less than 110 milliseconds was found more accurate in identifying orthodromic AVRT from AVNRT than the uncorrected [PPI – SVT CL] difference. The use of change in VA interval is of course not influenced by prolongation of the AV interval during pacing and does not require correction.[15,17,18]

Differential Right Ventricular Entrainment

Differential-site RV entrainment (from RV apex versus RV base) can help distinguish AVNRT from orthodromic AVRT. As discussed in Chapter 17, after entrainment of AVNRT, the PPI following entrainment from the RV base is longer than that post entrainment from the RV apex. Conversely, in orthodromic AVRT, the PPI tends to be similar, irrespective of the site of RV pacing.[19] To avoid potential errors introduced by decremental conduction within the AVN during RV pacing, it is preferable to perform correction of the PPI (by subtracting any increase in the AV interval of the return cycle beat, as compared with the AV interval during SVT). A differential corrected [PPI – SVT CL] of more than 30 milliseconds after transient entrainment (i.e., corrected PPI following pacing from the RV base being consistently ≥30 milliseconds longer than that following pacing from the RV apex) is consistent with AVNRT, whereas a differential corrected [PPI – SVT CL] of less than 30 milliseconds is consistent with orthodromic AVRT. Additionally, a differential VA interval (ventricular stimulus-to-atrial interval during entrainment from RV base versus RV septum) of more than 20 milliseconds is consistent with AVNRT, whereas a differential VA interval of less than 20 milliseconds is consistent with orthodromic AVRT.[19]

Entrainment with Manifest Ventricular Fusion

Manifest ventricular fusion during entrainment of SVT indicates that the circuit includes ventricular tissue (i.e., AVRT), excluding both AVNRT and AT (see Fig. 18-30).

Length of Pacing Drive Required for Entrainment

As discussed in Chapter 17, assessing the timing and type of response of SVT to RV pacing can help differentiate orthodromic AVRT from AVNRT. Because the RV pacing site is closer to the reentrant circuit in AVRT than to the AVNRT circuit, RV pacing resets the tachycardia in the setting of AVRT once ventricular capture is achieved, whereas the resetting response is delayed in the setting of AVNRT. Consequently, when resetting of the SVT occurs after a single paced QRS complex, orthodromic AVRT is suggested and AVNRT is generally excluded. On the contrary, if resetting occurs only after at least two beats AVNRT is suggested (Fig. 20-9).[20]

Atrial Resetting during the Transition Zone

In patients with AVNRT or AT, acceleration of the timing of atrial activation cannot occur via the AVN during the transition zone on initiation of RV pacing (during which the pacing train fuses with anterograde ventricular activation), because the HB is expected to be refractory, as indicated by ventricular activation still occurring via anterograde conduction over the HPS. If perturbation (≥15 milliseconds) of atrial timing occurs during the transition zone, it indicates the presence of a retrogradely conducting BT, which can be an integral part of the SVT circuit (i.e., orthodromic AVRT) or a bystander (as discussed in Chap. 17).[21]

Atrial and Ventricular Electrogram Sequence Following Cessation of Ventricular Pacing

As discussed in Chapter 11, the sequence of atrial and ventricular electrograms following cessation of overdrive ventricular pacing during SVT (without tachycardia termination) can help distinguish between the different mechanisms of SVT. It is necessary to verify the presence of 1:1 VA conduction during ventricular pacing before analyzing electrogram sequence. In the setting of AVNRT and orthodromic AVRT, the electrogram sequence immediately after the last paced QRS complex is atrial-ventricular (i.e., "A-V response"; see

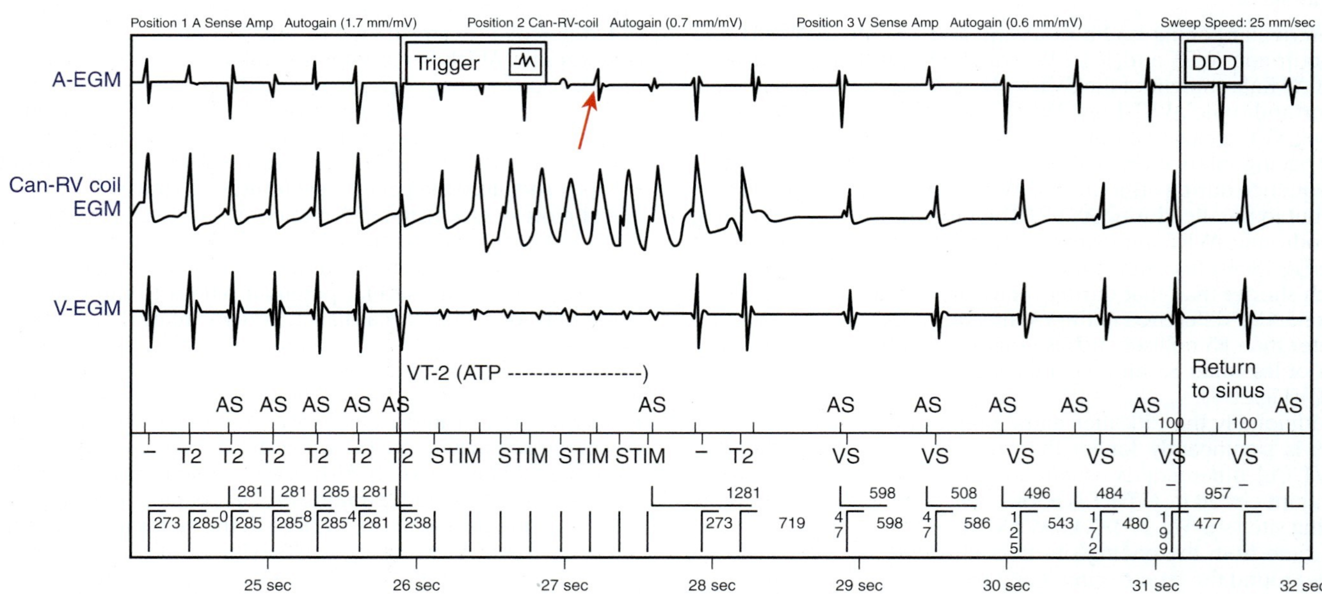

FIGURE 20-9 Intracardiac atrial, shock lead, and ventricular electrograms (A-EGM, Can-RV coil EGM, and V-EGM, respectively) stored by the ICD during an episode of tachycardia at a cycle length (CL) of 275 to 285 milliseconds and a 1:1 AV relationship. The supraventricular tachycardia (SVT) triggered antitachycardia pacing (ATP) therapy by the ICD with a burst of eight ventricular paced beats. ATP terminates the tachycardia, and sinus rhythm is restored. Note that the first three captured complexes during ATP failed to conduct to the atrium, and atrial activity continued unperturbed, which excludes VT as the mechanism of the tachycardia. Furthermore, the first reset (accelerated) atrial complex occurs after the fourth captured paced ventricular complex (red arrow), which is inconsistent with atrioventricular reentrant tachycardia (AVRT) and favors atrioventricular nodal reentrant tachycardia (AVNRT) or atrial tachycardia. The simultaneous atrial and ventricular activation during the tachycardia at baseline line also excludes AVRT and favors AVNRT.

Fig. 11-14). In contrast, in the setting of AT, cessation of overdrive ventricular pacing is followed by an atrial-atrial-ventricular electrogram sequence (i.e., an "A-A-V response"; see Fig. 11-14).[22]

Importantly, a pseudo–A-A-V response can occur: (1) during atypical AVNRT, (2) when 1:1 VA conduction is absent during overdrive ventricular pacing, (3) during typical AVNRT with long His bundle–ventricular (HV) or short HA intervals whereby atrial activation may precede ventricular activation, and (4) in patients with a bystander BT (Fig. 20-10). Replacing ventricular activation with HB activation (i.e., characterizing the response as A-A-H or A-H

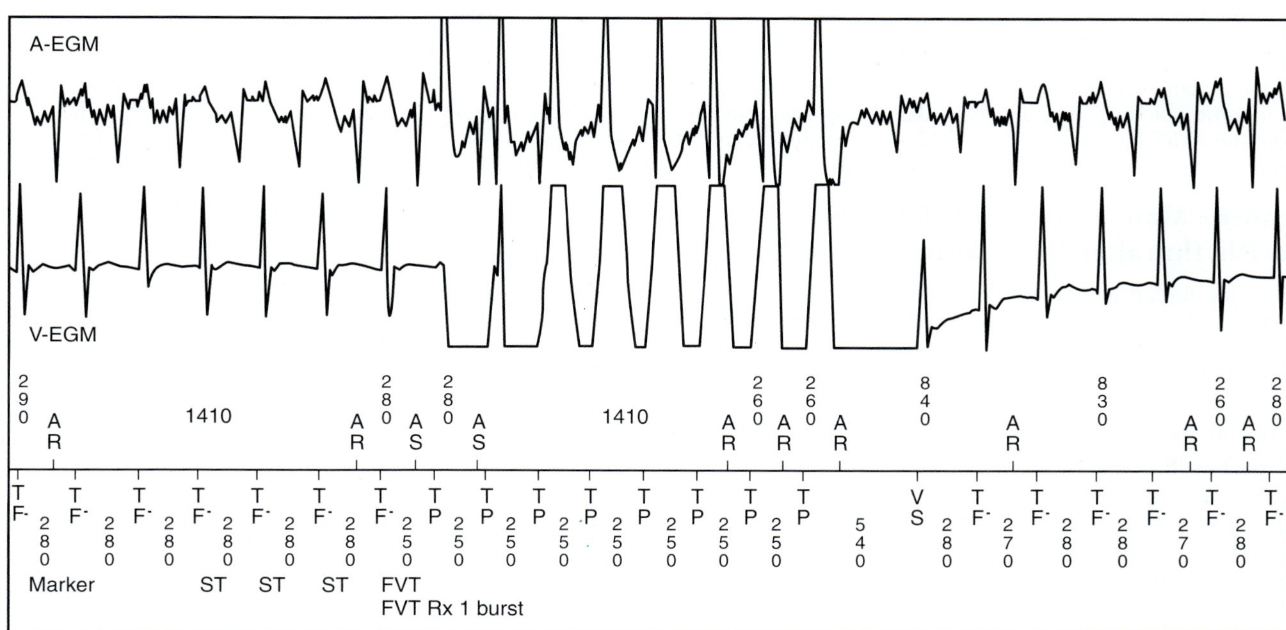

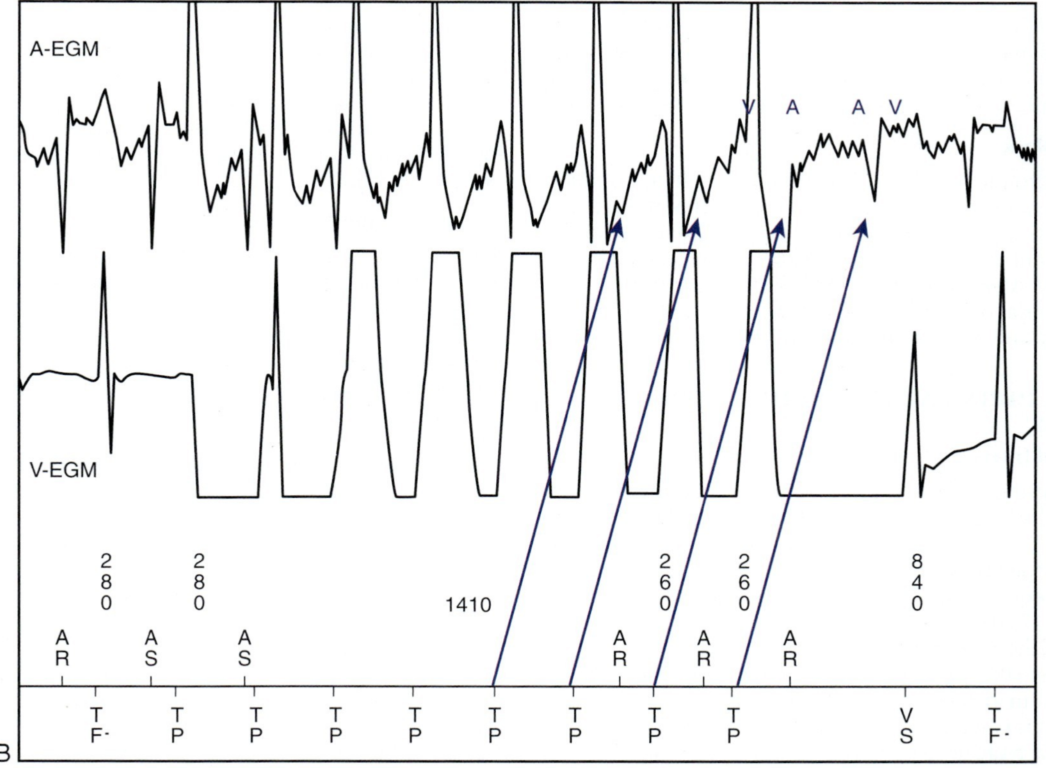

FIGURE 20-10 A, Intracardiac atrial and ventricular electrograms (A-EGM and V-EGM, respectively) stored by the ICD during an episode of supraventricular tachycardia (SVT) at a cycle length (CL) of 280 to 290 milliseconds and a 1:1 AV relationship. The SVT inappropriately triggered antitachycardia pacing (ATP) therapy by the ICD with a burst of eight ventricular paced beats at a CL of 250 milliseconds. ATP fails to terminate the tachycardia, which resumes at the baseline CL. **B**, Magnification of a portion of the *upper panel* showing atrial and ventricular intracardiac electrograms during ATP. Arrows track VA conduction following the last four paced ventricular complexes. VA conduction during ATP is present and can be verified by demonstrating acceleration of the atrial rate to that of the paced ventricular rate. After cessation of ATP, the tachycardia resumes with an A-A-V sequence, which is evident on interrogation of the atrial and ventricular channel electrograms *(lower panel)*. However, careful analysis to identify the last reset atrial complex (occurring at a CL similar to the pacing CL) indicates a pseudo–A-A-V response rather than an A-A-V response, which is consistent with atypical AV nodal reentrant tachycardia as the mechanism of the SVT. See text for discussion.

instead of A-A-V or A-V, respectively) can be more accurate and can help eliminate the pseudo–A-A-V response in patients with AVNRT and long HV intervals, short HA intervals, or both (see Fig. 20-8). On the other hand, a pseudo–A-V response can occur with automatic AT when the maneuver is performed during isoproterenol infusion, and can theoretically occur when AT coexists with retrograde dual AVN pathways or bystander BT (see Chap. 11).[22]

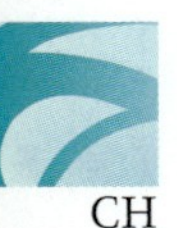

Termination

Ventricular pacing can easily terminate orthodromic AVRT, and failure to terminate the SVT with ventricular pacing argues against orthodromic AVRT. Termination of AVNRT is also common, but AT is less likely to be terminated by ventricular pacing.

Diagnostic Maneuvers during Normal Sinus Rhythm after Tachycardia Termination

When pacing the atrium or ventricle at the tachycardia CL, it is important that the autonomic tone be similar to its state during the tachycardia, because alterations of autonomic tone can independently influence AV or VA conduction.

ATRIAL PACING AT THE TACHYCARDIA CYCLE LENGTH

Atrial–His Bundle Interval

During AT and orthodromic AVRT, the AH interval during SVT is comparable to that during atrial pacing at a CL similar to the tachycardia CL because the activation wavefront propagates through a similar pathway during both the SVT and atrial pacing. On the other hand, the AH interval during AVNRT is shorter than that during atrial pacing, because the atrium and HB are activated in parallel during AVNRT (because of the presence of an upper common pathway) but in sequence during atrial pacing. Therefore, a ΔAH ($AH_{atrial\ pacing} - AH_{SVT}$) greater than 40 milliseconds is consistent with AVNRT. However, a ΔAH of less than 20 milliseconds favors AT and orthodromic AVRT. This has only been tested with RA pacing during right ATs and should be applied with caution when a left AT is suspected.

Atrioventricular Block

For AT and orthodromic AVRT, the AVN should be able to conduct 1:1 during atrial pacing and during the SVT, given that the pacing CL is equal to the tachycardia CL and that the same degree of autonomic tone is maintained, as would be expected when pacing is performed shortly after termination of SVT. Therefore, if AV block develops during atrial pacing, it suggests the presence of an upper common pathway and is consistent with AVNRT.

VENTRICULAR PACING AT THE TACHYCARDIA CYCLE LENGTH

His Bundle–Atrial Interval

Ventricular pacing during NSR at a CL similar to the tachycardia results in HA and VA intervals that are shorter than those during orthodromic AVRT (see Fig. 18-30). Contrariwise, in the setting of AVNRT, ventricular pacing at the tachycardia CL results in HA and VA intervals that are equal or longer during pacing than those during the SVT (see Fig. 17-20). To help distinguish between orthodromic AVRT and AVNRT, the HA interval is measured from the *end* of the His potential (where the impulse leaves the HB to enter the AVN) to the atrial electrogram in the high RA recording and the ΔHA interval ($HA_{pacing} - HA_{SVT}$) is calculated. In the setting of orthodromic AVRT, the ΔHA interval is typically less than −10 milliseconds; whereas, in the setting of AVNRT, the ΔHA interval is more than −10 milliseconds. When the retrograde His potential is not visualized, using the ΔVA interval instead of the ΔHA interval is not as accurate in discriminating orthodromic AVRT from AVNRT (see Chap. 17).[23]

Ventriculoatrial Block

In the setting of AT and AVNRT, and under comparable autonomic tone, 1:1 VA conduction over the AVN may or may not be maintained during ventricular pacing at a CL similar to the tachycardia CL because of possible retrograde block in the AVN or the lower common pathway. Anterograde conduction properties of the AVN or the lower common pathway may allow 1:1 conduction from the AT or AVNRT circuit down to the ventricle, but its retrograde conduction properties may not allow 1:1 retrograde conduction from the ventricle up to the atrium during ventricular pacing at a CL similar to the tachycardia CL. On the contrary, in the setting of orthodromic AVRT, 1:1 VA conduction is expected to be maintained because of the presence of an AV BT that was capable of mediating VA conduction at a similar rate during the AVRT. Therefore, if VA block is observed during ventricular pacing at the tachycardia CL, orthodromic AVRT is excluded (with the exception of orthodromic AVRT using a slowly conducting AV BT), and AT or AVNRT with lower common pathway physiology is more likely.

Atrial Activation Sequence

The retrograde atrial activation sequence during ventricular pacing is usually similar to that during SVT in the setting of AVNRT, but can be similar to or different from that during orthodromic AVRT, depending on whether retrograde VA conduction during ventricular pacing propagates over the AVN, the BT, or both. However, for AT, the retrograde atrial activation sequence during ventricular pacing is usually different from that during AT, except for ATs originating close to the AV junction.

DIFFERENTIAL RIGHT VENTRICULAR PACING

The response to differential-site RV pacing can be evaluated by comparing the VA interval and atrial activation sequence during pacing at the RV base versus the RV apex (see Chap. 18).

Ventriculoatrial Interval

When the VA interval during RV apical pacing is shorter than that during RV basal pacing, a retrogradely conducting septal BT is excluded. However, this maneuver may not exclude the presence of a free wall or a slowly conducting BT. On the other hand, when the VA interval during RV apical pacing is longer than that during RV basal pacing, a retrogradely conducting AV BT is diagnosed (see Fig. 18-33).

Atrial Activation Sequence

A retrograde atrial activation sequence that is different depending on the site of ventricular pacing indicates the presence of a BT. However, a constant atrial activation sequence does not help exclude or prove the presence of an AV BT.

Importantly, this maneuver does not exclude the presence of a distant right or left free wall AV BT, because the site of pacing is far from the AV BT; as a consequence, pacing from the RV apex or RV base may result in preferential VA conduction exclusively over the AVN and a constant atrial activation sequence. Similarly, this maneuver does not exclude the presence of a slowly conducting BT.

PARA-HISIAN PACING

The response to para-Hisian pacing can be determined by comparing the following four variables between HB-RB capture and noncapture while maintaining local ventricular capture and no atrial capture: (1) atrial activation sequence, (2) S-A interval, (3) local VA interval, and (4) HA interval (see Figs. 18-31 and 18-32).[24] Seven patterns of response to para-Hisian pacing can be observed (see Table 18-3). Please refer to Chapter 18 for a more detailed discussion of para-Hisian pacing.

Atrial Activation Sequence

An identical retrograde atrial activation sequence, with and without HB capture, indicates that retrograde conduction is occurring over the same system during HB-RB capture and noncapture (either the BT or the AVN) and does not help prove or exclude the presence of a BT. On the other hand, a retrograde atrial activation sequence that is different depending on whether the HB is captured indicates the presence of a BT.

His Bundle–Atrial and Ventriculoatrial Intervals

The HA and S-A (VA) intervals are recorded at multiple sites, including close to the site of earliest atrial activation during SVT. An S-A (VA) interval that is constant regardless of whether the HB-RB is being captured indicates the presence of a BT, whereas prolongation of the S-A (VA) interval on loss of HB capture, compared with that during HB capture, excludes the presence of a retrogradely conducting BT, except for slowly conducting and far free wall BTs.[24]

DUAL-CHAMBER SEQUENTIAL EXTRASTIMULATION

Dual-chamber sequential extrastimulation is a useful maneuver for identifying concealed slowly conducting BTs not revealed with standard pacing maneuvers. This maneuver involves the delivery of an eight-beat drive train of simultaneous atrial and RV pacing at a CL of 600 milliseconds, followed by an AES (A_2) delivered at a coupling interval equal to the predetermined AVN ERP, followed by a VES (V_2) delivered at a coupling interval equal to the drive train CL (600 milliseconds). Repeat drives are then performed with decrements of 10 milliseconds for V_2 until VA block is observed.[25]

The critically timed A_2 prolongs the AVN refractory period via concealed anterograde conduction, causing the V_2 to block retrogradely in the AVN when it would have conducted had the A_2 not been delivered (analogous to delivering a VES during SVT while the HB is refractory). If a BT is present, the V_2 conducts back to the atrium while the AVN remains refractory, resulting in a retrograde atrial activation pattern consistent with exclusive BT conduction. Please refer to Chapter 18 for a more detailed discussion on dual-chamber sequential extrastimulation.

Practical Approach to Electrophysiological Diagnosis of Supraventricular Tachycardia

It is important to understand that there is no single diagnostic maneuver or algorithm that is adequate in distinguishing between the different types of SVTs in all cases. Each maneuver has its own applications and limitations. Although several diagnostic criteria were found to have high specificity, sensitivity is frequently limited. Therefore, the investigator will often need to use a combination of SVT features and pacing maneuvers to establish an accurate diagnosis. Systematic evaluation of all possibilities and adherence to fundamental EP principles will help establish the correct diagnosis. Each step during the EP study in these patients can offer valuable information to the vigilant investigator that, if recognized, can potentially reduce procedure time and improve outcome.

Tables 20-1, 20-2, and 20-3 and Figure 20-11 outline some of the proposed strategies for the EP diagnosis of narrow complex SVTs. Baseline tachycardia features, atrial and ventricular programmed stimulation during the tachycardia and then during sinus rhythm after tachycardia termination, provide a diagnosis of the mechanism of SVT in the vast majority of cases.

When sustained SVT is inducible, overdrive pacing from the RV apex and base is performed at a CL 10 to 30 milliseconds shorter than the tachycardia CL; the pacing CL is then progressively reduced by 10 to 20 milliseconds in a stepwise fashion with discontinuation of ventricular pacing after each pacing CL to verify continuation versus termination of the SVT. When acceleration of the atrial CL to the pacing CL during ventricular pacing (with 1:1 VA conduction) is verified, several diagnostic criteria can be applied (see Table 20-2). Overdrive ventricular pacing during the SVT represents the single most important diagnostic maneuver that can provide several clues to the diagnosis of most SVTs. Therefore, it is preferable to employ this maneuver as an initial step in the diagnostic approach.[26]

TABLE 20-1 Diagnostic Strategy for Narrow QRS Supraventricular Tachycardia: Tachycardia Features

Atrial activation sequence	• Eccentric atrial activation sequence excludes AVNRT (except for the left variant of AVNRT). • An initial atrial activation site away from the AV groove and AV junction is diagnostic of AT and excludes both AVNRT and orthodromic AVRT.
VA interval	• VA interval of <70 msec or a ventricular-to-high RA interval of <95 msec during SVT excludes orthodromic AVRT, and is consistent with AVNRT, but can occur during AT with a long PR interval.
AV block	• Spontaneous or induced AV block with continuation of the tachycardia is consistent with AT, excludes AVRT, and is uncommon in AVNRT.
VA block	• VA block can rarely occur during AVNRT because of block in an upper common pathway. • Other potential mechanisms of SVT with VA block include automatic junctional tachycardia with retrograde VA block and orthodromic AVRT using a nodofascicular or nodoventricular BT for retrograde conduction.
Effects of BBB	• BBB does not affect the tachycardia CL or VA interval in AT, AVNRT, or orthodromic AVRT using a BT contralateral to the BBB. • BBB that prolongs the VA interval, with or without affecting the tachycardia CL, is diagnostic of orthodromic AVRT using an AV BT ipsilateral to the BBB and excludes AT and AVNRT.
Tachycardia CL variations	• Spontaneous changes in PR and RP intervals with a fixed A-A interval is consistent with AT, and excludes orthodromic AVRT. • Spontaneous changes in the tachycardia CL accompanied by a constant VA interval favor orthodromic AVRT. • Changes in atrial CL preceding similar changes in subsequent ventricular CL strongly favor AT or atypical AVNRT. • Changes in ventricular CL preceded by similar changes in the atrial CL favor typical AVNRT or orthodromic AVRT.
Tachycardia termination	• Spontaneous termination of SVT with a P wave not followed by a QRS practically excludes AT, except in the case of a nonconducted PAC terminating the AT. • Reproducible SVT termination in response to adenosine with a QRS not followed by a P wave excludes orthodromic AVRT using a rapidly conducting AV BT as the retrograde limb, is unusual in typical AVNRT, and is consistent with AT, PJRT, or atypical AVNRT.

A-A = atrial-atrial; AT = atrial tachycardia; AV = atrioventricular; AVNRT = atrioventricular nodal reentrant tachycardia; AVRT = atrioventricular reentrant tachycardia; BBB = bundle branch block; BT = bypass tract; CL = cycle length; PAC = premature atrial complex; PJRT = permanent junctional reciprocating tachycardia; RA = right atrium; SVT = supraventricular tachycardia; VA = ventriculoatrial.

Subsequently, a VES is delivered when the HB is refractory and then at progressively shorter VES coupling intervals (approximately 10-millisecond stepwise shortening of the VES coupling interval) so as to scan all of diastole. First, ventricular capture of the VES should be verified, and then the effect of the VES on the following atrial activation (advancement, delay, termination, or no effect) should be evaluated, as well as the timing of the VES in relation to the expected His potential during the SVT. Furthermore, conduction of the VES to the atrium and sequence of atrial activation following the VES should be carefully examined (see Fig. 20-6).

Atrial pacing is then performed at a CL 10 to 20 milliseconds shorter than the tachycardia CL. The pacing CL is then progressively reduced by 10 to 20 milliseconds in a stepwise fashion, with discontinuation of atrial pacing after each pacing CL to

TABLE 20-2 Diagnostic Strategy for Narrow QRS Supraventricular Tachycardia: Programmed Electrical Stimulation during Tachycardia

Ventricular Extrastimulation	
When the VES advances the next atrial activation	• Advancement of the next atrial impulse occurring with a VES delivered when the HB is not refractory usually does not help differentiate among the different types of SVTs. • If the advanced atrial activation occurs with similar prematurity (i.e., same coupling interval) to that of the VES (exact coupling phenomenon) or with more prematurity (i.e., shorter coupling interval) than that of the VES (paradoxical coupling phenomenon), orthodromic AVRT is diagnosed. • If advancement occurs when the HB is refractory, AVNRT is excluded. • If advancement occurs with an atrial activation sequence similar to that during SVT, regardless of the timing of the VES, AT is less likely than AVNRT or orthodromic AVRT. • When advancement occurs when the HB is refractory, with an atrial activation sequence similar to that during SVT, AVNRT is excluded, AT is unlikely, and orthodromic AVRT is the most likely diagnosis. • Resetting with manifest QRS fusion is consistent with orthodromic AVRT and excludes both AVNRT and focal AT.
When the VES delays the next atrial activation	• When the VES causes delay in the next atrial activation, regardless of the timing of the VES, AT is excluded, and when such delay occurs with a VES delivered when the HB is refractory, both AVNRT and AT are excluded.
When the VES terminates the SVT	• When termination occurs reproducibly with a VES delivered when the HB is refractory, AVNRT is excluded, and the presence of a retrogradely conducting AV BT is diagnosed. • If the atrial activation sequence following the VES is similar to that during the SVT, orthodromic AVRT is indicated and AT is practically excluded, except for the rare case in which AT originates close to the atrial insertion site of an innocent bystander AV BT. • When termination occurs reproducibly with a VES that does not activate the atrium, regardless of the timing of the VES in relation to the HB, AT is excluded; when this phenomenon is observed with a VES delivered when the HB is refractory, both AT and AVNRT are excluded and orthodromic AVRT is diagnosed.
When the VES fails to affect the next atrial activation	• If resetting does not occur with a relatively late VES, this usually does not help in the differential diagnosis of SVT. • If resetting does not occur with an early VES, despite advancement of the local ventricular activation at ventricular sites near the site of earliest atrial activation by >30 msec, orthodromic AVRT and the presence of a retrogradely conducting AV BT are excluded.
Ventricular Pacing	
VA dissociation	• When overdrive ventricular pacing during SVT fails to accelerate atrial CL to the pacing CL (i.e., the ventricles are dissociated from the tachycardia), AVRT is excluded, AT is the most likely diagnosis, but AVNRT is still possible.
VA interval	• ΔVA interval ($VA_{pacing} - VA_{SVT}$) >85 msec is consistent with AVNRT. • ΔVA of <85 msec is consistent with orthodromic AVRT.
Post-pacing interval	• [PPI – SVT CL] difference >115 msec is consistent with AVNRT. • [PPI – SVT CL] difference <115 msec is consistent with orthodromic AVRT.
Entrainment with ventricular fusion	• Ventricular fusion during entrainment indicates AVRT and excludes both AVNRT and AT.
Differential right ventricular entrainment	• Differential corrected [PPI – SVT CL] of >30 msec after transient entrainment from the RV apex versus the RV base is consistent with AVNRT. • Differential corrected [PPI – SVT CL] of <30 msec is consistent with orthodromic AVRT. • Differential VA interval (ventricular stimulus-to-atrial interval during entrainment from RV base versus RV septum) of >20 msec is consistent with AVNRT. • Differential VA interval of <20 msec is consistent with orthodromic AVRT.
Length of pacing drive required for entrainment	• Acceleration of the SVT to the pacing CL occurring after a single captured paced QRS complex is consistent with orthodromic AVRT and essentially excludes AVNRT. • Acceleration of the SVT to the pacing CL occurring only after ≥2 captured paced QRS complexes is consistent with AVNRT and excludes orthodromic AVRT.
Atrial activation sequence during ventricular pacing	• Atrial activation sequence during pacing different from that during the SVT is consistent with AT and practically excludes both orthodromic AVRT and AVNRT. • Atrial activation sequence during pacing similar to that during the SVT favors orthodromic AVRT or AVNRT over AT.
Atrial and ventricular electrogram sequence following cessation of ventricular pacing	• A-A-V response is consistent with AT (as long as pseudo–A-A-V response is excluded). • A-V response is consistent with AVNRT and orthodromic AVRT.
Atrial Pacing	
Entrainment during atrial pacing	• Demonstration of entrainment excludes automatic and triggered activity ATs.
Entrainment with atrial fusion	• Demonstration of entrainment with manifest atrial fusion excludes AVNRT and focal AT.
Overdrive suppression	• Overdrive suppression of the SVT favors automatic AT and excludes AVNRT and orthodromic AVRT.
AH interval	• ΔAH interval ($AH_{atrial\ pacing} - AH_{SVT}$) of >40 msec favors AVNRT over AT and orthodromic AVRT. • ΔAH interval of <20 msec favors AT and orthodromic AVRT over AVNRT.
VA linking	• On cessation of overdrive atrial pacing (with 1:1 AV conduction), if the VA interval following the last entrained QRS is reproducibly constant (<10 msec variation), despite pacing at different CLs or for different durations (VA linking) and similar to that during SVT, AT is unlikely. • If no VA linking is demonstrable, AT is more likely than other types of SVT.
Differential site atrial pacing	• On cessation of overdrive atrial pacing (with 1:1 AV conduction) from different atrial sites (high RA and proximal CS) at the same pacing CL, a maximal difference in the post-pacing VA intervals (the interval from last captured ventricular electrogram to the earliest atrial electrogram of the initial tachycardia beat after pacing) among the different atrial pacing sites (ΔVA interval) of >14 msec is consistent with AT. • ΔVA interval of <14 msec favors AVNRT or orthodromic AVRT over AT.

A-A = atrial-atrial; A-A-V = atrial-atrial-ventricular; AH = atrial-His bundle interval; AT = atrial tachycardia; AV = atrioventricular; AVNRT = atrioventricular nodal reentrant tachycardia; AVRT = atrioventricular reentrant tachycardia; BT = bypass tract; CL = cycle length; CS = coronary sinus; HB = His bundle; PPI = post-pacing interval; RA = right atrium; RV = right ventricle; SVT = supraventricular tachycardia; VA = ventriculoatrial; VES = ventricular extrastimulus.

TABLE 20-3 Diagnostic Strategy for Narrow QRS Supraventricular Tachycardia: Programmed Electrical Stimulation during Sinus Rhythm

Ventricular Pacing from Right Ventricular Apex at Tachycardia Cycle Length	
HA interval	• ΔHA interval ($HA_{pacing} - HA_{SVT}$) of more than −10 msec favors AVNRT. • ΔHA interval of less than −10 msec favors orthodromic AVRT.
Retrograde atrial activation sequence	• A retrograde atrial activation sequence during ventricular pacing similar to that during SVT favors orthodromic AVRT and AVNRT over AT.
VA block	• The presence of VA block or decremental VA conduction during ventricular pacing at a CL similar to the tachycardia CL and under comparable autonomic tone argues against orthodromic AVRT and favors AT and AVNRT.
Atrial Pacing from High Right Atrium at Tachycardia Cycle Length	
AH interval	• ΔAH interval ($AH_{atrial\ pacing} - AH_{SVT}$) of >40 msec favors AVNRT over AT and orthodromic AVRT. • ΔAH interval of <20 msec favors AT and orthodromic AVRT over AVNRT.
AV block	• Development of AV block during atrial pacing argues against AT and orthodromic AVRT, and favors AVNRT, given that the same degree of autonomic tone is maintained.
Differential Right Ventricular Pacing	
VA interval	• When the VA interval during RV apical pacing is shorter than that during RV basal pacing, a retrogradely conducting septal BT is excluded. • When the VA interval during RV apical pacing is longer than that during RV basal pacing, a retrogradely conducting AV BT is diagnosed.
Atrial activation sequence	• A retrograde atrial activation sequence that is different depending on the site of ventricular pacing indicates the presence of a BT. • A constant atrial activation sequence does not help exclude or prove the presence of an AV BT.
Para-Hisian Pacing	
Atrial activation sequence	• An identical retrograde atrial activation sequence, with and without HB capture, indicates that retrograde conduction is occurring over the same system during HB-RB capture and noncapture (either the BT or AVN) and does not help prove or exclude the presence of BT. • A retrograde atrial activation sequence that is different depending on whether HB is captured indicates the presence of a BT.
HA and VA intervals	• S-A (VA) interval (recorded at multiple sites, including close to the site of earliest atrial activation during SVT) that is constant regardless of whether the HB-RB is being captured indicates the presence of a BT. • Prolongation of the S-A (VA) interval on loss of HB capture, compared with that during HB capture, excludes the presence of a retrogradely conducting BT, except for slowly conducting and far free wall BTs.

AH = atrial-His bundle interval; AT = atrial tachycardia; AV = atrioventricular; AVN = atrioventricular node; AVNRT = atrioventricular nodal reentrant tachycardia; AVRT = atrioventricular reentrant tachycardia; BT = bypass tract; CL = cycle length; HA = His bundle–atrial interval; RB = right bundle branch; RV = right ventricle; S-A = stimulus-atrial interval; SVT = supraventricular tachycardia; VA = ventriculoatrial.

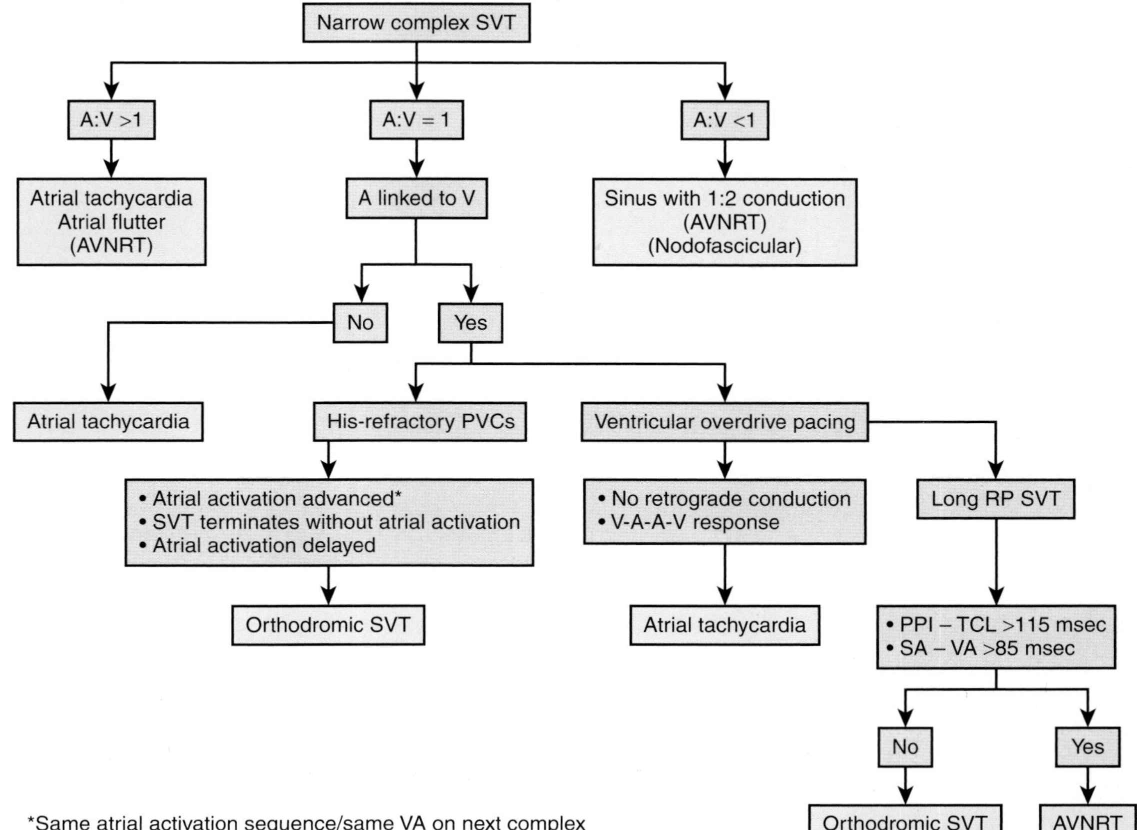

FIGURE 20-11 Algorithm for diagnosis of narrow complex supraventricular tachycardia (SVT). Items in parentheses are rarely seen. AVNRT = atrioventricular nodal reentry; CL = cycle length; PPI = post-pacing interval; PVC = premature ventricular complex; SA = stimulus-to-atrial interval; TCL = tachycardia cycle length; VA = ventriculoatrial interval.

ensure continuation versus termination of the SVT. The presence of entrainment, atrial fusion, AH interval, and VA linking should be evaluated (see Table 20-2).

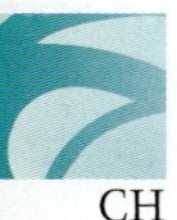

After tachycardia termination, ventricular and atrial pacing at the tachycardia CL, differential site RV pacing (RV apex versus base), and para-Hisian pacing maneuvers are performed (see Table 20-3).

REFERENCES

1. Lau EW: Infraatrial supraventricular tachycardias: mechanisms, diagnosis, and management, *Pacing Clin Electrophysiol* 31:490–498, 2008.
2. Porter MJ, Morton JB, Denman R, et al: Influence of age and gender on the mechanism of supraventricular tachycardia, *Heart Rhythm* 1:393–396, 2004.
3. Gonzalez-Torrecilla E, Almendral J, Arenal A, et al: Combined evaluation of bedside clinical variables and the electrocardiogram for the differential diagnosis of paroxysmal atrioventricular reciprocating tachycardias in patients without pre-excitation, *J Am Coll Cardiol* 53:2353–2358, 2009.
4. Ballo P, Bernabo D, Faraguti SA: Heart rate is a predictor of success in the treatment of adults with symptomatic paroxysmal supraventricular tachycardia, *Eur Heart J* 25:1310–1317, 2004.
5. Blomstrom-Lundqvist C, Scheinman MM, Aliot EM, et al: ACC/AHA/ESC guidelines for the management of patients with supraventricular arrhythmias—executive summary: a report of the American College of Cardiology/American Heart Association Task Force on Practice Guidelines and the European Society of Cardiology Committee for Practice Guidelines (Writing Committee to Develop Guidelines for the Management of Patients with Supraventricular Arrhythmias) developed in collaboration with NASPE-Heart Rhythm Society, *J Am Coll Cardiol* 42:1493–1531, 2003.
6. Knight BP, Ebinger M, Oral H, et al: Diagnostic value of tachycardia features and pacing maneuvers during paroxysmal supraventricular tachycardia, *J Am Coll Cardiol* 36:574–582, 2000.
7. Kertesz NJ, Fogel RI, Prystowsky EN: Mechanism of induction of atrioventricular node reentry by simultaneous anterograde conduction over the fast and slow pathways, *J Cardiovasc Electrophysiol* 16:251–255, 2005.
8. Kapa S, Henz BD, Dib C, et al: Utilization of retrograde right bundle branch block to differentiate atrioventricular nodal from accessory pathway conduction, *J Cardiovasc Electrophysiol* 20:751–758, 2009.
9. Josephson ME: Supraventricular tachycardias. In Josephson ME, editor: *Clinical cardiac electrophysiology*, ed 4, Philadelphia, 2008, Lippincott Williams & Wilkins, pp 175–284.
10. Lockwood D, Nakagawa H, Jackman W: Electrophysiological characteristics of atrioventricular nodal reentrant tachycardia: implications for the reentrant circuit. In Zipes DP, Jalife J, editors: *Cardiac electrophysiology: from cell to bedside*, ed 5, Philadelphia, 2009, WB Saunders, pp 615–646.
11. Issa ZF: Mechanism of paroxysmal supraventricular tachycardia with ventriculoatrial conduction block, *Europace* 11:1235–1237, 2009.
12. Morihisa K, Yamabe H, Uemura T, et al: Analysis of atrioventricular nodal reentrant tachycardia with variable ventriculoatrial block: characteristics of the upper common pathway, *Pacing Clin Electrophysiol* 32:484–493, 2009.
13. Srivathsan K, Gami AS, Barrett R, et al: Differentiating atrioventricular nodal reentrant tachycardia from junctional tachycardia: novel application of the delta H-A interval, *J Cardiovasc Electrophysiol* 19:1–6, 2008.
14. Maruyama M, Kobayashi Y, Miyauchi Y, et al: The VA relationship after differential atrial overdrive pacing: a novel tool for the diagnosis of atrial tachycardia in the electrophysiologic laboratory, *J Cardiovasc Electrophysiol* 18:1127–1133, 2007.
15. Kannankeril PJ, Bonney WJ, Dzurik MV, Fish FA: Entrainment to distinguish orthodromic reciprocating tachycardia from atrioventricular nodal reentry tachycardia in children, *Pacing Clin Electrophysiol* 33:469–474, 2010.
16. Platonov M, Schroeder K, Veenhuyzen GD: Differential entrainment: beware from where you pace, *Heart Rhythm* 4:1097–1099, 2007.
17. Gonzalez-Torrecilla E, Arenal A, Atienza F, et al: First postpacing interval after tachycardia entrainment with correction for atrioventricular node delay: a simple maneuver for differential diagnosis of atrioventricular nodal reentrant tachycardias versus orthodromic reciprocating tachycardias, *Heart Rhythm* 3:674–679, 2006.
18. Veenhuyzen GD, Stuglin C, Zimola KG, Mitchell LB: A tale of two post pacing intervals, *J Cardiovasc Electrophysiol* 17:687–689, 2006.
19. Segal OR, Gula LJ, Skanes AC, et al: Differential ventricular entrainment: a maneuver to differentiate AV node reentrant tachycardia from orthodromic reciprocating tachycardia, *Heart Rhythm* 6:493–500, 2009.
20. Dandamudi G, Mokabberi R, Assal C, et al: A novel approach to differentiating orthodromic reciprocating tachycardia from atrioventricular nodal reentrant tachycardia, *Heart Rhythm* 7:1326–1329, 2010.
21. AlMahameed ST, Buxton AE, Michaud GF: New criteria during right ventricular pacing to determine the mechanism of supraventricular tachycardia, *Circ Arrhythm Electrophysiol* 3:578–584, 2010.
22. Vijayaraman P, Lee BP, Kalahasty G, Wood MA, Ellenbogen KA: Reanalysis of the "pseudo A-A-V" response to ventricular entrainment of supraventricular tachycardia: importance of His-bundle timing, *J Cardiovasc Electrophysiol* 17:25–28, 2006.
23. Miller JM, Rosenthal ME, Gottlieb CD, et al: Usefulness of the delta HA interval to accurately distinguish atrioventricular nodal reentry from orthodromic septal bypass tract tachycardias, *Am J Cardiol* 68:1037–1044, 1991.
24. Nakagawa H, Jackman WM: Para-Hisian pacing: useful clinical technique to differentiate retrograde conduction between accessory atrioventricular pathways and atrioventricular nodal pathways, *Heart Rhythm* 2:667–672, 2005.
25. Sauer WH, Lowery CM, Cooper JM, Lewkowiez L: Sequential dual chamber extrastimulation: a novel pacing maneuver to identify the presence of a slowly conducting concealed accessory pathway, *Heart Rhythm* 5:248–252, 2008.
26. Veenhuyzen GD, Coverett K, Quinn FR, et al: Single diagnostic pacing maneuver for supraventricular tachycardia, *Heart Rhythm* 5:1152–1158, 2008.

CHAPTER 21 Approach to Wide QRS Complex Tachycardias

Clinical Considerations

Causes of Wide Complex Tachycardias

A narrow QRS complex requires rapid, highly synchronous electrical activation of the right ventricular (RV) and left ventricular (LV) myocardium, which can only be achieved through the specialized, rapidly conducting His-Purkinje system (HPS). A wide QRS complex implies less synchronous ventricular activation of longer duration, which can be due to intraventricular conduction disturbances (IVCDs), or ventricular activation not mediated by the His bundle (HB) but by a bypass tract (BT; preexcitation) or from a site within a ventricle (ventricular arrhythmias). IVCDs may be fixed and present at all heart rates, or they may be intermittent and related to either tachycardia or bradycardia. IVCDs can be caused by structural abnormalities in the HPS or ventricular myocardium or by functional refractoriness in a portion of the conduction system (i.e., aberrant ventricular conduction).[1]

Wide QRS complex tachycardia (WCT) is a rhythm with a rate of more than 100 beats/min and a QRS duration of more than 120 milliseconds. Several arrhythmias can manifest as WCTs (Table 21-1); the most common is ventricular tachycardia (VT), which accounts for 80% of all cases of WCT. Supraventricular tachycardia (SVT) with aberrancy accounts for 15% to 20% of WCTs. SVTs with bystander preexcitation and antidromic atrioventricular reentrant tachycardia (AVRT) account for 1% to 6% of WCTs.

In the stable patient who will undergo a more detailed assessment, the goal of evaluation should include determination of the cause of the WCT (particularly distinguishing between VT and SVT). Accurate diagnosis of the WCT requires information obtained from the history, physical examination, response to certain maneuvers, and careful inspection of the electrocardiogram (ECG), including rhythm strips and 12-lead tracings. Comparison of the ECG during the tachycardia with that recorded during sinus rhythm, if available, can also provide useful information.[2]

Clinical History

AGE

WCT in a patient older than 35 years is likely to be VT (positive predictive value of up to 85%). SVT is more likely in the younger patient (positive predictive value of 70%).

SYMPTOMS

Some patients with tachycardia can have few or no symptoms (e.g., palpitations, lightheadedness, diaphoresis), whereas others can have severe manifestations, including chest pain, dyspnea, syncope, seizures, and cardiac arrest. The severity of symptoms during a WCT is not useful in determining the tachycardia mechanism because symptoms are primarily related to the fast heart rate, associated heart disease, and the presence and extent of LV dysfunction, rather than to the mechanism of the tachycardia. It is important to recognize that VT does not necessarily result in hemodynamic compromise or collapse. Misdiagnosis of VT as SVT on the basis of hemodynamic stability is a common error that can lead to inappropriate and potentially dangerous therapy.[2]

DURATION OF THE ARRHYTHMIA

SVT is more likely if the tachycardia has recurred over a period of more than 3 years. The first occurrence of a WCT after myocardial infarction (MI) strongly implies VT.

PRESENCE OF UNDERLYING HEART DISEASE

The presence of structural heart disease, especially coronary heart disease and a previous MI, strongly suggests VT as the cause of WCT. In one report, over 98% of patients with a previous MI had VT as the cause of WCT, whereas only 7% of those with SVT had had an MI. It should be realized, however, that VT can occur in patients with no apparent heart disease, and SVT can occur in those with structural heart disease.[2]

PACEMAKER OR IMPLANTABLE CARDIOVERTER-DEFIBRILLATOR IMPLANTATION

A history of pacemaker or implantable cardioverter-defibrillator (ICD) implantation should raise the possibility of a device-associated tachycardia. Ventricular pacing can be associated with a small and almost imperceptible stimulus artifact on the ECG. The presence of an ICD is also of importance because such a device should identify and treat a sustained tachyarrhythmia, depending on device programming, and because the presence of an ICD implies that the patient is known to have an increased risk of ventricular tachyarrhythmias.

MEDICATIONS

Many different medications have proarrhythmic effects. The most common drug-induced tachyarrhythmia is torsades de pointes. Frequently implicated agents include antiarrhythmic drugs such as sotalol and quinidine, and certain antimicrobial drugs such as erythromycin. Diuretics are a common cause of hypokalemia and hypomagnesemia, which can predispose to ventricular tachyarrhythmias, particularly torsades de pointes in patients taking antiarrhythmic drugs. Furthermore, class I antiarrhythmic drugs, especially class IC agents, slow conduction and have a property of use dependency, a progressive decrease in impulse conduction velocity at faster heart rates. As a result, these drugs can cause rate-related aberration and a wide QRS complex during any tachyarrhythmia. Digoxin can cause almost any cardiac arrhythmia, especially with increasing plasma digoxin concentrations above 2.0 ng/mL (2.6 mmol/L). Digoxin-induced arrhythmias are more frequent at any given plasma concentration if hypokalemia is also present. The most common digoxin-induced arrhythmias include monomorphic VT (often with a relatively narrow QRS complex), bidirectional VT (a regular alternation of two wide QRS morphologies, each with a different axis), and nonparoxysmal junctional tachycardia.[2]

Physical Examination

Most of the elements of the physical examination, including the blood pressure and heart rate, are of importance primarily in determining how severe the patient's hemodynamic instability is and thus how urgently a therapeutic intervention is required. In patients with significant hemodynamic compromise, a thorough diagnostic evaluation should be postponed until acute management has been addressed. In this setting, emergency cardioversion is the treatment of choice and does not require knowledge of the mechanism of the arrhythmia.

Evidence of underlying cardiovascular disease should be sought, including the sequelae of peripheral vascular disease or stroke. A healed sternal incision is obvious evidence of previous cardiothoracic surgery. A pacemaker or defibrillator, if present, can typically be palpated in the left or, less commonly, right pectoral area below the clavicle, although some older devices are found in the anterior abdominal wall.

An important objective of the physical examination in the stable patient is to attempt to document the presence of atrioventricular (AV) dissociation. AV dissociation is present, although not always evident, in approximately 20% to 50% of patients with VT, but it is very rarely seen in SVT. Thus, the presence of AV dissociation strongly suggests VT, although its absence is less helpful. AV dissociation, if present, is typically diagnosed on ECG; however, it can produce a number of characteristic findings on physical examination. Intermittent cannon A waves may be observed on examination of the jugular pulsation in the neck, and they reflect simultaneous atrial and ventricular contraction; contraction of the right atrium (RA) against a closed tricuspid valve produces a transient increase in RA and jugular venous pressure. Cannon A waves must be distinguished from the continuous and regular prominent A waves seen during some SVTs. Such prominent waves result from simultaneous atrial and ventricular contraction occurring with every beat. Additionally, highly inconsistent fluctuations in the blood pressure can occur because of the variability in the degree of left atrial (LA) contribution to LV filling, stroke volume, and cardiac output. Moreover, variability in the occurrence and intensity of heart sounds (especially S_1) can also be observed and is heard more frequently when the rate of the tachycardia is slower.[2]

The response to carotid sinus massage can suggest the cause of the WCT. The heart rate during sinus tachycardia and automatic atrial tachycardia (AT) will gradually slow with carotid sinus massage and then accelerate on release. The ventricular rate during AT and atrial flutter (AFL) can transiently slow with carotid sinus massage because of increased atrioventricular node (AVN) blockade. The arrhythmia itself, however, is unaffected. Atrioventricular reentrant nodal tachycardia (AVRNT) and AVRT will either terminate or remain unaltered with carotid sinus massage. VTs are generally unaffected by carotid sinus massage, although this maneuver may slow the atrial rate and, in some cases, expose AV dissociation. Some VTs, such as idiopathic outflow tract VT, can rarely terminate in response to carotid sinus massage.

TABLE 21-1 Causes of Wide QRS Complex Tachycardia

CAUSE	DESCRIPTION, EXAMPLES
VT	Macroreentrant VT Focal VT
SVT with aberrancy	Functional BBB Preexistent BBB
Preexcited SVT	Antidromic AVRT AT or AVNRT with bystander BT
Antiarrhythmic drugs	Class IA and IC agents, amiodarone
Electrolyte abnormalities	Hyperkalemia
Ventricular pacing	

AT = atrial tachycardia; AVNRT = atrioventricular nodal reentrant tachycardia; AVRT = atrioventricular reentrant tachycardia; BBB = bundle branch block; BT = bypass tract; SVT = supraventricular tachycardia; VT = ventricular tachycardia.

Laboratory Tests

The plasma potassium and magnesium concentrations should be measured as part of the laboratory evaluation. Hypokalemia and hypomagnesemia can predispose to the development of ventricular tachyarrhythmias. Hyperkalemia can cause a wide QRS complex rhythm, usually with a slow rate, with loss of a detectable P wave (the so-called sinoventricular rhythm; Fig. 21-1) or abnormalities of AVN conduction. In patients taking digoxin, quinidine, or procainamide, plasma concentrations of these drugs should be measured to assist in evaluating possible drug toxicity.

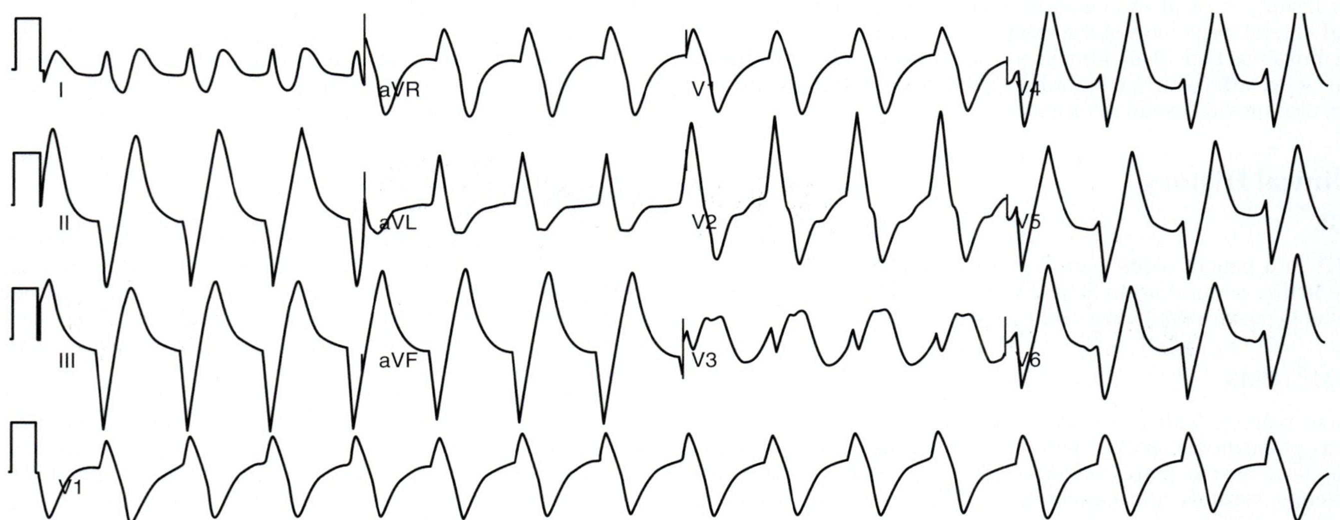

FIGURE 21-1 Wide QRS complex rhythm caused by hyperkalemia. No P waves are visible.

Pharmacological Intervention

The administration of certain drugs can be useful for diagnostic, as opposed to therapeutic, purposes. Termination of the arrhythmia with lidocaine suggests, but does not prove, that VT is the mechanism. Infrequently an SVT, especially AVRT, can terminate with lidocaine. On the other hand, termination of the tachycardia with procainamide or amiodarone does not distinguish between VT and SVT. Termination of the arrhythmia with digoxin, verapamil, diltiazem, or adenosine strongly implies SVT. However, VT can also occasionally terminate after the administration of these drugs.

Unless the cause for the WCT is definitely established, however, verapamil, diltiazem, and probably adenosine should not be administered, because they have been reported to cause severe hemodynamic deterioration in patients with VT and can even provoke ventricular fibrillation (VF) and cardiac arrest. Direct current (DC) cardioversion in unstable patients and intravenous procainamide or amiodarone in hemodynamically stable patients are the appropriate management approach.[2]

Electrocardiographic Features

Ventricular Tachycardia Versus Aberrantly Conducted Supraventricular Tachycardia

Because the diagnosis of a WCT cannot always be made with complete certainty, the unknown rhythm should be presumed to be VT in the absence of contrary evidence. This conclusion is appropriate both because VT accounts for up to 80% of cases of WCT, and because making this assumption guards against inappropriate and potentially dangerous therapy. As noted, the intravenous administration of drugs used for the treatment of SVT (verapamil, adenosine, or beta blockers) can cause severe hemodynamic deterioration in patients with VT and can even provoke VF and cardiac arrest. Therefore, these drugs should not be used when the diagnosis is uncertain.

In general, most WCTs can be classified as having one of two patterns: a right bundle branch block (RBBB)–like pattern (QRS polarity is predominantly positive in leads V_1 and V_2) or a left bundle branch block (LBBB)–like pattern (QRS polarity is predominantly negative in leads V_1 and V_2). The determination that the WCT has an RBBB-like pattern or an LBBB-like pattern does not, by itself, assist in making a diagnosis; however, this assessment should be made initially because it is useful in evaluating several other features on the ECG, including the QRS axis, the QRS duration, and the QRS morphology (Table 21-2).

RATE

The rate of the WCT is of limited value in distinguishing VT from SVT because there is wide overlap in the distribution of heart rates for SVT and VT. When the rate is around 150 beats/min, AFL with 2:1 AV conduction and aberrancy should be considered.

REGULARITY

Regularity of the WCT is not helpful in distinguishing VT from SVT because both are regular. However, VT is often associated with slight irregularity of the RR intervals, QRS morphology, and ST-T waves. Although marked irregularity strongly suggests atrial fibrillation (AF), VTs can be particularly irregular within the first 30 seconds of onset and in patients treated with antiarrhythmic drugs.

QRS DURATION

In general, a wider QRS duration favors VT. In the setting of RBBB-like WCT, a QRS duration more than 140 milliseconds suggests VT, whereas for LBBB-like WCT, a QRS duration more than 160 milliseconds suggests VT. In an analysis of several studies, a QRS duration more than 160 milliseconds overall was a strong predictor of VT (likelihood ratio > 20:1). On the other hand, a QRS duration less than 140 milliseconds is not helpful for excluding VT, because VT can sometimes be associated with a relatively narrow QRS complex.

A QRS duration more than 160 milliseconds is not helpful in identifying VT in several settings, including preexisting bundle branch block (BBB), although it is uncommon for the QRS to be wider than 160 milliseconds in this situation, preexcited SVT, and the presence of drugs capable of slowing intraventricular conduction (e.g., class IA and IC drugs). Of note, a QRS complex that is narrower during WCT than during normal sinus rhythm (NSR) suggests VT. However, this is rare, occurring in less than 1% of VTs.[2]

Rarely (4% in one series), VT can have a relatively narrow QRS duration (<120 to 140 milliseconds). This can be observed in VTs of septal origin or those with early penetration into the His-Purkinje system (HPS), as occurs with fascicular (verapamil-sensitive) VT.

A recent report found that the QRS onset-to-peak time (also termed "R wave peak time" or "intrinsicoid deflection") in lead II (measured from the beginning of the QRS to the first change of the polarity, independent of whether the QRS deflection is positive or negative) was significantly wider in VT compared with SVT with aberrancy, and a cutoff value of 50 milliseconds or greater identified VT with high sensitivity, specificity, and positive predictive values (93%, 99%, and 98%, respectively). However, this criterion has not been tested prospectively or validated in patients with preexisting conduction system disease, antiarrhythmic drug therapy, electrolyte imbalance, prior MI, and preexcited tachycardias. Additionally, certain types of VTs such as fascicular VT, bundle branch reentrant (BBR) VT, and septal myocardial VT, can have a shorter QRS onset-to-peak time because of their origin within or in close proximity to the His-Purkinje network.[1,3]

TABLE 21-2 Electrocardiographic Criteria Favoring Ventricular Tachycardia

AV Relationship

- Dissociated P waves
- Fusion beats
- Capture beats
- A/V ratio <1

QRS Duration

- >160 msec with LBBB pattern
- >140 msec with RBBB pattern
- QRS during WCT is narrower than in NSR
- Onset QRS to peak (+ or −) in lead II >50 msec

QRS Axis

- Axis shift of >40 degrees between NSR and WCT
- Right superior (northwest) axis
- Left axis deviation with RBBB morphology
- Right axis deviation with LBBB morphology

Precordial QRS Concordance

- Positive concordance
- Negative concordance

QRS Morphology in RBBB Pattern WCT

- Monophasic R, biphasic qR complex, or broad R (>40 msec) in lead V_1
- Rabbit ear sign: Double-peaked R wave in lead V_1 with the left peak taller than the right peak
- rS complex in lead V_6
- Contralateral BBB in WCT and NSR

QRS Morphology in LBBB Pattern WCT

- Broad initial R wave of ≥40 msec in lead V_1 or V_2
- R wave in lead V_1 during WCT taller than the R wave during NSR
- Slow descent to the nadir of the S, notching in the downstroke of the S wave in lead V_1
- RS interval >70 msec in lead V_1 or V_2
- Q or QS wave in lead V_6

AV = atrioventricular; BBB = bundle branch block; LBBB = left bundle branch block; NSR = normal sinus rhythm; RBBB = right bundle branch block; WCT = wide complex tachycardia.

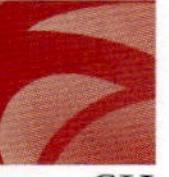

QRS AXIS

Generally, the more leftward the axis, the greater the likelihood of VT. A significant axis shift (>40 degrees) between the baseline NSR and WCT is suggestive of VT (Fig. 21-2A). A right superior ("northwest") axis (axis from −90 degrees to ±180 degrees) is rare in SVT and strongly suggests VT (see Fig. 21-2B).[2]

In a patient with an RBBB-like WCT, a QRS axis to the left of −30 degrees suggests VT (see Fig. 21-2A) and, in a patient with an LBBB-like WCT, a QRS axis to the right of +90 degrees suggests VT. Additionally, RBBB with a normal axis is uncommon in VT (<3%) and is suggestive of SVT.

PRECORDIAL QRS CONCORDANCE

Concordance is present when the QRS complexes in the six precordial leads (V_1 through V_6) are either all positive in polarity (tall R waves) or all negative in polarity (deep QS complexes). Negative concordance is strongly suggestive of VT (see Fig. 21-2D). Rarely, SVT with LBBB aberrancy will demonstrate negative concordance, but there is almost always some evidence of an R wave in the lateral precordial leads. Positive concordance is most often caused by VT (see Fig. 21-2A); however, this pattern may also be caused by preexcited SVT using a left posterior BT. Although the presence of precordial QRS concordance strongly suggests VT (>90% specificity), its absence is not helpful diagnostically (approximately 20% sensitivity).

ATRIOVENTRICULAR DISSOCIATION

AV dissociation is characterized by atrial activity (P waves) that is completely independent of ventricular activity (QRS complexes). The atrial rate is usually slower than the ventricular rate. Detection of AV dissociation is obviously impossible if AF is the underlying supraventricular rhythm.

AV dissociation is the hallmark of VT (specificity is almost 100%). However, although the presence of AV dissociation establishes VT as the cause, its absence is not as helpful (sensitivity is 20% to 50%). AV dissociation can be present but not obvious on the surface ECG because of a rapid ventricular rate. Additionally, AV dissociation is absent in a large subset of VTs; in fact, approximately 30% of VTs have 1:1 retrograde ventriculoatrial (VA) conduction (see Fig. 21-2D) and an additional 15% to 20% have second-degree (2:1 or Wenckebach) VA block (Fig. 21-3).[2]

Several ECG findings are helpful in establishing the presence of AV dissociation, including the presence of dissociated P waves, fusion beats, or capture beats.

DISSOCIATED P WAVES. When the P waves can be clearly seen and the atrial rate is unrelated to and slower than the ventricular rate, AV dissociation consistent with VT is present (Fig. 21-4). An atrial rate faster than the ventricular rate is more often seen with SVT having AV conduction block. However, during a WCT, the P waves are often difficult to identify; they can be superimposed on the ST segment or T wave (resulting in altered morphology). Sometimes, the T waves and initial or terminal QRS portions can

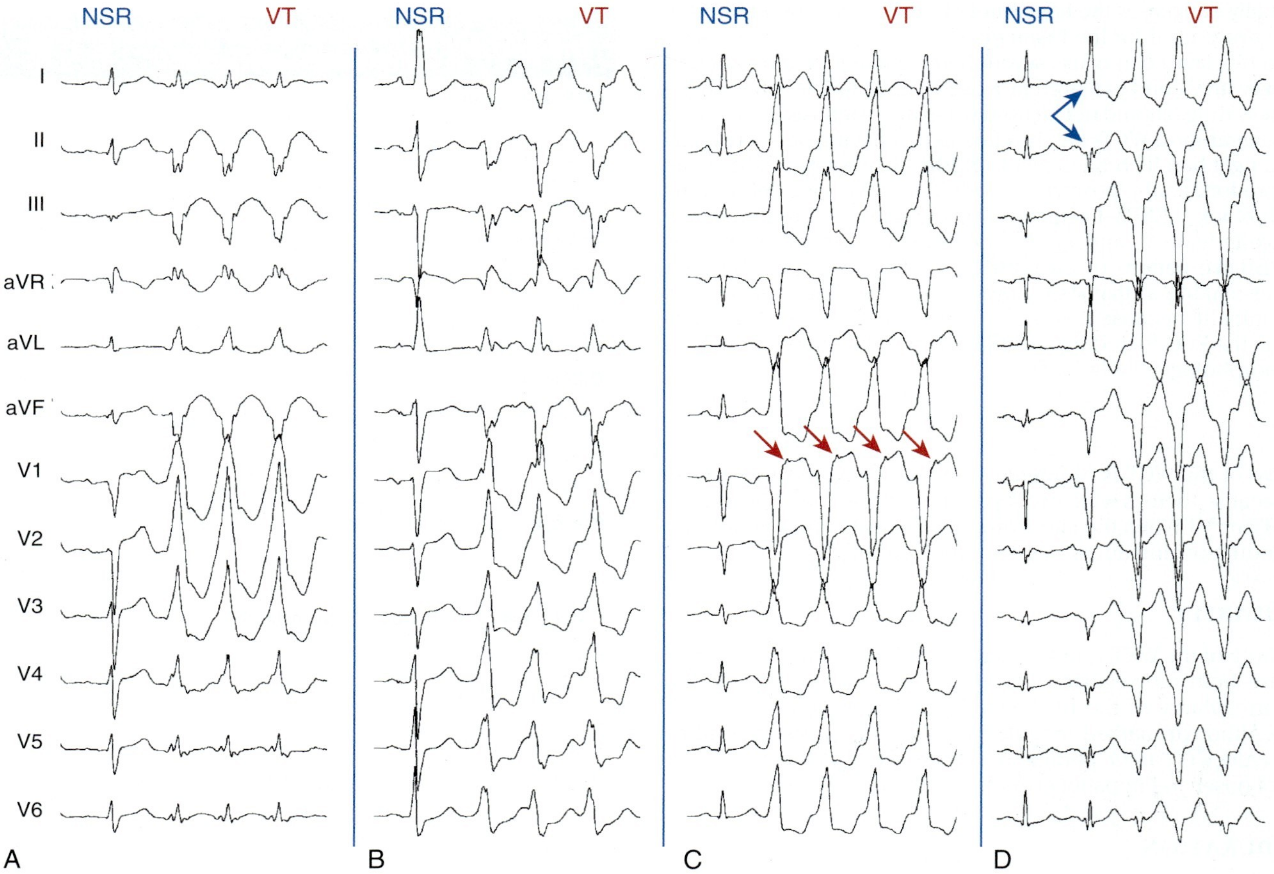

FIGURE 21-2 Surface ECG of four different patients illustrating ECG morphology during normal sinus rhythm (NSR) versus ventricular tachycardia (VT). **A,** VT with right bundle branch block (RBBB) pattern, positive concordance, and long RS interval. Note the monophasic R in lead V_1 during VT and the significant shift in the frontal plane axis in VT versus NSR. **B,** VT with an RBBB pattern and long RS interval. Note the superior ("northwest") frontal plane axis during VT. **C,** VT with a left bundle branch block (LBBB) pattern, long RS interval, and 1:1 ventriculoatrial conduction. Retrograde P waves (red arrows) are visible following the QRSs during VT. **D,** VT with LBBB pattern and negative concordance. Note that the second QRS (blue arrows) is a fusion between the sinus beat and the VT beat.

resemble atrial activity. Furthermore, artifacts can be mistaken for P waves. If the P waves are not obvious or suggested on the ECG, several alternative leads or modalities can help in their identification, including a modified chest lead placement (Lewis leads), an esophageal lead (using an electrode wire or nasogastric tube), a right atrial recording (obtained by an electrode catheter in the RA), carotid sinus pressure (to slow VA conduction and therefore change the atrial rate in the case of VT), or invasive electrophysiological (EP) testing.

FUSION BEATS. Ventricular fusion occurs when a ventricular ectopic beat and a supraventricular beat (conducted via the AVN and HPS) simultaneously activate the ventricular myocardium. The resulting QRS complex has a morphology intermediate between the appearance of a sinus QRS complex and that of a purely ventricular complex. Intermittent fusion beats during a WCT are diagnostic of AV dissociation and therefore of VT (see Fig. 21-4). It is also possible for premature ventricular complexes (PVCs) during SVT with aberration to produce fusion beats, which would erroneously be interpreted as evidence of AV dissociation and VT.

DRESSLER BEATS. A Dressler beat (capture beat) is a normal QRS complex identical to the sinus QRS complex, occurring during the VT at a rate *faster* than the VT. The term *capture beat* indicates that the normal conduction system has momentarily captured control of ventricular activation from the VT focus (see Fig. 21-4). Fusion and capture beats are more commonly seen when the tachycardia rate is slower. These beats do not alter the rate of the VT, although a change in the preceding and subsequent RR intervals may be observed.

QRS MORPHOLOGY

As a rule, if the WCT is caused by SVT with aberration, then the QRS complex during the WCT must be compatible with some form of BBB that could result in that QRS configuration. If there is no combination of bundle branch or fascicular blocks that could result in such a QRS configuration, then the diagnosis by default is VT or preexcited SVT.

As noted, WCTs can be classified as having an RBBB-like pattern or an LBBB-like pattern. Certain features of the QRS complex have been described that favor VT in RBBB-like or LBBB-like WCTs (Fig. 21-5).[2]

In the patient with a WCT and positive QRS polarity in lead V_1 (RBBB pattern), a monophasic R, biphasic qR complex, or broad R (>40 milliseconds) in lead V_1 favors VT (Fig. 21-6), whereas a triphasic RSR′, rSr′, rR′, or rSR′ complex in lead V_1 favors SVT (where the capital letter indicates large-wave amplitude, duration, or both; and the lowercase letter indicates small-wave amplitude, duration, or both; see Fig. 21-5). Additionally, a double-peaked R wave in lead V_1 favors VT if the left peak is taller than the right peak (the so-called rabbit ear sign; likelihood ratio > 50:1). A taller right rabbit ear does not help in distinguishing SVT from VT. On the other hand, an rS complex in lead V_6 is a strong predictor of VT (likelihood ratio > 50:1), whereas an Rs complex in lead V_6 favors SVT (see Fig. 21-6).

In the patient with a WCT and a negative QRS polarity in lead V_1 (LBBB pattern), a broad initial R wave of 40 milliseconds or more in lead V_1 or V_2 favors VT, whereas the absence of an initial R wave (or a small initial R wave of < 40 milliseconds) in lead V_1 or V_2

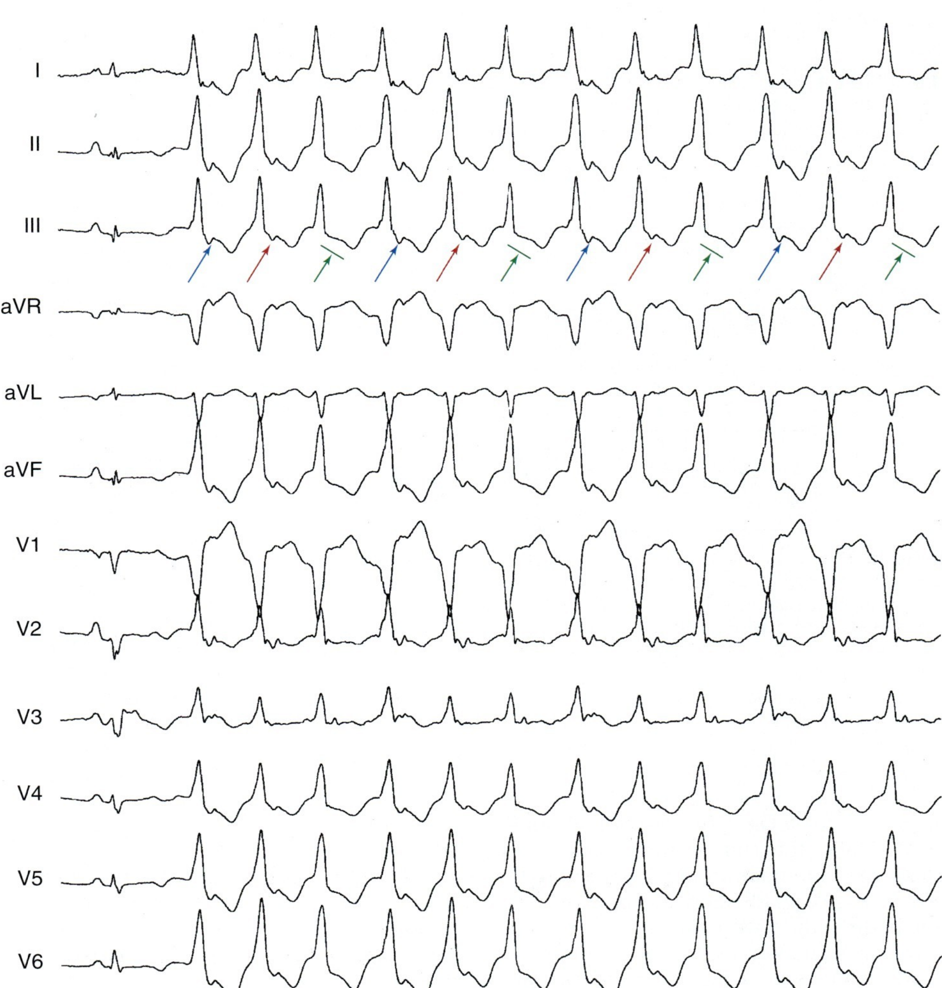

FIGURE 21-3 Ventricular tachycardia (VT) with type 1 second-degree (Wenckebach) ventriculoatrial (VA) block. The first beat is sinus with normal atrioventricular (AV) conduction. VT develops with an initially short VA interval (blue arrows), which then slightly prolongs (red arrows), and then VA block occurs (green arrows). Note that the VT has a right bundle branch block with long RS interval (in lead V_2).

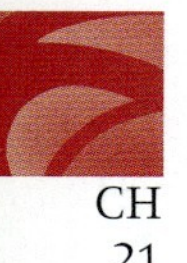

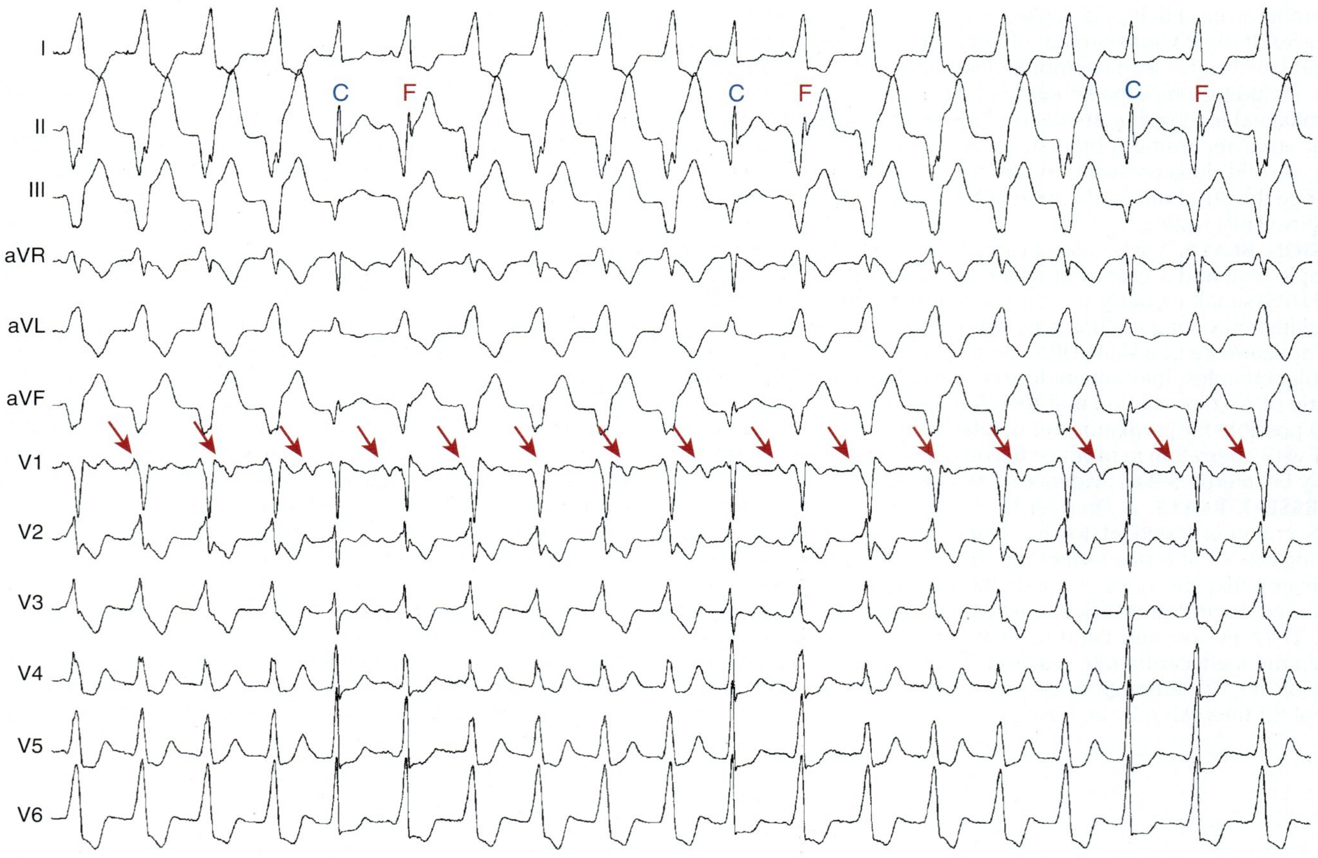

FIGURE 21-4 Ventricular tachycardia (VT) with atrioventricular (AV) dissociation. Sustained monomorphic VT with a cycle length (CL) of 488 milliseconds with AV dissociation coexists with sinus rhythm with a CL of 616 milliseconds. The sinus P waves can be clearly seen (arrows) marching throughout the different phases of the VT QRS complexes, and the atrial rate is unrelated to and slower than the ventricular rate. Because of the relatively slow VT rate, capture (C) and fusion (F) beats are observed frequently.

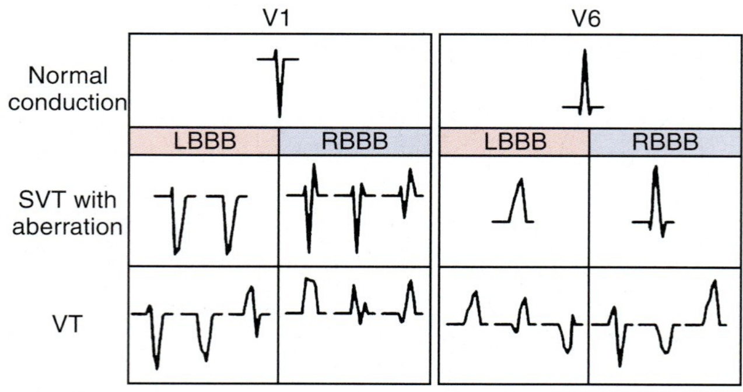

FIGURE 21-5 Diagrammatic representation of common QRS morphologies encountered in ventricular tachycardia (VT) and supraventricular tachycardia (SVT) with aberration in leads V_1 and V_6 for both left bundle branch block (LBBB) and right bundle branch block (RBBB) patterns. Note the initial portions of the QRS complex in normal and aberrant QRS complexes, contrasted with the initial QRS forces in VT complexes. The RS configurations can be designated as an RBBB or LBBB type (grouped with LBBB-type morphologies). *(From Miller JM, Das MK, Arora R, Alberte-Lista C: Differential diagnosis of wide QRS complex tachycardia. In Zipes DP, Jalife J, editors: Cardiac electrophysiology: from cell to bedside, ed 4, Philadelphia, 2004, WB Saunders, pp 747-757.)*

favors SVT (see Fig. 21-6). Additionally, an R wave in lead V_1 during a WCT taller than that during NSR favors VT. Furthermore, a slow descent to the nadir of the S wave, notching in the downstroke of the S wave, or an RS interval (from the onset of the QRS complex to the nadir of the S wave) of more than 70 milliseconds in lead V_1 or V_2 favors VT. In contrast, a swift, smooth downstroke of the S wave in lead V_1 or V_2 with an RS interval of less than 70 milliseconds favors SVT. In an analysis of several studies, the presence of any of these three criteria in lead V_1 (broad R wave, slurred or notched downstroke of the S wave, and delayed nadir of S wave) was a strong predictor of VT (likelihood ratio > 50:1). The QRS morphology in lead V_6 is also of value; the presence of any Q or QS wave in lead V_6 favors VT (likelihood ratio > 50:1; see Fig. 21-2D), whereas the absence of a Q wave in lead V_6 favors SVT.

When an old 12-lead surface ECG is available, comparison of the QRS morphology during NSR and WCT is helpful. Contralateral BBB in WCT and NSR strongly favors VT (see Fig. 21-6C and D). It is important to note that identical QRS morphology during NSR and WCT, although strongly suggestive of SVT, can also occur in bundle branch reentrant (BBR) and interfascicular reentrant VTs.

Unfortunately, the value of QRS morphological criteria in the diagnosis of a WCT is subject to several limitations. Most of the associations between the QRS morphology and tachycardia origin are based on statistical correlations, with substantial overlap. Moreover, most of the morphological criteria favoring VT are also present in a substantial number of patients with intraventricular conduction delay present during sinus rhythm, limiting their applicability in these cases. Additionally, morphological criteria tend to misclassify SVTs with preexcitation as VT. However, preexcitation is an uncommon cause of WCT (1% to 6% in most series), particularly if other factors (e.g., age, history) suggest another diagnosis.

VARIATION IN QRS AND ST-T MORPHOLOGY

Subtle, non–rate-related fluctuations or variations in the QRS and ST-T wave configuration suggest VT and reflect variations in the VT reentrant circuit within the myocardium. In contrast, because most SVTs follow fixed conduction pathways, they are generally characterized by complete uniformity of QRS and ST-T shape, unless the tachycardia rate changes.

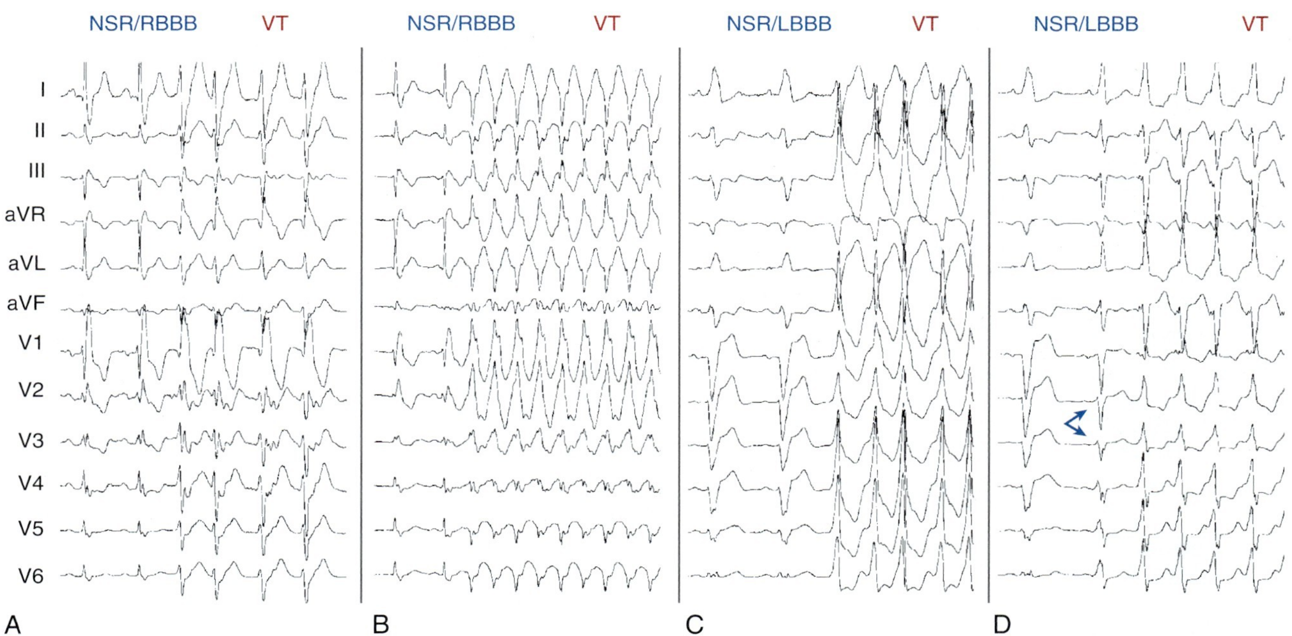

FIGURE 21-6 Surface ECG of four different patients illustrating ECG morphology during normal sinus rhythm (NSR) with bundle branch block (BBB) versus ventricular tachycardia (VT). **A,** NSR with right bundle branch block (RBBB) and VT with RBBB pattern. Note the loss of the initial r wave in V_1 and the larger S wave in V_6 during VT compared with NSR with RBBB. Additionally, note the shift in the frontal plane QRS axis from +90 degrees during NSR with RBBB to the northwest quadrant during VT. **B,** NSR with RBBB and VT with RBBB pattern. Note the change in QRS morphology in lead V_1 (from rsR during NSR with RBBB to monophasic R during VT) and lead V_6 (from RS during NSR with RBBB to QS during VT). Additionally, no RS complexes are observed in the precordial leads during VT. **C,** NSR with LBBB and VT with RBBB pattern. Note the positive precordial concordance during VT. **D,** NSR with LBBB and VT with RBBB pattern. Note the positive precordial concordance during VT. The second QRS (blue arrows) is a fusion between the sinus beat and the VT beat, and the fusion QRS is narrower than both the sinus and VT complexes.

Algorithms for the ECG Diagnosis of Wide Complex Tachycardia

The various criteria for the diagnosis of WCT listed are difficult to apply in isolation, because most patients will have some, but not all, of the features described. Several algorithms have been proposed to guide integrating ECG findings into a diagnostic strategy. Figure 21-7 illustrates an example of one approach. The effect of history of prior MI, preexcited tachycardias, antiarrhythmic medication usage, precordial lead placement, heart transplantation status, and the presence of congenital heart disease on QRS morphology criteria should be taken into account while applying these elements. Preexcited tachycardias may not be differentiated consistently with the proposed criteria, especially those using epicardial left-sided paraseptal or left-sided inferoposterior BTs.

ALGORITHM 1

The most commonly used algorithm is the so-called Brugada algorithm or Brugada criteria. The Brugada algorithm consists of four steps (Fig. 21-8). First, all precordial leads are inspected to detect the presence or absence of an RS complex (with R and S waves of any amplitude). If an RS complex cannot be identified in any precordial lead, the diagnosis of VT can be made with 100% specificity. Second, if an RS complex is clearly identified in one or more precordial leads, the interval between the onset of the R wave and the nadir of the S wave (the RS interval) is measured. The longest RS interval is considered if RS complexes are present in multiple precordial leads. If the longest RS interval is more than 100 milliseconds, the diagnosis of VT can be made with a specificity of 98% (see Fig. 21-8). Third, if the longest RS interval is less than 100 milliseconds, either VT or SVT still is possible and the presence or absence of AV dissociation must therefore be determined. Evidence of AV dissociation is 100% specific for the diagnosis of VT, but this finding has a low sensitivity. Fourth, if the RS interval is less than 100 milliseconds and AV dissociation cannot clearly be demonstrated, the QRS morphology criteria for V_1-positive and V_1-negative WCTs are considered. The QRS morphology criteria consistent with VT must be present in lead V_1 or V_2 and in lead V_6 to diagnose VT. A supraventricular origin of the tachycardia is assumed if either the V_1 and V_2 or V_6 criteria are not consistent with VT.

The Brugada algorithm was originally prospectively applied to 554 patients with electrophysiologically diagnosed WCTs. The reported sensitivity and specificity were 98.7% and 96.5%, respectively. Other authors also found the Brugada criteria useful, although they reported a lower sensitivity (79% to 92%) and specificity (43% to 70%).

ALGORITHM 2

A newer algorithm for differential diagnosis of WCT was analyzed in 453 monomorphic WCTs recorded from 287 patients, based on the following: (1) the presence of AV dissociation; (2) the presence of an initial R wave in lead aVR; (3) QRS morphology; and (4) estimation of the initial (V_i) and terminal (V_t) ventricular activation velocity ratio (V_i/V_t), determined by measuring the voltage change on the ECG tracing during the initial 40 milliseconds (V_i) and the terminal 40 milliseconds (V_t) of the same biphasic or multiphasic QRS complex (Fig. 21-9).[4,5]

This algorithm had superior overall total accuracy than that of the Brugada algorithm (90.3% versus 84.8%). The total accuracy of the fourth Brugada criterion was significantly lower (68% versus 82.2%) than that of the V_i/V_t criterion in the fourth step, accounting for most of the difference in outcome between the two methods.

The rationale proposed for the V_i/V_t criterion is that during WCT caused by SVT, the initial activation of the septum should be invariably rapid and the intraventricular conduction delay causing the wide QRS complex occurs in the mid to terminal part of the QRS. In contrast, in WCT caused by VT, there is initial slower muscle-to-muscle spread of activation until the impulse reaches the HPS, after which the rest of the ventricular muscle is more rapidly activated.

Antiarrhythmic drugs that impair conduction in the HPS, ventricular myocardium, or both (e.g., class I drugs and amiodarone) would be expected to decrease the V_i and V_t approximately to

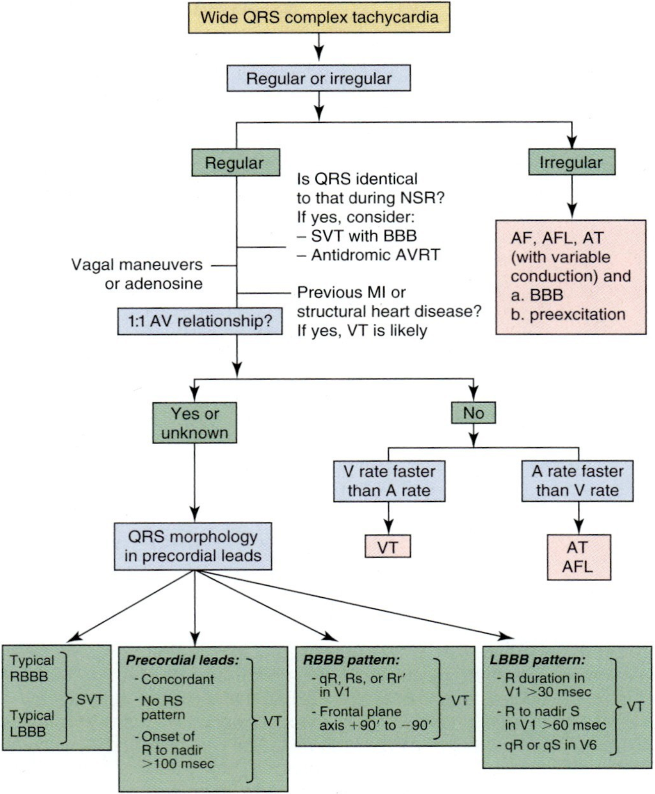

FIGURE 21-7 Differential diagnosis for wide QRS complex tachycardia. A = atrial; AF = atrial fibrillation; AFL = atrial flutter; AT = atrial tachycardia; AV = atrioventricular; AVRT = atrioventricular reentrant tachycardia; BBB = bundle branch block; LBBB = left bundle branch block; MI = myocardial infarction; NSR = normal sinus rhythm; RBBB = right bundle branch block; SVT = supraventricular tachycardia; V = ventricular; VT = ventricular tachycardia. *(From Blomström-Lundqvist C, Scheinman MM, Aliot EM, et al: American College of Cardiology; American Heart Association Task Force on Practice Guidelines; European Society of Cardiology Committee for Practice Guidelines [Writing Committee to Develop Guidelines for the Management of Patients with Supraventricular Arrhythmias]: ACC/AHA/ESC guidelines for the management of patients with supraventricular arrhythmias—executive summary: a report of the American College of Cardiology/American Heart Association Task Force on Practice Guidelines and the European Society of Cardiology Committee for Practice Guidelines [Writing Committee to Develop Guidelines for the Management of Patients with Supraventricular Arrhythmias], Circulation 108: 1871, 2003.)*

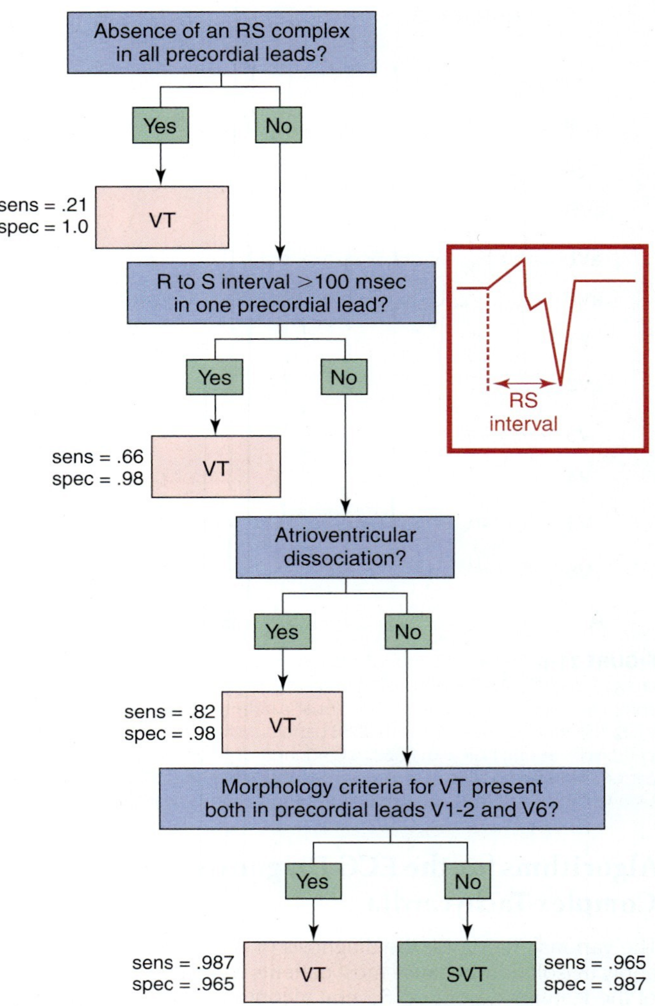

FIGURE 21-8 Brugada algorithm for distinguishing ventricular tachycardia (VT) from supraventricular tachycardia (SVT). As indicated in the inset, the RS interval is between the onset of the R wave and the nadir of the S wave. sens = sensitivity; spec = specificity. *(From Brugada P, Brugada J, Mont L, et al: A new approach to the differential diagnosis of a regular tachycardia with a wide QRS complex, Circulation 83:1649, 1991.)*

the same degree; therefore, the V_i/V_t ratio should not change significantly. Although the V_i/V_t ratio reflects the electrophysiology of many VTs, there are a number of exceptions to these criteria. First, disorders involving the myocardium locally can alter the V_i or V_t. For example, a decreased V_i with unchanged V_t can be present in the case of an SVT occurring in the presence of an anteroseptal MI, leading to the misdiagnosis of VT. Similarly, a scar situated at a late activated ventricular site can result in a decreased V_t in the presence of VT, leading to the misdiagnosis of SVT. Second, in the case of a fascicular VT, the V_i is not slower than the V_t. Third, if the exit site of the VT reentry circuit is very close to the HPS, it might result in a relatively narrow QRS complex and the slowing of the V_i can last for such a short time that it cannot be detected by the surface ECG.

ALGORITHM 3

The positive aVR criterion in algorithm 2 suggesting VT was further tested in 483 WCTs in 313 patients, and another algorithm based solely on QRS morphology in lead aVR was developed for distinguishing VT from SVT (Fig. 21-10).[6] The new aVR algorithm is based solely on the principle of differences in the direction and velocity of the initial and terminal ventricular activation during WCT caused by VT and SVT. During SVT with BBB, both the initial rapid septal activation, which can be either left to right or right to left, and the later main ventricular activation wavefront proceed in a direction away from lead aVR, yielding a negative QRS complex in lead aVR. An exception to this generalization occurs in the presence of an inferior MI; an initial r wave (Rs complex) may be seen in lead aVR during NSR or SVT because of the loss of initial inferiorly directed forces. An rS complex also may be present as a normal variant in lead aVR, but with an R/S ratio less than 1. With these considerations, an initial dominant R wave should not be present in SVT with BBB, and its presence suggests VT, typically arising from the inferior or apical region of the ventricles.

Furthermore, VTs originating from sites other than the inferior or apical wall of the ventricles, but not showing an initial R wave in aVR, should yield a slow, initially upward vector component of variable size pointing toward lead aVR (absent in SVT), even if the main vector in these VTs points downward, yielding a totally or predominantly negative QRS in lead aVR. Thus, in VT without an initial R wave in lead aVR, the initial part of the QRS in lead aVR should be less steep because of the slower initial ventricular activation having an initially upward vector component, which may be manifested as an initial r or q wave with a width more than 40 milliseconds, a notch on the downstroke of the QRS, or a slower ventricular activation during the initial 40 milliseconds

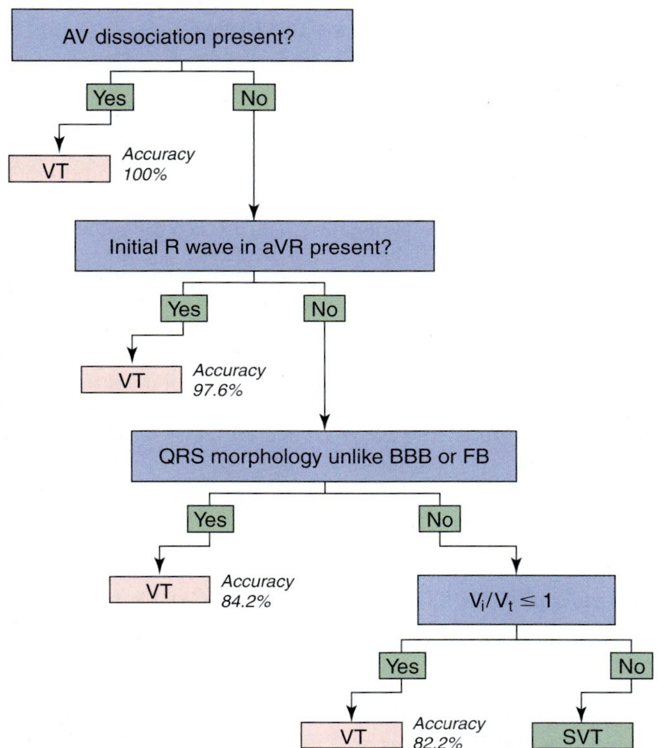

FIGURE 21-9 Stepwise algorithm for distinguishing ventricular tachycardia (VT) from supraventricular tachycardia (SVT). AV = atrioventricular; BBB = bundle branch block; FB = fascicular block; V_i/V_t = ratio of initial (V_i) to terminal (V_t) ventricular activation velocity. *(From Vereckei A, Duray G, Szénási G, et al: Application of a new algorithm in the differential diagnosis of wide QRS complex tachycardia, Eur Heart J 28:589, 2007.)*

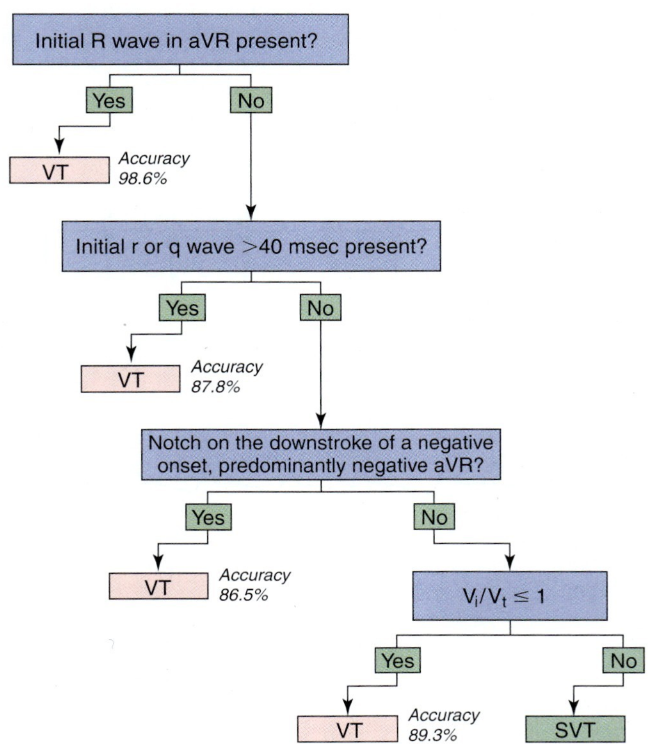

FIGURE 21-10 New algorithm using only lead aVR for differential diagnosis of wide QRS complex tachycardia. SVT = supraventricular tachycardia; V_i/V_t = ratio of initial (V_i) to terminal (V_t) ventricular activation velocity; VT = ventricular tachycardia. *(From Vereckei A, Duray G, Szénási G, et al: New algorithm using only lead aVR for differential diagnosis of wide QRS complex tachycardia, Heart Rhythm 5:89, 2008.)*

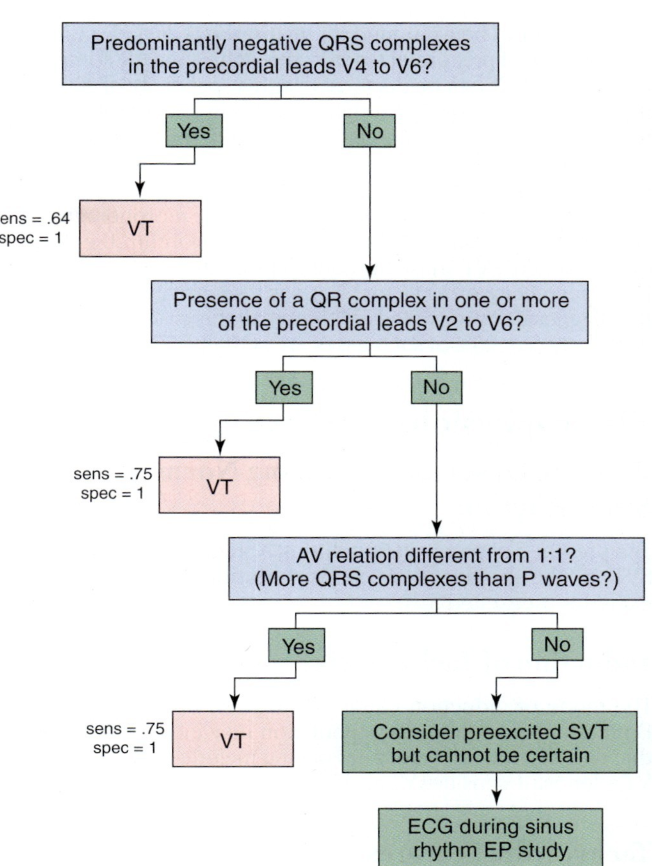

FIGURE 21-11 Brugada algorithm for distinguishing ventricular tachycardia (VT) from preexcited supraventricular tachycardia (SVT). AV = atrioventricular; EP = electrophysiology; sens = sensitivity; spec = specificity. *(From Antunes E, Brugada J, Steurer G, et al: The differential diagnosis of a regular tachycardia with a wide QRS complex on the 12-lead ECG, Pacing Clin Electrophysiol17,1515-1524, 1994.)*

than during the terminal 40 milliseconds of the QRS ($V_i/V_t \leq 1$) in lead aVR. In contrast, in SVT with BBB, the initial part of the QRS in lead aVR is steeper (fast) because of the invariably rapid septal activation going away from lead aVR, resulting in a narrow (≤40 milliseconds) initial r or q wave and V_i/V_t more than 1.[6]

The overall accuracy of the aVR algorithm was 91.5%, which is similar to algorithm 2 and superior to the Brugada algorithm (90.3% and 84.8%, respectively). The inability of the aVR algorithm to differentiate preexcited tachycardias from VTs, with the possible exception of the presence of an initial R wave in lead aVR, is a limitation of the algorithm.[6]

Ventricular Tachycardia Versus Preexcited Supraventricular Tachycardia

Differentiation between VT and preexcited SVT is particularly difficult, because ventricular activation begins outside the normal intraventricular conduction system in both tachycardias (see Fig. 12-6). As a result, algorithms for WCT, like QRS morphology criteria, tend to misclassify SVTs with preexcitation as VT. However, preexcitation is an uncommon cause of WCT, particularly if other factors, such as age and past medical history, suggest another diagnosis. For cases in which preexcitation is thought to be likely, such as a young patient without structural heart disease, or a patient with a known BT, a separate algorithm has been developed by Brugada and colleagues (Fig. 21-11). This algorithm consists of three steps. First, the predominant polarity of the QRS complex in leads V_4 through V_6 is defined as positive or negative. If predominantly negative, the diagnosis of VT can be made with 100% specificity. Second, if the polarity of the QRS complex is predominantly positive in V_4 through V_6, the ECG should be examined for the presence of a qR complex in one or more of precordial leads V_2 through V_6. If a qR complex can be identified, VT can be diagnosed with a specificity of 100%. Third, if a qR wave in leads V_2 through V_6 is absent, the AV relationship is then evaluated. If a 1:1 AV relationship is not present and there are more QRS complexes present than P waves, VT can be diagnosed with a specificity of 100%.

If the ECG of the WCT does not display any morphological characteristics diagnostic of VT after using this algorithm, the diagnosis of preexcited SVT must be considered. Although this algorithm has a specificity of 100% for VT, it has a sensitivity of only 75% for the diagnosis of preexcited SVT when all three steps are answered negatively (i.e., 25% of such cases are actually VT).

Electrophysiological Testing

Baseline Observations during Normal Sinus Rhythm

The presence of preexcitation during NSR or atrial pacing suggests SVT, and the absence of preexcitation during NSR and atrial pacing excludes preexcited SVT.

Induction of Tachycardia

The mode of induction cannot distinguish between SVT and VT. Both atrial and ventricular stimulation may induce SVT or VT. VTs that can be induced with atrial pacing include verapamil-sensitive VT, adenosine-sensitive VT, and BBR VT.[7]

Tachycardia Features

QRS MORPHOLOGY

As noted, when the QRS configuration of the WCT is not compatible with any known form of aberration, the rhythm is likely to be VT or preexcited SVT. QRS morphology during WCT that is identical to that during NSR may occur in SVT with BBB, preexcited SVT (when NSR is also fully preexcited), BBR VT, and interfascicular VT.

HIS BUNDLE–VENTRICULAR INTERVAL

When the His bundle–ventricular (HV) interval is positive (i.e., the His potential precedes the QRS onset), an HV interval during the WCT shorter than that during NSR ($HV_{WCT} < HV_{NSR}$) indicates VT or preexcited SVT. In contrast, an HV_{WCT} equal to or longer than HV_{NSR} indicates SVT with aberrancy, BBR VT, or (rarely) other VTs (see Figs. 18-24 and 26-3).[7,8]

When the HV interval is negative (i.e., the His potential follows the QRS onset), BBR VT and SVT with aberrancy are excluded. However, myocardial VTs and preexcited SVT generally have negative HV intervals (see Figs. 18-3 and 22-10).

Prolongation of the VA (and VH) interval and tachycardia cycle length (CL) with transient RBBB (caused by catheter-induced trauma or introduction of a ventricular extrastimulus [VES]) is diagnostic of antidromic AVRT using a right-sided BT and excludes preexcited AVNRT, but can theoretically occur in VT originating in the right ventricle (RV; with LBBB-like morphology). However, continuation of the WCT after development of RBBB excludes BBR VT except for the rare case of intrafascicular reentry.

OSCILLATION IN THE TACHYCARDIA CYCLE LENGTH

Variations in the tachycardia CL (the V-V intervals) that are dictated and preceded by similar variations in the A-A or H-H intervals are suggestive of SVT with aberrancy or BBR VT (Fig. 21-12). In contrast, variations in the V-V intervals that predict the subsequent H-H interval changes are consistent with myocardial VT or preexcited SVT.

HIS BUNDLE–RIGHT BUNDLE BRANCH POTENTIAL SEQUENCE

When both the HB and right bundle branch (RB) potentials are recorded, an HB-RB-V activation sequence occurs in SVT with aberrancy and BBR VT with an LBBB pattern. In either case, the HB-RB interval during WCT is equal to or longer than that in NSR. On the other hand, an RB-HB-V activation sequence occurs in antidromic AVRT using an atriofascicular or right-sided BT, the uncommon type of BBR VT with RBBB pattern, or myocardial VT originating

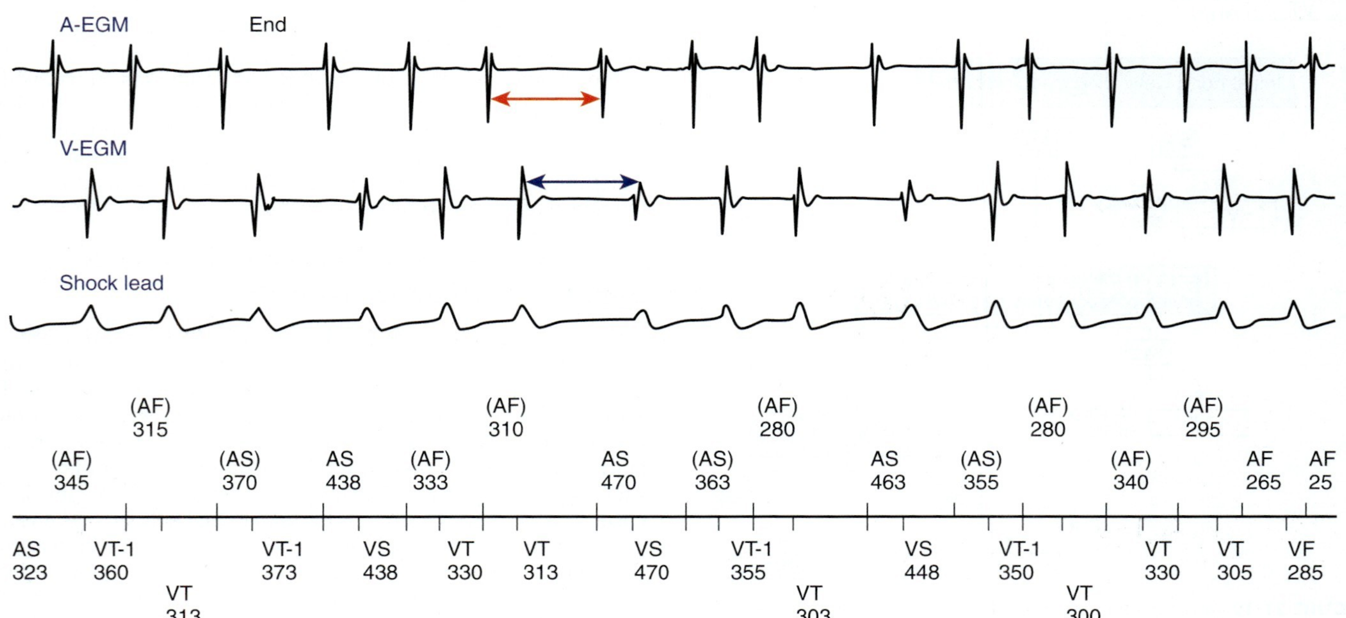

FIGURE 21-12 Intracardiac atrial (A-EGM) and ventricular (V-EGM) and shock lead electrograms stored by the implantable cardioverter-defibrillator during an episode of tachycardia with a 1:1 AV relationship. Note that variations in the tachycardia cycle length (the V-V intervals; blue double-headed arrow) are dictated and preceded by similar variations in the A-A intervals (red double-headed arrow), which is consistent with supraventricular tachycardia rather than ventricular tachycardia.

in the RV. An RB-V-HB activation sequence occurs in antidromic AVRT using atriofascicular BT, and a V-RB-HB or a V-HB-RB activation sequence can occur in VT.[7]

ATRIOVENTRICULAR RELATIONSHIP

A 1:1 AV relationship can occur in VT and SVT. When the atrial rate is faster than the ventricular rate, VT is unlikely, except in the rare case of coexistent atrial and ventricular tachycardias (Fig. 21-13). In contrast, when the ventricular rate is faster than the atrial rate, VT is more likely, except for the rare case of junctional tachycardia or AVNRT with VA block in an upper common pathway.

ATRIAL ACTIVATION SEQUENCE

A concentric atrial activation sequence can occur in SVT and VT, whereas an eccentric atrial activation sequence practically excludes VT.

EFFECTS OF ADENOSINE

Termination of WCT with adenosine can occur in SVT and adenosine-sensitive VT. AV block with continuation of the WCT can occur in aberrantly conducted AFL, AF, or AT. Adenosine can also have no effect on the WCT, whether it is a VT or SVT.

Diagnostic Maneuvers during Tachycardia

ATRIAL EXTRASTIMULATION

An atrial extrastimulus (AES), regardless of its timing, that advances the next ventricular activation with similar QRS morphology to that of the WCT excludes VT (see Fig. 18-28). Also, an AES (regardless of its timing) that delays the next ventricular activation excludes VT (see Fig. 19-4).

With a late-coupled AES delivered when the AV junctional portion of the atrium is refractory, if the AES advances the next ventricular activation, it proves the presence of an anterogradely conducting AV BT and excludes any arrhythmia mechanism that involves anterograde conduction over the AVN in the absence of a bystander BT. Moreover, if the AES advances the next ventricular activation with similar QRS morphology as that of the WCT, it proves that the BT is mediating ventricular activation during the WCT (as an integral part of the SVT circuit or as a bystander) and that the WCT is a preexcited SVT, and VT is excluded. Additionally, if the AES advances the timing of both the next ventricular activation and the subsequent atrial activation, it proves that the SVT is an antidromic AVRT using an atrioventricular or atriofascicular BT anterogradely, and excludes preexcited AVNRT and VT (see Fig. 18-28). Also, if the AES delays the next ventricular activation, it proves that the SVT is an antidromic AVRT using an atrioventricular or atriofascicular BT anterogradely, and excludes preexcited AVNRT and VT (see Fig. 19-4).[7,9,10]

ATRIAL PACING

The ability to entrain the WCT with atrial pacing can occur in VT and SVT. However, the ability to entrain the WCT with similar QRS morphology to that of the WCT (i.e., entrainment with concealed QRS fusion) excludes myocardial VT, but can occur in BBR VT and is typical for SVT. Additionally, atrial entrainment of WCT with manifest QRS fusion can occur in VT in the presence of a bystander BT, or in AVRT with multiple BTs, but not in antidromic AVRT without another BT, nor in SVT with aberrancy.[9]

The ability to dissociate the atrium with rapid atrial pacing without influencing the tachycardia CL (V-V interval) or QRS morphology suggests VT and excludes preexcited SVTs, AT with aberrancy,

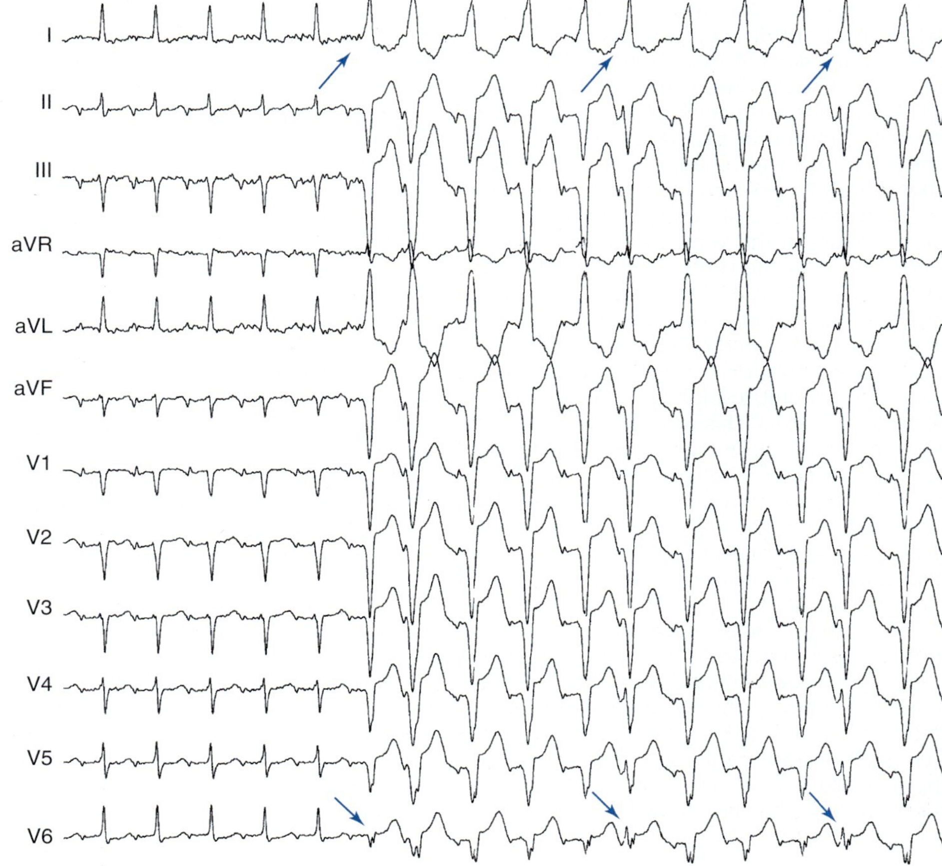

FIGURE 21-13 Surface ECG of atrial tachycardia (AT) with a narrow QRS complex with the development of ventricular tachycardia (VT) with a left bundle branch block (LBBB)–like pattern. Although the atrial rate is faster than the ventricular rate, aberrant conduction during AT as the mechanism of the widening of the QRS can be excluded by observation of QRS morphology in lead V_6 (QS) inconsistent with LBBB aberrancy, a significant shift in the frontal plane QRS axis between AT and VT, and the presence of fusion beats (arrows). Additionally, the atrial rate continues unperturbed, whereas the ventricular rate is slightly irregular.

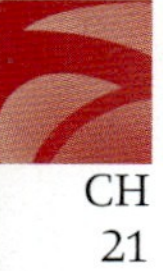

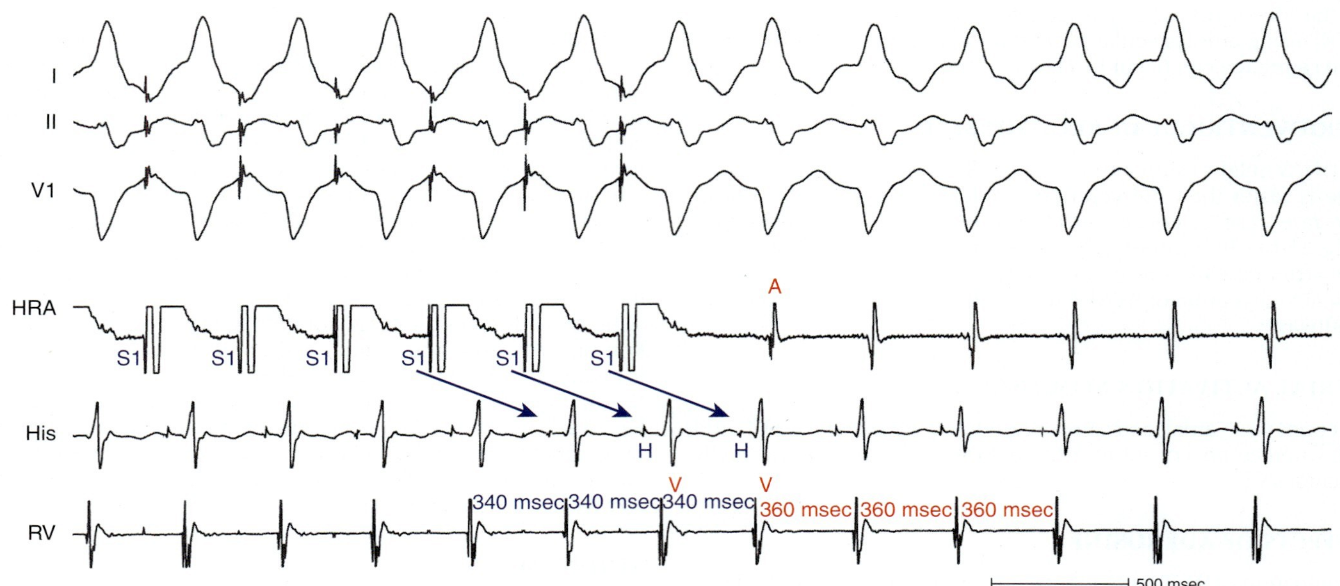

FIGURE 21-14 Pseudo–V-V-A response to atrial overdrive pacing (at a cycle length [CL] of 340 milliseconds) during wide QRS complex tachycardia (WCT) (tachycardia CL, 360 milliseconds). The QRS morphology and His bundle–ventricular (HV) interval (45 milliseconds) during atrial pacing are similar to those during tachycardia. On cessation of pacing, the last atrial-paced beat is followed by a "V-V-A response" suggestive of ventricular tachycardia as the mechanism. However, although the last atrial-paced beat is followed by two QRS complexes, the last captured QRS complex (which characteristically occurs at an R-R interval equal to the atrial pacing CL) is actually the second one (as indicated by blue arrows) due to anterograde conduction over the slow atrioventricular (AV) nodal pathway, resulting in an AV interval longer than the pacing CL. Therefore, the actual response is a "V-A response" consistent with supraventricular tachycardia. This supraventricular tachycardia was atrioventricular nodal tachycardia with left bundle branch block aberrancy.

and orthodromic AVRT with aberrancy. However, it does not exclude the rare case of AVNRT with aberrancy associated with anterograde block in an upper common pathway during rapid atrial pacing.

The response to atrial overdrive pacing during WCTs with a 1:1 AV relationship can help distinguish VT from SVT. The concept is analogous to examination of the response to ventricular overdrive pacing during narrow complex tachycardia. During VT, atrial overdrive pacing at a CL 20 to 60 milliseconds shorter than the tachycardia CL with 1:1 AV conduction results in anterograde capture with changing or narrowing of the tachycardia QRS morphology. When the tachycardia resumes after cessation of pacing, the earliest event (after the last reset ventricular complex) occurs in the ventricle because the atrium is being passively driven by the ventricle during the tachycardia. This results in a "V-V-A response." On the contrary, during antidromic AVRT or aberrantly conducted SVT, anterograde conduction occurs over a BT or AVN; and on cessation of atrial pacing, the last reset ventricular activation conducts to the atrium over the retrograde limb of the circuit, resulting in a "V-A response" and continuation of the tachycardia. This pacing maneuver is not useful when 1:1 AV conduction during atrial pacing is absent. Thus, when determining the response after atrial pacing during WCT, the presence of 1:1 VA conduction must be confirmed. Isorhythmic AV dissociation can mimic 1:1 AV conduction, especially when the pacing train is not long enough or the pacing CL is too slow. It is also important to ensure that atrial pacing does not terminate the tachycardia.[9,10]

A "pseudo–V-V-A response" can occur during SVTs associated with a long AV interval during atrial pacing (Fig. 21-14). Because anterograde conduction during atrial pacing occurs through the slow AVN pathway, the AV interval can be longer than the pacing CL (A-A interval), so that the last paced P wave is followed first by the QRS complex resulting from slow AV conduction of the preceding paced atrial beat, and then by the QRS complex resulting from the last paced P wave. Careful examination of the last QRS complex that resulted from AV conduction during atrial pacing helps avoid this potential pitfall; the last reset QRS complex characteristically occurs at an R-R interval equal to the atrial pacing CL, whereas the first tachycardia QRS complex usually occurs at a different return CL. Furthermore, a "pseudo–A-V response" can theoretically occur in the setting BBR VT or in those with intra- or interfascicular reentrant VT, whereby the return atrial impulse may precede the first non-reset QRS complex.[9,10]

VENTRICULAR EXTRASTIMULATION

A VES that resets (advances or delays) the next QRS without affecting the A-A interval is consistent with VT and practically excludes SVT. Furthermore, a VES that terminates the WCT without conduction to the atrium excludes AT and AVRT, is consistent with VT, but can also occur in AVNRT. In addition, a VES delivered when the HB is refractory and that terminates the WCT without atrial activation excludes SVT and is consistent with VT, although it can occur in orthodromic AVRT with aberrant conduction or in antidromic AVRT using a second BT as the retrograde limb of the circuit.[7]

VENTRICULAR PACING

When overdrive ventricular pacing during the WCT fails to accelerate the atrial CL to the pacing CL (i.e., the ventricles are dissociated from the tachycardia), VT and AVRT are excluded, AT is the most likely diagnosis, but AVNRT is still possible (Fig. 21-15). Additionally, entrainment with manifest QRS fusion can occur in VT or AVRT but excludes AT and AVNRT, whereas entrainment with concealed fusion excludes SVT with aberrancy. Additionally, entrainment from the RV apex followed by a post-pacing interval (PPI) that is equal (within 30 milliseconds) to the tachycardia CL excludes AVNRT, AT, and myocardial VT, but can occur with BBR VT and AVRT using a right-sided BT.

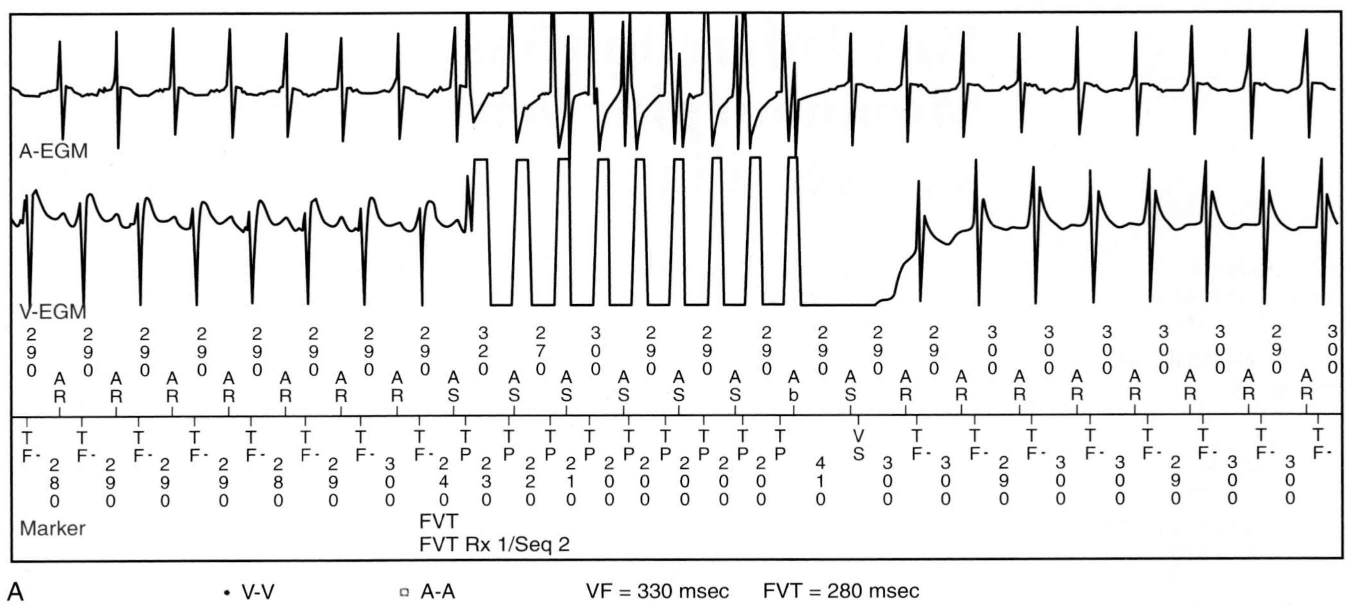

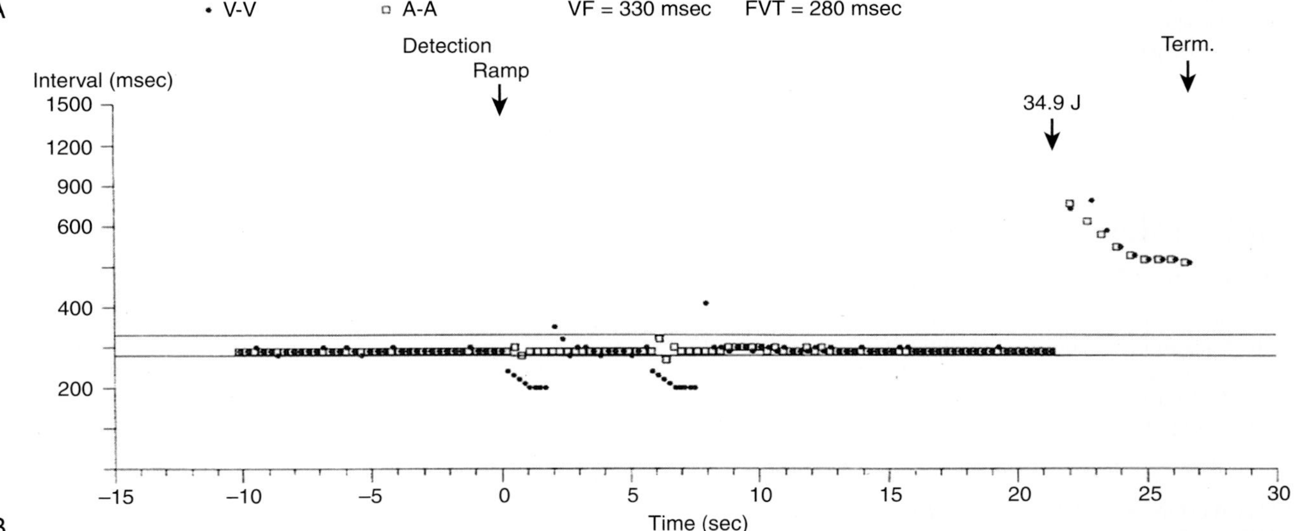

FIGURE 21-15 **A,** Intracardiac atrial and ventricular electrograms (A-EGM and V-EGM, respectively) stored by the implantable cardioverter-defibrillator (ICD) during an episode of tachycardia at a cycle length (CL) of 290 milliseconds and a 1:1 AV relationship. The tachycardia triggered antitachycardia pacing (ATP) therapy by the ICD with a ramp of nine ventricular paced beats. ATP fails to terminate the tachycardia, which resumes at the baseline CL. **B,** A plot of atrial versus ventricular CLs during the tachycardia and two sequences of ramp ATP. Note that the atrial rate continues unperturbed during ventricular pacing (i.e., ventriculoatrial dissociation was evident during ATP), which excludes ventricular tachycardia and orthodromic atrioventricular reentrant tachycardia and is consistent with either atrial tachycardia or atrioventricular nodal reentrant tachycardia.

REFERENCES

1. Surawicz B, Childers R, Deal BJ, et al: AHA/ACCF/HRS recommendations for the standardization and interpretation of the electrocardiogram. III. Intraventricular conduction disturbances: a scientific statement from the American Heart Association Electrocardiography and Arrhythmias Committee, Council on Clinical Cardiology; the American College of Cardiology Foundation; and the Heart Rhythm Society. Endorsed by the International Society for Computerized Electrocardiology, *J Am Coll Cardiol* 53:976–981, 2009.
2. Miller JM, Das MK: Differential diagnosis of wide QRS complex tachycardia. In Zipes DP, Jalife J, editors: *Cardiac electrophysiology: from cell to bedside*, ed 5, Philadelphia, 2009, WB Saunders, pp 823–830.
3. Pava LF, Perafan P, Badiel M, et al: R-wave peak time at DII: a new criterion for differentiating between wide complex QRS tachycardias, *Heart Rhythm* 7:922–926, 2010.
4. Vereckei A, Duray G, Szénási G, et al: Application of a new algorithm in the differential diagnosis of wide QRS complex tachycardia, *Eur Heart J* 28:589–600, 2007.
5. Dendi R, Josephson ME: A new algorithm in the differential diagnosis of wide complex tachycardia, *Eur Heart J* 28:525–526, 2007.
6. Vereckei A, Duray G, Szénási G, et al: New algorithm using only lead aV_R for differential diagnosis of wide QRS complex tachycardia, *Heart Rhythm* 5:89–98, 2008.
7. Josephson ME: Recurrent ventricular tachycardia. In Josephson ME, editor: *Clinical cardiac electrophysiology*, ed 4, Philadelphia, 2008, Lippincott Williams & Wilkins, pp 446–642.
8. Daoud EG: Bundle branch reentry. In Zipes DP, Jalife J, editors: *Cardiac electrophysiology: from cell to bedside*, ed 4, Philadelphia, 2004, WB Saunders, pp 683–686.
9. Abdelwahab A, Gardner MJ, Basta MN, et al: A technique for the rapid diagnosis of wide complex tachycardia with 1:1 AV relationship in the electrophysiology laboratory, *Pacing Clin Electrophysiol* 32:475–483, 2009.
10. Badhwar N, Scheinman MM: Electrophysiological diagnosis of wide complex tachycardia, *Pacing Clin Electrophysiol* 32:473–474, 2009.

CHAPTER 22 Post-Infarction Sustained Monomorphic Ventricular Tachycardia

Pathophysiology

Classification of Ventricular Tachycardia

Ventricular tachycardia (VT) is defined as a tachycardia (rate >100 beats/min) with three or more consecutive beats that originates below the bifurcation of the His bundle (HB), in the specialized conduction system, the ventricular muscle, or in a combination of both tissues, independent of atrial or atrioventricular nodal (AVN) conduction.[1,2]

CLASSIFICATION ACCORDING TO TACHYCARDIA MORPHOLOGY

Monomorphic VT has a single stable QRS morphology from beat to beat, indicating repetitive ventricular depolarization in the same sequence (Fig. 22-1). *Multiple monomorphic VTs* refers to more than one morphologically distinct monomorphic VT, occurring as different episodes or induced at different times. *Polymorphic VT* has a continuously changing or multiform QRS morphology (i.e., no constant morphology for more than five complexes, no clear isoelectric baseline between QRS complexes, or QRS complexes that have different morphologies in multiple simultaneously recorded leads), indicating a variable sequence of ventricular activation and no single site of origin (see Fig. 22-1).[3] *Torsades de pointes* is a polymorphic VT associated with a long QT interval, and is electrocardiographically characterized by twisting of the peaks of the QRS complexes around the isoelectric line during the arrhythmia. *Pleomorphic VT* has more than one morphologically distinct QRS complex occurring during the same episode of VT, but the QRS morphology is not continuously changing. *Bidirectional VT* is associated with a beat-to-beat alternans in the QRS frontal plane axis, often associated with digitalis toxicity or catecholaminergic VT. *Ventricular flutter* is a term that has been applied to a rapid (250 to 350 beats/min) VT that has a sinusoidal QRS configuration that prevents identification of the QRS morphology (see Fig. 22-1). *Ventricular fibrillation* (VF) is a rapid (usually >350 beats/min), grossly irregular ventricular rhythm with marked variability in QRS amplitude and cycle length (CL), and a changing morphology (see Fig. 22-1).[1,2]

CLASSIFICATION ACCORDING TO TACHYCARDIA DURATION

Sustained VT lasts for more than 30 seconds or requires termination (e.g., cardioversion) in less than 30 seconds because of hemodynamic compromise, whereas *nonsustained VT* is a tachycardia at more than 100 beats/min lasting for three or more complexes but for less than 30 seconds.[3] However, during electrophysiological (EP) testing, nonsustained VT is defined as more than five or six complexes of non–bundle branch reentrant (BBR) VT, regardless of morphology. BBR complexes are frequent (50%) in normal individuals in response to a ventricular extrastimulation (VES) and have no relevance to clinical nonsustained VT. Repetitive polymorphic responses are also common (up to 50%), especially in response to multiple (three or more) VESs with very short coupling intervals (less than 180 milliseconds). The clinical significance of induced polymorphic nonsustained VT is questionable.[3] *Incessant VT* is a continuous sustained VT that recurs promptly over several hours despite repeated interventions (e.g., electrical cardioversion) for termination.[4] Less commonly, incessant VT manifests as repeated bursts of VT that spontaneously terminate for a few intervening sinus beats, followed by the next tachycardia burst. The latter form is more common with the idiopathic VTs (see Fig. 23-1).[1,2]

CLASSIFICATION ACCORDING TO QRS MORPHOLOGY IN V_1

VT with a left bundle branch block (LBBB)-like pattern has a predominantly negative QRS polarity in lead V_1 (QS, rS, qrS), whereas VT with a right bundle branch block (RBBB)-like pattern has a predominantly positive QRS polarity in lead V_1 (rsR′, qR, RR, R, RS). However, the VT may not show features characteristic of the same bundle branch block (BBB)-like morphology in other leads.[1,3]

CLASSIFICATION ACCORDING TO TACHYCARDIA MECHANISM

Focal VT has a point source of earliest ventricular activation with a centrifugal spread of activation from that site. The mechanism can be automaticity, triggered activity, or microreentry. *Scar-related*

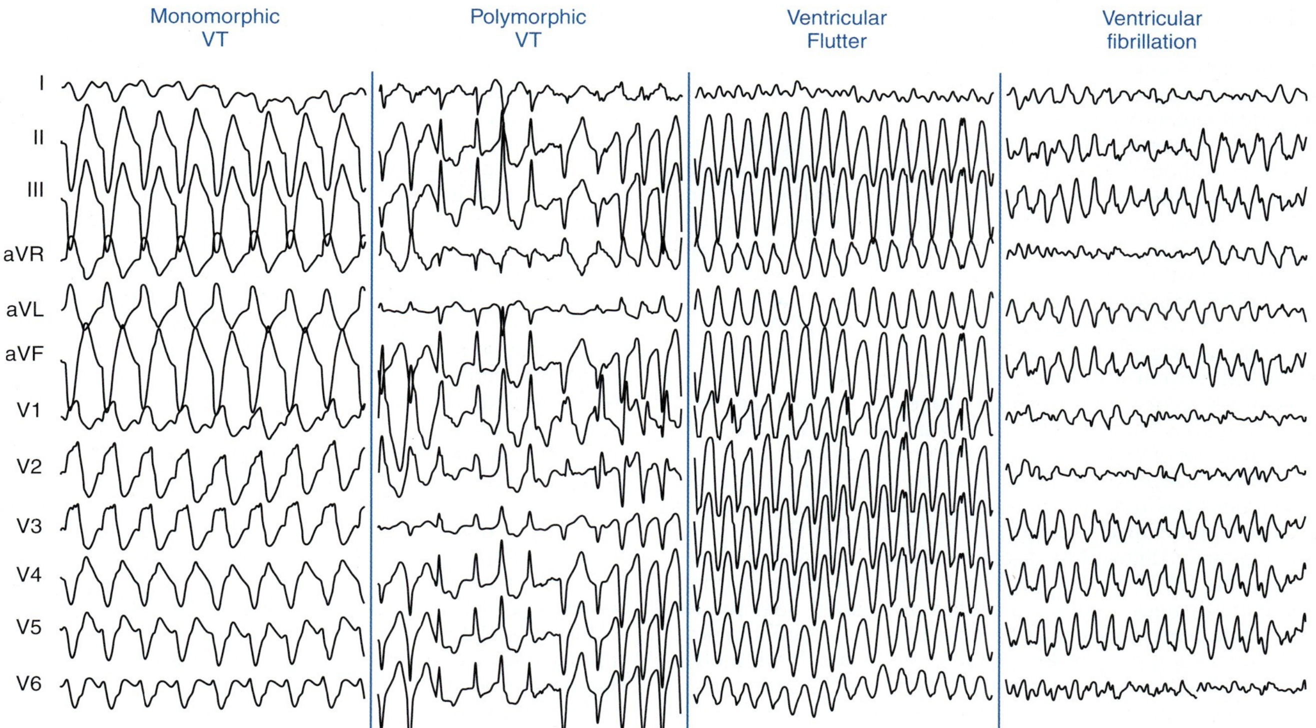

FIGURE 22-1 Surface ECG of different types of ventricular tachycardias. VT = ventricular tachycardia.

reentrant VT describes arrhythmias that have characteristics of reentry and originate from an area of myocardial scar identified from electrogram characteristics or myocardial imaging. Large reentry circuits that can be defined over several centimeters are commonly referred to as "macroreentry" circuits.[1,2]

Mechanism of Post-Infarction Ventricular Tachycardia

The majority of sustained monomorphic VTs (SMVTs) are caused by reentry involving a region of ventricular scar. The scar is most commonly caused by an old myocardial infarction (MI), but right ventricular (RV) dysplasia, sarcoidosis, Chagas disease, other nonischemic cardiomyopathies, surgical ventricular incisions for repair of tetralogy of Fallot, other congenital heart diseases, or ventricular volume reduction surgery (Batista procedure) can also cause scar-related reentry. Dense fibrotic scar creates areas of anatomical conduction block, and fibrosis between surviving myocyte bundles decreases cell-cell coupling and distorts the path of propagation, causing areas of slow conduction and block, which promotes reentry. In post-MI VT, a variety of different circuit configurations are possible. Generally, the reentrant circuit arises in areas of fibrosis interspersed with bundles of viable myocytes, producing a zigzag course of activation of and transverse conduction along a pathway lengthened by branching and merging bundles of surviving myocytes, leading to inhomogeneous anisotropy (see Fig. 3-18). Heterogeneity in tissue composition and autonomic innervations in these regions may create areas of aberrant conduction that generate the substrate for reentrant arrhythmias. Buried in the arrhythmogenic area is the common central pathway, the critical isthmus, causing slowing of impulse conduction, allowing reentry to occur. The isthmus itself can be surrounded by dead ends or branches that do not participate in the common pathway of the main reentrant circuit (bystander).[4,5]

Although previous data suggested that most isthmuses are anatomically determined by heterogeneous scar geometry, a recent study found that the diastolic pathway critical to post-MI VT reentrant circuits is typically protected by a boundary of fixed and functional block. In the majority of cases, development of functional unidirectional block was a prerequisite for initiation of VT, by protecting a region of myocardium that subsequently forms at least one border of the diastolic pathway. Evidence indicates that formation of functional block leading to reentry is associated with large dispersion in refractory periods over short anatomical distances.[6]

The critical isthmus contained in these reentry circuits often is a narrow path of tissue with abnormal conduction properties. Depolarization of the small mass of tissue in the isthmus is usually not detectable on the surface electrocardiogram (ECG) and constitutes the electrical diastole between QRS complexes during VT. The wavefront leaves the isthmus at the exit site and propagates out to depolarize the remainder of the ventricles, producing the QRS complex. After leaving the exit of the isthmus, the reentrant wavefront can return back to the entrance of the isthmus through an outer loop or an inner loop (see Fig. 5-14).[4] An outer loop is a broad sheet of myocardium along the border of the infarct. Depolarization of the outer loop can be detectable on the surface ECG. Reentrant circuits can have one or more outer loops. An inner loop is contained within the scar. Inner loop pathways can serve as potential components of a new reentrant circuit should the central common pathway be ablated. If multiple loops exist, the loop with the shortest conduction time generally determines the VT CL and is therefore the dominant loop. Any loop with a longer conduction time behaves as a bystander. Those bystander loops can serve as a potential component of a new reentrant circuit if the dominant loop is ablated.

The critical isthmus in post-MI VT is typically bounded by two approximately parallel conduction barriers that consist of a line of double potentials, a scar area, or the mitral annulus. The endocardial reentrant VT rotates around the isthmus boundaries and propagates slowly through the critical isthmus, which harbors diastolic potentials and measures, on average, approximately 30 mm long by 16 mm wide. The axis of a critical isthmus is typically oriented parallel to the mitral annulus plane in perimitral circuits and perpendicular to the mitral annulus plane in other circuits.[4] Ablation lesions produced with standard radiofrequency (RF) ablation catheters are usually less than 8 mm in diameter, relatively small in relation to the entire reentry circuit, and can be smaller than the width of the reentry path at different points in the circuit. Successful ablation of a large circuit is achieved by targeting an isthmus where the circuit can be interrupted with one or a small number of RF lesions, or by creating a line of RF lesions through a region containing the reentry circuit.

A recent study using electroanatomical substrate mapping found that patients without clinical SMVT had markedly smaller endocardial low-voltage areas, fewer scar-related electrograms (i.e., fractionated, isolated, and very late potentials, which represent electrically viable sites within the scar), and fewer putative conducting channels compared with similar ischemic cardiomyopathy patients with spontaneous SMVT, despite equally severe left ventricular (LV) dysfunction as well as similar infarct age and distribution. These differences in the endocardial EP substrate can play an important role in VT arrhythmogenesis in the chronic post-MI context. Both the extent of the scar areas (electrogram voltage <0.5 mV) and the presence of numerous channels within this zone seem to be critical to the development of VT. Although the border zone region of the scar (electrogram voltage, 0.5 to 1.5 mV) did not differ in area between the two groups, this zone also had a significantly higher prevalence of putative conducting channels in the SMVT patients. This suggests a fundamentally different scar composition (more "arrhythmogenic") in the SMVT patients. As noted, inhomogeneous scarring with varying degrees of subendocardial myocardial fiber preservation within dense zones of fibrosis leads to slowed conduction, nonuniform anisotropy, and the potential for channels within the scar zone—conditions necessary for the development of reentry.[7]

It is not uncommon for patients with post-MI VT to have more than one VT morphology. Even in patients presenting with a single SMVT, multiple distinct uniform VTs may be induced in the EP laboratory, especially during antiarrhythmic therapy. The induction of multiple VT morphologies during an ablation procedure suggests that the arrhythmogenic substrate has the capability to support multiple reentrant circuits or different exit sites from a single circuit. Distinct VT morphologies (as defined by the 12-lead ECG and tachycardia CL) often share a common isthmus but differ in propagation direction, location, or both across the isthmus perimeter during reentry, but can also arise from distinct, usually adjacent, circuits.

A focal mechanism of VT (abnormal automaticity or triggered activity) has been implicated in the settings of acute ischemia. Focal VT may also occur in the absence of an acute ischemic event in patients with chronic ischemic heart disease. A recent study found that a focal mechanism was present in up to 9% of VTs that were induced in patients with ischemic heart disease during EP study for RF ablation.[8]

Cardiac arrest and sudden cardiac death (SCD) in post-MI patients are predominantly caused by VT or VF. Bradyarrhythmias, including heart block, as well as electromechanical dissociation contribute to SCD, although they seem to account for a minority of events.

Clinical Considerations

Epidemiology

Coronary heart disease is the most frequent cause of clinically documented VT and VF (76% to 82% of patients). The incidence of SMVT in patients with an acute MI varies with the type of MI. Among almost 41,000 patients with an ST elevation (Q wave) MI treated with thrombolysis in the GUSTO-1 trial, 3.5% developed VT alone and 2.7% developed both VT and VF. A pooled analysis of four major trials of almost 25,000 patients with a non–ST elevation acute coronary syndrome (non–ST elevation MI and unstable angina) noted a lower incidence of VT—0.8% developed VT alone and 0.3% developed both VT and VF.[1,9]

SMVT within the first 2 days of acute MI is uncommon, occurring in up to 3% of patients as a primary arrhythmia and with VF in up to 2%, and is associated with an increase in in-hospital mortality compared with those without this arrhythmia. However, among 21- to 30-day survivors, mortality at 1 year is not increased, suggesting that the arrhythmogenic mechanisms can be transient in early post-MI SMVT. On the other hand, the typical patient with SMVT occurring during the subacute and healing phases, beginning more than 48 hours after an acute MI, has had a large, often complicated infarct with a reduced LV ejection fraction (LVEF), and such VT is a predictor of a worse prognosis.[9] SMVT within 3 months of an MI is associated with a 2-year mortality rate of 40% to 50%, with most deaths being sudden. Predictors of increased mortality in these patients are anterior wall MI; frequent episodes of sustained VT, nonsustained VT, or both; heart failure; and multivessel coronary disease, particularly in individuals with residual ischemia.

Early reperfusion of infarct-related arteries results in less aneurysm formation, smaller scars, and less extensive EP abnormalities, although a significant risk of late VT (often with rapid CLs) persists.[2,10] In patients with ST elevation MI treated with primary percutaneous coronary intervention, delayed reperfusion (>5 hours after MI) was associated with a sixfold increase in the odds of inducible SMVT by programmed electrical stimulation (performed 6 to 10 days post-MI) as well as an increased risk of spontaneous ventricular arrhythmias and SCD (after a mean follow-up of 28 ± 13 months) compared with early reperfusion (≤3 hours) independent of LVEF. It was estimated that each 1-hour delay in reperfusion conferred a 10.4% increase in the odds of inducible VT.[11]

Most episodes of SMVT associated with MI occur during the chronic phase. VT occurs in 1% to 2% of patients late after MI. The first episode can be seen within the first year post-MI, but the median time of occurrence is about 3 years and SMVT can occur as late as 10 to 15 years after an MI. Late SMVT often reflects significant LV dysfunction and the presence of a ventricular aneurysm or scarring. Late arrhythmias can also result from new cardiac events. The annual mortality rate for SMVT that occurs after the first 3 months following acute MI is approximately 5% to 15%. Predictors of VF include residual ischemia in the setting of damaged myocardium, LVEF less than 40%, and electrical instability, including inducible or spontaneous VT, particularly in those who present with cardiac arrest.

Recent evidence suggests that coronary revascularization before or shortly after implantable cardioverter-defibrillator (ICD) placement in high-risk post-MI patients with LV dysfunction and wide QRS duration can potentially reduce the risk for life-threatening ventricular arrhythmias and appropriate ICD shocks, and, hence, improve quality of life and reduce mortality.[12]

The relationship between SMVT and VF is uncertain, and it is not clear how often VF is triggered by SMVT rather than occurring de novo. SMVT can simply be the company kept by VF in a number of patients or, in the appropriate setting such as recurrent ischemia, a rapid VT can develop a wavefront that becomes fractionated, leading to VF.

SCD accounts for up to 15% of total mortality in industrialized countries and claims the lives of more than 300,000 people per year in the United States. Approximately 50% of deaths in patients with prior MI occur suddenly and unexpectedly. Ventricular arrhythmias are responsible for most of these deaths in stable ambulatory populations. Most SCD victims have known heart disease—most frequently coronary artery disease or prior MI. Cardiac arrest is the initial manifestation of heart disease in approximately 50% of cases. Such patients are more likely to have single-vessel coronary disease and normal or mildly abnormal LV systolic function than cardiac arrest victims with prior MI. Although heart failure increases risk for both sudden and nonsudden death, a history of heart failure is present in only approximately 10% of arrest victims.[13]

The risk for total and arrhythmic mortality is highest in the first month after an acute MI and stays high during the first 6 months after acute MI. After the first year post-MI, there appears to be a relatively quiescent period of relatively low rates of SCD, followed by a second peak 4 to 10 years after acute MI. The later occurrence of SCD may result from delayed ventricular remodeling resulting in the creation or activation of reentrant VT circuits on the infarct border as well as from heart failure developing late after MI.[14]

Several studies in patients with cardiac arrest have shown that VF as the causative rhythm appears to be decreasing, being replaced by pulseless electrical activity and asystole. Although the cause of this change is unknown, it may reflect patients with sicker hearts who are living longer due to better therapy. Hearts with advanced disease may be more likely to develop pulseless electrical activity and asystole than VF.[15]

Clinical Presentation

In chronic ischemic heart disease, VT results in a wide spectrum of clinical presentations, ranging from mild symptoms (palpitations) to symptoms of hypoperfusion (lightheadedness, altered mental status, presyncope, and syncope), exacerbation of heart failure and angina, and cardiovascular collapse. Hemodynamic consequences associated with VT are related to ventricular rate, duration of VT, presence and extent of LV dysfunction, ventricular activation sequence (i.e., ventricular dyssynchrony), and loss of atrioventricular (AV) synchrony.

Initial Evaluation

EVALUATION OF TYPE AND BURDEN OF VENTRICULAR ARRHYTHMIAS

Identifying and quantifying the types and burden of sustained and nonsustained VT are necessary. Ideally, a 12-lead ECG should be obtained. In patients with ICDs, stored device data such as electrogram morphology and CL can be used to identify the clinical VT.[2]

EVALUATION OF THE TRIGGERS OF VENTRICULAR ARRHYTHMIAS

Initial testing in patients with post-MI VT should evaluate for reversible causes of the arrhythmia. These include electrolyte imbalances, acute ischemia, heart failure, hypoxia, hypotension, drug effects, and anemia.

EVALUATION OF MYOCARDIAL ISCHEMIA

Although recurrent SMVT is rarely due to acute myocardial ischemia in patients with known coronary artery disease, diagnostic evaluation for acute or persistent ischemia is warranted to improve patient outcome, especially if the severity of coronary artery disease has not been previously established or prior episodes of VT caused hemodynamic compromise. This may include echocardiographic examination, exercise testing, and cardiac catheterization. In patients with reversible myocardial ischemia, coronary revascularization may be warranted, and can potentially reduce the risk of life-threatening ventricular arrhythmias.[12] However, if the severity of coronary disease has been recently defined and symptoms and hemodynamic tolerance of VT do not suggest significant ischemia, further evaluation may not be required.[1,2]

PREABLATION EVALUATION

Patients with post-MI VT should be evaluated for comorbidities that can alter the approach to mapping and ablation. Treatment of congestive heart failure and myocardial ischemia should be optimized. Coronary revascularization should be considered in patients with reversible ischemia, because substantial ischemic burden can often be aggravated by the potential induction of prolonged periods of tachycardia or hemodynamically unstable arrhythmias during the ablation procedure. In patients with frequent or incessant VT, however, catheter ablation may be required on an urgent basis before the assessment for coronary artery disease in order to gain prompt control of the ventricular arrhythmia.[1,2]

Mobile LV thrombus is an absolute contraindication to endocardial catheter ablation. In contrast, LV catheter ablation may be performed despite the presence of laminated thrombus, if the patient has been therapeutically anticoagulated with warfarin for at least 4 weeks prior to ablation. Similarly, the presence of intraatrial clots should be excluded in patients with inadequately anticoagulated persistent atrial fibrillation (AF) to reduce the risk of thromboembolism in the event of AF termination following electrical shocks for termination of unstable ventricular arrhythmias.

In patients with suspected peripheral vascular disease, evaluation of the presence of severe arterial disease is warranted, as it can affect the approach to LV access (atrial transseptal versus retrograde transaortic versus epicardial).[16] Similarly, an atrial transseptal approach allowing access to the LV through the mitral valve can be considered in the presence of a mechanical aortic valve or severe aortic valve disease.[2]

Assessment of the risks for sedation and anesthesia must be performed prior to the procedure, because these patients are likely to require deep sedation or general anesthesia.[2]

ARRHYTHMOGENIC SUBSTRATE IMAGING

In patients with ventricular dysfunction, tissue heterogeneity with inexcitable myocardial fibrous scar and surviving myocardium may provide a potential substrate for reentry circuits. Several noninvasive methodologies have been used to assess the substrate and identify patients at high risk for ventricular arrhythmias.

VENTRICULOGRAPHY. Left ventriculography provides valuable information about LV function and ventricular thrombi, representing a relative contraindication to catheter manipulation. Additionally, regions of wall motion abnormalities and aneurysms can be identified that likely harbor the VT substrate.

ECHOCARDIOGRAPHY. Transthoracic echocardiography is routinely performed to evaluate LV systolic function, LVEF, and wall motion abnormalities that may contain the potential VT substrate. Transthoracic echocardiography also serves as a reliable tool to rule out ventricular thrombi before LV procedures. Additionally, it helps to identify relatively infrequent cardiomyopathies associated with VT, for example, arrhythmogenic right ventricular dysplasia-cardiomyopathy and hypertrophic cardiomyopathy. Although echocardiography can provide anatomical and contractile parameters, it cannot provide relevant clinical information about transmural extent and intramyocardial location of the scar.[17]

Transesophageal echocardiography can be used in patients with AF or atrial flutter (AFL) to detect thrombi within the left atrium (LA) and LA appendage to prevent thromboembolic events when a transseptal access to the LV or cardioversion is required. Severe atheroma in the aorta detected on transesophageal echocardiography may encourage the operator to avoid the retrograde approach to the LV.

Intracardiac echocardiography (ICE) applied from the right atrium (RA) and the RV has been used for real-time imaging during VT ablation procedures. ICE provides both an anatomical and a functional assessment of the LV, allowing for real-time identification of wall motion abnormalities. ICE also allows for visualization of scarred tissue and thus may help to identify the VT substrate and facilitate mapping and ablation (see later).

DELAYED CONTRAST-ENHANCED CARDIAC MAGNETIC RESONANCE. Cardiac magnetic resonance (MR) imaging is a valuable tool for assessing cardiac anatomy and function and for identifying structural abnormalities serving as arrhythmia substrate. Delayed contrast-enhanced MR imaging delineates regions of scar tissue potentially forming part of the arrhythmia substrate in patients with ischemic cardiomyopathy (CMP).

Cardiac MR is extremely valuable for assessing viable and nonviable myocardium in infarcted and poorly contracting myocardial areas, and enables the depiction of transmural and nontransmural infarctions with high spatial resolution and better accuracy than scintigraphic techniques. Assessing the characteristics and distribution of myocardial scar by cardiac MR can potentially help identify patients at high risk of VT. In patients with ischemic CMP, the nontransmural hyperenhanced areas, but not the transmural hyperenhanced areas, were found to predict higher risk of sustained VT.[18]

Additionally, delayed enhancement cardiac MR imaging can potentially predict the approach required for successful VT ablation (endocardial versus epicardial) by visualizing the location of the scar (endocardial, intramyocardial, or epicardial). In a recent report, the presence of epicardial or intramyocardial scar on preprocedure MR was associated with a 0% procedural success rate when the operator limited ablation to the endocardium.

Recently, registration of preacquired MR images with real-time electroanatomical mapping has successfully been used to facilitate and guide catheter navigation and ablation in the LV. Visualization of ventricular anatomy and obstacles to procedural success, for example, epicardial fat in the case of epicardial mapping approaches, and the possibility of navigation and ablation in the ventricular chambers have the potential to reduce procedure time, decrease the rate of complications, and increase success rates.

One potential disadvantage concerns the safety of MR imaging in patients with implanted devices. Evolving technologies have improved the MR imaging compatibility of some devices.

POSITRON EMISSION TOMOGRAPHY. Currently, positron emission tomography (PET) is considered the gold standard for tissue viability assessment. In patients with scar-related VT, PET can accurately detect myocardial scar within the LV and provide additional tissue characterization by displaying metabolic and morphological information of the VT substrate. Its spatial resolution of 4 to 6 mm can delineate scar in any wall segment with good correlation between areas of endocardial voltage less than 0.5 mV and PET-defined myocardial scar.

Because PET scans alone do not provide the necessary anatomical information required for integration with electroanatomical maps, a computed tomography (CT) angiography scan is required to provide an anatomical skeleton onto which the biological information acquired from the PET scan would be superimposed on its precise anatomical location. Fusion of multimodality imaging sets derived from PET/CT allows accurate, simultaneous display of LV anatomy and myocardial scar and can facilitate an image-guided approach to substrate-based VT ablations.

CARDIAC CONTRAST-ENHANCED COMPUTED TOMOGRAPHY. Cardiac contrast-enhanced CT scanning enables a detailed and comprehensive evaluation of LV myocardium using multimodality imaging based on anatomical, dynamic, and perfusion parameters to identify abnormal substrate (myocardial scar and border zone) with high spatial (≤1 mm) and temporal resolution, which can be derived from a single CT scan. Areas of CT hypoperfusion correlate best with areas of abnormal voltage (<1.5 mV) rather than scar alone (<0.5 mV). Perfusion imaging from CT can indicate scar transmurality and intramyocardial scar location.[17]

The ability of contrast-enhanced CT to characterize the transmural extent and intramyocardial location of scar tissue and to visualize surviving mid- and epicardial myocardium at sites of endocardial scar can potentially help identify areas involved in myocardial reentry representing appropriate ablation targets and help to overcome one of the significant limitations of endocardial voltage mapping. Additionally, the presence of an epicardial VT substrate can facilitate planning of VT ablations, such as for a combined endocardial and epicardial approach.[17] When compared with contrast-enhanced MR, absolute sizes of early hypoperfused and late hyperenhanced regions were similar on contrast-enhanced CT and contrast-enhanced MR.[17]

The three-dimensional (3-D) CT-defined image of abnormal myocardium can be accurately extracted and embedded in clinical mapping systems displaying areas of abnormal anatomical, dynamic, and perfusion parameters for substrate-guided VT ablations.[17]

ROLE OF ELECTROPHYSIOLOGICAL TESTING

In patients with sustained monomorphic VT, EP testing is not recommended unless catheter ablation is planned. However, EP testing is useful in patients with coronary heart disease for the diagnostic evaluation of wide QRS complex tachycardias of unclear mechanism and in those with unexplained syncope. Additionally, EP testing can be used for risk stratification late after MI in patients with ischemic CMP and nonsustained VT (see below).[19]

Programmed stimulation induces VT in over 90% of patients with a history of VT. Although the rate and QRS morphology of induced VT may differ from that observed during spontaneous tachycardia, the induction of VT signifies the presence of a fixed anatomical substrate associated with an increased likelihood of future spontaneous events.[2]

Risk Stratification

There are more than 50 million North American adults with coronary artery disease and more than 7 million have had an MI. However, only a fraction of these patients will suffer a cardiac arrest. Therefore, noninvasive risk assessment after MI is required to identify patients at risk of SCD. Various tests assessing the extent of myocardial damage and scarring, myocardial conduction disorders, dispersion of repolarization, and autonomic imbalance have been proposed to identify patients at high risk of SCD who are likely to benefit from prophylactic ICD therapy. Some of these techniques potentially identify the underlying substrate (e.g., myocardial scar, intramyocardial conduction abnormalities) or triggers (e.g., autonomic imbalance, nonsustained VT) of malignant ventricular arrhythmias. However, most of these techniques have not been validated in independent populations and, although they can predict higher risk of total mortality, their ability to predict arrhythmic death is uncertain. Additionally, the majority of conventional risk stratifiers of SCD have a relatively low positive predictive value that would preclude their wide application as guidelines for ICD implantation in patients known to be at risk for SCD.[14,20]

To date, only two approaches have been proven useful in guiding prophylactic ICD therapy in post-MI patients: the presence of significant LV dysfunction alone or in combination with the inducibility of sustained VT/VF during programmed electrical stimulation beyond the early phase after MI. It should be recognized, however, that the development of SCD in post-MI patients is multifactorial, and multiple events need to coincide for a cardiac arrest to ensue; therefore, no one risk stratification test alone will be sufficient for all patients. Rather, combining multiple tests screening for the different potential mechanisms of SCD may be necessary. Furthermore, because progression of ischemic heart disease can result in the evolution of new mechanisms of SCD in individual patients, repetition of risk stratification tests at certain intervals may be required. It would seem reasonable (in the absence of data) to retest every 2 years in apparently stable patients to detect potential changes in substrate, regardless of which tests appear to have the highest yield.[14,20]

LEFT VENTRICULAR EJECTION FRACTION

Multiple studies evaluating survival of patients with prior MI established a clear relationship between reduced LVEF and increased mortality. LVEF behaves as a continuous variable, with gradually increasing mortality risk until the LVEF declines to 40% and then markedly increasing risk for values less than 40%. Nevertheless, the exact mechanisms involved in the strong correlation between decreased LV systolic function and increased incidence of SCD are not clearly defined.[14]

Although low LVEF identifies one patient population at relatively increased risk for SCD, there are clear limitations to LVEF as the ideal risk-stratification test for deciding whether to implant an ICD for primary prevention of SCD. LV systolic dysfunction lacks specificity. There is no evidence of any direct mechanistic link between low LVEF and mechanisms responsible for ventricular tachyarrhythmias and no study has demonstrated that reduced LVEF is specifically related to SCD. In fact, in studies that enrolled all patients after MI, patients with LVEF less than 30% to 35% account for no more than 50% of sudden cardiac arrest victims. Thus, although LVEF is a good marker of risk for *total* mortality, it does not provide insight into how patients are likely to die (sudden versus nonsudden).

Another limitation of LVEF is its poor sensitivity. Although most studies have focused on patients with markedly reduced LVEF, this group currently accounts for only 10% to 15% of MI survivors. Furthermore, patients with low LVEF are not uniform with regard to other prognostic markers, and not all are at high risk for SCD. In fact, most contemporary managed post-MI patients who suffer a cardiac arrest have better-preserved LV systolic function (i.e., LVEF ≥35%).

It is also recognized that methods of LVEF determination lack precision. Different imaging modalities can produce significantly different LVEF values and the accuracy of techniques varies among laboratories and institutions, and there is evidence that prognosis, and hence risk, depends on the method by which the LVEF is measured. It is therefore recommended to use the LVEF determination that clinicians believe is the most clinically accurate and appropriate in their institution.

INVASIVE ELECTROPHYSIOLOGICAL TESTING

Inducibility of VT/VF during invasive EP testing can enhance the predictive accuracy of reduced LVEF for post-MI patients with high mortality risk. The first Multicenter Automatic Defibrillator Implantation Trial (MADIT I) study demonstrated that those patients with inducible VT/VF and LVEF values less than or equal to 35% late after MI are likely to benefit from prophylactic ICD therapy. Moreover, the absolute mortality reduction in MADIT I (26.2% over 27 months) was substantially greater than what was found in either the second MADIT (MADIT II) or SCD Heart Failure Trial (SCD-HeFT). Similar results were found in the Multicenter UnSustained Tachycardia Trial (MUSTT).[19,21]

However, secondary analysis from MUSTT revealed that despite the significant difference in outcome between inducible patients enrolled in the trial and noninducible patients enrolled in a registry, EP inducibility was of limited value because the 5-year mortality rate in inducible patients was 48% compared with 44% in noninducible patients. Later, data from MADIT II showed that there is no need for additional risk stratifiers (including EP testing) when LVEF is so low. In more than 80% of patients randomized to the ICD arm of MADIT II, invasive EP testing with an attempt to induce tachyarrhythmias was performed at the time of ICD placement. VT inducibility, observed in 40% of studied patients, was not effective in identifying patients with cardiac events defined as VT, VF, or death. These observations from both MUSTT and MADIT II subanalyses suggest that in patients with substantially depressed LV function, EP inducibility should not be considered a useful predictor of outcome. It is possible, however, that inducibility might have much better predictive value in post-MI patients with LVEF greater than 30% or greater than 35%.[19,21]

Furthermore, using inducible VT/VF to guide prophylactic ICD therapy is limited by low sensitivity. Patients with LVEF values not exceeding 35% after MI and no inducible VT/VF still appear to have a substantial (>25%) risk of serious events over the near term.[21]

There are also no data to support the use of invasive EP testing in post-MI patients with LVEF values more than 40% or in the early post-MI period. In fact, the Beta-blocker Strategy plus Implantable Cardioverter-Defibrillator (BEST-ICD) trial found that inducible VT/VF early after MI does not predict benefit from ICD therapy. In contrast, the Cardiac Arrhythmias and Risk Stratification after Acute Myocardial Infarction (CARISMA) study found that inducible VT identified 6 weeks following an acute MI was a strong predictor of future life-threatening arrhythmias.[19,21]

Additionally, EP testing is invasive and not practical for broad application as a screening tool. Nonetheless, it can be valuable when used in patients in whom the risk of sustained arrhythmias and SCD is intermediate, and the potential benefit of ICD therapy uncertain. Current guidelines recommend prophylactic ICD therapy in post-MI patients with nonsustained VT and LVEF less than 40% if sustained VT/VF is inducible at EP study.[14]

MEASURES OF CARDIAC REPOLARIZATION

Microvolt-level T wave alternans (TWA) has emerged as a promising noninvasive marker of risk for SCD. TWA, measured on the surface ECG, detects subtle beat-to-beat oscillations in cardiac repolarization and has been linked to cellular mechanisms of arrhythmogenesis. Initial clinical studies of TWA demonstrated a high negative predictive value (≥95%). Additionally, an abnormal TWA was associated with significantly increased mortality risk as well as risk of arrhythmic events, although the positive predictive values were far more variable, depending on the characteristics of the study populations and pretest probability. Although those studies suggested that TWA could potentially provide prognostically useful information beyond the LVEF and help guide selection of appropriate patients for prophylactic ICD therapy, more recently, several large multicenter studies of TWA failed to support these findings and, in contrast, strongly suggested that a negative TWA result should not be used to withhold ICD therapy among patients who meet other standard criteria. Other noninvasive measures of dispersion of repolarization, including QT dispersion, QT variability, and QT dynamics, have had similar mixed predictive results in studies with limited clinical applicability.

MEASURES OF AUTONOMIC IMBALANCE

Methods to assess the autonomic nervous system, which has been thought to be a modulator between triggers of ventricular tachyarrhythmias and the underlying substrate, including heart rate variability, baroreflex sensitivity, heart rate turbulence, and deceleration capacity, have been evaluated for risk stratification of SCD. Multiple studies have correlated relative excess of sympathetic tone (or deficient parasympathetic tone) with increased mortality in post-MI patients as well as increased propensity for VF during acute ischemia. However, the majority of studies showed no significant difference in relative risk for SCD versus total mortality. Thus, these measures do not appear to provide a reliable measure of SCD risk and there is no evidence to support their use in guiding prophylactic ICD therapy.[22]

MEASURES OF MYOCARDIAL CONDUCTION DISORDERS

Increased QRS duration on a surface ECG has been associated with a higher risk of death after MI and appears to reflect greater LV dysfunction, but association with SCD has not been proven. Similarly, the presence of late potentials on signal-averaged ECG failed to identify patients likely to benefit from ICD therapy.[22] Recently, fragmentation of the QRS complex on the 12-lead surface ECG (filter range, 0.15 to 100 Hz; AC filter, 60 Hz, 25 mm/sec, 10 mm/mV), which likely signifies inhomogeneous ventricular activation due to myocardial scar, ischemia, or both in patients with coronary artery disease, has been found to potentially predict increased risk of appropriate ICD therapies in patients who received an ICD for primary and secondary prevention. The usefulness of this parameter needs further evaluation.[23,24]

GENETIC TESTING

There is compelling evidence that a genetic mechanism may increase patient susceptibility to SCD following MI, and genetic assessment may play a role in the future. However, there is presently no evidence for using genetic testing to identify post-MI patients at risk.[14,20]

CARDIAC MAGNETIC RESONANCE IMAGING

Characteristics of myocardial scar architecture and tissue heterogeneity in the periinfarct zone, as defined by contrast-enhanced cardiac MR, can potentially identify a proarrhythmic substrate and appears to be a strong predictor of ventricular arrhythmias and appropriate ICD therapies. In patients with ischemic CMP, the nontransmural, but not the transmural, hyperenhanced areas were found to predict higher risk of sustained VT.[18] However, large prospective trials are still required to evaluate the reliability of these techniques for risk stratification.[25]

RISK STRATIFICATION EARLY POST-INFARCTION

The risk of SCD is greatest in the first month after MI and appears to decline in the first year after MI. Nevertheless, both prospective and retrospective studies of prophylactic ICD therapy have failed to show a reduction in all-cause mortality in early post-MI patients. The reduction in the rate of death due to arrhythmia associated with ICD therapy was offset by an increase in the rate of death from nonarrhythmic cardiac causes in the ICD groups. This discrepancy not only highlights the limitations of current risk stratification techniques, but also reflects relative differences in the risk factors for SCD at different time points after MI and the fact that nonarrhythmic death accounts for an appreciable percentage of deaths during that time. Heart rate and creatinine clearance measured at baseline are strongly associated with SCD during the in-hospital period, whereas recurrent cardiovascular events (including heart failure, MI, and rehospitalization) and a baseline LVEF of 40% or less are more strongly associated with the occurrence of SCD after discharge.[21,26]

Whereas the cumulative incidence of SCD is greatest in post-MI patients with an LVEF of 30% or less, the incidence of SCD is greater in patients with an LVEF greater than 40% in the first 30 days after MI when compared with patients with an LVEF of 30% or less after 90 days. The strength of the association between LVEF and survival free from SCD appears to be greatest in long-term follow-up (>6 months). Currently, there is no strategy (invasive or noninvasive) that can reliably predict the risk for SCD or guide empiric ICD implantation soon after an MI. Data suggest it is best to wait 2 to 3 months after acute MI before performing risk stratification.[14,21,26]

Recent data suggest a potential benefit of EP testing in risk stratification in patients with ST elevation MI and LVEF less than 40% treated with primary percutaneous coronary intervention. Inducible SMVT by programmed electrical stimulation performed 6 to 10 days post-MI was associated with an increased risk of spontaneous VT/VF and SCD (after a mean follow-up of 28 ± 13 months). However, further evaluation in randomized clinical trials is required before adoption of this approach.[11]

Principles of Management

PHARMACOLOGICAL THERAPY

ACUTE THERAPY. The degree of hemodynamic tolerance should dictate the initial therapeutic strategy. VTs causing severe symptoms of angina or hemodynamic collapse almost always respond to synchronized electrical cardioversion. Treatment of pulseless VT is the same as that for VF and should follow the ACLS protocol. In patients with difficult-to-control or recurrent VT, intravenous amiodarone is the drug of choice. Intravenous procainamide and sotalol are alternatives. Lidocaine is less effective in the absence of acute ischemia; however, it can be considered in combination with either procainamide or amiodarone if the latter drugs are ineffective alone. Beta blockers offer additional benefit in patients with ischemic heart disease. Treatment of underlying conditions (e.g., acute ischemia, decompensated heart failure, electrolyte abnormalities) is also necessary.[19] For refractory VT storm, general anesthesia, sympathetic neural blockade, catheter ablation, and intraaortic balloon counterpulsation have been used.

CHRONIC THERAPY. Antiarrhythmic drugs can be considered in two main settings: as adjunctive therapy in patients with an ICD and as preventive therapy in patients who do not want or are not candidates for an ICD (e.g., because of marked comorbidities). Because an ICD does not prevent arrhythmias, patients who have frequent symptoms or device discharges triggered by VT/VF may benefit from adjunctive drug therapy. There are three main indications for antiarrhythmic drug therapy along with an ICD: to reduce the frequency of ventricular arrhythmias in patients with unacceptably frequent ICD therapies, to reduce the rate of VT so that it is better tolerated hemodynamically and more amenable to pace termination or low-energy cardioversion, and to suppress other arrhythmias (e.g., sinus tachycardia, AF, nonsustained VT) that cause symptoms or interfere with ICD function or cause inappropriate discharges.[19,27]

When ICD patients need drugs because of frequent shocks, the weight of evidence supports optimizing beta blocker therapy. When long-term antiarrhythmic therapy is required, amiodarone is the drug of choice. Sotalol is less effective than amiodarone and can cause torsades de pointes. Azimilide may be effective with fewer side effects (except torsades de pointes), but is not approved by the U.S. Food and Drug Administration or European authorities, and experience is limited. No comparative data for amiodarone and azimilide are available. For patients who cannot tolerate amiodarone or sotalol, dofetilide has been suggested as an alternative.[27]

Although some reports suggested the early use of antiarrhythmic drugs (prophylactically or after a single ICD shock), early prophylactic use may overtreat a large group of patients who will never have an ICD intervention but are exposed to drug side effects; or the drug may elicit an ICD intervention due to proarrhythmia. At this point, the decision as to when to start adjuvant antiarrhythmic drug therapy in patients who receive an ICD for secondary prevention should be individualized, with the expectation that well-designed therapy can reduce ICD shocks and improve quality of life. Until more data are available, routine use of prophylactic antiarrhythmic drugs in device patients does not appear to be warranted.[27]

IMPLANTABLE CARDIOVERTER-DEFIBRILLATOR

SECONDARY PREVENTION. ICD therapy has a proven mortality benefit among patients with structural heart disease and a history of VT or VF, with an absolute reduction in all-cause mortality of 7% and a significant 25% relative reduction in mortality compared with amiodarone therapy, due entirely to a 50% reduction in SCD. Implantation of an ICD is recommended for secondary prevention in patients with prior cardiac arrest or sustained VT, even in patients undergoing successful catheter ablation of the VT or responding to antiarrhythmic therapy, because the latter two approaches do not sufficiently reduce residual risk of SCD.[28]

Although one report has questioned the benefit from an ICD compared with pharmacological therapy in patients with VT and LVEF exceeding 40%, the guidelines did not stratify recommendations based on the LVEF.[29] This seems appropriate for two reasons: the prognostic importance of the LVEF was based on subset analysis and, given the current ease of ICD implantation, the potential adverse consequences of choosing a possibly less effective therapy are too great.[19]

PRIMARY PREVENTION. Current guidelines recommend prophylactic ICD implantation in patients with prior MI and reduced LVEF (<35%) who are on optimal medical management. These recommendations are based on the fundamental relationship that exists between reduced LVEF and cardiovascular mortality and the findings of MADIT II and SCD-HeFT. Both MADIT II and SCD-HeFT clearly demonstrated a mortality benefit from prophylactic ICD therapy in patients with a history of MI and severely reduced LVEF (≤ 30% and ≤ 35%, respectively). However, the absolute mortality reduction in these trials was modest: 5.6% over 27 months in MADIT II and 7.3% over 60 months in SCD-HeFT. Fewer than one in five ICD recipients in MADIT II and SCD-HeFT received appropriate ICD therapies over average follow-up periods of 20 and 60 months, respectively. Therefore, because appropriate ICD therapies overestimate the mortality benefit of ICD therapy by at least twofold, fewer than 1 in 10 patients who receive a prophylactic ICD for an LVEF of 35% or less post-MI are likely to receive a survival benefit in the near term.[19]

EP testing appears most useful as an adjunct test in patients having equivocal results after noninvasive testing and in whom the potential benefit of ICD therapy is uncertain. Examples include patients with remote MI, nonsustained VT, and an LVEF between 30% and 40%, as suggested by the recent American College of Cardiology/American Heart Association/European Society of Cardiology (ACC/AHA/ESC) guidelines, or in combination with other clinical risk factors or symptoms suggestive of ventricular tachyarrhythmias including palpitations, presyncope, and syncope. Patients with coronary artery disease who are found to have inducible monomorphic VT during programmed stimulation should be treated for the prevention of SCD. The mode of stimulation (burst pacing, single, or double VESs versus triple VESs) of sustained VT does not influence prognosis and should not influence treatment decisions.[19,21]

Although the risk of SCD is highest in the first month after MI, there is currently no reliable risk stratification strategy that can guide prophylactic ICD implantation, and primary prevention trials with ICD have failed to show a reduction in all-cause mortality in early post-MI patients identified on the basis of the current risk stratifiers. Therefore, in the early post-MI period, medical therapy and coronary revascularization, when feasible, should be optimized. The LVEF should then be measured at least 40 days post-MI and, if the LVEF is not more than 35%, the patient should be considered for ICD implantation.[21,26]

CATHETER ABLATION

Catheter ablation of post-MI VT is generally indicated as a *palliative* and *adjunctive* therapy in post-MI patients with ICD who experience frequent recurrences of VT or ICD therapies. Recurrences of VT/VF causing frequent ICD therapies (including ICD shocks) are relatively common. Approximately 20% to 35% of ICD recipients for primary SCD prevention and up to 45% of those who receive an ICD for secondary SCD prevention will receive an appropriate shock within 3 years of implantation. ICD therapy acting via such appropriate ICD shocks reduces the risk of SCD by approximately 60%, but the occurrence of shocks is associated with progressive heart failure symptoms, a significant decline in psychosocial quality of life, and a two- to fivefold increase in mortality. The incidence of appropriate shocks can be reduced by using antitachycardia pacing in the VT or VF detection zones, or with up-titration of medical therapies. If optimization of pharmacological therapies and device programming fails to suppress appropriate ICD shocks for VT, patients are eligible for catheter ablation. Catheter ablation reduces VT/VF recurrences and thereby ICD interventions by more than 75% in patients after multiple ICD shocks. In this patient population, the incidence of procedure-related death ranges from 0% to 3%, and the incidence of major complications from 3.6% to 10%.[19,30,31] Nonetheless, most patients with post-MI VT have multiple types of monomorphic VTs, and elimination of all VTs is often not feasible, and because the recurrence of an ablated VT or the onset of a new VT can be fatal, RF ablation is rarely used as the sole therapy for VT. Instead, it is typically used for patients with coronary artery disease as an adjunct to an implantable ICD or, less commonly, to antiarrhythmic drug therapy.[2]

Additionally, catheter ablation is necessary and can be life-saving in patients with electrical storm and incessant VT without any apparent correctable cause and despite adequate medical treatment. Repeated ICD shocks within a short time interval, known as an ICD "storm," occur in 10% to 25% of patients. Catheter ablation has a high acute success rate in eliminating the dominant type of VT. Accumulated evidence suggests that acute suppression of clinical VT in electrical storm can be achieved in approximately 90% of patients. However, arrhythmic recurrences are frequent during follow-up.

Catheter ablation also should be considered for patients with frequent premature ventricular complexes (PVCs), nonsustained VTs, or VT that is presumed to cause ventricular dysfunction.[2]

The optimal time of catheter ablation in ICD patients (after multiple ICD interventions or before any ICD intervention) remains unclear. In clinical practice, VT ablation is often not considered until pharmacological options have been exhausted, often after the patient has suffered substantial morbidity from recurrent episodes of VT and ICD shocks. However, recent studies suggest that catheter ablation for VT should generally be considered early in the treatment of patients with recurrent VT, even before initiating antiarrhythmic drug therapy. In fact, catheter ablation was found to reduce VT/VF recurrences and thereby ICD shocks by 43% to 73% when applied prophylactically, that is, before any ICD shock has been delivered. Interestingly, in this patient population the ablation-related mortality rate was 0%, and major complications occurred in 3.8% to 4.7%. Catheter ablation also significantly reduced the rate of hospitalizations for cardiac reasons, and was associated with a trend to fewer deaths in the ablation group during follow-up. The benefit was more pronounced in patients with LVEF of 30% or less.[2,19,30,31]

Table 22-1 lists the indications of ablation for ischemic VT, in accordance with the ACC/AHA/ESC 2006 guidelines for management of patients with ventricular arrhythmias and the prevention of sudden death.[19]

TABLE 22-1 Indications for Ablation of Ischemic Ventricular Tachycardia*

Class I	Patients after MI with an ICD who present with repetitive monomorphic VT that leads to multiple shocks or who present with drug-refractory incessant VT or "electrical storms" that cannot be prevented despite adequate reprogramming of the antitachycardia pacing mode, beta blocker and/or antiarrhythmic drug therapy, or when patients are intolerant of these drugs or do not wish to take them (level C)
	Patients after MI with an ICD who present with repetitive sustained VT, which made mandatory therapy with antiarrhythmic drugs that decreased the rate of VT below an acceptable intervention rate into the range of exercise-induced sinus rhythm despite concomitant beta blocker therapy (level C)
	Patients with bundle branch reentry after MI (level C)
Class IIa	Patients after MI with an ICD who present with infrequent monomorphic VT that has been terminated successfully by more than one electrical shock and that most probably cannot be avoided in the future despite adequate reprogramming of the antitachycardia pacing mode, and where it is difficult to predict whether future events can be avoided by beta blocker and/or antiarrhythmic drug therapy or when patients are not willing to take long-term drugs (level C)
Class IIb	As the sole procedure, that is, without an ICD, in patients after MI who have relatively well-preserved LV function (above 35% to 40%) and in whom VT is monomorphic, relatively slow, and well tolerated; who are considered to have a good long-term prognosis; and who are drug resistant, do not tolerate an antiarrhythmic drug, or do not accept long-term therapy (level C)
	Patients after MI who present with frequent self-terminating monomorphic VT that may cause ICD shock intervention that potentially cannot be avoided by changing the intervention rate of the ICD (level C)
	Patients with markedly reduced longevity and comorbidities (e.g., heart failure, reduced renal function) where VT can either not be prevented by antiarrhythmic drug therapy or drugs have not been tolerated and for whom an ICD would not be indicated because of the overall condition of the patient
	Patients with more than one ICD shock that is causing severe anxiety and psychological distress

*In accordance with the ACC/AHA/ESC 2006 guidelines for management of patients with ventricular arrhythmias and the prevention of sudden death.

ICD = implantable cardioverter-defibrillator; LV = left ventricular; MI = myocardial infarction; VT = ventricular tachycardia.

From Zipes DP, Camm AJ, Borggrefe M, et al: ACC/AHA/ESC 2006 guidelines for management of patients with ventricular arrhythmias and the prevention of sudden cardiac death: a report of the American College of Cardiology/American Heart Association Task Force and the European Society of Cardiology Committee for Practice Guidelines (Writing Committee to Develop Guidelines for Management of Patients with Ventricular Arrhythmias and the Prevention of Sudden Cardiac Death), *J Am Coll Cardiol* 48:e247-e346, 2006.

Electrocardiographic Features

In general, QRS patterns are less accurate in localizing the site of origin of reentrant VTs in patients with prior MI and wall motion abnormalities than they are for focal VTs in patients with normal hearts.[3,32] Nonetheless, the ECG is capable of regionalizing the VT to areas smaller than 15 to 20 cm^2, even in the most abnormal hearts.

The site of origin of VT is the source of electrical activity producing the VT QRS. Although this is a discrete site of impulse formation in automatic and triggered (i.e., focal) rhythms, during reentrant VT it represents the exit site from the diastolic pathway (isthmus) to the myocardium giving rise to the QRS. The pattern of ventricular activation and hence the resultant QRS depends on how the wavefront propagates from the site of origin to the remainder of the heart; this can be totally different during VT than during pacing from the same site in normal sinus rhythm (NSR).

A sophisticated algorithm has been developed using eight different patterns of R wave progression in the precordium in addition to the relationship with prior anterior or inferior MI, axis deviation, and BBB morphology. This algorithm has a predictive accuracy of more than 70% for a specific QRS morphology to identify for a particular endocardial region of 10 cm^2 or less (Fig. 22-2). A recent report indicated that the 12-lead surface ECG characteristics could reliably predict the LV VT exit site region in 71% of clinical VTs without prior knowledge of infarct location. That report described a new algorithm that was used independently of the sustainability of VT and could be applied over a wide range of tachycardia CLs and to patients with posterior or multiple sites of infarction (Figs. 22-3 and 22-4).[33]

ECG Clues to the Underlying Substrate

VTs arising from normal myocardium typically have rapid initial forces, whereas slurring of the initial forces is frequently seen when the VT arises from an area of scar or from the epicardium. Additionally, VTs originating from very diseased hearts usually have lower amplitude complexes than those arising in normal hearts, and the presence of notching of the QRS can be a sign of scar tissue.[3,32]

Whereas QS complexes can be seen in a variety of disorders, the presence of qR, QR, or Qr complexes in related leads is highly suggestive of the presence of an infarct. Sometimes it is easier to recognize the presence of MI during VT than during NSR.

General Principles in Localizing the Origin of Post-Infarction Ventricular Tachycardias

QRS DURATION. QRS duration is affected by the proximity of the VT origin to the septum. Post-MI VTs almost always arise in the LV or interventricular septum.[1,3,12] Septal VTs generally have QRS durations that are narrower than free wall VTs. Additionally, QRS width during VT is affected by the amount of myocardial disease, being wider with poor overall ventricular conduction.[1]

QRS AXIS. A right superior QRS axis suggests apical septal or apical lateral sites of origin, often demonstrating QS in leads I, II, and III and QS or rS in leads V_5 and V_6. A right inferior axis suggests a high basal origin (high LV septum, or high lateral LV). A left inferior axis is occasionally associated with VTs arising from the top of the LV septum. Sometimes, the QRS axis is inappropriate for the exit site. This almost always occurs with large apical infarcts. Typically, discrepancies occur in VTs with LBBB or RBBB with a right or left superior axis. Such discrepancies can be related to abnormalities of conduction out of the area of the reentrant circuit toward the rest of the myocardium.[32]

BUNDLE BRANCH BLOCK PATTERN. VTs with RBBB patterns always arise in the LV, and VTs with LBBB patterns almost always arise in or adjacent to the LV septum. Therefore, LBBB patterns, which all cluster on or adjacent to the septum, have a higher predictive accuracy (regardless of the presence of anterior versus

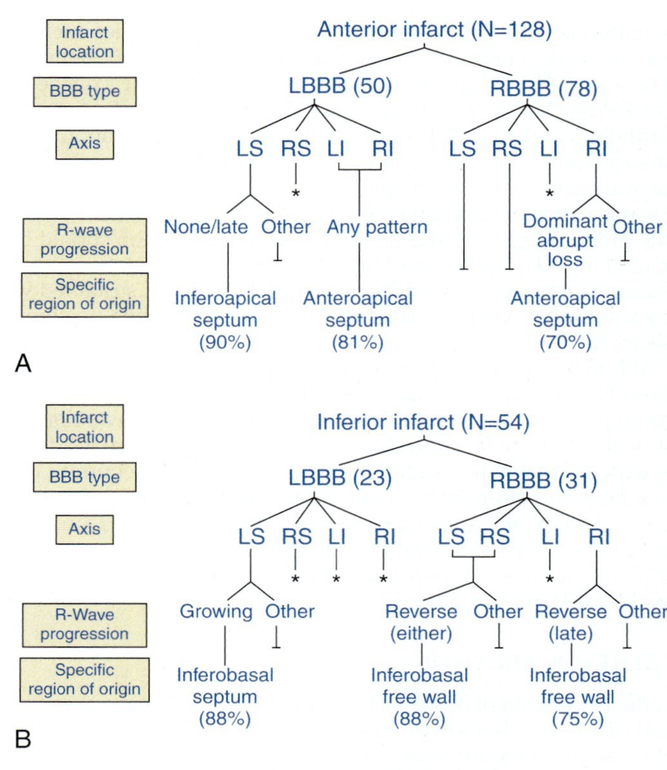

Precordial R-wave progression patterns

PATTERN	V1	V2	V3	V4	V5	V6
Increasing						
None or late						
Regression/growth (not QS)						
Regression/growth (QS)						
Dominant						
Abrupt loss						
Late reverse						
Early reverse						

C

FIGURE 22-2 Algorithm correlating region of origin to 12-lead ECG of ventricular tachycardia (VT), derived from the retrospective analysis. **A,** Anterior infarct-associated VTs. **B,** Inferior infarct-associated VTs. The first branch point is bundle branch block (BBB) configuration, followed by QRS axis and R wave progression. When possible, a specific region of origin is indicated. The number of VTs in each group is indicated in parentheses. A vertical line ending in an asterisk indicates inadequate numbers of VT for analysis; a vertical line terminating in a horizontal bar indicates adequate numbers for analysis, but no specific patterns. **C,** Precordial R wave progression patterns. Eight different patterns are listed, with the number of examples in parentheses. Typical R wave patterns for V_1 through V_6 are shown. I = inferior; L = left; LBBB = left bundle branch block; R = right; RBBB = right bundle branch block; S = superior. *(From Miller JM, Marchlinski FE, Buxton AE, Josephson ME: Relationship between the 12-lead electrocardiogram during ventricular tachycardia and endocardial site of origin in patients with coronary artery disease, Circulation 77:759, 1988.)*

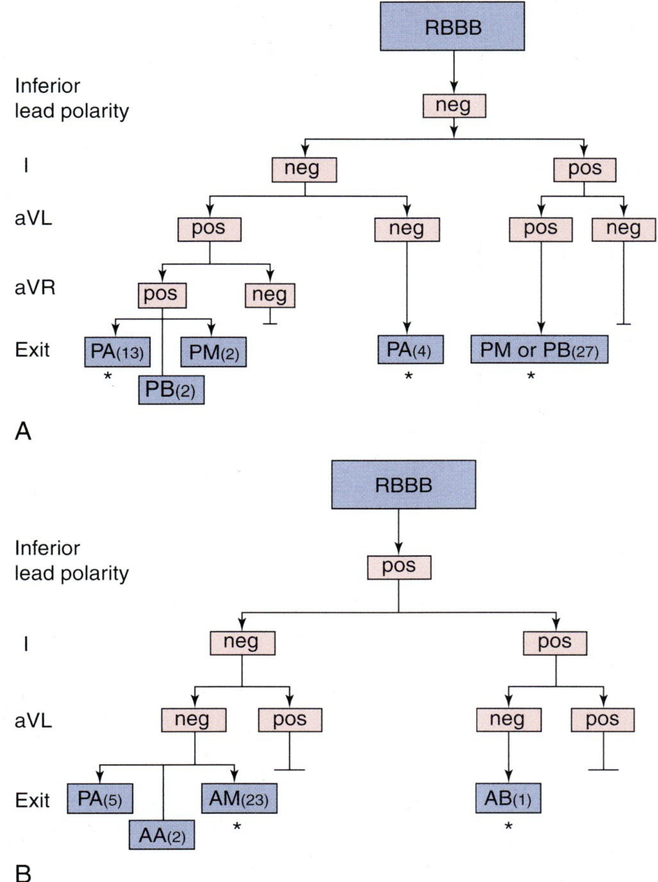

FIGURE 22-3 Algorithm correlating 12-lead ECG morphology of right bundle branch block (RBBB) ventricular tachycardia (VT) with exit site region, derived from retrospective analysis. **A,** VT with negative (neg) polarity in the inferior leads. **B,** VT with positive (pos) polarity in the inferior leads. A vertical line ending a horizontal bar indicates that no VT with this ECG pattern was identified. Exit sites with a positive predictive value (PPV) of at least 70% are marked by asterisks. The numbers of VTs for each ECG pattern and exit site region identified in retrospective analysis are shown in parentheses. AA = anteroapical; AB = anterobasal; AM = midanterior; PA = posteroapical; PB = posterobasal; PM = midposterior. *(From Segal OR, Chow AW, Wong T, et al: A novel algorithm for determining endocardial VT exit site from 12-lead surface ECG characteristics in human, infarct-related ventricular tachycardia, J Cardiovasc Electrophysiol 18:161, 2007.)*

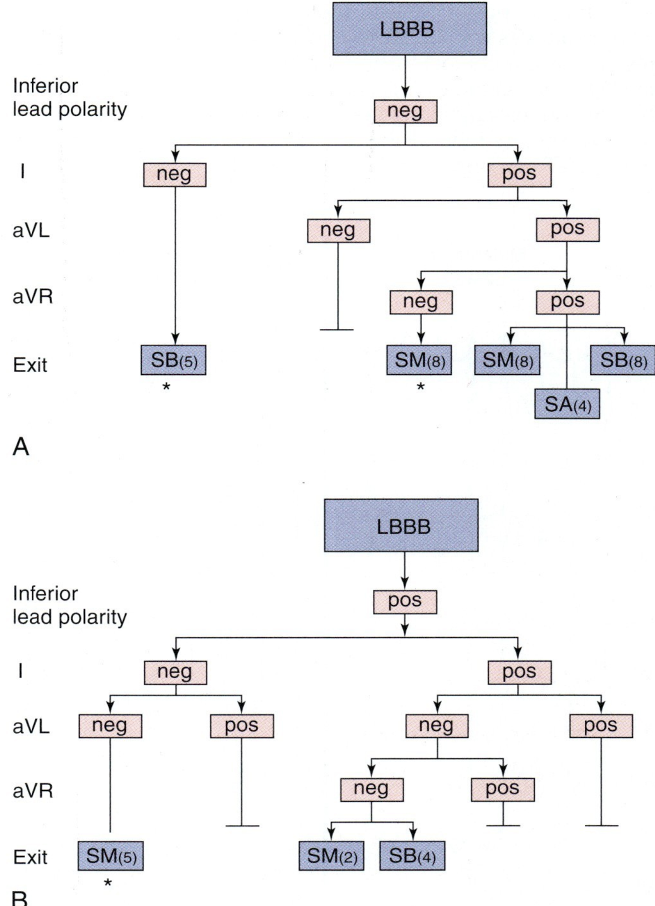

FIGURE 22-4 Algorithm correlating 12-lead ECG morphology of left bundle branch block (LBBB) ventricular tachycardia (VT) with exit site region, derived from retrospective analysis. **A,** VT with negative (neg) polarity in the inferior leads. **B,** VT with positive (pos) polarity in the inferior leads. A vertical line ending with a horizontal bar indicates that no VTs with this ECG pattern were identified. SA = anteroseptal; SB = basal septum; SM = midseptum. Exit sites with a positive predictive value (PPV) of at least 70% are marked by asterisks. Numbers of VTs for each ECG pattern and exit site region identified in retrospective analysis are shown in parentheses. *(From Segal OR, Chow AW, Wong T, et al: A novel algorithm for determining endocardial VT exit site from 12-lead surface ECG characteristics in human, infarct-related ventricular tachycardia, J Cardiovasc Electrophysiol 18:161, 2007.)*

inferior MI) than RBBB patterns, which could be septal or located on the free wall. Most VTs with RBBB patterns associated with inferior MI are clustered in a small region, but are more widely disparate with anterior MI (Figs. 22-5 and 22-6).[3,32]

CONCORDANCE. VTs with positive concordance in all precordial leads arise only at the base of the heart (LV outflow region [LVOT], along the mitral or aortic valves, or in the basal septum), whereas negative concordance is seen only in VTs originating near the apical septum, most commonly seen with anteroseptal MI.[3]

PRESENCE OF QS COMPLEXES. The presence of a QS complex in any lead suggests that the wavefront is propagating away from that site. Therefore, QS complexes in the inferior leads suggest that the activation is originating in the inferior wall, whereas QS complexes in the precordial leads suggest activation moving away from the anterior wall. QS complexes in leads V_2 to V_4 suggest anterior wall origin, QS complexes in leads V_3 to V_5 suggest apical location, and QS complexes in leads V_5 and V_6 suggest lateral wall. The presence of Q waves in leads I, V_1, V_2, and V_6 is seen in VTs with an RBBB pattern originating near the apex, but not those originating in the inferobasal parts of the LV. R waves in leads I, V_1, V_2, and V_6 are specific for VTs with an RBBB or LBBB pattern of posterior origin. Additionally, the presence of Q waves in leads I and V_6 in VTs with an LBBB pattern is seen with apical septal locations, whereas the presence of R waves in leads I and V_6 is associated with inferobasal septal locations.[3,32]

INFERIOR MYOCARDIAL INFARCTION VENTRICULAR TACHYCARDIAS

With inferior MI, most VTs have basal exit sites and thus have relatively preserved precordial R waves (that usually are present in leads V_2 to V_4 with the persistence of an r or R wave through lead V_6), although apical exit sites also occur (Fig. 22-7).[16] In VTs with RBBB, the R waves can persist across the precordium (positive concordance). When the VT originates near the posterior basal septum and when it arises more laterally (or posteriorly), there can be a decrease in the R wave amplitude across the precordium because the infarct can extend to the posterolateral areas (see Fig. 22-5).[34]

Left axis deviation is seen in inferior MI VTs when the exit site is near the septum. The more the VT moves from the midline toward the lateral (i.e., posterior) wall, the more right or superior the axis will become. VTs with LBBB (especially when left axis deviation is present) have a characteristic location at the inferobasal septum (see Fig. 22-6). As the VT axis shifts to a more normal axis, the exit site moves higher up along the septum. Rarely, inferior MI VTs can have exit sites as high as the aortic valve along the septum. Very rarely, the VT can only be ablated from the RV.

The mitral isthmus (between the mitral annulus and inferior infarct scar) contains a critical region of slow conduction in some patients with VT following inferior MI, providing a vulnerable and anatomically localized target for catheter ablation. This critical zone of slow conduction is activated parallel to the mitral annulus in either direction, resulting in two distinct QRS configurations not seen in VTs arising from other sites: LBBB pattern (rS in lead V_1, R

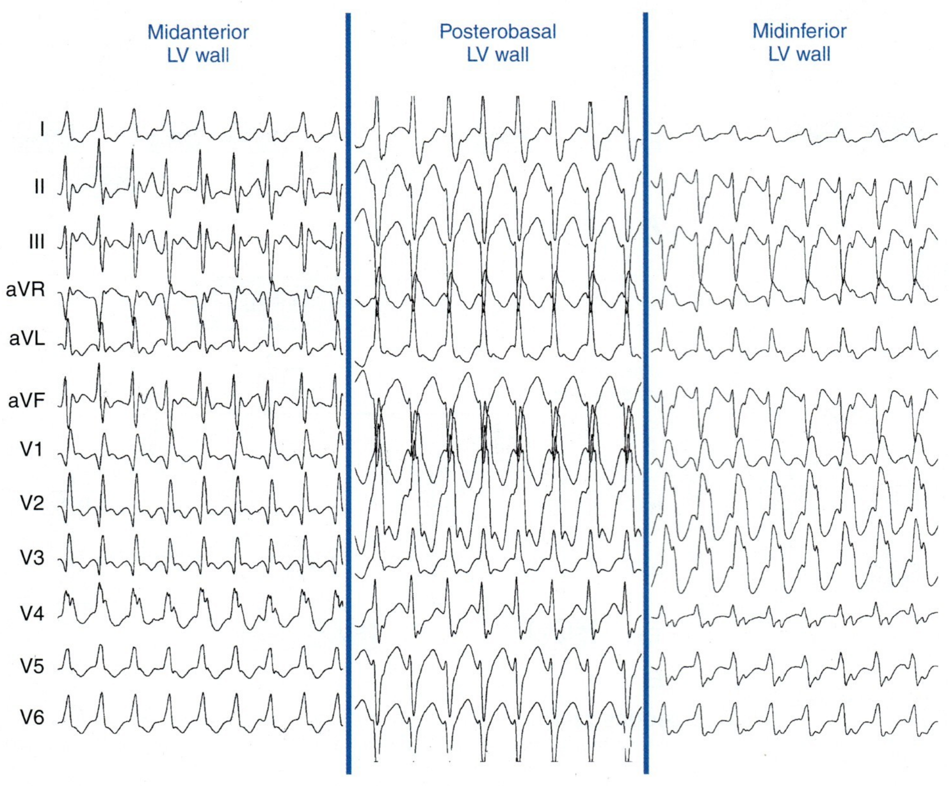

FIGURE 22-5 Surface ECG of sustained monomorphic ventricular tachycardia (SMVT) with right bundle branch block (RBBB) pattern. **Left panel,** Ventricular tachycardia (VT) with RBBB pattern and normal axis in a patient with prior anterior myocardial infarction (MI). The site of origin was mapped to the midanterior left ventricular (LV) wall. Note the qR pattern in leads V_1 to V_3, consistent with anterior infarct. **Middle panel,** VT with RBBB pattern and left superior axis in a patient with prior inferior MI. The site of origin was mapped to the posterobasal LV free wall. **Right panel,** VT with left bundle branch block (LBBB) pattern and left superior axis in a patient with prior inferior MI. The site of origin was mapped to the midinferior LV wall.

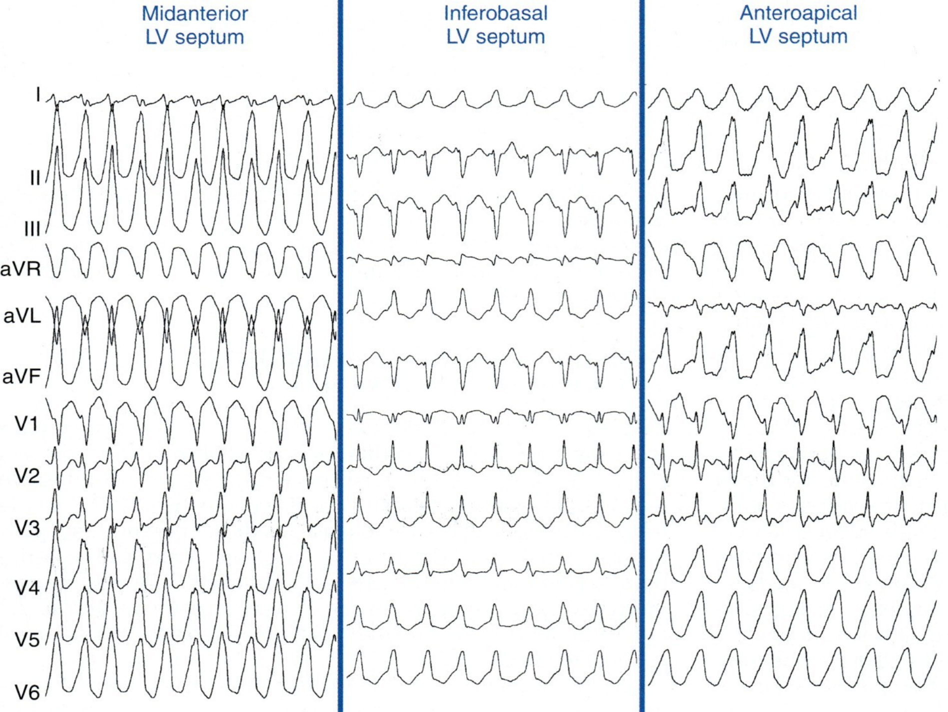

FIGURE 22-6 Surface ECG of sustained monomorphic ventricular tachycardia (SMVT) with left bundle branch block (LBBB) pattern. **Left panel,** Ventricular tachycardia (VT) with LBBB pattern and right inferior axis in a patient with prior anterior myocardial infarction (MI). The site of origin was mapped to the midanterior left ventricular (LV) septum. **Middle panel,** VT with LBBB pattern and left superior axis in a patient with prior inferior MI. The site of origin was mapped to the inferobasal LV septum. **Right panel,** VT with LBBB pattern and left inferior axis in a patient with prior anterior MI. The site of origin was mapped to the anteroapical LV septum.

in lead V_6) with left superior axis, and RBBB pattern (R in lead V_1, QS in lead V_6) and right superior axis.[3,32]

ANTERIOR MYOCARDIAL INFARCTION VENTRICULAR TACHYCARDIAS

Anterior MIs are usually associated with more extensive myocardial damage. Therefore, the accuracy of the ECG in localizing the origin of VTs associated with anterior MI is less than in those with inferior MI.[34]

VTs with LBBB and left axis deviation usually originate from the inferoapical septum, but occasionally there is a discrepancy, with the exit site being more superior than expected for the QRS axis. LBBB VTs associated with anteroseptal MI can present with QS complexes across the precordium (i.e., negative concordance), and they are always associated with a Q wave in leads I and aVL. If an R wave is seen in lead V_1 along with the Q wave in lead aVL, the location of the exit site is more posterior on the septum, closer to the middle third (see Fig. 22-6). VTs with LBBB and right inferior axis arise on the upper half of the mid- or apical septum but occasionally can be off the septum (see Fig. 22-7).[16,32]

RBBB VTs originating from the apex usually have a right and superior axis. Lead V_1 usually has a qR or, occasionally, a monophasic R wave, but there is almost always a QS or QR complex in leads V_2, V_3, and/or V_4. More commonly, when there are QS complexes in leads I, II, and III, there are also QS complexes across the precordium from lead V_2 through V_6. VTs with RBBB and right inferior axis arise on the septum but also can be seen across the apex superiorly on the free wall. In both cases, there is a negative deflection in leads aVR and aVL. VTs with LBBB or RBBB patterns and a marked inferior right axis arise superiorly on what usually is the edge of an anterior aneurysm.[32]

The most difficult VTs to localize are VTs with RBBB and right superior axis associated with anterior MI. QS complexes in the lateral leads (V_4 to V_6) reflect an origin near the apex, regardless of whether it is septal or lateral. It is almost impossible to distinguish VTs arising from the apical septum and the apical free wall based on the ECG alone. It is only when the VT location moves more posterolaterally that a difference can be appreciated as the R wave in lead aVR becomes dominant over the R wave in lead aVF. This is usually associated with a large apical aneurysm, but occasionally can also be seen with a posterolateral MI.[32]

HIGH POSTEROLATERAL MYOCARDIAL INFARCTION VENTRICULAR TACHYCARDIAS

VTs associated with high posterior MI (left circumflex artery territory) are characterized by a prominent R wave in leads V_1 to V_4 and right inferior axis.[32]

Epicardial Ventricular Tachycardias

With all other factors being equal, the epicardial origin of ventricular activation widens the initial part of the QRS complex (pseudo-delta wave). When the initial activation starts in the endocardium, rapid depolarization of the ventricles occurs along the specialized conducting system, resulting in a relatively narrower QRS on the surface ECG and the absence of a pseudo-delta wave. In contrast, when the initial ventricular activation occurs in the epicardium, the intramyocardial delay of conduction produces a slurred initial part of the QRS complex.

Several ECG findings suggest an epicardial origin of the LV VT with an RBBB pattern, and all generally rely on the late engagement of rapidly conducting His-Purkinje fibers by exits on the epicardium: (1) a pseudo-delta wave (measured from the earliest ventricular activation to the earliest fast deflection in any precordial lead) of 34 milliseconds or more has a sensitivity of 83% and a specificity of 95%; (2) a long R-wave peak time in lead V_2 (i.e., an interval from the beginning of the QRS complex to the time of initial downstroke of the R wave after it has peaked [previously known as the *intrinsicoid deflection*]) of at least 85 milliseconds has a sensitivity of 87% and a specificity of 90%; (3) a shortest RS complex duration (measured from the earliest ventricular activation to the nadir of the first S wave in any precordial lead) of 121 milliseconds or more has a sensitivity of 76% and a specificity of 85%; and (4) a QRS duration of more than

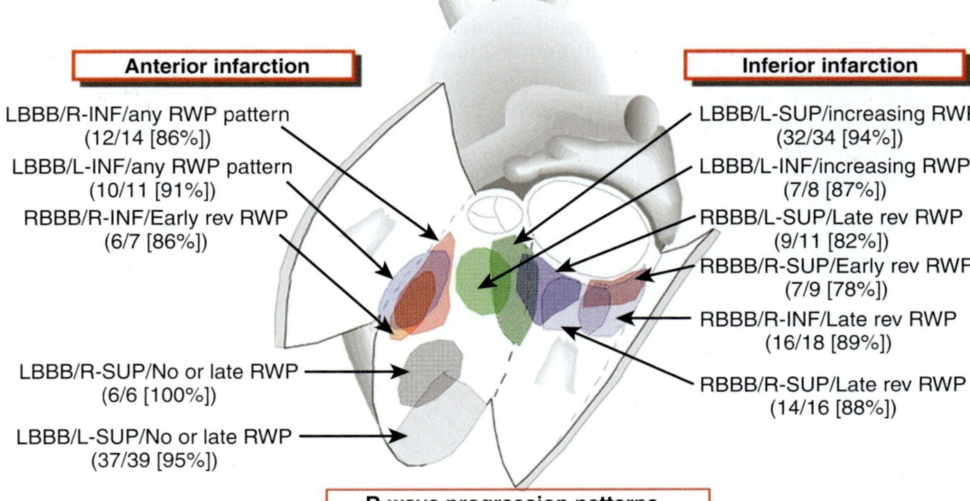

FIGURE 22-7 Scheme of regions of ventricular tachycardia exit sites in post-infarction patients. INF = inferior axis; L = left; LBBB = left bundle branch block; R = right; RBBB = right bundle branch block; RWP = precordial R-wave progression pattern (diagrammed in table at bottom); SUP = superior axis. *(From Miller JM, Scherschel JA: Catheter ablation of ventricular tachycardia: skill versus technology, Heart Rhythm 6:S86-S90, 2009, with permission.)*

200 milliseconds (Fig. 22-8). These parameters were assessed in patients without MI, however.[34]

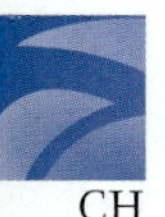

CH 22

Electrophysiological Testing

Induction of Tachycardia

RECOMMENDED STIMULATION PROTOCOLS

For evaluation of ventricular arrhythmias, multipolar catheters are typically positioned in the high RA, the HB position, and the RV apex. Recording the His potential during VT is important to differential BBR VT from myocardial VT. The most commonly used stimulation protocol applies pacing output at twice the diastolic threshold current and a pulse width of 1 to 2 milliseconds. Single VESs during NSR and at pacing drive CLs of 600 and 400 milliseconds are delivered, first from the RV apex and then from the RV outflow tract (RVOT). The prematurity of extrastimuli is increased until refractoriness or induction of sustained VT is achieved. Long-short cycle sequences may be tested. If these measures fail to induce VT, double and then triple VESs are used in the same manner. Because a VES with a very short coupling interval is more likely to induce VF as opposed to monomorphic VT, it may be reasonable to limit the prematurity of the VESs to a minimum of 180 milliseconds when studying patients for whom only inducible SMVT would be considered a positive endpoint. If VT still cannot be induced, rapid ventricular pacing is started at a CL of 400 milliseconds, gradually decreasing the pacing CL until 1:1 ventricular capture is lost or a pacing CL of 220 milliseconds is reached. Repeating the protocol at other pacing drive CLs, at other RV or LV stimulation sites, and/or after administration of isoproterenol or procainamide is then attempted.[3,19]

An alternative stimulation protocol uses a shorter pacing drive CL (350 milliseconds) and a reverse order of the pacing drive CL (i.e., starting the stimulation protocol at 350, then 400, and then 600 milliseconds). This *accelerated protocol* has been shown in one report to reduce the number of protocol steps and duration of time required to induce monomorphic VT by an average of more than 50% and improves the specificity of programmed electrical stimulation without impairing the yield of monomorphic VT.

Another proposed stimulation protocol exclusively uses four VESs; at no point are one, two, or three VESs used. At each basic drive train pacing CL, programmed electrical stimulation is initiated with coupling intervals of 290, 280, 270, and 260 milliseconds for the first through fourth VES. The coupling intervals of the VESs are then shortened simultaneously in 10-millisecond steps until S_2 (the first VES) falls during the refractory period or a 200-millisecond coupling interval is reached. If S_2 is refractory at 290 milliseconds, all extrastimuli are lengthened by 30 milliseconds, and programmed electrical stimulation is then initiated. This *six-step protocol* was tested in a single report and was shown to improve the specificity and efficiency of programmed electrical stimulation without compromising the yield of inducibility of monomorphic VT in patients with coronary artery disease.

NUMBER OF VENTRICULAR EXTRASTIMULI. The sensitivity of programmed electrical stimulation to initiate SMVT increases with increasing the number of VESs used, but at the expense of decreasing specificity. The use of three VESs seems optimal because it offers the highest sensitivity associated with an acceptable specificity. More aggressive stimulation is likely to produce nonspecific responses, usually polymorphic VT or VF.

In the majority of patients with coronary artery disease undergoing EP testing for risk stratification for SCD, triple VESs are typically required for VT induction. Sustained VT induced with triple VESs is usually faster and more likely to result in hemodynamic compromise. Despite these differences, long-term prognosis does not appear to be affected by the mode of induction. In a recent report, there was no difference in the incidence of arrhythmic death or all-cause mortality at 2 years between patients induced with burst pacing, one or two VESs, and those induced with three VESs.[21]

When SMVT is studied, the use of four VESs may be considered. However, when a patient resuscitated from cardiac arrest is studied, four VESs should not be used because the likelihood of inducing a nonspecific response (polymorphic VT/VF) is far higher than that of inducing SMVT (10:1). Triple VESs are required to induce SMVT in 20% to 40% of patients presenting with SMVT and in 40% to 60% of patients presenting with cardiac arrest.[3]

PACING DRIVE CYCLE LENGTH. The use of at least two pacing drive CLs (typically 600 and 400 milliseconds) is required to enhance the sensitivity of induction of SMVT in patients presenting with sustained VT of any morphology or those with cardiac arrest. VES at shorter or longer CLs or even in NSR may be necessary to initiate VT in some patients. Abrupt changes in CL can also facilitate VT induction. The CL used can also influence the number and prematurity of VESs required to initiate VT. Rapid ventricular pacing has a low yield in VT initiation.[3]

In 5% of patients with SMVT, and in less than 5% of those with cardiac arrest, VT can be initiated only with VES during NSR. On the other hand, most VTs that can be induced during NSR can also be induced during ventricular pacing or VESs delivered after a pacing drive.

SITE OF VENTRICULAR STIMULATION. In contrast to automatic or triggered activity VT, in which the stimulation site has no effect on VT inducibility, reentrant VT can demonstrate absolute or relative site specificity for initiation. In the majority of cases, development of functional unidirectional block is a prerequisite for initiation of macroreentrant VT; however, during VES, functional block may not always develop despite short coupling intervals, suggesting that formation of functional block is dependent on direction of activation following stimulation.[6] Therefore, the use of at least two sites of stimulation enhances the ability to induce VT.

If triple VESs are delivered only from the RV apex, 10% to 20% of patients will require the use of a second RV or LV pacing site for initiation of SMVT (less than 5% require an LV site). If double

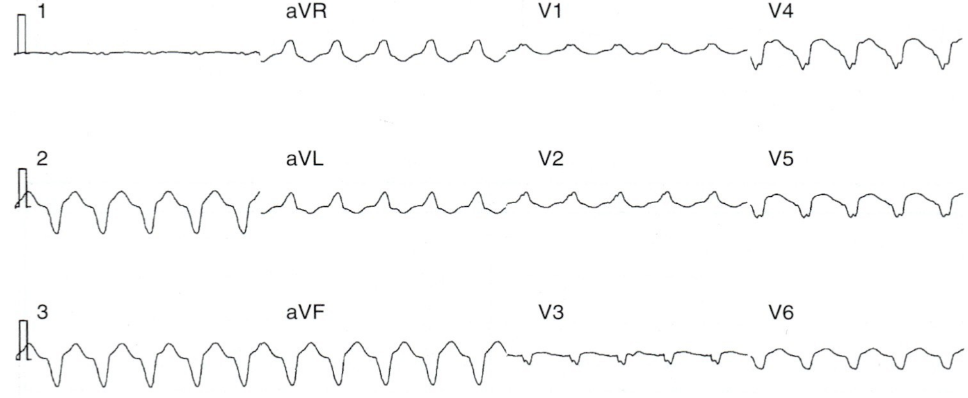

FIGURE 22-8 ECG of post-myocardial infarction ventricular tachycardia that required epicardial ablation. Note delayed QRS upstroke in V_2 and delayed S wave downstroke (pseudo-delta wave) and long RS interval in V_3 and V_4.

VESs are used, 20% to 30% will require a second pacing site (10% require an LV site). Because the number of VESs required for initiation can differ depending on the site of stimulation, which occurs in approximately 20% of patients with SMVT, the site that allows the use of the fewest number of VESs is preferred to avoid nonspecific responses. Thus, it is preferable to stimulate from both the RV apex and the RVOT at each drive CL and with the number of VESs before proceeding to more aggressive stimulation.[3]

If stimulation from the RV apex and RVOT fails to initiate VT, stimulation from the LV may be used. However, the yield is low (2% to 5%) for patients with SMVT and somewhat higher in patients with cardiac arrest.

Atrial extrastimulation (AES) can initiate VT in approximately 5% of patients with SMVT. Usually, those VTs can also be initiated by VES, are usually slower, and are reproducibly initiated over a broad zone of VES coupling intervals. Initiation with AES is more common in patients without coronary artery disease.

PACING CURRENT OUTPUT. Increasing the current (more than twice the diastolic threshold current or pulse width more than 2 milliseconds) produces only a small increase in sensitivity of initiating SMVT (more than 5%), but this is outweighed by a significant decrease in specificity and increase in the incidence of VF. The use of currents more than 5 mA is not recommended.[3]

ISOPROTERENOL. Isoproterenol has a low yield in facilitating induction in patients with coronary artery disease and SMVT and is more useful in initiation of exercise-related VTs or triggered activity outflow tract VTs.

REPRODUCIBILITY OF VENTRICULAR TACHYCARDIA INITIATION

More than 90% of patients with clinical SMVT will have inducible VT, regardless of the underlying pathology, with the exception of exercise-induced VT. Patients with cardiac arrest or nonsustained VT have a lower incidence of inducibility; inducibility is higher in patients with coronary artery disease.

SMVT can be reproducibly initiated from day to day and year to year, especially in patients with coronary artery disease. However, the exact mode of initiation is not necessarily reproducible. Once SMVT is initiated, it is easier to reinitiate by repeating the same stimulation protocol that was initially successful, either longitudinally (by repeating the entire protocol) or horizontally (by repeating each coupling interval).[3]

While reproducibility of sustained VT can be variable when comparing induction during the initial month post-MI with subsequent months, induction of any sustained VT in the more chronic phase of MI is highly reproducible over both short-term and extended time intervals. However, a change in the number of extrastimuli required for VT reinduction is reported in 30% to 70% of patients, and is more common as the time interval between studies increases. Similar inconsistencies are reported in the exact QRS morphology and CL of induced VTs during repeated testing. These data confirm that the substrate for chronic post-MI inducible VT per se can be highly stable for up to several years in the absence of major changes in clinical status. However, the mode of induction and VT characteristics demonstrate substantial variability; therefore, it is improbable that such features would predict long-term outcome.[35]

RELATIONSHIP OF VENTRICULAR EXTRASTIMULUS COUPLING INTERVAL AND PACING CYCLE LENGTH TO THE ONSET OF VENTRICULAR TACHYCARDIA

Conduction delay is required for the initiation of reentrant rhythms; thus, an inverse relationship between the coupling interval of the VES initiating the VT or the pacing train CL and the interval from the VES to the first VT complex favors reentry. In contrast, a linear relationship of the pacing CL or VES coupling interval to the interval to the first VT complex and initial CL of the VT favors triggered activity. In reentrant VT, the initial CL reflects conduction through the VT circuit, which in the absence of exit block should demonstrate the same or longer CL as the remaining VT cycles, depending on whether any conduction delay is produced in the circuit on initiation.[3]

ENDPOINTS OF PROGRAMMED ELECTRICAL STIMULATION

INDUCTION OF CLINICAL SUSTAINED MONOMORPHIC VENTRICULAR TACHYCARDIA. Induction of SMVT is very specific, especially with a VES coupling interval of more than 240 milliseconds, and only occurs in patients with spontaneous VT, cardiac arrest, or an arrhythmogenic substrate. In patients who had spontaneous VT prior to the EP study, the endpoint of programmed electrical stimulation should be induction of the clinical arrhythmia or the assumed arrhythmia. Clinical VT is defined as an inducible SMVT that matches the 12-lead ECG QRS morphology and approximate CL of the patient's documented, spontaneously occurring SMVT. Nonclinical VTs are defined as inducible SMVTs that were not previously known to have occurred spontaneously.[2]

INDUCTION OF MULTIPLE SUSTAINED MONOMORPHIC VENTRICULAR TACHYCARDIAS. The majority (85%) of patients with post-MI VT have more than one VT morphology. Even in patients presenting with a single SMVT, multiple distinct uniform VTs may be induced in the EP laboratory, especially during antiarrhythmic therapy. Multiple VT morphologies are defined as two or more inducible VTs having at least one of the following: (1) contralateral BBB patterns; (2) a frontal plane axis of 30 degrees or more divergent; (3) marked differences in individual ECG leads recorded from the same electrode locations; (4) a precordial transition zone in one or more leads or a different dominant deflection in more than one precordial lead; and/or (5) a different tachycardia CL (more than 100 milliseconds for VTs with a similar morphology). A change in VT morphology need not reflect a change in a reentrant circuit or site of impulse formation but may merely reflect a change in the overall pattern of ventricular activation. In some cases, pacing can reverse the direction of wavefront propagation within the same reentrant loop. Approximately 85% of multiple morphologically distinct SMVTs arise from the same region of the heart (i.e., have closely located exit sites or shared components of an isthmus or diastolic pathway).[3]

Multiple uniform VTs inducible in the EP laboratory are of clinical significance because the distinction between clinical and nonclinical is often uncertain. Clinically, the ECG of spontaneous VTs terminated by an ICD or emergency medical technicians is often not available. Even when available, differences in ECG lead placement, patient position, and antiarrhythmic drugs can influence the similarity between two episodes of VT that arise from the same circuit. Additionally, the presence of multiple VT morphologies might have been overlooked because of the lack of 12-lead ECGs obtained during multiple spontaneous episodes on a variety of different antiarrhythmic agents. The use of single-lead rhythm strips to record VT has been a major misleading factor suggesting that there is only one VT. The minimal number of ECG leads required to discern differences between different VT origins or circuits is not clear. The VT CL alone is influenced by antiarrhythmic drugs and can be similar for different VTs or may be different for VTs originating from the same region, and is therefore unreliable as a sole indicator of clinical VT. Of note, inducible VTs never seen spontaneously in the preablation state can occur spontaneously following ablation of the clinical VT.

Therefore, the term *clinical VT* should be reserved for induced VTs that are known to have the same 12-lead ECG QRS morphology and approximate CL as a spontaneous VT. Other VTs should be designated as *presumptive clinical* or *previously undocumented* VT morphology.[2]

INDUCTION OF POLYMORPHIC VENTRICULAR TACHYCARDIA OR VENTRICULAR FIBRILLATION. When EP testing is performed in patients presenting with SMVT, polymorphic VT and VF must be considered as nonspecific responses. Both sustained and nonsustained polymorphic VT and VF can be induced, even

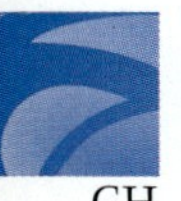

in normal subjects. In general, induction of VF requires multiple VESs delivered at shorter coupling intervals (usually less than 180 milliseconds) than induction of SMVT. On the other hand, induction of polymorphic VT or VF in a patient who presents with cardiac arrest can have a different implication. Because cardiac arrest can be initiated by a polymorphic VT, the induction of polymorphic VT in this patient population can be significant. Therefore, although doubt will always exist, reproducible polymorphic VT induction is treated as a possible indicator of the clinical arrhythmia. Features that suggest that a polymorphic VT can be mechanistically meaningful are reproducible initiation of the same polymorphic VT template, especially from different stimulation sites; inducibility with relatively mild stimulation (single or double VESs); and transformation of the polymorphic VT to SMVT by procainamide. The induction of any arrhythmia (SMVT, polymorphic VT, or VF) in the setting of a recent MI (less than 1 month) may not have clinical significance.[3]

INDUCTION OF VERY FAST VENTRICULAR TACHYCARDIA. The induction of VT with a CL longer than 230 milliseconds is predictive of recurrent ventricular arrhythmia in high-risk patients, such as those with prior MI and reduced LVEF (≤40%), ischemic cardiomyopathy presenting with syncope, resuscitated cardiac arrest, or asymptomatic nonsustained VT. In up to 20% of patients undergoing EP testing, VT with a CL ranging from 200 to 250 milliseconds may be inducible. Although a limited number of studies have closely and specifically examined long-term outcomes of this group of patients, and although previous large ICD trials, such as MADIT and MUSTT, excluded such patients if this arrhythmia was induced by more than two VESs, there is a growing body of evidence that this induced arrhythmia is of sufficient clinical importance that it should no longer be considered a nonspecific finding of EP testing, as it poses a significant risk of spontaneous ventricular arrhythmia or SCD over long-term follow-up. This risk appears equivalent to that of patients with inducible VT with a CL of 251 to 320 milliseconds, and markedly worse than that of patients who are noninducible, have inducible VF, or ventricular flutter (CL <200 milliseconds). These findings seem to be consistent regardless of the mode of induction of VT (with two or fewer, three or fewer, or four extrastimuli), or measured LVEF (≤30% or between 31% and 40%).[35]

Tachycardia Features

HIS BUNDLE ACTIVATION

NO VISIBLE HIS POTENTIAL DURING VENTRICULAR TACHYCARDIA. The His potential cannot be observed during VT in many patients, likely because the retrograde His potential is masked by ventricular activation or because of suboptimal catheter position. A proper HB catheter position can be verified by observation of the immediate appearance of the His potential on termination of the VT, the disappearance of the His potential on initiation of VT, or the sudden appearance of the His potential when spontaneous or induced supraventricular beats capture the HB (with or without ventricular capture) during VT. Additionally, when complete ventricular–His bundle (VH) block is present, dissociated His potentials will be observed.[3]

VISIBLE HIS POTENTIAL DURING VENTRICULAR TACHYCARDIA. His potentials can be recorded during VT in approximately 80% of patients. When the His potential is visible during VT, it is often difficult to determine whether the recorded His potential is anterograde or retrograde, and whether an apparent His potential is actually a right bundle branch (RB) potential. Recording the RB or left bundle branch (LB) potentials to demonstrate that their activation precedes HB activation during VT, and HB pacing producing a longer HV interval than the one noted during VT, usually helps clarify the situation.[3]

In patients with coronary artery disease, the relative timing of the retrograde His potential in the QRS depends on how quickly the His-Purkinje system (HPS) is engaged and how slowly the impulse reaches the ventricle to produce the QRS. Thus, depending on the relative conduction time up the HPS versus through the slowly conducting muscle to give rise to the QRS, the His potential can occur before, during, or after the QRS. The His potential can occasionally occur before ventricular activation (with a His bundle–ventricular [HV] interval during VT shorter than that during NSR; Fig. 22-9) and can also occur just after the onset of ventricular activation (with a VH interval; Fig. 22-10). The occurrence of an HV interval (i.e., with the His potential preceding the QRS onset) shorter than that during NSR (in the absence of preexcitation) or a VH interval (i.e., with the His potential following the QRS onset) implies the presence of retrograde HB activation; it further implies that retrograde conduction from the exit of VT (defined by the onset of the QRS) to the HB is less than the anterograde conduction time over the HPS to activate the ventricle.[1] Engagement of the HPS, when present, can allow for more rapid activation of the myocardium, which in turn results in a narrower QRS. Some have suggested that the site of origin of such VTs is within the HPS (i.e., fascicular VTs), although proof that such VTs originate from the fascicles and differ from other forms of VT is often lacking. The retrograde His potential appears to reflect passive activation of the HPS, rather than involvement of the HPS in the reentrant circuit. This concept is supported by several observations. HB deflections can appear intermittently (typically in a 2:1 or 3:2 fashion, and occasionally in a Wenckebach periodicity), and changes in the VH interval can occur without changes in the tachycardia

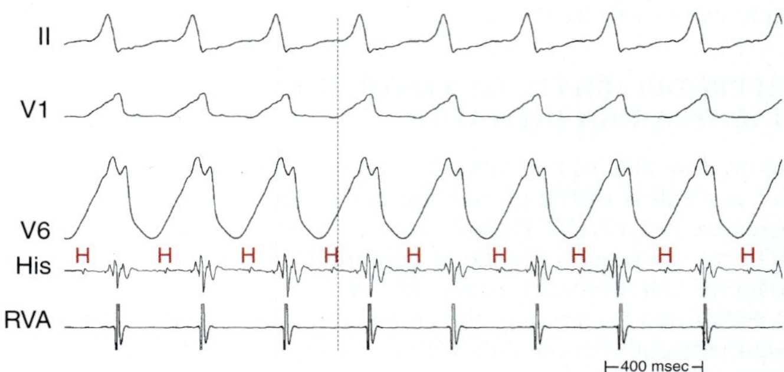

FIGURE 22-9 Ventricular tachycardia with short constant His bundle (HB)–ventricular (HV) interval, consistent with early retrograde activation of the HB.

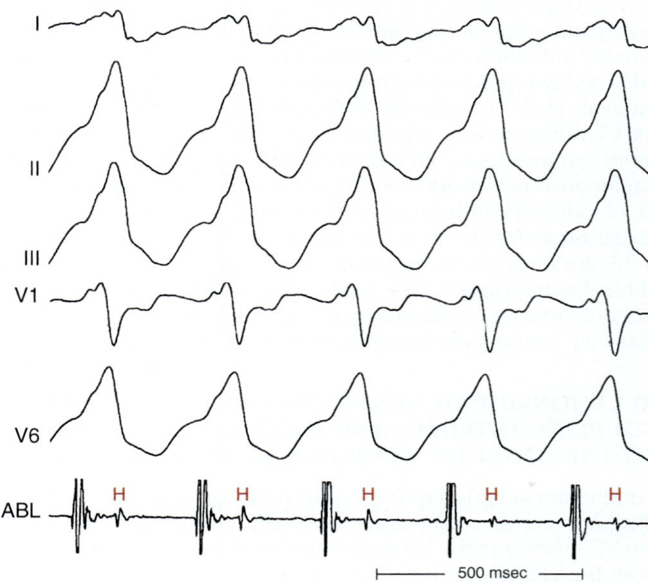

FIGURE 22-10 Ventricular tachycardia with a constant ventricular–His bundle (VH) interval, consistent with retrograde activation of the His bundle (HB). HB activation is recorded by the ablation catheter positioned in the left ventricular outflow tract.

CL (Fig. 22-11). In fact, marked changes in the tachycardia CL can be present with no changes in the VH interval. Furthermore, AES or atrial pacing can result in anterograde capture of the HB in the presence or absence of ventricular capture or fusion beats. Such an event, linking atrial activation to the HB deflection, proves that HB deflections are caused by anterograde activation and are unrelated to maintenance of the VT in the vast majority of cases.[3]

The mere presence of a His potential before the QRS with a normal HV interval is not absolutely reliable evidence that the tachycardia is a supraventricular tachycardia (SVT). The HV interval during VT is usually less than that during NSR; hence, if infranodal conduction delay is present during NSR, the VT can exist in the presence of an apparently normal HV interval (i.e., 35 to 55 milliseconds), but will be less than that during NSR. In post-MI VT, because ventricular activation is occurring in diastole (albeit slow enough not to be apparent on the surface ECG), the HPS could be activated during this time, giving rise to a short or possibly normal HV interval during the VT. The time to conduct retrogradely to the HB can theoretically be less than the time required to exit from the VT circuit and produce the onset of the QRS, thereby producing an HV interval. Such VTs, which are rare, have a narrow QRS. BBR VT can also give rise to an HV interval that is longer than that during NSR.

For wide complex tachycardias with the His potential preceding the QRS, an HV interval that is shorter during tachycardia than during NSR suggests VT or preexcited SVT (see Fig. 18-3), whereas an HV interval during tachycardia that is equal to or longer than that during NSR suggests SVT with aberrancy (see Fig. 18-24), BBR VT (see Fig. 26-3), or, rarely, other VTs. A changing AH interval, failure to observe anterograde His potential during VT with AV dissociation, or both suggests the presence of retrograde conduction with concealment in the AVN.

RIGHT VENTRICULAR APICAL LOCAL ACTIVATION TIME

In the setting of apical MI, VT with an RBBB pattern and R/S ratio in lead V_1 more than 1 is common, but lateral versus septal surface ECG QRS morphologies significantly overlap, with variable early R wave progression and a similar frontal plane axis. Assessing the activation time to a fixed reference endocardial recording at the RV apex can help regionalize a septal versus lateral origin for such VTs. For RBBB-type VT in the setting of an apical infarct, the QRS-to-RV apical activation time is consistently less than 100 milliseconds for an apical LV septal origin and more than 125 milliseconds for a lateral apical origin. The same values for the QRS-to-RV apical activation time will also help identify a septal versus lateral wall origin in the setting of prior nonapical infarcts.

Diagnostic Maneuvers during Tachycardia

The response of VT to programmed stimulation can be studied only for SMVT. Nonsustained VT is too short and unpredictable in duration to allow reliable evaluation. Polymorphic VT is invariably associated with rapid hemodynamic collapse. Also, SMVT must be well tolerated (tachycardia CL usually longer than 280 milliseconds) and must have a stable CL to evaluate the response to stimulation. Fast, unstable SMVT usually can be slowed by antiarrhythmic drugs (e.g., procainamide) to permit evaluation by programmed stimulation.

VENTRICULAR EXTRASTIMULATION DURING VENTRICULAR TACHYCARDIA

Initially, a single VES is delivered at a coupling interval 10 to 20 milliseconds shorter than the tachycardia CL. The coupling interval is then gradually decreased by 5- to 10-millisecond decrements, until the local effective refractory period (ERP) is reached. The RV apex is used as the initial site of stimulation. Stimulation from other sites (RVOT and LV) also can be used to gain information regarding the site specificity of a given response. The return CL is analyzed to evaluate whether the VES has influenced the VT in terms of resetting, ability and pattern of termination, and site specificity for stimulation affecting the VT.[3]

If resetting or termination of VT is not observed with single VESs, stimulation is repeated using double VESs. The first VES is delivered at a coupling interval 20 milliseconds greater than the longest coupling interval at which a single VES resets the VT, or 20 milliseconds above the local ERP if a single VES fails to interact with the VT. The second VES is delivered at a coupling interval equal to the tachycardia CL, and then this coupling interval is progressively decreased in 5- to 10-millisecond decrements until the local ERP is reached. The use of double VESs allows comparable coupling intervals to reach the circuit at a greater relative degree of prematurity and ability to influence the VT than if the same coupling interval were used for a single VES. By this methodology, only a single VES interacts with the circuit; if the two VESs are delivered such that each VES interacts with the site of impulse formation, interpretation of the response would then be difficult. Thus, the first VES is delivered so that it would not interact with the circuit but would help the second VES to do so.[3]

The response of VT to VES is evaluated for manifest or concealed perpetuation, resetting with or without fusion, and termination.

MANIFEST PERPETUATION. Manifest perpetuation is said to be present when the VES fails to influence the VT, resulting in a full compensatory pause surrounding the VES. Factors influencing the ability of the VES to interact with the VT include tachycardia CL, local ventricular ERP at the stimulation site, and distance between the stimulation site and VT circuit. The tachycardia CL and duration of the excitable gap are the most important factors; the faster the VT (especially with CLs less than 300 milliseconds) and the shorter the duration of the reentrant circuit excitable gap, the more difficult it is for the VES to enter the VT circuit. Local ERP at the stimulation site and at the site of impulse formation also can limit the prematurity with which the VES can be introduced.

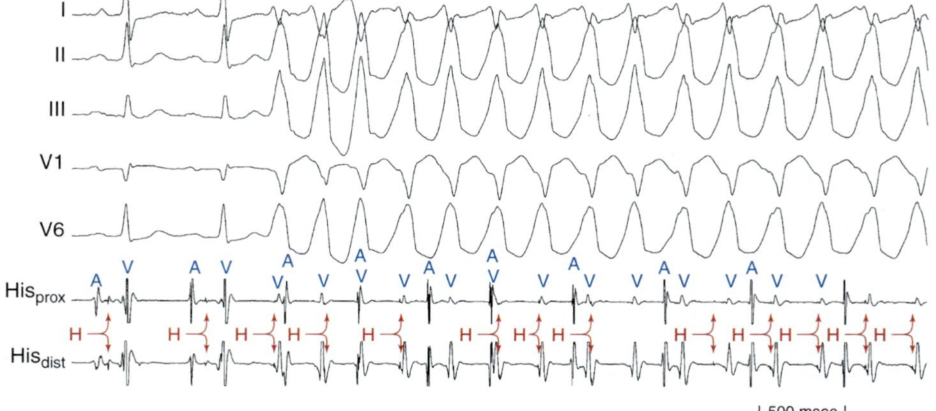

FIGURE 22-11 Ventricular tachycardia (VT) with variable relationship between ventricular and His bundle (HB) activation. HB catheter position is verified by observation of His potentials during normal sinus rhythm (NSR) at left. His potentials are observed intermittently during VT, with variable relationship to the QRS complexes, suggesting that the His-Purkinje system is not an essential part of the VT circuit.

Also, the farther the stimulation site is from the VT circuit, the more difficult it is for the VES to reach the circuit with adequate prematurity.

Failure of a VES to affect the VT circuit helps demonstrate the extent of the ventricular myocardium that is *not* required for the VT. Thus, the ability to capture significant portions of the ventricle by the VES without affecting the VT suggests that those captured areas are not required for the VT circuit. Similarly, intermittent capture of the HPS during VT suggests that it also is not necessary to maintain the VT, regardless of where the His potential is located relative to the QRS during the VT. In an analogous fashion, sinus captures (occurring spontaneously or in response to atrial stimulation) may occur without influencing the VT. The demonstration that neither the proximal HPS nor the majority of the ventricles are required to sustain the VT suggests that the VT circuit must occupy a relatively small and electrocardiographically silent area of the heart.[3]

CONCEALED PERPETUATION. Concealed perpetuation implies that the VES not only fails to influence the VT circuit, but also is followed by a pause that exceeds the tachycardia CL or that is occasionally interrupted by a sinus capture before the next VT beat. Such pauses are a form of functional exit block, because the VT impulse is unable to exit the circuit and depolarize the ventricles that have just been activated by the VES (Fig. 22-12).[3]

RESETTING. Resetting is the advancement (acceleration) of VT by a timed VES with a pause that is less than fully compensatory before resumption of the VT (Fig. 22-13). The first return VT complexes should have the same morphology and CL as the VT before the VES, regardless of whether a single or multiple extrastimuli are used.

The introduction of a single VES (S_2) during VT yields a return cycle (S_2-V_3) if the VT is not terminated. If S_2 does not affect the VT circuit, the coupling interval (V_1-S_2) plus the return cycle (S_2-V_3) will be equal to twice the VT cycle ($2 \times V_1V_1$)—that is, a fully compensatory pause will occur (see Fig. 3-14). Resetting of VT occurs when a less than fully compensatory pause occurs (by at least 20 milliseconds). In this situation, V_1-S_2 + S_2-V_3 will be less than $2 \times V_1V_1$, as measured from the surface ECG. Tachycardia CL oscillation should be taken into account when the return cycle is evaluated. To account for any tachycardia CL oscillation, at least a 20-millisecond shortening of the return cycle is required to demonstrate resetting. When more than a single VES is used, the relative prematurity should be corrected by subtracting the coupling interval(s) from the spontaneous tachycardia cycles when the VESs are delivered.[3]

To reset a reentrant VT, the stimulated wavefront must reach the reentrant circuit, encounter excitable tissue within the circuit (i.e., enter the excitable gap of the reentrant circuit), collide in the antidromic (retrograde) direction with the previous tachycardia beat, and continue in the orthodromic (anterograde) direction to exit at an earlier than expected time and perpetuate the tachycardia (see Fig. 3-15). If the VES encounters a fully excitable tissue, which commonly occurs in reentrant tachycardias with large excitable gaps, the tachycardia is advanced (i.e., made to occur earlier) by the extent to which the stimulated wavefront arrives at the entrance site prematurely. If the tissue is partially excitable, which can occur in reentrant tachycardias with small or partially excitable gaps, or even in circuits with large excitable gaps when the VES is very premature, the stimulated wavefront will encounter some conduction delay in the orthodromic direction within the circuit. As a consequence, the degree of advancement of the next tachycardia beat will depend on both the degree of prematurity of the VES and the degree of slowing of its conduction within the circuit. Therefore, the reset tachycardia beat can be early, on time, or later than expected.

EFFECT OF NUMBER OF VENTRICULAR EXTRASTIMULI. Approximately 60% of VTs can be reset with a single VES and 85% with double VESs using RV pacing. All VTs reset by a single VES can also be reset by double VESs. Double VESs produce resetting over a longer range of coupling intervals and should therefore be used to characterize the excitable gap of the VT more fully. The resetting zone is approximately 70 milliseconds for most VTs, but is usually longer in those VTs reset by both single and double VESs than those requiring double VESs. Resetting zones in response to single VESs usually occupy 10% to 20% of the VT cycle. This is increased to approximately 25% in response to double VESs, but occasionally can exceed 30%, even in response to a single VES. VTs with LBBB morphology are less likely to require double VESs for resetting than VTs with RBBB morphology, regardless of the

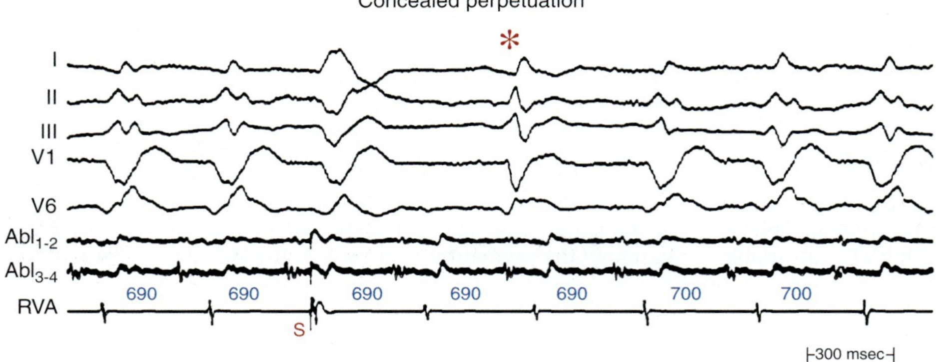

FIGURE 22-12 Concealed perpetuation in ventricular tachycardia (VT). For reentrant slow VT (cycle length = 690 milliseconds), a single ventricular extrastimulus (VES) is introduced (S) that seems to terminate the VT; a conducted sinus complex (*) follows and then VT recurs. However, inspection of the distal ablation (Abl_{1-2}) electrogram shows that VT never actually terminated, because the mid-diastolic electrogram continues unperturbed by the VES.

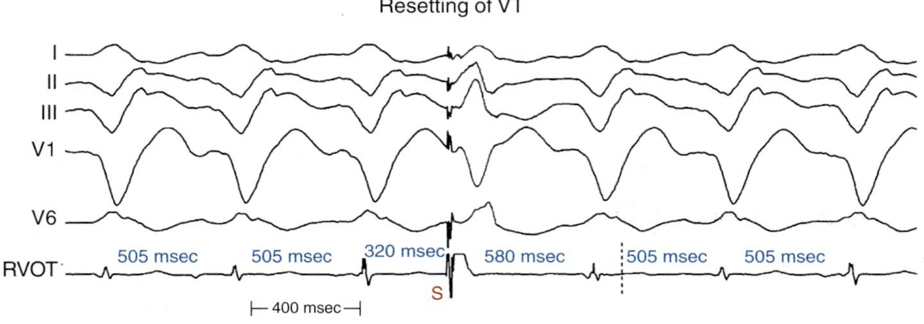

FIGURE 22-13 Resetting of ventricular tachycardia (VT). A single ventricular extrastimulus from the right ventricular outflow tract (RVOT) captures the ventricle during VT and causes the subsequent QRS to occur earlier than anticipated (dashed line), indicating resetting.

frontal plane axis, because VTs with LBBB arise in or adjacent to the septum, closer to the RV stimulation site.[3]

EFFECT OF SITE OF STIMULATION. Resetting does not require that the pacing site be located in the reentrant circuit. The closer the pacing site to the circuit, however, the less premature a single VES can be and reach the circuit without being extinguished by collision with the tachycardia wavefront emerging from the VT circuit. The longest coupling interval for a VES to be able to reset a reentrant tachycardia will depend on the tachycardia CL, the duration of the excitable gap of the tachycardia, local refractoriness at the pacing site, and conduction time from the stimulation site to the reentrant circuit. Neither local ventricular ERP nor local activation time influences the number of VESs required for resetting. Approximately 10% to 20% of VTs demonstrate site specificity in response to VES. Using double VESs reduces this site specificity. Approximately 70% of VTs can be reset with a single VES delivered to the RV apex or RVOT. Resetting of VT by a single VES can always be achieved from some site in the LV, even when resetting cannot be achieved from RV sites.[3]

RETURN CYCLE. The return cycle is the time interval from the resetting VES to the next excitation of the pacing site by the new orthodromic VT wavefront. This corresponds to the time required for the stimulated impulse to reach the circuit, conduct through the circuit, and exit. The noncompensatory pause following the VES and the return cycle are typically measured at the pacing site; however, they can also be measured to the onset of the surface ECG complex. Conduction time between the pacing site and the VT circuit may or may not be equal to that from the VT circuit to the pacing site. Differences in the VT circuit entrance and exit can result in differences in conduction time to and from the pacing site. These differences depend on the site of stimulation and VT site of origin. In VTs reset by both single and double VESs, the shortest return cycle seen by both methods is usually the same. If the return cycle is measured from the VES producing resetting to the onset of the first return VT QRS complex on the surface ECG, the shortest return cycle will be less than the tachycardia CL in more than 40% of VTs. Because stimulation is usually performed from the RV, conduction time into the VT circuit is incorporated into that measurement. If one considers conduction time between the pacing site and the circuit to be equal to that from the circuit to the pacing site (i.e., local activation time) and subtracts this value from the return cycle as measured to the surface ECG QRS, the resultant value for the return cycle is less than the tachycardia CL in 80% of VTs.[3]

RESETTING RESPONSE CURVES. Flat or mixed (flat, and then increasing) response curves characterize reentrant VTs. A flat curve is noted in approximately two-thirds of VTs, suggesting that a fully excitable gap is present. It also signifies anatomically separate entrance and exit sites of the circuit (see Fig. 3-16). In approximately 40% of VTs, the types of resetting curves can vary, depending on the site of ventricular stimulation. VESs from different pacing sites likely engage different sites in the VT circuit that are in different states of excitability or refractoriness and, therefore, result in different conduction velocities and resetting patterns.[3]

RESETTING WITH FUSION. The ability to reset a tachycardia after it has begun activating the myocardium (i.e., resetting with fusion) excludes automatic and triggered mechanisms and is diagnostic of reentry. Resetting with ECG fusion requires wide separation (in time, distance, or both) of entry and exit sites of the VT circuit, with the stimulus wavefront preferentially engaging the entrance. For resetting with fusion to occur, the premature paced wavefront has to reach the entrance of the reentrant circuit before it reaches the exit, and, at the same time, allow for the VT wavefront to exit the reentrant circuit, while the VT wavefront is unable to reach the entrance of the circuit before the paced wavefront (Fig. 22-14). Fusion of the stimulated impulse can be observed on the surface ECG and/or intracardiac recordings if the stimulated impulse is intermediate in morphology between a fully paced complex and the tachycardia complex. The ability to recognize surface ECG fusion requires a significant mass of myocardium to be depolarized by both the VES and VT. If presystolic activity in the reentrant circuit is present before delivery of the VES that resets the VT, this must be considered to represent local fusion. Thus, a VES delivered after the onset of the tachycardia QRS on the surface ECG that enters and resets the VT circuit will always demonstrate local fusion. Resetting with local fusion and a totally paced surface QRS complex suggests that the reentrant circuit is physically small. The farther the stimulation site is from the reentrant circuit, the less likely resetting with ECG fusion will occur. In this setting, the VES should be delivered at a shorter coupling interval to enable the paced wavefront to reach the VT circuit with sufficient prematurity; hence, the stimulated impulse will reflect a purely paced QRS without ECG fusion.

Resetting with surface ECG fusion of the QRS during RV stimulation is observed in 60% of VTs, 40% of which are usually reset with a VES delivered after the onset of the VT QRS. VTs reset with fusion have a higher incidence of flat resetting curves, longer resetting zones, and significantly shorter return cycle, measured from the stimulus to the onset of the VT QRS, than VTs not reset with fusion. The return cycle corrected to the tachycardia CL is shorter with VTs reset with fusion (0.89 versus 1.12). In 80% of VTs reset with fusion, the return cycle is shorter than the tachycardia CL measured at the onset of the QRS (versus only 4% of VTs reset without fusion). The return cycle minus local activation time is equal to the time for the wavefront to traverse the distance from the entrance to the exit of the circuit. This interval is less than the tachycardia CL in 100% of VTs reset with fusion. These findings are consistent with widely separate entrance and exit sites of the VT circuit.[3]

TERMINATION. Termination of VT by a VES occurs when the VES collides with the preceding tachycardia impulse antidromically and blocks in the reentrant circuit orthodromically (see Fig. 3-15). This occurs when the VES enters the reentrant circuit early enough in the relative refractory period, because it fails to propagate in the anterograde direction and encounters absolutely refractory tissue. In the retrograde direction, it confronts increasingly recovered tissue and is able to propagate until it collides with the circulating wavefront and terminates the arrhythmia.

Termination of VT by a single VES is uncommon, occurring in 10% to 46% of VTs. The closer the stimulation site to the circuit, the more prematurely a VES can engage the VT circuit, because the refractoriness and conduction delay in intervening myocardial tissue are avoided. The success of termination, however, is directly related to the number of VESs used. Occasionally, when stimulation is performed at the critical isthmus of the VT circuit, termination can occur with a nonpropagated VES that fails to depolarize the bulk of the myocardium but is adequate to depolarize the isthmus and make it refractory to the incoming VT wavefront, resulting in termination of the VT (Fig. 22-15).[3]

VENTRICULAR PACING DURING VENTRICULAR TACHYCARDIA

Rapid ventricular pacing is performed during VT at a pacing CL 10 to 20 milliseconds shorter than the tachycardia CL. The pacing CL is then decreased in 10-millisecond decrements in a stepwise fashion until the VT is terminated. Pacing is stopped after each pacing CL and the response of VT to pacing is assessed. It is important to ensure that termination and reinitiation of the VT have not occurred during the pacing train, which would then affect the interpretation of the VT response.

It is critical to synchronize the initiation of pacing to the electrogram at the pacing site, because absence of synchronization will lead to a variable coupling interval of the first paced impulse to the VT. It is also important to perform overdrive ventricular pacing at each pacing CL for sufficiently long duration to allow the pacing drive to penetrate and affect the VT circuit. Pacing for a short period is a common mistake; it results in erroneous evaluation of the VT response. For VTs that are not stable enough to allow completion of an entire stimulation protocol,

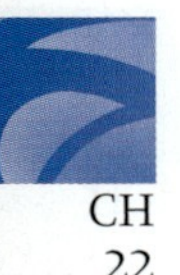

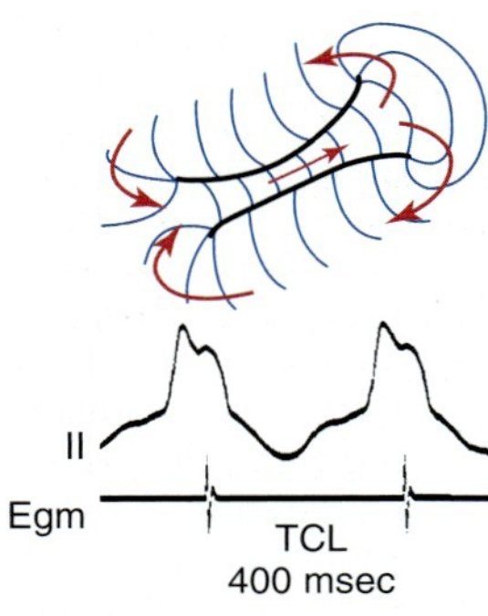

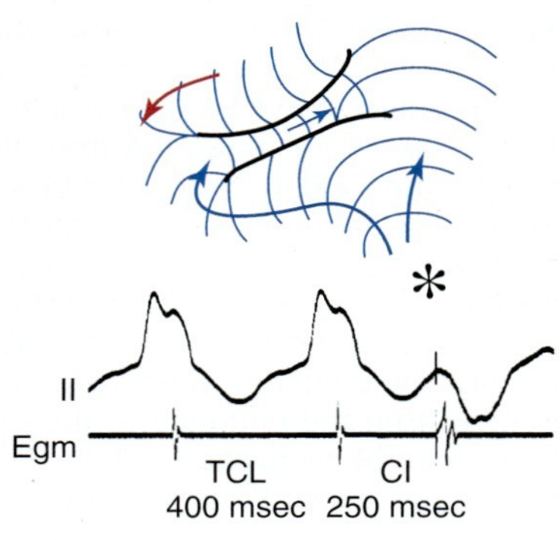

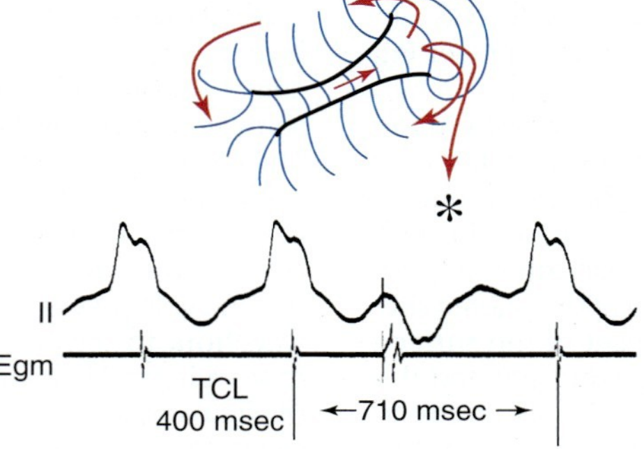

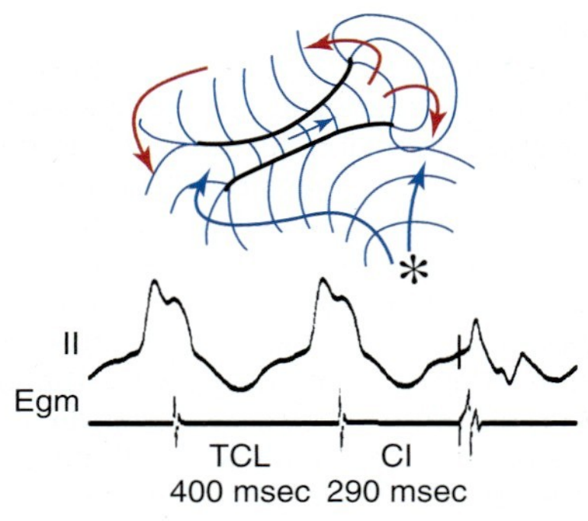

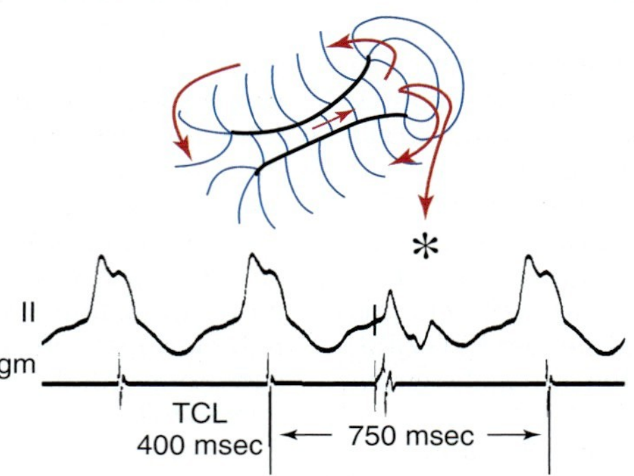

FIGURE 22-14 Schematic representation of the relationship of the return cycle during resetting of ventricular tachycardia (VT) to the absence or presence of surface ECG fusion. **A,** Stylized VT circuit, with direction of propagation as shown; electrogram is from a remote site. **B,** Single ventricular extrastimulus (VES) is introduced during VT at a coupling interval of 250 milliseconds. **Left panel,** The VES occurs early enough that the circuit's exit site is captured; thus, there is no fusion. Meanwhile, the paced wavefront (blue arrows) enters the entrance of the diastolic corridor before the approaching wavefront of the prior VT cycle (red arrow), allowing resetting. **Right panel,** Resetting is demonstrated in that the first VT cycle after the VES occurs at less than twice the tachycardia cycle length (TCL). **C,** A slightly later VES is introduced, with a paced wavefront (blue arrows) approaching the diastolic pathway's exit after the VT wavefront (red arrows) has already left; this results in ECG fusion. Meanwhile, as before, the paced wavefront arrives at the entrance site before the VT wavefront, allowing resetting. The **right panel** again shows resetting, this time with fusion. Asterisks = pacing site; CI = coupling interval; Egm = intracardiac electrogram.

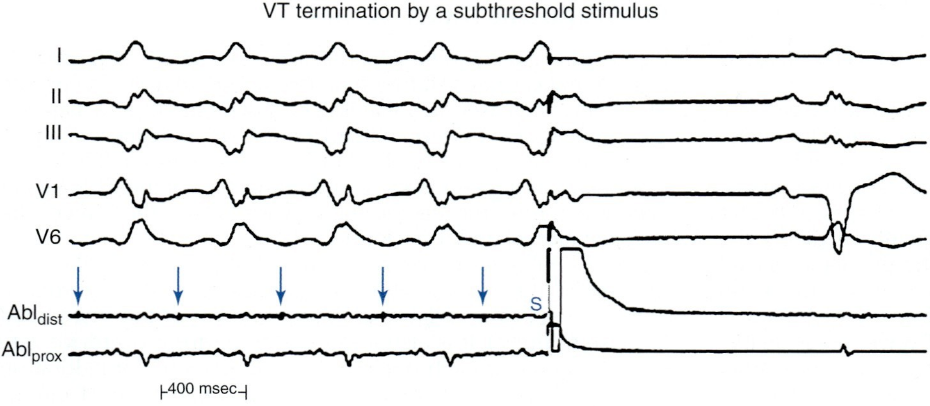

FIGURE 22-15 Ventricular tachycardia (VT) termination by a subthreshold ventricular extrastimulus (VES). VT is shown with the ablation electrode recording a small mid-diastolic potential (arrows). A single VES (S) is delivered during VT that does not appear to capture myocardium, yet terminates the tachycardia.

synchronized bursts of pacing at variable pacing CLs for a specified but variable number of beats, can usually be performed and can provide information about resetting or entrainment, overdrive suppression, and termination.

The response of VT to overdrive pacing is evaluated for overdrive suppression, acceleration, transformation into distinct uniform VT morphologies, entrainment, ability and pattern of termination, and site specificity for stimulation affecting the VT.

OVERDRIVE SUPPRESSION. Overdrive suppression analogous to that seen with automatic rhythms has not been observed in post-MI VTs, although prolonged return cycles can be seen at rapid pacing rates.

ACCELERATION. Acceleration by overdrive pacing refers to sustained shortening of the tachycardia CL following cessation of pacing. Acceleration occurs in 25% of VTs, and is more common with ventricular pacing than with VES (35% versus 5%). However, overdrive acceleration of VT analogous to that seen in triggered rhythms (i.e., linear relation of pacing CL to early acceleration of the tachycardia CL) is uncommon in post-MI VT. Because rapid ventricular pacing is usually required to terminate faster VTs, these VTs have a higher incidence of acceleration (40% of VTs with CL < 300 milliseconds with rapid ventricular pacing). Approximately 50% of the accelerated VTs can be terminated with even faster ventricular pacing; the other 50% (which can be polymorphic VT or ventricular flutter) require electrical cardioversion.

Acceleration is classified according to the morphology of the accelerated tachycardia: VT morphology identical to or different from the original VT, or polymorphic VT. An accelerated VT with a QRS morphology identical to the original VT suggests that the accelerated VT is using the same exit of the original VT circuit. The most likely mechanism underlying this form of VT acceleration is an area of block that determines the size of the reentrant circuit, which is determined to some extent by refractoriness. Rapid pacing can shorten the refractoriness in a proximal region of the arc of block, which would in turn shorten the length of the reentrant pathway. If the distal component of the arc of block remains unchanged, acceleration of the VT will occur with the same exit site and hence the same QRS morphology. Alternatively, rapid pacing can remove block in a shorter potential pathway, creating a smaller circuit.[3]

On the other hand, a VT morphology different from the original VT can be secondary to a change in the exit site from the same circuit, a reversal of the reentrant circuit, or the termination of the initial VT and initiation of a different VT elsewhere. Polymorphic VT with or without degeneration to VF can occur because of the inability of the myocardium to respond to the pacing CL with the development of changing activation wavefronts, leading to multiple reentrant wavelets that can degenerate into VF. There is no way to predict which type of acceleration will occur. However, in the presence of antiarrhythmic drugs, acceleration to different morphologically distinct VTs is common.

TRANSFORMATION. Transformation of the index VT into multiple distinct uniform VT morphologies can occur in response to overdrive pacing. It is not infrequent for stimulation during one VT to induce another VT of different morphology and CL, only to be changed to a third or fourth one by continued stimulation. The significance of all these multiple morphologically distinct VTs induced during overdrive pacing of the spontaneous VT is uncertain if they were never seen before spontaneously or induced by programmed stimulation. Usually, however, these VTs can also be induced by programmed electrical stimulation. Nevertheless, any VT (even if not seen before) that is uniform and has a CL longer than 250 milliseconds is clinically important. Those VTs may not have been observed previously because the original VT dominates because it is more readily inducible. Induction of rapid unstable VTs (CL <250 milliseconds) in patients who presented with only stable VT does not have prognostic value.[3]

The ability to change from one VT to another with a different CL using single or double VESs is infrequent during triggered rhythms (other than those because of digitalis), and is another observation that is most compatible with a reentrant mechanism.

ENTRAINMENT. Overdrive ventricular pacing at long CLs (i.e., 10 to 30 milliseconds shorter than the tachycardia CL) can almost always entrain reentrant VTs. The slower the pacing rate and the farther the pacing site from the reentrant circuit, the longer the pacing drive required to penetrate and entrain the tachycardia.

Following the first beat of the pacing train that penetrates and resets the reentrant circuit, the subsequent stimuli will interact with the reset circuit, which has an abbreviated excitable gap. Depending on the degree that the excitable gap is preexcited by that first resetting stimulus, subsequent stimuli fall on fully or partially excitable tissue. Entrainment is said to be present when two consecutive extrastimuli conduct orthodromically through the circuit with the same conduction time while colliding antidromically with the preceding paced wavefront. During entrainment, the paced stimuli enter the reentrant circuit, block with the existing tachycardia wavefront in the antidromic direction, and conduct through the circuit in the orthodromic direction to produce the return cycle beat.

ENTRAINMENT CRITERIA. Classic criteria for recognition of entrainment are the following: (1) fixed fusion of the paced complexes at any single pacing CL; (2) progressive fusion as the pacing CL decreases (i.e., the surface ECG progressively looks more like the purely paced QRS complex than a pure tachycardia QRS complex); and (3) resumption of the same VT morphology following pacing with a nonfused tachycardia QRS complex at a return cycle equal to the pacing CL (see Figs. 5-15 and 5-16). The return cycle is defined as the interval from the last paced beat to the first VT beat, and is measured from the surface QRS or RV electrograms.[36,37]

ENTRAINMENT WITH FUSION. As noted, fusion of the stimulated impulse can be observed on the surface ECG, intracardiac recordings, or both. The stimulated impulse will have hybrid morphology between the fully paced QRS and the tachycardia QRS (Fig. 22-16; and see Figs. 5-15 and 5-16). The ability to demonstrate surface ECG fusion requires a significant mass of myocardium to be depolarized by both the extrastimulus and the tachycardia. The farther the stimulation site from the reentrant circuit, the less likely entrainment with ECG fusion will occur. Overdrive pacing of a tachycardia of any mechanism can result in a certain degree of fusion, especially when the pacing CL is only slightly shorter than the tachycardia CL. Such fusion, however, is unstable during the same pacing drive at the same pacing CL, because pacing stimuli fall on a progressively earlier portion of the tachycardia cycle, producing progressively less fusion and more fully paced morphology. Such phenomena should be distinguished from entrainment, and sometimes this requires pacing for long intervals to demonstrate variable degrees of fusion. Focal tachycardias (automatic, triggered activity, or microreentrant) cannot manifest fixed or progressive fusion during overdrive pacing (Fig. 22-17). Moreover, overdrive pacing frequently results in suppression (automatic) or acceleration (triggered activity) of focal VTs rather than resumption of the original tachycardia with an unchanged tachycardia CL.[36,37]

ENTRAINMENT WITH MANIFEST FUSION. Entrainment of reentrant tachycardias commonly produces manifest fusion that is stable (fixed) during the pacing drive at a given pacing CL; repeated entrainment at pacing CLs progressively shorter than the tachycardia CL results in different degrees of QRS fusion, with the resultant QRS configuration looking more like a fully paced configuration (see Figs. 5-15 and 5-16).

ENTRAINMENT WITH INAPPARENT FUSION. Entrainment with inapparent fusion (also referred to as local or intracardiac fusion) is said to be present when a fully paced QRS morphology (with no ECG fusion) is observed during entrainment, even when the tachycardia impulse exits the reentrant circuit (orthodromic activation of the presystolic electrogram is present). In this setting, fusion is limited to a small area and does not produce surface ECG fusion, and only intracardiac (local) fusion can be recognized (see Fig. 5-18). Local fusion can only occur when the presystolic electrogram

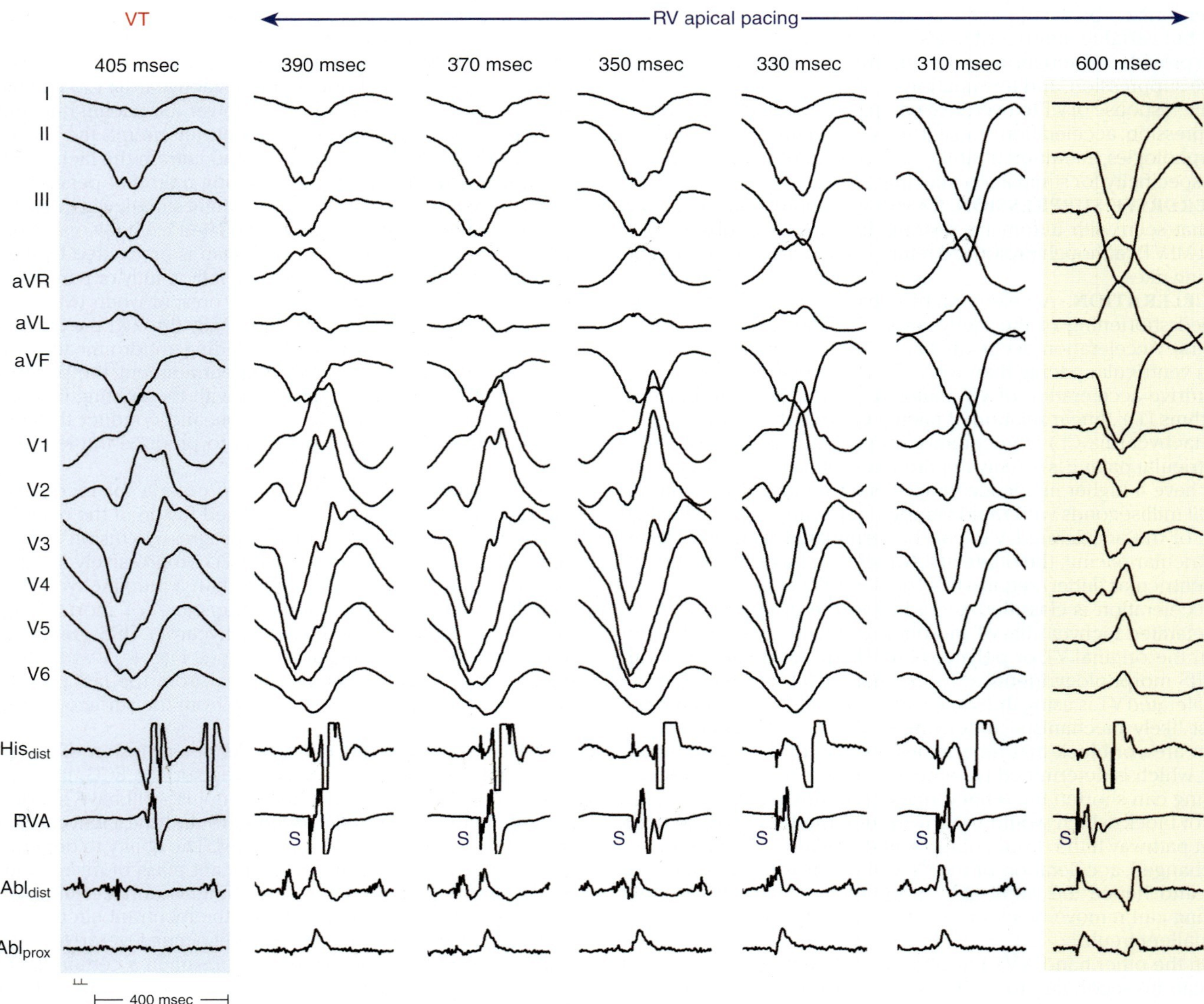

FIGURE 22-16 Fusion with ventricular pacing during macroreentrant post-infarction ventricular tachycardia (VT). VT with a right bundle branch block pattern and right superior axis is shown at left (cycle length [CL], 405 milliseconds, in blue shading). In the panels at right, pacing during VT over a range of CLs from the right ventricular (RV) apex (with a left bundle branch block pattern and left superior axis) is shown. Pure RV pacing during sinus rhythm at CL of 600 milliseconds is shown at far right (yellow shading). It is evident that while pacing during VT, QRS complexes at each paced CL are different from both VT and pure pacing, indicating contribution of both the VT and paced wavefronts to the QRS complexes (fusion, most evident in leads III, aVL, aVF, and V_1 and V_2).

is activated orthodromically. Collision with the last paced impulse must occur distal to the presystolic electrogram, either at the exit from the circuit or outside the circuit. In such cases, the return cycle measured at this local electrogram will equal the pacing CL. Therefore, a stimulus delivered after the onset of the surface ECG QRS during entrainment will always demonstrate local fusion. This is to be distinguished from entrainment with antidromic capture. When pacing is performed at a CL significantly shorter than the tachycardia CL, the paced impulse can penetrate the circuit antidromically and retrogradely (antidromically) capture the presystolic electrogram so that no exit from the tachycardia circuit is possible. Consequently, the surface QRS appears fully paced. When pacing is stopped, the impulse that conducts antidromically also conducts orthodromically to reset the reentrant circuit with orthodromic activation of the presystolic electrogram. When antidromic (retrograde) capture of the local presystolic electrogram occurs, the return cycle, even when measured at the site of the presystolic electrogram, will exceed the pacing CL by the difference in time between when the electrogram is activated retrogradely (i.e., preexcited antidromically) and when it would have been activated orthodromically (see Fig. 5-15).[36]

ENTRAINMENT WITH CONCEALED FUSION. Entrainment with concealed fusion (sometimes also referred to as "concealed entrainment") is defined as entrainment with orthodromic capture and a surface ECG complex identical to that of the tachycardia (Fig. 22-18). Entrainment with concealed fusion suggests that the pacing site is within a protected isthmus inside or outside the reentrant circuit, but attached to the circuit (i.e., the pacing site can be in, attached to, or at the entrance to a protected isthmus that forms the diastolic pathway of the circuit). In this setting, transient entrainment is achieved when the orthodromically directed stimulated wavefront resets the tachycardia, but an antidromically stimulated wavefront collides with the tachycardia wavefront in or near the reentry circuit and fails to exit the slow conduction zone. Only tissue near the pacing site within the critical isthmus is antidromically activated; hence, there is no evidence of fusion. Compared with the intrinsic tachycardia, this antidromic capture may result in earlier intracardiac recordings from bipole sites located adjacent to the pacing region. The morphological appearance of the ECG, however, is the same during entrainment as during the tachycardia. Entrainment with concealed fusion can occur by pacing from bystander pathways, such as a blind alley, alternate

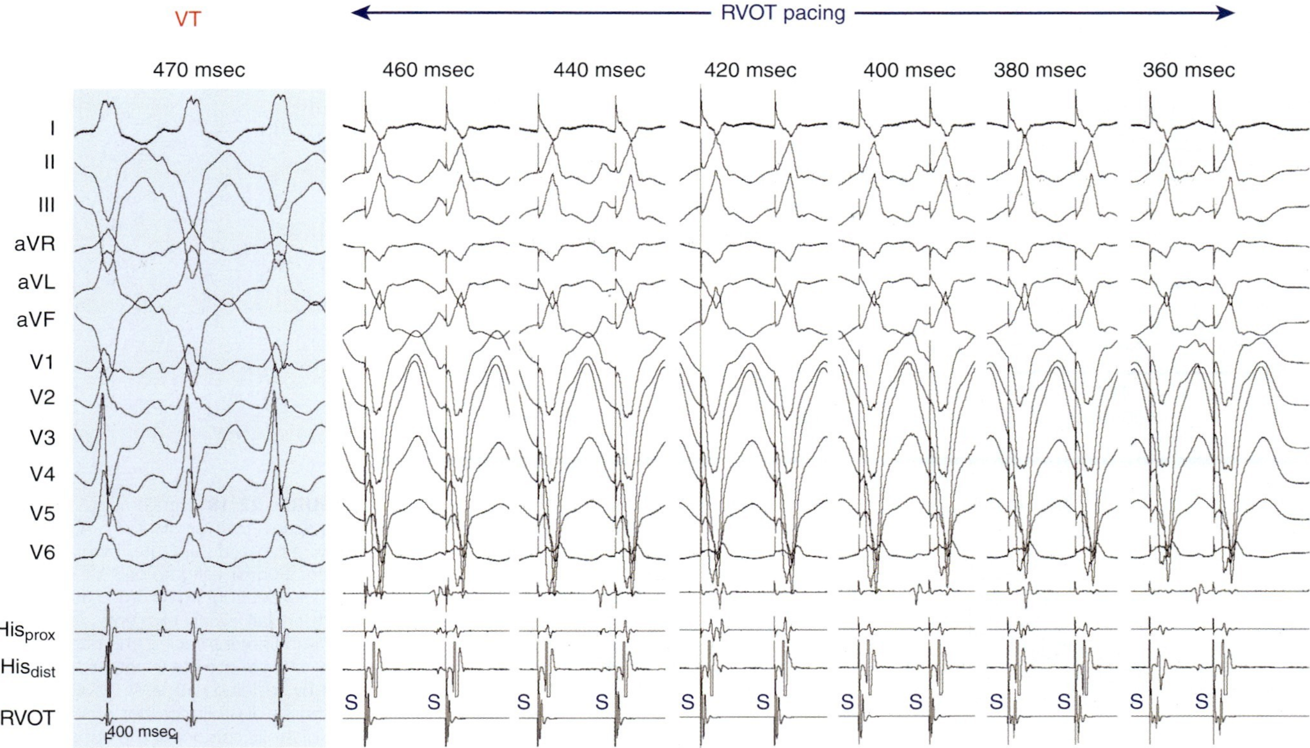

FIGURE 22-17 Lack of fusion with ventricular pacing during focal ventricular tachycardia (VT) in a patient with cardiomyopathy. VT with a right bundle branch block pattern and left superior axis is shown at left in blue shading (cycle length [CL], 470 milliseconds). In the panels at right, pacing during VT over a range of CLs from the right ventricular outflow tract (RVOT, with a left bundle branch block pattern and right inferior axis) is shown. It is clear that while pacing during VT, all QRS complexes are identical, indicating no contribution of the VT to the QRS complexes (thus no fusion).

pathway, or inner loop, that are not critical to the maintenance of reentry. In this situation, activation propagates from the main circuit loop but is constrained by block lines having the shape of a cul-de-sac; ablation at these sites does not terminate reentry.[36]

Occasionally, one of the first few stimuli of a drive train intended to entrain VT terminates VT without propagation. Subsequent stimuli often result in QRS complexes that do not resemble VT, leading the operator to conclude that the site is far from the isthmus. Review of the first few stimuli of pacing may show that the site actually was very attractive for ablation (Fig. 22-19).

POST-PACING INTERVAL. The post-pacing interval (PPI) is the interval from the last pacing stimulus that entrained the tachycardia to the next recorded electrogram at the pacing site (see Fig. 22-18). The PPI should be measured to the near-field potential that indicates depolarization of tissue at the pacing site. The PPI remains relatively stable when entrainment of VT is performed at the same site, regardless of the length of the pacing drive. This is in contrast to overdrive suppression seen in automatic arrhythmias, which would be associated with progressive delay of the first tachycardia beat return cycle with progressively longer overdrive pacing drives.[36-38]

TERMINATION. The ability to terminate SMVT by rapid ventricular pacing, VES, or both is influenced most importantly by the tachycardia CL (50% of VTs with CLs <300 milliseconds will require electrical cardioversion), but also by the local ERP at the pacing site, conduction time from the stimulation site to the site of origin of the VT, duration of the excitable gap, and presence of antiarrhythmic agents.

Failure of rapid ventricular pacing or VES to terminate VT has several potential explanations: the reentrant circuit being a protected focus; inability of VES to access the reentrant circuit because of local myocardial refractoriness; absence of an accessible excitable gap; termination of VT followed by reinitiation by a subsequent pacing impulse in the same pacing drive; and/or failure of conduction block to occur within the reentrant circuit, despite accelerating the VT to the faster pacing rate.

Factors influencing termination of VT can be modified. Refractoriness at the site of stimulation can be modified by the use of multiple VESs or a higher pacing current. The distance, conduction time, or both from the site of stimulation to the VT site can be modified by changing the site of stimulation. The tachycardia CL can be increased by antiarrhythmic agents, but the response is unpredictable. However, two problems are frequently encountered in attempts to terminate VT—acceleration of the VT by overdrive pacing and the appearance of multiple distinct uniform VT morphologies.[3]

Regardless of the mode of stimulation used, termination is usually abrupt, which distinguishes reentrant VTs from triggered VTs. In reentrant VTs, termination must occur when an impulse penetrates the circuit and blocks in both directions. Rapid ventricular pacing is the most efficacious way of VT termination, regardless of the tachycardia CL. Approximately 80% of VTs terminated by a single VES have a tachycardia CL longer than 400 milliseconds. All VTs terminated by single or double VESs can also be terminated by ventricular pacing. Termination is less likely to occur when the VT cannot be reset with very premature VES (i.e., the VES coupling interval is more than 75% of the tachycardia CL).[3]

A single VES delivered during entrainment of VT can facilitate termination of VT by allowing easier access to the excitable gap. Even when a single VES or overdrive pacing alone fails to terminate the VT, the combination of both may be successful. Overdrive pacing ensures stable resetting of the VT circuit, allowing a single VES to interact with the circuit much more prematurely than it could in the absence of entrainment. Overdrive pacing also shortens the excitable gap of tissue in the reset circuit, making it possible for a single VES to terminate the VT. This technique avoids the need for multiple VESs, which can increase the heterogeneity of conduction and refractoriness in the intervening tissue and produce polymorphic VT, and the need for rapid pacing, which might induce acceleration of the VT. This method is especially helpful in VTs that were accelerated by rapid pacing and especially in those VTs for which antiarrhythmic agents have made the tachycardia more difficult to terminate.[3]

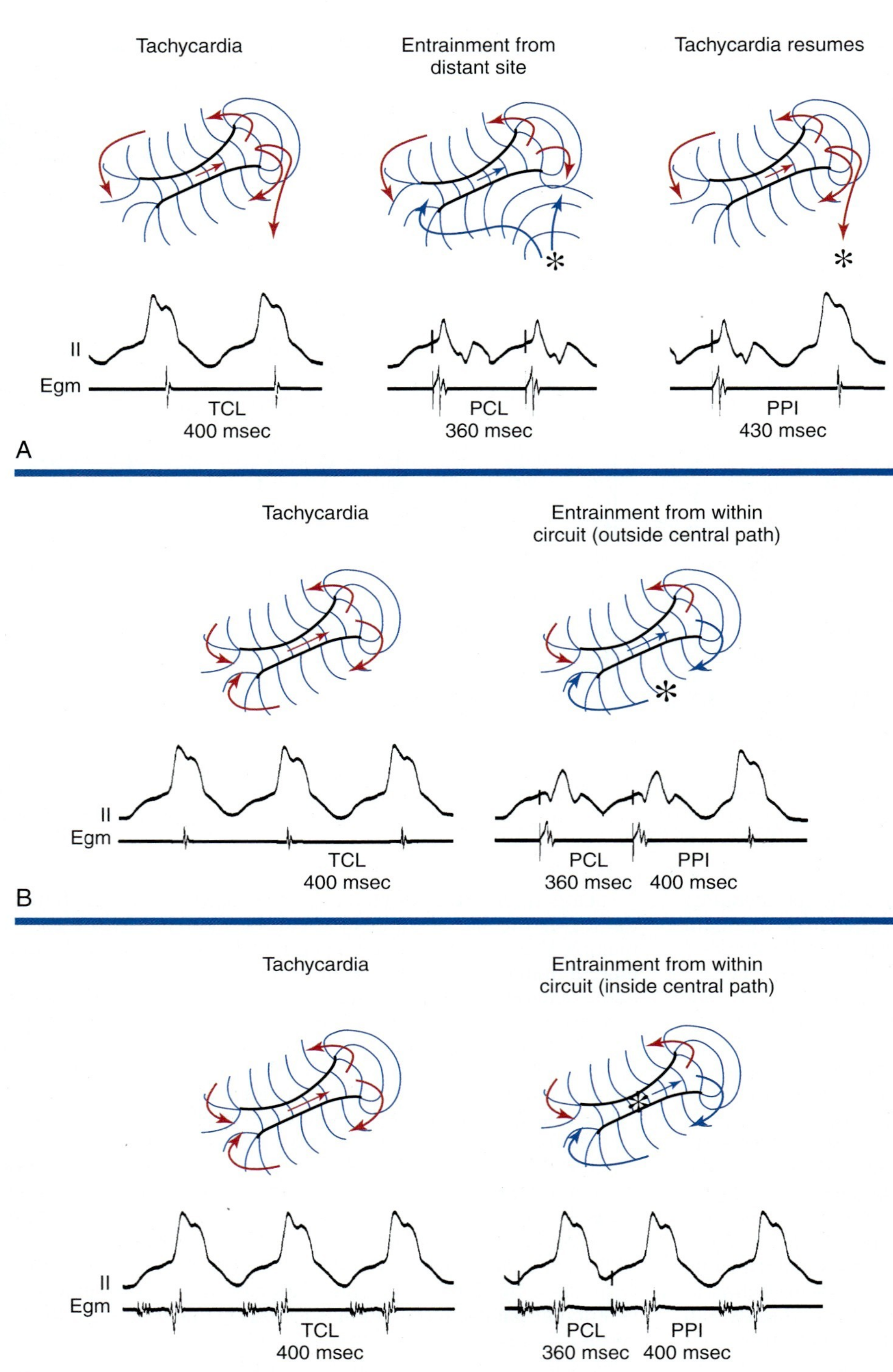

FIGURE 22-18 Entrainment mapping of ventricular tachycardia (VT). **A,** Entrainment of VT from a distant site. Diagrammatic representation of a figure-of-8 VT circuit at left, with an electrogram recorded at a site remote from critical circuit elements. At center, during entrainment pacing, the paced wavefront from this remote site (*) interacts with the circuit by colliding with a VT wavefront that has exited the diastolic corridor while also entering the diastolic corridor at the opposite end. This results in fusion (part of the ventricle depolarized by the VT wavefront, part by the paced wavefront). For as long as pacing continues, this fusion of ventricular activation remains stable. With cessation of pacing (right figure), the last paced wavefront enters the diastolic corridor as on other cycles but there is no subsequent paced wavefront to collide with the wavefront that is exiting the corridor; thus the first return cycle complex is entrained, but not fused. The post-pacing interval (PPI) measured at the site of pacing reflects the time it takes to make one complete revolution around the circuit plus any time required to get from the pacing site to the circuit and back from the circuit to the pacing site. **B,** Entrainment of VT from a site within the circuit. The pacing site (*) is within the circuit but outside the diastolic corridor. As a result, the entrained QRS complex shows fusion and the PPI equals the VT cycle length (CL). **C,** Entrainment of VT from a site within the critical isthmus. The pacing site (*) is within the circuit and inside the diastolic corridor, recording the mid-diastolic electrogram. As a result, the entrained QRS complex shows no fusion and the PPI equals the VT CL. The S-QRS interval equals the electrogram-to-QRS interval during VT. This is the ideal ablation site. Egm = intracardiac electrogram; PCL = pacing cycle length; TCL = tachycardia cycle length.

EFFECTS OF DRUGS ON VENTRICULAR TACHYCARDIA

Class I agents are the most uniformly successful drugs for slowing the rate of or terminating SMVT. These drugs can also facilitate the induction of SMVT in patients in whom SMVT cannot be induced by the standard programmed electrical stimulation protocol and in patients with coronary artery disease and nonsustained VT. These drugs can also occasionally produce incessant SMVT in patients who, before therapy, only had paroxysmal events. This phenomenon, almost always associated with a slower VT and prolongation of conduction by the agent, would not be expected if the mechanism were triggered activity or abnormal automaticity. Adenosine, beta blockers, and calcium channel blockers are ineffective for termination of post-MI VT.[3]

Exclusion of Other Arrhythmia Mechanisms

EXCLUSION OF TRIGGERED ACTIVITY VENTRICULAR TACHYCARDIA

STIMULATION SITE SPECIFICITY. The site of ventricular stimulation should have no effect on the initiation of triggered activity VT as long as the impulse reaches the focus of the VT. Reentrant

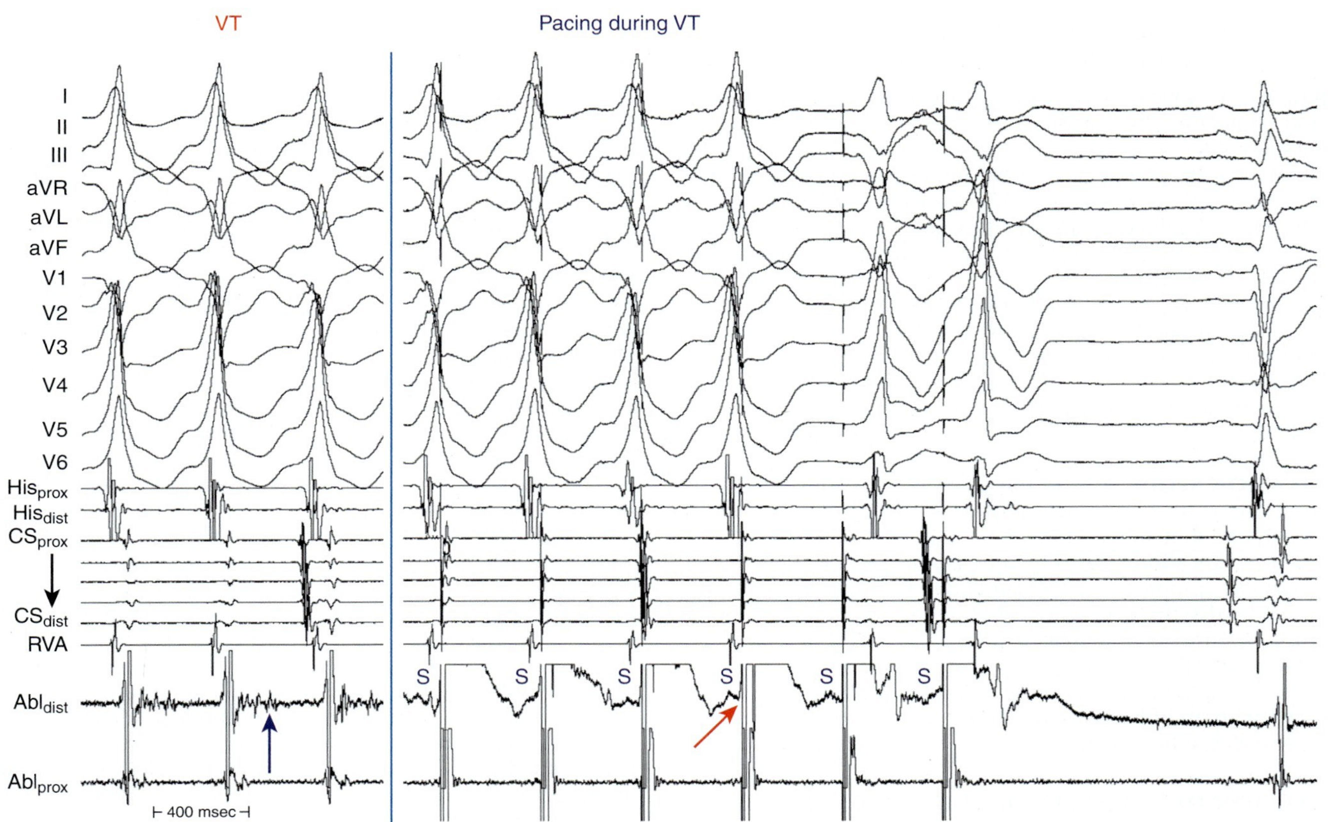

FIGURE 22-19 Nonpropagated ventricular tachycardia (VT) termination during attempted entrainment. VT is shown with a diastolic potential (blue arrow); during attempted stimulation at this site during VT, the first several stimuli (S) have no effect but the fifth stimulus (red arrow) results in VT termination without propagation of the impulse (no subsequent QRS). Subsequent stimuli capture the site but result in a very different QRS configuration.

VT, on the other hand, can demonstrate absolute or relative site specificity for initiation.

INDUCIBILITY WITH PROGRAMMED ELECTRICAL STIMULATION. Ventricular stimulation can initiate triggered activity VT in less than 65% of cases. Rapid ventricular pacing to initiate triggered VT should be more effective than VES, whereas it has a low yield in initiating reentrant VT. Multiple VESs during NSR or following a drive train of fewer than 8 to 10 beats usually fail to initiate triggered activity VT. Most episodes of triggered activity VT induced by ventricular stimulation are usually nonsustained. Induction of triggered activity VT with atrial pacing is not uncommon.[3]

REPRODUCIBILITY OF INITIATION. Reproducibility of triggered activity VT induction using all methods is less than 50%. Reproducibility of induction with single or double VESs is approximately 25%. Reproducibility is markedly affected by quiescence. Once a triggered rhythm is initiated, a period of quiescence is necessary to reinitiate the rhythm. Thus, the ability to initiate, terminate, and reinitiate sequence is uncommon, in contrast to reentrant VT.[3]

RELATIONSHIP OF PACING CYCLE LENGTH AND VENTRICULAR EXTRASTIMULUS COUPLING INTERVAL TO VENTRICULAR TACHYCARDIA. Typically, both the initial cycle of the triggered activity VT (the return cycle) and the tachycardia CL following cessation of pacing bear a direct relationship to the pacing CL, and a direct relationship to the coupling interval of the VES, when used. Thus, the shorter the initiating ventricular pacing CL, or the shorter the initiating VES coupling interval, the shorter the interval to the first VT beat and the shorter the initial VT CL. Occasionally, with early VESs, a jump in the interval to the onset of the VT complex occurs, so that it is approximately twice the interval to the onset of the VT initiated by later coupled VESs. This is secondary to failure of the initial delayed afterdepolarization (DAD) to reach threshold while the second DAD reaches threshold. Thus, in triggered activity VTs caused by DADs, the coupling interval of the initial VT complex shortens or suddenly increases in response to progressively premature VES. It would not be expected to demonstrate an inverse or gradually increasing relationship, in contrast to reentrant VT. Only with the addition of very early VESs or, occasionally, very rapid ventricular pacing (CL <300 milliseconds) can a sudden jump in the interval to the first VT complex be observed. Furthermore, ventricular pacing CLs longer or shorter than the critical CL window fail to induce triggered activity VT. This critical window may shift with changing autonomic tone.[3]

EFFECTS OF CATECHOLAMINE. Inducibility of triggered activity VT is facilitated by catecholamines, whereas in the setting of reentrant VT, isoproterenol facilitates VT induction in only 5% of cases. However, induction of triggered activity VT can be inconsistent and is exquisitely sensitive to the immediate autonomic status of the patient. Therefore, noninducibility during a single EP study is not enough evidence to attribute the arrhythmia to a nontriggered activity mechanism.

RESPONSE TO ANTIARRHYTHMIC DRUGS. Triggered activity VTs respond favorably to calcium channel blockers and beta blockers. Conversely, those drugs fail to terminate more than 95% of VTs associated with coronary artery disease.

DIASTOLIC ELECTRICAL ACTIVITY. In reentrant VT, electrical activity occurs throughout the VT cycle. Thus, during diastole, conduction is extremely slow and in a small enough area that it is not recorded on the surface ECG. Demonstration that the VT initiation is dependent on a critical degree of slow conduction, manifested by fragmented electrograms spanning diastole, and that maintenance of the VT is associated with repetitive continuous activity is consistent with a reentrant mechanism.

EXCLUSION OF BUNDLE BRANCH REENTRANT VENTRICULAR TACHYCARDIA

HIS BUNDLE–VENTRICULAR INTERVAL. BBR should be suspected when the His potential precedes ventricular activation and the HV interval during VT is longer than that during NSR. In other VTs, the His potential is usually immediately before or after, or obscured within, the local ventricular electrogram. Occasionally, the His potential can precede the onset of the QRS in post-MI VT; however, in contrast to BBR VT, the HV interval in those VTs is shorter than that during NSR.

OSCILLATION OF TACHYCARDIA CYCLE LENGTH. Spontaneous variation in the V-V intervals during BBR VT is dictated and preceded by similar changes in the H-H intervals. These changes can be demonstrated by ventricular stimulation during VT or can occur spontaneously following initiation. In other VTs, in contrast to BBR VT, the V-V interval variation usually dictates the subsequent H-H interval changes.

ACTIVATION SEQUENCE. In the common type of BBR (LBBB pattern), the activation wavefront travels retrogradely up the LB to the HB and then anterogradely down the RB, with subsequent ventricular activation. This sequence is reversed in BBR with an RBBB pattern. Unfortunately, RB and LB potentials are not always recorded, so that the typical activation sequences (LB-HB-RB-V or RB-HB-LB-V) are not available for analysis. Even if either sequence is present, the HPS (usually the LB) could be activated passively in the retrograde fashion to produce an HB-RB-V sequence during a VT with an LBBB pattern without reentry requiring the LB. In these cases, other diagnostic criteria for BBR should be used.

EXCLUSION OF SUPRAVENTRICULAR TACHYCARDIA

SUPRAVENTRICULAR TACHYCARDIA WITH ABERRANCY. If VT exhibits 1:1 VA conduction, it can mimic SVT with aberrancy. Surface QRS morphology usually helps distinguish SVT with typical RBBB or LBBB from VT. In VT, the atrium is not part of the tachycardia circuit and can be dissociated by atrial pacing. The HV interval in aberrantly conducted SVT is always equal to or longer than that during NSR, which is in contrast to intramyocardial VTs. Additionally, tachycardia response to VES and atrial pacing can be useful for distinguishing SVT from VT, as discussed in detail in Chapter 21.[39,40]

PREEXCITED SUPRAVENTRICULAR TACHYCARDIA. Differentiation between VT and preexcited SVT (i.e., an SVT with anterograde conduction over an AV bypass tract [BT]) is particularly difficult on the surface ECG, because ventricular activation begins outside the normal intraventricular conduction system in both tachycardias. As a result, many of the standard criteria cannot discriminate between preexcited SVT and VT. The HV interval is usually short or negative in both preexcited SVT and VT, and does not help in the differential diagnosis.

As noted, because the atrium is not part of the VT circuit, the ability to dissociate the atrium with rapid atrial pacing without influencing the tachycardia CL (V-V interval) or QRS morphology suggests VT and excludes preexcited SVTs. Other pacing maneuvers used for differential diagnosis are discussed in Chapter 21.[39,40]

Mapping

The main goal of VT mapping is identification of the site of origin or critical isthmus of the VT. The site of origin of the tachycardia is the source of electrical activity producing the QRS. Although this is a discrete site of impulse formation in automatic and triggered rhythms, during macroreentrant VT it represents the exit site from the diastolic pathway (the critical isthmus) to the myocardium giving rise to the QRS. An isthmus is defined as a conductive myocardial tissue bounded by nonconductive tissue (conduction barriers). This nonconductive tissue can be a scar area surrounding a corridor of surviving myocardium (indicated by double potentials), or an anatomical obstacle, such as the mitral annulus. The critical isthmus is a narrow segment of muscle cells connecting larger masses of myocardium that the depolarization wavefront must traverse to perpetuate the tachycardia. As a consequence, ablation of the critical isthmus should interrupt the tachycardia and prevent its inducibility.

Mapping of post-MI VT has several prerequisites, including inducibility of VT at the time of EP testing, hemodynamic stability of the VT (which usually requires a relatively slow VT rate), and stability of the VT reentry circuit (i.e., stable VT morphology and CL). If the tachycardia is not stable (morphologically or hemodynamically), mapping can still be performed by starting and stopping the VT after data acquisition at each site. Additionally, poorly tolerated rapid VTs sometimes can be slowed by antiarrhythmic drugs to allow for mapping. Antiarrhythmic drugs do not alter the sequence of activation, despite slowing of the VT and widening of the QRS and, although the electrogram at the site of origin can widen, its relationship to the onset of the QRS remains unchanged. Newer techniques such as basket catheter and noncontact mapping can also provide large amounts of activation mapping data during nonsustained or unstable VT.[2]

Mapping of VT circuits and identification of critical isthmuses are often challenging. The abnormal area of scarring, where the isthmus is located, is often large and contains false isthmuses (bystanders) that confuse mapping. Although in the majority of cases a portion of the VT isthmus is located in the subendocardium, where it can be ablated, in some cases the isthmuses or even the entire circuits are deep in the endocardium or even in the epicardium and cannot be identified or ablated from the endocardium. Additionally, multiple potential reentry circuits are frequently present, giving rise to multiple different monomorphic VTs in a single patient. Ablation in one area may abolish more than one VT or leave VT circuits in other locations intact.

When multiple VTs are inducible, it is recommended that all mappable VTs be completely mapped and targeted. However, some recommend targeting only the clinical VT, especially in very ill patients in whom the goal is to decrease the frequency of ICD shocks. It is important to have a 12-lead ECG of the clinical VTs available, if possible, for review at the time of the EP procedure. This information can be used to focus on the exit region suggested by the VT morphology to limit the extent of detailed mapping, particularly when the clinical VT is hemodynamically unstable. In patients with ICDs, VT is usually terminated promptly and a 12-lead ECG is often not available. Nonetheless, comparing the VT CL and ICD electrogram morphology during spontaneous and induced VTs can be helpful, particularly when trying to limit ablation targeting presumptive clinical VT.[2]

Activation Mapping

The main goal of activation mapping of post-MI VT is to seek sites with continuous activity spanning diastole, isolated diastolic potentials, or both. Typically, bipolar electrogram recordings are used for activation mapping, as they provide an improved signal-to-noise ratio and more clearly defined high-frequency components. In contrast, unipolar recordings in scar areas have very low amplitudes with a poor signal-to-noise ratio and distant activity can be difficult to separate from local activity. This is especially true when recording from areas of prior MI, where the QS potentials are ubiquitous and it is often impossible to select a rapid negative dV/dt when the entire QS potential is slowly inscribed. Therefore, unipolar electrograms are typically filtered at comparable settings to those of bipolar electrograms (30 to 300 Hz or more) when scar-related VT is studied. Filtering gives reasonably clean signals; however, the signal is often of very low amplitude. Therefore, bipolar recordings are preferred for activation mapping; filtered unipolar electrograms can be used to help ensure that the tip electrode, which is the ablation electrode, is responsible for the early component of the bipolar electrograms.[41]

Endocardial activation time is the timing of the local electrogram measured relative to the earliest onset of the QRS complex in the 12-lead ECG. Local activation time is best taken from the onset of the high-frequency bipolar electrogram as it leaves the baseline. Using the peak deflection or the point of the most rapid deflection as it crosses the baseline is of less value in multicomponent fractionated electrograms. The distal pole of the mapping catheter should be used for mapping of the earliest activation site, because it is the pole through which RF energy is delivered.

Contact is critical when standard quadripolar catheters are used. The degree of contact can be assessed by pacing threshold or impedance measurements at the recording electrode pair. Recording from multiple bipolar pairs from a multipolar electrode catheter in the LV is helpful in that if the proximal pair has a more attractive electrogram than the distal pair, the catheter can be withdrawn slightly to achieve the same position with the distal electrode. Using standard equipment, mapping a single SMVT requires recording and mapping performed at a number of sites, based on the ability of the investigator to recognize the mapping sites of interest from the morphology of the VT on the surface ECG.

CONTINUOUS ACTIVITY

Theoretically, if reentry is the mechanism of VT, electrical activity should occur throughout the VT cycle. Thus, during diastole, conduction should be extremely slow and in a small enough area such that it is not recorded on surface ECG. The QRS complex is caused by propagation of the wavefront from the exit of that diastolic isthmus to the surrounding myocardium. Demonstration that VT initiation is dependent on a critical degree of slow conduction, manifested by fragmented electrograms spanning diastole, and that maintenance of the VT is associated with repetitive continuous activity, would be compatible with reentry.

In post-MI VT, continuous activity, when observed, invariably occurs at sites that demonstrate markedly abnormal electrograms during NSR (Fig. 22-20). However, continuous diastolic activity can be recorded in only 5% to 10% of post-MI VTs with detailed mapping using standard equipment. The ability to record continuous activity depends on the spatial and geometric arrangement of the involved tissue, the position of the catheter, and the interelectrode distance. Thus, continuous diastolic activity is likely to be recorded only if a bipolar pair records a short isthmus. If a longer isthmus is recorded (i.e., the isthmus is larger than the recording area of the catheter, the catheter is not covering it completely, or both), a nonholodiastolic electrogram will be recorded. In such VTs, when nonholodiastolic electrical activity is recorded at the site of origin, repositioning of the catheter to other sites can allow recording of the bridging of diastole (electrical activity in these adjacent sites spans diastole) (Fig. 22-21). Failure to record continuous activity is then not surprising, because catheter and intraoperative VT mapping suggest that most post-MI VTs incorporate a diastolic pathway 1 to 3 cm long and a few millimeters to 1 cm wide, with a circuit area probably larger than 4 cm^2.

All areas from which diastolic activity is recorded are not necessarily part of the reentrant circuit. Such sites may reflect late activation and may not be related to the VT critical isthmus. Analysis of the response of these electrograms to spontaneous or induced changes in tachycardia CL is critical in deciding their relationship to the VT circuit. Electrical signals that come and go throughout diastole should not be considered continuous. For continuous activity to be consistent with reentry, the following must be demonstrated: (1) VT initiation is dependent on continuous activity (i.e., broadening of electrograms that span diastole); (2) VT maintenance is dependent on continuous activity, so that termination of continuous activity, either spontaneously or following stimulation, without affecting the VT would exclude such continuous activity as requisite for sustaining the VT; (3) the recorded continuous diastolic activity is not just a broad electrogram whose duration equals the diastolic interval, which can be verified by analyzing the local electrogram while pacing during sinus rhythm at a CL comparable to VT CL—if pacing produces continuous diastolic activity in the absence of VT, the continuous electrogram has no mechanistic significance; (4) motion artifact should be excluded (this is easiest because such electrograms are recorded only in infarcted areas and never from moving, contractile normal areas); (5) the continuous activity should be recorded from a circumscribed area; and (6) if possible, ablation of the area from which continuous activity is recorded will terminate the VT.

MID-DIASTOLIC ACTIVITY

An isolated mid-diastolic potential is defined as a low-amplitude, high-frequency diastolic potential separated from the preceding and subsequent ventricular electrograms by an isoelectric segment (Fig. 22-22). It is likely that isolated mid-diastolic potentials that cannot be dissociated from the VT are generated in segments of the zone of slow conduction or critical isthmus, which are integral components of the reentry circuit. The earliest presystolic electrogram closest to mid-diastole is the most commonly observed indicator of an isthmus site in a VT circuit; however, continuous diastolic activity and/or bridging of diastole at adjacent sites or mapping a discrete diastolic pathway would be most consistent with a reentrant circuit (see Fig. 22-20).

In post-MI reentrant VT, the earliest presystolic electrogram is invariably abnormal and frequently fractionated, split, or both, regardless of the QRS morphology of the VT or the location of the isthmus. Thus, a normal presystolic bipolar electrogram (amplitude >3 mV, duration <70 milliseconds) should prompt further search for earlier activity. The early activity often appears focal, with propagation from the early site to the remainder of the heart.

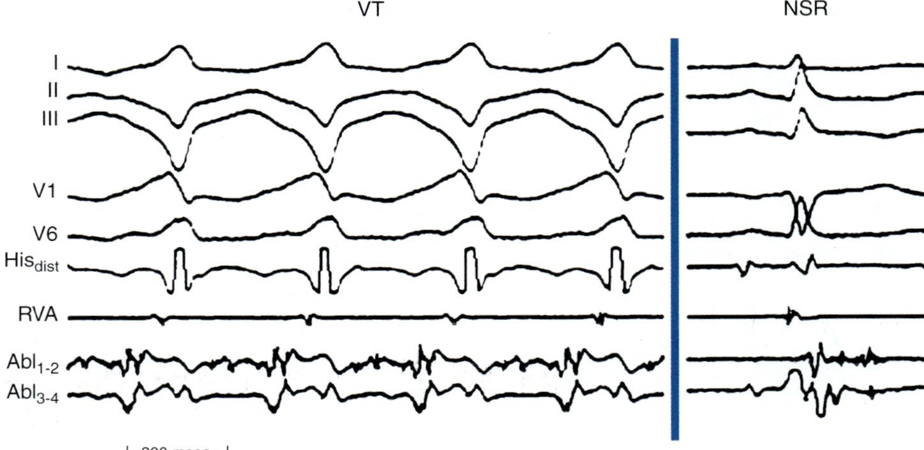

FIGURE 22-20 Continuous diastolic electrical activity during reentrant ventricular tachycardia (VT). VT is shown with almost continuous electrical activity in the distal ablation recording. During sinus rhythm (right), the electrogram is very fragmented and outlasts the surface QRS complex. NSR = normal sinus rhythm.

The earliest electrogram in post-MI VT not infrequently has diastolic and systolic components separated by an isoelectric component (see Fig. 22-22). Detailed mapping will usually reveal more than one site of diastolic activity. It is therefore essential to demonstrate that the diastolic site recorded is in fact the earliest site. This can be done by demonstrating that sites surrounding the assumed earliest site are activated later than that site, even though they may be diastolic in timing. If, after very detailed mapping, the earliest recorded site is not at least 50 milliseconds presystolic, this suggests that either the map is inadequate (most common) or the VT arises deeper than the subendocardium, in the midmyocardium, or even incorporating the subepicardium.

It is important to recognize that mid-diastolic sites also can be part of a larger area of abnormal slow conduction unrelated to the VT circuit (i.e., a dead-end pathway), and can be recorded from a bystander site attached to the isthmus. Therefore, regardless of where in diastole the presystolic electrogram occurs (early, mid, or late), its appearance on initiation of VT and diastolic timing, although necessary, does not confirm its relevance to the VT mechanism. One must always confirm that the electrogram cannot be

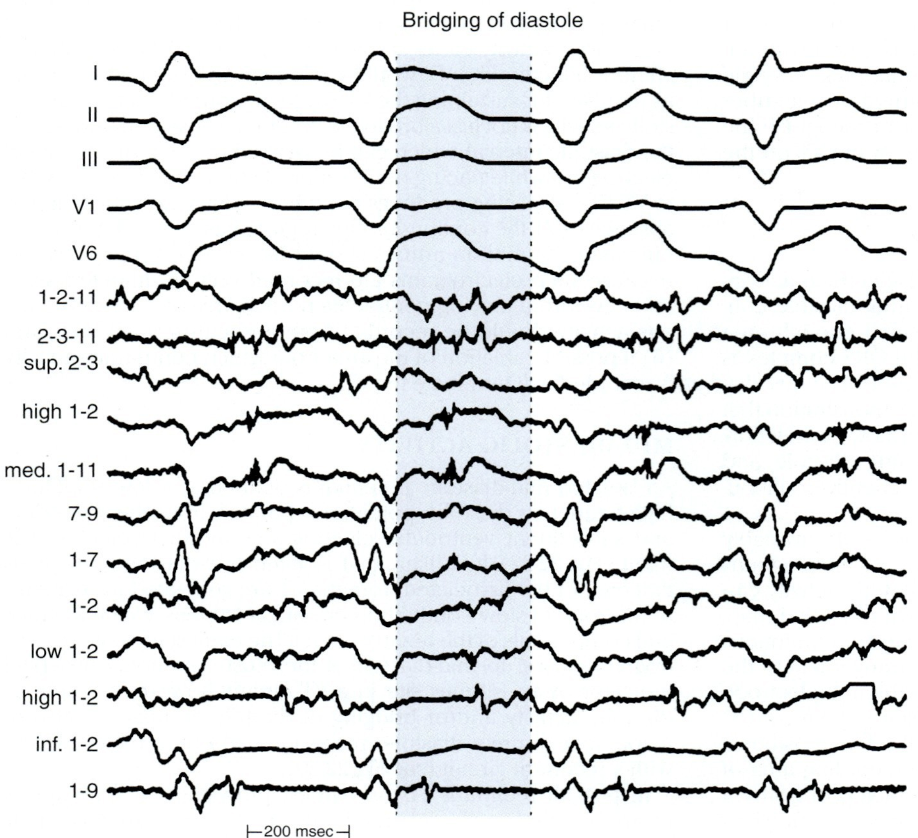

FIGURE 22-21 Bridging of diastole during reentrant ventricular tachycardia (VT). Shown is the compilation of numerous mapping sites around the left ventricular apical region during VT; diastole is shaded, showing progression of activation from early to mid to late diastole.

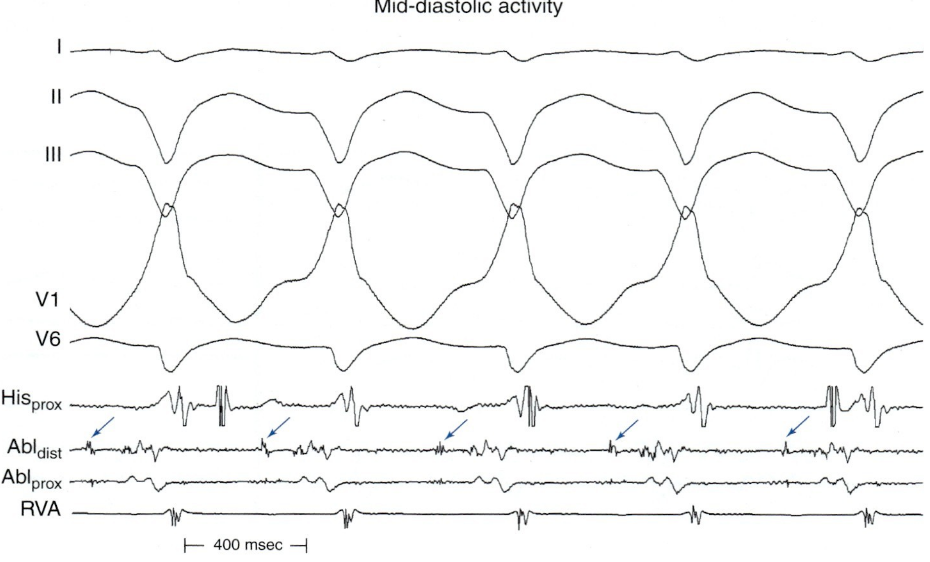

FIGURE 22-22 Mid-diastolic electrical activity during reentrant ventricular tachycardia (VT). VT is shown with small mid-diastolic potentials (arrows) on the ablation recording.

dissociated from the VT and is required for VT maintenance (see Fig. 5-12). Thus, during spontaneous changes in the tachycardia CL or those produced by programmed electrical stimulation, the electrogram, regardless of its position in diastole, should show a fixed relationship to the subsequent QRS and not the preceding QRS. Very early diastolic potentials, in the first half of diastole, can represent an area of slow conduction at the entrance of a protected isthmus. Such potentials will remain fixed to the prior QRS (exit site from the isthmus), and delay between it and the subsequent QRS would reflect delay entering or propagating through the protected diastolic pathway. This phenomenon is an uncommon response of presystolic electrograms occurring in the second half of diastole to pacing at rates slightly faster than the VT rate in post-MI VTs, but has been described in idiopathic and verapamil-sensitive VTs. Theoretically, such electrical activity may also arise from tissue between the site of impulse formation (the reentrant circuit) and the muscle mass that gives rise to the surface ECG. This response is also uncommon.

LIMITATIONS OF ACTIVATION MAPPING

Standard transcatheter endocardial mapping as performed in the EP laboratory is limited by the number, size, and types of electrodes that can be placed within the heart. Because these methods cover only a small portion of the endocardial surface, time-consuming point-by-point maneuvering of the catheter is required to trace the origin of an arrhythmic event and its activation sequence in the neighboring areas.

The success of roving point mapping is predicated on the sequential beat-by-beat stability of the activation sequence being mapped and the ability of the patient to tolerate the sustained arrhythmia. Therefore, it can be difficult to perform activation mapping in the case of poorly inducible VT at the time of EP testing, hemodynamically unstable VT, and unstable VT morphology. Extensive mapping is not possible when the VT repeatedly changes, causing multiple different morphologies. However, as noted, mapping can still be facilitated by starting and stopping the tachycardia after data acquisition at each site, slowing the VT rate by antiarrhythmic agents, or the use of multipolar basket catheters or noncontact mapping arrays.

Although activation mapping is adequate for defining the site of origin of focal tachycardias, it is deficient by itself in defining the critical isthmus of macroreentrant tachycardias. Adjunctive mapping modalities (e.g., entrainment mapping, pace mapping) are required for this.

Finally, using conventional activation mapping techniques, it is difficult to conceive the 3-D orientation of cardiac structures because these use a limited number of recording electrodes guided by fluoroscopy. Although catheters using multiple electrodes to acquire data points are available, the exact location of an acquired unit of EP data is difficult to ascertain because of inaccurate delineation of the location of anatomical structures. The inability to associate the intracardiac electrogram accurately with a specific endocardial site also limits the reliability with which the roving catheter tip can be placed at a site that was previously mapped. This results in limitations when the creation of long linear lesions is required to modify the substrate, and when multiple isthmuses, or channels, are present. This inability to identify, for example, the site of a previous ablation increases the risk of repeated ablation of areas already dealt with and the likelihood that new sites can be missed.

Entrainment Mapping

Focal ablation of multiple sites defined as in the reentrant circuit may not result in elimination of VT; that instead requires ablation of an isthmus bordered by barriers on either side, which is critical to the reentrant circuit. Because the circuit incorporates sites outside this critical isthmus, ablation of these external sites will eliminate VT, although it may slightly alter the tachycardia CL or morphology. Stimulation at sites recording diastolic activity can provide evidence of its relationship to the VT circuit. Entrainment mapping is used to verify whether a diastolic electrogram (regardless of where in diastole it occurs, its position, and appearance on initiation of VT) is part of the VT circuit, focusing ablation efforts in areas likely to eliminate VT (see Fig. 22-18).[42]

Pacing is usually started at a CL just shorter than the tachycardia CL. Pacing should be continued for a sufficiently long duration to allow for entrainment; short pacing trains are usually not helpful. Pacing is then repeated at progressively shorter pacing CLs. After cessation of each pacing drive, the presence of entrainment should be verified by the presence of fixed fusion of the paced complexes at a given pacing CL, progressive fusion at faster pacing CLs, and resumption of the same tachycardia morphology following cessation of pacing with a nonfused complex at a return cycle that is equal to the pacing CL (see Figs. 5-15 and 5-16). The mere acceleration of the tachycardia to the pacing rate and then resumption of the original tachycardia after cessation of pacing does not establish the presence of entrainment, and evaluation of the PPI or other criteria is meaningless when the presence of true entrainment has not been verified. Moreover, it is important to verify the absence of termination and reinitiation of the tachycardia during the same pacing train. Once the presence of entrainment has been verified, several criteria can be used to indicate the relation of the pacing site to the reentrant circuit, as listed in Table 22-2 (Fig. 22-23; and see Fig. 5-14).[42]

There are several limitations to the entrainment mapping technique. Entrainment requires the presence of sustained, hemodynamically well-tolerated tachycardia of stable morphology and CL. Furthermore, overdrive pacing can result in termination, acceleration, or transformation of the index tachycardia into a different one, making further mapping challenging. Additionally, pacing and recording from the same area is required for entrainment mapping. This is usually satisfied by pacing from electrodes 1 and 3 and recording from electrodes 2 and 4 of the mapping catheter. However, this technique has its own limitations. Differences, albeit slight, exist in the area from which electrodes 2 and 4 record as compared with electrodes 1 and 3, as do differences in the relationship of the site of stimulation from poles 1 and 3 to the recorded electrogram from poles 2 and 4 (i.e., proximal or distal to the recording site). Furthermore, the total area affected by the pacing stimulus can exceed the local area, especially when high currents (more than 10 mA) are required for stimulation, in addition to the fact that the pacing artifact can obscure the early part of the captured local electrogram. In such a case, a comparable component of the electrogram can be used to measure the PPI.

TABLE 22-2 Entrainment Mapping Reentrant Ventricular Tachycardia

Pacing from Sites Outside VT Circuit
• Manifest fusion on surface ECG and/or intracardiac recordings • PPI – tachycardia CL > 30 msec • S-QRS interval > local electrogram to QRS interval
Pacing from Sites Inside VT Circuit but Outside Protected Isthmus
• Manifest fusion on surface ECG and/or intracardiac recordings • PPI – tachycardia CL < 30 msec • S-QRS interval = local electrogram-to-QRS interval
Pacing from Protected Isthmus Outside VT Circuit
• Concealed fusion • PPI – tachycardia CL > 30 msec • S-QRS interval > local electrogram to QRS interval
Pacing from Protected Isthmus Inside VT Circuit
• Concealed fusion • PPI – tachycardia CL < 30 msec • S-QRS interval = local electrogram to QRS interval (±20 msec)

CL = cycle length; PPI = post-pacing interval; VT = ventricular tachycardia.

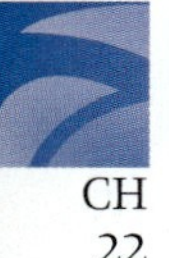

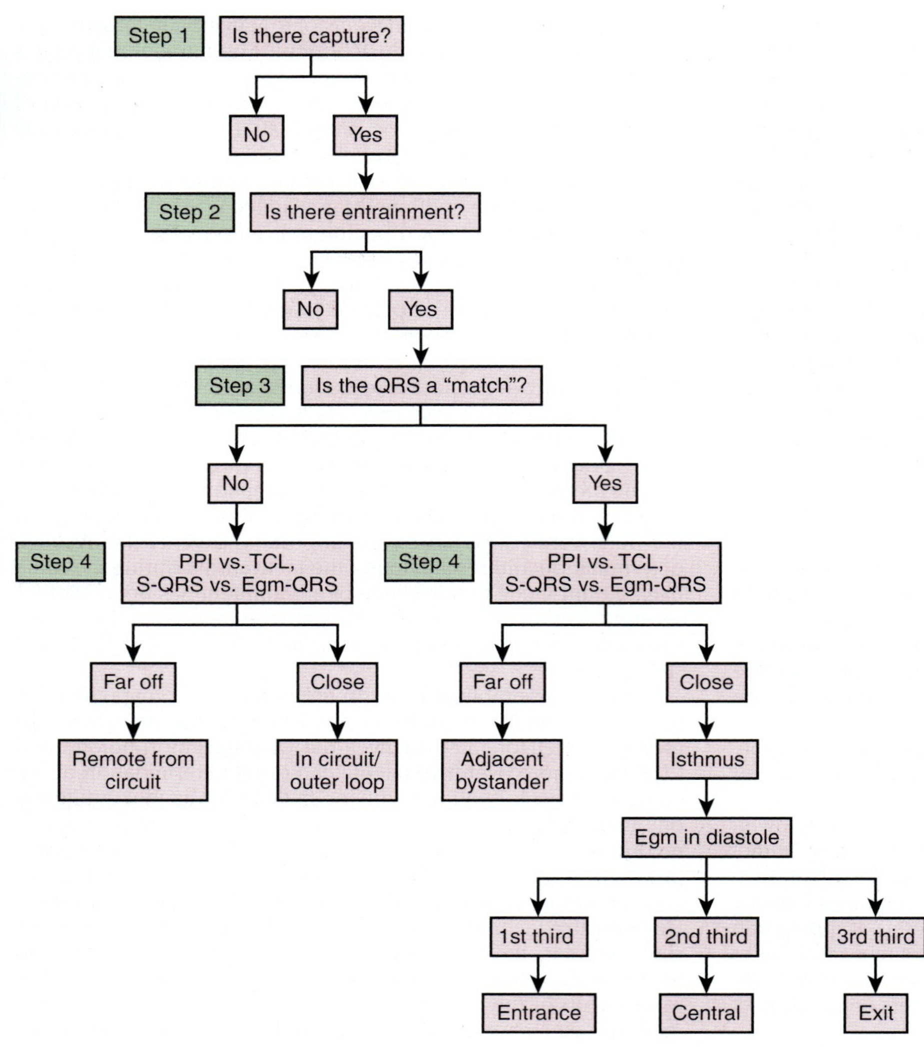

FIGURE 22-23 An algorithmic approach to entrainment in ventricular tachycardia. See text for details. Egm = electrogram; PPI = post- pacing interval; TCL = tachycardia cycle length.

The RV electrogram can also be used because it should have the same relationship to the paced site as it does from the electrogram during VT if the paced site is in the circuit. In both cases, these measurements provide indirect evidence of events in the circuit (i.e., the PPI will approximate the tachycardia CL if the stimulation site is in the circuit).

ENTRAINMENT WITH CONCEALED FUSION

Entrainment with concealed fusion (sometimes also referred to as "concealed entrainment" or "exact entrainment") is defined as entrainment with orthodromic capture and a QRS complex on the 12-lead surface ECG identical to that of the VT, and it suggests that the pacing site is within, attached to, or at the entrance to a protected isthmus that forms the diastolic pathway of the circuit (Fig. 22-24; and see Fig. 22-18). However, the positive predictive value of entrainment with concealed fusion in identifying effective ablation sites is only 50% to 60%, indicating that entrainment with concealed fusion can often occur at sites that are not critical to the maintenance of reentry (bystander pathway), such as a blind alley, alternate pathway, or inner loop. Even when such sites are believed to reside within the reentrant circuit isthmus, ablation can fail if lesions are too small to interrupt the circuit completely.[36]

Other mapping criteria can be helpful in increasing the probability of identifying an effective site for ablation of VT in combination with entrainment with concealed fusion (Table 22-3). If the S-QRS interval–to–tachycardia CL ratio is less than 0.7, the positive predictive value for successful ablation is approximately 70%. Furthermore, if the electrogram-QRS interval is equal to the S-QRS interval at a site at which there is entrainment with concealed fusion, the positive predictive value increases to approximately 80%. Finally, an isolated mid-diastolic potential that cannot be dissociated from VT increases the positive predictive value for identifying an effective ablation site to approximately 90%.[36,43,44]

POST-PACING INTERVAL

Assessment of the PPI helps differentiate early presystolic electrical activity from late diastolic activity that can be unrelated to the tachycardia circuit (see Fig. 22-24). During entrainment from sites within the reentrant circuit, the orthodromic wavefront from the last stimulus propagates through the reentry circuit and returns to the pacing site following the same path as the circulating reentry wavefront. The conduction time required is the revolution time through the circuit. Thus, the PPI, measured from the pacing site recording, should be equal (within 20 to 30 milliseconds) to the tachycardia CL. At sites distant from the circuit, stimulated wavefronts propagate to the circuit, then through the circuit, and finally back to the pacing site. Thus, the PPI should be equal to the tachycardia CL, plus the time required for the stimulus to propagate from the pacing site to the tachycardia circuit and back (see Fig. 5-14). The greater the difference between the PPI and the tachycardia CL, the longer the conduction time and distance between the pacing site and the reentry circuit.[36,43]

TABLE 22-3 Sensitivity, Specificity, and Predictive Values of Analyzed Mapping Criteria in Association with Concealed Entrainment for Effective Ablation Sites

MAPPING CRITERION	SENSITIVITY (%)	SPECIFICITY (%)	POSITIVE PREDICTIVE VALUE (%)	NEGATIVE PREDICTIVE VALUE (%)
Concealed entrainment	—	—	54	—
IMDP				
Overall	40	76	67	53
Not dissociable from VT	32	95	89	54
PPI = VT CL	58	19	45	29
S-QRS/VT CL <0.7	96	52	71	92
S-QRS = EGM-QRS				
Excluding IMDP	32	86	73	51
Including IMDP	56	86	82	62

CL = cycle length; EGM = electrogram; IMDP = isolated mid-diastolic potential; PPI = post-pacing interval; S-QRS = stimulus-to-QRS interval; VT = ventricular tachycardia.
From Bogun F, Bahu M, Knight BP, et al: Comparison of effective and ineffective target sites that demonstrate concealed entrainment in patients with coronary artery disease undergoing radiofrequency ablation of ventricular tachycardia, *Circulation* 95:183, 1997.

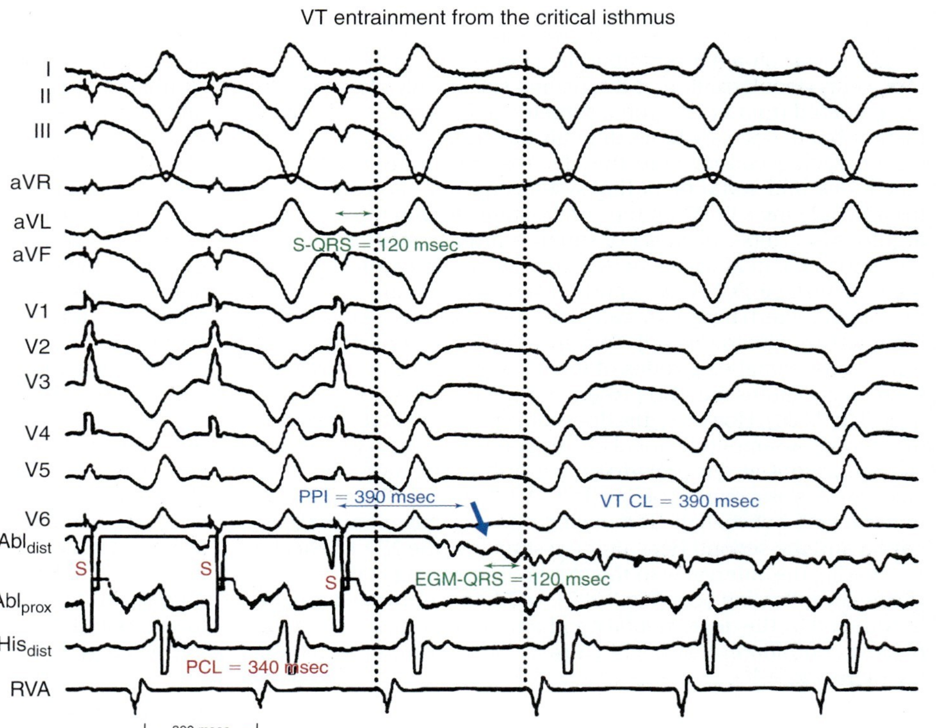

FIGURE 22-24 Entrainment during post-myocardial infarction ventricular tachycardia (VT) from the critical isthmus. The mid-diastolic potential (arrow) is present at the pacing site. Dashed lines denote QRS onset. Each stimulated complex is identical to that of VT at right (entrainment with concealed fusion). This, and findings that the stimulus-QRS (S-QRS) interval with pacing equals the electrogram-QRS (EGM-QRS) interval in VT and that the post-pacing interval (PPI) equals the VT cycle length (CL), indicates that pacing is from the protected diastolic corridor. Radiofrequency delivery at this site terminated VT in 4 seconds. PCL = pacing cycle length.

The PPI should be measured to the near-field potential that indicates depolarization of tissue at the pacing site (see Figs. 22-18 and 22-24). In regions of scar, electrode catheters often record multiple potentials separated in time, some of which are far-field potentials that are caused by depolarization of adjacent myocardium. Far-field potentials are common during catheter mapping of infarct-related VT and can confound interpretation of the PPI. Assignment of an incorrect time of activation will render activation sequence maps misleading. The presence of far-field potentials also reduces the accuracy of entrainment mapping using the PPI. Measurement of the PPI to a far-field potential introduces an error, the magnitude of which is related to the conduction time between the pacing site and the source of the far-field potential (Fig. 22-25). When the PPI appears to be shorter than the tachycardia CL, the potential used for measurement is likely a far-field potential. Analysis of the potentials recorded during entrainment often allows identification of the far-field potential so that it can be excluded from activation maps and the PPI measurement and, hence, improves the accuracy of mapping scar-related arrhythmias. The stimulus artifact obscures the potential produced in the tissue immediately at the stimulation site (i.e., near-field potentials). Thus, the local potential is not visible during pacing, but reappears after the last entrained QRS complex. On the other hand, far-field potentials usually fall sufficiently late after the pacing stimulus to be visible, and remain undisturbed during entrainment (see Fig. 22-25). These far-field potentials are accelerated to the pacing rate, but are not changed in morphology compared with those observed during tachycardia. The far-field potentials often precede the next stimulus by a short interval so that the tissue generating the far-field potential is probably refractory at the time of the next stimulus. Hence, the stimulus is not directly depolarizing the tissue generating the far-field potential. That these potentials are distant from the distal recording electrode is further supported by the lack of effect of RF ablation on the far-field potential.[36]

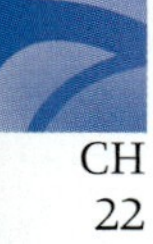

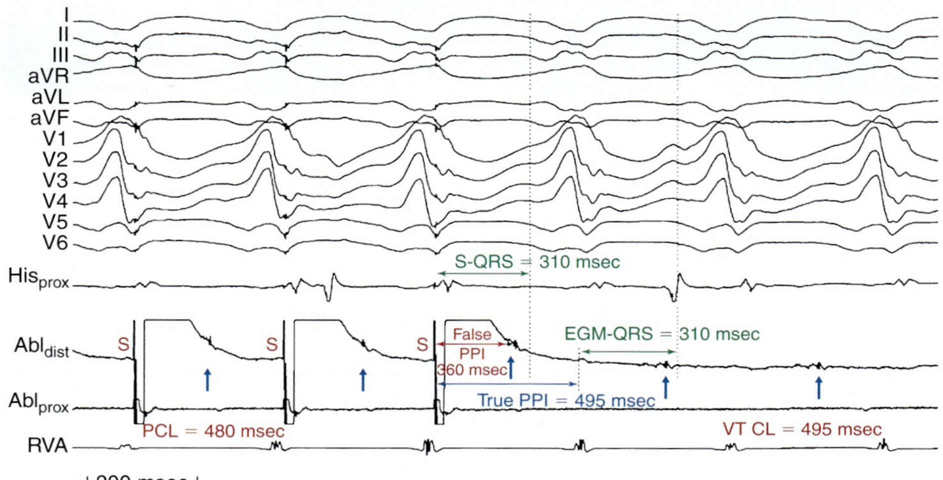

FIGURE 22-25 Entrainment during post-myocardial infarction ventricular tachycardia (VT) at a site with both systolic and late diastolic (arrows) potentials. Stimulation (S) entrains VT with an identical QRS configuration (concealed fusion) and a very long S-QRS interval, suggesting pacing at the entrance of the protected isthmus. The sharp electrogram (arrows) at this site is present and accelerated to the pacing cycle length (PCL), suggesting that the tissue generating this potential is not directly depolarized by the pacing stimulus and is, therefore, a far-field potential. The post-pacing interval (PPI) measured from the last stimulus to this far-field potential is falsely short. The local potential (red arrow) is not discernible during pacing, consistent with direct capture, but reappears after the last stimulus. The true PPI is measured from the last stimulus to this local potential.

The validity of the difference between the PPI and VT CL (PPI – VT CL) is based on the assumption that the recorded electrogram represents depolarization at the pacing site. Ideally, electrograms are recorded from the mapping catheter electrodes used for stimulation, but this is sometimes difficult. Electrical noise introduced during pacing can obscure the electrograms at the stimulating electrodes, and some recording systems do not allow recording from the pacing site. When the electrograms from the pacing site are not discernible because of stimulus artifact, relating the timing of the near-field potential to a consistent intracardiac electrogram or surface ECG wave can be used to determine the PPI. A reasonable alternative is to calculate the PPI from electrograms recorded by electrodes adjacent to those used for pacing (i.e., from the proximal electrodes of the mapping catheter), provided such electrograms are also present in the distal electrode recordings (Fig. 22-26). However, this does introduce potential error, particularly if low-amplitude local electrograms present at the pacing site are absent at the proximal recording site. A more accurate alternative is assessment of the [PPI – VT CL] value from the conduction time between the last pacing stimulus that entrains tachycardia and the second beat after the stimulus (the N + 1 beat) by comparing this interval with the electrogram timing at the pacing site in any following beat (Fig. 22-27). Additional errors can also be introduced by the decremental conduction properties of the zone of slow conduction that might cause a rate-dependent lengthening of the PPI.[36,44]

ELECTROGRAM-TO-QRS INTERVAL VERSUS STIMULUS-TO-QR INTERVAL

This criterion is helpful in differentiating a critical component of the zone of slow conduction from a blind alley or noncritical alternate (bystander) pathway, in a manner analogous to that of the [PPI – VT CL] method (see Fig. 5-14). An electrogram-QRS interval equal to the S-QRS interval (±20 milliseconds) suggests that the pacing site lies within the reentry circuit and not in a dead-end bystander pathway attached to the circuit (see Figs. 22-24 and 22-25). This method requires that the stimulated orthodromic wavefronts exit from the circuit at the same site as the tachycardia wavefronts (i.e., presence of entrainment with concealed fusion). Any degree of QRS fusion indicates that the stimulated wavefronts could be exiting from another route, invalidating this analysis. However, QRS fusion is often difficult to detect when less than 22% of the QRS is fused, which poses a major limitation to the S-QRS method.

To avoid this limitation, a modification of the S-QRS interval method has been proposed whereby the S-QRS interval is measured to the second beat, which unquestionably results from a wavefront that has emerged from the tachycardia circuit and is not fused. The QRS complex and electrogram inscribed during or immediately after the pacing stimulus are defined as $QRS_{(N)}$ and $electrogram_{(N)}$, respectively; the following QRS and electrogram are defined as $QRS_{(N+1)}$ and $electrogram_{(N+1)}$, respectively. The $S\text{-}QRS_{(N+1)}$ interval and $electrogram_{(N+1)}\text{-}QRS_{(N+2)}$ interval are then determined; the difference between these two intervals is defined as the N + 1 difference. Because the $S\text{-}QRS_{(N+1)}$ interval is not influenced by QRS fusion during entrainment, an endocardial electrogram that is remote from the pacing site can potentially be used as the timing reference, instead of the QRS onset. Often, the endocardial recording is more precise and easily used for the fiducial point.[44]

The S-QRS criterion increases the positive predictive value of successful ablation outcome at sites demonstrating entrainment with concealed fusion to 80% (see Table 22-3). However, the electrogram-QRS interval may not be equal to the S-QRS interval at sites within the reentrant circuit. Several factors can explain this. Decremental conduction properties of the zone of slow conduction can potentially lengthen the S-QRS interval during pacing, and stimulus latency in an area of diseased tissue can also account for a delay in the S-QRS interval compared with the electrogram-QRS interval. In addition, failure of the recording electrodes to detect low-amplitude depolarizations at the pacing site can account for a mismatch of the S-QRS and electrogram-QRS intervals (Fig. 22-28).

RATIO OF STIMULUS-TO-QRS INTERVAL TO TACHYCARDIA CYCLE LENGTH

Some investigators have proposed that critical areas of slow conduction within the reentrant circuit could be identified by overdrive pacing from LV sites associated with prolonged conduction times from the pacing site to the exit from the infarct scar, as reflected by the S-QRS interval. Although sites requisite for the reentrant circuit that exhibit slow conduction can behave in this manner, the mere presence of prolonged conduction from the S-QRS interval does not prove that the slow conduction is part of a reentrant circuit pathway. Multiple areas within the infarct zone can exhibit fractionated or abnormal electrograms and reduced excitability, which are associated with increased S-QRS intervals, yet may have nothing to do with the VT circuit itself.

Others have used a prolonged stimulus to local electrogram time during entrainment to identify pathways containing slow conduction. This again does not prove that the electrogram at the recording site has anything to do with the VT, because slow conduction involved in the orthodromic capture of this electrogram can occur inside or outside the circuit. In fact, whenever ECG fusion occurs, some electrograms outside the circuit (i.e., those activated after

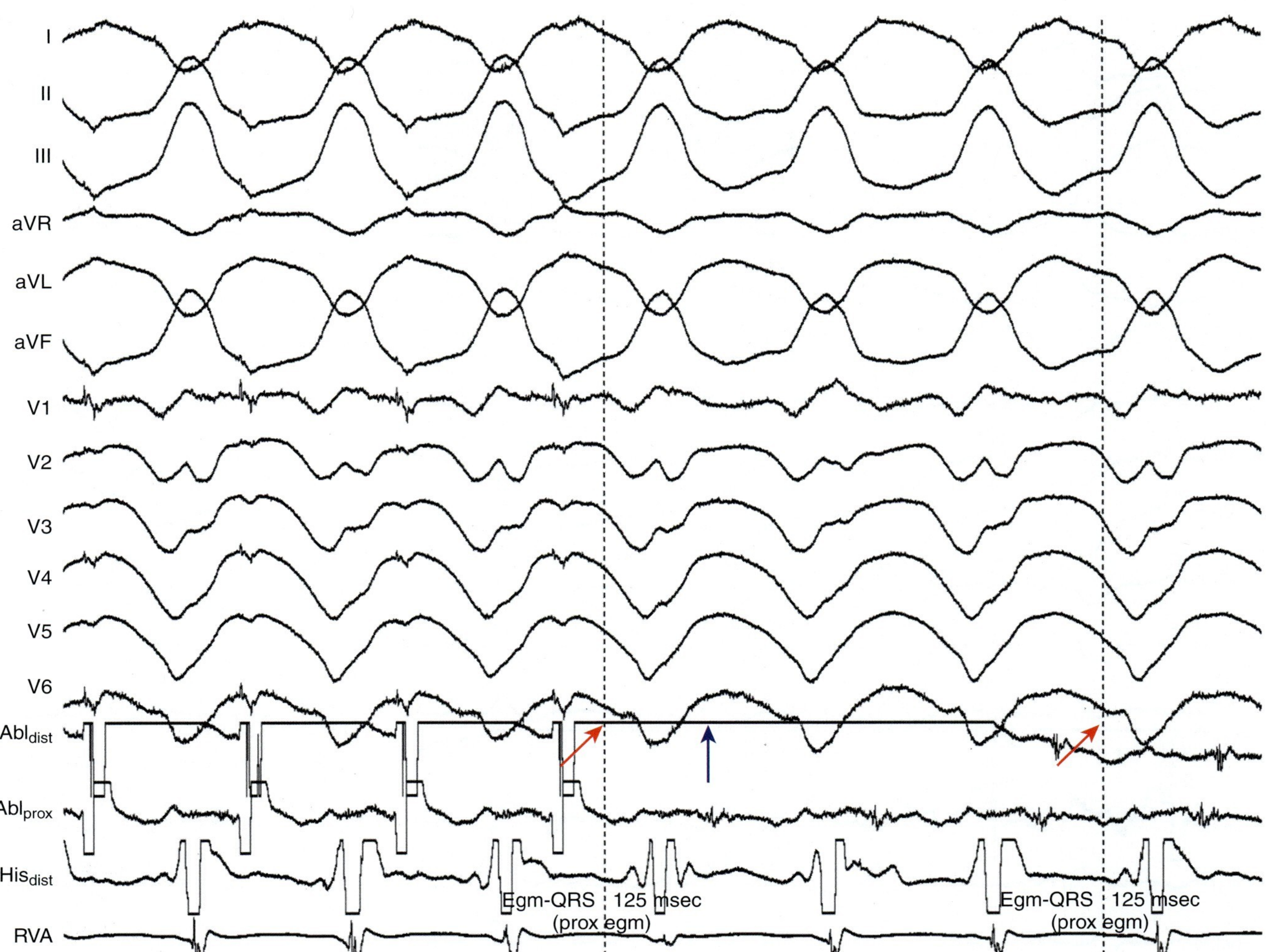

FIGURE 22-26 Using the proximal electrogram recording as a surrogate for the distal electrogram. Entrainment of ventricular tachycardia (VT) is shown. The post-pacing interval cannot be directly assessed owing to saturation of the distal ablation electrode (Abl_{dist}) recording (blue arrow). The interval from the proximal ablation electrode (Abl_{prox}) recording electrogram to QRS can be compared with the same interval during VT (red arrows) to serve as a surrogate for the distal ablation recording electrogram, as long as there is minimal disparity in the timing of these two recordings. Egm = electrogram.

leaving the exit that is part of the VT wavefront) will be orthodromically activated and will fulfill the requirements for entrainment. For the same reason, termination with block before this orthodromically entrained electrogram does not mean that it was a critical component of the circuit.

On the other hand, during entrainment with concealed fusion, the S-QRS interval is an approximate indication of the location of the pacing site relative to the reentry circuit exit. A short S-QRS interval (<30% of the tachycardia CL) suggests a site near the exit. Long S-QRS intervals (>70% of the tachycardia CL) suggest bystander sites rather than a critical isthmus. Therefore, at sites demonstrating entrainment with concealed fusion, an S-QRS interval–to–tachycardia CL ratio not exceeding 0.7 suggests that the sites lie within the common pathway (isthmus) of the reentrant circuit, and sites at which the ratio is equal to or more than 0.7 are considered to lie outside the common pathway (see Fig. 5-14). The S-QRS interval–to–VT CL ratio not greater than 0.7 criterion improves the positive predictive value of entrainment with concealed fusion to approximately 70%. Moreover, the negative predictive value of this criterion is 92%, indicating that ablation at sites with entrainment with concealed fusion at which the S-QRS interval–to–VT CL ratio is more than 0.7 is unlikely to be successful (see Table 22-3).

Pace Mapping

QRS MORPHOLOGY DURING PACING VERSUS VENTRICULAR TACHYCARDIA

When ventricular activation originates from a pointlike source (e.g., during focal VT or during pacing from an electrode catheter), the QRS configuration recorded in the surface ECG is determined by the sequence of ventricular activation, which is largely determined by the initial site of ventricular depolarization. Analysis of specific QRS configurations in multiple leads allows estimation of the pacing site location to within several square centimeters (see Figs. 5-21 and 5-22). Therefore, comparing the paced QRS configuration with that of VT is particularly useful for locating a small arrhythmia focus in a structurally normal heart (e.g., idiopathic RVOT VT), whereas pace mapping has been less useful for guiding the ablation of post-MI VT.[44]

Reentry circuits in healed infarct scars often extend over several square centimeters and can have a variety of configurations. In many circuits, the excitation wavefront circulates through surviving myocytes within the scar, the depolarization of which is not detectable on the standard surface ECG. The QRS complex is then inscribed after the reentry wavefront exits the scar and propagates across the

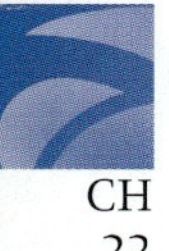

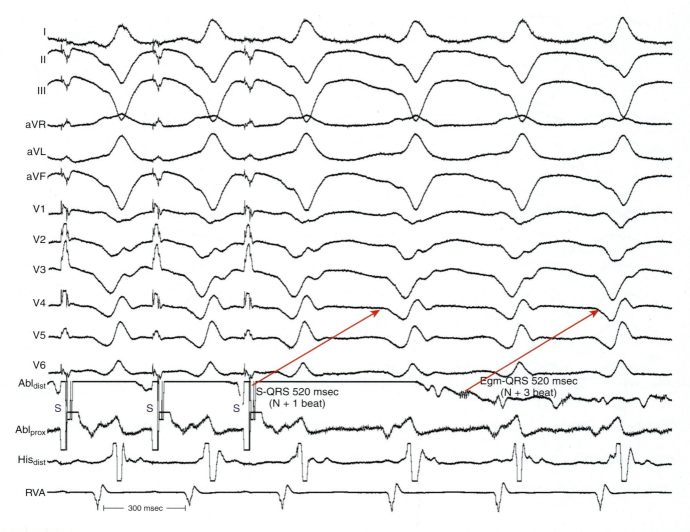

FIGURE 22-27 The "N + 1" rule. Entrainment of ventricular tachycardia (VT) is shown. The post-pacing interval cannot be directly assessed because of saturation of the distal ablation electrode (Abl_{dist}) recording. The interval from stimulus (S) to the next VT complex ("N + 1") can be compared with the interval from the electrogram after it is again visible, to a subsequent VT complex ("N + 3" in this case). If the difference between these intervals is less than 20 milliseconds, the site of stimulation is likely in the circuit.

ventricles. At sites at which the reentrant wavefront exits the scar, pace mapping is expected to produce a QRS configuration similar to that of the VT (see Fig. 5-23). Pace mapping at sites more proximally located in the isthmus should also produce a similar QRS complex, but with a longer S-QRS interval. The S-QRS interval lengthens progressively as the pacing site is moved along the isthmus, consistent with pacing progressively farther from the exit (see Fig. 5-23).[44]

In infarct-related VT, however, a paced QRS configuration different from that during VT does not reliably indicate that the pacing site is distant from the reentry circuit. At many reentry circuit sites, pacing during NSR can produce a QRS configuration different from that during VT. In fact, it is uncommon to have similar or even almost identical morphology result from pacing from a known isthmus determined by mapping. Several factors can explain this mismatch.[45] First, the pattern of ventricular activation and hence resultant QRS depends on how the wavefront propagates from the exit of the isthmus to the remainder of the heart, which can be totally different during VT than during pacing from the same site during NSR (see Fig. 5-23). In fact, such pacing would be expected to produce a different QRS than the VT because the paced wavefront spreads centrifugally to the heart while the VT wavefront spreads in one direction (i.e., orthodromically). This observation is one of the important limitations of the use of pace mapping to identify the critical isthmus of post-MI VT. Propagation in the diseased myocardium is not homogeneous, and small differences in catheter location can cause grossly different propagation wavefronts and resultant QRS complexes. Even small differences in the angle of contact of catheter to the ventricular wall and site of initial ventricular activation can alter the precise QRS configuration. The relationship between conduction time, pacing site location in the isthmus, and conduction block determines whether pace mapping in an isthmus produces a QRS that resembles that of VT. When pace mapping in a defined isthmus is performed, the stimulated wavefront can only follow along its course, which occurs in at least two directions—orthodromic and antidromic (relative to the direction of VT propagation). The wavefront is only detected on the surface ECG when it leaves this protected channel. If the isthmus is long and the catheter is positioned in the distal part, near the exit, the orthodromic wavefront leaves the exit and rapidly depolarizes the region along the infarct, colliding with and preventing emergence of the antidromic wavefront from the infarct region. The resulting QRS complex is then similar to that of VT. If the isthmus is short, or the catheter is positioned more proximally, the stimulated antidromic wavefront leaves the protected isthmus at the entrance, propagating to the surrounding myocardium and producing a different QRS morphology (see Fig. 5-23). If the orthodromic wavefront reaches the exit, a fusion QRS is produced that includes depolarization from both the antidromic and orthodromic wavefronts.

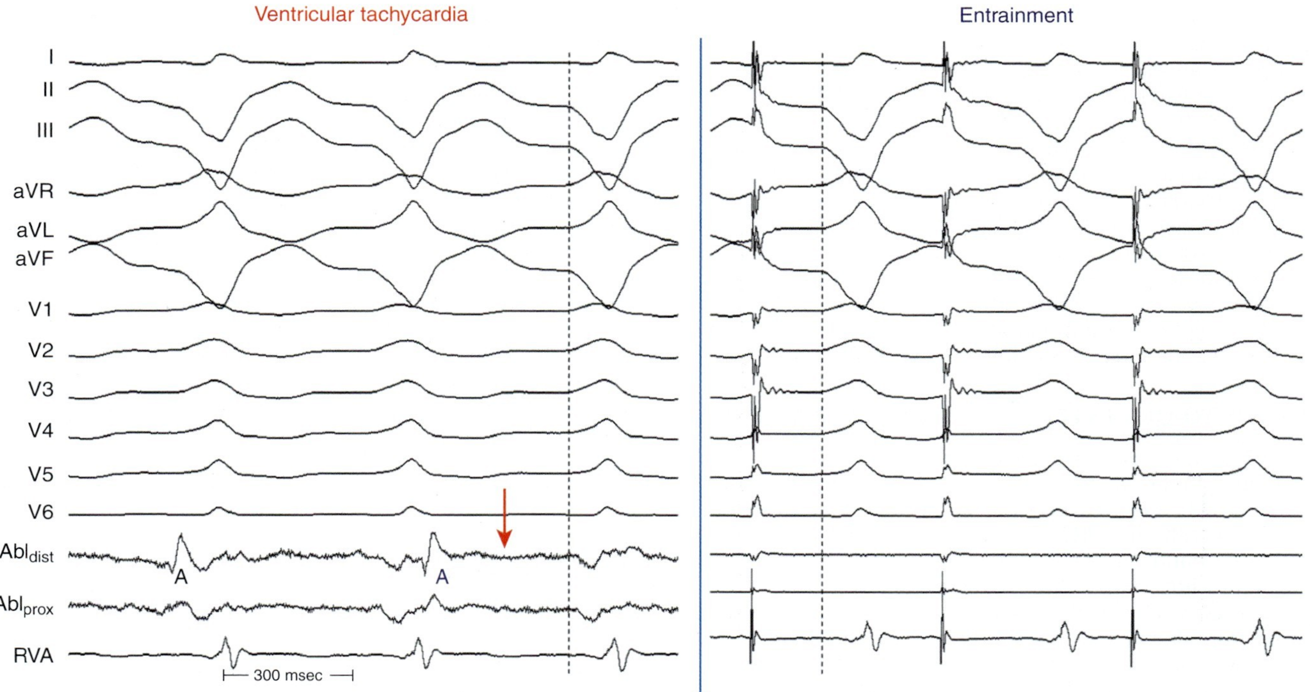

FIGURE 22-28 Capture during inferobasal post-infarct ventricular tachycardia (VT) without recorded electrogram. At left is VT during which the distal ablation electrode (Abl$_{dist}$) recording shows no clear diastolic activity; however, stimulation at this site readily captures the ventricle. The red arrow shows the timing during VT equal to the stimulus-QRS interval during pacing. A = atrial recording.

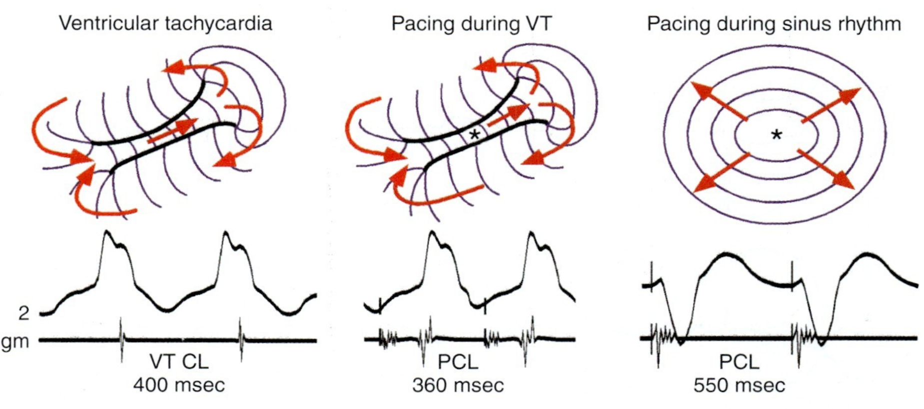

FIGURE 22-29 Functional block during ventricular tachycardia (VT). At left, VT propagates through a diastolic corridor maintained by lines of block. At center, pacing during VT within the diastolic corridor (asterisk) propagates in the same manner as VT because of maintenance of lines of block. At right, pacing during sinus rhythm at the same site results in a completely different activation pattern and QRS complex if the lines of block during VT were functionally, rather than anatomically, determined. CL = cycle length; Egm = intracardiac electrogram; PCL = pacing CL.

A second explanation is that the process whereby VT is generated in patients with structural heart disease usually involves the development of an area of functional block to conduction. Such functional block is not fixed, not anatomical, and variable in its extent. When formed, it combines with an area of fixed conduction block caused by, for example, the infarct scar, to create a protected channel for conduction that allows reentry to occur. Regions of functional block, present during VT, can define propagation paths during tachycardia but not during pace mapping in NSR. Therefore, if block defining an isthmus is present only during VT and is absent during pace mapping in NSR, the stimulated wavefront produced by pacing at the isthmus site would propagate in all directions, resulting in a different QRS morphology (Fig. 22-29). This is further exaggerated by the fact that pace mapping is usually performed at rates slower than the VT to avoid VT induction during the mapping process, which can reduce the likelihood of development of a line of functional block. Additionally, the area over which the current is delivered, especially where high current is required for relatively inexcitable tissue, can influence the pattern of subsequent ventricular activation, presumably by capturing more distant (i.e., far-field) tissue. When this occurs, it can indicate pacing in a region of a protected isthmus, where pacing at low output would capture only the isthmus, whereas pacing at a higher output can capture both the isthmus and far-field tissue, resulting in different QRS morphologies and S-QRS intervals (Fig. 22-30). Finally, some circuits can have more than one exit, with wavefronts emerging from the scar at multiple locations. Different exits can participate preferentially during VT but not during pace mapping, and vice versa.

On the other hand, pacing during NSR from sites attached to the reentrant circuit but not part of the circuit can occasionally produce QRS morphology identical to that of the VT, because the stimulated wavefront can be physiologically forced to follow the same route of activation as the VT as long as pacing is carried out between the entrance and exit of the protected isthmus. Although this strategy can result in the identification of irrelevant inner loop and adjacent bystander sites as well as the desired isthmus sites, it still can be helpful in gross identification of the region of the VT circuit.[2]

Conduction away from the pacing site (and the resultant QRS morphology) can potentially be influenced by the pacing output, pacing rate, and antiarrhythmic drugs. To minimize the impact of rate-related changes in conduction, pacing is performed at a relatively slow rate. Pacing slower than the rate of the VT, however, can further reduce the relationship of the paced QRS morphology to that of the VT target area. During bipolar pacing, capture at the proximal electrode rather than the distal electrode can also modify the QRS morphology. The sequence of ventricular activation can vary during pacing at different stimulus strengths. This phenomenon is more pronounced with bipolar than unipolar pacing, likely because of anodal capture at higher stimulus strengths (Fig. 22-31). This potential problem can be avoided by using unipolar pacing and by limiting the current output to 10 mA and 2 milliseconds, which is within the range of routine programmed stimulation.[46]

STIMULUS-TO-QRS INTERVAL DURING PACE MAPPING

Parts of VT reentry circuit isthmuses can be traced during NSR by combining both the QRS morphology and the S-QRS delay during pace mapping in anatomical maps. Pacing in normal myocardium is associated with an S-QRS interval of less than 40 milliseconds. On the other hand, an S-QRS interval more than 40 milliseconds is consistent with slow conduction away from the pacing site, and is typically associated with abnormal fractionated electrograms recorded from that site. Thus, pace mapping can provide a measure of slow conduction, as indicated by the S-QRS interval, which can indicate a greater likelihood that the pacing site is in a reentry circuit. Creating a latency map using an electroanatomical mapping system to represent the regions of S-QRS latency graphically also can be a useful method for initially screening sites during NSR (see Fig. 5-23). It is likely that pacing sites with long S-QRS delays are in a potential isthmus, adjacent to regions of conduction block. However, this isthmus can be part of the reentrant circuit (i.e., critical isthmus) or a bystander (see Fig. 5-14).

The reentry circuit exit, which is more likely to be at the border of the infarct and close to the normal myocardium, often has no delay during pace mapping during NSR, even though it may be reasonable to target for ablation. Sites with long S-QRS intervals can be more proximal in the isthmuses; therefore, they are more likely to be associated with propagation of the paced wavefront in the antidromic direction away from the reentry circuit, producing a QRS different from that of the VT (see Fig. 5-23). Sites with prolonged S-QRS intervals during pace mapping are frequently associated with other markers of reentry circuit sites; however, this can be a somewhat limited mapping guide. Approximately 25% of likely reentry circuit sites have short S-QRS intervals during pace mapping, and more than 20% of sites with long S-QRS intervals do not appear to be in the reentry circuit.[2]

VALUE OF PACE MAPPING

At best, a pace map that matches the VT would only identify the exit site to the normal myocardium, which can be distant from the critical sites of the circuit required for ablation. Thus, pace mapping remains only a corroborative method of localizing reentrant

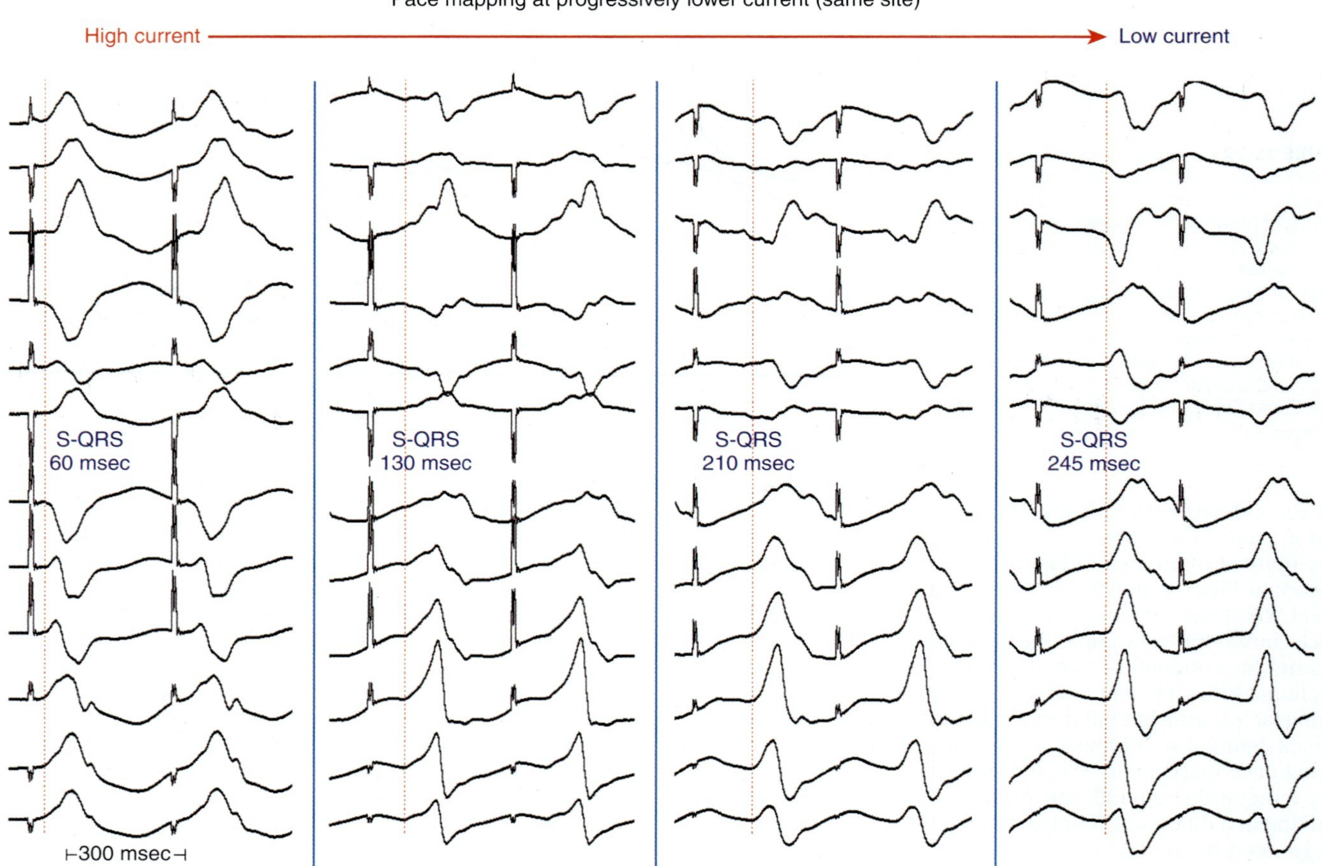

FIGURE 22-30 Effect of stimulus strength on QRS complex and stimulus (S)-QRS during pace mapping. QRS complexes resulting from pacing from the same site, but at different current strength, are shown from higher (left) to lower (right) output. Note the dramatic changes in QRS configuration as well as the progressively longer S-QRS interval. This was easily reproducible; increasing output reversed the ECG and S-QRS interval findings, and lowering output again recapitulated the data shown here.

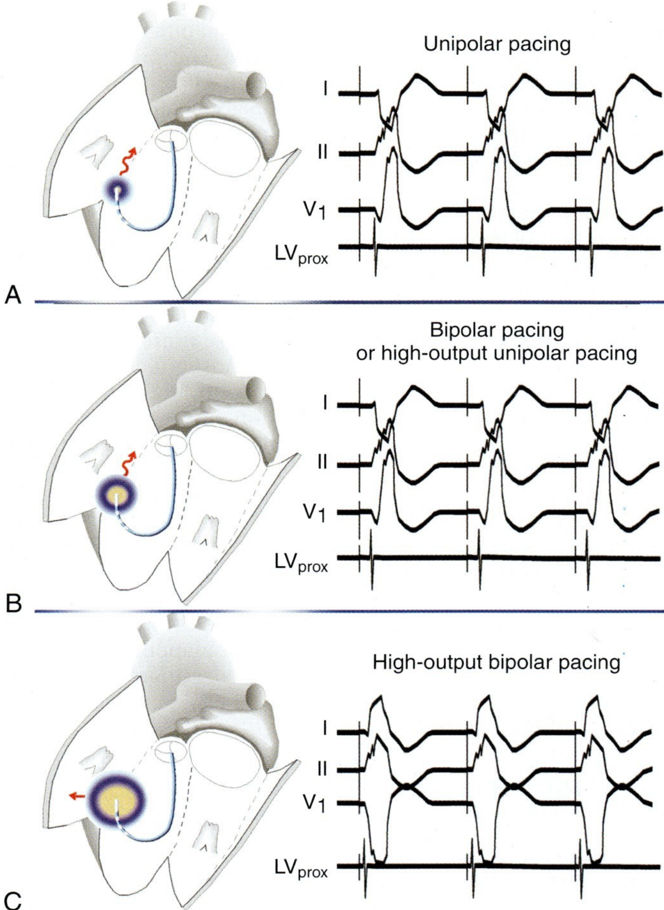

FIGURE 22-31 Effect of bipolar and high-output stimulation on the paced QRS complex morphology in scarred myocardium. The diagram illustrates a catheter stimulating a site within scar tissue on the left ventricular (LV) anterior septum. **A,** With low-output unipolar pacing, a relatively small zone is captured (blue halo) resulting in a long stimulus (S)-QRS interval because the impulse must travel through scar until it encounters enough tissue to generate a QRS complex. **B,** Bipolar or higher output unipolar pacing captures a larger area, resulting in a shorter S-QRS but using the same path, resulting in the same QRS morphology as at lower output unipolar pacing. **C,** High-output bipolar pacing captures a much larger area and can now activate normal myocardium directly, bypassing the slow conduction zone in scar tissue. This results in a very short S-QRS and a very different QRS complex morphology than previously, despite pacing at the same site.

VT. It can be used to focus initial mapping to regions likely to contain the reentrant circuit exit or abnormal conduction but is not sufficiently specific or sensitive to be the sole guide for ablation. Pace mapping can also be used in conjunction with substrate mapping when other mapping techniques are not feasible, so that it can provide information on where ablation can be directed.[2]

TECHNIQUE OF PACE MAPPING

At isthmus sites, as identified by activation and entrainment mapping during VT, pace mapping in NSR is attempted after VT termination. Either bipolar or unipolar pacing may be used. Pace mapping is preferably performed with unipolar stimuli (10 mA, 2 milliseconds) from the distal electrode of the mapping catheter (cathode) and an electrode in the inferior vena cava (IVC; anode). Bipolar pacing produces a smaller stimulus artifact; however, there is the possibility of capture at the proximal ring electrode as well as at the tip electrode that may reduce accuracy, particularly if larger interelectrode distances (8 to 10 mm) and high-current strength is used. Pacing only slightly above threshold is likely to improve accuracy. The pacing CL is usually the same for each site in an individual patient (500 to 700 milliseconds), faster than the sinus rate and slower than the rate of the induced VTs.[2]

The resulting 12-lead ECG morphology is compared with that of the VT. ECG recordings should be reviewed at the same gain and filter settings and at a paper-sweep speed of 100 mm/sec. It is often helpful to have a split-screen display of the target VT in one panel, comparing this with all 12 leads of the paced QRS complexes brought into another panel, as well as with print regular 12-lead ECGs for side-by-side comparison on paper. The greater the degree of concordance between the morphology during pacing and tachycardia, the closer the catheter is to the site of origin of the tachycardia (see Fig. 5-22).

Evaluation of the S-QRS also is of value. The S-QRS interval is measured to the onset of the earliest QRS on the 12-lead ECG. Sites from which pace mapping produces the same QRS as that of the initial isthmus site with different S-QRS delays are identified in an attempt to trace the course of the VT isthmus (see Figs. 5-14 and 5-23).

Substrate Mapping during Baseline Rhythm

Substrate mapping refers to delineation of the infarcted myocardium (VT substrate) based on the identification of abnormal local electrogram configuration (fractionated electrograms, multipotential electrograms, and/or electrograms with isolated delayed components) and abnormal local electrogram amplitude (voltage mapping) during the baseline rhythm (NSR, AF, ventricular pacing; Fig. 22-32). Post-MI VTs can be unstable or unsustainable and therefore not approachable by conventional point-by-point activation

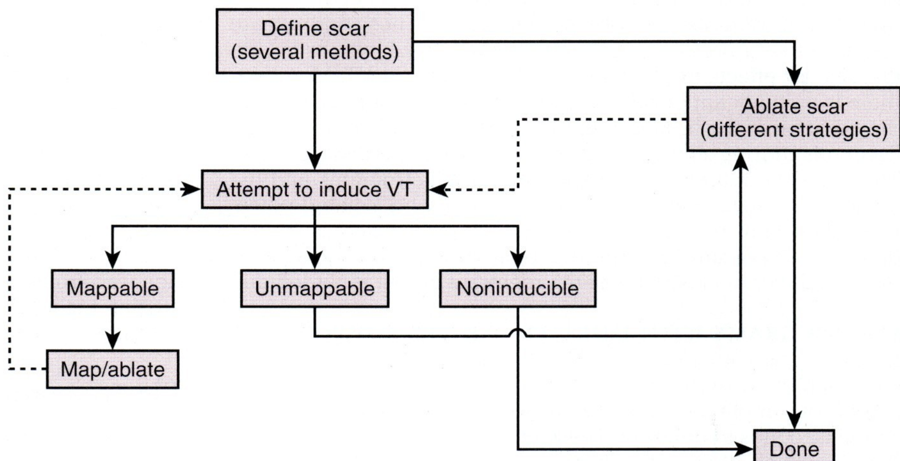

FIGURE 22-32 An algorithmic approach to treatment of scar-based ventricular tachycardia, consisting of an iterative process. See text for details.

mapping and entrainment maneuvers. Therefore, mapping during the baseline rhythm rather than during VT is of significant value. Substrate mapping helps identify the VT substrate and facilitates ablation of multiple VTs, pleomorphic VTs, and VTs that are unmappable because of hemodynamic instability or that are not reliably inducible. Substrate mapping is also of value in ablation of stable VTs, because it can help focus activation and entrainment mapping efforts on a small region harboring the VT substrate, and therefore help minimize how long the patient is actually in VT.[2]

ABNORMAL ELECTROGRAMS DURING THE BASELINE RHYTHM

The vast majority (approximately 85%) of post-MI VTs occurs at sites that have abnormal and/or late electrograms during NSR (see Fig. 22-20). Infarct regions are well delineated as areas of low-amplitude abnormal electrograms. Therefore, potential arrhythmogenic areas can be identified in the presence of abnormalities, late electrograms, or both, which are associated with arrhythmogenic tissue. However, abnormal sinus rhythm electrograms with multiple potentials are also frequently seen in bystander regions that are not integral parts of the reentrant circuit. Recording of simply abnormal low-voltage electrograms is highly nonspecific because the extensive areas in which they are located are not sufficiently specific to be the sole guide for ablation if the ablation approach seeks to target a small focal region. Therefore, additional electrogram characteristics have been proposed to improve the accuracy of sinus rhythm mapping.

FRACTIONATED ELECTROGRAMS. Reentry circuit isthmuses consist of a proximal part (entrance), a central part, and an exit from which the wavefront leaves the abnormal region and rapidly depolarizes the normal myocardium, resulting in the formation of the QRS complex. Conduction through the isthmus or at its entrance, exit, or both is often slow and nonuniformly anisotropic because of the transverse uncoupling of myocytes by fibrosis; hence electrogram fractionation is a common finding in areas of scar and VT substrate. Additionally, during NSR, a typical local electrogram in the border of an infarct has a low voltage but is adjacent to more normal myocardium in the border, causing a multipotential electrogram that has markedly different amplitudes, with a large rounded potential (reflecting a far-field signal from activation of the large mass of surrounding tissue) and a small sharp potential (reflecting local depolarization of a small mass of fibers in the infarct). These electrograms are common in the infarct region, may be found throughout the scar, and are not specific for the critical isthmus of the reentry circuit. Therefore targeting of fractionated electrograms has never been shown to be an effective ablation strategy.[4,7]

WIDE ELECTROGRAMS. Critical isthmus sites in the VT reentry circuit are likely to be located at sites with the latest activation during NSR. Most critical isthmus sites display electrograms that have a duration of more than 200 milliseconds, isolated diastolic potentials during NSR, or both (see Fig. 22-20). These findings are consistent with post-infarction remodeling, which results in progressive EP effects in the anatomical substrate for VT. Moreover, there is a significant positive correlation between infarct age and the duration of the broadest endocardial electrograms (>200 milliseconds) during sinus rhythm mapping in the peri-infarct zone. The older the infarct, the broader are the electrograms and the longer is the delay between the electrogram and isolated potentials. Sites with the broadest electrograms or isolated potentials detected during sinus rhythm mapping are typically identical to those at the critical isthmus of the reentrant circuit recorded during induced VT.[47]

ELECTROGRAMS WITH ISOLATED DELAYED COMPONENTS. Electrograms with isolated delayed components are defined as electrograms with double or multiple components separated by a very low-amplitude signal or an isoelectric interval more than 50 milliseconds in duration. These electrograms can reflect local depolarization of surviving fiber bundles that are well insulated by dense scar, where local activation is recorded late, well after the higher amplitude far-field electrogram and often well after the end of the surface QRS complex or T wave. Late isolated potentials during NSR are relatively uncommon (15% of all multiple potentials) but can be markers of an anatomically constrained, slowly conducting critical diastolic isthmus during VT.[47] However, isolated potential mapping is limited by the imperfect specificity due to bystander cul-de-sacs or nonspecific slowed conduction as well as imperfect sensitivity due to low-amplitude local signals or the direction of wavefront propagation obscuring isolated potentials. Nevertheless, this type of electrogram, although unable to differentiate the central isthmus from a close bystander, can help refine the area of interest. The areas demonstrating such electrograms are relatively small compared with scar areas; therefore, this method permits a focus on the diagnostic techniques and ablation in defined areas. Furthermore, recording of these electrograms before and during VT induction serves to relate them and VT within seconds, provided that the isolated diastolic component of the electrogram precedes the first VT beat and then becomes mid-diastolic. Additionally, pacing at these sites may capture the local potential and conduct slowly out of the scar, resulting in a long S-QRS interval and, if sharing an exit of a targeted VT, a good or excellent pace map.[4] The ablation of all sites demonstrating electrograms with isolated diastolic components can overcome the lack of specificity of the selection of a single site as an ablation target when entrainment mapping criteria are not fulfilled (Fig. 22-33). Ablation of these electrograms can also eliminate the substrate for different VTs otherwise not ablated by limited, conventional strategies.[7]

CHANGING DIRECTION OF VENTRICULAR ACTIVATION WAVEFRONT

Electrogram amplitude is in part a reflection of the depolarizing muscle mass as well as wavefront direction. Multipotential electrograms are sometimes detectable during NSR, but low-amplitude potentials can be obscured by the signal from the surrounding larger mass of myocardium. In regions of block, changing the direction of depolarization can produce greater separation between activation of adjacent bundles, altering the separation of multipotential electrograms. Regions containing isthmuses and conduction block can be detected by analyzing electrograms recorded during two different ventricular activation sequences, such as sinus rhythm (or atrial pacing) and then RV pacing.

Theoretically, a wavefront propagating parallel to the long axis of adjacent but separate fiber bundles would activate adjacent bundles simultaneously, reducing the time between potentials. Consequently, multiple potentials can become superimposed on each other, preventing their detection. On the other hand, a wavefront traveling perpendicular to a fiber long axis that encounters bundles would be expected to result in greater temporal separation of potentials in these regions (Fig. 22-34). Conversely, multipotential electrograms that persist in both activation sequences are more likely to be associated with the reentry circuit isthmuses. Persistent multipotential electrograms may indicate greater separation from surrounding muscle, with fixed block and disordered conduction, regardless of the direction of activation. Therefore, changing the direction of the activation wavefront can unmask some areas of block and slow conduction. Multipotential electrograms with more than two deflections, highly predictive of a reentry substrate, are more frequently recorded during RV pacing. Theoretically, this can be related to the fact that during NSR several simultaneous activation wavefronts can coexist, making the probability of electrogram overlap higher than during RV pacing, when only one activation wavefront is present.

Electroanatomical Mapping

Electroanatomical mapping can help in the precise description of VT reentrant circuits, sequence of ventricular activation during the

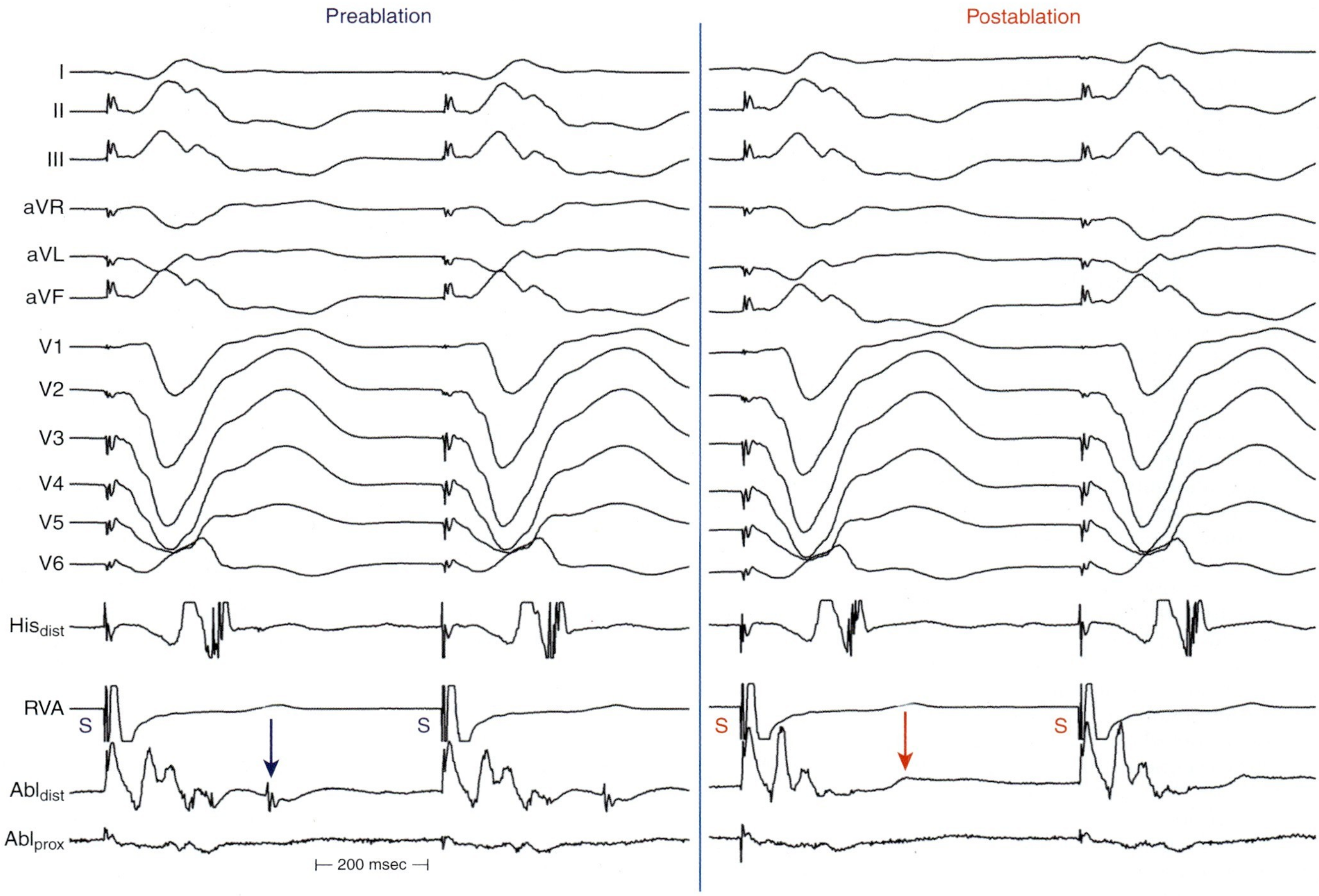

FIGURE 22-33 Elimination of endocardial late potentials with ablation. At left, a very delayed potential is seen during ventricular pacing (blue arrow); after ablation at this site (right panel), the potential has been eliminated (red arrow).

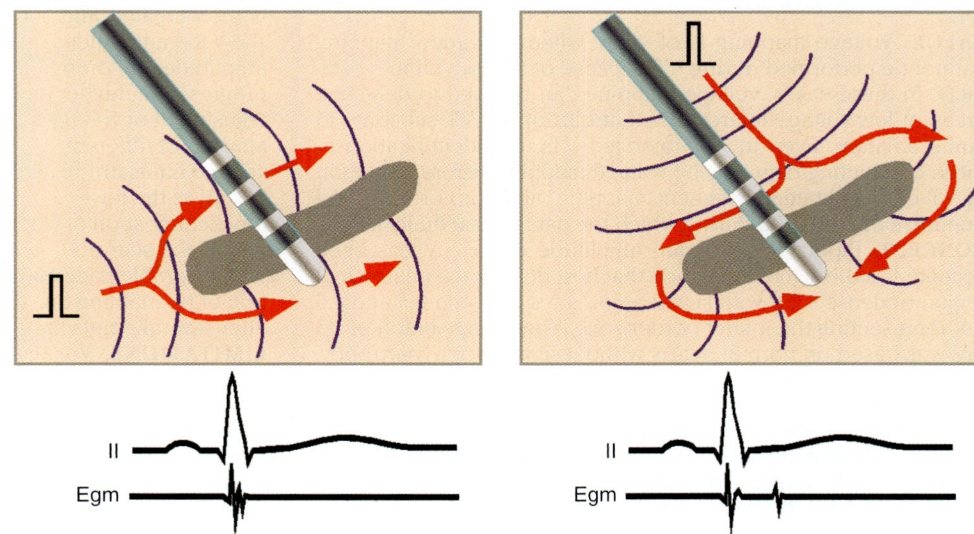

FIGURE 22-34 Effect of direction of wavefront propagation on electrogram (Egm) configuration. A catheter is recording over an island of scar surrounded by normal tissue. At left, a wavefront arriving from the left side is split by the scar, but tissue on each side of the scar is activated at about the same time, resulting in a relatively normal Egm. At right, a wavefront arriving from right angles to the prior one is split by the scar, with tissue on the near side activated early and that on the opposite side activated much later, resulting in a markedly split recording.

VT, rapid visualization of the activation wavefront, and identification of slow-conducting pathways and appropriate sites for entrainment mapping. These systems also help navigation of the ablation catheter, planning of ablation lines, and maintaining a log of sites of interest (e.g., sites with favorable entrainment or pace mapping findings), which can then be revisited with precision. Additionally, voltage (scar) mapping is a helpful feature of the current electroanatomical mapping systems.[2]

The CARTO electroanatomical mapping system (Biosense Webster, Diamond Bar, Calif.) has been extensively used in mapping and ablation of post-MI VT, and is described here as a model for 3-D mapping. The ESI-NavX (St. Jude Medical, St. Paul, Minn.)

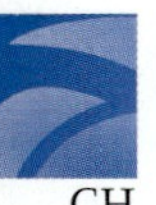

has also been successfully used for mapping and ablation of scar-related VT.

ELECTROANATOMICAL ACTIVATION MAPPING

The electrical reference is chosen as a morphologically stable and regular electrogram obtained from an endocardial (e.g., RV apical electrogram) or surface lead (e.g., surface ECG lead with a QRS complex during VT demonstrating a sharp apex and a strong positive or negative deflection). The width of the window of interest is adjusted to approximate, usually 20 milliseconds less than, the VT CL. The middle of the window of interest is selected to coincide with the electrical reference.

Activation mapping is performed to define the ventricular activation sequence during VT. A reasonable number of points have to be recorded. The LV is plotted during VT by dragging the mapping catheter over the endocardium. Stability is assessed by monitoring position on biplane fluoroscopy and on the electroanatomical mapping system and by continuous monitoring of electrogram morphology and timing. Points are added to the map only if stability criteria in space and local activation time are met. The local activation time at each site should have a beat-to-beat variability of less than 5 milliseconds. The local activation time for each endocardial position under the mapping catheter is calculated as the interval between the electrical reference and the onset of the high-frequency bipolar electrogram as it leaves the baseline. Infarct regions are sought first and more data points are acquired around these areas, as identified by low-amplitude potentials, with diastolic electrograms, or double potentials. The resulting reentrant circuit is considered to be the spatially shortest route of unidirectional activation encompassing a full range of mapped activation times (>90% of the tachycardia CL) and returning to the site of earliest activation.

The activation map can also be used to catalogue sites at which pacing maneuvers are performed during assessment of the VT. Silent areas are defined as ventricular potential amplitude of less than 0.05 mV, which is the baseline noise in the Biosense Webster system, and the absence of ventricular capture at 20 mA. Such areas are tagged as scar and therefore appear in gray on the 3-D maps.

VOLTAGE (SCAR) MAPPING

VALUE. Voltage mapping is of value when activation mapping cannot be performed during VT because of hemodynamic instability. In these cases, voltage mapping can be used to delineate areas of low-voltage infarct scar that harbor the VT substrate to guide ablation. Even in well-tolerated VTs, the identification of these conducting channels by voltage mapping before induction of VT can facilitate subsequent mapping, ablation, or both and minimize the duration during which the patient is actually in VT.

CONCEPT. Bipolar electrogram amplitude of 0.5 mV has been accepted as the signal amplitude that best defines the anatomical region of dense scar, with signal amplitudes between 0.5 and 1.5 mV representing the infarct border zone. The voltage cutoff of 1.5 mV was based on normal hearts without significant hypertrophy. Therefore, cutoff values of 2.0 mV or even 2.2 mV will better define the substrate in the setting of markedly hypertrophied ventricles, especially given the fact that the distinction between normal and abnormal bipolar signals in most patients with prior MI tends to be very discrete and dramatic and, as a consequence, altering the upper limit of the color range to 2.0 mV will do little to alter the bipolar voltage map. On the other hand, whereas bipolar voltages less than 1.5 mV likely represent underlying myocardial fibrosis, further subdivision of voltage zones below this value is perhaps somewhat arbitrary, with human validation data presently lacking. The border zone at the margins of confluent post-infarct scarring do, however, tend to have relatively more preserved voltages (in the range from 0.5 to 1.5 mV), and some data suggest that the majority of rapid unmappable VTs have critical circuit components located in this zone.[4] Additionally, pacing provides complementary information to electrogram amplitude; only 2% of sites with amplitude more than 0.5 mV have a pacing threshold more than 10 mA, whereas a substantial number of very low-amplitude sites have high pacing thresholds, and many sites in reentry circuit isthmuses have very low amplitudes.

In patients with post-MI VT, the low-voltage infarct areas are relatively large (average area, 38.6 ± 34.6 cm^2; range, 6.4 to 205.4 cm^2), so that complete encirclement with RF ablation lesions is likely to be difficult, although linear ablation to join areas of electrically unexcitable scar to each other or to other conduction barriers can be associated with good ablation outcomes.[4] On the other hand, identification of the conducting channels within the infarct region, which are relatively small bundles of viable tissue compared with the scar areas, can permit focus on the diagnostic techniques and ablation to defined areas that potentially harbor the VT substrate. In one study, 86% of such channels were related to induced or clinical VT, which implies high arrhythmogenic potential. This procedure can also allow the ablation of some nontolerated or noninducible VTs not approachable by conventional entrainment and activation mapping methods.[4]

Relative voltage preservation within denser regions of scar is a hallmark of central conducting channels that may form anatomically constrained diastolic isthmuses during VT, and adjusting the voltage representation on the isopotential map can help visualize these zones. Another operational definition of dense scar is based on its electrical inexcitability. Anatomical isthmuses are identified on the basis of voltage mapping as regions where the pacing threshold is less than 10 mA, located between two areas of electrically unexcitable scar or between electrically unexcitable scar and an anatomical obstacle, such as the mitral or aortic valve annulus.[4]

TECHNIQUE. The LV is mapped during NSR to construct a voltage map displaying peak-to-peak electrogram amplitude, with the color range set between 0.5 and 1.5 mV. Thus, purple areas represent normal-amplitude electrograms, and electrogram amplitude progressively diminishes as colors proceed to blue, green, yellow, and red. At low-amplitude (<0.5 mV) sites, pacing is performed with 10-mA, 2-millisecond pulse width stimuli. If pacing does not capture, the contact of the catheter is confirmed by observing the response to gentle manipulation. Sites with a pacing threshold greater than 10 mA are tagged as electrically unexcitable scar, marked as gray regions (see Fig. 6-14). A color-coded voltage map is then created and superimposed on the anatomical model to show the amplitudes of all selected points, with red as the lowest amplitude and orange, yellow, green, blue, and purple indicating progressively higher amplitudes (Fig. 22-35). Careful step-by-step adjustment of voltage scar definition on the isopotential map and analysis of different voltage levels within the 0.5-mV scar (i.e., the voltage limits are reset to 0.3 to 0.5 mV as the upper limit and to 0.1 mV as the lower, representing dense scar) may be required for the identification of viable myocardium and conducting channels within the scar area (Fig. 22-36).[48] Points of interest (e.g., those with favorable pace maps) can also be marked or tagged as location only, enabling one to return precisely to the region of interest after several points have been investigated.

LIMITATIONS. Voltage mapping relies heavily on the correct interpretation of electrograms. Because voltage is used to define scar, consistent catheter contact is necessary. If catheter contact is not sufficient, the voltage map will suggest an erroneous scar. Although an electrogram amplitude of 0.5 mV has been used to identify electrical scars, a minimal amplitude that distinguishes excitable tissue from unexcitable scar has not been established.[4] Additionally, although voltage mapping likely identifies large unexcitable areas of scar, small strands of fibrosis, which may still create important conduction block, may escape detection amidst the background of high-amplitude far-field signals. Furthermore, it is likely that large sheets of surviving endocardial myocardium occur in some patients with circuits created by functional block during VT and no endocardial electrically unexcitable scar. When the boundaries of the isthmus are functional lines of block, they cannot be detected during NSR. The dispersion of voltage in some

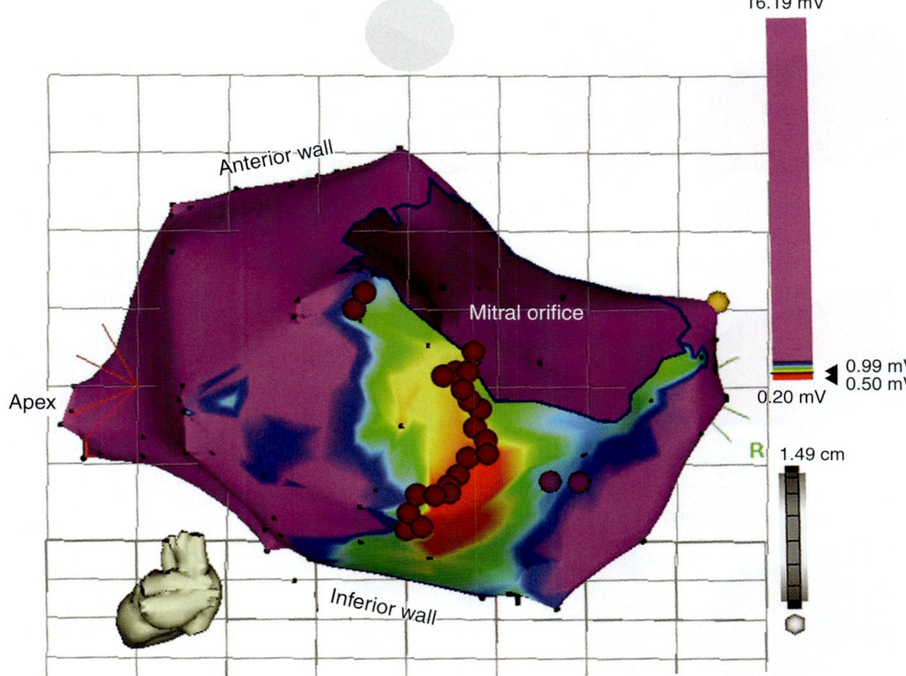

FIGURE 22-35 Electroanatomical voltage map of scar-based ventricular tachycardia (VT) in a patient with a prior inferior wall myocardial infarction (posterior view). The scale at right shows bipolar voltage; the red area denotes a very low-voltage (<0.5 mV) infarct zone with a small isthmus of higher voltage between this area and the mitral annulus. Red dots indicate a line of radiofrequency applications to transect this isthmus (additional red dots denote ablation at other sites that terminated VT).

scar areas can appear only when activated at the VT rate. Even when conducting channels within the scar area can be identified by voltage mapping, their relationship to the VT circuit remains to be assessed by other mapping methods (e.g., entrainment mapping); plots of electrogram amplitude alone do not adequately identify VT circuit isthmuses. In well-tolerated VT, no more than 50% of proven isthmus sites will be revealed by this approach.[4] Also, differences in wavefront direction, such as seen with RV pacing, may obscure the presence of double potentials or higher voltage local channel signals. Finally, electrogram amplitude is influenced by the particular recording methods, and these values may differ with other electrode spacings and filter settings.

SUBSTRATE IMAGE INTEGRATION

LV scar and its border zone represent the target of "substrate modification" VT ablations; therefore, an exact anatomical delineation is critical. However, the current gold standard of voltage mapping has several limitations—a single endocardial voltage measurement only incompletely describes a complex intramural scar anatomy. Detailed voltage maps prolong the procedure time and falsely low voltage measurements (caused by suboptimal catheter contact) can lead to incorrect scar definition. Additionally, small areas of scar may not be detected, given the spatial resolution of at least 5 mm, covered by the 3.5- or 4-mm catheter tip/proximal ring distance.

Many of these limitations can be overcome by integrating scar imaging into the VT ablation. Multiple imaging modalities detailing the LV substrate in a 3-D format can be visualized and displayed simultaneously with the electroanatomical 3-D LV voltage map. These imaging approaches can be used to correctly predict abnormal voltage locations in advance of the mapping procedure, which may allow the electrophysiologist to concentrate on areas of likely myocardial scar, obviate the need to perform a complete point-by-point voltage mapping, identify falsely low-voltage recordings in areas of normal perfusion due to suboptimal catheter contact, as well as reduce procedure time and fluoroscopic exposure. Additionally, some imaging modalities are able to characterize the transmural extent and intramyocardial location of scar tissue, which can potentially help to identify intramural and epicardial arrhythmia substrate, overcoming a limitation of endocardial voltage mapping.

IMAGE INTEGRATION USING POSITRON EMISSION TOMOGRAPHY-COMPUTED TOMOGRAPHY. Because PET scans alone do not provide the necessary anatomical information required for integration with electroanatomical maps, a CT angiography scan is required to provide an anatomical skeleton onto which the biological information acquired from the PET scan would be superimposed on its precise anatomical location.

Both PET and CT images can be spatially aligned using an automatic registration algorithm. All regions in the PET image with uptake greater than a threshold (50% of maximal uptake) are overlaid at the corresponding location on the CT image. Thus a fused image can be created having accurate anatomical information at the spatial resolution of the original CT with accurate metabolic information for the LV myocardium from the registered PET. The regions in the fused image showing [18F]fluorodeoxyglucose (FDG) uptake represent non-scarred myocardium, and regions with no uptake indicate scarred myocardium.[49] Myocardial scar is displayed as an area of absent voxels ("hole in the wall") within the reconstructed LV wall to indicate scar location and size. The use of PET 3-D reconstructions at multiple metabolic thresholds allows the characterization of the scar border zone and simultaneous 3-D display of myocardial scar and border zone embedded into the LV anatomy as well as the display of detailed scar anatomy which can be targeted during the VT ablation.[50]

The fused "anatomical-metabolic" PET-CT image is imported into the CARTO system using the commercially available CARTOMerge software (Biosense Webster). To merge the PET-CT image, landmark points at the coronary ostia or in the coronary cusps and at the apical septum are usually acquired (guided by ICE; see below). The corresponding points are matched on the fused PET-CT image. Once the 3-D voltage map is created, surface registration is performed. Alternatively, multiple points can be acquired at different planes of the aorta as the catheter is dragged along the descending aorta, arch, and ascending aorta. Using an automated program available in the mapping system, the electroanatomical map and the fused PET-CT image are then aligned.[49]

IMAGE INTEGRATION USING MAGNETIC RESONANCE. The spatial resolution of PET/CT imaging is limited to 4 to 6 mm, which does not allow for determination of complex scar anatomy and

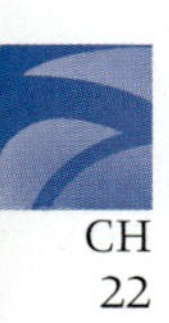

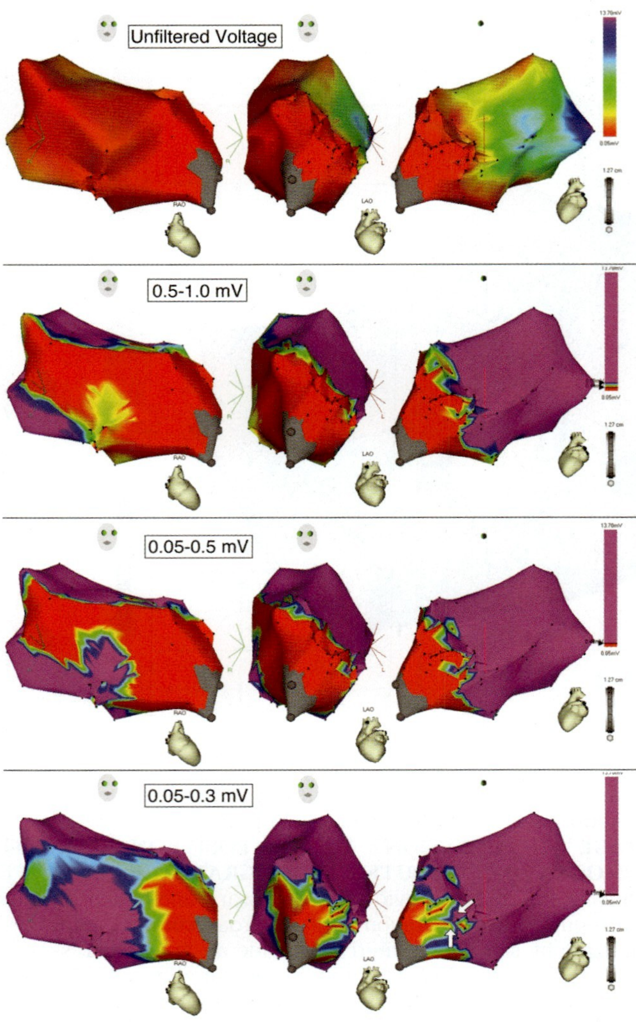

FIGURE 22-36 Filtering voltage maps to expose conduction channels. Right and left anterior oblique (RAO and LAO, respectively) and left lateral views of endocardial left ventricular voltage maps are shown (higher, normal voltages are purple, low voltages red; dense scar is gray). At top is the "raw," unfiltered voltage. Successive panels beneath show different bandwidths of filtering as indicated at the top of each panel, revealing possible "channels" of viable tissue coursing with scar areas (white arrows in bottom panel). Ablation lines to transect these channels (which would not otherwise be evident) can then be performed.

mural location. Epicardial scar may have low PET signal, but normal endocardial voltage. In contrast, delayed-enhancement MR imaging provides excellent detail and is quickly becoming the gold standard for scar determination and is currently the only modality that can assess the transmurality of the infarct (i.e., can determine whether the scar is endocardial, intramyocardial, or epicardial).

The MR image can be merged with the 3-D electroanatomical voltage map, using CARTOMerge software, employing landmark and surface registration (as discussed above).[18]

IMAGE INTEGRATION USING CONTRAST-ENHANCED CARDIAC TOMOGRAPHY. Cardiac contrast-enhanced CT scanning enables a comprehensive three-modality characterization (anatomical, dynamic, and perfusion) of LV scar from a single contrast-enhanced CT with high spatial (≤1 mm) and temporal resolution. Areas of CT hypoperfusion correlate best with areas of abnormal voltage (<1.5 mV) rather than scar alone (<0.5 mV). Perfusion imaging from CT can indicate scar transmurality and intramyocardial scar location. The 3-D CT scan can be integrated into clinical mapping systems to guide VT ablation. Primary registration is performed with landmark points and visual alignments, as previously discussed.[17]

IMAGE INTEGRATION USING INTRACARDIAC ULTRASOUND. Although preacquired MR, PET, and CT imaging have been used to define LV scar and guide mapping and ablation in post-MI VT, registration is often difficult, unfortunately, and may be imprecise. Additionally, images obtained on different days may confound registration if LV geometry changes because of loading conditions.

ICE has been recently used to guide catheter navigation. Real-time ICE images can provide accurate chamber geometries and scar boundaries of the LV. Additionally, ICE provides both an anatomical and a functional assessment of the LV, allowing for real-time identification of wall motion abnormalities. Unlike PET/CT and MR imaging, ICE imaging does not require potentially toxic contrast agents, nor does it expose the patient to ionizing radiation.

The CARTOSound image integration module (Biosense Webster) incorporates the electroanatomical map into a map derived from ICE and allows for 3-D reconstruction of the LV from real-time 2-D ICE images, facilitating interventional navigation within the LV. ICE imaging is performed using a 10 Fr phased-array transducer-catheter incorporating a navigation sensor (SoundStar; Biosense Webster), which records individual 90-degree sector image planes of the cardiac chamber of interest, including their location and orientation, to the CARTO workspace. A 3-D volume rendered image is created by obtaining electrocardiogram-gated ICE images of the endocardial surface of the LV.[51,52]

To create the CARTOSound volume map of the LV, the ICE catheter is manipulated in the RA, RV, and RVOT to visualize all parts of the LV. The LVOT, the aortic root, and the mitral valve are mapped with the probe positioned in the RA, whereas the body of the LV is mapped with the probe positioned in the RV, against the interventricular septum. The latter position provides a longitudinal view of the LV cavity. Lateral tilt allows base-to-apex scanning through the body of the LV with deeper insertion, withdrawal, or rotation of the probe used as necessary to complete the map. Short-axis cross-sectional views of the LV can be obtained with the ICE probe positioned in the RVOT. Images are acquired in end expiration and gated to the R wave or the pacing spike. Ultrasound imaging in which the wall segment is well visualized can reliably identify scar both by wall thickness and motion, a process that does not require wall contact. Akinetic and thinned wall segments are marked in a separate volume and labeled as scar on the ultrasound volume map. Normal or hypokinetic segments are labeled as nonscar. Separate geometries (scar and nonscar) are made of the LV and each of the papillary muscles. Once the ultrasound map is completed, a distinct CARTO voltage map is created (as described above).[51]

The area of scar identified using ICE was found to correspond accurately to that defined using standard bipolar voltage settings during point-by-point mapping. This may help limit catheter manipulation in the LV by focusing effort on the potential substrate regions identified by ICE. Real-time monitoring of the endocardial-catheter interface also helps direct the catheter to the important anatomical structures that can be critical to the VT circuit, such as crypts and trabeculations, which may otherwise be missed.[51,52] Additionally, the CARTOSound volume map of the LV can also be used as a facilitator of CT/MR image integration.[49,53]

Noncontact Mapping

When VT is short-lived, hemodynamically unstable, or cannot be reproducibly initiated, simultaneous multisite data acquisition using a noncontact mapping system (EnSite 3000; St. Jude Medical) can help localize the VT site of origin. The system has been shown to reliably identify presystolic endocardial activation sites (potential exits) for reentrant VTs and thus starting points for conventional mapping. It may also help identify VT isthmuses and therefore suitable targets for ablation.

Substrate mapping based on scar or diseased tissue, which has been recently introduced to noncontact mapping technology, can be particularly helpful when the VT is not inducible during the procedure. Dynamic substrate mapping allows the creation of voltage

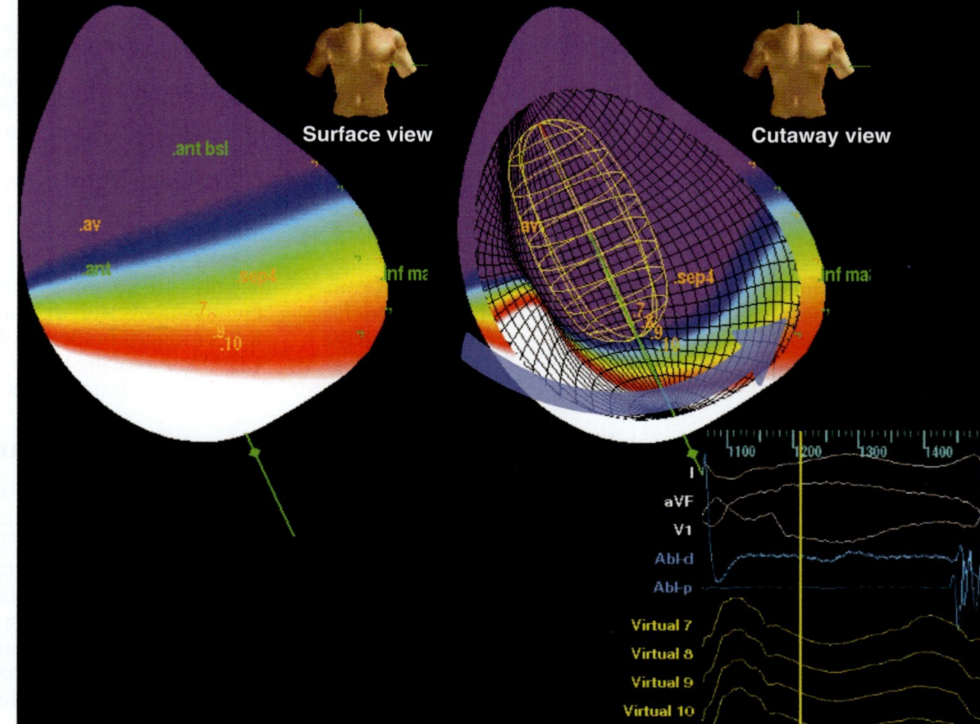

FIGURE 22-37 Use of multipolar electrode array for ventricular tachycardia (VT) mapping. Maps from the EnSite system are shown in a patient with inferior wall infarction. At left is a snapshot of the activation wavefront projected on the endocardial surface (white = activation). At right is the same instant of activation in a cutaway view, showing the wireframe of the endocardial balloon-based electrode array. At bottom right are contact and virtual electrograms from the array during VT; the wavefront propagates from left to right, along the mitral annulus (curved blue arrow).

maps from a single cardiac cycle and provides the ability to identify low-voltage areas, as well as fixed and functional block, on the virtual endocardium through noncontact methodology.[54]

CONCEPT

The noncontact mapping system records electrical potentials from a multielectrode array (MEA) surrounding a 7.5-mL balloon within the LV cavity. Electrical potentials at the LV endocardial surface some distance away are calculated. Sites of mid-diastolic endocardial activity, which are likely adjacent to reentry circuit exits, are usually identifiable; in some cases, isthmuses can be identified (Fig. 22-37).

Voltages are displayed as a colored isopotential map on the virtual endocardium. The color scale is adjusted to create a binary display, with negative unipolar potentials in white on a purple background, producing a unipolar activation map. Diastolic depolarization is defined as activity on the isopotential map that can be continuously tracked back in time from VT exit sites, defined on the map as synchronous with the QRS onset. Diastolic activity and exit sites are then marked on the virtual endocardium, and the mapping catheter is navigated to them by the locator.[54]

The dynamic substrate mapping algorithm allows the creation of unipolar noncontact voltage maps from a single cardiac cycle, defined as the percentages of the maximal voltage recorded in the entire chamber. Until further studies define the correct dynamic substrate mapping percentage that can be compared with the scar and scar border zone defined by contact mapping, areas having values less than 50% may be defined as "abnormal myocardium." A recent report assessed the relationship between successful ablation sites determined by noncontact mapping and concealed entrainment as well as the region of "abnormal myocardium" defined by the dynamic substrate mapping: 85% of VTs arose from the border defined by the dynamic substrate mapping 30% area.[54]

TECHNIQUE

The EnSite 3000 system requires a 9 Fr MEA and a 7 Fr conventional (roving) deflectable mapping-ablation catheter. A standard ablation catheter is placed in the LV by a retrograde transaortic route. Using a separate arterial access site, the MEA catheter is advanced to the LV apex over a 0.032-inch J-tipped guidewire. The right anterior oblique (RAO) and left anterior oblique (LAO) views are used to assess the correct position of the balloon catheter, placed parallel to the long axis and with the pigtail end as close as possible to the LV apex. The guidewire is then withdrawn and the balloon inflated with a contrast-saline mixture. The balloon is positioned in the center of the LV and does not come in contact with the LV wall. Care is taken in order to have a distance between the MEA catheter and the region of interest less than 40 mm; if necessary the catheter can be repositioned.

Construction of the virtual endocardium model is preliminarily obtained during sinus rhythm by moving the ablation catheter along the LV endocardial surface to collect a series of geometric points during NSR or VT. Using this geometric information, the computer creates a model of the LV. After the LV geometry is reconstructed, 5 seconds of NSR is recorded by the system, and the substrate map is superimposed on the anatomy. High-pass filters are adjusted at the lowest value that minimizes the shift of the isoelectric baseline to avoid confusing depolarization with repolarization.[54]

Subsequently, VT is induced by programmed stimulation and mapping of the arrhythmia can begin. A 5- to 10-second segment of any induced VT is recorded with the noncontact system and the VT may then be terminated by overdrive pacing or electrical shock. The data acquisition process is performed automatically by the system, and all data for the entire LV are acquired simultaneously.

VT circuit exit points and potential ablation targets can be identified as sites where a QS unipolar electrogram morphology is recorded, which, on the color-coded isopotential map, corresponded to the site of earliest activation followed by a rapid activation wavefront. Projection of the virtual endocardial electrograms over this area is performed at different high-pass filter settings (1, 2, 4, 8, 16, and 32 Hz) to avoid misinterpretation with repolarization waveforms. This region is searched starting from the abnormal myocardium defined by dynamic substrate mapping and is considered a good target site for ablation when confirmed by EP criteria (contact activation mapping, entrainment mapping, and/or pace mapping).[54]

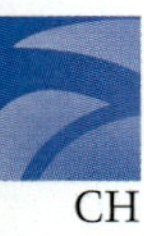

The locator technology is used to guide the ablation catheter to the proper location in the heart. The system allows the operator to create linear ablation lesions that transect critical regions and then return precisely to areas of interest, visualizing lines of ablation as they are being created and performing the ablation during NSR.

LIMITATIONS

The most important shortcoming of the noncontact mapping system is the deterioration in the accuracy of noncontact electrograms for distances greater than 40 mm between the MEA catheter and the recording site, which can occur in dilated ventricles. Very low-amplitude signals may not be detected, particularly if the distance between the center of the balloon catheter and endocardial surface exceeds 40 mm, limiting the accurate identification of diastolic signals.

Because the geometry of the cardiac chamber is contoured at the beginning of the study during NSR, changes in chamber size and in contraction pattern during tachycardia can adversely affect the accuracy of the location of the endocardial electrograms. Additionally, detection and display of activation from two adjacent structures, such as the papillary muscle and subjacent myocardium, is problematic.[2]

Moreover, because isopotential maps are predominantly used, ventricular repolarization must be distinguished from atrial depolarization and diastolic activity. Early diastole can be especially challenging to map during VT. Care has to be taken to confirm that the virtual electrogram is related to local activation and not baseline drift or repolarization.[2]

Because of the potential for thrombus formation, the use of this system requires the maintenance of a greater degree of anticoagulation (activated clotting time [ACT] >350 seconds) while the mapping balloon is in place than is generally required for the point-by-point mapping techniques. Additionally, positioning of the MEA catheter in the LV can be difficult in the setting of atherosclerotic aorta or tortuous peripheral arteries, requiring a transseptal approach.[54] The mapping sheath is 9 Fr in diameter; femoral hematomas and pseudoaneurysms are the most frequently encountered complications.[2]

Mapping Post-Infarction Premature Ventricular Complexes

A recent study found that in post-MI patients with frequent PVCs, the PVCs originated at sites of low voltage corresponding with the infarct location in approximately 85% of patients, similar to patients with post-MI VT. Additionally, in patients with ischemic CMP and VT that matches the PVC morphology, both types of arrhythmias have critical target sites within areas of low voltage, and the site of origin of PVCs often corresponds with the exit site of the VT reentrant circuit.[55] Furthermore, as is the case with VT, late potentials can be detected during diastole at the site of origin of most of the PVCs. The late potentials follow the ventricular electrogram during sinus rhythm and precede the ventricular electrogram during PVCs. Slight differences in morphology between PVCs and VT may be observed and may be rate-related.[56]

Possible mechanisms of PVCs in post-MI patients include reentry, triggered activity, and abnormal automaticity. Because of several features in common with post-MI VT, reentry may play a principal role in post-MI PVCs; however, this has not been confirmed by high-resolution mapping. Nevertheless, in a small percentage of patients, PVCs do not originate from scar tissue. In those patients, the PVCs can be due to triggered activity or abnormal automaticity, similar to idiopathic PVCs.[56]

Because post-MI PVCs and VT often share critical areas, mapping of the PVCs can be used as a surrogate for mapping of the VT. Ablation of frequent PVCs can potentially eliminate VT in these patients. However, the sensitivity and specificity of this approach in a nonselected population are not known, nor is the prevalence of PVCs indicating VT exit sites. If this concept is confirmed in larger series, PVC mapping can be used to identify exit sites of PVCs and to search for diastolic potentials prior to PVCs that may indicate areas of slow conduction relevant for the VT. Targeting the PVCs alone may be sufficient to eliminate the VTs that had an exit site near or at the PVC site of origin, obviating the need for induction of VT, which can be of great value in patients with unstable or unmappable VTs.[57] Voltage mapping in these patients can be helpful in focusing the mapping procedure to the low-voltage areas, because this area contains the arrhythmogenic substrate in most patients.[56]

Furthermore, in post-MI patients with frequent PVCs, PVC ablation may result in an improvement in the LVEF. It may be appropriate to screen patients with ischemic CMP for frequent PVCs with a 24-hour Holter monitor before implanting an ICD for primary prevention of SCD. Ablation of the frequent PVCs may improve the LVEF such that the patient no longer meets the LVEF criterion for an ICD.[55]

Mapping of Intramural and Epicardial Circuits

A significant proportion of VT circuits have one or more critical components located in the epicardium. This is particularly true in nonischemic substrates. VT originating from the subepicardium is an important cause of failure of endocardial ablation approaches. In tertiary centers, epicardial ablation has been required in approximately 10% to 25% of post-MI VTs, and seems to be more common with inferior rather than anterior wall infarctions.

Various ECG characteristics have been used to predict whether an epicardial approach may be required based on the VT morphology; however, the surface ECG alone is not reliably predictive of the need for epicardial access and mapping for any given VT. QRS morphology is related solely to the VT exit site and this does not imply that some other component of the circuit (such as the critical isthmus or entrance site) cannot be ablated from the endocardium, even when an epicardial exit is implied by the ECG characteristics.[34,43]

Additionally, contrast-enhanced CT and delayed enhancement cardiac MR can identify areas of myocardial scar that correlate with VT substrate and can determine whether the scar is endocardial, intramyocardial, or epicardial. In a recent report, the presence of epicardial or intramyocardial scar on preprocedure delayed enhancement MR was associated with a 0% procedural success rate when the operator limited ablation to the endocardium. Having this MR imaging information before entering the procedure permits the operator to plan an appropriate mapping and ablation strategy and to better inform the patient about the risks, benefits, and chances of procedural success.

During endocardial mapping of post-MI VT, inability to identify the reentry circuit isthmus on the endocardium can suggest that the isthmus is epicardial or intramural. In these cases, endocardial activation mapping can demonstrate a focal point of earliest endocardial activation where entrainment indicates a potential exit or outer loop site, but ablation fails to interrupt VT, suggesting that there is an epicardial or intramural circuit with a broad endocardial exit.

Mapping arrhythmia foci or circuits that are deep within the myocardium or in the epicardium can be performed via the coronary sinus (CS) or pericardial space, and is discussed in detail in Chapter 27.

Practical Approach to Ventricular Tachycardia Mapping

EVALUATION PRIOR TO MAPPING

Evaluation of potential ischemia, which could contribute to instability during the ablation procedure, is necessary. Echocardiography; ventriculography; or nuclear, PET, and/or MR imaging may be used to identify the size and location of the infarct that potentially contains the arrhythmogenic scars (Fig. 22-38). These tests also help exclude the presence of LV thrombus, which can increase the risk of embolization during mapping. Organized thrombus

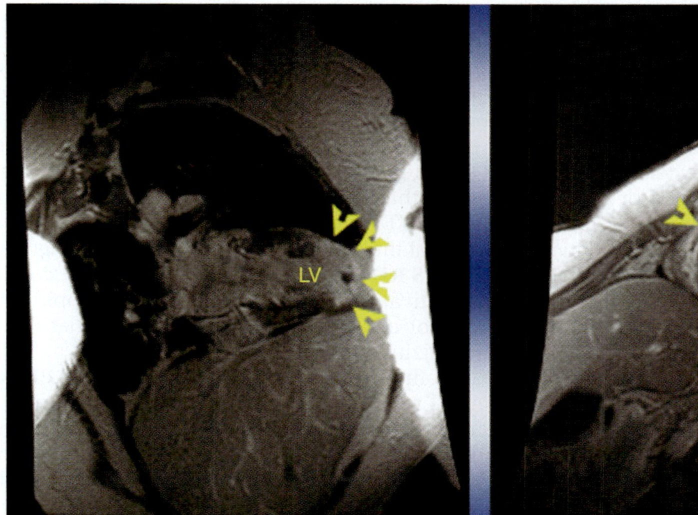

FIGURE 22-38 Magnetic resonance scans of the left ventricle (LV) in a patient with an old anterior myocardial infarction. Long axis (at left) and short axis (at right) views of the LV show a dense anteroapical scar (arrowheads), which can be visualized as a white thin area of the LV wall. *(Courtesy of Dr. Nasar Nallamothu, Prairie Cardiovascular Consultants, Springfield, Ill.)*

can overlie the area of interest for ablation and prevent effective energy delivery to target sites.

MAPPING HEMODYNAMICALLY STABLE SUSTAINED MONOMORPHIC VENTRICULAR TACHYCARDIA

LEFT VENTRICULAR ACCESS. The LV is accessed through the retrograde transaortic approach, usually via a femoral arterial access. An atrial transseptal approach may also be used, although accessing the entire LV is then more difficult. Both transseptal and retrograde approaches may be used concomitantly, so when a particular region of the LV cannot be mapped using one approach, it may be mapped using the other approach. Anticoagulation (with intravenous heparin) is started once the LV is accessed to maintain the ACT between 250 and 350 seconds. Certain electrode arrays with high thrombogenicity may require an ACT of at least 300 seconds.[1]

A standard 4-mm- or 8-mm-tip or, preferably, an irrigated-tip ablation catheter with 2-5-2–mm spacing for proximal electrodes is used. Poles 1 to 3 (distal) and 2 to 4 (proximal) of the ablation catheter are used for recording, and poles 1 to 3 are used for stimulation. Catheter position is identified fluoroscopically in the RAO and LAO views. Three-dimensional electroanatomical mapping is usually used to aid mapping and ablation.

STEP 1: SUBSTRATE MAPPING DURING BASELINE RHYTHM. Infarct regions are sought first and more data points are acquired around these areas. Refining the area under investigation relies on the usual clinical indicators, such as echocardiographic, ventriculographic, PET, or MR imaging findings (e.g., regions of wall motion abnormalities, areas of scars), and 12-lead ECG recordings of spontaneous and induced VT are analyzed to regionalize the site of origin of the VT. Also, ICE can be of value for real-time identification of scar regions as well as for facilitation of atrial septal puncture if required. Additionally, integration of those imaging modalities into the 3-D electroanatomical mapping can help visualize and display the LV substrate in a 3-D format and focus initial mapping efforts to those regions.

Substrate mapping may be attempted initially during NSR or ventricular pacing (unless VT is incessant), targeting the LV scar and its border zone as identified by scar imaging modalities, to help refine the area of interest and identify potential targets for further activation and entrainment mapping. Goals of substrate mapping are the identification of abnormal local electrogram configuration during NSR and/or RV pacing and voltage mapping. Sites with fractionated electrograms, multipotential electrograms, and/or isolated diastolic electrograms are tagged and catalogued on the 3-D mapping system for future revisiting and guidance. Voltage mapping is performed using a 3-D mapping system to identify areas of abnormal low-amplitude local electrograms during NSR.

STEP 2: ACTIVATION MAPPING DURING VENTRICULAR TACHYCARDIA. Programmed stimulation is used to induce VT and to ascertain the ease of inducibility for subsequent testing, unless the VT is incessant. Activation mapping during VT is then carried out, initially focusing mapping to regions of VT substrate as identified during substrate mapping.

During activation mapping, particular sites of interest are sought, including the following: (1) sites with abnormal local bipolar electrogram (amplitude ≤0.5 mV; duration ≥60 milliseconds); (2) sites at which the local electrogram precedes the QRS complex by at least 50 milliseconds (activation times are taken from the onset of the bipolar electrogram); and (3) sites with the earliest local activation closest to mid-diastole, isolated mid-diastolic potentials, or continuous activity. Filtered unipolar electrograms can help ensure that the tip electrode, which is the ablation electrode, is responsible for the early component of the bipolar electrograms. In addition, demonstration of a fixed relationship of the diastolic electrograms to the subsequent VT QRS, despite spontaneous or induced oscillations of the tachycardia CL, is important to exclude the possibility that those electrograms do not reflect late activation from unrelated dead-end pathways.

STEP 3: ENTRAINMENT MAPPING DURING VENTRICULAR TACHYCARDIA. Pacing is performed during VT at selected LV sites, as identified during activation and substrate mapping. Pacing trains at CLs 10 to 30 milliseconds shorter than the tachycardia CL are introduced using the least pacing output that captures the ventricle. Pacing should be continued for sufficiently long durations to ensure entrainment of the VT.

The presence of entrainment should be confirmed by the demonstration of fixed fusion of the paced QRS at any single pacing CL, progressive fusion (i.e., the surface ECG progressively looks more like the VT QRS than a purely paced QRS) as the pacing CL decreases, and resumption of the VT following pacing with a nonfused VT QRS at a return cycle equal to the pacing CL. Once the presence of entrainment is confirmed, three parameters should be evaluated—the presence of manifest or concealed fusion, the PPI, and the local electrogram-QRS interval during VT versus the S-QRS interval during entrainment. The 12-lead ECGs during pacing and during VT are compared to evaluate whether manifest or concealed fusion is present. The PPI is measured from the stimulus artifact to the onset of the local electrogram of the first VT (unpaced) beat at the pacing site. Finally, the local electrogram-QRS interval during VT and the S-QRS interval during entrainment are measured on the distal bipolar pair recording of the mapping catheter or with the use of the proximal bipolar pair when the presence of artifacts in the distal pole recording prevents reliable measurement.

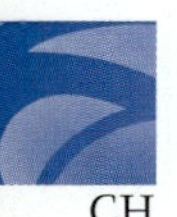

The following three criteria are used to define the critical isthmus and predict the success of RF application in elimination of the VT: (1) entrainment with concealed fusion; (2) PPI minus tachycardia CL not exceeding 30 milliseconds; and (3) S-QRS interval minus local electrogram to QRS interval not exceeding 20 milliseconds. Other predictors of successful ablation sites include an S-QRS interval to VT CL ratio not exceeding 0.7, long S-QRS interval, alteration of the tachycardia CL and/or termination by subthreshold or nonpropagated stimuli (see Fig. 22-19), and repeated VT termination occurring with catheter manipulation or pacing at the site.

STEP 4: PACE MAPPING DURING NORMAL SINUS RHYTHM. Pace mapping can be used to complement activation and entrainment mapping findings, although it may not always be necessary, especially when several criteria localizing the VT isthmus have been identified. At isthmus sites defined during VT, pace mapping during NSR is attempted after VT termination, with the mapping catheter being kept at the isthmus location. Pace mapping is preferably performed with unipolar stimuli (10 mA, 2 milliseconds) from the distal electrode of the mapping catheter (cathode) and an electrode in the IVC (anode). The same pacing CL is usually used for each site in an individual patient (500 to 700 milliseconds), slightly faster than the sinus rate and slower than the rate of the induced VTs. The resulting 12-lead ECG morphology is compared with that of the tachycardia. ECG recordings should be reviewed at the same gain and filter settings. It is often helpful to have the 12-lead ECGs of the VT and paced QRS complexes displayed side-by-side on split screens of the recording system for comparison. The greater the degree of concordance between the morphology during pacing and tachycardia, the closer is the catheter to the exit site of the tachycardia isthmus. It is important to recall that pace mapping at an isthmus may not produce a QRS identical to VT for reasons discussed above.

Evaluation of the S-QRS interval during pace mapping is of interest. The S-QRS interval is measured to the onset of the earliest QRS on the 12-lead ECG. Sites from which pace mapping produces the same QRS as that of the initial isthmus site with different S-QRS delays are identified in an attempt to trace the course of the VT isthmus.

MAPPING HEMODYNAMICALLY UNSTABLE OR UNSUSTAINABLE MONOMORPHIC VENTRICULAR TACHYCARDIA

Only 30% of patients referred for treatment of VT are suitable for ablation guided only by mapping during VT. Most patients have VTs that are too unstable to allow extensive mapping during the arrhythmia because of hemodynamic collapse, frequent changes from one VT to another, or inability to reproducibly induce the VT. In patients in whom the induced VT is only marginally tolerated (hypotension without syncope), circulatory support can be achieved with an intravenous infusion of dopamine, dobutamine, or phenylephrine; intraaortic balloon counterpulsation; partial or complete cardiopulmonary bypass; or LV assist device. Additionally, intravenous procainamide (infused with a maximal loading dose of 15 mg/kg at a rate of 50 mg/min, followed by a continuous infusion at a maximal rate of 0.11 mg/kg/min) can help slow and stabilize the VT rate.[43]

When the VT is unstable or unsustainable and, therefore, not approachable by conventional entrainment maneuvers and point-by-point activation mapping techniques, substrate mapping during NSR rather than during VT is of significant value, and can help delineate the infarcted myocardium (VT substrate) as well as help focus limited activation-entrainment mapping efforts on small predefined regions harboring the VT substrate and, therefore, help minimize how long the patient is actually in VT, which may be feasible even for poorly tolerated VT.

STEP 1: SUBSTRATE MAPPING DURING BASELINE RHYTHM. Infarct regions that potentially harbor the VT substrate (as identified on preacquired imaging techniques and VT morphology on 12-lead ECG) are sought first and more data points are acquired around these areas. Sites are identified to represent VT substrate based on their amplitude and configuration. Activation mapping is used to identify sites with abnormal local electrogram configuration (fractionated electrograms, multipotential electrograms, and isolated diastolic electrograms) during NSR, RV pacing, or both. These sites are tagged and catalogued by the 3-D mapping system for future revisiting and guidance. Voltage mapping (using a 3-D mapping system) is used to identify areas of abnormal low-amplitude local electrograms during NSR. These sites are then used to guide designing linear ablation lesions targeting the VT exit sites or slow conducting channels within scar areas, or to guide other mapping maneuvers (activation, entrainment mapping, or both) that then can be performed quickly during short periods of VT.

STEP 2: PACE MAPPING DURING NORMAL SINUS RHYTHM. Pace mapping during NSR is performed at the border zone between scar and normal tissue to approximate the exit site of each inducible VT. Pacing at each site is evaluated for two criteria: paced QRS morphology matching that of the VT and long S-QRS interval. The resulting 12-lead ECG pace QRS morphology is compared with that of the VT. The greater the degree of concordance between the morphology during pacing and tachycardia, the closer is the catheter to the site of origin of the tachycardia. Sites with S-QRS latency are also sought, which may correlate with slow channels and isthmuses within the infarct area that may be in or close to the VT circuit.

STEP 3: LIMITED ACTIVATION AND ENTRAINMENT MAPPING DURING VENTRICULAR TACHYCARDIA. When hemodynamic compromise during the VT is the main limitation for conventional activation and entrainment mapping methods, inductions of brief episodes of VT (with the mapping catheter at the optimal site, as identified by substrate and pace mapping approaches) can allow assessment of the relationship of the abnormal electrograms to the VT circuit. This can also allow entrainment maneuvers to be performed at those sites to help distinguish sites critical to the VT circuit from bystander sites. VT is then quickly terminated before significant hemodynamic compromise ensues. This approach can be facilitated by hemodynamic support with the use of intravenous vasopressors, intraaortic balloon pump, or both. However, it requires being able to reproducibly induce the same VT morphology.

STEP 4: MULTISITE DATA ACQUISITION MAPPING. This approach uses a system that simultaneously records electrograms throughout the ventricle during one or a few beats of the unstable VT, following which the VT can be terminated to allow ablation during stable sinus rhythm. Simultaneous multisite data acquisition using the noncontact mapping system (EnSite 3000) may rapidly identify VT exit sites and thus starting points for conventional mapping. It can also help identify VT isthmuses and therefore suitable targets for ablation.

STEP 5: ACTIVATION MAPPING OF PREMATURE VENTRICULAR COMPLEXES. In post-MI patients with frequent PVCs and VT, these arrhythmias can share an anatomically preformed reentrant circuit or at least a common exit site. Therefore, mapping the PVCs (rather than the VT) can be a helpful additional technique for identifying critical areas, especially exit sites, in scar-related VT.

Ablation

Target of Ablation

HEMODYNAMICALLY STABLE VENTRICULAR TACHYCARDIA

As noted, focal ablation of multiple sites defined as in the reentrant circuit may not eliminate VT. Elimination requires ablation of an isthmus bordered by barriers on either side. These isthmuses are usually found at the border zone of the infarct and are defined as conductive myocardial tissue delineated by nonconductive tissue. The nonconductive tissue can be a scar area or an anatomical obstacle, such as the mitral annulus. The isthmuses are the preferred targets for VT ablation because they are usually narrow and critical parts of the VT reentry circuit, allowing ablation with a small set of RF lesions.

Results of ablation of infarct-related VTs have been improving over the past decade because of better understanding and selection of ablation sites. Initial attempts at ablation targeted early presystolic potentials, followed by the use of mid-diastolic potentials; both approaches yielded unsatisfactory results. Presystolic potentials were found to be nonspecific, because they might be in an area of scar tissue—for example, inner loop, bystander (inner sites attached to the central pathway), or not related to the VT circuit. Mid-diastolic potentials, which cannot be dissociated from the VT during entrainment, are uncommon (30% of patients) and can be related to a bystander site. Demonstration of entrainment of VT with concealed fusion as a guide to VT ablation has increased ablation success rates. However, entrainment with concealed fusion alone to guide VT ablation has only a 50% positive predictive value for terminating VT, because concealed entrainment can be observed during pacing from bystander sites connected to, but not integral parts of, the reentrant circuit. Multiple criteria (e.g., S-QRS latency, mid-diastolic potentials) have been suggested, alone or in combination, to improve identification of the critical zone of the VT. These criteria have a different sensitivity and specificity with variable positive predictive values whenever they are used in different combinations. Recent data have shown that sites where the three entrainment criteria described (concealed fusion, PPI equal to the VT CL, and S-QRS interval <70% of the VT CL) are met have the highest ablation success rates, with a positive predictive value of 100% and negative predictive value of 96% (see Table 22-3).

The inability to find the appropriate target site can be caused by inadequate density of mapping points; the presence of a large amount of scar tissue; intramyocardial or epicardial location of the VT isthmus; technical difficulty in catheter manipulation; and acceleration, termination, or changing of VT to a different arrhythmia during attempts at entrainment limiting mapping of the VT.

STABLE SUSTAINED VENTRICULAR TACHYCARDIA

For stable VTs, reentry circuit isthmuses are defined by activation and entrainment mapping as sites with continuous activity or isolated mid-diastolic potentials, entrainment with concealed fusion, PPI equal to the VT CL, and S-QRS interval less than 70% of the VT CL. Additionally, there are other criteria that can identify the location of the critical isthmus. Reproducible alteration of the tachycardia CL or termination of VT by subthreshold or nonpropagated pacing stimuli is also an indication that the pacing site is in a circuit isthmus (see Fig. 22-19). The stimulus likely captures locally, but the propagated impulse blocks before exiting the scar region and creates bidirectional conduction block in the reentry circuit. Alternatively, the stimulus prolongs refractoriness at the site through an electrotonic effect. This finding is specific for predicting a successful ablation site, but is observed infrequently, with a sensitivity of only 16%.[43] Furthermore, mild mechanical trauma caused by the mapping catheter occasionally terminates the VT and may render the tachycardia noninducible for a variable period of time, preventing further mapping. This event suggests that the vulnerable region for the VT is small as well as superficial, and ablation at the site can be successful.[16,43] Empiric thermal mapping (RF application for 10 seconds to assess VT termination) can also help confirm sites within the VT isthmus. VT termination during short RF applications without induction of PVCs suggests an isthmus location. When RF application fails to terminate the VT at a site that appears to be in the circuit, catheter-tissue contact may be inadequate, the site may be a bystander, or the isthmus may consist of a broad band.[43]

MULTIPLE INDUCIBLE VENTRICULAR TACHYCARDIAS

In patients referred for post-MI VT ablation, an average of three to four VTs is commonly inducible by programmed electrical stimulation. When multiple VTs are inducible during EP testing, several investigators have targeted the predominant morphology of VT. Ablation that focused on the clinical VT but did not target other inducible VTs successfully abolished the clinical VT in 71% to 76% of cases. However, during follow-up, approximately one-third of patients with acutely successful ablation of the clinical VT had arrhythmia recurrences, some of which occurred because of a VT different from that initially targeted for ablation. Furthermore, there are several difficulties with selecting a dominant, clinical VT for ablation. Often, it is not possible to determine which VT is the one that has occurred spontaneously. Only a limited recording of one or a few ECG leads may be available. In patients with an ICD, the device typically terminates VT before an ECG is obtained, and VT is documented only on intracardiac recordings. Even if one VT is identified as predominant, other VTs that are inducible can subsequently occur spontaneously.

An alternative approach is to attempt ablation of all inducible VTs that are sufficiently tolerated to allow mapping. The 3-year risk of recurrent VT after such an approach is 33%.

At present, the clinical endpoint for VT ablation remains unclear. Although the targeting of all induced VTs is a prevalent strategy, the level of aggressiveness to achieve this endpoint must be weighed against hemodynamic stability, volume shifts, and prolonged anesthesia in tenuous patients.[58] The goal(s) of ablation, however, should be individualized. In patients undergoing ablation because of frequent ICD shocks or tachycardia-induced CMP, elimination of problematic VT morphologies is appropriate. On the other hand, elimination of all inducible VTs should be considered especially for patients who cannot undergo or decline ICD implantation.

UNMAPPABLE VENTRICULAR TACHYCARDIA

Over the past three decades, two effective surgical strategies have been developed for treatment of post-MI VT. Subendocardial resection, guided by the presence of the endocardial scar and involving removal of the subendocardial layer containing the arrhythmogenic tissue, is associated with a 70% to 80% arrhythmia cure rate. Such surgical therapy is performed when uniform sustained VT cannot be initiated at the time of surgery. The second technique is encircling endocardial ventriculotomy, whereby circumferential surgical lesions are placed through the border zone, presumably interrupting potential VT circuits. This experience was critical in establishing the concepts on which substrate-based ablation is based; the arrhythmogenic substrate is predominantly located in the subendocardium and resides, at least partly, in the border zone between densely infarcted or fibrotic tissue and normal tissue. This substrate has distinguishing electrogram characteristics, and removal or interruption of this arrhythmogenic tissue can abolish the VT.

Catheter ablation of post-MI VT during stable sinus rhythm, guided by delineation of the infarct region from sinus rhythm electrograms, maintains hemodynamic stability while ablation of unstable VTs and multiple VTs can potentially be achieved. However, how best to guide placement of ablation lesions is unclear. Single-point ablation guided by analysis of individual electrograms during NSR (used to identify surviving myocardial strands in the infarcted area that can be relevant for a VT reentrant circuit) or pace mapping (used to identify potential exit sites of the VT circuit) has proved insufficient to guide VT ablation and carries a risk of unnecessary ablation at ineffective sites (e.g., in dead-end pathways not integral to the tachycardia circuit). Ablation over the entire infarct region or around the entire infarct border zone (as identified by LV scar imaging modalities and voltage mapping) is often not feasible, nor necessarily desirable. The infarct size or area of low-voltage electrograms is usually large (averaging 21 cm in circumference in one study), necessitating extensive and transmural ablation lesions, which is difficult to achieve using the current catheter-based ablative techniques and can result in increased risk of complications, including damage to functioning myocardium.

Currently, ablation strategies are guided by the identification of potential reentry circuit isthmuses and exit sites based on substrate, pace, and entrainment mapping. Given the less precise localization of the reentry circuit, a more extensive ablation approach involving the delivery of energy over a relatively large area within the scar is commonly employed.[2] Linear RF lesions are placed using one of several guiding principles:

- Ablation lines extending across the borders of the endocardium that demonstrate abnormal bipolar electrogram voltage.[1]
- Focal ablation lesions delivered at sites demonstrating delayed electrograms ("late potentials") during substrate mapping, to eliminate these electrograms (see Fig. 22-33).
- Ablation lines extending perpendicular to the scar border, from the area of dense scar (i.e., areas demonstrating the lowest amplitude signals [<0.5 mV]) across the border zone and connecting out to normal myocardium (i.e., areas demonstrating a distinctly normal signal [>1.5 to 2.0 mV]) or to anatomical barriers (e.g., mitral annulus) (see Fig. 22-35). This approach represents the closest approximation achieved by endocardial catheter ablation to subendocardial surgical resection of the VT substrate.[1]
- Ablation lines extending parallel to the scar edge in the border zone of the scar and intersecting sites where pace mapping approximates the QRS morphology of VT. The ablation lines should be deployed within the border zone defined by voltage mapping (0.5 to 1.0 mV) to avoid damaging normal myocardium.[1]
- Ablation lines extending perpendicular to all defined isthmuses (channels of surviving myocardium) within the scar areas or between islands of unexcitable segments within the infarct (identified as a region of relatively larger voltage bordered by low voltage within the scar and abnormal electrograms during NSR).
- Focal ablation lesions delivered at sites demonstrating electrograms with isolated diastolic components, provided that pace mapping at those sites reproduces target VT QRS morphology, with an S-QRS interval of more than 40 milliseconds, the electrogram at those sites becomes mid-diastolic during VT induction, and entrainment maneuvers during brief inductions of VT have confirmed relationship of those sites to the VT circuit.

These different substrate ablation strategies have not been directly compared and differences in outcomes are not apparent in the literature. Variations in anatomy may also influence the effectiveness of the different methods. In many patients, a combination of these techniques is needed for successful identification and ablation of critical sites of the reentrant circuit.

Ablation Technique

Catheter ablation of scar-related VT usually requires relatively extensive tissue injury to abolish the arrhythmia substrate, which can be facilitated by the use of larger electrodes or irrigated electrodes. For ablation of scar-related VT, irrigated RF electrodes are preferred to large (8-mm)-tip electrodes. Cooled RF ablation allows increased power delivery, deeper lesions in myocardial scar, and potentially improved outcomes. In contrast, increasing the size of the electrode both reduces the spatial resolution of mapping and increases the disparity in temperatures across the surface of the electrode such that hot regions can lead to coagulum formation despite relatively low temperatures recorded from the electrode. On the other hand, external irrigation involves administration of potentially large amounts of intravascular saline, which can cause acute heart failure; therefore, careful monitoring of fluid balance is required and a urinary catheter and diuretic administration may be needed during the procedure. Internal irrigation catheters or large-tip catheters should be considered if intravascular volume administration will be difficult to manage, as in patients with renal failure, severe heart failure, or both.[2]

Once a target is selected, cooled RF ablation may be performed using an external or internal irrigation system. The external irrigation system (ThermoCool; Biosense Webster) uses an 8 Fr catheter that has an electrode 3.5 mm in length with six holes in the tip through which saline flows at 30 mL/min during RF application. In the internal irrigation system (Chilli; Boston Scientific, Natick, Mass.), saline flows at 36 mL/min through the electrode and returns through a second lumen to be discarded outside the patient. For both cooled RF systems, RF application is initiated at a power output of 20 to 30 W; the power is gradually increased to achieve a fall in impedance of 5 to 10 Ω or a maximal measured electrode tip temperature of 40°C to 45°C. Energy application is continued for 30 to 120 seconds. RF current application is discontinued if measured impedance increases by more than 10 Ω, the catheter changes position, or VT fails to terminate after 30 to 60 seconds.

Alternatively, RF current can be delivered generally during VT from a mapping catheter with a solid 8-mm tip. RF energy is delivered in a temperature-controlled mode for 60 to 120 seconds at each ablation target site, with a maximal temperature target of 60°C to 70°C and 50-70 W of maximal power delivered. Alternatively, RF energy is delivered at an initial power of 10 W and the power is titrated upward, as guided by temperature monitoring, to attain a temperature of 60°C. Once this endpoint is reached, the application of energy is continued for 20 seconds or longer. If VT fails to terminate, the energy application is discontinued and mapping is continued at other sites; if VT does terminate, the RF application is continued for a total of 60 seconds at the final power setting. Ablation can also be performed with a 4-mm-tip electrode with power titrated to a 5- to 10-Ω drop in impedance or a maximal temperature of 60°C to 65°C. Impedance is monitored during RF delivery. In case of an impedance rise, the ablation catheter is removed from the body and the distal electrode is wiped clean of the coagulum before continuing with the procedure.

At isthmus sites identified by entrainment, RF ablation typically terminates VT within 20 seconds. A second RF application is typically given at successful target sites if VT cannot immediately be reinitiated and the catheter has not moved. Successful ablation sites usually result in VT termination within 5 to 15 seconds of the RF application. Therefore, if there is no termination of VT by 30 seconds, it is suggested to discontinue RF energy application to decrease the likelihood of ablation of noninvolved myocardial tissue, with potential impairment of LV function. However, assuring adequate catheter-tissue contact is important before abandoning what appeared to be a good target site. This can be done with monitoring the catheter tip on fluoroscopy or on ICE and observing the rise in temperature or drop in impedance during RF application.

For ablation of unstable VT, RF energy is delivered during NSR. A series of ablation lesions are made to transect the critical isthmus in the most convenient area, targeting the narrowest portion of the isthmus when allowed by catheter positioning and stability. To join the isthmus boundaries, RF lines are usually drawn perpendicular to the mitral annulus plane in perimitral circuits (see Fig. 22-35) and parallel to the mitral annulus plane in all other circuits. RF lesions are applied to the region until pacing with 10-mA, 2-millisecond strength stimuli fails to capture, or reversal of ventricular electrograms in CS recordings occurs (Fig. 22-39). After completion of each set of RF lesions, programmed electrical stimulation is repeated.

Application of RF energy at successful exit, central, or entry VT circuit sites usually results in termination of the VT within a mean time of 10 ± 11 seconds. When RF application at other sites terminates the VT, the average time to termination is 19 ± 16 seconds, which suggests that a larger region must be heated for interruption of reentry. Persistence of inducibility of VT after successful termination with a single RF application, despite further applications of RF energy at the same site, is probably secondary to inadequate lesion size because of a wide isthmus, epicardial location, and/or significant fibrosis, thrombus, or calcification. In some cases, lack of consistent electrode-tissue contact can result from dislodgment of the electrode when a sudden change in rhythm occurs (such as VT termination).

When RF application fails to terminate the VT at a site that appears to be in the circuit, the site may be a bystander. Failure of ablation has been attributed to a number of factors, including inaccurate mapping because of failure to apply appropriate criteria for localizing a protected isthmus and/or inability to find such a site,

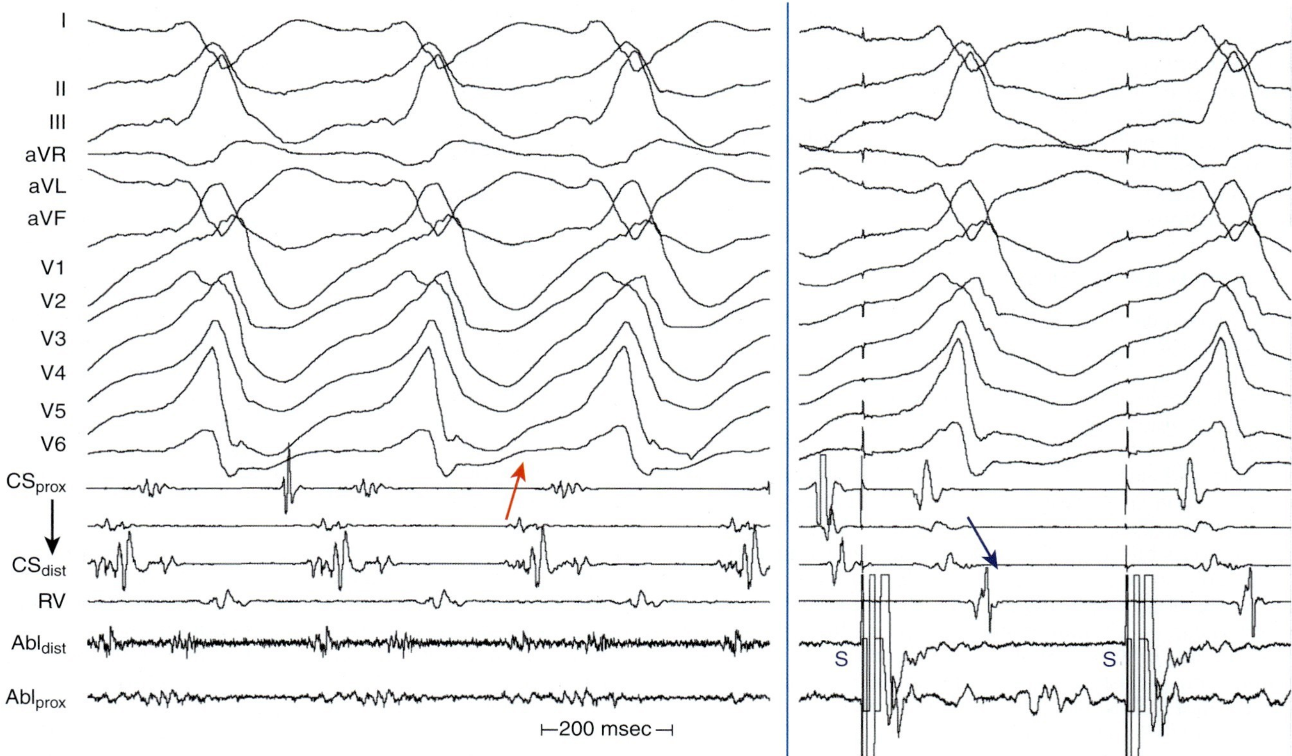

FIGURE 22-39 Mitral isthmus block in inferior wall post-infarction ventricular tachycardia (VT). During VT, shown in the **left panel** (as well as sinus rhythm and right ventricular pacing [data not shown]), ventricular electrograms in the coronary sinus (CS) recordings propagate from distal to proximal (red arrow). After ablation to the mitral annulus, pacing from a coronary vein branch distal to the ablation line **(right panel)** shows propagation now from proximal to distal CS (blue arrow), indicating conduction block in the mitral isthmus.

and also to inadequate lesion size produced by the RF application. Occasionally, successful termination of VT is achieved with RF application at a site at which failure is predicted. This may occur if the site is not at the isthmus region but in the nearby vicinity, with good conduction of temperature to the isthmus.

Endpoints of Ablation

At effective target sites, RF energy terminates VT and prevents reinduction of the targeted VT using the entire programmed electrical stimulation protocol. An ablation target site is deemed ineffective when the application of RF energy does not terminate or prevent the reinduction of VT despite an electrode-tissue interface temperature of more than 55°C.

Successful VT ablation is defined as noninducibility of any VT (excluding polymorphic VT, ventricular flutter, and VF). When clinical or presumed clinical VTs have been adequately documented previously and can be induced at the outset of the procedure, the minimal endpoint of ablation should be to eliminate the induction of that VT during postprocedure programmed stimulation. The entire programmed electrical stimulation protocol should be performed and should include up to three VESs delivered from at least two ventricular sites (one of which may be LV), with the shortest coupling intervals of 180 to 200 milliseconds or to refractoriness. If the initial stimulation protocol required additional LV pacing sites or catecholamine infusion to induce VT, then that protocol should be repeated following ablation. The complete protocol of programmed electrical stimulation is again repeated after a 30-minute waiting period, unless such aggressive stimulation places the patient at risk of cardiopulmonary deterioration.[2]

VT modification is defined as noninducibility of all clinical VTs (i.e., all inducible VTs that are known to have the same 12-lead ECG QRS morphology and approximate CL as spontaneous VTs), but with other monomorphic VTs remaining inducible. Following ablation of one or more reentry circuits, the remaining inducible VTs are often faster, suggesting that regions of slow conduction have been ablated; the remaining circuits that can form have a shorter revolution time. Thus, the arrhythmia substrate appears to have been modified. Modification of the reentry substrate is a common outcome of ablation, and is usually associated with a favorable outcome and a relatively low risk of arrhythmia recurrence.

On the other hand, the mere change in the "intensity" of stimulation required to induce VT (greater number of extrastimuli and alternative stimulation sites) is not a reliable endpoint.[2] In one report, induction of any VT post ablation was associated with a significantly greater risk of VT recurrence (nearly twofold), whereas persistent induction of only more rapid "nonclinical" VTs did not predict recurrence.[59]

In patients who present with incessant VT, restoration of stable sinus rhythm may represent a reasonable clinical endpoint, irrespective of the outcome of subsequent programmed stimulation.

Outcome

MANAGEMENT AFTER ABLATION

Following successful catheter ablation, antiarrhythmic drugs may be discontinued. Nonetheless, because of the relatively high risk of VT recurrence and the progressive nature of the VT substrate, antiarrhythmic drug therapy is often continued in most patients following VT ablation. In some cases, cessation of antiarrhythmic drugs that had suppressed some VTs may allow them to occur; therefore, freedom from antiarrhythmic drugs may not be a reasonable goal of ablation; instead, dose reduction may be an important goal, particularly for amiodarone, for which the incidence of side effects is closely related to daily dose. In various trials, dose reduction of amiodarone is reported and doses may be reduced in a progressive manner starting within the first 3 to 6 months post ablation.[1,2]

Within the first 3 months post ablation in the LV, there may be a risk of systemic thromboembolism, particularly if extensive ablation lesions were applied. Antiplatelet agents (aspirin, clopidogrel, or both) are typically used in all patients with ischemic heart disease. Additionally, warfarin may be used for higher risk patients (documented thrombus, previous stroke or transient ischemic attack, AF, severe LV dysfunction). Short-term (6 to 12 weeks) warfarin therapy may also be considered in patients who received extensive ablation over large areas (e.g., several centimeters).[1,2]

SUCCESS AND RECURRENCE

Catheter ablation generally results in improved arrhythmia control in the majority (50% to 83%) of patients who have a mappable scar-related VT and can also decrease the frequency of VT episodes triggering ICD therapies. The variable success of post-MI VT ablation has been attributed to a number of factors, including inaccurate mapping because of failure to apply appropriate criteria for localizing a protected isthmus and/or inability to find such a site, and inadequate lesion size produced by RF. Outcome appears to be improved with irrigated ablation techniques.[1] Ablation targeting critical isthmuses for stable VTs is successful, abolishing the inducible "targeted" or "clinical" VT in 71% to 86% of selected patients. During average follow-ups ranging from 9 to 42 months, noninducibility of the clinical VT immediately postprocedure is associated with a lower risk of VT recurrence and nonfatal VT (13% to 46%), compared with persistent inducibility of the clinical VT (up to 80%); the risk of SCD is low (0% to 6%), reflecting common use of ICDs for patients felt to be at risk.[43]

Also, substrate-guided ablation generally achieves a marked reduction in VT episodes and ICD shocks in patients with scar-related VT, even if occasional recurrences of VT persist during follow-up. It is a reasonable approach for patients with unmappable VT and may be combined with other mapping approaches in patients with mappable VTs.[1] In patients with a single stable spontaneous VT morphology well documented prior to the procedure, the persistent induction of "nonclinical" VTs that are faster than the targeted VT was reported to have little influence on subsequent spontaneous recurrence rates. Although the occasional spontaneous occurrence of these "nonclinical" VTs during follow-up is well documented, ablation of clinical VT (but not necessarily all VTs) can be associated with a lower incidence of electrical storm and cardiac death, despite a high likelihood of sporadic VT recurrence.[2,59] Nonetheless, lack of inducible ventricular arrhythmias following VT ablation is associated with improved survival.[60] In patients with failure of ablation or another VT inducible, the 3- to 4-year risk of VT recurrence is much higher (60% to 64%) as compared with patients with no inducible monomorphic VT of any morphology (recurrence, 14% to 20%). Additionally, induction of multiple VT morphologies during the procedure may predict higher risk of arrhythmia recurrence post ablation.[58] In patients with incessant VT or VT storm, catheter ablation can be life-saving and can acutely control the arrhythmia in over 90% of patients. Although single episodes of VT recur in approximately one-third of patients, 74% to 92% remain free of incessant VT or VT storm.[2]

Recurrence of the patient's initial spontaneous VT is usually presumed to occur if either the 12-lead ECG demonstrates the same VT morphology as the initial VT, or the VT CL as recorded from the ICD is within 20 milliseconds of the initial VT CL (if there has been no change in antiarrhythmic drug therapy). When the clinical VT recurs, it generally has a longer CL. This occurs because (1) the RF lesion might have produced slowing of conduction, and not block, in the critical isthmus, possibly because the width of the isthmus exceeds the size of the ablation lesion; (2) the RF lesion might have increased the length of the central common pathway by increasing the barrier around which the impulse circulated, without changing the circuit exit; and/or (3) the RF lesion might actually have been successful in eliminating the critical isthmus of the VT circuit, but an inner loop, which was present and not part of the primary reentry circuit, became an active participant in a new longer circuit that had the same exit site as the original VT.

When a VT with different morphology occurs, it is usually one of the inducible VTs from the same region. This likely reflects different exit sites or different potential reentrant circuits in the same area of the infarct.

COMPLICATIONS

Patients with post-MI VT typically have depressed LV function and concomitant illnesses. Ablation is often a late attempt in controlling refractory arrhythmias, sometimes after significant hemodynamic compromise has developed. Therefore, significant complications (e.g., worsened heart failure, stroke, transient ischemic attack, MI, cardiac perforation, or heart block) occur in approximately 3.6% to 10% of patients. Procedure-related mortality ranges from 0% to 3%. Local hemorrhagic complications (large hematomas or arterial pseudoaneurysms, arteriovenous fistula) occur in more than 2% of patients. Strokes and transient ischemic attacks occur in approximately 1%, and cardiac tamponade in 1%.[1]

Exacerbation of heart failure can develop in the acute phase post ablation. Extensive ablation in viable myocardium, injury to the aortic or mitral valves during LV catheter manipulation, repeated hemodynamically unstable VT episodes, and saline administration from externally irrigated ablation catheters are procedural complications that can potentially exacerbate heart failure and myocardial ischemia. Therefore, it is prudent to restrict ablation lesions to areas of infarction, as identified from low-amplitude electrograms in regions observed to have little contractility on echocardiography or ventriculography.[1,2]

On the other hand, coronary artery injury is not common during endocardial RF application of post-MI VT. Larger coronary vessels are less susceptible to injury than small vessels, likely due to the greater cooling effect of blood flow. Additionally, ablation in infarct-related areas is likely to involve territories of occluded infarct arteries. Of 215 patients in one series, only a single patient suffered MI from occlusion of a marginal artery.

Although ablation guided by substrate mapping avoids the hemodynamic consequences of prolonged mapping during VT, the lack of a precise reentry circuit target is compensated by extensive ablation lesion sets, which increases the potential for complications. In a recent multicenter study, major complications including worsening heart failure were observed in 7.3% of patients, and 3.0% died within 7 days of ablation.[1]

During follow-up later after ablation, the largest source of mortality was death from heart failure, accounting for more than one third of mortality and exceeding 10% per year in some studies. Although this risk of death is not unexpected in this population, because the mere occurrence of VT is a marker for increased heart failure and mortality, ablation of VT can potentially contribute to progression of heart failure.

In a recent meta-analysis of five studies including 457 participants with structural heart disease (predominantly ischemic CMP), complications of catheter ablation occurred in 6.3% of patients, including death (1%), stroke (1%), cardiac perforation (1%), and complete heart block (1.6%). There was no statistically significant difference in mortality compared with patients treated with antiarrhythmic medications.[61]

Before considering VT ablation, possible aggravating factors should be addressed to reduce the risks of procedural complications. Although myocardial ischemia by itself does not generally cause recurrent monomorphic VT, it can be a trigger in patients with scar-related reentry circuits. Furthermore, severe ischemia during induced VT increases the risk of mapping and ablation procedures. An assessment of the potential for ischemia is generally warranted in these patients. Patients with LV dysfunction should also have an echocardiogram to assess the possible presence of LV thrombus that could be dislodged and embolize during catheter manipulation in the LV. Scar-related VTs are often associated with poor LV function and multiple inducible VTs; most patients will remain candidates for an ICD, with ablation used for control of symptoms caused by frequent arrhythmia recurrences.

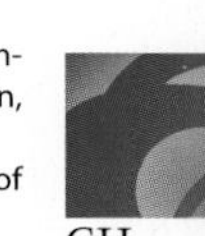

REFERENCES

1. Natale A, Raviele A, Al-Ahmad A, et al: Venice Chart International Consensus document on ventricular tachycardia/ventricular fibrillation ablation, *J Cardiovasc Electrophysiol* 21:339–379, 2010.
2. Aliot EM, Stevenson WG, Mendral-Garrote JM, et al: EHRA/HRS Expert Consensus on Catheter Ablation of Ventricular Arrhythmias: developed in a partnership with the European Heart Rhythm Association (EHRA), a Registered Branch of the European Society of Cardiology (ESC), and the Heart Rhythm Society (HRS); in collaboration with the American College of Cardiology (ACC) and the American Heart Association (AHA), *Heart Rhythm* 6:886–933, 2009.
3. Josephson ME: Recurrent ventricular tachycardia. In Josephson ME, editor: *Clinical cardiac electrophysiology*, ed 4, Philadelphia, 2008, Lippincott Williams & Wilkins, pp 446–642.
4. Haqqani HM, Marchlinski FE: Electrophysiologic substrate underlying postinfarction ventricular tachycardia: characterization and role in catheter ablation, *Heart Rhythm* 6(Suppl 8):S70–S76, 2009.
5. Klein HU, Reek S: "The older the broader": electrogram characteristics help identify the critical isthmus during catheter ablation of postinfarct ventricular tachycardia, *J Am Coll Cardiol* 46:675–677, 2005.
6. Segal OR, Chow AW, Peters NS, Davies DW: Mechanisms that initiate ventricular tachycardia in the infarcted human heart, *Heart Rhythm* 7:57–64, 2010.
7. Haqqani HM, Kalman JM, Roberts-Thomson KC, et al: Fundamental differences in electrophysiologic and electroanatomic substrate between ischemic cardiomyopathy patients with and without clinical ventricular tachycardia, *J Am Coll Cardiol* 54:166–173, 2009.
8. Das MK, Scott LR, Miller JM: Focal mechanism of ventricular tachycardia in coronary artery disease, *Heart Rhythm* 7:305–311, 2010.
9. Gupta S, Pressman GS, Figueredo VM: Incidence of, predictors for, and mortality associated with malignant ventricular arrhythmias in non-ST elevation myocardial infarction patients, *Coron Artery Dis* 21:460–465, 2010.
10. Piers SR, Wijnmaalen AP, Borleffs CJ, et al: Early reperfusion therapy affects inducibility, cycle length, and occurrence of ventricular tachycardia late after myocardial infarction, *Circ Arrhythm Electrophysiol* 4:195–201, 2011.
11. Kumar S, Sivagangabalan G, Thiagalingam A, et al: Effect of reperfusion time on inducible ventricular tachycardia early and spontaneous ventricular arrhythmias late after ST elevation myocardial infarction treated with primary percutaneous coronary intervention, *Heart Rhythm* 8:493–499, 2011.
12. Barsheshet A, Goldenberg I, Narins CR, et al: Time dependence of life-threatening ventricular tachyarrhythmias after coronary revascularization in MADIT-CRT, *Heart Rhythm* 7:1421–1427, 2010.
13. Vest RN III, Gold MR: Risk stratification of ventricular arrhythmias in patients with systolic heart failure, *Curr Opin Cardiol* 25:268–275, 2010.
14. Buxton AE: Risk stratification for sudden death in patients with coronary artery disease, *Heart Rhythm* 6:836–847, 2009.
15. Dukkipati SR, d'Avila A, Soejima K, et al: Long-term outcomes of combined epicardial and endocardial ablation of monomorphic ventricular tachycardia related to hypertrophic cardiomyopathy, *Circ Arrhythm Electrophysiol* 4:185–194, 2011.
16. Miller JM, Scherschel JA: Catheter ablation of ventricular tachycardia: skill versus technology, *Heart Rhythm* 6(Suppl 8):S86–S90, 2009.
17. Tian J, Jeudy J, Smith MF, et al: Three-dimensional contrast-enhanced multidetector CT for anatomic, dynamic, and perfusion characterization of abnormal myocardium to guide ventricular tachycardia ablations, *Circ Arrhythm Electrophysiol* 3:496–504, 2010.
18. Yokokawa M, Tada H, Koyama K, et al: The characteristics and distribution of the scar tissue predict ventricular tachycardia in patients with advanced heart failure, *Pacing Clin Electrophysiol* 32:314–322, 2009.
19. Zipes DP, Camm AJ, Borggrefe M, et al: ACC/AHA/ESC 2006 guidelines for management of patients with ventricular arrhythmias and the prevention of sudden cardiac death: a report of the American College of Cardiology/American Heart Association Task Force and the European Society of Cardiology Committee for Practice Guidelines (Writing Committee to Develop Guidelines for Management of Patients With Ventricular Arrhythmias and the Prevention of Sudden Cardiac Death), *J Am Coll Cardiol* 48:e247–e346, 2006.
20. Goldberger JJ: Evidence-based analysis of risk factors for sudden cardiac death, *Heart Rhythm* 6(Suppl 3):S2–S7, 2009.
21. Piccini JP, Zhang M, Pieper K, et al: Predictors of sudden cardiac death change with time after myocardial infarction: results from the VALIANT trial, *Eur Heart J* 31:211–221, 2010.
22. Hamilton RM, Azevedo ER: Sudden cardiac death in dilated cardiomyopathies, *Pacing Clin Electrophysiol* 32(Suppl 2):S32–S40, 2009.
23. Das MK, Zipes DP, Fragmented QRS: a predictor of mortality and sudden cardiac death, *Heart Rhythm* 6(Suppl 3):S8–S14, 2009.
24. Das MK, Maskoun W, Shen C, et al: Fragmented QRS on twelve-lead electrocardiogram predicts arrhythmic events in patients with ischemic and nonischemic cardiomyopathy, *Heart Rhythm* 7:74–80, 2010.
25. Crawford T, Cowger J, Desjardins B, et al: Determinants of postinfarction ventricular tachycardia, *Circ Arrhythm Electrophysiol* 3:624–631, 2010.
26. Solomon SD, Zelenkofske S, McMurray JJ, et al: Sudden death in patients with myocardial infarction and left ventricular dysfunction, heart failure, or both, *N Engl J Med* 352:2581–2588, 2005.
27. Patel C, Yan GX, Kocovic D, Kowey PR: Should catheter ablation be the preferred therapy for reducing ICD shocks? Ventricular tachycardia ablation versus drugs for preventing ICD shocks: role of adjuvant antiarrhythmic drug therapy, *Circ Arrhythm Electrophysiol* 2:705–711, 2009.
28. Callans DJ: Patients with hemodynamically tolerated ventricular tachycardia require implantable cardioverter defibrillators, *Circulation* 116:1196–1203, 2007.
29. Passman R, Kadish A: Sudden death prevention with implantable devices, *Circulation* 116:561–571, 2007.
30. Reddy VY, Reynolds MR, Neuzil P, et al: Prophylactic catheter ablation for the prevention of defibrillator therapy, *N Engl J Med* 357:2657–2665, 2007.
31. Kuck KH: Should catheter ablation be the preferred therapy for reducing ICD shocks? Ventricular tachycardia in patients with an implantable defibrillator warrants catheter ablation, *Circ Arrhythm Electrophysiol* 2:713–720, 2009.
32. Josephson ME, Callans DJ: Using the twelve-lead electrocardiogram to localize the site of origin of ventricular tachycardia, *Heart Rhythm* 2:443–446, 2005.
33. Segal OR, Chow AW, Wong T, et al: A novel algorithm for determining endocardial VT exit site from 12-lead surface ECG characteristics in human, infarct-related ventricular tachycardia, *J Cardiovasc Electrophysiol* 18:161–168, 2007.
34. Haqqani HM, Morton JB, Kalman JM: Using the 12-lead ECG to localize the origin of atrial and ventricular tachycardias. 2. Ventricular tachycardia, *J Cardiovasc Electrophysiol* 20:825–832, 2009.
35. Kumar S, Sivagangabalan G, Choi MC, et al: Long-term outcomes of inducible very fast ventricular tachycardia (cycle length 200-250 ms) in patients with ischemic cardiomyopathy, *J Cardiovasc Electrophysiol* 21:262–269, 2010.
36. Deo R, Berger R: The clinical utility of entrainment pacing, *J Cardiovasc Electrophysiol* 20:466–470, 2009.
37. Waldo AL: From bedside to bench: entrainment and other stories, *Heart Rhythm* 1:94–106, 2004.
38. Colombowala IK, Massumi A, Rasekh A, et al: Variability in postpacing intervals predicts global ventricular activation pattern during tachycardia, *Pacing Clin Electrophysiol* 33:129–134, 2010.
39. Abdelwahab A, Gardner MJ, Basta MN, et al: A technique for the rapid diagnosis of wide complex tachycardia with 1:1 AV relationship in the electrophysiology laboratory, *Pacing Clin Electrophysiol* 32:475–483, 2009.
40. Badhwar N, Scheinman MM: Electrophysiological diagnosis of wide complex tachycardia, *Pacing Clin Electrophysiol* 32:473–474, 2009.
41. Stevenson WG, Soejima K: Recording techniques for clinical electrophysiology, *J Cardiovasc Electrophysiol* 16:1017–1022, 2005.
42. Derejko P, Szumowski LJ, Sanders P, et al: Clinical validation and comparison of alternative methods for evaluation of entrainment mapping, *J Cardiovasc Electrophysiol* 20:741–748, 2009.
43. Zeppenfeld K, Stevenson WG: Ablation of ventricular tachycardia in patients with structural heart disease, *Pacing Clin Electrophysiol* 31:358–374, 2008.
44. Khairy P, Balaji S: Cardiac arrhythmias in congenital heart diseases, *Indian Pacing Electrophysiol J* 9:299–317, 2009.
45. Kanter RJ: Pearls for ablation in congenital heart disease, *J Cardiovasc Electrophysiol* 21:223–230, 2010.
46. Brunckhorst CB, Delacretaz E, Soejima K, et al: Identification of the ventricular tachycardia isthmus after infarction by pace mapping, *Circulation* 110:652–659, 2004.
47. Bogun F, Krishnan S, Siddiqui M, et al: Electrogram characteristics in postinfarction ventricular tachycardia: effect of infarct age, *J Am Coll Cardiol* 46:667–674, 2005.
48. Arbelo E, Josephson ME: Ablation of ventricular arrhythmias in arrhythmogenic right ventricular dysplasia, *J Cardiovasc Electrophysiol* 21:473–486, 2010.
49. Fahmy TS, Wazni OM, Jaber WA, et al: Integration of positron emission tomography/computed tomography with electroanatomical mapping: a novel approach for ablation of scar-related ventricular tachycardia, *Heart Rhythm* 5:1538–1545, 2008.
50. Tian J, Smith MF, Chinnadurai P, et al: Clinical application of PET/CT fusion imaging for three-dimensional myocardial scar and left ventricular anatomy during ventricular tachycardia ablation, *J Cardiovasc Electrophysiol* 20:597–604, 2009.
51. Bunch TJ, Weiss JP, Crandall BG, et al: Image integration using intracardiac ultrasound and 3D reconstruction for scar mapping and ablation of ventricular tachycardia, *J Cardiovasc Electrophysiol* 21:678–684, 2010.
52. Khaykin Y, Skanes A, Whaley B, et al: Real-time integration of 2D intracardiac echocardiography and 3D electroanatomical mapping to guide ventricular tachycardia ablation, *Heart Rhythm* 5:1396–1402, 2008.
53. Bogun FM, Desjardins B, Good E, et al: Delayed-enhanced magnetic resonance imaging in nonischemic cardiomyopathy: utility for identifying the ventricular arrhythmia substrate, *J Am Coll Cardiol* 53:1138–1145, 2009.
54. Pratola C, Baldo E, Toselli T, et al: Contact versus noncontact mapping for ablation of ventricular tachycardia in patients with previous myocardial infarction, *Pacing Clin Electrophysiol* 32:842–850, 2009.
55. Sarrazin JF, Labounty T, Kuhne M, et al: Impact of radiofrequency ablation of frequent post-infarction premature ventricular complexes on left ventricular ejection fraction, *Heart Rhythm* 6:1543–1549, 2009.
56. Sarrazin JF, Good E, Kuhne M, et al: Mapping and ablation of frequent post-infarction premature ventricular complexes, *J Cardiovasc Electrophysiol* 21:1002–1008, 2010.
57. Bogun F, Crawford T, Chalfoun N, et al: Relationship of frequent postinfarction premature ventricular complexes to the reentry circuit of scar-related ventricular tachycardia, *Heart Rhythm* 5:367–374, 2008.
58. Tung R, Josephson ME, Reddy V, Reynolds MR: Influence of clinical and procedural predictors on ventricular tachycardia ablation outcomes: an analysis from the substrate mapping and ablation in Sinus Rhythm to Halt Ventricular Tachycardia Trial (SMASH-VT), *J Cardiovasc Electrophysiol* 21:799–803, 2010.
59. Stevenson WG, Wilber DJ, Natale A, et al: Irrigated radiofrequency catheter ablation guided by electroanatomic mapping for recurrent ventricular tachycardia after myocardial infarction: the multicenter thermocool ventricular tachycardia ablation trial, *Circulation* 118:2773–2782, 2008.
60. Sauer WH, Zado E, Gerstenfeld EP, et al: Incidence and predictors of mortality following ablation of ventricular tachycardia in patients with an implantable cardioverter-defibrillator, *Heart Rhythm* 7:9–14, 2010.
61. Mallidi J, Nadkarni GN, Berger RD, et al: Meta-analysis of catheter ablation as an adjunct to medical therapy for treatment of ventricular tachycardia in patients with structural heart disease, *Heart Rhythm* 8:503–510, 2011.

CHAPTER 23 Adenosine-Sensitive (Outflow Tract) Ventricular Tachycardia

Classification

Ventricular tachycardia (VT) is usually associated with structural heart disease, with coronary artery disease and cardiomyopathy (CMP) being the most common causes. However, about 10% of patients who present with VT have no obvious structural heart disease (idiopathic VT).[1] Absence of structural heart disease is usually suggested if the electrocardiogram (ECG) (except in Brugada syndrome and long QT syndrome), echocardiogram, and coronary arteriogram collectively are normal. Nevertheless, magnetic resonance (MR) imaging may demonstrate mild structural abnormalities and subtle areas of diminished wall motion in some patients with idiopathic VT, even if all other test results are normal. In addition, focal dysautonomia in the form of localized sympathetic denervation has been reported in patients with VT and no other obvious structural heart disease. Of note, idiopathic VT occasionally occurs in patients with structural heart disease, in whom the structural heart disease is not related to the VT. Furthermore, frequent or incessant idiopathic VT can be a cause of tachycardia-induced CMP.[2]

Several distinct types of idiopathic VT have been recognized and classified with respect to the origin of VT (right ventricle [RV] versus left ventricle [LV]), VT morphology (left bundle branch block [LBBB] versus right bundle branch block [RBBB] pattern), response to exercise testing, response to pharmacological agents (adenosine-sensitive versus verapamil-sensitive versus propranolol-sensitive VT), and behavior of VT (repetitive salvos versus sustained).[3]

Pathophysiology

Mechanism of Adenosine-Sensitive Ventricular Tachycardia

Most forms of outflow tract VTs are adenosine-sensitive and are thought to be caused by catecholamine-induced, cyclic adenosine monophosphate (cAMP)–mediated delayed afterdepolarizations (DADs) and triggered activity, which is supported by several tachycardia features (see Chap. 4).[4] Heart rate acceleration facilitates VT initiation. This can be achieved by programmed stimulation, rapid pacing from either the ventricle or the atrium, or infusion of a catecholamine alone or during concurrent rapid pacing. Additionally, termination of the VT is dependent on direct blockade of the dihydropyridine receptor by calcium channel blockers or by agents or maneuvers that lower cAMP levels (e.g., by activation of the M_2 muscarinic receptor with edrophonium or vagal maneuvers, inhibition of the beta-adrenergic receptor with beta blockers, or activation of the A_1 adenosine receptor with adenosine). Furthermore, a direct relationship exists between the coupling interval of the initiating ventricular extrastimulus (VES) or ventricular pacing cycle length (CL) and the coupling interval of the first VT beat. Additionally, VT initiation is CL-dependent; pacing CLs longer or shorter than a critical CL window fail to induce VT. This critical window can shift with changing autonomic tone.[1,5,6]

Types of Adenosine-Sensitive Ventricular Tachycardia

Approximately 90% of idiopathic VTs are caused by one of two phenotypic forms of adenosine-sensitive VT. Repetitive monomorphic VT is the most common form (60% to 90%) and is characterized by frequent premature ventricular complexes (PVCs), couplets, and salvos of nonsustained VT, interrupted by brief periods of normal sinus rhythm (NSR; Fig. 23-1). This form of VT usually occurs at rest or following a period of exercise, and typically decreases during exercise, but can be incessant.[1] On the other hand, paroxysmal exercise-induced VT is characterized by sustained episodes of VT precipitated by exercise or emotional stress, separated by long intervals of NSR with infrequent PVCs (Fig. 23-2).[1] Evidence has suggested that both types represent polar ends of the spectrum of idiopathic VT caused by cAMP-mediated triggered activity, and there is considerable overlap between the two types. Furthermore, this subtype classification, although useful, is not necessarily precise and depends on the means and duration of rhythm recordings. Patients are typically categorized based on their presenting or index arrhythmia. Prolonged telemetry and long-term ambulatory ECG recordings have demonstrated that most patients with one subtype of outflow tract VT show evidence for at least one other subtype with an identical morphology. Almost all patients with nonsustained VT have high-density repetitive runs and frequent PVCs. In patients who present with repetitive PVCs, nonsustained VT can also be observed in approximately 70%; however, only 20% of these patients develop runs of more than five beats.[7]

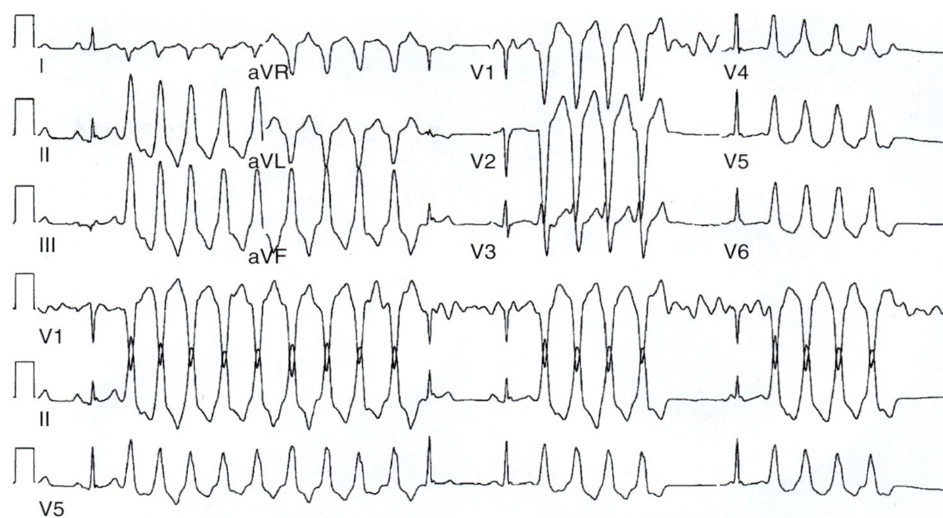

FIGURE 23-1 Surface ECG of repetitive monomorphic right ventricular outflow tract tachycardia. Repetitive bursts of ventricular tachycardia are present, with occasional sinus complexes.

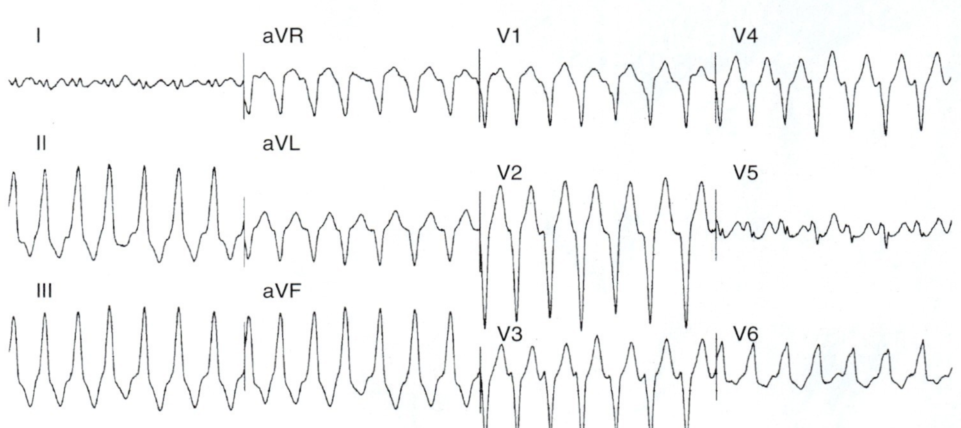

FIGURE 23-2 Surface ECG of sustained right ventricular outflow tract tachycardia.

Anatomical Considerations

Adenosine-sensitive idiopathic VT usually arises from outflow tracts (most frequently from the RV outflow tract [RVOT]). Other variants of outflow tract VT (with similar underlying electrophysiological [EP] mechanism) include ventricular arrhythmias arising from the aortic cusps, pulmonary artery, mitral or tricuspid inflow tracts, papillary muscles, and epicardial foci in close proximity to the coronary venous system.[3] Understanding the unique and complex anatomical relationships of the outflow tracts is critical for analyzing the ECG and mapping findings during outflow tract VT as well as for safe catheter maneuvering and ablation.

RIGHT VENTRICULAR OUTFLOW TRACT

The RVOT is the tubelike portion of the RV cavity above the supraventricular crest, and is defined superiorly by the pulmonic valve and inferiorly by the RV inflow tract and the top of the tricuspid annulus (the region of the His bundle [HB] and proximal right bundle branch). The lateral aspect of the RVOT region is the RV free wall. The RVOT passes cephalad in a posterior and slightly leftward direction. The medial aspect is formed by the anterior interventricular septum at the base of the RVOT and RV musculature opposite to the anterior LV outflow region (LVOT) (as a cephalad continuation of the interventricular septum) and the root of the aorta (immediately adjacent to the right coronary cusp) at the region just inferior to the pulmonic valve (Fig. 23-3).[8]

Although the medial aspect of the RVOT is frequently referred to as the "septal" wall, it should be noted that the outflow tract per se is not part of the interventricular septum, and the septum is a component only of the most proximal part of the RVOT at the branch point of the septomarginal trabeculation. Above this area, the RVOT curves to pass anterior and cephalad to the LVOT, and, therefore, any perforation in the septal part is more likely to go outside the heart than into the LV (Fig. 23-4).

From the coronal view above the pulmonic valve, the RVOT region is seen wrapping around the LVOT and the root of the aorta and extending leftward (see Fig. 23-3). Whereas the inflow portion of the RV lies to the right and anterior to the inflow portion of the LV, the RVOT courses anterior to the LVOT such that the distal RVOT and pulmonic valve are located to the left side of the body in relationship to the aortic valve and the distal LVOT. The pulmonic valve is typically placed approximately 5 to 10 mm cephalad and to the left of the aortic valve such that the supravalvular portion of the aorta lies in immediate proximity to the portions of the pulmonic valve; immediately anterior to the aortic valve is the posterior muscular infundibular portion of the RVOT.[8,9]

The top of the RVOT can be convex or crescent-shaped, with the posteromedial region directed rightward and the anterolateral region directed leftward. The anteromedial aspect of the RVOT actually is located in close proximity to the LV epicardium, adjacent to the anterior interventricular vein and in proximity to the left anterior descending coronary artery. The aortic valve

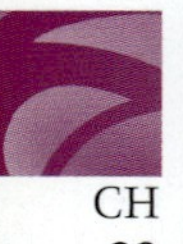

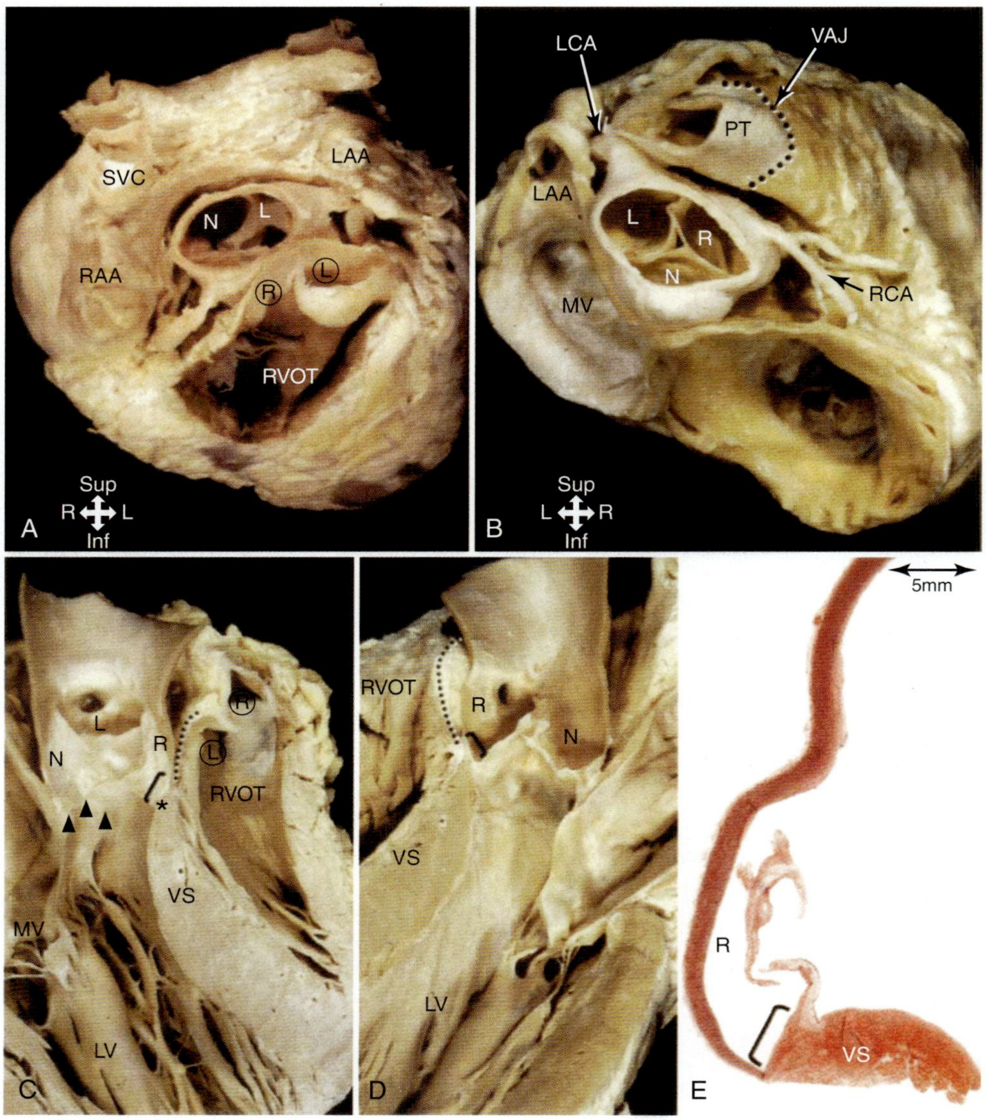

FIGURE 23-3 Anatomy of the outflow tracts and aortic sinuses. These heart specimens illustrate the anatomical arrangement between the right ventricular outflow tract (RVOT) and the aortic sinuses. **A,** Viewed superoanterioly the RVOT passes leftward and superior to the aortic valve. **B,** The superoposterior view shows the left (L) and right (R) coronary aortic sinuses adjacent to the pulmonary infundibulum. The noncoronary (N) aortic sinus is remote from the RVOT, but is related to the mitral valve (MV) and central fibrous body. The dotted line marks the ventriculoarterial junction (VAJ) between the wall of the pulmonary trunk (PT) and right ventricular muscle. Note the cleavage plane behind the pulmonary infundibulum and in front of the aortic root. **C** and **D,** These simulated parasternal long-axis sections show two halves of the same heart and display the left and right coronary orifices. The right- and left-facing pulmonary sinuses (R and L in circles, respectively) are situated superior to the aortic sinuses. The dotted line marks the epicardial aspect of the subpulmonary infundibulum in the so-called "septal" area (as illustrated in **E**). Inf = inferior; LAA = left atrial appendage; LCA = left coronary artery; LV = left ventricle; RAA = right atrial appendage; RCA = right coronary artery; SVC = superior vena cava; Sup = superior; TV = tricuspid valve; VS = ventricular septum. *(From Ouyang F, Fotuhi P, Ho SY, et al: Repetitive monomorphic ventricular tachycardia originating from the aortic sinus cusp: electrocardiographic characterization for guiding catheter ablation. J Am Coll Cardiol 39:500, 2002.)*

cusps sit squarely within the crescent-shaped posterior region of the RVOT and are inferior to the pulmonic valve (see Fig. 23-3). The most posterior aspect of the RVOT is adjacent to the region of the right coronary cusp, and the posteromedial (leftward) surface is adjacent to the anterior margin of the right coronary cusp or the medial aspect of the left coronary cusp.[10] The thickness of the RVOT wall is variable, ranging from approximately 3 to 6 mm, and is thinnest in the rightward, anterior, and subpulmonic valve portions, and thickest in the posterior infundibular part that is adherent to the anterior LVOT as a cephalad continuation of the interventricular septum.[8]

LEFT VENTRICULAR OUTFLOW REGION

Unlike the RV, the inflow and outflow tracts of the LV are at an acute angle to one another. The central location of the aortic valve places the LVOT between the mitral valve and the ventricular septum. In turn, approximately half of the aortic outlet is muscular and the other half (being the area of valvular continuity between the mitral and aortic valves) is fibrous. The curvature of the ventricular septum continuing into the free wall forms the anterosuperior wall of the LVOT. It is the deep anterior (aortic) leaflet of the mitral valve that forms the aortic-mitral curtain. The extremities of the fibrous continuity are the left and right fibrous trigones, the right trigone forming the central fibrous body. The LVOT passes underneath the RVOT in a rightward and cephalad direction pointing toward the right shoulder (see Fig. 23-4).[11]

AORTIC CUSPS

The aortic root is defined as the interface between the LV and the ascending aorta, extending from the sinotubular junction in the aorta to the basal valvular leaflets with their attachment within the LV (see Fig. 23-3). Approximately two-thirds of the circumference of the lower part of the aortic root is connected to the muscular ventricular septum, with the remaining one-third in fibrous continuity with the aortic leaflet of the mitral valve. Its components are the sinuses of Valsalva, the fibrous interleaflet triangles, and the valvular leaflets themselves. The aortic valve is composed of three symmetric, semilunar-shaped cusps. The recess of each cusp is called the "sinus of Valsalva." The aortic (coronary) cusps are firmly anchored to the fibrous skeleton within the root of the aorta. A circular ridge on the innermost aspect of the aortic wall, at the upper margin of each sinus, is the sinotubular ridge—the junction of the sinuses and the aorta. The aortic cusps are named according to their orientation in the body—left and right (both facing the pulmonic valve anteriorly) and posterior. The left aortic sinus gives rise to the left coronary artery, and the right aortic sinus gives rise to the right coronary artery. Usually, no vessels arise from the posterior aortic sinus, which is therefore known as the noncoronary

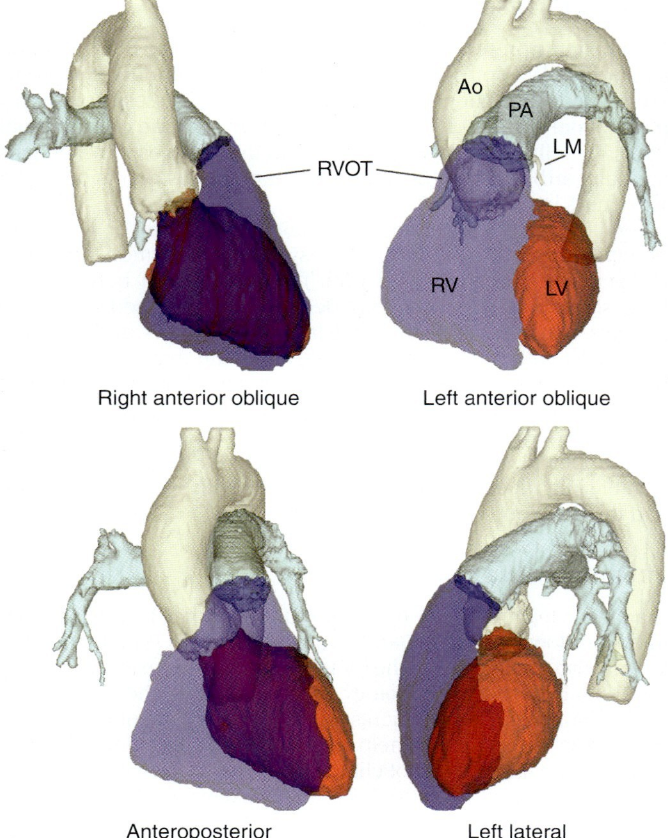

FIGURE 23-4 Anatomical relationships for ablation of outflow tract ventricular tachycardia (VT). Most RVOT VTs arise from just proximal to the pulmonic valve; note that the RVOT in this region is all free wall (not septal wall) and the leftward aspect of the RVOT is very near the LM, making it vulnerable to injury. Note also the close relationships between RVOT, aortic sinuses of Valsalva, and subaortic left ventricle (LV), explaining why VTs from this general region can have similar ECG morphologies. Ao = aorta; LM = left main coronary artery; PA = pulmonary artery; RVOT = right ventricular outflow tract.

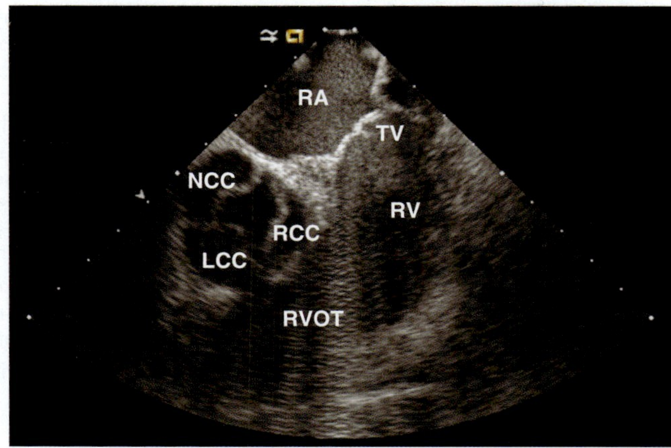

FIGURE 23-5 Intracardiac echocardiography (ICE) cross-sectional image of the aortic valve acquired with the ICE catheter positioned at the His bundle region of the RV septum. LCC = left coronary cusp; NCC = noncoronary cusp; RA = right atrium; RCC = right coronary cusp; RV = right ventricle; RVOT = right ventricular outflow tract; TV = tricuspid valve.

sinus. Three equally spaced sites of minimal tethering within the aortic root mark the junctions of the sinuses of Valsalva. Each sinus is associated with a leaflet of the aortic valve, whereas the junctions between the adjacent sinuses are aligned with the commissures between the aortic valve leaflets.[12-14]

The aortic valve is the cardiac centerpiece; it lies in contact or continuity with all four cardiac chambers and shares important proximate relationships with each of the other cardiac valves (Video 20). It comes into contact with the right atrium (RA), left atrium (LA), interatrial septum, RVOT, mitral valve (aortomitral continuity), pulmonic valve, tricuspid valve, and conduction system (see Fig. 23-3).[8,9]

The aortic root is inferior, posterior, and somewhat rightward compared with the RVOT. As noted, the posterior subpulmonic valve portions of the RVOT are immediately anterior and more proximally continuous with the anterior myocardial subaortic LVOT and more distally to the right coronary cusp. The lateral and more distal portions of the left coronary cusp lie immediately subjacent to the peripulmonic valve portions of the RVOT. In some instances, the supravalvular myocardial fibers of one outflow tract may be continuous with the other outflow tract's infravalvular myocardium, thus forming a functional syncytium.[8]

The left coronary cusp lies to the left of the right coronary cusp and is related to the posterior wall of the RVOT (Fig. 23-5). The commissure between the right and left coronary cusps is just posterior to the distal RVOT and is close but caudal to the posterior pulmonic valve annulus. More leftward and posteriorly, the left coronary cusp lies in continuity with the anterior leaflet of the mitral valve (aortomitral continuity). Adjacent to this site lies the peripulmonic valve myocardium and, more laterally, the posterior lobe of the LA appendage (when present).[8,9]

The right coronary cusp lies immediately posterior to the relatively thick posterior infundibular portion of the RVOT. Caudally, there is continuity with the anterior LVOT, and at the level of valve insertion there is either physical continuity or very close proximity between myocardium that extends above this valve cusp, the LVOT, and the posterior RVOT. The posterior part of the right coronary cusp is adjacent to the central fibrous body, which carries within it the penetrating portion of the HB. Anteriorly, the right coronary cusp is related to the bifurcating atrioventricular (AV) bundle and the origin of the left bundle branch. The right coronary cusp does not have a direct relationship with either atrium, but lateral to the commissure with the noncoronary cusp lies the RA appendage, trunk of the right coronary artery, and a variable amount of fat.[8,9]

The noncoronary cusp is the most posterior of the aortic cusps, and lies immediately anterior to the interatrial septum and superior to the central fibrous body, and has the RA and LA as the posterior right and left relations, respectively (see Fig. 23-5). In fact, atrial tachycardias have reportedly been ablated from within the noncoronary cusp because of its close relationship to the atria. Caudally, like the other cusps, the noncoronary cusp is in continuity with the LVOT myocardium. Other than this site, however, it has no anatomical relationship with any other ventricular myocardium. The triangle between the noncoronary and the right coronary sinuses incorporates within it the membranous part of the septum (the location of the penetrating HB). This fibrous part of the septum is crossed on its right side by the hinge of the tricuspid valve, which divides the septum into *atrioventricular* and *interventricular* components.[8,9,12,13]

Because of the semilunar nature of the attachments of the aortic valvular leaflets, there are three triangular extensions of the LVOT that reach to the level of the sinotubular junction. These triangles, however, are formed not of ventricular myocardium but of the thinned fibrous walls of the aorta between the expanded sinuses of Valsalva.[14]

For the greater part, the aortic sinuses are made up of the wall of the aorta. However, sleeves of ventricular myocardium extend beyond the aortic valve attachments for variable distances (analogous to atrial myocardial extensions in the pulmonary veins). Whereas the right coronary cusp and the anterior portions of the left coronary cusp frequently exhibit these myocardial sleeves, the posterior portions of the left coronary cusp and the noncoronary cusp, particularly in relation to the fibrous continuity with the anterior leaflet of the mitral valve (the aortomitral continuity), are exclusively fibrous and usually devoid of myocardium.[8,9,15] The noncoronary cusp at its junction of the right coronary cusp may have sleeves of ventricular myocardium and, at present, it is not clearly known whether myocardial extensions into the noncoronary cusp represent atrial or ventricular myocardium.[8]

Idiopathic VT can originate from the right or, more commonly, left coronary cusp, as well as from the junction of the left and right coronary cusps. The substrate of this VT likely originates from the strands of ventricular myocardium present at the bases of those cusps. In contrast, the base of the noncoronary cusp is composed of fibrous tissue and, thus, is an extremely rare site of origin of VT.[16,17] However, the nature of the actual substrate being ablated has not been clearly defined. For example, the ablation electrode placed in the depth of the right coronary cusp may be mapping and ablating a focus arising from the supravalvular extension into the cusp, LVOT myocardium, or a deeper posterior RVOT myocardium.[9]

PULMONARY ARTERY

The pulmonary sinuses are not as prominent as the aortic sinuses. Nevertheless, owing to the semilunar configuration of the valvular leaflets, the hinge line of each leaflet crosses the ventriculoarterial junction at two points. Consequently, there are always small segments of myocardium of the infundibulum at the nadirs of the three sinuses. Between adjacent sinuses, the wall comprises small triangles of fibrous tissue that become incorporated into the RV when the valve closes. On the epicardial aspect, the ventriculoarterial junction is not always a sharply defined line. Extensions of ventricular myocardium into the adventitia occur in approximately 20% of individuals and have been traced to a maximal distance of 6 mm beyond the junction.[11]

As noted, the pulmonic and aortic valves are not at the same level (see Fig. 23-3). The pulmonic valve, the most superiorly situated of the cardiac valves, lies at the level corresponding to the third left costal cartilage at its junction with the sternum. The transverse plane of the aortic valve slopes inferiorly, away from the plane of the pulmonic valve, such that the orifice of the aortic valve faces rightward at an angle of at least 45 degrees from the median plane.[11]

Because of its anterior and leftward location, only the posterior and rightward parts of the pulmonary artery have important relations with other cardiac structures. Of the three cusps of the pulmonic valve, the septal (right) pulmonic cusp lies at variable distances from and sometimes adjacent to the distal portions of the RA appendage. The left pulmonic cusp, being the most superficial, lies immediately beneath the pericardium and has no other cardiac structures related to it. The posterior pulmonary cusp externally lies in the proximal portion of the left main coronary artery and the distal portions in the LA appendage. The supravalvular portion of the aorta lies close to and in some cases adjacent to the junction and surrounding parts of the right and posterior pulmonic cusps.[8,9]

The pulmonic valve and supravalvular portion of the pulmonary artery are well-established locations of origin for ventricular arrhythmias. As noted, ventricular myocardial sleeves extend above the semilunar valves for a variable distance (a few millimeters and up to more than 2 centimeters). Whereas the myocardial sleeves typically extend circumferentially around the pulmonic valve between and above all three cusps just above the annulus, more distally the extension is patchy and generally asymmetrical. Myocardial extensions also occur in the intercuspal clefts in addition to within the cusps.[8]

Clinical Considerations

Epidemiology

Approximately 60% to 80% of idiopathic VTs arise from the RV (most commonly the RVOT). RVOT VT comprises 10% of all VTs referred to an electrophysiologist. Age at presentation is usually 30 to 50 years (range, 6 to 80 years). Women are more commonly affected.[1,5]

Clinical Presentation

Most patients present with palpitations, 50% develop dizziness, and a minority (10%) present with syncope. Most commonly, symptoms are related to frequent PVCs or nonsustained VT. Less commonly, paroxysmal sustained VT is precipitated by exercise or emotional stress. The clinical course is benign and the prognosis is excellent. Sudden cardiac death (SCD) is rare. Spontaneous remission of the VT occurs in 5% to 20%.

Very frequent idiopathic nonsustained VT, PVCs, or both can precipitate a reversible form of LV systolic dysfunction, similar to tachycardia-induced dilated CMP. The relationship between the LV dysfunction and VT may not be initially recognized, and those patients can present with heart failure symptoms and become diagnosed with nonischemic dilated CMP and may even undergo prophylactic implantation of a defibrillator, which unfortunately often results in delivery of inappropriate shocks triggered by frequent nonsustained episodes of idiopathic VT.[2] Interpolation of the PVCs appears to predict an increased risk of PVC-induced CMP.[18] Notably, in a recent report, 20% of patients with PVC-induced CMP had the PVC focus in one of the aortic cusps.[19]

Initial Evaluation

Diagnostic features include (1) structurally normal heart; (2) origin in the outflow tract (RVOT and, less commonly, LVOT), although the VT can also originate from the RV inflow tract, RV apex, or LV; and (3) QRS with LBBB-like morphology and inferior axis. The echocardiogram is normal in most patients. Slight RV enlargement is observed rarely. Exercise testing can help reproduce patients' clinical VT 25% to 50% of the time, but is not clinically helpful in most cases.

The diagnosis of idiopathic VT is one of exclusion; structural heart disease, CMP, and coronary artery disease have to be excluded, usually by cardiac stress testing and echocardiography. Left heart catheterization, right heart catheterization, or both may be warranted.

Additionally, it is important to differentiate idiopathic VT from other potentially malignant forms of VT that may also arise from the outflow tract region, including VT in arrhythmogenic RV dysplasia-cardiomyopathy (ARVD), catecholaminergic polymorphic VT (CPVT), Brugada syndrome, and idiopathic polymorphic VT and ventricular fibrillation (VF). A Brugada ECG pattern, findings of reduced LV or RV function, polymorphic VT or multiple VT morphologies, a history of recurrent syncope, or a family history of SCD mandates further detailed evaluation.

The diagnosis of ARVD should be carefully considered. Signal-averaged ECG, MR imaging of the RV, RV biopsy, and RV angiography are all unremarkable in idiopathic RVOT VT and help exclude ARVD. An invasive EP study is usually not necessary to establish a diagnosis, although it can occasionally help exclude other forms of tachyarrhythmias (see later).[2]

It is important to recognize that, in some patients, idiopathic VT can coexist with structural heart disease, including CMP, in which setting the VT is not related to the cardiac disease. On the other hand, very frequent idiopathic nonsustained VT, PVCs, or both can precipitate dilated CMP. The responsible ectopy can arise from any ventricular site, but the RVOT, being the most common type of idiopathic ventricular ectopy, is more commonly associated with ectopy-related CMP. Therefore, in patients who present with a dilated CMP of unclear etiology and who have frequent PVCs or nonsustained VT, it is important to assess the contribution of PVCs or VT to LV systolic dysfunction. A reversible form of dilated nonischemic CMP precipitated by idiopathic VT should be suspected when very frequent PVCs, nonsustained VT, or both are observed on a 24-hour Holter recording, especially when the QRS morphology is monomorphic and is suggestive of origin from the outflow tract. A PVC burden of more than 20% is present in most of those patients with tachycardia-induced CMP, but some patients have as few as 5% PVCs. In a recent report, a cutoff PVC burden of more than 24% was strongly associated with the presence of CMP. However, this cutoff value failed to identify every patient at risk of CMP, and for individual patients, the critical PVC burden can be lower. A cutoff PVC burden of more than 16% would result in a sensitivity of 90% for CMP, but the specificity would be reduced to 58%.[20] Although pharmacological suppression of the PVCs, such as by amiodarone therapy, may help evaluate the relationship between the arrhythmia and CMP, the usefulness of this approach and duration of therapy required have not been defined. Often, elimination of the PVCs by catheter ablation results in improvement and resolution of LV dysfunction within a few months. Therefore, catheter ablation of the PVCs is appropriate prior to implantable cardioverter-defibrillator (ICD) implantation for primary prevention of SCD; successful elimination of the PVCs may result in improvement in LV function such that the patient no longer qualifies for an ICD.[2,21]

Principles of Management

ACUTE MANAGEMENT

Acute termination of outflow tract VT can be achieved by vagal maneuvers or intravenous administration of adenosine (6 mg, titrated up to 24 mg as needed). Intravenous verapamil (10 mg given over 1 minute) is an alternative, provided the patient has adequate blood pressure and has a previously established diagnosis of a VT that is sensitive to verapamil. Hemodynamic instability warrants emergency cardioversion.

CHRONIC MANAGEMENT

Long-term treatment options for outflow tract VT include medical therapy and catheter ablation. Medical therapy may be indicated in patients with mild to moderate symptoms. For patients with symptomatic, drug-refractory VT or those who are drug intolerant or who do not desire long-term drug therapy, catheter ablation is the treatment of choice. Catheter ablation is also recommended for patients with frequent PVCs or nonsustained VT when they are presumed to cause LV dysfunction, even in otherwise asymptomatic patients.[2]

Medications, including beta blockers, verapamil, and diltiazem, have a 25% to 50% rate of efficacy. Alternative therapy includes class IA, IC, and III agents. Radiofrequency (RF) ablation now has cure rates of over 90%, which makes it a preferable option, given the young age of most patients with outflow tract VT.

Electrocardiographic Features

Surface Electrocardiogram

ECG DURING NORMAL SINUS RHYTHM

The surface ECG during NSR is usually normal. Up to 10% of patients have complete or incomplete RBBB.

ECG DURING VENTRICULAR TACHYCARDIA

Repetitive monomorphic VT is characterized by frequent PVCs, couplets, and salvos of nonsustained VT, interrupted by brief periods of NSR (see Fig. 23-1). Paroxysmal exercise-induced VT is characterized by sustained episodes of VT precipitated by exercise or emotional stress (see Fig. 23-2). Both types characteristically have an LBBB pattern with a right inferior (more common) or left inferior axis. The tachycardia rate is frequently rapid (CL < 300 milliseconds), but can be highly variable. A single morphology for the VT or PVCs is characteristic.[1,6]

Exercise Electrocardiogram

Exercise testing reproduces VT in less than 25% to 50% of patients with clinical VT. The VT can manifest as nonsustained or, less commonly, sustained. There are two general positive response patterns: initiation of VT during the exercise test and initiation of VT during the recovery period. Both scenarios likely represent examples of the dependence of VT on a critical window of heart rates for induction. This window can be narrow and only transiently present during exercise, resulting in induction of VT only during recovery. In patients with repetitive monomorphic VT, the VT is often suppressed during exercise. CPVT, also exercise dependent, can be distinguished by the alternating QRS axis with 180-degree rotation on a beat-to-beat basis (bidirectional VT) or polymorphic VT, which can degenerate into VF.

Ambulatory Monitoring

Several VT characteristics can be observed on ambulatory monitoring recordings. Ventricular ectopy typically occurs at a critical range of heart rates (CL dependence). The coupling interval of the first PVC is relatively long (approximately 60% of the baseline sinus CL). A positive correlation exists between the sinus rate preceding the VT and the VT duration. Additionally, the VT occurs in clusters, and is most prevalent on waking and during the morning and later afternoon hours. The VT is extremely sensitive to autonomic influences, resulting in poor day-to-day reproducibility.[1,6]

Electrocardiographic Localization of Outflow Tract Ventricular Tachycardia

VTs originating from the RVOT typically display LBBB morphology with a precordial QRS transition (first precordial lead with R/S ratio >1) that begins no earlier than lead V_3 and more typically occurs in lead V_4. The frontal plane axis, precordial R/S transition, QRS width, and complexity of the QRS morphology in the inferior leads can more precisely indicate the origin of VT within the RVOT. Most RVOT VTs originate from the anterosuperior aspect of the leftward ("septal") aspects, just under the pulmonic valve. These tachycardias produce a characteristic 12-lead ECG appearance with tall positive QRS complexes in leads II, III, and aVF and large negative complexes in leads aVR and aVL. The QRS morphology in lead I typically is multiphasic and has a net QRS vector of zero or is only modestly positive (see Fig. 23-2).

However, not all VTs with a QRS morphology of LBBB and inferior or normal axis can be ablated successfully from the RVOT. Some VTs originate in the subaortic LV (LVOT, 10% to 15% of adenosine-sensitive VTs), above the pulmonic valve (i.e., from muscle tracts in the pulmonary artery), and occasionally in the aortic root. Idiopathic RV VTs with a superior QRS axis generally originate in the body of the RV on the anterior free wall, or in the mid- and distal septum (Table 23-1).

It is important to recognize that the prediction of the precise origin of outflow tract VT can still be challenging because of the close anatomical relationship of the different anatomical compartments of the outflow tract area. For example, an R/S transition zone in precordial lead V_3 is common in patients with idiopathic outflow tract VT, with a prevalence of up to 58%. The prevalence of R/S transition in lead V_3 in RVOT VT is not statistically different from VT originating outside the RVOT; therefore, the predictive value for this ECG criterion is low. Approximately 50% of outflow tract tachycardias with an R/S transition in V_3 could be successfully ablated from the RVOT; however, one study has shown that a significant proportion of patients need different anatomical approaches for successful RF catheter ablation using up to six different anatomical accesses, including the LV, the aortic sinus of Valsalva, the coronary sinus (CS), the pulmonary artery, and the epicardium via a percutaneous pericardial puncture.[22]

RIGHT VENTRICULAR OUTFLOW TRACT VERSUS LEFT VENTRICULAR OUTFLOW REGION

The absence of an R wave in lead V_1 and precordial transition zone in lead V_4, V_5, or V_6 predicts an RVOT origin. On the other hand, the presence of an R wave in leads V_1 and V_2 and RS transition in leads V_1 or V_2 are characteristic of an LVOT origin (Figs. 23-6 and 23-7). Because of the continuity between the posterior RVOT and the anterior LVOT, a very similar R wave in lead V_3 may be seen with arrhythmia that originates in either structure, and R/S transition in lead V_3 is not specific.

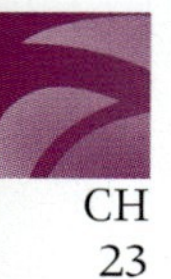

TABLE 23-1 Estimation Indexes of Right Ventricular Outflow Tract Ventricular Tachycardia Origins by 12-Lead ECG*

Anterior Versus Posterior: QRS Duration, Leads II and III R Wave Pattern				
QRS duration	>140 msec	≤140 msec	Rr′ or rr′ in II and III	R in II and III
Free wall side	7	1	0	8
"Septal"	6	21	5	22
Left Versus Right: Leads aVR and aVL QS Wave Amplitude, Lead I Polarity				
QS amplitude	aVR < aVL	aVR ≥ aVL	Lead I negative	Lead I positive
Left side	18	5	20	3
Right side	2	10	3	9
Superior Versus Inferior: Leads V_1 and V_2 Initial r Wave Amplitude				
V_1 and V_2	High r*	Low r†		
Proximal side below pulmonic valve	14	8		
Distal side below pulmonic valve		4	9	
LVOT Versus RVOT: Lead V_3 R/S Ratio				
V_3	R/S ≥ 1	R/S < 1		
LVOT side	4	1		
RVOT side	6	29		

*High r means initial r wave amplitude greater than 0.2 mV in both leads.
†Low r means r wave amplitude less than 0.2 mV in one or both leads.
LVOT = left ventricular outflow region; RVOT = right ventricular outflow tract.
From Kottkamp H, Chen X, Hindricks G, et al: Idiopathic left ventricular tachycardia: new insights into electrophysiological characteristics and radiofrequency catheter ablation, *Pacing Clin Electrophysiol* 18:1285, 1995.

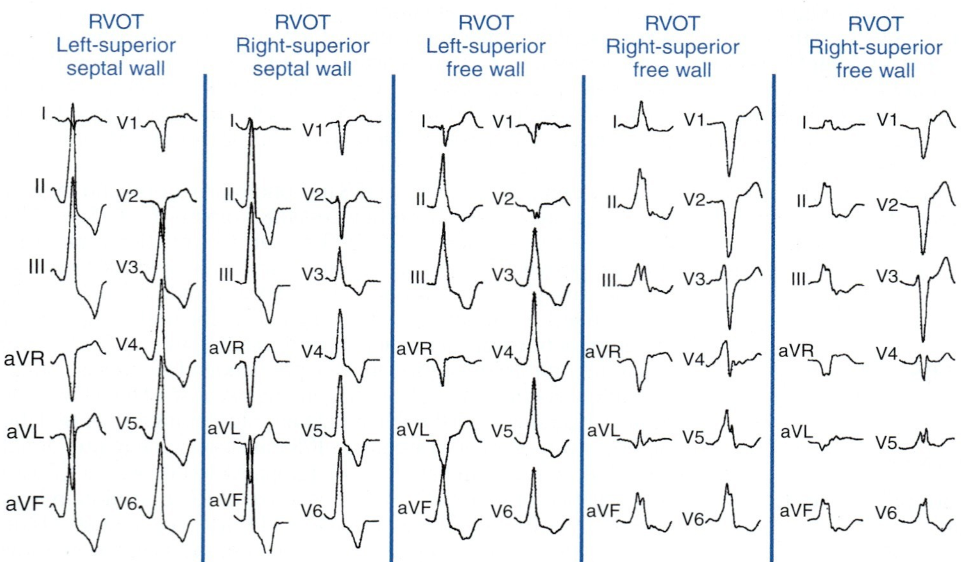

FIGURE 23-6 ECG of premature ventricular complexes from the right ventricular outflow tract (RVOT).

In the latter setting, a precordial R/S transition during VT that is earlier than that during NSR argues against an LVOT origin. Additionally, comparing the R wave amplitude divided by total QRS amplitude (i.e., R/[R + S]) in lead V_2 during VT with that during NSR can help distinguish between LVOT and RVOT origins in patients with lead V_3 precordial transition. A transition ratio $(R/[R + S]_{VT} \div R/[R + S]_{NSR})$ of at least 0.60 is highly suggestive of an LVOT origin.[23] Furthermore, a QS complex in lead I is also suggestive of subaortic LV origin.[8,22]

"SEPTAL" VERSUS FREE WALL RIGHT VENTRICULAR OUTFLOW TRACT

QRS duration less than 140 milliseconds, monophasic R wave without notching (i.e., no RR′ or Rr′) in leads II and III, and early precordial transition (by lead V_4) suggest a septal origin. On the other hand, the triphasic RR′ or Rr′ waves in VT of free wall origin probably reflect the longer QRS duration and the phased excitation from the RV free wall to the LV (see Fig. 23-6).

LEFT (ANTEROMEDIAL ATTACHMENT) VERSUS RIGHT (POSTEROLATERAL ATTACHMENT) SIDE OF THE RIGHT VENTRICULAR OUTFLOW TRACT

In general, a QS complex in lead I is generated from sites at or near the anterior medial aspect of the RVOT (the most leftward portion of the RVOT in the supine anteroposterior orientation). As the site of origin moves rightward, on either the posterior or the anterior wall, R waves appear in lead I and become progressively dominant and the QRS axis becomes more leftward. Similarly, a QS amplitude in aVL greater than that in aVR suggests an origin in the left side of the RVOT; a QS amplitude in aVR greater than that in aVL suggests an origin in the right side (see Fig. 23-6).

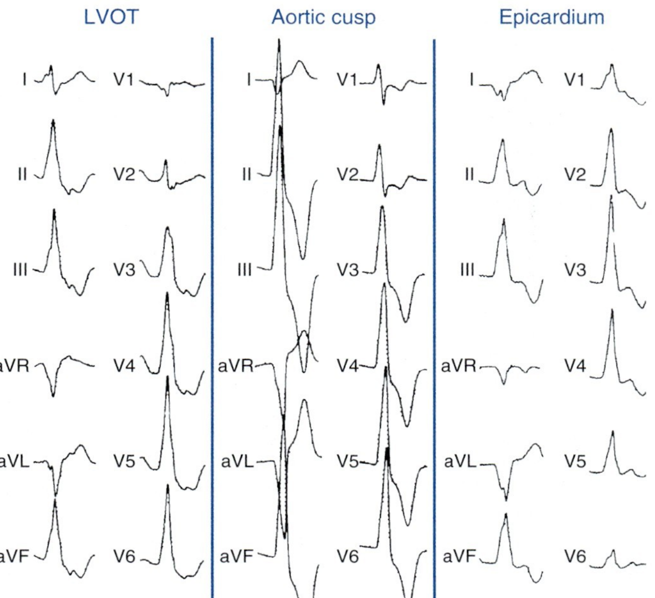

FIGURE 23-7 ECG of premature ventricular complexes from the left ventricular outflow region (LVOT), aortic cusp, and epicardium.

SUPERIOR VERSUS INFERIOR RIGHT VENTRICULAR OUTFLOW TRACT

The R wave amplitude tends to be larger in leads V_1 and V_2 at superior and leftward sites; as the site of origin shifts to the right or inferiorly, there is a trend toward lower right precordial R wave amplitude and a shift in the precordial transition zone to the left. Furthermore, R wave amplitude in lead V_2 or "r" wave amplitude in leads V_1 and V_2 greater than 0.2 mV suggests a superior origin. Additionally, the closer the origin to the pulmonic valve, the more rightward and inferior the axis (i.e., R wave taller in lead III than in lead II) because of the anatomical leftward location of the pulmonic valve and lead III being an inferior *and* rightward lead; the more posterior and inferior the origin, the more leftward the axis (see Fig. 23-6). Also, lead aVL (being a left-sided lead) becomes isoelectric or slightly positive as the site of origin moves inferiorly (close to the HB region), whereas aVR (being a right-sided lead) remains negative.[8]

VENTRICULAR TACHYCARDIAS ARISING ABOVE THE PULMONIC VALVE

Because of the superior and leftward location of these sites, VTs arising above the pulmonic valve are associated with a small but definite vector toward the right, resulting in a small initial R wave in lead V_1. Additionally, suprapulmonic origins exhibit a strong right inferior frontal plane axis (a QS or rS wave in lead I, large R waves in II, III, aVF, and deep QS complexes in aVR and aVL, with the R wave being taller in lead III than in lead II and the S wave being deeper in aVL than in aVR). Those VTs also tend to display an R/S ratio in lead V_2 and R wave amplitude in inferior leads that are significantly larger than those in RVOT VT.[8,9,24] However, moderate overlap exists between VTs originating above the pulmonic valve and RVOT VTs, and because the RVOT is the exit site of VT arising from the pulmonary artery, discriminating between the two groups using ECG parameters can be difficult.[25]

VENTRICULAR TACHYCARDIAS ARISING FROM THE TRICUSPID ANNULUS

VTs arising from the tricuspid annulus demonstrate LBBB morphology and positive QRS polarity in leads I, V_5, and V_6. In contrast to VTs arising from the RVOT, no positive QRS polarities in any of the inferior leads characterize VTs arising from the tricuspid annulus. No negative component of the QRS complex is found in lead I, and the R wave magnitude in lead I is typically greater in VTs arising from the tricuspid annulus than those arising from the RVOT.[26] Additionally, VTs arising from the tricuspid annulus have an rS or QS pattern in lead aVR, just as those arising from the RVOT; however, in lead aVL, a QS or rS pattern is rare (8%), and the QRS polarity in lead aVL is positive in almost all VTs arising from the annulus (89%), in contrast to those arising from the RVOT.[26]

VENTRICULAR TACHYCARDIAS ARISING FROM THE RIGHT VENTRICULAR PAPILLARY MUSCLES

RV papillary muscle VTs display LBBB morphology with a QS or rS pattern in lead V_1 and a wider QRS complex and more prevalent notching than in RVOT VT. VTs arising from the anterior and posterior papillary muscles are frequently associated with a superior axis and a late R wave transition in the precordial leads (later than lead V_4), whereas septal papillary muscle VTs more often display an earlier precordial transition (in lead V_4 or earlier) and an inferior axis (due to the more basal insertion of the septal compared with the anterior and posterior papillary muscles). More than one PVC or VT morphology can be present in a significant proportion of patients with papillary muscle VTs.[27] Compared with origins from the septum, VTs from the free wall exhibit longer QRS duration and deeper S waves in leads V_2 and V_3.[28]

VENTRICULAR TACHYCARDIAS ARISING FROM THE LEFT VENTRICULAR PAPILLARY MUSCLES

VT can also arise from posterior or anterior papillary muscles. The QRS morphology during VT has an RBBB pattern with either left superior (posterior papillary muscle) or rightward inferior (anterior papillary muscle) axis.[29,30] The ECG features are very similar in the LV papillary muscle and fascicular VTs; nonetheless, in contrast to fascicular VT, papillary muscle VT has a broader QRS complex (150 ± 15 milliseconds versus 127 ± 11 milliseconds). Additionally, all fascicular VTs, versus none of papillary muscle VTs, had an rsR′ pattern in lead V_1. An R/S ratio not exceeding 1 in lead V_6 for VTs in the LV anterolateral region also suggests papillary muscle VT.[31] Furthermore, spontaneous variations in QRS morphology occur relatively frequently during VTs originating from the LV papillary muscles, a feature that can help distinguish these VTs from LV fascicular VT, the latter being a reentrant tachycardia with a consistent QRS morphology.[32]

OTHER LEFT VENTRICULAR SITES OF ORIGIN

VT can originate from multiple LV sites, including the subaortic LV, the superior basal region of the left interventricular septum, papillary muscle, aortomitral continuity, mitral annulus, aortic cusps, and epicardial sites in the region of the great cardiac and anterior interventricular veins. Most of these sites of origin are associated with an LBBB pattern and inferior axis. A basal LV septal origin is suggested by LBBB morphology associated with an early precordial transition in lead V_1 or V_2. An origin from the aortomitral continuity is associated with RBBB morphology and broad monophasic R waves across the precordial leads. As the origin moves laterally along the mitral annulus, the R wave in lead I and in the inferior leads decreases in amplitude. LVOT free-wall VTs have an early transition and persistent dominant R wave across the precordium, with a small or absent S wave out to the apex (see Fig. 23-7). The R wave in V_2 is broad and occupies a greater percentage of the QRS width than RVOT VTs. LVOT VT can occasionally have an epicardial site of origin. This form is associated with an R wave in lead V_1, S wave in lead V_2, precordial transition in leads V_2 to V_4, deep QS in lead aVL, and tall R wave in the inferior leads. Contrariwise, an R wave in lead V_2 taller than in leads V_1 or V_3 suggests an origin in the so-called crux of the heart, near the posterior descending artery.[1,33]

VENTRICULAR TACHYCARDIAS ARISING FROM THE AORTIC CUSPS

For LVOT VT, the absence of an S wave in leads V_5 or V_6 suggests a supravalvular origin, whereas the presence of such waves is consistent with an infravalvular origin (see Fig. 23-7). An R wave in lead aVL may exclude an origin in the left or right aortic cusp.[16]

Origin from the aortic cusp is also strongly suggested by a longer duration and greater amplitude of the R wave in leads V_1 and V_2 (R/QRS duration >50% and R/S amplitude >30%) as compared with VT originating from the RVOT, because the aortic valve lies to the right and posterior to the RVOT. Correction of the transitional zone to cardiac rotation (i.e., comparing the R/S transitional zone in precordial leads during VT with that during NSR) can be a useful marker for differentiating an RVOT origin from an aortic cusp origin. When the transitional zone during VT occurs in one or more precordial leads earlier than during NSR, an aortic cusp origin is favored, even when the transitional zone during VT occurs later than lead V_2 (Fig. 23-8).[34]

Left aortic cusp VTs initially depolarize the LV and typically have a multiphasic QRS complex such as an M or W pattern in lead V_1, suggesting transseptal activation (see Fig. 23-7). A simple qR complex or a monophasic R wave suggests an origin near the aortomitral continuity.[15] The R wave is positive by lead V_2 or V_3 with VT from the right aortic cusp and by lead V_1 or V_2 from the left aortic cusp.[10] Additionally, left aortic cusp VTs tend to have a QS or rS complex in lead I, whereas right aortic cusp VTs have a greater R wave amplitude in lead I based on how posterior and rightward the right aortic cusp is positioned. In young patients with a vertical heart, the QRS complex in lead I can be negative in and around both the left and right aortic cusp regions. In patients with a horizontal heart, the area surrounding the aortic valve will be directed rightward relative to the LV apex–lateral wall, and a positive QRS complex in lead I can be seen.[10]

When comparing origins from the right versus the left aortic cusps, RBBB morphology may exclude origins from the right coronary cusp. Additionally, the ratio of the R wave amplitude in leads II and III (III/II ratio) is significantly greater (>0.9) for VTs with a left coronary cusp origin than for those with a right coronary cusp origin.[16]

A common site of origin is just between the right and left commissures. This site is often recognized by a notch on the downstroke in V_1 with an intermediate (relative to the right and left cusps) precordial transition. A qrS pattern in leads V_1 to V_3 is very helpful for predicting an origin in the junction between the right and left coronary cusps.[35]

VTs originating from the aortic cusp often (25%) show preferential conduction to the RVOT, which can render some algorithms using the ECG characteristics less reliable. In fact, 20% of the VTs with an aortic cusp origin in that report showed a late QRS transition after V_3. In some of those cases, an insulated myocardial fiber across the ventricular outflow septum may exist.[36]

EPICARDIAL VENTRICULAR TACHYCARDIA

Several QRS characteristics suggest an epicardial VT origin of LV VTs, including the presence of a very slurred upstroke (pseudo-delta wave ≥34 milliseconds), long R-wave peak time (i.e., the interval from the beginning of the QRS complex to the time of initial downstroke of the R wave after it has peaked [previously known as the *intrinsicoid deflection*] ≥85 milliseconds) in lead V_2, and shortest precordial RS complex of at least 121 milliseconds (see Fig. 23-7).

These criteria, however, do not seem to apply uniformly to all LV regions or to VTs originating from the RV. Other site-specific criteria have been suggested for identifying an epicardial origin for LV VTs: the presence of a Q wave in lead I for basal superior and apical superior VTs; the absence of a Q wave in any of the inferior leads for basal superior VTs; and the presence of a Q wave in the inferior leads for basal inferior and apical inferior VTs.[37] Also, measurement of the *maximal deflection index* (defined as the product of the time to maximal deflection in precordial leads divided by the QRS duration) can help identify epicardial LVOT VT. A delayed shortest precordial maximal deflection index (≥0.55) identifies epicardial VT remote from the aortic sinus of Valsalva with high sensitivity and specificity. This observation is consistent with slower spread of activation from a focus on the epicardial surface relative to the endocardium and delayed global ventricular activation resulting from later engagement of the His-Purkinje network.[3,38]

Epicardial VTs originating close to the proximal segment of the great cardiac vein typically display RBBB morphology, whereas VTs originating close to the distal segment have LBBB morphology. This can be explained by a location within the basal-lateral myocardium for the former and a more anterobasal location for the latter arrhythmias. If the site of origin is in the proximal segment of the great cardiac vein, the initial vector is directed toward lead V_1, accounting for the RBBB morphology. As the site of origin moves toward the distal part of the great cardiac vein, closer to the anteroseptal myocardium, the initial vector is directed away from V_1, resulting in LBBB morphology. An R-wave width greater than 75 milliseconds in lead V_1 is useful for differentiating epicardial idiopathic VTs from endocardial arrhythmias. The broader R wave is explained by a more posterior position relative to lead V_1 compared with the RVOT. However, because of a more anterior position relative to lead V_1, the epicardial arrhythmias that are located within the distal part of the great cardiac vein have a narrow R wave in lead V_1, making them impossible to distinguish from RVOT VT.[38,39] Epicardial VTs that appear to follow the anterior interventricular vein often have a characteristic loss of R wave from leads V_1 and V_2, with broad R waves in leads V_3 through V_6.

For VTs originating from the RV, the presence of an initial Q wave in lead I and QS in lead V_2 for anterior sites in the RV strongly predicts an epicardial origin. Similarly, an initial Q wave in leads II, III, and aV_F is observed with pace mapping from the inferior epicardial locations in the RV.[40]

Electrophysiological Testing

Induction of Tachycardia

Frequently, VT foci can become inactive in the EP laboratory environment, caused by sedative medications or deviation from daily activities (e.g., exercise or caffeine intake) that can affect VT activity. Thus, in preparation for a VT ablation procedure, antiarrhythmic drugs should be withheld for at least five half-lives before the EP study and minimal sedation should be used throughout the procedure if possible. Additionally, it may be appropriate to monitor the patient in the EP laboratory initially without sedation. If no spontaneous tachycardia is observed, isoproterenol is administered. If no VT can be induced, a single quadripolar catheter is placed in the RV, and programmed electrical stimulation is performed. If VT focus remains quiescent, the procedure may be aborted and retried at a future date. If VT is inducible at any step, the full EP catheter arrangement and EP study are undertaken.[6]

The programmed electrical stimulation protocol usually includes incremental ventricular burst pacing from the RV apex and RVOT (until 1:1 capture is lost or a pacing CL of 220 milliseconds is reached) and single, double, and triple VESs at multiple CLs (600 and 400 milliseconds) from the RV apex and RVOT. Additionally, VT inducibility can be facilitated by catecholamines.[1,6] Isoproterenol infusion (up to 4 μg/min, or 30% increase in heart rate) is frequently used. If VT is not induced with isoproterenol, rapid ventricular pacing and VES should be repeated. If VT is still noninducible, isoproterenol is discontinued because VT can develop during the washout phase, analogous to VT occurring during the recovery phase post-exercise. If VT is still not inducible, isoproterenol is restarted and atropine (0.04 μg/kg) and aminophylline (2.8 mg/kg) may be sequentially administered (with and without programmed electrical stimulation) to attenuate the potential antiarrhythmic effects of endogenous acetylcholine and adenosine, which inhibit cAMP.[6]

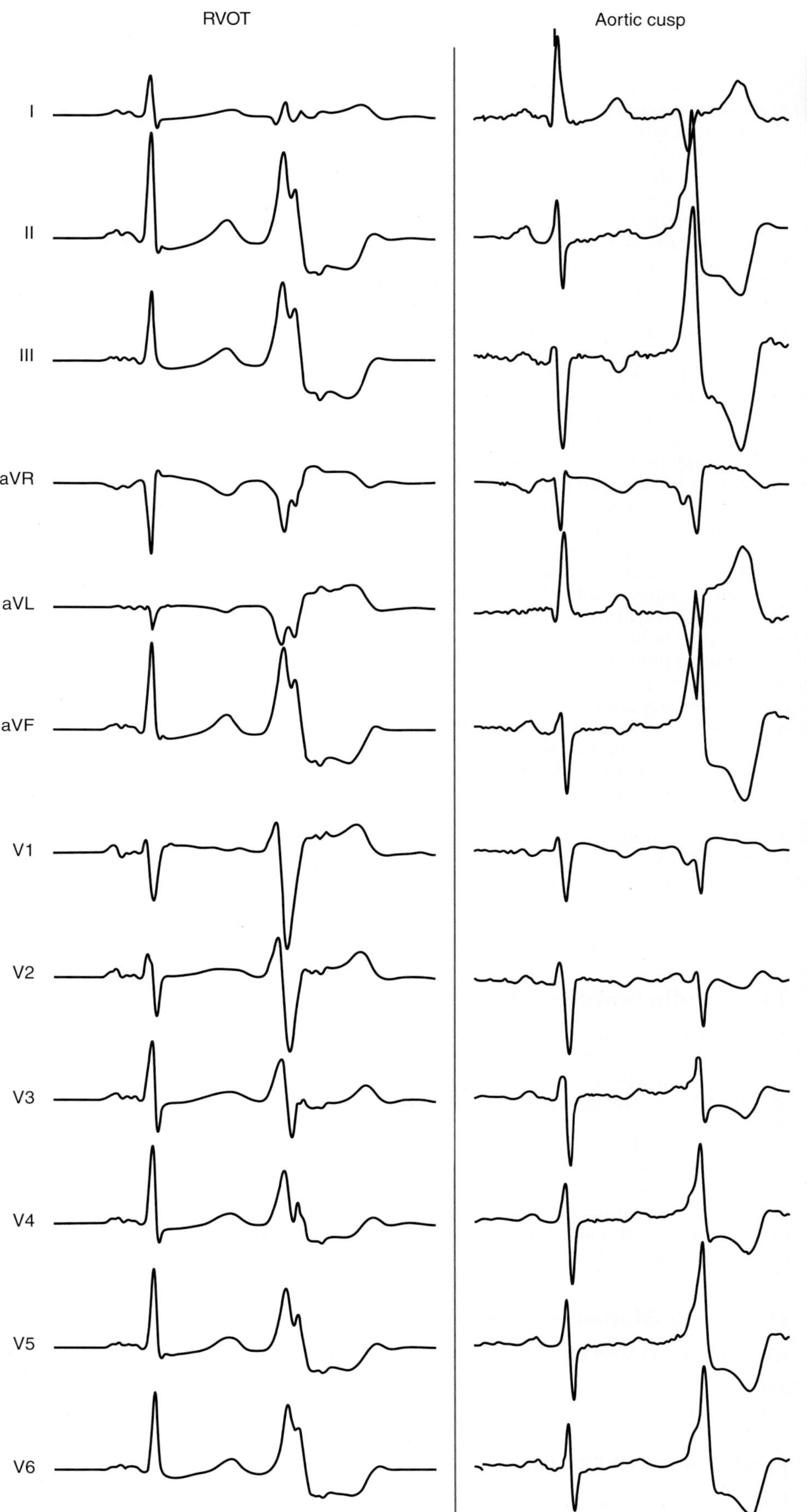

FIGURE 23-8 Correction of the precordial R/S transitional zone to cardiac rotation for differentiation between right ventricular outflow (RVOT) origins and aortic cusp origins of premature ventricular complexes (PVCs). At left, the transitional zone occurs between leads V_2 and V_3 during both normal sinus rhythm (NSR) and PVC, but slightly earlier in NSR, suggestive of RVOT origin of the PVC. At right, the transitional zone during PVC occurs in lead V_3, earlier than that during NSR (occurring in V_6), which is suggestive of an aortic cusp origin of the PVC. Note that although the transitional zone during the PVC at left occurs earlier than during the PVC at right, correction of the transitional zone to cardiac rotation (i.e., comparing the R/S transitional zone in precordial leads during VT with that during NSR) demonstrates that the transitional zone during the PVC at right occurs much earlier than during NSR, consistent with aortic cusp origin, whereas the transitional zone occurs during the PVC at left slightly later than during NSR, suggesting an RVOT origin.

Ventricular stimulation can initiate the VT in less than 65% of patients and, in contrast to reentrant VT, rapid ventricular pacing is usually more effective than VES. Induction of sustained VT is less common in patients with repetitive monomorphic VT than in those with paroxysmal sustained VT. In one report, sustained VT was inducible during EP testing in 78% of patients who presented clinically with sustained VT, in 48% of patients who presented with nonsustained VT, and in 4% of those with PVCs only.[7] Most episodes of triggered activity VT induced by ventricular stimulation are usually nonsustained. Reproducibility of VT induction using all methods is less than 50%, whereas reproducibility of induction with single or double VESs is approximately 25%. Induction with atrial pacing is not uncommon. Of note, in contrast to reentrant VT, initiation of outflow tract VT does not require associated ventricular conduction delay or block for initiation.[6]

Typically, the initial cycle of the VT bears a direct relationship to the pacing CL (whether or not VESs are delivered following the pacing drive). Thus, the shorter the initiating pacing CL, the shorter the interval to the first VT beat and the shorter the initial VT CL. Similarly, the initial cycle of the VT bears a direct relationship to the coupling interval of the VES initiating the VT.[1,6] Occasionally, with the addition of very early VESs or with very rapid ventricular pacing (CL <300 milliseconds), a sudden jump in the interval to the first VT complex may be observed, such that it is approximately twice the interval to the onset of the VT initiated by later coupled VESs. This can be caused by failure of the initial DAD to reach threshold, whereas the second DAD reaches threshold. Thus, in triggered activity VTs caused by DADs, the coupling interval of the initial VT complex either shortens or suddenly increases in response to progressively premature VES; it usually does not demonstrate an inverse or gradually increasing relationship (in contrast to reentrant VT).[6]

Ventricular pacing CLs longer or shorter than the critical CL window may fail to induce VT. This critical window can shift with changing autonomic tone. The site of ventricular stimulation has no effect on the initiation of triggered activity VT as long as the paced impulse reaches the focus of the VT (in contrast to reentrant VT).[6]

VT induction can be inconsistent. Induction is exquisitely sensitive to the immediate autonomic status of the patient. Therefore, noninducibility during a single EP study is not enough evidence to attribute the arrhythmia to a nontriggered activity mechanism.[1,6]

Tachycardia Features

As noted, the VT can be sustained or in the form of frequent monomorphic PVCs, couplets, and salvos of nonsustained VT. QRS morphology has an LBBB pattern with a right inferior or left inferior axis. The VT rate is frequently rapid (CL <300 milliseconds) but can be highly variable.[1,6]

During VT, the His potential follows the onset of the QRS (i.e., negative His bundle–ventricular [HV] interval) and is usually buried inside the local ventricular electrogram. Ventriculoatrial (VA) conduction may or may not be present. The VT is very sensitive to adenosine, Valsalva maneuvers, carotid sinus massage, edrophonium, verapamil, and beta blockers.[1]

Diagnostic Maneuvers during Tachycardia

RESPONSE TO VENTRICULAR EXTRASTIMULATION

VES results in a decreasing resetting response curve characteristic of DAD-related triggered activity.[6]

RESPONSE TO OVERDRIVE PACING

The VT cannot be entrained by ventricular pacing (i.e., no fusion demonstrable). Rapid ventricular pacing during the VT can result in acceleration in the VT. There is a direct relationship between the overdrive pacing CL and the coupling interval and CL of the VT resuming after cessation of pacing.[1]

Exclusion of Other Arrhythmia Mechanisms

Idiopathic outflow tract VT should be differentiated from other forms of VT with an LBBB pattern, including VT in ARVD, bundle branch reentrant VT, reentrant VT following surgical repair of congenital heart disease, and post-infarction VT originating from the LV septum. In addition, antidromic atrioventricular reentrant tachycardia using an atriofascicular bypass tract also presents with wide complex tachycardia with an LBBB pattern.

RVOT VT should, in particular, be distinguished from ARVD, a disorder with a more serious clinical outcome. Although RVOT VT is associated with a benign prognosis with no familial basis, it can be extremely difficult to distinguish from the concealed phase of ARVD, in which typical ECG and imaging abnormalities are absent. The VT in ARVD also affects young adults, is commonly catecholamine-facilitated, and can originate from the RVOT.

Although the VT in ARVD can have morphological features similar to RVOT VT (LBBB with inferior axis), several ECG criteria during VT can help distinguish between the two arrhythmias. Longer QRS duration (≥120 milliseconds), precordial transition at lead V_6, and the presence of notching in the QRS in one or more leads all favor ARVD over RVOT VT. Additionally, the presence of an LBBB morphology with a superior axis is very unlikely in idiopathic RVOT VT. Also, VTs in ARVD patients generally have lower QRS amplitude and more fragmentation, but these are qualitative differences and not always present.[41]

In ARVD, the resting 12-lead ECG in NSR typically shows inverted T waves in the right precordial leads. When present, RV conduction delay with an epsilon wave (best seen in leads V_1 and V_2) is helpful in the diagnosis of ARVD. The resting surface ECG in NSR is typically normal in patients with idiopathic VT, with no epsilon wave, QRS widening or fragmentation, or other markers of delayed activation of the RV. Nevertheless, the ECG can also be normal in up to 40% to 50% of patients with ARVD at presentation, but in almost no patient after 6 years. Furthermore, approximately 10% of patients with idiopathic VT can have complete or incomplete RBBB during NSR.[2,42]

Although the induction of multiple VT morphologies is very unlikely in idiopathic RVOT VT, patients with several idiopathic VT morphologies have been reported. On the other hand, patients with ARVD may initially present with only one VT morphology consistent with an RVOT origin.

Patients with idiopathic VT have a normal signal-averaged ECG when in NSR and normal imaging studies (echocardiography, MR imaging, contrast ventriculography) of RV size and function. In contrast, the presence of RV dilation, aneurysm, or both is consistent with ARVD.

The response of VT during EP testing is also helpful in distinguishing idiopathic RVOT VT from ARVD. The repetitive initiation of these VTs by programmed ventricular stimulation suggests a reentrant mechanism, and is much more common in ARVD than idiopathic outflow tract VT (93% versus 3%).[42] Additionally, recording fractionated diastolic electrograms during VT or NSR at the site of origin of VT or other RV sites is inconsistent with idiopathic RVOT VT, but is typical for ARVD. As noted, the induction of VTs with different QRS morphologies is common in ARVD (observed in 73% of patients in one report) and is inconsistent with RVOT VT. Although isoproterenol infusion can induce VT in patients with idiopathic RVOT VT, it has a similar effect in ARVD and therefore does not help distinguish between these disorders. Reentry is the mechanism of VT in the majority of the ARVD patients, whereas RVOT VT almost always displays features of triggered activity. The VT in ARVD does not terminate with adenosine.

Additionally, electroanatomical voltage mapping can help distinguish early or concealed ARVD from idiopathic VT by detecting RV electroanatomical scars that correlate with the histopathological features pathognomonic of ARVD.[43]

Malignant ventricular arrhythmias (VF or polymorphic VT) are sometimes associated with idiopathic VT or PVCs originating from the outflow tract, even in patients with no established diagnosis of ARVD. It is of particular importance to distinguish the malignant form from the benign form of idiopathic outflow tract VT, because the malignant form of idiopathic VT or PVCs often leads to unexpected SCD. Data suggest that a shorter CL during monomorphic VT, when present, as well as a history of syncope with malignant characteristics, may be a predictor of the coexistence of VF or polymorphic VT in patients with idiopathic VT originating from RVOT. Holter monitoring to record spontaneous episodes of RVOT VT and obtaining detailed previous history of syncope with malignant characteristics are useful to differentiate the malignant form from the benign form of RVOT VT.[42]

Mapping

VT origins in the RVOT are anatomically classified into three-dimensional (3-D) directions: anterior and posterior, right and left, and superior and inferior. The anterior half of the RVOT by fluoroscopy in the 60-degree left anterior oblique (LAO) projection is defined as the anterior side (or free wall side) and the posterior half is defined as the posterior side (or "septal" side; see Fig. 23-4). When viewed by fluoroscopy in the 30-degree right anterior oblique (RAO) projection, the posterior half of the outflow is defined as the right (or posterolateral) side, and the anterior half is defined as the left (or anterolateral) side. The area within 1 cm just below the pulmonic valve is defined as the superior (or distal) side, and the area more than 1 cm away is defined as the inferior (or proximal) side.

The prediction of the precise origin of outflow tract tachycardias can be challenging because of the close anatomical relationship of the different anatomical compartments of the outflow tract area. Therefore, a stepwise mapping procedure has been proposed, especially when the ECG does not provide clear criteria to guide localization of the VT site of origin.[22] Because most VTs originate from the RVOT, mapping is started there and, if that fails to identify the origin of the VT, mapping is extended to involve the pulmonary artery, although this site of origin is rare, because no additional anatomical access is required.[24] If activation mapping and pace mapping suggest a focus outside the RVOT and pulmonary artery, mapping of the CS can add useful information as to whether a left-sided epicardial origin is present.[22] If a transvenous access is not successful, mapping the LVOT and aortic cusps via a retrograde arterial access is usually the next step.

Finally, if all previous anatomical accesses are unsuccessful, epicardial mapping via a percutaneous pericardial access should be considered. Mapping findings suggestive of epicardial origin include suboptimal pace maps generated from the ventricular endocardial surface, absence of sharp potentials greater than 15 milliseconds prior to QRS onset, low-amplitude far-field potentials at the earliest endocardial sites, the occurrence of a very slurred upstroke and wide QS complex, and a large area of equally (and minimally) presystolic sites on the activation map.

Activation Mapping

Activation mapping is the method of choice for identifying a hemodynamically stable, focal VT. It may be performed by point-by-point mapping with a roving mapping catheter, with the use of multiple catheters, or with multielectrode arrays. Initially, one should seek the general region of the origin of ectopy as indicated by the surface ECG. All 12 leads should be inspected and the lead showing the earliest and most discernible onset of the QRS during VT or PVCs should be selected as the reference point for subsequent mapping. Subsequently, a single mapping catheter is moved under the guidance of fluoroscopy into the RVOT, and the bipolar signals are sampled from several endocardial sites.

Endocardial activation mapping is performed during VT or PVCs to identify the site of earliest activation relative to the onset of the QRS. It is important to record examples of VT or PVCs prior to inserting catheters, because the catheters can cause ectopic complexes

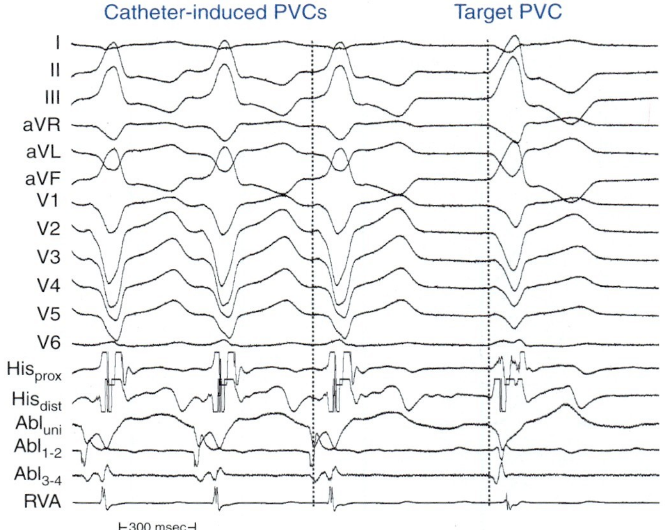

FIGURE 23-9 Catheter-induced premature ventricular complexes (PVCs) versus target spontaneous PVCs. Three complexes of catheter-induced PVCs are seen at left, during which both unipolar and bipolar signals are very early (as would be expected, because catheter tip irritation is causing these complexes). During the actual target PVC, however, this site is not early at all. This illustrates the need to be certain of the characteristics of the target PVC or ventricular tachycardia complex before beginning mapping.

that resemble the target VT or PVCs (Fig. 23-9). The site of origin of the VT is defined as the site with the earliest bipolar recording in which the distal tip shows the earliest intrinsic deflection and QS unipolar electrogram configuration.

Activation times are generally measured from the onset or the first rapid deflection of the bipolar electrogram to the earliest onset of the QRS on the surface ECG during VT or PVCs. The distal pole of the mapping catheter should be used for searching for the earliest activation site, because it is the pole through which RF energy is delivered. Once an area of relatively early local activation is found, small movements of the catheter tip in that region are undertaken until the site is identified with the earliest possible local activation relative to the tachycardia complex.

Bipolar electrograms at the site of origin are modestly early (preceding the surface QRS by 10 to 45 milliseconds) and have high-amplitude and rapid slew rates. Fractionated complex electrograms and mid-diastolic potentials are rarely, if ever, seen and should raise suspicion of underlying heart disease.[1]

Once the site with the earliest bipolar signal is identified, the unipolar signal from the distal ablation electrode should be used to supplement conventional bipolar mapping (Fig. 23-10). The unfiltered (0.05 to >300 Hz) unipolar signal morphology should show a monophasic QS complex with a rapid negative deflection. Although this electrogram configuration is very sensitive for successful ablation sites, it is not specific (70% of unsuccessful ablation sites also manifest a QS complex). The size of the area with a QS complex can be larger than the VT site of origin, exceeding 1 cm or more in diameter. Additionally, because the entirety of the heart is directed away from most positions in the RVOT, a QS can be observed with unipolar recordings from most locations in the outflow tract. The timing of the unipolar electrograms recorded at sites distant from the VT focus, however, does not precede the onset of the VT QRS.[44] Thus, a QS complex should not be the only mapping finding used to guide ablation (see Fig. 23-10). Nonetheless, successful ablation is unusual at sites with an RS complex, because these are generally distant from the VT focus. Concordance of the timing of the onset of the bipolar electrogram with that of the filtered or unfiltered unipolar electrogram, with the rapid downslope of the S wave of the unipolar QS complex coinciding with the initial peak of the bipolar signal, helps ensure that the tip electrode,

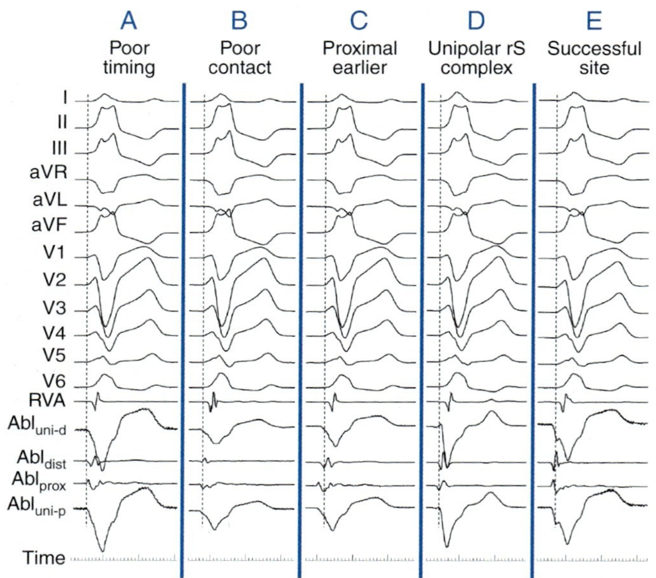

FIGURE 23-10 Activation mapping results from five sites are shown with 12 leads of a single ventricular tachycardia (VT) complex, as well as intracardiac recordings from the right ventricular apex, proximal and distal ablation electrode bipolar recordings, and unipolar recordings from the tip electrode (uni-d) and the second electrode (uni-p). A vertical dashed line denotes QRS onset. Sites A to D are suboptimal ablation sites for the reasons noted. Site E was where ablation terminated VT.

which is the ablation electrode, is responsible for the early component of the bipolar electrogram (see Fig. 23-10).[6] Additionally, the presence of slight ST elevation on the unipolar recording and the ability to capture the site with unipolar pacing are used to indicate good electrode contact.

It is important to recognize that some myocardial fibers in the RVOT can potentially be in continuity with those in the LVOT. As a consequence, what mapping defines as the earliest site of activation relative to neighboring myocardium can be misleading. For example, if the true origin of an arrhythmia in the supravalvular aortic cusps then exits both to the infravalvular LVOT myocardium and to the posterolateral subpulmonic RVOT, an early site relative to all neighboring RVOT myocardium may be found in the RVOT.[44]

Careful catheter manipulation during mapping should seek to avoid mechanical trauma that can transiently abolish the arrhythmia. On the other hand, catheter manipulation frequently induces PVCs that can closely mimic target PVCs. The findings on the mapping catheter during these catheter-induced complexes are invariably excellent (e.g., substantial presystolic activation time, sharp QS on the unipolar recording). These complexes must be analyzed and carefully compared with prerecorded VT or PVC complexes to avoid delivery of RF energy at sites with no relevance to actual VT.

When mapping above the aortic or pulmonic valve, near- and far-field potentials are typically recorded. The exact nature and cause of these spikes are unknown but are thought to be analogous to PV potentials, that is, they represent electrical activation of myocardial sleeves distal to valve attachment. Because of the overlapping nature of the outflow tract and supravalvular region, when two potentials are seen, only the near-field potential should be used for activation timing. In addition to noting the actual timing of activation, the timing of the near-field electrogram relative to the far-field electrogram should be evaluated.[9] Typically, in sinus rhythm, the near-field potential (representing local supravalvular myocardial activation) is seen after the far-field ventricular electrogram (likely representing outflow tract activation) separated by an isoelectric period (presumably from conduction delay across the site of valve insertion). If during VT or PVC, the sequence of activation is reversed, that is, the near-field electrogram precedes the far-field electrogram by a similar or greater isoelectric period duration, an etiological role for the supravalvular myocardium can be inferred. This finding alone, however, does not suggest that ablation at this particular site will be successful because (as with PV phenomena) other supravalvular locations may show earlier activation than the site being mapped. On the other hand, if the near-field electrogram still succeeds the far-field ventricular electrogram during VT or PVC, then the supravalvular tissue, although present, is a bystander being passively activated during arrhythmia originating in the outflow tract myocardium below the valve. In some cases, the near-field electrogram is fused with the far-field electrogram during tachycardia. This suggests an origin of arrhythmia exactly at the cusp or passive activation from a true distant site of origin to both the supravalvular and infravalvular myocardium.[8]

Pace Mapping

Pace mapping is pacing during or in the absence of tachycardia to assess the possible relation of the pacing site to a tachycardia focus or a reentry circuit. Pace mapping is used to confirm the results of activation mapping and can be of great value, especially when the VT is scarcely inducible. Although there are some limitations to this technique, several studies have demonstrated efficacy using pace mapping to choose ablation target sites for idiopathic VT.[45]

TECHNIQUE

Pace mapping during VT (at pacing CL 20 to 40 milliseconds shorter than the tachycardia CL) is preferable whenever possible, because it facilitates rapid comparison of VT and paced QRS complexes at the end of a pacing train in simultaneously displayed 12-lead ECGs. If sustained VT cannot be induced, mapping is performed during spontaneous nonsustained VT or PVCs. In this setting, the pacing CL and coupling intervals of the VES should match those of spontaneous ectopy. Pace mapping is preferably performed with unipolar stimuli (≤10 mA, 2 milliseconds) from the distal electrode of the mapping catheter (cathode) and an electrode in the inferior vena cava (IVC) (anode). Unipolar pacing, however, causes a large stimulus artifact in the surface ECG. Bipolar pacing from the closely spaced distal electrodes of the mapping catheter is more commonly used. Although the possibility for capture at either the distal or proximal bipolar electrodes can reduce spatial accuracy, this does not appear to be a major limitation. Use of current strengths near threshold should improve accuracy by limiting the size of the virtual electrode in the tissue and preventing capture of myocardium distant from the pacing site. Pacing thresholds of at least 5 to 10 mA typically indicate insufficient electrode-tissue contact or inexcitable areas.[3]

INTERPRETATION

Pace maps with identical or near-identical matches of VT morphology in all 12 surface ECG leads can be indicative of the site of origin of VT (see Fig. 5-22). ECG recordings should be reviewed at the same gain and filter settings and at a paper-sweep speed of 100 mm/sec. It is often helpful to have a split-screen display of the target VT in one panel, comparing this with all 12 leads of the paced QRS complexes brought into another panel, as well as with printed regular 12-lead ECGs for side-by-side comparison on paper. Differences in the QRS morphology between pacing and spontaneous VT in a single lead can be critical. Pacing at a site 5 mm from the index pacing site can result in minor differences in QRS configuration (notching, new small component, change in amplitude of individual component, or overall change in QRS shape) in at least one lead in most patients. In contrast, if only major changes in QRS morphology are considered, pacing sites separated by as much as 15 mm can appear similar.

Although qualitative comparison of the 12-lead ECG morphology between a pace map and VT is frequently performed, there are few objective criteria for quantifying the similarity between two 12-lead ECG waveform morphologies. Such comparisons are

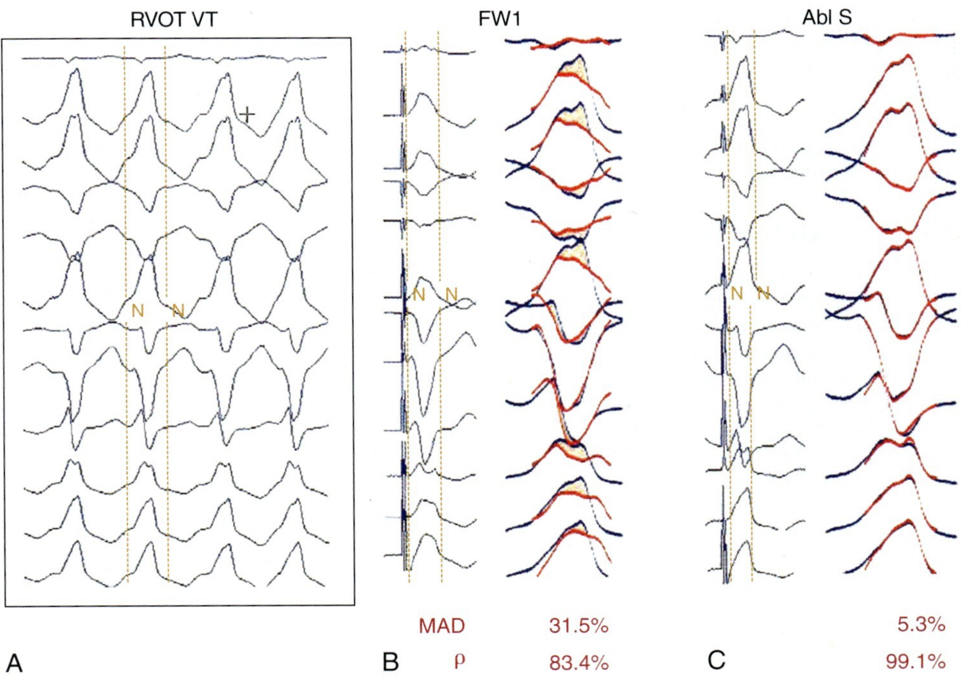

FIGURE 23-11 The mean absolute deviation (MAD) score. **A,** Example of right ventricular outflow tract (RVOT) ventricular tachycardia (VT). The second VT complex has been identified as the target waveform by the annotation markers placed on either side of this complex. **B,** Pace map from a free wall site 1 (FW1) next to the superimposed VT and pace map waveforms after automatic computer alignment. There are substantial differences between these two waveforms (highlighted in gray), resulting in an MAD score of 31.5%. **C,** Pace map from the successful ablation site (Abl S) near the posterior septum and the superimposed pace map and VT waveform. Note in the Abl S panel that when these two waveforms are aligned they are nearly superimposable, and result in a very low MAD score of 5.3%. Correlation coefficients for these comparisons are also shown. *(From Gerstenfeld EP, Dixit S, Callans DJ, et al: Quantitative comparison of spontaneous and paced 12-lead electrocardiogram during right ventricular outflow tract ventricular tachycardia, J Am Coll Cardiol 41:2046, 2003).*

frequently completely subjective or semiquantitative, such as a "10/12 lead match." Discrepancies in ablation outcome can result, in part, from subjective differences in opinion regarding the closeness of a pace map match to the clinical VT. On the other hand, automated objective interpretation can offer some advantage to human interpretation. Template matching processes digital images to match the target QRS complex (template signal) and the paced QRS complex (test signal), and provides a score according to the similarity between the two QRS morphologies.[46] The most common human error in analyzing a pace map is not appreciating subtle amplitude or precordial lead transition differences between two ECG patterns, and such subtle differences can be reflected in a single quantitative number calculated by an automated metric.

Two waveform comparison metrics, the correlation coefficient (CORR) and the mean absolute deviation (MAD), have been evaluated to calculate the template-matching score. Although both metrics quantitatively compare the waveforms, MAD tends to be more sensitive to differences in waveform amplitude than CORR. Successful ablation sites were associated with significantly lower MAD score than were unsuccessful sites, but only a trend toward a higher CORR at the successful ablation sites was observed. The MAD score grades 12-lead ECG waveform similarity as a single number, ranging from 0% (identical) to 100% (completely different). An MAD score less than or equal to 12% was found to be 93% sensitive and 75% specific for a successful ablation site (Fig. 23-11). It is not surprising that the MAD score is more sensitive than specific; characteristics other than a 12-lead ECG match are necessary for a successful ablation, including catheter-tissue contact, catheter orientation, and tissue heating. An MAD score greater than 12%, and certainly greater than 15% (100% negative predictive value), suggests sufficient dissimilarity between pace map and clinical tachycardia to dissuade ablation at that site. An MAD score less than or equal to 12% is considered an excellent match, and ablation at these sites is warranted if catheter contact and stability are adequate (see Fig. 23-11). The MAD score is computationally simple and should be easy to incorporate into current EP recording systems, allowing feedback to the physician of pace map comparison before turning on the RF energy. The MAD score can also be used to standardize 12-lead ECG waveform morphology comparisons among different laboratories, and can be useful for guiding ablation of RVOT VT.[46]

Studies using the CORR have found that the spatial resolution of a good pace map for targeting RVOT VT was 1.8 cm^2 in diameter and therefore was inferior to the spatial resolution of activation mapping. Of note, in almost 20% of patients in this report, pace maps failed to reproduce adequate correlation coefficients to identify the site of origin of all PVCs/VT. Nonetheless, the effective ablation sites had a high degree of correlation with pace mapping at effective ablation sites. Another metric, root-mean-square error, also was found to be a better discriminator of differences among individual lead waveforms than CORR.[46]

PITFALLS

Current strengths up to 10 mA have little effect on unipolar paced ECG configuration. In contrast, bipolar pacing can introduce some variability in the paced ECG, which can be minimized by low pacing outputs and small interelectrode distance (≤5 mm). Additionally, the morphology of single paced QRS complexes can vary depending on coupling interval, and the QRS morphology during overdrive pacing is affected by the pacing CL. Therefore, the coupling interval or CL of the template arrhythmia should be matched during pace mapping; otherwise, rate-dependent changes in QRS morphology independent of the pacing site can confound mapping results. Similarly, spontaneous couplets from the same focus may have slight variations in QRS morphology that must be considered when seeking a pace match. Of note, isoproterenol infusion has no significant effect on the QRS configuration.

Pace mapping can be difficult to perform above the semilunar valves (in the aortic cusps or pulmonary artery) and can require high pacing current strengths. Because of the close anatomical proximity of the various structures in the supravalvular outflow tract region, high-output pacing may reproduce the ECG or clinical arrhythmia even when the origin is in a different cardiac chamber. For example, high-output pace mapping from the right coronary cusp may reproduce the ECG even when the origin is in the posterior RVOT or subvalvular anterior LVOT.[9] Additionally, supravalvular arrhythmia origin may exit to the ventricular

myocardium below the valve. Thus, pace mapping above the valve and at the exit site may be similar. For example, if pace mapping is performed during aortic cusp VT at a breakthrough site on the posterior RVOT, a perfect result (despite supraaortic origin) will be obtained. Yet, ablation energy delivered there typically fails in terminating the arrhythmia and may result in a change in VT morphology resulting now from a different exit of the cuspal arrhythmogenic focus.[8]

Electroanatomical Mapping

Propagation of activation during RVOT VT is so rapid that minor differences between adjacent sites become difficult to detect, leading to a large number of sites with clinically indistinguishable activation times when examined on a site-by-site basis. However, when displayed simultaneously on a spatially precise electroanatomical reconstruction, the centers of the early activation area and the presumed site of VT origin become easy to identify (Fig. 23-12).[45] Electroanatomical 3-D mapping (CARTO mapping system [Biosense Webster, Diamond Bar, Calif.] or EnSite NavX system [St. Jude Medical, St. Paul, Minn.]) uses a single mapping catheter attached to a system that can precisely localize the catheter tip in 3-D space and store activation time on a 3-D anatomical reconstruction.[1,45] Electroanatomical mapping permits spatial discrimination between sites separated by less than 1 mm.

Initially, a stable reference electrogram is selected. This is the fiducial marker on which the entire mapping procedure is based. Preferably, a QRS on the surface ECG is selected as the reference signal. Alternatively, an intracardiac electrogram (e.g., RV apex) can be selected as the reference point, in which case care must be taken to avoid dislodging this catheter because, if it moves, timing of mapping catheter activations will not be comparable to previously mapped sites. Following selection of the reference electrogram, positioning of the anatomical reference, and determination of the window of interest, the mapping catheter is positioned in the RVOT under fluoroscopic guidance.

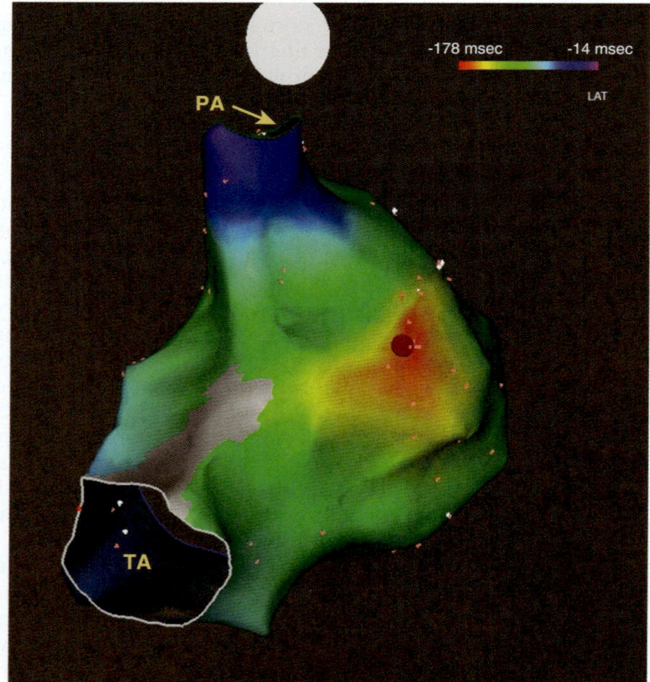

FIGURE 23-12 Electroanatomical (CARTO 3) activation map (posterior view) of ventricular ectopy originating from the right ventricular outflow tract (RVOT). The site of impulse origin during ectopy was in the posterolateral aspect of the RVOT (red area), at which point ablation eliminated the ventricular tachycardia (red dot). PA = pulmonic valve annulus; TA = tricuspid annulus.

At the outset, the plane of the HB location and pulmonic valve are defined and tagged to outline the superior and inferior limits of the RVOT. The mapping catheter is advanced superiorly in the RVOT until no discrete bipolar electrograms are seen in the distal electrode pair. The catheter then is retracted until electrograms in the distal electrode pair reappear and pacing results in capture of the RVOT endocardium. This marks the level of the pulmonic valve. At least three points are acquired and tagged to construct the pulmonic valve.[22] Next, a detailed electroanatomical activation map of the RVOT is constructed by acquiring multiple points during PVCs or VT. The local activation time at each site is determined from the intracardiac bipolar electrogram and is measured in relation to the fixed reference electrogram (surface QRS or intracardiac electrogram). Points are added to the map only if stability criteria in space and local activation time are met. The end-diastolic location stability criterion is less than 2 mm and the local activation time stability criterion is less than 2 milliseconds. Activation maps display the local activation time by a color-coded overlay on the reconstructed 3-D geometry (see Fig. 23-12). The electroanatomical maps of focal VT demonstrate radial spreading of activation, from the earliest local activation site (red in CARTO, white in NavX) in all directions (a well-defined early activation site surrounded by later activation sites).

The principles used for conventional activation mapping discussed above are also used here to define the site of origin of VT. Although the traditional single-catheter mapping of the region of interest is still required, the ability to use the catheter localization system to steer precisely back to previously obtained sites of earliest activation greatly facilitates the ablation process. Display of activation times facilitates comparison of data from nearby sites, overcoming the imprecision of assigned activation times at single points, and permits rapid identification of a putative site of origin. The activation map can also be used to catalogue sites at which pacing maneuvers are performed during assessment of the tachycardia (e.g., sites with a good pace map).

When using a 3-D electroanatomical mapping system, it is important to understand that a change in rhythm during the mapping procedure can alter cardiac geometry to the extent that anatomical points acquired during one rhythm cannot be relied on after a change in rhythm. This is relevant during mapping of isolated PVCs or nonsustained VT, because locations assigned to early activation sites during the arrhythmia can potentially be removed from the same locations when assigned during normal rhythm (e.g., at the time of RF delivery after tachycardia termination). Therefore, after termination of the arrhythmia, "revisiting" the site of early activation tagged during PVCs or tachycardia may be unfeasible or even misleading as a target for ablation.

Noncontact Mapping

The spatial and temporal resolution of point-by-point activation mapping is limited by the number of contact electrodes and the time required. When VT is hard to induce or of short duration, simultaneous multisite data acquisition can help map the VT focus. The biggest advantage of noncontact endocardial mapping is its ability to recreate the endocardial activation sequence from simultaneously acquired multiple data points over a few (theoretically one) tachycardia beats, without requiring sequential point-to-point acquisitions. More detailed mapping, however, is necessary to find the precise site to ablate.[3,47]

The EnSite 3000 noncontact mapping system (St. Jude Medical, St. Paul, Minn.) consists of a noncontact catheter (9 Fr) with a multielectrode array (MEA) surrounding a 7.5-mL balloon mounted at the distal end. To create a map, the balloon catheter is advanced over a 0.035-inch guidewire under fluoroscopic guidance and positioned in the RVOT. The balloon is then deployed; it may be filled with contrast dye, permitting it to be visualized fluoroscopically (Fig. 23-13). The balloon is positioned in the center of the RVOT and does not come in contact with the endocardial walls being mapped. Systemic anticoagulation is critical to prevent thromboembolic complications; intravenous heparin is usually administered to maintain the activated clotting time (ACT) at 250 to 300 seconds.[3]

A conventional (roving) deflectable mapping catheter is also positioned in the RVOT and used to collect geometry information. The tricuspid annulus, HB, and pulmonic valve are initially tagged and a detailed 3-D geometry of the RVOT ("virtual" endocardium) is reconstructed by moving the mapping catheter around the RVOT.

The MEA simultaneously acquires multiple data points over a few tachycardia beats or PVCs. The system then reconstructs over 3360 unipolar electrograms simultaneously and superimposes them onto the computer-generated model of the RVOT, producing isopotential maps with a color range representing voltage amplitude. The highest chamber voltage is at the site of origin of the electrical impulse (see Video 8). Color settings are adjusted so that the color range matches 1 to 1 with the millivolt range of the electrogram deflection of interest. The color scale for each isopotential map is set so that white indicates the most negative potential and blue indicates the least negative potential. Activation can be tracked on the isopotential map throughout the cycle to the onset of the tachycardia beat. Wavefront propagation can be displayed as a user-controlled 3-D movie (Fig. 23-14).[3,47]

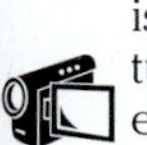

Additionally, the system can simultaneously display as many as 32 electrograms as waveforms. Unipolar or bipolar electrograms (virtual electrograms) are then reconstructed at sites of earliest activation on the isopotential maps to look for a unipolar QS pattern. The origin of VT is defined as the earliest site showing a single spot of isopotential mapping and a QS pattern of the noncontact unipolar electrogram. Isochronal maps can also be created, which represent progression of activation throughout the chamber relative to a user-defined electrical reference timing point.

Contact mapping using the conventional ablation catheter may also be performed at sites of interest to supplement noncontact mapping findings, and color-coded contact activation maps can be displayed on the same 3-D geometry. Once the earliest activation is identified, the site is labeled on the 3-D map and the locator signal is used to navigate the ablation catheter to it in real time during tachycardia or during normal rhythm when sustained tachycardia is not inducible.

Although noncontact mapping can rapidly identify VT foci, a second catheter is still required for precise localization of the target site and delivery of RF energy. Thus, noncontact mapping helps identify starting points for conventional activation mapping. Additionally, manipulation of the array into the RVOT can be difficult and contact of some portions of the area with myocardium may induce PVCs that appear similar to clinical PVCs or VT.

Basket Catheter Mapping

Basket catheters have been used successfully to guide ablation of idiopathic VT arising from the RVOT, and are of particular interest in patients with infrequent arrhythmia that limits mapping. This

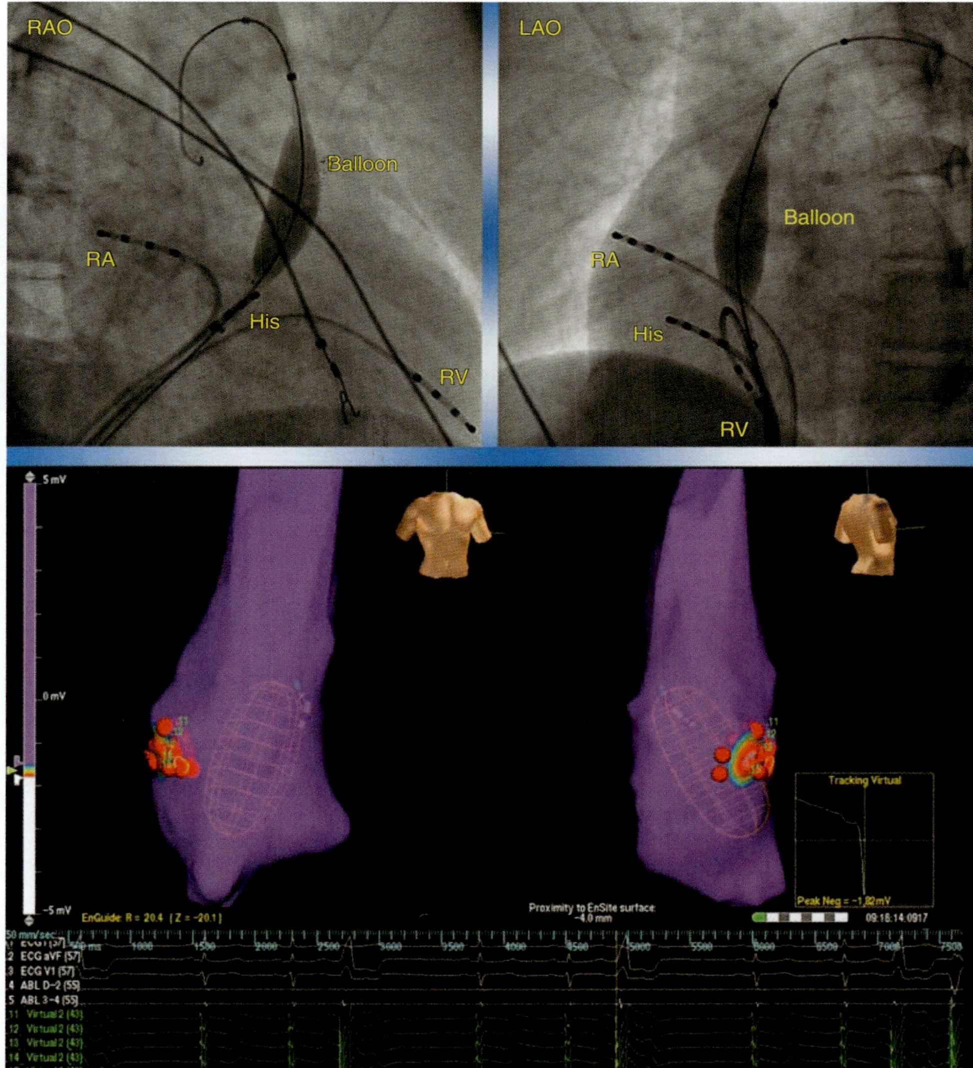

FIGURE 23-13 Noncontact mapping of idiopathic right ventricular outflow tract (RVOT) ventricular tachycardia. **Upper panel,** Fluoroscopic (right anterior oblique [RAO] and left anterior oblique [LAO]) views of the EnSite balloon catheter positioned in the RVOT. **Middle panel,** Color-coded isopotential map of RVOT activation during a single premature ventricular complex (PVC). The inset shows a virtual electrogram at the site of earliest activation (note the QS pattern). Red dots indicate radiofrequency applications. Further detailed mapping using a standard mapping catheter localized the PVC focus to a site adjacent to the site, with the earliest local activation identified by the balloon catheter. **Lower panel,** Surface ECG and intracardiac contact (ABL) and virtual noncontact (green) electrograms are shown during mapping of PVCs. *(Courtesy of Dr. James Mullin, Prairie Cardiovascular Consultants, Springfield, Ill.)*

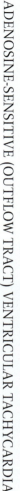

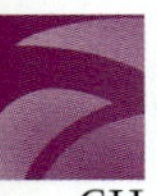

mapping catheter consists of an open-lumen catheter shaft with a collapsible, basket-shaped distal end, which is composed of 64 electrodes mounted on eight flexible, self-expanding, equidistant metallic splines (each spline carrying eight ring electrodes; see Fig. 4-4). The electrodes are equally spaced 4 or 5 mm apart, depending on the size of the basket catheter used (with diameters of 48 or 60 mm, respectively). Each spline is identified by a letter (from A to H) and each electrode by a number (from 1 to 8), with electrode 1 having the distal position on the splines.[3]

The size of the RV is initially evaluated (usually with echocardiography) to help select the appropriate size of the basket catheter. The collapsed basket catheter is advanced under fluoroscopic guidance through an 11 Fr long sheath into the RV; the basket is then expanded. After basket catheter deployment, the conventional catheters are introduced and positioned in standard positions (Fig. 23-15). Several observations can help determine electrical-anatomical relations of the basket catheter electrodes, including fluoroscopically identifiable markers (spline A has one marker and spline B has two markers located near the shaft of the basket catheter) and electrical signals recorded from certain electrodes (e.g., ventricular, atrial, or HB electrograms), which can help identify the location of those particular splines.

From the 64 electrodes, 64 unipolar signals and 32 to 56 bipolar signals can be recorded, by combining 1-2, 3-4, 5-6, 7-8, or by combining 1-2, 2-3, until 7-8 electrodes are on each spline. The color-coded animation images simplify the analysis of multielectrode recordings and help in establishing the relation between activation patterns and anatomical structures. The degree of resolution is lower than that in 3-D mapping systems but appears satisfactory for clinical purposes.

The concepts of conventional activation mapping discussed above are then used to determine the site of origin of the tachycardia. The ablation catheter is placed in the region of earliest activity and is used for more detailed mapping of the site of origin of the VT. The Astronomer navigation system (Boston Scientific, Natick, Mass.) permits precise and reproducible guidance of the ablation catheter tip electrode to targets identified by the basket catheter. Without the use of this navigation system, it can be difficult to identify the alphabetical order of the splines by fluoroscopic guidance. The capacity of pacing from most basket electrodes allows the evaluation of activation patterns and pace mapping.

Basket catheter mapping is not commonly used because of several limitations. Most basket catheters are difficult, if not impossible, to steer; thus, positioning in the RVOT can be challenging. In addition, firm contact with the tip of the basket and RVOT myocardium can induce ectopic complexes that mimic spontaneous VT or PVCs. Spatial sampling is limited by the interspline and interelectrode distances, and endocardial contact is often limited because of the complex geometry of the ventricles. A second catheter is still required to be manipulated to the site identified for more precise localization of the target for ablation as well as RF energy delivery.[3]

Ablation

Target of Ablation

The ablation target site is defined as the site where the earliest endocardial activation time during VT or PVCs and exact or best pace map matches can be obtained. Activation mapping and pace mapping are highly correlated techniques and both methods are

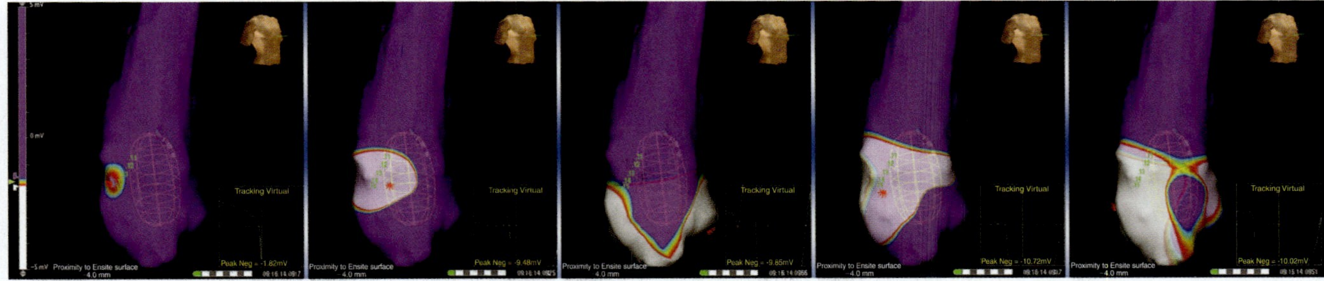

FIGURE 23-14 Noncontact color-coded propagation maps during a premature ventricular complex (PVC) originating from the right ventricular outflow tract. Wavefront propagation spreads radially from a small focus (from left to right). The insets show a virtual electrogram with the bar indicating the timing of activation during the PVC.

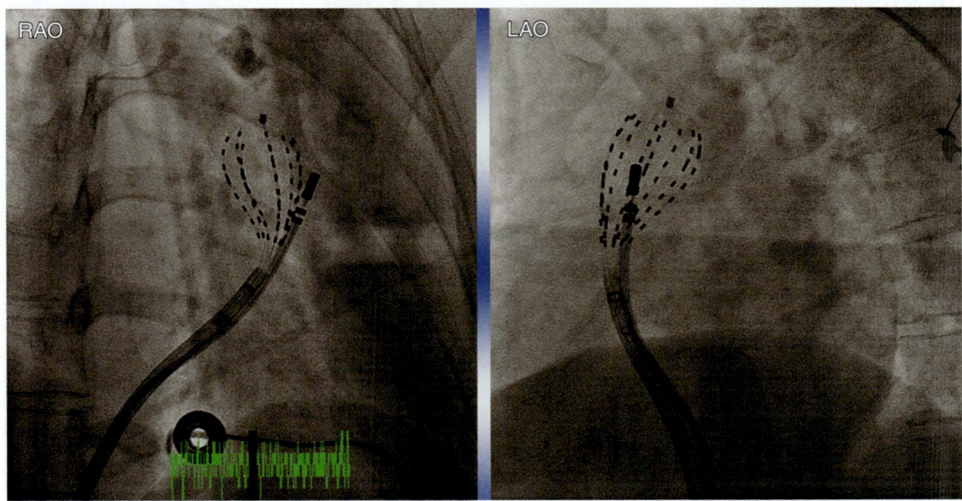

FIGURE 23-15 Fluoroscopic (right anterior oblique [RAO] and left anterior oblique [LAO]) views of a basket catheter positioned in the right ventricular outflow tract for mapping of idiopathic outflow tract ventricular tachycardia. A second catheter is used for further mapping and ablation.

typically used to select ablation sites—the more confirmatory information, the more likely the site of origin will fall within the range of the RF lesion produced (see Fig. 23-10). There is little objective evidence to support the widely held notion that pace mapping provides superior spatial resolution for localizing idiopathic outflow tract VT, compared with activation mapping.[3,45]

Ventricular Tachycardias Originating in the Right Ventricular Outflow Tract

To map the RVOT via the femoral vein, the mapping catheter is advanced into the mid-RV. From there, a sharp clockwise torque directs the catheter toward the anterior portion of the RVOT. The mapping catheter is then advanced into the proximal pulmonary artery and slowly withdrawn into the RVOT until the first local endocardial electrogram is recorded. This site is just below the pulmonic valve, and is at the level where most RVOT VTs originate.[1,6] It is important to avoid trying to advance the catheter when its tip is perpendicular to the RVOT, because this can result in perforation and cardiac tamponade. Torque is applied to the catheter for circumferential mapping of the RVOT within 1 cm of the pulmonic valve. The plane of the septum in the LAO view is nearly perpendicular to the imaging plane. Delineating the boundaries within which mapping will be carried out is useful, rather than discovering after several minutes of mapping that more tissue lies in one direction or another from where efforts had previously been concentrated. A second catheter positioned at the proximal HB, midanterior septum, or both helps in accurate localization, because "septal" sites are almost always within the same vertical plane or further rightward relative to these catheter positions in the LAO view.

For mapping of the posterior portion of the RVOT, the catheter needs to be flexed posteriorly and counterclockwise torque applied. Such application of counterclockwise torque, however, will tend to pull the electrodes back into the RV inflow portion. Using a long guiding sheath in the RV may offer adequate catheter stability. Additionally, mapping of the posterior RVOT wall can be facilitated by advancing the mapping catheter retrogradely into the right aortic sinus (see below), which lies immediately anterior to the RVOT (see Fig. 23-3).[8,9] Also, it is important to carefully analyze the electrogram at the site of early activation on the RVOT to see if a far-field pattern is seen. Mapping the supravalvular aortic cusp can be necessary if the earliest signal is far field in character near the posterior portion of the pulmonic valve.[8]

Based on the results of activation and pace mapping at these initial sites, and guided by surface QRS morphology, attention is then directed to sites of early activation and best pace map matches. If very thorough mapping in the RVOT fails to localize the VT site of origin, mapping is extended into the pulmonary artery. It is important to resist the temptation to ablate the earliest site in a given chamber unless all of the different chambers have been mapped or unless the unipolar electrogram displays a QS morphology concordant with the earliest bipolar electrogram and the pace map at the site of earliest activation matches perfectly.[44]

Ventricular Tachycardias Originating in the Left Ventricular Outflow Region

If very thorough mapping and ablation in the RVOT and pulmonary artery fail to localize or terminate the tachycardia, and recordings from distal CS or great cardiac or anterior interventricular veins suggest LV origin, the femoral artery is cannulated. The catheter is advanced to the descending aorta and, in this position, a tight J curve is formed with the catheter tip before passage to the aortic root to minimize catheter manipulation in the arch. In a 30-degree RAO view, the curved catheter is advanced through the aortic valve with the J curve opening to the right, so the catheter passes into the LV oriented anterolaterally (see Fig. 4-9). The straight catheter tip must never be used to cross the aortic valve because of the risk of leaflet damage or perforation, and also because the catheter tip can slip into the left or right coronary artery or a coronary bypass graft, mimicking entry to the LV and causing damage to these structures. A long vascular sheath can provide added catheter stability. Anticoagulation should be started once the LV is accessed (intravenous heparin, 5000-unit bolus followed by a 1000-unit infusion is usually used), to maintain the ACT between 250 and 300 seconds.[3]

The catheter is carefully manipulated in the LVOT until an early ventricular electrogram is recorded and pace mapping shows a QRS identical to the clinical VT morphology. Pace mapping at these sites often requires high output pacing. Other parts of the LV can occasionally harbor the focus of the VT (Fig. 23-16).

Ventricular Tachycardias Originating in the Aortic Cusps

When mapping the sinuses of Valsalva, it is important to consider the entire surface of each of the cusps as well as the corresponding area just beneath the valve, as distinct activation times and pace maps are obtained from each point. Additionally, myocardial extensions can exist between the right and left cusps, and mapping and ablation of these sites usually require the catheter prolapsed below the valve and flexed onto the great arterial wall for contact and then gently pulled up into this intercuspal region.[8,44]

Fluoroscopy alone or in combination with a 3-D electroanatomical mapping system may not be sufficient to facilitate comprehensive mapping of the supravalvular region, and intracardiac echocardiographic (ICE) imaging or contrast aortography is typically used. ICE imaging can be particularly useful in identifying mapping-ablation catheter location (see Video 20). Longitudinal

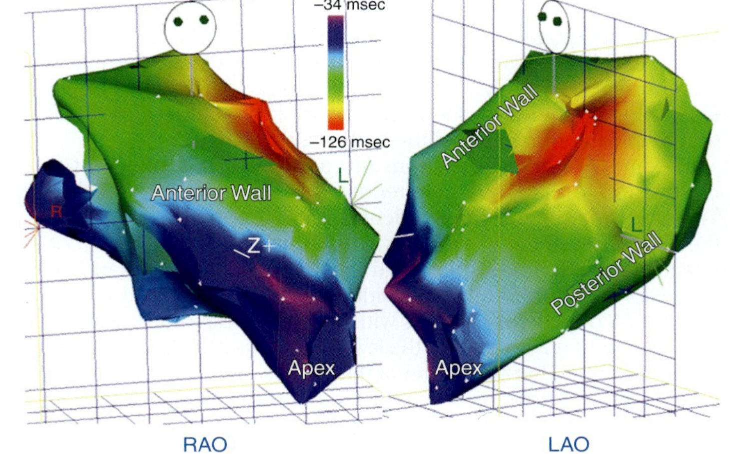

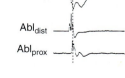

FIGURE 23-16 Focal left ventricle ventricular tachycardia (LV VT)—intracardiac recordings during VT and electroanatomical map of focal anterior wall LV VT. Note electrogram features of focality (QS on unipolar and slight presystolic timing of unipolar and bipolar electrograms during VT) as well as centrifugal spread of activation on the color map. LAO = left anterior oblique; RAO = right anterior oblique.

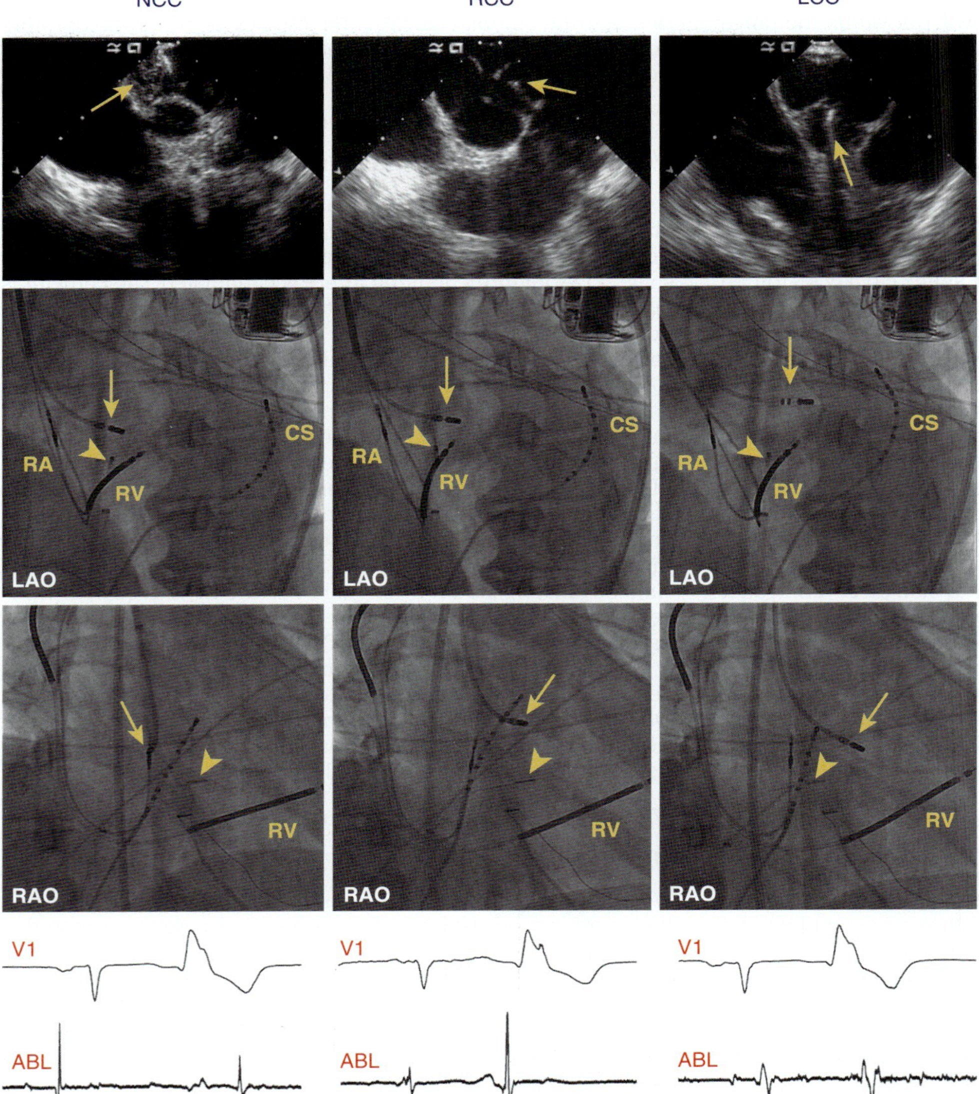

FIGURE 23-17 Top, Intracardiac echocardiography (ICE) images (top row) and left anterior oblique (LAO) and right anterior oblique (LAO) fluoroscopic views (middle and bottom rows, respectively). **Bottom,** Intracardiac recordings. Images and recordings were obtained during mapping in the noncoronary cusp (NCC, left panels), right coronary cusp (RCC, middle panels), and left coronary cusp (LCC, left panels). The ablation catheter tip on ICE and fluoroscopic images is marked by yellow arrows. Cross-sectional ICE images of the aortic valve were obtained with the ICE catheter (arrowheads) positioned at the His bundle region of the right ventricular (RV) septum. Right atrial (RA) and RV leads of an implantable cardioverter-defibrillator and a decapolar catheter positioned in the coronary sinus (CS) are marked. In the NCC, large near-field atrial and small far-field ventricular electrograms are recorded. The recorded electrograms from the RCC show a large ventricular electrogram and far-field atrial electrogram. In the LCC, large ventricular and small, far-field atrial electrograms are recorded. See text for discussion.

views are best to appreciate the relationship of the RVOT and LVOT and for identifying the ostia of the coronary arteries. A cross-sectional view is of most value in identifying the cusps themselves (Fig. 23-17). Once the three cusps are visualized, the interatrial septum will be seen in immediate relationship to the noncoronary cusp. Rightward and anterior to the noncoronary cusp and immediately behind the RVOT lies the right coronary cusp. Another landmark for the right coronary cusp is that the septal and anterior leaflets of the tricuspid valve will meet at the junction between the right and noncoronary cusps. The left coronary cusp is identified as being leftward and anterior to the noncoronary cusp and in close relation to the anterior leaflet of the mitral valve.[8,44]

In some VTs originating from the aortic cusps, a preferential conduction to the RVOT may render pace mapping less reliable. Therefore, when the local ventricular activation does not precede the QRS onset of the VT or PVCs adequately or RF ablation is not effective in the RVOT, despite obtaining a good pace map, mapping of the aortic cusp should be considered. On the other hand, in one report, 27% of patients with VTs with an aortic cusp origin had the local ventricular activation in the RVOT preceding the QRS onset of the VT or PVCs. Therefore, when a good pace map is not obtained or RF ablation is not effective in the RVOT, despite the fact that local ventricular activation adequately precedes the QRS onset of the VT or PVCs, mapping of the aortic cusp should be considered.[36]

A catheter positioned at the RV HB region can be very useful in catheter ablation of aortic cusp VTs. It can be used as a landmark for mapping within the noncoronary and right coronary cusps, where the proximity of the to the HB should be kept in mind to avoid inadvertent damage to the AV conduction system. Additionally, the local ventricular activation time relative to the QRS onset at the HB region in the RV can be an electrophysiological clue for differentiating VT origins in the aortic root. The activation time in the HB region is usually significantly earlier during PVCs originating from the right versus the left coronary cusp, suggesting that the activation from the right coronary cusp may propagate to the ventricular septum and RV before the LV free wall, whereas that from the left coronary cusp may do so after part of the LV free wall activates (Fig. 23-18). The local ventricular activation time relative to the QRS onset at the RV HB region is typically significantly greater for the VTs with origins from left coronary cusp and the junction of the right and left coronary cusps than for those from the noncoronary and right coronary cusps.[16]

When the left coronary cusp site appears early but ablation is unsuccessful, the posterior supravalvular pulmonary artery region and the anterior interventricular ring and branches should be mapped. Sometimes the LA appendage, which lies close to the posterior pulmonary artery laterally, can be mapped and in rare instances ablated for supravalvular tachycardia. Similarly, the

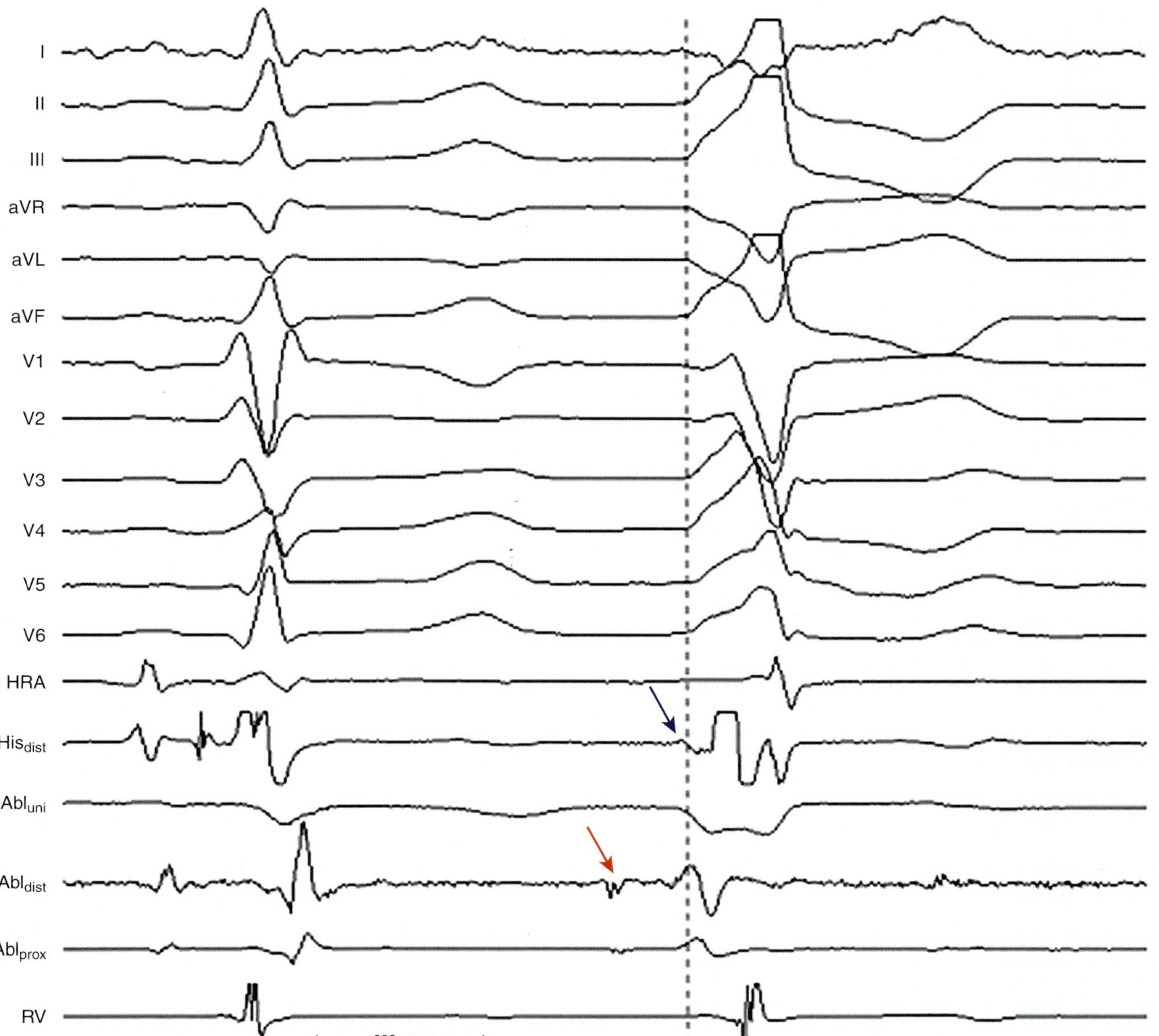

FIGURE 23-18 Recordings from a patient with premature ventricular complexes (PVCs) originating from the right aortic cusp. A sinus rhythm complex as well as the PVC is shown; the vertical line denotes the onset of the PVC QRS. The blue arrow shows that the His bundle ventricular electrogram is slightly presystolic, whereas the red arrow shows the electrogram at the site of origin of the PVC in the sinus of Valsalva, occurring about 100 milliseconds prior to the QRS onset.

superior vena cava medially lies close to the supravalvular portions of the ascending aorta above the right coronary cusp.[9]

When the earliest ventricular activation is identified in an aortic cusp, it is preferable to insert a 5 Fr pigtail catheter into the aortic root through the left femoral artery. The aortic root and the ostia of the right coronary artery and left main coronary artery are visualized by aortic root angiography.[9,22] Selective angiography of the coronary arteries may also be performed with the ablation catheter positioned at the desired location so as to assess the anatomical relationships between these structures and the location of the ablation catheter. If the origin of VT is in the left coronary cusp, it is preferable to cannulate the left main coronary artery with a 5 Fr left Judkin catheter, which serves as a marker and for protection of the left main coronary artery in case of ablation catheter dislodgment during RF application.[48] Alternatively, a combination of electroanatomical mapping and ICE imaging (usually appreciated in the longitudinal view of the LVOT) may be used to confirm anatomical location, catheter tip position and contact, and distance to coronary vasculature and to monitor RF delivery.[35,44]

RIGHT CORONARY CUSP

The recorded electrogram from the right coronary cusp typically shows a large ventricular electrogram, which represents activation of the overlying relatively thick posterior wall of the RVOT infundibulum (see Fig. 23-17). Because this tissue is immediately adjacent to the anterior portion of the right coronary cusp, the electrogram may appear near field, and the site of early activation can be difficult to distinguish between arrhythmia origination from the myocardium extending above this cusp.[8] Nonetheless, during PVCs originating from the right coronary cusp itself, a smaller and relatively fragmented but near-field electrogram will be observed to precede the large ventricular electrogram and results from activation of the small myocardial sleeve extending into the cusp.

A far-field atrial electrogram may also be recorded in the right coronary cusp, particularly at more posterior locations (closer to the noncoronary cusp), and represents atrial activation of the anteroseptal tricuspid annulus, the RA appendage, or both.[8,49]

On fluoroscopy, a catheter positioned in the right coronary cusp (using the retrograde approach) will point rightward in the LAO projection and anterior in the RAO projection. When the fluoroscopic view appears to suggest right cusp position but a large atrial electrogram is noted, the catheter should be manipulated with clockwise torque to see whether the atrial electrogram becomes larger. If so, the catheter is likely to be in the noncoronary cusp and the fluoroscopic images are misleading, perhaps because of atrial enlargement or counterclockwise rotation of the heart. In this setting, withdrawal of the catheter followed by application of counterclockwise torque and then advancing the catheter again will move the catheter from the noncoronary cusp to the right coronary cusp.[8]

LEFT CORONARY CUSP

Electrograms obtained in the left coronary cusp are the most variable of the aortic cusps, but typically the ventricular electrogram amplitude is larger than that of the atrial electrogram. More anteriorly close to the commissure with the right coronary cusp, a large ventricular electrogram, again originating in the posterior RVOT, can be recorded (see Fig. 23-17). More leftward and posteriorly, however, because of the aortomitral continuity, recorded ventricular electrograms are small and far field in nature. In the RAO fluoroscopic view, as the catheter is rotated counterclockwise in the left coronary cusp, a relatively larger but usually far-field atrial electrogram is located representing LA activation close to the anteroseptal mitral annulus.[49]

NONCORONARY CUSP

A large near-field atrial electrogram is typically recorded in the noncoronary cusp, which represents activation of the thick myocardium of the interatrial septum located immediately posterior to the midportion of the noncoronary cusp (see Fig. 23-17).[49] When the catheter is rotated leftward and rightward from the interatrial septum, electrograms from the LA and RA, respectively, are recorded. A far-field ventricular electrogram may also be recorded from the noncoronary cusp and, depending on the exact catheter location, this smaller electrogram may reflect ventricular activation of the posterior LVOT, anteroseptal tricuspid annulus, or supravalvular myocardial activation.[8]

On fluoroscopy, a catheter positioned in the noncoronary cusp will point posteriorly in the RAO projection. In the LAO projection, however, the noncoronary cusp can be difficult to distinguish from the left coronary cusp because both appear to be somewhat leftward. When counterclockwise torque is applied and a large near-field atrial electrogram is seen, catheter location in the noncoronary cusp is verified. As discussed previously, ICE imaging can also help to clarify catheter location. The probe should be placed close to the tricuspid annulus and directed leftward. If the catheter tip is located in a cusp and the interatrial septum can be visualized in the same plane, noncoronary cusp location can be determined. If the tricuspid valve anterior leaflet is visualized along with the RVOT, then the catheter tip is probably in the right coronary cusp and simply directed posteriorly. Again, a simple maneuver of counterclockwise torque on the catheter while visualizing fluoroscopically and with ICE will result in a large ventricular electrogram being recorded and thus identifying catheter location in the right coronary cusp.[9]

Ventricular Tachycardias Originating from the Left Ventricular Papillary Muscles

The anterolateral (or anterior) and posteromedial (or posterior) LV papillary muscles are thick, finger-like processes attached to the ventricular wall at one end and to the mitral leaflets by multiple tendons (chordae tendineae) on the other end. The anterior papillary muscle originates from the middle to apical site of the LV ventral wall, whereas the posterior papillary muscle arises from the inferior wall of the LV. VTs generally originate from the base of the papillary muscle.

RF catheter ablation of these VTs is particularly challenging, likely secondary to the complex structure of the papillary muscles as well as the relatively deep VT origins within the thick muscle.[32]

Generally, large-tip (8-mm) or irrigated-tip ablation catheters and RF lesions in a relatively wide area and, not infrequently, on both sides of the papillary muscle are required to completely eliminate the VT. This is likely related to either poor catheter contact with the tissue or a relatively deep focus of the VT. ICE can be helpful in these cases and can facilitate catheter navigation and positioning.[32]

Sites with the earliest endocardial activation and matching pace maps are targeted by ablation. Purkinje potentials often (in 40% of patients) can be observed at successful ablation sites. However, pace mapping alone is usually insufficient to guide successful ablation. The site of origin of VT can be located deep within the papillary muscle and away from the breakout site; although the latter site can be recognized as the site with the best pace map, ablation there may not eliminate the VT.[31,32,50]

In up to 50% of patients, LV papillary muscle VTs exhibit variable QRS morphologies spontaneously, after the initial RF ablation lesions, or both, likely related to different directions of propagation of the wavefront exiting the papillary muscle.[32]

Epicardial Idiopathic Ventricular Tachycardias

The anterior and lateral portions of the RVOT are fairly thin. Thus, ablation from the endocardium is usually effective, even when VT foci occur on the epicardial surface. The posterior RVOT (infundibulum) is much thicker, but the epicardial surface of the posterior infundibulum is the LVOT, and thus ablation may be effective from either the LVOT or the RVOT for arrhythmias arising deep in the myocardium of the posterior RVOT.[15]

For the supravalvular aortic region there is no true epicardial location because the RVOT lies anterior to the right and left coronary cusps and the atria lie posterior to the noncoronary cusp.[15]

On the other hand, idiopathic VTs can originate from the LV epicardium in up to 14% of patients with idiopathic VT. Epicardial idiopathic VTs typically arise in close proximity to the coronary venous system, including the anterior interventricular vein (which runs in the anterior interventricular sulcus parallel to the left anterior descending coronary artery), the great cardiac vein (which runs in the left AV groove parallel to the left circumflex coronary artery and forms the CS once it is joined by the left atrial oblique vein of Marshall and the posterolateral vein of the LV), the junction of the anterior interventricular and great cardiac veins (near the bifurcation of the left coronary artery), and less commonly the middle cardiac vein (which runs with the posterior descending coronary artery in the posterior interventricular groove).[3,39]

The region of the epicardial surface of the LV near the bifurcation of the left main coronary artery that is bounded by an arc from the left anterior descending coronary artery (superior to the first septal perforating branch) and the left circumflex coronary artery occupies the most superior portion of the LV and has been termed the LV summit (Fig. 23-19). This region is the most common site of idiopathic epicardial LV VT origins. The LV summit is bisected by the great cardiac vein into an inferior portion, lateral to this structure (which is accessible to epicardial catheter ablation) and a superior region that is inaccessible to catheter ablation because of the close proximity of the coronary arteries and the thick layer of epicardial fat that overlies the proximal portion of these vessels.[51]

LV summit VTs are most commonly ablated within the great cardiac or anterior interventricular veins.[8] Epicardial mapping via the coronary venous system can be achieved with small (2.5 Fr), flexible, multipolar electrode catheters introduced through a guiding catheter positioned at the CS ostium. CS venography is typically required to help delineate its anatomy and to visualize the great

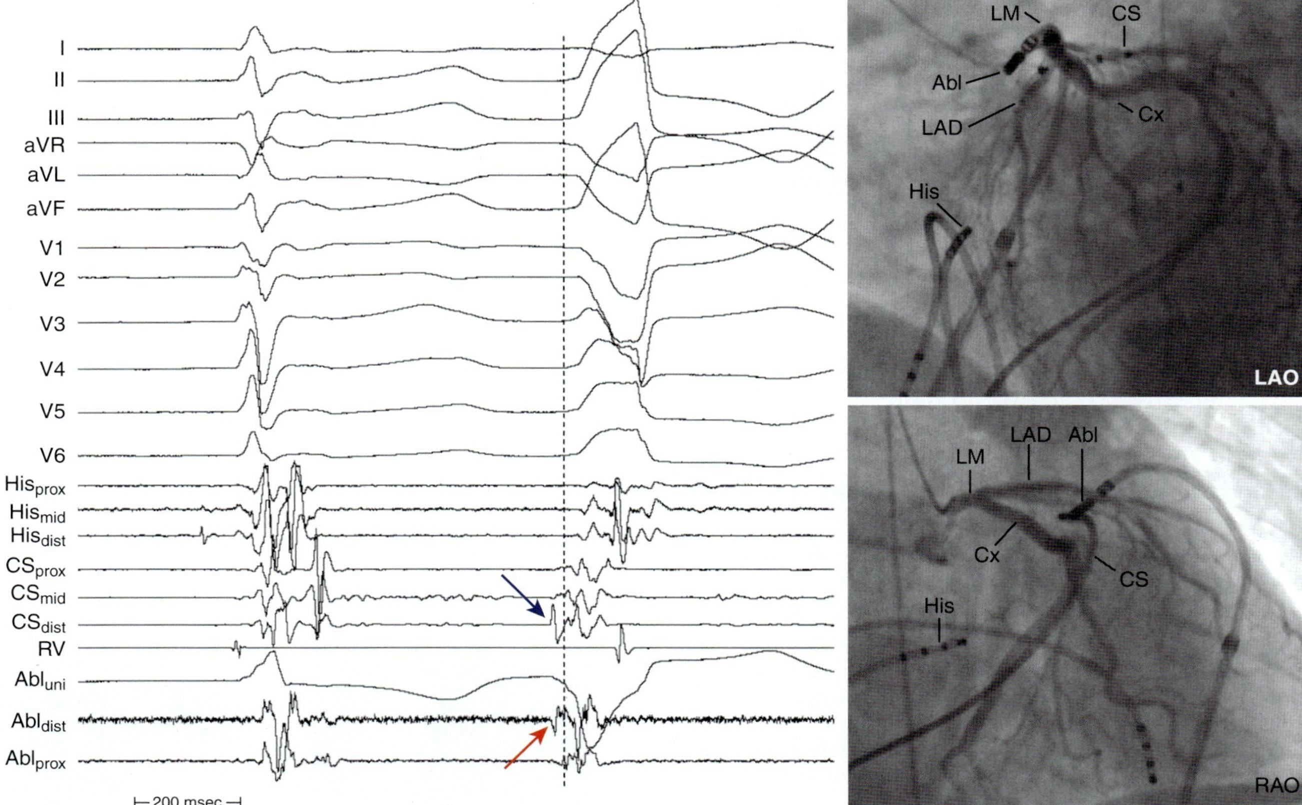

FIGURE 23-19 Recordings from a patient with premature ventricular complexes (PVCs) originating on the left ventricular (LV) summit. The dashed line denotes the onset of the PVC QRS complex. Note that the distal coronary sinus electrogram (CS_{dist}) occurs well before the onset of the QRS, similar to the ablation catheter recording in the pericardial space; the location is shown in the fluoroscopic views at right (Abl). Cx = circumflex coronary artery; LAD = left anterior descending artery; LAO = left anterior oblique; LM = left main coronary artery; RAO = right anterior oblique.

cardiac and anterior interventricular veins. Once the catheter is positioned at the target site, and before RF energy delivery, coronary arteriography should be performed to outline the spatial relationship between the target vein and the adjacent coronary artery (see Fig. 23-19). After ablation, coronary arteriography should be performed to rule out damage to coronary arteries. Additionally, pacing from the distal ablation electrode should be performed at an output of 20 mA. If diaphragmatic capture can be demonstrated, then ablation should not be attempted to avoid phrenic nerve injury.[38,39]

However, epicardial mapping and ablation via the coronary venous system can be challenging. Currently available ablation catheters often are difficult to advance beyond the distal great cardiac vein or the proximal portions of the middle cardiac vein because of the tortuosity, sharp angulation, and small caliber of the distal veins. Additionally, with conventional 4-mm electrodes, delivery of more than 10 to 15 W seldom is possible because of limited electrode cooling, leading to a rapid rise in electrode temperature, although even low power often is sufficient. Given those difficulties, the percutaneous epicardial approach may offer potential advantages for mapping and ablation of those VTs. The latter approach provides access to the entire epicardial surface and the deployment of a greater range of ablation catheters and energy sources, although technical challenges related to access and the insulating effects of epicardial fat remain.[38,39] Nonetheless, despite these technical challenges, ablation of idiopathic VT via the coronary venous system appears to be at least as effective as with a percutaneous transthoracic approach, which has a reported success rate of approximately 70%. Using the coronary venous system for mapping and ablation may result in a lower complication rate because damage to the RV or extracardiac structures is less likely to occur. Percutaneous epicardial mapping and ablation may be considered in patients with epicardial VTs when ablation from within the coronary venous system in not feasible (see Chap. 27 for detailed discussion).

Radiofrequency Energy Delivery

Because outflow tract VTs are focal in nature and the target tissue consists of structurally nondiseased myocardium, extensive tissue injury is usually not necessary for successful ablation. Steerable catheters with 4- or 5-mm-tip electrodes and conventional nonirrigated energy application are generally used. RF applications at moderate temperatures (target temperature, 55°C) and a maximal power output of 30 to 40 W seem to be safe and effective. Duration of energy application should not exceed 30 to 60 seconds.[13] Rarely, if ever, does one need more than 50 W or use of irrigated or large-tip electrodes to ablate outflow tract VTs successfully, and it is preferable to avoid those ablation approaches to prevent cardiac perforation. Some investigators recommend the use of lower target temperatures and irrigated electrodes for left-sided idiopathic focal VT, assuming a higher risk of coagulum formation and thromboembolic complications compared with ablation in the RV.[3,44]

Several measures must be taken to avoid injuring the coronary arteries during ablation of VTs arising from the coronary cusps. RF energy delivery in the aortic sinuses is preferably started at a low power output (15 W) and then increased to no more than 30 W to achieve a target temperature of approximately 50°C. Ablation should also be performed during continuous fluoroscopy to observe for catheter dislodgment, and energy delivery should be discontinued in case of even minimal dislodgment from the site showing the best mapping findings. RF application should also be

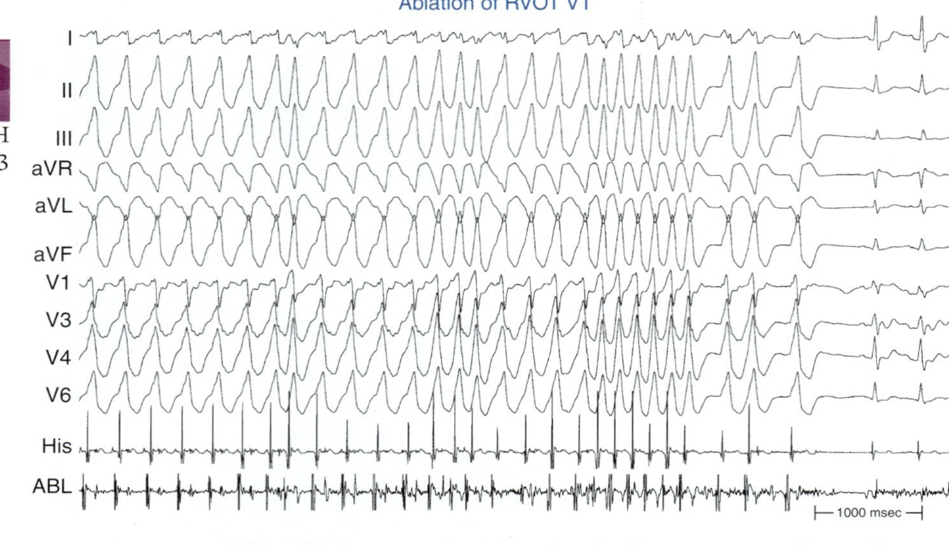

FIGURE 23-20 Ablation of right ventricular outflow tract (RVOT) ventricular tachycardia (VT). Radiofrequency energy delivery is started during sustained VT. Acceleration of the VT is observed within a few seconds, followed by slowing and termination of the VT.

stopped if the repetitive or sustained VT cannot be terminated after 10 seconds. Coronary angiography is often performed immediately after the ablative procedure to exclude coronary artery spasm, dissection, or thrombus.

RF delivery at successful ablation sites often can result in a rapid ventricular response (identical QRS morphology to that of VT), followed by gradual slowing and complete resolution (Fig. 23-20). This finding has a high specificity, but low sensitivity, for successful ablation sites.[1] When RF is delivered during VT, termination of VT at successful sites usually occurs within 10 seconds.

Typically, a few (range, 2 to 11; mean, 5) RF applications are required. Occasionally, following several RF applications, the first VT morphology is no longer seen but a second, similar one is now observed. This can be caused by an actual second focus near the first or modification of the exit site from the first focus (Fig. 23-21). In this situation, ablation within 1 to 2 cm of the first site eliminates the second VT morphology.

Endpoints of Ablation

Successful ablation is defined as the lack of spontaneous or inducible PVCs and VT, with and without isoproterenol administration (using the best method for induction documented before ablation), at least 30 minutes after ablation.

Outcome

The acute success rate is greater than 90%. The recurrence rate is approximately 7% to 10%. Of these, 40% recur during the first 24 to 48 hours after the ablation procedure. Recurrence of VT beyond the first year post ablation is rare. The success of ablation depends on the presence of spontaneous or inducible VT or PVCs at the time of the procedure. Predictors of recurrences include poor pace map, late activation at target sites, reliance on pace mapping alone, and termination of VT inducibility with mechanical trauma by the mapping-ablation catheter before RF delivery.

Complications are rare. RBBB develops in 2% and cardiac tamponade is rare. Systemic thromboembolism and damage to the aortic valve can occur during ablation of LVOT or aortic cusp VTs.[3]

The potential for acute coronary artery occlusion is a major risk consideration with catheter manipulation within the aortic cusps. Damage to the coronary arteries can result from catheter manipulation and ablation in the aortic root, secondary to RF energy delivery in close proximity to the ostia of the right or left coronary arteries as well as inadvertent catheter engagement of the left main

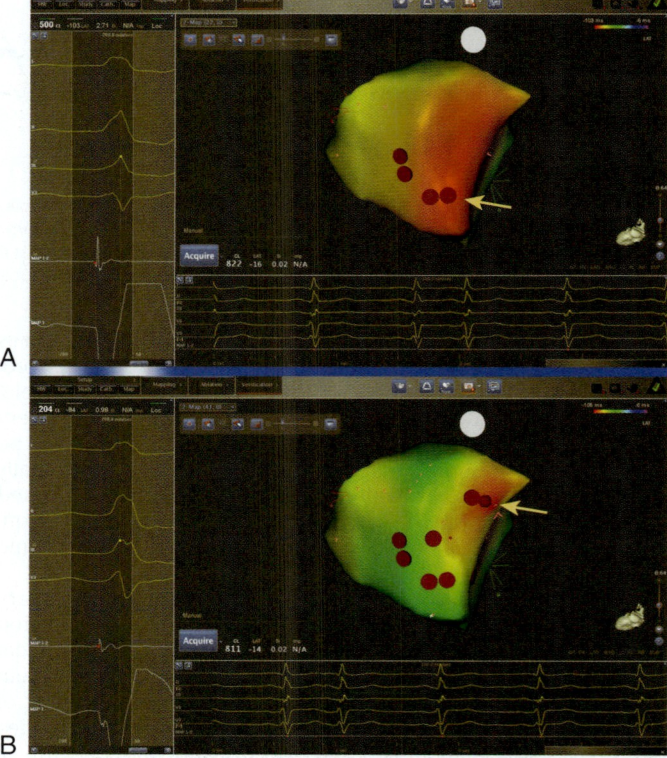

FIGURE 23-21 Electroanatomical (CARTO) activation map (posterior views) of premature ventricular complexes (PVCs) originating from the right ventricular outflow tract (RVOT). Left panels show (in order from top to bottom) surface ECG leads (I, II, III, V_1) and bipolar and unipolar recording of the distal ablation electrodes during the PVCs. **A,** The site of impulse origin during ectopy is in the posterolateral aspect of the RVOT (red area, arrow) at which intracardiac recordings show early bipolar electrogram concordant with a QS-unipolar electrogram; ablation (red dots) at this site eliminated VT. **B,** PVCs with slightly different QRS morphology (note the notching in the QRS in ECG leads II and III) emerged after initial ablation. Mapping revealed the focus of the latter PVCs (note intracardiac recordings) at a close but different location from the site targeted by initial ablation, at which ablation (red area, arrow) eliminated all PVCs.

coronary artery when ablating in the left coronary cusp. It is also important to recognize the potential risk of coronary artery damage when ablating in the RVOT and pulmonary artery. The right coronary artery is typically 4 to 5 mm away from the proximal part of the RVOT near the free wall, and is separated by a variable amount of fat. Additionally, the cephalocaudal separation of the pulmonic and aortic valve results in close proximity of the pulmonic valve to the origin of the right coronary artery, and the left main coronary artery lies in immediate posterior proximity to the subvalvular RVOT near the pulmonic valve as well as the supravalvular pulmonary artery. Thus, when concern exists about possibly damaging the artery, the ablation catheter should be kept where energy delivery is to be given, and either a root aortogram, coronary angiography, or careful ICE imaging should be performed.[9]

The penetrating HB lies at the membranous septum formed in part by the commissure between the right coronary and noncoronary cusps. Ablation at this site could potentially damage the HB. The HB electrogram can be obtained at several supravalvular locations including the right coronary cusp posteriorly, the noncoronary cusp anteriorly, and when the electrode has been prolapsed below the plane of the semilunar valve in between these two cusps. During VT, however, the His potential can be inscribed within the ventricular electrogram as a result of retrograde activation to the HB.[9] Therefore, when ablating in the depths of the noncoronary cusp, particularly toward the junction with the right coronary cusp, monitoring for fast pathway damage (AH interval prolongation, junctional beats) is advisable.

Cryoablation

Initial experience suggests cryocatheter techniques to be a potent tool in treating idiopathic RVOT VT.[52] A major advantage of cryoablation is the virtual absence of pain, which makes the use of analgesia unnecessary. Moreover, reasonable fluoroscopy and procedure times can be achieved by an experienced investigator. Stability of the catheter during cryoablation can be advantageous because monitoring of catheter position by fluoroscopy is not necessary. Adhesion of the catheter, however, requires precise positioning before the start of cryoablation. Slight dislocations, as may easily occur with breathing, can delay ablation success. Furthermore, brushing of the catheter within a small, defined area, as often observed with RF ablations, cannot occur; therefore, repositioning of the catheter to adjust for a dislocation is not possible during cryoablation. The cryocatheter differs substantially in size and rigidity from standard RF catheters and requires some experience in handling.

Complete disappearance of the arrhythmia is typically observed within 20 seconds of cryoablation. Therefore, cryoablation is stopped after 60 seconds if no positive effect is observed.

Given the high success rate and low risk of RF ablation of outflow tract VT, it may be difficult to demonstrate a clinical advantage of cryoablation over RF ablation. Cryoablation can be useful in difficult or atypical sites when a maximal stability of the catheter is necessary—for example, to avoid dislodgment of the catheter into the coronary arteries during ablation of idiopathic VT originating from the aortic cusps. Additionally, cryoablation may be considered for elimination of epicardial VTs from within the coronary venous system, when RF energy delivery is limited. Also, the absence of pain during ablation may render the procedure more comfortable for the patient, especially when the use of sedative medications suppresses inducibility of the VT.[38,39]

REFERENCES

1. Lerman BB: Ventricular tachycardia in patients with structurally normal hearts. In Zipes DP, Jalife J, editors: *Cardiac electrophysiology: from cell to bedside*, ed 5, Philadelphia, 2009, WB Saunders, pp 657–668.
2. Aliot EM, Stevenson WG, Mendral-Garrote JM, et al: EHRA/HRS Expert Consensus on Catheter Ablation of Ventricular Arrhythmias: developed in a partnership with the European Heart*Rhythm* Association (EHRA), a Registered Branch of the European Society of Cardiology (ESC), and the Heart*Rhythm* Society (HRS); in collaboration with the American College of Cardiology (ACC) and the American Heart Association (AHA), *Heart Rhythm* 6:886–933, 2009.
3. Natale A, Raviele A, Al-Ahmad A, et al: Venice Chart International Consensus document on ventricular tachycardia/ventricular fibrillation ablation, *J Cardiovasc Electrophysiol* 21:339–379, 2010.
4. Markowitz SM, Lerman BB: Mechanisms of focal ventricular tachycardia in humans, *Heart Rhythm* 6(Suppl 8):S81–S85, 2009.
5. Iwai S, Cantillon DJ, Kim RJ, et al: Right and left ventricular outflow tract tachycardias: evidence for a common electrophysiologic mechanism, *J Cardiovasc Electrophysiol* 17:1052–1058, 2006.
6. Josephson ME: Recurrent ventricular tachycardia. In Josephson ME, editor: *Clinical cardiac electrophysiology*, ed 4, Philadelphia, 2008, Lippincott Williams & Wilkins, pp 446–642.
7. Kim RJ, Iwai S, Markowitz SM, et al: Clinical and electrophysiological spectrum of idiopathic ventricular outflow tract arrhythmias, *J Am Coll Cardiol* 49:2035–2043, 2007.
8. Asirvatham SJ: Correlative anatomy for the invasive electrophysiologist: outflow tract and supravalvar arrhythmia, *J Cardiovasc Electrophysiol* 20:955–968, 2009.
9. Tabatabaei N, Asirvatham SJ: Supravalvular arrhythmia: identifying and ablating the substrate, *Circ Arrhythm Electrophysiol* 2:316–326, 2009.
10. Bala R, Marchlinski FE: Electrocardiographic recognition and ablation of outflow tract ventricular tachycardia, *Heart Rhythm* 4:366–370, 2007.
11. Ho SY: Anatomic insights for catheter ablation of ventricular tachycardia, *Heart Rhythm* 6(Suppl 8):S77–S80, 2009.
12. Anderson RH: Clinical anatomy of the aortic root, *Heart* 84:670–673, 2000.
13. Rillig A, Meyerfeldt U, Birkemeyer R, et al: Catheter ablation within the sinus of Valsalva—a safe and effective approach for treatment of atrial and ventricular tachycardias, *Heart Rhythm* 5:1265–1272, 2008.
14. Piazza N, de Jaegere P, Schultz C, et al: Anatomy of the aortic valvar complex and its implications for transcatheter implantation of the aortic valve, *Circ Cardiovasc Interv* 1:74–81, 2008.
15. Suleiman M, Asirvatham SJ: Ablation above the semilunar valves: when, why, and how? Part I, *Heart Rhythm* 5:1485–1492, 2008.
16. Yamada T, McElderry HT, Doppalapudi H, et al: Idiopathic ventricular arrhythmias originating from the aortic root prevalence, electrocardiographic and electrophysiologic characteristics, and results of radiofrequency catheter ablation, *J Am Coll Cardiol* 52:139–147, 2008.
17. Alasady M, Singleton CB, McGavigan AD: Left ventricular outflow tract ventricular tachycardia originating from the noncoronary cusp: electrocardiographic and electrophysiological characterization and radiofrequency ablation, *J Cardiovasc Electrophysiol* 20:1287–1290, 2009.
18. Olgun H, Yokokawa M, Baman T, et al: The role of interpolation in PVC-induced cardiomyopathy, *Heart Rhythm* 8:1046–1049, 2011.
19. Yokokawa M, Good E, Crawford T, et al: Ventricular tachycardia originating from the aortic sinus cusp in patients with idiopathic dilated cardiomyopathy, *Heart Rhythm* 8:357–360, 2011.
20. Baman TS, Lange DC, Ilg KJ, et al: Relationship between burden of premature ventricular complexes and left ventricular function, *Heart Rhythm* 7:865–869, 2010.
21. Bogun F, Morady F: Ablation of ventricular tachycardia in patients with nonischemic cardiomyopathy, *J Cardiovasc Electrophysiol* 19:1227–1230, 2008.
22. Tanner H, Hindricks G, Schirdewahn P, et al: Outflow tract tachycardia with R/S transition in lead V_3: six different anatomic approaches for successful ablation, *J Am Coll Cardiol* 45: 418–423, 2005.
23. Betensky BP, Park RE, Marchlinski FE, et al: The V_2 transition ratio: a new electrocardiographic criterion for distinguishing left from right ventricular outflow tract tachycardia origin, *J Am Coll Cardiol* 57:2255–2262, 2011.
24. Sekiguchi Y, Aonuma K, Takahashi A, et al: Electrocardiographic and electrophysiologic characteristics of ventricular tachycardia originating within the pulmonary artery, *J Am Coll Cardiol* 45:887–895, 2005.
25. Tada H, Tadokoro K, Miyaji K, et al: Idiopathic ventricular arrhythmias arising from the pulmonary artery: prevalence, characteristics, and topography of the arrhythmia origin, *Heart Rhythm* 5:419–426, 2008.
26. Tada H, Tadokoro K, Ito S, et al: Idiopathic ventricular arrhythmias originating from the tricuspid annulus: prevalence, electrocardiographic characteristics, and results of radiofrequency catheter ablation, *Heart Rhythm* 4:7–16, 2007.
27. Crawford T, Mueller G, Good E, et al: Ventricular arrhythmias originating from papillary muscles in the right ventricle, *Heart Rhythm* 7:725–730, 2010.
28. Van HH, Garcia F, Lin D, et al: Idiopathic right ventricular arrhythmias not arising from the outflow tract: prevalence, electrocardiographic characteristics, and outcome of catheter ablation, *Heart Rhythm* 8:511–518, 2011.
29. Doppalapudi H, Yamada T, McElderry HT, et al: Ventricular tachycardia originating from the posterior papillary muscle in the left ventricle: a distinct clinical syndrome, *Circ Arrhythm Electrophysiol* 1:23–29, 2008.
30. Yamada T, McElderry HT, Okada T, et al: Idiopathic focal ventricular arrhythmias originating from the anterior papillary muscle in the left ventricle, *J Cardiovasc Electrophysiol* 20:866–872, 2009.
31. Yamada T, Doppalapudi H, McElderry HT, et al: Idiopathic ventricular arrhythmias originating from the papillary muscles in the left ventricle: prevalence, electrocardiographic and electrophysiological characteristics, and results of the radiofrequency catheter ablation, *J Cardiovasc Electrophysiol* 21:62–69, 2010.
32. Yamada T, Doppalapudi H, McElderry HT, et al: Electrocardiographic and electrophysiological characteristics in idiopathic ventricular arrhythmias originating from the papillary muscles in the left ventricle: relevance for catheter ablation, *Circ Arrhythm Electrophysiol* 3:324–331, 2010.
33. Tada H, Ito S, Naito S, et al: Idiopathic ventricular arrhythmia arising from the mitral annulus: a distinct subgroup of idiopathic ventricular arrhythmias, *J Am Coll Cardiol* 45:877–886, 2005.
34. Yoshida N, Inden Y, Uchikawa T, et al: Novel transitional zone index allows more accurate differentiation between idiopathic right ventricular outflow tract and aortic sinus cusp ventricular arrhythmias, *Heart Rhythm* 8:349–356, 2011.
35. Bala R, Garcia FC, Hutchinson MD, et al: Electrocardiographic and electrophysiologic features of ventricular arrhythmias originating from the right/left coronary cusp commissure, *Heart Rhythm* 7:312–322, 2010.

36. Yamada T, Murakami Y, Yoshida N, et al: Preferential conduction across the ventricular outflow septum in ventricular arrhythmias originating from the aortic sinus cusp, *J Am Coll Cardiol* 50:884–891, 2007.
37. Bazan V, Gerstenfeld EP, Garcia FC, et al: Site-specific twelve-lead ECG features to identify an epicardial origin for left ventricular tachycardia in the absence of myocardial infarction, *Heart Rhythm* 4:1403–1410, 2007.
38. Daniels DV, Lu YY, Morton JB, et al: Idiopathic epicardial left ventricular tachycardia originating remote from the sinus of Valsalva: electrophysiological characteristics, catheter ablation, and identification from the 12-lead electrocardiogram, *Circulation* 113:1659–1666, 2006.
39. Baman TS, Ilg KJ, Gupta SK, et al: Mapping and ablation of epicardial idiopathic ventricular arrhythmias from within the coronary venous system, *Circ Arrhythm Electrophysiol* 3:274–279, 2010.
40. Bazan V, Bala R, Garcia FC, et al: Twelve-lead ECG features to identify ventricular tachycardia arising from the epicardial right ventricle, *Heart Rhythm* 3:1132–1139, 2006.
41. Hoffmayer KS, Machado ON, Marcus GM, et al: Electrocardiographic comparison of ventricular arrhythmias in patients with arrhythmogenic right ventricular cardiomyopathy and right ventricular outflow tract tachycardia, *J Am Coll Cardiol* 58:831–838, 2011.
42. Shimizu W: Arrhythmias originating from the right ventricular outflow tract: how to distinguish "malignant" from "benign"? *Heart Rhythm* 6:1507–1511, 2009.
43. Corrado D, Basso C, Leoni L, et al: Three-dimensional electroanatomical voltage mapping and histologic evaluation of myocardial substrate in right ventricular outflow tract tachycardia, *J Am Coll Cardiol* 51:731–739, 2008.
44. Callans DJ: Catheter ablation of idiopathic ventricular tachycardia arising from the aortic root, *J Cardiovasc Electrophysiol* 20:969–972, 2009.
45. Azegami K, Wilber DJ, Arruda M, et al: Spatial resolution of pacemapping and activation mapping in patients with idiopathic right ventricular outflow tract tachycardia, *J Cardiovasc Electrophysiol* 16:823–829, 2005.
46. Kurosaki K, Nogami A, Sakamaki M, et al: Automated template matching to pinpoint the origin of right ventricular outflow tract tachycardia, *Pacing Clin Electrophysiol* 32(Suppl 1): S47–S51, 2009.
47. Bai R, Napolitano C, Bloise R, et al: Yield of genetic screening in inherited cardiac channelopathies: how to prioritize access to genetic testing, *Circ Arrhythm Electrophysiol* 2:6–15, 2009.
48. Yamada T, McElderry HT, Okada T, et al: Idiopathic left ventricular arrhythmias originating adjacent to the left aortic sinus of valsalva: electrophysiological rationale for the surface electrocardiogram, *J Cardiovasc Electrophysiol* 21:170–176, 2010.
49. Sasaki T, Hachiya H, Hirao K, et al: Utility of distinctive local electrogram pattern and aortographic anatomical position in catheter manipulation at coronary cusps, *J Cardiovasc Electrophysiol* 22:521–529, 2011.
50. Yokokawa M, Good E, Desjardins B, et al: Predictors of successful catheter ablation of ventricular arrhythmias arising from the papillary muscles, *Heart Rhythm* 7:1654–1659, 2010.
51. Yamada T, McElderry HT, Doppalapudi H, et al: Idiopathic ventricular arrhythmias originating from the left ventricular summit: anatomical concepts relevant to ablation, *Circ Arrhythm Electrophysiol* 3:616–623, 2010.
52. Kurzidim K, Schneider HJ, Kuniss M, et al: Cryocatheter ablation of right ventricular outflow tract tachycardia, *J Cardiovasc Electrophysiol* 16:366–369, 2005.

CHAPTER 24 Verapamil-Sensitive (Fascicular) Ventricular Tachycardia

Pathophysiology

Verapamil-sensitive left ventricular tachycardia (LV VT) is a reentrant tachycardia. The diagnosis of reentry as the mechanism of fascicular VT is supported by several observations. The VT can reproducibly be initiated and terminated by programmed electrical stimulation, entrainment and resetting with fusion can be demonstrated, and an inverse relationship between the coupling interval of the initiating ventricular extrastimulus (VES) or ventricular pacing cycle length (CL) and the first VT beat can be observed.

The exact nature of the reentry circuit in verapamil-sensitive VT has provoked considerable interest. Some investigators have suggested that it is a microreentry circuit in the territory of the left posterior fascicle (LPF). Others have suggested that the circuit is confined to the Purkinje system, which is insulated from the underlying ventricular myocardium. False tendons or fibromuscular bands that extend from the posteroinferior LV to the basal septum have also been implicated in the anatomical substrate of this tachycardia. Less often, the reentry circuit is located in fibers distal to the left anterior fascicle (LAF) or may arise from fascicular locations high in the septum.[1]

Currently, overwhelming evidence suggests that the VT is caused by a reentrant circuit incorporating the posterior Purkinje system with an excitable gap and a slow conduction area.[2-4] The VT substrate can be a small macroreentrant circuit consisting of the LPF serving as one limb and abnormal Purkinje tissue with slow, decremental conduction serving as the other limb. The anterograde limb may be associated with longitudinal dissociation of the LPF or contiguous tissue that is directly coupled to the LPF (such as a false tendon) or, alternatively, has ventricular myocardium interposed. The zone of slow conduction appears to depend on the slow inward calcium current, because the degree of slowing of tachycardia CL in response to verapamil is entirely attributed to its negative dromotropic effects on the area of slow conduction.

The entrance site to the slow conduction zone is thought to be located closer to the base of the LV septum. From there, activation propagates anterogradely (from basal to apical along the LV septum) over the abnormal Purkinje tissue with decremental conduction properties and verapamil sensitivity, which serves as the anterograde limb of the circuit and appears to be insulated from the nearby ventricular myocardium. The lower turnaround point of the reentrant circuit is located in the lower third of the septum, where the wavefront captures the fast conduction Purkinje tissue from or contiguous to the LPF, and retrograde activation occurs over the LPF from the apical to basal septum forming the retrograde limb of the reentrant circuit. Also, at the lower turnaround point anterograde activation occurs down the septum to break through (at the exit of the tachycardia circuit) in the posterior septal myocardium below. The upper turnaround point of the reentrant circuit occurs over a zone of slow conduction located close to the main trunk of the left bundle branch (LB) in the basal interventricular septum (Fig. 24-1). The estimated distance between the entrance and exit of the circuit is approximately 2 cm.[3,5]

Clinical Considerations

Epidemiology

Age at presentation is typically 15 to 40 years (unusual after 55 years). Males are more commonly affected (60% to 80%). Verapamil-sensitive VT is the most common form of idiopathic LV VT, and it accounts for 10% to 15% of all idiopathic VTs.[2,6]

Clinical Presentation

Most patients present with mild to moderate symptoms of palpitations and lightheadedness. Occasionally, symptoms are debilitating, and include fatigue, dyspnea, and presyncope. Syncope and sudden cardiac death are very rare. The VT is typically paroxysmal and can last for minutes to hours. Although idiopathic LV VT can occur at rest, it is sensitive to catecholamines and often occurs during exercise, after exercise, or emotional distress. Occasionally, the VT can be incessant, may be sustained for a long period (days), and does not revert spontaneously to normal sinus rhythm (NSR). Patients with incessant tachycardia can develop cardiomyopathy.[7] The clinical course is benign and the prognosis is excellent. Spontaneous remission of the VT may occur with time.

Initial Evaluation

Diagnostic features of fascicular VT include induction with atrial pacing, right bundle branch block (RBBB) with left (or, less commonly, right) axis deviation, structurally normal heart, and verapamil sensitivity. Evaluation to exclude structural heart disease is necessary and typically includes echocardiographic examination, stress testing, and/or cardiac catheterization, depending on patient age and risk factors.

Principles of Management

ACUTE MANAGEMENT

Intravenous verapamil is typically successful in acutely terminating the VT. Termination with adenosine is rare, except for patients in whom isoproterenol is used for induction of the tachycardia in the EP laboratory.

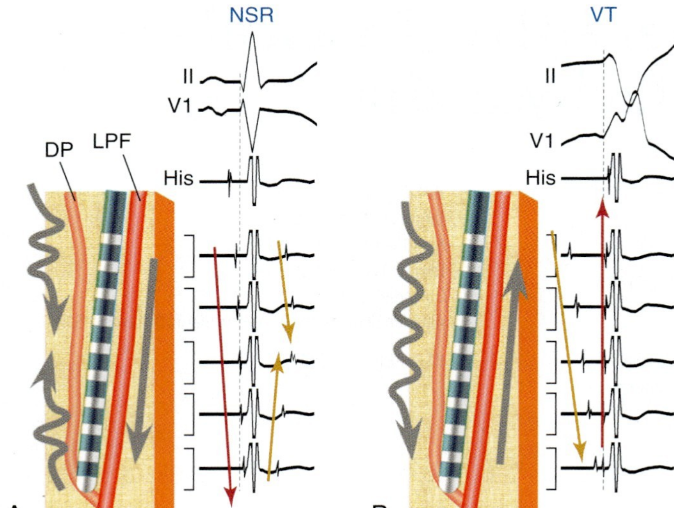

FIGURE 24-1 Schematic illustration of the reentrant circuit in verapamil-sensitive left ventricular tachycardia (LV VT). A block of the LV septum is depicted with the left posterior fascicle (LPF) and diastolic pathway (DP) running in parallel until they intersect at the bottom. A 10-pole catheter is shown recording between pathways; electrograms from each pair are shown along with surface ECG leads and His bundle recordings. **A,** A sinus rhythm complex is shown; the dashed line denotes QRS onset. Note the direction and speed of propagation over the LPF while the DP is activated after the QRS and in both directions (arrows). **B,** During a VT complex, the DP is activated anterogradely and the LPF retrogradely (arrows). NSR = normal sinus rhythm. See text for discussion.

CHRONIC MANAGEMENT

Long-term therapy with verapamil is useful in mild cases; however, it has little effect in patients with severe symptoms and the efficacy of oral verapamil in preventing tachycardia relapse is variable. Radiofrequency (RF) ablation is highly effective (success rate of 85% to 90%) and is recommended for patients with severe symptoms.[2]

Electrocardiographic Features

ECG during Normal Sinus Rhythm

The resting ECG is usually normal. Symmetrical, inferolateral T wave inversion can be present after termination of the VT.

ECG during Ventricular Tachycardia

The QRS during VT typically has RBBB with LAF block configuration. The R/S ratio is less than 1 in leads V_1 and V_2 (Fig. 24-2).[3] VTs arising more toward the middle at the region of the posterior papillary muscle have a left superior axis and RS in leads V_5 and V_6, whereas those arising closer to the apex have a right superior axis with a small "r" and deep S (or even QS) in leads V_5 and V_6. In contrast to VT associated with structural heart disease, the QRS duration during fascicular VT is relatively narrow (<140 to 150 milliseconds), and the RS interval (the duration from the beginning of the QRS to the nadir of the S wave) in the precordial leads is relatively short (60 to 80 milliseconds); thus, the VT is frequently called "fascicular" VT. The VT rate is approximately 150 to 200 beats/min (range, 120 to 250 beats/min). Alternans in the CL is frequently noted during the VT; otherwise, the VT rate is stable.

Fascicular VT can be classified into three subtypes: (1) left posterior fascicular VT with an RBBB and superior axis configuration (common form); (2) left anterior fascicular VT with RBBB and right-axis deviation configuration (uncommon form); and (3) upper septal fascicular VT with a narrow QRS and normal axis configuration (rare form).[1]

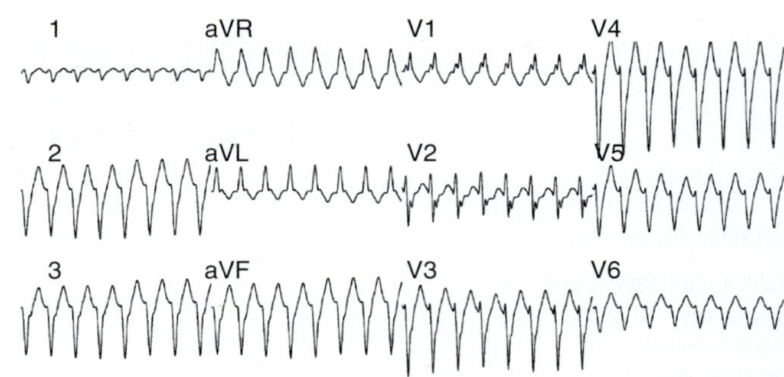

FIGURE 24-2 Surface ECGs of verapamil-sensitive left ventricular tachycardia (LV VT). Note the right bundle branch block and left anterior fascicle block pattern characteristic of these VTs.

Electrophysiological Testing

Induction of Tachycardia

Fascicular VT can usually be initiated with atrial extrastimulation (AES), VES, atrial pacing, or ventricular pacing. Often, isoproterenol alone, or during concurrent programmed stimulation, facilitates induction. An inverse relationship is observed between the coupling interval of the initiating VES or ventricular pacing CL and the first VT beat.

Tachycardia Features

SITE OF EARLIEST VENTRICULAR ACTIVATION

The site of earliest ventricular activation during VT (which represents the exit of the reentrant circuit) is in the region of the LPF (inferoposterior LV septum) in 90% to 95% of LV VTs (explaining the RBBB–superior axis configuration of the QRS), and in the region of the LAF (anterosuperior LV septum) in 5% to 10% of LV VTs (explaining the RBBB–right axis configuration of the QRS). In most cases, ventricular electrograms are discrete during both NSR and VT. The His bundle (HB) is not a component of the reentrant circuit, because a retrograde His potential is often recorded 20 to 40 milliseconds after the earliest ventricular activation (Fig. 24-3).

PURKINJE POTENTIAL

The Purkinje potential (PP or P2) is a discrete, high-frequency potential that precedes the site of earliest ventricular activation by 15 to 42 milliseconds and is recorded in the posterior third of the LV septum during VT and NSR (Fig. 24-4; see also Fig. 24-3).[3,4] Because this potential also precedes ventricular activation during NSR, it is believed to originate from activation of a segment of the LPF, and to represent the lower turnaround point in the reentrant circuit. The earliest ventricular activation site (exit) during VT is identified more apically in the septum than the region with the earliest recorded PP.

LATE DIASTOLIC POTENTIAL

The late diastolic potential (LDP, P1, or pre-PP) is a discrete potential that precedes the PP during VT, and is recorded at the basal, middle, or apical LV septum. The LDP is thought to originate from activation at the entrance to the abnormal Purkinje tissue (the specialized, verapamil-sensitive zone), which is thought to serve as the anterograde limb of the reentrant circuit. The LDP differs in morphology from the PP and has a relatively small amplitude and low-frequency component. The area with LDP recording is confined to a small region (0.5 to 1.0 cm^2) and is included in the larger area where the PP is recorded (2 to 3 cm^2); hence, the LDP often is recorded simultaneously with the PP by the same electrode. The LDP is recorded within an area proximal to the earliest PP recording

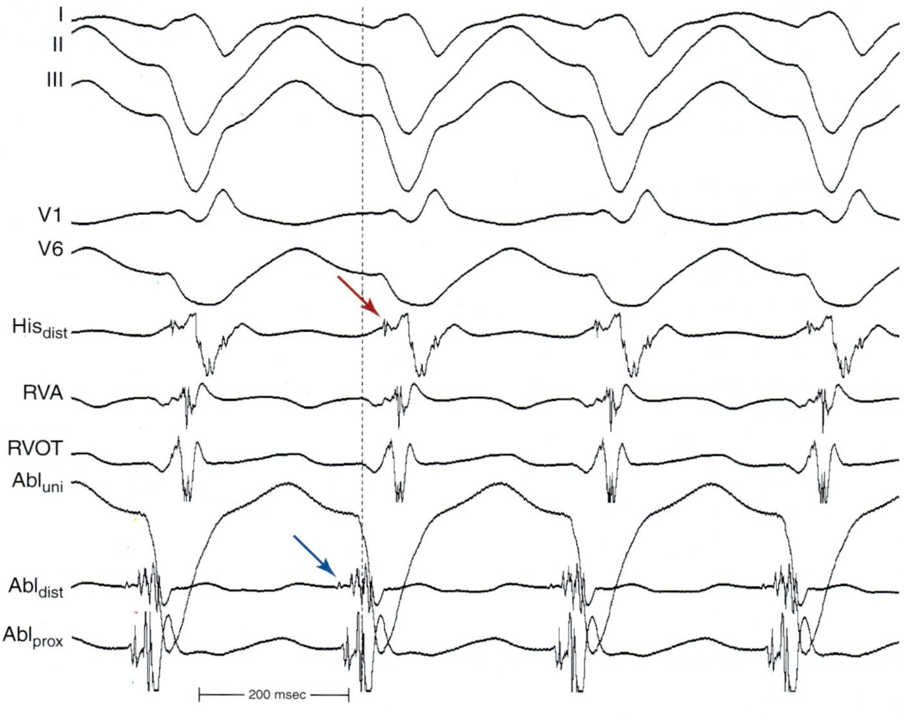

FIGURE 24-3 Idiopathic (fascicular) left ventricular tachycardia. The blue arrow shows late diastolic small potential, 45 milliseconds prior to QRS onset. Distinct Purkinje-like potentials (blue arrow) are evident before the dotted line denoting QRS onset, as well as in the proximal ablation electrogram. The red arrow indicates retrograde His potential. Note the unipolar QS configuration just coinciding with QRS onset.

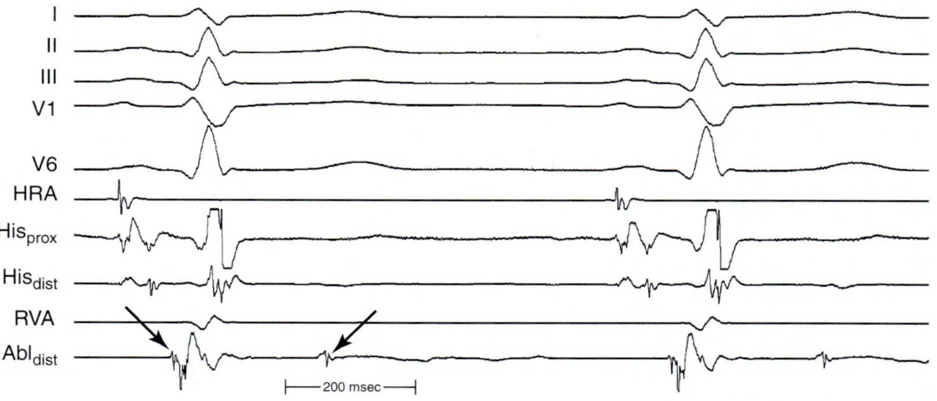

FIGURE 24-4 Sinus rhythm recordings at a successful ablation site for idiopathic (fascicular) left ventricular tachycardia. The left arrow points to a Purkinje-like potential just prior to the local electrogram (also slightly preceding the onset of the QRS); the right arrow shows a sharp, delayed diastolic potential, purportedly from the slow-conducting limb of the circuit.

site, and is activated from the basal to apical septum toward the earliest PP site. The relative activation times of the LDP, PP, and local ventricular potential at the LDP recording site to the onset of QRS complex are −50.4 ± 18.9, −15.2 ± 9.6, and 3.0 ± 13.3 milliseconds, respectively (see Fig. 24-3). The earliest ventricular activation site (exit) during VT is identified at the posteroapical septum and is more apical in the septum than the region with LDP.[3,4]

VENTRICULAR ACTIVATION SEQUENCE

During NSR, conduction propagates anterogradely (proximal to distal or basal to apical) and rapidly down the LPF, generating an anterograde PP followed by ventricular activation (see Fig. 24-1). In parallel, the impulse slowly conducts anterogradely over the abnormal Purkinje tissue, and such slow conduction, block in the proximal segment, or both allow the anterograde wavefront traveling rapidly over the LPF to conduct retrogradely up the slow pathway, resulting in fusion of delayed (late) ascending and descending potentials that follow or are buried in local ventricular depolarization, which likely represent the LDPs recorded during VT (see Fig. 24-4). Those late potentials have been found only in patients with idiopathic LV VT and not in control subjects, and have been recorded in the midinferior septum within or contiguous to the LPF.[3]

During ventricular pacing, the LPF is activated retrogradely, generating a retrograde PP. In parallel, the impulse produces bidirectional activation of the abnormal Purkinje pathway in a manner similar, but in reverse direction, to that during NSR.[2]

During VT, activation propagates anterogradely (from the basal to the apical site of the LV septum) over the abnormal Purkinje tissue, giving rise to an anterograde LDP; hence, the earliest LDP is seen in the basal septum and the latest LDP is seen in the apical septum. The reentrant wavefront then turns around in the lower third of the septum and activates the fast conduction Purkinje fibers along the LPF, generating a retrograde PP. Subsequently, the wavefront propagates anterogradely down the septum to exit the reentrant circuit and activate the posterior septal myocardium, and retrogradely over the LPF from apical to basal septum, forming the retrograde limb of the tachycardia, with an upper turnaround point of the reentrant wavefront occurring over a zone of slow conduction (between LDP and PP areas) located close to the main trunk of the LB (see Fig. 24-1).[3,5]

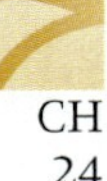

For a VES to initiate VT, retrograde block has to occur in the abnormal Purkinje tissue with retrograde conduction of the paced wavefront up the LPF (generating a retrograde PP) with some delay, and then down the abnormal Purkinje tissue (generating an anterograde LDP) to initiate reentry. Thus, during VT, the LDP precedes PP, which in turn precedes ventricular activation.

RESPONSE TO PHARMACOLOGICAL AND PHYSIOLOGICAL MANEUVERS

Intravenous verapamil slows the rate of VT progressively and then terminates it. Diltiazem is equally effective. Nonsustained VT may continue to occur for a while after termination. VT is usually rendered noninducible after verapamil. Verapamil significantly prolongs the VT CL, LDP-PP interval, and PP-LDP interval during VT. However, the interval from PP to the onset of the QRS complex remains unchanged.[3,7]

Response of VT to lidocaine, procainamide, amiodarone, sotalol, and propranolol is less consistent, and these drugs are usually ineffective. Carotid sinus massage and Valsalva maneuvers have no effect on the VT. Fascicular VT is generally unresponsive to adenosine; however, when catecholamine stimulation (isoproterenol infusion) is required for the initiation of VT, the VT can become adenosine-sensitive.

Diagnostic Maneuvers during Tachycardia

ENTRAINMENT

Ventricular pacing can entrain the VT with antidromic or orthodromic capture.[3] Manifest entrainment is more frequently achieved when pacing is performed from the right ventricular outflow tract (RVOT), because the RVOT is closer to the entrance site of the area of slow conduction in the reentrant circuit, located near the base of the LV septum. On the other hand, pacing from the RV apex is less likely to demonstrate entrainment and, when it does, it is unlikely to demonstrate manifest fusion because of the distance from the entrance site of the circuit and because of the narrow excitable gap of the reentrant circuit. During entrainment, the LDP (representing the entrance of the circuit) is orthodromically captured and, as the pacing rate is increased, the LDP-PP interval (representing an area of decremental Purkinje tissue) prolongs, whereas the stimulus-to-LDP and PP-QRS intervals typically remain constant. Entrainment can usually be demonstrated with ventricular pacing at a CL approximately 10 to 30 milliseconds shorter than the tachycardia CL.[2,3] Analysis of entrainment from different ventricular sites helps identify the relationship of those sites to the VT circuit (Table 24-1).

RESETTING

VT can be reset by VES, with an increasing or mixed resetting response (characteristic of reentrant circuit with an excitable gap).[3]

TERMINATION

VT can be reproducibly terminated with programmed electrical stimulation.[3]

Exclusion of Other Arrhythmia Mechanisms

The differential diagnosis of idiopathic LV VT should include interfascicular VT, which has several characteristic features: (1) bifascicular block QRS morphology during VT, which is identical to that during NSR; (2) reversal of activation sequence of the HB and LB during VT; and (3) spontaneous oscillations in the VT CL caused by changes in the LB-LB interval that precede and drive the VT CL. Interfascicular VT terminates with VES or RF ablation that produces block in LAF or LPF.

TABLE 24-1 Entrainment Mapping of Verapamil-Sensitive Left Ventricle Ventricular Tachycardia

Pacing from Sites Outside VT Circuit (RV Apex or RVOT)
• Manifest ventricular fusion on the surface ECG (fixed fusion at a single pacing CL and progressive fusion on progressively shorter pacing CLs) or fully paced QRS morphology • PPI – tachycardia CL >30 msec • Interval between stimulus artifact to onset of QRS on surface ECG is greater than the interval between local ventricular electrogram on pacing lead to onset of QRS on surface ECG
Pacing from Sites Inside VT Circuit (Posteroinferior LV Septum)
• Manifest ventricular fusion on the surface ECG (fixed fusion at a single pacing CL and progressive fusion on progressively shorter pacing CLs) • PPI – tachycardia CL <30 msec • Interval between stimulus artifact to onset of QRS on surface ECG equals the interval between local ventricular electrogram on pacing lead to onset of QRS on surface ECG (±20 msec)
Pacing from Protected Isthmus Inside VT Circuit (Site Where Both PP and LDP Are Recorded)
• Concealed ventricular fusion (i.e., paced QRS is identical to the VT QRS) • PPI – tachycardia CL <30 msec • Interval between stimulus artifact to onset of QRS on surface ECG equals the interval between PP to onset of QRS on surface ECG (±20 msec) • Stimulus-to-LDP interval is long and LDP is orthodromically captured from proximal to distal sites during activation

CL = cycle length; LDP = late diastolic potential; LV = left ventricle; PP = Purkinje potential; PPI = post-pacing interval; RV = right ventricle; RVOT = right ventricular outflow tract; VT = ventricular tachycardia.

When fascicular VT is associated with 1:1 ventriculoatrial (VA) conduction, and because of its responsiveness to verapamil and inducibility by atrial pacing, it can be misdiagnosed as supraventricular tachycardia (SVT) with bifascicular block aberrancy. The His bundle–ventricular (HV) interval during SVT with aberrancy is equal to or slightly longer than that during NSR. In contrast, the HV interval during fascicular VT is negative or shorter than that during NSR. Furthermore, the HB is activated in an anterograde direction during SVT but in a retrograde direction during fascicular VT.

Recently, VT originating from the LV papillary muscles in patients with or without prior myocardial infarction has been described. In contrast to fascicular VT, papillary muscle VT has a broader QRS complex (150 ± 15 milliseconds versus 127 ± 11 milliseconds). Additionally, all fascicular VTs, versus none of papillary muscle VTs, had an rsR′ pattern in lead V_1. An R/S ratio less than or equal to 1 in lead V_6 for VTs in the LV anterolateral region also suggests papillary muscle VT.[8] Furthermore, spontaneous variations in QRS morphology occur relatively frequently during VTs originating from the LV papillary muscles, a feature that can help distinguish these VTs from LV fascicular VT; the latter being a reentrant tachycardia with a consistent QRS morphology.[9-11]

Ablation

Target of Ablation

Definition of the appropriate ablation target has evolved with better understanding of the anatomical substrate of the VT. Initially, the ablation target site was defined as the site where the best pace map and the earliest endocardial ventricular activation time could be obtained during VT. Subsequently, in combination with pace mapping, the earliest PP potential preceding QRS onset during VT (considered to be the lower turnaround point of the reentrant circuit) in the posterior third of the LV septum was reported to be a marker for successful ablation. Successful ablation is achieved at sites where PP is recorded 30 to 40 milliseconds before QRS onset (Fig. 24-5). Entrainment mapping at this location helps confirm the relationship to the reentrant circuit. Of note, this area is located

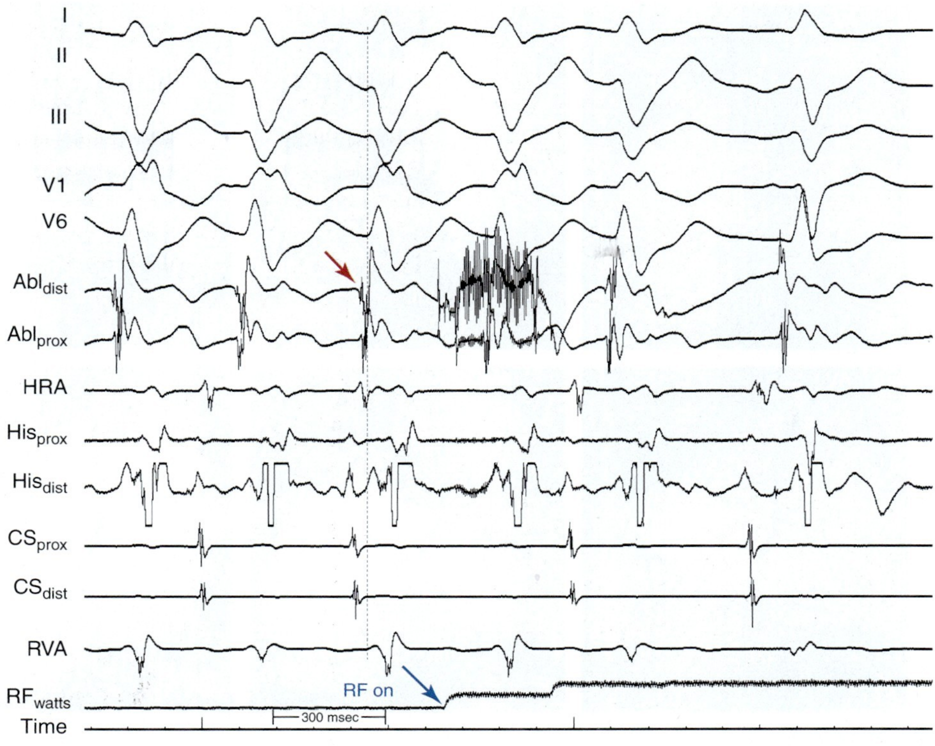

FIGURE 24-5 Ablation of idiopathic (fascicular) left ventricular tachycardia (LV VT). Radiofrequency (RF) delivery is begun (blue arrow) at the site of the diastolic Purkinje potential during idiopathic LV VT. Within less than 1 second, VT terminates. The red arrow indicates probable Purkinje potentials.

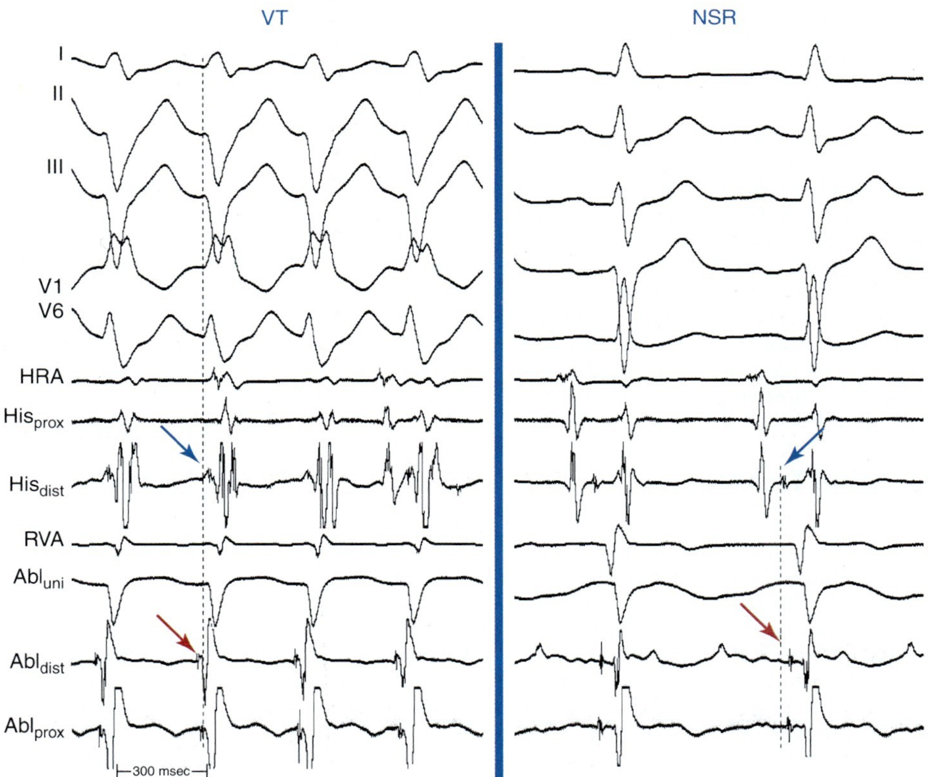

FIGURE 24-6 Ablation of idiopathic (fascicular) left ventricular tachycardia (LV VT). Shown are recordings during VT (left) and normal sinus rhythm (NSR; right) from a successful ablation site for idiopathic LV VT. Red arrows indicate probable Purkinje potentials, activated distal-to-proximal during VT and proximal-to-distal during sinus. Blue arrows show His potentials, occurring after QRS onset during VT.

more basally than the LV area that shows the earliest ventricular activation during VT (the exit point of the circuit into the ventricular septum), suggesting that the location of the earliest ventricular activation during tachycardia is not an ideal site for ablation of this arrhythmia.

Later on, the LDP recorded during VT, which likely reflects the excitation within the critical slow conduction area participating in the reentry circuit, was reported to be a useful marker in guiding successful ablation.[3,4]

Currently, ablation is targeted to a site over the middle or inferoapical portion of the LV septum where the earliest PP and LDP are recorded (Fig. 24-6). Verification of these sites can be achieved with entrainment mapping demonstrating concealed fusion and progressive prolongation of the LDP-PP interval with increasing

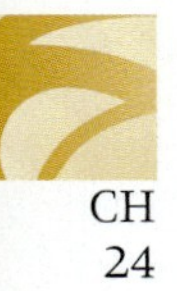

CH 24

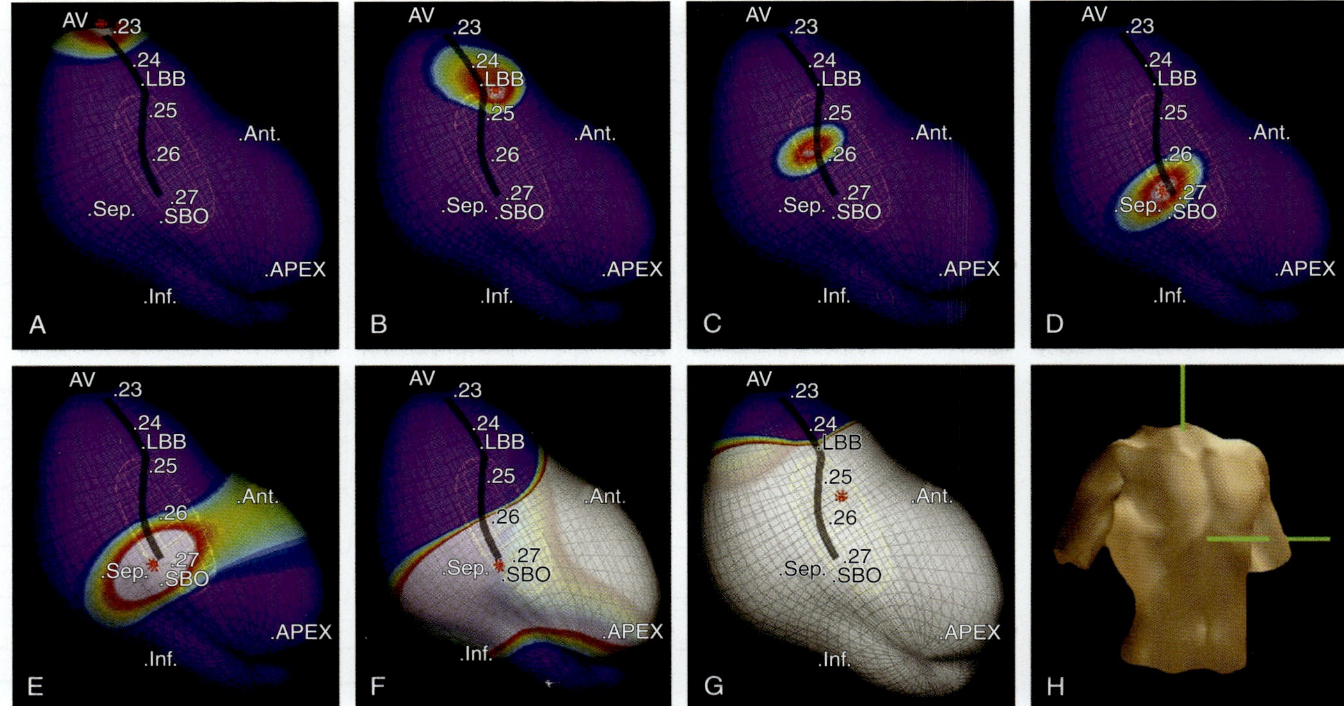

FIGURE 24-7 Noncontact mapping during normal sinus rhythm (NSR). Shown is an animated propagation map of the left ventricle (LV) from frames A to G in the right anterior oblique view during NSR. Note that the sinus activation propagates down from the His bundle (AV) to the left bundle branch (LBB), and then bifurcates into left anterior and left posterior fascicles before the entire LV is finally activated. The activation breakout point is at the midposterior septum and marked sinus breakout point (SBO) on the map. The thick black line indicates the propagation direction of the wavefronts from AV down to SBO. Ant = anterior; Inf = inferior; Sep = septal. *(From Chen M, Yang B, Zou J, et al: Non-contact mapping and linear ablation of the left posterior fascicle during sinus rhythm in the treatment of idiopathic left ventricular tachycardia, Europace 7:138, 2005.)*

pacing rate. In addition, pressure applied to the catheter tip at the LDP region occasionally results in VT termination with conduction block between LDP and PP. Pace mapping can also be used as an adjunct to verify this site, but because of poor sensitivity, is less helpful than in focal VTs.

It is important to recognize that successful ablation is not necessarily predicted by targeting the earliest (most proximal) LDP. Success can actually be achieved by ablating an LDP distal to the earliest potential. This approach helps reduce the risk of damaging the trunk of the LB. If such an LDP cannot be detected, the site with the earliest ventricular activation with a fused PP may then be targeted.[3]

Ablation Technique

It is helpful to initiate the VT reproducibly prior to entering the LV; if VT is not inducible, LV mapping may not be warranted. If VT can be readily initiated before but not after entering the LV, a portion of the circuit has probably been traumatized and one should wait several minutes and try to reinitiate before mapping any further.

Ablation is performed through the retrograde transaortic approach using a deflectable 4-mm-tip catheter. The catheter is advanced by prolapsing into the LV and directed to the LV septum. Mapping is initially concentrated at the inferoapical septum. If an ideal site is not found in this area, the ablation catheter is moved upward to the midseptal area. It is important to move the catheter slowly and carefully to avoid mechanical trauma to the circuit. Endocardial activation mapping and entrainment mapping are performed to define the target site of ablation.

Once the target site is identified, a test RF current is applied for 20 seconds with an initial power of 20 to 35 W, targeting a temperature of 60°C.[3,12] If the VT is terminated or slowed within 15 seconds, additional current is applied for another 60 to 120 seconds and power is increased up to 40 W to reach the target temperature if necessary. If the test RF current is ineffective despite adequate catheter contact, ablation should be directed to another site after additional mapping. This approach helps limit RF damage to the area of LPF and LB.

Successful ablation sites are often associated with progressive prolongation of the LDP-PP interval, with termination of VT coincident with conduction block between the two potentials.[3] Rarely, if ever, does one need more than 50 W or the use of irrigated or large-tip electrodes to ablate these VTs successfully. After successful ablation, the LDP appears after the QRS complex during sinus rhythm.

Endpoints of Ablation

Successful ablation is defined as the lack of inducibility of VT, with and without isoproterenol administration (using the best method for induction documented before ablation), at least 30 minutes after ablation.

Outcome

The acute success rate is more than 90%, even when different mapping methods are used. The recurrence rate is approximately 7% to 10%, with most recurrences occurring in the first 24 to 48 hours after the ablation procedure. Complications are rare and include different degrees of fascicular block, LBBB, cardiac tamponade, aortic regurgitation, and mitral regurgitation caused by torn chordae that may result from entrapment of the ablation catheter in a chorda of the mitral leaflet.[12]

Ablation of Noninducible Ventricular Tachycardia

Conventional activation mapping, guided by either the earliest PP or the LDP, although effective, depends on the inducibility and

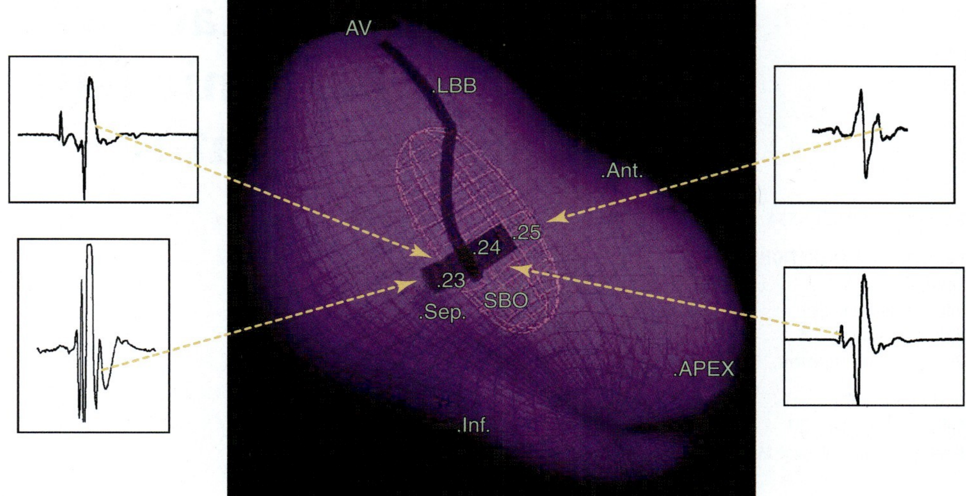

FIGURE 24-8 Noncontact mapping during normal sinus rhythm (NSR). A linear ablation lesion was created perpendicular to the wavefront propagation direction and 1 cm above the sinus breakout point (SBO). Both the starting and ending lesion points have a small Purkinje potential preceding the ventricular activation. Ant = anterior; AV = His recording area; Inf = inferior; LBB = left bundle branch; Sep = septal. *(From Chen M, Yang B, Zou J, et al: Non-contact mapping and linear ablation of the left posterior fascicle during sinus rhythm in the treatment of idiopathic left ventricular tachycardia, Europace 7:138, 2005.)*

endurance of fascicular VT. However, the VT may not be inducible in the EP laboratory. Additionally, the critical substrate of LV VT is amenable to mechanical injury because of catheter manipulation, which will render the tachycardia noninducible. In these cases, substrate mapping and ablation during NSR have been suggested to eradicate LV VT.

Two approaches have been used for substrate mapping during sinus rhythm: (1) ablation of the site where the earliest LDP is recorded during sinus rhythm (occurring 15 to 45 milliseconds after the PP). The PP-QRS interval at the successful ablation site with LDP is relatively short (mean, 13 ± 8 milliseconds); and (2) anatomical linear ablation to transect the involved middle to distal LPF and destroy the substrate of LV VT.[3,13]

The EnSite 3000 noncontact mapping system (St. Jude Medical, St. Paul, Minn.) has been used to identify the sinus breakout point (i.e., the LV site with the earliest local activation during NSR), and that point has been used to guide linear ablation perpendicular to the conduction direction of LPF.[13,14] Particular attention is paid to the geometric detail in the areas of the HB, septum, and apex of the LV. Once the ventricular geometry has been generated, the system can then calculate electrograms from more than 3000 endocardial points simultaneously by reconstructing far-field signals to create the isopotential map of sinus rhythm using a single cardiac cycle. The HB, LB, fascicles, and sinus breakout point are tagged as special landmarks in the geometry. The sinus breakout point is located in the midposterior septum and the local virtual electrogram presents with QS morphology (Fig. 24-7). Virtual electrograms at points from the HB down to the sinus breakout point show a sharp, low-amplitude potential preceding the ventricular potential. The interval between these two potentials becomes progressively shorter as the activation propagates from the HB to the sinus breakout point, until the two potentials finally fuse together at the sinus breakout point. Virtual electrograms recorded from the points placed in the pattern of block above the sinus breakout point show the whole Purkinje network in the LPF area. An ablation line is created perpendicular to the activation direction of LPF and 1 cm above the sinus breakout point (Fig. 24-8). A small Purkinje potential preceding the ventricular activation is observed at its starting and ending points (see Fig. 24-8). The mean length of the deployed line is usually 2.0 ± 0. 4 cm, requiring a mean of 5.5 ± 1.6 RF applications. A significant rightward shift of the QRS axis in the surface limb leads can be observed after the ablation procedure.[13,14]

REFERENCES

1. Nogami A: Idiopathic left ventricular tachycardia: assessment and treatment, *Card Electrophysiol Rev* 6:448–457, 2002.
2. Lerman BB: Ventricular tachycardia in patients with structurally normal hearts. In Zipes DP, Jalife J, editors: *Cardiac electrophysiology: from cell to bedside*, ed 5, Philadelphia, 2009, WB Saunders, pp 657–668.
3. Nogami A, Naito S, Tada H, et al: Demonstration of diastolic and presystolic Purkinje potentials as critical potentials in a macroreentry circuit of verapamil-sensitive idiopathic left ventricular tachycardia, *J Am Coll Cardiol* 36:811–823, 2000.
4. Tsuchiya T, Okumura K, Honda T, et al: Effects of verapamil and lidocaine on two components of the re-entry circuit of verapamil-sensitive idiopathic left ventricular tachycardia, *J Am Coll Cardiol* 37:1415–1421, 2001.
5. Ramprakash B, Jaishankar S, Rao HB, Narasimhan C: Catheter ablation of fascicular ventricular tachycardia, *Indian Pacing Electrophysiol J* 8:193–202, 2008.
6. Iwai S, Lerman BB: Management of ventricular tachycardia in patients with clinically normal hearts, *Curr Cardiol Rep* 2:515–521, 2000.
7. Wu D, Wen MS, Yeh SJ: Ablation of idiopathic left ventricular tachycardia. In Huang SKS, Wilber DJ, editors: *Radiofrequency catheter ablation of cardiac arrhythmias: basic concepts and clinical applications*, ed 2, Armonk, NY, 2000, Futura, pp 601–620.
8. Yamada T, McElderry HT, Doppalapudi H, et al: Idiopathic ventricular arrhythmias originating from the aortic root prevalence, electrocardiographic and electrophysiologic characteristics, and results of radiofrequency catheter ablation, *J Am Coll Cardiol* 52:139–147, 2008.
9. Yamada T, Doppalapudi H, McElderry HT, et al: Electrocardiographic and electrophysiological characteristics in idiopathic ventricular arrhythmias originating from the papillary muscles in the left ventricle: relevance for catheter ablation, *Circ Arrhythm Electrophysiol* 3:324–331, 2010.
10. Bogun F, Desjardins B, Crawford T, et al: Post-infarction ventricular arrhythmias originating in papillary muscles, *J Am Coll Cardiol* 51:1794–1802, 2008.
11. Good E, Desjardins B, Jongnarangsin K, et al: Ventricular arrhythmias originating from a papillary muscle in patients without prior infarction: a comparison with fascicular arrhythmias, *Heart Rhythm* 5:1530–1537, 2008.
12. Li D, Guo J, Xu Y, Li X: The surface electrocardiographic changes after radiofrequency catheter ablation in patients with idiopathic left ventricular tachycardia, *Int J Clin Pract* 58:11–18, 2004.
13. Chen M, Yang B, Zou J, et al: Non-contact mapping and linear ablation of the left posterior fascicle during sinus rhythm in the treatment of idiopathic left ventricular tachycardia, *Europace* 7:138–144, 2005.
14. Friedman PA, Asirvatham SJ, Grice S, et al: Noncontact mapping to guide ablation of right ventricular outflow tract tachycardia, *J Am Coll Cardiol* 39:1808–1812, 2002.

CHAPTER 25 Ventricular Tachycardia in Nonischemic Dilated Cardiomyopathy

Pathophysiology

Cardiomyopathies are traditionally defined on the basis of structural and functional phenotypes, notably dilated, hypertrophic, and restrictive. The dilated cardiomyopathy (CMP) phenotype is the most common and is often viewed as a "final common pathway" of numerous types of cardiac injuries.

The diagnosis of nonischemic dilated CMP is established by the absence of significant (>75% stenosis) coronary artery disease and prior myocardial infarction (MI). Nonischemic dilated CMP is not a single disease entity. Valvular heart disease, hypertension, sarcoidosis, amyloidosis, Chagas disease, alcohol abuse, infections, and pregnancy, among others, need to be considered as possible etiologies. An underlying etiology for adult dilated CMP is found in only 50% of patients. The remaining 50% are considered idiopathic. Idiopathic dilated CMP is characterized by an increase in myocardial mass and a reduction in ventricular wall thickness. The heart assumes a globular shape, and there is a pronounced ventricular chamber dilation and atrial enlargement.[1]

There is increasing evidence that a significant portion (35%) of idiopathic dilated CMP is secondary to familial forms of dilated CMP. Familial dilated CMP is clinically and genetically heterogeneous and it exhibits various patterns of hereditary transmission, including autosomal dominant with variable penetrance (most common, accounting for about 90% of cases), X-linked (5% to 10%), autosomal recessive (rare), and maternal transmission through mitochondrial DNA (rare).

To date, 33 genes have been linked to nonsyndromic familial dilated CMP. Notably, the frequencies of dilated CMP mutations in any one gene are low (<1% to 8%), and a genetic cause is identified in only 30% to 35% of familial dilated CMP cases. Although usually nonsyndromic, dilated CMP can be included in syndromic disease involving various organ systems, most commonly skeletal muscle disease (muscular dystrophy).[2]

Mutations in the genes responsible for sarcomere and cytoskeletal protein synthesis have been identified as the cause of familial dilated CMP, and several hypotheses have been put forward to explain the etiology and pathology of the disease. Several gene mutations have been identified in the autosomal form of familial dilated CMP, including those encoding Z-disc proteins (alpha-actin-2, muscle LIM protein, titin-cap), costameres, adherens junctions, desmosomes, intermediate filaments, sarcomere proteins (cardiac alpha-actin, beta-myosin heavy chain, cardiac troponin T, alpha-tropomyosin, titin), sarcoplasmic reticulum proteins (phospho-lamban), and ion channel (SUR2A). Of note, different mutations in the sarcomere genes can cause hypertrophic CMP. Mutations in lamin A/C also cause Emery-Dreifuss muscular dystrophy. Autosomal dominant dilated CMP can exhibit either a pure CMP phenotype or dilated CMP with cardiac conduction system disease. X-linked familial CMP is usually caused by defects in the dystrophin gene and is typically associated with skeletal muscle involvement (Duchenne and Becker muscular dystrophy). The infantile form of X-linked dilated CMP or Barth syndrome typically affects male infants (characterized by neutropenia and growth retardation).

As compared with sporadic cases of idiopathic dilated CMP, familial CMP patients are younger and tend to have higher left ventricular ejection fraction (LVEF) and more significant myocardial fibrosis. In patients with idiopathic dilated CMP, the proposed diagnostic criteria for the familial form of the disease are the existence of two or more affected family members, or of one first-degree relative with a documented history of unexplained sudden death before 35 years of age. In most cases, proof of a genetic cause of a CMP has a limited impact on the treatment of the index patient, but can have important implications in regard to family screening and genetic counseling. Dilated CMP in patients who do not have a known family history may also have a genetic basis.[3]

In contrast to ischemic heart disease, the electrophysiological (EP) substrate for sustained monomorphic ventricular tachycardia (VT) in patients with nonischemic dilated CMP is not clearly defined. Although bundle branch reentry (BBR) VT is identified as the VT mechanism in a significant percentage of patients with monomorphic VT in the setting of nonischemic CMP, the majority (80%) of VTs appear to originate from the myocardium and are due to scar-related reentry rather than BBR.[4] BBR VT is discussed separately in Chapter 26.

On the other hand, premature ventricular complexes (PVCs) and nonsustained VTs induced by programmed electrical stimulation or occurring spontaneously in patients with end-stage idiopathic dilated CMP initiate primarily in the subendocardium by a focal mechanism without evidence of macroreentry. The nature of the focal mechanism remains unknown; triggered activity arising from early or delayed afterdepolarizations seems to be more likely than microreentry.

Myocardial fibrosis, myocyte disarray, and membrane abnormalities are important factors in the substrate causing VT in patients with dilated CMP. Sustained VT is associated with more extensive myocardial fibrosis and nonuniform anisotropy involving both the endocardium and epicardium, compared with patients without sustained reentry. The reentry circuits are typically associated with regions of low-voltage electrograms, consistent with scar. Catheter mapping studies of patients with nonischemic CMP point to reentry around scar deep in the myocardium, near the ventricular base and in the perivalvular region, as the underlying mechanism for VT.

Studies of explanted hearts with dilated nonischemic CMP have found inexcitable fibrosis creating regions of conduction block and surviving myocardium providing the substrate for potential reentry circuits. Slow conduction through muscle bundles separated by interstitial fibrosis can cause a zigzag path and promote reentry. Furthermore, patients with nonischemic CMP and predominance of scar distribution involving 26% to 75% of wall thickness (as quantified by magnetic resonance [MR] imaging) are more likely to have inducible VT. Delayed-enhancement MR imaging typically reveals nontransmural scar areas often distributed in the basal portion of the ventricular free wall or basal to midportion of the septum. Sustained VTs are observed more frequently in patients having a greater volume of hyperenhanced areas and greater number of hyperenhanced segments, and nontransmural scar tissue was present at the VT circuit exit site in the majority of patients.[5,6]

The cause of fibrosis in CMP is not well defined. Scattered regions of replacement fibrosis are commonly seen at autopsy, but confluent regions of scar are not common. The unique propensity for abnormal basal endocardial voltage and VT site of origin in patients with nonischemic CMP remains unexplained. Low-voltage areas have also been observed during electroanatomical mapping in patients with focal VT and BBR VT, although the scar areas appeared to be smaller.

The scar and fibrosis resulting from nonischemic etiologies are distinctly different from post-MI scar; hence, the reentrant circuit may have different anatomical and functional properties that affect propagation. Compared with post-MI VT, the scar tends to be smaller and less confluent, the total number of the transmural scar segments is significantly smaller, and with less endocardial involvement in nonischemic CMP.[4] Whereas ischemia produces a predictable wavefront of necrosis progressing from subendocardium to epicardium (and scar areas larger endocardially than epicardially), usually confined to a specific coronary vascular territory, scars in nonischemic CMP have been shown to have a predilection for the midmyocardium and epicardium. In contrast to the dense scar with isolated surviving myocardial bundles, scar in nonischemic CMP is patchy and may have fewer fixed boundaries and protected channels or isthmuses, which can alter the extent of local conduction slowing.[7]

Nonetheless, several similarities of the arrhythmia substrate exist in myocardial reentry VT in patients with dilated nonischemic CMP compared with that in patients with previous MI. Low-voltage areas are observed in all patients, and the regions of scar are frequently adjacent to a valve annulus, as is often the case in VT after inferior wall MI. The annulus often seems to form a border for an isthmus in the reentry path, which suggests the formation of a long channel, or isthmus, along an annulus contributing to the formation of reentry circuits that can support VT.

Clinical Considerations

Epidemiology

The incidence of nonischemic dilated CMP in adults in Western countries varies from 5 to 8 per 100,000 person-years, with a prevalence of 36 to 40 per 100,000 individuals. The 5-year mortality for dilated CMP has been estimated at 20%, with sudden cardiac death (SCD) accounting for approximately 30% (8% to 51%) of deaths. Nonetheless, nonischemic dilated CMP patients may represent a low arrhythmic death risk subgroup among all CMP patients.

Ventricular arrhythmias, both symptomatic and asymptomatic, are common in patients with nonischemic dilated CMP. Nonsustained VT can be observed in 30% to 50% of patients, but its incidence decreases significantly after optimization of medical treatment.[8] However, syncope and SCD are infrequent initial manifestations of the disease. The incidence of SCD is highest among patients with indicators of more advanced cardiac disease who are also at highest risk of all-cause mortality. Although VT, ventricular fibrillation (VF), or both are considered the most common mechanism of SCD, bradycardia, pulmonary embolism, electromechanical dissociation, and other causes account for up to 50% of SCDs in patients with advanced heart failure.

Initial Evaluation

Transthoracic echocardiography is the usual modality for diagnosis of dilated CMP. Cardiac stress testing, coronary angiography, or both are typically performed in patients with coronary risk factors. Ambulatory cardiac monitoring is required for patients with symptoms suggestive of arrhythmias, but not for screening purposes. Cardiac MR is a useful tool for detecting and assessing the characteristics and heterogeneous distribution of scar tissue in its composition of the wall layer, as well as its precise location within the ventricle. The location of scar tissue often corresponds to areas critical for VT circuits in these patients. Unfortunately, most patients presenting with appropriate implantable cardioverter-defibrillator (ICD) shocks currently cannot undergo MR imaging because of the device. New ICD technology will eliminate that restriction in the future.

Risk Stratification

Risk stratification is difficult in dilated CMP. Although SCD occurs less frequently in patients with less advanced cardiac disease, the proportion of SCD to all-cause death is higher in this group.

Predictors of overall outcome (such as LVEF, end-diastolic LV volume, older age, hyponatremia, pulmonary capillary wedge pressure, systemic hypotension, atrial fibrillation) also predict SCD and generally reflect severity of disease. Unfortunately, they do not specifically predict arrhythmic death and are not useful in the patient with less severe disease.

LVEF has remained the most studied and the most powerful predictor and is the primary method currently used in clinical decisions for the prevention of SCD in patients with heart failure. Depressed LVEF is also a powerful predictor of cardiac mortality. On the basis of the results of large clinical trials, in clinical practice an LVEF of 35% or less has become the primary criterion used for prophylactic ICD placement. The use of LVEF as the predominant risk stratifier has serious limitations, however, because LVEF lacks sensitivity for prediction of SCD. Even a low LVEF (<20%) may not have high positive predictive value for SCD. Clinical factors such as functional class, history of heart failure, nonsustained VT, age, LV conduction abnormalities, inducible sustained VT, and atrial fibrillation influence arrhythmic death and total mortality risk and, consequently, potentially influence the prognostic value of a depressed LVEF. Therefore, patients with an LVEF greater than 30% and other risk factors may have a higher mortality and a higher risk of SCD than those with an LVEF less than 30% but no other risk factors.[9]

Syncope has been associated with a higher risk of SCD regardless of the proven etiology of the syncope, and ICD recipients with syncope receive appropriate shocks at a rate comparable to a secondary prevention cohort.

PVCs and nonsustained VT correlate with the severity of cardiac disease and occur in the majority of patients with severe LV dysfunction. This limits the usefulness of ventricular arrhythmias as risk stratifiers as they would be expected to be sensitive but not specific. Additionally, the presence and characteristics (frequency, length, and rate) of nonsustained VT do not appear to predict increased risk of subsequent life-threatening ventricular arrhythmias in patients with severe LV impairment receiving optimal medical treatment. Nevertheless, it has been suggested that the presence of nonsustained VT may be more specific in the individual with better LV systolic function. Nonsustained VT significantly increases the risk of malignant ventricular arrhythmias in the subgroup with an LVEF greater than 35%. In these patients, even without worsening LV systolic function and symptoms, survival free from malignant ventricular arrhythmias is similar to that of patients with an LVEF less than 35% with or without nonsustained VT.[8]

Cardiac MR can be used to evaluate the presence and magnitude of nontransmural scar tissue. Patients with nonischemic CMP and sustained VT typically have a greater volume and number of hyperenhanced (scar) areas compared with those without sustained VT.[5]

Patients typically have wide QRS complexes during the baseline rhythm, often with left bundle branch block or a nonspecific intraventricular conduction defect. Prolonged QRS duration has been associated with increased mortality in heart failure patients, but association with SCD has not been proven. Recently, fragmentation of the QRS complex on the 12-lead surface electrocardiogram (ECG) (filter range, 0.15 to 100 Hz; AC filter, 60 Hz, 25 mm/sec, 10 mm/mV) has been found to potentially predict increased risk of appropriate ICD therapies as well as a higher combined endpoint of ICD therapy and mortality in nonischemic CMP patients who received an ICD for primary and secondary prevention. The usefulness of this parameter needs further evaluation.[10] During VT, QRS complexes are typically very wide and fragmented; most patients have multiple QRS morphologies of VT (Fig. 25-1).[11]

Prolongation of the QT interval, QT dispersion, and QT variability have had mixed predictive results with limited clinical applicability at present. Furthermore, studies evaluating the association of abnormal heart rate turbulence and reduced heart rate variability and SCD in heart failure patients have had conflicting results.[9]

Microvolt T-wave alternans has relatively modest (0.22) positive predictive value for SCD in patients with dilated CMP. Previous studies suggested a high negative predictive value for primary prevention of SCD, and T-wave alternans was hypothesized to be a useful tool to differentiate between patients who would benefit from ICD implantation and those who would not. However, results from recent studies failed to support this hypothesis and strongly suggested that a negative microvolt T-wave alternans result should not be used to withhold ICD therapy among patients who meet standard criteria.[9]

EP testing plays a minor role in risk stratification because of low VT inducibility, low reproducibility, and poor predictive value of induced VT. Although induction of VT by EP testing has been shown to predict SCD, unfortunately failure to induce VT misses most individuals destined to die suddenly.[1]

Principles of Management

PHARMACOLOGICAL THERAPY

Drug therapy, such as beta blockers and angiotensin-converting enzyme inhibitors, improves overall mortality in patients with heart failure and reduces the risk of SCD. In contrast, the use of antiarrhythmic drugs for primary prevention in patients with nonischemic CMP does not improve survival and is not recommended.[1]

In patients with symptomatic ventricular arrhythmias, amiodarone is generally the preferred antiarrhythmic agent because of the absence of significant negative hemodynamic effects and low proarrhythmic potential, although controlled comparative trials of drugs are not available. Antiarrhythmic drug therapy can help improve quality of life in ICD patients receiving frequent appropriate shocks. Although amiodarone can potentially improve mortality and reduce the incidence of SCD in patients with nonischemic dilated CMP, it is inferior to ICD therapy for secondary prevention of VT and VF.[1,12]

IMPLANTABLE CARDIOVERTER-DEFIBRILLATOR

The benefit of ICD therapy in secondary prevention of SCD in nonischemic dilated CMP has been well established and is superior to amiodarone or any other drug therapy. ICD implantation is recommended in patients with prior cardiac arrest or sustained VT, even in those undergoing catheter ablation of the VT or responding to antiarrhythmic therapy.

On the other hand, the benefit of ICD treatment for primary prevention of nonischemic CMP is still uncertain. Whereas prophylactic ICD implantation is of significant benefit in ischemic CMP patients, the magnitude of absolute benefit in nonischemic CMP patients is relatively small (1.4% per year; cumulative, 7% over 5 years), but there is a relative risk reduction of 23%, as nonischemic CMP patients have a better prognosis and a lower mortality rate than patients with ischemic CMP.

Vigorous efforts have been made in developing noninvasive stratification methods to identify the subgroup of nonischemic CMP patients at high risk for SCD. However, the best approach to

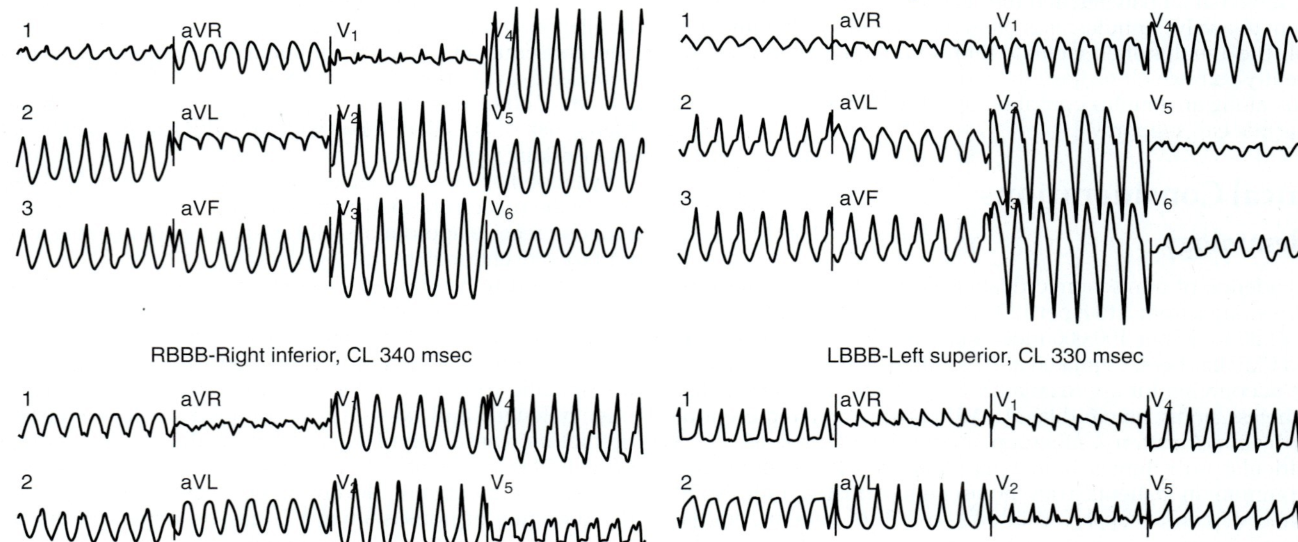

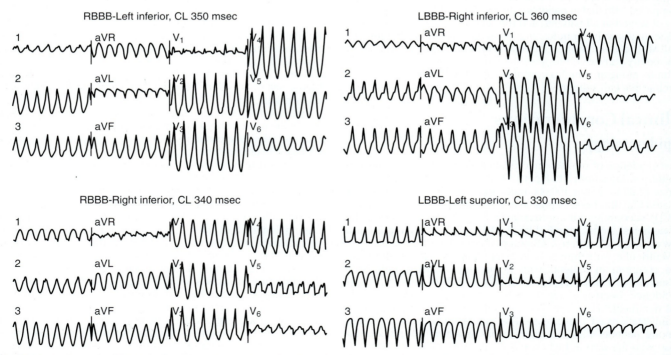

FIGURE 25-1 Surface 12-lead ECGs of different ventricular tachycardia (VT) configurations in a patient with dilated cardiomyopathy. VTs were mapped to sites on the anteroapical, anterobasal, and inferobasal septum. CL = cycle length; LBBB = left bundle branch block; RBBB = right bundle branch block.

identifying patients and the value of various risk stratification tools are not entirely clear. Currently, there is no coherent strategy for intervention based on data integrating the results of these techniques. Many of the identified risk factors are also associated with increased risk for nonsudden death. At the present time, LVEF remains the single most important risk stratification tool to identify individuals with a high risk of SCD, again emphasizing that it predicts all-cause mortality and not necessarily arrhythmic risk. Despite some uncertainty regarding ICD benefit for nonischemic CMP patients without heart failure, regardless of LVEF, the cumulative information available from clinical trials and observational data, in conjunction with opinions of experts in the field, supports prophylactic ICD therapy among the subgroup of patients with nonischemic CMP and LVEF less than 35% who remain in NYHA functional class II or III heart failure on optimal medical therapy.[12]

The appropriate timing to perform ICD implantation in dilated CMP is still controversial. It is important to understand that medical management with angiotensin-converting enzyme inhibitors and beta blockers with or without aldosterone antagonists has proven mortality benefit in these patients and should be optimized as much as possible before ICD placement. Many patients significantly improve their clinical status, and may be excluded as candidates for an ICD after optimization of medical treatment. The most recent European Society of Cardiology (ESC)/American College of Cardiology (ACC)/American Heart Association (AHA) guidelines suggest ICD implantation for primary prevention only in patients with dilated CMP receiving chronic optimal medical therapy. How long it takes to reach optimal medical treatment can be debatable.[8]

CATHETER ABLATION

The most common indication for catheter ablation of VT in patients with nonischemic CMP is frequent ICD discharges (or electrical storm) that are refractory to antiarrhythmic drug therapy. However, because of the future risk of life-threatening VT due to progression of the myopathic process, catheter ablation is not a substitute for an ICD, even when excellent short-term results are achieved.

Additionally, some investigators have suggested consideration of catheter ablation as a therapeutic option in conjunction with ICD implantation in patients with nonischemic CMP who present with a first documented episode of sustained monomorphic VT, with the goal of avoiding future ICD shocks.

Mapping

After exclusion of BBR, mapping of sustained VT in nonischemic CMP employs the approaches for scar-related VT (see Chap. 22). QRS morphology during VT can be used to regionalize the site of origin of the VT. Endocardial activation mapping is performed in patients with stable VTs. Most VTs are localized to the area around the mitral annulus. Entrainment and pace mapping are used to define the relationship of different endocardial sites to the circuit of the VT. Furthermore, the relationship of reentry circuits to regions of scar supports the feasibility of a substrate mapping approach, targeting the abnormal area based on voltage mapping during sinus rhythm, to guide ablation of unstable VT, similar to that described for patients with post-MI VT.

Substrate Mapping

Patients with nonischemic CMP frequently have VTs that are unstable or unsustainable and therefore not approachable by conventional entrainment maneuvers and point-by-point activation mapping. Therefore, mapping during the baseline rhythm (substrate mapping) rather than during VT is of significant value. *Substrate mapping* refers to delineation of the VT substrate based on the identification of abnormal local electrogram configuration (fractionated electrograms, multipotential electrograms, and/or electrograms with isolated delayed components) and the identification of abnormal local electrogram amplitude during sinus rhythm (voltage mapping). Substrate mapping is also of value in ablation of stable VTs, because it can help focus activation-entrainment mapping efforts on a small region harboring the VT substrate, and therefore help minimize how long the patient is actually in VT.[4]

Isolated potentials during sinus rhythm likely reflect fixed scar tissue. Although large areas of scar are uncommon in patients with nonischemic CMP, extensive interstitial fibrosis is frequently seen histologically. Strands of fibrous tissue may serve as electrical barriers and result in electrogram fragmentation. Isolated potentials can be identified in many, but not all, patients with nonischemic CMP. Additionally, isolated potentials are not present to the same extent in all forms of nonischemic CMP. They could be identified in all patients with ARVD and most patients with cardiac sarcoidosis but not in all patients with idiopathic dilated CMP. Patients in whom isolated potentials can be identified at critical ablation sites appear to have a better short- and mid-term prognosis after catheter ablation than patients in whom the arrhythmogenic substrate is not characterized by isolated potentials.[8]

Electroanatomical Voltage Mapping

Voltage mapping during sinus rhythm (or ventricular pacing) in patients with nonischemic CMP typically demonstrates a modest-sized area of endocardial electrogram abnormalities (ranging from 6% to 48% of the LV endocardial surface, but uncommonly involving more than 25% of the total endocardial surface area) located near the ventricular base, frequently surrounding the aortic and mitral valve region and then extending apically. The amount of dense scar (<0.5 mV) accounts for approximately 27% ± 20% (range, 0% to 64%) of the overall abnormal low-voltage endocardial substrate. The exit site of a VT circuit corresponds to these basal electrogram abnormalities. Therefore, voltage mapping during sinus rhythm can be used to guide further mapping techniques (entrainment and pace mapping) and also to guide ablation lesions (especially in patients with unmappable VTs).

Frequently, the VT substrate may be solely or predominantly intramural or epicardial. Because of the frequent presence of an epicardial substrate, some experienced operators use a simultaneous endocardial and epicardial mapping approach.[13]

Activation Mapping

After construction of an endocardial voltage map during the baseline rhythm, VT is induced by programmed ventricular stimulation. The average number of induced VT morphologies is 3 ± 1 per patient, with a range of one to six VTs. Because surface ECG documentation of the presenting arrhythmia is often not available, clinical versus nonclinical VT is difficult to define with certainty. Mapping is therefore directed at all sustained monomorphic VTs induced by programmed stimulation. For hemodynamically tolerated sustained VT, activation mapping is performed to identify sites with early presystolic or mid-diastolic activity (Fig. 25-2).[14]

Entrainment Mapping

Entrainment can be demonstrated in most patients with sustained monomorphic VT. The critical isthmus for hemodynamically tolerated VT is defined as the site of entrainment with concealed fusion and a return cycle length equal to the VT cycle length (see Fig. 25-2). For unstable VT, limited entrainment mapping can be feasible with brief induction and termination of the tachycardia.[14]

Pace Mapping

Pace mapping has been shown to be an effective corroborative method to regionalize the VT circuit and define potential exit sites along the border zone of any low-voltage region. Pace mapping with the paced QRS morphology mimicking that of VT on the 12-lead ECG can help identify the exit site of the VT circuit.

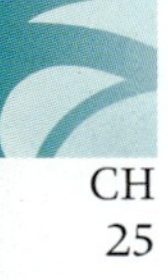

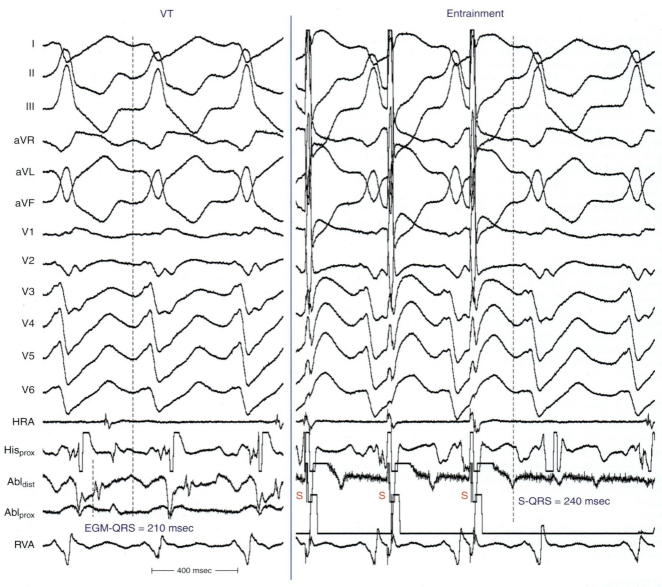

FIGURE 25-2 Entrainment mapping of ventricular tachycardia (VT) in dilated nonischemic cardiomyopathy. VT is shown at left, with the ablation catheter at a site with an early diastolic recording; entrainment at this site has a stimulus-QRS interval similar to that of the electrogram-QRS during VT, with a perfect pace match. Ablation at this site eliminated VT.

Additionally, pace mapping can identify regions of slow conduction with a stimulus-QRS interval (S-QRS) greater than 40 milliseconds and a pace map match consistent with the exit region from an isthmus. For the unmappable VT (because of hemodynamic intolerance, inconsistent induction, altering QRS morphology, and/or nonsustained duration), pace mapping is the predominant mapping technique and is directed to the scar border zone as defined by voltage mapping.[14]

Epicardial Mapping

When endocardial mapping and ablation fail, the epicardial approach should be considered. Mapping is initially attempted within the coronary venous system, and if no suitable ablation sites are identified, mapping within the pericardial space is then performed. However, if there are clues on the ECG that suggest an epicardial VT or if there is documentation by MR imaging of largely epicardial scar, performing percutaneous epicardial mapping as the first step (before the administration of heparin) may be considered.[15]

The importance of epicardial reentry circuits in CMP has been demonstrated for patients with Chagas disease and, more recently, for patients with dilated CMP unrelated to Chagas disease (see Fig. 27-1). In fact, the epicardial approach may be required in about 30% of patients with nonischemic CMP and VT.[15] Percutaneous epicardial ablation of VT can be guided by activation, entrainment, and pace mapping (see Chap. 27).

Ablation

For patients with mappable VTs, focal ablation targets the critical isthmus of the reentrant circuit as defined by activation, entrainment, and pace mapping techniques. For unmappable VTs, linear ablation lesions are guided by substrate mapping and pace mapping in the scar border zone. Linear lesions are created in regions that cross the border zone and intersect the best pace map site, which approximates the exit site of the VT circuit, similar to strategies described for unmappable post-MI VT (see Chap. 22).

An irrigated-tip ablation catheter is preferred for ablation because it can create larger lesions and also can be used for radiofrequency (RF) energy delivery within the coronary venous system if needed. The power setting is adjusted to an impedance drop of 10 Ω starting with 30 to 35 W. If RF energy is applied during VT, it is applied for 30 seconds and, if VT does not terminate, the catheter is moved to an alternate site. If VT terminates during the energy application, the application is continued for a total of 120 milliseconds. In the setting of nontolerated VTs, RF energy is delivered for 60 to 120 milliseconds at each site to create ablation lines as guided by substrate mapping.[15]

The endpoint of the procedure is noninducibility of all the VTs for which an appropriate target site can be identified. Induction of multiple VTs is not uncommon in patients with dilated CMP. Whether targeting all inducible VTs is superior to targeting only the VTs that have been clinically documented is still unclear.[15]

There are only a few single-center reports on acute outcome of VT ablation in the setting of nonischemic CMP, with short- to intermediate-term follow-up in relatively small numbers of patients. Acute success in eliminating inducible VT has varied from 56% to 74% with VT recurrence of 42% to 75% with endocardial ablation. Satisfactory control of VTs previously refractory to medical treatment can be achieved in a majority of patients (60% to 70%) with continuing antiarrhythmic medications, if tolerated. Outcome appears to be somewhat improved with epicardial ablation, but long-term follow-up in a large cohort of patients is lacking.[13,15]

The success of endocardial ablation of VTs associated with nonischemic CMP is lower than that observed for post-MI VTs. Reentry circuits deep to the endocardium and in the epicardium appear to be a likely explanation. Combined endocardial and epicardial mapping approaches are likely to improve the success of ablation.[7]

Less than 5% of patients have major complications, such as cardiac tamponade, thromboembolic events, or death. Electromechanical dissociation after multiple VT inductions can occur in patients with very low ejection fractions. Limiting the number of inductions of VT may help to prevent this life-threatening complication.[15]

Sarcoid Cardiomyopathy

Pathophysiology

Sarcoidosis is an inflammatory noncaseating (nonnecrotizing) granulomatous disease characterized histologically by epithelioid cells and multinucleated giant cells. It is thought to represent a T cell–mediated immune process, but the etiology remains unknown. The main organ systems involved by sarcoidosis are the lungs and thoracic lymph nodes, although virtually no organ systems are spared, including the central nervous system and the skin. Clinical cardiac involvement occurs in approximately 4% to 5% of patients, whereas at autopsy 20% to 25% are found to have some cardiac involvement. Importantly, pulmonary involvement may be minimal or even clinically absent; extensive cardiac sarcoid may be present as the only disease manifestation.

Cardiac sarcoidosis is an infiltrative disease and has a predilection for involving the base of the interventricular septum and cardiac conduction system. Patients can develop various degrees of heart block and tachyarrhythmias. A dilated CMP can occur, with the LV and the interventricular septum primarily involved. Two patterns of regional wall motion abnormalities are frequently observed, involving the basal free wall and the anteroapical septum. Mitral valve abnormalities, papillary muscle dysfunction, LV aneurysm formation, and pericardial effusions are also seen. Cor pulmonale can develop due to chronic pulmonary fibrotic disease.

The inflammatory process in cardiac sarcoidosis often is initiated in the myocardium, creating lesions (granulomas) that then extend to the epicardium, endocardium, or both. Inflammation and fibrosis participate in ventricular arrhythmogenesis, one of the hallmarks of cardiac sarcoidosis. Surviving muscle bundles within scar tissue most likely form the substrate for reentry.[16]

Multiple, monomorphic VTs, which are common in cardiac sarcoidosis, are predominantly due to a scar-related, reentrant mechanism. Low-amplitude and fragmented potentials are recorded both in the endocardial and epicardial regions of both ventricles. The presence of isolated potentials during sinus rhythm at most effective ablation sites suggests that a process similar to post-MI VT is responsible for VTs in patients with cardiac sarcoidosis. The most common site of VT circuit is the peritricuspid area, which is consistent with the predominance of basal involvement of the right ventricular septum in cardiac sarcoidosis. The disease process can be located intramurally and may be reachable by neither the endocardial nor the epicardial approach.[13,16]

Clinical Considerations

Determining cardiac involvement in patients with sarcoidosis is difficult because granulomas may be present without clinical dysfunction. Patients with cardiac sarcoidosis can present with congestive heart failure, atrioventricular block, supraventricular arrhythmia, and/or ventricular tachyarrhythmia. Importantly, cardiac involvement of sarcoidosis is associated with a mortality rate greater than 40% at 5 years, and many of the deaths are caused by ventricular tachyarrhythmias. Approximately 50% of patients with cardiac sarcoidosis require treatment for ventricular arrhythmias. These patients usually have multiple monomorphic VTs, with either left or right bundle branch block morphology. Arrhythmias can be refractory to a combination of steroids and antiarrhythmic drugs in almost half of the patients. ICD implantation is the mainstay therapy in these patients. Nonetheless, RF catheter ablation as an adjunct therapy to ICD can be effective in eliminating VT or in markedly reducing the VT burden, with success rates in a recently reported registry ranging from 25% to 70%, depending on the location of the reentrant circuit.[13,16]

EP testing can potentially provide prognostic information in asymptomatic patients with cardiac sarcoidosis. VT inducibility may help to identify those at risk for ventricular arrhythmia. A negative EP study appears to predict a benign course within the first several years after diagnosis. More studies are needed to guide prophylactic ICD therapy in this population.[17]

For cardiac sarcoidosis, cardiac biopsy is one of the few ways to confirm the diagnosis, although cardiac MR imaging with delayed enhancement can sometimes detect the granular cells, which resemble clumps of sand or salt grains, and help to regionalize the disease process and indicate whether scarring is located intramurally, epicardially, endocardially, or transmurally.[18] About one-third of the patients with cardiac sarcoidosis have detectable abnormalities visible in an echocardiogram.[16]

Chagas Cardiomyopathy

Pathophysiology

Chagas disease is an endemic disease in Latin America caused by a unicellular parasite, *Trypanosoma cruzi*. Almost 18 million people are infected and almost 25% of them will develop chronic myocardial disease in the following years or decades.[19]

Chronic Chagas heart disease, the most serious manifestation of Chagas disease, is an inflammatory form of dilated CMP. The panmyocarditis of Chagas heart disease progressively involves the various cardiac tissues and results in extensive cardiac fibrosis. When the extent of myocardial damage is severe, the disease manifests as myocardial dysfunction that may be segmental, typically a ventricular aneurysm, or global, resembling a dilated CMP.[19,20]

Myocardial damage can occur in various areas of both ventricles, but the inferolateral segment of the LV is the most commonly involved site, with frequently observed wall motion abnormalities. Apical, septal, and apical inferior aneurysms have also been described. The classic lesion of Chagas disease is a localized aneurysm of the LV apex, with relatively normal surrounding wall motion. This results in a narrow neck when visualized by echocardiography or ventriculography; when present, this can usually distinguish an aneurysm of Chagas heart disease from one due to coronary artery disease. The aneurysms and segmental abnormalities are thought to result from localized destruction of extracellular matrix collagen along with myocyte loss, which leads to focal weakening of the ventricular wall. The apical location is particularly vulnerable because of the nature of the collagen structure at this location, normal apical thinning, and a relatively increased wall stress, which would promote the gradual development of aneurysmal dilation of the weakened segment. Regional dyssynergy caused by segmental conduction abnormalities could also contribute to aneurysm formation.[19,21]

Histological examination reveals focal and diffuse myocardial fibrosis, predominantly in the subepicardium, interspersed with viable but often damaged myocardial fibers. VT can arise from various regions in both ventricles, but LV inferolateral scar is the main source of sustained VT reentrant circuits. In theses areas, endocardial mapping frequently shows fragmented and late potentials during sinus rhythm as well as continuous or diastolic activity during VT. Histological analysis of those segments has shown focal and diffuse fibrosis that is predominantly subepicardial with nonuniform anisotropy of the surviving fibers. Epicardial VT reentrant circuits occur frequently in Chagas CMP; approximately 70% of VTs are epicardial in origin.[19,20]

Clinical Considerations

Cardiac abnormalities can be detected in all phases or forms of Chagas disease. The natural history and the type of cardiac involvement can vary widely in patients with Chagas disease. Patients can present with a wide variety of clinical manifestations; the most important of these are ventricular arrhythmias, sudden death, congestive heart failure, thromboembolism, stroke, and heart block.[20,21]

VT in Chagas disease can have heterogeneous presentations. SCD, usually due to VF and VT, is the most common cause of death, occurring more often than in other types of dilated CMP, with an incidence ranging from 51% to 65%. Frequently, the arrhythmic episodes are clustered in short periods, causing electrical storms ("chagasic storm"). Ventricular ectopy is remarkably frequent in all stages of the disease, even when there is no other evidence of cardiac involvement. Ectopy is dense and temporally unvarying, with patients often having tens of thousands of ectopic beats per day. In one report, 14% of patients presented with aborted sudden death, and sustained VT or sudden death occurred subsequently in 39% of patients with LV aneurysm or dysfunction. Nonsustained VT has been found by ambulatory monitoring in 10% of patients with mild wall motion abnormalities, in 56% of those with severe wall motion abnormalities or aneurysms without heart failure, and in 87% of those with advanced congestive heart failure.[19,20]

The presence of nonsustained VT detected during ambulatory Holter monitoring and particularly during stress testing is a strong predictor of SCD. LV dysfunction is also a predictor of poor outcome, particularly if associated with ventricular arrhythmias.

Sustained VT is inducible with programmed ventricular stimulation in most patients who present with sustained ventricular arrhythmias and in half of those who have symptomatic nonsustained VT. EP testing in asymptomatic patients with cardiac involvement has shown that sinus node dysfunction is present in 18%, pacing-induced atrioventricular block in 41%, and multiple sites of conducting system dysfunction often coexist.

Ventricular tachyarrhythmias in the setting of Chagas disease are very difficult to treat. Antiarrhythmic drug therapy is frequently ineffective. Limited data exist on the catheter ablation of VTs associated with Chagas CMP. Success rates are limited when only endocardial mapping and ablation techniques are used. Epicardial ablation has been shown to improve outcome and should be considered in these cases, perhaps as the initial ablation strategy. ICDs are generally the treatment of choice.

Because of the high incidence of thromboembolic phenomena, oral anticoagulants are recommended for patients with atrial fibrillation, previous embolism, and apical aneurysm with thrombus, even in the absence of controlled clinical trials demonstrating their efficacy.[20,21]

REFERENCES

1. Hamilton RM, Azevedo ER: Sudden cardiac death in dilated cardiomyopathies, *Pacing Clin Electrophysiol* 32(Suppl 2):S32–S40, 2009.
2. Kleber AG, Rudy Y: Basic mechanisms of cardiac impulse propagation and associated arrhythmias, *Physiol Rev* 84:431–488, 2004.
3. Boussy T, Paparella G, de Asmundis C, et al: Genetic basis of ventricular arrhythmias, *Heart Fail Clin* 6:249–266, 2010.
4. Aliot EM, Stevenson WG, Mendral-Garrote JM, et al: EHRA/HRS Expert Consensus on Catheter Ablation of Ventricular Arrhythmias: developed in a partnership with the European Heart Rhythm Association (EHRA), a Registered Branch of the European Society of Cardiology (ESC), and the Heart Rhythm Society (HRS); in collaboration with the American College of Cardiology (ACC) and the American Heart Association (AHA), *Heart Rhythm* 6:886–933, 2009.
5. Yokokawa M, Tada H, Koyama K, et al: The characteristics and distribution of the scar tissue predict ventricular tachycardia in patients with advanced heart failure, *Pacing Clin Electrophysiol* 32:314–322, 2009.
6. Yokokawa M, Tada H, Koyama K, et al: Nontransmural scar detected by magnetic resonance imaging and origin of ventricular tachycardia in structural heart disease, *Pacing Clin Electrophysiol* 32(Suppl 1):S52–S56, 2009.
7. Nakahara S, Tung R, Ramirez RJ, et al: Characterization of the arrhythmogenic substrate in ischemic and nonischemic cardiomyopathy implications for catheter ablation of hemodynamically unstable ventricular tachycardia, *J Am Coll Cardiol* 55:2355–2365, 2010.
8. Kuhne M, Abrams G, Sarrazin JF, et al: Isolated potentials and pace-mapping as guides for ablation of ventricular tachycardia in various types of nonischemic cardiomyopathy, *J Cardiovasc Electrophysiol* 21:1017–1023, 2010.
9. Vest RN III, Gold MR: Risk stratification of ventricular arrhythmias in patients with systolic heart failure, *Curr Opin Cardiol* 25:268–275, 2010.
10. Das MK, Zipes DP: Fragmented QRS: a predictor of mortality and sudden cardiac death, *Heart Rhythm* 6(Suppl 3):S8–S14, 2009.
11. Das MK, Maskoun W, Shen C, et al: Fragmented QRS on twelve-lead electrocardiogram predicts arrhythmic events in patients with ischemic and nonischemic cardiomyopathy, *Heart Rhythm* 7:74–80, 2010.
12. Myerburg RJ, Reddy V, Castellanos A: Indications for implantable cardioverter-defibrillators based on evidence and judgment, *J Am Coll Cardiol* 54:747–763, 2009.
13. Natale A, Raviele A, Al-Ahmad A, et al: Venice Chart International Consensus document on ventricular tachycardia/ventricular fibrillation ablation, *J Cardiovasc Electrophysiol* 21: 339–379, 2010.
14. Josephson ME: Catheter and surgical ablation in the therapy of arrhythmias. In Josephson ME, editor: *Clinical cardiac electrophysiology*, ed 4, Philadelphia, 2008, Lippincott Williams & Wilkins, pp 746–888.
15. Bogun F, Morady F: Ablation of ventricular tachycardia in patients with nonischemic cardiomyopathy, *J Cardiovasc Electrophysiol* 19:1227–1230, 2008.
16. Jefic D, Joel B, Good E, et al: Role of radiofrequency catheter ablation of ventricular tachycardia in cardiac sarcoidosis: report from a multicenter registry, *Heart Rhythm* 6:189–195, 2009.
17. Mehta D, Mori N, Goldbarg SH, et al: Primary prevention of sudden cardiac death in silent cardiac sarcoidosis: role of programmed ventricular stimulation, *Circ Arrhythm Electrophysiol* 4:43–48, 2011.
18. Cheong BY, Muthupillai R, Nemeth M, et al: The utility of delayed-enhancement magnetic resonance imaging for identifying nonischemic myocardial fibrosis in asymptomatic patients with biopsy-proven systemic sarcoidosis, *Sarcoidosis Vasc Diffuse Lung Dis* 26: 39–46, 2009.
19. Rassi A Jr, Rassi A, Marin-Neto JA: Chagas disease, *Lancet* 375:1388–1402, 2010.
20. Rassi A Jr, Rassi A, Rassi SG: Predictors of mortality in chronic Chagas disease: a systematic review of observational studies, *Circulation* 115:1101–1108, 2007.
21. Bern C, Montgomery SP, Herwaldt BL, et al: Evaluation and treatment of Chagas disease in the United States: a systematic review, *JAMA* 298:2171–2181, 2007.

CHAPTER 26 Bundle Branch Reentrant Ventricular Tachycardia

Pathophysiology

Bundle branch reentrant (BBR) ventricular tachycardia (VT) is a reentrant VT with a well-defined reentry circuit, incorporating the right bundle branch (RB) and left bundle branch (LB) as obligatory limbs of the circuit, connected proximally by the His bundle (HB) and distally by the ventricular septal myocardium (Fig. 26-1).

Single BBR beats can be induced in up to 50% of patients with normal intraventricular conduction undergoing electrophysiological (EP) study. The QRS during BBR can display either left bundle branch block (LBBB) or right bundle branch block (RBBB) when anterograde ventricular activation occurs over the RB or LB, respectively. The vast majority have LBBB configuration. BBR with an LBBB pattern can also occur occasionally during right ventricular (RV) pacing. This requires that the effective refractory period of the LB be longer than that of the RB, or that retrograde conduction over the RB be resumed after an initial bilateral block in the His-Purkinje system (HPS) (i.e., gap phenomenon). Left ventricular (LV) pacing does not seem to increase the yield of induction of BBR with RBBB morphology.[1]

In patients with normal intraventricular conduction, BBR is a self-limited phenomenon. The rapid conduction and long refractory period of the HPS prevent sustained BBR in normal hearts. Spontaneous termination of BBR most commonly occurs in the retrograde limb between the ventricular muscle and the HB.[1] Sometimes, anterograde block can also occur, making refractoriness in the RB-Purkinje system the limiting factor. Continuation of BBR as a tachycardia is critically dependent on the interplay between conduction velocity and recovery of the tissue ahead of the reentrant wavefront. Two changes from normal physiology must occur for BBR to become sustained: (1) an anatomically longer reentrant pathway caused by a dilated heart, providing sufficiently longer conduction time around the HPS; and (2) slow conduction in the HPS caused by HPS disease.[1] These two factors are responsible for sufficient prolongation of conduction time to permit expiration of the refractory period of the HPS ahead of the propagating reentrant wavefront.

Rarely, self-terminating BBR can occur with a narrow QRS during ventricular extrastimulation (VES) in the setting of normal intraventricular conduction. After retrograde conduction via the left anterior fascicle (LAF) or left posterior fascicle (LPF), anterograde propagation occurs over the RB and the remaining LB fascicle, resulting in a narrow QRS with either LAF or LPF block.

Clinical Considerations

Epidemiology

Sustained BBR VT usually occurs in patients with structural heart disease, especially dilated cardiomyopathy. Idiopathic dilated cardiomyopathy is the anatomical substrate for BBR VT in 45% of cases, and BBR VT accounts for up to 41% of all inducible sustained VTs in this population. BBR VT can also be associated with cardiomyopathy secondary to valvular or ischemic heart disease, and has been reported with Ebstein anomaly, hypertrophic cardiomyopathy, and even in patients without structural heart disease other than intraventricular conduction abnormalities.[2]

In patients with spontaneous sustained monomorphic VT, the incidence of inducible BBR VT ranges from 4.5% to 6% in patients with ischemic heart disease to 16.7% to 41% in patients with nonischemic cardiomyopathy. BBR VT accounts for up to 6% of all forms of induced sustained monomorphic VT. Importantly, in patients with BBR VT, additional myocardial VTs occur in 25%.[3] Of note, BBR VT is more frequently found in patients with VT clusters (up to 12.5%) than in patients with less frequent episodes of VT.[4]

Clinical Presentation

Sustained BBR VT is typically unstable secondary to very rapid ventricular rates (often 200 to 300 beats/min) and poor underlying ventricular function; 75% of patients present with syncope or cardiac arrest.

Initial Evaluation

BBR VT should be suspected in the presence of typical electrocardiogram (ECG) QRS morphology during normal sinus rhythm (NSR) and VT (see later), especially in a patient with dilated cardiomyopathy. Echocardiographic examination and coronary arteriography are required in most patients to evaluate for structural heart disease.

Principles of Management

Pharmacological antiarrhythmic therapy is usually ineffective. Radiofrequency (RF) catheter ablation of a bundle branch (typically the RB) can cure BBR VT and is currently regarded as first-line therapy.

Associated myocardial VT occurs in approximately 25% of patients post ablation, and these patients continue to be at a high risk of sudden cardiac death. Therefore, implantable cardioverter-defibrillator (ICD) therapy is indicated for secondary prevention, and additional antiarrhythmic therapy is required for some patients. ICD implantation will also provide back-up pacing, which is frequently required post ablation secondary to the development of atrioventricular (AV) block or an excessively prolonged His bundle–ventricular (HV) interval. Implantation of a dual-chamber or biventricular ICD should be considered in these patients.

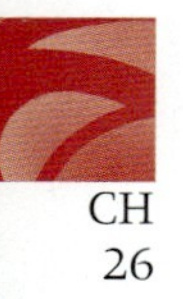

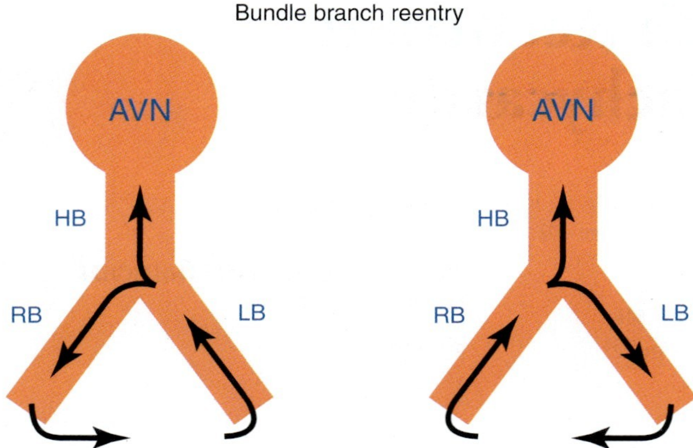

FIGURE 26-1 Schematic illustration of the two types of bundle branch reentry (BBR) circuits. At left is the most commonly seen type of BBR ventricular tachycardia (VT). Retrograde conduction occurs via the left bundle branch (LB) and anterograde conduction occurs via the right bundle branch (RB). This yields a VT in which the QRS has a left bundle branch block (LBBB) pattern. At right is the uncommon type of BBR VT. Retrograde conduction occurs via the RB and anterograde conduction occurs via the LB, which yields a VT in which the QRS has an RBBB pattern. AVN = atrioventricular node; HB = His bundle.

Because BBR VT has a limited response to antiarrhythmic drugs and can be an important cause of repetitive ICD therapies, catheter ablation of the arrhythmia should always be considered as an important adjunct to the device therapy.

EP testing should be considered in patients with repetitive episodes of VT and dilated cardiomyopathy, history of cardiac valve repair or replacement, or QRS morphology during VT similar to sinus rhythm QRS. If sustained BBR VT is inducible during programmed stimulation, catheter ablation is recommended.[4]

Electrocardiographic Features

Baseline ECG

The baseline rhythm is usually NSR or atrial fibrillation (AF). Almost all patients with BBR VT demonstrate intraventricular conduction abnormalities. The most common ECG abnormality is nonspecific intraventricular conduction delay (IVCD) with an LBBB pattern and PR interval prolongation (Fig. 26-2). Complete RBBB is rare but does not preclude BBR as the mechanism of VT. Although total interruption of conduction in one of the bundle branches would theoretically prevent occurrence of BBR, an ECG pattern of complete BBB may not be an accurate marker of *complete* conduction block; a similar QRS configuration can be caused by conduction delay, rather than block, in the bundle branch. Occasionally, complete AV block may be observed.[2]

ECG during Ventricular Tachycardia

Twelve-lead ECG documentation of BBR VT is usually unavailable because the VT is rapid and hemodynamically unstable. The VT rate is usually 180 to 300 beats/min. QRS morphology during VT is a typical BBB pattern and can be identical to that in NSR. BBR VT with an LBBB pattern is the most common VT morphology, and it usually has normal or left axis deviation (see Fig. 26-2). In contrast to VT of myocardial origin, BBR with an LBBB pattern characteristically shows a rapid intrinsicoid deflection in the right precordial leads, suggesting that initial ventricular activation occurs through the HPS and not ventricular muscle. BBR VT with an RBBB pattern usually has a leftward axis, but it can have a normal or rightward axis, depending on which fascicle is used for anterograde propagation.[1]

Electrophysiological Testing

Baseline Observations during Normal Sinus Rhythm

Conduction abnormalities in the HPS are almost invariably present and are a critical prerequisite for the development of sustained BBR, regardless of the underlying anatomical substrate (Fig. 26-3).[5] The average HV interval is about 80 milliseconds (range, 60 to 110 milliseconds). Although some patients can have the HV interval in NSR within normal limits, functional HPS impairment in these patients manifests as HV interval prolongation or split HB potentials, commonly becoming evident during atrial programmed stimulation or burst pacing. Nonspecific IVCD with an LBBB pattern and PR interval prolongation are the most common abnormalities.[2]

Induction of Tachycardia

VES from the RV apex is the usual method used to induce BBR with an LBBB pattern. Induction is consistently dependent on the achievement of a critical conduction delay in the HPS (i.e., critical ventricular–His bundle [VH] interval) following the VES.

During RV pacing at a constant cycle length (CL) and during introduction of VES at relatively long coupling intervals, retrograde conduction to the HB occurs via the RB. At shorter VES coupling intervals, retrograde delay and block occur in the RB when its relative and effective refractory periods are encountered, respectively. When retrograde block occurs in the RB, the impulse propagates across the septum and retrogradely up the LB to the HB, producing a long V_2-H_2 interval. The LB would still be capable of retrograde conduction because of its shorter refractoriness and because of the delay associated with transseptal propagation. Further shortening of the coupling intervals is associated with increasing delay in LB conduction (i.e., increasing V_2-H_2 interval). Within a certain range of coupling intervals, increasing retrograde LB delay allows for the recovery of anterograde conduction via the RB, and another ventricular activation ensues, displaying a wide QRS with an LBBB pattern. This beat is called the "BBR beat" or "V_3 phenomenon."[2]

An inverse relationship exists between retrograde conduction delay in the LB (V_2-H_2 interval) and the time of anterograde conduction in the RB (H_2-V_3 interval). This is because the faster the impulse propagates transseptally and up the LB, the more likely it will reach the RB while it is still refractory from the previous retrograde activation (concealment) by the VES, resulting in slower anterograde conduction down the RB.

BBR is more likely to occur when the VES is delivered following pacing drives incorporating long to short CL changes as compared with constant CL drives, because of CL dependency of the HPS refractoriness. An abrupt change in CL (i.e., long to short) can result in a more distal site of retrograde block, and less concealment, along the myocardium-Purkinje-RB axis, which can allow sufficient recovery of excitability in the anterograde limb of the circuit (i.e., the RB-Purkinje-myocardium axis) for reentry to develop. In addition, earlier recovery of excitability along this axis, because of the more distal site of block and less concealment, is associated with a shorter H_2-V_3 interval in this reentrant beat.[1]

Procainamide, which increases conduction time within the HPS, especially in the diseased HPS, and, potentially, isoproterenol can facilitate induction of sustained BBR. In some patients, the arrhythmia can be inducible only with atrial pacing.[2]

Tachycardia Features

BBR VT can only be diagnosed using intracardiac recording (Table 26-1). AV dissociation is typically present, during the tachycardia, but 1:1 ventriculoatrial (VA) conduction can occur. BBR VT is characterized by inscription of the His potential before the QRS complex, with the HV interval during BBR with an LBBB pattern generally being similar to or longer than that during baseline

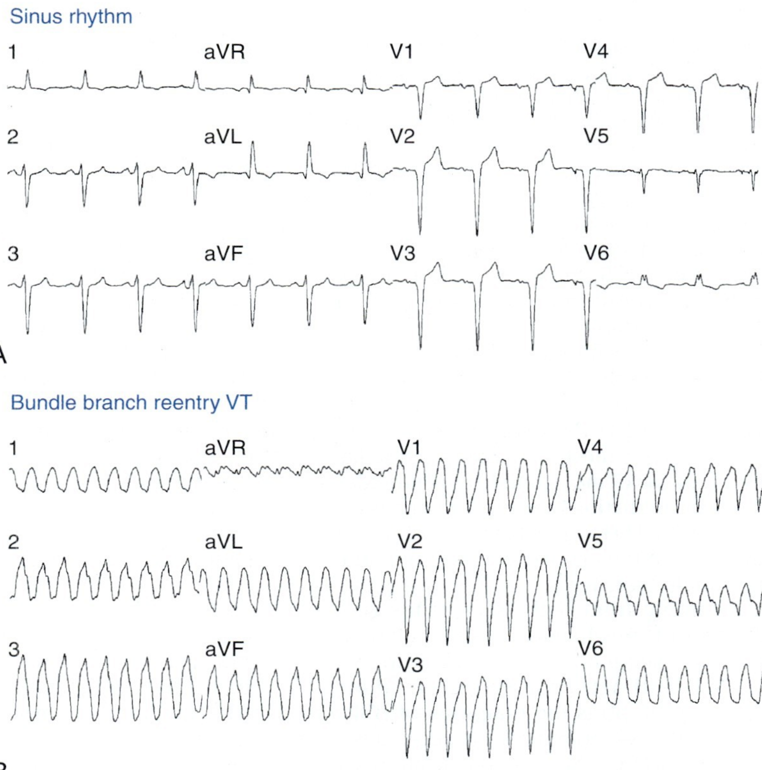

FIGURE 26-2 ECG of bundle branch reentrant (BBR) ventricular tachycardia (VT). **A,** Normal sinus rhythm baseline with intraventricular conduction delay resembling left bundle branch block. **B,** BBR VT. Note typical-appearing complete LBBB in this rapid VT.

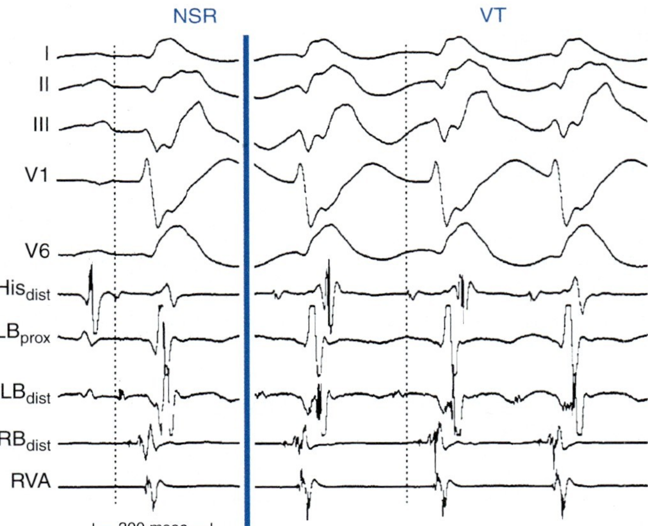

FIGURE 26-3 Bundle branch reentrant (BBR) ventricular tachycardia (VT) versus normal sinus rhythm (NSR). Sinus and BBR VT with His, left bundle branch (LB), and right bundle branch (RB) recordings in a patient with a prior septal myocardial infarction. Dashed lines mark the onset of His deflection. During NSR, the His potential is followed first by the LB potential; RB activation is further delayed. The fact that left bundle branch block (LBBB) is present on the ECG suggests that, although the LB is activated prior to the RB, delay is encountered more distally in the left ventricular His-Purkinje system such that LBBB is evident on the ECG. During BBR VT, activation propagates in an LB-His-RB sequence. Retrograde LB activation is very delayed, most likely because of the same factors responsible for the ECG in NSR.

TABLE 26-1 Diagnostic Criteria of Bundle Branch Reentrant Ventricular Tachycardia

- The QRS morphology of the tachycardia shows a typical RBBB or LBBB pattern.
- The onset of ventricular depolarization is preceded by HB, RB, or LB potentials with an appropriate sequence of H-RB-LB activation and relatively stable HV, RB-V, or LB-V intervals.
- Spontaneous variations in V-V intervals are preceded by similar changes in H-H/RB-RB/LB-LB intervals.
- The induction of tachycardia during programmed stimulation is consistently dependent on achieving a critical conduction delay in the HPS.
- Tachycardia termination is preceded by a spontaneous or pacing-induced block in the HPS.
- The HV during tachycardia is longer than HV during sinus rhythm.
- BBR is noninducible after successful ablation of the RB.

BBR = bundle branch reentry; HB = His bundle; HPS = His–Purkinje system; HV = His bundle–ventricular; LB = left bundle branch; LBBB = left bundle branch block; LB-V = left bundle–ventricular; RB = right bundle branch; RBBB = right bundle branch block; RB-V = right bundle–ventricular.

rhythm (the HV interval is usually 55 to 160 milliseconds; see Fig. 26-3). However, in rare cases, the HV interval during BBR VT can be slightly shorter (by less than 15 milliseconds) than the HV interval in NSR, because during BBR the HB is activated in the retrograde direction simultaneously (in parallel) with the proximal part of the bundle branch serving as the anterograde limb of the reentry circuit, whereas during NSR, activation of the HB and activation of the bundle branch occur in sequence.[1]

The relative duration of the HV interval recorded during VT as compared with NSR would depend on two factors: the balance between anterograde and retrograde conduction times from the upper turnaround point of the reentry circuit, and the site of HB recording relative to the upper turnaround point (i.e., the HB catheter electrode positioned at the proximal versus distal HB). Conduction delay in the bundle branch used as the anterograde limb of the circuit tends to prolong the HV interval during VT, whereas retrograde conduction delay to the HB recording site, as well as the use of a relatively proximal HB recording site (far from the turnaround point), tend to shorten the HV interval. The right bundle–ventricular (RB-V) interval during VT with LBBB morphology must always be longer than that recorded in sinus rhythm, emphasizing the importance of recording the RB potential during VT.[1]

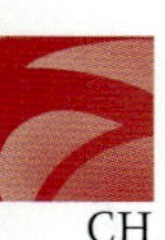

The HV interval during BBR with an RBBB pattern can be significantly different from that during NSR (HV interval, 65 to 250 milliseconds). During NSR, the HV interval is usually determined by conduction over whichever bundle branch conducts most rapidly, whereas during BBR it is determined by conduction over the typically diseased LB.

In the common type of BBR VT (LBBB pattern), the activation wavefront propagates retrogradely up the LB to the HB and then anterogradely down the RB, with subsequent ventricular activation. This sequence is reversed in BBR with an RBBB pattern. The HV and RB-V (during VT with LBBB morphology) or left bundle–ventricular (LB-V) intervals (during VT with RBBB morphology) are relatively stable.

During BBR VT, spontaneous variations in the V-V intervals are preceded and dictated by similar changes in the H-H (and RB-RB or LB-LB) intervals. In other words, the VT CL is affected by variation in the V-H (V-RB or V-LB) intervals. These changes can occur spontaneously, most commonly immediately after induction of the VT, or be demonstrated by ventricular stimulation during VT. However, oscillations in the V-V intervals can occasionally precede those of the H-H intervals during BBR VT because of conduction variations in the anterograde, rather than the retrograde, conducting bundle branch.[3]

Recording from both sides of the septum can help to identify the BBR mechanism. Documentation of a typical H-RB-V-LB activation sequence (during VT with LBBB morphology), or of an H-LB-V-RB activation sequence (during VT with RBBB morphology), supports the diagnosis of BBR (see Fig. 26-3).[1] Unfortunately, the RB potentials, LB potentials, or both are not always recorded, so that the typical activation sequences (LB-H-RB-V or RB-H-LB-V) are not available for analysis. Even if either activation sequence is present, the HPS (usually the LB) could be activated passively in a retrograde fashion to produce an H-RB-V sequence during a VT with LBBB pattern without reentry requiring the LB. In these cases, other diagnostic criteria for BBR should be used. In addition, during VT with LBBB morphology, RV activation must precede the LV activation. The opposite is true for the VT with RBBB morphology.

BBR can be terminated by block in the HPS—spontaneous, pacing-induced, secondary to catheter trauma, or caused by ablation.

Diagnostic Maneuvers during Tachycardia

Pacing maneuvers can be extremely helpful to establish the diagnosis of BBR; however, application of the pacing maneuvers during BBR is often not feasible because of the hemodynamic compromise commonly associated with these VTs.

ENTRAINMENT

BBR VT can be entrained by ventricular pacing. Entrainment with manifest QRS fusion during ventricular pacing is classic for BBR VT. Entrainment with concealed fusion can be demonstrated by pacing at the LB or RB (i.e., within the reentrant circuit). During entrainment from the RV apex, a post-pacing interval (PPI) – VT CL difference of greater than 30 milliseconds excludes a BBR mechanism, provided that the RV apex catheter is correctly positioned. The greater this value is, the more reliable is the certainty of exclusion. Conversely, a p[PPI – VT CL] difference of less than 30 milliseconds is consistent with, but not diagnostic of, a BBR mechanism.[3]

Entrainment of BBR VT with concealed QRS fusion can also occur during atrial pacing. This approach, however, demands that the patient not be in AF and usually requires the infusion of atropine, isoproterenol, or both to avoid AV block during rapid atrial pacing. The combination of entrainment with concealed QRS fusion during atrial pacing and entrainment with manifest QRS fusion during ventricular pacing has been recently proposed as a useful diagnostic criterion for BBR VT with LBBB QRS morphology.

RESETTING

VES can reset the VT by advancing the HB or bundle branch potential. In addition, VES can reverse the direction of impulse propagation during BBR. Theoretically this requires double VESs, with the first VES producing block and the second initiating the reentry in the opposite direction.

OTHER PACING MANEUVERS

The ability to dissociate the HB or, particularly, a bundle branch (RB or LB) potential strongly argues against a BBR mechanism. An atrial extrastimulus (AES) that blocks below the HB deflection should terminate BBR. Additionally, simultaneous LV and RV pacing should prevent BBR.[2]

Exclusion of Other Arrhythmia Mechanisms

MYOCARDIAL VENTRICULAR TACHYCARDIAS

Myocardial VTs are rarely associated with classic LBBB (or RBBB) QRS morphology, as is expected with BBR VT. Additionally, in myocardial VTs, the His potential is often obscured within the local ventricular electrogram. Occasionally, the His potential may precede the onset of the QRS, thus resembling BBR VT; however, the HV interval in myocardial VTs is usually shorter than that during NSR. In contrast to BBR VT, spontaneous or induced tachycardia CL variations during myocardial VTs usually precede and dictate H-H interval changes.[3]

Entrainment with concealed QRS fusion during atrial pacing excludes myocardial VT and should be expected in BBR VT. When entrainment with concealed fusion can be demonstrated by pacing at the LB or RB, BBR VT is very likely. In addition, a [PPI – VT CL] difference of less than 30 milliseconds after entrainment of the VT from the RV apex is suggestive of BBR VT; in contrast, in myocardial VTs, the [PPI – VT CL] difference is greater than 30 milliseconds, unless the VT originates in the apex.

IDIOPATHIC (FASCICULAR) LEFT VENTRICULAR TACHYCARDIA

The QRS and HV interval are normal during NSR in idiopathic VT. In contrast, BBR VT is rare in the absence of baseline HPS conduction abnormalities. Additionally, the His potential falls within or before the QRS in idiopathic LV VT, producing a negative or short HV interval, and HB activation follows activation of the left fascicles, which is inconsistent with RBBB-type BBR VT.

SUPRAVENTRICULAR TACHYCARDIA WITH ABERRANCY

BBR VT typically exhibits AV dissociation, which excludes atrial tachycardia (AT) and atrioventricular reentrant tachycardia (AVRT). Occasionally, BBR VT can be associated with 1:1 VA conduction, and it can then mimic supraventricular tachycardia (SVT) with aberrancy.

Multiple HB recordings, using a hexapolar or octapolar catheter, can help demonstrate the direction of HB depolarization—anterograde during SVT and retrograde during BBR VT. Also, recording of LB and RB potentials in addition to the HB potential can be helpful; activation of the HB occurs anterogradely via the atrioventricular node (AVN) during SVT and precedes the RB potential by an interval equal to or longer that that during NSR.

The atrium is not part of the circuit in the BBR VT and can be dissociated by atrial pacing, which excludes AT and AVRT as the mechanism of wide complex tachycardia. Moreover, during entrainment from the RV apex, a [PPI – tachycardia CL] difference of greater than 30 milliseconds excludes a BBR mechanism. Conversely, a [PPI – tachycardia CL] difference of less than 30 milliseconds excludes atrioventricular nodal reentrant tachycardia (AVNRT). Additionally, entrainment with manifest fusion during ventricular pacing excludes AVNRT and AT and should be expected in BBR VT.

Furthermore, the ability to terminate or reset the tachycardia with a VES introduced when HB is refractory excludes AT and AVNRT.

ANTIDROMIC ATRIOVENTRICULAR REENTRANT TACHYCARDIA USING AN ATRIOFASCICULAR BYPASS TRACT

During antidromic AVRT, the impulse propagates retrogradely over the RB to the HB, a sequence inconsistent with BBR with an LBBB pattern. The AV relationship is always 1:1 during AVRT and rarely so during BBR VT. Because the atrium is not part of the circuit in BBR VT, it can be dissociated by atrial pacing, which excludes AVRT. Moreover, resetting the tachycardia with an AES from the right atrial (RA) free wall, timed when the AV junctional atrium is refractory, excludes VT. Similarly, the ability of an AES to terminate the tachycardia without conduction to the ventricle or to retard (delay) the following ventricular activation excludes VT (see Figs. 18-28 and 19-4).

Ablation

Target of Ablation

The ablation target is either the RB or the LB; however, RB ablation is easier and usually is the method of choice. In most patients with BBR VT, although diffuse conduction system disease is present, the conduction abnormality in the LB is more severe than that in the RB. Nonetheless, preserved slow conduction over the LB can be demonstrated in the majority of patients, and the LB can still maintain 1:1 AV conduction during NSR.[6] For the occasional patients in whom anterograde conduction down the LB is known to be inadequate for maintaining AV conduction, ablation of the RB will commit the patient to a permanent pacemaker. Therefore, ablation of the LB in these patients is preferable because it can prevent BBR and still preserve anterograde conduction.

The mere presence of LBBB on the surface ECG does not mean complete block in the LB. Signs that can indicate that conduction down the LB may be inadequate in maintaining 1:1 AV conduction and favor ablation of the LB over the RB include (1) development of high-grade AV block below the HB on transient RBBB that can occur secondary to RV catheter manipulation, and (2) observation of an LB potential following the ventricular electrogram either intermittently or during every sinus beat.

Ablation Technique

ABLATION OF THE RIGHT BUNDLE BRANCH

The HB divides at the junction of the fibrous and muscular boundaries of the intraventricular septum into the RB and LB. The RB is an anatomically compact unit that travels as the extension of the HB after the origin of the LB. The RB courses down the right side of interventricular septum near the endocardium in its upper third, deeper in the muscular portion of the septum in the middle third, and then again near the endocardium in its lower third. The RB is a long, thin, discrete structure; it does not divide throughout most of its course, and begins to ramify as it approaches the base of the right anterior papillary muscle, with fascicles going to the septal and free walls of the RV.

A quadripolar catheter is positioned at the HB region and maintained as a reference. The ablation catheter is initially positioned in the HB region and the area of the septum at which the largest His potential is recorded. The catheter is then advanced gradually (in the right anterior oblique [RAO] view) superiorly and to the patient's left side, with clockwise torque to ensure adequate catheter tip contact with the septum and RB and continuous adjustment of the catheter's curvature until the RB potential is recorded. Attempts should be made to obtain the distal RB recording to ensure that the catheter tip is away from the HB and LB.

The RB potential can be distinguished from the HB potential by the absence of or minimal atrial electrogram on the recording and presence of a sharp deflection inscribed at least 15 to 20 milliseconds later than the His potential (Fig. 26-4). An RB-V interval value of less than 30 milliseconds may not be a reliable marker of the RB potential in these patients because disease of the HPS can cause prolongation of the RB-V conduction time.

When there is RB conduction delay at baseline, the RB potential can become hidden within the ventricular electrogram, and it may be impossible to map during NSR, especially when the surface ECG shows complete or incomplete RBBB. However, the RB potential should be readily observed during BBR beats induced by RV stimulation or during BBR VT. In this setting, anatomically guided lesions or a linear ablation perpendicular to the axis of the RB distal to the HB recording may be effective.

A 4-mm-tip ablation catheter is typically used for RB ablation. RF application is usually started at low levels (5 W) and gradually increased every 10 seconds, targeting a temperature of 60°C. In general, RBBB develops at 15 to 20 W. Successful ablation will result in clear development of RBBB in lead V_1 (Fig. 26-5; and see Fig. 26-4). Occasionally, an accelerated rhythm from the RB is observed during ablation (analogous to accelerated junctional rhythm with HB ablation; see Fig. 26-5).

ABLATION OF THE LEFT BUNDLE BRANCH

Whereas the RB is anatomically a continuation of the HB, the LB arises as a broad band of fibers from the HB in a perpendicular direction toward the inferior septum. The main LB penetrates the membranous portion of the interventricular septum under the

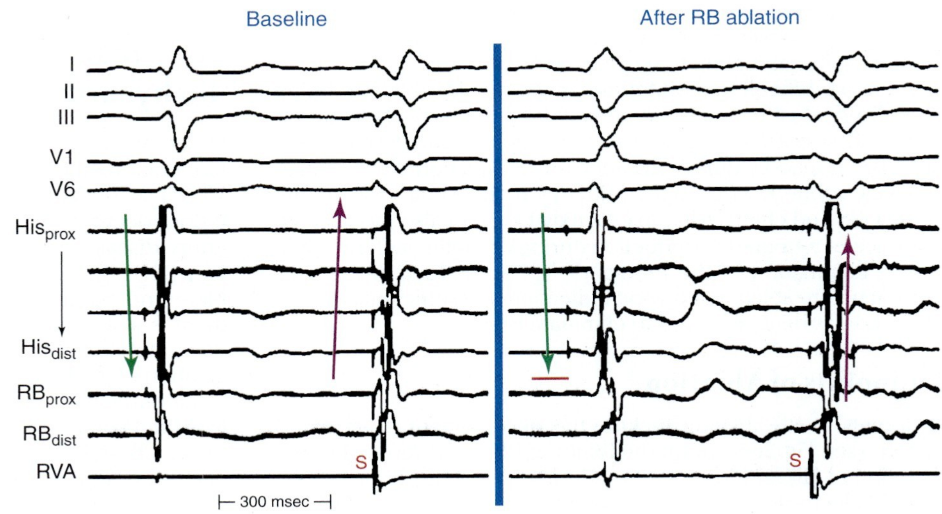

FIGURE 26-4 Ablation of bundle branch reentry (BBR). Sinus and right ventricular apical paced complexes from before (left) and after (right) catheter ablation of the right bundle branch (RB) in a patient with BBR VT. Four bipolar recordings from a catheter at the His position and RB are shown. Prior to RB ablation, propagation along the His-RB axis is linear, anterograde during sinus rhythm (green arrow), and retrograde during RV pacing (purple arrow). After RB ablation, anterograde propagation is interrupted (green arrow, red line) and retrograde activation of the His electrograms occurs after the local ventricular electrogram (purple arrow), indicating block in the RB with transseptal propagation, then up the left bundle.

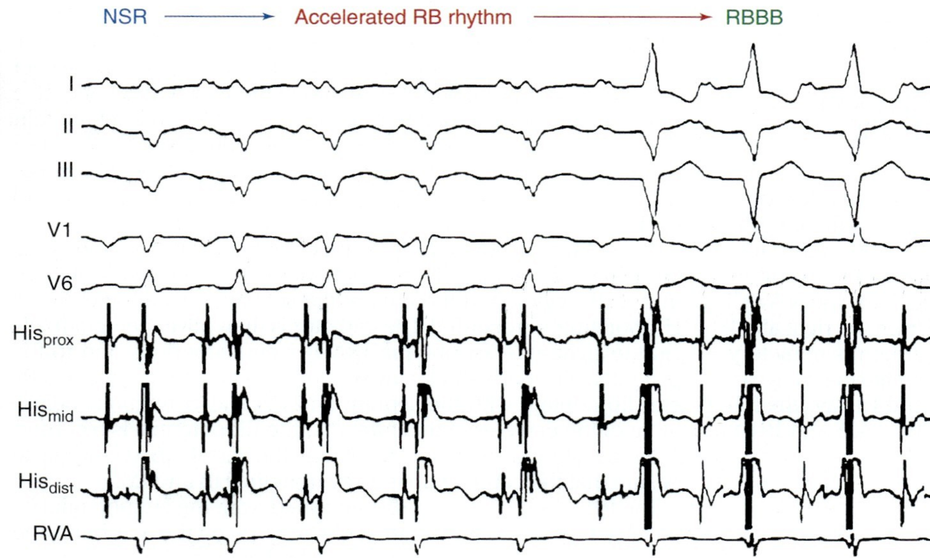

FIGURE 26-5 Right bundle branch (RB) ablation. During RB ablation, delivery of radiofrequency current causes accelerated rhythm from the RB until complete block occurs (note lead V_1). The His bundle–ventricular interval after ablation is 145 milliseconds (baseline, 80 milliseconds). NSR = normal sinus rhythm; RBBB = right bundle branch block.

aortic ring and then divides into several fairly discrete branches.The LPF arises more proximally than the LAF, appears as an extension of the main LB, and is large in its initial course. It then fans out extensively posteriorly toward the papillary muscle and inferoposteriorly to the free wall of the LV. The LAF crosses the LV outflow region and terminates in the Purkinje system of the anterolateral wall of the LV. In the RAO view, the LPF extends from the HB region toward the inferior diaphragmatic wall and the LAF extends toward the apex of the heart. However, considerable variability exists.

The mapping catheter is placed via a transaortic approach into the LV. The inferoapical septum is a starting point. The catheter is then gradually withdrawn toward the HB until a discrete LB potential is recorded. The LB-V interval should be less than or equal to 20 milliseconds, and the AV electrogram amplitude ratio should be less than or equal to 1:10. At this position, the tip of the catheter typically is 1 to 1.5 cm inferior to the optimal HB recording site near the distal portion of the common LB. On the other hand, the disease process that results in LBBB in patients with BBR probably leaves only a remnant of conducting tissue that may be more readily ablated than a normal LB would be.

Because the LB is a broad band of fibers (typically 1 to 3 cm long and 1 cm wide), it can be difficult to ablate with a single RF application. Furthermore, the fascicles can diverge proximally; thus, ablation of the LB can be difficult without harming the HB. In these situations, it may be necessary to deliver several lesions along the left side of the septum in an arc distal to the HB, extending from the anterior superior septum (a point near the RB in the RAO view) to the inferior basal septum to transect both fascicles.

It is more difficult to monitor the progress of LB ablation during RF delivery. Most patients will already have some IVCD localized to the LB system. As opposed to the usually clear development of RBBB in lead V_1 during RB ablation, LB ablation can produce relatively subtle ECG changes, primarily manifesting as widening of the QRS and changes in the QRS axis. One can also monitor the presence of retrograde conduction during VES after each RF application. Elimination of the retrograde V_2-H_2 conduction that was present before ablation is a good indication that sufficient ablation of the LB has been achieved to eliminate BBR.

Endpoints of Ablation

Endpoints of RB ablation include the development of an RBBB pattern (see Fig. 26-5), noninducibility of BBR, and reversal of the direction of HB and RB activation during RV pacing. Prior to ablation, HB electrodes are depolarized during RV pacing from distal to proximal (RB-HB); after RB ablation, HB activation is delayed and reversed (HB-RB; see Fig. 26-4).

Endpoints of LB ablation include elimination of retrograde conduction of VESs over the LB and noninducibility of BBR.

After ablation, aggressive ventricular stimulation should be performed to evaluate the inducibility of VT. Also, decremental atrial pacing should be performed to evaluate the conduction properties of the HPS and the propensity for infra-Hisian AV block. It is advisable to stress the HPS with intravenous procainamide and ensure that anterograde conduction is preserved.[3]

Outcome

Recurrence of BBR VT after successful ablation is extremely rare. The reported incidence of clinically significant conduction system impairment requiring implantation of a permanent pacemaker varies from 10% to 30%.[2]

Pacemaker implantation is indicated when infra-Hisian AV block is demonstrated with atrial pacing, or when the post-ablation HV interval is 100 milliseconds or greater. As noted, associated myocardial VT is observed in approximately 25% of patients post ablation, and these patients continue to be at a high risk of sudden cardiac death. Therefore, ICD implantation is indicated for secondary prevention, and additional antiarrhythmic therapy is required for some patients.

Interfascicular Reentrant Ventricular Tachycardia

Of the two types of macroreentry in the HPS (i.e., BBR and interfascicular reentry), BBR is by far the most common mechanism of VT.[7] VT secondary to interfascicular reentry is extremely rare; when it does occur, it is most commonly seen in patients with coronary artery disease, specifically those with anterior myocardial infarction (MI) with LAF or LPF block. In these patients, RBBB is complete and bidirectional, so true BBR cannot occur. Additionally, there is slow conduction in the apparently blocked fascicle.[2] Of note, interfascicular reentrant VT can develop in patients following ablation of the RB for the treatment of BBR VT.[7]

Interfascicular reentry incorporates the LAF and LPF as obligatory limbs of the circuit, connected proximally by the main trunk of the LB and distally by the ventricular myocardium (Fig. 26-6). The tachycardia usually has an RBBB morphology. The orientation of the frontal plane axis is variable and depends on the direction

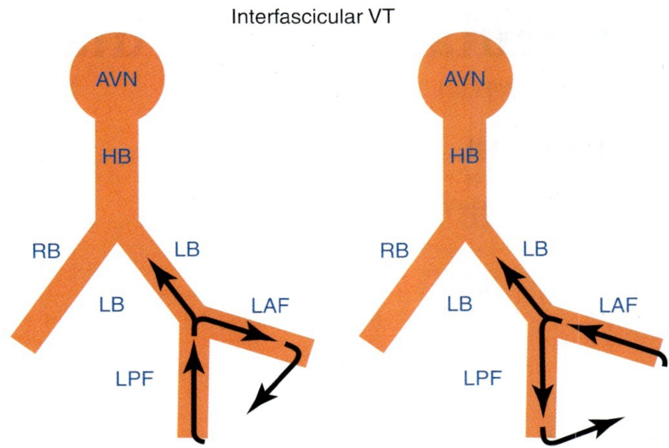

FIGURE 26-6 Schematic illustration of the two types of interfascicular ventricular tachycardia (VT) circuits. **Left:** The interfascicular reentrant VT uses the left posterior fascicle (LPF) as the retrograde limb of the reentrant circuit and the left anterior fascicle (LAF) as the anterograde limb. **Right:** The interfascicular reentrant VT uses the LAF as the retrograde limb of the reentrant circuit and the LPF as the anterograde limb. In both types, because the ventricle is activated via the left bundle branch (LB), the QRS has right bundle branch block morphology. The QRS axis will depend on which fascicle serves as the anterograde route of ventricular activation. The right bundle branch (RB) is activated in a bystander fashion and is not necessary for sustaining the tachycardia. AVN = atrioventricular node; HB = His bundle.

of propagation in the reentrant circuit. Anterograde activation over the LAF and retrograde through the LPF would be associated with right axis deviation, whereas the reversed activation sequence shows left axis deviation (see Fig. 26-6).[1,2]

In contrast to BBR VT, the HV interval during interfascicular VT is usually shorter by more than 40 milliseconds than that recorded in NSR.[1] This is because the upper turnaround point of the circuit, the distal end of the LB bifurcation point, is relatively far from the retrogradely activated HB. During interfascicular VT, the LB potential should be inscribed before the His potential. In contrast, during BBR VT with RBBB morphology, the His potential usually precedes the LB potential, although the reverse is theoretically possible if the retrograde conduction time to the HB recording point is significantly prolonged. Interfascicular reentry also demonstrates variations in the V-V interval preceded by similar changes in the H-H interval.

Atrial pacing, AES, VES, and ventricular pacing can initiate interfascicular reentry by producing transient anterograde block in the slowly conducting fascicle (LAF or LPF), with subsequent impulse anterograde conduction over the healthy fascicle, giving rise to a QRS morphology identical to that during NSR, and then retrogradely in the initially blocked fascicle to initiate reentry. Compared with BBR VT, interfascicular VT can be more difficult to induce by ventricular pacing, because of the inability to create the necessary EP conditions for this type of reentry during ventricular stimulation (i.e., retrograde block in the distal LAF and slow conduction via the LPF, or vice versa), although this may occur during anterograde penetration of the HPS by supraventricular impulses (i.e., anterograde block in the LPF and slow conduction in the LAF, or vice versa).[7]

Successful ablation of the arrhythmia can be performed by targeting the diseased fascicle (LAF or LPF), guided by fascicular potentials.[2] When interfascicular reentry occurs in the setting of an anterior MI, complete cure by ablation is usually not possible because other myocardial VTs are almost always present, and the LV ejection fraction is usually poor, thereby mandating ICD implantation for improved survival. When interfascicular reentry occurs without coronary artery disease, in association with degenerative disease of the conduction system, LV systolic function is usually normal and cure of the VT is possible by ablation of the diseased fascicle, although implantation of a permanent pacemaker will likely be required.

REFERENCES

1. Josephson ME: Recurrent ventricular tachycardia. In Josephson ME, editor: *Clinical cardiac electrophysiology*, ed 4, Philadelphia, 2008, Lippincott Williams & Wilkins, pp 446–642.
2. Daoud EG: Bundle branch reentry. In Zipes D, Jalife J, editors: *Cardiac electrophysiology: from cell to bedside*, ed 4, Philadelphia, 2004, WB Saunders, pp 683–688.
3. Balasundaram R, Rao HB, Kalavakolanu S, Narasimhan C: Catheter ablation of bundle branch reentrant ventricular tachycardia, *Heart Rhythm* 5(6 Suppl):S68–S72, 2008.
4. Sakata T, Tanner H, Stuber T, Delacretaz E: His-Purkinje system re-entry in patients with clustering ventricular tachycardia episodes, *Europace* 10:289–293, 2008.
5. Lopera G, Stevenson WG, Soejima K, et al: Identification and ablation of three types of ventricular tachycardia involving the His-Purkinje system in patients with heart disease, *J Cardiovasc Electrophysiol* 15:52–58, 2004.
6. Schmidt B, Tang M, Chun KR, et al: Left bundle branch–Purkinje system in patients with bundle branch reentrant tachycardia: lessons from catheter ablation and electroanatomic mapping, *Heart Rhythm* 6:51–58, 2009.
7. Blanck Z, Sra J, Akhtar M: Incessant interfascicular reentrant ventricular tachycardia as a result of catheter ablation of the right bundle branch: case report and review of the literature, *J Cardiovasc Electrophysiol* 20:1279–1283, 2009.

CHAPTER 27 Epicardial Ventricular Tachycardia

Electrophysiological Substrate

Mapping and ablation of arrhythmogenic substrates have traditionally been performed via the endocardial approach. Not infrequently, however, the site of origin of a focal tachycardia or a portion of the critical isthmus or even the entire circuit of a macroreentrant tachycardia is located deep in the endocardium or even in the subepicardium and cannot be identified or ablated from the endocardium. In these settings, the epicardial approach to mapping and ablation can be a valuable strategy for elimination of the arrhythmia.

The importance of epicardial ventricular tachycardia (VT) circuits was first highlighted in Chagas disease, which classically results in an epicardial involvement in approximately 70% of patients. Epicardial substrates also have recently been increasingly recognized in the setting of scar-related VT in patients with nonischemic cardiomyopathy (CMP), arrhythmogenic right ventricular cardiomyopathy-dysplasia (ARVD), and prior myocardial infarction (MI, "ischemic CMP"), as well as in patients with idiopathic VT.

Patients with ischemic heart disease tend to have larger endocardial than epicardial scars, usually confined to a specific coronary vascular territory. Although there is a predilection for a subendocardial location of the VT substrate, epicardial circuits can be observed in a significant portion of patients. In tertiary centers, epicardial ablation has been required in up to 10% of post-MI VTs, and appears to be more frequently required for inferior wall infarct VTs than for those with anterior wall infarcts.

In patients with nonischemic CMP, detailed epicardial electroanatomical substrate mapping has identified large confluent low-voltage areas consistent with myocardial scar. The epicardial scar areas are typically larger than the endocardial left ventricular (LV) scar areas and have a typical distribution similar to that for endocardial LV scars, usually located in basal lateral areas of the LV adjacent to the mitral valve annulus. Epicardial ablation is needed more often in patients with sustained monomorphic VT associated with dilated, nonischemic CMP than in patients with prior MI.[1]

In patients with ARVD, sizable low-voltage areas often involve the infundibulum, free wall, and basal perivalvular regions, constituting the endocardial substrate. More recently, extensive epicardial low-voltage areas, often with fractionated and late electrographic recordings, have been identified. The epicardial scar is consistently larger than that on the endocardial surface. In patients with ARVD and VT refractory to endocardial ablation, the origin of VT defined on the epicardium is frequently noted beyond the endocardial-defined scar.[2] In a recent report, the highest prevalence of epicardial VTs was observed in patients with ARVD (41%) and nonischemic CMP (35%), followed by patients with ischemic heart disease (16%).[3]

Small series have also reported successful ablation of epicardial VTs following a failed endocardial ablation in patients with idiopathic outflow tract VTs. Often underrecognized, the incidence of an epicardial origin in idiopathic VT may be as high as 14%. Idiopathic outflow tract VTs with epicardial origins can originate close to the anterior interventricular vein, great cardiac vein, and middle cardiac vein; and successful ablation from within these structures has been reported. When this approach fails, percutaneous epicardial mapping and ablation have been reported to be feasible and successful.[4]

Electrocardiographic Features

Several ECG findings can suggest an epicardial origin of the VT with right bundle branch block (RBBB)–like configuration, all of which generally rely on the late engagement of His-Purkinje fibers by exits on the epicardium, resulting in intramyocardial delay of conduction and a slurred initial part of the QRS complex: (1) pseudo-delta wave (so called because of its similarity to the slurred upstroke delta wave observed during ventricular preexcitation) greater than 34 milliseconds (measured from the earliest ventricular activation to the earliest fast deflection in any precordial lead) has a sensitivity of 83% and a specificity of 95%; (2) long R-wave peak time in lead V_2 (i.e., interval from the beginning of the QRS complex to the time of initial downstroke of the R wave after it has peaked [previously known as the *intrinsicoid deflection*]) greater than 85 milliseconds has a sensitivity of 87% and a specificity of 90%; (3) shortest RS complex duration (measured from the earliest ventricular activation to the nadir of the first S wave in any precordial lead) equal to or greater than 121 milliseconds has a sensitivity of 76% and a specificity of 85%; and (4) QRS duration greater than 200 milliseconds (see Fig. 22-8).[4,5]

These criteria, however, do not seem to apply uniformly to all LV regions or to VTs originating from the right ventricle (RV). Other site-specific criteria have been suggested for identifying an epicardial origin for LV VTs: (1) the presence of a Q wave in lead I for basal superior and apical superior VTs; (2) the absence of a Q wave in any of the inferior leads for basal superior VTs; and (3) the presence of a Q wave in the inferior leads for basal inferior and apical inferior VTs. Also, measurement of the *maximal deflection index* (defined as the time from QRS onset to maximal deflection in precordial leads divided by the QRS duration) can help identify epicardial VT originating in the LV outflow region. A delayed shortest precordial maximal deflection index (≥0.55) identifies epicardial VT remote from the aortic sinus of Valsalva with high sensitivity and specificity. This observation is consistent with slower spread of activation from a focus on the epicardial surface relative to the endocardium and delayed global ventricular activation resulting from later engagement of the His-Purkinje network.[6,7]

Epicardial VTs originating close to the proximal segment of the great cardiac vein typically display RBBB morphology, whereas VTs originating close to the distal segment have left bundle branch block (LBBB) morphology. This may be explained by a location within the basal-lateral myocardium for the former and a more anterobasal location for the latter arrhythmias. If the site of origin is in the proximal segment of the great cardiac vein, the initial vector is directed toward lead V_1, accounting for the RBBB morphology. As the site of origin moves toward the distal part of the great cardiac vein, closer to the anteroseptal myocardium, the initial vector is directed away from V_1, resulting in LBBB morphology. An R-wave width greater than 75 milliseconds in lead V_1 is useful for differentiating epicardial idiopathic VTs from endocardial arrhythmias. The broader R wave is explained by a more posterior position relative to lead V_1 compared with the RV outflow tract (RVOT). However, because of a more anterior position relative to lead V_1, the epicardial arrhythmias that are located within the distal part of the great cardiac vein have a narrow R wave in lead V_1, making them impossible to distinguish from RVOT VT.[7,8] Epicardial VTs that appear to follow the anterior interventricular vein often have a characteristic loss of R wave from leads V_1 and V_2 with broad R waves in leads V_3 through V_6.

For VTs originating from the RV, the presence of an initial Q wave in lead I and QS in lead V_2 for anterior sites in the RV strongly predicts an epicardial origin. Similarly, an initial Q wave in leads II, III, and aVF is observed with pace mapping from the inferior epicardial locations in the RV.

Although various ECG characteristics have been used to predict whether an epicardial approach may be required based on the VT morphology, it is important to understand that the QRS morphology is related solely to the VT exit site and this does not imply that some other component of the circuit (such as the critical isthmus or entrance site) cannot be ablated from the endocardium, even when an epicardial exit is implied by the ECG characteristics. Therefore, it is unlikely that the surface ECG by itself will ever be entirely predictive of the need for epicardial access for mapping and ablation for any given VT.[5] Additionally, large areas of conduction delay often present in patients with myocardial scar can produce misleading activation sequences and confound ECG prediction.[9]

Percutaneous Epicardial Approach

Clinical Considerations

VT originating from the subepicardium is an important cause of failure of endocardial ablation approaches. Mapping arrhythmia foci or circuits that are deep within the myocardium or in the epicardium can be attempted via the coronary sinus (CS) or pericardial space. The CS approach, however, has important limitations. Catheter manipulation is limited by the anatomical distribution of the cardiac veins, and epicardial circuits may be identified only when the vessel cannulated happens to be in the region of the circuit. An alternative epicardial approach involves inserting an introducer sheath percutaneously into the pericardial space in the manner used for pericardiocentesis. The subxiphoid approach to the epicardial space allows extensive and unrestricted mapping of the epicardial surface of both ventricles, and has been used most commonly for VT mapping and ablation (far less so for supraventricular arrhythmias). Nonetheless, mapping of the CS and accessible coronary venous branches can be performed prior to the percutaneous epicardial approach to look for clues of an epicardial origin of the VT circuit, and has been particularly useful in idiopathic outflow tract VTs.[4,9]

Catheter ablation from the epicardium is often required for elimination of VTs due to nonischemic CMP and is occasionally useful for VTs in a variety of other diseases, as well as some idiopathic VTs. Nonetheless, despite the increasing recognition that ventricular arrhythmias may originate from epicardial foci, epicardial VT ablation remains a specialized procedure and is performed at relatively few centers. In the majority of reported cases, percutaneous epicardial VT ablation has been performed only after failure of a thorough endocardial mapping and ablation session, at a separate setting or during the same setting after exhausting endocardial mapping efforts. Simultaneous endocardial and epicardial mapping can have several advantages (Fig. 27-1), such as a better chance to map and ablate all inducible VTs, reduce the number of procedures required for patients with suspected epicardial VTs, and an opportunity to acquire more expertise with the technique.[4] Also, epicardial mapping and ablation may be useful as a first procedure when endocardial mapping is not an option because of intraventricular thrombi or in patients with metallic prostheses in the aortic and mitral valves.[4]

There are several conditions that can significantly limit the feasibility of percutaneous epicardial mapping and ablation. Previous cardiac surgery usually results in significant pericardial fibrosis, and the pericardial space is often, but not always, virtually replaced by fibrotic adhesions. In this setting, percutaneous cannulation of the pericardial sac is very difficult; even when percutaneous cannulation is successful, manipulation of the instruments is extremely limited and difficult. Additionally, pericardial venous varices have been reported in patients with SVC and azygous venous occlusion. Thus, catheter manipulation and ablation inside the pericardial space of a patient with pericardial varices can result in severe bleeding complications. When pericardial varices are suspected, the diagnosis can be made by three-dimensional (3-D) computed tomography (CT) angiography. Also, the presence of a large hiatal hernia can predispose to inadvertent perforation (and subsequent mediastinal infections) during cannulation attempts. Congenital

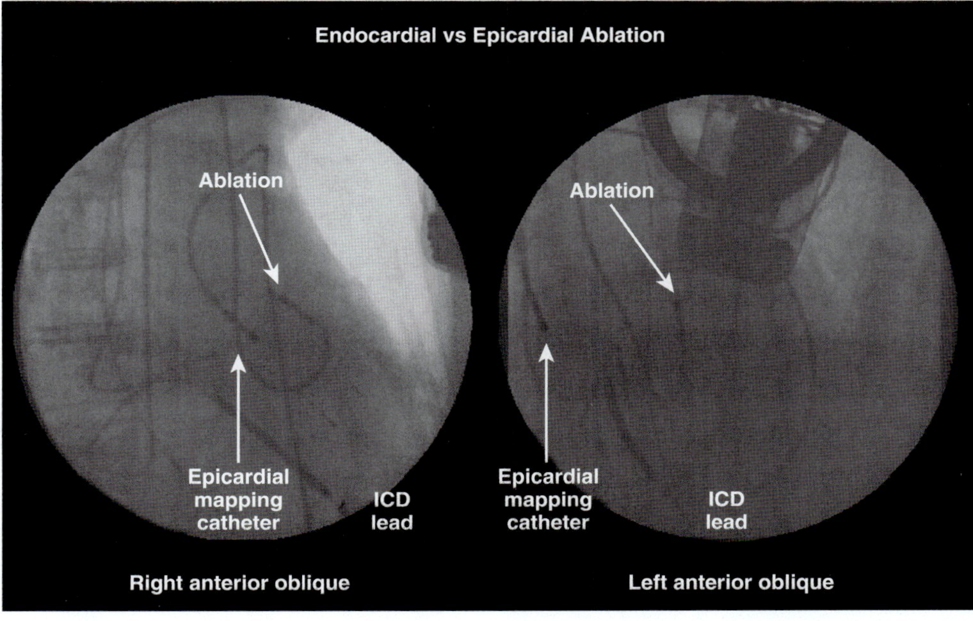

FIGURE 27-1 Combined endocardial and epicardial mapping of ventricular tachycardia (VT) in dilated nonischemic cardiomyopathy. Shown are fluoroscopic views of endocardial and epicardial ablation catheter positions. VT was eventually eliminated with endocardial ablation at the site shown (basal left ventricle). ICD = implantable cardioverter-defibrillator.

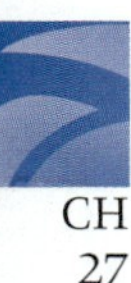

absence of the pericardium is a rare congenital anomaly (approximately 1 in every 10,000 autopsies) that is most often asymptomatic and can be an incidental finding after the patient is referred for a pericardial procedure. In the preprocedural evaluation, this rare anomaly may be suspected by an abnormal cardiac rotation or silhouette on the chest x-ray film. Definitive diagnosis can be made by CT or magnetic resonance (MR) imaging.[10]

Preablation Evaluation

Epicardial access should be obtained only when an epicardial origin of the VT circuit is strongly suspected based on a thorough preprocedural assessment. In a recent study employing simultaneous endocardial and epicardial mapping, the endocardium was ultimately thought to be a better target than the epicardium in up to 21% of patients. This highlights the importance of preoperative evaluations and procedure planning.

Careful analysis of the ECG during VT or premature ventricle complexes (PVCs) is essential. As noted, different ECG criteria for recognizing an epicardial origin of arrhythmia have been proposed. Additionally, MR imaging can help identify epicardial substrate in cardiomyopathies.[3] Furthermore, evaluation should include comprehensive clinical assessment and imaging studies to recognize any preexisting contraindications, and to minimize complications. Chest radiograph, echocardiography, and cardiac CT or MR imaging have proven to be useful for screening these patients.

CONTRAST-ENHANCED MAGNETIC RESONANCE IMAGING

Delayed contrast-enhanced MR imaging delineates regions of scar tissue potentially forming part of the arrhythmia substrate in patients with ischemic and nonischemic CMP, and enables the depiction of transmural and nontransmural scars with high spatial resolution, allowing determination of whether the scar is endocardial, intramyocardial, or epicardial (Fig. 27-2).

The suspicion of an epicardial VT substrate can facilitate planning of VT ablations, such as for a combined endocardial and epicardial approach, especially given the fact that visualization of epicardial or intramyocardial scar on preprocedure delayed enhancement MR imaging was found to be predictive of failure of the endocardial approach and of the need for the epicardial approach for VT ablation.[11]

Cardiac MR imaging can also help determine the underlying etiology of nonischemic CMP in some patients, such as myocarditis, sarcoidosis, and ARVD, which can be associated with a higher susceptibility for VT. Furthermore, in patients undergoing epicardial mapping and ablation procedures, registration of preacquired MR images with real-time electroanatomical mapping allows visualization of ventricular anatomy and obstacles to procedural success, such as epicardial fat, which can be helpful during the mapping procedure in differentiating the cause of low epicardial voltages (fat versus scar).[11]

One potential disadvantage concerns the safety of MR imaging in patients with implantable cardioverter-defibrillators (ICDs). In these patients, cardiac CT may be used for scar and fat imaging.

CONTRAST-ENHANCED COMPUTED TOMOGRAPHY

A contrast-enhanced CT scan enables detailed and comprehensive evaluation of LV myocardium using triple, multimodality imaging based on anatomical, dynamic, and perfusion parameters to identify abnormal substrate (myocardial scar and border zone) with high spatial (≤1 mm) and temporal resolution, which can be derived from a single CT scan. Areas of CT hypoperfusion correlate best with areas of abnormal voltage (<1.5 mV) rather than scar alone (<0.5 mV). Perfusion imaging from CT enables characterization of the transmural extent and intramyocardial location of scar tissue and visualization of surviving mid- and epicardial myocardium in the regions of scar, which can help identify areas potentially involved in the VT substrate. Such preprocedural information can help the operator plan an appropriate mapping and ablation strategy and better inform the patient about the risks, benefits, and chances of procedural success.[12]

The 3-D CT-defined abnormal myocardium can be accurately extracted and embedded in clinical mapping systems displaying areas of abnormal anatomical, dynamic, and perfusion parameters for substrate-guided VT ablations.[12] Additionally, CT epicardial fat imaging can be used to characterize the extent of fat tissue by extracting and integrating epicardial fat information into the 3-D electroanatomical voltage map, thereby helping to distinguish epicardial fat from scar tissue.[13]

Anatomical Considerations

The pericardium is a double-walled, flask-shaped sac that contains the heart and the roots of the great vessels, superior vena cava (SVC), and pulmonary veins (PVs). By separating the heart from its surroundings—the descending aorta, lungs, diaphragm, esophagus, trachea, and tracheobronchial lymph nodes—the pericardial space allows complete freedom of cardiac motion within this sac.[10]

The pericardium consists of two sacs intimately connected with one another: an outer fibrous envelope (the fibrous pericardium) and an inner serous sac (the serous pericardium). The fibrous pericardium consists of fibrous tissue and forms a flask-shaped bag, the neck of which is closed by its fusion with the external coats of the great vessels, while its base is attached by loose fibroareolar tissue to the central tendon and to the muscular fibers of the left side of the diaphragm. The fibrous pericardium is also attached to the

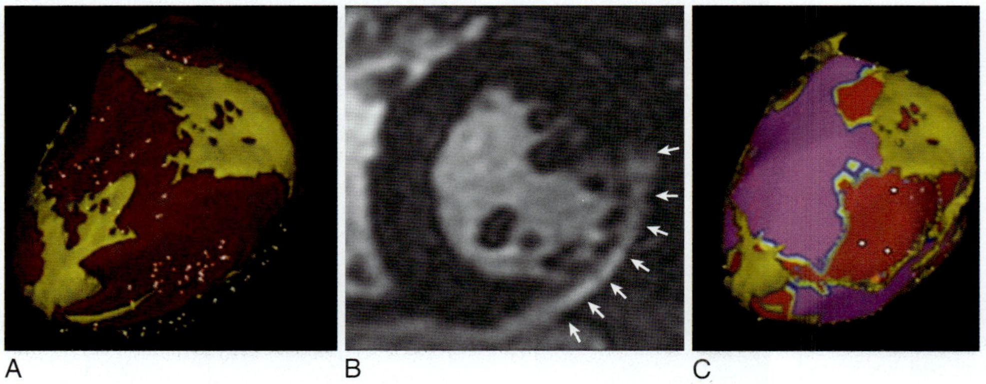

FIGURE 27-2 Epicardial fat and scar. **A,** Extracted epicardial fat (yellow) together with the epicardium (dark red) in a patient with nonischemic cardiomyopathy. **B,** Short-axis magnetic resonance imaging indicates an epicardial scar in the inferolateral left ventricular area (white arrows). **C,** Voltage map in the same patient, indicating an area of low voltage extending from the basolateral free wall of the left ventricle to the left ventricular apex. The epicardial fat (yellow) is merged with the electroanatomical voltage map. The low-voltage area projects on the left ventricular epicardium that is devoid of fat. *(From Desjardins B, Morady F, Bogun F: Effect of epicardial fat on electroanatomical mapping and epicardial catheter ablation, J Am Coll Cardiol 56:1320-1327, 2010.)*

posterior sternal surface by superior and inferior sternopericardial ligaments.[10] These attachments are essential to maintain the normal cardiac position in relation to the surrounding structures, to restrict the volume of the thin-walled cardiac chambers (right atrium and ventricle), and also to serve as direct protection against injuries.

The vessels receiving fibrous prolongations from the fibrous pericardium are the aorta, the SVC, the right and left pulmonary arteries, and the four PVs. The inferior vena cava (IVC) enters the pericardium through the central tendon of the diaphragm, and receives no covering from the fibrous layer.

The serous pericardium is a delicate membrane that lies within the fibrous pericardium and lines its walls; it is composed of two layers: the parietal pericardium and the visceral pericardium. The parietal pericardium is fused to and inseparable from the fibrous pericardium. On the other hand, the visceral pericardium, which is composed of a single layer of mesothelial cells, is part of the epicardium (i.e., the layer immediately outside of the myocardium) and covers the heart and the great vessels except for a small area on the posterior wall of the atria. The visceral layer extends to the beginning of the great vessels, and is reflected from the heart onto the parietal layer of the serous pericardium along the great vessels in tubelike extensions. This happens at two areas: where the aorta and pulmonary trunk leave the heart and where the SVC, IVC, and PVs enter the heart.[10] The serous pericardium is also metabolically active.

At the pericardial reflections and at the posterior wall between the great vessels, the pericardial space is divided up into a contiguous network of recesses and sinuses. There are three sinuses in the pericardial space: the superior sinus, the transverse sinus, and the oblique sinus. The superior sinus (superior aortic recess) lies anterior to the upper ascending aorta and main pulmonary artery. The transverse sinus is limited by a pericardial reflection between the superior PVs and contains the right pulmonary artery. The oblique sinus is confined by the pericardial reflections around the PVs and the IVC. The postcaval recess lies behind the SVC, the right pulmonary artery, and the right superior PV. The right and left PV recesses extend between their respective superior and inferior PVs.[10]

The pericardial cavity or sac is a continuous virtual space that lies between the parietal and visceral layers of serous pericardium. The heart invaginates the wall of the serous sac from above and behind, and practically obliterates its cavity, the space being merely a potential one. The sac normally contains 20 to 40 mL of clear fluid that occupies the virtual space between the two layers. Because all pericardial reflections are located basally in relation to the great vessels, the entire epicardial surface is accessible from the pericardial space, except for the atrial and ventricular septa, which are not in direct contact with the pericardium. Unlike the endovascular approach, the pericardial space is notable for the absence of obstacles and the relative ease with which catheter manipulation can be performed.[10] By the same token, achieving firm, stable contact with the catheter tip at the target site may be difficult.

Technical Considerations

Although the procedure is usually performed in the electrophysiological (EP) laboratory, it is more ideal to perform percutaneous pericardial procedures in a hybrid laboratory where cardiac surgery can be performed promptly.

The subxiphoid approach procedure may be performed under conscious sedation, deep sedation with the support of an anesthesiologist, or general anesthesia. Deep sedation or general anesthesia allows better control of respiratory motion, which can potentially reduce the chance of unintentional RV puncture, as well as better pain control, given the fact that epicardial radiofrequency (RF) ablation is usually associated with significant pain and patient discomfort. On the other hand, if patients are paralyzed under general anesthesia, diaphragmatic motion with phrenic nerve stimulation during pacing may not occur to warn of proximity of RF applications.[4] Intravenous antibiotics should be routinely administered within an hour prior to the procedure. Previous heparin administration should be reversed before pericardial access; this is accomplished by protamine infusion to decrease the activated clotting time to less than 150 seconds.

Initially, catheters are positioned in the CS and RV apex through the femoral approach. The pericardial space is accessed using a 17- or 19-gauge Tuohy needle (Codman Inc., Raynham, Mass.), which is also used to enter the epidural space when administering epidural anesthesia (typically approximately 100 mm in overall length and a 1.5-mm outer diameter). The puncture is performed at the angle between the left border of the subxiphoid process and the lower left rib, with the needle pointing to the left shoulder. The puncture needle approaches the site with a shallow angle in order to penetrate the skin and slide under the rib cage. After crossing the subcutaneous tissue, the stylet is removed, and a 10-mL syringe containing 1% lidocaine or a nonionic contrast agent is attached to the proximal port of the needle. The needle is then advanced under fluoroscopic guidance (40-degree left anterior oblique [LAO] view or, preferably, biplane right anterior oblique [RAO] and LAO projections) until close to the cardiac silhouette. The needle angle is adjusted according to the region that the operator wishes to access. Directing the needle superiorly at a relatively shallow angle, aiming for the RV apex in the RAO projection, generally allows entry into the pericardial space anteriorly over the RV and facilitates access to the anterior aspect of the RV and LV. Directing the needle more posteriorly and toward the left shoulder allows it to enter the pericardium over the diaphragmatic portion of the heart, such that the sheath typically tracks along the posterior aspect of the LV, as observed in the LAO projection. The medial third of the RV is the preferred entry region because of the absence of major coronary vessels in this region.[9,14]

In the 40-degree LAO view, injection of a small amount of contrast (approximately 1 mL) can help assess the relation of the needle to the parietal pericardium (Video 21). If the diaphragm has not been reached, the contrast will be seen in the subdiaphragmatic area. Once tenting of the pericardium is seen, a slight advance achieves entry into the space, and often one can feel the "pop" as the needle penetrates the fibrotic parietal pericardial wall. Contact of needle with the myocardium can be suggested by tactile feedback, occurrence of ventricular ectopy, or observation of a current of injury from a crocodile clip attached to the shaft of the needle. In this setting, further advancement of the needle can result in ventricular puncture and should be avoided.[15]

When the needle reaches the pericardial sac, aspiration without blood indicates that the needle has not entered the RV, and injected contrast will spread around the heart, restricted to its silhouette. In some cases, the needle will get close enough to the heart, but the contrast will not be clearly identified in the pericardial sac. In this situation, despite the needle being out of the pericardial sac, it is likely that a defect has been created in the membrane, through which it is possible to advance a soft-tipped guidewire and enter the pericardial sac. If the needle is not close enough to the pericardial membrane, the guidewire will move toward the subdiaphragmatic area. In these cases, the wire must be pulled back and small movements with the needle and the wire must be performed until the pericardial space is reached.[9]

Confirmation that the wire is intrapericardial and has not been inadvertently inserted into a cardiac chamber is obtained by observing the course of the wire in multiple fluoroscopic projections confirming that it crosses multiple cardiac chambers, hugging the edge of the cardiac silhouette in the 40-degree LAO view, circumferential to both the right and left heart, and without induction of PVCs. Observation in the RAO or anterior-posterior projection alone can be misleading, as a wire that enters the RV and passes into the right atrium (RA) or pulmonary artery can be misinterpreted as intrapericardial.[9,15]

Inadvertent RV puncture is not rare, but is usually benign if only the needle or wire has entered the chamber in a patient who is not anticoagulated. When the RV is inadvertently entered with the needle (indicated by aspiration of blood or contrast injection passing to the pulmonary artery), the needle can be withdrawn slightly (reentering the pericardial space after exiting the ventricle); contrast injection can then show silhouetting of the heart, and at that point the guidewire is advanced into the pericardial space. The small hole in the RV generally seals without incident. If the dilator and sheath have been passed into the RV, the larger hole may require surgical repair.[4]

Attempted epicardial access fails in approximately 10% of patients. The percutaneous approach to the pericardial space can be difficult in patients with pericardial adhesions (e.g., following cardiac surgery or pericarditis). In postsurgical patients, the adhesions are mostly concentrated in the anterior portion of the heart; therefore, the puncture must be directed toward the diaphragmatic area. In contrast, adhesion can be more diffuse in postpericarditis patients. Surgical creation of a subxiphoid pericardial window and manual dissection and lysis of the lesions to allow catheter mapping and ablation in the EP laboratory have been shown to be feasible in a small series.[4]

After reaching the pericardial space, a long soft "J" tip guidewire is advanced far enough to silhouette the pericardial space. The puncture needle is then withdrawn and an 8 Fr dilator is advanced over the guidewire under fluoroscopic guidance for predilation, followed by insertion of a standard 8 Fr sheath (see Video 21). If it is necessary to insert another catheter, a second guidewire can be advanced through the sheath, which should be removed, leaving two wires inside the pericardial space. Subsequently, a separate sheath is introduced over each of the guidewires. Alternatively, a second puncture of the pericardial sac may be performed, using the same steps described for the first puncture. Before removing the dilator out of the sheath, the sheath must be pushed against the chest to ensure that the tip of the sheath is placed inside the pericardial sac. Although using a standard 15 cm, 8 Fr sheath may suffice for inferior wall VT circuits, the use of longer sheaths (e.g., Agilis; St. Jude Medical, St. Paul, Minn.) should be considered, especially in patients with a larger thoracic anteroposterior dimension.

There is concern that abrasion or laceration of pericardial structures can occur by the edges of a stiff sheath if the sheath is left in the pericardium without a catheter protruding from the lumen. Therefore, it is recommended not to leave a large sheath in the pericardial space without a catheter in place. Also, it is important to lead with a wire or ablation catheter before advancing or moving the curl of the sheath to avoid damaging epicardial structures.[9]

Before introducing the mapping-ablation catheter, the sheath must be aspirated to check for bleeding. Approximately 10% to 20% of patients experience pericardial bleeding, particularly if inadvertent RV puncture has occurred. Bleeding is managed by frequent aspiration from the pericardial access sheath. It is not uncommon to aspirate 10 to 30 mL of bloody drainage from the pericardial sheath early in the procedure. At this point, anticoagulation should not have been administered; therefore, any bleeding should be self-limited and is generally considered a minor complication because it is not necessary to interrupt the procedure. Major bleeding is rare, and it can be related to the learning curve. Systemic anticoagulation with intravenous heparin is started when subsequent LV endocardial mapping, coronary angiography, or both are desired only after verifying the absence of continued pericardial bleeding.[9]

When bleeding is under control, the mapping-ablation catheter can be introduced. Once it is inside the pericardial sac, the catheter can be easily moved, allowing exploration of the entire epicardial surface. In patients with pericardial adhesions, the catheter can be used to perform blunt dissection of the adhesions; however, care must be taken to avoid cardiac perforation with the catheter tip in these cases. If the area of interest is too close to the tip of the sheath, a simple pull-back in the catheter can lead to the loss of pericardial access. Therefore, it is preferable to advance the catheter inside the pericardial space and return to the point of interest by deflecting the tip of the catheter back toward it.

Percutaneous Epicardial Mapping

Once an introducer sheath and catheter are in place, the catheter can be moved freely in the pericardial sac, constrained only by the reflections of the pericardial membrane located around the PVs and great vessels. Catheter mapping of the epicardium can be performed using fluoroscopy, an electroanatomical mapping system, or both. Atrial surface mapping can be limited by the normal pericardial reflections and by the atrial irregular anatomy (right and left atrial appendages). Ventricular surface mapping, however, can be performed more easily. During manipulation of the sheath, small amounts of air can reach the pericardial space, which can easily be detected by fluoroscopy. The presence of air can induce instability to the catheter secondary to the lack of contact between the parietal and visceral membranes of the pericardial sac. Aspiration of air will restore contact characteristic of the pericardial space.

The approach to epicardial mapping is essentially the same as for endocardial ablation, including activation mapping, entrainment mapping, substrate mapping, and pace mapping, discussed in detail in Chapter 22. The following discussion highlights certain peculiarities pertaining to the percutaneous epicardial approach to mapping.

ACTIVATION MAPPING

In scar-related VTs, inability to identify the reentry circuit isthmus on the endocardium can suggest that the isthmus is epicardial or intramural. In these cases, endocardial activation mapping can demonstrate a focal point of earliest endocardial activation where entrainment mapping indicates a potential exit or outer loop site, but ablation fails to interrupt VT, suggesting that there is an epicardial or intramural circuit with a broad endocardial exit. Some idiopathic VTs that have a focal origin also have a point of earliest endocardial breakthrough, but typically activation is not presystolic.[9]

If an appropriate target site for VT ablation cannot be identified despite extensive endocardial and epicardial mapping, an epicardial VT circuit sheltered by epicardial fat or an intramural circuit should be suspected. Cardiac MR imaging can potentially help delineate the extent of epicardial fat as well as intramural scarring suggestive of an intramural circuit.[13]

ENTRAINMENT AND PACE MAPPING

Entrainment and pace mapping maneuvers are usually difficult to perform using bipolar pacing because of a very high epicardial stimulation threshold (>15 mA) in approximately 70% of cases, likely related to the presence of epicardial fat and/or poor catheter contact due to freedom of catheter movement in the pericardial space.[4] With unipolar pacing, the pacing threshold generally is less than 10 mA at 2 milliseconds in normal tissue.[9] Epicardial fat less than 5 mm in thickness interposed between the ablating catheter and the epicardium usually does not modify the epicardial ventricular stimulation threshold.[14] Of note, ablation with irrigated RF generally renders the pacing threshold at the target area greater than 10 mA secondary, in part, to introduction of the irrigant fluid into the pericardial space.[9] This fluid can potentially result in decreased physical contact between the electrode and epicardial surface.

ELECTROANATOMICAL SUBSTRATE MAPPING

Substrate and VT mapping approaches are similar to those described for the endocardium. Areas of infarction or scar have low-amplitude electrograms similar to findings during endocardial mapping. However, epicardial fat, which is concentrated along the coronary sulcus and the interventricular grooves, can cause low-amplitude electrograms, falsely suggesting scar in voltage maps. Normal epicardial electrograms demonstrate bipolar signal amplitude typically above 0.94 to 1.5 mV; whereas signal amplitude associated with fat, large vessel coronary anatomy, or both might demonstrate significantly lower amplitude.[4,9,13,16]

As noted, epicardial fat less than 0.8 to 5 mm in thickness interposed between the ablating catheter and the epicardium usually does not modify the amplitude or duration of the bipolar epicardial electrogram. However, in areas with a layer of epicardial fat greater than 5 mm in thickness the amplitude of the bipolar epicardial electrogram can decrease, resulting in ventricular noncapture, which may confound the ability to discriminate between fat and scar. Importantly, despite the lower electrogram amplitude, epicardial fat will not produce "abnormal" (fractionated and split) electrograms. Therefore, to avoid a misclassification of low-voltage areas due to epicardial fat or major coronary vasculature as abnormal, it is important to analyze the location and extent of the confluent voltage abnormality as well as the electrogram signal characteristics. The presence of abnormal electrograms (fractionated, split, or late potentials) is usually a more reliable indicator of scar.[1,13,14]

Registration of preacquired CT or MR images detailing the LV substrate with the real-time 3-D electroanatomical voltage map allows visualization of regions of scar tissue and can potentially facilitate mapping and ablation (see Fig. 27-2). CT and MR imaging can also be used to characterize the extent of fat tissue by extracting and integrating epicardial fat information into the electroanatomical voltage maps, thereby helping to distinguish epicardial fat from scar tissue and identify areas that are difficult to penetrate because of extensive epicardial fat (Fig. 27-3).[13]

Percutaneous Epicardial Ablation

RADIOFREQUENCY ABLATION

The target for ablation is selected exactly like the endocardial target is selected. RF energy remains the primary ablative energy source for epicardial ablation. During standard RF energy application in the pericardial space, heating to the point of thrombus formation and charring is of less concern, because there is no potential for arterial embolization from the epicardial space; therefore, higher temperatures (>60°C) can be tolerated. However, standard RF ablation may not be as effective when delivered to the epicardium compared with lesions delivered to the endocardium because of the lack of convective cooling of the ablation electrode by the circulating blood. This results in high electrode temperatures at low-power settings (≤10 W), limiting power delivery in the pericardial space and impairing lesion formation. Additionally, the presence of epicardial fat (≥3.5 to 10 mm in thickness) between the ablation catheter and the targeted area can also represent an important obstacle to the effectiveness of VT ablation.[4,9,13,14]

On the other hand, open and closed loop irrigated catheters allow the delivery of energy at power settings capable of creating larger and deeper (up to 5 mm) epicardial lesions than standard RF ablation, even in the absence of circulating blood in the pericardial space. Additionally, the presence of epicardial fat interposed between the catheter tip and the myocardial tissue only moderately attenuates the efficacy of cooled-tip ablation.[4]

Optimal parameters for RF power titration and irrigation are not completely defined. With external irrigation, it is desirable to use lower flow rates, as compared with those used during endocardial mapping and ablation, to limit infusion of fluid into the pericardial space, because thrombus formation in the epicardium does not pose a risk of embolization. Commonly, the flow rate is set at 0 to 2 mL/min during mapping and at 10 to 20 mL/min during ablation, and is titrated as required to maintain electrode temperature at less than 50°C. RF energy is commonly delivered at a power output of 30 to 50 W for 60 to 120 seconds. Monitoring for an impedance fall is commonly used to assess likely adequate power delivery.[9]

With open irrigation, an obligatory fluid volume will enter the pericardial sac and, unless intermittently or continuously evacuated, it gradually results in cardiac tamponade. Therefore, intrapericardial fluid must be periodically drained after every few RF applications or every 15 to 20 minutes. This can be accomplished by intermittently removing the ablation catheter to allow aspiration from the pericardial sheath or placing a second pericardial catheter for drainage purposes. Alternatively, using a single sheath that is larger than the ablation catheter allows aspiration of fluid around the catheter from the side port, either intermittently or continuously (via attaching the side port to a suction bottle or gravity drain) without withdrawing the ablation catheter.[4,9,17]

Internally cooled RF ablation is an attractive choice for pericardial ablation as no fluid is infused and one need not worry about monitoring pericardial fluid throughout the ablation procedure.[18]

At the completion of the mapping-ablation procedure, the ablation catheter is replaced by a pigtail catheter, which is gently aspirated to remove excess intrapericardial fluid, and to confirm the absence of bleeding. Evaluation of the pericardial space can be performed by transthoracic echocardiography and by injecting 2 to 3 mL of contrast under fluoroscopy, to confirm complete drainage before removing the sheath. Methylprednisolone at 0.5 to 1.0 mg can be injected into the pericardial space prior to removal of the pigtail catheter to decrease the likelihood of postprocedure pericarditis. Generally, no major reaccumulation of pericardial fluid is observed following postprocedure draining of the pericardial fluid. The pigtail catheter may be kept inside the pericardial sac for as long as it is considered necessary. After controlling the bleeding, monitoring the patient with serial transthoracic echocardiography 24 hours later is recommended. Intravenous antibiotic therapy is administered postprocedure and follow-up echocardiogram should be performed.

PREVENTION OF CORONARY ARTERY INJURY

Coronary artery injury, severe spasm, or both can occur during epicardial mapping and RF ablation. The base and the anterior and posterior septal areas are the more dangerous zones. Prior to ablation, direct visualization of the relation between the ablation site and

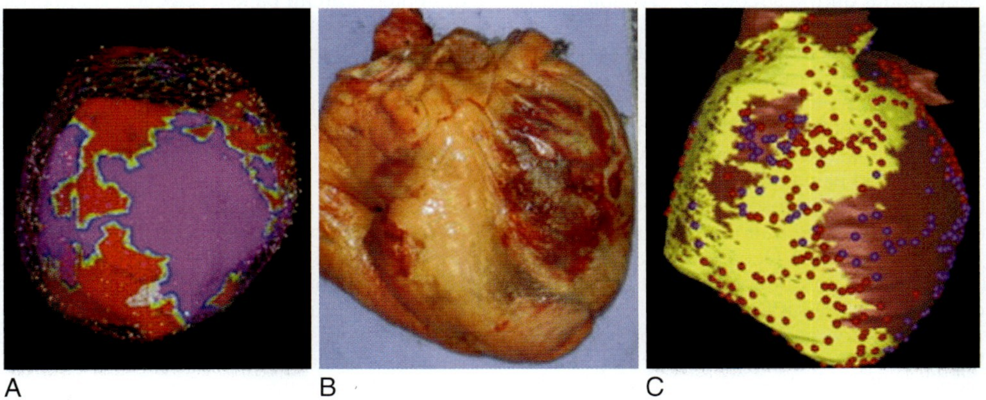

FIGURE 27-3 Distribution of epicardial fat and electroanatomical mapping. **A,** Epicardial voltage map of a patient with nonischemic cardiomyopathy. The voltage map shows surface reconstruction of the anterior surface of the heart. There is a low-voltage area (red) extending from the right ventricular outflow tract to the apex and following the lateral inferior margin to the base of the right ventricle. **B,** Gross pathology of the same heart after cardiac transplantation illustrating that the area of low voltage on the left largely corresponds to an area of epicardial fat. **C,** The extracted epicardial fat from the computed tomography data in this patient is shown in yellow. The remaining epicardial surface (dark red) is devoid of fat. The three-dimensional epicardial fat map was integrated with the voltage map. Low-voltage points are bright red and normal voltage points are purple. *(From Desjardins B, Morady F, Bogun F: Effect of epicardial fat on electroanatomical mapping and epicardial catheter ablation, J Am Coll Cardiol 56:1320-1327, 2010.)*

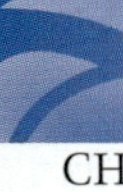

adjacent coronary arteries must be obtained, usually by coronary angiography performed with the ablation catheter on the target site. An absolute safe distance between the ablation site and epicardial artery has not been defined, and likely varies depending on the RF energy applied, coronary artery diameter and flow, and the presence of overlying fat. Based on available data and experience, a distance of at least 5 mm between the ablation electrode and an epicardial artery is commonly accepted. It is also important to ensure that the catheter is not touching the vessel at any point of the cardiac cycle during angiography. Coronary artery spasm has been reported during mapping in the pericardial space and could occur as a result of ablation close to the artery; extrinsic compression of a coronary artery can also result from edema caused by nearby ablation. Cryoablation appears to have less risk of coronary injury in animal models, but can still create occlusion and intimal damage when in close proximity, particularly to small vessels. Further confirmatory studies are warranted.[4]

PREVENTION OF PHRENIC NERVE INJURY

The left phrenic nerve is potentially susceptible to injury along its epicardial course adjacent to the lateral LV wall. The left phrenic nerve descends behind the left brachiocephalic vein and passes over the aortic arch, pulmonary trunk, and then with the pericardium over the left atrial (LA) appendage. From there it descends along the pericardium over the LV and frequently passes laterally over the obtuse margin of the LV, close to the lateral vein and the left marginal artery and, in only a small percentage of cases, close to the left main coronary artery and great cardiac vein. Not infrequently, the phrenic nerve courses through sites that might be considered appropriate target ablation sites, potentially limiting the safety and efficacy of ablation.[19]

Proximity to the nerve can be detected by high-output pacing (typically at more than 10 mA) to detect diaphragmatic stimulation on fluoroscopy, allowing its course to be marked on a 3-D map. The nerve can branch over the LV, so simply noting sites at which phrenic capture occurred does not necessarily delineate the course of all branches. It is important to recognize that detection by phrenic nerve capture is prevented by the use of paralytic agents during general anesthesia. However, these drugs are typically used during induction of anesthesia and their effects have dissipated by the time ablation is being performed.

Catheter ablation should be avoided at sites adjacent to the phrenic nerve. Alternatively moving the nerve away from the myocardium by injection of air into the pericardium or placement of a balloon catheter between the ablation target site and nerve can allow safe RF ablation. Alternative energy sources such as cryoenergy have been used to prevent phrenic nerve injury. Cryomapping uses temporary phrenic nerve injury to determine when to avoid full cryoablation. However, data on the success of cryoablation in the pericardial space are limited.[4,19,20]

Mechanical separation of the phrenic nerve from adjacent structures, using a large balloon, involves insertion of a wire though one of the existing pericardial sheaths to the vicinity of the ablation catheter positioned at the target epicardial site. A 25 mm × 40 mm peripheral angioplasty balloon is advanced over the wire to these locations. The balloon is inflated using an insufflator and contrast until complete inflation is seen on fluoroscopy. This technique can be limited by the inability to steer the balloon catheter and position it in the desired epicardial location. Occasionally, a deflectable sheath can be required to direct the balloon to the appropriate location and provide additional support and stability.[19]

Another method is to introduce a combination of saline and air into the pericardium to achieve a "controlled" hydropneumopericardium to increase the distance between the phrenic nerve and the ablation target area. This involves using a 20-mL syringe to introduce saline and air alternately in 20-mL increments under careful monitoring of arterial pressure and fluoroscopy. At each step, epicardial pacing is performed to assess phrenic nerve capture and diaphragmatic stimulation. Instillation of air and/or saline is performed slowly until phrenic nerve capture is lost or systolic arterial pressure drops to 60 mm Hg. Although cardiac tamponade can develop secondary to sudden accumulation of fluid or air in the pericardial space, controlled and progressive introduction of fluid and air with careful hemodynamic monitoring usually allows separation of the phrenic nerve from the epicardial surface without causing clinically significant tamponade.[19]

The combination of air and fluid appears to be more successful in preventing phrenic nerve injury during epicardial ablation than injecting air alone or fluid alone. In contrast to injection of fluid alone, the combination of air and fluid allows injection of a higher volume in the pericardial space with a lower impact on blood pressure than use of fluid alone. With air only, a significant resistance can be felt in most patients after injections of more than 300 mL despite stable blood pressure. Of note, air in the pericardial space can increase the defibrillation threshold, requiring emergency evacuation if defibrillation is required.[19]

CRYOABLATION

Cryoablation is an alternative to RF ablation that is not limited by absence of cooling blood flow in the pericardial space and is less prone to cause coronary artery injury in animal models. In fact, the absence of circulating blood in the pericardial space theoretically should favor creation of cryolesion. However, human experience is limited, and more studies are needed to assess safety and efficacy. Cryoablation did not produce significantly larger lesions than irrigated RF in an animal model.[4] Cryoablation is commonly used in the operating room. Surgical cryoablation with hand held surgical probes achieves much lower temperatures (less than −150°C) and generates larger lesions than small EP catheters.[9]

Outcome

Percutaneous epicardial catheter techniques have expanded the options for investigating and treating arrhythmias. Percutaneous pericardial access can be obtained in more than 90% of patients who have not had prior cardiac surgery or clinical pericarditis, even in those who required repeated epicardial procedures. However, pericardial adhesions after cardiac surgery often prevent percutaneous access, although limited access is possible in some patients. A direct surgical approach to the pericardial space via a subxiphoid pericardial window or thoracotomy can achieve access in most patients.[9,21]

Percutaneous access to the pericardial space has improved the outcome of catheter ablation in patients with scar-related VT. In several reports, arrhythmia control with epicardial ablation was achieved in 63% to 78% of patients.[3,9] However, it is important to note that these findings reflect practices at centers that specialize in arrhythmia management and may not be applicable to less experienced operators or centers. Careful patient selection is important, and the procedure should be performed by experienced operators with surgical backup.[3]

The transthoracic epicardial mapping and ablation technique is a relatively safe procedure. Severe complications have been relatively infrequent (approximately 5%), but several potential risks require attention. RV perforation and hemopericardium can be observed in up to 30% of cases. The amount of blood drained from the pericardial space usually ranges from 20 to 300 mL. Thus, most of the time, the occurrence of hemopericardium does not preclude the continuation of the procedure, although repeated aspiration of the pericardial space may be required throughout the procedure. However, major pericardial bleeding remains the most common complication (4.5%), occasionally requiring surgical intervention. Therefore, precautions must be in place for managing severe bleeding, including availability of appropriate surgical expertise.[3]

Several precautions are important to avoid injury to adjacent structures. RF injury to coronary arteries can cause acute thrombosis or damage to the arterial wall. Coronary angiography must be performed immediately before ablation to select a safe area for RF applications.[4]

Left phrenic nerve injury and diaphragmatic paralysis can result from RF ablation over the lateral LV wall. As noted, different strategies have been proposed with the aim of localizing the nerve, defining the nerve course, and then increasing the distance between the ablation site and the nerve itself.[20]

Infrequently, hemoperitoneum can result after injuring a subdiaphragmatic vessel during the puncture, and these patients may require surgery to control the intraabdominal bleeding. Hepatic laceration and bleeding are also potential risks.[4,14]

Symptomatic pericarditis is common after the procedure, occurring in approximately 30% of patients. In the majority of cases, pericardial inflammation is mild and resolves within a few days with nonsteroidal antiinflammatory medications. Administration of methylprednisolone at 0.5 to 1 mg/kg into the epicardial space at the end of the procedure can potentially help reduce the pericardial inflammatory reaction. It is important to note that inflammatory pericarditis can render the epicardial space percutaneously inaccessible for repeat procedures because of the development of adhesions.[4,9,14]

Transvenous Epicardial Mapping and Ablation

Clinical Considerations

Coronary veins provide endovascular access to the epicardial regions of the ventricles, and have been used for mapping and ablation of arrhythmia foci or circuits that are deep within the myocardium or in the epicardium without having to access the epicardium percutaneously. Access through the great cardiac and anterior interventricular veins allows mapping over a wide area of the anterolateral LV wall, whereas access through the middle cardiac vein allows mapping over the inferior wall of the ventricles and posterior aspect of the interventricular septum.

Up to 14% of patients with idiopathic PVCs can have an epicardial site of origin identified within the coronary venous system, most often in the great cardiac vein. Successful long-term ablation of these arrhythmias was achieved from within the coronary venous system in approximately 70% of patients.[8]

However, epicardial mapping and ablation via the coronary venous system has important limitations. Epicardial circuits may be identified only when the cannulated vessel happens to be in the region of the circuit. Additionally, catheter manipulation is limited by the anatomical distribution and size of these vessels. Currently available ablation catheters often are difficult to advance beyond the distal great cardiac vein or the proximal portions of the middle cardiac vein because of the tortuosity, sharp angulation, and small caliber of the distal veins. Furthermore, a conventional ablation catheter may completely occlude a branch of the CS, preventing cooling of the ablation electrode and resulting in high impedance when RF energy is delivered. This markedly reduces the amount of power that can be delivered and may result in adherence of the ablation electrode to the wall of the vein. In fact, delivery of more than 10 to 15 W seldom is possible. An external saline-cooled ablation catheter allows more consistent delivery of RF energy, with less heating at the electrode-tissue interface.[7]

Anatomical Considerations

The myocardium drains mainly by three groups of veins: (1) the CS and its tributaries, which return blood from almost the whole heart; (2) the anterior cardiac veins, which primarily drain the anterior regions of the RV and the right cardiac border, ending principally in the RA; and (3) the Thebesian venous network (venae cordis minimae), which is the smaller cardiac venous system and is composed of small venous branches made primarily of endothelial cells, which are continuous with the lining of the cardiac chambers, and drains the subendocardium. The Thebesian veins open directly into any of the four chambers but are more prominent on the right and, to a lesser extent, the LA and sometimes the LV.[22-24]

Normally, the CS has five first-order tributaries: the great cardiac vein, the middle cardiac vein, the small cardiac vein, the posterior cardiac vein of the LV, and the oblique vein of the LA (oblique vein of Marshall). These tributaries then branch into second- and third-order tributaries. The CS returns the blood to the RA from the whole heart (including its septa) except the anterior region of the RV and small, variable parts of both atria and the LV.

The CS begins as a continuation of the great cardiac vein, extending from the valve of Vieussens (which often marks the junction of the CS with the great cardiac vein) to the ostium of the CS as it terminates in the RA. The length of the CS varies from 30 to 55 mm and its diameter varies from 6 to 16 mm in its middle portion (depending on the loading conditions and the presence of underlying cardiac disease or prior cardiac surgery).[22,23]

The CS invariably lies in the posterior aspect of the atrioventricular (AV) groove in the sulcus between the LA and LV and opens into the RA. The CS ostium (CS os) is 5 to 15 mm in diameter and is located on the posterior interatrial septum anterior to the Eustachian ridge and valve and posterior to the tricuspid annulus. The CS os is guarded by the highly variable, crescent-shaped Thebesian valve. This valve usually covers the superior and posterior surfaces of the CS os, but may nearly completely cover the os with formation of fenestrations and can hinder cannulation of the CS.[22-24]

The anterior interventricular vein is the largest and most consistent of the cardiac veins. It drains a significant portion of the LV anterior wall and the interventricular septum, begins at the cardiac apex, and ascends toward the base of the heart in the anterior interventricular sulcus, parallel to the left anterior descending coronary artery. The phrenic nerve may lie close to lateral branches of this vein. The anterior interventricular vein is the most anterior vein seen in the RAO projection. At the base of the heart, near the bifurcation of the left coronary artery, the anterior interventricular vein turns laterally and becomes the "great cardiac vein," which courses along the left AV groove (parallel to the left circumflex coronary artery) and wraps around the left side of the heart.[22-24]

The great cardiac vein is joined by the LA oblique vein of Marshall and the posterolateral vein of the LV to form the CS. In addition to several smaller tributaries from the LA and ventricles, the great cardiac vein receives two main branches, namely, the large left marginal vein (along the lateral border of the heart) and the posterior cardiac vein of the LV (also known as the posterolateral vein).[22-24]

The middle (or "posterior interventricular") cardiac vein is the largest proximal tributary of the CS and is present in nearly all hearts. This vein drains the inferior walls of both ventricles and interventricular septum and courses with the posterior descending coronary artery in the posterior interventricular groove, joining the CS close to the RA orifice or, rarely, entering the RA directly.

The small cardiac vein is an inconstant vessel that receives blood from the back of the RA and RV, runs in the coronary sulcus between the RA and RV parallel to the right coronary artery, and empties into either the CS, the middle cardiac vein, or the RA.

Of all of the branches of the coronary venous system, the great cardiac and middle cardiac veins are the two most consistently present branches. Unlike the middle cardiac vein, the great cardiac vein varies considerably in its course. Lateral and posterior venous branches together are seen in approximately 50% of human hearts, unlike the anterior interventricular and middle cardiac veins, which are seen in more than 90%.

The venous valves can hinder catheter access within the coronary venous system, especially the Thebesian valve, which may completely cover the CS os in a variety of forms or be imperforate. Other venous valves, like the valve of Vieussens, are often present at the entrances of the ventricular veins into the great cardiac vein, or at the entrance of a smaller vein into a larger vein. These tend to be flimsy endothelial ridges but can present some resistance on probing or when trying to pass a catheter.[22-24]

Technical Considerations

CS venography is typically required to help delineate its anatomy and guide ablation. The great cardiac and the anterior interventricular veins allow epicardial access to the anterior basal ventricular surface. The middle cardiac vein allows epicardial access to the inferior ventricular surface.

Small electrode catheters (e.g., the 2.5 Fr multipolar catheter Pathfinder; Cardima, Inc., Fremont, Calif.) can be introduced into the CS and advanced out into the cardiac veins. The catheter can be positioned in different coronary venous branches to map different regions of the epicardial surface of the ventricles.[8]

Once the ablation catheter is positioned at the target site, and before energy delivery, coronary angiography should be performed to assess the distance of the catheter tip to a major epicardial coronary artery (see Fig. 23-19). If this distance is less than 4 mm ablation should not be attempted. In this situation, cryoablation can be performed with little or no risk of coronary artery injury. Additionally, pacing from the distal ablation electrode should be performed at an output of 20 mA. If diaphragmatic capture can be demonstrated, then ablation should not be attempted to avoid phrenic nerve injury.

RF ablation within the coronary venous system is usually performed with a 3.5-mm open-irrigated-tip catheter at a power output of 15 to 25 W for up to 60 seconds (Fig. 27-4). If this catheter cannot

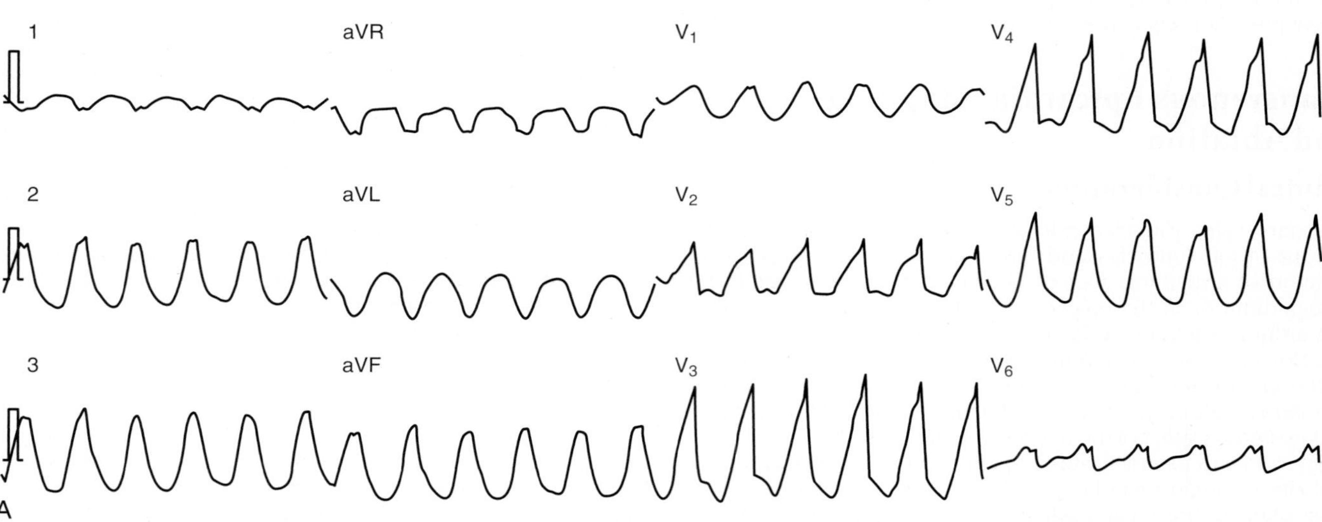

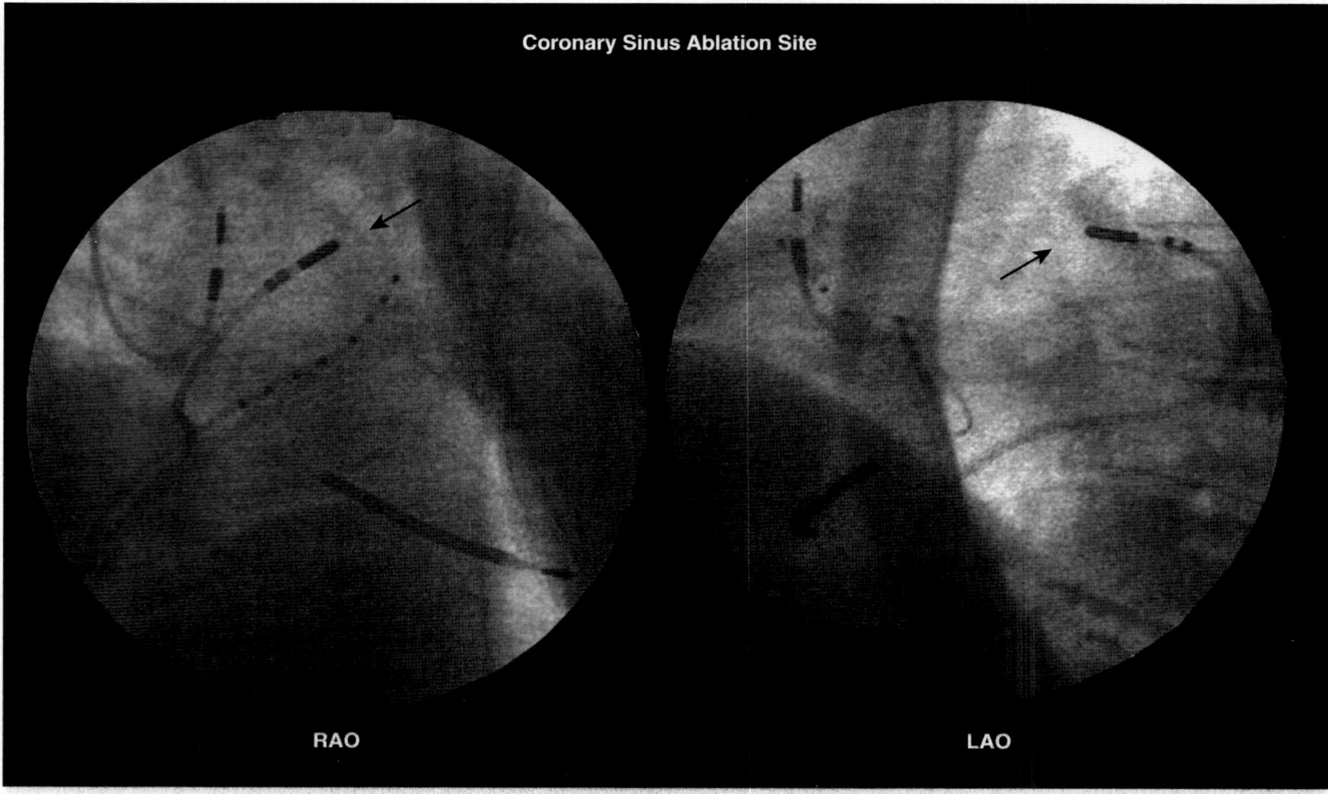

FIGURE 27-4 Idiopathic epicardial ventricular tachycardia (VT). **A,** Surface ECG of a slow VT that was ablated from the coronary sinus (CS) after both endocardial and epicardial mapping failed to eliminate the VT. **B,** Right anterior oblique (RAO) and left anterior oblique (LAO) fluoroscopic views of catheter location for VT ablation from the CS.

be maneuvered to the ablation target site, a 5 Fr, 6 Fr, or 7 Fr ablation catheter may be used. For nonirrigated-tip catheters, the target temperature is usually set to 55°C to 60°C with a power output of 15 to 30 W. Impedance should be monitored during RF applications, and RF energy delivery should be stopped if impedance rises significantly. If RF energy delivery is limited, cryoablation using a 6-mm CryoAblation catheter (Medtronic, Minneapolis, Minn.) may be considered, although this catheter is less maneuverable than an RF catheter.[8]

Outcome

The outcome of the ablation procedure is a function of the proximity of the ideal target site to accessible portions of the coronary venous system as well as the ability to deliver an effective amount of ablative energy to the target site. Despite the anatomical constraints, ablation via the coronary venous system has yielded success rates of approximately 70%. Using the coronary venous system for mapping and ablation can potentially result in a lower complication rate than the percutaneous pericardial approach because damage to the RV or extracardiac structures is less likely to occur.[7]

Coronary artery injury is an ever-present risk, especially near the proximal part of the anterior interventricular vein. Arterial injury, including thrombosis, medial necrosis, and hyperplasia, is inversely proportional to vessel diameter; there is little evidence of injury when vessel diameter exceeds 0.5 to 1.0 mm. Similar findings were reported for cryoablation. As noted, coronary angiography should be performed before delivering RF energy near or within a branch of the CS to determine whether there are any branches of the right or left coronary artery in proximity to the ablation site.[7]

REFERENCES

1. Cano O, Hutchinson M, Lin D, et al: Electroanatomic substrate and ablation outcome for suspected epicardial ventricular tachycardia in left ventricular nonischemic cardiomyopathy, *J Am Coll Cardiol* 54:799–808, 2009.
2. Garcia FC, Bazan V, Zado ES, et al: Epicardial substrate and outcome with epicardial ablation of ventricular tachycardia in arrhythmogenic right ventricular cardiomyopathy/dysplasia, *Circulation* 120:366–375, 2009.
3. Sacher F, Roberts-Thomson K, Maury P, et al: Epicardial ventricular tachycardia ablation a multicenter safety study, *J Am Coll Cardiol* 55:2366–2372, 2010.
4. Aliot EM, Stevenson WG, Mendral-Garrote JM, et al: EHRA/HRS Expert Consensus on Catheter Ablation of Ventricular Arrhythmias: developed in a partnership with the European Heart Rhythm Association (EHRA), a Registered Branch of the European Society of Cardiology (ESC), and the Heart Rhythm Society (HRS); in collaboration with the American College of Cardiology (ACC) and the American Heart Association (AHA), *Heart Rhythm* 6:886–933, 2009.
5. Haqqani HM, Morton JB, Kalman JM: Using the 12-lead ECG to localize the origin of atrial and ventricular tachycardias. 2. Ventricular tachycardia, *J Cardiovasc Electrophysiol* 20:825–832, 2009.
6. Natale A, Raviele A, Al-Ahmad A, et al: Venice Chart International Consensus document on ventricular tachycardia/ventricular fibrillation ablation, *J Cardiovasc Electrophysiol* 21:339–379, 2010.
7. Daniels DV, Lu YY, Morton JB, et al: Idiopathic epicardial left ventricular tachycardia originating remote from the sinus of Valsalva: electrophysiological characteristics, catheter ablation, and identification from the 12-lead electrocardiogram, *Circulation* 113:1659–1666, 2006.
8. Baman TS, Ilg KJ, Gupta SK, et al: Mapping and ablation of epicardial idiopathic ventricular arrhythmias from within the coronary venous system, *Circ Arrhythm Electrophysiol* 3:274–279, 2010.
9. Tedrow U, Stevenson WG: Strategies for epicardial mapping and ablation of ventricular tachycardia, *J Cardiovasc Electrophysiol* 20:710–713, 2009.
10. d'Avila A, Scanavacca M, Sosa E, et al: Pericardial anatomy for the interventional electrophysiologist, *J Cardiovasc Electrophysiol* 14:422–430, 2003.
11. Yokokawa M, Tada H, Koyama K, et al: The characteristics and distribution of the scar tissue predict ventricular tachycardia in patients with advanced heart failure, *Pacing Clin Electrophysiol* 32:314–322, 2009.
12. Tian J, Jeudy J, Smith MF, et al: Three-dimensional contrast-enhanced multidetector CT for anatomic, dynamic, and perfusion characterization of abnormal myocardium to guide ventricular tachycardia ablations, *Circ Arrhythm Electrophysiol* 3:496–504, 2010.
13. Desjardins B, Morady F, Bogun F: Effect of epicardial fat on electroanatomical mapping and epicardial catheter ablation, *J Am Coll Cardiol* 56:1320–1327, 2010.
14. d'Avila A: Epicardial catheter ablation of ventricular tachycardia, *Heart Rhythm* 5(6 Suppl):S73–S75, 2008.
15. Lachman N, Syed FF, Habib A, et al: Correlative anatomy for the electrophysiologist. I. The pericardial space, oblique sinus, transverse sinus, *J Cardiovasc Electrophysiol* 21:1421–1426, 2010.
16. Zeppenfeld K, Stevenson WG: Ablation of ventricular tachycardia in patients with structural heart disease, *Pacing Clin Electrophysiol* 31:358–374, 2008.
17. Vest JA, Seiler J, Stevenson WG: Clinical use of cooled radiofrequency ablation, *J Cardiovasc Electrophysiol* 19:769–773, 2008.
18. Lustgarten DL, Spector PS: Ablation using irrigated radiofrequency: a hands-on guide, *Heart Rhythm* 5:899–902, 2008.
19. Di Biase L, Burkhardt JD, Pelargonio G, et al: Prevention of phrenic nerve injury during epicardial ablation: comparison of methods for separating the phrenic nerve from the epicardial surface, *Heart Rhythm* 6:957–961, 2009.
20. Fan R, Cano O, Ho SY, et al: Characterization of the phrenic nerve course within the epicardial substrate of patients with nonischemic cardiomyopathy and ventricular tachycardia, *Heart Rhythm* 6:59–64, 2009.
21. Michowitz Y, Mathuria N, Tung R, et al: Hybrid procedures for epicardial catheter ablation of ventricular tachycardia: value of surgical access, *Heart Rhythm* 7:1635–1643, 2010.
22. Habib A, Lachman N, Christensen KN, Asirvatham SJ: The anatomy of the coronary sinus venous system for the cardiac electrophysiologist, *Europace* 11(Suppl 5):v15–v21, 2009.
23. Ho SY, Sanchez-Quintana D, Becker AE: A review of the coronary venous system: a road less traveled, *Heart Rhythm* 1:107–112, 2004.
24. Singh JP, Houser S, Heist EK, Ruskin JN: The coronary venous anatomy: a segmental approach to aid cardiac resynchronization therapy, *J Am Coll Cardiol* 46:68–74, 2005.

CHAPTER 28 Ventricular Arrhythmias in Hypertrophic Cardiomyopathy

Pathophysiology

Hypertrophic cardiomyopathy (CMP) is characterized by an otherwise unexplained thickened but nondilated left ventricle (LV) in the absence of any other cardiac or systemic condition capable of producing the magnitude of hypertrophy evident (e.g., aortic valve stenosis, systemic hypertension, some expressions of athlete's heart, infiltrative or storage disorders), independent of whether obstruction to LV outflow is present.

Hypertrophic CMP is characterized by myocyte disarray. Cardiomyocytes in hypertrophic CMP become hypertrophied, enlarged, and distorted, which leads to disorientation of adjacent cells and arrangement in chaotic disorganized patterns (instead of the normal parallel cellular arrangement), forming circles or whorls around foci of connective tissue. Although the disorganized architecture is evident in the majority (95%) of patients dying of hypertrophic CMP, it is not specific to hypertrophic CMP, and it occurs in other syndromic causes of LV hypertrophy such as Noonan syndrome and Friedreich ataxia, congenital heart disease, hypertension, and aortic stenosis. Nevertheless, myocyte disarray in hypertrophic CMP is typically more extensive, occupying more than 5% of the total myocardium, including substantial portions of hypertrophied as well as nonhypertrophied LV myocardium, 33% of the ventricular septum, and 25% of the free wall.

Changes in myocyte architecture lead to ventricular hypertrophy (Fig. 28-1). The degree and distribution of LV hypertrophy vary markedly. LV hypertrophy can be asymmetrical or symmetrical. The symmetrical form of hypertrophic CMP accounts for more than one-third of cases and is characterized by concentric thickening of the LV with a small ventricular cavity dimension. Asymmetrical septal hypertrophy is the most common variant, which is associated with thickening of the basal anterior septum, which bulges beneath the aortic valve and causes narrowing of the LV outflow region. However, isolated segmental hypertrophy may affect the LV apex (apical hypertrophic CMP) or any portion of the LV. The morphological pattern of LV hypertrophy is not closely predictive of the severity of symptoms or prognosis. Although LV apical aneurysms are observed only rarely (2%), they are associated with a higher rate of adverse disease consequences (10.5% per year) as compared with the general hypertrophic CMP population.[1]

Hypertrophic CMP is a complex and clinically heterogeneous disease that demonstrates remarkable diversity in disease course, age of onset, severity of symptoms, LV outflow obstruction, and risk for sudden cardiac death (SCD). The characteristic diversity of the hypertrophic CMP phenotype is attributable to the intergenetic heterogeneity (with a variety of mutations encoding protein components of the cardiac sarcomere), the intragenetic heterogeneity (with multiple different mutations identified in each gene), as well as the potential influence of modifier genes and environmental factors.

The arrhythmogenic substrate responsible for ventricular tachycardia (VT) occurrence in hypertrophic CMP has not been completely defined. Myofibrillar disarray as well as diffuse interstitial myocardial fibrosis or extensive scarring (likely caused by abnormalities of intramural coronary arteries and focal ischemia), which potentially predispose to disordered conduction patterns and increased dispersion of electrical depolarization and repolarization, have been suggested as factors contributing to ventricular arrhythmogenesis.[2]

Molecular Genetics

Hypertrophic CMP is familial in approximately half the cases and sporadic in the other half. The disease is transmitted as a Mendelian trait with an autosomal dominant pattern of inheritance and variable clinical penetrance. There is substantial diversity in the genetic causes of hypertrophic CMP. To date, nearly 900 different mutations have been reported in at least 24 genes encoding eight sarcomere proteins, including cardiac alpha- and beta-myosin heavy chains; cardiac troponins T, I, and C; cardiac myosin-binding protein C; alpha-tropomyosin; actin; titin; and essential and regulatory myosin light chains. Among these genes, mutations in *MYH7,* encoding beta-myosin heavy chain, and *MYBPC3,* encoding cardiac myosin binding protein-C, are the most common, each accounting for one-quarter to one-third of all cases.[3,4] For each gene, several different mutations have been identified, and specific mutations are associated with different disease severity and prognosis.[5]

In addition, nonsarcomeric protein mutations in genes involved in cardiac metabolism (e.g., the gamma subunit of adenosine monophosphate [AMP]–activated protein kinase, PRKAG2, and lysosome-associated membrane protein 2 [LAMP-2], as in Danon disease), which are responsible for primary cardiac glycogen storage cardiomyopathies in older children and young adults, can be associated with a clinical presentation mimicking or indistinguishable from sarcomeric hypertrophic CMP. A high prevalence of conduction system dysfunction (with the requirement of permanent pacing in 30% of patients) characterizes PRKAG2 mutations. These diseases are often associated with ventricular preexcitation (Wolff-Parkinson-White syndrome). LAMP2 mutations are associated with early-onset LV hypertrophy (often in childhood) with rapid progression of heart failure and poor prognosis. These clinical entities are distinct from hypertrophic CMP caused by sarcomere protein mutations, despite the shared feature of LV hypertrophy. In addition, there can be genetic overlap between hypertrophic CMP and LV noncompaction.[4]

In infants and children, LV hypertrophy mimicking typical hypertrophic CMP caused by sarcomere protein mutations is often associated with congenital malformations and syndromes, inherited disorders of metabolism, and neuromuscular diseases, such as Fabry disease, Pompe disease, amyloidosis, carnitine deficiency, mitochondrial diseases, Friedreich ataxia, Noonan syndrome, and

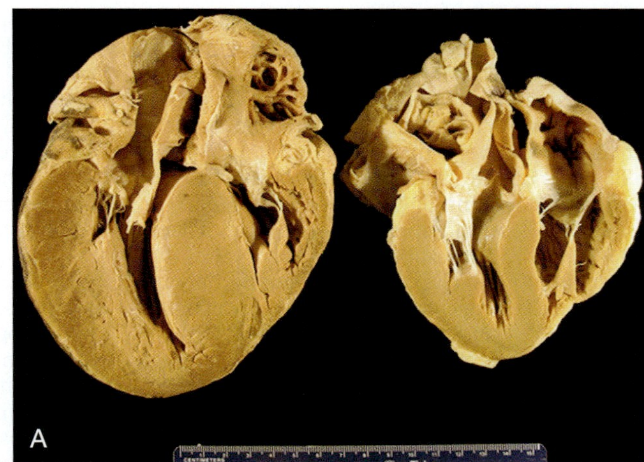

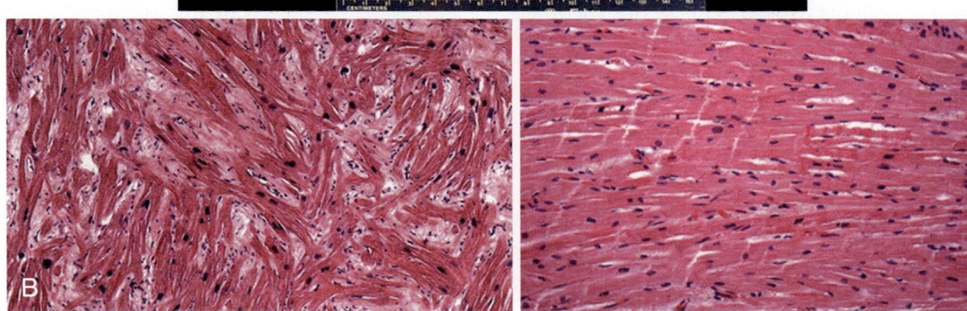

FIGURE 28-1 Pathological features of hypertrophic cardiomyopathy (CMP). **A,** Gross pathology showing markedly increased LV wall thickness associated with hypertrophic CMP (left) as compared with normal cardiac morphology (right). **B,** Histological sections stained with hematoxylin and eosin demonstrate myocyte disarray, where myocytes are oriented at bizarre and variable angles to each other, and increased myocardial fibrosis (left), the pathognomonic features of hypertrophic CMP. In contrast, normal myocardium demonstrates a very orderly arrangement of myocytes (right). Images are shown at ×10 magnification. *(From Ho CY: Hypertrophic cardiomyopathy, Heart Fail Clin 6:141-159, 2010.)*

LEOPARD syndrome. Hypertrophic CMP can be distinguished from these disorders by dysmorphological examination, neuromuscular examination, metabolic screening, family information, and genetic testing.[3,6]

Clinical Considerations

Epidemiology

Hypertrophic CMP is the most common genetic cardiovascular disease, with a prevalence of approximately 0.2% of the general population for the disease phenotype recognized by echocardiography.

Approximately 10% to 20% of individuals with hypertrophic CMP have a lifetime-increased risk for SCD, most likely resulting from VT and ventricular fibrillation (VF). Hypertrophic CMP is the leading single cause of SCD in competitive athletes in the United States, accounting for approximately one-third of such deaths. Although SCD occurs most often in adolescents or young adults, it can occur at any age. However, SCD is uncommon in young children.

SCD can be the first manifestation of disease. Individuals with hypertrophic CMP who are at the highest risk for SCD can have an at least 3% to 5% annual risk for SCD, whereas individuals in the general hypertrophic CMP population have a 1% annual risk for SCD.

Early studies based on tertiary referral-based populations with hypertrophic CMP suggested a poor prognosis with estimated annual mortality rates of 4% to 6%; however, subsequent studies on broader-based populations suggest that prognosis is typically more favorable with estimated annual mortality rates of 1% to 3% and a normal life expectancy of 75 years or more in about 25% of individuals, the majority of whom have little functional disability.

Clinical Presentation

The clinical presentation of hypertrophic CMP is characterized by extreme variability in disease course, age of onset, severity of symptoms, and risk for SCD. Many patients are either asymptomatic or mildly symptomatic. The majority of patients present during adolescence or young adulthood, but symptoms can develop at any age. Symptomatic patients typically present with dyspnea, chest pain, palpitations, fatigue, orthostatic lightheadedness, presyncope, and syncope. Other complications include atrial and ventricular arrhythmias, infective endocarditis, and congestive heart failure. As noted, SCD can be the first manifestation of the disease.[7]

Shortness of breath, particularly exertional, is the most common symptom of hypertrophic CMP, occurring in up to 90% of patients, typically secondary to diastolic LV dysfunction. Syncope occurs in approximately 15% to 25% of patients, typically secondary to abnormal hemodynamic function (i.e., dynamic LV outflow obstruction) or, infrequently, secondary to cardiac arrhythmias.[7,8] Atrial fibrillation (AF) is the most common arrhythmia observed in hypertrophic CMP, occurring in approximately 20% to 25% of patients, and is associated with an increased risk of stroke and thromboembolic complications.

LV outflow obstruction, when present, can produce a characteristic dynamic systolic ejection murmur and bifid pulse. About 25% of individuals with hypertrophic CMP demonstrate LV outflow obstruction at rest, but in many patients the obstruction is variable, occurring in response to exercise or maneuvers that decrease LV preload or afterload or increase contractility or heart rate (dynamic outflow obstruction).

Although LV ejection fraction (LVEF) is typically preserved or even hyperdynamic, up to 5% to 10% of patients may progress to the "burned-out" or end-stage phase of hypertrophic CMP, marked by LV systolic dysfunction, and occasionally progressive LV dilatation and wall thinning. These patients may develop refractory symptoms or end-stage heart failure requiring cardiac transplantation.

Ventricular Arrhythmias

The predominant arrhythmia syndrome associated with hypertrophic CMP is sudden cardiac arrest, presumably due to polymorphic VT or VF. SCD occurs with an annual mortality rate of approximately 6% in referral-based populations and 1% in community-based studies. However, certain patient subgroups can have much higher rates, surpassing the American College of Cardiology/American Heart Association (ACC/AHA) guideline document definition of high risk for SCD (≥2% annual risk).[9]

Hypertrophic CMP is the most common cause of SCD in young people, including competitive athletes, in the United States. SCD occurs throughout life, with a peak in adolescence and young adulthood (<30 to 35 years of age), and can be the initial disease presentation. SCD occurs most commonly during mild exertion or sedentary activities; nonetheless, an important proportion of such events is associated with vigorous exertion.

Ambulatory electrocardiogram (ECG) monitoring frequently reveals premature ventricular complexes (in 88% of patients), nonsustained VT (25% to 30%), and supraventricular tachyarrhythmias such as AF and atrial flutter (30% to 40%). The frequency of all arrhythmias during 48-hour ambulatory ECG monitoring is age related. Nonsustained VT is associated with severity of hypertrophy and symptom class; supraventricular arrhythmias are more common in patients with LV outflow obstruction.

Stable sustained monomorphic VT (SMVT) is rare, but can occur in patients with midventricular obstruction or apical LV aneurysms. The recurrence rate of VT is relatively high (56%) in hypertrophic CMP patients, and electrical storm can occur. During electrophysiological (EP) testing, induction of SMVT has a low reproducibility, and polymorphic VT and VF are often induced. The VT is commonly associated with a superior axis on the frontal plane, suggesting LV apical origins. An arrhythmic substrate, such as an aneurysm, can be important for the occurrence of stable SMVT.[1,10]

Appropriate implantable cardioverter-defibrillator (ICD) discharges in hypertrophic CMP patients occur annually in 10.6% of ICD recipients for secondary prevention after cardiac arrest (5-year cumulative probability, 39%), and in 3.6% of ICD recipients for primary prevention (5-year probability, 17%).[11] Of note, arrhythmogenic events do not necessarily portend other adverse clinical outcomes. Specifically, appropriate ICD discharges do not appear to predict the occurrence of heart failure or the need for other invasive therapies (e.g., surgical myectomy, septal ablation).[12]

Initial Evaluation

Clinical diagnosis is generally made with transthoracic echocardiography, demonstrating LV hypertrophy in a nondilated ventricle (Fig. 28-2). Cardiac magnetic resonance (MR) imaging also can provide very valuable additional information in the diagnosis of hypertrophic CMP and in differentiating it from other disorders. Marked ECG abnormalities are typically present in the majority of patients.

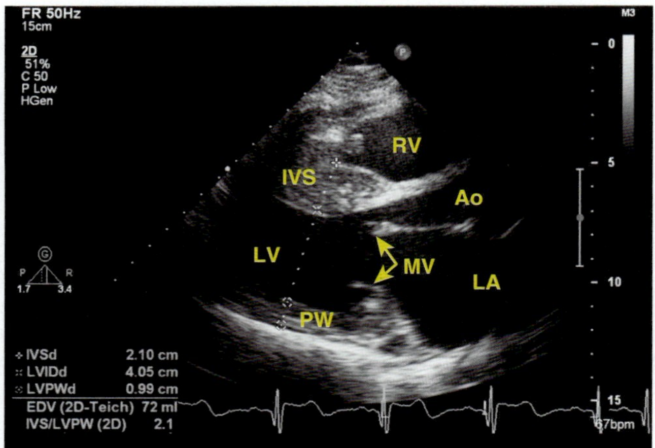

FIGURE 28-2 Echocardiographic appearance of hypertrophic cardiomyopathy. Parasternal long-axis view from a patient with hypertrophic cardiomyopathy demonstrating asymmetrical septal hypertrophy. The interventricular septum (marked by arrow) measures 2.1 cm, the posterior wall measures 0.99 cm. Ao = aorta; IVS = interventricular septum; LA = left atrium; LV = left ventricle; MV = mitral valve; PW = posterior wall; RV = right ventricle.

In addition to clinical history, risk stratification for SCD in hypertrophic CMP patients requires family pedigree analysis (premature sudden death), echocardiogram (hypertrophy, LV outflow gradient), 48-hour ambulatory ECG (nonsustained VT), and a symptom-limited exercise test with careful measurement of blood pressure (abnormal blood pressure response).

Clinical genetic testing for hypertrophic CMP comprising the eight most common disease-causing genes is now commercially available. Overall, the yield of genetic testing in probands with hypertrophic CMP is approximately 60%, but it depends on patient selection, falling to approximately 30% in sporadic disease.[13,14] Although the knowledge of the underlying gene and mutation has a limited role in risk stratification and management of the individual patient, genetic testing is recommended for patients with an established clinical diagnosis of hypertrophic CMP in whom mutation-specific confirmatory testing would benefit, confirm, or exclude the diagnosis in at-risk family members. Once a pathogenic mutation has been detected, cascade screening of the relatives is indicated. On the other hand, genetic testing is not recommended for diagnosis of hypertrophic CMP in patients with nondiagnostic clinical features because the absence of a sarcomere mutation cannot rule out familial hypertrophic CMP. Furthermore, variants of uncertain significance can pose a problem in subjects with lower clinical pretest probability of a pathogenic sarcomere mutation.[4]

Risk Stratification

The traditionally acknowledged noninvasive risk stratification strategy for primary prevention uses five clinical markers that have been defined in several retrospective and observational studies. These primary prevention risk factors (applicable to hypertrophic CMP patients without prior cardiac arrest) are: (1) premature hypertrophic CMP-related sudden death in one or more relatives; (2) unexplained syncope (especially in the young and related to exertion); (3) multiple, repetitive (or prolonged) nonsustained VT on ambulatory (Holter) monitoring; (4) severe LV hypertrophy (maximal wall thickness of ≥30 mm); and (5) an abnormal blood pressure response during upright exercise (i.e., failure of blood pressure to rise appropriately by more than 20 to 30 mm Hg from baseline).[8,15,16]

The risk associated with each of these factors is greatest in younger patients; hence, this risk stratification approach is generally employed in patients younger than 50 years. However, it is important to understand that even achieving this measure of longevity does not confer immunity to SCD.

The relative weight that can be assigned to each of the traditional risk markers has not been defined. A consensus document on hypertrophic CMP from the ACC and European Society of Cardiology (ESC) categorized known risk factors for SCD as "major" and "possible in individual patients" (Table 28-1). Although the absence of risk factors identifies a low-risk group, the positive predictive value of any single risk factor is limited. Risk stratification based on incorporation of multiple risk factors would likely improve positive predictive accuracy.[9]

It is also important to note that the traditional risk stratification strategy in hypertrophic CMP remains imprecise and a few SCDs have been reported in young hypertrophic CMP patients judged to be at low risk without any of the acknowledged risk markers.[17]

In addition to the five traditional risk factors, other features of hypertrophic CMP may increase SCD risk for patients in selected subgroups. LV apical aneurysm (which is observed only in 2% of hypertrophic CMP patients) has been associated with a substantial (10%) annual event rate, largely because of the arrhythmogenic substrate created by the fibrotic thin-walled aneurysm.[1,18] Similarly, patients in the end-stage phase of the disease (characterized by LV systolic dysfunction, wall thinning, and chamber enlargement) awaiting heart transplantation have a substantial arrhythmia-related event rate of 10% per year.[17]

Although LV outflow obstruction (subaortic gradient ≥30 mm Hg at rest) is a determinant of progressive heart failure and cardiovascular death (particularly from stroke), the specific relationship to SCD is weak and insufficient to regard LV outflow obstruction as a primary SCD risk marker.[19] Reduction of obstruction by myotomy/myectomy (or alcohol ablation) is not considered a primary strategy for mitigating SCD risk. Similarly, the severity of clinical symptoms such as dyspnea, chest pain, and effort intolerance has not been correlated with increased risk of SCD.[9]

Currently, genetic testing appears to have little clinical application to the assessment of prognosis. Although certain mutations (e.g., some beta-myosin heavy chain and troponin T mutations) responsible for hypertrophic CMP can be associated with a higher risk for SCD compared with other mutations, there is substantial overlap between different disease gene groups, and exceptions are common.[4] Hence, the prognostic value of disease-causing mutations in hypertrophic CMP for risk stratification is questionable, and the clinical course of individual patients cannot be reliably predicted based solely on particular genetic substrates and disease-causing mutations.[17]

Percutaneous alcohol septal ablation appears to augment the risk of SCD in patients with hypertrophic CMP. Alcohol septal ablation typically creates a sizable transmural scar occupying on average 30% of the ventricular septum and 10% of the overall LV chamber. Alcohol-induced infarcts can potentially compound preexisting and underlying myocardial electrical instability resulting in increased arrhythmogenicity and higher risk of malignant ventricular arrhythmias. Several studies have documented the occurrence of sustained ventricular arrhythmias and SCD following septal ablation in approximately 10% to 20% of patients with or without SCD risk factors. Long-term outcome and survival following alcohol ablation is fourfold less favorable compared with myotomy/myectomy (which leaves no intramyocardial septal scar), and the rate of appropriate ICD therapy among alcohol ablation patients with primary prevention ICDs is threefold more frequent than in other patients (10.3% per year versus 3.6% per year).

Invasive EP testing has little predictive value for SCD in hypertrophic CMP, and has proved an impractical and nonspecific prognostic strategy, and without advantage over the traditional noninvasive risk stratification. In addition, it may be difficult to defibrillate hypertrophic CMP patients if rapid VT or VF is initiated.

Similarly, there is insufficient evidence to regard specific 12-lead ECG patterns, T wave alternans, heart rate variability, QT interval prolongation and dispersion, or coronary arterial bridging as risk markers in hypertrophic CMP patients.[17,20]

The role of cardiac MR imaging in risk stratification in patients with hypertrophic CMP is being evaluated. Cardiac MR imaging can help determine the severity and distribution of LV hypertrophy. Detection of myocardial fibrosis by gadolinium cardiac MR imaging (i.e., delayed enhancement) may have a role as a clinical predictor for increased risk of SCD. Up to 80% of patients with hypertrophic CMP have some degree of myocardial gadolinium hyperenhancement (the presumptive imaging correlate of increased myocardial fibrosis or scar) on cardiac MR (Fig. 28-3). However, the extent of hyperenhancement is greater in patients with progressive disease (28.5% versus 8.7%) and in patients with two or more risk factors for SCD (15.7% versus 8.6%).[21] Additionally, patients with diffuse rather than confluent enhancement had two or more risk factors for SCD (87% versus 33%).[17]

TABLE 28-1 Risk Factors for Sudden Cardiac Death in Hypertrophic Cardiomyopathy

MAJOR RISK FACTORS	POSSIBLE IN INDIVIDUAL PATIENTS
• Cardiac arrest (ventricular fibrillation)	• Atrial fibrillation
• Spontaneous sustained ventricular tachycardia	• Myocardial ischemia
• Family history of premature sudden death	• Left ventricular outflow obstruction
• Unexplained syncope	• High-risk mutation
• Left ventricular thickness ≥30 mm	• Intense (competitive) physical exertion
• Abnormal exercise blood pressure	
• Nonsustained spontaneous ventricular tachycardia	

From Zipes DP, Camm AJ, Borggrefe M, et al: ACC/AHA/ESC 2006 guidelines for management of patients with ventricular arrhythmias and the prevention of sudden cardiac death: a report of the American College of Cardiology/American Heart Association Task Force and the European Society of Cardiology Committee for Practice Guidelines, *J Am Coll Cardiol* 48:e247-e346, 2006.

Electrocardiographic Features

The ECG is abnormal in more than 90% of patients with hypertrophic CMP and in 75% of asymptomatic relatives. An abnormal ECG in the young is a sensitive marker of early disease expression. ECGs show a wide variety of abnormal patterns; however, no particular ECG pattern is characteristic or predictive of future events. Left atrial enlargement, repolarization abnormalities (ST-T changes including marked T wave inversion), and deep and narrow Q waves (most commonly in the inferolateral leads) are the most frequent ECG findings (Fig. 28-4). Voltage criteria for LV hypertrophy alone are nonspecific and are often seen in normal young adults. Giant negative T waves in the midprecordial leads are characteristic of hypertrophy confined to the LV apex.

Principles of Management

No treatments to prevent or modify disease progression currently exist. Therefore current treatment focuses on symptom management, assessment for risk of SCD, and family screening. Patients

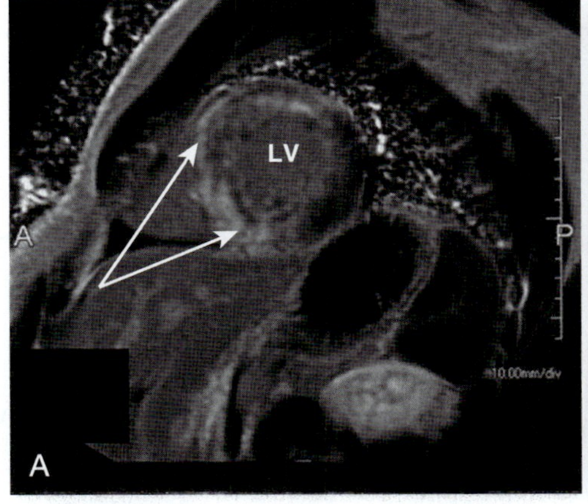

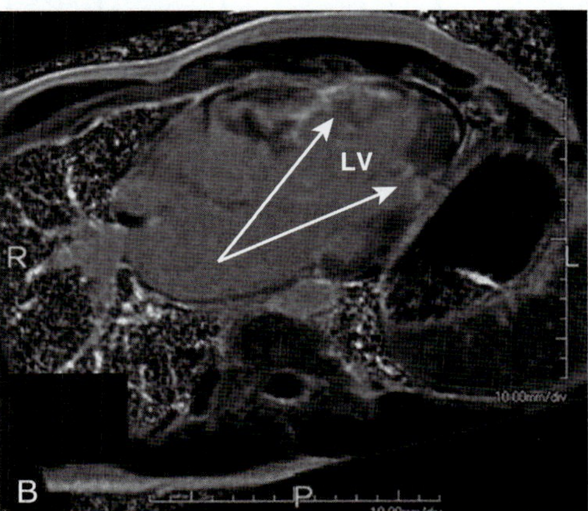

FIGURE 28-3 Delayed hyperenhancement magnetic resonance images from a patient with symptomatic hypertrophic obstructive cardiomyopathy, demonstrating areas of extensive scarring in the basal interventricular septum (**A**, arrow). Notice also the areas of patchy scarring in the posterior wall (**B**, arrow). The image on the left is a short-axis view, and the image on the right is a three-chamber view. LV = left ventricle. *(From Kwon DH, Smedira NG, Rodriguez ER, et al: Cardiac magnetic resonance detection of myocardial scarring in hypertrophic cardiomyopathy: correlation with histopathology and prevalence of ventricular tachycardia, J Am Coll Cardiol 54:242-249, 2009.)*

with LV outflow obstructive symptoms or heart failure are treated with beta blockers, verapamil, and disopyramide. Reduced heart rate and decreased contractility resulting from their action can potentially alleviate symptoms related to LV outflow obstruction. In cases that are unresponsive to drugs, septal surgical myotomy/myectomy or percutaneous alcohol septal ablation (Fig. 28-5) should be considered.

For AF the goal is to restore and maintain sinus rhythm. Anticoagulation is also required because of the high risk for thromboembolic complications.

Dual-chamber pacing modifies the LV excitation pattern by changing the depolarization synchrony of the LV contraction, and can potentially be useful in a subset of symptomatic patients who have substantial LV outflow gradients (>30 mm Hg at rest or >50 mm Hg provoked) refractory to medical therapy and are not candidates for surgical myotomy/myectomy or alcohol septal ablation (Fig. 28-6). Although the initial observational studies in patients with hypertrophic CMP showed promising results, subsequent randomized clinical studies failed to show a significant benefit of dual-chamber pacing, and there are currently no data available to support the contention that pacing alters the clinical course of the disease or improves survival or long-term quality of life in hypertrophic CMP. Hence, routine implantation of dual-chamber pacemakers is no longer used, except in rare situations.[22]

Implantable Cardioverter-Defibrillator

ICD therapy is the most effective and reliable approach for reduction of the risk of SCD in patients with hypertrophic CMP, both for secondary prevention and altering the natural history of this disease. Of note, the interval from ICD implantation to first appropriate device intervention is quite variable, and often considerable in length. Even ICD recipients for secondary prevention after a cardiac arrest can survive for many years with or without the aid of ICD discharge.[17] On the other hand, prophylactic pharmacological treatment alone (amiodarone, beta blockers, or verapamil) does not offer hypertrophic CMP patients reliable protection against SCD and is generally not indicated.

ICD implantation is recommended for secondary prevention in patients with prior cardiac arrest or sustained VT, because of the relatively high recurrence rates in this subgroup. ICD implantation is also recommended for primary prevention in patients with multiple risk factors (two or more) for SCD. However, ICD implantation for primary prevention in patients with only one risk factor is controversial. In this subgroup, management decisions should be individualized, taking into consideration other markers of disease severity, other less established risk factors (e.g., prior alcohol septal ablation, LV aneurysm), as well as the desires of the fully informed patient and family.

It is important to note that the number of risk factors in ICD recipients for primary prevention is unrelated to the likelihood of an appropriate therapy; about 35% of patients with appropriate ICD interventions for VT/VF had undergone implantation for only a single risk factor; and the likelihood of appropriate discharge was similar in patients with one, two, or three or more risk markers.[11] Therefore, a single marker of high risk may represent sufficient evidence to justify the recommendation for a prophylactic ICD in selected patients with hypertrophic CMP. Indeed, the most recent ACC/AHA/ESC practice guidelines make primary prevention with the ICD a class IIa indication, based on the presence of one or more risk factors.[9,22] Whether hypertrophic CMP patients should have ICDs implanted routinely following alcohol septal ablation is presently unresolved.

The absence of risk factors for SCD accurately identifies a cohort of patients with a low risk of SCD. Nevertheless, regular periodic reassessment of low-risk adults with Holter monitoring, exercise testing, and echocardiography is recommended. Changes in symptoms, particularly sustained palpitations or syncope, warrant urgent reevaluation at any age.

Catheter Ablation

In patients with apical aneurysms and SMVT, recurrence is quite high and antiarrhythmic drug therapy or catheter ablation should be considered. Antiarrhythmic medications have limited efficacy. When catheter ablation is undertaken, it should be appreciated that an epicardial approach may be warranted in a significant number of patients; in a recent report, an electrophysiologically identifiable epicardial scar was present in 80% of patients compared with 60% with an endocardial scar.[1,2,18,23,24]

Participation in Sports

Participation in intense competitive sports can represent a potential risk factor in athletes with hypertrophic CMP, even when conventional markers are absent, and exclusion from most participation in contact and most organized competitive sports is recommended

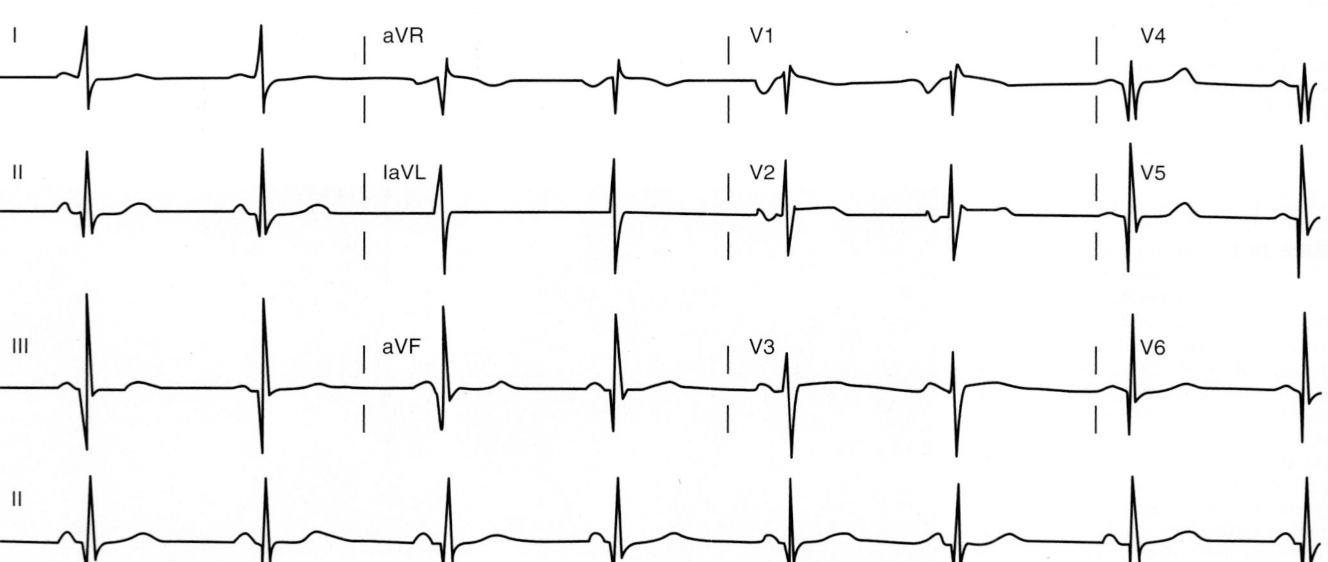

FIGURE 28-4 Surface ECG in a patient with hypertrophic cardiomyopathy. Note the deep narrow Q waves in the inferolateral leads.

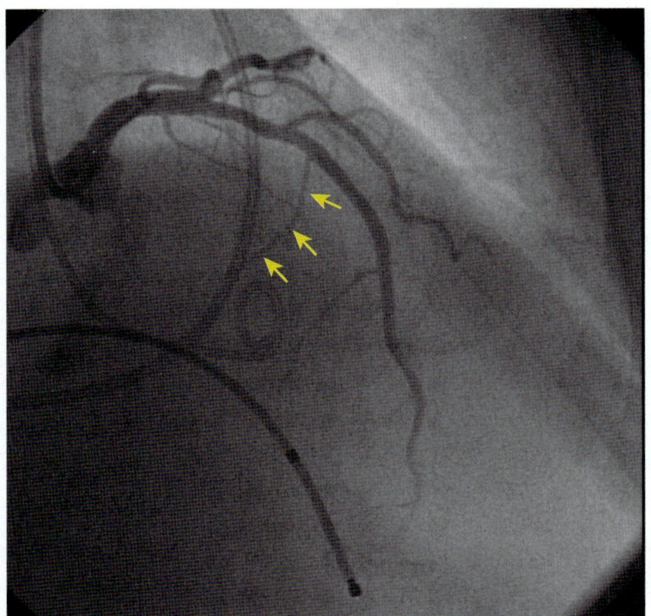

FIGURE 28-5 Left coronary angiography in a patient with asymmetrical septal hypertrophic cardiomyopathy. A right lateral oblique view is shown. The septal perforator branch (marked by arrows) of the left anterior descending artery is the target for alcohol septal ablation. A temporary pacing wire is positioned in the right ventricle and a pigtail catheter is positioned in the left ventricle.

(even in patients with ICDs), with the exception of low-intensity, class 1A sports (e.g., golf, bowling, billiards).

Family Screening

As expected in an autosomal dominant disease, every offspring has a 50% chance of inheriting the mutation and therefore of developing hypertrophic CMP. However, because of age dependence of penetrance, many mutation carriers may not exhibit phenotypic expression early in life, and many others may express the phenotype, but remain asymptomatic and, hence, remain undiagnosed unless screened. Therefore, it is generally considered that all first- and second-degree genetically related family members of patients with hypertrophic CMP should undergo screening with detailed history and physical examination, 12-lead ECG, and echocardiogram.

Because penetrance is age dependent, many family members may not express the phenotype at the time of examination and may be falsely considered "unaffected." Thus, periodic evaluation of the "unaffected" family members is necessary, as some may develop hypertrophic CMP later in life. Annual screening should be considered in adolescents and young adults (ages 12 to 25 years), in athletes, and in those with a family history of early-onset disease. Screening every 3 to 5 years in other individuals may be adequate (Table 28-2).[13]

When the causative mutation in the index patient is identified, genetic testing is recommended for all first-degree relatives and can have particular advantages over clinical screening, as ECG or echocardiographic abnormalities may be absent or subtle, or develop late in life. Furthermore, genetic testing affords permanent reassurance to those family members who test gene-negative,

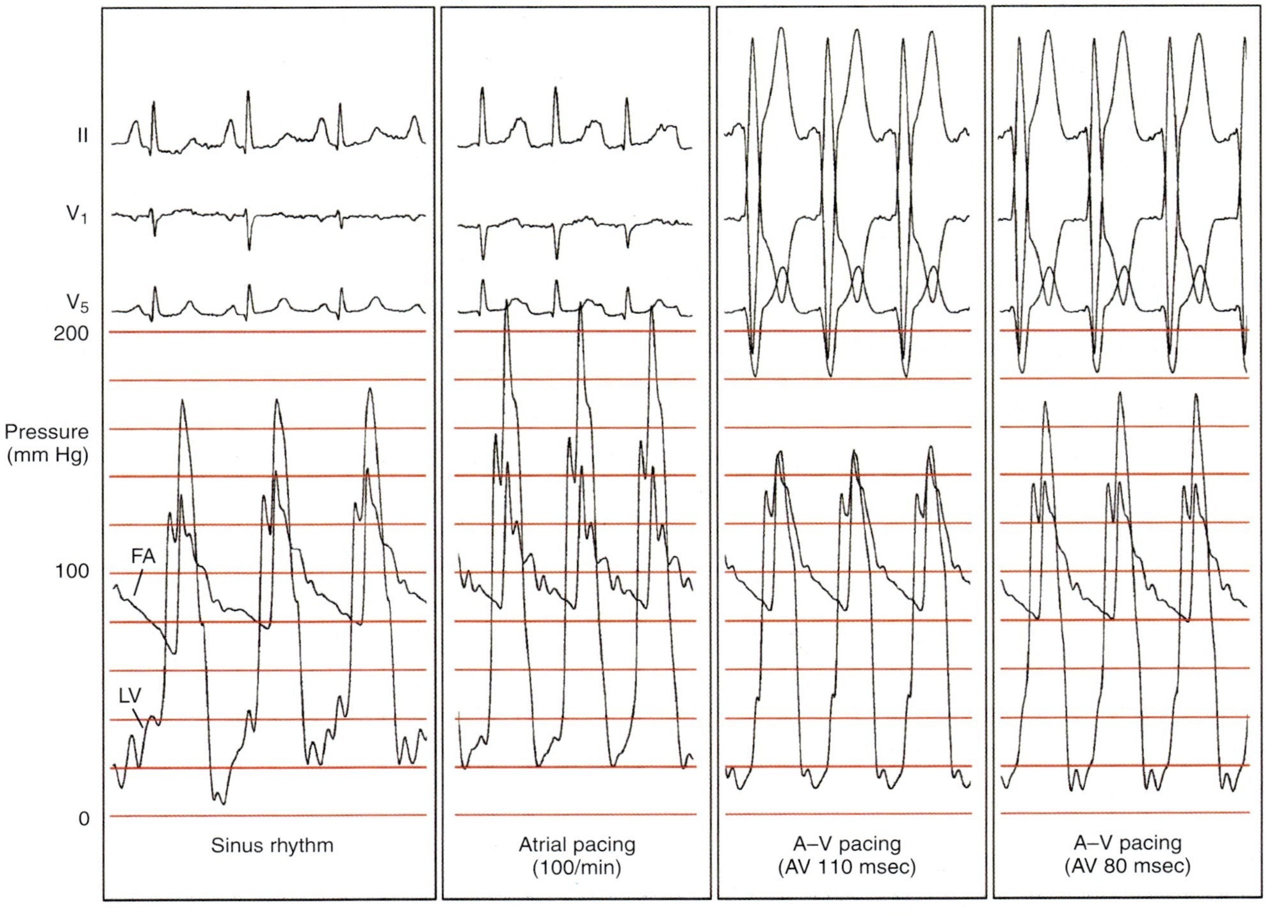

II
V1
V5
200
Pressure (mm Hg)
FA
100
LV
0
Sinus rhythm
Atrial pacing (100/min)
A–V pacing (AV 110 msec)
A–V pacing (AV 80 msec)

FIGURE 28-6 Reduction of left ventricular (LV) outflow obstruction by ventricular pacing. The four panels show ECG and hemodynamics (femoral arterial [FA] and LV) under different conditions in a patient with hypertrophic cardiomyopathy and dynamic LV outflow obstruction. Panels from left to right: Baseline sinus rhythm showing a peak LV-FA gradient of almost 40 mm Hg. During atrial pacing at 100/min, the gradient increases to 50 mm Hg. With addition of right ventricular pacing at 100/min and an atrioventricular (AV) interval of 110 milliseconds, the gradient is almost eliminated; finally, when the AV interval is shortened, the gradient increases again to about 30 mm Hg.

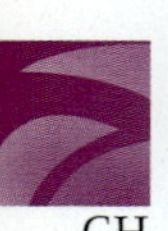

TABLE 28-2 Clinical Screening Strategies with Echocardiography and 12-Lead ECG for Detection of Hypertrophic Cardiomyopathy in Families

AGE OF FAMILY MEMBER	SCREENING STRATEGY
<12 yr old	Optional unless: • Family history of premature hypertrophic CMP death or other adverse complications • Competitive athlete in an intense training program • Onset of symptoms • Other clinical suspicion of early left ventricular hypertrophy
12 to ~18–21 yr old	Every 12–18 mo
>18–21 yr old	Probably about every 5 yr, or more frequent intervals with a family history of late-onset hypertrophic CMP and/or malignant clinical course

CMP = cardiomyopathy.

obviating the need for clinical investigations or long-term follow-up and screening of their offspring.[4,14]

Athletes with a family history of hypertrophic CMP should probably undergo annual ECG, echocardiography, 24-hour Holter monitoring, exercise testing, and genetic testing before being allowed to participate in competitive sports.

Asymptomatic individuals found to carry a hypertrophic CMP mutation on genetic screening should undergo a comprehensive cardiac evaluation and risk stratification similar to patients with known hypertrophic CMP. Additionally, genotype-positive athletes should be excluded from most competitive sports, even when they are asymptomatic and have no abnormalities on echocardiogram and ECG.

Prophylactic pharmacological therapy in asymptomatic carriers of hypertrophic CMP genes is ineffective and not recommended.

REFERENCES

1. Furushima H, Chinushi M, Iijima K, et al: Ventricular tachyarrhythmia associated with hypertrophic cardiomyopathy: incidence, prognosis, and relation to type of hypertrophy, *J Cardiovasc Electrophysiol* 21:991–999, 2010.
2. Santangeli P, Di Biase L, Lakkireddy D, et al: Radiofrequency catheter ablation of ventricular arrhythmias in patients with hypertrophic cardiomyopathy: safety and feasibility, *Heart Rhythm* 7:1036–1042, 2010.
3. Morita H, Rehm HL, Menesses A, et al: Shared genetic causes of cardiac hypertrophy in children and adults, *N Engl J Med* 358:1899–1908, 2008.
4. Ackerman MJ, Priori SG, Willems S, et al: HRS/EHRA Expert Consensus Statement on the state of genetic testing for the channelopathies and cardiomyopathies, *Heart Rhythm* 8:1308–1339, 2011.
5. Boussy T, Paparella G, de Asmundis C, et al: Genetic basis of ventricular arrhythmias, *Heart Fail Clin* 6:249–266, 2010.
6. Pinto JR, Parvatiyar MS, Jones MA, et al: A functional and structural study of troponin C mutations related to hypertrophic cardiomyopathy, *J Biol Chem* 284:19090–19100, 2009.
7. Williams L, Frenneaux M: Syncope in hypertrophic cardiomyopathy: mechanisms and consequences for treatment, *Europace* 9:817–822, 2007.
8. Spirito P, Autore C, Rapezzi C, et al: Syncope and risk of sudden death in hypertrophic cardiomyopathy, *Circulation* 119:1703–1710, 2009.
9. Zipes DP, Camm AJ, Borggrefe M, et al: ACC/AHA/ESC 2006 guidelines for management of patients with ventricular arrhythmias and the prevention of sudden cardiac death: a report of the American College of Cardiology/American Heart Association Task Force and the European Society of Cardiology Committee for Practice Guidelines (Writing Committee to Develop Guidelines for Management of Patients With Ventricular Arrhythmias and the Prevention of Sudden Cardiac Death), *J Am Coll Cardiol* 48:e247–e346, 2006.
10. Lim KK, Maron BJ, Knight BP: Successful catheter ablation of hemodynamically unstable monomorphic ventricular tachycardia in a patient with hypertrophic cardiomyopathy and apical aneurysm, *J Cardiovasc Electrophysiol* 20:445–447, 2009.
11. Maron BJ, Spirito P, Shen WK, et al: Implantable cardioverter-defibrillators and prevention of sudden cardiac death in hypertrophic cardiomyopathy, *JAMA* 298:405–412, 2007.
12. Maron BJ, Haas TS, Shannon KM, et al: Long-term survival after cardiac arrest in hypertrophic cardiomyopathy, *Heart Rhythm* 6:993–997, 2009.
13. Maron BJ, Seidman JG, Seidman CE: Proposal for contemporary screening strategies in families with hypertrophic cardiomyopathy, *J Am Coll Cardiol* 44:2125–2132, 2004.
14. Bos JM, Towbin JA, Ackerman MJ: Diagnostic, prognostic, and therapeutic implications of genetic testing for hypertrophic cardiomyopathy, *J Am Coll Cardiol* 54:201–211, 2009.
15. Miller MA, Gomes JA, Fuster V: Risk stratification of sudden cardiac death in hypertrophic cardiomyopathy, *Nat Clin Pract Cardiovasc Med* 4:667–676, 2007.
16. Christiaans I, van Engelen K, van Langen IM, et al: Risk stratification for sudden cardiac death in hypertrophic cardiomyopathy: systematic review of clinical risk markers, *Europace* 12:313–321, 2010.
17. Maron BJ, Spirito P: Implantable defibrillators and prevention of sudden death in hypertrophic cardiomyopathy, *J Cardiovasc Electrophysiol* 19:1118–1126, 2008.
18. Maron MS, Finley JJ, Bos JM, et al: Prevalence, clinical significance, and natural history of left ventricular apical aneurysms in hypertrophic cardiomyopathy, *Circulation* 118:1541–1549, 2008.
19. Efthimiadis GK, Parcharidou DG, Giannakoulas G, et al: Left ventricular outflow tract obstruction as a risk factor for sudden cardiac death in hypertrophic cardiomyopathy, *Am J Cardiol* 104:695–699, 2009.
20. Sherrid MV, Cotiga D, Hart D, et al: Relation of 12-lead electrocardiogram patterns to implanted defibrillator-terminated ventricular tachyarrhythmias in hypertrophic cardiomyopathy, *Am J Cardiol* 104:1722–1726, 2009.
21. Adabag AS, Maron BJ, Appelbaum E, et al: Occurrence and frequency of arrhythmias in hypertrophic cardiomyopathy in relation to delayed enhancement on cardiovascular magnetic resonance, *J Am Coll Cardiol* 51:1369–1374, 2008.
22. Epstein AE, DiMarco JP, Ellenbogen KA, et al: ACC/AHA/HRS 2008 guidelines for device-based therapy of cardiac rhythm abnormalities: executive summary, *Heart Rhythm* 5: 934–955, 2008.
23. Dukkipati SR, d'Avila A, Soejima K, et al: Long-term outcomes of combined epicardial and endocardial ablation of monomorphic ventricular tachycardia related to hypertrophic cardiomyopathy, *Circ Arrhythm Electrophysiol* 4:185–194, 2011.
24. Dukkipati SR, d'Avila A, Soejima K, et al: Long-term outcomes of combined epicardial and endocardial ablation of monomorphic ventricular tachycardia related to hypertrophic cardiomyopathy, *Circ Arrhythm Electrophysiol* 4:185–194, 2011.

CHAPTER 29 Ventricular Tachycardia in Arrhythmogenic Right Ventricular Cardiomyopathy-Dysplasia

Pathophysiology

Arrhythmogenic right ventricular cardiomyopathy-dysplasia (ARVD) is an inherited primary disease of the myocardium characterized by ventricular arrhythmias and structural abnormalities of the right ventricle (RV). The hallmark pathological findings are progressive myocyte loss and fibrofatty (fibrous and adipose) tissue replacement, with a predilection for the RV, but the left ventricle (LV) and septum also can be affected. Fibrofatty replacement of the myocardium produces "islands" of scar that can lead to reentrant VTs, and these patients have an increased risk of sudden cardiac death (SCD), mostly secondary to ventricular tachycardia (VT).[1]

The exact cause of ARVD is not fully understood. Several theories for the pathogenesis of ARVD have been proposed, some of which reflect acquired rather than familial disease: dysontogenic, degenerative, inflammatory, and apoptotic. Progressive myocyte replacement can be secondary to a metabolic disorder affecting the RV. This process would be analogous to the situation involving skeletal muscle in patients with muscular dystrophy, in whom progressive degeneration of muscle occurs with time. The loss of myocardial tissue also can reflect increased apoptosis (programmed cell death) of myocardial cells. A possible infectious or immunological cause resulting in post-inflammatory RV fibrofatty cardiomyopathy has also been suggested—up to 80% of hearts at autopsy documenting inflammatory infiltrates. In recent years, research has focused on identifying the genetic basis for ARVD.

Molecular Genetics

Familial disease occurs in approximately 30% to 50% of cases of ARVD, and two patterns of inheritance have been described: autosomal dominant disease with incomplete penetrance (most common) and autosomal recessive disease (rare). Autosomal recessive forms of ARVD include Naxos disease (also known as familial palmoplantar keratosis and "mal de Meleda" disease) and Carvajal syndrome (a disorder of LV cardiomyopathy), both of which are associated with skin and hair abnormalities.

The autosomal dominant nonsyndromic ARVD-1 to ARVD-12 as well as the two rare recessive forms (Naxos disease and Carvajal syndrome) have been mapped to 12 genetic loci, with mutations in eight gene loci identified (Table 29-1). Although some identified gene mutations such as RYR2 may be phenocopies of ARVD, a common theme of desmosomal protein mutations has been emerging. In fact, five of the eight gene loci encode desmosomal proteins (desmoplakin [DSP], plakophilin-2 [PKP2], desmoglein-2 [DSG2], desmocollin-2 [DSC2], junctional plakoglobin [JUP]) and have been found in association with the ARVD phenotype in up to 50% of cases. Among the known genes, mutations in PKP2 appear to be the most common causes of ARVD, accounting for approximately 20% of cases. Mutations in DSG2 and DSP each account for approximately 10% to 15% of cases. Therefore, ARVD is currently considered, at least in a subset, a disease of the cardiac desmosome.[2,3] The majority of these mutations are insertion/deletion or nonsense mutations, which are expected to cause premature termination of the encoded proteins.[1]

Mutations in genes encoding nondesmosomal proteins also can potentially cause ARVD. Alterations of the 5′ and 3′ regulatory elements of *TGFB3*, encoding transforming growth factor-β_3, have each been reported. More recently, a mutation in *TMEM43*, encoding a transmembrane protein with ties to an adipogenic transcription factor, was reported as the cause for ARVD-5, a subtype of ARVD with prominent LV involvement. Mutations in *RYR2*, encoding the

TABLE 29-1 Known Genetic Loci for Arrhythmogenic Right Ventricular Cardiomyopathy-Dysplasia

LOCUS NAME	CAUSATIVE GENE	MODE OF INHERITANCE
ARVD-1	Transforming growth factor-β_3	Autosomal dominant
ARVD-2	Cardiac ryanodine receptor (RYR2)	Autosomal dominant
ARVD-3	Unknown	Autosomal dominant
ARVD-4	Unknown	Autosomal dominant
ARVD-5	Transmembrane protein-43	Autosomal dominant
ARVD-6	Unknown	Autosomal dominant
ARVD-7	Unknown	Autosomal dominant
ARVD-8	Desmoplakin (DSP)	Autosomal dominant
ARVD-9	Plakophilin-2 (PKP2)	Autosomal dominant
ARVD-10	Desmoglein-2	Autosomal dominant
ARVD-11	Desmocollin-2	Autosomal dominant
ARVD-12	Plakoglobin (JUP)	Autosomal dominant
Naxos disease	Plakoglobin (JUP)	Autosomal recessive
Carvajal syndrome	Desmoplakin (DSP)	Autosomal recessive

cardiac ryanodine receptor (the major calcium release channel of the sarcoplasmic reticulum in cardiomyocytes, also implicated in familial catecholaminergic polymorphic VT), result in a form of arrhythmogenic cardiomyopathy (ARVD-2) characterized by exercise-induced polymorphic VT that does not appear to have a reentrant mechanism, occurring in the absence of significant structural abnormalities. Patients do not develop characteristic features of ARVD on the 12-lead electrocardiogram (ECG) or signal-averaged ECG, and global RV function remains unaffected. ARVD-2 shows a closer resemblance to familial catecholaminergic polymorphic VT in both etiology and phenotype; its inclusion under the umbrella term of ARVD remains controversial.[2-4]

Pathogenesis

Cardiac desmosomes are specialized, multiprotein complexes in the intercalated disks that anchor intermediate filaments to the cytoplasmic membrane in adjacent cardiomyocytes, thereby forming a three-dimensional (3-D) scaffolding and providing mechanical strength and cohesion of cardiomyocytes in the beating heart (Fig. 29-1). Cardiac desmosomes are also responsible for regulating transcription of genes involved in adipogenesis and apoptosis as well as maintaining proper electrical conductivity through regulation of gap junctions and calcium homeostasis. Cardiac desmosomes are composed of three groups of proteins: the cadherin family, the Armadillo family, and the plakin family. The cadherin family is composed of three desmocollins and three desmogleins, which are primarily responsible for anchoring the structure to the membrane. The Armadillo family is composed of plakoglobin and three plakophilins, which form the core structure and possess signaling capabilities. The plakin family is composed of DSP, envoplakin, periplakin, plectin, and pinin, which are responsible for the attachment of the desmosomes to intermediary filaments.[1,5]

The mechanisms by which the affected desmosomes cause myocyte apoptosis, fibrogenesis, adipogenesis, and slow ventricular conduction, thus leading to impaired RV function and increased arrhythmogenicity, remain to be determined. Mutations in desmosomal genes alter the number or integrity of desmosomes and thereby lead to impaired mechanical coupling and failure of cell-to-cell adhesion structures during exposure to physical strain, resulting in cardiomyocyte detachment and degeneration, with subsequent inflammation and replacement by fibrofatty

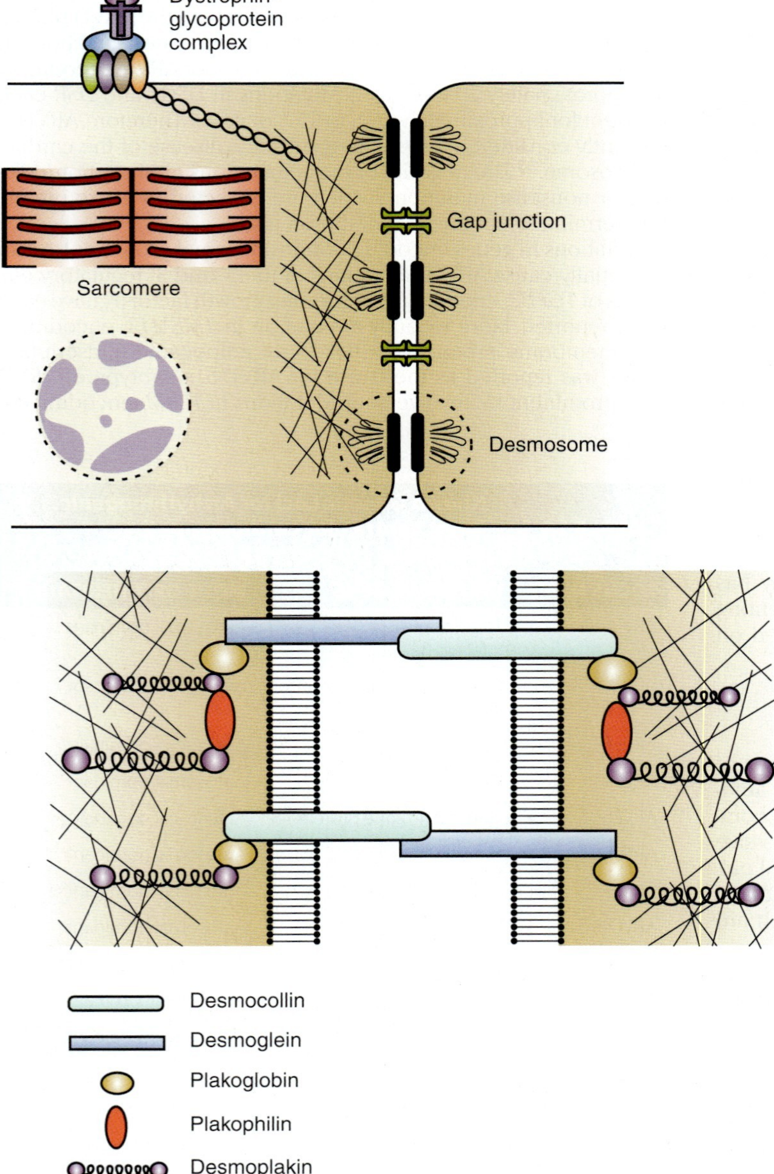

FIGURE 29-1 Molecular structure of the cardiac desmosome. The desmosomal cadherins desmocollin and desmoglein form classic homotypic and heterotypic interactions between cells. These membrane-bound proteins are linked through the Armadillo family members, plakoglobin, and plakophilin to the intermediate filament–binding protein desmoplakin. This complex anchors the desmosome to the cytoskeleton of the cell, and thus indirectly to the sarcomere, nuclear membrane, and the dystrophin-associated glycoproteins. *(From Ellinor PT, MacRae CA, Thierfelder L: Arrhythmogenic right ventricular cardiomyopathy, Heart Fail Clin 6:161-177, 2010.)*

tissue. Fibrofatty replacement is a nonspecific repair process also observed in the muscular dystrophies. The architecture of thin surviving myocardial bundles within the fibrofatty tissue creates lengthened conduction pathways, conduction slowing at pivotal points, and conduction block. All factors contribute to activation delay and can create an electrophysiological (EP) substrate for reentry and VT. Ventricular dysfunction can ensue in the later stages owing to progressive myocyte detachment and death.[6]

Additionally, mutations in desmosomal proteins can impair expression of interacting proteins at the intercalated disk (e.g., gap junction or ion channel proteins), giving rise to impairment of intercellular conductance and promoting ventricular arrhythmogenesis, even in the absence of fibrofatty tissue replacement. Impaired desmosomal structure and function also can affect other cell-to-cell contact structures in the myocardium. In particular, connexin-43 remodeling in the gap junctions, which contributes to delayed conduction and ventricular arrhythmogenesis, is often observed in ARVD patients, and these potential electrical conduction abnormalities may favor arrhythmic events that characterize the disease and predispose patients to high risk of SCD.[2-4]

Pathology

Regardless of the mechanism, the patchy replacement of the RV myocardium by fibrofatty tissue provides a substrate for reentrant ventricular arrhythmias. The most striking morphological feature of the disease is the diffuse or segmental loss of RV myocytes, with replacement by fibrofatty tissue and thinning of the RV wall. Patchy inflammatory infiltrates can be present in areas of myocardial damage. Fibrofatty replacement usually begins in the subepicardium or midmural layers and progresses to the subendocardium. Only the endocardium and myocardium of the trabeculae may be spared. The sites of involvement can be localized and in early disease are often confined to the so-called "triangle of dysplasia"—namely, the RV outflow tract (RVOT), RV apex, and inferolateral wall near the tricuspid valve. RV aneurysms (Fig. 29-2), and segmental RV hypokinesia are typical. Diffuse myocardial involvement leads to global RV dilation. However, the fibrofatty pattern of ARVD is limited not only to the RV; the disease also can migrate to the LV free wall (commonly observed in advanced disease), with a predilection for the posteroseptal and posterolateral areas, with relative sparing of the septum.[2-4]

In ARVD, the regions of abnormal myocardium do not always follow the pattern of dense scar surrounded by a ring of abnormal myocardium, often referred to as the scar border zone. Sometimes, abnormal voltages are found alone, without dense scar defining the regions. This is because ARVD is a different process from scarring caused by myocardial infarction (MI). Infarction causes dense scar surrounded by a border zone because of the ischemic penumbra that surrounds the infarcted territory. In ARVD, however, the process is patchy and can cause inhomogeneous scarring in anatomically disparate areas. Nonetheless, previous data have shown that it is still possible to identify well-demarcated borders around these abnormal regions.

Despite the widespread impression that ARVD is universally a progressive disease process, a recent report found that the extent of the endocardial scar as measured by bipolar voltage mapping in patients with ARVD and VT remained relatively stable, despite progressive RV dilation.[7]

A monomorphic VT in the setting of ARVD is associated with a predominantly perivalvular distribution of endocardial electrogram abnormalities and arrhythmia origin. Reentry in areas of abnormal myocardium is the most likely mechanism of VT in ARVD. Most reentrant circuits cluster around the tricuspid annulus and the RVOT. The critical isthmus contained in these reentry circuits often is a narrow path of tissue with abnormal conduction properties, typically bounded by two approximately parallel conduction barriers that consist of scar areas, the tricuspid annulus, or both. Depolarization of the small mass of tissue in the isthmus is usually not detectable on the surface ECG and constitutes the electrical diastole between QRS complexes.

Clinical Considerations

Epidemiology

ARVD occurs in young adults (80% are younger than 40 years) and is more common in men. The mean age at diagnosis of familial ARVD is approximately 31 years. The disease is almost never diagnosed in infancy and rarely before the age of 10.

The incidence and prevalence of ARVD are uncertain and may vary regionally. The prevalence of the disease in the general population is estimated at 0.02% to 0.1% but is dependent on geographic circumstances. In certain regions of Italy (Padua, Venice) and Greece (island of Naxos), an increased prevalence of 0.4% to 0.8% for ARVD has been reported. Others estimate the prevalence in Europe and North America to be 1 per 5000 individuals.

Clinical Presentation

The clinical presentation varies widely because ARVD includes a spectrum of different conditions rather than a single entity. Different pathological processes can manifest a diversity of symptoms. Additionally, ARVD can have a temporal progression and can present differently according to the time of presentation.

Four clinicopathological stages of ARVD can be considered: the early "concealed" phase, followed by the "overt electrical disorder," the "phase of RV failure," and finally, the phase of

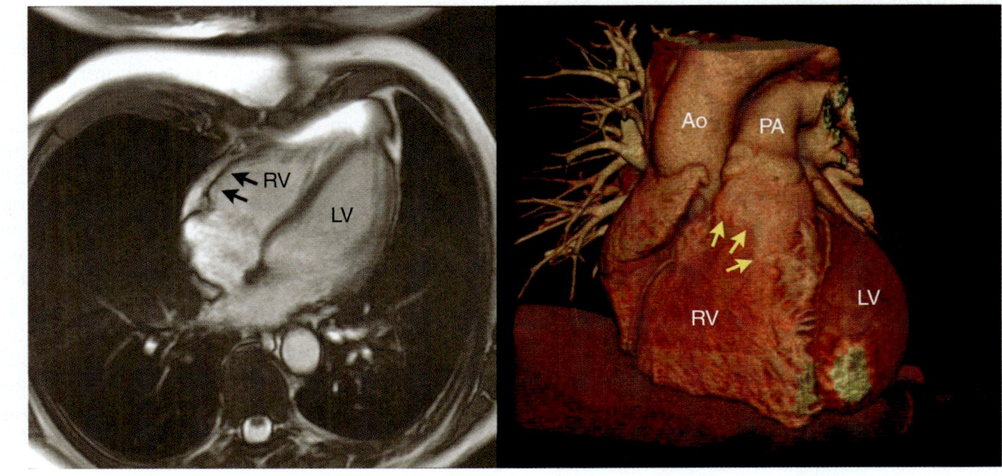

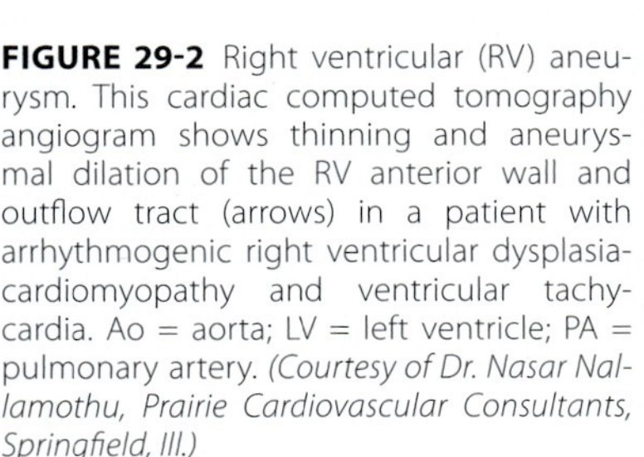

FIGURE 29-2 Right ventricular (RV) aneurysm. This cardiac computed tomography angiogram shows thinning and aneurysmal dilation of the RV anterior wall and outflow tract (arrows) in a patient with arrhythmogenic right ventricular dysplasia-cardiomyopathy and ventricular tachycardia. Ao = aorta; LV = left ventricle; PA = pulmonary artery. *(Courtesy of Dr. Nasar Nallamothu, Prairie Cardiovascular Consultants, Springfield, Ill.)*

"biventricular failure." Although ARVD is a genetically transmitted disease, it is associated with a long asymptomatic lead time and individuals in their teens may not have any characteristics of ARVD clinically or on screening tests. Early ARVD is often asymptomatic (the "concealed" phase), occasionally associated with minor ventricular arrhythmias and subtle structural changes. Nonetheless, these patients are still at risk of SCD, especially during intense physical exertion. With disease progression, the "overt electrical disorder" typically causes symptomatic ventricular arrhythmia and more obvious morphological abnormalities detectable by imaging. Further disease extension results in RV dilation and dysfunction (the "phase of RV failure"), precipitating symptoms and signs of right heart failure. Unless SCD occurs, progressive impairment of cardiac function can result in biventricular heart failure late in the evolution of ARVD, usually within 4 to 8 years after typical development of complete right bundle branch block (RBBB). End-stage disease is often indistinguishable from dilated cardiomyopathy and manifests with congestive heart failure, atrial fibrillation, and an increased incidence of thromboembolic events. Overall, judging the accurate position of the patient on the time scale of the spectrum can be difficult, and some patients may remain stable in the same phase of the disease for several decades.[8]

ARVD is one of the most arrhythmogenic human heart diseases known. Electrical instability is present at the very early stages of ARVD. Ventricular arrhythmias range from isolated ectopy to sustained VT or ventricular fibrillation (VF).[8] Approximately 50% of patients with ARVD present with symptomatic ventricular arrhythmias, most commonly sustained and nonsustained VT, manifested by palpitations, dizziness, and/or syncope. The frequency of ventricular arrhythmias in ARVD varies with the severity of the disease, ranging from 23% in patients with mild disease to almost 100% in patients with severe disease. Ventricular arrhythmias characteristically occur during exercise; up to 50% to 60% of patients with ARVD show monomorphic VT during exercise testing.

One of the unfortunate features of ARVD is SCD, which is the first clinical manifestation of ARVD in 50% of afflicted individuals. In fact, up to 5% of SCDs in young adults in the United States are attributed to ARVD. In northeast Italy, ARVD was found to be responsible for 22.4% of SCDs in young athletes and in 8.2% of SCDs in nonathletes. In most patients, the mechanism of SCD in ARVD is acceleration of VT, with ultimate degeneration into VF. Generally, RV failure and LV dysfunction are independently associated with cardiovascular mortality.

Supraventricular tachycardias are observed in approximately 25% of patients with ARVD referred for treatment of ventricular arrhythmias; less often, they are the only arrhythmia present. In decreasing order of frequency, supraventricular tachycardias in these patients include atrial fibrillation, atrial tachycardia, and atrial flutter.

Some patients are asymptomatic and ARVD is only suspected by the finding of ventricular ectopy and other abnormalities on routine ECG or other testing because of a positive family history. In a review of 37 families, only 17 of 168 patients with ARVD (10%) were healthy carriers. In one report, 9.6% of those initially unaffected subjects developed structural signs of disease on echocardiography during a mean follow-up of 8.5 years; almost 50% had symptomatic ventricular arrhythmias. Progression from mild to moderate disease occurred in 5% of patients, and progression from moderate to severe disease occurred in 8%.

Initial Evaluation

The noninvasive diagnosis of ARVD can be exceedingly difficult. Several factors, including marked phenotypic variation, incomplete and low (30%) penetrance, and age-related disease development and progression contribute to the complexity of the clinical diagnosis. Particularly problematic is recognition of the early stages of ARVD, when overall RV function may be normal, with local or regional wall-motion abnormalities that are difficult to quantify; nonetheless, the absence of clinical features does not necessarily confer low risk.

Definitive diagnosis of ARVD requires histological confirmation. A myocardial biopsy showing myocyte loss (<45% residual myocytes) with fibrosis and fatty infiltration (>40% fibrous tissue and >3% fat) confirms the diagnosis. However, myocardial biopsy lacks sufficient sensitivity (67% in one report) owing to the patchy nature of the disease. For safety reasons, the biopsy is performed mostly in the interventricular septum, which is histopathologically rarely involved in the disease process. Biopsy sampling performed on the RV free wall may improve the ability to diagnose ARVD. Nevertheless, because of the frequently observed wall thinning with aneurysms or diverticula, free wall sampling is associated with risk of perforation, particularly when performed at random sites. Therefore, the role of endomyocardial biopsy in the diagnosis of ARVD remains controversial.

Electroanatomical voltage mapping, which seems to be an effective technique to detect RV low-voltage regions reflecting fibrofatty myocardial atrophy in patients with ARVD, has been shown to improve the diagnostic accuracy of myocardial biopsy by reducing the sampling errors. Endomyocardial biopsies are obtained from low-voltage areas, preferably from the border zone, in order to minimize the risk of perforation.[9]

Additionally, immunohistochemical analysis of conventional biopsy samples to detect a change in the distribution of desmosomal proteins can also improve the sensitivity and specificity of this diagnostic tool. Reduced immunoreactive signal levels of plakoglobin at intercalated disks were found to be a consistent feature in patients with ARVD but not seen in other forms of myocardial disease.[10]

Recognition of the problems in diagnosing ARVD and the fact that there is no "gold standard" or single test that is diagnostic of ARVD led to the formation of a task force in 1994 that proposed major and minor criteria to aid in the diagnosis, based on family history as well as structural, histological, functional, arrhythmic, and ECG abnormalities (Table 29-2).[11] The diagnosis of ARVD is based on the presence of two major criteria, one major plus two minor criteria, or four minor criteria. It is important to recognize, however, that these criteria were defined retrospectively from aggregated series of referrals to tertiary care institutions dominated by the overt or severe end of the disease spectrum (i.e., symptomatic index cases and SCD victims) and have never been prospectively validated; therefore, their applicability is limited in situations where the prior probability of ARVD is different from the initial derivation set of patients. Consequently, the original task force criteria are highly specific but lacked sensitivity for early and familial disease. Furthermore, this diagnostic approach does not specify the preferred order of imaging techniques to examine and score RV morphology and function.[5,11]

A recent study of a large number (108) of newly diagnosed patients suspected of having ARVD found that a combination of diagnostic imaging tests is needed to evaluate the presence of RV structural, functional, and electrical abnormalities. ECG, echocardiography, RV angiography, signal-averaged ECG (SAECG), and Holter monitoring provide optimal clinical evaluation of patients suspected of having ARVD. The diagnostic performance of MR imaging and RV biopsy seemed to be inferior in comparison with the five tests recommended.[12] Based on these findings, the original task force criteria have been recently modified to incorporate the emerging diagnostic modalities and advances in the genetics of ARVD to improve diagnostic sensitivity while maintaining diagnostic specificity. In this modification of the task force criteria, quantitative criteria were proposed and abnormalities were defined on the basis of comparison with normal subject data.[11] Scoring by major and minor criteria was maintained, structural abnormalities were quantified, and task force criteria highly specific for ARVD were upgraded to major. Furthermore, new criteria were added: terminal activation duration of QRS equal to or greater than 55 milliseconds, VT with left bundle branch block (LBBB) morphology and superior axis, and genetic criteria.[13]

A recent study found that the new task force criteria are increasing the diagnostic yield of ARVD when applied to patients with suspected disease.[13] When performing and analyzing imaging studies,

TABLE 29-2 Original and Revised Task Force Diagnostic Criteria for Arrhythmogenic Right Ventricular Cardiomyopathy-Dysplasia

	ORIGINAL TASK FORCE CRITERIA	REVISED TASK FORCE CRITERIA
I. Global or Regional Dysfunction and Structural Alterations*		
Major	• Severe dilation and reduction of RV ejection fraction with no (or only mild) LV impairment • Localized RV aneurysms (akinetic or dyskinetic areas with diastolic bulging) • Severe segmental dilation of the RV	By 2-D echo: • Regional RV akinesia, dyskinesia, or aneurysm *and* one of the following (end diastole): • PLAX RVOT ≥ 32 mm (corrected for body size [PLAX/BSA] ≥ 19 mm/m^2) • PSAX RVOT ≥ 36 mm (corrected for body size [PSAX/BSA] ≥ 21 mm/m^2) • *or* fractional area change ≤ 33% By MRI: • Regional RV akinesia or dyskinesia or dyssynchronous RV contraction *and* one of the following: • Ratio of RV end-diastolic volume to BSA ≥ 110 mL/m^2 (men) or ≥ 100 mL/m^2 (women) • *or* RV ejection fraction ≤ 40% By RV angiography: • Regional RV akinesia, dyskinesia, or aneurysm
Minor	• Mild global RV dilation and/or ejection fraction reduction with normal LV • Mild segmental dilation of the RV • Regional RV hypokinesia	By 2-D echo: • Regional RV akinesia or dyskinesia *and* one of the following (end diastole): • PLAX RVOT ≥ 29 to < 32 mm (corrected for body size [PLAX/BSA] ≥ 16 to < 19 mm/m^2) • PSAX RVOT ≥ 32 to < 36 mm (corrected for body size [PSAX/BSA] ≥ 18 to < 21 mm/m^2) • *or* fractional area change > 33% to ≤ 40% By MRI: • Regional RV akinesia or dyskinesia or dyssynchronous RV contraction *and* one of the following: • Ratio of RV end-diastolic volume to BSA ≥ 100 to < 110 mL/m^2 (men) or ≥ 90 to < 100 mL/m^2 (women) • *or* RV ejection fraction > 40% to ≤ 45%
II. Tissue Characterization of Wall		
Major	• Fibrofatty replacement of myocardium on endomyocardial biopsy	• Residual myocytes < 60% by morphometric analysis (or < 50% if estimated) with fibrous replacement of the RV free wall myocardium in at least one sample, with or without fatty replacement of tissue on endomyocardial biopsy
Minor		• Residual myocytes < 60% by morphometric analysis (or < 50% if estimated) with fibrous replacement of the RV free wall myocardium in at least one sample, with or without fatty replacement of tissue on endomyocardial biopsy
III. Repolarization Abnormalities		
Major		• Inverted T waves in right precordial leads (V_1, V_2, and V_3) or beyond in individuals >14 yr of age (in the absence of complete right bundle branch block QRS ≥ 120 msec)
Minor	• Inverted T waves in right precordial leads (V_2 and V_3) (people age >12 yr, in absence of right bundle branch block)	• Inverted T waves in leads V_1 and V_2 in individuals >14 yr of age (in the absence of complete right bundle branch block) or in V_4, V_5, or V_6 • Inverted T waves in leads V_1, V_2, V_3, and V_4 in individuals >14 yr of age in the presence of complete right bundle branch block
IV. Depolarization/Conduction Abnormalities		
Major	• Epsilon waves or localized prolongation (>110 msec) of the QRS complex in right precordial leads (V_1 to V_3)	• Epsilon wave (reproducible low-amplitude signals between end of QRS complex to onset of the T wave) in the right precordial leads (V_1 to V_3)
Minor	• Late potentials (SAECG)	• Late potentials by SAECG in at least one of three parameters in the absence of a QRS duration ≥ 110 msec on the standard ECG • Filtered QRS duration (fQRS) ≥ 114 msec • Duration of terminal QRS < 40 µV (low-amplitude signal duration) ≥ 38 msec • Root-mean-square voltage of terminal 40 msec ≥ 20 µV • Terminal activation duration of QRS ≥ 55 msec measured from the nadir of the S wave to the end of the QRS, including R′, in V_1, V_2, or V_3, in the absence of complete right bundle branch block
V. Arrhythmias		
Major		• Nonsustained or sustained ventricular tachycardia of left bundle branch morphology with superior axis (negative or indeterminate QRS in leads II, III, and aVF and positive in lead aVL)
Minor	• Left bundle branch block–type ventricular tachycardia (sustained and nonsustained) (ECG, Holter, exercise) • Frequent ventricular extrasystoles (>1000 per 24 hr) (Holter)	• Nonsustained or sustained ventricular tachycardia of RV outflow configuration, left bundle branch block morphology with inferior axis (positive QRS in leads II, III, and aVF and negative in lead aVL) or of unknown axis • >500 ventricular extrasystoles per 24 hr (Holter)

Continued

TABLE 29-2 Original and Revised Task Force Diagnostic Criteria for Arrhythmogenic Right Ventricular Cardiomyopathy-Dysplasia—cont'd

	ORIGINAL TASK FORCE CRITERIA	REVISED TASK FORCE CRITERIA
VI. Family History		
Major	• Familial disease confirmed at necropsy or surgery	• ARVC/D confirmed in a first-degree relative who meets current task force criteria • ARVC/D confirmed pathologically at autopsy or surgery in a first-degree relative • Identification of a pathogenic mutation† categorized as associated or probably associated with ARVC/D in the patient under evaluation
Minor	• Family history of premature sudden death (<35 yr of age) due to suspected ARVC/D • Familial history (clinical diagnosis based on present criteria)	• History of ARVC/D in a first-degree relative in whom it is not possible or practical to determine whether the family member meets current task force criteria • Premature sudden death (<35 yr of age) due to suspected ARVC/D in a first-degree relative • ARVC/D confirmed pathologically or by current task force criteria in second-degree relative

*Hypokinesis is not included in this or subsequent definitions of RV regional wall motion abnormalities for the proposed modified criteria.

†A pathogenic mutation is a DNA alteration associated with ARVC/D that alters or is expected to alter the encoded protein, is unobserved or rare in a large non-ARVC/D control population, and either alters or is predicted to alter the structure or function of the protein or has demonstrated linkage to the disease phenotype in a conclusive pedigree.

Diagnostic terminology for original criteria: This diagnosis is fulfilled by the presence of two major, or one major plus two minor, criteria or by four minor criteria from different groups. Diagnostic terminology for revised criteria: definite diagnosis: two major or one major and two minor criteria, or four minor from different categories; borderline: one major and one minor or three minor criteria from different categories; possible: one major or two minor criteria from different categories.

2-D = two-dimensional; ARVC/D = arrhythmogenic right ventricular cardiomyopathy/dysplasia; aVF = augmented voltage unipolar left foot lead; aVL = augmented voltage unipolar left arm lead; BSA = body surface area; LV = left ventricle; MRI = magnetic resonance imaging; PLAX = parasternal long-axis view; PSAX = parasternal short-axis view; RVOT = right ventricular outflow tract; RV = right ventricle; SAECG = signal-averaged ECG.

Adapted with permission from Marcus FI, McKenna WJ, Sherrill D, et al: Diagnosis of arrhythmogenic right ventricular cardiomyopathy/dysplasia: proposed modification of the task force criteria, *Circulation* 121:1533-1541, 2010.

it is important to recognize, because ARVD is a rare disease, the importance of expert interpretation of the complex-shaped RV and the need for quantitation of RV structure and function as well as specific protocols for optimal evaluation. Referral to centers with expertise in this field should be considered.

Molecular genetic analysis can potentially facilitate timely diagnosis, guiding interpretation of borderline investigations, and enabling cascade screening of relatives. Unfortunately, sequence analysis of the known desmosomal ARVD-related genes only identifies a responsible mutation in approximately 50% of ARVD probands. Nevertheless, recent studies support the use of genetic testing as a new diagnostic tool in ARVD and also suggest a prognostic impact, as the severity of the disease appears different according to the underlying gene or the presence of multiple mutations.[8,14] In a substantial number of probands, more than one disease-causing mutation can be found (mostly in different genes).[15] Therefore, it is recommended that all desmosome genes be tested simultaneously in the proband. Whenever a pathogenic mutation is identified, it becomes possible to establish a presymptomatic diagnosis of the disease among family members and to provide them with genetic counseling to monitor the development of the disease and to assess the risk of transmitting the disease to offspring.[16] Importantly, genetic testing is not recommended for patients with only a single minor criterion according to the 2010 task force criteria.[17]

ARVD is distinguished from dilated cardiomyopathy by the greater degree of arrhythmogenicity. Although ventricular arrhythmia is a relatively common finding in dilated cardiomyopathy, it is rare in the absence of significant ventricular dysfunction, and SCD is seldom the mode of presentation. In contrast, ARVD is associated with a propensity toward ventricular arrhythmia even in the absence of significant ventricular dysfunction. SCD is the first clinical manifestation of the disease in more than 50% of probands with ARVD. Additionally, regional involvement and aneurysm formation, characteristic of ARVD, argue against the diagnosis of dilated cardiomyopathy.

Risk Stratification

Factors identifying patients with ARVD who are at risk for SCD have not yet been defined in large prospective studies focusing on survival. Nonetheless, several markers of increased risk for life-threatening ventricular arrhythmias have been described, including (1) previous history of cardiac arrest or a history of VT with hemodynamic compromise; (2) history of unexplained syncope (when VT or VF has not been excluded as the cause of syncope); (3) extensive RV disease; (4) LV involvement; (5) family history of cardiac arrest in first-degree relatives; (6) genotypes of ARVD associated with a high risk for SCD (e.g., patients with ARVD2, who can develop polymorphic VT and juvenile SCD associated with sympathetic stimulation); (7) increased QRS dispersion (maximal measured QRS duration minus minimal measured QRS duration is 40 milliseconds or more); (8) S wave upstroke equal to or greater than 0 milliseconds on the 12-lead ECG; (9) patients with Naxos disease; (10) induction of VT during EP testing; (11) detection of nonsustained VT on noninvasive monitoring; (12) male gender; and (13) young age at presentation (<5 years).[18]

Principles of Management

PHARMACOLOGICAL THERAPY

Beta blockers, sotalol, and amiodarone have been used to reduce the risk of recurrence of ventricular arrhythmias in ARVD patients. The usefulness of antiarrhythmic drugs for primary prevention, however, is less well established.

Previous studies, which determined selection of antiarrhythmic therapy based on suppression of VT in the EP laboratory, found that sotalol was more effective than beta blockers and amiodarone in patients with inducible VT and in those with noninducible VT. Thus, sotalol was considered as a first-line antiarrhythmic agent in ARVD both for primary and secondary prevention. However, this was questioned in a recent study of a cohort of rigorously characterized ARVD population treated with empirically prescribed antiarrhythmic agents. In this study, beta blockers were neither protective nor harmful, sotalol was not effective, and amiodarone, although only received by a relatively small number of patients, showed superior efficacy in preventing sustained VT and implantable cardioverter-defibrillator (ICD) therapies.[19]

Therefore, among asymptomatic patients and those with mild disease, beta blockers may still be a reasonable recommendation to reduce the possibility of adrenergically induced arrhythmia. Patients with well-tolerated and non–life-threatening ventricular arrhythmias are at relatively low risk for SCD and can be treated with antiarrhythmic drugs, guided either noninvasively with ambulatory monitoring or with EP testing.[20] Recent data argue against the empirical use of sotalol therapy, especially when permitting additional episodes of VT/VF is highly undesirable. It appears that,

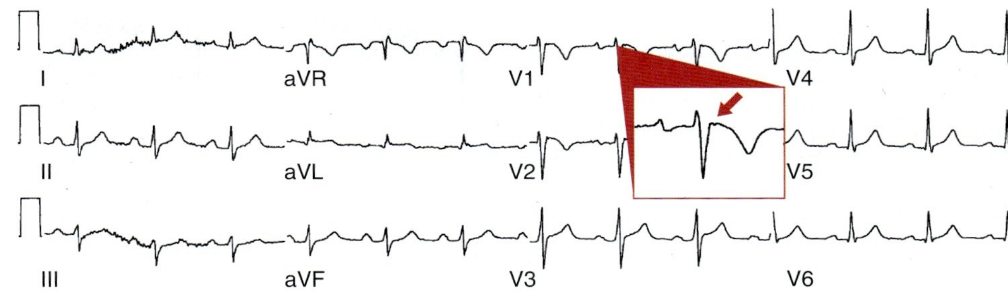

FIGURE 29-3 Surface ECG of sinus rhythm in a patient with arrhythmogenic right ventricular dysplasia-cardiomyopathy. Inset, Magnified view of a single complex in V_1 showing epsilon waves (arrow).

as in other settings, amiodarone is the most effective empirical antiarrhythmic drug therapy in patients with ARVD.[19]

Antiarrhythmic drugs can also be given to reduce the frequency of ventricular arrhythmia in patients with unacceptably frequent ICD therapies.

When the disease has progressed to right or biventricular failure, treatment consists of the current therapy for heart failure, including diuretics, beta blockers, and angiotensin-converting enzyme inhibitors. Although angiotensin-converting enzyme inhibitors are well known for slowing progression in other cardiomyopathies, they have not been proven to be helpful in ARVD. Individuals with reduced RV ejection fraction with dyskinetic portions of the RV may benefit from long-term anticoagulation with warfarin to prevent thrombus formation and subsequent pulmonary embolism. For intractable RV failure, cardiac transplantation can be the only remaining alternative.[20]

IMPLANTABLE CARDIOVERTER-DEFIBRILLATOR

An ICD is the most effective prevention against SCD. For secondary prevention, ICD implantation is recommended in patients with prior cardiac arrest and those with poorly tolerated arrhythmias that are not completely suppressed by antiarrhythmic drug therapy. During a mean follow-up of 39 months, nearly one-half of these patients had an appropriate ICD therapy, 16% had an inappropriate therapy, and 14% had a device-related complication.[5,21]

ICD implantation is also recommended for primary prevention in patients who are considered to be at high risk for SCD (see above). It is important to recognize, however, that there is not yet clear consensus on the specific risk factors that identify those patients with ARVD in whom the probability of SCD is sufficiently high to warrant an ICD for primary prevention.[18]

Importantly, ICD implantation in ARVD patients is associated with several risks. Areas of the RV myocardium in patients with ARVD may be thin and noncontractile and can be penetrated during placement of the RV leads, with subsequent cardiac tamponade. Also, the fibrofatty nature of the RV can lead to difficulty in attaining a location with acceptable R wave amplitude and pacing threshold. Marginal parameters may prevent adequate sensing of arrhythmias, resulting in improper ICD function or failure. A separate pace-sense lead may be necessary, positioned in the RV septum or outflow tract.[20]

CATHETER ABLATION

Catheter ablation of monomorphic VT has a 60% to 90% success rate in patients with ARVD. However, given the chance of long-term recurrence, ablation is not considered curative. Therefore, catheter ablation of VT has been considered mainly in patients with recurrent VT causing frequent ICD shocks and refractory to antiarrhythmic medications and those with VT storm or incessant VT refractory to antiarrhythmic medications. Nonetheless, with the recent advances in mapping and ablation techniques and the improved safety and success of the ablation procedures, as well as the lack of highly effective antiarrhythmic drug therapy, some investigators recommend catheter ablation as a first-line approach in patients presenting with recurrent monomorphic VT.[8,22] ICD implantation is recommended as well, because of the unpredictability of recurrences.

Patients with limited endocardial substrate, those with late VT termination with RF delivery, and certainly those with persistent VT despite aggressive endocardial ablation should be considered for an epicardial approach.[23]

PARTICIPATION IN SPORTS

Because of the association between exercise and the induction of ventricular tachyarrhythmias, a diagnosis of ARVD is generally considered incompatible with competitive sports and moderate- to high-intensity-level recreational activities. Furthermore, any activity, competitive or not, that causes symptoms of palpitations, presyncope, or syncope should be avoided.[20]

FAMILY SCREENING

First-degree relatives should be screened clinically with 12-lead ECG, echocardiography, and cardiac MR imaging. Given the low penetrance observed in most families, screening should be extended throughout the kindred to at least one generation beyond the last affected individual. Asymptomatic family members with a normal comprehensive evaluation are less likely to have inherited the gene defect, but should undergo follow-up at regular intervals (every 2 to 3 years) until definitive diagnostic tools are available.[5] When the causative mutation in the index patient is identified, genetic testing is recommended in family members. A negative genetic test result for the familial mutation would obviate the need for repeated follow-up examinations.

Electrocardiographic Features

ECG during Sinus Rhythm

Approximately 40% to 50% of patients with ARVD have a normal ECG at presentation. However, by 6 years, almost all patients have one or more of several findings on ECG during normal sinus rhythm (NSR), including epsilon wave, T wave inversion, QRS duration equal to or greater than 110 milliseconds in leads V_1 through V_3, and RBBB. Significant differences exist in most ECG features among ARVD patients according to the degree of RV involvement, and they are more prevalent in diffuse ARVD than in the localized form of the disease.[6,8]

The hallmark feature of ARVD, the epsilon wave, is a marker of delayed activation of the RV free wall and outflow tract and is considered a major diagnostic criterion for ARVD. The epsilon wave has the appearance of a distinct wave just beyond the QRS, in the ST segment, in the right precordial leads, particularly in lead V_1, and represents low-amplitude potentials caused by delayed activation of some portion of the RV (Fig. 29-3). Although the epsilon wave has been considered highly specific for ARVD, ECG markers that reflect ventricular conduction delay in ARVD (including the epsilon wave) are frequently observed in subjects with a spontaneous or drug-induced type 1 ECG pattern of Brugada syndrome.[24] Additionally, this criterion is of limited sensitivity, observed in only 10% to 37% of ARVD patients when evaluated by standard ECG. The use of highly amplified (20 mV) precordial leads and modified limb leads can increase the detection of epsilon potentials to 75% but is rarely utilized.[6,8]

Other markers of delayed activation of the RV include prolongation of the QRS duration to at least 110 milliseconds in leads V_1 through V_3, and a ratio of the sum of the QRS duration in leads $(V_1 + V_2 + V_3)/(V_4 + V_5 + V_6) \geq 1.2$ (sensitivity of 35% to 98%). In fact, a QRS duration greater than 110 milliseconds in lead V_1 has a sensitivity of 26% to 75% and a specificity of 100% in patients suspected of having ARVD based on historical features. Additionally, incomplete or complete RBBB can be observed in 18% and 15% of patients, respectively. Epicardial mapping suggests that these patterns are usually caused by parietal block, rather than by disease of the bundle branch itself. In the presence of an RBBB pattern, selective prolongation of the QRS duration in leads V_1 to V_3 compared with lead V_6 (>25 milliseconds, parietal block) is an important hallmark of ARVD (sensitivity of 52% to 64%).[6,8,11,12] Furthermore, T wave inversion in leads V_1 through V_3 in the absence of RBBB is considered a minor diagnostic criterion for ARVD and its prevalence in ARVD has been reported as 55% to 94% in different series. The extent of right precordial T wave inversion relates to the degree of RV involvement. Increased QT dispersion (i.e., inter-lead variability of the QT interval) has been observed in ARVD.

Prolongation of the upstroke of the S wave (≥55 milliseconds from the nadir of the S wave to the isoelectric line) in leads V_1 through V_3 in the absence of RBBB, which presumably represents altered depolarization, was found in the original report to be a very sensitive ECG criterion for ARVD (present in all cases with diffuse ARVD and in 90% in the localized form of the disease). However, the sensitivity of this criterion was less than 60% in several other reports. This measurement has the highest diagnostic usefulness for differentiating the localized form of ARVD from idiopathic RVOT VT, correlates with the degree of RV involvement, and is an independent predictor of VT induction. It is recognized that a prolonged S wave upstroke directly relates to QRS width in the right precordial leads; nonetheless, it is superior to localized QRS prolongation in distinguishing the mild form of ARVD from idiopathic RVOT VT.[6,11,12]

Another ECG marker of ARVD described recently is the "terminal activation delay." This parameter is measured from the nadir of the S wave to the end of all depolarization deflections, thereby including not only the S wave upstroke but also both late fractionated signals and epsilon waves, to the completion of the QRS complex. A prolonged terminal activation delay (≥55 milliseconds) was observed in 71% of ARVD patients and only 4% of controls.[6,25]

QRS fragmentation in standard ECG leads, defined as deflections at the beginning of the QRS complex, on top of the R wave or in the nadir of the S wave, has a sensitivity of 85% for the diagnosis of ARVD.[26]

The SAECG is a highly amplified and signal-processed ECG that can detect microvolt-level electrical potentials in the terminal QRS complex, known as late potentials. Late potentials, which reflect the slow conduction in the ventricular myocardium and electrical potentials that extend beyond the activation time of normal myocardium, typically arise from scarred myocardium, an anatomical substrate potentially responsible for reentrant ventricular arrhythmias. The SAECG and its three components (filtered QRS duration, low-amplitude signal duration, and root-mean-square voltage of the last 40 milliseconds of the QRS) are highly associated with the diagnosis of ARVD. Late potentials and fragmented electrical activity can be detected by signal-averaged ECG in 50% to 80% of patients with ARVD. Although there are no guidelines for abnormal SAECG in patients with ARVD, it is common practice to categorize the SAECG as abnormal if two or more of these parameters are abnormal. In a recent report, the sensitivity of using SAECG for diagnosis of ARVD was increased from 47% using two of the three criteria to 69% by using any one of the three criteria, while maintaining a high specificity of 90% to 95%. Abnormal SAECG was strongly associated with dilated RV volumes and decreased RV ejection fraction detected by cardiac MR imaging. SAECG abnormalities did not vary with clinical presentation or reliably predict spontaneous or inducible VT, and had limited correlation with ECG findings.[11,24,27] Additionally, SAECG abnormalities appear to correlate with the presence of low-voltage areas selectively in the RVOT as observed during electroanatomical voltage mapping, whereas surface ECG abnormalities are associated with a more diffuse RV involvement.[28] The usefulness of SAECG for predicting inducible VT in ARVD remains uncertain.[24]

ECG during Ventricular Tachycardia

Ventricular ectopy in ARVD usually arises from the RV and therefore has an LBBB pattern similar to that seen in idiopathic RVOT VT. The ECG morphology of the VT is predominantly LBBB, but RBBB can be observed and does not exclude an RV origin (Fig. 29-4). The QRS axis during VT is typically between −90 and +110 degrees; an extreme rightward direction of the QRS axis is uncommon.[29] No correlation has been observed between any specific ECG morphology and a particular activation pattern, although all RBBB morphology VTs exhibit a peritricuspid circuit.

Additionally, patients with ARVD frequently demonstrate the presence of more than one VT morphology, either spontaneously (64%) or during an EP study (88%).[6]

Electrophysiological Features

Tachycardia Features

Tachycardia is inducible with programmed electrical stimulation in the majority of ARVD patients with clinical VT. Isoproterenol infusion facilitates VT induction in many patients.

Reentry in areas of abnormal myocardium is the most likely mechanism of VT in ARVD. Most reentrant circuits cluster around the tricuspid annulus and the RVOT. Multiple morphologies of inducible VT are common. A variety of different reentry circuit sites can be identified with entrainment mapping. A single region can give rise to multiple VT morphologies. Previous studies showed mean numbers of different VT morphologies per patient ranging from 1.8 to 3.8.[6]

Overdrive pacing during VT at cycle lengths (CLs) 20 to 50 milliseconds shorter than the tachycardia CL typically results in entrainment of the tachycardia. The presence of entrainment should be confirmed by the demonstration of fixed fusion of the paced QRS at any single pacing CL, progressive fusion as the pacing CL decreases (i.e., the surface ECG progressively looks more like the VT QRS than a purely paced QRS), and resumption of the VT following pacing with a nonfused VT QRS at a return cycle equal to the pacing CL. Once the presence of entrainment is confirmed, three parameters should be evaluated—the presence of manifest or concealed fusion, the post-pacing interval (PPI), and the local electrogram-to-QRS interval during VT versus the stimulus-to-QRS (S-QRS) interval during entrainment. The 12-lead ECGs during pacing and during VT are compared to evaluate whether manifest or concealed fusion is present. The PPI is measured from the stimulus artifact to the onset of the local electrogram of the first VT (unpaced) beat in the pacing lead recording. Finally, the local electrogram-to-QRS interval during VT and the S-QRS interval during entrainment are measured on the distal bipolar pair recording of the mapping catheter or with the use of the proximal bipolar pair when the presence of artifacts in the distal pole recording prevents reliable measurement.

Exclusion of Other Arrhythmia Mechanisms

In clinical practice, the disease that most frequently mimics ARVD is idiopathic RVOT VT. Although RVOT VT is associated with a benign prognosis with no familial basis, it can be extremely difficult to distinguish from the concealed phase of ARVD, in which typical ECG and imaging abnormalities are absent.

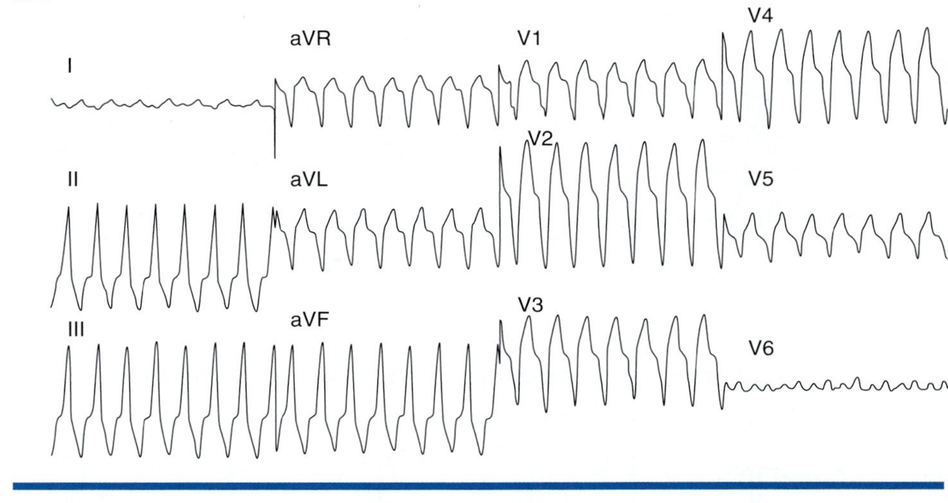

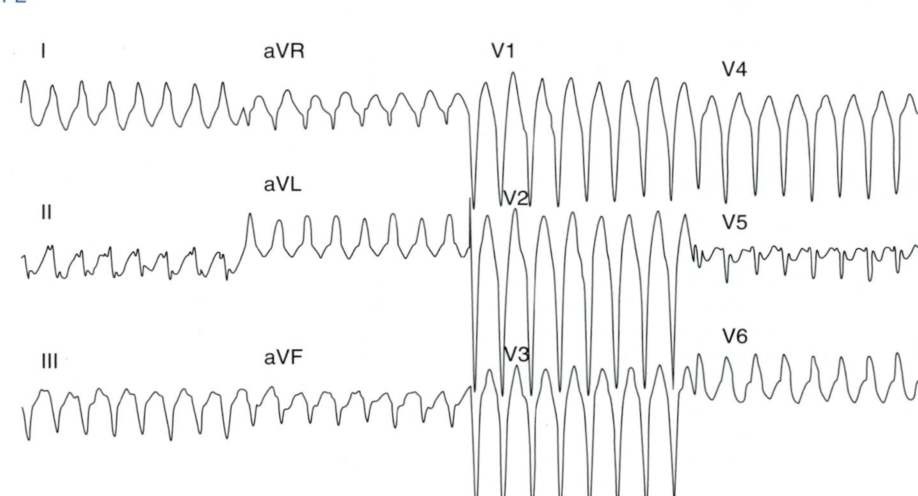

FIGURE 29-4 Surface lead ECGs of ventricular tachycardia (VT) in a patient with arrhythmogenic right ventricular dysplasia-cardiomyopathy. Both have left bundle branch block–type morphology but with very different frontal axes.

The resting surface ECG in NSR is typically normal in patients with idiopathic VT, with no epsilon wave, QRS widening or fragmentation, or other markers of delayed activation of the RV typically observed in ARVD patients. However, the ECG is also normal in 40% to 50% of patients with ARVD at presentation, but in almost no patient after 6 years.[30]

Both idiopathic RVOT VT and VT caused by ARVD generally have LBBB morphology. However, the presence of an LBBB morphology VT with a superior axis is very unlikely in idiopathic RVOT VT. Additionally, VTs in ARVD patients generally have lower QRS amplitude and more fragmentation, but these qualitative differences are not always present.

Patients with idiopathic VT have a normal SAECG when in NSR and normal imaging studies (echocardiography, MR imaging, contrast ventriculography) of RV size and function. Other clues suggesting the presence of an RV cardiomyopathy include the presence of RV dilation, multiple VT morphologies, and a well-defined anatomical substrate.

The response during EP testing is also helpful in distinguishing idiopathic RVOT VT from ARVD. The repetitive initiation of VT by programmed stimulation suggests a reentrant mechanism. In one report, programmed electrical stimulation induced VT in all but 1 of 15 patients with ARVD compared with only 2 patients with idiopathic RVOT VT (93% versus 3%). Additionally, fractionated diastolic electrograms recorded during VT or NSR at the VT site of origin or other RV sites were present in all but one patient with ARVD, but were not seen in any patient with idiopathic RVOT VT. Furthermore, the induction of VTs with different QRS morphologies was seen only in ARVD (73% versus 0%). Although isoproterenol infusion can induce VT in patients with idiopathic RVOT VT, it has a similar effect in ARVD and therefore does not help distinguish between these disorders. Reentry was the mechanism of tachycardia in 80% of the ARVD group, whereas 97% of RVOT VT had features of triggered activity.

Electroanatomical voltage mapping appears to be an effective way of distinguishing early or concealed ARVD from idiopathic VT by detecting RV electroanatomical scars that correlate with the histopathological features pathognomonic of the disease.[31]

Mapping

VTs in ARVD share many features observed in post-MI VTs. First, the tachycardias typically are monomorphic and have a macroreentrant mechanism. Second, the circuits are composed of zones of abnormal conduction, characterized by low-amplitude abnormal electrograms, with identifiable exit regions to the surrounding myocardium. Third, outer loops, which can be broad portions of the reentry circuit in communication with the surrounding myocardium, have also been observed. Fourth, the same types of targets for ablation previously identified in post-MI VT (critical isthmus) can also be useful for targeting VT in ARVD. Therefore, mapping techniques for ARVD-related VT are similar to those used for post-MI VT (see Chap. 22).[8]

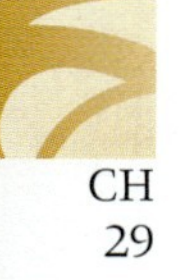

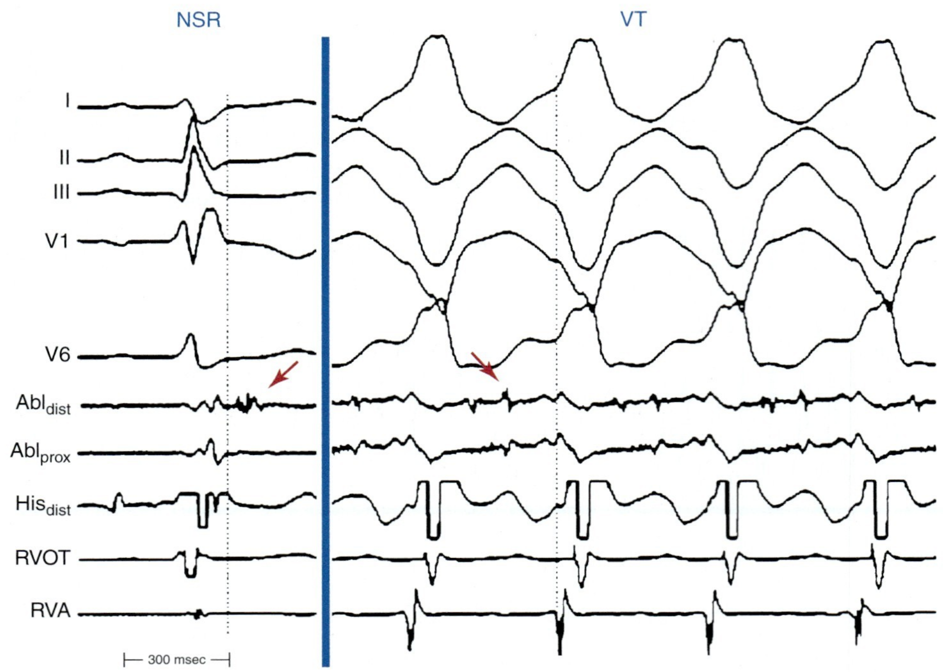

FIGURE 29-5 ECG and intracardiac recordings during normal sinus rhythm (NSR; left) and ventricular tachycardia (VT; right) in a patient with arrhythmogenic right ventricular dysplasia-cardiomyopathy. During NSR, a late potential is present (arrow); the same potential occurs during mid-diastole during VT. RVOT = right ventricular outflow tract.

Activation Mapping

Most reentrant circuits cluster around the inferolateral tricuspid annulus, the RVOT, and the RV apex, which are the typical areas of fibrous and fatty infiltration in ARVD. Hence, these areas are targeted first by activation mapping. Because the VT circuit is composed of zones of abnormal conduction, characterized by low-amplitude abnormal electrograms, with identifiable exit regions to the surrounding myocardium, endocardial activation mapping during VT typically detects abnormal fragmented or split low-voltage electrograms, with diastolic potentials (Fig. 29-5).[8]

During activation mapping, particular sites of interest include: (1) sites with abnormal local bipolar electrogram (amplitude, ≤0.5 mV; duration, ≥60 milliseconds); (2) sites at which the local electrogram precedes the QRS complex by at least 50 milliseconds (activation times are taken from the onset of the bipolar electrogram); and (3) sites with the earliest local activation closest to mid-diastole, isolated mid-diastolic potentials, or continuous activity. Once identified, these sites are targeted by entrainment mapping (see later) to establish their relationship to the tachycardia circuit.

Detailed mapping will usually reveal more than one site of presystolic activity. It is therefore essential to demonstrate that the presystolic site recorded is in fact the earliest site. A normal presystolic bipolar electrogram (amplitude, >3 mV; duration, <70 milliseconds) should prompt further search for earlier activity. If, after very detailed mapping, the earliest recorded site is not at least 50 milliseconds presystolic, this suggests that either the map is inadequate (most common) or the VT arises deeper than the subendocardium, in the midmyocardium, or even incorporating the subepicardium. VTs in patients with ARVD exhibiting a focal activation pattern have also been described; however, an epicardial reentrant circuit with a defined endocardial exit may explain the focal activation pattern of the RV endocardium.[8,29]

An isolated mid-diastolic potential is defined as a low-amplitude, high-frequency diastolic potential separated from the preceding and subsequent ventricular electrograms by an isoelectric segment. It is likely that isolated mid-diastolic potentials that cannot be dissociated from the VT are generated in segments of the zone of slow conduction or common pathway (isthmus), which are integral components of the reentry circuit. It is important to recognize that not all presystolic activity recorded during VT is related to the mechanism; it could represent delayed activity not related to the tachycardia mechanism, dead-end pathways, or even an artifact. Therefore, it is important to confirm that presystolic activity is related to the reentrant circuit. Demonstration of a fixed relationship of the diastolic electrograms to the subsequent VT QRS, despite spontaneous or induced oscillations of the tachycardia CL, helps exclude the possibility that those electrograms reflect late activation from unrelated dead-end pathways.[8]

Additionally, 3-D electroanatomical mapping can help in the precise description of VT reentrant circuits, sequence of ventricular activation during the VT and rapid visualization of the activation wavefront, and identification of slow-conducting pathways and appropriate sites for entrainment mapping. Local activation times are assigned according to the onset of the bipolar electrogram registered at the tip of the mapping catheter and are color-coded. These systems also help in navigation of the ablation catheter, planning of ablation lines, and maintaining a log of sites of interest (e.g., sites with favorable entrainment or pace mapping findings), which can then be revisited with precision. Additionally, voltage (scar) mapping is a helpful feature of some of the electroanatomical mapping systems (see later).[8]

Entrainment Mapping

Entrainment mapping is used to characterize reentry circuits in ARVD, identify critical isthmuses, and guide ablation. Pacing is performed during VT at a CL 10 to 30 milliseconds shorter than the VT CL, at RV sites identified during activation mapping, demonstrating continuous activity or isolated mid-diastolic potentials. For stable VTs, the following three criteria are used to define the critical isthmus and predict the success of RF application in termination of the VT: (1) entrainment with concealed fusion; (2) PPI equal to the tachycardia CL (within 20 to 30 milliseconds); (3) and S-QRS interval equal to the local electrogram-to-QRS interval (±20 milliseconds). Other predictors of successful ablation sites include S-QRS interval–to–VT CL ratio less than 0.7, long S-QRS interval, and alteration of the tachycardia CL and/or termination by subthreshold or nonpropagated stimuli. However, because of the diffuse nature of the disease in ARVD, isthmuses may sometimes be wide and good entrainment maps can be obtained from a rather large area. In this case, linear lesions across the diastolic pathway may be necessary.[8]

Pace Mapping

Pace mapping can be used to complement activation and entrainment mapping findings and to confirm ablation target sites, although it may not be always necessary, especially when several criteria localizing the VT isthmus have been identified. At isthmus sites defined during VT, pace mapping during NSR is attempted after VT termination, with the mapping catheter being kept at the same location. Pace mapping is preferably performed with unipolar stimuli (10 mA, 2 milliseconds) from the distal electrode of the mapping catheter (cathode) and an electrode in the inferior vena cava (anode).

The resulting 12-lead ECG morphology is compared with that of the tachycardia. ECG recordings should be reviewed at the same gain and filter settings. The greater the degree of concordance between the morphology during pacing and tachycardia, the closer is the catheter to the site of origin of the tachycardia.

At best, a pace map that matches the VT would only identify the exit site to the normal myocardium, and can be distant from the critical sites of the circuit required for ablation. Thus, pace mapping remains only a corroborative method of localizing VT. It can be used to focus initial mapping to regions likely to contain the reentrant circuit exit or abnormal conduction but is not sufficiently specific or sensitive to be the sole guide for ablation.

Pace mapping can also be used in conjunction with substrate mapping when other mapping techniques are not feasible, so that it can provide information on where ablation can be directed. The VT circuit's exit site is approximated by the site of pace mapping that generates QRS complexes similar to those of VT. From that point, evaluation of the S-QRS interval (measured to the onset of the earliest QRS on the 12-lead ECG) can help trace the course of the VT isthmus. Sites along the VT isthmus are associated with good pace maps but with progressively longer S-QRS intervals.[8]

Electroanatomical Substrate Mapping

Electroanatomical substrate mapping provides a helpful tool in reconstructing the VT circuit in patients with ARVD and hemodynamically stable VTs, in conjunction with activation and entrainment mapping techniques.[29] Additionally, in a subset of ARVD patients, conventional mapping during VT can be limited by changing multiple morphologies, nonsustainability, or hemodynamic instability. Substrate-based voltage mapping during sinus rhythm can be used in these cases to identify regions of scar and abnormal myocardium and guide, in conjunction with pace mapping, ablation of linear lesions to connect or encircle the abnormal regions.[22]

The dysplastic regions can be identified, quantified, and differentiated from healthy myocardium by the presence of electrograms with low amplitudes and longer durations, reflecting replaced myocardial tissue. Voltage mapping is performed during sinus rhythm, atrial pacing, or ventricular pacing. The peak-to-peak signal amplitude of the bipolar electrogram is measured automatically. Endocardial regions with a bipolar electrogram amplitude greater than 1.5 mV are defined as normal, and dense scar areas are defined as those with an amplitude less than 0.5 mV. Abnormal myocardium is defined as an area of contiguous recordings with a bipolar electrogram amplitude between 0.5 and 1.5 mV.

As noted, in ARVD, the normal myocardium is replaced by fatty and then fibrous tissue, causing thinning and scarring, predominantly in the RV. Studies have found that regions of abnormal voltage suggestive of scar were observed in all ARVD patients. The endocardial bipolar voltage abnormalities tend to be perivalvular and, although affecting predominantly the RV free wall, involve some aspect of the septum in most (76%) patients. This pattern is consistent with pathological studies demonstrating a predilection for scar to occur in these particular areas in ARVD. Whether an extensive perivalvular fibrotic process is specific for patients who present with sustained monomorphic VT in the setting of ARVD is yet to be determined.[22,29] In contrast to the post-MI pattern of dense scar surrounded by a border zone, the regions of abnormal myocardium in ARVD are commonly patchy and inhomogeneous, occurring in anatomically disparate areas. As a consequence, low-voltage identification in ARVD is less useful as a marker for ablation because it is very widespread. Nonetheless, evaluating the existence of different voltage areas within the 0.5-mV scar (i.e., the voltage limits are reset to 0.3 to 0.5 mV as the upper limit and to 0.1 mV as the lower, representing dense scar) can potentially help visualize channels of slow conduction within scar tissue.[8] The critical isthmus of each of the reentrant circuit typically is bounded by an area of low-voltage scar on one side and an anatomical barrier (tricuspid annulus) on the other side, or by two parallel lines of double potentials.[29]

A recent report found that identifying ventricular electrograms with an isolated delayed component during sinus rhythm (defined as a distinct electrogram after the QRS separated [by ≥40 milliseconds] by an isoelectric interval or very low-amplitude signal of <0.1 mV) can be used to define the substrate for the VT circuit and, when combined with other mapping maneuvers, can help guide catheter ablation in ARVD patients with noninducible or unmappable VTs.[32]

Importantly, the disease in ARVD has been reported to begin epicardially and progress to the endocardium; therefore, endocardial fibrosis, as reflected by the voltage map findings, can be a manifestation of more extensive disease involvement and can be anticipated to be the more common substrate for uniform sustained VT (Fig. 29-6).[23]

Endocardial *unipolar* voltage mapping (with a cutoff of 5.5 mV) can potentially provide a more global assessment of myocardial voltage and more closely approximate the degree and location of epicardial bipolar voltage abnormalities that serve as a substrate for VT in ARVD patients with no or limited endocardial bipolar voltage abnormalities. Therefore, endocardial *unipolar* voltage mapping may help in decision making related to proceeding to epicardial substrate mapping and ablation (Fig. 29-7).[33]

Noncontact Mapping

When VT is short-lived, hemodynamically unstable, or cannot be reproducibly initiated, simultaneous multisite data acquisition using a noncontact mapping system (EnSite 3000; St. Jude Medical, St. Paul, Minn.) can help localize the VT site of origin. The system can help identify presystolic endocardial activation sites (potential exits) for reentrant VTs and thus starting points for conventional mapping. It may also help identify VT isthmuses and therefore suitable targets for ablation.

The EnSite 3000 noncontact mapping system consists of a noncontact catheter (9 Fr) with a multielectrode array surrounding a 7.5-mL balloon mounted at the distal end. To create a map, the balloon catheter is positioned in the RV through the left subclavian vein approach with a 260-cm-long 0.035-inch guidewire. The distal tip is placed at the RV apex. The balloon is then deployed, and it can be filled with a mixture of contrast and saline to be visualized fluoroscopically. The balloon is positioned in the center of the RV cavity and does not come into physical contact with the atrial walls being mapped. Systemic anticoagulation is critical to avoid thromboembolic complications. Intravenous heparin is usually given to maintain the activated clotting time (ACT) at 250 to 300 seconds.

A conventional deflectable mapping-ablation catheter is also positioned in the RV and used to collect geometry information. The tricuspid annulus, His bundle, and pulmonic valve are initially tagged and a detailed geometry of the RV and RVOT is reconstructed by moving the mapping catheter around the RV. Subsequently, a detailed geometry of the RV is reconstructed by moving the mapping catheter around the endocardium. Using this information, the computer creates a model, called a convex hull, of the chamber during diastole. The patient may be in NSR or tachycardia during creation of the geometry.

Once chamber geometry has been delineated, VT is induced and mapping can begin. The data acquisition process is performed

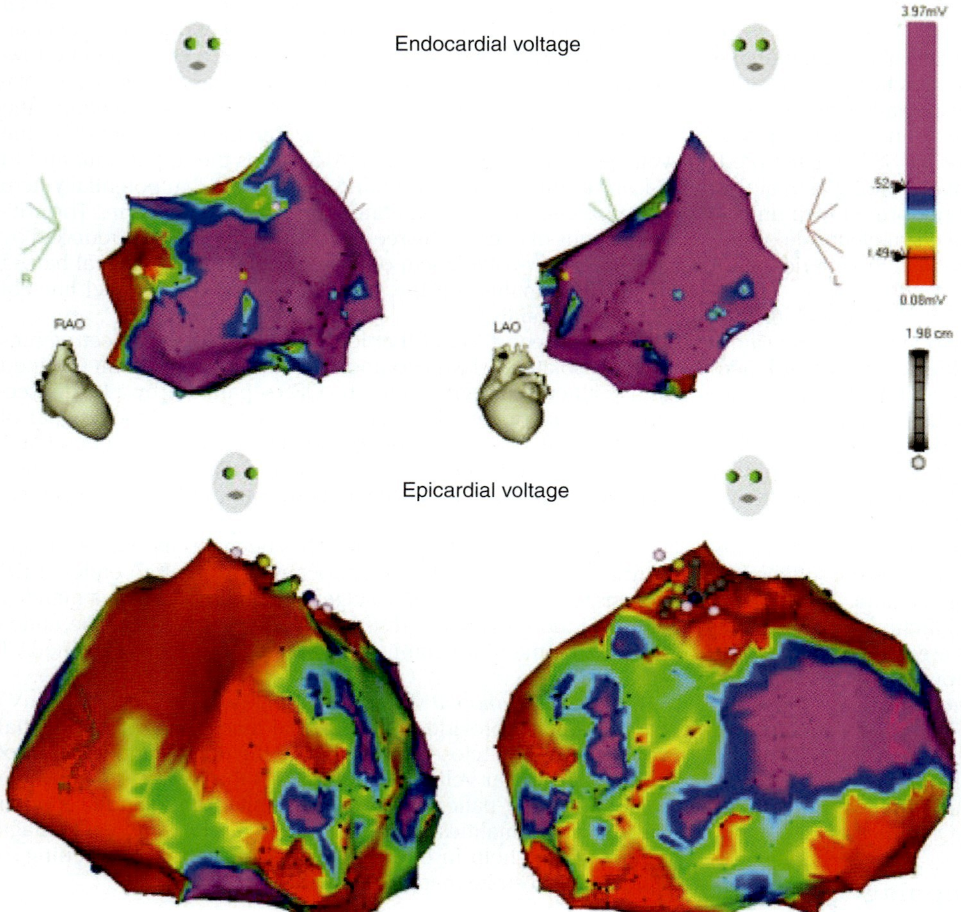

FIGURE 29-6 Right and left anterior oblique electroanatomical endocardial (top) and epicardial (bottom) voltage maps in a patient with ARVD. Red areas denote low voltage/scar. On the endocardial map, only a small area shows abnormal voltage (near lateral tricuspid valve, red area); however, on the epicardial map, substantially larger areas show abnormal low voltage. LAO = left anterior oblique; RAO = right anterior oblique.

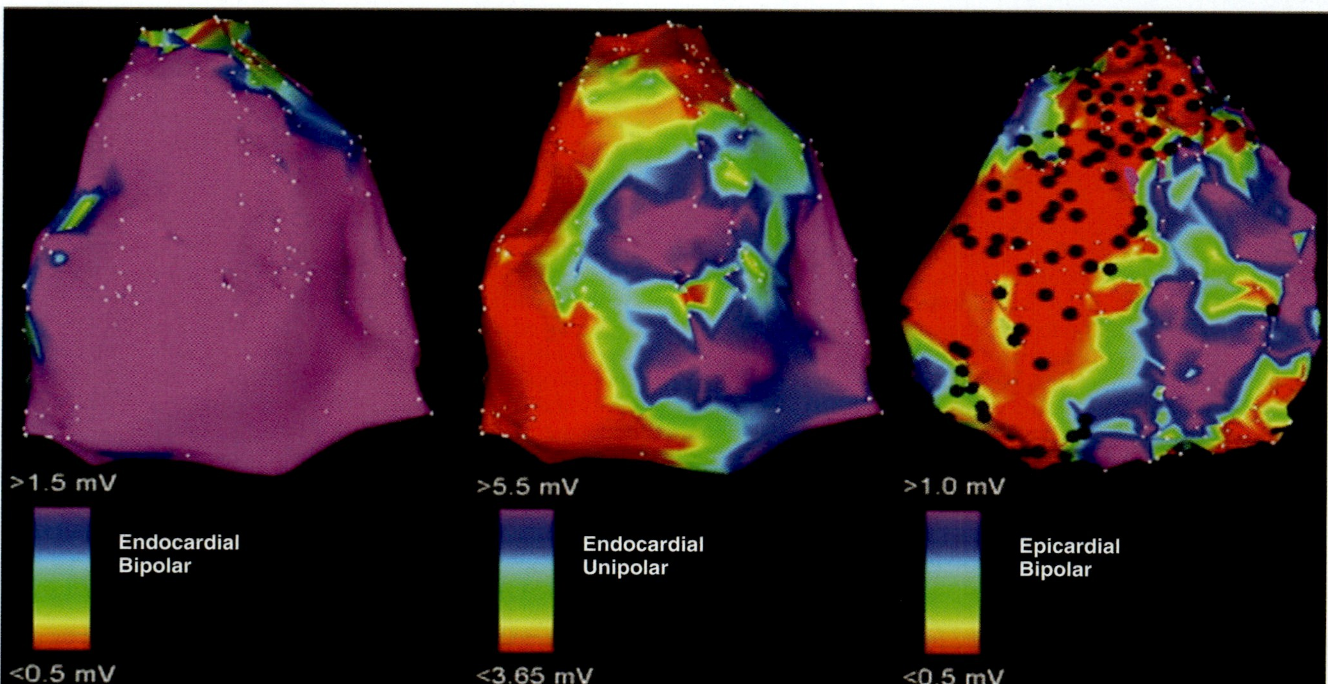

FIGURE 29-7 Unipolar endocardial electrograms defining the location and greater extent of epicardial bipolar electrogram abnormalities in a patient with arrhythmogenic right ventricular cardiomyopathy-dysplasia. **Left:** Endocardial bipolar voltage map demonstrates a paucity of low-voltage regions. **Center:** Endocardial unipolar voltage mapping reveals a much greater burden of abnormal myocardium (<5.5 mV) extending from the lateral tricuspid valve up to the pulmonic valve region and inferiorly across the right ventricular free wall. **Right:** Epicardial bipolar voltage map confirms the extensive area of abnormal epicardium. Black dots represent wide, split, and/or late epicardial electrograms and help to identify low-voltage areas consistent with scar versus fat. *(From Polin GM, Haqqani H, Tzou W, et al: Endocardial unipolar voltage mapping to identify epicardial substrate in arrhythmogenic right ventricular cardiomyopathy/dysplasia, Heart Rhythm 8:76-83, 2011.)*

automatically by the system, and all data for the entire chamber are acquired simultaneously. The system then reconstructs more than 3000 unipolar electrograms simultaneously and superimposes them onto the virtual endocardium, producing color-coded isopotential maps to depict graphically regions that are depolarized. Activation can be tracked on the isopotential map throughout the tachycardia cycle and wavefront propagation can be displayed as a user-controlled 3-D "movie." The color range represents voltage or timing of onset. Sites of early (presystolic) endocardial activity, which are likely adjacent to reentry circuit exits, are usually identifiable; in some cases, isthmuses can be identified. Diastolic depolarization is defined as activity on the isopotential map that can be continuously tracked back in time from VT exit sites, defined on the map as synchronous with the QRS onset. Diastolic activity and exit sites are then marked on the virtual endocardium, and a mapping catheter is navigated to them by the locator technology. Ablation lesions can be tagged, facilitating performing linear ablation devoid of gaps across the tachycardia critical isthmus.

Unless the multielectrode array position is significantly changed, the accepted geometry can be applicable during the entire procedure, and the same geometry can be used for mapping different VT morphologies as well as for substrate mapping.

Substrate mapping based on scar or diseased tissue, which has been recently introduced to the noncontact mapping technology, can be particularly helpful when the VT is not inducible during the procedure. Dynamic substrate mapping allows the creation of voltage maps from a single cardiac cycle and provides the ability to identify low-voltage areas, as well as fixed and functional block, on the virtual endocardium through noncontact methodology.[34]

Percutaneous Epicardial Mapping

A recent report found that, in patients with ARVD and VT who failed endocardial ablation, low-voltage areas consistent with scar were more extensive on the epicardium than the endocardium and uniformly included wide, split, and late electrograms consistent with abnormal conduction. The origin of VT defined by activation/entrainment mapping and suggested by the detailed substrate mapping observations and targeted for ablation was also frequently noted beyond the endocardially defined scar. Successful epicardial ablation sites were often opposite endocardia[l] normal voltage or where ablation had been ineffective.[23]

Therefore, patients with limited endocardial substrate, those late VT termination with endocardial RF delivery, and certa[in] those with persistent VT despite aggressive endocardial ablati[on] should be considered for an epicardial approach. Additionall[y] surface ECG criteria identifying a QS complex in lead V_2 or leads III and aVF during VT can be helpful in identifying patients who should be considered for an epicardial approach with the initial procedure.[23]

The approach to epicardial mapping is essentially the same as for endocardial ablation, including activation mapping, entrainment mapping, substrate mapping, and pace mapping, and is discussed in detail in Chapter 27.

Ablation

Target of Ablation

For stable VTs, reentry circuit isthmuses are the target of ablation and are defined by activation and entrainment mapping as sites with continuous activity or isolated mid-diastolic potentials, entrainment with concealed fusion, PPI equal to the VT CL, and S-QRS interval less than 70% of the VT CL. Alteration of the tachycardia CL or termination of VT by subthreshold or nonpropagated stimuli, and repeated VT termination occurring with catheter manipulation or pacing at the site, also suggest an isthmus location (Fig. 29-8).[29]

For hemodynamically unstable VTs, substrate mapping during sinus rhythm followed by brief inductions of VT (with the mapping catheter at the optimal site, as identified by substrate and pace mapping) can allow assessment of the relationship of the abnormal electrograms to the VT circuit. This can also allow entrainment maneuvers to be performed at those sites to help distinguish sites critical to the VT circuit from bystander sites. VT is then quickly terminated before significant hemodynamic compromise ensues. This approach can be facilitated by hemodynamic support with the use of intravenous vasopressors, intraaortic balloon pump, or both. This approach, however, requires being able to induce the same VT reproducibly. The use of noncontact mapping can be of value in these cases.

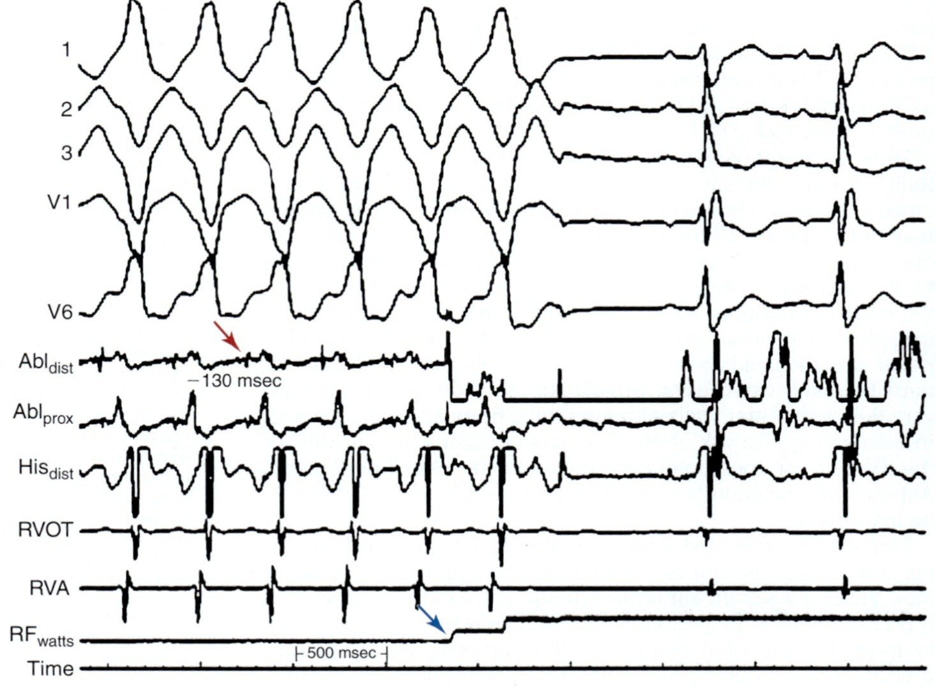

FIGURE 29-8 Ablation of arrhythmogenic right ventricular dysplasia-cardiomyopathy (ARVD) ventricular tachycardia. Shown is radiofrequency (RF) energy delivery in the basal lateral right ventricle in a patient with ARVD. Note the mid-diastolic potential (red arrow) 130 milliseconds prior to QRS onset and almost immediate cessation of ventricular tachycardia on RF delivery. Blue arrow marks initiation of RF energy delivery.

ne critical isthmuses of the reentrant circuit(s) can be ...ed, linear ablation lesions are delivered to sever those ...nuses. For unmappable VTs (due to poor inducibility or ...nging VT morphology), RF ablation can be performed as ...ear lesions targeting potential exit sites and isthmuses of VT ...ircuits based on the location of the best pace map, location of valvular anatomical boundaries, and the substrate defined by the voltage mapping. Typically, linear lesions are created over target regions by sequential point lesions designed to: (1) connect scar or abnormal myocardium to a valve continuity; (2) connect scar or abnormal myocardium to another scar; (3) extend from the most abnormal endocardium (<0.5 mV) to normal myocardium (>1.5 mV); or (4) encircle the scar or abnormal region, depending on the scar location and size.[22,32]

Ablation Technique

Ablation may be performed with a 4-mm-tip (maximal target temperature of 60°C and maximal power of 50 W), an 8-mm-tip (maximal temperature of 65°C and maximal power of 75 W), or an irrigated-tip catheter (maximal temperature of 40-45°C and maximal power of 50 W). Irrigated RF ablation catheters are preferred, because power delivery can be limited in the trabeculated and annular regions where cooling from circulating blood flow is low. However, careful attention to power titration and monitoring impedance is necessary to reduce the risk of perforation when ablating in the free wall of the RV.[35] Ablation is usually maintained for 60 to 120 seconds at the site where the tachycardia is terminated (in ablation during stable VT) or at each point along the linear ablation.[8]

Endpoints of Ablation

Lack of inducibility of VT is the endpoint of the ablation procedure. When the VT is scarcely inducible at baseline, the disappearance of all the isolated delayed components of the VT-related area can be used as an endpoint for the substrate-based ablation approach.

Outcome

Ablation of VT in ARVD remains a clinical challenge and should be viewed as a potential palliative procedure in selected patients. Although VT ablation has been reported to successfully eliminate inducible VT acutely in 41% to 88% of patients, long-term success is low, and during average follow-ups of 11 to 24 months, VT recurs in 11% to 83% of patients, even following extensive or repeated ablation attempts.[22,29,36] Recurrences usually manifest as nonsustained VT, a slower monomorphic sustained VT, or a new monomorphic VT.[8,35]

Multiple morphologies, hemodynamic instability, or noninducibility can limit the success of VT ablation. Additionally, ARVD can create a large number of potential circuits; an empirical approach may not eliminate all the possible pathways. Achieving adequate energy delivery can also be a problem, especially in regions difficult to access by catheter—in particular, abnormal regions along the tricuspid annulus, which can require the use of 8-mm-tip or irrigation-tip ablation catheters to achieve effective lesions underneath the tricuspid valve. It must be emphasized that caution must be taken when using irrigated-tip ablation in patients with very thin ventricular walls, although thick fibrous tissue is present in many areas. The risk of creating deeper lesions in thin walls of the RV body or apex potentially increases the risk of perforation. Although the magnitude of this risk is not well known, it seems to be infrequent.[8]

Furthermore, recent studies have shown a high prevalence of epicardial isthmuses in ARVD. Epicardial mapping and ablation have yielded a significant improvement in ablation efficacy; thus, it is reasonable to begin mapping endocardially, but be prepared to move to epicardial mapping following pericardial puncture if endocardial mapping and ablation do not quickly yield good results. In a recent report, percutaneous epicardial mapping and ablation were performed in 13 consecutive patients with ARVD after failed endocardial VT ablation. Twenty-seven distinct VTs were targeted for ablation from the epicardium; during 18 ± 13 months of follow-up, 77% of patients were free of VT.[23]

The discrepancy between the good acute results and the unfavorable long-term outcome may be explained by the progressive nature of ARVD, which predisposes to the occurrence of new and malignant arrhythmogenic substrates over time. This hypothesis, however, has been questioned by a recent study that demonstrated the absence of progression of the area of the endocardial scar as measured by voltage mapping in patients with ARVD and VT, despite demonstrating progressive RV dilation in these patients.[7]

REFERENCES

1. Lombardi R, Marian AJ: Arrhythmogenic right ventricular cardiomyopathy is a disease of cardiac stem cells, *Curr Opin Cardiol* 25:222–228, 2010.
2. Otten E, Asimaki A, Maass A, et al: Desmin mutations as a cause of right ventricular heart failure affect the intercalated disks, *Heart Rhythm* 7:1058–1064, 2010.
3. Hamilton RM, Fidler L: Right ventricular cardiomyopathy in the young: an emerging challenge, *Heart Rhythm* 6:571–575, 2009.
4. Maass K: Arrhythmogenic right ventricular cardiomyopathy and desmin: another gene fits the shoe, *Heart Rhythm* 7:1065–1066, 2010.
5. Boussy T, Paparella G, de Asmundis C, et al: Genetic basis of ventricular arrhythmias, *Heart Fail Clin* 6:249–266, 2010.
6. Cox MG, Nelen MR, Wilde AA, et al: Activation delay and VT parameters in arrhythmogenic right ventricular dysplasia/cardiomyopathy: toward improvement of diagnostic ECG criteria, *J Cardiovasc Electrophysiol* 19:775–781, 2008.
7. Riley MP, Zado E, Bala R, et al: Lack of uniform progression of endocardial scar in patients with arrhythmogenic right ventricular dysplasia/cardiomyopathy and ventricular tachycardia, *Circ Arrhythm Electrophysiol* 3:332–338, 2010.
8. Arbelo E, Josephson ME: Ablation of ventricular arrhythmias in arrhythmogenic right ventricular dysplasia, *J Cardiovasc Electrophysiol* 21:473–486, 2010.
9. Avella A, d'Amati G, Pappalardo A, et al: Diagnostic value of endomyocardial biopsy guided by electroanatomic voltage mapping in arrhythmogenic right ventricular cardiomyopathy/dysplasia, *J Cardiovasc Electrophysiol* 19:1127–1134, 2008.
10. Asimaki A, Tandri H, Huang H, et al: A new diagnostic test for arrhythmogenic right ventricular cardiomyopathy, *N Engl J Med* 360:1075–1084, 2009.
11. Marcus FI, McKenna WJ, Sherrill D, et al: Diagnosis of arrhythmogenic right ventricular cardiomyopathy/dysplasia: proposed modification of the task force criteria, *Circulation* 121:1533–1541, 2010.
12. Marcus FI, Zareba W, Calkins H, et al: Arrhythmogenic right ventricular cardiomyopathy/dysplasia clinical presentation and diagnostic evaluation: results from the North American Multidisciplinary Study, *Heart Rhythm* 6:984–992, 2009.
13. Cox MG, van der Smagt JJ, Noorman M, et al: Arrhythmogenic right ventricular dysplasia/cardiomyopathy diagnostic task force criteria: impact of new task force criteria, *Circ Arrhythm Electrophysiol* 3:126–133, 2010.
14. Fressart V, Duthoit G, Donal E, et al: Desmosomal gene analysis in arrhythmogenic right ventricular dysplasia/cardiomyopathy: spectrum of mutations and clinical impact in practice, *Europace* 12:861–868, 2010.
15. Bauce B, Nava A, Beffagna G, et al: Multiple mutations in desmosomal proteins encoding genes in arrhythmogenic right ventricular cardiomyopathy/dysplasia, *Heart Rhythm* 7: 22–29, 2010.
16. Zipes DP, Camm AJ, Borggrefe M, et al: ACC/AHA/ESC 2006 guidelines for management of patients with ventricular arrhythmias and the prevention of sudden cardiac death: a report of the American College of Cardiology/American Heart Association Task Force and the European Society of Cardiology Committee for Practice Guidelines (Writing Committee to Develop Guidelines for Management of Patients With Ventricular Arrhythmias and the Prevention of Sudden Cardiac Death), *J Am Coll Cardiol* 48:e247–e346, 2006.
17. Ackerman MJ, Priori SG, Willems S, et al: HRS/EHRA expert consensus statement on the state of genetic testing for the channelopathies and cardiomyopathies, *Heart Rhythm* 8:1308–1339, 2011.
18. Epstein AE, DiMarco JP, Ellenbogen KA, et al: ACC/AHA/HRS 2008 guidelines for device-based therapy of cardiac rhythm abnormalities: executive summary, *Heart Rhythm* 5: 934–955, 2008.
19. Marcus GM, Glidden DV, Polonsky B, et al: Efficacy of antiarrhythmic drugs in arrhythmogenic right ventricular cardiomyopathy: a report from the North American ARVC Registry, *J Am Coll Cardiol* 54:609–615, 2009.
20. Kies P, Bootsma M, Bax J, et al: Arrhythmogenic right ventricular dysplasia/cardiomyopathy: screening, diagnosis, and treatment, *Heart Rhythm* 3:225–234, 2006.
21. Hodgkinson KA, Parfrey PS, Bassett AS, et al: The impact of implantable cardioverter-defibrillator therapy on survival in autosomal-dominant arrhythmogenic right ventricular cardiomyopathy (ARVD5), *J Am Coll Cardiol* 45:400–408, 2005.
22. Verma A, Kilicaslan F, Schweikert RA, et al: Short- and long-term success of substrate-based mapping and ablation of ventricular tachycardia in arrhythmogenic right ventricular dysplasia, *Circulation* 111:3209–3216, 2005.
23. Garcia FC, Bazan V, Zado ES, et al: Epicardial substrate and outcome with epicardial ablation of ventricular tachycardia in arrhythmogenic right ventricular cardiomyopathy/dysplasia, *Circulation* 120:366–375, 2009.
24. Letsas KP, Efremidis M, Weber R, et al: Epsilon-like waves and ventricular conduction abnormalities in subjects with type 1 ECG pattern of Brugada syndrome, *Heart Rhythm* 8: 874–878, 2011.

25. Cox MG, van der Smagt JJ, Wilde AA, et al: New ECG criteria in arrhythmogenic right ventricular dysplasia/cardiomyopathy, *Circ Arrhythm Electrophysiol* 2:524–530, 2009.
26. Peters S, Trummel M, Koehler B: QRS fragmentation in standard ECG as a diagnostic marker of arrhythmogenic right ventricular dysplasia-cardiomyopathy, *Heart Rhythm* 5:1417–1421, 2008.
27. Folino AF, Bauce B, Frigo G, Nava A: Long-term follow-up of the signal-averaged ECG in arrhythmogenic right ventricular cardiomyopathy: correlation with arrhythmic events and echocardiographic findings, *Europace* 8:423–429, 2006.
28. Santangeli P, Pieroni M, Dello RA, et al: Noninvasive diagnosis of electroanatomic abnormalities in arrhythmogenic right ventricular cardiomyopathy, *Circ Arrhythm Electrophysiol* 3:632–638, 2010.
29. Miljoen H, State S, De Chillou CC, et al: Electroanatomic mapping characteristics of ventricular tachycardia in patients with arrhythmogenic right ventricular cardiomyopathy/dysplasia, *Europace* 7:516–524, 2005.
30. Shimizu W: Arrhythmias originating from the right ventricular outflow tract: how to distinguish "malignant" from "benign"? *Heart Rhythm* 6:1507–1511, 2009.
31. Corrado D, Basso C, Leoni L, et al: Three-dimensional electroanatomical voltage mapping and histologic evaluation of myocardial substrate in right ventricular outflow tract tachycardia, *J Am Coll Cardiol* 51:731–739, 2008.
32. Nogami A, Sugiyasu A, Tada H, et al: Changes in the isolated delayed component as an endpoint of catheter ablation in arrhythmogenic right ventricular cardiomyopathy: predictor for long-term success, *J Cardiovasc Electrophysiol* 19:681–688, 2008.
33. Polin GM, Haqqani H, Tzou W, et al: Endocardial unipolar voltage mapping to identify epicardial substrate in arrhythmogenic right ventricular cardiomyopathy/dysplasia, *Heart Rhythm* 8:76–83, 2011.
34. Yao Y, Zhang S, He DS, et al: Radiofrequency ablation of the ventricular tachycardia with arrhythmogenic right ventricular cardiomyopathy using non-contact mapping, *Pacing Clin Electrophysiol* 30:526–533, 2007.
35. Aliot EM, Stevenson WG, Mendral-Garrote JM, et al: EHRA/HRS expert consensus on catheter ablation of ventricular arrhythmias: developed in a partnership with the European Heart Rhythm Association (EHRA), a Registered Branch of the European Society of Cardiology (ESC), and the Heart Rhythm Society (HRS); in collaboration with the American College of Cardiology (ACC) and the American Heart Association (AHA), *Heart Rhythm* 6:886–933, 2009.
36. Dalal D, Jain R, Tandri H, et al: Long-term efficacy of catheter ablation of ventricular tachycardia in patients with arrhythmogenic right ventricular dysplasia/cardiomyopathy, *J Am Coll Cardiol* 50:432–440, 2007.

CHAPTER 30 Ventricular Arrhythmias in Congenital Heart Disease

Pathophysiology

Most information concerning patients with ventricular tachycardia (VT) and congenital heart disease pertains to tetralogy of Fallot, as compared with other forms of congenital heart disease. Tetralogy of Fallot is the most common cyanotic congenital cardiac malformation. The core lesion is an underdeveloped subpulmonary infundibulum, which is superiorly and anteriorly displaced, resulting in the well-known tetrad of pulmonary stenosis, ventricular septal defect, aortic override, and right ventricular (RV) hypertrophy. Correction of the defect involves patch closure of the ventricular septal defect and relief of RV outflow tract (RVOT) obstruction, which typically requires resection of a large amount of RV muscle. When the procedure was first performed, it was not done through the tricuspid valve but required a ventriculotomy. The pulmonic valve annulus is usually small, and repair with a transannular patch leads to chronic pulmonic insufficiency, which can be severe if associated with downstream obstruction caused by significant pulmonary arterial stenosis. It has been hypothesized that ventricular arrhythmias in these patients are of the result of years of chronic cyanosis, followed by the placement of a ventriculotomy, increased RV pressures caused by inadequate relief of obstruction, and severe pulmonic regurgitation with RV dysfunction. Such factors can lead to myocardial fibrosis and result in the substrate for reentrant ventricular arrhythmias.[1]

Using intraoperative mapping, VT after surgical correction of tetralogy of Fallot has been classified into two types: VT originating from the RVOT, which is considered to be related to prior right ventriculotomy or reconstruction of the RVOT (Fig. 30-1); and VT originating from the RV inflow tract septum, which is thought to be related to closure of the ventricular septal defect.

The electrophysiological (EP) mechanism responsible for VT after surgical correction of congenital heart disease is typically a macroreentrant circuit within the RV around a scar or prosthetic materials used during surgical repair. Reentry circuit isthmuses are located within anatomically defined pathways bordered by unexcitable tissue. Four discrete anatomical isthmuses that often support VT have been identified. The most common isthmus is between the superior aspect of the tricuspid annulus and unexcitable scar/patch in the free wall of the RVOT. The other isthmuses exist between the pulmonic valve and RV free wall scar (in the absence of a transannular patch), between the septal patch and tricuspid annulus through the region of the ventriculo-infundibular fold, and between the septal patch and pulmonic valve.[2,3]

The sites of the diastolic activation and delayed conduction along the reentrant circuit have been shown to have significant abnormalities such as fibrosis, adiposis, and degeneration of the myocardium. The scattered surviving myocyte islets embedded in the extensive adiposis and/or fibrosis can form an electrical maze around the surgical suture area, resembling the histological findings in the border zone of infarcted myocardium. Furthermore, RV remodeling induced by pressure or volume load promotes hypertrophy and fibrosis, which can potentially result in slow conduction, providing the link between impaired hemodynamics and VT.[3]

Clinical Considerations

Epidemiology

Congenital heart disease is the most common form of birth defect, with an estimated 1% to 2% of live newborns afflicted by moderate or severe types. Ventricular arrhythmias late after repair of congenital heart disease are a common finding, predominantly in those with tetralogy of Fallot, and potentially contribute to sudden cardiac death (SCD) in this population. The incidence of late SCD has been debated but ranges from 1% to 5% during a follow-up period of 7 to 20 years after surgery. The incidence of arrhythmias generally increases as the patient with congenital heart disease ages. Patients with surgical correction of ventricular septal defect or pulmonary stenosis also have a higher than normal risk of serious ventricular arrhythmias and SCD.[1] SCD is the most common cause of death in patients after repair of congenital heart disease, with a 25- to 100-fold increased risk compared with the general population.[4]

In patients with tetralogy of Fallot, serious ventricular arrhythmias are rare during the first 10 to 15 years following corrective surgery. This is followed by a steady increase in the incidence of ventricular arrhythmias, primarily VT, which are prevalent in 15% of adult patients late after surgery. The incidence of VT in this population is 11.9%, with an 8.3% risk of SCD by 35 years of follow-up.[3-7]

Although tetralogy of Fallot is typically cited as the archetypal lesion when VT in the adult congenital heart disease patient population is discussed, serious ventricular arrhythmias can also develop in other types of congenital heart malformations, even in the absence of direct surgical scarring to ventricular muscle, including congenital aortic stenosis, transposition of the great arteries when the RV supports the systemic circulation, severe Ebstein anomaly, certain forms of single ventricle, and ventricular septal defect with pulmonary arterial hypertension. The appearance of ventricular arrhythmias in these cases commonly coincides with deterioration in overall hemodynamic status.[8] In the past 20 years, many patients with tetralogy of Fallot have undergone transatrial repair, operating on the RV through the tricuspid valve after right atriotomy. In these cases, there is no incision in the RV free wall around which reentry can occur, although reentry around the ventricular septal defect patch can still take place.

Risk Stratification

NONINVASIVE RISK STRATIFICATION

Although controversy still exits, considerable progress has been made toward identifying noninvasive risk factors for VT and SCD in congenital heart disease patients. Tetralogy of Fallot is perhaps the one condition for which such data are fairly extensive. Independent predictors of clinical VT include QRS duration equal to or greater than 180 milliseconds, late and rapid increase in QRS

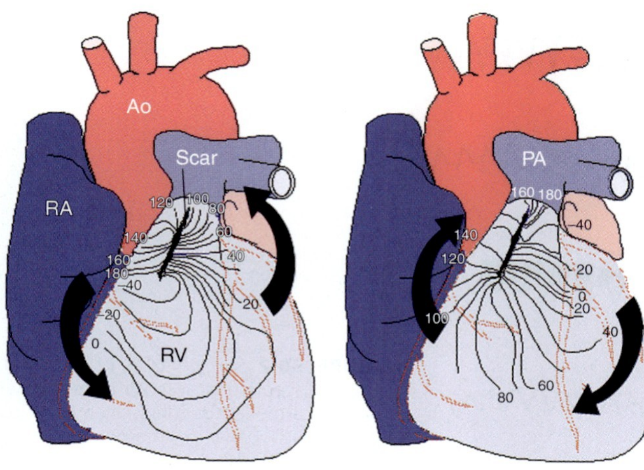

FIGURE 30-1 Ventricular tachycardia (VT) postsurgical repair of tetralogy of Fallot. Illustrated is scar-based reentry in surgically repaired tetralogy of Fallot with a right ventriculotomy. The incision heals as a nonconductive scar, leaving a small rim of muscle between the pulmonic valve annulus and scar. This is the diastolic corridor for rotation in either direction as shown, giving rise to VT with left bundle branch block–like QRS morphology and left superior axis or, in the opposite direction of rotation, right bundle branch block–like QRS morphology and right inferior axis. Ao = aorta; CL = cycle length; LBBB = left bundle branch block; LS = left superior; PA = pulmonary artery; RA = right atrium; RI = right inferior; RV = right ventricle.

duration after surgery, dispersion of QRS duration on the surface electrocardiogram (ECG), increased QT interval dispersion, high-grade ventricular ectopy on Holter monitoring, complete heart block, older age at surgery (especially older than 10 years), presence of a transannular RVOT patch, increased RV systolic pressures, RVOT aneurysm, pulmonic and tricuspid regurgitation, and left ventricular diastolic dysfunction.[1,6,7]

ELECTROPHYSIOLOGICAL TESTING

Despite advances in noninvasive risk stratification, identification of high-risk subgroups has not been sufficiently accurate to guide management decisions reliably. More recently, in patients with repaired tetralogy of Fallot, inducible monomorphic or polymorphic sustained VT by programmed ventricular stimulation was found to be a significant independent predictor of subsequent clinical sustained VT or SCD in patients with and without antiarrhythmic drug therapy, VT ablation, or implantable cardioverter-defibrillator (ICD). In this patient population, the rate of inducible sustained VT is approximately 35%, which is similar to that reported in patients with prior myocardial infarction (MI) and left ventricular ejection fractions less than 40% and spontaneous nonsustained VT. Additionally, the diagnostic value of EP testing (sensitivity, 77%; specificity, 80%; diagnostic accuracy, 79%) and prognostic significance (relative ratio, 4.7 for subsequent clinical VT or SCD) compares favorably with programmed ventricular stimulation in post-MI patients. Independent risk factors for inducible sustained VT were age greater than 18 years at the time of testing, palpitations, prior palliative surgery, frequent or complex ventricular ectopy, or nonsustained VT, and a cardiothoracic ratio of 0.6 or more on chest radiograph.[7]

Nonetheless, EP testing yield remains too imperfect and too impractical to be recommended as a general screening tool and is usually reserved for selected patients with concerning symptoms (e.g., palpitations, dizziness, or unexplained syncope) or Holter findings, when VT is suspected but not yet proven. Additionally, the subpopulation of patients deemed at intermediate risk of SCD based on a combination of other parameters may benefit most from risk stratification with an EP study.[7,8]

TABLE 30-1 Risk Score for Appropriate Defibrillator Shocks in Primary Prevention in Patients with Tetralogy of Fallot

VARIABLE	EXPONENTIAL VALUES OF BETA COEFFICIENTS	POINTS ATTRIBUTED
Prior palliative shunt	3.2	2
Inducible sustained ventricular tachycardia	2.6	2
QRS duration ≥180 msec	1.4	1
Ventriculotomy incision	3.4	2
Nonsustained ventricular tachycardia	3.7	2
Left ventricular end-diastolic pressure ≥12 mm Hg	4.9	3
Total points		0–12

From Khairy P, Harris L, Landzberg MJ, et al: Implantable cardioverter-defibrillators in tetralogy of Fallot, *Circulation* 117:363-370, 2008.

Principles of Management

IMPLANTABLE CARDIOVERTER-DEFIBRILLATOR

ICDs play an important role in the primary and secondary prevention of SCD in this patient population. In a recent prevalence study, ICDs were implanted in 10% of the adult population with tetralogy of Fallot repair for either primary (59%) or secondary (41%) prevention indications. Both groups experienced high rates of appropriate therapies.

SECONDARY PREVENTION. ICD implantation is recommended in patients who have survived cardiac arrest or an episode of sustained VT with hemodynamic compromise.[9] The most common anatomical diagnosis among device recipients is tetralogy of Fallot, followed by transposition of the great arteries and aortic stenosis. The rate of appropriate therapies for VT or ventricular fibrillation (VF) events in this patient population averages 9.8% per year and about 35% over a follow-up period of 5 years, with the median time to first shock less than 1 year.[5,6,9,10]

PRIMARY PREVENTION. Some subgroups of patients with congenital heart disease are recognized as being at risk for life-threatening ventricular arrhythmias and SCD, including those with large scars from a prior ventriculotomy (e.g., tetralogy of Fallot repair), and those who develop advanced degrees of ventricular dysfunction from long-standing hemodynamic burdens (e.g., congenital aortic stenosis, single ventricle). Recent data support the benefit of ICD implantation for primary prevention in patients deemed to be at high risk for SCD. Up to 44% of patients with tetralogy of Fallot repair who received prophylactic ICDs experience sustained ventricular tachyarrhythmias, and appropriate therapies occur in 7.7% of patients per year. These annual rates are comparable to those of other high-risk populations, including patients with primary prevention ICDs for ischemic, dilated, or hypertrophic cardiomyopathy. A combination of surgical, hemodynamic, ECG, and EP factors modulates the risk of appropriate shocks.[5,6]

As noted, multiple risk factors for VT and SCD in congenital heart disease patients have been identified in an effort to better define which are most likely to benefit from a primary prevention ICD. Recently, a risk score to predict appropriate ICD shocks in tetralogy patients with ICDs for primary prevention indications was derived from six clinical variables (surgical, hemodynamic, electrocardiographic, and EP factors) identified by multivariate analyses (Table 30-1). Patients with fewer than 3 points (low risk) experienced no appropriate shocks. In patients with 3 to 5 points (intermediate risk) and more than 5 points (high risk), appropriate shocks were received by 3.8% and 17.5% of patients per year, respectively.[5] Although these risk-stratification schemes can provide reasonable sensitivity, they have suboptimal specificity for patients at highest risk because of

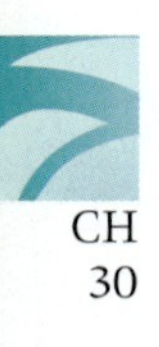

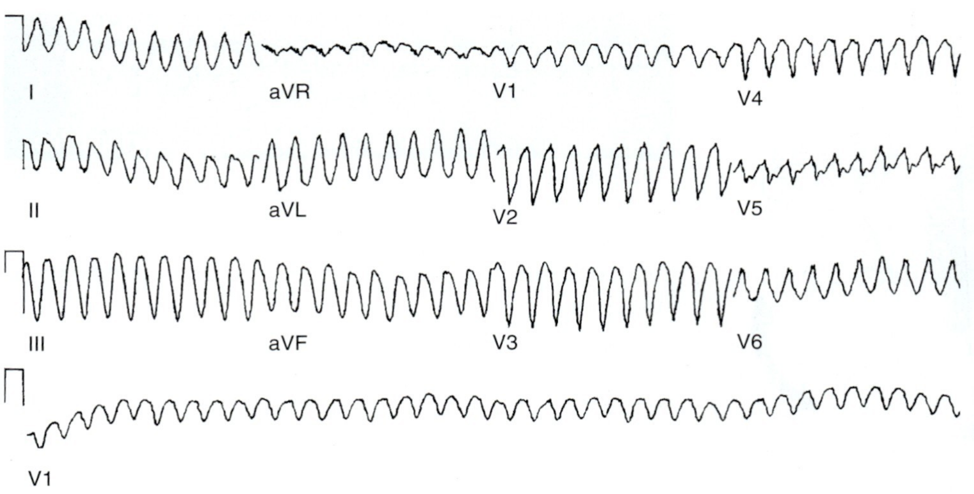

FIGURE 30-2 Surface ECG of ventricular tachycardia postsurgical repair of tetralogy of Fallot. Note the left bundle branch block pattern and left superior axis morphology characteristic of clockwise macroreentry around the right ventriculotomy scar.

the small population size and the relatively low incidence of SCD in congenital heart disease patients (approximately 2% per decade of follow-up in patients with tetralogy of Fallot repair).[9] EP testing can potentially help to identify patients at risk for malignant ventricular arrhythmias; however, patient selection for screening with EP testing and the timing and frequency of testing remain to be elucidated. At present, there is no generally accepted scheme for rhythm surveillance in asymptomatic tetralogy patients.[5,7,8]

Even in patients considered at risk for malignant ventricular arrhythmias, the benefit of ICD implantation should be carefully weighed against the risks of such a procedure in this unique group of patients. Transvenous implantation of the ICD may not be feasible in patients with the more complex varieties of congenital heart disease, necessitating epicardial insertion of the ICD leads with the added morbidity of a sternotomy or thoracotomy for epicardial electrodes. Even when transvenous implantation procedures are feasible, they can be very challenging in patients with distorted anatomy, requiring that the implanting physician be well acquainted with the details of congenital heart lesions and the types of surgical repairs. Because of the considerable variation in surgical techniques and individual anatomy, careful review of detailed operative reports is essential in these cases. Additionally, the ICD lead failure rate from both insulation breaches and conductor breaks is high in this patient population, exceeding 20% over 5 years (likely due to the young age and high activity level of this patient group), which results in added morbidity of corrective procedures. Moreover, the negative psychological impact of an implanted device and inappropriate shocks (occurring in up to 47%, predominantly caused by supraventricular tachycardias and lead failures) in a relatively young patient should not be underestimated.[5,9,10]

For all these reasons, ICD decisions in congenital heart disease patients should be individualized, taking into account the various risk factors, all of which must then be viewed in the context of the individual patient's history and general hemodynamic status to refine the selection process.[8-10]

ANTIARRHYTHMIC DRUG THERAPY

Similar to patients with post-MI VT, antiarrhythmic agents are generally not considered a stand-alone therapy in congenital heart disease patients with sustained ventricular arrhythmias or cardiac arrest, but can be considered in two main settings: as adjunctive therapy in patients with an ICD and as preventive therapy in patients who do not want or are not candidates for an ICD. ICD patients who experience frequent symptoms or device discharges triggered by ventricular arrhythmias may benefit from adjunctive drug therapy. When antiarrhythmic drug therapy is required, beta blockers and sotalol are commonly used. Amiodarone can carry significant long-term risk of adverse events given the young age of the patient population. The efficacy of dofetilide and dronedarone has not been adequately evaluated.[7,8]

SURGICAL REPAIR

Surgical interventions to improve cardiac status and alleviate residual hemodynamic problems (such as septal defect or valvular regurgitation) may play a role in reducing arrhythmia risk in certain carefully selected congenital heart disease patients, especially those with new-onset or worsening arrhythmias. Furthermore, VT mapping and ablation can be performed intraoperatively at the time of cardiac surgery. Nonetheless, the impact of surgery on modifying the risk for SCD remains controversial.[5,7,8]

CATHETER ABLATION

Catheter ablation for VT in tetralogy of Fallot generally is not considered as a stand-alone therapy, given the potential risk of recurrences of the same or new ventricular arrhythmias, and is primarily performed in patients with recurrent sustained monomorphic VT that is causing frequent ICD shocks or significant symptoms. Catheter ablation can also be considered in patients with symptomatic spontaneous sustained VT in whom ICD implantation is not recommended or not feasible.

Additionally, catheter ablation can be considered as isolated VT therapy for those patients with hemodynamically stable monomorphic and slow VT, and even then, follow-up EP studies are necessary to ensure that the same or different circuits cannot be induced before dismissing the need for an ICD.[8]

Furthermore, patients after tetralogy repair with a history of syncope and induced monomorphic VT during EP testing may be considered for either ICD placement or an attempt at catheter ablation of the VT with or without backup ICD implantation.[2,7]

Electrocardiographic Features

During normal sinus rhythm (NSR), QRS widening after tetralogy of Fallot repair is probably the result of a combined effect of the surgical injury to the myocardium and the right bundle branch, and from the RV enlargement. Therefore, a prolonged QRS duration cannot be considered the specific expression of delayed intraventricular conduction from an arrhythmogenic substrate, but a nonspecific marker of electrical instability.[11]

The VT is most commonly monomorphic and macroreentrant, rotating clockwise or counterclockwise around myotomy scars or surgical patches. QRS morphology during VT is determined by the pattern of ventricular activation around the scar. Most commonly, left or right bundle branch block with right inferior axis morphology is seen during clockwise rotation around the scar. Less commonly, left bundle branch block with left axis morphology is observed (Fig. 30-2).[12] Right bundle branch block–like morphology can be present if the tachycardia exits on the septal aspect of the RV free wall.

Mapping

Detailed knowledge of the congenital and surgical anatomy, including all available operative reports, is essential before ablation. Transthoracic and transesophageal echocardiography, right heart catheterization, computed tomography, and/or magnetic resonance imaging should be considered to clarify the anatomical landmarks for mapping.

As noted, in patients with repaired tetralogy of Fallot, the mechanism of VT is macroreentry involving the RV, either at the site of anterior right ventriculotomy or at the site of a ventricular septal defect patch. Once sustained and stable monomorphic VT is induced, endocardial activation mapping and entrainment mapping are performed to detect an adequate site for ablation. Activation mapping during VT is used to identify sites with mid-diastolic activity. Entrainment mapping is performed in a manner analogous to that used for post-MI VT, and is used to characterize the relationship of ventricular sites to the reentrant circuit and to verify that a diastolic electrogram, regardless of where in diastole it occurs and its position and appearance on initiation of VT, is part of the VT circuit. Entrainment with concealed fusion and a difference between the post-pacing interval and the VT cycle length not exceeding 30 milliseconds and a stimulus-to-QRS (S-QRS) interval not exceeding 70% of the VT cycle length helps identify the critical isthmus of the reentrant circuit to be targeted by catheter ablation.

For VTs that are not mappable because of hemodynamic instability or termination during catheter manipulation or entrainment mapping, pace mapping during sinus rhythm is used to identify exit sites of the reentrant circuit. Reentry circuit isthmuses can be approximated by pace mapping at sites where the QRS morphology matches that of the VT with an S-QRS interval of at least 40 milliseconds. If the VT can be briefly tolerated, the catheter is moved to the presumed isthmus site during NSR, and the VT is reinduced to confirm the position within the circuit either by entrainment mapping or by termination during radiofrequency (RF) energy application.[3]

Electroanatomical mapping can be of value because the presence of multiple circuits and the complexity of anatomical alteration, particularly in the vicinity of surgical scar, can pose significant challenges to mapping and ablation procedures. Additionally, voltage mapping of the area of interest can help identify the area of scar and border zone and guide conventional mapping techniques. Furthermore, most reentrant circuit isthmuses are located within anatomically defined isthmuses bordered by unexcitable tissue. These boundaries can be identified by three-dimensional mapping during normal NSR. Transecting anatomical isthmuses by linear RF lesions during NSR can potentially eliminate the tachycardia, even when conventional mapping is not feasible because of poorly tolerated or noninducible tachycardia.[1,3,11]

When VT is short-lived, hemodynamically unstable, or cannot be reproducibly initiated, simultaneous multisite data acquisition using a noncontact mapping system (EnSite 3000; St. Jude Medical, St. Paul, Minn.) can help localize the VT site of origin. Propagation of activation within the RV can be traced throughout the whole tachycardia cycle by analyzing color-coded isopotential maps to identify the protected zone of the reentrant circuit between surgical barriers, anatomical barriers, or both. Additionally, dynamic substrate mapping allows the creation of voltage maps from a single cardiac cycle and provides the ability to identify low-voltage areas, as well as fixed and functional block, on the virtual endocardium through noncontact methodology.[13]

Ablation

The critical isthmus of the VT circuit is the usual target of ablation. A good pace map and entrainment with concealed QRS fusion and a prolonged S-QRS interval indicate more precisely an adequate site for ablation. Linear ablation lesions can also be performed using data obtained from substrate mapping to target anatomical isthmuses between surgical and structural lines of block. In tetralogy of Fallot patients, most VT circuits use the anatomical isthmus between the RVOT free wall scar or patch and the tricuspid annulus or pulmonic valve, and/or the septal scar or patch and either the tricuspid annulus or the pulmonic valve. Ablation lines transecting these anatomical isthmuses eliminate the VT in most patients. In one report, all of the ablation lines that needed to be created extended from 10 to 40 mm.[3,14]

RF ablation is usually performed with an open saline-irrigated catheter (power limit, 50 W), a closed irrigation catheter, or an 8-mm-tip catheter (power limit, 70 W). Ablation is performed during VT when possible. If VT is terminated or slowed during RF application, additional lesions are placed to connect the adjoining anatomical boundaries across the VT circuit isthmus, as defined by voltage mapping and pace mapping techniques, and RF lesions are placed during NSR until unipolar pacing fails to capture. After completion of the lesions, programmed stimulation is repeated to reassess tachycardia inducibility.[3]

Ablation success for any particular VT is defined by lack of reinducibility. Completeness of linear RF lesion lines can be validated by demonstrating absence of capture during pacing along the line, double potentials, and activation mapping during pacing from above or below the line.[14]

The experience with catheter ablation of VT in congenital heart disease is limited. Several reports have described single-center experiences spanning several eras of technological advances. In a report of 20 patients with VT and congenital heart disease, 50% of patients were unable to undergo ablation because of VT noninducibility, hemodynamic instability, access or anatomical problems, or proximity of the ablation target to the His bundle. The acute success rate for mappable VTs was 83%, with a long-term recurrence rate of 40%. In another report, immediate noninducibility of sustained or nonsustained VT was achieved in 15 of 16 patients (94%) after the ablation procedure. Repeat ventricular stimulation 5 to 7 days later revealed noninducibility in 14 patients (88%). At successful ablation sites, a good pace map during sinus rhythm could be found in 15 of the 16 patients (94%). However, an area of slow conduction, defined as mid-diastolic low-amplitude endocardial potential, could be found in only 3 patients (19%). The mean activation time of the endocardial electrogram preceding the QRS complex on the surface ECG at the ablation site was −69 ± 16 milliseconds. In 9 of 11 patients with inducible sustained VT (82%), entrainment with concealed fusion and a prolonged S-QRS interval (10 to 120 milliseconds) could be demonstrated. A recent report of 11 patients with VT after repair of congenital heart disease used electroanatomical substrate mapping during NSR in addition to conventional mapping, when feasible. RF ablation eliminated VT in all patients, with 91% remaining free of VT at a follow-up time of 30 ± 29 months. In another report, noncontact mapping facilitated successful ablation in 8 of 10 patients (80%).[1,3,14]

REFERENCES

1. Walsh EP: Interventional electrophysiology in patients with congenital heart disease, *Circulation* 115:3224–3234, 2007.
2. Khairy P, Stevenson WG: Catheter ablation in tetralogy of Fallot, *Heart Rhythm* 6:1069–1074, 2009.
3. Zeppenfeld K, Schalij MJ, Bartelings MM, et al: Catheter ablation of ventricular tachycardia after repair of congenital heart disease: electroanatomic identification of the critical right ventricular isthmus, *Circulation* 116:2241–2252, 2007.
4. Roos-Hesselink JW, Karamermer Y: Significance of postoperative arrhythmias in congenital heart disease, *Pacing Clin Electrophysiol* 31(Suppl 1):S2–S6, 2008.
5. Khairy P, Harris L, Landzberg MJ, et al: Implantable cardioverter-defibrillators in tetralogy of Fallot, *Circulation* 117:363–370, 2008.
6. Khairy P, Aboulhosn J, Gurvitz MZ, et al: Arrhythmia burden in adults with surgically repaired tetralogy of Fallot: a multi-institutional study, *Circulation* 122:868–875, 2010.
7. Le Gloan L, Khairy P: Management of arrhythmias in patients with tetralogy of Fallot, *Curr Opin Cardiol* 26:60–65, 2010.
8. Warnes CA, Williams RG, Bashore TM, et al: ACC/AHA 2008 Guidelines for the Management of Adults with Congenital Heart Disease: a report of the American College of Cardiology/American Heart Association Task Force on Practice Guidelines (writing committee to develop guidelines on the management of adults with congenital heart disease), *Circulation* 118:e714–e833, 2008.
9. Walsh EP: Practical aspects of implantable defibrillator therapy in patients with congenital heart disease, *Pacing Clin Electrophysiol* 31(Suppl 1):S38–S40, 2008.

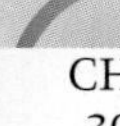

10. Tomaske M, Bauersfeld U: Experience with implantable cardioverter-defibrillator therapy in grown-ups with congenital heart disease, *Pacing Clin Electrophysiol* 31(Suppl 1):S35–S37, 2008.
11. Folino AF, Daliento L: Arrhythmias after tetralogy of Fallot repair, *Indian Pacing Electrophysiol J* 5:312–324, 2005.
12. Josephson ME: Catheter and surgical ablation in the therapy of arrhythmias. In Josephson ME, editor: *Clinical cardiac electrophysiology*, ed 4, Philadelphia, 2008, Lippincott Williams & Wilkins, pp 746–888.
13. Pratola C, Baldo E, Toselli T, et al: Contact versus noncontact mapping for ablation of ventricular tachycardia in patients with previous myocardial infarction, *Pacing Clin Electrophysiol* 32:842–850, 2009.
14. Kriebel T, Saul JP, Schneider H, et al: Noncontact mapping and radiofrequency catheter ablation of fast and hemodynamically unstable ventricular tachycardia after surgical repair of tetralogy of Fallot, *J Am Coll Cardiol* 50:2162–2168, 2007.

CHAPTER 31 Ventricular Arrhythmias in Inherited Channelopathies

Sudden cardiac death (SCD) is a major contributor to population mortality, with an overall incidence in the United States estimated to be between 0.1% and 0.2%, resulting in approximately 300,000 to 350,000 deaths annually.

Ventricular fibrillation (VF) or pulseless ventricular tachycardia (VT) is the initial rhythm recorded in 25% to 36% of witnessed cardiac arrests occurring at home, but in a much higher proportion (38% to 79%) of witnessed cardiac arrests occurring in a public setting.[1] The majority of SCD events are associated with structural heart disease, with coronary artery disease and its complications being involved in up to 60% to 80% of cases, followed by other cardiomyopathies. However, in 10% to 20% of SCDs, no cardiac structural abnormalities are detectable. The lack of an apparent cause in many of those cases initially led to the classification as "sudden unexplained death syndrome" (SUDS) or "sudden infant death syndrome" (SIDS). Many of these are caused by primary electrical disorders, including long QT syndrome (LQTS), catecholaminergic polymorphic VT (CPVT), Brugada syndrome, and short QT syndrome (SQTS), as well as cases identified as "idiopathic VF" when the underlying cause often remains unknown.[2]

SCD may originate from a variety of arrhythmias, as a wide spectrum of pathogenic mechanisms has been identified over the years. VT degenerating first to VF and later to asystole appears to be the most common pathophysiological cascade involved in fatal arrhythmias recorded as the primary electrical event at the time of SCD, particularly in patients with advanced heart disease. In patients without structural heart disease, polymorphic VT and torsades de pointes caused by various genetic or acquired cardiac abnormalities, such as ion channel abnormalities, or acquired LQTS commonly contribute to the initiation of life-threatening arrhythmias.

Long QT Syndrome

The LQTS is a rare inherited cardiac channelopathy with variable penetrance that is associated with an abnormally prolonged QT interval and an increased propensity to life-threatening ventricular arrhythmias in the presence of a structurally normal heart.[3-5]

In 1957, Anton Jervell and Fred Lange-Nielsen published the first report on a familial (autosomal recessive) disorder characterized by the presence of a striking prolongation of the QT interval, congenital deafness, and a high incidence of SCD at a young age. Subsequently, Romano and Ward independently identified an almost identical, but autosomal dominant, disorder that is not associated with deafness. A genetic relationship between the two was then proposed and the two syndromes were considered variants of one disease under the unifying name of "LQTS."

The progressive unraveling of the molecular basis of LQTS has disclosed that whereas the autosomal dominant Romano-Ward syndrome depends on mutations affecting at least five genes encoding sodium (Na^+) and potassium (K^+) channels, the autosomal recessive Jervell and Lange-Nielsen syndrome depends on homozygous or compound heterozygous mutations of either one of the two genes encoding the subunits forming the channel conducting the slowly activating delayed rectifier K^+ current (I_{Ks}). Being a recessive disease, the Jervell and Lange-Nielsen syndrome is far less common than the Romano-Ward syndrome.[3,6,7]

The initial molecular studies suggested that all genes linked to the LQTS phenotype encode for various subunits of cardiac ion channels. Subsequent findings, however, revealed that LQTS could also be caused by mutations of genes coding for channel-associated cellular structural proteins as well. Nonetheless, the concept that LQTS genes ultimately affect cardiac ion currents, either directly (ion channel mutations) or indirectly (modulators), still holds true.[3]

In the contemporary literature, Romano-Ward syndrome is used interchangeably with LQTS, but is now less commonly used in favor of the LQT1 to LQT13 scheme according to the underlying genetic mutation (see below).

Epidemiology

There are no systematic studies on LQTS prevalence in the general population. A recent estimate of the prevalence of LQTS is 1:2000 based on the results of genetic screening in families and the incidence of compound heterozygotes (i.e., persons with two

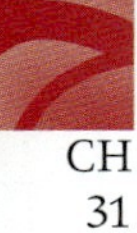

TABLE 31-1 Common Types of the Long QT Syndrome

	LQT1	LQT2	LQT3
Pathophysiology			
Gene	*KCNQ1 (K_vLQT1)*	*KCNH2 (HERG)*	*SCN5A*
Protein	$K_v7.1$	$K_v11.1$	$Na_v1.5$
Ionic current	Decreased I_{Ks}	Decreased I_{Kr}	Increased late I_{Na}
Clinical Presentation			
Incidence of cardiac events	63%	46%	18%
Incidence of SCD	4%	4%	4%
Arrhythmia triggers	Emotional/physical stress (swimming, diving)	Emotional stress, arousal (alarm clock, telephone), rest	Sleep/rest
ECG	Broad-based T wave	Low-amplitude, bifid T wave	Long isoelectric ST segment
QT response to exercise	Attenuated QTc shortening and an exaggerated QTc prolongation during early and peak exercise	Normal QT during exercise but with exaggerated QT hysteresis	Supernormal QT shortening
Management			
Exercise restriction	+++	++	?
Response to beta blockers	+++	+++	?
Potassium supplement	+	++	+
Left cervicothoracic sympathectomy	++	++	++
Response to mexiletine	+	+	++

I_{Kr} = rapidly activating delayed rectifier K^+ current; I_{Ks} = slowly activating delayed rectifier potassium current; I_{Na} = sodium current; QTc = corrected QT interval; SCD = sudden cardiac death.

mutations). However, the clinical disease is less common (approximately 1 in 5000) because most mutation carriers remain asymptomatic.[8] The usual mode of inheritance is autosomal dominant, with the exception of the autosomal recessive Jervell and Lange-Nielsen type.[6]

The most frequent clinical types of LQTS are LQT1 to LQT3. The remaining 10 types (LQT4 to LQT13) make up less than 5% of the genotype-identified LQTS.

Clinical Presentation and Natural Course

ROMANO-WARD SYNDROME

Most information regarding the clinical features of LQTS have been derived from analysis of data from large series of LQTS patients, the largest of which is the International LQTS Registry. LQTS probands are diagnosed at an average age of 21 years. The clinical course of patients with LQTS is variable, owing to incomplete penetrance. It is influenced by age, genotype, gender, environmental factors, therapy, and possibly other modifier genes. At least 37% of individuals with the LQT1 phenotype, 54% with the LQT2 phenotype, and 82% with the LQT3 phenotype remain asymptomatic and many are referred for evaluation because of the diagnosis of LQTS of a family member or the identification of long QT interval on surface electrocardiogram (ECG) obtained for unrelated reasons.[5]

Symptomatic patients can present with palpitations, presyncope, syncope, or cardiac arrest. Recurrent syncope can mimic primary seizure disorders. Syncope in patients with LQTS is generally attributed to polymorphic VT (torsades de pointes), but can also be precipitated by severe bradycardia in some patients with LQT3. Death is usually due to VF.

Syncope is the most frequent symptom, occurring in 50% of symptomatic probands by the age of 12 years, and in 90% by the age of 40 years. The incidence of syncope in LQTS patients is approximately 5% per year, but can vary depending on the LQTS genotype. On the other hand, the incidence of SCD is much lower, approximately 1.9% per year. Nonfatal events (syncope and aborted cardiac arrest) in LQTS patients remain the strongest predictors of subsequent LQTS-related fatal events. The overall risk of subsequent SCD in an LQTS patient who has experienced a previous episode of syncope is approximately 5% per year.[9]

LQT1, LQT2, and LQT3 comprise more than 90% of all genotyped LQTS cases. LQT1 is the most frequent genetic form of LQTS, accounting for 42% to 45% of genotyped LQTS cases. LQT2 is the second most prevalent form of the disease and accounts for 35% to 45% of genotyped LQTS cases (Table 31-1).[5,10]

Of individuals who die of complications of Romano-Ward syndrome, SCD is the first sign of the disorder in an estimated 10% to 15%. The risk for SCD from birth to age 40 years has been reported as approximately 4% in each of the phenotypes.

Risk and lethality of cardiac events among untreated individuals are strongly influenced by the genotype. The frequency of cardiac events is significantly higher among LQT1 (63%) and LQT2 (46%) patients than among patients with the LQT3 genotype (18%). However, the likelihood of dying during a cardiac event is significantly higher among LQT3 patients (20%) than among those with the LQT1 (4%) or the LQT2 (4%) genotype.[10-12]

Cardiac events (syncope, cardiac arrest, SCD) in LQTS patients do not occur at random; the factors precipitating cardiac events seem to be specific for each genetic variant. LQT1 patients present an increased risk during physical or emotional stress (90%), and only 3% of the arrhythmic episodes occur during rest/sleep. Swimming and diving appear as highly specific triggers in LQT1 patients. LQT2 patients are at higher risk for lethal events during arousal (44%), but are also at risk during sleep and at rest (43%). Only 13% of cardiac events occur during exercise. Cardiac events in LQT2 patients are typically associated with arousal and auditory stimulation. In fact, the triggering of events by startling, sudden awakening, or sudden loud noises (such as a telephone or alarm clock ring) is virtually diagnostic of LQT2. Notably, individual factors such as gender, location and type of mutation, and QTc prolongation appear to be associated with trigger-specific events; female adolescents with LQT2 appear to experience a greater than ninefold increase in the risk for arousal-triggered cardiac events compared with male adolescents in the same age group. In contrast, gender does not seem to be a significant risk factor for exercise-triggered events among carriers of the same genotype (Fig. 31-1).[13]

On the other hand, LQT3 patients experience cardiac events largely while asleep or at rest (65%) without emotional arousal,

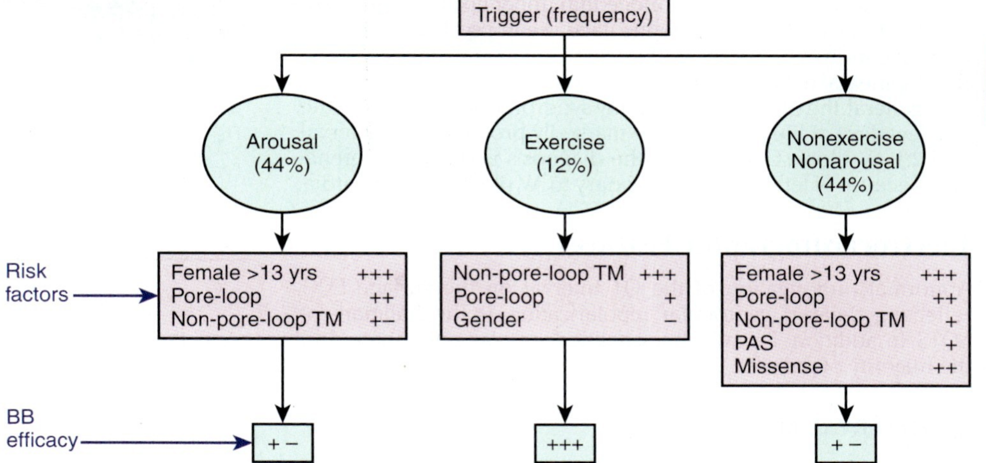

FIGURE 31-1 Trigger-specific risk factors and response to therapy in long QT syndrome type 2 (LQT2). Plus and minus signs are approximate representations of the risk/response based on the hazard ratios and associated *p* values from the multivariate models. BB = beta blocker; PAS = Per-Arnt-Sim domain of the HERG channel; TM = transmembrane. *(Reproduced with permission from Kim JA, Lopes CM, Moss AJ, et al: Trigger-specific risk factors and response to therapy in long QT syndrome type 2, HeartRhythm 7:1797-1805, 2010.)*

and only occasionally during exercise (4%). Notably, the majority of patients continue to experience their cardiac events under conditions similar to their first classified event.[10,11]

The effect of gender on outcome is age-dependent, with boys being at higher risk than girls during childhood and early adolescence, but no significant difference in gender-related risk being observed between 13 and 20 years. The gender-related risk reverses afterward, and female patients maintain higher risk than male patients throughout adulthood.[14]

The genotype can potentially affect the clinical course of the LQTS and modulate the effects of age and gender on clinical manifestations.[15] Although the three major LQTS genotypes (LQT1, LQT2, or LQT3) are associated with similar risks for life-threatening cardiac events in children and adolescents after adjustment for clinical risk factors (including gender, QTc duration, and time-dependent syncope), the risk for cardiac events is augmented in LQT2 women aged 21 to 40 years and in LQT3 patients greater than 40 years of age. The risk of syncope and SCD decreases during pregnancy but increases in the postpartum period, especially among LQT2 women.[10-12]

JERVELL AND LANGE-NIELSEN SYNDROME

The Jervell and Lange-Nielsen syndrome is the recessive variant of the LQTS, characterized by congenital deafness and cardiac phenotype (QT prolongation, ventricular arrhythmias, and SCD). The Jervell and Lange-Nielsen syndrome is caused by two homozygous or compound heterozygous mutations of either one of the two genes (*KCNQ1* and *KCNE1*) that encode components of the I_{Ks} channel.

Patients with Jervell and Lange-Nielsen syndrome have a more severe cardiac phenotype than those with Romano-Ward syndrome. Complete loss of I_{Ks} in hair cells and endolymph of the inner ear results in congenital bilateral sensorineural deafness. Patients begin to experience cardiac events very early in life; 15% suffer a cardiac event during the first year of life, 50% by age 3 years, and 90% by age 18 years. In untreated patients, approximately 50% die of ventricular arrhythmias by the age of 15 years. Furthermore, SCD occurs in more than 25% of patients despite medical therapy.[6]

The conditions that trigger the cardiac events are, overall, very similar to those described for LQT1. Up to 95% of events occur during sympathetic activation (exercise and emotions), and only 5% of the events occur at rest or during sleep.[6]

ANDERSEN-TAWIL SYNDROME

Andersen-Tawil syndrome (LQT7) is a rare autosomal dominant disorder caused by mutations of the gene *KCNJ2,* which encodes the inward rectifier potassium channel, Kir2.1. This syndrome is characterized by a triad of a skeletal muscle phenotype (periodic paralysis caused by abnormal muscle relaxation), a cardiac phenotype (borderline or mildly prolonged QT interval, prominent U waves, and adrenergically mediated ventricular arrhythmias), and distinctive skeletal dysmorphic features (low-set ears, ocular hypertelorism, small mandible, fifth-digit clinodactyly, syndactyly, short stature, scoliosis, and a broad forehead).[16-18]

Affected individuals present initially with either periodic paralysis or cardiac symptoms (palpitations, syncope, or both) in the first or second decade. The arrhythmias displayed by affected patients are generally more benign compared with other types of LQTS and rarely degenerate into hemodynamically compromising rhythms like torsades de pointes, as ultimately evidenced by the lack of SCD cases so far.[17] Intermittent weakness occurs spontaneously, or may be triggered by prolonged rest or rest following exertion; however, the frequency, duration, and severity of symptoms are variable between and within affected individuals, and are often linked to fluctuations in plasma potassium levels. Mild permanent weakness is common.

There is a high degree of variability in penetrance and phenotypic expression. Approximately 60% of affected individuals manifest the complete triad and up to 80% express two of the three cardinal features.

TIMOTHY SYNDROME

Timothy syndrome (LQT8) is a rare multisystem disorder caused by mutations of the *CACNA1C* gene, which encodes the L-type Ca^{2+} channel, $Ca_V1.2$, and is characterized by syndactyly, QT prolongation, congenital heart disease, cognitive and behavioral problems, musculoskeletal diseases, immune dysfunction, and more sporadically autism.

Timothy syndrome is characterized by a remarkable prolongation of the QTc interval, functional 2:1 atrioventricular (AV) block (observed in up to 85% of patients, and likely caused by the extremely prolonged ventricular repolarization and refractory periods), and macroscopic T wave alternans (positive and negative T waves alternating on a beat-to-beat basis). Additionally, congenital heart defects are observed in approximately 60% of patients and include patent ductus arteriosus, patent foramen ovale, ventricular septal defect, tetralogy of Fallot, and hypertrophic cardiomyopathy. Timothy syndrome is highly malignant; the majority of patients seldom survive beyond 3 years of age. Polymorphic VT and VF occur in 80% of patients (commonly triggered by an increase in sympathetic tone) and are the leading cause of death, followed by infection and complications of intractable hypoglycemia.

Extracardiac features include cutaneous syndactyly (variably involving the fingers and toes), which is observed in almost all patients. Facial findings (observed in approximately 85% of individuals) include low-set ears, flat nasal bridge, thin upper lip, small upper jaw, small, misplaced teeth, and round face. Neuropsychiatric involvement occurs in approximately 80% of individuals and includes global developmental delays and autism spectrum disorders.

In general, the diagnosis of Timothy syndrome is made within the first few days of life based on the markedly prolonged QT interval and 2:1 AV block. Occasionally, the diagnosis is suspected prenatally because of fetal distress secondary to AV block or bradycardia.

Electrocardiographic Features

Abnormal prolongation of the QT interval on the surface ECG, reflecting delayed ventricular repolarization, is the hallmark of LQTS. In addition, T wave abnormalities are also encountered in the majority of patients.

QT INTERVAL MEASUREMENT

QT interval is the body surface representation of the duration of ventricular depolarization and subsequent repolarization. Any deviation or dispersion of either depolarization (e.g., bundle branch block) or repolarization (e.g., prolongation or dispersion of the action potential duration) prolongs the QT interval.[19]

An accurate measurement of the QT interval is important for the diagnosis of LQTS. A 12-lead ECG tracing at a paper speed of 25 mm/sec at 10 mm/mV is usually adequate to make accurate measurements of the QT interval. The QT interval is measured as the interval from the onset of the QRS complex, that is, the earliest indication of ventricular depolarization, to the end of the T wave, that is, the latest indication of ventricular repolarization. The QT interval is measured in all ECG leads where the end of the T wave can be clearly defined (preferably leads II and V_5 or V_6), with the longest value being used. The end of the T wave is the point at which the descending limb of the T wave intersects the isoelectric line. Three to five consecutive cardiac cycles are taken to derive average values for R-R, QRS, and QT intervals.[5,20-23]

When the end of the T wave is indistinct, or if a U wave is superimposed or inseparable from the T wave, it is recommended that the QT be measured in the leads not showing U waves (often aVR and aVL) or that the downslope of the T wave be extended by drawing a tangent to the steepest proportion of the downward limb of the T wave until it crosses the baseline (i.e., the T-P segment). Nonetheless, it should be recognized that defining the end of the T wave in these ways might underestimate the QT interval.[22] Some investigators advocate measurement of both the QT interval and the QTU interval (with the latter measurement taken to the end of the U wave as it intersects the isoelectric line) because the QTU interval probably reflects the total duration of ventricular depolarization.[20]

The highest diagnostic and prognostic value in LQTS families has been observed for QTc in leads II and V_5 of the 12-lead ECG. Thus, QTc should be obtained in one of these leads if measured in only one ECG lead. However, other leads presented with similar diagnostic (aVR) or prognostic (V_2/V_3) value alone, and, in general, the lead with the longest QT interval is used for measurement.[23]

QT INTERVAL CORRECTION FOR GENDER

The QT interval shortens after puberty in men but not women, resulting in a longer QT in women than in men. The reported gender difference in various studies varies from 6 to 10 milliseconds in older age groups and from 12 to 15 milliseconds in younger adults. Overall, the gender difference in the rate-corrected QT interval becomes small after 40 years of age and practically disappears in older men and women. Separate gender- and age-specific QT adjustment formulas have been proposed to accommodate these differences.[22]

QT INTERVAL CORRECTION FOR HEART RATE

Because the heart rate (R-R cycle length) is the primary modifier of ventricular action potential, QT interval measurements must be corrected for the individual's R-R interval (QTc) to allow for comparisons. Various correction formulas have been developed (Table 31-2), the most widely used being the formula derived by Bazett in 1920 from a graphic plot of measured QT intervals in 39 young subjects. The Bazett correction, however, performs less well at high and low heart rates (undercorrects at fast heart rates and overcorrects at slow heart rates).[20] Therefore, it was recommended by the American Heart Association/American College of Cardiology Foundation/Heart Rhythm Society (AHA/ACC/HRS) in 2009 that linear regression functions rather than the Bazett formula be used for QT rate correction. In addition to the Bazett formula, many other correction formulas, such as the Framingham-Sagie, Fridericia, Hodges, and Nomogram-Karjalainen formulas, have been proposed.[5,21,22]

TABLE 31-2 Formulas for Heart Rate Correction of the QT Interval

Bazett	$QTcB = QT/(\text{R-R interval})^{1/2}$ (all intervals in seconds)
Framingham-Sagie	$QTcFa = QT + 154(1 - 60/\text{heart rate})$
Fridericia	$QTcFi = QT/(\text{R-R interval})^{1/3}$
Hodges	$QTcH = QT + 1.75(\text{heart rate} - 60)$
Nomogram-Karjalainen	$QTcN = QT + \text{nomogram correction factor}$

In a recent report, the accuracy of five different QT correction formulas was evaluated for determining drug-induced QT interval prolongation. The Bazett correction formula provided the most marked QTc variations at heart rates distant from 60 beats/min. The Fridericia formula was found to overestimate QTc at faster heart rates, being more reliable at slower heart rates. Conversely, the Hodges, Nomogram, and Framingham formulas demonstrated less QTc variability over the whole range of the investigated heart rates and seemed to be similarly satisfactory at heart rates of up to 100 beats/min. Among them, the Hodges method, followed by the Nomogram-Karjalainen method, appeared to be the most accurate in determining the correct QTc and subsequently in guiding clinical decisions.[21]

Importantly, there exists a substantial interindividual variability of the QT/R-R relationship, which represents the relationship between QT duration and heart rate. In contrast, a high intraindividual stability of the QT/R-R pattern has been shown, suggesting that a genetic component might partly determine individual QT length. Therefore, population-based and averaged QT correction cannot accurately predict a normal QT interval at a given R-R interval in a *given* patient. Individual-specific QT/R-R hysteresis correction in combination with individualized heart rate correction can potentially reduce intrasubject QTc variability.[19,24]

QT INTERVAL CORRECTION TO QRS DURATION

The QT interval prolongs in ventricular conduction defects, and an adjustment for QRS duration becomes necessary. This can be accomplished best by incorporating QRS duration and R-R interval as covariates into the QT adjustment formula or by using the JT interval (QT duration minus QRS duration). If the JT interval is chosen, normal standards established specifically for the JT interval should be used. QT and JT adjustment formulas have recently been introduced for use in the setting of prolonged ventricular conduction. With confirmation, they may be incorporated into automated algorithms to provide appropriate correction factors.[22]

QT INTERVAL PROLONGATION

The diagnosis of QT interval prolongation can be challenging because of the difficulty in defining the "end" of the T wave and the need for correction for heart rate, age, and gender. This is further complicated by the lack of linear behavior of the Bazett formula at slower and faster heart rates as well as the arbitrary definition

TABLE 31-3 Suggested Bazett-Corrected QT Interval Values for Diagnosis of QT Prolongation

RATING	1-15 YEARS	ADULT MAN	ADULT WOMAN
Normal	<440	<430	<450
Borderline	440-460	430-450	450-470
Prolonged	>460	>450	>470

Values given in milliseconds.
From Goldenberg I, Moss AJ: Long QT syndrome, *J Am Coll Cardiol* 51:2291-2300, 2008.

of the gender-based diagnostic cut-off values that define an abnormally prolonged QTc (QTc of 450 milliseconds for men and QTc of 460 milliseconds for women; Table 31-3).

Furthermore, no single QTc value separates all LQTS patients from healthy controls. The QT interval is subject to large variations even in healthy individuals, and substantial overlap exists with QTc values obtained from LQTS mutation carriers in the range between 410 and 470 milliseconds. In up to 40% of LQTS patients QTc intervals fall in the normal range. Nevertheless, QTc values greater than 470 milliseconds in men and greater than 480 milliseconds in women are practically never seen among healthy individuals (especially when their heart rate is 60 to 70 beats/min), but LQTS cannot be excluded merely by the presence of a normal QTc interval.[25] Therefore, unless excessive QTc prolongation (>500 milliseconds, corresponding to the upper quartile among affected genotyped individuals) is present, the QTc interval should always be evaluated in conjunction with the other diagnostic criteria. In the case of borderline QTc prolongation, serial ECG and 24-hour Holter recordings can potentially assist in establishing QT prolongation, as can various challenge tests.[7]

Of note, a considerable variability in QTc interval duration can be observed in patients with LQTS when serial ECGs are recorded during follow-up. This time-dependent change in QTc duration is an important determinant of the phenotypic expression of the disease. Up to 40% of patients with LQTS will have QTc greater than 500 milliseconds at least once during long-term follow-up, but only 25% will have that degree of QT prolongation during their initial evaluation. The maximal QTc duration measured at any time before age 10 years was shown to be the most powerful predictor of cardiac events during adolescence, regardless of baseline, mean, or most recent QTc values. In addition, the QT interval normally may exhibit individual variations during the day.[25,26]

T WAVE MORPHOLOGY

ST-T wave abnormalities are common among LQTS patients, and some of the ST-T anomalies are characteristic for a specific genotype. Patients with LQT1 commonly exhibit a smooth, broad-based T wave that is present in most leads, particularly evident in the precordial leads. The T wave generally has a normal to relatively high amplitude and often no distinct onset. LQT2 patients generally present with low-amplitude T waves, which are notched or bifid in approximately 60% of carriers. The bifid T wave can be confused with a T-U complex; however, unlike the U waves, the bifid T waves are usually present in most of the 12 ECG leads. LQT3 patients often show late-onset, narrow, peaked, and/or biphasic T waves with a prolonged isoelectric ST segment. Occasionally, the T wave is peaked and asymmetrical with a steep downslope. These ST-T wave patterns can be seen in 88% of LQT1 and LQT2 carriers and in 65% of LQT3 carriers. However, exceptions are present in all three genotypes, and the T wave pattern can vary with time, even in the same patient with a specific mutation.[27,28]

No specific T wave pattern has been suggested in the LQT5 and LQT6 syndromes. T-U wave abnormalities such as biphasic T waves following long pauses like those found in the LQT2 syndrome are commonly observed in the LQT4 syndrome. Enlarged U waves separated from the T wave are reported to be characteristic ECG features in the LQT7 syndrome. Severe QT interval prolongation and macroscopic T wave alternans can be observed in LQT8.[27]

Despite the initial enthusiasm in achieving a genotype-phenotype correlation for specific LQT-associated genes, this approach failed to provide a high diagnostic yield because of the frequent exceptions in T wave morphology presentation. Therefore, other T wave parameters, such as duration, amplitude, asymmetry, and flatness, as well as the T wave peak–to–T wave end interval, have been used as highly specific quantitative descriptors (see below).[28]

TORSADES DE POINTES

Torsades de pointes is a polymorphic VT occurring in the setting of QT interval prolongation (acquired or congenital LQTS) and is characterized by a progressive change of the electrical axis, typically rotating 180 degrees in approximately 10 to 12 cycles. This results in the characteristic sinusoidal twisting of the peaks of the QRS complexes around the isoelectric line of the recording; hence, the name *torsades de points* or "twisting of the points."

The tachycardia rate typically is in the range of 150 to 300 beats/min. In many cases, torsades de pointes is a self-limiting arrhythmia that spontaneously dies out after a few tens of cycles; however, most patients experience multiple episodes of the VT occurring in rapid succession. Only in a minority of cases does torsades de pointes degenerate into VF, which almost without exception leads to SCD if immediate rescue intervention is unavailable.[7]

DISPERSION OF REPOLARIZATION

In experimental models of the LQTS, prolonged repolarization, transmural dispersion of repolarization, and early afterdepolarizations (EADs) are the three EP components linked to the genesis of torsades de pointes. Prolongation of the action potential duration (and QT interval) per se is not pathogenic, as demonstrated by the fact that a homogeneous action potential duration prolongation (such as occurs following amiodarone therapy) fails to generate reentry. Several ECG indices have been proposed in recent years as noninvasive surrogates for transmural dispersion of repolarization. Transmural dispersion of repolarization arises from repolarization heterogeneity that exists between the epicardial and putative midmyocardial (M) cells that lie toward the endocardium of the left ventricular (LV) wall. These midmyocardial cells are especially sensitive to a repolarization challenge and exhibit significant prolongation of the action potential duration compared with other transmural cell types.[7,29,30]

Although some controversy exists, some experimental models suggest that the peak of the T wave coincides with the end of epicardial repolarization (the shortest action potentials), whereas the end of the T wave coincides with the end of repolarization of the M cells (the longest action potentials). Hence, the interval from the peak of the T wave to the end of the T wave ($T_{peak\text{-}to\text{-}end}$) in each surface ECG lead has been proposed as an index of transmural repolarization, which can potentially be a more sensitive predictor of arrhythmogenic risk than the QT interval, because the latter represents the total duration of electrical ventricular activation) and not necessarily the dispersion of transmural repolarization.[7,29,30]

Although changes in the $T_{peak\text{-}to\text{-}end}$ interval can potentially show the dynamicity of the transmural dispersion of repolarization in clinical settings in LQTS patients, the role of measuring the $T_{peak\text{-}to\text{-}end}$ interval in these patients is not clearly defined yet. In fact, the normal value of the $T_{peak\text{-}to\text{-}end}$ interval on the ECG has not been established. Nonetheless, an interval of more than 100 milliseconds is uncommon in normal subjects compared with that in subjects with LQTS (9% versus 55%).[30]

LQT2 exhibits a larger-degree transmural dispersion of repolarization, as measured by the $T_{peak\text{-}to\text{-}end}$ interval, compared with LQT1 and normal hearts. In fact, the $T_{peak\text{-}to\text{-}end}$ interval has been proposed as a diagnostic criterion in differentiation between LQT2 and LQT1 patients. Additionally, whereas LQT1 patients and normal subjects demonstrate stable $T_{peak\text{-}to\text{-}end}$ intervals independent

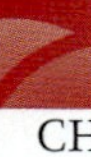

of heart rates, LQT2 patients exhibit a trend to decreased $T_{peak\text{-}to\text{-}end}$ intervals at fast heart rates and to increased $T_{peak\text{-}to\text{-}end}$ durations at slow heart rates. In both LQT1 and LQT2 patients, the longest $T_{peak\text{-}to\text{-}end}$ intervals are associated with sudden changes in the heart rate trend. Importantly, the magnitude of transmural dispersion of the repolarization interval does not seem to differ between asymptomatic and symptomatic patients in either LQT1 or LQT2. Conversely, symptomatic LQT2 patients exhibit a trend toward longer QT intervals than do asymptomatic patients.[29]

On ambulatory monitoring, transmural dispersion of repolarization, measured as $T_{peak\text{-}to\text{-}end}$ intervals during normal daily activities, appears to be greater in LQT2 than in LQT1 patients. LQT1 patients exhibit abrupt increases in $T_{peak\text{-}to\text{-}end}$ intervals at elevated heart rates, whereas LQT2 patients exhibit increases in transmural dispersion of repolarization at a much wider range of rates. In addition, beta-adrenergic stimulation (exercise or epinephrine infusion) increases transmural dispersion of repolarization in both LQTS models, transiently in LQT2 and persistently in LQT1.[29]

An alternate approach to determine repolarization heterogeneity is provided by the QT interval dispersion. The QT dispersion index is obtained by the difference between the maximal and minimal QT intervals ($QT_{max} - QT_{min}$) measured on a 12-lead ECG. It reflects the spatial heterogeneity of myocardial refractoriness more accurately than single QT values. Visualization of the differences in QT interval in the different ECG leads is facilitated by the display of a suitable subset of temporally aligned simultaneous leads with a slight separation on the amplitude scale.[22] However, QT interval dispersion measurements are subject to similar shortcomings encountered with the QT interval assessment, as a large overlap between affected and healthy individuals is observed.[7] Further, accurate measurement on the scalar ECG at a paper speed of 25 mm/sec is difficult. The same caveat applies to measuring $T_{peak\text{-}to\text{-}end}$.

The ratio of the amplitudes of the U and T waves has been suggested as the clinical counterpart of EADs, and a progressive increase in this ratio was found to precede the onset of torsades de pointes in an experimental model of LQTS. In addition, the increment in U wave amplitude after a premature ventricular complex (PVC) has been suggested as a marker for arrhythmia risk in "pause-dependent" LQTS. In patients with bifid T waves, some investigators used the late component of the T wave, rather than the U wave. The diurnal maximal ratio between late and early T wave peak amplitude correlates with a history of LQTS-related symptoms better than the baseline QTc interval in both LQT1 and LQT2 patients. In LQT1 and LQT2 patients, diurnal distributions of maximal T2-to-T1 wave amplitude ratios are similar to reported corresponding distributions of cardiac events, and can potentially be used as a predictor of the arrhythmia risk for asymptomatic patients with known type 1 or 2 LQT genotype.[31]

Diagnosis of the Long QT Syndrome

The LQTS is a clinical diagnosis, primarily based on the clinical presentation, personal and family history, and ECG findings. A detailed family history of syncope and SCD is essential, not only in first-degree relatives (mother, father, siblings, children), but also in more distant relatives. Importantly, family history should also be investigated for other potential manifestations of malignant arrhythmias that might not have been classified as cardiac in origin, such as drowning, death while driving, epileptic seizures, as well as SIDS. Data on comorbidities in evaluated individuals or family members (such as congenital deafness) should also be acquired. Clinical features such as triggers of syncope and specific QT morphological attributes in patients in whom the clinical diagnosis has been made can suggest the affected gene in 70% to 90% of patients.[5,32]

The QTc interval is the most common standardized parameter used for diagnosing LQTS and quantifying ventricular repolarization. As noted, QTc values greater than 470 milliseconds in men and greater than 480 milliseconds in women are practically never seen among healthy individuals (especially at heart rates of 60 to 70 beats/min) and are considered diagnostic of LQTS (as long as acquired forms of LQTS are excluded) even in asymptomatic subjects and those having a negative family history. When a prolonged QTc is observed during faster heart rates (>90 beats/min), it is important to repeat the ECG once the heart rate slows down, to minimize the error that can potentially be introduced by heart rate correction formulas.[25]

Additionally, LQTS can be suspected in individuals with QTc values exceeding 450 milliseconds for men and exceeding 460 milliseconds for women; these subjects are considered to have "high probability for LQTS" if they have a history of syncope and familial SCD. On the other hand, LQTS is very unlikely among men with QTc less than 390 milliseconds and among women with QTc less than 400 milliseconds.[25]

Importantly, a significant proportion (20% to 40%) of patients with genetically proven LQTS have normal or borderline QTc measurements at rest ("concealed" LQTS). Therefore, the diagnosis of LQTS should not be excluded based solely on a QTc interval in the normal range (400 to 450 milliseconds), and additional testing is indicated whenever the clinical history requires exclusion of LQTS. In this setting, obtaining a resting ECG periodically sometimes can uncover an abnormal prolongation of the QTc interval, given the considerable day-to-day variability in QTc of patients with LQTS. Additionally, reviewing the ECGs of all family members can be valuable, because some family members can have obvious QT prolongation. Several additional clinical tests and tools have been used in the clinical evaluation of LQTS, including ambulatory ECG recordings, exercise stress testing, epinephrine QT stress testing, and genetic testing. Although these diagnostic tools can all contribute to identifying patients with LQTS, a "gold standard" diagnostic tool is still lacking. Invasive EP testing is generally not useful in the diagnosis of LQTS.[33,34]

CLINICAL SCORING SYSTEMS

When the diagnosis is not clear, two clinical scoring systems have been developed to enhance the diagnostic reliability of clinical parameters and to estimate the probability of LQTS: the Keating criteria and the Schwartz score. The Keating criteria are a binary combination of QTc values with LQTS-related symptoms. According to these criteria, individuals are affected if they have a QTc interval greater than 470 milliseconds even in the absence of symptoms, or if they have typical symptoms with a QTc interval greater than or equal to 450 milliseconds. The Schwartz score incorporates ECG features in combination with personal clinical history and family history. Scores were arbitrarily divided into three probability categories, providing a quantitative estimate of the risk for LQTS (Table 31-4).[35,36]

When applied to family members of positively genotyped patients, these systems demonstrated excellent high specificity (99%) but very low sensitivity (19% for the Schwartz "high probability" score and 36% for the Keating criteria), and severely underdiagnosed disease carriers (false negatives). Significant underdiagnosis was also found among probands, despite the fact that probands are generally more seriously affected than their relatives. A high probability of LQTS (Schwartz criteria) was found only in 57% of probands with a confirmed molecular diagnosis. The performance of QTc interval measurement alone (with a cut-off value of 430 milliseconds) is superior to the Schwartz and Keating criteria when DNA testing is available for the confirmation of disease carriership, as it has far better sensitivity (72%) while retaining reasonable specificity (86%). Thus, in families with known causal gene mutations, genetic analysis is the method of choice to identify the relatively high proportion of silent carriers of disease-causing mutations.[35,36]

AMBULATORY CARDIAC MONITORING

Holter monitoring is not sufficiently well standardized to serve in the primary assessment for ventricular repolarization analysis, and only rarely will show spontaneous arrhythmias in LQTS patients.

TABLE 31-4 Diagnostic Criteria for the Long QT Syndrome

FINDING	SCORE
ECG*	
QTc† ≥ 480 msec	3
QTc† = 460-470 msec	2
QTc† = 450 msec (in men)	1
Torsades de pointes‡	2
T wave alternans	1
Notched T wave in three leads	1
Low heart rate for age§	0.5
Clinical History	
Syncope with stress‡	2
Syncope without stress‡	1
Congenital deafness	0.5
Family History¶	
Family members with definite LQTS	1
Unexplained SCD in immediate family members <30 yr of age	0.5

*Findings in the absence of medications or disorders known to affect these ECG findings.
†The corrected QT interval (QTc) is calculated by the Bazett formula.
‡Torsades de pointes and syncope are mutually exclusive.
§Resting heart rate below the second percentile for age.
¶The same family member cannot be counted in both categories.
Scoring: 1 point, low probability of LQTS; 2 or 3 points, intermediate probability of LQTS; 4 or more points, high probability of LQTS.
LQTS = long QT syndrome; SCD = sudden cardiac death.
Modified from Goldenberg I, Moss AJ: Long QT syndrome, *J Am Coll Cardiol* 51:2291-2300, 2008.

However, this method can sometimes be used for the detection of extreme QT interval events that occur infrequently during the day. Characteristic T wave changes may be revealed during sleep or following post-extrasystolic pauses.[25,32]

EXERCISE STRESS TESTING

Exercise testing can be useful to assess QT adaptation to heart rate, a measure of the integrity of the I_{Ks} channels. Postural changes in QTc and prolonged QT hysteresis during exercise testing can be helpful in identifying patients with LQTS and even in predicting the genotype and can potentially help direct genetic testing. Gradual supine bicycle testing can help minimize signal artifact from upper body motion observed during treadmill exercise.

Attenuated QTc shortening and an exaggerated QTc prolongation during early and peak exercise are characteristic of LQT1. As will be discussed later, genetic mutations in LQT1 result in reduction of the amplitude of I_{Ks}, one of the dominant K^+ currents responsible for repolarization especially at rapid heart rates (during sympathetic stimulation). Attenuation of I_{Ks} results in failure of the QT to adapt (i.e., shorten) in response to increasing heart rate. Unlike LQT1 patients, normal subjects, LQT2 patients, and LQT3 patients decrease their respective QTc intervals from rest at peak exercise. A maladaptive paradoxical QTc prolongation during the recovery phase (QTc >460 milliseconds or a ΔQTc [QTc at 3 minutes of recovery minus the baseline supine QTc] >30 milliseconds) was found to distinguish patients with either manifest or concealed LQT1 from normal subjects and those with LQT2 and LQT3 genotypes.[37]

In contrast, patients with LQT2 mutations have normal QT shortening and minimal QTc prolongation during exercise, but they characteristically demonstrate an exaggerated QT hysteresis compared with LQT1 patients and normal subjects. QT hysteresis is normally measured by comparing the QT intervals during exercise versus the recovery period at comparable heart rates (e.g., when the heart rate accelerates to approximately 100 beats/min during early exercise and 1 to 2 minutes into the recovery phase, when the heart rate typically decelerates to approximately 100 beats/min). In LQT2 patients, the QT fails to shorten at these intermediate heart rates in early exercise because of attenuated I_{Kr} (rapidly activating delayed rectifier potassium current; a so-called I_{Kr} zone). This is followed by recruitment of the unimpaired, sympathetically responsive I_{Ks}, resulting in appropriate QT shortening at faster heart rates through to peak exercise, which persists into the recovery phase. This consequently leads to an exaggerated QT difference between exercise and recovery at comparable heart rates, which is manifested as increased QT hysteresis.[34,38]

The LQT3 phenotype is characterized by a constant shortening of the action potential duration (and QT interval) with exercise because of stimulation of the intact I_{Ks} channel and augmentation of a late inward Na^+ current.[38]

QTc prolongation when comparing lying with standing positions at the beginning of exercise testing also can be useful in identifying LQTS patients and predicting genotype. In a recent report, postural QTc increase was more than 30 milliseconds in 68% of "concealed" LQTS patients, and QT hysteresis was more than 25 milliseconds in 67% of concealed LQT2 patients.

Postural and exercise-induced QTc prolongation and QT hysteresis can be attenuated with beta blockade; therefore, beta blocker therapy should be discontinued before exercise testing. Additionally, exercise treadmill testing can also reveal the characteristic T wave morphology in patients with LQT1 and LQT2 syndromes.[7]

Importantly, induction of arrhythmias during exercise is very rare in LQTS patients. Exercise-induced ventricular ectopy exceeding isolated PVCs is observed in less than 10% of patients.[7,32] The presence of exercise-induced ventricular ectopy beyond single, isolated PVCs must prompt intense evaluation because it was found to have a positive predictive value exceeding 90% for the presence of significant cardiac pathology. However, CPVT, rather than LQTS, is the far more likely diagnosis.[39]

EPINEPHRINE QT STRESS TEST

Catecholamine provocation testing can help diagnose patients with concealed LQT1, with a positive predictive value approaching 75% and a negative predictive value of 96%. Furthermore, epinephrine provocation testing was found to be a powerful test to predict the genotype of LQT1, LQT2, and LQT3 syndromes.[32,38,40]

Two major protocols have been developed for epinephrine infusion. Using the "escalating-dose infusion protocol," epinephrine infusion is initiated at 0.025 μg/kg/min and then increased sequentially every 10 minutes to 0.05, 0.1, and 0.2 μg/kg/min. The 12-lead ECG is continuously recorded during sinus rhythm under baseline conditions and during epinephrine infusion. The QT interval is measured 5 minutes after each dose increase. Epinephrine infusion should be stopped for systolic blood pressure greater than 200 mm Hg, nonsustained VT or polymorphic VT, frequent PVCs (>10 per minute), T wave alternans, or patient intolerance. A paradoxical QT interval response (prolongation of the absolute QT interval of ≥30 milliseconds) during low-dose epinephrine infusion provides a presumptive clinical diagnosis of LQT1, with a positive predictive value of 75%. The diagnostic accuracy can be reduced in patients receiving beta blockers.[38]

Using the "bolus and infusion protocol," an epinephrine bolus (0.1 μg/kg) is administered and immediately followed by continuous infusion (0.1 μg/kg/min) for 5 minutes. The QT interval is measured 1 to 2 minutes after the start of epinephrine infusion when the R-R interval is the shortest (which represents the peak epinephrine effect) and 3 to 5 minutes after the start of epinephrine infusion (which represents the steady-state epinephrine effect).[40]

During the epinephrine test, patients with LQT1 manifest prolongation of the QTc at the peak of the epinephrine effect, which is maintained under steady-state conditions of epinephrine. In contrast, epinephrine prolongs the QTc more dramatically at the peak of epinephrine infusion in LQT2 patients, but the QTc returns to baseline levels under steady-state conditions. A much

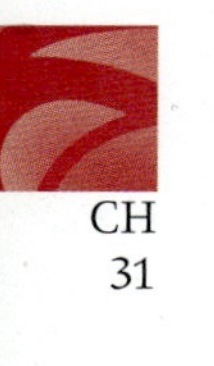

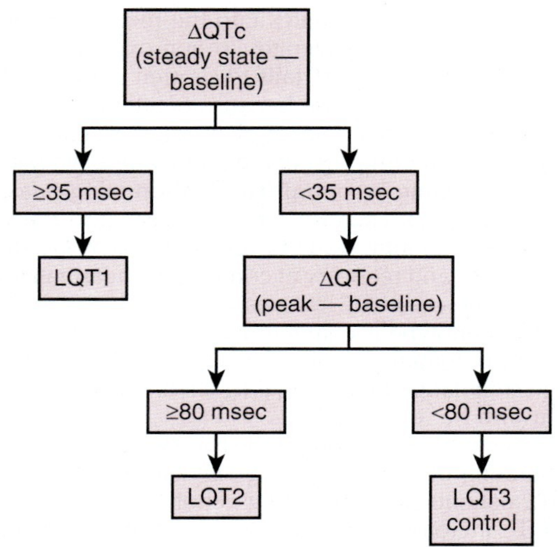

FIGURE 31-2 Epinephrine provocative testing for the diagnosis of LQTS. Control = normal subjects; LQT = long QT syndrome genotype; QTc = corrected QT interval.

milder prolongation of QTc at the peak of epinephrine has been described in LQT3 patients and in healthy subjects, and it returns to the baseline levels under steady-state conditions. A subject is considered to have an LQT1 response if the QTc increase in the peak phase is greater than 35 milliseconds and is maintained throughout the steady-state phase (Fig. 31-2). LQT2 response is likely if the peak QTc increase of greater than 80 milliseconds is not maintained in the steady-state phase. In one report, the sensitivity and specificity of the epinephrine test to differentiate LQT1 from LQT2 were 97% and 96%, those from LQT3 were 97% and 100%, and those from healthy subjects were 97% and 100%, respectively, when ΔQTc greater than 35 milliseconds at steady state was used. The sensitivity and specificity to differentiate LQT2 from LQT3 or healthy subjects were 100% and 100%, respectively, when ΔQTc greater than 80 milliseconds at peak was used.[40]

The escalating-dose infusion protocol is generally better tolerated by the patient and carries a lower incidence of false-positive responses. On the other hand, the bolus and infusion protocol offers the ability to monitor the temporal course of the epinephrine response at peak dose (during the bolus) and during steady state (during the infusion), which is particularly important in individuals with LQT2 in whom transient prolongation of the uncorrected QT interval can occur, followed by subsequent shortening.[38]

GENETIC TESTING

Although the diagnosis of LQTS frequently can be certain based on clinical diagnostic measures, in which setting molecular screening may not be necessary, genetic testing can still be of value; identification of the specific gene affected (or the site of the mutation within the gene) can potentially guide therapeutic choice and enhance risk stratification. Importantly, identification of the disease-causing mutation in the proband provides the ability to easily identify affected family members and implement lifestyle adjustment and presymptomatic treatment, and is thereby potentially lifesaving. Furthermore, genetic testing may be important in the identification of concealed LQTS, because a significant minority (25% to 50%) of individuals with genetically proven LQTS have a nondiagnostic QTc.[3,5,7,32]

Genetic testing is a powerful tool to identify patients with LQTS. Yet, it remains expensive and unavailable to many centers. Depending on the stringency of clinical phenotype assessment, the yield for positive genetic results in LQTS ranges from 50% to 78%, and is highest among tested individuals with the highest clinical probability (i.e., those with longer QTc intervals and more severe symptoms). The remaining probands with a strong clinical probability of LQTS will have a negative genetic test result, probably because of technical difficulties with genotyping, noncoding variants, or as yet unidentified disease-associated genes. Therefore, a negative genetic test in a subject with clinical LQTS (i.e., genotype-negative/phenotype-positive LQTS) does not provide a basis to exclude the diagnosis.[3,32-34]

There is also the potential for false-positive results; genetic testing may identify novel mutations of unclear significance, which could represent normal variants, and require validation and further analysis (e.g., linkage within a family or in vitro studies).[32-34]

Currently, comprehensive or LQT1 to LQT3 (*KCNQ1*, *KCNH2*, and *SCN5A*)-targeted LQTS genetic testing is recommended for symptomatic patients with a strong clinical index of suspicion for LQTS as well as for asymptomatic patients with QT prolongation (QTc ≥480 milliseconds [prepuberty] or ≥500 milliseconds [adults]) in the absence of other clinical conditions that might prolong the QT interval.[41]

Genetics of the Long QT Syndrome

To date, more than 500 mutations of 13 different genes responsible for a hereditary form of LQTS have been identified (Table 31-5), with the majority of the known mutations located in the first three: LQT1 (*KCNQ1*) mutations account for 42% to 45% of genetically positive LQTS, LQT2 (*KCNH2*) for 35% to 45%, and LQT3 (*SCN5A*) for 8% to 10%.

Overall, nine of these genes encode ion channel subunits that are specifically involved in cardiac action potential generation. LQT4 (*ANK2*), LQT9 (*CAV3*), LQT11 (*AKAP9*), and LQT12 (*SNTA1*) are caused by mutations in a family of versatile membrane adapters other than ion channel subunits. Nonetheless, the concept that LQTS genes ultimately affect ionic currents, either directly (ion channel mutations) or indirectly (modulators), still holds true.

Two modes of inheritance are involved in the LQTS: an autosomal dominant pattern and an autosomal recessive pattern. The majority of LQTS cases are inherited in an autosomal dominant fashion. Conversely, Jervell and Lange-Nielsen syndrome, which is inherited in an autosomal recessive fashion, is very rare, affecting less than 1% of LQTS cases.

Genetic analysis reveals two or more mutations in 5% to 10% of LQTS patients with clinical phenotypes of Romano-Ward syndrome. These compound mutations (so-called double hits) appear to be associated with a more severe phenotype than that associated with a single hit.[42]

Most reported mutations are in coding regions, although noncoding mutations (resulting in the loss of allele expression) have also been described. Most LQTS families have their own mutations, which are often termed "private" mutations.[32]

Several genetic mechanisms have been implicated in the development of LQTS including abnormalities in protein synthesis (transcription, translation), posttranslational protein processing resulting in abnormal transport to the cell surface membrane (protein trafficking, folding, assembly of subunits, glycosylation), ion channel gating (biophysical and kinetic properties), or permeation (ion selectivity, unitary conductance).

The majority of LQTS cases are caused by heterozygous disease; thus, mutations causing abnormalities in channel coassembly or trafficking result in up to 50% maximal reduction in the number of functional channels (haplotype insufficiency), because the gene product from the healthy allele remains intact. On the other hand, mutations that abolish channel function while preserving subunit assembly can result in dominant-negative suppression of the healthy allele as well, causing a more severe reduction (up to 94%) of the total amount of functional protein (dominant-negative effect) and favoring a more severe clinical course and a higher frequency of arrhythmia-related cardiac events.[7,12]

TABLE 31-5 Molecular Basis of the Congenital Long QT Syndrome

DISEASE	GENE	PROTEIN	IONIC CURRENT	FUNCTION	FREQUENCY	INHERITANCE
LQT1	*KCNQ1* (*K_vLQT1*)	K_v7.1	Subunit alpha I_{Ks}	Loss	42%-45%	Autosomal dominant
LQT2	*KCNH2* (*HERG*)	K_v11.1	Subunit alpha I_{Kr}	Loss	35%-45%	Autosomal dominant
LQT3	*SCN5A*	Na_v1.5	Subunit alpha I_{Na}	Gain	8%-10%	Autosomal dominant
LQT4 (ankyrin-B syndrome)	*ANKB*	ANK2	Adaptor I_{Na}	Loss	<1%	Autosomal dominant
LQT5	*KCNE1*	MinK	Subunit beta I_{Ks}	Loss	<1%	Autosomal dominant
LQT6	*KCNE2*	MiRP1	Subunit alpha I_{Kr}	Loss	<1%	Autosomal dominant
LQT7 (Andersen-Tawil syndrome)	*KCNJ2*	Kir2.1	Subunit alpha I_{K1}	Loss	<1%	Autosomal dominant
LQT8 (Timothy syndrome)	*CACNA1C*	Ca_v1.2	Subunit alpha I_{CaL}	Gain	<1%	Autosomal dominant
LQT9	*CAV3*	Caveolin-3	Adaptor I_{Na}	Gain	<1%	Autosomal dominant
LQT10	*SCN4B*	$Na_v\beta_4$	Subunit beta I_{Na}	Gain	<1%	Autosomal dominant
LQT11	*AKAP9*	Yotiao	Regulatory adaptor I_{Ks}	Loss	<1%	Autosomal dominant
LQT12	*SNTA1*	$Alpha_1$-syntrophin	Scaffolding protein I_{Na}	Gain	<1%	Autosomal dominant
LQT13	*KCNJ5*	Kir3.4 (GIRK4)	Subunit alpha I_{KACh}	Loss	<1%	Autosomal dominant
JLN1	*KCNQ1* (*K_vLQT1*)	K_v7.1	Subunit alpha I_{Ks}	Loss	99.5%	Autosomal recessive
JLN2	*KCNE1*	MinK	Subunit beta I_{Ks}	Loss	0.5%	Autosomal recessive

I_{CaL} = L-type Ca^{2+} current; I_{K1} = inward rectifier K^+ current; I_{KACh} = acetylcholine-activated inward rectifier K^+ current; I_{Kr} = rapidly activating delayed rectifier K^+ current; I_{Ks} = slowly activating delayed rectifier K^+ current; I_{Na} = Na^+ current; JLN1 and JLN 2 = Jervell and Lange-Nielsen syndrome types 1 and 2, respectively; LQT1 to LTQ13 = long QT syndrome types 1 to 13, respectively.

MUTATIONS RELATED TO THE SLOWLY ACTIVATING DELAYED RECTIFIER POTASSIUM CURRENT (I_{Ks})

I_{Ks} contributes to human atrial and ventricular repolarization, particularly during action potentials of long duration, and plays an important role in determining the rate-dependent shortening of the cardiac action potential. As heart rate increases, I_{Ks} increases because channel deactivation is slow and incomplete during the shortened diastole. This allows I_{Ks} channels to accumulate in the open state during rapid heart rates and contribute to the faster rate of repolarization.[43,44] Importantly, I_{Ks} is functionally upregulated when other repolarizing currents (such as I_{Kr}) are reduced, potentially serving as a "repolarization reserve" and a safeguard against loss of repolarizing power (see Chap. 2). Mutations in LQT1, LQT5, and LQT11 result in attenuation of I_{Ks} and, as a consequence, prolongation of repolarization, action potential duration, and QT interval.[7,43] LQT1 is caused by loss-of-function mutations of the *KCNQ1* (*K_vLQT1*) gene, which encodes the alpha subunit (K_v7.1) of the inward I_{Ks}. More than 170 mutations of this gene have been reported, comprising many Romano-Ward (autosomal dominant) syndromes and accounting for approximately 45% of all genotyped LQT families.[12] Of note, mutations involving the transmembrane domain of *KCNQ1* result in more severe disease compared with C-terminal mutations.

LQT5 is caused by loss-of-function mutations of the *KCNE1* gene, which encodes the beta subunit (MinK) that modulates I_{Ks}.[7]

Homozygous or compound heterozygous loss-of-function mutations of either the *KCNQ1* or *KCNE1* gene cause the autosomal recessive form of LQTS (the Jervell and Lange-Nielsen syndrome). Patients with *KCNQ1* mutations (type 1 Jervell and Lange-Nielsen syndrome) have an almost sixfold greater risk of arrhythmic events, whereas patients with *KCNE1* mutations (type 2 Jervell and Lange-Nielsen syndrome) appear to be at lower risk. Although the Jervell and Lange-Nielsen syndrome is the most severe among the major variants of LQTS, the parents of Jervell and Lange-Nielsen syndrome patients are generally less symptomatic than other LQT1 patients, despite the fact that they all are heterozygous for the same gene. This is likely related to the observation that most of the LQT1 genetic variants are missense mutations exerting a dominant-negative effect, whereas most (74%) Jervell and Lange-Nielsen mutations of *KCNQ1* are frame-shift/truncating mutations that are unable to cause dominant-negative suppression but are likely to interfere with subunit assembly. Jervell and Lange-Nielsen syndrome accompanies complete loss of I_{Ks} in hair cells and endolymph of the inner ear, which results in congenital deafness.[6]

LQT11 is caused by loss-of-function mutations of the *AKAP9* gene, which encodes an A-kinase anchoring protein (Yotiao), shown to be an integral part of the I_{Ks} macromolecular complex. The presence of Yotiao is necessary for the physiological response of the I_{Ks} to beta-adrenergic stimulation. LQT11 mutations reduce the interaction between Yotiao and the I_{Ks} channel (K_v7.1), preventing the functional response of I_{Ks} to cyclic adenosine monophosphate (cAMP) and adrenergic stimulation and causing an attenuation of I_{Ks}.[3]

MUTATIONS RELATED TO THE RAPIDLY ACTIVATING DELAYED RECTIFIER POTASSIUM CURRENT (I_{Kr})

I_{Kr} is largely responsible for repolarization of most cardiac cells and plays an important role in governing the cardiac action potential duration and refractoriness. Mutations in LQT2 and LQT6 result in attenuation of I_{Kr} and cause a decrease in the K^+ outward current and prolongation of repolarization, action potential duration, and QT interval.[44]

LQT2 is caused by loss-of-function mutations of the *KCNH2* (*HERG*) gene, which encodes the alpha subunit (K_v11.1) of the inward I_{Kr}. LQT2 syndrome accounts for almost 45% of all genotyped congenital LQTS cases. Approximately 200 mutations in this gene have been identified, which result in rapid closure of the HERG channels and decrease the normal rise in I_{Kr}, leading to delayed ventricular repolarization and QT prolongation. Mutations

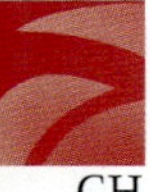

involving the pore region of the HERG channel are associated with a significantly more severe clinical course than nonpore mutations; most pore mutations are missense mutations with a dominant-negative effect.[12]

LQT6 is caused by loss-of-function mutations of the *KCNE2* gene, which encodes the accessory beta subunit (MiRP1) of the HERG channel. LQT6 displays clinical resemblance to LQT2.[7]

MUTATIONS RELATED TO THE INWARD RECTIFIER POTASSIUM CURRENT (I_{K1})

Andersen-Tawil syndrome (LQT7) is caused by loss-of-function mutations of the *KCNJ2* gene, which encodes the voltage-dependent K^+ channel (Kir2.1) that contributes to the inward I_{K1}. Kir2.1 channels are expressed primarily in skeletal muscle, heart, and brain. The majority of mutations exerts a dominant-negative effect on channel current.[7,16,17]

Disruption of the I_{K1} function can potentially lead to prolongation of the terminal repolarization phase and QT interval, which can predispose to the generation of EADs and diastolic membrane depolarizations (DADs) causing ventricular arrhythmias. However, unlike other types of LQTS, where the afterdepolarizations arise from reactivation of L-type Ca^{2+} channels, the EADs/DADs generated in LQT7 are likely secondary to Na^+-Ca^{2+} exchanger-driven depolarization. It is believed that the differential origin of the triggering beat is responsible for the observed discrepancy in arrhythmogenesis and the clinical features compared with other types of LQTS. Additionally, it is likely that prolongation of the action potential duration in LQT7 is somewhat homogeneous across the ventricular wall (i.e., transmural dispersion of repolarization is less prominent than in other types of LQTSs), which can potentially explain the low frequency of torsades de pointes. Flaccid paralysis results from failure to propagate action potentials in the muscle membrane as a result of sustained membrane depolarization.[7,16,17]

MUTATIONS RELATED TO THE ACETYLCHOLINE-ACTIVATED POTASSIUM CURRENT (I_{KACh})

LQT13 is caused by loss-of-function mutations of the *KCNJ5* gene, which encodes the alpha subunit (Kir3.4, GIRK4) of the inward I_{KACh}. The Kir3.4 mutation is the most recently identified LQT-associated gene, and it exerts dominant-negative effects on Kir3.1/Kir3.4 channel complexes by disrupting membrane targeting and stability of Kir3.4.[45]

MUTATIONS RELATED TO THE SODIUM CURRENT (I_{Na})

LQT3 is caused by gain-of-function mutations of the *SCN5A* gene, which encodes the alpha subunit ($Na_v1.5$) of the cardiac voltage-gated Na^+ channel that is responsible for the I_{Na}. LQT3 accounts for approximately 8% of the congenital LQTS cases. More than 80 mutations have been identified in the *SCN5A* gene, with the majority being missense mutations mainly clustered in $Na_v1.5$ regions that are involved in fast inactivation (i.e., S4 segment of DIV, the DIII-DIV linker, and the cytoplasmic loops between the S4 and S5 segments of DIII and DIV), or in regions that stabilize fast inactivation (e.g., the C-terminus).[12,46,47]

Several mechanisms have been identified to underlie ionic effects of *SCN5A* mutations in LQT3. Most of the *SCN5A* mutations cause a gain of function through disruption of fast inactivation, allowing repeated reopening during sustained depolarization and resulting in an abnormal, small but functionally important sustained (or persistent) noninactivating Na^+ current (I_{sus}) during the action potential plateau. Other, less common mechanisms include increased window current, which results from delayed inactivation of mutant Na^+ channels, occurring at more positive potentials and widening the voltage range during which the Na^+ channel may reactivate without inactivation. Additionally, some mutations cause slower inactivation, which allows longer channel openings, and causes a slowly inactivating Na^+ current (the late Na^+ current, I_{NaL}). Because the general membrane conductance is small during the action potential plateau, the presence of a persistent inward Na^+ current, even of small amplitude, can potentially have a major impact on the plateau duration and can be sufficient to prolong repolarization and QT interval. QT prolongation and the risk of developing arrhythmia is more pronounced at slow heart rates, when the action potential duration is longer, allowing more Na^+ current to enter the cell.[12,46]

Regardless of the mechanism, increased Na^+ current (I_{sus}, window current, I_{NaL}, or peak I_{Na}) upsets the balance between depolarizing and repolarizing currents in favor of depolarization. The resulting delay in the repolarization process triggers EADs (i.e., reactivation of the L-type Ca^{2+} channel during phase 2 or 3 of the action potential), especially in Purkinje fiber myocytes where action potential durations are intrinsically longer.[47]

LQT9 is caused by gain-of-function mutations of the *CAV3* gene, which encodes caveolin-3, a plasma membrane scaffolding protein that interacts with $Na_v1.5$ and plays a role in compartmentalization and regulation of channel function. Mutations in caveolin-3 induce kinetic alterations of the Na^+ channel that result in persistent late Na^+ current (I_{sus}) and have been reported in cases of SIDS.[7,47]

LQT10 is caused by gain-of-function mutations of the *SCN4B* gene, which encodes the beta subunit ($Na_v\beta_4$) of the $Na_v1.5$ ion channel. To date, only a single mutation in one patient has been described, which resulted in a shift in the inactivation of the Na^+ current toward more positive potentials, but did not change the activation. This resulted in increased window currents at membrane potentials corresponding to phase 3 of the action potential.[7,47]

LQT12 is caused by mutations of the *SNTA1* gene, which encodes alpha$_1$-syntrophin, a cytoplasmic adaptor protein that enables the interaction between $Na_v1.5$, nitric oxide synthase, and sarcolemmal Ca^{2+} ATPase complex that appears to regulate ion channel function. By disrupting the interaction between $Na_v1.5$ and sarcolemmal calcium ATPase complex, *SNTA1* mutations cause increased $Na_v1.5$ nitrosylation with consequent reduction of channel inactivation and increased I_{sus} densities.[3,47]

MUTATIONS RELATED TO THE L-TYPE CALCIUM CURRENT (I_{CaL})

Timothy syndrome (LQT8) is caused by gain-of-function mutations of the *CACNA1C* gene, which encodes the alpha subunit ($Ca_v1.2$) of the voltage-dependent L-type Ca^{2+} channel that contributes to I_{CaL}.

The inward I_{CaL} sustains depolarization and gives rise to the plateau phase essential for excitation-contraction coupling. Gain-of-function mutations of *CACNA1C* result in near complete elimination of voltage-dependent inactivation of $Ca_v1.2$ channels, leading to inappropriate continuation of the depolarizing I_{CaL} and lengthening of the plateau phase.

MUTATIONS IN THE ANKYRIN-B GENE

LQT4 is caused by loss-of-function mutations of the *ANK2* gene, which encodes ankyrin-B, a structural membrane adapter protein that anchors ion channels to specific domains in the plasma membrane. Functionally, ankyrins bind to several ion channel proteins, targeting these proteins to specialized membrane domains, such as the anion exchanger (chloride-bicarbonate exchanger), Na^+-K^+ adenosine triphosphatase (ATPase), I_{Na}, the Na^+-Ca^{2+} exchanger ($I_{Na\text{-}Ca}$), and Ca^{2+} release channels (including those mediated by the receptors for inositol triphosphate [IP_3] or ryanodine [RyR2]). Hence, *ANK2* mutations can potentially result in improper localization and activity of ion-conducting proteins. Five mutations of this gene have been reported, resulting in increased intracellular concentration of Ca^{2+} and, sometimes, fatal arrhythmia. However, QT interval prolongation is not a consistent feature in patients with ankyrin-B dysfunction; instead, varying degrees of cardiac dysfunction are observed including bradycardia, sinus arrhythmia, idiopathic VF, CPVT, and SCD. Therefore, ankyrin-B dysfunction is now regarded as a clinical entity distinct from classic LQTS (referred to as the "ankyrin-B syndrome").

Pathophysiology of the Long QT Syndrome

MECHANISM OF QT INTERVAL PROLONGATION

Any factor that evokes lengthening of the action potential duration holds the potential of causing an LQTS phenotype, especially if it does it heterogeneously. Electrophysiologically, prolongation of the action potential duration and QT interval can arise from either a decrease in the outward repolarizing current (K^+ currents: I_{Kr}, I_{Ks}, I_{K1}, I_{KACh}) or an increase in inward depolarizing membrane current (Na^+ current, Ca^{2+} current, or both) during phases 2 and 3 of the action potentials (Fig. 31-3).

Most commonly, QTc prolongation is produced by delayed repolarization due to attenuation of I_{Ks} (LQT1, LQT5, LQT11), I_{Kr} (LQT2, LQT6), I_{K1} (LQT7), or I_{KACh} (LQT13). Less commonly, QT prolongation results from prolonged depolarization due to an increase in I_{Na} (LQT3, LQT4, LQT9, LQT10, LQT12) or I_{CaL} (LQT8).[7]

MECHANISM OF DISPERSION OF REPOLARIZATION

The LQTS is caused by an excessive and heterogeneous prolongation of the repolarization phase of the ventricular action potential. In the normal ventricle, there are heterogeneous cell types with different action potential morphologies and durations, mainly attributed to cell-specific and regional variability in the functional expression of different populations of ion channels (transient outward K^+ channels [I_{to}], I_{Ks}), and the Na^+ window current (I_{Na}) and/or their accessory proteins. Some experimental studies proposed the presence of three irregular cell layers in the ventricle with distinct electrical properties: endocardial, midmyocardial (M cells), and epicardial cells. Overall, the putative midmyocardial cells (which have a smaller I_{Ks}, a larger late I_{Na}, and a larger Na^+-Ca^{2+} exchange current [$I_{Na\text{-}Ca}$]) appear to generate longer action potential durations that are more susceptible to modification compared with the endocardium and epicardium. The epicardial cells have the shortest action potential durations because of a prominent I_{to}. Repolarization of endocardial cells usually occurs between repolarization of the epicardial and midmyocardial cells. Notably, factors that prolong the action potential appear to elicit a disproportionate prolongation of the action potential duration in midmyocardial cells. As a result, dispersion of the action potential duration becomes irregularly exaggerated across the ventricular wall, yielding an increase in the action potential duration heterogeneity.[7]

Conditions leading to a reduction in I_{Kr} (e.g., LQT2) or augmentation of late I_{Na} (e.g., LQT3) produce a preferential prolongation of the M cell action potential. Consequently, QT interval prolongation is accompanied by a dramatic increase in transmural dispersion of repolarization. In contrast, conditions leading to a reduction in I_{Ks} alone (e.g., LQT1) result in a homogeneous prolongation of action potential duration across the ventricular wall with little increase in transmural dispersion of repolarization. However, concurrent beta-adrenergic stimulation (e.g., exercise, isoproterenol) results in abbreviation of epicardial and endocardial action potential duration with little or no change in the M cell action potential, resulting in marked augmentation of transmural dispersion of repolarization and arrhythmogenesis (see Fig. 31-3).[27]

On the surface ECG, the peak of the normal T wave coincides with repolarization of the epicardial action potential (the shortest action potential) whereas repolarization of the longest action potential in the midmyocardial cells coincides with the end of the T wave. Hence, the increased dispersion of transmural repolarization results in prolongation of the interval from the peak of the T wave to the end of the T wave ($T_{peak\text{-}to\text{-}end}$) on the surface ECG.[7,29,30]

MECHANISM OF TORSADES DE POINTES

The excessive increase in the spatial and/or temporal action potential duration heterogeneity favors the generation of EADs because of reactivation of L-type Ca^{2+} channels, and on some occasions the late I_{Na} or Na^+-Ca^{2+} exchanger. The EADs can cause PVCs that can potentially trigger the initiation of ventricular arrhythmias. Furthermore, excessive transmural heterogeneity of the action potential duration provides the substrate for unidirectional block and functional reentry circuits to propagate torsades de pointes.[7]

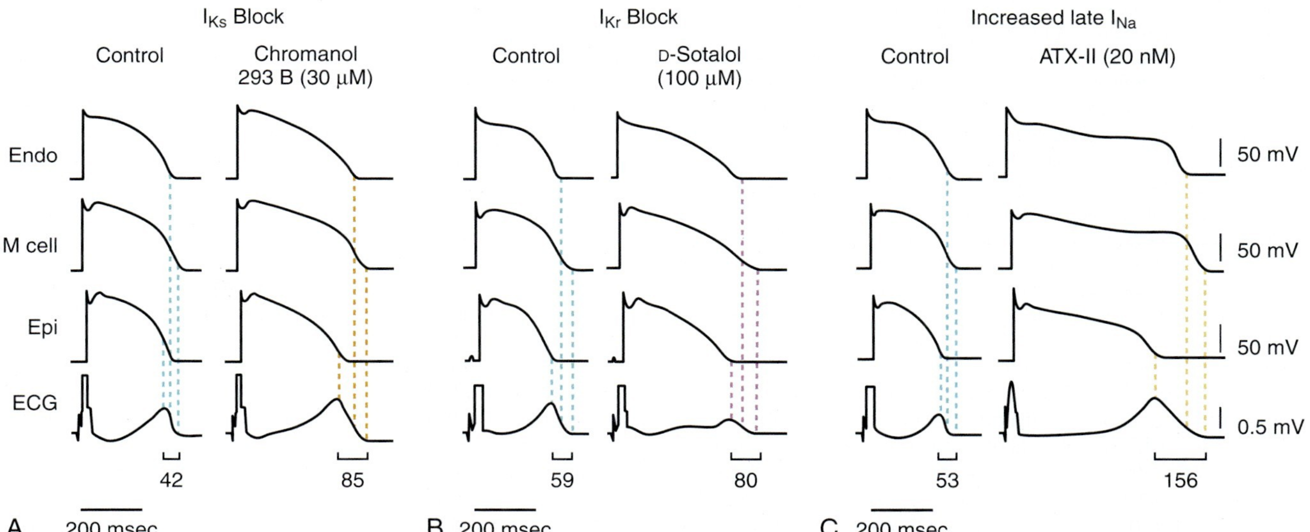

FIGURE 31-3 Pathophysiology of long QT syndrome. Transmembrane action potentials and transmural electrocardiogram (ECG) traces in control and after I_{Ks} block **(A)**, I_{Kr} block **(B)**, and increase in late I_{Na} **(C)**, in arterially perfused canine left ventricular wedge preparations. **A** to **C** depict action potentials simultaneously recorded from endocardial (Endo), M cell, and epicardial (Epi) sites, together with a transmural ECG trace. Basic cycle length, 2000 milliseconds. In all cases, the peak of the T wave in the ECG is coincident with the repolarization of the epicardial action potential, whereas the end of the T wave is coincident with the repolarization of the M cell action potential. Repolarization of the endocardial cell is intermediate between that of the M cell and epicardial cell. Transmural dispersion of repolarization across the ventricular wall, defined as the difference in the repolarization time between M and epicardial cells, is denoted below the ECG traces. ATX-II = sea anemone toxin; I_{Na} = sodium current; I_{Kr} = rapidly activating delayed rectifier K^+ current; I_{Ks} = slowly activating delayed rectifier potassium current. *(From Antzelevitch C: Drug-induced channelopathies. In Zipes DP, Jalife J, editors: Cardiac electrophysiology: from cell to bedside, ed 5, Philadelphia, 2009, WB Saunders, pp 195-203.)*

Although torsades de pointes is presumably often initiated by EAD-triggered PVCs, its propagation likely is due to intramural reentrant mechanisms, giving rise to one or more intramural rotors that impose a rapid ectopic ventricular rhythm (typically 150 to 300 beats/min) while migrating inside the ventricular wall. Hence, with each new cycle the principal depolarization focus migrates accordingly, resulting in a progressive change of the electrical axis, typically rotating 180 degrees in approximately 10 to 12 cycles. This results in a polymorphic VT with the characteristic sinusoidal "twisting of the points" pattern on the 12-lead ECG.[7]

Notably, although the atrium seems to be resistant to generating EADs in response to agents that prolong repolarization, atrial EADs and "atrial torsades de pointes" have been reported in some LQTS patients as well as cesium-treated dogs.[48]

MECHANISM OF EXERCISE-INDUCED CHANGES

Patients with LQT1 and LQT2 genotypes have differing patterns of QT adaptation during beta-adrenergic stimulation (e.g., during stress, exercise, epinephrine infusion). Patients with LQT1 appear to have less repolarization reserve during exercise as evidenced by a progressive or persistent pattern of QTc prolongation at faster heart rates, compared with patients with LQT2, in whom maximal QTc prolongation occurs at submaximal heart rates in the early phase of sympathetic stimulation with subsequent fall toward baseline values at faster heart rates.[10]

I_{Ks} is markedly enhanced by beta-adrenergic stimulation through G-protein/cAMP-mediated channel phosphorylation by protein kinase A (PKA) (requiring AKAP9 [Yotiao]) and PKC (requiring MinK). This produces a rate-dependent shortening of the action potential duration in normal hearts. Importantly, I_{Ks} is functionally upregulated when other repolarizing currents (such as I_{Kr}) are reduced, potentially serving as a "repolarization reserve" and a safeguard against loss of repolarizing power, especially when beta-adrenergic stimulation is present.[44,49]

LQT1 subjects have compromised I_{Ks} channels that are not as responsive to sympathetic stimulation, and phase 3 repolarization in these individuals is retarded. Consequently, during beta-adrenergic stimulation, there are relatively more unopposed depolarizing forces via the L-type Ca^{2+} channel and the Na^+-Ca^{2+} exchanger that prolong the action potential duration and hence the QT interval.

In contrast, subjects with LQT2 have dysfunctional I_{Kr} channels, which represent a smaller fraction of the K^+ channels responsible for phase 3 repolarization and are not as sympathetically responsive as I_{Ks} channels. Therefore, in LQT2 patients, the QT fails to shorten at the intermediate heart rates in the early phase of exercise or epinephrine infusion because of attenuation of I_{Kr}. This is followed by recruitment of I_{Ks} ("repolarization reserve") at faster heart rates during continuing exercise or epinephrine infusion, with concomitant appropriate abbreviation of the action potential duration and QT shortening, which persists into the recovery phase. This consequently leads to an exaggerated QT difference between the exercise and recovery QT/R-R curves that is manifested as increased QT hysteresis, which appears to be a characteristic feature of the LQT2 phenotype.[34]

The LQT3 phenotype is characterized by a constant reduction of the action potential duration with epinephrine because of stimulation of the intact I_{Ks} channel and augmentation of the late inward Na^+ current. In fact, LQT3 patients may have supranormal QT adaptation in response to exercise compared with control subjects. *SCN5A* mutations in LQT3 cause a gain of function through disruption of fast channel inactivation, allowing repeated reopening during sustained depolarization and resulting in a small but functionally important enhancement of the I_{Na} during action potential plateau. As a consequence, the risk of developing arrhythmia will be expected to be particularly high at slow heart rates, when the action potential duration is longer, allowing more Na^+ current to enter the cell.[38]

The differences in the dynamic response of ventricular repolarization to sympathetic stimulation may explain the epidemiological observation that patients with LQT1 are more likely to have life-threatening events during sympathetic activation compared with patients with other genotypes and also may underlie the responsiveness of LQT1 patients to beta blocker therapy.[10]

MECHANISM OF GENOTYPE-PHENOTYPE VARIABILITY

The LQTS is a complex and multifactorial disorder characterized by a broad phenotypic heterogeneity. The clinical phenotype (QTc values, arrhythmia-related symptoms, and outcomes) is highly variable, not only between families carrying different causal mutations, but also among family members carrying an identical mutation, with a broad continuous spectrum of clinical or subclinical phenotypes. One end of this spectrum is concealed LQTS (silent carriers of disease-causing mutations), whereby no QT prolongation or related symptoms are observed. At the other end of the spectrum are the severe symptomatic LQTS cases, these often representing the index cases easily identified in families. In between are patients with different degrees of QT prolongation and different levels of severity of arrhythmias.[7]

A multitude of genetic and acquired interacting factors (some defined but many still unknown) influence the pathophysiology and clinical course of each person and ultimately determine a spectrum of phenotypes. Among these factors is the fact that action potential generation is a polygenic process; different LQTS genes affect different ion current mechanisms. Even mutations in the same gene can affect gene expression levels and ionic current activity to different extents and via different mechanisms. As noted above, mutations located in the transmembrane segment (for LQT1) or pore region (for LQT2) generally result in more malignant disease compared with mutations in other locations. Similarly, mutations causing a dominant-negative effect (e.g., missense mutations involving the pore region of the channel) result in more profound channel dysfunction and more severe clinical disease that those associated with haplotype insufficiency (e.g., mutations causing coassembly or trafficking abnormalities).[7,12]

The "repolarization reserve" hypothesis, whereby multiple hits to repolarization are required to compromise repolarization and surpass the threshold for developing clinical QT prolongation and torsades de pointes, can underlie, at least in part, the phenotypic heterogeneity in LQTS. In this setting, a mutation in one of the LQT-linked genes causing an attenuation of a cardiac ionic current may result in only a limited disruption of the repolarization process, which can be clinically concealed and become unmasked (manifesting as QT prolongation and arrhythmias) only when accompanied by another insult to the same or a different ionic current (e.g., drugs or electrolyte abnormalities). In fact, it has been suggested that some cases of acquired LQTS represent inadvertent "unmasking" of subclinical congenital LQTS.[7,30]

Adding to the complexity is the "double-hit" phenomenon, secondary to either two mutations in the same gene (compound heterozygosity) or mutations in two different LQT genes (digenic heterozygosity). Double hits occur in 5% to 10% of LQTS patients and the resulting phenotype is more severe than with a single hit.[7]

Genetic factors are also involved in the control of cardiac repolarization at the population level. The heritability of the QTc interval has been estimated as between 25% and 52%. Ventricular action potential is under the joint control of multiple ionic currents, and the activity and expression levels of the channels underlying each of these currents establish a subtle equilibrium between depolarizing and repolarizing currents determining the action potential duration in each individual. Common genetic variants differing from the ancestor sequence by one nucleotide (i.e., single nucleotide polymorphism) in genes coding for proteins that are known or suggested to affect ion channel function appear to influence this equilibrium even via weak effects on activity and/or expression level of channel subunits and can potentially play a role in determining cardiac repolarization duration and QTc length in healthy individuals.[50] Therefore, apart from the known LQT-linked genetic mutations, allelic variation elsewhere in the genome, most often single nucleotide polymorphisms, in the same disease-causing gene or in other genes can amplify otherwise subclinical disturbances of the repolarization into overt LQTS and potentially contribute to the variable penetrance and clinical phenotype heterogeneity.[50,51]

Furthermore, the genetic constitution is dynamic over time; the resultant intrinsic risk for arrhythmias can change according to age, LV hypertrophy, and heart failure resulting in structural and electrical remodeling of the heart.[7]

In summary, the cardiac repolarization process is strongly dependent on various parameters, among them heart rate, age, gender, sympathetic tone, electrolyte balance, and medications, as well as inherited and acquired pathological conditions. The interaction of the underlying LQTS genetic mutation with other genetic factors in the same gene or elsewhere in the host genome, as well as with multiple superimposed acquired risk determinants ("disease modifiers"), has a substantial impact on the expressivity of the phenotype of the LQT genotype.

Differential Diagnosis

Typical cases of LQTS are so characteristic that differential diagnosis is not even considered. When dealing with borderline cases, several conditions should be considered including vasovagal syncope, orthostatic hypotension, arrhythmogenic right ventricular cardiomyopathy/dysplasia (ARVD), CPVT, hypertrophic cardiomyopathy, and epilepsy.

It is especially important to distinguish acquired factors that result in QT prolongation from the inherited form of LQTS. The acquired form of LQTS is far more prevalent than the congenital form. Causes of abnormal prolongation of the QT interval include myocardial ischemia, cardiomyopathies, hypokalemia, hypocalcemia, hypomagnesemia, autonomic influences, drugs, and hypothermia.[5] Hypokalemia causes prolongation of the action potential duration because of reduced K^+ conductance. Low extracellular K^+ levels accelerate fast inactivation of the HERG channel and further decrease I_{Kr}.

By far, the most common environmental stressor resulting in acquired LQTS is drug therapy, including antiarrhythmic drugs, some antihistaminics, antipsychotics, and antibiotics. Noncardiovascular drugs that can potentially precipitate QT interval prolongation and arrhythmias comprise approximately 2% to 3% of total prescribed medications. Indeed, the risk of acquired LQTS is the most common cause of withdrawal or restriction of drugs that have already been marketed. The vast majority of drugs associated with the acquired form of LQTS are known to interact with the HERG channel (which mediates I_{Kr}), likely because of unique structural properties rendering this channel unusually susceptible to blockade by a wide range of different drugs. Compared with other cardiac K^+ channels, the HERG channel has a large, funnel-like vestibule that allows many small-sized molecules to enter and block the channel (see Chap. 2). The more spacious inner cavity is due to the lack of the Pro-X-Pro sequence motif in the S6 segment (which is present in most other voltage-gated K^+ channels and is believed to induce a sharp bend in the inner S6 helices of voltage-gated K^+ channels, reducing the inner vestibule), which presumably facilitates access of drugs to the pore region from the intracellular side of the channel to block the channel current. Additionally, the HERG channel contains two aromatic sites inside its pore (not present in most other K^+ channels), which provide high-affinity binding sites for aromatic moieties of a wide range of structurally diverse compounds. Interaction of these compounds with the channel's pore causes functional alteration of its biophysical properties, occlusion of the permeation pathway, or both.[7,44,52]

Other mechanisms underlying drug-induced LQTS have been recently described, including disruption of HERG channel protein trafficking, with consequent reduction of surface membrane expression of otherwise functional channels (e.g., pentamidine), or folding and assembly of channel subunits. The accessory beta subunit (MiRP1, *KCNE2*) also determines the drug sensitivity.[7]

Several factors can potentially increase the risk of susceptibility of acquired LQTS as a complication of drug therapy, including female gender (70% of patients with drug-induced torsades de pointes are women), hypokalemia, hypomagnesemia, hypocalcemia, bradycardia, congestive heart failure, LV hypertrophy, recent conversion from atrial fibrillation (AF), and the degree of QT interval prolongation on baseline ECG. Other risk factors include high drug doses, rapid intravenous infusion, and concurrent use of drugs that prolong the QT interval or that slow drug metabolism. Additionally, genetically determined variability in pharmacodynamics (e.g., polymorphisms and mutations of the cytochrome system) can be responsible for significant variations in drug response. Most patients with drug-induced torsades de pointes have one or more risk factors.[44,49,53]

Furthermore, mutations of ion channel genes responsible for LQTS have been implicated as a risk factor. In fact, previously unrecognized congenital LQTS, of any subtype, can be identified in 5% to 20% of patients with drug-induced torsades de pointes. Therefore, it might be useful to screen for genetic variations in patients with overt drug-induced LQTS.[41] In addition, polymorphisms (i.e., common genetic variations present in >1% of the population) in cardiac ion channels can potentially increase the risk for the development of drug-induced torsades de pointes. In these patients, drug-induced LQTS appears to represent a "forme fruste" of congenital LQTS. This is likely related to a redundancy in repolarizing currents; normal repolarization is accomplished by multiple ion channels, providing a safety reserve for repolarization. As a result, a mutation or polymorphism in one of the LQTS genes can be clinically inapparent until another insult to repolarization, such as a drug, hypokalemia, or hypomagnesemia, is superimposed.[7,32]

In contrast to the most common types of congenital LQTS (LQT1 and LQT2), a short-long-short cycle length sequence constitutes the typical pattern of initiation of torsades de pointes in acquired LQTS. The short-long R-R intervals are usually caused by a PVC followed by a compensatory pause. Torsades de pointes also can occur in association with bradycardia or frequent pauses (sometimes referred to as "pause-dependent LQTS").

Risk Stratification

The clinical course in LQTS patients is not uniform and is influenced by many factors, including age, gender, genotype, environmental factors, therapy, and possibly other modifier genes.

GENETIC MARKERS OF RISK

The genotype has been shown to be an important predictor of LQTS-related cardiac events. The risk of cardiac events has been shown to be significantly higher in LQT1 and LQT2 when compared with LQT3, with events occurring at a younger age. The cumulative mortality, however, appears to be similar regardless of the genotype, as patients with LQT3 exhibit a higher percentage of potentially lethal events.

LQT1 patients exhibit a 49% increase in the risk of cardiac events as compared with LQT2 patients. However, in the 15- through 40-year age group, the risk of a first cardiac event is significantly higher among LQT2 patients (67% increase in the risk as compared with LQT1 patients).[15] Among LQTS patients receiving beta blocker therapy, the LQT2 and LQT3 genotypes are associated with increased risk of arrhythmic events as compared with LQT1.[10]

In addition to identifying the LQT genotype, knowing the specific mutation and its biophysical function can help improve risk stratification. For LQT1, patients with mutations in the transmembrane domain of the KCNQ1 ion channel had more frequent cardiac events (syncope, aborted cardiac arrest, or SCD) and a greater risk of the first cardiac event occurring at a younger age than did patients with C-terminal mutations. For LQT2, pore mutations have a more severe clinical course and a higher frequency of arrhythmic events occurring at a younger age when compared with nonpore mutations. In particular, missense mutations in the transmembrane pore (S5-loop-S6) region appear to be associated with the highest risk of clinical arrhythmia. Preliminary data for LQT3 patients also suggest that the location of the mutation can play a role in determining the severity of the clinical phenotype. Furthermore, the biophysical function of the mutation is also important in determining the phenotype. Mutations with a dominant-negative effect on ion channel function (>50% reduction in function) have a more severe phenotype compared with mutations exhibiting haploinsufficiency (≤50% reduction in function). These genetic risks were independent of traditional clinical risk factors such as the manifest QTc interval on the ECG, suggesting that variability in the electrophysiological effects of the different mutations contributes to the variability in the risk of life-threatening cardiac events.[10,15]

Patients with the Jervell and Lange-Nielsen and Timothy syndromes have poor prognosis and are less likely to respond to beta blocker therapy alone. In contrast, the Andersen-Tawil syndrome has a generally more benign clinical course in terms of arrhythmic death.

ELECTROCARDIOGRAPHIC MARKERS OF RISK

QT INTERVAL PROLONGATION. The QTc interval is the best prognostic ECG parameter in LQTS families. A QTc interval of at least 470 milliseconds is a predictor for increased risk for symptoms, whereas a QTc of at least 500 milliseconds predicts an increased risk of life-threatening cardiac events. The risk for cardiac events demonstrates a nearly exponential increase for the QTc interval decile. The maximal QTc duration measured at any time before age 10 was shown to be the most powerful predictor of cardiac events during adolescence, regardless of baseline, mean, or most recent QTc values.[23,26]

T-U WAVE MORPHOLOGY. The ratio of amplitude of the U wave to that of the T wave has been suggested as the clinical counterpart of EADs; a progressive increase in the ratio of the U wave to the T wave preceded the onset of torsades de pointes in an experimental model of LQT. In addition, the increment in U wave amplitude after a PVC has been suggested as a marker for arrhythmia risk in "pause-dependent" LQT.

Furthermore, in patients with bifid T waves, the diurnal maximal ratio between late and early T wave peak amplitude was found to correlate with a history of LQTS-related symptoms better than the baseline QTc interval in both LQT1 and LQT2 patients, and can potentially be used to assess the risk of symptoms in asymptomatic patients with known type 1 or 2 LQTS genotype. In LQT1 patients, a ratio of at least 3 suggests a high probability of being symptomatic whereas a ratio not exceeding 2 suggests a low probability. Among LQT2 patients, ratios suggestive of being symptomatic or asymptomatic are, respectively, at least 2.4 and not more than 1.5.[31]

CLINICAL MARKERS OF RISK

SYNCOPE. Nonfatal events (syncope and aborted cardiac arrest) in LQTS patients remain the strongest predictor of subsequent LQTS-related fatal events, and the overall risk of subsequent SCD in an LQTS patient who has experienced a previous episode of syncope is approximately 5% per year.[9]

The risk of subsequent syncopal episodes can be reduced with beta blocker therapy; however, patients experiencing syncope while receiving beta blockers are at high risk of subsequent cardiac events, a risk similar to that observed in patients who are not treated with beta blockers.[9]

Both the timing and frequency of syncopal events are related to the subsequent risk of cardiac events. Patients with recent (within the past 2 years) syncope and a higher number of syncopal events during this period carry a higher risk of cardiac events.[54]

FAMILY HISTORY. The incomplete penetrance and variable expressivity in LQTS preclude predicting severity of symptoms in relatives of a symptomatic LQTS patient. In fact, SCD of a sibling (at any age) does not seem to contribute to increased personal risk of LQTS-related life-threatening cardiac events. Instead, the risk of adverse events in relatives appears to be determined more by the individual's own risk factors (QTc duration, personal history of syncope, and gender).[55]

GENDER. The effect of gender on outcome is age-dependent, with boys exhibiting a significant (71% to 85%) increase in risk for syncope, aborted cardiac arrest, or SCD as compared with girls during childhood and early adolescence. However, a gender risk reversal occurs after age 14 years, in which girls exhibit an 87% increase in the risk of cardiac events compared with boys among probands and a 3.3-fold increase in the risk among affected family members. When only life-threatening cardiac events (aborted cardiac arrest or SCD) are considered, the onset of gender risk reversal occurs at a later age. The cumulative probability of a first life-threatening cardiac event from age 1 to 12 years is 5% in boys compared with only 1% among girls, whereas in the age range of 12 to 20 years, there is no significant gender difference in risk. Risk reversal for the endpoint of aborted cardiac arrest or SCD occurs after the age of 20 years, and female patients maintain higher risk than male patients throughout adulthood.[14]

Importantly, the effect of gender on outcome appears to be genotype-dependent. Among those not more than 14 years of age, male LQT1 patients exhibit the highest risk of cardiac events; female LQT1 patients had intermediate risk; and both male and female LQT2 patients had the lowest risk. No significant gender-related difference in risk was shown among LQT2 and LQT3 children. In contrast, in the 15- through 40-year age group, risk is highest among LQT2 women, intermediate among LQT1 women, and lowest among LQT1 and LQT2 men.[15]

The mechanisms behind these age-dependent differences in gender-related risk are unknown. Environmental (increased physical activity), hormonal (opposing effects of estrogens and androgens on ventricular repolarization), and/or genetic (modifier genes not shared by boys and girls) factors can potentially play a role.[14]

AGE. Risk factors in LQTS are time-dependent and age-specific (Table 31-6). LQTS patients who experience an aborted cardiac arrest during the first year of life are at a very high risk for subsequent life-threatening cardiac events during the first decade of life. The risk factors for a cardiac event in LQTS infants also include a QTc of at least 500 milliseconds, a heart rate not exceeding 100 beats/min, and female gender.[56] In LQTS children, risk factors for life-threatening cardiac events include male gender, a history of syncope at any time during childhood, and a QTc duration greater than 500 milliseconds.[14] Among adolescent patients with suspected LQTS, recent episodes of syncope (in particular within the past 2 years) and QTc greater than 530 milliseconds predict increased risk of LQTS-related cardiac events.[54] Although LQT1 genotype predicts higher risk in patients not more than 14 years of age (especially boys), the risk is higher for LQT2 in patients 15 years of age or older (especially women). In adult patients, predictors of worse outcome include a QTc greater than 500 milliseconds, female gender, and history of syncope before age 18 years. Additionally, patients with LQT2 mutations appear to be at a greater risk for a cardiac event than patients with LQT1 or LQT3 genotypes.[4]

Beyond 40 years of age, recent syncope (within the past 2 years) appears to be the predominant risk factor in affected subjects, and those with a positive mutation had a significantly higher mortality, particularly those with an LQT3 mutation. Furthermore, women with a QTc greater than 470 milliseconds are at a higher risk of LQTS-related cardiac events, whereas in men event rates are similar in the various QTc categories. After the age of 60 years, the risk of death due to LQTS competes with other disease entities that may lead to death.

Principles of Management

The main therapeutic modalities for the prevention of life-threatening cardiac events include beta blockers, left cervicothoracic sympathetic denervation, and ICD implantation. In nongenotyped patients, beta blockers comprise the mainstay therapy, whereas

TABLE 31-6 Age-Specific Risk Factors for Life-Threatening Cardiac Events in Long QT Syndrome Patients*

AGE GROUP	RISK FACTOR	HAZARD RATIO (P VALUE)	BETA BLOCKER EFFICACY, % REDUCTION (P VALUE)
Childhood (1-12 yr)	Male gender	3.96 (<0.001)	73% (0.002)
	QTc > 500 msec	2.12 (0.02)	
	Prior syncope		
	Recent (<2 yr)	14.34 (<0.001)	
	Remote (≥2 yr)	6.45 (<0.001)	
Adolescence (10-20 yr)	QTc > 530 msec	2.3 (<0.001)	64% (0.01)
	Syncope		
	≥2 syncopal events in past 2 yr	18.1 (<0.001)	
	1 syncopal event in past 2 yr	11.7 (<0.001)	
	≥2 syncopal events in past 2-10 yr	5.8 (<0.001)	
	1 syncopal events in past 2-10 yr	2.7 (<0.001)	
Adulthood (18-40 yr)	Female gender	2.68 (<0.05)	60% (<0.01)
	QTc duration		
	QTc ≥ 500 msec	6.35 (<0.01)	
	QTc = 500-549 msec	3.34 (<0.01)	
	Prior syncope	5.10 (<0.01)	
Adulthood (41-60 yr)†	Recent syncope (<2 yr)	9.92 (<0.001)	42% (0.40)‡
	QTc > 530 msec	1.68 (0.06)	
	LQT3 genotype	4.76 (0.02)	

*Findings are from separate multivariable Cox models in each age group for the endpoint of aborted cardiac arrest or sudden cardiac death.
†Because long QT syndrome (LQTS)–related events are more difficult to delineate in the older age group, the endpoint in the 41- to 60-year age group comprised aborted cardiac arrest or death from any cause.
‡Lack of a statistically significant beta blocker effect in this age group may relate to the broad endpoint of death from any cause.
QTc = corrected QT interval.
From Goldenberg I, Moss AJ: Long QT syndrome, *J Am Coll Cardiol* 51:2291-2300, 2008.

cervicothoracic sympathetic denervation and implantation of an ICD are therapeutic options in high-risk LQTS patients who experience recurrent cardiac events despite beta blocker therapy.[12]

PHARMACOLOGICAL THERAPY

Treatment with beta blockers is associated with a significant (53% to 64%) reduction in risk of LQTS-related life-threatening events (syncope, cardiac arrest, and SCD), regardless of age (see Table 31-6). The benefit appears to be most substantial in patients at highest risk for cardiac events. On the other hand, very low-risk patients (no history of syncope, QTc <500 milliseconds, girls <age 14, LQT2 men of any age, and LQT1 women >age 14) have such a small frequency of events that beta blockers may not provide a significant benefit.[15]

Genetic data can be used to guide the therapeutic management plan. Given the critical role of catecholamines in precipitating arrhythmias in LQT1, beta blocker therapy is particularly effective for this group of patients; approximately 90% of LQT1 patients treated with beta blockers remained free from syncope and cardiac arrest after a mean follow-up time of 5.4 years and showed a total mortality rate of 1%. Although beta blockers were generally considered to have lower efficacy in LQT2 patients as compared with LQT1 patients, recent data argue for a similar magnitude of risk reduction in LQT2 patients (beta blocker therapy decreased cardiac events from 58% to 23% after an average follow-up of 4.9 years on therapy). The higher residual event rate in LQT2 patients while receiving beta blocker therapy is likely due to a higher overall event rate in patients with this genotype, rather than to an attenuated efficacy of medical therapy in this high-risk population.[10,15] A recent report found that a trigger-specific response to beta blocker therapy exists within the LQT2 population. Beta blockers appear to be more protective against exercise-triggered cardiac events than arousal- or non–exercise-related events (see Fig. 31-1).[13]

On the other hand, LQT3 patients were not shown to have a significant benefit from beta blockers; in these patients, prolongation of the QT intervals is aggravated at slow heart rates. Thus, a reduction in heart rate with beta blockers can potentially pose a therapeutic problem in these patients. Among LQT3 patients receiving beta blocker therapy, the adjusted risk for a cardiac event is fourfold higher than among LQT1 patients.[12]

In summary, beta blockers comprise the mainstay therapy for the prevention of life-threatening cardiac events and, given the approximately 12% risk of SCD as the first manifestation of LQTS, they should be considered the first-line measure in all nongenotyped patients and in patients with LQT1 or LQT2 genotypes, regardless of their symptomatic or risk status. Recent data have argued against the routine empirical administration of beta blockers to all patients and advocated limiting therapy to high-risk patients (including LQT1 boys in the ≤14-year group, LQT2 women in the 15- to 40-year age group, patients with a history of syncope and/or documented torsades de pointes, and patients with a QTc ≥500 milliseconds), whereas low-risk LQT1 and LQT2 patients (including female LQT1 patients and LQT2 patients in the 0- to 14-year age group and LQT1 patients and LQT2 men in the 15- to 50-year age group, without prior syncope and with a QTc <500 milliseconds) are treated with beta blocker therapy on an individual basis, and routine initiation of medical therapy if they become symptomatic or if follow-up ECGs show an increase in QTc duration. That said, it is important to understand that all these recommendations are based on observational studies and not randomized clinical trials.[15]

Propranolol and nadolol are the beta blockers most frequently used, although different beta blockers (including atenolol and metoprolol) demonstrate similar effectiveness in preventing cardiac events in patients with LQTS. The protective effect of beta blockers is related to their adrenergic blockade that diminishes the risk of cardiac arrhythmias; hence, the goal of beta blocker therapy is to blunt the maximal heart rate during exercise, and the adequacy of beta blockade can be assessed by exercise testing or ambulatory monitoring. Beta blockers do not substantially shorten the QT interval.[32]

Despite the beneficial effects of beta blockers, a high rate of residual cardiac events has been reported in patients receiving beta blocker therapy, occurring in 10%, 23%, and 32% of LQT1, LQT2, and LQT3 patients, respectively, after a mean follow-up time of 5.4 years. Therefore, patients who remain symptomatic despite treatment with beta blockers should be considered for other therapeutic modalities.[57] Interestingly, it has been reported that lack of compliance can be an important cause of events occurring during beta blocker treatment in LQT1 patients.[10]

IMPLANTABLE CARDIOVERTER-DEFIBRILLATOR

ICD therapy is highly effective to prevent SCD in high-risk LQTS patients (mortality of 1.3% in high-risk ICD patients compared with 16% in non-ICD patients during a mean follow-up time of 8 years) and should be considered for secondary prevention in patients with prior cardiac arrest and for primary prevention in those who experience syncope and/or ventricular tachyarrhythmias while receiving beta blocker therapy.[4,14,54]

Although prophylactic ICD therapy can be considered for LQTS patients with risk factors for SCD (see Table 31-6) regardless of medical therapy, recent data suggest that high-risk LQT1 and LQT2 patients should be considered for prophylactic ICD implantation only if they develop recurrent cardiac events (e.g., syncope or torsades de pointes) despite beta blocker therapy or when compliance with or intolerance to medical therapy is a concern. Clear understanding by the patient and/or family of the relative merits of each strategy is essential. Although beta blocker therapy significantly reduces the risk of SCD in this population, it is not completely protective, and residual cardiac events still occur. On the other hand, data suggest that syncopal episodes almost always precede cardiac arrest in patients receiving beta blockers, allowing for institution of other therapeutic modalities, such as ICD implantation. Additionally, ICD therapy is not without complications. Infection, lead malfunction, inappropriate shocks, psychiatric sequelae, as well as device and lead longevity, especially in the young patient, have to be taken into consideration.[9,15,32,58]

Early ICD therapy should be considered in patients with the LQT3 genotype, Jervell and Lange-Nielsen syndrome, or Timothy syndrome because the lethality among these patients is high and the efficacy of beta blockers appears to be more limited.

It is important to recognize that a strong family history of SCD is not an independent risk factor for LQTS patients. Although prophylactic ICD implantation is a class IIb indication in these patients, personal risk factors should be considered before recommending prophylactic ICD implantation.

Importantly, because ICD therapy does not prevent the occurrence of arrhythmias, the concurrent administration of beta blockers is recommended for symptomatic and high-risk patients.

LEFT CERVICOTHORACIC SYMPATHECTOMY

Left cervicothoracic sympathectomy, which involves resection of the left stellate ganglion and the first two to four thoracic ganglia, is another antiadrenergic therapeutic measure used in high-risk patients with LQTS, especially in those with recurrent cardiac events despite beta blocker therapy. In addition to beta-adrenergic inhibition, cervicothoracic sympathetic denervation provides alpha-adrenergic inhibition, which may be important for some patients.

Although left cardiac sympathetic denervation is associated with a significant long-term reduction in the frequency of aborted cardiac arrest and syncope, it is not completely protective against SCD, with a residual mortality rate of 5% at 5 years. Therefore, ICD is superior therapy to cervicothoracic sympathectomy. Left cardiac sympathetic denervation is more effective in patients with LQT1 than in those with other types of LQTS.[12]

Cervicothoracic sympathectomy may be indicated in some high-risk patients with recurrent symptoms while receiving a full dose of beta blocker or those intolerant to beta blocker therapy, especially those in whom ICD implantation is not feasible (e.g., small infants). Additionally, cervicothoracic sympathectomy can be of value in ICD patients experiencing frequent shocks despite receiving adequate doses of beta blockers.[12]

PERMANENT PACEMAKER

Cardiac pacing, in conjunction with beta blocker therapy, can potentially reduce the risk of bradycardia-dependent QT prolongation, decrease heart-rate irregularities (eliminating short-long-short sequences), and reduce repolarization heterogeneity. Permanent pacemakers can be of value especially in patients who continue to be symptomatic despite beta blocker therapy or those in whom bradycardia or AV block limits the use of such therapy. In particular, patients with documented pause- or bradycardia-induced torsades de pointes and those with LQT3 genotype may derive significant benefit from cardiac pacing.[12]

Nevertheless, the high mortality in patients with recurrent symptoms (syncope or torsades de pointes) while receiving beta blocker therapy is not adequately attenuated by the addition of cardiac pacing. Therefore, if cardiac pacing is being considered, the use of an ICD is more logical, because it provides protection from SCD as well as the benefit of cardiac pacing.

When cardiac pacing is employed, atrial pacing is preferred, at a rate that shortens the QTc to less than 440 milliseconds. It is recommended to minimize ventricular pacing as much as possible, because it can potentially increase the heterogeneity of ventricular repolarization. However, in patients with AV block, ventricular pacing is important to maintain AV synchrony and elimination of ventricular pauses and long-short cycles.

CATHETER ABLATION

In LQTS patients, frequent episodes of torsades de pointes are occasionally triggered by focal, monomorphic PVCs. In this setting, focal radiofrequency (RF) ablation of the PVCs can be valuable in reducing the burden of arrhythmias and the frequency of ICD therapies.

LIFESTYLE MODIFICATIONS

Physical activity and stress-related emotions frequently trigger cardiac events in patients with LQTS, especially patients with LQT1 or LQT2. Therefore, all competitive sports (except those in the class IA category, such as billiards, bowling, cricket, and golf) should be restricted in symptomatic LQTS patients (regardless of the QTc duration or underlying genotype) as well as asymptomatic patients with baseline QT prolongation (QTc ≥470 milliseconds in men, ≥480 milliseconds in women). Swimming is particularly hazardous in LQT1 patients and should therefore be limited or performed under appropriate supervision, even in subjects with genotype-positive/phenotype-negative LQT1.[59]

Because many first cardiac events occur before the age of 15 years in male patients, particularly those with the LQT1 genotype, whereas female patients may experience first cardiac events after the age of 20 years, LQT1 men require stricter exercise restriction before the age of 15, but less restriction after age 15 years.[59]

The restriction limiting participation to class IA activities may be liberalized for the asymptomatic patient with genetically proven LQT3 genotype and those with genotype-positive/phenotype-negative LQTS (i.e., identification of an LQTS-associated mutation in an asymptomatic individual with a nondiagnostic QTc).[59]

Preventive measures in LQTS patients in general and LQT2 patients in particular include avoidance of unexpected auditory stimuli (such as alarm clocks and telephones), especially during rest or sleep.

All patients with LQTS should avoid drugs that prolong the QT interval or reduce their serum potassium or magnesium levels. Patients should consult with their physician before taking any medications or over-the-counter supplements. Families with LQTS may also consider basic life support training and operation of an automated external defibrillator.

GENE-SPECIFIC THERAPY

The standard therapeutic options for LQTS (including beta blockers, cardiac sympathetic denervation, ICD) rely on genotype to only a minor degree, yet are quite effective. Nevertheless, beta blockers and left cervicothoracic sympathectomy have some degree of genotype specificity, being quite effective in LQT1 and LQT2 and less effective in LQT3 (see Table 31-1). Similarly, behavior modification is most helpful in LQT1 and LQT2. For practical purposes, however, this apparent genotype specificity influences therapy decisions in only a very small number of patients.[12,27]

Gene-specific LQTS therapy is an area under investigation and appears to be promising, including Na^+ channel blockers, K^+ channel activators, alpha-adrenergic receptor blockers, protein-kinase inhibitors, and atropine. However, current experience with these drugs is limited.[12]

Intravenous nicorandil, an agent that promotes ATP-dependent K^+ channel (I_{KATP}) opening, has been shown to improve repolarization abnormalities and can potentially be of therapeutic value in suppressing repetitive episodes of torsades de pointes in the LQT1 and LQT2 patients and less efficiently in LQT3 patients. Unfortunately, oral administration of nicorandil reaches much lower plasma concentrations than those used in the experimental setting, thus limiting the potential for its clinical use.[27]

Mexiletine, a class IB Na^+ channel blocker, was shown to shorten the QT interval and was suggested as gene-specific therapy for patients with the LQT3 genotype, in whom enhanced late Na^+ inward current underlies prolongation of the QT interval. However, the response to mexiletine was not consistent and was shown to be mutation-specific. Furthermore, there is no conclusive evidence that shortening of the QT interval in these patients translates into a clinical benefit. Until prospective clinical trials confirm the effectiveness of mexiletine, it should be used in LQT3 patients only in conjunction with beta blockers or with the backup of an ICD. In addition, some investigators recommend testing the effectiveness of mexiletine by the administration of half the daily dose during continuous ECG monitoring. Only if the QTc is shortened by more than 40 milliseconds within 90 minutes of drug administration (when the peak plasma concentration is reached) should mexiletine be added to beta blocker therapy.[12,27]

Similarly, the antianginal agent ranolazine reduces late Na^+ current, shortens the action potential duration, and suppresses EAD-triggered arrhythmias in animal models of LQT3, and can potentially offer a therapeutic benefit in LQT3 patients.[12]

Additionally, flecainide, a class IC Na^+ channel blocker, was shown to shorten the QT interval in LQT3 patients with a specific mutation (D1790G) in the *SCN5A* gene. However, flecainide is reported to elicit a Brugada phenotype in some LQT3 patients; therefore, this drug should not be used in LQT3 patients except for those with this specific *SCN5A* mutation.[12]

Potassium supplements can be of value especially in LQT2 patients, who are particularly sensitive to low K^+ levels because the conductance of KCNH2 channels is directly related to extracellular K^+ concentrations. Therefore, efforts should be made to maintain a serum K^+ level greater than or equal to 4 mEq/L in patients with this genotype. Acute intravenous treatment with K^+ can be effective in suppressing torsades de pointes. Furthermore, long-term oral potassium supplements, even in patients with normal K^+ levels at baseline, can potentially reduce repolarization abnormalities in LQT2. Increasing extracellular K^+ concentrations enhances I_{Kr} and at least partially compensates for the loss of I_{Kr} in LQT2 and can potentially limit the development of an arrhythmogenic substrate under long QT conditions. Whether these effects translate into clinical benefit in reduction of the risk of cardiac events is still unclear.[12,15]

FAMILY SCREENING

Timely (often presymptomatic) identification of disease carriers is important because preventive measures and therapies can effectively avert SCD.[27] Therefore, when a patient is diagnosed with LQTS, ECGs should be obtained on all first-degree family members (i.e., parents, siblings, offspring) to determine whether others are affected. Unexplained sudden death in a young individual should trigger a similar evaluation to determine if LQTS is present in the family.[5]

When the causal mutation has been identified in the proband, first-degree relatives should be offered genetic screening, even those with a negative clinical and ECG phenotype.[36,41] Genotyping of family members can help exclude the diagnosis in some persons as well as identify silent mutation carriers and allow prophylactic treatment.[7] However, detailed genetic counseling is warranted before proceeding to this testing, particularly for asymptomatic persons for whom the option of not testing must also be recognized.[32]

Brugada Syndrome

The Brugada syndrome is an autosomal dominant inherited channelopathy characterized by ST segment elevation or J wave in the right precordial leads. First described in 1992, the syndrome is associated with a high incidence of SCD secondary to a rapid polymorphic VT or VF in patients with structurally normal hearts.

Epidemiology

The prevalence of the Brugada ECG pattern in an apparently healthy population is varied, ranging from 0.14% in the Japanese population to 0.61% in Europeans, and may reach as high as 3% in endemic areas of Southeast Asia. In the United States, the prevalence ranges from 0.012% to 0.43%, depending on the demographics of the patient population studied. However, because the aberrant ECG pattern can be intermittently present or concealed, it is difficult to estimate the true prevalence of the disease in the general population.[60,61] For unclear reasons, the Brugada syndrome is either more prevalent or more penetrant in Eastern countries (mainly in Southeast Asia), where the disease occurs endemically.[62]

The Brugada syndrome exhibits an autosomal dominant pattern of transmission and variable penetrance. In up to 60% of patients the disease can be sporadic, that is, absent in parents and other relatives. A family history of unexplained SCD is present in approximately 20% to 40% of Brugada probands in Western countries and in a lower percentage of probands (15% to 20%) in Japan.

Although the disease is inherited as an autosomal dominant trait, there is a striking male predominance in its phenotype (ratio of men to women, 8:1). It remains unknown why men have a more penetrant form of the disease. Although gene mutations provide a proarrhythmic substrate, the adult male dominance of clinical manifestation suggests that gender- and age-related factors (e.g., sex hormones) may play a role in triggering the arrhythmia in Brugada syndrome.[61,63,64]

The age of onset of clinical manifestations (syncope or cardiac arrest) is the third to fourth decade of life (mean age of SCD occurrence, 41 ± 15 years), but cases have been diagnosed in infancy and in patients in their 80s.[61,65]

Clinical Presentation

Patients with Brugada syndrome are at high risk of rapid polymorphic VT, VF, and SCD. Syncope, agonal respirations, nocturnal labored respiration with agitation, and "seizures" are the only symptoms the patient may have before SCD occurs.

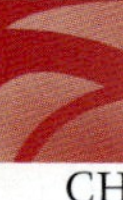

The Brugada syndrome is the leading cause of death in men not more than 40 years of age, particularly in countries in which the syndrome is endemic. The Brugada syndrome is believed to be responsible for 4% to 12% of all SCDs, and at least 20% of those occurring in patients with structurally normal hearts. The Brugada syndrome has even been described as responsible for SIDS as well as the sudden unexplained nocturnal death syndrome (SUNDS; also known as SUDS).[62,65] Nevertheless, the majority of Brugada syndrome patients do not manifest life-threatening events; approximately 10% to 15% of clinically affected patients experience one or more cardiac arrests before age 60.[61] In a meta-analysis of prognostic studies, patients with Brugada ECG pattern have an approximately 10% risk of SCD, syncope, or ICD shock at an average follow-up time of 2.5 years, or approximately 3.8% per year.[66]

Cardiac arrhythmia and death in the Brugada syndrome seem to occur largely in the early morning hours during sleep and in the setting of bradycardia. Circadian variation of sympathovagal balance, hormones, and other metabolic factors are likely to contribute to this circadian pattern. Bradycardia resulting from altered autonomic balance or other factors likely contributes to the initiation of arrhythmia.[65]

Some episodes of syncope or SCD can be triggered by fever, large meals (gastric distention), alcohol and cocaine toxicity, and drugs.[62] In fact, it now appears that many previously described episodes of "febrile seizures" may in fact represent bouts of polymorphic VT in patients with temperature-sensitive mutations.[67,68] Some patients with the Brugada syndrome experience an electrical storm of VF, but with no obvious precipitating factors.

Approximately 20% of patients with Brugada syndrome develop supraventricular arrhythmias. AF is observed in 10% to 20% of patients. Atrioventricular nodal reentrant tachycardia and Wolff-Parkinson-White syndrome also have been reported. A recent study reported that inducibility of ventricular arrhythmias is positively correlated with a history of atrial arrhythmias. In patients with an indication for an ICD, the incidence of atrial arrhythmias was 27% versus 13% in patients without an indication for an ICD, which suggests a more advanced disease process in patients with Brugada syndrome and spontaneous atrial arrhythmias.[65]

The identification of concomitant conduction defects (PR interval ≥210 milliseconds and His bundle–ventricular [HV] interval ≥60 milliseconds) has been shown to correlate with the presence of *SCN5A* mutations. Therefore, all *SCN5A*-positive patients should be closely monitored for the onset of conduction block.

Electrocardiographic Features

BRUGADA ST SEGMENT ELEVATION

Three ECG repolarization patterns in the right precordial leads are recognized (Fig. 31-4). Type 1 is characterized by ST segment elevation of at least 2 mm (0.2 mV) with a coved (downward convex) morphology, associated with an incomplete or complete right bundle branch block (RBBB) pattern and followed by a descending negative T wave, with little or no isoelectric separation. The type 2 pattern has a "saddleback" appearance with a high take-off ST segment elevation of at least 2 mm, a trough displaying an ST elevation greater than or equal to 1 mm, and then either a positive or biphasic T wave. The type 3 pattern has either a saddleback or coved appearance with an ST segment elevation of less than 1 mm. These three patterns can be observed spontaneously in serial ECG tracings from the same patient or after the introduction of specific drugs. Only the type 1 ECG pattern is diagnostic of the Brugada syndrome, with type 2 and type 3 ECG patterns being suggestive but not specific.[62,65]

The use of more cephalad placement of the right precordial leads in a superior position (up to the second intercostal space above normal) can increase the sensitivity for detecting the Brugada ECG pattern in some patients, both in the presence or absence of a drug

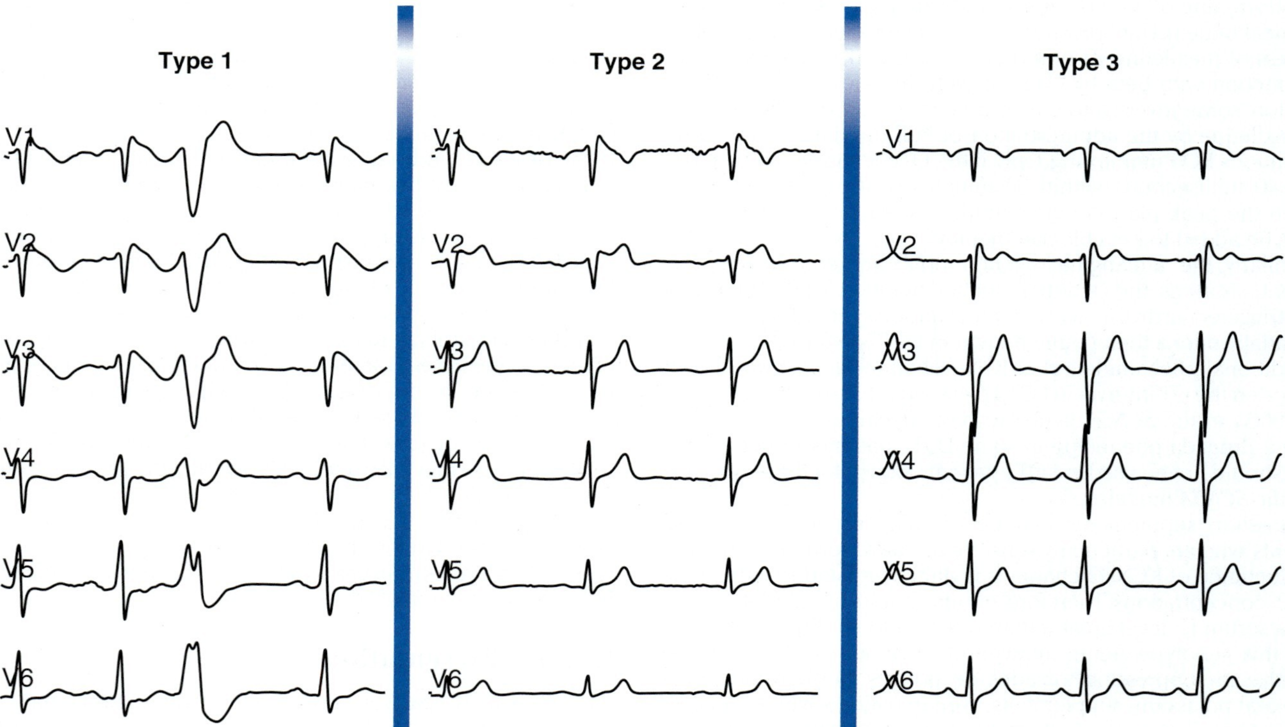

FIGURE 31-4 Brugada ECG patterns. Note the ventricular ectopic beat in the left panel with a QRS morphology consistent with origin from the right ventricular outflow tract. See text for discussion.

challenge. Recent data suggest that patients with a diagnostic ECG with the leads positioned at a higher position have a prognosis similar to that of individuals with a type 1 ECG recorded using the standard position.[65,69]

The presence of the type 1 pattern is dynamic, and it is rare for patients to present with uniformly diagnostic tracings. Therefore, serial ECGs can be necessary for diagnostic evaluation in high-risk patients. Continuous Holter monitoring also can help assess ST segment elevation at nighttime, because such changes can be modified by autonomic tone.[61]

The ECG manifestations of the Brugada syndrome, when concealed, can be unmasked by stress, fever, various vagal stimuli (including gastric distention), vagotonic agents, a combination of glucose and insulin, hyperkalemia, hypokalemia, hypercalcemia, alcohol and cocaine toxicity, class I antiarrhythmic medications, as well as a number of other noncardiac medications.[65]

Furthermore, the ECG phenotype in the Brugada syndrome can be modified by autonomic changes. Adrenergic stimulation attenuates whereas acetylcholine accentuates the ECG abnormalities in affected individuals. Clinically, this correlates well with the propensity for cardiac events to occur at rest or during sleep.[61]

QT INTERVAL PROLONGATION

A slight prolongation of the QT interval is sometimes observed in association with ST segment elevation in patients with the Brugada syndrome. The QT interval is prolonged more in the right precordial leads than it is in the left precordial leads, presumably because of a preferential prolongation of action potential duration in right ventricular (RV) epicardium secondary to accentuation of the action potential notch.

QRS FRAGMENTATION

In addition to the repolarization abnormality, the Brugada syndrome is associated with depolarization abnormalities and conduction disturbances. Fragmentation of the QRS complex (manifesting as multiple small spikes within the QRS complex) has been recently observed in 40% of patients with the Brugada syndrome and in the majority (85%) of those who had VF episodes. It has been proposed that the multiple spikes within the fragmented QRS complex suggest the presence of an arrhythmogenic substrate that has multiple areas of conduction slowing, and can potentially predict a high risk of life-threatening ventricular arrhythmias. Notably, fragmentation of the QRS occurs preferentially in the right precordial leads, especially in the higher intercostal spaces, suggesting a localized conduction abnormality within the RV outflow tract (RVOT) region. The use of a low-pass filter with a low cutoff frequency (>25 Hz), as commonly employed to remove the electromyogram signal, can eliminate the QRS fragmentation. Thus, low-noise amplifier and a relatively high cutoff low-pass filter frequency (150 Hz) need to be used.[70]

Epsilon-like waves and localized prolongation of the QRS complex in the right precordial leads have been observed in some patients with a spontaneous or drug-induced type 1 Brugada ECG pattern, likely reflecting RV activation delay.[71]

CONDUCTION ABNORMALITIES

Depolarization abnormalities, including prolongation of P wave duration, PR interval, and QRS duration, are frequently observed, particularly in patients linked to *SCN5A* mutations. PR interval prolongation likely reflects HV conduction delay. Of note, loss-of-function *SCN5A* mutations can lead to isolated cardiac conduction defects or Lev-Lenègre disease, characterized by disturbances in any part of the conduction system without QT interval prolongation or Brugada ST segment elevation. Additionally, prolonged sinus node recovery time and sinoatrial conduction time, slowed atrial conduction, and atrial standstill have been reported in association with the syndrome.[61,65]

SIGNAL-AVERAGED ELECTROCARDIOGRAPHY

Signal-averaged ECG demonstrates late potentials in approximately 60% to 70% of clinically affected Brugada syndrome patients. In this setting, late potentials can be a clinical marker of the disease, representing the delayed second upstroke of the epicardial action potential, a local phase 2 reentry (failing to trigger transmural reentry), or an intraventricular conduction delay.[61,65]

EXERCISE TESTING

Treadmill exercise testing can potentially aggravate the ECG abnormalities in the Brugada syndrome, including widening of the QRS, prolongation of the QTc duration, and augmentation of precordial peak ST segment elevation (which reaches its maximal amplitude during the early phase of recovery from exercise). Nonetheless, exercise was not found to induce ventricular arrhythmia in Brugada patients.[72]

Diagnosis of the Brugada Syndrome

DIAGNOSTIC CRITERIA

The diagnosis of Brugada syndrome is based on clinical diagnostic criteria. The Brugada syndrome is definitively diagnosed when type 1 ST segment elevation is observed in more than one right precordial lead (V_1 to V_3), in conjunction with one of the following: (1) documented VF; (2) polymorphic VT; (3) a family history of SCD at age less than 45 years; (4) coved-type ECGs in family members; (5) inducibility of VT with programmed electrical stimulation; (6) syncope; or (7) nocturnal agonal respiration.[65]

The diagnosis of Brugada syndrome is also considered positive when type 2 (saddleback pattern) or type 3 ST segment elevation is observed in more than one right precordial lead under baseline conditions and conversion to the diagnostic type 1 pattern occurs after administration of a Na^+ channel blocker. One or more of the clinical criteria described above also should be present. Drug-induced conversion of type 3 to type 2 ST segment elevation is considered inconclusive for a diagnosis of Brugada syndrome.[65,73]

PROVOCATIVE DRUG TESTING

When concealed, the ECG characteristics of the Brugada syndrome can be unmasked by potent Na^+ channel blockers (class IA or IC agents). Provocative drug testing is generally not performed if a patient displays an intermittently spontaneous type 1 ECG, because the test does not offer additional diagnostic or prognostic value in these patients, and it is not devoid of risk for provoking arrhythmic events.

The drug challenge test involves administration of ajmaline, flecainide, procainamide, or pilsicainide (Table 31-7) under close cardiac monitoring and in a setting that is fully equipped for resuscitation. Procainamide remains the only choice for intravenous pharmacological induction protocols in the United States, despite consensus that both ajmaline and flecainide are more efficacious and are likely safer because of shorter half-life.[74]

TABLE 31-7 Drugs Used to Unmask Brugada ECG Pattern

DRUG	DOSE
Ajmaline	1-mg/kg IV infusion over 5 min
Flecainide	2-mg/kg IV infusion over 10 min, maximum 150 mg; or 400 mg oral
Procainamide	10-mg/kg IV infusion over 10 min
Pilsicainide	1-mg/kg IV infusion over 10 min

IV = intravenous.

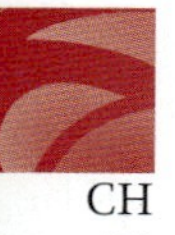

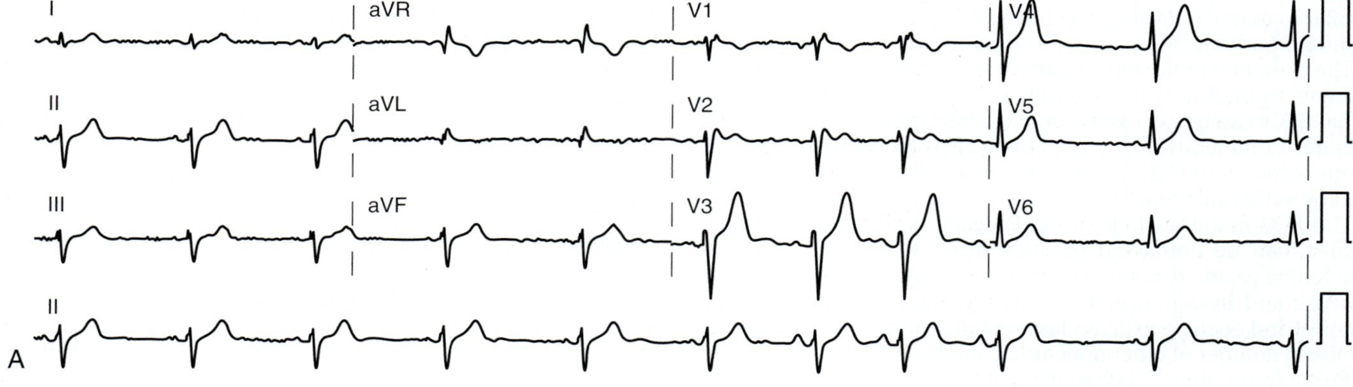

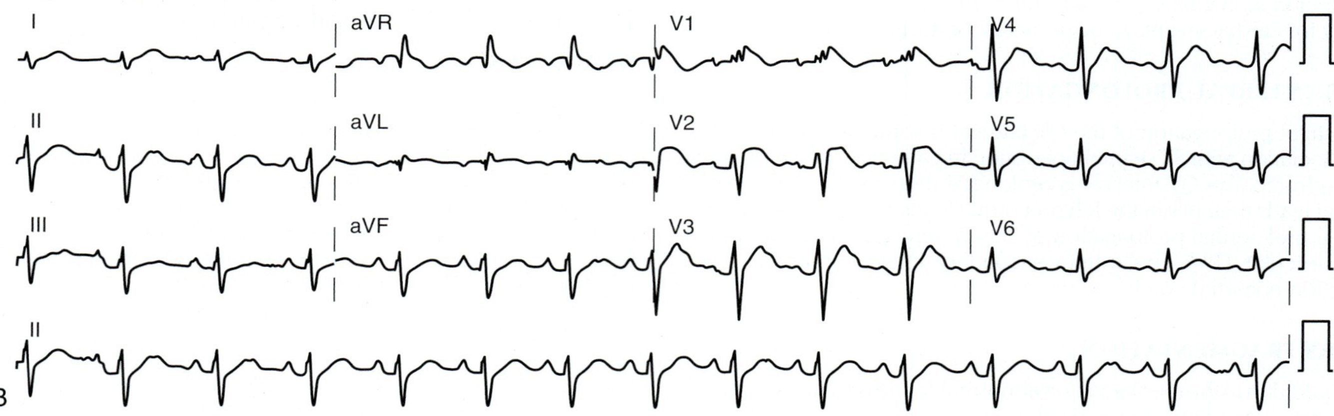

FIGURE 31-5 Brugada ECG patterns. **A,** ECG showing type 3 Brugada ECG pattern at baseline. **B,** Type 1 Brugada ECG pattern developed post administration of flecainide.

The drug challenge test is terminated when (1) the diagnostic type 1 ST segment elevation develops (Fig. 31-5), (2) the ST segment elevation in type 2 ECG pattern increases by at least 2 mm, (3) PVCs or other arrhythmias develop, or (4) the QRS widens by 30% or more. Although the drug challenge test is generally safe, it can potentially precipitate malignant cardiac arrhythmias or advanced AV block, particularly in patients with preexisting intraventricular conduction disturbances (wide QRS complex) or infranodal AV conduction delay. Isoproterenol and sodium lactate can be effective antidotes in this setting. The sensitivity and specificity of flecainide testing have recently been estimated at 77% and 80%, respectively. Of note, quinidine, a class IA antiarrhythmic and a Na^+ channel blocker, generally normalizes ST elevation in Brugada syndrome patients owing to its potent I_{to}-blocking effect.[61,65,69,73]

GENETIC TESTING

Diagnostic genetic testing may be considered for patients who clinically manifest with symptoms of the Brugada syndrome. Although the knowledge of a specific mutation may not provide guidance for determining prognosis or treatment, identification of a disease-causing mutation in the family can lead to genetic identification of at-risk family members who are clinically asymptomatic and who may have normal ECG. However, it is important to remember that a negative result of genetic testing does not exclude the presence of the disease and, therefore, only a positive genetic diagnosis is informative.[65,75] Genetic screening of *SCN5A* in unselected patients with diagnosis of Brugada syndrome has low yield and may not be cost-effective. Only 13% of patients with spontaneous or drug-induced type 1 Brugada ECG pattern, 4% of those with type 2 or 3 Brugada ECG pattern, and 2% of individuals with idiopathic VF or family history of SCD are genotyped on *SCN5A*. The yield of genotyping increases substantially in patients with type 1 Brugada ECG pattern and prolonged PR interval, suggesting that this subset of patients with Brugada syndrome should be screened.[75] Genetic testing is not indicated in the setting of an isolated type 2 or type 3 Brugada ECG pattern.[41]

Genetics of the Brugada Syndrome

The Brugada syndrome is a channelopathy that causes current dysfunction in those channels participating in the generation of the cardiac action potential. *SCN5A*, the gene that encodes the alpha subunit ($Na_v1.5$) of the cardiac Na^+ channel, was the first gene linked to Brugada syndrome. Although most mutations occur in *SCN5A*, mutations in other genes related to the Na^+ current as well as genes that affect L-type Ca^{2+} channels (I_{CaL}) or transient outward K^+ channels (I_{to}) have been identified in patients with the Brugada syndrome (Table 31-8). These channelopathies cause Brugada syndrome phenotype by attenuating I_{Na}, attenuating I_{CaL}, and/or enhancing I_{to}. However, the relationships between genotype and phenotype are not always predictive. Mutations in different genes can express similar Brugada syndrome phenotypes. Conversely, mutations in the same gene can lead to different syndromes.[62,63,65]

On the other hand, the failure to identify gene mutations in most patients with the Brugada syndrome suggests that unknown mutations or pathophysiological cellular regulations (such as post-translational modulations, phosphorylation, glycosylation) may also cause similar ion current defects and clinical manifestations.[63]

TABLE 31-8 Molecular Basis of the Brugada Syndrome

DISEASE	GENE	PROTEIN	IONIC CURRENT	FUNCTION	INHERITANCE
BrS type 1	*SCN5A*	$Na_v1.5$	Subunit alpha I_{Na}	Loss	Autosomal dominant
BrS type 2	*GPD1L*	G3PD1L	Interaction subunit alpha I_{Na}	Loss	Autosomal dominant
BrS type 3	*CACNA1C*	$Ca_v1.2$	Subunit alpha I_{CaL}	Loss	Autosomal dominant
BrS type 4	*CACNB2B*	$Ca_v\beta_2$	Subunit beta I_{CaL}	Loss	Autosomal dominant
BrS type 5	*SCN1B*	$Na_v\beta_1/\beta_{1b}$	Subunit beta I_{Na}	Loss	Autosomal dominant
BrS type 6	*KCNE3*	MiRP2	Subunit beta I_{Ks}/I_{to}	Gain	Autosomal dominant
BrS type 7	*SCN3B*	$Na_v\beta_3$	Subunit beta I_{Na}	Loss	Autosomal dominant

BrS = Brugada syndrome; I_{CaL} = L-type Ca^{2+} current; I_{Ks} = slowly activating delayed rectifier K^+ current; I_{Na} = Na^+ current; I_{to} = transient outward K^+ current.

MUTATIONS RELATED TO THE SODIUM CURRENT

On average 18% to 30% of cases of the Brugada syndrome can be attributed to loss-of-function mutations in the *SCN5A* gene, which encodes the alpha subunit ($Na_v1.5$) of the cardiac voltage-gated Na^+ channel, resulting in a reduction of the depolarizing inward sodium current (I_{Na}). A higher incidence of *SCN5A* mutations has been reported in familial than in sporadic cases. I_{Na} initiates the ventricular action potential, thereby controlling cardiac excitability and electric conduction velocity.[62]

So far, more than 200 Brugada syndrome-associated mutations have been described in the *SCN5A* gene. Some of these mutations result in loss of function due to impaired channel trafficking to the cell membrane, disrupted ion conductance, or altered gating function. Most of the mutations are missense mutations, whereby a single amino acid is replaced by a different amino acid. Missense mutations commonly alter the gating properties of mutant channels. Because virtually all reported *SCN5A* mutation carriers are heterozygous, mutant channels with altered gating can result in an up to 50% reduction of I_{Na}. Different *SCN5A* mutations can cause different degrees of I_{Na} reduction and, hence, different levels of severity of the clinical phenotype of the Brugada syndrome.[62,65,66]

SCN5A loss-of-function mutations have also been linked to patients with progressive cardiac conduction system disease (Lev-Lenègre disease). Mutated *SCN5A* can also impede the closure (gain of function) of the Na^+ channel, leading to type 3 LQTS (LQT3). It was reported that all three syndromes (Brugada syndrome, LQT3, and Lev-Lenègre disease) occurred within a single family because of a single mutated *SCN5A* gene. Approximately 65% of mutations identified in the *SCN5A* gene are associated with the Brugada syndrome phenotype.[63]

Compared with Brugada patients without an *SCN5A* mutation, those with *SCN5A* mutations generally exhibit longer and progressive conduction delays (PQ, QRS, and HV intervals), frequent occurrences of fragmented QRS complex, and ventricular arrhythmias of extra-RVOT origin.[63]

In addition to *SCN5A* mutations, reduction in I_{Na} can be caused by mutations in the *SCN1B* gene (encoding the beta$_1$ and beta$_{1b}$ subunits of the Na^+ channel) and the *SCN3B* gene (encoding the beta$_3$ subunit of the Na^+ channel), resulting in Brugada syndrome type 5 and type 7, respectively.[62,63]

Furthermore, mutations in the *GPD1L* (glycerol-3-phosphate dehydrogenase 1-like) gene, which encodes the protein glycerol-3-phosphate dehydrogenase 1-like (G3PD1L), affect the trafficking of the cardiac Na^+ channel to the cell surface, resulting in reduction of I_{Na} and "type 2" Brugada syndrome.[62] Brugada syndrome associated with *GPD1L* gene mutations is characterized by progressive conduction disease, low sensitivity to procainamide, and a relatively good prognosis.[63]

MUTATIONS RELATED TO THE CALCIUM CURRENT

Approximately 11% to 12% of cases of the Brugada syndrome are attributable to loss-of-function mutations in the cardiac Ca^{2+} channel resulting in a reduction of the depolarizing I_{CaL}. Brugada syndrome type 3 is caused by mutations in the *CACNA1C* gene, which encodes the pore-forming alpha$_1$ subunit ($Ca_v1.2$) of the L-type voltage-gated Ca^{2+} channel. Brugada syndrome type 4 is caused by mutations in the *CACNB2* gene, which encodes for the regulatory beta$_2$ subunit ($Ca_v\beta_2$) of $Ca_v1.2$, which modifies gating of I_{CaL}. The mechanism of Brugada syndrome type 3 and type 4 involves a reduction of the depolarizing I_{CaL}. Mutations in the alpha and beta subunits of the Ca^{2+} channel can also lead to a shorter than normal QT interval, creating a new clinical entity consisting of combined Brugada/SQTS.[62]

MUTATIONS RELATED TO THE POTASSIUM CURRENT

Gain-of-function mutations in the *KCNE3* gene, which encodes the auxiliary beta subunit (MiRP2) of the transient outward K^+ channel ($K_v4.3$), results in an increase in I_{to} density and causes Brugada syndrome type 6.[53,62,63]

Pathophysiology of the Brugada Syndrome

MECHANISM OF BRUGADA ECG PATTERN

The ST-T wave changes in Brugada syndrome likely reflect a profound change in the process of ventricular repolarization, particularly in the relationship between the endocardial and epicardial repolarization processes. The cellular basis for this phenomenon is thought to be the result of loss of function of Na^+ channels (reduced I_{Na}) that differentially alters the action potential morphology in epicardial versus endocardial cells.[47,63]

I_{to} is a prominent repolarizing current; it partially repolarizes the membrane, shaping rapid (phase 1) repolarization of the action potential, setting the height of the initial plateau (phase 2), and resulting in a pronounced action potential notch and, in combination with depolarizing Ca^{2+} currents, in a "spike-and-dome" morphology. I_{to} channel densities are heterogeneously distributed across the myocardial wall and in different regions of the heart, being much higher in the RV than in the LV, in the epicardium than in the endocardium, and nearer the base than the apex of the ventricles. These regional differences are responsible for the shorter duration, the prominent phase 1 notch, and the "spike and dome" morphology of RV epicardial and midmyocardial action potentials compared with endocardium and LV. A prominent I_{to}-mediated action potential notch in ventricular epicardium but not endocardium produces a transmural voltage gradient during early ventricular repolarization that registers as a J wave or J point elevation on the ECG (Fig. 31-6).[76,77]

Na^+ channel malfunction and reduction of I_{Na} associated with the Brugada syndrome accentuate the notch produced by I_{to}, leading to partial or complete loss of the action potential dome, premature repolarization, and significant action potential shortening, presumably by deactivation or voltage modulation that reduces I_{CaL}. These changes occur predominantly in regions where I_{to} is abundant (such as RVOT epicardium). In contrast, endocardial

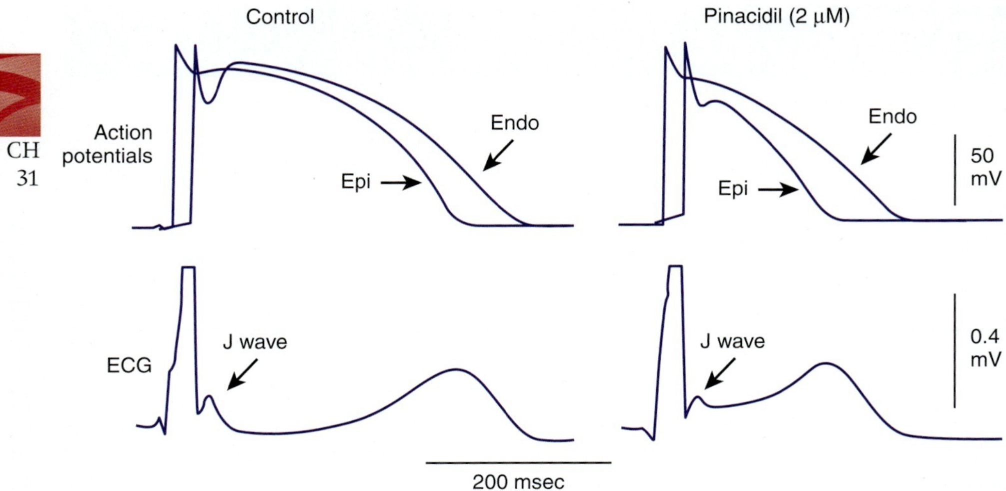

FIGURE 31-6 Cellular basis for the early repolarization syndrome. Shown are a simultaneous recording of transmembrane action potentials from epicardial (Epi) and endocardial (Endo) regions and a transmural ECG in an isolated arterially perfused canine left ventricular wedge. The J wave on the transmural ECG is manifest because of the presence of an action potential notch in epicardium but not endocardium. Pinacidil, an ATP-sensitive K^+ channel opener, causes depression of the action potential dome in epicardium, resulting in ST segment elevation on the ECG resembling the early repolarization syndrome. *(Reproduced with permission from Yan GX, Lankipalli RS, Burke JF, et al: Ventricular repolarization components on the electrocardiogram: cellular basis and clinical significance, J Am Coll Cardiol 42:401-409, 2003.)*

cells display a much smaller I_{to} and, consequently, I_{Na} reduction would not significantly affect action potential morphology and duration.[62] This is likely to manifest on the ECG as an early repolarization pattern consisting of a J point elevation, slurring of the terminal part of the QRS, and mild ST segment elevation. A further increase in net repolarizing current can result in complete loss of the action potential dome in the RVOT epicardium, leading to more pronounced dispersion of repolarization (epicardial repolarization precedes repolarization in endocardial regions) and a transmural voltage gradient that manifests as greater ST segment elevation.[62,76]

Additionally, the reduction in I_{Na} observed in Brugada syndrome linked to an *SCN5A* mutation leads to a reduction in the upstroke velocity of action potential phase 0, and, as a result, slowing in atrial and ventricular electrical conduction. Conduction slowing preferentially involves the RVOT. This often is reflected by prolongation in atrioventricular and intraventricular conduction intervals (PR and HV intervals and QRS duration) on the ECGs of Brugada syndrome patients with an *SCN5A* mutation. Slowed transmural conduction (which preferentially involves the RVOT) likely contributes to ST elevation by delaying epicardial activation, thus increasing the transmural gradient of the membrane potential.[47,63]

MECHANISM OF VENTRICULAR ARRHYTHMIAS

The excessive increase in intramural dispersion of repolarization (between epicardium and endocardium) facilitates reentrant excitation waves between depolarized endocardium and prematurely repolarized epicardium. A significant outward shift in current can cause a prominent action potential notch causing more negative potentials during phase 1 of the action potential and loss of activation of I_{CaL}. As a consequence, loss of the action potential dome and marked abbreviation of the action potential develop in regions where I_{to} is prominent (epicardium) but not in other locations. The dome then can propagate from regions where it is maintained to regions where it is lost, giving rise to a very closely coupled extrasystole (phase 2 reentry) that in turn can initiate polymorphic VT or VF (Fig. 31-7).

Although the repolarization abnormalities facilitate the onset of polymorphic VT, it is the depolarization disturbance (conduction slowing leading to wave break of the reentrant wave) that allows the VT to become sustained and to degenerate to VF. Because the RVOT is the critical area associated with depolarization and repolarization abnormalities, it is a frequent origin of VT and VF in the setting of Brugada syndrome (see Fig. 31-4).[47,62,78]

MECHANISM OF AGE AND GENDER EFFECTS

The effects of gender on the Brugada syndrome phenotype (being more prevalent in men) may be due to intrinsic differences in Na^+ channel expression between men and women (e.g., higher I_{to} densities in men) or due to differences in hormone levels (e.g., higher testosterone levels in men). The phase 1 notch potentially mediates the effects of sex hormones on the phenotypic expressions of Na^+ channel dysfunction, thus contributing to the male predominance of Brugada syndrome. Estrogen suppresses the expression of the $K_v4.3$ channel, resulting in reduced I_{to} and a shallow phase 1 notch, whereas testosterone enhances the outward currents (I_{Kr}, I_{Ks}, I_{K1}) and reduces the inward current (I_{CaL}), thus deepening the phase 1 notch.[47,63,64]

MECHANISM OF TEMPERATURE SENSITIVITY

The exact mechanism by which fever triggers arrhythmias in Brugada syndrome remains unknown. Mutations responsible for Brugada syndrome can potentially alter the temperature sensitivity of fast inactivation of the Na^+ channel (e.g., more slow inactivation at higher temperatures). Alternatively, temperature elevation can potentially result in a positive shift of steady-state activation, acceleration of inactivation, and slow recovery from inactivation in both wild and mutant Na^+ channels, resulting in I_{Na} reduction, deepening of the phase 1 notch of the action potential, and aggravation of the Brugada syndrome.[47,63,68,79]

MECHANISM OF EXERCISE-INDUCED CHANGES

Mechanisms that underlie ECG responses in the Brugada syndrome to exercise are complex, which may be related to different molecular-genetic mutations underlying the Brugada syndrome phenotype. Exercise testing can potentially aggravate the ECG abnormalities in the Brugada syndrome. However, other factors (e.g., autonomic nervous system, ion current imbalances) also play a role. Nonetheless, exercise was not found to induce ventricular arrhythmia in Brugada patients.[47,72]

Brugada syndrome–linked loss-of-function mutations in *SCN5A* reduce I_{Na} more during tachycardia, likely secondary to accumulation of mutant Na^+ channels in the slow inactivated state. Na^+ channels activate on depolarization and inactivate within milliseconds thereafter. Before reopening, channels must recover from inactivation during diastole. At fast heart rates, the diastolic interval becomes too short for mutant channels to completely recover from the slow inactivated state, resulting in decreased availability of open channels and, as a consequence, accentuation of Na^+ channel loss of function produced by *SCN5A* mutations.[47,72]

MECHANISM OF DRUG EFFECTS

Pharmacological agents that primarily block I_{Na} but not I_{to} (flecainide, ajmaline, and procainamide) can further diminish I_{Na} that is already reduced by the Brugada mutations. This may explain the

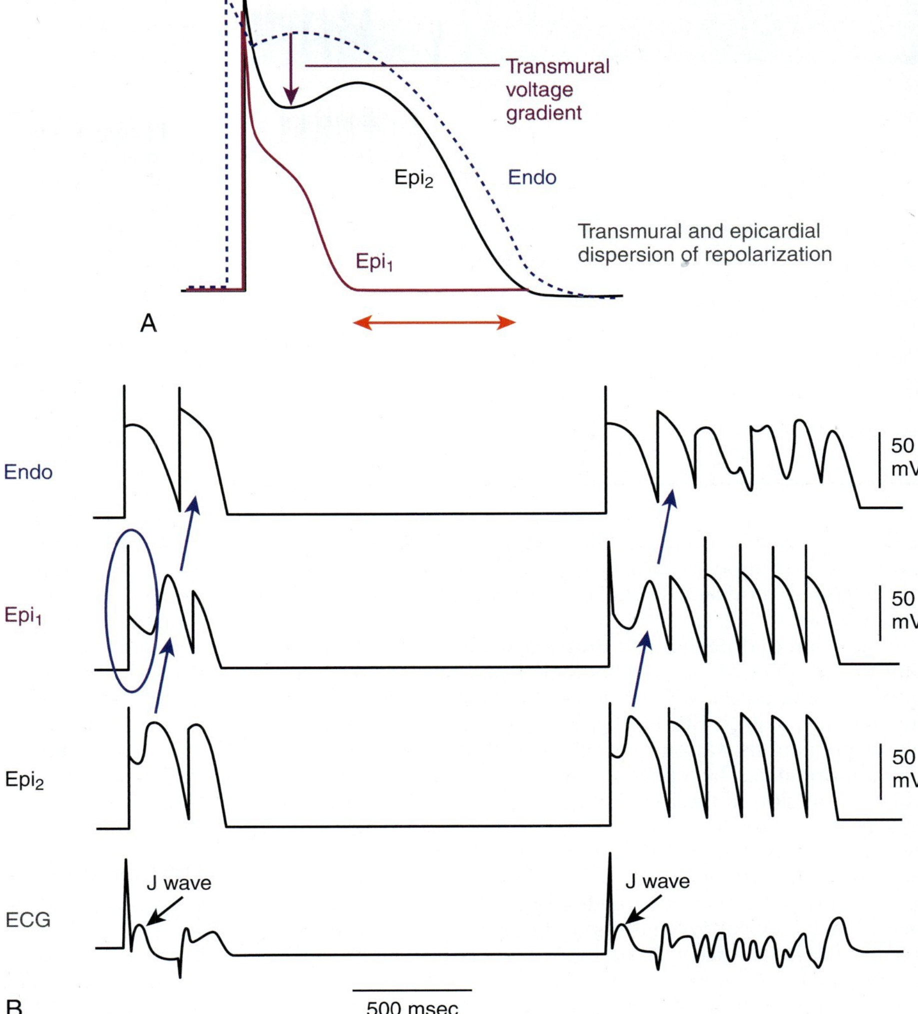

FIGURE 31-7 Potential mechanism for arrhythmogenesis in the Brugada and early repolarization syndromes. **A,** With enhanced repolarization in regions with prominent transient outward current (I_{to}), all-or-none repolarization can occur, creating a substrate for arrhythmias. **B,** Simultaneous action potentials from two epicardial sites (Epi_1 and Epi_2) and one endocardial site (Endo), and surface ECG. A loss of the action potential dome in Epi_1, but not in Epi_2, leads to apparent propagation of the dome from Epi_2 to Epi_1, inducing reentry. *(Reproduced with permission from Benito B, Guasch E, Rivard L, Nattel S: Clinical and mechanistic issues in early repolarization of normal variants and lethal arrhythmia syndromes, J Am Coll Cardiol 56:1177-1186, 2010.)*

use of Na^+ channel blockers to unmask concealed forms of the Brugada syndrome and the potential proarrhythmic adverse effects of these and other pharmacological agents. In contrast, quinidine, in addition to blocking I_{Na}, has a relatively strong effect in blocking I_{to}. Hence, quinidine can effectively suppress ST elevation and ventricular arrhythmias in patients with the Brugada syndrome.[64]

Beta-adrenergic stimulation induces increased inward I_{CaL} and attenuates the excess of outward current, resulting in reduction of ST segment elevation in right precordial leads and potentially underlying the therapeutic benefit observed for isoproterenol infusion for prevention of ventricular arrhythmias in Brugada syndrome patients with electrical storm. In contrast, acetylcholine facilitates the loss of the action potential dome by suppressing I_{CaL} and/or augmenting K^+ current.[80]

Differential Diagnosis

A variety of pharmacological agents and conditions have been reported to produce a Brugada-like ST segment elevation, although the likelihood of arrhythmias is unclear. In general, factors that increase outward currents (e.g., I_{to}, I_{KATP}, I_{Kr}, I_{Ks}) or decrease inward currents (e.g., I_{Na}, I_{CaL}) at the end of phase 1 of the action potential can potentially accentuate or unmask ST segment elevation similar to the ECG pattern observed in patients with the Brugada syndrome.

Among antiarrhythmic drugs, class IC agents (flecainide, propafenone, pilsicainide) most effectively amplify or unmask ST segment elevation, owing to their strong use-dependent blocking effect of the fast I_{Na}. Pilsicainide, a pure class IC drug, is likely to more strongly induce ST segment elevation than flecainide, because the latter also mildly blocks I_{to}.

On the other hand, class IA drugs (ajmaline, procainamide, disopyramide) exhibit less use-dependent block of fast I_{Na} and, consequently, induce a weaker ST segment elevation than class IC drugs. Additionally, the degree of I_{to} blockade inflected by class IA agents can ameliorate their I_{Na}-blocking effect and, as a consequence, influence the degree of ST elevation. Ajmaline exhibits less inhibition of I_{to} and induces more pronounced ST segment elevation than flecainide. In contrast, quinidine generally normalizes ST segment elevation, despite its I_{Na}-blocking effect, owing to its relatively strong I_{to}-blocking effect.

Class IB antiarrhythmic drugs (lidocaine, mexiletine) block fast I_{Na} primarily at fast heart rates (because of the rapid dissociation of these drugs from Na^+ channels). Therefore, these drugs have little or no effect on fast I_{Na} at moderate or slow heart rates.

Several psychotropic drugs have been reported to unmask Brugada-like ST segment elevation, secondary to block of fast I_{Na} usually with drug overdose. Other drugs that can potentially unmask a Brugada-like ECG pattern include verapamil, lithium, H_1 antihistamines, propofol, alcohol intoxication, cocaine intoxication, and potentially nitrates, vagomimetic agents, and beta blockers (Table 31-9).[64]

Whether this "acquired" form of Brugada syndrome unmasks clinically inapparent Brugada syndrome ("forme fruste") or merely represents one end of a broad spectrum of responses to Na^+ channel blockers is not known. The prognosis of asymptomatic patients

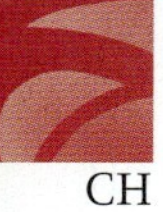

TABLE 31-9 Drug-Induced Brugada Syndrome

DRUG GROUP	EXAMPLE(S)
Class IC antiarrhythmic drugs	Flecainide, propafenone, pilsicainide
Class IA antiarrhythmic drugs	Ajmaline, procainamide, disopyramide
Calcium channel blockers	Verapamil, diltiazem, nifedipine
Beta blockers	Propranolol
H_1-Antihistamines	Dimenhydrinate
Tricyclic antidepressants	Amitriptyline, nortriptyline, desipramine
Tetracyclic antidepressants	Maprotiline
Selective serotonin reuptake inhibitors	Fluoxetine
Phenothiazines	Perphenazine, trifluoperazine
Local anesthetics	Bupivacaine
Other drugs	Lithium, nitrates, propofol

with drug-induced Brugada ECG pattern, but without a family history of SCD, appears to be benign once the offending agent is discontinued, provided the full-blown Brugada syndrome is not uncovered.[64]

In addition to drug-induced Brugada syndrome, it is also important to exclude a variety of pathological and physiological conditions that can potentially mimic the Brugada ECG pattern. These include atypical RBBB, LV hypertrophy, pulmonary embolism, acute pericarditis, various central and autonomic nervous system abnormalities, hyperkalemia, hypercalcemia, ARVD, mechanical compression of the RVOT (e.g., by tumor), pectus excavatum, hyperthermia, and hypothermia. Acute myocardial infarction or ischemia involving the RVOT can produce Brugada-like ST elevation, likely because of the attenuation of I_{CaL} and enhancement of I_{KATP} during ischemia. Additionally, a Brugada-like ST elevation can occasionally appear for a brief period after direct-current cardioversion; it is not known whether these patients are gene carriers for the Brugada syndrome.[61,65]

Early repolarization syndromes (J wave syndromes) can mimic Brugada ECG pattern (see later discussion). ST segment elevation encountered in healthy well-trained athletes is usually distinguished from Brugada ECG pattern by an upslope rather than a downslope of the ST segment and by remaining largely unaffected by challenge with a Na^+ channel blocker.[61,65]

Risk Stratification

Brugada syndrome patients initially presenting with aborted SCD are at the highest risk for a recurrence (69% at 54 ± 54 months of follow-up), whereas patients presenting with syncope and a spontaneously appearing type 1 ECG have a recurrence rate of 19% at 26 ± 36 months of follow-up.[65,69]

On the other hand, risk stratification in asymptomatic patients with Brugada syndrome has been a matter of continuous controversy in recent years. Multiple reports suggested that male gender and spontaneous occurrence of type 1 ST elevation predict higher risk for cardiac events (syncope, aborted cardiac arrest, SCD; odds ratios, 3.47 and 4.65, respectively), whereas asymptomatic patients in whom ST segment elevation appeared only after provocation with Na^+ channel blockers appear to be at minimal risk for arrhythmic events.

Importantly, familial forms of the Brugada syndrome do not appear to be associated with a worse prognosis than are sporadic cases; in other words, a positive family history of Brugada syndrome does not predict outcome. Similarly, a positive family history for SCD and the identification of an *SCN5A* genotype are not reliable predictors for poor outcome in asymptomatic patients.[66,69,81]

The usefulness of inducibility of ventricular arrhythmias by programmed stimulation as a predictor for poor outcome has been debated and is unresolved. VF or sustained polymorphic VT can be induced in approximately 50% to 70% of Brugada patients during EP testing. Whereas some investigators found programmed stimulation to be a useful discriminator of risk, others have not found it to be predictive. These discrepancies are likely the result of differences in patient characteristics, subtle differences in the diagnostic criteria, and the use of nonstandardized or noncomparable stimulation protocols. It is important to recognize that VF can be induced by programmed electrical stimulation in 6% to 9% of apparently healthy individuals and can represent a false-positive and nonspecific response, particularly when aggressive stimulation protocols are used.[65,66,69]

Patients with a type 2 or 3 ECG pattern that did not convert to type 1 during drug challenge testing were found to have a good prognosis and noninducible ventricular arrhythmias during programmed electrical stimulation. However, in a recent report, the prognosis of probands with non–type 1 Brugada-pattern ECG (even after challenge with a Na^+ channel blocker) was similar to that of patients with spontaneous or drug-induced type 1 ST elevation. Patients presenting with aborted cardiac arrest had a grim prognosis (annual rate of arrhythmic events of 10.6%), whereas those presenting with syncope or no symptoms had an excellent prognosis (annual rate of arrhythmic events ≤1.2%) irrespective of their ECG pattern (that is, type 1 versus non–type 1). Also, a family history of SCD at age less than 45 years and coexistence of early repolarization in the inferolateral leads (observed in 8% to 11% of Brugada patients) were predictors of poor outcome. In contrast, VT/VF inducibility during programmed stimulation was not a predictor of outcome. Furthermore, men with a spontaneous type 1 ECG recorded only at the higher leads V_1 and V_2 showed a prognosis similar to that of men with a type 1 ECG when using standard leads.[73,81]

Principles of Management

IMPLANTABLE CARDIOVERTER-DEFIBRILLATOR

Currently, an ICD is the only proven effective treatment for the Brugada syndrome. There is general consensus that ICD implantation is recommended in patients with type 1 Brugada ECG (either spontaneously or after Na^+ channel blockade) and a history of aborted SCD or related symptoms such as syncope, seizure, or nocturnal agonal respiration, given that noncardiac causes of these symptoms have been carefully excluded. The cumulative efficacy of ICD therapy (at least one appropriate defibrillation) in these patients is 18%, 24%, 32%, 36%, and 38% at 1, 2, 3, 4, and 5 years of follow-up, respectively. ICD devices need to be carefully programmed in Brugada syndrome patients in order to avoid inappropriate shocks, given the high incidence of supraventricular arrhythmias (especially AF) in this population. Programming a single VF zone of more than 210 beats/min with or without a monitoring zone of more than 180 beats/min is preferable.[65,82]

On the other hand, there is no similar consensus regarding the management of asymptomatic patients with the Brugada syndrome. Whereas some experts advocate close follow-up, others propose the evaluation of VT/VF inducibility by programmed stimulation for risk stratification and to decide on ICD implantation in patients with spontaneous type 1 Brugada ECG. It is important to recognize that ICD therapy is not without complications. A recent study of ICD use in 220 patients with the Brugada syndrome, of whom nearly 50% were symptomatic, showed that during a 3-year follow-up inappropriate shocks occurred 2.5 times more frequently (20%) than appropriate shocks (8%), and other procedure-related complications occurred in 8% of patients. Therefore, more studies are needed to define further the risk stratification strategy in these patients.[82]

For asymptomatic patients with normal baseline ECG and those with spontaneous type 1 Brugada ECG but noninducible VT/VF during programmed stimulation, reassurance is adequate management.[65,69]

CATHETER ABLATION

In Brugada syndrome patients with frequent episodes of VT/VF, monomorphic PVCs originating predominantly in the RVOT or RV Purkinje network are often the trigger for VT, and focal RF ablation of the PVCs can be valuable in reducing the burden of arrhythmias and ICD therapies. Furthermore, recent work suggests that extensive ablation over the RVOT epicardium can revert the ECG pattern to normal and eliminate episodes of VT/VF.

PHARMACOLOGICAL THERAPY

At present, there is no specific pharmacological treatment to prevent SCD in patients with Brugada syndrome. Because of the critical role of I_{to} in the arrhythmogenesis in the Brugada syndrome, I_{to} blockade may be protective. Additionally, agents that augment I_{CaL} have been shown to have a therapeutic value. Both groups of drugs can potentially restore the RV epicardial action potential dome, thus normalizing the ST segment and preventing phase 2 reentry and polymorphic VT in the Brugada syndrome. Although clinical evidence of the long-term efficacy in the prevention of SCD is limited, the use of I_{to} blockers and agents that augment I_{CaL} may be considered in high-risk patients who are not candidates for ICD implantation, as adjunctive chronic treatment in ICD patients with frequent appropriate ICD therapies, as well as in patients with VF storm.[65,67] Additionally, these agents may be considered as an alternative therapeutic strategy to early ICD implant if an acceptable therapeutic response (i.e., ECG normalization and noninducibility of ventricular arrhythmia on programmed stimulation) can be achieved. Further systematic evaluation of the usefulness of these oral agents in larger numbers of Brugada patients is required to make a definitive conclusion.[67,69]

Quinidine, a class IA Na^+ channel blocker, has a relatively strong effect in blocking I_{to} and has been found effective in suppressing arrhythmia inducibility on EP testing in up to 76% of Brugada syndrome patients as well as in preventing the occurrence of spontaneous arrhythmias. Relatively high doses (1200 to 1500 mg/day) of quinidine are recommended.

Denopamine, an alpha/beta-adrenergic stimulant, also can potentially be effective as a chronic treatment, probably by increasing I_{CaL}. Also, cilostazol, a phosphodiesterase III inhibitor that increases I_{CaL}, has been reported to be effective in suppressing VF in Brugada syndrome. More recently, bepridil was shown to suppress the incidence of VF episodes, probably by blocking I_{to}. Tedisamil, an experimental potent I_{to} blocker without the relatively strong inward current-blocking actions of quinidine, may become a therapeutic option.

In patients with Brugada syndrome and electrical storm of VF, isoproterenol, a beta-adrenergic agonist, is reported to decrease ST elevation and suppress repetitive episodes of VF, likely via augmentation of I_{CaL}. In one report, five of seven patients with VF storm were successfully treated with isoproterenol infusion (dose titrated to achieve a 20% increase in heart rate). However, discontinuation or decrease in the infusion rate often resulted in recurrence of arrhythmias, and the total duration of intravenous therapy was quite long (average, 20 days). Eventually, all patients were successfully switched to oral medications (denopamine, quinidine, cilostazol, bepridil, or a combination thereof). Before consideration of isoproterenol therapy, however, it is critical that the diagnosis of Brugada syndrome be clearly established as the underlying etiology of VF storm. Isoproterenol infusion can be devastating in patients with VF due to other mechanisms, especially CPVT. This is especially important to recognize because a Brugada-like ST segment elevation can occasionally appear for a brief period in a patient successfully defibrillated from VF.[67]

Interestingly, in some *SCN5A* mutations that impair protein trafficking to the cell membrane, mexiletine (a class IB Na^+ channel blocker) has the potential to serve as a mutation-specific therapy. Mexiletine binds to mutant proteins and acts as a molecular chaperone to rescue their trafficking to the sarcolemma and restore I_{Na}. However, it is questionable whether such drugs can be used as therapy because (once expressed on the sarcolemma) the mutant proteins can potentially display arrhythmia-causing gating defects. Moreover, Na^+ channel–blocking effects of the drug reduce I_{Na} and, hence, can potentially aggravate the ECG changes or trigger arrhythmias in the Brugada syndrome.[47]

Finally, several drugs have been reported to exacerbate the ECG pattern of ST segment elevation in the Brugada syndrome and to trigger arrhythmias, and should be avoided. These drugs include antiarrhythmics (class IA, IC), beta blockers, tricyclic antidepressants, local anesthetics (bupivacaine), opioid analgesics (propoxyphene), propofol, K^+ channel activators (pinacidil), lithium, cocaine, alpha-adrenergic agonists (methoxamine), and vagomimetic agents. Furthermore, fever, which can potentially trigger fatal events, should be treated promptly.[65] It should be stressed that ventricular arrhythmias in Brugada syndrome respond differently from most other VTs in that they are suppressed by sympathomimetic agents and enhanced by vagomimetic agents.

PARTICIPATION IN SPORTS

Although a clear association between exercise and SCD has not been established, restriction to participation in class IA sports seems advisable, especially given the potential impact of hyperthermia on triggering cardiac events in patients with the Brugada syndrome. The presence of an ICD device warrants the same restrictions to class IA sports.[59,83]

FAMILY SCREENING

Most individuals diagnosed with the Brugada syndrome have inherited the disease-causing mutation from a parent. Although a proband with the Brugada syndrome may have the disorder as the result of a de novo gene mutation, this is very rare (approximately 1%). Because the disease is inherited as autosomal dominant, each child of an individual with Brugada syndrome has a 50% chance of inheriting the mutation. Nonetheless, the family history may appear to be negative because of failure to recognize the disorder in family members, decreased penetrance, early death of the parent before the onset of warning symptoms, or late onset of symptoms in the affected parent. Therefore, the lack of a family history does not rule out a heritable disease.

It is recommended that at-risk individuals with a family history of Brugada syndrome should undergo ECG monitoring every 1 to 2 years. The presence of type 1 ST elevation should be further investigated.

Given the insensitivity of ECG changes in establishing the diagnosis, molecular genetic testing of at-risk asymptomatic family members of a patient with Brugada syndrome should be considered if the disease-causing mutation has been identified in the proband. Family members who test positive for the familial mutation should receive baseline ECG and annual ECG screening examinations, and should be instructed to avoid medications that can induce ventricular arrhythmias and to seek medical attention immediately on occurrence of symptoms.[41] On the other hand, a negative genetic test result for the familial mutation would obviate the need for repeated follow-up examinations. Genetic testing also can be used for prenatal diagnosis. All patients who undergo genetic testing should receive pretest and post-test genetic counseling to understand the implications of testing.

Short QT Syndrome

The SQTS is a recently recognized inherited channelopathy, first described in 2000, occurring in young individuals with structurally normal hearts. Affected patients are characterized by constantly short QT intervals (QTc <360 milliseconds) associated with AF, syncope, and/or SCD.[84]

Epidemiology

SQTS has been described in very few families worldwide; therefore, all the information available is based on small numbers of cases.

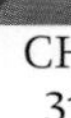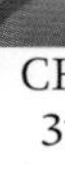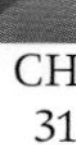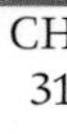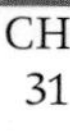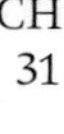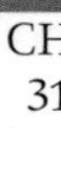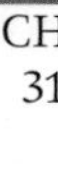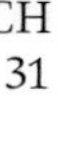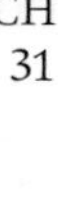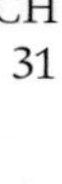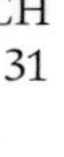

The majority (75.4%) of affected subjects have been men. The age of presentation is quite variable, ranging from infancy to the eighth decade of life, with a mean age of 20 to 30 years. Up to 72% of patients with SQTS have a family history of SQTS or SCD.[84,85]

Clinical Presentation

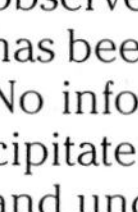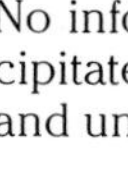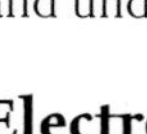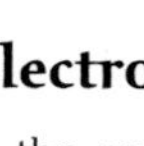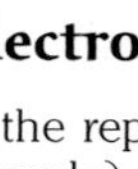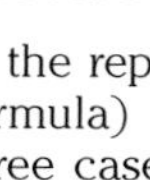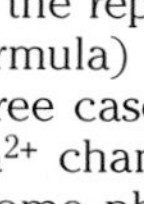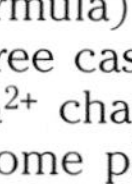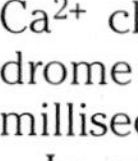

More than 60% of the subjects have symptoms at presentation, with cardiac arrest being the most frequent symptom, representing the first clinical manifestation in one-third of patients. Syncope is observed as a first clinical presentation less frequently (14%). AF has been documented in approximately 30% of patients with SQTS. No information is available on whether specific triggers may precipitate cardiac events, as cardiac arrest has occurred both at rest and under stress.[84,85]

Electrocardiographic Features

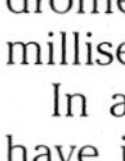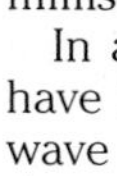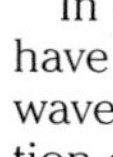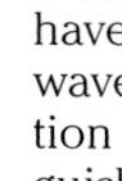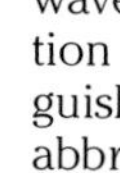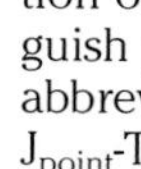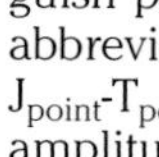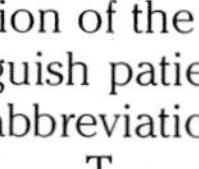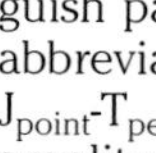

In the reported cases of SQTS, the QTc interval (using the Bazett formula) was always less than 320 milliseconds, except for the three cases with loss-of-function mutations of the cardiac L-type Ca^{2+} channel associated with familial SCD and a Brugada syndrome phenotype, in whom the QTc interval was less than 360 milliseconds.

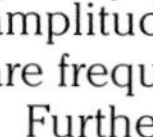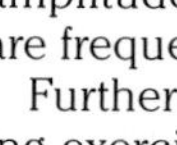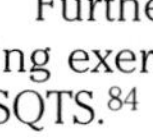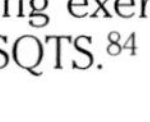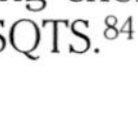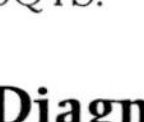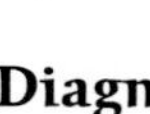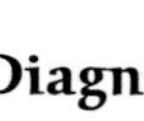

In addition to constantly short QTc intervals, affected patients have in common a short or even absent ST segment, with the T wave initiating immediately from the S wave. Extreme abbreviation of the J_{point}-T_{peak} interval (<120 milliseconds) can help distinguish patients with SQTS from healthy subjects with an apparent abbreviation of the ST segment and shortened QT intervals (mean J_{point}-T_{peak} interval of 188 ± 11 milliseconds). Additionally, high-amplitude, narrow, and symmetrical T waves in the precordial leads are frequently observed in SQTS patients.[84]

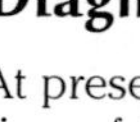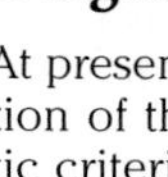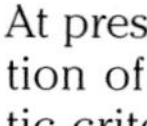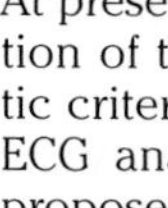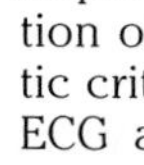

Furthermore, the physiological shortening of the QT interval during exercise-induced tachycardia can be blunted in patients with SQTS.[84]

Diagnosis of the Short QT Syndrome

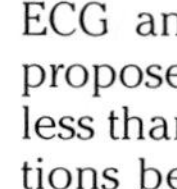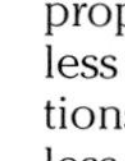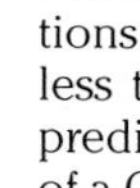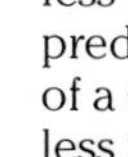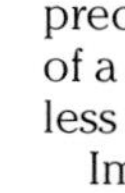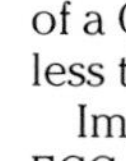

At present, there is still no clear consensus concerning the definition of the lower limit of a "normal" QT interval or the diagnostic criteria sufficient to establish the diagnosis of SQTS. Based on ECG analysis of 14,379 healthy individuals, some investigators proposed that a QTc interval less than 350 milliseconds, which is less than 88% of the mean predicted value (i.e., >2 standard deviations below the mean), be considered short, and a QTc interval less than 320 milliseconds, which is less than 80% of the mean predicted value, be considered abnormally short. The prevalence of a QTc interval less than 88% was 2.5% and that of a QTc interval less than 80% was 0.03%.

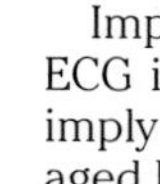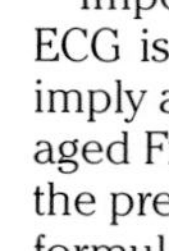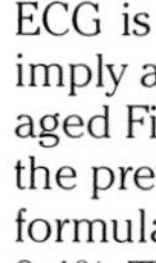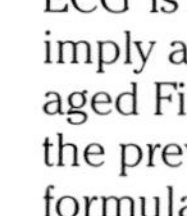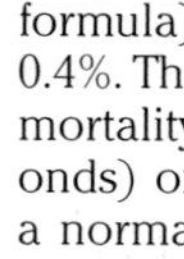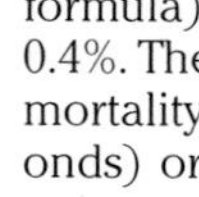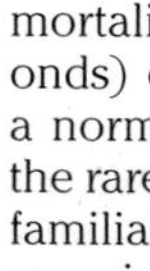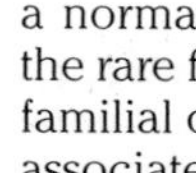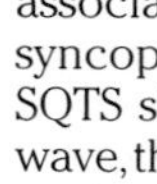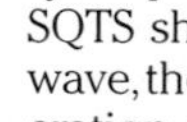

Importantly, the presence of a short QT interval on the surface ECG is not sufficient to make a diagnosis of SQTS and does not imply a significant risk of SCD. In fact, in a recent study in a middle-aged Finnish population (n = 10,822) followed up for 29 ± 10 years, the prevalence of QTc less than 320 milliseconds (using the Bazett formula) was 0.1% and that of QTc less than 340 milliseconds was 0.4%. There was no difference in the all-cause or cardiovascular mortality between subjects with a very short QTc (≤320 milliseconds) or short QTc (≤340 milliseconds) and those subjects with a normal QTc interval (360 to 450 milliseconds).[86] Nevertheless, the rare finding of a short QT interval should initiate exclusion of a familial occurrence. When the occurrence of a short QT interval is associated with episodes of AF, sustained palpitation, unexplained syncope, VF, and/or a positive family history for premature SCD, SQTS should be suspected. Additionally, the morphology of the T wave, the J_{point}-T_{peak} interval, and QT adaptation to heart rate acceleration can potentially help distinguish patients with SQTS from healthy patients with shortened QT intervals.

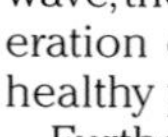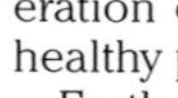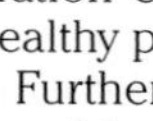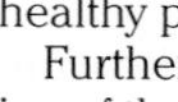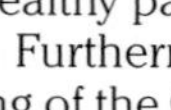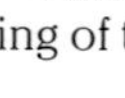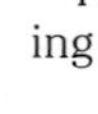

Furthermore, other potential underlying etiologies for shortening of the QT interval should be excluded, including hyperkalemia, hypercalcemia, hyperthermia, acidosis, digitalis overdose, and/or administration of acetylcholine and catecholamines.[84]

TABLE 31-10 Diagnostic Criteria of the Short QT Syndrome

QTc	
<370 msec	1
<350 msec	2
<330 msec	3
J_{point}-T_{peak} Interval < 120 msec	1
Clinical History*	
History of sudden cardiac arrest	2
Documented polymorphic VT or VF	2
Unexplained syncope	1
Atrial fibrillation	1
Family History*	
First- or second-degree relative with high-probability SQTS	2
First- or second-degree relative with autopsy-negative sudden cardiac death	1
Sudden infant death syndrome	1
Genotype*	
Genotype positive	2
Mutation of undetermined significance in a culprit gene	1

Notes:

- High-probability SQTS, ≥4 points; intermediate-probability SQTS, 3 points; low-probability SQTS, ≤2 points.
- ECG: Must be recorded in the absence of modifiers known to shorten the QT.
- J_{point}-T_{peak} interval must be measured in the precordial lead with the greatest amplitude T wave.
- Clinical history: Events must occur in the absence of an identifiable etiology, including structural heart disease.
- Points cannot be combined for the following three markers: cardiac arrest, documented polymorphic VT, and unexplained syncope.
- Family history: Points can only be received once in this section.
- A minimum of 1 point must be obtained in the electrocardiographic section in order to obtain additional points.

QTc = corrected QT interval; SQTS = short QT syndrome; VF = ventricular fibrillation; VT = ventricular tachycardia.

The role of EP study in diagnosis and risk stratification is not yet fully defined. During EP testing, atrial and ventricular effective refractory periods are significantly shortened, and VT/VF is inducible in 60% to 91% of patients. However, whether inducibility of ventricular arrhythmias is predictive of adverse clinical outcome remains unclear.[84]

Genetic analysis may be considered for patients with a strong clinical index of suspicion for SQTS based on the personal and family history, and ECG phenotype.[41] A mutation in genes related to SQTS is observed in 23% of probands.[85] Genetic testing can help identify silent carriers of SQTS-related mutations; however, the risk of cardiac events in genetically affected individuals with a normal ECG is currently not known. Similarly, given the limited number of patients with SQTS so far identified, genetic analysis at present does not contribute to risk stratification.

A diagnostic scoring system to facilitate diagnosis of SQTS has been proposed recently, based on a comprehensive review of 61 reported cases of the SQTS. The diagnostic criteria incorporate the ECG findings, clinical history, family history, as well as genotype findings (Table 31-10). In this system, all patients should have a QTc interval (using the Bazett formula) of no more than 370 milliseconds. Clinical events (cardiac arrest, nonsustained polymorphic VT or VF, syncope, AF) must occur in the absence of other identified clinical pathologies. Although these diagnostic criteria can potentially facilitate evaluation in suspected cases of SQTS, their value for evaluation of family members can potentially be

TABLE 31-11 Molecular Basis of the Short QT Syndrome

DISEASE	GENE	PROTEIN	IONIC CURRENT	FUNCTION	INHERITANCE
SQT1	*KCNH2 (HERG)*	$K_v11.1$	Subunit alpha I_{Kr}	Gain	Autosomal dominant
SQT2	*KCNQ1 (K_vLQT1)*	$K_v7.1$	Subunit alpha I_{Ks}	Gain	Autosomal dominant
SQT3	*KCNJ2*	Kir2.1	Subunit alpha I_{K1}	Gain	Autosomal dominant
SQT4	*CACNA1C*	$Ca_v1.2$	Subunit alpha I_{CaL}	Loss	Autosomal dominant
SQT5	*CACNB2B*	$Ca_v\beta_{2b}$	Subunit beta I_{CaL}	Loss	Autosomal dominant

I_{CaL} = L-type Ca^{2+} current; I_{K1} = inward rectifier K^+ current; I_{Kr} = rapidly activating delayed rectifier K^+ current; I_{Ks} = slowly activating delayed rectifier K^+ current; SQT1 to SQT5 = short QT syndrome types 1 to 5, respectively.

limited because of incomplete disease penetrance. Importantly, treatment considerations should be reserved for subjects receiving a high-probability score, whereas medical surveillance or expert opinion should be considered for intermediate- or low-probability cases.[87]

Genetics of the Short QT Syndrome

To date, mutation analysis has implicated five distinct genes in the etiology of a proportion of patients diagnosed with SQTS, although the majority of diagnosed cases do not have reported genetic associations. It is expected that further genes will be identified. Genetic studies reveal a genetically heterogeneous disease with gain-of-function mutations of voltage-gated K^+ channel genes and loss-of-function mutation in the L-type Ca^{2+} channel genes (Table 31-11). These mutations cause either an increase in the outward repolarizing K^+ currents or a decrease in the inward depolarizing currents, leading to shortening of the action potential duration, the QT interval, and the effective refractory period. Shortening of refractoriness is a key mechanism predisposing to increased atrial and ventricular susceptibility to premature stimulation, leading to AF and VF.[84]

SQT1, the most common genotype, is caused by mutations of the *KCNH2* gene (*HERG*, encoding the alpha subunit $K_v11.1$ of the I_{Kr}). A gain-of-function mutation on *KCNH2* causes a shift of voltage dependence of inactivation of I_{Kr} by +90 mV out of the range of the action potential, which results in a significant increase in I_{Kr} during the action potential plateau. The resulting I_{Kr} increase achieved by altered gating hastens repolarization, thereby shortening action potential duration and facilitating reentrant excitation waves to induce atrial and/or ventricular arrhythmia. Additionally, gain-of-function mutations in *KCNE2* (MiRP1) have been found in two families with AF. In contrast, loss-of-function mutations in the *KCNH2* gene are responsible for LQT2.[11,49,53,85]

SQT2 is caused by mutations of the *KCNQ1* gene (*K_vLQT1*, encoding the alpha subunit $K_v7.1$ of the I_{Ks}). A gain-of-function mutation of *KCNQ1* causes a shift in the voltage dependence of I_{Ks} activation by −20 mV and acceleration of activation kinetics, leading to enhancement of I_{Ks} and of the action potential duration and shortening of the QT interval. Loss-of-function mutations in the *KCNQ1* gene are responsible for LQT1.

SQT3 is caused by a mutation in the *KCNJ2* gene (encoding for the strong inwardly rectifying channel protein Kir2.1 of the I_{K1}). A gain-of-function mutation causes a significant increase in the outward I_{K1} at potentials between −75 and −45 mV, leading to shortening of the QT interval and asymmetrical T waves with a rapid terminal phase. On the other hand, loss-of-function mutations in the *KCNJ2* gene, identified in patients with the Andersen syndrome, generate prolongation of the QT intervals (LQT7).[84]

SQT4 is caused by mutations of the *CACNA1C* gene (encoding the alpha$_1$ subunit $Ca_v1.2$ of the cardiac L-type Ca^{2+} channel) and SQT5 is caused by mutations of the *CACNB2* gene (encoding the beta$_{2b}$ subunit of the cardiac L-type Ca^{2+} channel). Loss-of-function mutations of those genes result in major attenuation in I_{CaL} amplitude, leading to shortening of the action potential duration, and are associated with asymmetrical T waves, attenuated QT–heart rate relationship, and AF. The three patients reported to harbor these mutations had a Brugada type 1 phenotype. Additionally, loss-of-function mutations of the *CACNA1C* and *CACNB2* genes have recently been linked to a sudden death syndrome that combines the features of Brugada syndrome, including the characteristic ECG pattern, and a short QT interval. It was speculated that these mutations cause Brugada syndrome by aggravating transmural voltage gradients. Conversely, a gain-of-function mutation of the Ca^{2+} channel is known to generate the LQT8 (Timothy syndrome).[88,89]

Principles of Management

IMPLANTABLE CARDIOVERTER-DEFIBRILLATOR

At present, ICD implantation is the therapy of choice for the prevention of SCD in symptomatic patients with SQTS. Importantly, patients with SQTS are potentially susceptible to inappropriate shocks because of the tall, narrow T waves and the high prevalence of AF.[84,90]

PHARMACOLOGICAL THERAPY

Quinidine was shown to prolong the QT interval, normalize atrial and ventricular effective refractory periods, and prevent inducibility of ventricular arrhythmias during EP testing in patients with SQT1. In a recent report, the incidence of arrhythmic events during the follow-up was 4.9% per year in the patients without pharmacological prophylaxis, whereas no arrhythmic events occurred in those receiving hydroquinidine (even if previously symptomatic).[85]

Hence, quinidine can potentially serve as an adjunct to ICD therapy in the treatment of paroxysmal AF or recurrent ventricular tachyarrhythmias in this subgroup of patients or as an alternative option to ICD in patients who cannot receive it (children) or who decline the implant.[84,85]

PARTICIPATION IN SPORTS

Until the phenotype of SQTS is better understood, a universal restriction from competitive sports with the possible exception of class IA activities seems to represent the most prudent recommendation.[59]

Catecholaminergic Polymorphic Ventricular Tachycardia

CPVT, also known as familial polymorphic VT, is a rare but highly malignant inherited arrhythmia disorder characterized by exercise- and stress-induced polymorphic or bidirectional VT, which is an important cause of syncope and SCD in individuals with a structurally normal heart.[91,92]

Epidemiology

The prevalence of CPVT has been estimated to be 1:10,000. The mean age of onset is between 7 and 9 years, although later onset has been reported. Approximately 30% of probands have a family history of stress-related syncope, seizure, or SCD before age 40 years. There is a high level of penetrance of the disease (75% to 80%).[93]

Clinical Presentation

CPVT patients typically present with syncope triggered by exercise or emotion, and a distinctive pattern of reproducible, stress-related, bidirectional VT in the absence of structural heart disease or QT interval prolongation.

CPVT is one of the most malignant forms of ventricular arrhythmia. Approximately 80% of untreated CPVT patients develop symptoms (syncope, VT or VF) by age 40 and overall mortality is 30% to 50%.[91] SCD can be the first manifestation of the disease in a significant proportion of cases.[94]

Electrocardiographic Features

The resting ECG of patients with CPVT is often normal, without prolongation or shortening of the QT interval, atrioventricular and intraventricular conduction defects, or Brugada-like ST elevation. Sinus bradycardia and prominent U waves can be observed in some patients.

The distinguishing ventricular arrhythmia of CPVT ("bidirectional VT") is characterized by alternating QRS axis with 180-degree rotation on a beat-to-beat basis. However, the typical bidirectional VT is not observed in all patients. In one report, bidirectional VT was documented in only 35% of probands, whereas the remaining patients showed polymorphic VT or VF. Importantly, the morphology of VT, which is polymorphic or bidirectional, is strongly dependent on the ECG recording lead. When the maximal QRS vector changes in one lead during bidirectional VT, the axis perpendicular to the former lead shows polymorphic VT. However, unlike other polymorphic VTs, such as torsades de pointes, the QRS morphology is not chaotic but has some regularity.[94,95]

A characteristic feature of CPVT is the progressive worsening of arrhythmias with increasing exercise workload. Ventricular arrhythmias during exercise stress testing appear quite consistently at a heart rate of 110 to 130 beats/min; initially, polymorphic PVCs appear. The complexity and frequency of arrhythmias progressively worsen as workload increases: ventricular bigeminy, salvoes of polymorphic PVCs, and polymorphic or bidirectional VT, often appearing in this order. If exercise is not promptly discontinued, bidirectional VT may degenerate into polymorphic VT and VF. On termination of exercise, arrhythmias progressively diminish in term of VT rate and VT duration until they disappear. Isolated premature atrial complexes, nonsustained supraventricular tachycardia, and short runs of AF usually are observed during exercise, with an onset at a range of heart rates similar to or slower than that of ventricular arrhythmias.[94,95]

Diagnosis of Catecholaminergic Polymorphic Ventricular Tachycardia

Diagnosing CPVT patients may be challenging because the resting ECG, echocardiography, signal-averaging ECG, and EP testing frequently are completely normal. Clinical diagnosis is made based on symptoms (syncope or aborted SCD), family history, and response to exercise or isoproterenol infusion. Ventricular arrhythmias can be observed with a combination of Holter monitoring, exercise, and drug provocation in more than 80% of patients.

CPVT diagnosis is frequently missed or delayed, unless exercise stress testing or ambulatory cardiac monitoring is performed to document ventricular arrhythmias. Not infrequently, syncopal episodes are considered as vasovagal in origin, and no further workup is performed. If the loss of consciousness is associated with convulsions, it may be misdiagnosed as epileptic seizures if a prolonged circulatory arrest resulted in brain ischemia. Unexplained cardiac arrest also is frequently misdiagnosed as idiopathic VF.[93] CPVT should be suspected when a syncopal episode induced by exercise or emotion occurs in a child or in a young patient with a normal resting ECG and no structural heart disease. Additionally, CPVT should be considered in all cases of idiopathic VF and unexplained cardiac arrest (normal coronary arteries, normal ventricular function, and normal ECG), especially if an adrenergic trigger is present.[93,94]

A standardized exercise stress test is the most important step for diagnosis of CPVT. In at least 80% of CPVT patients, exercise stress testing induces ventricular arrhythmias, which typically appear when the sinus rate exceeds an individual threshold rate (usually at 110 to 130 beats/min). As noted, the progressive worsening of arrhythmias during exercise is highly reproducible and is a diagnostic marker of CPVT. Progressive ventricular arrhythmias can also be provoked by intravenous infusion of catecholamines (e.g., isoproterenol or epinephrine).[91,95]

Sometimes, the exercise-provoked arrhythmias can be demonstrated only after a delay of months or more after the first syncopal episode has occurred, emphasizing the necessity of repeated exercise stress tests when there is a high suspicion of CPVT.[95]

Additionally, continuous ambulatory monitoring may reveal arrhythmias typical for CPVT if the sinus rate of the patient exceeds the individual arrhythmia-inducing threshold during monitoring, and can be very useful in young children, whenever performing a maximal exercise stress test is difficult. Implantation of a loop recorder can also be valuable in some cases.[93-95]

Invasive EP testing is of no value in the diagnosis or risk stratification in patients with CPVT. Arrhythmias are seldom inducible by programmed electrical stimulation.[93,95]

Genetic testing should be performed in all definitive CPVT probands and also considered in subjects with idiopathic VF when an adrenergic trigger is identified.[41] Using a comprehensive screening approach, the percentage of successfully genotyped CPVT patients is approximately 55% to 60%. However, because the cardiac ryanodine receptor gene (*RyR2*, which underlies the most common form of CPVT) is one of the largest genes in the human genome, genetic testing is usually time-consuming and costly. Genetic screening for disease-causing mutations in the calsequestrin gene (*CASQ2*, which underlies the autosomal recessive form of CPVT) is advisable in all pedigrees compatible with a recessive pattern of inheritance but also in all apparently sporadic CPVT cases with negative *RyR2* screening even in the absence of parental consanguinity.[93,94]

Genetics of Catecholaminergic Polymorphic Ventricular Tachycardia

CPVT is caused by mutations in genes that encode for key Ca^{2+} regulatory proteins. Two genetic variants of CPVT have been described: an autosomal dominant trait (CPVT1; most common) caused by mutations in the *RyR2* gene, and a recessive form (CPVT2; rare) associated with homozygous mutations in the *CASQ2* gene. Heterozygous carriers of one *CASQ2* mutation are usually healthy.[93]

RyR2 is the major calcium release channel of the sarcoplasmic reticulum, mediating excitation-contraction coupling. Approximately 50% to 70% of patients with CPVT harbor *RyR2* mutations. To date, more than 70 *RyR2* mutations linked to CPVT have been identified. CPVT mutant RyR2s typically show gain-of-function defects following channel activation by PKA phosphorylation (in response to beta-adrenergic stimulation or caffeine), resulting in uncontrolled Ca^{2+} release from the sarcoplasmic reticulum during electrical diastole, which facilitates the development of DADs and triggered arrhythmias.[91,96,97]

CASQ2 is a sarcoplasmic reticulum Ca^{2+} buffering protein associated with RyR2. CASQ2 plays an active role in the control of Ca^{2+} release from the sarcoplasmic reticulum to the cytosol. So far, seven *CASQ2* mutations linked to CPVT have been reported. Whereas some of these mutations are thought to compromise CASQ2 synthesis and result in reduced expression or complete absence of CASQ2 in the heart, other mutations seem to cause expression of defective CASQ2 proteins with abnormal regulation of cellular Ca^{2+} homeostasis.[91,94,96]

Missense mutations in *RyR2* also have been linked to a form of arrhythmogenic cardiomyopathy (ARVD-2) characterized by exercise-induced polymorphic VT that does not appear to have a reentrant mechanism, occurring in the absence of significant structural abnormalities. Patients do not develop characteristic features of ARVD on the 12-lead ECG or signal-averaged ECG, and global RV function remains unaffected. ARVD-2 shows a closer resemblance to familial CPVT in both etiology and phenotype; its inclusion under the umbrella term of ARVD remains controversial.[98-100]

Recently, three novel loss-of-function mutations of the *KCNJ2* gene (encoding for the strong inwardly rectifying channel protein Kir2.1 of the I_{K1}) have been found in patients with CPVT. These patients had prominent U waves, ventricular ectopy, and polymorphic VT, but no dysmorphic features or skeletal muscle abnormalities.[101] I_{K1} reduction may trigger arrhythmia by allowing inward currents, which are no longer counterbalanced by the strong outward I_{K1}, to gradually depolarize the membrane potential during phase 4. Membrane depolarization during phase 4 induces arrhythmia by facilitating spontaneous excitability.[53]

Pathophysiology of Catecholaminergic Polymorphic Ventricular Tachycardia

MECHANISM OF VENTRICULAR ARRHYTHMIAS

Abnormalities in the control of sarcoplasmic reticulum Ca^{2+} release constitute the central pathogenic abnormality in CPVT, although considerable controversy exists about the molecular mechanisms causing these defects. RyR2 and CASQ2 are both critically involved in the regulation of cardiac excitation-contraction coupling. Ca^{2+} influx via the L-type Ca^{2+} channels in the cell membrane during the action potential plateau triggers more massive Ca^{2+} release (Ca^{2+} transients) from the sarcoplasmic reticulum into the cytosol via activation of Ca^{2+} release channels (RyR2). This amplifying process, termed Ca^{2+}-induced Ca^{2+} release (CICR), causes a rapid increase in cytosolic Ca^{2+} concentration to a level required for optimal binding of Ca^{2+} to troponin C and induction of contraction.[89,97,102] During diastole, most of the surplus Ca^{2+} in the cytosol is resequestered into the sarcoplasmic reticulum by the sarcoplasmic/endoplasmic reticulum calcium adenosine triphosphatase (SERCA), the activity of which is controlled by the phosphoprotein phospholamban. Additionally, some of the Ca^{2+} is extruded from the cell by the Na^+-Ca^{2+} exchanger to balance the Ca^{2+} that enters with the Ca^{2+} current. Recurring Ca^{2+} release-uptake cycles provide the basis for periodic elevations of the cytosolic Ca^{2+} concentration and contractions of myocytes, and hence for the orderly beating of the heart (see Fig. 3-6).[96,103,104]

The molecular mechanisms by which *RyR2* mutations alter the physiological properties and function of RyR2 are not completely defined. It has been suggested that CPVT mutations in *RyR2* reduce the binding affinity of RyR2 for the regulatory protein FKBP12.6 (calstabin-2) that stabilizes the closed conformational state of the RyR2 channel, thus enabling the channel to close completely during diastole (at low intracellular Ca^{2+} concentrations) and preventing aberrant Ca^{2+} leakage from the sarcoplasmic reticulum, ensuring muscle relaxation. PKA phosphorylation (induced by beta-adrenergic stimulation) of the mutant channels results in further worsening of the binding affinity of FKBP12.6 for the mutant RyR2, thus increasing the probability of an open state at diastolic Ca^{2+} concentrations. As a consequence, the mutant RyR2 channel fails to completely close during diastole, resulting in diastolic Ca^{2+} leak from the sarcoplasmic reticulum during stress or exercise.[91,96,105]

An alternative hypothesis is that CPVT mutations in *RyR2* sensitize the channel to luminal (sarcoplasmic reticulum) Ca^{2+} such that under baseline conditions, where sarcoplasmic reticulum load is normal, there is no Ca^{2+} leak. Under beta-adrenergic (sympathetic) stimulation, sarcoplasmic reticulum Ca^{2+} concentration becomes elevated above the reduced threshold, causing Ca^{2+} to leak out of the sarcoplasmic reticulum. A third hypothesis for *RyR2*-related CPVT is that mutations in *RyR2* impair the intermolecular interactions between discrete *RyR2* domains necessary for proper folding of the channel and self-regulation of channel gating.[96,105]

Calsequestrin is the most important Ca^{2+} storage protein in the sarcoplasmic reticulum and it forms a part of a large quaternary complex with RyR2, triadin, and junctin; all together, these proteins play a major role in regulating intracellular Ca^{2+}. Calsequestrin represents a high-capacity, low-affinity Ca^{2+}-binding protein that is able to bind luminal Ca^{2+} (40 to 50 Ca^{2+} ions per molecule) during diastole, buffering Ca^{2+} within the sarcoplasmic reticulum and preventing diastolic Ca^{2+} release via RyR2 to the cytosol. CASQ2 mutations result in disruption of the control of RyR2s by luminal Ca^{2+} required for effective termination of sarcoplasmic reticulum Ca^{2+} release and prevention of spontaneous Ca^{2+} release during diastole, leading to diminished Ca^{2+} signaling refractoriness and generation of arrhythmogenic spontaneous Ca^{2+} releases (Fig. 31-8).[96]

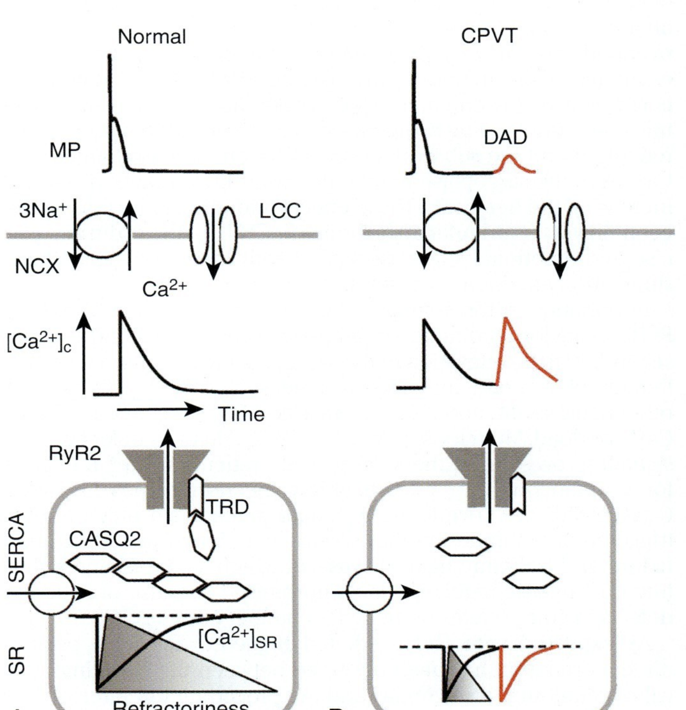

FIGURE 31-8 Calcium cycling in normal myocytes and myocytes harboring catecholaminergic polymorphic ventricular tachycardia (CPVT) *CASQ2* mutations. **A,** In normal myocytes, Ca^{2+} influx through L-type Ca^{2+} channels during the action potential activates RyR2s and initiates the release of Ca^{2+} stored in the sarcoplasmic reticulum (SR) on CASQ2 polymers. SR Ca^{2+} release terminates when the drop in intra-SR $[Ca^{2+}]$ causes RyR2s to close because of inhibition by CASQ2 monomers at reduced $[Ca^{2+}]_{SR}$. The RyR2s stay refractory until $[Ca^{2+}]_{SR}$ is restored by SERCA. The rate of $[Ca^{2+}]_{SR}$ recovery and thus the rate of restitution from luminal Ca^{2+}-dependent refractoriness depends on both SERCA activity and the Ca^{2+}-binding capacity of CASQ2. Ca^{2+} signaling refractoriness prevents spontaneous Ca^{2+} release during diastole. **B,** Arrhythmogenic *CASQ2* mutations disrupt Ca^{2+} handling through either one or a combination of decreased *CASQ2* expression, reduced CASQ2 Ca^{2+} binding capacity (via disruption of CASQ2 polymerization), and impaired CASQ2 interaction with the RyR2 complex (via TRD). Alterations in CASQ2 abundance and/or behavior result in diminished and shortened Ca^{2+} signaling refractoriness after each release through accelerating recovery of $[Ca^{2+}]_{SR}$, altering RyR2 gating dependency on $[Ca^{2+}]_{SR}$, or both. PKA-mediated stimulation of SERCA (via PLB) further accelerates SR refilling, accounting for the dependency of CPVT on adrenergic stimulation. Compromised RyR2 refractoriness results in spontaneous SR Ca^{2+} release, which in turn elicits DADs through stimulation of NCX. CASQ2 = calsequestrin; DAD = delayed afterdepolarization; LCC = L-type Ca^{2+} channel; NCX = Na^+-Ca^{2+} exchange; PKA = protein kinase A; PLB = phospholamban; RyR2 = ryanodine receptor type 2; SERCA = sarcoplasmic/endoplasmic reticulum calcium ATPase; TRD = triadin. *(Reproduced with permission from Györke S: Molecular basis of catecholaminergic polymorphic ventricular tachycardia, Heart Rhythm 6:123-129, 2009.)*

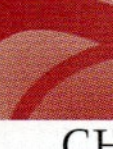

DADs and triggered activity have been proposed as the arrhythmogenic mechanism in CPVT because the bidirectional ECG pattern of this VT closely resembles the arrhythmias associated with intracellular Ca^{2+} overload and the DADs observed during digitalis toxicity. Mutations in *RyR2* or *CASQ2* lead to cytosolic Ca^{2+} overload that results in activation of the Na^+-Ca^{2+} exchanger, which in turn generates a net inward current (the so-called transient inward current [I_{Ti}]). I_{Ti} underlies diastolic membrane depolarizations (DADs), which may reach the threshold for Na^+ channel activation and trigger abnormal beats.[91,93]

When the DADs are of low amplitude, they usually are not apparent or clinically significant. Probably the most important influence that causes subthreshold DADs to reach threshold is a decrease in the initiating cycle length; fast heart rates increase both the amplitude and rate of the DADs. Additionally, catecholamines can facilitate the development of DADs by several mechanisms, including (1) increasing the L-type Ca^{2+} current through stimulation of beta-adrenergic receptors and increasing cAMP, which results in an increase in transsarcolemmal Ca^{2+} influx and intracellular Ca^{2+} overload (see Fig. 3-6); (2) enhancing the activity of the Na^+-Ca^{2+} exchanger, thus increasing the likelihood of DAD-mediated triggered activity; (3) enhancing the uptake of Ca^{2+} by the sarcoplasmic reticulum, leading to increased Ca^{2+} stored in the sarcoplasmic reticulum and the subsequent release of an increased amount of Ca^{2+} from the sarcoplasmic reticulum during contraction; and (4) increasing the heart rate. These effects underlie the increased susceptibility to ventricular arrhythmias in CPVT patients during exercise and emotional stress associated with increased sympathetic stimulation and increased heart rates.

Importantly, in the setting of digitalis poisoning, the abnormal RyR2 behavior leading to spontaneous Ca^{2+} release and DADs is secondary to the elevation of the sarcoplasmic reticulum Ca^{2+} content (store overload–induced Ca^{2+} release, SOICR). In CPVT, on the other hand, spontaneous Ca^{2+} release and DADs can occur without Ca^{2+} overload. Mutations in *RyR2* or *CASQ2* lead to defective Ca^{2+} signaling lowering of the sarcoplasmic reticulum Ca^{2+} threshold for spontaneous Ca^{2+} release below the normal baseline level ("perceived" Ca^{2+} overload). A similar mechanism may underlie triggered arrhythmias in other disease conditions, including heart failure and ischemic heart disease, in which sarcoplasmic reticulum Ca^{2+} release regulation is compromised because of acquired defects in components of the RyR2 channel complex.[96]

As expected with DAD-mediated triggered activity, a positive direct correlation has been observed between the coupling interval of ventricular arrhythmias and the preceding R-R interval. This observation may also suggest that supraventricular arrhythmias commonly observed prior to the onset of ventricular arrhythmias during exercise in CPVT patients may act as a trigger for the development of DADs and triggered activity in the ventricle.[93]

MECHANISM OF THE BIDIRECTIONAL MORPHOLOGY OF VENTRICULAR TACHYCARDIA

The EP mechanisms leading to the characteristic bidirectional morphology of the VT are not clear. Changes in conduction direction from a single ventricular focus with every other beat, VT originating from one focus that triggers another focus, and double ventricular foci (from the right and left apical portions of the heart) are some of the proposed mechanisms. The QRS morphology of bidirectional VT is inconsistent in the same recording lead, suggesting that the focus of the arrhythmia can vary to some extent.[93,96] Some investigators suggested that CPVT starts from a single focus or double foci, usually originating from the RVOT, whereas the ensuing beats tend to originate from the LV. Others found that a left posterior inferior origin accounts for the majority of cases. Additionally, the Purkinje network has been suggested as the site of origin of bidirectional VT, with alternating firing from the right and left branches of the Purkinje fibers.[94]

A recent experimental model suggested a "ping-pong" mechanism may underlie ventricular arrhythmias in CPVT, whereby DAD-induced triggered activity develops at different heart rate thresholds in different regions of the His-Purkinje system (HPS) or ventricles. First, once the heart rate exceeds a certain threshold, ventricular bigeminy develops from a single site in the HPS or ventricular myocardium. The shortened R-R cycle length due to ventricular bigeminy induces DAD-triggered beats from a second focus within the HPS, with the latter reciprocally activating PVCs from the first focus; a process that is repeated back and forth, in a ping-pong pattern. "Reciprocating bigeminy" from the two sites produces the bidirectional VT characteristic of CPVT. Polymorphic VT results when three or more sites concurrently develop bigeminy, whereas monomorphic VT develops when repetitive DADs generate a run of triggered activity from a single site.[106]

MECHANISM OF DRUG EFFECTS

The demonstration that DADs are the initiating mechanism for arrhythmogenesis in CPVT provides a twofold rationale for the use of beta blockers for the treatment of CPVT. Antiadrenergic therapy is a logical therapy to attenuate the effect of adrenergic stimulation induced by exercise or emotion. In addition to this effect, the bradycardia induced by beta blockers is likely to exert an additional antiarrhythmic action by reducing the probability that a DAD would reach the threshold for triggering premature beats. Accordingly, the lower the heart rate achieved with beta blocker therapy, the higher the probability of preventing malignant arrhythmias.[91]

Flecainide (a Na^+ channel blocker) has recently been demonstrated to prevent lethal ventricular arrhythmias in CPVT, an effect likely mediated by inducing brief closures of open RyR2 to subconductance states and, thus, reducing Ca^{2+} spark amplitude.[105]

Differential Diagnosis

Other inherited arrhythmogenic cardiac disorders that can cause malignant ventricular tachyarrhythmias should also be excluded. A QTc interval less than 320 milliseconds should raise a suspicion of SQTS. On the other hand, a prolonged QTc suggests LQTS. Whereas the onset of clinical symptoms of LQTS is often around puberty, the first syncopal events in CPVT patients tend to occur during childhood. Importantly, induction of arrhythmias during exercise is very rare in LQTS patients. Furthermore, LQTS patients develop torsades de pointes (characterized by the twisting of the points of the QRS complexes), in contrast to CPVT patients, who manifest with the typical bidirectional VT with a beat-to-beat 180-degree rotation of the QRS complex.[91,93,94]

Bidirectional VT can also occur in patients with type 7 LQTS (LQT7, Andersen-Tawil syndrome) linked to mutations in the *KCNJ2* gene, which may be considered a CPVT phenocopy, particularly in patients with Andersen-Tawil syndrome having borderline QT interval prolongation. SCD is exceptional among Andersen-Tawil syndrome and *KCNJ2* mutation carriers.[16,17] Furthermore, unlike CPVT, Andersen-Tawil syndrome is characterized by extracardiac features such as periodic paralysis and facial dysmorphism.[91,93,94]

Ankyrin-B syndrome can also manifest with catecholamine-mediated ventricular arrhythmias. Loss-of-function mutations in the *ANK2* gene (encoding cardiac ankyrin-B, a structural membrane adapter protein) result in increased intracellular concentration of Ca^{2+} and, sometimes, fatal arrhythmia. Although this syndrome has been categorized under LQTS (LQT4), the inconsistent QT interval prolongation and the varying degrees of cardiac dysfunction and arrhythmias observed (including bradycardia, sinus arrhythmia, idiopathic VF, adrenergically mediated VT, and SCD) distinguishes ankyrin-B syndrome as a clinical entity distinct from classic LQTS.

Exercise-provoked arrhythmias also can develop in ARVD, but the typical ECG pattern of ARVD and the structural abnormalities of the RV separate ARVD from CPVT. The typical arrhythmia in ARVD, monomorphic VT with a left bundle branch block (LBBB) pattern, is clearly different from the polymorphic PVCs or VT in CPVT.[95]

In contrast to CPVT, patients with Brugada syndrome do not manifest polymorphic PVCs on physical effort; rather, arrhythmias in Brugada syndrome appear usually at rest or during sleep. Furthermore, the absence of ST segment elevation in the precordial ECG leads at baseline and after provocation testing with Na^+ channel blockers helps distinguish CPVT from Brugada syndrome.[95]

Risk Stratification

Risk stratification for SCD in CPVT is not possible because of the relatively small number of patients reported. As noted, CPVT is one of the most malignant forms of ventricular arrhythmias, with a high mortality rate. CPVT patients with prior cardiac arrest and those in whom symptoms are not completely suppressed by pharmacological therapy are considered at high risk for SCD. Programmed electrical stimulation typically fails in inducing ventricular arrhythmias, and is of no value for risk stratification. Furthermore, the predictive value of inducibility of ventricular arrhythmias by catecholamine infusion or exercise for risk stratification has not been demonstrated.

Principles of Management

PHARMACOLOGICAL THERAPY

Beta blockers are the first line of treatment for CPVT and should be promptly initiated to prevent occurrence of ventricular tachyarrhythmias. Because of the poor prognosis of untreated CPVT, drug therapy is indicated for all clinically diagnosed patients and usually also for all silent carriers of a CPVT mutation. The most widely used beta blockers are nadolol (1 to 2.5 mg/kg per day) and propranolol (2.5 to 3.5 mg/kg per day). Intravenous propranolol is the treatment of choice for acute management of CPVT.

Whereas some studies have reported an almost complete prevention of cardiac events during beta blocker therapy, other studies found a high recurrence rate (up to 30% to 50%) of symptoms and even SCD despite the drug therapy, and the efficacy of beta blockers in CPVT appears to be lower than that seen in the LQT1 variant of LQTS.[93,95]

Exercise stress testing and Holter monitoring can help determine the adequate beta blocker dosage for arrhythmia control. It should be noted, however, that the absence of exercise-provoked arrhythmias does not completely exclude the risk of arrhythmia recurrence, and the maximal tolerated dose of beta blockers should be prescribed to maximize control of arrhythmias with a goal to avoid the heart rate exceeding the threshold rate for CPVT. Furthermore, compliance with regular therapy is extremely important, because missing even a single dose can potentially lead to arrhythmias and increase the risk of SCD.[93,95]

Recent studies show that the addition of flecainide to beta blocker therapy can effectively reduce exercise-induced ventricular arrhythmias in CPVT patients not controlled by beta blocker therapy alone.[107] As noted, flecainide effects are mediated by direct blockade of RyR2 channels and reduction of Ca^{2+} spark amplitude rather than Na^+ channel blockade.[108-110]

Limited data suggest that verapamil (an inhibitor of RyR2) can be an alternative option for treatment of CPVT. Also, verapamil can potentially provide additional protection when used in combination with beta blockers. However, because of the small number of patients and the limited follow-up, there is no conclusive evidence for recommending verapamil alone or in combination with beta blockers, and its impact on prognosis is not known.[95]

IMPLANTABLE CARDIOVERTER-DEFIBRILLATOR

Given that no drugs can be effective in providing complete protection from SCD, ICD therapy is recommended for CPVT patients who have survived a cardiac arrest, as well as those who continue to have symptoms (syncope or sustained or hemodynamically unstable VT) despite adequate beta blocker therapy.[58]

Approximately half of ICD recipients experience an appropriate shock to terminate VT during 2 years of follow-up. It is important to maintain the maximal tolerated dose of beta blockers in ICD patients to help reduce the risk of arrhythmic storms and ICD shocks.[91,93]

CATHETER ABLATION

When ventricular arrhythmias are triggered by monomorphic PVCs, catheter ablation of the focus of PVCs may be attempted to help reduce the frequency and burden of arrhythmias and ICD shocks. Not infrequently, the initiating beat of VT exhibits an LBBB–inferior axis pattern, suggestive of a ventricular outflow tract origin.[111]

SYMPATHETIC DENERVATION

Small case series suggest the effectiveness of left cardiac sympathetic denervation in patients with recurrent symptoms despite beta blocker therapy or those experiencing frequent ICD shocks or intractable arrhythmic storms.[93]

PARTICIPATION IN SPORTS

Symptomatic CPVT patients as well as asymptomatic patients (detected as part of familial screening) with documented exercise- or isoproterenol-induced VT should refrain from all competitive sports with the possible exception of minimal contact, class IA activities. A less restrictive approach may be possible for the genotype-positive/phenotype-negative (asymptomatic, no inducible VT) athlete.[59]

FAMILY SCREENING

Given the severe clinical manifestations and poor prognosis of CPVT, once CPVT diagnosis is made in a proband, it is essential to expand the evaluation to both first- and second-degree relatives to find other potential CPVT patients.[41] Exercise testing, Holter monitoring, or both are used for screening family members. Importantly, some CPVT patients may not have arrhythmias in the exercise stress test during early childhood, but a change in the phenotype occurs later in life. Therefore, regular follow-up with repeated exercise stress tests is indicated, for example, for younger siblings of a CPVT patient.

Screening of family members by genetic testing is recommended when a gene mutation has been identified in the proband.[94] Considering the early age of manifestation of CPVT and its association with SIDS, confirmatory genetic testing should be performed at birth. Genetic evaluation facilitates diagnosis in silent carriers and allows implementation of preventive pharmacological therapy and reproductive risk assessment.[41,75,112]

Early Repolarization Syndromes

Early repolarization ECG patterns, consisting of a distinct J wave or J point elevation, a notch or slur of the terminal part of the QRS, and an ST segment elevation, are predominantly found in healthy young men and have traditionally been viewed as totally benign, "normal variants." However, this concept has been challenged by several recent studies, which suggested that early repolarization patterns in apparently healthy subjects could represent a marker of increased dispersion of repolarization and arrhythmogenesis, and of the presence of a relationship between certain repolarization patterns and some cases of idiopathic VF and SCD.[113,114]

Epidemiology

The prevalence of early repolarization in the general population varies from 1% to 9%, depending on age (predominant in young adults), race (highest among black populations), gender (predominant in men), and the criterion for J point elevation (0.05 mV versus 0.1 mV).[2,115] In a study of a community-based general population of 10,864 middle-aged subjects, the prevalence of early repolarization

(J point elevation >0.1 mV) was 5.8%, including 3.5% in the inferior leads, 2.4% in the lateral leads, and 0.1% in both. With J point elevation greater than 0.2 mV, the prevalence dropped to 0.33%.[116] The ST segment after the J point was horizontal or descending in approximately 71.5% and rapidly ascending in 28.5%. In young athletes, early repolarization in the inferior and/or lateral leads was observed in up to 44%, with the majority of subjects having ascending ST segment patterns after J point elevation.[117]

Early repolarization is more frequent in patients with idiopathic VF than in control subjects (31% versus 5% in one report, 42% versus 13% in a second report). Moreover, among patients with idiopathic VF, those with early repolarization are more likely to have a history of syncope or SCD than those without early repolarization.[115,118]

The presence of an early repolarization pattern, especially in the inferior or lateral leads, has recently been recognized in some studies as associated with vulnerability to VF and a 4- to 10-fold increase in the risk for SCD.[115] In the 35- to 45-year age range of maximal early repolarization-related SCD incidence, a J wave is estimated to increase idiopathic VF risk from 3.4 per 100,000 to 11 per 100,000.[118] The prevalence of inferolateral J-point elevation is higher in the family members of sudden arrhythmic death syndrome probands compared with the general population (23% versus 11%).[119] Furthermore, J point elevation of more than 0.2 mV in inferior leads appears to be a stronger predictor of death from cardiac causes than other well-known ECG risk markers, such as the QTc interval and signs of LV hypertrophy.[116]

It is important to recognize, however, that the interrelations between epidemiological factors predisposing to early repolarization per se and SCD-associated early repolarization are still unclear.[2]

Electrocardiographic Features

The early repolarization pattern is a common ECG variant characterized by an elevation of the J point, ST segment elevation with upper concavity, and tall/symmetric T waves in at least two contiguous leads. The J point marks the junction between the end of the QRS complex and the beginning of the ST segment on the surface ECG. Elevation of the J point, the so-called J wave, is defined as a positive "humplike" deflection at the onset of the ST segment immediately after a positive QRS complex. In most studies, elevation of the J point and/or ST segment from the baseline by at least 0.1 mV was considered definitive of early repolarization.[115,116] The pattern of ST segment elevation after the J point can be classified as horizontal/descending (≤0.1-mV elevation of the ST segment within 100 milliseconds after the J point), or concave/rapidly ascending (>0.1-mV elevation of ST segment within 100 milliseconds after the J point or a persistently elevated ST segment of >0.1 mV throughout the ST segment).[117]

The early repolarization pattern can vary in response to autonomic tone and heart rate. Bradycardia and increased vagal tone (e.g., during sleep) accentuate ST segment elevation. Contrariwise, tachycardia and adrenergic stimulation (e.g., exercise testing or the infusion of isoproterenol) suppress J wave amplitude and ST segment elevation. Additionally, hypothermia can induce prominent J waves ("Osborn waves").[2,115]

Pathophysiology of Early Repolarization Syndromes

MECHANISM OF EARLY REPOLARIZATION AND J WAVES

The exact ionic and cellular mechanisms for the J wave and early repolarization pattern are still unknown. Heterogeneity in the distribution of I_{to} channels across the myocardial wall, being more prominent in ventricular epicardium than endocardium, results in the shorter duration, prominent phase 1 notch, and "spike and dome" morphology of the epicardial action potential as compared with the endocardium. The resultant transmural voltage gradient during the early phases (phases 1 and 2) of the action potential is thought to be responsible for the inscription of the J wave on the surface ECG (see Fig. 31-6).[76,77]

An outward shift of currents, secondary to a decrease in the inward currents (I_{Na} and I_{CaL}), an increase in the outward K^+ currents (I_{to}, I_{Kr}, I_{Ks}, I_{KACh}, I_{KATP}), or both, can cause accentuation of the action potential notch, leading to augmentation of the J wave or the appearance of ST segment elevation on the surface ECG. An outward shift of currents that extends beyond the action potential notch not only can accentuate the J wave but also can lead to partial or complete loss of the dome of the action potential, leading to a protracted transmural voltage gradient that manifests as greater ST segment elevation and gives rise to J wave syndromes. The type of ion current affected and its regional distribution in the ventricles determines the particular phenotype (including the Brugada syndrome, early repolarization syndrome, hypothermia-induced ST segment elevation, and infarction-induced ST segment elevation).[2,76,77]

In this context, factors that influence the kinetics of I_{to} or the other repolarization currents can modify the manifestation of the J wave on the ECG. Na^+ channel blockers (procainamide, pilsicainide, propafenone, flecainide, and disopyramide), which reduce the inward I_{Na}, can accentuate the J wave and ST segment elevation in patients with concealed J wave syndromes. Quinidine, which inhibits both I_{to} and I_{Na}, reduces the magnitude of the J wave and normalizes ST segment elevation. Additionally, acceleration of the heart rate, which is associated with reduction of I_{to} (because of the slow recovery of I_{to} from inactivation), results in a decrease in the magnitude of the J wave. Male predominance can potentially result from larger epicardial I_{to} density versus that in women.[2,76]

MECHANISM OF ARRHYTHMOGENESIS

The exact relationship of an early repolarization pattern and malignant ventricular arrhythmias remains unclear. It is likely that the increased transmural heterogeneity of ventricular repolarization (i.e., dispersion of repolarization between epicardium and endocardium), which is responsible for J point elevation and the early repolarization pattern on the surface ECG, is also responsible for the increased vulnerability to ventricular tachyarrhythmias. A significant outward shift in current can cause partial or complete loss of the dome of the action potential in regions where I_{to} is prominent (epicardium), with the consequent loss of activation of I_{CaL}. The dome of the action potential then can propagate from regions where it is preserved (midmyocardium and endocardium) to regions where it is lost (epicardium), giving rise to phase 2 reentry, which can generate PVCs that in turn can initiate polymorphic VT or VF (see Fig. 31-7).[2,76,116]

Differential Diagnosis

Based on the localization of the early repolarization pattern on the 12-lead surface ECG and its potential association with risk for life-threatening arrhythmias, some investigators classified early repolarization patterns into three types. In type 1, the early repolarization pattern manifests predominantly in the lateral precordial leads; this form is very prevalent among healthy male athletes and is thought to be associated with a relatively low level of risk for arrhythmic events. In type 2, the early repolarization pattern is localized to the inferior or inferolateral leads; this form is associated with a moderate level of risk. In type 3, early repolarization is more global, involving the inferior, lateral, and right precordial leads. Type 3 is associated with the highest level of risk (Table 31-12).[76]

Early repolarization ECG patterns can also be observed during hypothermia, with cocaine abuse, in patients with Brugada syndrome, and with hypertrophic cardiomyopathy. In the Brugada syndrome, ST segment elevation is limited to the right precordial leads (see Table 31-12). In hypothermia, J waves (Osborne waves) can manifest diffusely in all leads or be confined to selected leads. Rarely, hypothermia can induce ECG changes that mimic those of Brugada syndrome. Although Brugada and early repolarization syndromes

TABLE 31-12 J Wave Syndromes

	Inherited				Acquired	
	EARLY REPOLARIZATION IN LATERAL LEADS (ERS TYPE 1)	EARLY REPOLARIZATION IN INFERIOR OR INFEROLATERAL LEADS (ERS TYPE 2)	GLOBAL EARLY REPOLARIZATION (ERS TYPE 3)	BRUGADA SYNDROME	ISCHEMIA-MEDIATED VT/VF	HYPOTHERMIA-MEDIATED VT/VF
Anatomical location responsible for chief electrophysiological manifestations	Anterolateral left ventricle	Inferior left ventricle	Left and right ventricles	Right ventricle	Left and right ventricles	Left and right ventricles
Leads displaying J point/J wave abnormalities	I, V_4-V_6	II, III, aVF	Global	V_1-V_3	Any of the 12 leads	Any of the 12 leads
Response of J wave amplitude/ ST elevation to:						
Bradycardia or pause	Increase	Increase	Increase	Increase	N/A	N/A
Sodium channel blockers	Little or no change	Little or no change	Little or no change	Increase	N/A	N/A
Gender dominance	Male	Male	Male	Male	Male	Either gender
VF	Rare; commonly seen in healthy men and athletes	Yes	Yes; electrical storms	Yes	Yes	Yes
Response to quinidine	Normalization of J point elevation and inhibition of VT/VF	Normalization of J point elevation and inhibition of VT/VF	Limited data; normalization of J point elevation and inhibition of VT/VF	Normalization of J point elevation and inhibition of VT/VF	Limited data	Inhibition of VT/VF
Response to isoproterenol	Normalization of J point elevation and inhibition of VT/VF	Normalization of J point elevation and inhibition of VT/VF	Limited data	Normalization of J point elevation and inhibition of VT/VF	N/A	N/A
Gene mutations	*CACNA1C, CACNB2B57*	*KCNJ8,56, CACNA1C, CACNB2B57*	*CACNA1C57*	*SCN5A, CACNA1C, CACNB2B, GPD1-L, SCN1B, KCNE3, SCN3B, KCNJ8*	*SCN5A72*	N/A

ERS = early repolarization syndrome; N/A = data not available; VF = ventricular fibrillation; VT = ventricular tachycardia.
From Antzelevitch C, Yan GX: J wave syndromes, *Heart Rhythm* 7:549-558, 2010.

differ with respect to the magnitude and lead location of abnormal J wave manifestation, they are thought to represent a continuous spectrum of phenotypic expression termed *J wave syndromes*.[114]

Risk Stratification

Although early repolarization is a common entity, unexplained SCD in young adults is very rare. Even in the 35- to 45-year age range of maximal early repolarization-related SCD incidence, a J wave is estimated to increase idiopathic VF risk from 3.4 per 100,000 to 11 per 100,000, which is still relatively low. Therefore, the incidental discovery of a J wave on routine screening should not be interpreted as a marker of "high risk" for SCD because the odds for this fatal disease would still be roughly 1:10,000. Nonetheless, the presence of early repolarization should attract careful attention in certain groups of patients. Additionally, several properties of the early repolarization pattern (location, magnitude of the J wave, and degree of ST elevation) can potentially have significant prognostic implications.[2,118]

J WAVE AMPLITUDE

Evidence suggests that the height of J point elevation, rather than its mere presence, can potentially provide important risk stratification information. J point elevation greater than 0.2 mV in the inferior leads predicts a 2.9-fold increase in SCD risk, whereas an elevation of at least 0.1 mV predicts a more modest (1.4-fold) increase in risk of arrhythmic death. A similar phenomenon was also observed in survivors of primary VF. It is worth noting that a J point elevation greater than 0.2 mV seems to be rare (0.3% to 0.7%) in the normal population, but was observed in 16% of patients with idiopathic VF.[2,115,116,120]

J WAVE DISTRIBUTION

A recent study found that 46.9% of patients with VF and early repolarization exhibited the early repolarization pattern in both inferior and lateral leads.[115] The early repolarization pattern in the inferior leads is a stronger predictor of death from cardiac causes or from arrhythmia than that localized to the lateral leads. Conversely, in asymptomatic individuals, early repolarization is most prominent in midprecordial leads (V_2 to V_4), a pattern that is especially predominant among athletes and is thought to entail a more benign prognosis.[2,120]

J WAVE FLUCTUATION

Although the pattern of J point elevation on baseline measurement remains constant during long-term follow-up in the majority of subjects, the magnitude of J point elevation can fluctuate even without drug provocation or exercise. Marked spontaneous accentuation of J wave amplitude as well as spontaneous beat-to-beat fluctuation in the morphological pattern of early repolarization can frequently be observed during periods of electrical storm (including frequent PVCs and episodes of VF). Therefore, transient and marked augmentation of J wave amplitude can potentially portend a high risk for VF in patients with early repolarization.[120,121]

ST SEGMENT PATTERN

For early repolarization patterns in the inferior or lateral leads, the presence of horizontal or descending ST segments after the J point predicts an increased risk for arrhythmic death, especially if accompanied by a high-amplitude (>0.2 mV) J point elevation. In contrast, the presence of rapidly upsloping ST segments after the J point (which is the most common pattern observed in young athletes) predicts a benign prognosis.[117]

OTHER REPOLARIZATION ABNORMALITIES

The presence of only ST segment elevation or R wave slurring, without J point elevation, does not appear to predict high risk of arrhythmic events. Moreover, the presence of QRS slurring does not add diagnostic value to the presence of J point elevation, regardless of its magnitude or the leads where it is observed.[118] Additionally, T wave alternans and QT dispersion do not appear to be useful for SCD risk stratification in early repolarization, although evidence is scarce.

EXERCISE TESTING

Exercise suppresses the early repolarization pattern both in symptomatic and asymptomatic subjects, irrespective of the location of early repolarization. Therefore, exercise testing does not seem to provide prognostic information.

INVASIVE ELECTROPHYSIOLOGICAL TESTING

Invasive EP testing is not helpful for risk stratification. Patients with early repolarization do not exhibit significantly higher inducibility with programmed ventricular stimulation than those without early repolarization. Furthermore, EP testing has limited sensitivity for risk stratification of symptomatic patients; VF is inducible by programmed stimulation in only 34% of the patients with a clinical history of VF.

GENETIC SCREENING

Genetic contributions to SCD-associated early repolarization are suggested by common familial SCD histories in symptomatic early repolarization patients. Early repolarization appears to be a heritable phenotype; offspring of early repolarization–positive parents have a 2.5-fold increased risk of presenting with early repolarization in their ECG.[122] Additionally, in a recent report, 16% of cases with VF and early repolarization had a family history of SCD. Geographic differences in distribution have also been described, with early repolarization–related SCD being particularly prevalent among Southeast Asians.[2] However, because early repolarization was not associated with an increased risk of SCD until recently, the genetic markers to differentiate benign and arrhythmic forms of early repolarization have not been identified. Recently, mutations of the *DPP6* gene, identified in a subset of patients with idiopathic VF, may prove valuable in the identification of asymptomatic subjects. However, at this time, the role of genetic screening for risk stratification has not been well characterized.[113]

Principles of Management

Management of VF associated with early repolarization is similar to that of idiopathic VF discussed below. There is not yet a clear consensus on the specific risk factors that identify asymptomatic early repolarization subjects in whom the probability of SCD is sufficiently high to warrant an ICD for primary prevention. Even the presence of unexplained syncope or family history of SCD in the context of early repolarization is not sufficient to recommend prophylactic ICD implantation, because those parameters have not been shown to reliably identify patients at risk for life-threatening arrhythmias. The latter group of patients, however, should be offered close follow-up and general guidelines for the management of syncope.[2,58]

On the other hand, the presence of an early repolarization pattern in the right precordial leads or the presence of a rapidly upsloping ST segment after the J point in patients with early repolarization in the inferior or lateral leads predicts a benign prognosis, at least in middle-aged subjects. These individuals should probably not be profiled as high risk if they are asymptomatic and have no family history of life-threatening arrhythmias or SCD.[117]

PARTICIPATION IN SPORTS

Restriction from competitive sports is appropriate in patients with idiopathic VF. However, no information is available about lifestyle modification in patients with early repolarization. Given the high prevalence of early repolarization patterns (especially in leads V_2 to V_6) in athletes, occurring in 20% of noncompetitive athletes and in up to 90% of high-performance athletes, and because the midprecordial early repolarization location is generally believed to be benign, and in the absence of reliable risk-stratifying parameters, a universal restriction from competitive sports in asymptomatic athletes with early repolarization, even at competitive levels, does not seem warranted. Nonetheless, certain restrictions may be considered in highly active patients with resting bradycardia and prominent early repolarization patterns localized to the inferior or inferolateral leads, although definitive guidelines are still lacking.[2]

Idiopathic Ventricular Fibrillation

Idiopathic VF is defined as spontaneous VF without any known *structural* or *electrical* heart disease.[113]

Epidemiology

Idiopathic VF accounts for up to 10% of victims of SCD, mainly in the young. The mean age at presentation is approximately 35 to 45 years, and two-thirds of patients are men. A family history of SCD or idiopathic VF is present in up to 20% of patients, suggesting that at least a subset of idiopathic VF is hereditary.[113]

Clinical Presentation

Idiopathic VF manifests as either syncope or cardiac arrest that is typically not related to physical or emotional stress. VF often occurs at night, when heart rate is slower and vagal tone is augmented. The recurrence of VF in patients with idiopathic VF is approximately 30%, and the proportion of patients presenting with cardiac arrest as opposed to syncope appears to be much higher in idiopathic VF than in other channelopathies, suggesting that ventricular arrhythmias in other channelopathies are more likely to terminate spontaneously whereas idiopathic VF tends to be sustained. Electrical storm occurs in approximately 10% of patients.[113,123]

Diagnosis of Idiopathic Ventricular Fibrillation

The diagnosis of idiopathic VF is based on exclusion of an underlying structural or primary electrical heart disease. Hence, a thorough cardiac evaluation is warranted. Echocardiography, stress testing, coronary angiography, and cardiac magnetic resonance imaging need to be considered to exclude structural cardiac disease, such as coronary artery disease, congenital coronary anomalies, dilated cardiomyopathy, hypertrophic cardiomyopathy, ARVD, cardiac sarcoidosis, myocarditis, and left apical ballooning. Metabolic disorders, electrolyte abnormalities, and drug intoxication also need to be excluded.[123]

Careful analysis of the surface 12-lead ECG is mandatory to exclude primary electrical heart disease. Abnormal shortening or prolongation of the QT interval can suggest SQTS or LQTS, respectively. Repolarization abnormalities in the right precordial leads can suggest the Brugada syndrome. The presence of ventricular preexcitation can suggest preexcited supraventricular tachyarrhythmias as the underlying cause of VF. It is important to understand that all these disorders can manifest with minor or borderline ECG abnormalities, and recording serial ECGs, recording of modified precordial leads (such as in the Brugada ECG pattern), ECG recording during exercise or after drug challenge, and/or continuous ambulatory cardiac monitoring can be necessary to unmask diagnostic ECG abnormalities.[123] Pharmacological drug challenge to exclude the Brugada syndrome, and exercise stress testing or catecholamine infusion to exclude CPVT, should be considered. Invasive EP testing may be considered, especially when sinus node dysfunction, AV conduction abnormalities, or the presence of a bypass tract is suspected.[123]

Genetics of Idiopathic Ventricular Fibrillation

A recent report provided evidence for a familial component in idiopathic VF and suggested a role for *DPP6* as the causal gene. Overexpression of *DPP6*, which encodes dipeptidyl-peptidase 6, a putative component of the transient outward current (I_{to}) channel complex in the heart, was proposed as the likely pathogenetic mechanism. *DPP6* significantly alters the inactivation kinetics of both $K_v4.2$ and $K_v4.3$ and promotes expression of these alpha subunits in the cell membrane. Clinical evaluation of 84 risk-haplotype carriers and 71 noncarriers revealed no ECG or structural parameters indicative of cardiac disease. Penetrance of idiopathic VF was high; 50% of risk-haplotype carriers experienced (aborted) SCD before the age of 58 years.[113]

The I_{to} current, which mediates phase 1 of the action potential, is distributed heterogeneously across the ventricular wall, being more prominent in epicardium compared with endocardium. An increase in I_{to} amplitude resulting from increased *DPP6* can potentially cause a deeper phase 1 in the epicardium with the appearance of a J wave on the surface ECG. An additional increase in I_{to} potentially leads to ST segment elevation. However, no EP abnormalities were observed on the baseline ECG in carriers of the risk haplotype and no differences in prevalence of early repolarization were observed between haplotype carriers and noncarriers. Importantly, arrhythmic episodes appeared not to be preceded by any discernable ECG abnormality. Any morphological action potential changes that might be present were apparently not sufficient to inscribe on the ECG and, therefore, are as yet obscuring the nature of the arrhythmogenic substrate, which in fact might be very local, in the lower part of the RV free wall.[113]

Principles of Management

PHARMACOLOGICAL THERAPY

Data from controlled trials or experimental studies are largely lacking. Preliminary clinical experience with quinidine is promising. Beta-adrenergic agonists are beneficial in idiopathic VF, particularly for arrhythmic storm. Amiodarone has limited efficacy. Beta blockers, lidocaine, mexiletine, and verapamil are usually not beneficial.

Acceleration of the heart rate (up to 120 beats/min) by isoproterenol infusion or by atrial or ventricular pacing can be very effective for the acute control of ventricular arrhythmias. Deep sedation may also be considered in refractory cases.[2,124]

IMPLANTABLE CARDIOVERTER-DEFIBRILLATOR

SECONDARY PREVENTION. For secondary prevention, ICD implantation is recommended in patients with prior cardiac arrest due to VF. In patients with ICDs and frequent nonsustained ventricular arrhythmias, recurrent sustained arrhythmias precipitating frequent ICD shocks, or both, adjuvant antiarrhythmic therapy with quinidine can be helpful.[58] Of note, patients with VF and early repolarization have shown a higher incidence of VF recurrence than VF patients without early repolarization (43% versus 23% during 5 years of follow-up).

PRIMARY PREVENTION. In view of the lack of specific risk factors or of ECG or imaging abnormalities in patients with idiopathic VF (apart from the early repolarization patterns discussed earlier), identification of at-risk subjects is currently not possible. The presence of unexplained syncope or family history of idiopathic VF or SCD is not sufficient to recommend prophylactic ICD implantation, because those parameters have not been shown to reliably identify patients at risk for life-threatening arrhythmias. Nevertheless, careful work-up of the cause of syncope and close follow-up should be undertaken.[2,58]

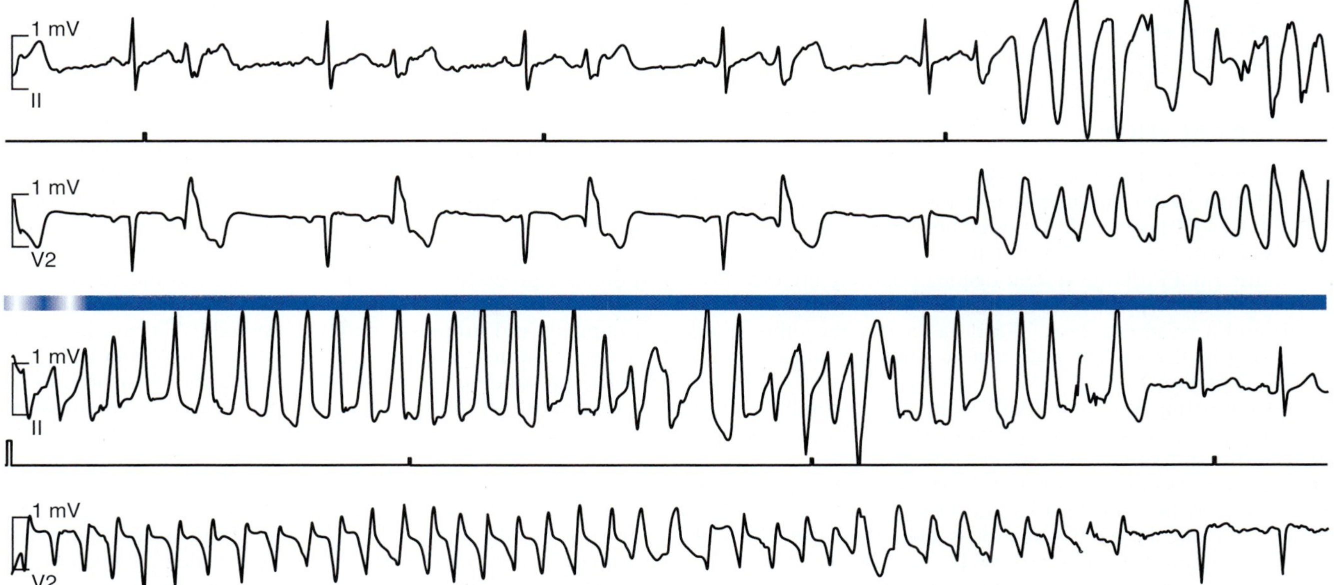

FIGURE 31-9 Polymorphic ventricular tachycardia (VT) triggered by premature ventricular complexes (PVCs). The telemetry rhythm strips show normal sinus rhythm with PVCs that trigger an episode of polymorphic VT. Note that the morphology of the triggering PVCs is similar to that of the isolated PVC.

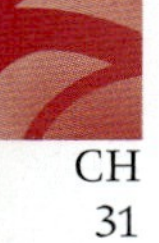

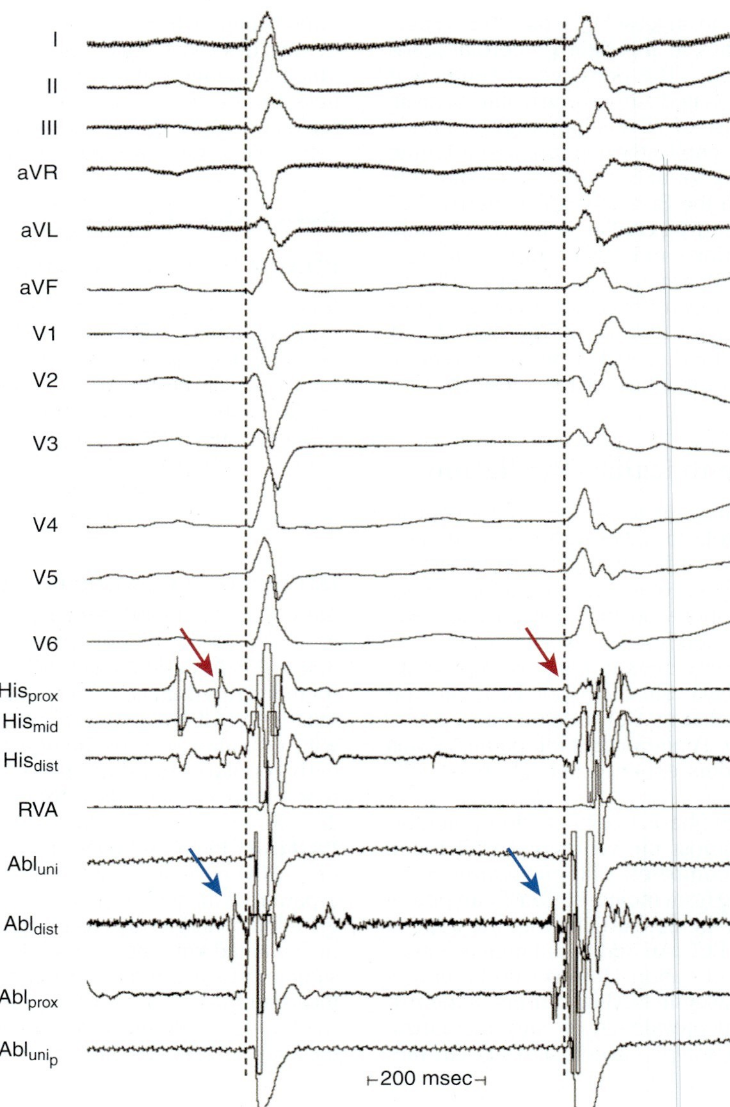

FIGURE 31-10 Sinus rhythm (left) and premature ventricular complexes (PVCs, right) in a patient with idiopathic ventricular fibrillation. Dashed lines denote the onset of QRS complexes. Blue arrows indicate Purkinje potentials, and red arrows indicate His potentials. During sinus rhythm, His potentials precede Purkinje potentials, the sequence of which is reversed in the PVCs.

CATHETER ABLATION

Recent evidence suggests an important role of specific triggers in the RVOT or in the Purkinje system for initiation of idiopathic VF (Fig. 31-9). VF-triggering PVCs originate from various locations within the Purkinje system in the majority of patients. PVCs originating in the right Purkinje system display relatively uniform ECG morphologies and typically have an LBBB pattern with a left superior axis and a relatively short QRS duration. On the other hand, PVCs arising in the left Purkinje system produce more variable 12-lead ECG patterns.

PVCs originating from the RVOT, although generally considered "benign," can also initiate polymorphic VT and VF in some patients with idiopathic VF. Distinguishing between the "malignant" forms and the benign form of RVOT PVCs is often challenging. Data suggest that shorter CLs during monomorphic VT, short coupling intervals of the PVCs, as well as a history of syncope with malignant characteristics, can potentially predict the coexistence of VF or polymorphic VT in patients with idiopathic RVOT VT/PVCs. However, significant overlap exists.[125]

When ventricular arrhythmias are triggered by monomorphic PVCs, catheter ablation of the PVC focus can potentially prevent further episodes of VF or reduce the burden of arrhythmias. In the setting of PVCs arising from the Purkinje network, a presystolic low-amplitude and high-frequency signal (Purkinje potential) is typically recorded at the successful ablation site, whereby the Purkinje potential precedes and is closely coupled to the ventricular signal of the culprit PVC (Fig. 31-10). Abolition of the local Purkinje potentials and suppression of the targeted PVCs have been shown in a small series to significantly reduce the frequency of VF.[126]

The presence of frequent PVCs during the ablation procedure can significantly improve the success of ablation. Not infrequently, the optimal time for ablation is at the time of an arrhythmic storm when the PVCs tend to be frequent. When the PVCs are absent at the time of the procedure, provocative maneuvers including the use of isoproterenol or programmed electrical stimulation are not usually helpful. Pace mapping can be used in cases of monomorphic ventricular ectopy when a clear 12-lead recording of the clinical PVCs initiating VF has been obtained (Figs. 31-11 and 31-12).[126,127]

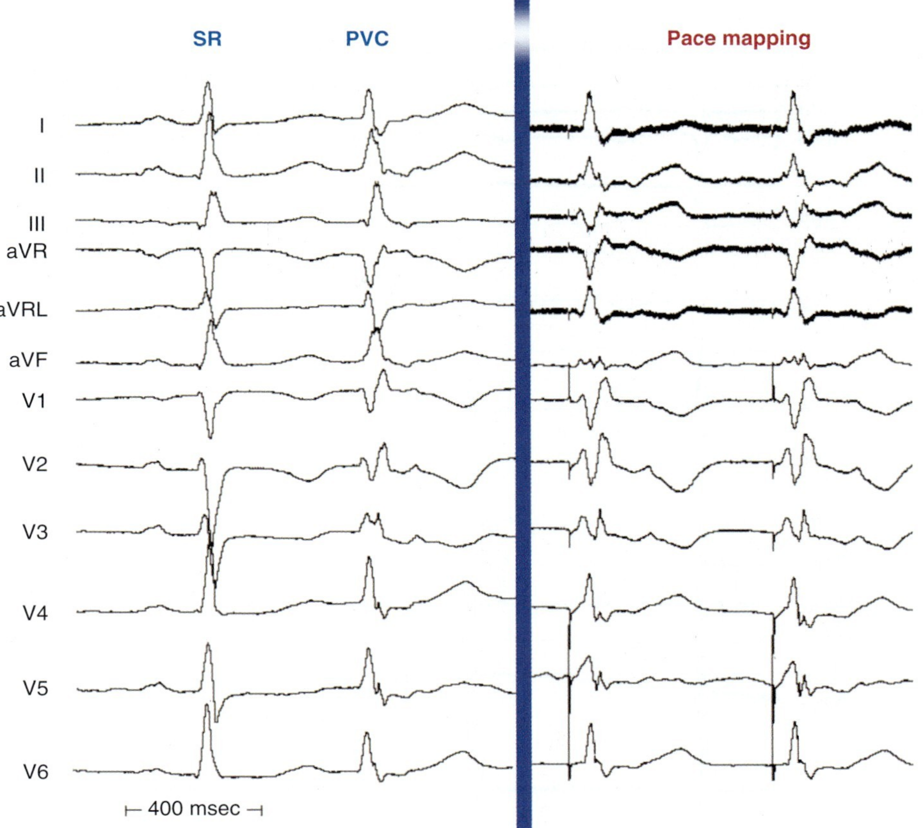

FIGURE 31-11 At left, sinus rhythm (SR) and a premature ventricular complex (PVC) in a patient with idiopathic VF are shown. At right, pacing at the PVC site of origin closely mimics the PVC.

Catheter ablation of focal PVCs may be considered especially in patients with frequent episodes of syncope or repeated ICD shocks refractory to drug therapy. Nonetheless, ablation therapy is not a substitute for ICD therapy because of the risk of recurrence of VF (in 18% of patients) triggered by PVCs either from the original focus or from new foci.[126,127]

It is worth noting that recent studies found a concordance between the site of origin of VF-triggering PVCs and the location of the early repolarization pattern on the surface ECG. Patients with early repolarization recorded in inferior leads alone had PVCs originating from the inferior LV wall, whereas those with early repolarization recorded in both inferior and lateral leads had PVCs originated from multiple regions.[115]

PARTICIPATION IN SPORTS

Restriction from competitive sports is appropriate in patients with idiopathic VF.

FAMILY SCREENING

Unlike other arrhythmia syndromes, such as Brugada syndrome or LQTS, no cardiac abnormalities are observed in idiopathic VF patients, apart from the early repolarization ECG pattern, which is also not infrequently observed in the general population. Hence, family members who may be at risk cannot be identified and the penetrance of idiopathic VF cannot be assessed on the basis of an ECG phenotype.

Elucidation of underlying genetic defects will provide more insight into the pathogenesis of the disorder and, crucially, will allow presymptomatic identification of individuals at risk. The recent identification of mutations of the *DPP6* gene as a potential familial component in idiopathic VF may prove valuable in the identification of presymptomatic subjects. However, at this time, the role of genetic screening has not been well characterized.[113]

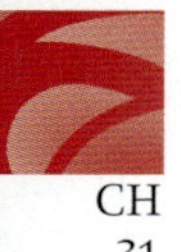

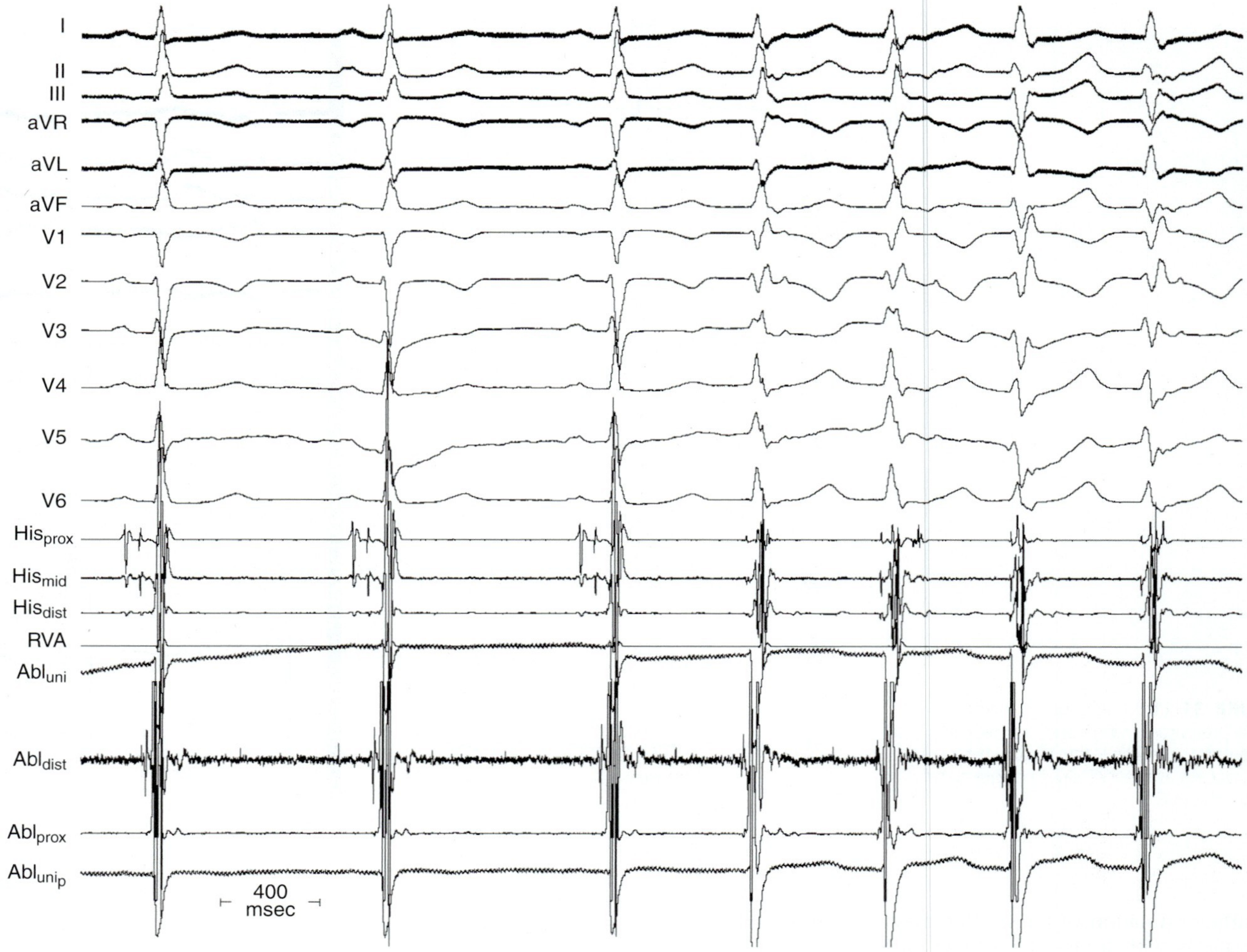

FIGURE 31-12 Three seconds after the onset of radiofrequency energy delivery at the site of premature ventricular complex (PVC) origin in a patient with idiopathic VF, a burst of ectopy occurs having the same QRS configuration as the spontaneously occurring PVC (see Figs. 31-10 and 31-11).

REFERENCES

1. Weisfeldt ML, Everson-Stewart S, Sitlani C, et al: Ventricular tachyarrhythmias after cardiac arrest in public versus at home, *N Engl J Med* 364:313–321, 2011.
2. Benito B, Guasch E, Rivard L, Nattel S: Clinical and mechanistic issues in early repolarization of normal variants and lethal arrhythmia syndromes, *J Am Coll Cardiol* 56:1177–1186, 2010.
3. Lu JT, Kass RS: Recent progress in congenital long QT syndrome, *Curr Opin Cardiol* 25:216–221, 2010.
4. Sauer AJ, Moss AJ, McNitt S, et al: Long QT syndrome in adults, *J Am Coll Cardiol* 49:329–337, 2007.
5. Goldenberg I, Moss AJ: Long QT syndrome, *J Am Coll Cardiol* 51:2291–2300, 2008.
6. Schwartz PJ, Spazzolini C, Crotti L, et al: The Jervell and Lange-Nielsen syndrome: natural history, molecular basis, and clinical outcome, *Circulation* 113:783–790, 2006.
7. Saenen JB, Vrints CJ: Molecular aspects of the congenital and acquired long QT syndrome: clinical implications, *J Mol Cell Cardiol* 44:633–646, 2008.
8. Crotti L, Stramba-Badiali M, Ferrandi C: Prevalence of the long QT syndrome, *Circulation* 112(Suppl II):II-660, 2005.
9. Jons C, Moss AJ, Goldenberg I, et al: Risk of fatal arrhythmic events in long QT syndrome patients after syncope, *J Am Coll Cardiol* 55:783–788, 2010.
10. Sy RW, Chattha IS, Klein GJ, et al: Repolarization dynamics during exercise discriminate between LQT1 and LQT2 genotypes, *J Cardiovasc Electrophysiol* 21:1242–1246, 2010.
11. Ruan Y, Liu N, Napolitano C, Priori SG: Therapeutic strategies for long-QT syndrome: does the molecular substrate matter? *Circ Arrhythm Electrophysiol* 1:290–297, 2008.
12. Moss AJ, Goldenberg I: Importance of knowing the genotype and the specific mutation when managing patients with long QT syndrome, *Circ Arrhythm Electrophysiol* 1:213–226, 2008.
13. Kim JA, Lopes CM, Moss AJ, et al: Trigger-specific risk factors and response to therapy in long QT syndrome type 2, *Heart Rhythm* 7:1797–1805, 2010.
14. Goldenberg I, Moss AJ, Peterson DR, et al: Risk factors for aborted cardiac arrest and sudden cardiac death in children with the congenital long-QT syndrome, *Circulation* 117:2184–2191, 2008.
15. Goldenberg I, Bradley J, Moss A, et al: Beta-blocker efficacy in high-risk patients with the congenital long-QT syndrome types 1 and 2: implications for patient management, *J Cardiovasc Electrophysiol* 21:893–901, 2010.
16. Lu CW, Lin JH, Rajawat YS, et al: Functional and clinical characterization of a mutation in KCNJ2 associated with Andersen-Tawil syndrome, *J Med Genet* 43:653–659, 2006.
17. Tsuboi M, Antzelevitch C: Cellular basis for electrocardiographic and arrhythmic manifestations of Andersen-Tawil syndrome (LQT7), *Heart Rhythm* 3:328–335, 2006.
18. Tristani-Firouzi M, Jensen JL, Donaldson MR, et al: Functional and clinical characterization of KCNJ2 mutations associated with LQT7 (Andersen syndrome), *J Clin Invest* 110:381–388, 2002.
19. Franz MR: Bazett, Fridericia, or Malik? *Heart Rhythm* 5:1432–1433, 2008.
20. Goldenberg I, Moss AJ, Zareba W: QT interval: how to measure it and what is "normal," *J Cardiovasc Electrophysiol* 17:333–336, 2006.
21. Chiladakis J, Kalogeropoulos A, Arvanitis P, et al: Preferred QT correction formula for the assessment of drug-induced QT interval prolongation, *J Cardiovasc Electrophysiol* 21:905–913, 2010.
22. Rautaharju PM, Surawicz B, Gettes LS, et al: AHA/ACCF/HRS recommendations for the standardization and interpretation of the electrocardiogram. IV. The ST segment, T and U waves, and the QT interval: a scientific statement from the American Heart Association Electrocardiography and Arrhythmias Committee, Council on Clinical Cardiology; the American College of Cardiology Foundation; and the Heart Rhythm Society, *J Am Coll Cardiol* 53:982–991, 2009.
23. Monnig G, Eckardt L, Wedekind H, et al: Electrocardiographic risk stratification in families with congenital long QT syndrome, *Eur Heart J* 27:2074–2080, 2006.
24. Malik M, Hnatkova K, Schmidt A, Smetana P: Accurately measured and properly heart-rate corrected QTc intervals show little daytime variability, *Heart Rhythm* 5:1424–1431, 2008.
25. Viskin S: The QT interval: too long, too short or just right, *Heart Rhythm* 6:711–715, 2009.
26. Goldenberg I, Mathew J, Moss AJ, et al: Corrected QT variability in serial electrocardiograms in long QT syndrome: the importance of the maximum corrected QT for risk stratification, *J Am Coll Cardiol* 48:1047–1052, 2006.
27. Shimizu W: The long QT syndrome: therapeutic implications of a genetic diagnosis, *Cardiovasc Res* 67:347–356, 2005.

28. Vatta M: Genetic variants and ECG pattern variability in long QT syndrome: how far are we? *Heart Rhythm* 7:904–905, 2010.
29. Viitasalo M, Oikarinen L, Swan H, et al: Ambulatory electrocardiographic evidence of transmural dispersion of repolarization in patients with long-QT syndrome type 1 and 2, *Circulation* 106:2473–2478, 2002.
30. Jeyaraj D, Abernethy DP, Natarajan RN, et al: I_{Kr} channel blockade to unmask occult congenital long QT syndrome, *Heart Rhythm* 5:2–7, 2008.
31. Viitasalo M, Oikarinen L, Swan H, et al: Ratio of late to early T-wave peak amplitude in 24-h electrocardiographic recordings as indicator of symptom history in patients with long-QT syndrome types 1 and 2, *J Am Coll Cardiol* 47:112–120, 2006.
32. Roden DM: Clinical practice. Long-QT syndrome, *N Engl J Med* 358:169–176, 2008.
33. Clur SA, Chockalingam P, Filippini LH, et al: The role of the epinephrine test in the diagnosis and management of children suspected of having congenital long QT syndrome, *Pediatr Cardiol* 31:462–468, 2010.
34. Wong JA, Gula LJ, Klein GJ, Yee R, et al: Utility of treadmill testing in identification and genotype prediction in long-QT syndrome, *Circ Arrhythm Electrophysiol* 3:120–125, 2010.
35. Hofman N, Wilde AA, Kaab S, et al: Diagnostic criteria for congenital long QT syndrome in the era of molecular genetics: do we need a scoring system? *Eur Heart J* 28:575–580, 2007.
36. Rossenbacker T, Priori SG: Clinical diagnosis of long QT syndrome: back to the caliper, *Eur Heart J* 28:527–528, 2007.
37. Horner JM, Horner MM, Ackerman MJ: The diagnostic utility of recovery phase QTc during treadmill exercise stress testing in the evaluation of long QT syndrome, *Heart Rhythm* 8:1698–1704, 2011.
38. Vyas H, Hejlik J, Ackerman MJ: Epinephrine QT stress testing in the evaluation of congenital long-QT syndrome: diagnostic accuracy of the paradoxical QT response, *Circulation* 113:1385–1392, 2006.
39. Horner JM, Ackerman MJ: Ventricular ectopy during treadmill exercise stress testing in the evaluation of long QT syndrome, *Heart Rhythm* 5:1690–1694, 2008.
40. Shimizu W, Noda T, Takaki H, et al: Diagnostic value of epinephrine test for genotyping LQT1, LQT2, and LQT3 forms of congenital long QT syndrome, *Heart Rhythm* 1:276–283, 2004.
41. Ackerman MJ, Priori SG, Willems S, et al: HRS/EHRA Expert Consensus Statement on the State of Genetic Testing for the Channelopathies and Cardiomyopathies, *Heart Rhythm* 8:1308–1339, 2011.
42. Itoh H, Shimizu W, Hayashi K, et al: Long QT syndrome with compound mutations is associated with a more severe phenotype: a Japanese multicenter study, *Heart Rhythm* 7:1411–1418, 2010.
43. Tristani-Firouzi M, Sanguinetti MC: Structural determinants and biophysical properties of HERG and KCNQ1 channel gating, *J Mol Cell Cardiol* 35:27–35, 2003.
44. Tamargo J, Caballero R, Gomez R, et al: Pharmacology of cardiac potassium channels, *Cardiovasc Res* 62:9–33, 2004.
45. Yang Y, Yang Y, Liang B, et al: Identification of a Kir3.4 mutation in congenital long QT syndrome, *Am J Hum Genet* 86:872–880, 2010.
46. Viswanathan PC, Balser JR: Biophysics of normal and abnormal cardiac sodium channel function. In Zipes DP, Jalife J, editors: *Cardiac electrophysiology: from cell to bedside*, ed 5, Philadelphia, 2009, WB Saunders, pp 93–104.
47. Amin AS, Sghari-Roodsari A, Tan HL: Cardiac sodium channelopathies, *Pflugers Arch* 460:223–237, 2010.
48. Burashnikov A, Antzelevitch C: Late-phase 3 EAD. A unique mechanism contributing to initiation of atrial fibrillation, *Pacing Clin Electrophysiol* 29:290–295, 2006.
49. Charpentier F, Merot J, Loussouarn G, Baro I: Delayed rectifier K^+ currents and cardiac repolarization, *J Mol Cell Cardiol* 48:37–44, 2010.
50. Gouas L, Nicaud V, Berthet M, et al: Association of KCNQ1, KCNE1, KCNH2 and SCN5A polymorphisms with QTc interval length in a healthy population, *Eur J Hum Genet* 13:1213–1222, 2005.
51. Pfeufer A, Jalilzadeh S, Perz S, et al: Common variants in myocardial ion channel genes modify the QT interval in the general population: results from the KORA study, *Circ Res* 96:693–701, 2005.
52. Smyth JW, Shaw RM: Forward trafficking of ion channels: what the clinician needs to know, *Heart Rhythm* 7:1135–1140, 2010.
53. Amin AS, Tan HL, Wilde AA: Cardiac ion channels in health and disease, *Heart Rhythm* 7:117–126, 2010.
54. Hobbs JB, Peterson DR, Moss AJ, et al: Risk of aborted cardiac arrest or sudden cardiac death during adolescence in the long-QT syndrome, *JAMA* 296:1249–1254, 2006.
55. Kaufman ES, McNitt S, Moss AJ, et al: Risk of death in the long QT syndrome when a sibling has died, *Heart Rhythm* 5:831–836, 2008.
56. Spazzolini C, Mullally J, Moss AJ, et al: Clinical implications for patients with long QT syndrome who experience a cardiac event during infancy, *J Am Coll Cardiol* 54:832–837, 2009.
57. Priori SG, Napolitano C, Schwartz PJ, et al: Association of long QT syndrome loci and cardiac events among patients treated with beta-blockers, *JAMA* 292:1341–1344, 2004.
58. Epstein AE, DiMarco JP, Ellenbogen KA, et al: ACC/AHA/HRS 2008 guidelines for device-based therapy of cardiac rhythm abnormalities: executive summary, *Heart Rhythm* 5:934–955, 2008.
59. Zipes DP, Ackerman MJ, Estes NA III, et al: Task Force 7: arrhythmias, *J Am Coll Cardiol* 45:1354–1363, 2005.
60. Patel SS, Anees S, Ferrick KJ: Prevalence of a Brugada pattern electrocardiogram in an urban population in the United States, *Pacing Clin Electrophysiol* 32:704–708, 2009.
61. Rossenbacker T, Priori SG: The Brugada syndrome, *Curr Opin Cardiol* 22:163–170, 2007.
62. Campuzano O, Brugada R, Iglesias A: Genetics of Brugada syndrome, *Curr Opin Cardiol* 25:210–215, 2010.
63. Morita H, Zipes DP, Wu J: Brugada syndrome: insights of ST elevation, arrhythmogenicity, and risk stratification from experimental observations, *Heart Rhythm* 6(Suppl 11):S34–S43, 2009.
64. Yap YG, Behr ER, Camm AJ: Drug-induced Brugada syndrome, *Europace* 11:989–994, 2009.
65. Antzelevitch C, Brugada P, Borggrefe M, et al: Brugada syndrome: report of the second consensus conference: endorsed by the Heart Rhythm Society and the European Heart Rhythm Association, *Circulation* 111:659–670, 2005.
66. Gehi AK, Duong TD, Metz LD, et al: Risk stratification of individuals with the Brugada electrocardiogram: a meta-analysis, *J Cardiovasc Electrophysiol* 17:577–583, 2006.
67. Ohgo T, Okamura H, Noda T, et al: Acute and chronic management in patients with Brugada syndrome associated with electrical storm of ventricular fibrillation, *Heart Rhythm* 4:695–700, 2007.
68. Probst V, Denjoy I, Meregalli PG, et al: Clinical aspects and prognosis of Brugada syndrome in children, *Circulation* 115:2042–2048, 2007.
69. Triedman JK: Brugada and short QT syndromes, *Pacing Clin Electrophysiol* 32(Suppl 2):S58–S62, 2009.
70. Morita H, Kusano KF, Miura D, et al: Fragmented QRS as a marker of conduction abnormality and a predictor of prognosis of Brugada syndrome, *Circulation* 118:1697–1704, 2008.
71. Letsas KP, Efremidis M, Weber R, et al: Epsilon-like waves and ventricular conduction abnormalities in subjects with type 1 ECG pattern of Brugada syndrome, *Heart Rhythm* 8:874–878, 2011.
72. Amin AS, de Groot EA, Ruijter JM, et al: Exercise-induced ECG changes in Brugada syndrome, *Circ Arrhythm Electrophysiol* 2:531–539, 2009.
73. Evain S, Briec F, Kyndt F, et al: Sodium channel blocker tests allow a clear distinction of electrophysiological characteristics and prognosis in patients with a type 2 or 3 Brugada electrocardiogram pattern, *Heart Rhythm* 5:1561–1564, 2008.
74. Antzelevitch C: Brugada syndrome, *Pacing Clin Electrophysiol* 29:1130–1159, 2006.
75. Bai R, Napolitano C, Bloise R, et al: Yield of genetic screening in inherited cardiac channelopathies: how to prioritize access to genetic testing, *Circ Arrhythm Electrophysiol* 2:6–15, 2009.
76. Antzelevitch C, Yan GX: J wave syndromes, *Heart Rhythm* 7:549–558, 2010.
77. Niwa N, Nerbonne JM: Molecular determinants of cardiac transient outward potassium current (I(to)) expression and regulation, *J Mol Cell Cardiol* 48:12–25, 2010.
78. Morita H, Zipes DP, Fukushima-Kusano K, et al: Repolarization heterogeneity in the right ventricular outflow tract: correlation with ventricular arrhythmias in Brugada patients and in an in vitro canine Brugada model, *Heart Rhythm* 5:725–733, 2008.
79. Morita H, Zipes DP, Morita ST, Wu J: Temperature modulation of ventricular arrhythmogenicity in a canine tissue model of Brugada syndrome, *Heart Rhythm* 4:188–197, 2007.
80. Watanabe A, Fukushima KK, Morita H, et al: Low-dose isoproterenol for repetitive ventricular arrhythmia in patients with Brugada syndrome, *Eur Heart J* 27:1579–1583, 2006.
81. Kamakura S, Ohe T, Nakazawa K, et al: Long-term prognosis of probands with Brugada-pattern ST-elevation in leads V_1-V_3, *Circ Arrhythm Electrophysiol* 2:495–503, 2009.
82. Sacher F, Probst V, Iesaka Y, et al: Outcome after implantation of a cardioverter-defibrillator in patients with Brugada syndrome: a multicenter study, *Circulation* 114:2317–2324, 2006.
83. Zipes DP, Camm AJ, Borggrefe M, et al: ACC/AHA/ESC 2006 guidelines for management of patients with ventricular arrhythmias and the prevention of sudden cardiac death: a report of the American College of Cardiology/American Heart Association Task Force and the European Society of Cardiology Committee for Practice Guidelines (Writing Committee to Develop Guidelines for Management of Patients With Ventricular Arrhythmias and the Prevention of Sudden Cardiac Death), *J Am Coll Cardiol* 48:e247–e346, 2006.
84. Schimpf R, Borggrefe M, Wolpert C: Clinical and molecular genetics of the short QT syndrome, *Curr Opin Cardiol* 23:192–198, 2008.
85. Giustetto C, Schimpf R, Mazzanti A, et al: Long-term follow-up of patients with short QT syndrome, *J Am Coll Cardiol* 58:587–595, 2011.
86. Anttonen O, Junttila MJ, Rissanen H, et al: Prevalence and prognostic significance of short QT interval in a middle-aged Finnish population, *Circulation* 116:714–720, 2007.
87. Gollob MH, Redpath CJ, Roberts JD: The short QT syndrome proposed diagnostic criteria, *J Am Coll Cardiol* 57:802–812, 2011.
88. Grant AO: Cardiac ion channels, *Circ Arrhythm Electrophysiol* 2:185–194, 2009.
89. van der Heyden MA, Wijnhoven TJ, Opthof T: Molecular aspects of adrenergic modulation of cardiac L-type Ca^{2+} channels, *Cardiovasc Res* 65:28–39, 2005.
90. Kaufman ES: Mechanisms and clinical management of inherited channelopathies: long QT syndrome, Brugada syndrome, catecholaminergic polymorphic ventricular tachycardia, and short QT syndrome, *Heart Rhythm* 6(Suppl 8):S51–S55, 2009.
91. Mohamed U, Napolitano C, Priori SG: Molecular and electrophysiological bases of catecholaminergic polymorphic ventricular tachycardia, *J Cardiovasc Electrophysiol* 18:791–797, 2007.
92. Kontula K, Laitinen PJ, Lehtonen A, et al: Catecholaminergic polymorphic ventricular tachycardia: recent mechanistic insights, *Cardiovasc Res* 67:379–387, 2005.
93. Liu N, Ruan Y, Priori SG: Catecholaminergic polymorphic ventricular tachycardia, *Prog Cardiovasc Dis* 51:23–30, 2008.
94. Napolitano C, Priori SG: Diagnosis and treatment of catecholaminergic polymorphic ventricular tachycardia, *Heart Rhythm* 4:675–678, 2007.
95. Ylanen K, Poutanen T, Hiippala A, et al: Catecholaminergic polymorphic ventricular tachycardia, *Eur J Pediatr* 169:535–542, 2010.
96. Gyorke S: Molecular basis of catecholaminergic polymorphic ventricular tachycardia, *Heart Rhythm* 6:123–129, 2009.
97. Wehrens XH: The molecular basis of catecholaminergic polymorphic ventricular tachycardia: what are the different hypotheses regarding mechanisms? *Heart Rhythm* 4:794–797, 2007.
98. Otten E, Asimaki A, Maass A, et al: Desmin mutations as a cause of right ventricular heart failure affect the intercalated disks, *Heart Rhythm* 7:1058–1064, 2010.
99. Maass K: Arrhythmogenic right ventricular cardiomyopathy and desmin: another gene fits the shoe, *Heart Rhythm* 7:1065–1066, 2010.
100. Hamilton RM, Fidler L: Right ventricular cardiomyopathy in the young: an emerging challenge, *Heart Rhythm* 6:571–575, 2009.
101. Anumonwo JM, Lopatin AN: Cardiac strong inward rectifier potassium channels, *J Mol Cell Cardiol* 48:45–54, 2010.
102. Bodi I, Mikala G, Koch SE, et al: The L-type calcium channel in the heart: the beat goes on, *J Clin Invest* 115:3306–3317, 2005.
103. Laurita KR, Rosenbaum DS: Mechanisms and potential therapeutic targets for ventricular arrhythmias associated with impaired cardiac calcium cycling, *J Mol Cell Cardiol* 44:31–43, 2008.

104. Ter Keurs HE, Boyden PA: Calcium and arrhythmogenesis, *Physiol Rev* 87:457–506, 2007.
105. Kushnir A, Marks AR: The ryanodine receptor in cardiac physiology and disease, *Adv Pharmacol* 59:1–30, 2010.
106. Baher AA, Uy M, Xie F, et al: Bidirectional ventricular tachycardia: ping pong in the His-Purkinje system, *Heart Rhythm* 8:599–605, 2011.
107. van der Werf C, Kannankeril PJ, Sacher F, et al: Flecainide therapy reduces exercise-induced ventricular arrhythmias in patients with catecholaminergic polymorphic ventricular tachycardia, *J Am Coll Cardiol* 57:2244–2254, 2011.
108. Cerrone M, Napolitano C, Priori SG: Catecholaminergic polymorphic ventricular tachycardia: a paradigm to understand mechanisms of arrhythmias associated to impaired Ca^{2+} regulation, *Heart Rhythm* 6:1652–1659, 2009.
109. Blayney LM, Lai FA: Ryanodine receptor–mediated arrhythmias and sudden cardiac death, *Pharmacol Ther* 123:151–177, 2009.
110. Hwang HS, Hasdemir C, Laver D, et al: Inhibition of cardiac Ca^{2+} release channels (RyR2) determines efficacy of class I antiarrhythmic drugs in catecholaminergic polymorphic ventricular tachycardia, *Circ Arrhythm Electrophysiol* 4:128–135, 2011.
111. Sy RW, Gollob MH, Klein GJ, et al: Arrhythmia characterization and long-term outcomes in catecholaminergic polymorphic ventricular tachycardia, *Heart Rhythm* 8:864–871, 2011.
112. Hofman N, van Langen I, Wilde AA: Genetic testing in cardiovascular diseases, *Curr Opin Cardiol* 25:243–248, 2010.
113. Alders M, Koopmann TT, Christiaans I, et al: Haplotype-sharing analysis implicates chromosome 7q36 harboring DPP6 in familial idiopathic ventricular fibrillation, *Am J Hum Genet* 84:468–476, 2009.
114. Antzelevitch C, Yan GX, Viskin S: Rationale for the use of the terms J-wave syndromes and early repolarization, *J Am Coll Cardiol* 57:1587–1590, 2011.
115. Haissaguerre M, Derval N, Sacher F, et al: Sudden cardiac arrest associated with early repolarization, *N Engl J Med* 358:2016–2023, 2008.
116. Tikkanen JT, Anttonen O, Junttila MJ, et al: Long-term outcome associated with early repolarization on electrocardiography, *N Engl J Med* 361:2529–2537, 2009.
117. Tikkanen JT, Junttila MJ, Anttonen O, et al: Early repolarization: electrocardiographic phenotypes associated with favorable long-term outcome, *Circulation* 123:2666–2673, 2011.
118. Rosso R, Kogan E, Belhassen B, et al: J-point elevation in survivors of primary ventricular fibrillation and matched control subjects: incidence and clinical significance, *J Am Coll Cardiol* 52:1231–1238, 2008.
119. Nunn LM, Bhar-Amato J, Lowe MD, et al: Prevalence of J-point elevation in sudden arrhythmic death syndrome families, *J Am Coll Cardiol* 58:286–290, 2011.
120. Derval N, Simpson CS, Birnie DH, et al: Prevalence and characteristics of early repolarization in the CASPER Registry: Cardiac Arrest Survivors With Preserved Ejection Fraction Registry, *J Am Coll Cardiol* 58:722–728, 2011.
121. Nam GB, Kim YH, Antzelevitch C: Augmentation of J waves and electrical storms in patients with early repolarization, *N Engl J Med* 358:2078–2079, 2008.
122. Reinhard W, Kaess BM, Debiec R, et al: Heritability of early repolarization: a population-based study, *Circ Cardiovasc Genet* 4:134–138, 2011.
123. Schimpé R, Wolpert C, Borggrefe M: Idiopathic ventricular fibrillation. In Zipes DP, Jalife J, editors: *Cardiac electrophysiology: from cell to bedside*, ed 5, Philadelphia, 2009, WB Saunders, pp 763–768.
124. Haissaguerre M, Sacher F, Nogami A, et al: Characteristics of recurrent ventricular fibrillation associated with inferolateral early repolarization role of drug therapy, *J Am Coll Cardiol* 53:612–619, 2009.
125. Shimizu W: Arrhythmias originating from the right ventricular outflow tract: how to distinguish "malignant" from "benign"? *Heart Rhythm* 6:1507–1511, 2009.
126. Aliot EM, Stevenson WG, Mendral-Garrote JM, et al: EHRA/HRS Expert Consensus on Catheter Ablation of Ventricular Arrhythmias: developed in a partnership with the European Heart Rhythm Association (EHRA), a Registered Branch of the European Society of Cardiology (ESC), and the Heart Rhythm Society (HRS); in collaboration with the American College of Cardiology (ACC) and the American Heart Association (AHA), *Heart Rhythm* 6:886–933, 2009.
127. Knecht S, Sacher F, Wright M, et al: Long-term follow-up of idiopathic ventricular fibrillation ablation: a multicenter study, *J Am Coll Cardiol* 54:522–528, 2009.

CHAPTER 32 Complications of Catheter Ablation of Cardiac Arrhythmias

Reported rates of major complications following contemporary catheter ablation procedures vary by as much as five- to eightfold between various types of ablation procedures, ranging from 0.8% for supraventricular tachycardia (SVT), 3.4% for idiopathic ventricular tachycardia (VT), 5.2% for atrial fibrillation (AF), and 6.0% for VT associated with structural heart disease. Death is a rare complication of catheter ablation, occurring in 0.11% to 0.30% of patients with regular SVT, and in 0.31% of those with VT. Transseptal catheterization appears to be the cause of death in 0.2% of procedures.[1]

Local Vascular Complications

Complications at the catheter insertion sites are among the most common problems observed following catheter ablation procedures, estimated to occur in about 2% to 6% of procedures, and can cause significant morbidity. Local vascular complications are higher among females, older adults, obese patients, and those with preexisting peripheral vascular disease. Additionally, the risk is related to the type of procedure performed (right or left heart catheterization), the size and number of sheaths and catheters used during the procedure, as well as the associated periprocedural use of anticoagulant or antiplatelet agents.[2] The rates of complications related to the site of vascular access are higher following catheter ablation of AF (1.8%) and VT in patients with structural heart disease (0.7% to 4.7%) compared with ablation of SVT (0.4%).[1]

Bleeding is the most common vascular complication. This can simply result in a local hematoma of little clinical significance. Vascular laceration can cause large hematomas in the groin and thigh. Acute bleeding generally can be controlled with prolonged manual compression. Groin hematomas usually resolve in 1 to 2 weeks if ongoing bleeding is stopped. Large hematomas can require blood transfusion, but surgical repair is rarely required. Arteriovenous fistulas and pseudoaneurysms need to be excluded in the setting of large or continually expanding hematomas. Retroperitoneal hematomas are often the result of arterial puncture above the inguinal ligament, allowing bleeding and hematoma to extend to the retroperitoneal space. Retroperitoneal hematomas should be suspected in the setting of a marked drop in hematocrit or unexplained hypotension or flank pain. Abdominal computed tomography (CT) scanning or ultrasound is required to confirm the diagnosis. Retroperitoneal bleeds are generally managed conservatively (bed rest, blood transfusion). Catheter or surgical interventions, however, can occasionally be required.[3]

Femoral artery pseudoaneurysms form when a tear through all the layers of the artery at the puncture site fails to seal, allowing persistent blood flow outside the vessel into a space contained by the surrounding tissue. This is in contrast to a hematoma, which has clotted blood outside the vessel with absence of flow. Pseudoaneurysms lack a fibrous wall and are contained by a surrounding shell of hematoma and the overlying soft tissues. Risk factors for pseudoaneurysm development include the use of large vascular sheaths, potent post-procedure anticoagulation, inadequacy of initial effort at hemostasis after removal of sheaths, and punctures of the femoral artery that are too distal, that is, at the level of bifurcation of the femoral artery or below. Also, multiple attempts at vascular access (arterial or venous) with inadvertent arterial puncture appear to increase the risk for pseudoaneurysm formation. Repeated damage to the arterial wall may result in weakening that leads to pseudoaneurysm development.

A pseudoaneurysm typically manifests a painful pulsatile mass with a systolic bruit or thrill, and the diagnosis is confirmed by duplex ultrasonography. Pseudoaneurysms can be complicated by rupture or distal embolization. Pseudoaneurysms that are less than 2 cm in size and not enlarging may resolve without intervention, with serial imaging to confirm spontaneous resolution; those that are enlarging or are greater than 2 cm in size can treated by ultrasound-guided compression of the "neck" connecting the pseudoaneurysm with the vessel or by percutaneous thrombin injection. Occasionally, surgical repair is required, especially for large pseudoaneurysms with a wide connection to the parent artery. Once diagnosed, a pseudoaneurysm should be treated rather than allowing the opportunity for spontaneous resolution.

Femoral arteriovenous fistulas commonly result when bleeding from the arterial puncture tracks into the adjacent venous puncture. Arteriovenous fistulas are more likely to arise when arterial and venous punctures are performed on the same side or when arterial puncture is performed below the common femoral artery, where several superficial branches of the femoral vein overlie the femoral artery. Diagnosis is made on examination with the finding of a pulsatile mass with a continuous "to and fro" bruit and confirmed by ultrasound. Many of the iatrogenic arteriovenous fistulas are small and close spontaneously within 1 year, but ultrasound-guided compression or surgical repair can be necessary. Because cardiac volume overload and limb damage are highly unlikely with persistent arteriovenous fistulas, conservative management for at least 1 year is reasonable.[2]

Deep venous thrombosis and pulmonary embolism are rare and can result from venous injury, especially during prolonged procedures requiring multiple venous lines, or in the setting of venous compression by a large arterial hematoma. Femoral arterial thrombosis is rare and occurs more commonly in the setting of a small vessel lumen, the use of a large-diameter sheath, preexisting peripheral vascular disease, diabetes mellitus, and female gender.

Accurate vascular puncture and effective initial control of bleeding after sheath removal are the best measures to prevent local vascular complications. Early diagnosis and management of local access-site complications are important to reduce morbidity and improve outcome.

Cardiac Perforation

Incidence

Previous studies reported the incidence of cardiac perforation with catheter-based interventions as follows: 0.8% for all procedures, 1.5% to 4.7% for valvuloplasty, 0.5% to 0.8% for angioplasty-atherectomy, 0.01% for diagnostic catheterization, 0.1% to 0.2% for electrophysiological (EP) studies, 0.2% for SVT ablation, 0.4% to 2.7% for VT ablation, and 0.5% to 4.0% for left atrial (LA) ablation.[1,4,5]

The incidence of procedure-related cardiac tamponade increases with the increasing number of catheter ablation procedures for the treatment of AF, which typically involves one or more atrial septal punctures, extensive intracardiac catheter manipulation and ablation within the thin-walled LA, and the need for high levels of systemic anticoagulation during the procedure.[2,6]

Mechanism

Cardiac perforation can be caused by mechanical trauma secondary to catheter manipulation, myocardial tissue rupture due to radiofrequency (RF) ablation, or inadvertent injury during atrial septal puncture. Extensive catheter manipulation, especially in areas with thin walls such as the LA roof, right ventricular (RV) free wall, RV outflow tract (RVOT), RV apex, and atrial appendages, can cause mechanical tear of the chamber wall. Cardiac perforation can also occur away from the area of mapping and ablation, usually caused by penetration of an unattended RV catheter in the setting of rapid and vigorous heart action because of high-dose isoproterenol infusion. Inadvertent puncture of the right atrial (RA) free wall or lateral LA wall can occur during transseptal catheterization. High RF power output, especially when using large- or irrigated-tip ablation catheters, can increase the risk of cardiac perforation. An audible pop associated with an abrupt rise in impedance is heard in many patients who develop tamponade. Popping occurs because of tissue boiling causing myocardial rupture, and is increased by irrigated-tip ablation, high tissue-catheter interface flow, poor or unstable tissue contact, and high catheter tip temperature.[2,6]

Detection

Prompt recognition and management of cardiac perforation are critical to prevent the development of cardiac tamponade and potentially life-threatening hemodynamic collapse. Although the presentation often is dramatic with abrupt hypotension, it can be insidious with a more gradual fall in blood pressure. The use of an arterial line that provides continuous blood pressure monitoring can help detect early hemodynamic compromise. Sinus tachycardia is common in the setting of cardiac tamponade that gradually develops. Nonetheless, the absence of tachycardia does not exclude cardiac tamponade; in fact sinus bradycardia can develop secondary to a vagal reflex in the setting of a rapidly developing cardiac tamponade. Any chest pain that persists beyond the completion of an ablation lesion, especially if associated with hypotension and diaphoresis, should alert the operator to the possible development of pericardial effusion.[2,6-8]

Assessment of the cardiac silhouette fluoroscopically can provide the first clue, especially if a similar assessment was made at baseline. Decreased excursion of the lateral heart border on fluoroscopy in the left anterior oblique (LAO) projection, indicating accumulating pericardial effusion, usually can be seen well before a drop in blood pressure and prior to progression to cardiac tamponade. Some operators obtain a baseline LAO cine image at the onset of a procedure to serve as a reference for comparison during the procedure, followed by intermittent evaluation of the same fluoroscopic projection during the procedure.[2,6-8]

Transthoracic echocardiography is the most definitive method for confirming the development of pericardial effusion. Intracardiac echocardiography (ICE), commonly used to guide transseptal puncture for LA procedures, also can facilitate the early detection of pericardial effusions before the emergence of tamponade physiology. Most of the pericardial space is not visualized from the RA imaging venue used to visualize the interatrial septum, and limited catheter rotation is usually required. Advancing the ICE catheter into the RV and rotating the transducer against the interventricular septum can readily identify pericardial effusions (Fig. 32-1).

Perforation without tamponade may occur during placement of diagnostic catheters or while accessing the LA by transseptal catheterization; detection at this time can prevent progression to tamponade but requires a high index of suspicion. Several clues should alert the operator to the possibility of cardiac perforation, including a ventricular catheter that reaches the edge of the cardiac silhouette, high pacing thresholds at sites despite normal electrograms and apparent good tissue contact on fluoroscopy, a right bundle branch block (RBBB) complex during "RV" pacing, and a catheter tip position discordant from where it should be (i.e., an RV catheter too far leftward with intended RV apical location; Fig. 32-2). With atrial septal puncture for accessing the left heart chambers, the aorta can be inadvertently entered; if only the needle enters the aorta and this is recognized before advancing the dilator and sheath, the needle can be withdrawn and the patient monitored for stability of vital signs and with echocardiography. The procedure can be continued if there is no accumulation of pericardial fluid after 15 to 30 minutes of monitoring. If the dilator and sheath have been advanced into the aortic root before the error is recognized, it is imperative that the sheath not be removed immediately, as this can result in immediate and perhaps irretrievable hemodynamic collapse due to intractable bleeding into the pericardial space.

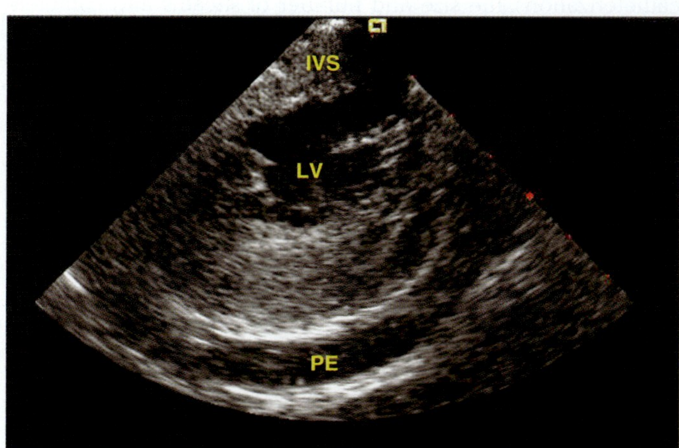

FIGURE 32-1 Intracardiac echocardiography (ICE) imaging of pericardial effusion. The phased-array ICE transducer is positioned in the right ventricle, showing a short-axis view of the left ventricle (LV) and a moderate pericardial effusion (PE). IVS = interventricular septum.

Management

The management of pericardial effusion is largely determined by its relative size and hemodynamic effect. Trivial pericardial effusions, if recognized early during the procedure, should be monitored continuously but do not warrant termination of the procedure. For larger effusions, the procedure should be terminated and anticoagulation, if administered, should be reversed. Protamine is used to reverse the effects of heparin, and activated factor VII, fresh frozen plasma, and vitamin K can be used in patients with therapeutic anticoagulation with warfarin. Intravenous fluids, vasopressors, and transfusion of blood products can be required, depending on the extent of the effusion and the severity of hemodynamic decompensation. Intravenous atropine can be of value in patients with increased vagal tone.[3,9]

If perforation without tamponade is recognized, an echocardiogram should be obtained as a baseline. If the offending catheter is a standard 5 or 6 Fr shaft, it can often be withdrawn back into the heart while monitoring the echocardiogram for accumulation of pericardial fluid. Most often, there will be no bleeding into the pericardial space and the procedure can be continued. If systemic anticoagulation is planned for left-sided catheterization, the operator must decide how important it is to continue the procedure with the risk of bleeding into the pericardium. If a larger catheter or large vascular sheath has been inadvertently placed in the pericardial space, echocardiography should be obtained along with cardiothoracic surgical consultation. In many if not most cases, the sheath may be safely withdrawn into the heart without adverse consequences, but the team must be ready to transport the patient to an operating room for repair of a hole or tear in the wall of the affected heart chamber. In some cases, especially when the patient is fully anticoagulated, it may be prudent to transport the patient to the operating room and prepare for urgent sternotomy before removing the catheter/sheath so as to be able to rapidly enter the chest if hemodynamic collapse occurs.

Although pericardiocentesis typically is required for large pericardial effusions, smaller effusions manifesting signs of cardiac tamponade, or both, and can effectively restore hemodynamic function, it carries the potential risk of cardiac chamber laceration, inadvertent puncture of the RV, pneumothorax, and infection. In a subset of patients (especially older female patients with a small to moderate amount of pericardial effusion who are not anticoagulated), a conservative approach incorporating administration of intravenous fluids and vasopressors to address the hemodynamic consequences of cardiac tamponade was found in a recent report a reasonable initial strategy and could obviate the need for emergency pericardiocentesis.[2,7]

Pericardiocentesis should be performed promptly when indicated, because there is usually a narrow therapeutic time window for intervention before critical hemodynamic compromise ensues. The procedure can be performed under fluoroscopic guidance (Video 22). Echocardiography can also be used to guide pericardiocentesis (Video 23). When echocardiography is not readily available, fluoroscopy is usually adequate to guide a safe procedure, and reliance on transthoracic echocardiography should not lead to unnecessary delay in diagnosis or therapy. The technique of percutaneous pericardiocentesis is discussed in Chapter 27. In most patients, an indwelling catheter is required for a short interval after initial drainage to confirm that the bleeding has stopped and that no effusion is reaccumulating. In the event of persistence or rapid reaccumulation of the effusion, exploration by thoracic surgery can be required. Up to 13.3% of LA perforations during AF ablation require surgical closure. Autotransfusion of blood removed from the pericardial space can be of value in patients with persistent bleeding, and is best done using an autologous blood recovery system, because direct autotransfusion can result in a systemic inflammatory response.[3,6,9]

Early pericarditis after cardiac perforation is common. In one report, 53.3% of such patients had persistent chest pain after effusion evacuation and removal of the pericardial catheter suggestive of pericardial inflammation. Nonsteroidal antiinflammatory agents are adequate in most patients. Additionally, intrapericardial steroids (triamcinolone, 20 mg) can help reduce pericardial inflammation. Subacute reaccumulation of pericardial fluid suggestive of postcardiac injury syndrome or inflammatory pericarditis can also occur, requiring repeat pericardiocentesis.[3,9]

Thromboembolism

Systemic thromboembolism can complicate EP procedures in the left side of the heart. The rate of thromboembolic events is 0.4% to 2.1% for AF ablation and up to 2.8% for ablation of VT originating in the left ventricle (LV).[1,4,10] In patients undergoing AF ablation, history of a prior cerebrovascular event is the most potent individual risk factor for post-ablation cerebrovascular events and is associated with a ninefold increased risk of periprocedural stroke. Additionally, the incidence of periprocedural stroke increases in

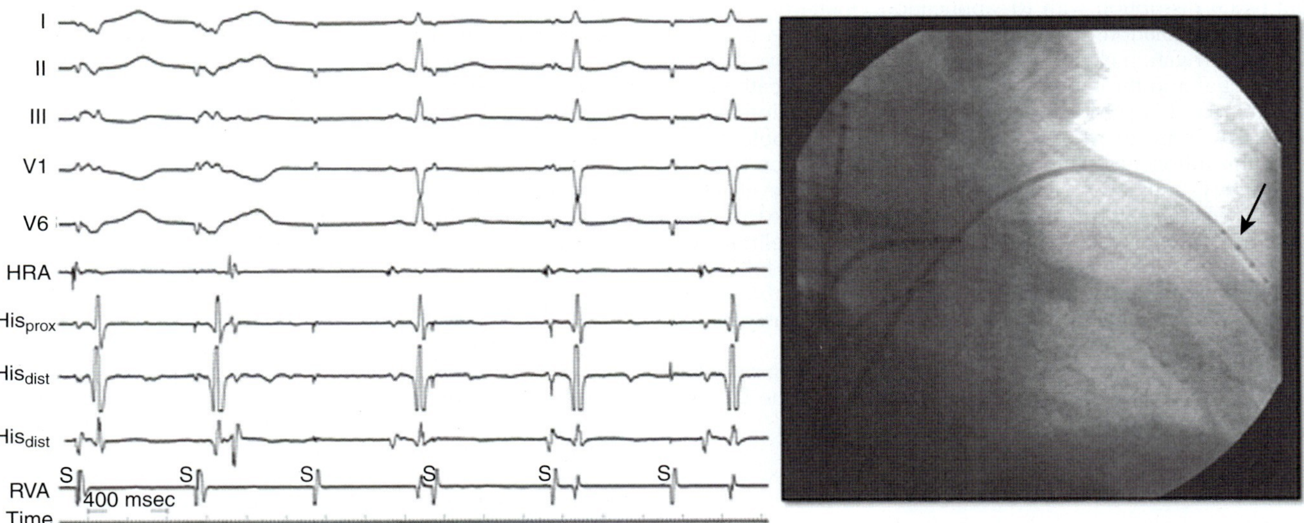

FIGURE 32-2 Cardiac perforation during electrophysiological study. Surface ECG and intracardiac recordings from a patient who was undergoing electrophysiological study. Recordings show poor capture from a catheter intended for the right ventricular apex (RVA); captured complexes have a right bundle branch block pattern. These features are explained by the accompanying right anterior oblique fluoroscopic image showing that the RVA catheter (arrow) has perforated the RV anterior wall and is pacing the anterolateral left ventricular epicardium.

a step-wise fashion with an increasing $CHADS_2$ score (congestive heart failure, hypertension, age >75 years, diabetes, and previous stroke/transient ischemic attack).[10]

Mechanism

Potential sources of emboli include thrombus formation on high-profile wires, catheters, and sheaths inserted in the LA or LV, char formation at the tip of the ablation catheter or at the site of ablation, thrombi or air passing through a patent foramen ovale or transseptal puncture, and dislodgment of a preexistent LA or LV thrombus by catheter manipulation. Additionally, new LA appendage thrombi may develop in patients with persistent AF after planned or inadvertent conversion to sinus rhythm, especially in the setting of insufficient levels of anticoagulation before, during, or after ablation. Furthermore, endocardial disruption from the ablation lesions can potentially become a nidus for thrombus formation. Also, aortic atheroembolism can occur during retrograde transaortic LV access for ablation of VTs or atrioventricular (AV) bypass tracts (BTs), and it tends to be associated with difficulty in manipulation of catheters within a severely diseased aorta.[10]

Thromboembolic events typically occur within 24 hours of the ablation procedure, with the high-risk period extending for the first 2 weeks following ablation. Cerebral thromboembolism is most common, but emboli can also involve the coronary, abdominal, or peripheral vascular circulations. Although silent cerebral thromboembolism has been reported, its incidence and clinical significance are unknown.[11]

Prevention

Prevention remains the best strategy in minimizing cerebrovascular events during left heart mapping and ablation, and this may be achieved by the following: (1) preprocedural transthoracic or transesophageal echocardiography (TEE) in patients with AF as well as those with ischemic VT with LV dysfunction; (2) aggressive intraprocedural anticoagulation, including early heparin administration (once vascular access is obtained), followed by continuous infusion to maintain the activated clotting time at greater than 300 seconds; (3) meticulous attention to sheath management, including constant infusion of heparinized saline and air filters; (4) minimizing char formation during lesion creation by regulating power delivery to prevent abrupt impedance rise; and (5) using ICE during AF ablation for early detection of intracardiac thrombi and accelerated bubble formation consistent with endocardial tissue disruption with RF application. Open-irrigation RF ablation or cryoablation, compared with standard 4- or 8-mm solid tip or closed irrigation electrodes, can potentially decrease the formation of char and thrombus at the tip of the ablation catheter.[10] Administration of large doses of protamine on completion of the ablation procedure to reverse heparin abruptly can potentially promote thrombogenesis and warrants further evaluation to confirm its safety. Continuation of warfarin at a therapeutic level at the time of AF ablation can potentially be a better alternative to strategies that use bridging with heparin or enoxaparin, as it eliminates a period of inadequate anticoagulation immediately following the ablation procedure, a critical period for thromboembolic risk because of the inflammation and irritation inherently associated with ablation.[12,13]

In patients with severe disease of the aorta, using a long vascular sheath to advance the ablation catheter directly into the LV can potentially reduce the risk of aortic atheroembolism.

Air Embolism

Vascular air embolism is a potentially life-threatening event that can occur during left and right heart procedures. Because many cases of venous air embolism go unnoticed, the true incidence of this complication is unknown. Air embolism has been reported in the interventional radiology literature at an incidence of 0.13%.[2,3,9]

Mechanism

Small amounts of air embolized in the venous circulation are generally broken up in the capillary bed and absorbed from the circulation without significant sequelae. Embolization of large volumes of air (>5 mL/kg) can cause severe complications (shock or cardiac arrest). However, complications have been reported with as little as 20 mL of air. On the other hand, embolization of as little as 2 or 3 mL of air into the arterial circulation can be fatal.

Paradoxical air embolization into the arterial circulation can occur through direct passage of air into the arterial system via anomalous structures such as an atrial or ventricular septal defect, a patent foramen ovale, or pulmonary arterial-venous malformations. Direct arterial air embolism is caused by the introduction of air into the LA via the transseptal sheath as well as via long vascular sheaths occasionally used for catheter stabilization during transaortic mapping and ablation in the LV.[3,9]

With the patient in the supine position, large volumes of air rapidly entering the venous circulation typically lodge in the RVOT or pulmonary artery, and can cause RVOT obstruction, marked reduction of cardiac output, and potentially hemodynamic collapse. Also, air embolization can lead to serious inflammatory changes in the pulmonary vessels including direct endothelial damage and accumulation of platelets and fibrin. Air in the systemic circulation can induce ischemia by various mechanisms, such as obstruction of the blood flow, vasospasm, and thrombus formation because of platelet activation.

Clinical Presentation

Most cases of venous air embolism are subclinical and do not result in untoward outcomes, and even when symptomatic, they go unrecognized because of the nonspecific nature of clinical presentation that can mimic other cardiac, pulmonary, and neurological dysfunctions. Therefore, a high index of suspicion is necessary to establish the diagnosis.[3]

The outcome of venous air embolism is directly related to the amount of air and the rate at which it enters the vein. Spontaneously breathing patients can experience more serious consequences than those under controlled positive-pressure ventilation because they generate negative intrathoracic pressure during the respiratory cycle, facilitating air entrainment. Awake patients typically manifest shortness of breath, continuous coughing, chest pain, and a sense of "impending doom." Jugular venous distention, hypotension, tachycardia, and electrocardiographic (ECG) signs of right heart strain (ST-T wave abnormalities) can be observed. Severe cases are characterized by cardiovascular collapse.[3,9]

Arterial air emboli can distribute to almost any organ and can have devastating clinical sequelae. Direct cerebral air embolism can be associated with altered mental status, seizures, and focal neurological signs. A common presentation of air embolism during LA mapping and ablation is acute inferior ischemia, heart block, or both (Fig. 32-3). This reflects preferential downstream migration of air emboli into the right coronary artery.

Detection

Routine diagnostic modalities to identify air embolism in the terminal arterial circulations lack sensitivity, and diagnosis is typically based on the appropriate clinical scenario, with possible air identified in cardiac chambers. Air in the RV or pulmonary artery can be visualized on fluoroscopy as well as transthoracic echocardiography. TEE is currently the most sensitive monitoring device for venous air embolism. Prompt CT or magnetic resonance (MR) imaging obtained before the intravascular air is absorbed may show multiple serpiginous hypodensities representing air in the cerebral vasculature, with or without acute infarction, but imaging later in the course of the disease shows diffuse acute infarcts (Fig. 32-4).[3,9]

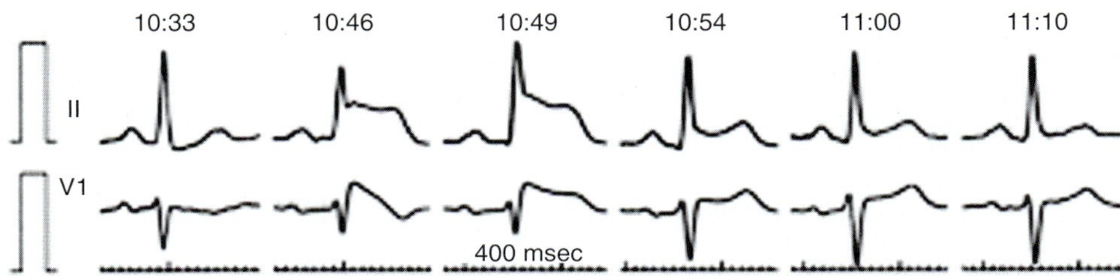

FIGURE 32-3 Coronary air embolism. Leads II and V_1 are shown from a patient with a left-sided bypass tract who suffered air embolism during transseptal catheterization and catheter advancement into the left atrium. Snapshots of ECGs taken at the designated times show the baseline (10:33) normal findings, dramatic ST elevation immediately following transseptal catheterization (10:46), and progressive resolution over the next 25 minutes. Time scale and 10-mV calibration marks are shown.

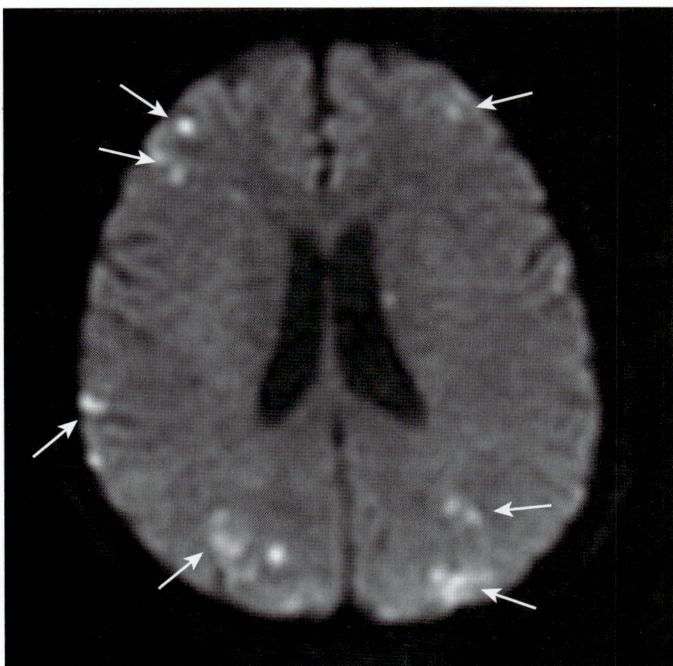

FIGURE 32-4 Cerebral air embolism. A transverse section of a magnetic resonance image of the brain in a patient who sustained cerebral air embolism during ablation of atrial fibrillation, showing many areas of diffusion restriction scattered throughout both hemispheres, representing acute infarcts.

Prevention

The optimal management of air embolism is prevention. Careful sheath management, including constant infusion of heparinized saline and air filters, should be observed. Although air can be introduced through the infusion line, it can also occur with suction when catheters are removed. Therefore, whenever catheters are removed, they need to be withdrawn slowly to minimize suction effects and the fluid column within the sheath should be aspirated simultaneously. The sheath should then be aspirated and irrigated to ascertain that neither air nor blood has collected in the sheath.[3] Importantly, the entire volume of the sheath should be aspirated after initial deployment as well as after each time a catheter is removed and reinserted, in order to ensure that a continuous column of fluid is present in the sheath and disallowing the possibility of trapped air that could otherwise be introduced when a catheter is advanced through the sheath. Testing to ascertain the sheath's capacity prior to insertion is a good practice.

Management

Initially, it is essential to take all measures necessary to prevent further air embolization. For venous air embolism, placing the patient in the left lateral decubitus and Trendelenburg position helps air remain in the RA, where it will not contribute to an "air lock" in the RVOT. Additionally, direct extraction of air from the venous circulation if localized in the RA or RV can be attempted by aspiration from a central venous or pulmonary artery catheter. Air aspiration should be performed with the patient supine or in a Trendelenburg position while holding his or her breath at the end of inspiration or during a Valsalva maneuver.[14]

Administration of intravenous fluids and vasopressors can be necessary for hemodynamic support. Supplemental 100% oxygen therapy can reduce the size of the air embolus by increasing the rate of nitrogen absorption from air bubbles. Because gas bubbles are not buoyant enough to counteract arterial blood flow, these measures are more suitable for treating venous and RV air emboli.[14]

When cerebral air embolism is suspected, it is important to maximize cerebral perfusion by administration of fluids and supplemental oxygen. Hyperbaric oxygen therapy is regarded as the treatment of choice in patients with cerebral air embolism and prompt transfer to a hyperbaric oxygen therapy center should be considered. When started within a few hours, hyperbaric oxygen therapy can potentially compress the existing bubbles, speed resolution of bubbles by establishing a high diffusion gradient, improve oxygenation of ischemic tissues, and reduce endothelial thromboinflammatory injury.[3,11,14]

Coronary Artery Injuries

The incidence of coronary artery injuries during ablation procedures is extremely low despite the close proximity of coronary arteries to common sites of ablation. The low incidence is likely due, at least in part, to the high-velocity blood flow within the epicardial coronary arteries, allowing these vessels to act as a heat sink; substantive heating of vascular endothelium is prevented by heat dissipation in the coronary blood flow (convective cooling), even when the catheter is positioned close to the vessel. However, high RF power delivery in small hearts, such as in pediatric patients, or in direct contact with the vessel can potentially cause coronary arterial injury.[15,16] Additionally, the rarity of coronary artery injury can be due to underrecognition, because its clinical presentation (e.g., chest discomfort and elevation in cardiac troponin levels) can easily be misdiagnosed as pericardial irritation, myocardial injury secondary to RF ablation, or both.

Mechanism

The potential for acute coronary artery occlusion is a significant risk consideration with catheter ablation within the aortic cusps. Damage to the coronary arteries can result from catheter manipulation and ablation in the aortic root, secondary to RF energy delivery in close proximity to the ostium of the right or left coronary artery, as well as inadvertent catheter engagement of the left main coronary artery when ablating in the left coronary cusp.[17,18]

It is also important to recognize the potential risk of coronary artery damage when ablating in the RVOT and pulmonary artery. The right coronary artery is typically 4 to 5 mm away from the proximal part of the RVOT near the free wall, and is separated by a variable amount of

fat. Additionally, the cephalocaudal separation of the pulmonic and aortic valves results in close proximity of the pulmonic valve to the origin of the right coronary artery, and the left main coronary artery lies in immediate posterior proximity to the subvalvular RVOT near the pulmonic valve as well as the supravalvular pulmonary artery.[17,18]

Because of the proximity of the right coronary artery to the cavotricuspid isthmus and the left circumflex artery to the lateral mitral annulus, coronary artery injury can potentially occur during ablation at mitral or tricuspid annuli.[15] Transient inferior ST segment elevation and acute occlusion of the right coronary artery have been reported following ablation of the cavotricuspid isthmus, and left circumflex artery injury has been reported following ablation of left-sided AV BTs. Also, late stenosis of the right coronary artery has been observed in children with Ebstein anomaly of the tricuspid valve who undergo ablation of a right-sided AV BT.[19]

Percutaneous epicardial ablation probably poses a greater risk of coronary artery injury, severe spasm, or both, whereby the large epicardial coronary arteries can be in direct contact with the ablation catheter and movement of the ablation catheter in the pericardial space can occur during ablation endangering adjacent coronary arteries. The coronary sinus (CS) and its branches are also in close relation to the distal circumflex and the posterolateral branches of the right coronary artery, and ablation within the coronary venous system (for AV BTs, lateral mitral isthmus, and VT) can cause coronary injuries.[5,15]

RF injury to coronary arteries can cause acute thrombosis or damage to the arterial wall. Arterial injury is inversely proportional to vessel diameter; there is little evidence of injury when vessel diameter exceeds 0.5 to 1.0 mm.[15]

Coronary artery spasm has been reported during mapping in the pericardial space and can occur as a result of ablation close to the artery. Extrinsic compression of a coronary artery can also result from edema caused by nearby ablation.

Clinical Presentation

Coronary arterial injury generally presents with acute coronary occlusion or spasm at the time of ablation associated with chest pain and ST elevation; nonetheless, delayed presentations can also occur.[15]

Importantly, RF ablation frequently (in 25% to 100% of cases) causes significant elevations in cardiac troponin levels that are not related to coronary arterial injury, with mean peak levels of 0.13 to 6 ng/mL for troponin I, and 0.20 to 2.41 ng/mL for troponin T. In contrast to acute coronary syndromes, troponin elevations observed following RF ablation typically peak early (2 to 8 hours versus 18 to 24 hours) and normalize early.[20] The levels of troponin elevation correlate with the number of RF lesions applied, the site of lesions (ventricular more than atrial more than annular), and the approach to the left side (transaortic more than transseptal). Ablation of focal lesions (atrioventricular nodal reentrant tachycardia [AVNRT], atrioventricular reentrant tachycardia [AVRT]) causes less frequent (in 25% to 88% of cases) elevation of troponin levels as compared with linear lesion ablation (typical and atypical atrial flutter [AFL], AF, and VT) where all patients are expected to have an increase in troponin levels. The prognostic significance of asymptomatic elevations of troponin I remains unclear.[20]

Prevention

Several precautions are important to avoid injury to coronary arteries during percutaneous epicardial ablation, ablation via the coronary venous system, and ablation in the coronary cusps. Prior to ablation near or within a branch of the CS or in the pericardial space, direct visualization of the relation between the ablation site and adjacent coronary arteries must be obtained, usually by coronary angiography performed with the ablation catheter on the target site. An absolute safe distance between the ablation site and epicardial artery has not been defined; nonetheless, a distance of at least 5 mm between the ablation catheter and an epicardial artery is commonly accepted. It is also important to ensure that the catheter is not touching the vessel at any point of the cardiac cycle during angiography. Cryoablation appears to have less risk of coronary injury in animal models, but can still create occlusion and intimal damage when in close proximity, particularly to small vessels.[5]

When ablation in the aortic cusp is planned, it is preferable to insert a 5 Fr pigtail catheter into the aortic root and obtain aortic root angiography to visualize the aortic root and the ostia of the right and left coronary arteries.[18] Selective angiography of the coronary arteries also can be performed with the ablation catheter positioned at the desired location so as to assess the anatomical relationships between these structures and the location of the ablation catheter. If the origin of VT is in the left coronary cusp, it is preferable to cannulate the left main coronary artery with a 5 Fr left Judkins catheter, which serves as a marker and for protection of the left main coronary artery in case of ablation catheter dislodgment during RF application. Alternatively, a combination of electroanatomical mapping and ICE imaging can be used to confirm anatomical location, catheter tip position and contact, and distance to coronary vasculature and to monitor RF delivery.[17]

To avoid injuring the coronary arteries during ablation of arrhythmias arising from the coronary cusps, it is preferable to start RF energy delivery at a low power output (15 W) and then increase to no more than 30 W to achieve a target temperature of approximately 50°C. Additionally, ablation should also be performed during continuous fluoroscopy to observe for catheter dislodgment, and energy delivery should be discontinued in case of even minimal dislodgment from the site showing the best mapping findings. RF application should also be stopped if the repetitive or sustained VT cannot be terminated after 10 seconds. Coronary angiography is often performed immediately after the ablation procedure to exclude coronary artery spasm, dissection, or thrombus.[18]

Iatrogenic Cardiac Arrhythmias

Atrioventricular Block

AV block is the most important complication of AVNRT ablation. AV block occurs in about 0.2% to 0.8% of slow pathway ablation using the posterior approach, generally occurs during RF delivery or within the first 24 hours postablation, and is almost always preceded by junctional ectopy with VA block. The level of block is usually in the atrioventricular node (AVN). Predictors of AV block include proximity of the anatomical ablation site to the compact AVN, occurrence of fast junctional tachycardia (cycle length <350 milliseconds) during RF application, occurrence of junctional rhythm with VA block, the number of RF applications (related to the amount of tissue damage), and significant worsening of anterograde AV conduction during the ablation procedure. The anterior approach for AVNRT ablation is associated with a higher risk of inadvertent complete AV block (approximately 10%, but ranging from 2% to 20%).[21] During ablation of AVNRT, careful monitoring of AV conduction during RF application and prompt discontinuation of energy delivery on evidence of AV block are the keys to minimize the incidence of AV block. RF delivery should be immediately discontinued when the following occur: (1) the impedance rises suddenly (>10 Ω); (2) the PR interval (during normal sinus rhythm [NSR] or atrial pacing) prolongs; (3) AV block develops; (4) retrograde conduction block is observed during junctional ectopy; or (5) fast junctional tachycardia (tachycardia cycle length <350 milliseconds) occurs, which can herald imminent heart block.

AV block can also occur when ablating along the interventricular septum in the close vicinity of the compact AVN or His bundle (HB), including ablation of superoparaseptal and midseptal AV BTs or ATs as well as para-Hisian VTs. Additionally, because the penetrating HB lies at the membranous septum formed in part by the commissure between the right coronary and noncoronary cusps, ablation of VTs originating in this region can potentially damage the HB (Fig. 32-5).

When a His potential is detectable at the ablation catheter location, titrated RF energy output and RF application for a short

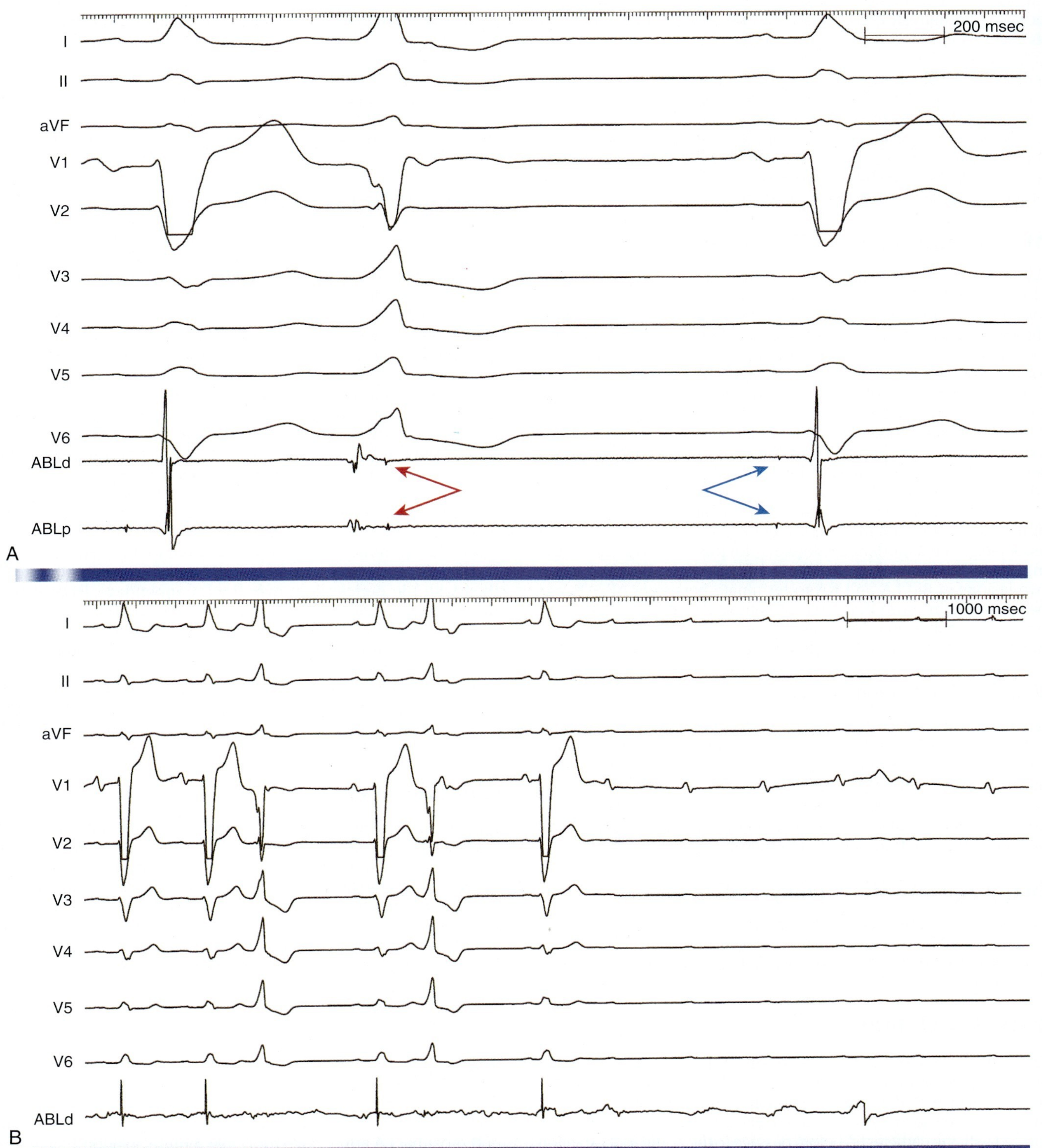

FIGURE 32-5 Atrioventricular (AV) block complicating catheter ablation of premature ventricular complexes (PVCs) originating from the para-Hisian region. In **A**, note the presence of anterograde His potentials on the proximal and distal ablation electrodes (ABLp and ABLd, respectively) during sinus rhythm (blue arrows) and retrograde His potentials during PVCs (red arrows) at the site of earliest ventricular activation during PVCs. In **B**, radiofrequency energy delivery results in complete AV block secondary to injury to the His bundle.

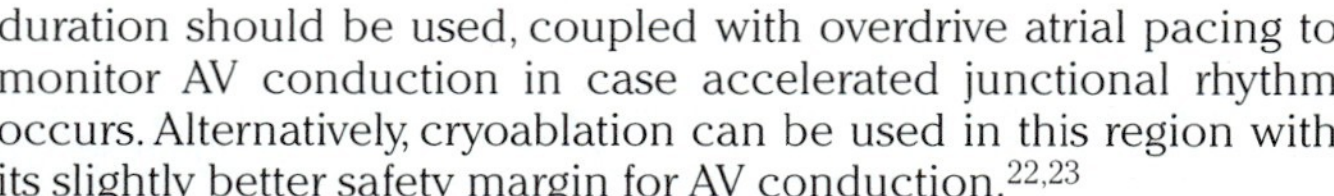

duration should be used, coupled with overdrive atrial pacing to monitor AV conduction in case accelerated junctional rhythm occurs. Alternatively, cryoablation can be used in this region with its slightly better safety margin for AV conduction.[22,23]

In some patients, mechanical trauma from the catheter induces temporary AV block. Also, catheter manipulation in the RV or LV can cause mechanical bundle branch block (often transient), which can potentially cause complete AV block in patients with preexisting block in the contralateral bundle branch. Furthermore, ablation of the right bundle branch in patients with bundle branch reentrant VT is commonly followed by complete AV block (in up to 30%) because of preexisting severe disease in the left bundle branch.

Macroreentrant Atrial Tachycardias

Whereas the occurrence of new arrhythmias following focal RF ablation has not been a clinical problem, linear ablation lesions, if incomplete, can promote reentry propagating through the gaps in the ablation lines. Even when conduction block across the ablation lines is verified, the ablation lines commonly performed in the LA for ablation of AF can still facilitate reentry by providing conduction obstacles and protected isthmuses with adjacent anatomical structures in the atrium.[24,25] In fact, LA macroreentry is a relatively common complication of catheter ablation of AF, occurring in up to 50% of cases. The incidence of ATs seems to be lower following segmental ostial pulmonary vein (PV) isolation (<5%) compared with circumferential PV isolation, and much higher following circumferential or linear LA ablation (>30%). Targeting complex fractionated atrial electrograms without linear lesions or PV isolation is associated with a moderate risk (8.3%) for post-ablation ATs. Following stepwise approaches of catheter ablation incorporating extensive lesions in the LA and RA to terminate persistent AF, ATs can be observed in more than 50% of patients.[26-28] Although ATs can occur at variable time intervals after AF ablation procedures, the most common timing appears to be 1 to 2 months postablation.[29,30]

Ventricular Arrhythmias

Ventricular fibrillation has been reported in up to 6% of patients with chronic AF after AVN ablation when the ventricular pacing rate is lower than 70 beats/min. This complication can be minimized by postablation pacing for 3 months at a higher rate—that is, 90 beats/min. A possible mechanism for postablation ventricular arrhythmia is activation of the sympathetic nervous system and a prolongation of action potential duration.

Inappropriate Sinus Tachycardia

Inappropriate sinus tachycardia can occur in some patients after posteroseptal BT or AVN ablation, suggesting disruption of the parasympathetic input and/or sympathetic input into the sinus node and AVN.

Valvular Damage

The aortic valve can be damaged during retrograde crossing of the ablation catheter for retrograde ablation of LV VTs and left-sided BTs. To prevent leaflet damage or perforation, the straight catheter tip must never be used to cross the aortic valve; instead, a tight J curve is formed with the catheter tip before passage to the aortic root. Ablation of arrhythmias originating from the aortic cusp can also result in valvular damage, and limiting RF power output and duration is necessary.

Damage to the mitral valve can result from entanglement of the ablation catheter within the mitral valve apparatus during transaortic or transseptal ablation procedures, but serious damage is unlikely. The risk of valvular damage (occasionally requiring thoracic surgery and valve replacement) is higher following entrapment of catheters with multiple splines or circular mapping catheters in the valvular apparatus (e.g., during AF ablation), which can be potentially difficult to free. Forcible traction of the catheter should be avoided as it can potentially damage the valve and ultimately lead to mitral valve replacement. To prevent injury to the papillary muscles or chordae tendineae, prior to pulling on the catheter, one may consider instead advancing the catheter toward the LV apex. Advancing the sheath over the catheter and withdrawing the catheter into the sheath followed by withdrawal of the whole assembly can facilitate the effort further. When gentle manipulation and moderate traction are unsuccessful, removing the catheter by thoracic surgery may be preferable; in this way the valve can potentially be spared significant damage.[3,31]

Phrenic Nerve Injury

Phrenic nerve damage and consequent diaphragmatic paralysis have been a long-recognized complication during endocardial ablation in the RA or LA as well as during percutaneous epicardial ablation procedures.

The intrathoracic course of the right phrenic nerve, especially as it approximates the superior vena cava (SVC) and RA (and not infrequently the right superior PV), is the principal reason for susceptibility to nerve damage from endocardial ablation. Injury to the right phrenic nerve has typically been reported during sinus node modification or ablation of ATs in the RA free wall, SVC, or right superior PV. Right phrenic nerve injury has become more frequent with the increasing number of AF ablation procedures that involve electrical isolation of the SVC as well as ablation around the right superior PV, especially when balloon ablation catheters are used. The reported incidence of phrenic nerve injury secondary to AF ablation varies from 0% to 0.48%.[32,33]

The left phrenic nerve descends behind the left brachiocephalic vein and passes over the aortic arch, pulmonary trunk, and then with the pericardium over the LA appendage. From there it descends along the pericardium over the LV and frequently passes laterally over the obtuse margin of the LV, close to the lateral vein and the left marginal artery and, in only a small percentage of cases, close to the left main coronary artery and great cardiac vein. Left phrenic nerve injury can occur during AF or AT ablation in the region of the proximal LA appendage roof, during ablation of left posterolateral BTs, as well as during percutaneous epicardial ablation adjacent to the lateral LV wall.[34,35]

Clinical Presentation

Phrenic nerve injury can be asymptomatic in about one-third of cases. The most frequent symptom is dyspnea. Other symptoms or clinical findings are cough or hiccup during ablation and the development of postablation pneumonia or pleural effusion. In asymptomatic patients, the diagnosis is made on the routine chest x-ray (Fig. 32-6) with hemidiaphragm paresis or paralysis (hemidiaphragm elevation with paradoxical movement). There is no active treatment known to aid phrenic nerve healing. Complete or partial recovery of diaphragmatic function can be observed in 66% and 17% of patients, respectively, sometimes not realized until several weeks or even months later.[36]

Prevention

In areas at high risk of phrenic nerve injury (RA free wall, posteroseptal part of the SVC, inferoanterior aspect of the right PV ostium, and proximal LA appendage roof) that require ablation, high-output (10 mA) pacing should be performed before energy delivery. The ability to pace the phrenic nerve should prompt attempting to find a slightly different site or, if this is not possible, applying RF energy at low power and/or for short duration. This technique can be combined with electroanatomical mapping of the RA, SVC, LA, and right PVs to reconstruct the anatomical course of the right phrenic nerve. Even when the phrenic nerve cannot be paced, intermittent fluoroscopic visualization of the ipsilateral diaphragm movement should be performed during RF application at high-risk sites, and RF delivery should be terminated if diaphragmatic excursion decreases.

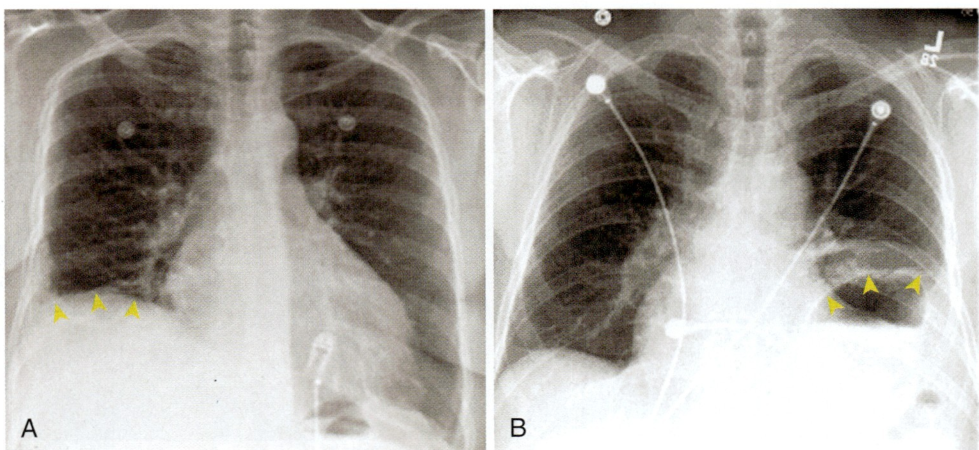

FIGURE 32-6 Chest x-rays (posteroanterior views) showing right hemidiaphragmatic paralysis (arrowheads) caused by right phrenic nerve injury **(A)**, and left hemidiaphragmatic paralysis caused by left phrenic nerve injury **(B)** during catheter ablation of atrial fibrillation.

An alternative technique is to position a catheter in the SVC at a site where the phrenic nerve can be consistently captured, and pace the phrenic nerve during ablation. RF energy delivery should be stopped immediately if diaphragmatic contraction becomes less vigorous or ceases.

Early recognition of phrenic nerve injury during RF delivery (which can be indicated by the development of hiccup, cough, or decrease in diaphragmatic excursion during energy delivery) allows immediate interruption of the application prior to the onset of permanent injury, which is associated with the rapid recovery of phrenic nerve function. This is not feasible in patients undergoing general anesthesia.

Recently, diaphragmatic electromyography has been used to monitor phrenic nerve integrity during ablation. A progressive decline in compound motor action potential amplitude heralded phrenic nerve palsy, with a 30% decrease yielding the best predictive value, preceding hemidiaphragmatic paralysis by about 30 seconds. To record right diaphragmatic compound motor action potentials, two standard surface electrodes are connected to a central computerized electrophysiology workstation. The recording electrode is placed on the thorax 5 cm superior to the tip of the xiphoid process and the reference electrode is positioned along the right costal margin with a 16-cm interelectrode distance. Diaphragmatic bipolar electromyographic signals are recorded during continuous pacing of the right phrenic nerve, using a catheter in the SVC. The clinical application of this approach to prevent phrenic nerve palsy induced by cryoballoon ablation of the right superior PV is still in its preliminary stages, and further evaluation is required to validate and optimize this approach.[37,38]

The use of a non-RF source of energy is unlikely to prevent this complication because phrenic nerve injury has been reported with ultrasound, laser, and cryotherapy. Furthermore, phrenic nerve injury occurs independently of the strategy of AF ablation used (PV isolation versus wide circumferential LA ablation).

During percutaneous epicardial ablation, proximity to the phrenic nerve can be detected by high-output pacing (typically at >10 mA) to detect diaphragmatic stimulation on fluoroscopy, allowing its course to be marked on a three-dimensional (3-D) map.[39] The nerve can branch over the LV, so simply noting sites at which phrenic nerve capture occurs does not necessarily delineate the course of all branches. It is important to recognize that detection by phrenic nerve capture is prevented by the use of paralytic agents during general anesthesia. However, these drugs are typically used during induction of anesthesia and their effects have dissipated by the time ablation is being performed. Catheter ablation should be avoided at sites adjacent to the phrenic nerve. Alternatively, moving the nerve away from the myocardium by injection of air into the pericardium or placement of a balloon catheter between the ablation target site and nerve can allow safe RF ablation. Alternative energy sources such as cryoenergy have been used to prevent phrenic nerve injury. Cryomapping uses temporary phrenic nerve injury to determine when to avoid full cryoablation. However, data on the success of cryoablation in the pericardial space are limited.[34,35]

Pulmonary Vein Stenosis

Incidence

PV stenosis is one of the most serious complications of AF ablation and has been reported with a wide range of incidence (0% to 42%), mainly because of different ablation strategies and differing methodology for estimating postablation PV ostia. The severity of PV stenosis is generally categorized as mild (<50%), moderate (50% to 70%), or severe (>70%). When moderate and mild lesions are included, the overall rate is as high as 15.5% (Fig. 32-7). However, the rate of severe PV stenosis has fallen to as low as 1.0% to 1.4% with increasing experience and improvements in technique, such as performing ablation outside the PVs and the use of ICE. Late progression of PV stenosis to severe stenosis or even complete occlusion can occur in up to 27% of patients (Fig. 32-8), particularly in the smaller PVs. Of note, stenosis seems to be more common in the left-sided PVs.[11]

Circumferential LA ablation, with ablation limited to atrial tissue outside the PV orifice, seems to have lower rates of PV stenosis, whereas focal ablation inside the PV has a higher risk. Moreover, with PV isolation techniques, the use of an individual encircling lesion set that requires RF ablation between the ipsilateral PVs carries a higher risk of PV stenosis. With the focal ablation approach, PV stenosis can occur at a rate up to 33% to 42%. Although this represents an overestimation of the problem because increased TEE flow velocity was used to establish the diagnosis, it remains a major concern. With PV isolation techniques, the incidence of severe PV stenosis is approximately 1% to 5%. MR and spiral CT scanning have shown that although current PV isolation techniques are associated with minimal reduction of the PV ostial diameter, stenosis exceeding 50% can occur in up to 18% of cases, whereas very severe stenosis (>90%) is found in up to 2% of cases. Following circumferential LA ablation, the prevalence of PV stenosis likely ranges between 2% and 7%. In one report, a detectable reduction in PV diameter was present in 38% of PVs; however, moderate and severe PV stenosis was observed in 3.2% and 0.6% of PVs, respectively.[3,9]

Mechanism

The mechanism of the development of PV stenosis remains unclear. Acute reduction of PV diameter (by approximately 30%) has been demonstrated during ablation. It was initially speculated that these changes are caused by edema and spasm. Thermal injury, induced by RF, has recently been shown to produce Ca^{2+}-mediated irreversible tissue contracture occurring with the production of most if not all RF lesions, and therefore almost certainly contributes to

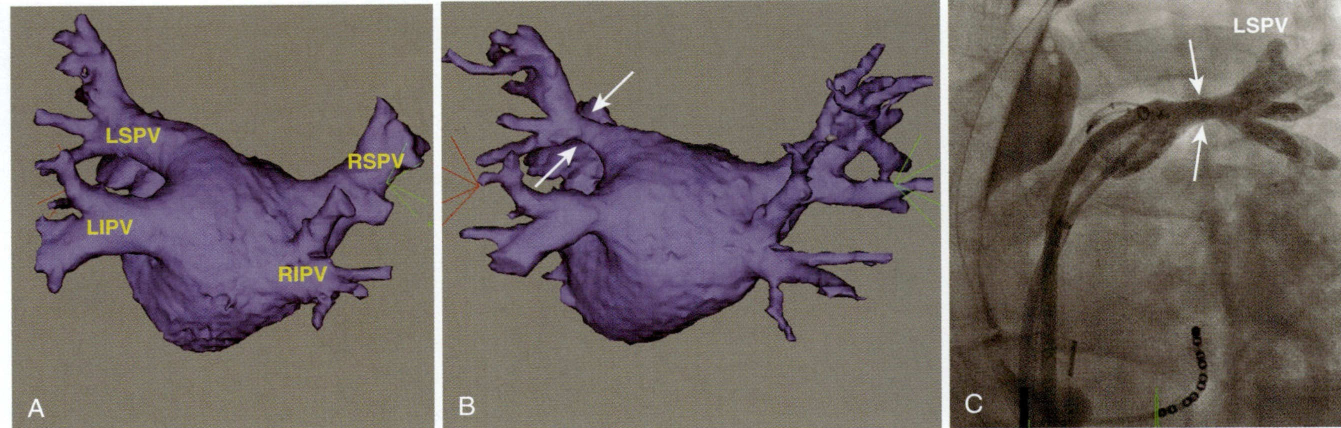

FIGURE 32-7 Pulmonary vein (PV) stenosis. **A,** CT image of the left atrium and PVs at baseline before segmental ostial PV isolation. **B,** CT image 3 months after the ablation procedure, showing moderate stenosis of the left superior pulmonary vein (LSPV; arrows) and mild stenosis of the left inferior pulmonary vein (LIPV). **C,** Angiogram (left anterior oblique view) of the LSPV, showing a moderate degree of stenosis (arrows). RIPV = right inferior pulmonary vein; RSPV = right superior pulmonary vein.

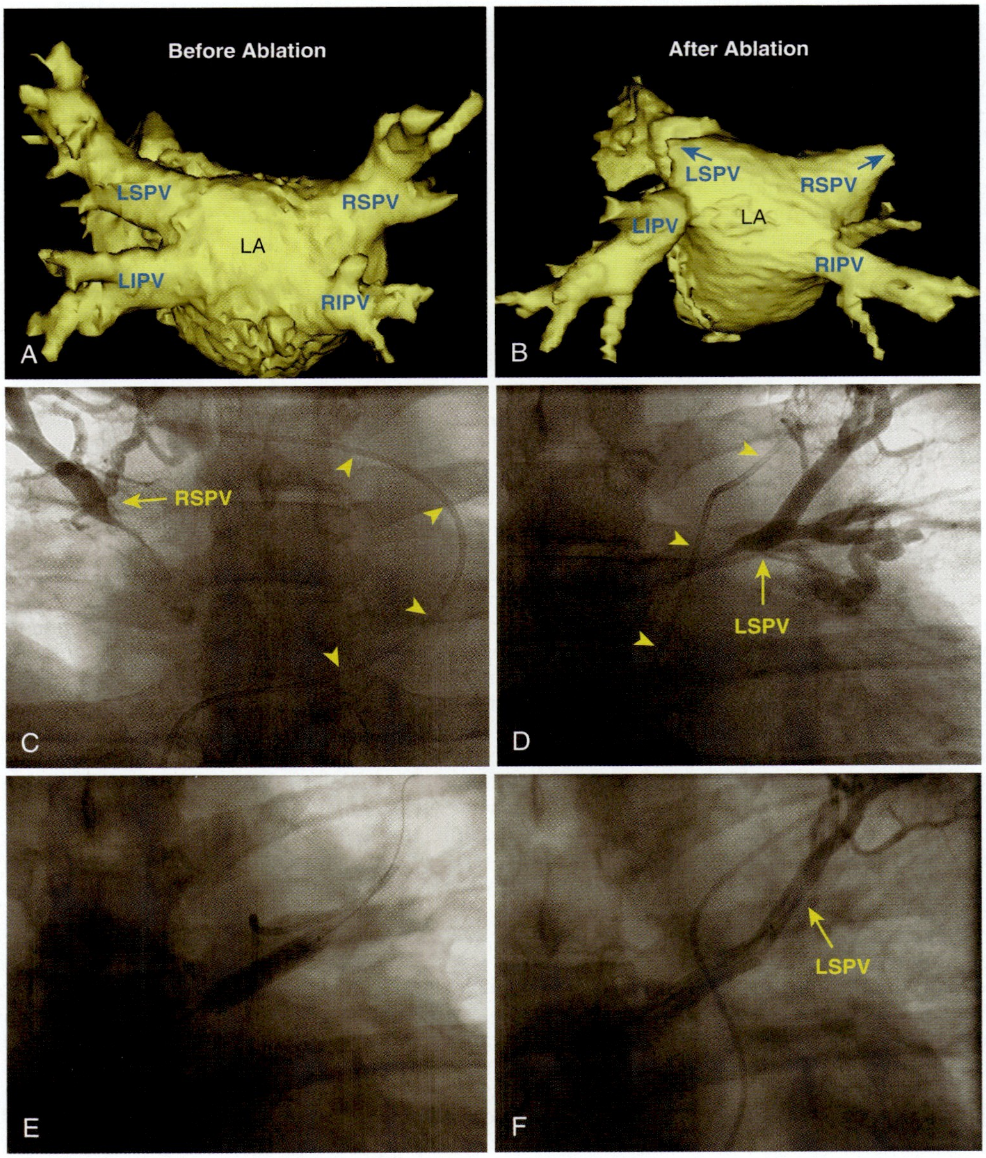

FIGURE 32-8 Pulmonary vein (PV) occlusion. **Upper panels,** CT image of the left atrium (LA) and PVs at baseline before segmental ostial PV isolation **(A)** and 5 months after ablation **(B).** Following ablation complete occlusion of both superior PVs is observed. **Middle panels,** Fluoroscopic (anteroposterior) views during angiography of the right superior pulmonary vein (RSPV) **(C)** and left superior pulmonary vein (LSPV) **(D),** showing severe stenosis-occlusion of both PVs at the ostia. PV angiography was performed with contrast injection via a catheter positioned in the pulmonary artery (arrowheads). **Lower panels,** Fluoroscopic (anteroposterior) views during stenting of the LSPV: **E,** Angioplasty balloon is inflated for stent deployment in the LSPV; **F,** angiogram of the left superior PV following stenting. LIPV = left inferior pulmonary vein; RIPV = right inferior pulmonary vein.

stenosis. It is well known that thermal injury produces denaturation of extracellular proteins, especially collagen. Thermally induced collagen shrinkage has been well documented in animal and human studies. When near-circumferential lesions are produced within the tubular confines of the PVs, the consequences can be easily demonstrated as PV contracture. Thus, PV stenosis likely results from a combination of endothelial disruption with platelet activation and later neointimal proliferation, reversible edema, collagen denaturation, and shrinkage and thermal contracture. The occurrence and degree of PV stenosis correlate with the amount of energy delivered and lesion extension. The high incidence of mild PV stenosis likely reflects PV reverse remodeling rather than pathological PV stenosis. This hypothesis is based on the observation that all the mild PV stenoses were concentric rather than eccentric.[3,9]

When severe stenosis or occlusion of a PV develops suddenly, gradual decline and then cessation of the arterial flow to the affected lung segment are observed. This is caused by a decline in the arteriovenous gradient as well as compression by the developing tissue edema. As a consequence, the involved alveoli are affected by the resulting ischemia and surrounding edema, leading to atelectasis, infarction, or susceptibility to infections. With the resulting alterations in pulmonary hemodynamics, redistribution of blood flow occurs with the opening of vascular channels or neovascularization in which tissue hypoxia is known to play a role. Hence, the venous drainage of the affected segment becomes mainly dependent on the ipsilateral veins draining the healthy lobes. If the ipsilateral vein(s) is also stenosed, the impedance to the pulmonary flow increases, adding to the hemodynamic burden. Symptoms attributable to PV stenosis are typically not seen unless the perfusion of the affected lobe falls below 20% or the perfusion of the entire lung on the affected side falls below 25%.[40]

Clinical Presentation

PV stenosis after ablation is frequently asymptomatic, especially when a mild or moderate degree of PV stenosis is present or a single vein is involved. Severe PV stenosis can be associated with various respiratory symptoms that frequently mimic more common lung diseases, such as asthma, pneumonia, lung cancer, and pulmonary embolism. A high degree of suspicion is necessary to avoid performing misleading diagnostic procedures and to allow proper and prompt management. The onset of symptoms is usually several months after ablation. The initial manifestation is generally dyspnea on exertion, which typically evolves over the course of 1 to 3 months. Persistent cough is a common symptom. Pleuritic chest pain is a late symptom, and hemoptysis is uncommon. Both pleuritic chest pain and hemoptysis are likely related to complete vessel or branch occlusion.[3,9]

It seems that symptom severity is related not only to the degree of stenosis but also to the number of PVs with stenosis. Symptoms may improve spontaneously over time in a significant percentage of patients. In one report, this improvement occurred in 50% of patients and was always related to improvement in the radiological abnormalities previously detected, although other hemodynamic compensatory mechanisms (e.g., development of collaterals) can also play a role.

Detection

To date, it remains unclear which is the best and most cost-effective noninvasive modality for detecting PV stenosis after ablation. TEE and CT scanning are most commonly used (Videos 24 and 25); however, no single imaging modality has been able to assess all relevant aspects of PV stenosis. Therefore, complementary methods are used (see Fig. 32-7). Although many investigators recommend routine follow-up CT or MR imaging for detection of asymptomatic PV stenosis 3 to 4 months after ablation of AF, it is unknown whether early diagnosis and treatment of asymptomatic PV stenosis provide any long-term advantage to the patient.[40] Nevertheless, it is recommended that follow-up PV imaging be performed to screen for PV stenosis during the initial experience of an AF ablation technique for quality control purposes.[3,9]

Spiral CT and MR imaging of the PVs are readily available and can reveal the correct diagnosis; they are probably the most helpful in identifying the location and extent of the stenosis (see Fig. 32-7). However, the sensitivity and specificity of these imaging modalities need to be studied further. Of note, the diagnosis of PV occlusion cannot be made reliably using CT or MR imaging, and pulmonary artery wedge angiography is the only method for confirming the diagnosis.[41]

TEE provides adequate visualization of the superior PVs, but imaging of the right and left inferior PVs is inconsistent. Hence, TEE is not typically used as a first-line imaging study for routine screening. Nonetheless, TEE provides additional functional data regarding the significance of PV stenosis.[40] On TEE, PV stenosis is usually indicated by an increased maximal PV Doppler flow velocity or by the presence of turbulence and deformity of the flow signal, as defined by a minimal flow between systolic and diastolic peak flow of 60% of the mean of both peaks. ICE allows straightforward imaging of all PVs and provides a good view into the first 1 to 3 cm of the vein. Color flow contrast imaging is also useful for identifying the location of the orifice of the most tightly stenotic vessels.

Blood gas assessment and pulmonary function testing do not seem to be useful as screening measures for early PV stenosis. Radiographic findings in PV stenosis are nonspecific. Chest radiography often reveals parenchymal consolidation, pleural effusion, or both. Ventilation/perfusion scanning can be done to characterize the functional significance of the stenosis. In the presence of significant PV stenosis, perfusion abnormalities are usually marked and appear similar to the changes seen in pulmonary embolism.

Prevention

The best way to manage PV stenosis is to avoid it. PV stenosis is independently related to RF lesion location, size, and distribution and to baseline PV diameter . The prevalence of this complication has decreased because of various factors, including abandonment of in-vein ablation at the site of the AF focus, limiting ablation to the extraostial portion of the PV or PV antrum, use of advanced imaging techniques to guide catheter placement and RF application, reduction in target ablation temperature and energy output, and increased operator experience.[11]

Cryothermal ablation has unique characteristics that may prove to be desirable when lesions are required within the PV. Specifically, there is less endothelial disruption, maintenance of extracellular collagen matrix without collagen denaturation, and no collagen contracture related to thermal effects. These characteristics may translate into a reduction in PV stenosis as compared with RF ablation.

Management

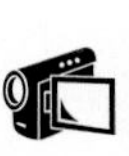

PV intervention is recommended in symptomatic patients. PV stenting appears to be associated with a lower restenosis rate compared with angioplasty (Video 26).[42] For asymptomatic patients with severe PV stenosis, some investigators have also suggested interventional therapy because lesions can progress and eventually lead to total occlusion, precluding dilation and potentially resulting in hemodynamic compromise (see Fig. 32-8).[11] Others have proposed regular clinical follow-up and intervention considered only when symptoms develop. However, it is important to understand that patients can become symptomatic only after the long-term sequelae of PV occlusion become manifest, at which time intervention may not be technically feasible or, even when successful, may not be associated with significant improvement in perfusion of the affected lung segments. It is also important to consider the age, functional capacity, and associated comorbidities as well as anatomical and technical factors pertaining to the stenotic vein when making a decision regarding interventional treatment in asymptomatic patients.[11]

TEE or ICE can facilitate accurate stent placement by reliably identifying the orifice of the tightly stenotic vein. Unfortunately, both in-stent and in-segment restenosis can recur in up to 61% of patients, and repeat intervention is warranted in symptomatic patients. Stenosis within the body of the stent is likely caused by neointimal hyperplasia and fibrosis. Out-of-stent restenosis is usually observed at bifurcation points beyond the stent into the vessel, also suggesting the progression of PV pathology, despite stent placement. There is no experience to date with the use of drug-eluting stents in this setting, but such a high restenosis rate makes a strong case for the investigation of those devices and larger diameter stents.[11]

Atrioesophageal Fistula

Incidence

The true incidence of atrioesophageal fistula after catheter ablation is unknown, but has been estimated to be between 0.03% and 0.2%, although underreporting is likely.[43,44] Despite its rarity, atrioesophageal fistula remains a devastating complication associated with high mortality, accounting for 15.6% of cases with fatal outcome (the second leading cause of death post AF ablation, following cardiac tamponade).[45]

On the other hand, esophageal mucosal changes consistent with thermal injury have been reported in up to 47% of the patients following AF ablation, and esophageal ulcerations confirmed by esophagogastroscopy or capsule endoscopy can be observed in 14% to 18%.[46,47]

Mechanism

The precise mechanism of atrioesophageal fistula formation has not yet been determined. Proposed potential mechanisms include direct thermal injury of the esophageal wall in immediate proximity to the posterior LA wall, thermal injury of the arterial blood supply to the esophagus, and mechanical injury to the esophagus during periprocedural TEE as a contributing or predisposing factor.[3]

The esophagus is located at the center of the posterior mediastinum and runs in close proximity to the posterior LA wall for about 5 cm of its course. In that region, the esophagus is separated from the LA only by the pericardial sac (the oblique sinus), which insinuates itself between the openings of the right and left PVs. The LA posterior wall thickness is 2 to 4 mm and the thickness of the esophageal wall is 2 to 3 mm in cross section at the LA-esophageal area of contact. During RF catheter ablation, lesion depth, extension, and volume are related to the design of the ablation electrode and RF power delivered. Theoretically, esophageal damage can occur, even during LA ablation using a standard 4-mm-tip ablation catheter. However, cooled and large-tip ablation catheters induce extended lesions. Thus, delivering high-power RF applications on the LA posterior wall between the left and right PVs can potentially deeply damage the esophagus, resulting in atrioesophageal fistula formation.[48,49]

The esophagus does not have a serosal layer and is fixed primarily in the pharynx and gastroesophageal junction. In the mediastinum, the esophageal position is dynamic because of peristalsis. In fact, the esophagus often shifts sideways by 2 cm or more in most patients undergoing catheter ablation for AF under conscious sedation. Additionally, the position of the esophagus in relation to the LA and PV demonstrates high variability. In many cases, the esophagus is very close to the ostia of the PVs and lies only a short distance from the LA wall. In most subjects (90%), the esophagus courses down beside the ostia of the left PVs with a mean distance of 10.1 mm to the left superior PV and 2.8 mm to the left inferior PV. Therefore, anatomical localization of the esophagus can be critical before or during AF ablation to prevent atrioesophageal fistula, especially as there is a need for transmural atrial lesions.

The risk of esophageal injury likely is enhanced by increasing the magnitude and duration of local tissue heating (i.e., the total ablation energy delivered to cardiac tissue near the esophagus), which is related to catheter tip size, contact pressure, catheter orientation, and power output and duration. In fact, all reported cases of atrioesophageal fistulas have in common attempts to perform deep RF lesions on the LA posterior wall. Additionally, ablation strategies incorporating extensive ablation in the LA posterior wall and the type of AF (persistent more than paroxysmal AF, possibly due to the additional linear ablation lesions) have been associated with an increased rate of esophageal ulcerations. A short LA-to-esophagus distance, the use of nasogastric tubes, and general anesthesia are other potential risk factors for esophageal injury during RF ablation.[49,50]

Cryoballoon ablation commonly causes significant decreases in esophageal temperature, especially during cryoablation of the inferior PVs, resulting in esophageal ulcerations. Although no instances of atrioesophageal fistula formation after cryoballoon PV isolation have yet been reported, the total number of cryoballoon ablation cases performed is relatively small to reliably detect this rare complication. Furthermore, esophageal ulcerations have been observed following cryoballoon ablation at rates (17% of patients) similar to those seen with RF ablation. Although there is no definitive proof that esophageal ulcer formation is predictive of fistulas, it is reasonable to assume that esophageal ulcerations may represent the first step on the way to atrioesophageal fistula. Therefore, until further experience indicates otherwise, cryoballoon ablation should not be considered completely safe in regard to atrioesophageal fistula formation.[51]

Excessive esophageal heating, esophageal ulcerations, and atrioesophageal fistula formation have been observed post PV isolation using high-intensity focused ultrasound (HIFU). In a recent study, elevated esophageal temperature prompting cessation of HIFU energy delivery occurred in 9% of PVs. Despite use of the safety algorithm, the occurrence of esophageal thermal damage and lethal atrioesophageal fistula could not be prevented, occurring in 1 of 28 patients. This safety concern argues against the clinical use of HIFU in its current iteration for PV isolation.[52]

Clinical Presentation

The clinical course of atrioesophageal fistula formation varies in abruptness of presentation and timing (ranging from 2 days to 4 weeks), and mostly is manifest after patient discharge from the hospital. The presenting symptoms can include hematemesis, sepsis, or air embolization and stroke. The leading symptom of esophageal perforation is high fever or severe chest or epigastric pain.

Leukocytosis is the earliest and most sensitive laboratory marker. Thoracic CT or MR imaging is the most valuable diagnostic examination (Fig. 32-9, Video 27). The dramatic neurological complications occur with a delay of at least a few hours after the first symptoms. Endoscopy is a diagnostic modality that should be avoided because insufflation of the esophagus with air can result in a devastating cerebrovascular accident and death secondary to a large air embolus. Immediate surgery (within a few hours after the first symptoms) can potentially prevent neurological complications and possibly result in a high survival rate, without residue. Delay of treatment seems to have devastating results.[3]

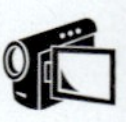

Prevention

Various strategies may be used to avoid the development of an atrioesophageal fistula, including the following: (1) assessment of esophageal position before and during ablation; (2) avoiding ablation in the vicinity of the esophagus; (3) mechanical displacement of the esophagus; (4) monitoring of the esophageal temperature during energy delivery; and (5) reduction of ablation energy power output and duration at sites close to the esophagus. However, because of the rarity of this complication, it remains unproven whether the use of these approaches lowers or eliminates the risk of esophageal perforation or fistula formation, and the optimal technique has not yet been determined. Therefore, it appears prudent to apply a combination of these preventive techniques during AF ablation. These strategies are discussed in detail in Chapter 11.[48-50,53-55]

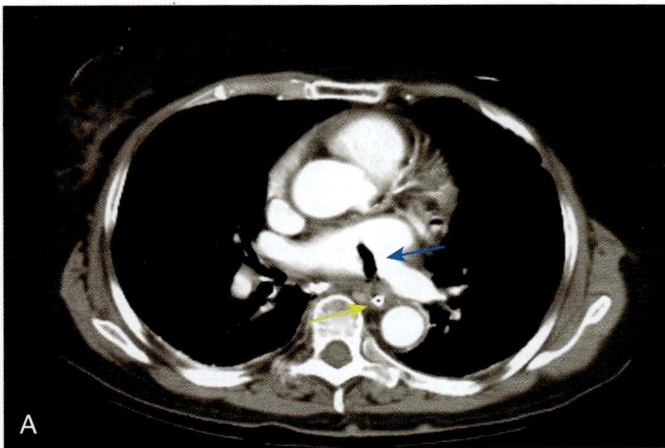

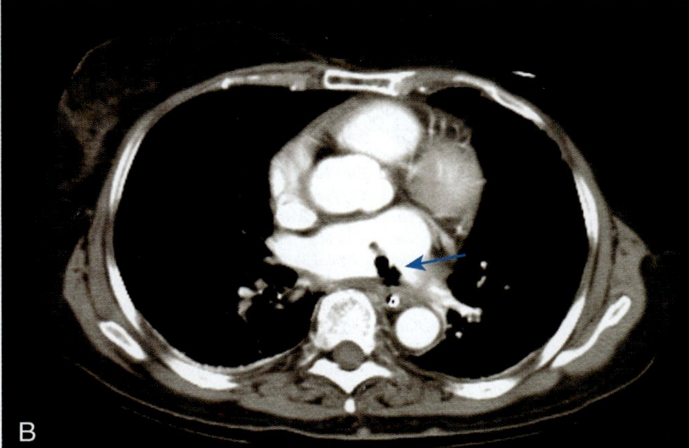

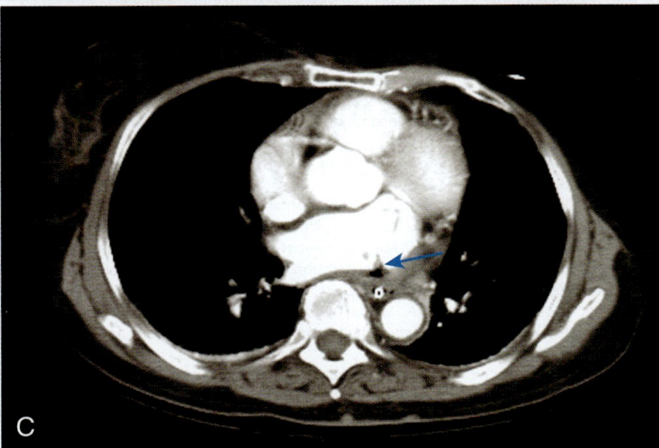

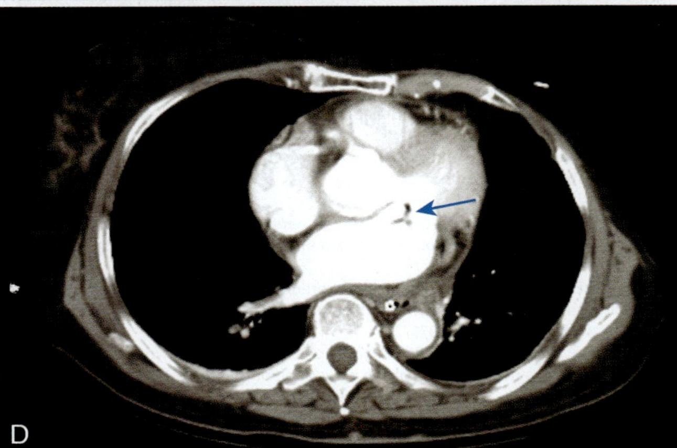

FIGURE 32-9 Atrioesophageal fistula postablation of atrial fibrillation. Multiple transverse sections of a chest computed tomography scan, revealing air bubbles (blue arrows) in the superior aspect of the left atrium **(A-C)** and at the level of the mitral valve **(D)**. Note that air appears to originate from the anterior esophageal wall **(B** and **C)**. Nasogastric tube is visualized in the esophagus (yellow arrow).

Radiation Exposure

Catheter ablation of complex cardiac arrhythmias, including AF, macroreentrant ATs, and reentrant VTs, can be associated with markedly prolonged fluoroscopy durations. The use of CT scanning before and after AF ablation procedures further increases patient exposure to radiation. Direct monitoring of patient skin doses during procedures is highly desirable.

Radiation exposures during the different interventional procedures are highly variable. Cardiac catheterizations generally expose patients to an average dose of 250 rad (2.5 Gy). Percutaneous coronary interventions are particularly dangerous (average dose, 640 rad [6.4 Gy]) because radiation is focused only on those vessels with stenosis. Although these represent standard exposure estimates, interventional procedures are highly variable.[56] In one report, only 1 of 15 patients undergoing AF ablation reached a peak skin dose of 2 Gy, despite prolonged fluoroscopy durations (up to 99 minutes). This finding is striking and speaks to the effectiveness of the systems that use several technologies to reduce radiation exposure, such as last image hold, pulsed fluoroscopy, and additional filters.[57]

With similar fluoroscopy durations in both projections, the radiation dose is higher in the LAO than in the right anterior oblique (RAO) projection, primarily because of a longer attenuation path for the x-ray beam entering in the LAO projection.

Clinical Presentation

In EP procedures, the patient tissue receiving the greatest radiation dose is the skin area of the back at the entrance point of the x-ray beam, and skin injuries are well-recognized complications for catheter ablation procedures. The threshold for transient erythema and epilation is 2 to 3 Gy, for acute skin injury is 2 to 8 Gy, and for chronic radiation injury is 10 Gy.[56] Obese patients, those with preexisting health conditions such as collagen vascular disease, diabetes mellitus, or ataxia telangiectasia, and those who received a high radiation dose from a previous procedure, can be at a greater risk for radiation skin damage.

Acute radiation injury (characterized by erythema with vesiculation, erosion, and pain) usually starts within days after exposure and persists up to several weeks (Fig. 32-10). Chronic radiation injury manifests months to years after exposure and presents clinically as permanent erythema, dermal atrophy, and ulceration.

Acute radiation-induced skin injury can be misdiagnosed as contact dermatitis, viral or bacterial infection, or a spider bite, and a high index of suspicion is required. Fluoroscopy-induced injuries affect an area congruent to the entrance of the x-ray beam that typically has well-defined borders (see Fig. 32-10), which occur when the beam is not moved or resized during prolonged fluoroscopy over one site. It is important to alert patients who had undergone prolonged procedures or known to have received a high skin radiation dose to examine him- or herself about 2 to 3 weeks after the procedure to look for skin changes and to contact the interventionalist if any are observed.

Skin biopsy is usually not necessary and not recommended, especially given the potential risk of a nonhealing ulcer at the site of biopsy in the radiation-damaged skin area. Furthermore, the findings on skin biopsy generally are not pathognomonic for radiation change.

The estimated lifetime risk of a fatal malignancy after AF ablation using a modern low-frame pulsed fluoroscopy system is relatively low (0.15% for women and 0.21% for men in one report) and is higher than, although within the range of, previously reported risk to result from the ablation of standard types of supraventricular

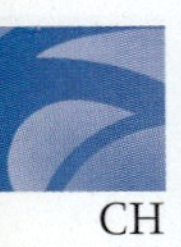

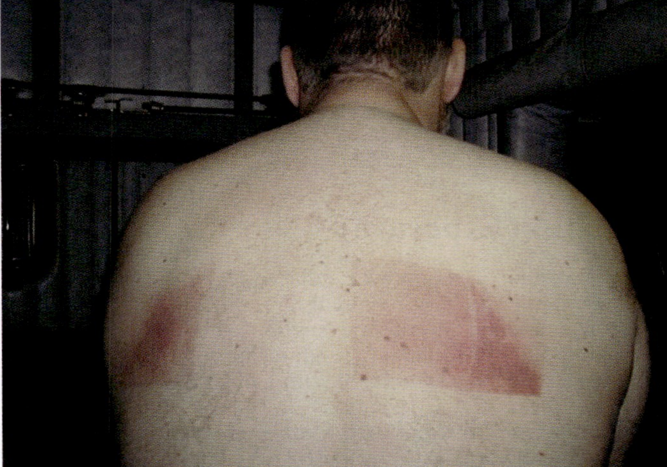

FIGURE 32-10 Acute radiation-induced skin injury (erythema) 2 to 3 weeks following radiofrequency ablation of atrial fibrillation using biplane fluoroscopy. The affected areas have well-defined borders congruent with the entrance of the x-ray beam.

arrhythmias (0.03% to 0.26%). It has been estimated that for every 60 minutes of fluoroscopy, the mean total lifetime excess risk of a fatal malignancy is 0.03% to 0.065%.

Prevention

Increasing availability and familiarity with 3-D mapping systems should significantly reduce fluoroscopy time and the need for biplane fluoroscopy. The use of remote navigation systems also is likely to reduce fluoroscopy exposure of the patient and operator.[57] Additionally, judicious and intermittent use of fluoroscopy, that is, keeping the x-rays on for only a few seconds at a time, long enough to view the current catheter position, can reduce total fluoroscopic times considerably. The presence of grids in x-ray systems primarily increases the contrast and hence the image quality; however, they increase the dose to the patient and staff by a factor of two or more, and removal of the grid can help reduce the dose of radiation. Additionally, periodically rotating the fluoroscope at different angles helps spread the total radiation dose over a broader area of the patient's skin so that no single region receives the entire dose. Other methods include adjustment of beam quality, using pulsed fluoroscopy, inserting appropriate metal filters (aluminum, copper, or other materials) into the beam at the collimator, and minimizing geometric magnification by keeping the image receptor close to the patient and the source away.

REFERENCES

1. Bohnen M, Stevenson WG, Tedrow UB, et al: Incidence and predictors of major complications from contemporary catheter ablation to treat cardiac arrhythmias, *Heart Rhythm* 8:1661–1666, 2011.
2. Doppalapudi H, Yamada T, Kay N: Complications during catheter ablation of atrial fibrillation: identification and prevention, *Heart Rhythm* 6:S18–S25, 2009.
3. Calkins H, Brugada J, Packer DL, et al: HRS/EHRA/ECAS Expert Consensus Statement on Catheter and Surgical Ablation of Atrial Fibrillation: recommendations for personnel, policy, procedures and follow-up. A report of the Heart Rhythm Society (HRS) Task Force on Catheter and Surgical Ablation of Atrial Fibrillation, *Heart Rhythm* 4:816–861, 2007.
4. Natale A, Raviele A, Al-Ahmad A, et al: Venice Chart International Consensus document on ventricular tachycardia/ventricular fibrillation ablation, *J Cardiovasc Electrophysiol* 21:339–379, 2010.
5. Aliot EM, Stevenson WG, Mendral-Garrote JM, et al: EHRA/HRS Expert Consensus on Catheter Ablation of Ventricular Arrhythmias: developed in a partnership with the European Heart Rhythm Association (EHRA), a Registered Branch of the European Society of Cardiology (ESC), and the Heart Rhythm Society (HRS); in collaboration with the American College of Cardiology (ACC) and the American Heart Association (AHA), *Heart Rhythm* 6:886–933, 2009.
6. McElderry HT, Yamada T: How to diagnose and treat cardiac tamponade in the electrophysiology laboratory, *Heart Rhythm* 6:1531–1535, 2009.
7. Kim RJ, Siouffi S, Silberstein TA, et al: Management and clinical outcomes of acute cardiac tamponade complicating electrophysiologic procedures: a single-center case series, *Pacing Clin Electrophysiol* 33:667–674, 2010.
8. Latchamsetty R, Gautam S, Bhakta D, et al: Management and outcomes of cardiac tamponade during atrial fibrillation ablation in the presence of therapeutic anticoagulation with warfarin, *Heart Rhythm* 8:805–808, 2011.
9. Dixit S, Marchlinski FE: How to recognize, manage, and prevent complications during atrial fibrillation ablation, *Heart Rhythm* 4:108–115, 2007.
10. Scherr D, Sharma K, Dalal D, et al: Incidence and predictors of periprocedural cerebrovascular accident in patients undergoing catheter ablation of atrial fibrillation, *J Cardiovasc Electrophysiol* 20:1357–1363, 2009.
11. Barrett CD, Di Biase L, Natale A: How to identify and treat patient with pulmonary vein stenosis post atrial fibrillation ablation, *Curr Opin Cardiol* 24:42–49, 2009.
12. Gautam S, John RM, Stevenson WG, et al: Effect of therapeutic INR on activated clotting times, heparin dosage, and bleeding risk during ablation of atrial fibrillation, *J Cardiovasc Electrophysiol* 22:248–254, 2011.
13. Hussein AA, Martin DO, Saliba W, et al: Radiofrequency ablation of atrial fibrillation under therapeutic international normalized ratio: a safe and efficacious periprocedural anticoagulation strategy, *Heart Rhythm* 6:1425–1429, 2009.
14. Mirski MA, Lele AV, Fitzsimmons L, Toung TJ: Diagnosis and treatment of vascular air embolism, *Anesthesiology* 106:164–177, 2007.
15. Roberts-Thomson KC, Steven D, Seiler J, et al: Coronary artery injury due to catheter ablation in adults: presentations and outcomes, *Circulation* 120:1465–1473, 2009.
16. Cesario D, Boyle N, Shivumar K: Lesion forming technologies for catheter ablation. In Zipes DP, Jalife J, editors: *Cardiac electrophysiology: from cell to bedside*, ed 5, Philadelphia, 2009, WB Saunders, pp 1051–1058.
17. Callans DJ: Catheter ablation of idiopathic ventricular tachycardia arising from the aortic root, *J Cardiovasc Electrophysiol* 20:969–972, 2009.
18. Tabatabaei N, Asirvatham SJ: Supravalvular arrhythmia: identifying and ablating the substrate, *Circ Arrhythm Electrophysiol* 2:316–326, 2009.
19. Mykytsey A, Kehoe R, Bharati S, et al: Right coronary artery occlusion during RF ablation of typical atrial flutter, *J Cardiovasc Electrophysiol* 21:818–821, 2010.
20. Alaiti MA, Maroo A, Edel TB: Troponin levels after cardiac electrophysiology procedures: review of the literature, *Pacing Clin Electrophysiol* 32:800–810, 2009.
21. Estner HL, Ndrepepa G, Dong J, et al: Acute and long-term results of slow pathway ablation in patients with atrioventricular nodal reentrant tachycardia—an analysis of the predictive factors for arrhythmia recurrence, *Pacing Clin Electrophysiol* 28:102–110, 2005.
22. Steven D, Rostock T, Hoffmann BA, et al: Favorable outcome using an abbreviated procedure for catheter ablation of AVNRT: results from a prospective randomized trial, *J Cardiovasc Electrophysiol* 20:522–525, 2009.
23. Opel A, Murray S, Kamath N, et al: Cryoablation versus radiofrequency ablation for treatment of atrioventricular nodal reentrant tachycardia: cryoablation with 6-mm-tip catheters is still less effective than radiofrequency ablation, *Heart Rhythm* 7:340–343, 2010.
24. Sawhney N, Anousheh R, Chen W, Feld GK: Circumferential pulmonary vein ablation with additional linear ablation results in an increased incidence of left atrial flutter compared with segmental pulmonary vein isolation as an initial approach to ablation of paroxysmal atrial fibrillation, *Circ Arrhythm Electrophysiol* 3:243–248, 2010.
25. Schmidt M, Daccarett M, Segerson N, et al: Atrial flutter ablation in inducible patients during pulmonary vein atrium isolation: a randomized comparison, *Pacing Clin Electrophysiol* 31:1592–1597, 2008.
26. Matsuo S, Lim KT, Haissaguerre M: Ablation of chronic atrial fibrillation, *Heart Rhythm* 4:1461–1463, 2007.
27. Morady F, Oral H, Chugh A: Diagnosis and ablation of atypical atrial tachycardia and flutter complicating atrial fibrillation ablation, *Heart Rhythm* 6(Suppl 8):S29–S32, 2009.
28. Kron J, Kasirajan V, Wood MA, et al: Management of recurrent atrial arrhythmias after minimally invasive surgical pulmonary vein isolation and ganglionic plexi ablation for atrial fibrillation, *Heart Rhythm* 7:445–451, 2010.
29. Themistoclakis S, Schweikert RA, Saliba WI, et al: Clinical predictors and relationship between early and late atrial tachyarrhythmias after pulmonary vein antrum isolation, *Heart Rhythm* 5:679–685, 2008.
30. Choi JI, Pak HN, Park JS, et al: Clinical significance of early recurrences of atrial tachycardia after atrial fibrillation ablation, *J Cardiovasc Electrophysiol* 21:1331–1337, 2010.
31. Kesek M, Englund A, Jensen SM, Jensen-Urstad M: Entrapment of circular mapping catheter in the mitral valve, *Heart Rhythm* 4:17–19, 2007.
32. Vatasescu R, Shalganov T, Kardos A, et al: Right diaphragmatic paralysis following endocardial cryothermal ablation of inappropriate sinus tachycardia, *Europace* 8:904–906, 2006.
33. Lachman N, Syed FF, Habib A, et al: Correlative anatomy for the electrophysiologist. II. Cardiac ganglia, phrenic nerve, coronary venous system, *J Cardiovasc Electrophysiol* 22:104–110, 2011.
34. Fan R, Cano O, Ho SY, et al: Characterization of the phrenic nerve course within the epicardial substrate of patients with nonischemic cardiomyopathy and ventricular tachycardia, *Heart Rhythm* 6:59–64, 2009.
35. Di Biase L, Burkhardt JD, Pelargonio G, et al: Prevention of phrenic nerve injury during epicardial ablation: comparison of methods for separating the phrenic nerve from the epicardial surface, *Heart Rhythm* 6:957–961, 2009.
36. Sacher F, Monahan KH, Thomas SP, et al: Phrenic nerve injury after atrial fibrillation catheter ablation: characterization and outcome in a multicenter study, *J Am Coll Cardiol* 47:2498–2503, 2006.
37. Franceschi F, Dubuc M, Guerra PG, Khairy P: Phrenic nerve monitoring with diaphragmatic electromyography during cryoballoon ablation for atrial fibrillation: the first human application, *Heart Rhythm* 8:1068–1071, 2011.
38. Franceschi F, Dubuc M, Guerra PG, et al: Diaphragmatic electromyography during cryoballoon ablation: a novel concept in the prevention of phrenic nerve palsy, *Heart Rhythm* 8:885–891, 2011.
39. Schmidt B, Chun KR, Ouyang F, et al: Three-dimensional reconstruction of the anatomic course of the right phrenic nerve in humans by pace mapping, *Heart Rhythm* 5:1120–1126, 2008.
40. Baranowski B, Saliba W: Our approach to management of patients with pulmonary vein stenosis following AF ablation, *J Cardiovasc Electrophysiol* 22:364–367, 2011.

41. Prieto LR, Kawai Y, Worley SE: Total pulmonary vein occlusion complicating pulmonary vein isolation: diagnosis and treatment, *Heart Rhythm* 7:1233–1239, 2010.
42. Neumann T, Kuniss M, Conradi G, et al: Pulmonary vein stenting for the treatment of acquired severe pulmonary vein stenosis after pulmonary vein isolation: clinical implications after long-term follow-up of 4 years, *J Cardiovasc Electrophysiol* 20:247–251, 2009.
43. Cappato R, Calkins H, Chen SA, et al: Updated worldwide survey on the methods, efficacy, and safety of catheter ablation for human atrial fibrillation, *Circ Arrhythm Electrophysiol* 3:32–38, 2010.
44. Dagres N, Hindricks G, Kottkamp H, et al: Complications of atrial fibrillation ablation in a high-volume center in 1,000 procedures: still cause for concern? *J Cardiovasc Electrophysiol* 20:1014–1019, 2009.
45. Cappato R, Calkins H, Chen SA, et al: Prevalence and causes of fatal outcome in catheter ablation of atrial fibrillation, *J Am Coll Cardiol* 53:1798–1803, 2009.
46. Halm U, Gaspar T, Zachaus M, et al: Thermal esophageal lesions after radiofrequency catheter ablation of left atrial arrhythmias, *Am J Gastroenterol* 105:551–556, 2010.
47. Schmidt M, Nolker G, Marschang H, et al: Incidence of oesophageal wall injury post-pulmonary vein antrum isolation for treatment of patients with atrial fibrillation, *Europace* 10:205–209, 2008.
48. Dagres N, Anastasiou-Nana M: Prevention of atrial-esophageal fistula after catheter ablation of atrial fibrillation, *Curr Opin Cardiol* 26:1–5, 2011.
49. Bahnson TD: Strategies to minimize the risk of esophageal injury during catheter ablation for atrial fibrillation, *Pacing Clin Electrophysiol* 32:248–260, 2009.
50. Martinek M, Bencsik G, Aichinger J, et al: Esophageal damage during radiofrequency ablation of atrial fibrillation: impact of energy settings, lesion sets, and esophageal visualization, *J Cardiovasc Electrophysiol* 20:726–733, 2009.
51. Ahmed H, Neuzil P, d'Avila A, et al: The esophageal effects of cryoenergy during cryoablation for atrial fibrillation, *Heart Rhythm* 6:962–969, 2009.
52. Neven K, Schmidt B, Metzner A, et al: Fatal end of a safety algorithm for pulmonary vein isolation with use of high-intensity focused ultrasound, *Circ Arrhythm Electrophysiol* 3:260–265, 2010.
53. Chugh A, Rubenstein J, Good E, et al: Mechanical displacement of the esophagus in patients undergoing left atrial ablation of atrial fibrillation, *Heart Rhythm* 6:319–322, 2009.
54. Bunch TJ, Day JD: Novel ablative approach for atrial fibrillation to decrease risk of esophageal injury, *Heart Rhythm* 5:624–627, 2008.
55. Tilz RR, Chun KR, Metzner A, et al: Unexpected high incidence of esophageal injury following pulmonary vein isolation using robotic navigation, *J Cardiovasc Electrophysiol* 21:853–858, 2010.
56. Frazier TH, Richardson JB, Fabre VC, Callen JP: Fluoroscopy-induced chronic radiation skin injury: a disease perhaps often overlooked, *Arch Dermatol* 143:637–640, 2007.
57. Lickfett L, Mahesh M, Vasamreddy C, et al: Radiation exposure during catheter ablation of atrial fibrillation, *Circulation* 110:3003–3010, 2004.

INDEX

Note: Page numbers followed by f and t indicate figures and tables, respectively.

C

D

E

F

G

J

INDEX

K

L

INDEX

M

N

O

P

Q

R

INDEX

S

W

Y

Z